SAUNDERS
Comprehensive Review for the
NCLEX-RN EXAMINATION

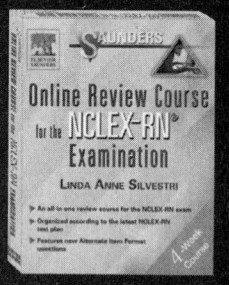
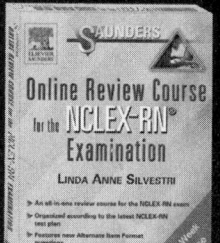
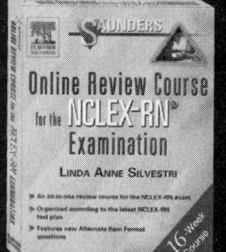
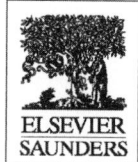

SAUNDERS

Comprehensive Review for the

NCLEX-RN EXAMINATION

LINDA ANNE SILVESTRI, MSN, RN

Instructor of Nursing, Salve Regina University
Newport, Rhode Island
President, Nursing Reviews, Inc., and
Professional Nursing Seminars, Inc.
Charlestown, Rhode Island

THIRD EDITION

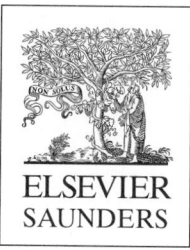

ELSEVIER
SAUNDERS

ELSEVIER
SAUNDERS

11830 Westline Industrial Drive
St. Louis, Missouri 63146

NOTICE

Pharmacology is an ever-changing field. Standard safety precautions must be followed, but as new
research and clinical experience broaden our knowledge, changes in treatment and drug therapy may
become necessary or appropriate. Readers are advised to check the most current product information
provided by the manufacturer of each drug to be administered to verify the recommended dose, the
method and duration of administration, and contraindications. It is the responsibility of the licensed
prescriber, relying on experience and knowledge of the patient, to determine dosages and the best
treatment for each individual patient. Neither the publisher nor the author assumes any liability for
any injury and/or damage to persons or property arising from this publication.

The Publisher

Previous editions copyrighted 1999, 2002

International Standard Book Number 0-7216-0347-5

Director, Review and Testing: Loren S. Wilson
Managing Editor: Michele D. Hayden
Publishing Services Manager: John Rogers
Senior Project Manager: Cheryl A. Abbott
Design Manager: Bill Drone

Printed in the United States of America

Last digit is the print number: 9 8 7 6 5 4 3 2 1

To my parents.
To my mother,
Frances Mary,
and in loving memory of my father,
Arnold Lawrence,
who taught me to always love, care, and be the best that I could be.

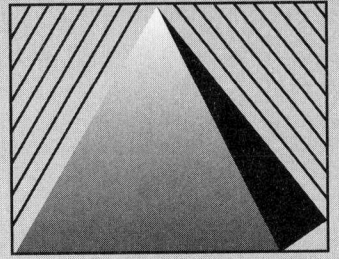

About the Author

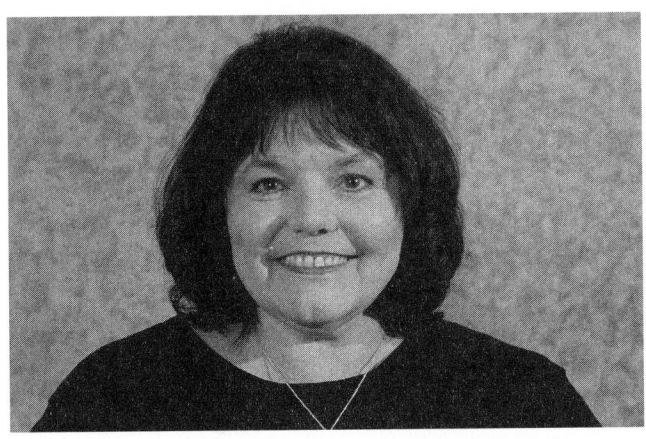

Linda Anne Silvestri received her diploma in nursing at Cooley Dickinson Hospital School of Nursing in Northampton, Massachusetts. Afterwards, she worked at Baystate Medical Center in Springfield, Massachusetts. At Baystate Medical Center, she worked in acute medical-surgical units, the intensive care unit, the emergency department, pediatric units, and other acute care units. She later received an associate degree from Holyoke Community College in Holyoke, Massachusetts, and then received her BSN from American International College in Springfield, Massachusetts.

A native of Springfield, Massachusetts, Linda began her teaching career as an instructor of medical-surgical nursing and leadership-management nursing at Baystate Medical Center School of Nursing in 1981. In 1985 she earned her MSN from Anna Maria College, Paxton, Massachusetts, with a dual major in Nursing Management and Patient Education. Linda is a member of Sigma Theta Tau.

Linda relocated to Rhode Island in 1989 and began teaching advanced medical-surgical nursing and psychiatric nursing to RN and LPN students at the Community College of Rhode Island. While teaching at the Community College of Rhode Island, a group of students approached Linda, asking her to help them prepare for the NCLEX examination. Based on her experience as a nursing educator and as an item writer for the NCLEX exams, she developed a comprehensive review course to prepare nursing graduates for the NCLEX examination. In 1994 Linda began teaching medical-surgical nursing at Salve Regina University in Newport, Rhode Island. She also prepares nursing students at Salve Regina University for the NCLEX-RN examination.

In 1991 Linda established Professional Nursing Seminars, Inc., and in 2000 she established Nursing Reviews, Inc. Both companies are dedicated to conducting review courses for the NCLEX-RN and the NCLEX-PN examinations and assisting nursing graduates to achieve their goals of becoming Registered Nurses and/or Licensed Practical/Vocational Nurses.

Today, Linda Silvestri's companies conduct review courses for the NCLEX examinations throughout New England. She is the successful author of numerous review products, including *Saunders Comprehensive Review for the NCLEX-RN Examination, Saunders Q&A Review for the NCLEX-RN Examination, Saunders Computerized Review for the NCLEX-RN Examination, Saunders Instructor's Resource Package for the NCLEX-RN Examination, Saunders Comprehensive Review for the NCLEX-PN Examination, Saunders Q&A Review for NCLEX-PN Examination, Saunders Review Cards for the NCLEX-PN Examination,* and *Saunders Instructor's Resource Package for the NCLEX-PN Examination.* Linda has also authored several online products including the online specialty tests titled *Adult Health, Mental Health, Maternal-Newborn, Pediatrics, and Pharmacology,* and the *Saunders Online Review Course for the NCLEX-RN Examination.*

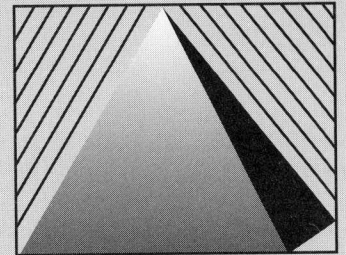

Contributors

Janice Almon Call, MSN, RN, C
Instructor, Department of Nursing
North Central Texas College
Gainesville, Texas

Elizabeth M. Carson, EdD, RN
Assistant Professor
Saint Anthony College of Nursing
Rockford, Illinois

Nancy Wilson Darland, MSN, RNC, CNS
Professor, Division of Nursing
College of Applied and Natural Sciences
Louisiana Tech University
Ruston, Louisiana

Kimberly Green, RN
Graduate, Department of Nursing
Salve Regina University
Newport, Rhode Island

Jo Ann Barnes Mullaney, PhD, RN, CS
Professor of Nursing
Salve Regina University
Newport, Rhode Island

Tina Nink, MSN, RN, FNP
Nursing Instructor
Illinois Valley Community College
Oglesby, Illinois

Tommie Wright Pniewski, MSN, RN, CNAA
Associate Professor of Nursing
Hopkinsville Community College;
President and CEO, Nursing Directions
Hopkinsville, Kentucky

Joan Schmitke, DSN, APRN, FNP, BC
Associate Professor
Eastern Kentucky University
Department of Baccalaureate and Graduate Nursing
Richmond, Kentucky

Geneva Scott, MSN, RN, BSS
Acting Director, ADN Programming
Weatherford College
Weatherford, Texas

Shirley Sherrick-Escamilla, MSN, RNC
Assistant Professor
McAuley School of Nursing
University of Detroit-Mercy
Detroit, Michigan

Bethany Hawes Sykes, EdD, RN, CEN
Nursing Instructor
Salve Regina University
Newport, Rhode Island

Laurent W. Valliere, BS
Vice President
Professional Nursing Seminars, Inc.
Charlestown, Rhode Island

Sheila E. Virgin, DSN, APRN, FNP
Associate Professor
Eastern Kentucky University
Richmond, Kentucky

Mary Hauser Whitaker, MSN, RN
Assistant Professor
Eastern Kentucky University
Department of Baccalaureate and Graduate Nursing
Richmond, Kentucky

Terry Yoesting, MS, RN
Professor
Grayson County College
Denison, Texas

The author and publisher would also like to acknowledge the following individuals for contributions to the previous editions of this book:

Marion G. Anema, PhD, RN
Dean, Nursing Program
Professor of Nursing
Tennessee State University
Nashville, Tennessee

Marianne P. Barba, MS, RN, CPC
Care New England
Coventry, Rhode Island

Carol A. Baxter, EdD, RN
CEO, Baxter Consulting
Lancaster, Pennsylvania

Eloise M. Brotzman, MSEd, MSN, RNC
Nursing Instructor
St. Luke's School of Nursing
Bethlehem, Pennsylvania

Reitha Cabaniss, MSN, RN
Nursing Faculty
Bevill State Community College
Sumiton, Alabama

Darlene Nebel Cantu, MSN, RNC
Assistant Director
School of Professional Nursing
Baptist Health System
San Antonio, Texas

Heather Carlson, RN
Graduate, Department of Nursing
Salve Regina University
Newport, Rhode Island

Shannon Chase, RN
Graduate, Department of Nursing
Salve Regina University
Newport, Rhode Island

Jane Anne Claffy, MSN, RNC
Assistant Professor of Nursing
Ulster County Community College
Stone Ridge, New York;
Adjunct Faculty, Avila Institute of Gerontology
Germantown, New York

Alice D. Coomes, MSN, RN
Assistant Professor of Nursing
Kentucky Wesleyan College
Owensboro, Kentucky

Gloria Coschigano, MSN, RN, CS
Assistant Professor of Nursing
Westchester Community College
Valhalla, New York

Jean W. Davis, EdD, RN, CS
Associate Professor of Nursing
Barry University School of Nursing
Miami Shores, Florida

Jean DeCoffe, MSN, RN
Assistant Professor of Nursing
Curry College
Milton, Massachusetts

Carole A. Devine, MSN, RN
Associate Professor of Nursing
Community College of Rhode Island
Newport, Rhode Island;
Associate Professor of Nursing
University of Rhode Island
College of Nursing
Kingston, Rhode Island

Kerry H. Fater, PhD, RN, CS
Associate Professor of Nursing
University of Massachusetts-Dartmouth
North Dartmouth, Massachusetts

Ginette G. Ferszt, PhD, RN, CS
Nursing Faculty
University of Rhode Island
College of Nursing
Kingston, Rhode Island

Cathy Fortenbaugh, MSN, RN, AOCN, CNS, C
Oncology Clinical Nurse Specialist
Pennsylvania Hospital
Philadelphia, Pennsylvania

Jane H. Freeman, EdD, RN
Professor of Nursing
Lurleen B. Wallace College of Nursing and Health Sciences
Jacksonville, Alabama

Rita S. Glazebrook, PhD, RN, CNP
Associate Professor of Nursing
St. Olaf College;
Director
Minnesota Intercollegiate Nursing Consortium
Northfield, Minnesota

Joyce Hammer, MSN, RN
Lecturer of Nursing
Wayne State University
Detroit, Michigan

Jacqueline Lynne Harris, MNSc, RN, ONC
Assistant Professor
Harding University
Searcy, Arkansas

Mary Ann Hogan, MSN, RN, CS
Instructor of Nursing
University of Massachusetts
Amherst, Massachusetts

Mary Kathleen Jackson, BSN, RN, CPN
Instructor of Nursing
Southeastern Community College
Whiteville, North Carolina

Gail M. Johnson, EdD, MSN, RN, CNAA, BC
Director, Professional Practice
Capital Health System
Trenton, New Jersey

Katherine Theresa Jorgensen, MSN, RN, MA
Associate Professor of Nursing
University of South Dakota
Vermillion, South Dakota

Elisa Mangosing Lemmon, MSN, RN, C
Program Coordinator
Riverside School of Professional Nursing
Riverside Regional Medical Center
Newport News, Virginia

Teresa Leonard, MSN, RN, CCRN
Assistant Professor of Nursing
University of North Alabama
Florence, Alabama

Carol O. Long, PhD, RN
Assistant Professor of Nursing
Arizona State University
Tempe, Arizona

Marilyn Lusk, MSN, MS, RN
Nursing Faculty
Mohave Community College
Kingman, Arizona

Linda Ann Martin, MSN, RN, APN-C
Faculty Coordinator
St. Francis Medical Center School of Nursing
Trenton, New Jersey

Dorothy Mae Mathers, MSN, RN
Assistant Professor of Nursing
Pennsylvania College of Technology
Williamsport, Pennsylvania

Betsy J. Nield, MS, RNC
Professor of Nursing
Community College of Rhode Island
Warwick, Rhode Island

Patricia A. Parsons, MSN, MS, RN
Instructor of Nursing
Riverland Community College
Austin, Minnesota

Elizabeth Phillip, MSN, RN
Nursing Faculty
St. Luke's School of Nursing
Bethlehem, Pennsylvania

Ethel Pruden, MSN, RN
Assistant Professor of Nursing
Armstrong Atlantic State University
Savannah, Georgia

Marion Sawyier, MSN, RN
Faculty
Albuquerque Technical-Vocational Institute
Albuquerque, New Mexico

Nancy Schlapman, PhD, RN
Associate Professor and Coordinator
Baccalaureate Nursing Program
Indiana University School of Nursing
Kokomo, Indiana

Jane Schlickau, MN, RN, ARNP, CTN
Associate Professor of Nursing
Southwestern College
Winfield, Kansas

Shellie Simons, MS, RN
Chairperson
Division of Nursing
Roxbury Community College
Boston, Massachusetts

Marian I. Stewart, MSN, RN
Associate Professor of Nursing
Level II Coordinator
Motlow State Community College
Lynchburg, Tennessee

Lynn Tesh, MSN, RN
Dean, Curriculum Programs
Randolph Community College
Asheboro, North Carolina

Cheryl J. Vitacco-Grab, MSN, RNC
Nursing Instructor
Lancaster Institute for Health Education
Lancaster, Pennsylvania

Loretta A. Wack, MSN, PNP, FNP
Associate Professor of Nursing
Nursing Program Coordinator
Blue Ridge Community College
Weyers Cave, Virginia

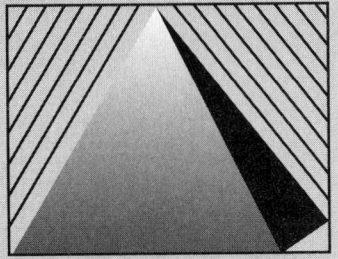

Reviewers

Karen A. Ahearn, BSN, RN, MPA
Director of Maternal Child Nursing
Saint Barnabas Medical Center
Livingston, New Jersey

Traudel B. Cline, MSN, RN
Nurse Educator
Milwaukee Area Technical College
Milwaukee, Wisconsin

Darlene DeWitt, RN, BS, CIC
Clinical Instructor, Practical Nursing
Meridian Technology Center
Stillwater, Oklahoma

Rebecca Gesler, MSN, RN
Director of Nursing
Saint Catharine College
Louisville, Kentucky

Margaret M. Gingrich, MSN, RN
Associate Professor
Harrisburg Area Community College
Harrisburg, Pennsylvania

Shari Gould, RN
Yoakum, Texas

Karen D. Hetzel, PhD, APRN, BC
Professor
Rhode Island College
Providence, Rhode Island

Elizabeth Kupczyk, MSN, RN
Assistant Professor of Nursing
Trinity Christian College
Palos Heights, Illinois

Rosemary Macy, MS, RN
Assistant Professor
Boise State University
Boise, Idaho

Cecilia Jane Maier, MS, RN, CCRN
Assistant Professor
Mount Carmel College of Nursing
Columbus, Ohio

Janet Tompkins McMahon, MSN, RN
Associate Professor of Nursing
Pennsylvania College of Technology
Williamsport, Pennsylvania

Lorene Payne, MSN, RN
Professor of Nursing
Tomball College
Tomball, Texas

Harriet Conley Wichowski, PhD, RN
Associate Professor
University of Tennessee at Chattanooga
Chattanooga, Tennessee

Linda S. Wood, MSN, RN
Director of Practical Nursing
Massanutten Technical Center
Harrisonburg, Virginia

Marguerite E. Wright, MSN, RN, RDMS
Assistant Professor
Gordon College
University System of Georgia
Barnesville, Georgia

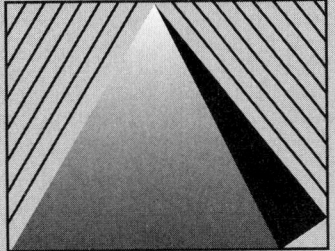

Preface

*"To know that even one life has breathed easier
because you have lived, this is to have succeeded."*

Ralph Waldo Emerson

Welcome to *Saunders Pyramid to Success!*
The *Saunders Comprehensive Review for the NCLEX-RN Examination* is one of a series of products designed to assist you in achieving your goal of becoming a registered nurse. The *Saunders Comprehensive Review for the NCLEX-RN Examination* will provide you with a comprehensive review of all of the nursing content areas specifically related to the new 2004 test plan for the NCLEX-RN exam, implemented by the National Council of State Boards of Nursing.

ORGANIZATION

The *Saunders Comprehensive Review for the NCLEX-RN Examination* contains 20 units and 76 chapters. The chapters are designed to identify specific components of nursing content. The chapters contain practice questions reflective of the chapter content and of the 2004 test plan for the NCLEX-RN exam.

The new test plan identifies a framework based on *Client Needs*. These Client Needs categories include Safe, Effective Care Environment; Health Promotion and Maintenance; Psychosocial Integrity; and Physiological Integrity. *Integrated Processes* are also identified as a component of the test plan. These include Caring, Communication and Documentation, Nursing Process, and Teaching/Learning. All of the chapters address the components of the test plan framework.

Unit I: NCLEX-RN Exam Preparation

Chapter 1 addresses all of the information about the 2004 test plan for the NCLEX-RN exam and the testing procedures related to the examination. This chapter answers all of those questions that you may have regarding the testing procedures.

Chapter 2 provides information to the foreign-educated nurse about the process of obtaining a license to practice as a registered nurse in the United States.

Chapter 3 discusses the issue of NCLEX-RN exam preparation from a nonacademic view and provides an emphasis on a holistic approach for your individual test preparation. This chapter identifies the components of a structured study plan and pattern, anxiety reduction techniques, and personal focus issues.

Nursing students want to hear what other students have to say about their experiences with the NCLEX-RN examination. Students seek a view of what it is really like to take an NCLEX-RN examination. Chapter 4 is written by a nursing student who recently took the NCLEX-RN examination. The chapter addresses the issue of what the examination is all about and includes the student's "story of success."

Test-taking strategies is a critical component of success in taking such an important examination. Chapter 5, *Test-Taking Strategies*, includes all of those important strategies that will assist in teaching you how to read a question, how not to read into a question, and how to use the process of elimination and various other strategies to select the correct response from the options presented.

Unit II: Issues in Nursing

Unit II addresses relevant nursing issues reflective of the components of the test plan for the NCLEX-RN exam. Chapter 6, *Cultural Diversity*, identifies cultures and the related factors that promote maintenance of cultural identity when caring for culturally diverse clients. Alternative and complementary therapies are also reviewed in this chapter. Chapter 7, *Ethical and Legal Issues*, provides a review of the ethical and legal considerations important to the practice of nursing and relevant to the components of the test plan. Chapter 8, *Leadership, Delegating, and Prioritizing Client Care*, identifies the leadership and management issues pertinent to the practice of nursing. This chapter emphasizes content related to time management, prioritizing, assignment-making, and the principles related to delegation. Disaster planning and triage are also reviewed.

Unit III: Nursing Sciences

The chapters in this unit specifically address areas that students have identified as areas of concern requiring review. Chapter 9, *Fluids and Electrolytes*, and Chapter 10, *Acid-Base Balance*, highlight the key components of physiology, then introduce the necessary nursing assessments and nursing interventions required in caring for a client with an alteration or imbalance. Chapter 11, *Laboratory Values*, identifies common laboratory studies, normal values, and significant information related to the specific laboratory test. Chapter 12, *Nutrition*, addresses the various food groups and important nutritional components of specific diet therapy. This chapter will assist in your review of the selection of the correct food or the foods to avoid with certain physiological conditions, because these types of questions are certainly addressed in the NCLEX-RN examination. Chapter 13, *Total Parenteral Nutrition;* Chapter 14, *Intravenous Therapy;* and Chapter 15, *Administration of Blood Products* stress all of the key components of nursing care for a client. These chapters focus on the nurse's role in the administration of these therapies and in monitoring for complications.

Unit IV: Fundamental Skills

Chapter 16, *Provision of a Safe Environment*, addresses nursing care specific to client safety and the measures that promote environmental safety. Standard precautions, transmission-based precautions, and radiation precautions are reviewed. In addition, chemical and biological warfare agents and their potentially fatal effects are reviewed. Chapter 17, *Administration of Medication and Intravenous Solutions*, includes the important components related to conversion tables and calculation of medication dosages, intravenous (IV) solutions and flow rates, IV medications, and unit doses, such as heparin and insulin. Chapter 18, *Basic Life Support*, has been included to assist you in reviewing the steps in cardiopulmonary resuscitation and the Heimlich maneuver and to refresh your memory on the priorities to be addressed in emergency situations. Chapter 19, *Perioperative Nursing Care*, addresses the key components related to caring for the client requiring surgery. Chapter 20, *Positioning Clients*, identifies safe client positions specific to various surgical and diagnostic procedures. Chapter 21, *Care of a Client with a Tube*, addresses the common types of tubes used in the clinical setting, such as chest, gastrointestinal, or renal tubes, which have always been very confusing to students, particularly in terms of their purpose and nursing care involved.

Units V through VII: Maternity Nursing, Growth and Development across the Life Span, and Pediatric Nursing

Unit V, *Maternity Nursing,* includes chapters that address maternity issues, the care of the newborn, and maternity and newborn medications. Unit VI, *Growth and Development across the Life Span,* addresses the common theories of growth and development used in the profession of nursing, developmental stages and transitions, and content related to caring for the older client. Unit VII, *Pediatric Nursing,* focuses on pediatric care and the specifics related to administering medication to the child.

Unit VIII through XVIII: Adult Health

Units VIII through XVIII address the components of adult health and are divided based on specific body systems including the integumentary, endocrine, gastrointestinal, respiratory, cardiovascular, renal, eye and ear, neurological, musculoskeletal, and immune system and oncology nursing. These chapters incorporate the Integrated Processes and all of the Client Needs components of the test plan for the NCLEX-RN exam, with a particular emphasis on Physiological Integrity. Each unit includes a pharmacology chapter that provides a comprehensive review of the medications specific to that body system.

Unit XIX: Mental Health Nursing

This unit primarily addresses the Psychosocial Integrity category of the Client Needs component of the test plan. Specific mental health disorders are addressed. This unit includes a chapter that provides a comprehensive review of the psychiatric medications.

Unit XX: Comprehensive Test

Unit XX contains a comprehensive examination and contains practice questions related to all of the content areas addressed in this book. It consists of 265 questions representative of the percentages identified in the test plan for the NCLEX-RN exam. Multiple response questions and questions in the alternate test question format are included in this test, as well as the practice tests found at the end of each chapter in this book.

SPECIAL FEATURES OF THE BOOK
Pyramid Terms

Each content area, either a chapter or unit, begins with *Pyramid Terms* and their definitions. These important terms are significant to the content contained in the chapter. In addition, the *Pyramid Terms* are in bold type throughout the content section.

◢ Pyramid to Success

The *Pyramid to Success*, a unit or chapter introduction, provides you with an overview of the chapter, guidance and direction regarding the focus of review in the particular content area, and its relative importance to the 2004 test plan for the NCLEX-RN exam. Specific nursing content areas as specified in the test plan are identified. The *Pyramid to Success* reviews the Client Needs and the Integrated Processes as they pertain to the content in that unit or chapter. These points are the specific components to keep in mind as you review the chapter outline.

◢ Pyramid Points

Pyramid Points ◢ are the bullets that are placed at specific content areas throughout the chapters. The *Pyramid Points* provide you with immediate recognition of content that is important in preparation for the NCLEX-RN examination. These bullets identify areas of content that typically appear on the NCLEX-RN examination.

Practice Questions

While preparing for the NCLEX-RN examination, it is crucial for students to practice questions. This book contains over 1800 practice questions in NCLEX-style format. The accompanying software includes all of the questions from the book, plus an additional 2200 questions for a total of over 4000 questions.

Multiple Response and Critical Thinking Questions

Each content chapter is followed by a practice test. Each practice test contains several *Multiple Response* questions and one *Critical Thinking* question. The *Critical Thinking* question may be presented as either a fill-in-the blank question, a multiple response question, or a prioritizing (ordered response) question. These questions provide you with practice in prioritizing, decision-making, and critical thinking skills.

Image Questions

The accompanying software contains *Image Questions* representative of the 2004 test plan for the NCLEX-RN exam. These questions are in NCLEX-style format and each question presents an image or picture as a component of the question.

Answer Section

The answer sections for each practice question include the correct answer, rationale, test-taking strategy, question categories, and reference source. The structure for the answer section is unique and provides the following information.

The Rationale: The rationale provides you with the significant information regarding both correct and incorrect options.

Test-Taking Strategy: The test-taking strategy provides you with the logical path in selecting the correct option and assists you in selecting an answer to a question on which you must guess. Specific suggestions for review are identified in the test-taking strategy.

Question Categories: Each question is identified based on the categories used by the test plan for the NCLEX-RN exam. Additional content categories are provided with each question to assist you in identifying areas in need of review. The categories identified with each practice question include Level of Cognitive Ability, Client Needs, Integrated Process, and the specific nursing Content Area. All categories are identified by their full names so that you do not need to memorize codes or abbreviations.

Reference: A reference, including the page number, is provided so you can easily find the information that you need to review in your undergraduate nursing textbooks.

PHARMACOLOGY AND MEDICATION CALCULATIONS REVIEW

Students consistently verbalize that pharmacology is an area in which they need assistance. The 2004 test plan for the NCLEX-RN exam incorporates pharmacology in the examination to a greater extent than in the past. Therefore, pharmacology chapters have been included for your review and practice. This book includes 13 pharmacology chapters, a medication and intravenous (IV) calculation chapter, and a pediatric medication calculation chapter. Each of these chapters is followed by a practice test using the same question format as described above. This book contains over 400 pharmacology questions. Additional pharmacology questions can be found on the accompanying software.

NCLEX-RN EXAM REVIEW SOFTWARE

Packaged in this book you will find a CD-ROM containing review software for the NCLEX-RN exam. This software contains over 4000 practice questions. It also includes the image practice questions and other alternative format questions. This Windows and Macintosh compatible program offers three testing modes for review.

Quiz—Ten randomly chosen questions in a specific selected content area. The answer, rationale, test-taking strategy, question categories, reference source, and results appear after you answer all 10 questions.

Study—All questions in a specific selected content area. The answer, rationale, test-taking strategy, question categories, and reference source appear after answering each question.

Examination—One hundred randomly chosen questions from the entire pool of more than 4000 questions. The answer, rationale, test-taking strategy, question categories, reference source, and results appear after you answer all 100 questions.

HOW TO USE THIS BOOK

Saunders Comprehensive Review for the NCLEX-RN Examination is especially designed to help you with your successful journey to the peak of the *Saunders Pyramid to Success*, becoming a registered nurse. As you begin your journey through this book, you will be introduced to all of the important points regarding the 2004 NCLEX-RN examination, the process of testing, and the unique and special tips regarding how to prepare yourself for this very important examination.

You should begin your process through the *Saunders Pyramid to Success* by reading all of Unit I in this book and becoming familiar with the important points regarding the NCLEX-RN examination. Read the chapter from the nursing graduate who recently passed the examination and note what this graduate has to say about the examination. The test-taking strategy chapter will provide you with those important strategies that will guide you in selecting the correct option or assist you in selecting an answer to a question you must guess. Read this chapter and practice these strategies as you proceed through your journey with this book. Continue your journey by reading each of the chapters and content areas. Review the Pyramid Terms and the Pyramid to Success and identify the Client Needs and Integrated Processes specific to the test plan in that area. Read each of the content areas focusing on the Pyramid Points that identify those areas most likely to be tested on the NCLEX-RN examination.

As you read each chapter, identify your strengths and those areas in need of further review. Highlight these areas and test your strengths and abilities by taking all of the practice tests provided at the end of the chapters. Be sure to read all of the rationales and the test-taking strategies. The rationales provide you with the significant information regarding both the correct and incorrect options. The test-taking strategy offers you the logical path to selecting the correct option. The strategy also identifies content area that you need to review if you had difficulty with the question. Use the reference source listed so you can easily find the information that you need to review.

After reviewing all of the chapters in the book, turn to Unit XX, the Comprehensive Test. Take this examination and then review each question, answer, and rationale. Identify any areas requiring further review; then take the time to review those areas again.

After using this book to review specific content areas, continue on your journey through the *Saunders Pyramid to Success* with the companion book, *Saunders Q&A Review for the NCLEX-RN Examination*, for additional practice questions. The companion book and its accompanying software offer you over 3500 practice questions on specific areas outlined by the 2004

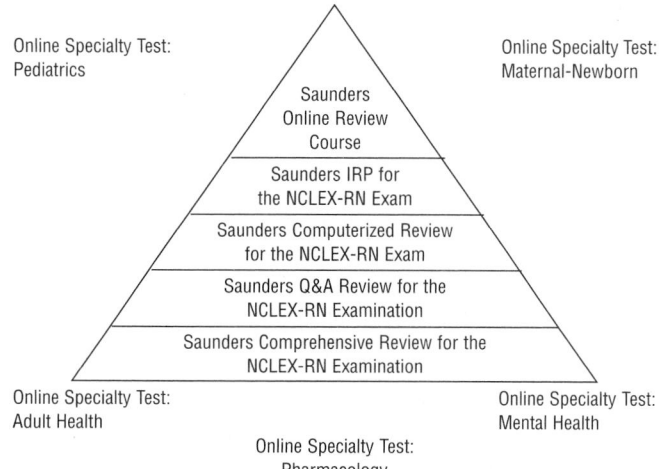

test plan for the NCLEX-RN exam. With practice questions uniquely focused on the Client Needs and the Integrated Processes, you can assess your level of competence. To determine your readiness for the NCLEX-RN examination, you will use the next step in the *Saunders Pyramid to Success, the Saunders Computerized Review for the NCLEX-RN Examination*. This unique software program contains 2000 NCLEX-RN style questions. The software provides a detailed analysis similar to that in standardized nursing examinations. To strengthen your abilities in a specific content area, use the online specialty tests. Online specialty tests are available in the following content areas: Adult Health, Mental Health, Maternal-Newborn, Pediatrics, and Pharmacology. Each specialty test provides you with 100 practice test questions in NCLEX-style format.

The *Saunders Online Review Course for the NCLEX-RN Examination* is another valuable resource to use in preparing for the examination. This course contains a total of 10 modules and 47 lessons. Every lesson contains content for review, illustrations, practice questions, and a case study followed by questions related to the case study. Each module is followed by a 100-question exam that contains questions representative of the content in the module lessons. There is also a Pretest Exam, a Comprehensive (Cumulative) Exam, and a CAT (computerized adaptive testing) Exam. The course provides you with a systematic and individualized method for preparing to take the NCLEX examination.

A final component of the *Saunders Pyramid to Success* is the *Saunders Instructor's Resource Package for the NCLEX-RN Examination*. This manual and CD-ROM accompany the Saunders program of review products. Be sure to ask your nursing program director and nursing faculty about this CD-ROM and its use for a review course or a self-paced review in your school's computer laboratory.

Good Luck with your journey through the *Saunders Pyramid to Success*. I wish you continued success throughout your new career as a registered nurse!

LINDA ANNE SILVESTRI, MSN, RN

To All Future Registered Nurses,

Congratulations to you!

You should be very proud and pleased with yourself on your most recent well-deserved accomplishment of completing your nursing program to become a registered nurse. I know that you have worked very hard to become successful and that you have proven to yourself that indeed you can achieve your goals.

In my opinion, you are about to enter the most wonderful and rewarding profession that exists. Your willingness, desire, and ability to assist those who need nursing care will bring great satisfaction to your life.

In the profession of nursing, your learning will be a lifelong process. This aspect of the profession makes it stimulating and dynamic. Your learning process will continue to expand and grow as the profession continues to evolve. Your next very important endeavor will be the learning process involved to achieve success in your examination to become a registered nurse.

I am excited and pleased to be able to provide you with the *Saunders Pyramid to Success* products that will prepare you for your next important professional goal, becoming a registered nurse. I want to thank all of my former nursing students whom I have assisted in preparing for the NCLEX-RN exam for their willingness to offer ideas regarding their needs in preparing for licensure. Student ideas have certainly added a special uniqueness to all of the products available in *Saunders Pyramid to Success*.

Saunders Pyramid to Success products provide you with everything that you need to prepare for the NCLEX-RN exam. These products include material that is required for the NCLEX-RN exam preparation for all nursing students regardless of educational background, specific strengths, areas in need of improvement, or clinical experience during the nursing program.

So, let's get started and begin our journey through the *Pyramid to Success* and welcome to the wonderful profession of nursing!

Sincerely,

Linda Anne Silvestri MSN, RN

Linda Anne Silvestri, MSN, RN

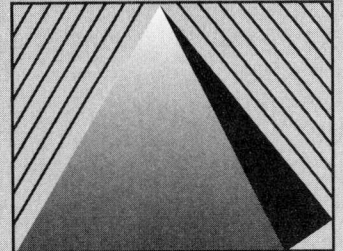

Acknowledgments

Sincere appreciation and warmest thanks are extended to the many individuals who in their own way have contributed to the publication of this book.

First, I want to thank all of my nursing students at the Community College of Rhode Island in Warwick who approached me in 1991 and persuaded me to assist them in preparing to take the NCLEX-RN examination. Their enthusiasm and inspiration led to the commencement of my professional endeavors in conducting review courses for the NCLEX-RN exam for nursing students. I also thank the numerous nursing students who have attended my review courses for their willingness to share their needs and ideas. Their input has certainly added a special uniqueness to this publication.

I wish to acknowledge the nursing faculty who taught in my review courses for the NCLEX-RN exam. Their commitment, dedication, and expertise have certainly assisted nursing students in achieving success with the NCLEX-RN exam. Additionally, I want to acknowledge Laurent W. Valliere for his contribution to this publication, for teaching in my review courses for the NCLEX-RN exam, and for his commitment and dedication in assisting my nursing students to prepare for the NCLEX-RN exam from a nonacademic point of view.

I sincerely acknowledge and thank two very important individuals from Elsevier Health Sciences. I thank Loren Wilson, Director, Review and Testing, for all of her assistance throughout the preparation of this edition and for her continuous enthusiasm, support, and expert professional guidance. And, I thank Shelly Hayden, Managing Editor, for her continuous assistance and for keeping me on track. Her expert organizational skills maintained order for all of the work that I submitted for manuscript production.

A special thank you and acknowledgment go to two important individuals, Dianne E. Ventrice and Lawrence Fiorentino. They provided continuous support and dedication to my work in both the NCLEX exam review courses and in reference support for the third edition of this book.

I want to acknowledge all of the staff at Elsevier Health Sciences for their tremendous assistance throughout the preparation and production of this publication. A special thank you to all of them.

I thank all of the special people in the production department who played important roles in finalizing this publication: Cheryl Abbott, Senior Project Manager; John Rogers, Publishing Services Manager; and Bill Drone, Design Manager.

I sincerely thank Bob Boehringer, Director of Nursing Marketing, and Karen McKie, Marketing Manager, from the Nursing Marketing Department, whose support, hard work, and special creativity assisted with this publication.

I would also like to acknowledge Patricia Mieg, Educational Sales Representative, who encouraged me to submit my ideas and initial work for the first edition of this book to the W.B. Saunders Company.

I want to acknowledge my parents who opened my door of opportunity in education. I thank my mother, Frances Mary, for all of her love, support, and assistance as I continuously worked to achieve my professional goals. I thank my father, Arnold Lawrence, who always provided insightful words of encouragement. My memories of his love and support will always remain in my heart.

I also thank my sister, Dianne Elodia, my brother, Lawrence Peter, and my niece, Gina Marie, who were continuously supportive, giving, and helpful during my research and preparation of this publication.

I want to acknowledge all of the contributors who provided many of the practice questions contained in this publication and the many faculty and student reviewers for their thoughts and ideas.

I sincerely thank Mary Ann Hogan, MSN, RN, from the University of Massachusetts in Amherst, Massachusetts, who has always encouraged and supported me through my professional endeavors. Her numerous contributions to this publication are a reflection of her dedication to the profession of nursing and to nursing students. A special thank you to Dr. JoAnn Mullaney from Salve Regina University in Newport, Rhode Island, for her numerous and expert contributions to this publication and to Kimberly Green, RN, for providing a chapter to this publication regarding her experiences with the NCLEX-RN exam.

I also need to thank Salve Regina University for the opportunity to educate nursing students in the baccalaureate nursing program and for its support during my research and writing of this publication. I would like to especially acknowledge my colleagues, Dr. Sandra Solem, Dr. Ellen McCarty, Dr. JoAnn Mullaney, Dr. Jane McCool, Dr. Peggy Matteson, and Dr. Bethany Sykes, for all of their support and encouragement.

I wish to acknowledge the Community College of Rhode Island for providing me the opportunity to educate nursing students in the Associate Degree of Nursing Program, and a special thank you to Patricia Miller, MSN, RN, and Michelina McClellan, MS, RN, from Baystate Medical Center School of Nursing in Springfield, Massachusetts, who were my very first mentors in nursing education.

Lastly, a very special thank you to all my nursing students, past, present, and future. Your love and dedication to the profession of nursing and your commitment to provide health care will bring never-ending rewards!

Linda Anne Silvestri, MSN, RN

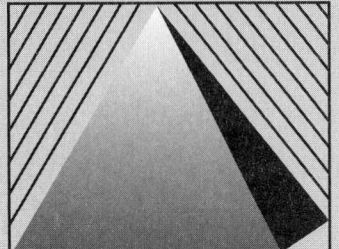

Contents

NCLEX-RN Exam Preparation

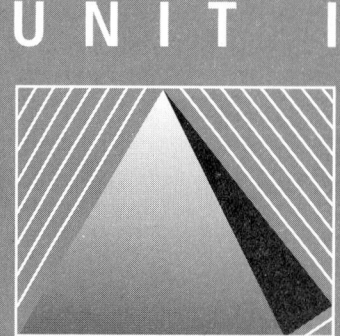

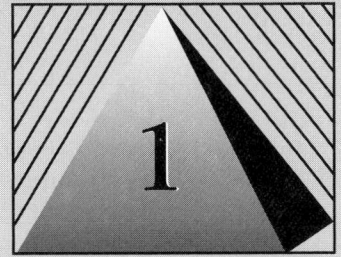

The NCLEX-RN Examination

▲ THE PYRAMID TO SUCCESS

Welcome to the Pyramid to Success.

Saunders Comprehensive Review for the NCLEX-RN Examination is specially designed to help you begin your successful journey to the peak of the pyramid, becoming a registered nurse. As you begin your journey, you will be introduced to all of the important points regarding the NCLEX-RN examination and the process of testing and to the unique and special tips regarding how to prepare yourself for this important examination. You will read what a nursing graduate who recently passed the NCLEX-RN exam has to say about the test. All those important test-taking strategies are detailed. These details will guide you in selecting the correct option or assist you in selecting an answer to a question at which you must guess.

Each of the content areas in this book begins with the Pyramid to Success. The Pyramid to Success addresses specific points related to the NCLEX-RN exam, including the Pyramid Terms and the Client Needs and the Integrated Processes as identified in the test plan framework for the examination. Pyramid Terms are key words that are defined and are boldfaced throughout each chapter to direct your attention to those significant points for the examination. The Client Needs and the Integrated Processes specific to the content of the chapter are identified.

Throughout each chapter, you will find Pyramid Point bullets that identify areas most likely to be tested on the NCLEX-RN examination. Read each chapter, and identify your strengths and areas that are in need of further review. Test your strengths and abilities by taking all the practice tests provided in this book. Be sure to read all the rationales and the test-taking strategies. The rationale provides you with significant information regarding the correct option and incorrect options. The test-taking strategy provides you with the logical path to selecting the correct option. The test-taking strategy also

identifies the content area to review, if required. The reference source and page number are provided so that you can find the information easily that you need to review. Each question is coded based on the level of cognitive ability, the Client Needs category, the Integrated Process, and the nursing content area.

Following the completion of your comprehensive review in this book, continue on your journey though the Pyramid to Success with the companion book, *Saunders Q & A Review for the NCLEX-RN Examination*, which provides you with more than 3500 practice questions based on the NCLEX-RN exam test plan. Then you are ready for the *Saunders Computerized Review*, a computer disk program that contains more than 2000 NCLEX-RN exam–style questions to help you determine your readiness for the NCLEX-RN exam. Additional resources to assist you in preparing for this examination include the online specialty tests titled Adult Health, Mental Health, Maternal-Newborn, Pediatrics, and Pharmacology and the online review course for the NCLEX-RN exam.

The online review course for the NCLEX-RN exam addresses all areas of the test plan identified by the National Council of State Boards of Nursing, Inc. The course contains a pretest that provides feedback regarding your strengths and weaknesses and that generates an individualized study schedule in a calendar format. Content review includes practice questions and case studies, figures and illustrations, a glossary, and animations and videos. A cumulative examination and a computer adaptive test are also key components of the online review course. The types of practice questions in this course include multiple choice, fill in the blank, multiple response, those that require you to prioritize (ordered response), and questions containing figures that may require you to use the computer mouse to answer. These additional products in Saunders Pyramid to Success, including the online specialty tests and the online review course, can be obtained online at *www.elsevierhealth.com/reviewandtesting*.

Let's begin our journey through the Pyramid to Success.

THE EXAMINATION PROCESS

An important step in the Pyramid to Success is to become as familiar as possible with the examination process. A significant amount of anxiety can occur in candidates facing the challenge of this examination. Knowing what the examination is all about and knowing what you will encounter during the process of testing will assist in alleviating fear and anxiety. The information contained in this chapter addresses the procedures related to the development of the NCLEX-RN exam test plan, the components of the test plan, and the answers to the questions most commonly asked by nursing students and graduates preparing to take the NCLEX-RN exam. The information contained in this chapter related to the test plan was obtained from the National Council of State Boards of Nursing (NCSBN) Web site (*www.ncsbn.org*) and from the *Test Plan for the National Council Licensure Examination for Registered Nurses* (effective date: April 2004), National Council of State Boards of Nursing, Chicago, 2003. You can obtain additional information regarding the test and its development by accessing the NCSBN Web site or by writing to the National Council of State Boards of Nursing, 111 E. Wacker Drive, Suite 2900, Chicago, IL 60601.

COMPUTER ADAPTIVE TESTING

The acronym *CAT* stands for computer adaptive test, which means that the examination is created as the test taker answers each question. All of the test questions are categorized based on the test plan structure and the level of difficulty of the question. As you answer a question, the computer determines your competency based on the answer you selected. If you selected a correct answer to a question, the computer scans the question bank and selects a more difficult question. If you selected an incorrect answer, the computer scans the question bank and selects an easier question. This process continues until the test plan requirements are met and a reliable pass or fail decision is made.

When a test question is presented on the computer screen, you must answer it or the test will not move on. This means that you will not be able to skip questions, go back and review questions, or go back and change answers. Remember, in a CAT, once an answer is recorded, all subsequent questions administered depend, to an extent, on the answer selected for that question. Skipping and returning to earlier questions are not compatible with the logical methodology of a CAT. The inability to skip questions or go back to change previous answers will not be a disadvantage to you. Actually, you will not fall into that "trap" of changing a correct answer to an incorrect one with CAT. If you are faced with a question that contains unfamiliar content, you may need to guess at the answer. There is no penalty for guessing on this examination. Remember, with the majority of the questions, the answer will be right there in front of you. If you need to guess, use your nursing knowledge to its fullest extent, as well as all of the test-taking strategies that you have practiced in this review program.

You do not need any computer experience to take this examination. A keyboard tutorial is provided and administered to all test takers at the start of the examination. The tutorial will instruct you on the use of the on-screen optional calculator, the use of the mouse, and how to record an answer. In addition to the traditional four-option multiple-choice question, the tutorial also provides instructions on how to respond to different question formats. A proctor is present to assist in explaining the use of the computer to ensure your full understanding of how to proceed.

DEVELOPMENT OF THE TEST PLAN

The test plan for the NCLEX-RN examination is developed by the National Council of State Boards of Nursing, Inc. As an initial step in the test development process, the NCSBN considers the legal scope of nursing practice as governed by state laws and regulations, including the nurse practice act, and uses these laws to define the areas on the examination that will assess the competence of a candidate (test taker) for licensure.

The NCSBN also conducts a practice analysis study to determine the framework for the test plan for the examination. The participants in this study include newly licensed registered nurses from all types of basic education programs. The NCSBN provides participants a list of nursing activities and asks them about the frequency of performing these specific activities, their impact on maintaining client safety, and the setting where the activities were performed. A panel of experts at the NCSBN analyzes the results of the study and makes decisions regarding the test plan framework. Because nursing practice continues to change, the NCSBN conducts this study every 3 years. The results of this study, most recently conducted in 2002, provided the structure for the test plan implemented in April 2004.

THE TEST PLAN

The content of the NCLEX-RN exam reflects the activities that a newly licensed, entry-level registered nurse must be able to perform to provide clients with safe and effective nursing care. The questions are written to address the levels of cognitive ability, Client Needs, and Integrated Processes as identified in the test plan developed by the NCSBN (Box 1-1).

Examination Questions

Each examination question addresses the following:
A level of cognitive ability
A Client Needs category
An Integrated Process

BOX 1-2

Level of Cognitive Ability

A nurse is caring for a client with a T5 spinal cord injury. The client complains of a severe headache and is feeling anxious. The nurse notes the client is sweating, is experiencing bradycardia, and is hypertensive. Which nursing intervention is most appropriate initially?
1. Check for bladder distention.
2. Notify the physician.
3. Medicate the client with an analgesic.
4. Discuss the client's feelings of anxiety.
Answer: 1
This question requires you to analyze the data provided in the question to determine the most appropriate initial nursing intervention. You need to know the signs and symptoms of autonomic dysreflexia and the potential causes, such as a full bladder or bowel, to determine the most appropriate initial action.
Level of cognitive ability: Analysis

Reference: Ignatavicius, D., & Workman, M. (2002). *Medical-surgical nursing: Critical thinking for collaborative care* (4th ed., p. 935). Philadelphia: W. B. Saunders.

Levels of Cognitive Ability

The examination for licensure as a registered nurse may include questions at the cognitive levels of knowledge, comprehension, application, and analysis. However, the majority of the questions are written at the application or higher levels of cognitive ability, such as the analysis level, because the practice of nursing requires critical thinking in decision making. This means that the test taker will be required to analyze and apply the information provided in the test question. Box 1-2 presents an example of a question that requires you to analyze data to determine the nursing intervention.

Client Needs

In the test plan implemented in April 2004 the NCSBN has identified a test plan framework based on Client Needs. The NCSBN identifies four major categories of Client Needs. Some of these categories are further divided into subcategories. The Client Needs categories include Safe, Effective Care Environment, Health Promotion and Maintenance, Psychosocial Integrity, and Physiological Integrity (Table 1-1).

TABLE 1-1

Client Needs Categories and Percent of Questions

Client Needs Category	Percent of Questions on NCLEX-RN Exam
SAFE, EFFECTIVE CARE ENVIRONMENT	
Management of Care	13%-19%
Safety and Infection Control	8%-14%
HEALTH PROMOTION AND MAINTENANCE	6%-12%
PSYCHOSOCIAL INTEGRITY	6%-12%
PHYSIOLOGICAL INTEGRITY	
Basic Care and Comfort	6%-12%
Pharmacological and Parenteral Therapies	13%-19%
Reduction of Risk Potential	13%-19%
Physiological Adaptation	11%-17%

Safe, Effective Care Environment

The Safe, Effective Care Environment category includes two subcategories: Management of Care and Safety and Infection Control. Management of Care (13% to 19%) addresses content that tests the knowledge, skills, and ability required to enhance the care delivery setting to protect clients, families, significant others, visitors, and health care personnel. Safety and Infection Control (8% to 14%) addresses content that tests the knowledge, skills, and ability required to protect clients, families, significant others, visitors, and health care personnel from health and environmental hazards. Box 1-3 presents examples of questions that address these two subcategories.

Health Promotion and Maintenance

The Health Promotion and Maintenance category (6% to 12%) addresses the principles related to growth and development. This Client Needs category also addresses content that tests the knowledge, skills, and ability required to assist the client, family members, and significant others to prevent health problems, to recognize alterations in health, and to develop health practices that promote and support wellness. See Box 1-4 for an example of a question in this Client Needs category.

Psychosocial Integrity

The Psychosocial Integrity category (6% to 12%) addresses content that tests the knowledge, skills, and ability required to promote and support the client, client's family, and significant other's ability to cope, adapt, and problem solve during stressful events. This Client Needs category also addresses the emotional, mental, and social well-being of the client, family, or significant other, and the knowledge, skills, and ability required to care for the client with an acute or chronic

---

BOX 1-3

Safe, Effective Care Environment

MANAGEMENT OF CARE

A nurse calls a physician to report that a client with congestive heart failure has developed increased wheezes on lung auscultation and dyspnea. The physician was in a hurry because of involvement in an emergency situation in the emergency room and gives the nurse an order for furosemide (Lasix) by telephone but was unclear about the route of the medication. The most appropriate action by the nurse would be what?

1. Administer the medication by the intravenous route because this route usually is used with clients with congestive heart failure.
2. Administer the medication by the oral route and clarify the order once the physician has finished caring for the client in the emergency room.
3. Call the nursing supervisor for assistance in determining the route of the medication.
4. Call the physician who gave the telephone order and clarify the order.

Answer: 4

This question is an example of a question that represents the subcategory Management of Care in the Client Needs category of Safe, Effective Care Environment. The nurse has the responsibility to protect the client from harm. Because the medication order is incomplete, the nurse must call the physician who gave the order by telephone and obtain an order for a medication route.

Reference: Potter, P., & Perry, A. (2001) *Fundamentals of nursing* (5th ed., p. 434). St. Louis: Mosby.

SAFETY AND INFECTION CONTROL

A nurse is caring for a client who is receiving total parenteral nutrition through a central vein. Which nursing action will decrease the client's risk of developing an infection from this therapy?

1. Assessing vital signs at 4-hour intervals
2. Instructing the client to perform a Valsalva's maneuver during intravenous tubing changes
3. Administering acetaminophen (Tylenol) before changing the central line dressing
4. Using aseptic technique in handling the total parenteral nutrition solution and tubing

Answer: 4

This question addresses the subcategory Safety and Infection Control in the Client Needs category Safe, Effective Care Environment. The question addresses content related to asepsis. Option 1 will detect signs of an infection but is not associated with prevention or decreasing the risk of infection. Options 2 and 3 do not relate to infection. Aseptic technique is critical to prevent infection.

Reference: Ignatavicius, D., & Workman, M. (2002). *Medical-surgical nursing: Critical thinking for collaborative care* (4th ed., pp. 208, 1370). Philadelphia: W. B. Saunders.

BOX 1-4

Health Promotion and Maintenance

A nurse in a day care center is planning play activities for a group of toddlers. The nurse selects which most appropriate play materials for the children?

1. Rattles, stuffed animals, squeaky dolls, soft mobiles
2. Videos, compact disc player, board games
3. Cards, Monopoly game, sewing kits, paint-by-number kits
4. Blocks, rocking horse, finger paints, wooden puzzles, thick crayons, paper

Answer: 4

This question addresses the Client Needs category Health Promotion and Maintenance and specifically relates to the principles of growth and development of a toddler. The toddler engages in parallel play, and appropriate toys promote increased locomotor skills, meet the need for tactile play, and are safe. Option 1 identifies toys appropriate for the infant. Option 2 identifies activities for an adolescent. Option 3 identifies activities appropriate for the school-age child.

Reference: James, S., Ashwill, J., & Droske, S. (2002). *Nursing care of children: Principles & practice* (2nd ed., pp. 154, 157). Philadelphia: W. B. Saunders.

mental illness. See Box 1-5 for an example of a question in this Client Needs category.

Physiological Integrity

The Physiological Integrity category includes four subcategories: Basic Care and Comfort, Pharmacological and Parenteral Therapies, Reduction of Risk Potential, and Physiological Adaptation. Basic Care and Comfort (6% to 12%) addresses content that tests the knowledge, skills, and ability required to provide comfort and assistance to the client in the performance of activities of daily living. Pharmacological and Parenteral Therapies (13% to 19%) addresses content that tests the knowledge, skills, and ability required to administer medications and parenteral therapies. Reduction of Risk Potential (13% to 19%) addresses content that tests the knowledge, skills, and ability required to prevent complications or health problems related to the client's condition or any prescribed treatments or procedures. Physiological Adaptation (11% to 17%) addresses content that tests the knowledge, skills, and ability required to provide care to clients with acute, chronic, or life-threatening conditions. See Box 1-6 for examples of questions in this Client Needs category.

BOX 1-5

Psychosocial Integrity

A nurse, providing information to the wife of a client who abuses alcohol, encourages the woman to attend an Al-Anon support group. The wife tells the nurse that she is embarrassed by her husband's behavior and that it would be difficult for her to face other persons. To help alleviate the wife's concern, the nurse would most appropriately tell the wife that

1. The support group is always led by a nurse and a physician.
2. The members of the group experience the same problem she is facing.
3. She will not know any of the members of the support group.
4. She does not need to provide her name or any other identifying information to the group.

Answer: 2

This question addresses the Client Needs category Psychosocial Integrity and specifically relates to supporting the client's significant other during a stressful event. Al-Anon is a support group for spouses and friends of alcoholics or addicts. Support groups are based on the premise that persons who have experienced a particular problem are able to help others with the same problem. Although a nurse or other health care professional may be asked to speak at a support group meeting, the members of the group lead the group. Option 3 is incorrect because the nurse cannot ensure that the spouse will not know any of the members. Although option 4 may be correct, it is not the most appropriate response to give the wife.

Reference: Stuart, G., & Laraia, M. (2001). *Principles and practice of psychiatric nursing* (7th ed., p. 499). St. Louis: Mosby.

BOX 1-6

Physiological Integrity

BASIC CARE AND COMFORT

A nurse provides instructions to a client about the use of a cane and watches as the client uses the device. Which observation by the nurse indicates the need to provide additional instructions to the client?

1. The client holds the cane on the strong side.
2. The client holds the cane about 6 inches to the side of the foot.
3. The client flexes the elbow at a 15- to 30-degree angle when holding the cane in place.
4. The client moves the cane and the stronger leg forward first and then moves the weaker leg forward.

Answer: 4

This question addresses the subcategory Basic Care and Comfort in the Client Needs category Physiological Integrity and addresses client mobility and promoting assistance in an activity of daily living. Note the issue of the question: the need for the nurse to provide additional instructions. Visualize each of the options in terms of their safety in performing ambulation regarding the use of a cane. This will direct you to the option that is unsafe.

Reference: Potter, P., & Perry, A. (2001). *Fundamentals of nursing* (5th ed., pp. 1007-1008). St. Louis: Mosby.

PHARMACOLOGICAL AND PARENTERAL THERAPIES

A client is taking capreomycin sulfate (Capastat), a second-line antituberculosis medication, as a component of pharmacological treatment for tuberculosis. The client calls the nurse at the physician's office and tells the nurse that he is experiencing ringing in the ears. The nurse most appropriately tells the client that

1. He should speak with the physician about the problem.
2. Ringing in the ears is an expected effect of the medication.
3. He should discontinue the medication.
4. Ringing in the ears is a harmless effect of the medication.

Answer: 1

This question addresses the subcategory of Pharmacological and Parenteral Therapies in the Client Needs category Physiological Integrity. Capreomycin is a second-line antituberculosis medication administered along with a first-line medication to treat tuberculosis. Capreomycin can cause damage to cranial nerve VIII (ototoxicity), resulting in hearing loss, tinnitus, and disturbance of balance. Ototoxicity is not an expected or harmless effect of the medication, and if it occurs, the physician needs to be notified. The nurse does not adjust a medication dosage or discontinue a medication.

Reference: Lehne, R. (2001). *Pharmacology for nursing care* (4th ed., pp. 988-999). Philadelphia: W. B. Saunders.

REDUCTION OF RISK POTENTIAL

A client with acute myocardial infarction receives therapy with alteplase, recombinant (t-PA). The nurse assesses for complications of this treatment. Which assessment data would the nurse document as indicating a possible complication?

1. Epistaxis
2. Vomiting
3. ST segment elevation on electrocardiogram
4. Absent pedal pulses

Answer: 1

This question addresses the subcategory of Reduction of Risk Potential in the Client Needs category Physiological Integrity. Bleeding is a major side effect of t-PA therapy. This question addresses content related to the complication of a treatment.

Reference: Hodgson, B., & Kizior, R. (2004). *Saunders nursing drug handbook 2004* (p. 33). Philadelphia: W. B. Saunders.

Continued

BOX 1-6

Physiological Integrity—cont'd

PHYSIOLOGICAL ADAPTATION

A nurse reviews the blood gas results of a client with pneumonia. The nurse analyzes the results and determines that the client is experiencing respiratory acidosis. Which of the following validates the nurse's findings?

1. pH 7.45, P_{CO_2} 52 mm Hg
2. pH 7.35, P_{CO_2} 40 mm Hg
3. pH 7.25, P_{CO_2} 50 mm Hg
4. pH 7.50, P_{CO_2} 30 mm Hg

Answer: 3

This question addresses the subcategory of Physiological Adaptation in the Client Needs category Physiological Integrity. The normal pH is 7.35 to 7.45. The normal P_{CO_2} is 35 to 45 mm Hg. In respiratory acidosis the pH is down and the P_{CO_2} is up. Options 1 and 4 reflect an elevated pH that indicates an alkalotic condition. Option 2 reflects a normal blood gas result. The content addressed in this question relates to an acid-base imbalance, an alteration in body systems.

Reference: Ignatavicius, D., & Workman, M. (2002). *Medical-surgical nursing: Critical thinking for collaborative care* (4th ed., p. 225). Philadelphia: W. B. Saunders.

BOX 1-7

Integrated Processes

A female client and her newborn infant have undergone testing for human immunodeficiency virus (HIV), and both clients have been found to be positive. The news is devastating, and the mother is crying. The most appropriate nursing action at this time is to

1. Call an HIV counselor and make an appointment for the mother and her newborn infant.
2. Describe the progressive stages and treatments for HIV to the mother.
3. Examine with the mother how she contracted HIV.
4. Listen quietly while the mother talks and cries.

Answer: 4

This question addresses the Integrated Process of Caring. The mother has just received devastating news and needs to have someone with her to cope with this issue. The nurse needs to sit with the mother and actively listen while she talks and cries. Calling an HIV counselor may be helpful but is not what she needs at this time. The other options are not appropriate for the mother at this time. The most caring action is to address the mother's feelings and to provide support to her.

Integrated Process: Caring

Reference: Potter, P., & Perry, A. (2001). *Fundamentals of nursing* (5th ed., pp. 459-462). St. Louis: Mosby.

Integrated Processes

The NCSBN identifies four processes that are fundamental to the practice of nursing. These processes are a component of the test plan and are incorporated throughout the major categories of Client Needs. The Integrated Processes include caring, communication and documentation, nursing process (assessment, analysis, planning, implementation, and evaluation), and teaching/learning. See Box 1-7 for an example of a question that incorporates the Integrated Process of caring.

TYPES OF QUESTIONS ON THE EXAMINATION

The types of questions you may find on the examination include multiple choice, fill in the blank, multiple response, prioritizing (ordered response), and questions that contain a figure or illustration. You also may encounter a question that may require you to use the mouse component of the computer system. For example, you may be presented with a visual that displays the arterial vessels of an adult client. In this visual, you may be asked to "point and click" (using the mouse) on the area where the dorsalis pedis pulse could be felt. The NCSBN provides specific directions for you to follow with these questions to guide you in your process of testing. Be sure to read these directions as they appear on the computer screen.

Multiple-Choice Questions

Most of the questions that you will be asked to answer will be in the multiple-choice format. These questions provide you with data about a particular client situation and four answers or options.

Fill in the Blank

Fill in the blank questions may ask you to perform a medication calculation or to calculate an intake or output record on a client. These questions also may ask you questions about other content, such as a major side effect of a medication or a specific nursing intervention. You will need to type in your answer. See Box 1-8 for an example.

Multiple Response

For a multiple response question, you will be asked to select or check all of the options, such as nursing

BOX 1-8

Fill in the Blank

A physician orders an intravenous dose of 200,000 units of penicillin G benzathine (Bicillin) for an adult client. The label on the 10-mL ampule sent from the pharmacy reads penicillin G benzathine (Bicillin), 300,000 units per mL. The nurse prepares how much medication to administer the correct dose? (Round to the nearest tenth.)

Answer: 0.7 mL (or 0.7)

In this question you need to use the formula for calculating a medication dose. Once you determine the dose, you will need to type in your answer. In this particular question, you are asked to round to the nearest tenth. Always follow the specific directions noted on the computer screen when answering the question. Also remember that there will be an onscreen calculator on the computer for your use if needed.

Reference: Potter, P., & Perry, A. (2001). *Fundamentals of nursing* (5th ed., pp. 897-898). St. Louis: Mosby.

BOX 1-9

Multiple Response

A hospitalized client who was diagnosed with a cerebral aneurysm is placed on aneurysm precautions. Select all nursing interventions that apply for these precautions.

Answer

___ Allow the client to perform activities of daily living independently, including bathing and dressing.

_X_ Encourage the client to dress in street clothes and shoes every day.

___ Encourage restful activities such as listening to quiet music.

___ Keep the room well lit, especially during the daytime hours.

_X_ Administer stool softeners to the client.

_X_ Restrict visitors and keep visits short.

In a multiple response question, you will be asked to select or check all of the options, such as nursing interventions, that relate to the information in the question. To answer this question, recalling the pathophysiology associated with a cerebral aneurysm and that a primary concern is rupture of the aneurysm will assist in identifying the appropriate nursing interventions. Remember, follow the specific directions given on the computer screen.

Reference: Phipps, W., Monahan, F., Sands, J., Marek, J., & Neighbors, M. (2003). *Medical-surgical nursing: Health and illness perspectives* (7th ed., p. 1385). St. Louis: Mosby.

interventions, that relate to the information in the question. No partial credit is given for correct selections. You need to do exactly as the question asks, which will be to select *all* that apply. See Box 1-9 for an example.

Prioritizing (Ordered Response)

In this type of question, you will be asked to use the computer mouse to drag and drop your nursing actions

BOX 1-10

Prioritizing (Ordered Response)

A nurse performs an assessment on an older client admitted to the hospital with a diagnosis of dehydration. On assessment the nurse notes that the client is weak when ambulating, is intermittently confused, and has dry skin. The client reports that she has been able to eat and drink small amounts but that the diarrhea will not stop. The client also tells the nurse that she lives alone and is not able to socialize much because she does not drive or have family close by that can visit her. The nurse develops a plan of care and identifies five nursing diagnoses. Prioritize the nursing diagnoses (using the numbers 1, 2, 3, 4, 5) from highest priority (number 1) to lowest priority (number 5).

___ Deficient fluid volume
___ Risk for impaired skin integrity
___ Acute confusion
___ Risk for injury
___ Risk for social isolation

Answer: 14235

This question asks you to prioritize in order of importance the nursing diagnoses identified for this client and provides you with directions regarding numbering from lowest priority to highest priority. Remember, read the directions on the computer screen to guide you in answering this type of question. The nursing diagnosis most appropriate (highest priority) for the client who is dehydrated is deficient fluid volume. Because the nursing diagnosis acute confusion is an actual client problem and because confusion could place the client at risk for injury, acute confusion would be the second priority. Risk for injury, risk for impaired skin integrity, and risk for social isolation are potential (at risk), not actual, problems. Risk for injury would be the third priority. Risk for impaired skin integrity is the fourth priority because it is a physiological need. This would be followed by risk for social isolation, a psychosocial need.

Reference: Ignatavicius, D., & Workman, M. (2002). *Medical-surgical nursing: Critical thinking for collaborative care* (4th ed., p. 164). Philadelphia: W. B. Saunders.

in order of priority. Information will be presented in a question and based on the data; you need to determine what you will do first, second, third, and so forth. See Box 1-10 for an example.

Figure or Illustration

A question with a figure or illustration will ask you to answer the question based on the figure or illustration. The question could contain a chart, table, or a figure or illustration. You also may be asked to use the computer mouse to "point and click" on a specific area in the visual. A visual or image may appear in any type of question, including a multiple-choice question. See Box 1-11 for an example.

BOX 1-11

Visual or Illustration

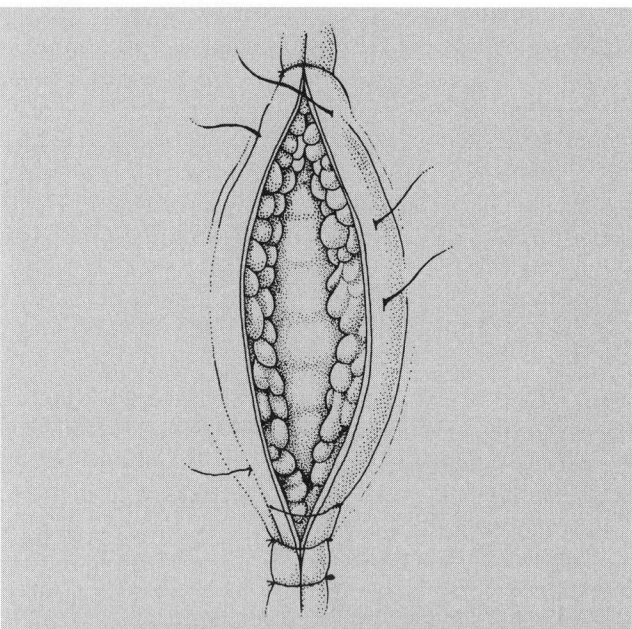

FIG. 1-1 Modified from Ignatavicius, D., & Workman, M. (2002). *Medical-surgical nursing: Critical thinking for collaborative care* (4th ed., p. 291). Philadelphia: W. B. Saunders.

A nurse is changing an abdominal dressing on a client who had abdominal surgery. After removing the old dressing, the nurse assesses the surgical site. The nurse takes which initial action if this wound appearance was observed?
1. Redress the wound with a dry, sterile dressing.
2. Document the findings.
3. Apply a sterile nonadherent dressing.
4. Ask the client to cough to assess for protrusion of the internal structures.

Answer: 3

In this question, you are provided with a figure and are asked for the initial nursing action based on your observation. Wound dehiscence is a partial or complete separation of the outer layers of the wound. From the options provided, the nurse would apply a sterile, nonadherent dressing to the wound. A dry dressing could disrupt the integrity of the underlying tissues. The nurse would document the findings, but this would not be the initial action. Asking the client to cough could cause an extension of the outer layers of the wound.

Reference: Ignatavicius, D., & Workman, M. (2002). *Medical-surgical nursing: Critical thinking for collaborative care* (4th ed., p. 291). Philadelphia: W. B. Saunders.

ITEM WRITERS

The NCSBN selects question (item) writers after an extensive application process. The writers are registered nurses who hold a master's degree or a higher degree. Many of the writers are nursing educators; however, a nurse currently employed in clinical nursing practice and working directly with nurses who have entered practice within the last 12 months may be selected to participate in this process. Question writers voluntarily submit an application to become a writer and must meet specific criteria established by the council to be accepted as participants in the process.

REGISTERING TO TAKE THE EXAMINATION

The initial step in the registration process is to submit an application to the state board of nursing in the state in which you intend to obtain licensure. You need to obtain information from the board of nursing regarding the specific registration process because the process may vary from state to state. In most states, you may register for the examination through the Web, by mail, or by telephone. The NCLEX candidate Web site is *www.vue.com/nclex*. Following the registration instructions and completing the registration forms precisely and accurately is important. Registration forms not properly completed or not accompanied by the proper fees in the required method of payment will be returned to you and will delay testing. You must pay a fee for taking the examination, and you also may have to pay additional fees to the board of nursing in the state in which you are applying. You will be sent a confirmation indicating that your registration was received. If you do not receive a confirmation within 4 weeks of submitting your registration, you should contact the candidate services. Information regarding this contact can be obtained at the NCLEX candidate Web site at *www.vue.com/nclex*.

AUTHORIZATION TO TEST

Once your eligibility to test has been determined by the board of nursing in the state in which licensure is requested, your registration form is processed and an Authorization to Test form will be sent to you. You cannot make an appointment until the board of nursing declares eligibility and you receive an Authorization to Test form. The examination will take place at Pearson Professional Centers, and you can make an appointment through the Web or by telephone. First-time test takers will be offered an appointment within 30 days of the call to schedule an appointment, and repeat test takers will be offered an appointment within 45 days. You can schedule an appointment at any Pearson Professional Centers. You do not have to take the examination in the same state in which you are seeking licensure. A confirmation of your appointment will be sent to you.

The Authorization to Test form contains important information, including your test authorization number, candidate identification number, and an expiration date. Note the expiration date on the form because you must test by this date. You also need to take your Authorization to Test form to the test center on the day of your examination or you will not be admitted to the examination.

If for any reason you need to cancel or reschedule your appointment to test, you can make the change on the candidate Web site (*www.vue.com/nclex*) or by calling candidate services. The change needs to be made 1 full business day (24 hours) before your scheduled appointment.

If you fail to arrive for the examination or fail to cancel your appointment to test without providing appropriate notice, you will forfeit your examination fee and your Authorization to Test will be invalidated. This information will be reported to the board of nursing in the state in which you have applied for licensure, and you will be required to register and pay the testing fees again.

You must arrive at the testing center at least 30 minutes before the test is scheduled. If you arrive late for the scheduled testing appointment, you may be required to forfeit your examination appointment. If forfeiture of the appointment is necessary, you will need to reregister for the examination and pay an additional fee. The board of nursing will be notified that you did not test. A few days before your scheduled date of testing, take the time to drive to the testing center to determine its exact location, the length of time required to arrive to that destination, and any potential obstacles that might delay you, such as road construction, traffic, or parking sites.

SPECIAL TESTING CIRCUMSTANCES

If you require special testing accommodations, you should contact the board of nursing before submitting a registration form. The board of nursing will provide the procedures for the request. The board of nursing must authorize special testing accommodations. Following board of nursing approval, the NCSNB reviews the requested accommodations and also must approve the request. If the request is approved, the testing appointment must be made by the NCLEX exam program coordinator, whom you can contact by calling NCLEX exam candidate services. You must cancel or reschedule an appointment through the NCLEX exam program coordinator.

THE TESTING CENTER

The test center is designed to ensure complete security of the testing process. Strict candidate identification requirements have been established. To be admitted to the testing center, you must bring the Authorization to Test form, along with two forms of identification. Both forms of identification must be signed and current or nonexpired, and one must contain a recent photograph of you.

The name on the photograph identification must be the same as the name on the Authorization to Test form. A digital fingerprint, signature, and photograph will be taken at the test center and will accompany the NCLEX exam results to confirm your identity. Additionally, if you leave the testing room for any reason, you will be required to have your fingerprint taken again to be readmitted to the room.

Personal belongings are not allowed in the testing room. Secure storage will be provided for you; however, storage space is limited, so you must plan accordingly. In addition, the testing center will not assume responsibility for your personal belongings. The testing waiting areas are generally small; therefore friends or family members who accompany you are not permitted to wait in the testing center while you are taking the examination.

Once you have completed the admission process and a brief orientation, the proctor will escort you to the assigned computer. You will be seated at an individual table area with an appropriate work space that includes computer equipment, appropriate lighting, an erasable note board, and a marker. No items, including unauthorized scratch paper, are allowed into the testing room. Electronic devices such as watches, beepers, or cell phones are not allowed in the testing room. Eating, drinking, or the use of tobacco is not allowed in the testing room. You will be observed at all times by the test proctor while taking the examination. Additionally, video and audio recording of all test sessions occurs. Pearson Professional Centers has no control over the sounds made by typing on the computer. If these sounds are distracting, raise your hand to summon the proctor. Earplugs are available on request.

You must follow the directions given by the test center staff and must remain seated during the test, except when authorized to leave. If you feel that you have a problem with the computer, need an additional note board, need to take a break, or need the test proctor for any reason, you must raise your hand.

TESTING TIME

The maximum testing time is 6 hours, and this period includes the tutorial, two preprogrammed optional breaks, and any unscheduled breaks that you may take. The computer screen will notify you of the time for these breaks. You must leave the testing room during breaks, and when you return, you will be required to provide a fingerprint to be readmitted to the testing room.

LENGTH OF THE EXAMINATION

The minimum number of questions that you will need to answer is 75. Of these 75 questions, 60 will be operational (scored) questions and 15 will be pretest (unscored) questions. The maximum number of questions in the test is 265. Fifteen of the total number of questions that you need to answer will be pretest (unscored) questions.

The pretest questions are questions that may be presented as scored questions on future examinations. These pretest questions are not identified as such. In other words, you do not know which questions are the pretest (unscored) questions.

PASS OR FAIL DECISIONS

All of the examination questions are categorized by test plan area and level of difficulty. This is an important point to keep in mind when you consider how the computer makes a pass or fail decision because a pass or fail decision is not based on a percentage of correctly answered questions. After the minimum number of questions have been answered (75 questions), the computer compares the test taker's ability level to the standard required for passing. The standard required for passing is set based on the expert judgment of several individuals appointed by the NCSBN. If the test taker is clearly above the passing standard, then the test taker passes the examination. If the test taker is clearly below the passing standard, then the test taker fails the examination. If the computer is not able to determine clearly whether the test taker has passed or failed because the test taker's ability is close to the passing standard, then the computer continues asking questions. After each question, the computer determines the test taker's ability, and when it becomes clear on which side of the passing standard the test taker falls (above the standard or below the standard), the examination ends. If the test taker is administered the maximum number of questions (265 questions), the computer will make a pass or fail decision by recomputing the test taker's final ability level, based on every question answered, and comparing it with the passing standard. If the ability level is above the passing standard, the test taker passes. If the ability level is not above the passing standard, the test taker fails.

If the examination ends because you have run out of time, the computer may not have enough information to make a clear pass or fail decision. If this is the situation, the computer will review the test taker's performance during testing and specifically at the performance with the last 60 questions answered. If the test taker's ability was consistently above the passing standard on the last 60 questions, the test taker passes. If the test taker's ability falls to or below the passing standard, even once, the test taker fails.

COMPLETING THE EXAMINATION

Once you complete the test, you will complete a brief computer-delivered questionnaire about your testing experience. After you complete this questionnaire, you need to raise your hand to summon the test proctor.

The test proctor will collect and inventory all note boards and then permit you to leave.

PROCESSING RESULTS

Every computerized examination is scored twice; once by the computer at the testing center and then again after the examination is transmitted to Pearson Professional Centers. No results are released at the test center. The board of nursing will mail your results to you about 1 month after you take the examination. You should not call Pearson Professional Centers, NCSBN, candidate services, or the state board of nursing for results.

CANDIDATE PERFORMANCE REPORT

A candidate performance report is provided to a test taker who failed the examination. This report provides the test taker with information about their strengths and weaknesses in relation to the test plan and provides a guide for studying and retaking the examination. In most states, the test taker must wait 45 days before retaking the examination.

INTERSTATE ENDORSEMENT

Because the NCLEX-RN examination is a national examination, you can apply to take the examination in any state. Once you receive licensure, you can apply for interstate endorsement. The procedures and requirements for interstate endorsement may vary from state to state, and you can obtain these procedures from the state board of nursing in the state in which you seek endorsement.

STATE BOARDS OF NURSING

Contact information was obtained from the National Council of State Boards of Nursing, Inc. Web site (*www.ncsbn.org/*). Because contact information may change, access this web site if necessary.

Alabama Board of Nursing
770 Washington Ave.
RSA Plaza, Suite 250
Montgomery, AL 36130-3900
(334) 242-4060
Web site: *www.abn.state.al.us/*

Alaska Board of Nursing
550 W. Seventh Ave., Suite 1500
Anchorage, AK 99501-3567
(907) 269-8161
Web site: *www.dced.state.ak.us/occ/pnur.htm*

American Samoa Health Services Regulatory Board
LBJ Tropical Medical Center
Pago Pago, AS 96799
(684) 633-1222

Arizona State Board of Nursing
1651 E. Morten Ave., Suite 210
Phoenix, AZ 85020
(602) 889-5150
Web site: *www.azboardofnursing.org/*

Arkansas State Board of Nursing
University Tower Building
1123 S. University, Suite 800
Little Rock, AR 72204-1619
(501) 686-2700
Web site: *www.state.ar.us/nurse*

California Board of Registered Nursing
400 R St., Suite 4030
Sacramento, CA 95814-6239
(916) 322-3350
Web site: *www.rn.ca.gov/*

Colorado Board of Nursing
1560 Broadway, Suite 880
Denver, CO 80202
(303) 894-2430
Web site: *www.dora.state.co.us/nursing/*

Connecticut Board of Examiners for Nursing
Department of Public Health
410 Capitol Ave., MS# 13PHO
P.O. Box 340308
Hartford, CT 06134-0328
(860) 509-7624
Web site: *www.state.ct.us/dph/*

Delaware Board of Nursing
861 Silver Lake Blvd.
Cannon Building, Suite 203
Dover, DE 19904
(302) 739-4522
Web site: *www.professionallicensing.state.de.us/boards/ nursing/index.shtml*

District of Columbia Board of Nursing
Department of Health
825 N. Capitol St., NE, 2nd Floor
Room 2224
Washington, DC 20002
(202) 442-4778
Web site: *www.dchealth.dc.gov*

Florida Board of Nursing
Mailing address
4052 Bald Cypress Way, BIN C02
Tallahassee, FL 32399-3252
Physical address
4042 Bald Cypress Way
Room 120
Tallahassee, FL 32399

(850) 245-4125
Web site: *www.doh.state.fl.us/mqa/*

Georgia Board of Nursing
237 Coliseum Drive
Macon, GA 31217-3858
(478) 207-1640
Web site: *www.sos.state.ga.us/plb/rn*

Guam Board of Nurse Examiners
Regular mailing address
P.O. Box 2816
Hagatna, GU 96932
Street address (for FedEx and UPS)
651 Legacy Square Commercial Complex
South Route 10
Suite 9
Mangilao, GU 96913
(671) 735-7406; (671) 725-7411

Hawaii Board of Nursing
King Kalakaua Building
335 Merchant St., 3rd Floor
Honolulu, HI 96813
(808) 586-3000
Web site: *www.state.hi.us/dcca/pvl/ areas_nurse.html*

Idaho Board of Nursing
280 N. 8th St., Suite 210
P.O. Box 83720
Boise, ID 83720
(208) 334-3110
Web site: *www.state.id.us/ibn/ibnhome.htm*

Illinois Department of Professional Regulation
James R. Thompson Center
100 W. Randolph, Suite 9-300
Chicago, IL 60601
(312) 814-2715
Web site: *www.dpr.state.il.us/*

Illinois Department of Professional Regulation
320 W. Washington St.
3rd Floor
Springfield, IL 62786
(217) 782-8556

Indiana State Board of Nursing
Health Professions Bureau
402 W. Washington St., Room W066
Indianapolis, IN 46204
(317) 234-2043
Web site: *www.state.in.us/hpb/boards/isbn/*

Iowa Board of Nursing
RiverPoint Business Park

400 S.W. 8th St.
Suite B
Des Moines, IA 50309-4685
(515) 281-3255
Web site: *www.state.ia.us/government/nursing/*

Kansas State Board of Nursing
Landon State Office Building
900 S.W. Jackson, Suite 1051
Topeka, KS 66612
(785) 296-4929
Web site: *www.ksbn.org*

Kentucky Board of Nursing
312 Whittington Pkwy., Suite 300
Louisville, KY 40222
(502) 329-7000
Web site: *www.kbn.ky.gov/*

Louisiana State Board of Nursing
3510 N. Causeway Blvd., Suite 501
Metairie, LA 70002
(504) 838-5332
Web site: *www.lsbn.state.la.us/*

Maine State Board of Nursing
158 State House Station
Augusta, ME 04333
(207) 287-1133
Web site: *www.maine.gov/boardofnursing/*

Maryland Board of Nursing
4140 Patterson Ave.
Baltimore, MD 21215
(410) 585-1900
Web site: *www.mbon.org*

Massachusetts Board of Registration in Nursing
Commonwealth of Massachusetts
239 Causeway St.
Boston, MA 02114
(617) 727-9961
Web site: *www.state.ma.us/reg/boards/rn/*

Michigan CIS/Bureau of Health Professions
Ottawa Towers North
611 W. Ottawa, 1st Floor
Lansing, MI 48933
(517) 335-0918
Web site: *www.michigan.gov/healthlicense*

Minnesota Board of Nursing
2829 University Ave. SE
Suite 500
Minneapolis, MN 55414
(612) 617-2270
Web site: *www.nursingboard.state.mn.us/*

Mississippi Board of Nursing
1935 Lakeland Drive, Suite B
Jackson, MS 39216-5014
(601) 987-4188
Web site: *www.msbn.state.ms.us/*

Missouri State Board of Nursing
3605 Missouri Blvd.
P.O. Box 656
Jefferson City, MO 65102-0656
(573) 751-0681
Web site: *www.ecodev.state.mo.us/pr/nursing/*

Montana State Board of Nursing
301 South Park
P.O. Box 200513
Helena, MT 59620-0513
(406) 841-2340
Web site: *www.discoveringmontana.com/dli/bsd/license/
bsd_boards/nur_board/board_page.htm*

Nebraska Health and Human Services System
Department of Regulation & Licensure,
    Nursing Section
301 Centennial Mall South
Lincoln, NE 68509-4986
(402) 471-4376
Web site: *www.hhs.state.ne.us/crl/nursing/
nursingindex.htm*

Nevada State Board of Nursing
Licensure and Certification
2500 W. Sahara Ave., Suite 207
Las Vegas, Nevada 89102-4293
(702) 486-5800
Web site: *www.nursingboard.state.nv.us/*

New Hampshire Board of Nursing
P.O. Box 3898
78 Regional Drive, BLDG B
Concord, NH 03302
(603) 271-2323
Web site: *www.state.nh.us/nursing/*

New Jersey Board of Nursing
P.O. Box 45010
124 Halsey St., 6th Floor
Newark, NJ 07101
(973) 504-6586
Web site: *www.state.nj.us/lps/ca/medical.htm*

New Mexico Board of Nursing
4206 Louisiana Blvd., NE
Suite A
Albuquerque, NM 87109
(505) 841-8340
Web site: *www.state.nm.us/clients/nursing*

New York State Board of Nursing
Education Bldg.
89 Washington Ave.
2nd Floor West Wing
Albany, NY 12234
(518) 474-3817, ext. 120
Web site: *www.nysed.gov/prof/nurse.htm*

North Carolina Board of Nursing
3724 National Drive, Suite 201
Raleigh, NC 27612
(919) 782-3211
Web site: *www.ncbon.com/*

North Dakota Board of Nursing
919 S. 7th St., Suite 504
Bismarck, ND 58504
(701) 328-9777
Web site: *www.ndbon.org/*

Northern Mariana Islands
Commonwealth Board of Nurse Examiners
P.O. Box 501458
Saipan, MP 96950
(670) 664-4812

Ohio Board of Nursing
17 S. High St., Suite 400
Columbus, OH 43215-3413
(614) 466-3947
Web site: *www.nursing.ohio.gov*

Oklahoma Board of Nursing
2915 N. Classen Blvd., Suite 524
Oklahoma City, OK 73106
(405) 962-1800
Web site: *www.youroklahoma.com/nursing*

Oregon State Board of Nursing
800 N.E. Oregon St., Box 25
Suite 465
Portland, OR 97232
(503) 731-4745
Web site: *www.osbn.state.or.us/*

Pennsylvania State Board of Nursing
P.O. 2649
Harrisburg, PA 17105-2649
(717) 783-7142
Web site: *www.dos.state.pa.us/bpoa/cwp/view.asp?a=1104*
    8q=432869

Commonwealth of Puerto Rico
Board of Nurse Examiners
800 Roberto H. Todd Ave.
Room 202, Stop 18
Santurce, PR 00908
(787) 725-7506

Rhode Island Board of Nurse Registration and Nursing
    Education
105 Cannon Building
Three Capitol Hill
Providence, RI 02908
(401) 222-5700
Web site: *www.healthri.org/hsr/professions/nurses.htm*

South Carolina State Board of Nursing
110 Centerview Drive
Suite 202
Columbia, SC 29210
(803) 896-4550
Web site: *www.llr.state.sc.us/pol/nursing*

South Dakota Board of Nursing
4305 S. Louise Ave., Suite 201
Sioux Falls, SD 57106-3115
(605) 362-2760
Web site: *www.state.sd.us/dcr/nursing/*

Tennessee State Board of Nursing
425 Fifth Ave. N
1st Floor—Cordell Hull Building
Nashville, TN 37247
(615) 532-5166
Web site: *www.tennessee.gov/health*

Texas Board of Nurse Examiners
333 Guadalupe, Suite 3-460
Austin, TX 78701
(512) 305-7400
Web site: *www.bne.state.tx.us/*

Utah State Board of Nursing
Heber M. Wells Bldg., 4th Floor
160 E. 300 S
Salt Lake City, UT 84111
(801) 530-6628
Web site: *www.commerce.state.ut.us/*

Vermont State Board of Nursing
81 River St.
Heritage Building
Montpelier, VT 05609-1106
(802) 828-2396
Web site: *www.vtprofessionals.org/opr1/nurses/*

Virgin Islands Board of Nurse Licensure
Veterans Drive Station
St. Thomas, VI 00803
(340) 776-7397

Virginia Board of Nursing
6603 W. Broad St., 5th Floor
Richmond, VA 23230-1712
(804) 662-9909
Web site: *www.dhp.state.va.us/*

Washington State Nursing Care Quality Assurance
  Commission
Department of Health
HPQA #6
310 Israel Road SE
Tumwater, WA 98501-7864
(360) 236-4700
Web site: *https://wws2.wa.gov/doh/hpqa-licensing/HPS6/
  Nursing/default.htm*

West Virginia Board of Examiners for Registered
  Professional Nurses
101 Dee Drive
Charleston, WV 25311
(304) 558-3596
Web site: *www.wvrnboard.com*

Wisconsin Department of Regulation and Licensing
1400 E. Washington Ave., RM 173
Madison, WI 53708
(608) 266-0145
Web site: *www.drl.state.wi.us/*

Wyoming State Board of Nursing
2020 Carey Ave., Suite 110
Cheyenne, WY 82001
(307) 777-7601
Web site: *nursing.state.wy.us/*

REFERENCES

Hodgson, B., & Kizior, R. (2004). *Saunders nursing drug handbook 2004.* Philadelphia: W. B. Saunders.

Ignatavicius, D., & Workman, M. (2002). *Medical-surgical nursing: Critical thinking for collaborative care* (4th ed.). Philadelphia: W. B. Saunders.

James, S., Ashwill, J., & Droske, S. (2002). *Nursing care of children: Principles & practice* (2nd ed.). Philadelphia: W. B. Saunders.

Lehne, R. (2001). *Pharmacology for nursing care* (4th ed.). Philadelphia: W. B. Saunders.

National Council of State Boards of Nursing. http://www.ncsbn.org/

National Council of State Boards of Nursing (Eds.) (2003). *Test Plan for the National Council Licensure Examination for Registered Nurses* (effective date: April 2004). Chicago: Author.

Phipps, W., Monahan, F., Sands, J., Marek, J., & Neighbors, M. (2003). *Medical-surgical nursing: Health and illness perspectives* (7th ed.). St. Louis: Mosby.

Potter, P., & Perry, A. (2001). *Fundamentals of nursing* (5th ed.). St. Louis: Mosby.

Stuart, G., & Laraia, M. (2001). *Principles and practice of psychiatric nursing* (7th ed.). St. Louis: Mosby.

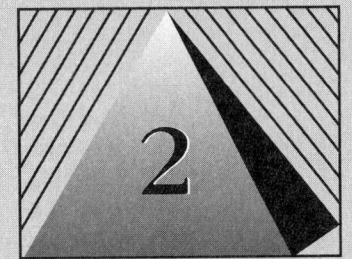

Preparation for the NCLEX Exam: Transitional Issues for the Foreign-Educated Nurse

This chapter provides you with information regarding the certification processes that you will have to pursue to become a registered nurse in the United States. An important factor to consider as you pursue this process is that some of the requirements may vary from state to state. Therefore, as a first step in the process, you must contact the board of nursing in the state in which you are planning to obtain licensure. To assist you in making a contact with the state board of nursing, refer to Chapter 1 in this book. At the end of the chapter you will find the addresses, telephone numbers, and Web site addresses for each state and for U.S. territories. You also can access this information through the National Council of State Boards of Nursing (NCSBN) Web site at *www.ncsbn.org*. Once you have accessed the NCSBN Web site, select the link titled "Boards of Nursing." Additionally, you can write to the NCSBN regarding the NCLEX exam. The address is 111 E. Wacker Drive, Suite 2900, Chicago, IL 60601. The telephone number for the NCSBN is (312) 525-3600; the fax number is (312) 279-1032.

VISASCREEN

United States immigration law requires certain health care professionals to successfully complete a screening program before receiving an occupational visa (Section 343 of the Illegal Immigration Reform and Immigration Responsibility Act of 1996). Therefore you are required to obtain a VisaScreen certificate.

The Commission on Graduates of Foreign Nursing Schools (CGFNS) is the organization that offers this federal screening program. The International Commission on Health Care Professions, a division of the CGFNS, administers the VisaScreen. The VisaScreen components include an educational analysis, license verification, assessment of proficiency in the English language, and an examination that tests nursing knowledge. This chapter describes each of these components. Once the applicant successfully achieves each of the components, the applicant is presented with a VisaScreen certificate. You can obtain information related to the VisaScreen through the CGFNS Web site at *www.cgfns.org*.

Educational Analysis

The educational analysis component requires the following:
1. Applicant must present proof of completion of senior secondary school education, separate from any professional certification.
2. Applicant must present proof of completion from a government-approved professional health care program of at least two years in length.
3. Applicant must provide documentation that he or she has completed a minimum number of clock and/or credit hours in specific theoretical and clinical areas while in nursing school.

Licensure Verification

The applicant must present all current and past licensure for review.

Proficiency in the English Language

The applicant must submit proof of a passing score on an approved U.S. Department of Education and Health and Human Services English language proficiency examination (Box 2-1 lists English proficiency examinations and testing organizations).

Testing Nursing Knowledge

An **examination to test nursing knowledge** includes the following:
1. The 1-day qualifying examination that is administered as part of the process for obtaining a CGFNS Certificate tests nursing knowledge; therefore a CGFNS Certificate provides proof of adequate nursing knowledge. This qualifying examination is described in Components of the CGFNS Certification Program.
2. A foreign-educated nurse who is licensed and practicing nursing in the United States also is required to obtain a VisaScreen; if the nurse does not have a CGFNS Certificate, the nurse may be granted eligibility to take the NCLEX exam to provide proof of nursing knowledge.

STATE REQUIREMENTS

Most states in the United States require that you receive certification from the CGFNS before you can be eligible to take the NCLEX exam. If the state in which you intend to obtain licensure does not require CGFNS Certification, it may require submission of some of the same documents that the CGFNS requires. Therefore in addition to what the CGFNS requires, a state may require the following:
1. Proof of citizenship or lawful alien status
2. Official transcripts of educational credentials sent directly to the board of nursing from the school of nursing
3. Validation of theoretical instruction and clinical practice in a variety of nursing areas including medical nursing, surgical nursing, pediatric nursing, maternity and newborn nursing, and mental health nursing
4. Copy of nursing license and/or diploma
5. Proof of proficiency in the English language
6. Photographs of the applicant
7. Application fees

THE COMMISSION ON GRADUATES OF FOREIGN NURSING SCHOOLS

The CGFNS provides a certification program for nurses educated and licensed outside of the United States.

The certificate program offered by the CGFNS is a requirement of most state boards of nursing, and the certificate may be required before you can take the NCLEX exam. The certificate program ensures that you are eligible and qualified to meet licensure and other practice requirements in the United States, and it also predicts your success on the NCLEX exam. This program also assists you in obtaining your VisaScreen certificate. You can obtain additional information relating to the CGFNS and its certification program through the CGFNS Web site at *www.cgfns.org*.

Eligibility for the CGFNS Certification Program

The CGFNS Certification Program is designed for nurses educated outside of the United States who hold an initial and current registration/licensure as a first-level general registered nurse. According to the CGFNS, a first-level nurse is called a registered nurse or professional nurse in most countries. As a general nurse, the foreign-educated nurse must have obtained theoretical instruction and clinical practice in a variety of nursing areas. These nursing areas include medical nursing, surgical nursing, pediatric nursing, maternity and newborn nursing, and mental health nursing. If the nurse educated outside of the United States does not meet these requirements, the nurse is not eligible for the certification program.

Components of the CGFNS Certification Program

The CGFNS Certification Program contains three parts, and you must complete all parts successfully to be awarded a CGFNS Certificate. The three parts include a credentials review, a 1-day qualifying examination that tests nursing knowledge, and an English language proficiency examination. You can take the qualifying and English language proficiency examinations at various locations throughout the world. This provides the applicant the opportunity to obtain the CGFNS Certificate before coming to the United States to take the NCLEX exam. These three parts of the certificate program are described next.

Credentials Review

The CGFNS requires validation of education and a licensing history of the applicant to ensure that the applicant has the appropriate credentials to seek certification. The CGFNS must receive transcripts and validation documents from the nursing program and licensing agency. The CGFNS does not accept transcripts and validation documents from the applicant. The specific credentialing requirements are similar to those needed for the VisaScreen certificate and include the following:

1. Completion of a senior secondary school education
2. Graduation from a government-approved nursing program of at least 2 years in length
3. Acquisition of theoretical instruction and clinical practice in the areas of medical nursing, surgical nursing, pediatric nursing, maternity/newborn nursing, and mental health nursing
4. Possession of a full and unrestricted license or registration to practice as a first-level general nurse in the country where he or she completed their general nursing education
5. Possession of a current license or registration as a first-level general nurse

Qualifying Examination

The qualifying examination tests the applicant's knowledge in nursing in the areas of adult health, pediatrics, maternity and newborn, mental health, and community health. The examination is designed to ensure that the applicant has the knowledge to provide nursing care to various client groups at the same level as recent U.S. nursing graduates.

English Language Proficiency Examination

The applicant must take and pass an English language proficiency examination. You can take the examination before or after the qualifying examination. The English language proficiency examination needs to be taken from a testing organization that is approved by the CGFNS, and the applicant must apply directly with the testing organization to take the examination. The scores must be sent directly to the CGFNS from the testing organization. The CGFNS will not accept test scores from the applicant. Box 2-1 lists the types of English proficiency examinations, approved testing organizations, and their contact information.

The CGFNS identifies certain applicants as exempt from the English language proficiency requirement. For an applicant to be exempt, the applicant must meet all of the following criteria: native language is English; country of nursing education was Australia, Canada (except Quebec), Ireland, New Zealand, or the United Kingdom; and language of instruction and language of textbooks was English.

Once you successfully have met each of the three required components of the CGFNS Certification Program, the CGFNS will issue a certificate of completion. Unless the state in which you intend to obtain licensure indicates additional requirements, and if you have received your VisaScreen certificate, you will be eligible to take the NCLEX exam.

REGISTERING TO TAKE THE NCLEX EXAM

If you are planning to take the examination in the United States, the initial step in the registration process is to submit an application to the state board of nursing in the state in which you intend to obtain licensure. You need to obtain information from the board of nursing regarding the specific registration process because the process may vary from state to state. In most states, you may register for the examination through the Web, by mail, or by telephone. The NCLEX candidate Web site is *www.vue.com/nclex*. You must follow the registration instructions and complete the registration forms precisely and accurately. Registration forms not properly completed or not accompanied by the proper fees in the required method of payment, will be returned to you and will delay testing. You must pay a fee for taking the examination, and you also may have to pay additional fees to the board of nursing in the state in which you are applying. You will be sent a confirmation indicating that your registration was received. If you do not receive a confirmation within 4 weeks of submitting your registration, you should contact the candidate services. You can obtain information regarding candidate services at the candidate Web site at *www.vue.com/nclex*.

Once the board of nursing in the state in which you request licensure has verified your eligibility to take the examination, the board will process your registration form and send you an Authorization to Test form. You cannot make an appointment until the board of nursing declares eligibility and you receive an Authorization to Test form. The examination will take place at Pearson Professional Centers, and you can make an appointment through the Web or by telephone. You can schedule an appointment at any Pearson Professional Centers. You do not have to take the examination in the same state in which you are seeking licensure. A confirmation of your appointment will be sent to you. For additional information regarding the NCLEX exam and testing procedures, refer to Chapter 1.

According to NCSBN, NCLEX examination testing abroad is expected to be available as of January 2005. The countries that will provide this testing are Seoul, South Korea; London, England; and Hong Kong. These testing sites provide the nurse who is interested in becoming a licensed nurse in the United States an opportunity to pass the NCLEX examination before traveling to the United States.

PREPARING TO TAKE THE NCLEX EXAM

The challenge that is presented to you is one that requires patience and endurance. The positive result of your endeavor certainly will reward you professionally and give you the personal satisfaction of knowing you have become part of a family of highly skilled professionals, the registered nurse. You have successfully completed the requirements to become eligible to take the NCLEX exam, and now you have one more important goal to achieve: to pass the exam.

I highly recommend adequate preparation for the NCLEX examination because the examination is difficult. An important step that you have taken in preparing is that you are using this book, *Saunders Comprehensive Review for the NCLEX-RN Examination*. Once you have reviewed the content and answered the practice questions, the next step in your journey to success is to use the companion book, *Saunders Q & A Review for the NCLEX-RN Examination*. This book also provides you with more than 3500 practice questions based on the NCLEX-RN exam test plan. Then you are ready for the *Saunders Computerized Review*, a computer disk program that contains more than 2000 NCLEX-RN–style questions to help you determine your readiness for the NCLEX-RN exam.

If you prefer to prepare by using online resources, access the *Saunders Online Review Course for the NCLEX-RN Examination* at *http://evolve.elsevier.com/reviewandtesting/*. Additional online specialty tests titled Adult Health, Mental Health, Maternal-Newborn, Pediatrics, and Pharmacology are also available.

Lastly, never lose sight of your goal. Patience and dedication will contribute significantly to your achieving the status of registered nurse. Remember, success is climbing a mountain, facing the challenge of obstacles, and reaching the top of the mountain. I wish you the best success in your career as a registered nurse in the United States of America.

REFERENCES

Commission on Graduates of Foreign Nursing Schools. http://www.cgfns.org.

Educational Testing Service, Princeton, New Jersey. toefl@ets.org.

International English Language Testing System. ielts@ceii.org; http://www.ielts.org.

National Council of State Boards of Nursing. http://www.ncsbn.org.

Pathways to Success

LAURENT W. VALLIERE

▲ THE PYRAMID TO SUCCESS

Preparing to take the NCLEX-RN exam can produce a great deal of anxiety. You may be thinking that this exam is the most important examination that you will ever have to take and that it reflects the culmination of everything that you have worked so hard to achieve. The NCLEX-RN exam is an important test because receiving that nursing license means that you can begin your career as a registered nurse. Your success on the NCLEX-RN exam involves expelling all thoughts that allow this examination to appear overwhelming and intimidating. Such thoughts will take complete control over your destiny. A positive attitude, a structured plan for preparation, and maintaining control in your pathway to success will ensure you reach the peak of the Pyramid to Success (Box 3-1).

THE FOUNDATION

The foundation of the Pyramid to Success begins with a positive attitude and developing short- and long-term goals. A positive attitude and a list of goals will lead you toward achievement and success. Without these components, the Pyramid to Success leads to nowhere and has no end point. You will expend energy and valuable time and will experience exhaustion without any accomplishment. Therefore taking the time to develop that positive attitude and to establish your short- and long-term goals is imperative.

BOX 3-1

Pathways to Success

THE FOUNDATION
Maintaining a positive attitude
Thinking about short- and long-term realistic goals
Developing control

THE LIST
Documenting short- and long-term realistic goals
Maintaining control

THE PLAN
Developing a study plan and schedule
Deciding on the place to study
Balancing personal and work obligations with the study schedule
Sharing the study schedule and personal needs with others
Implementing the study plan

POSITIVE PAMPERING
Establishing healthy eating habits
Planning time for exercise and fun activities

Including activities in the schedule that provide positive mental stimulation

FINAL PREPARATION
Reviewing goals
Identifying goals achieved
Remaining focused to complete the plan of study
Writing down the date and time of the examination and posting it next to your name with the letters *R.N.* following and the word *YES!*
Planning a test drive to the testing center
Relaxing activities on the day before the examination

THE DAY OF THE EXAMINATION
Grooming yourself for success
Eating a healthy and nutritious breakfast
Maintaining a confident and positive attitude
Maintaining control
Meeting the challenges of the day
Reaching the peak of the Pyramid to Success

Where do you start? To begin this process, find a location that offers solitude. Sit or lie in a comfortable position, close your eyes, relax, inhale deeply, hold your breath to a count of 4, exhale slowly, and again relax. Repeat this breathing exercise several times until you begin to feel relaxed and free from anxiety. Allow your mind to become void of all chatter. Now you are in control, and your mind can see for miles. Your highway of life has a multitude of destinations to which you may travel. Now is the time for you to plan the order of your journey to the Pyramid to Success.

THE LIST

Once you have relaxed, you can create "The List." The list is your set of goals. At this time, you may or may not have a scheduled date for taking the NCLEX-RN exam. Begin by developing the goals you wish to accomplish today, tomorrow, and in the future. Allow yourself the opportunity to list all that is flowing from your mind. Write your goals on a piece of paper. When the list is complete, set it aside for 2 or 3 days. After 2 or 3 days, retrieve and review the list and begin the process of planning for preparing for the NCLEX-RN exam.

THE PLAN

Now that you have the list in order, look at your goals that relate to studying for the licensing examination. The first task is to decide what study pattern works best for you. Take the time to review what has worked most successfully for you in the past. You have questions you must address to develop your plan for study (Box 3-2).

"The Plan" must include how you will manage your study needs and the demands of your family and friends. Take time to think about how you will balance your everyday commitments with your plan for study. Your family and friends are key players in your life and are going to become a part of your Pyramid to Success.

BOX 3-2

Developing a Plan for Study

Do I work better alone or in a group study environment?
If I work best in a group, does the group consist of one, two, or more study partners?
Who are these study partners?
How long should my study sessions last?
Does the time of day that I study make a difference for me?
Do I retain more if I study in the morning?
How does my work schedule affect my study pattern?
How do I balance my family obligations with my need to study?
Do I have a comfortable study area at home, or do I need to find another environment that is conducive to my study needs?

After you have established your study needs, communicate with your family and friends your needs and the importance of your study plan in achieving your goal of becoming a registered nurse.

The plan must include a schedule. Establish a realistic schedule that includes your daily, weekly, and future goals, and adhere to it. This consistency will provide advantages to you and to those supporting you. A daily schedule allows you to plan your topic areas for study more carefully. Adherence to the plan helps you develop a rhythm that can only enhance your retention and positive momentum. Those who are supporting you will share this rhythm and will be able to schedule their activities and life better because you are consistent with your study schedule. You are moving forward, and you are in control.

A difficult part of the plan may be how you will deal with those family members and friends who choose not to participate in your Pyramid to Success. What if an individual or individuals choose not to be part of the pyramid? For example, what do you do if a friend asks you to go to a movie and it is your scheduled study time? Your friend may say, "Come on. Take some time off. You have plenty of time to study. Study later when we get back!" Then you are faced with a decision. You must weigh all of the factors carefully. You must keep your goals in mind and remember that your need for positive momentum is critical. Your decision may not be an easy one but must be one that will help you ensure that you achieve your goal of becoming a registered nurse. Remember, a positive momentum and goal achievement need to be shared by all who support you.

POSITIVE PAMPERING

You can maintain positive momentum only if you are balanced properly. This means that you must continue to care for yourself. Proper exercise, diet, and positive mental stimulation are critical to achieving your goal of becoming a registered nurse. Just as you have developed a schedule for study, you should have a schedule that includes some fun and some form of physical activity. You have your choice—aerobics, running, weight lifting, bowling, or whatever makes you feel good about yourself. Time spent away from the hard study schedule and devoted to some form of fun and physical exercise pays its rewards 100-fold. You will feel alive and more energetic with a schedule that includes these activities.

Establish healthy eating habits. Stay away from fatty foods because they will slow you down. Eat lighter meals and eat more frequently. Include complex carbohydrates in your diet for energy, and be careful not to include too much caffeine in your daily diet. Continue to feel good about yourself because you are in control. Take the time to pamper yourself with activities that make you feel even better about who you are. Make dinner reservations at your favorite restaurant with someone who is special and is supporting your goal to become a registered nurse. Take walks in a place that has a particular tranquility that enables you to reflect on the positive momentum that you have achieved and maintained. Whatever it is, wherever it takes you, allow yourself the time to do some positive pampering.

FINAL PREPARATION

You have established the foundation of your pyramid. You have developed your list of goals and your study plan and have maintained your positive momentum. You are moving forward, and you are in control. When you receive your date and time for the NCLEX-RN exam, you may immediately think, "I am not ready!" Stop. Reflect on all that you have achieved. Think about your goal achievement and the organization of the positive life momentum with which you have surrounded yourself. Think about all those individuals who love and support your effort to become a registered nurse. Believe that the challenge that awaits you is one for which you have prepared successfully and will lead you to your goal: becoming a registered nurse.

Take a deep breath, and organize the remaining days so that they support your educational and personal needs. Support your positive momentum with a visual technique. Write your name in large letters, and write the letters *R.N.* after it. Post one or more of these visual reinforcements in areas that you frequent. This form of motivational technique works for many individuals preparing for this examination.

Through all that you have accomplished to this point, it is imperative that you not fall into the trap of expecting too much of yourself. The idea of perfection must not drive you to a point that causes your positive momentum to hesitate. You must believe in who you are, as you are, and stay focused on your goal. Allow yourself the opportunity to continue to carry out your plan in a manner that is most conducive to who you are, not someone else. The date and time are in hand. Write down the date and time, and underneath write the word *YES*. Post this next to your name along with *R.N.*

You must ensure that you have command over how to get to the testing center. A test run is a must. Time the drive, and allow for road construction or whatever may occur to slow the traffic down. On the test run, when you arrive at the test facility, you may want to walk into it. Walk in and become familiar with the lobby and the surroundings. This may help to alleviate some of the peripheral nervousness associated with entering an unknown building. Remember, you must do whatever it takes to keep yourself in control. If familiarizing yourself with the facility will help you to maintain positive momentum, by all means be sure to do so. Who is in control? You are.

At this time check your study plan and make the necessary adjustments now that a firm date and time are set. Adjust your review so that it flows to your needs and that your study plan ends 2 days before the examination. Remember that the mind is like a muscle. If you overwork it, it has no strength or stamina. Your strategy is to rest the body and the mind on the day before the examination. Your strategy is to stay in control and allow yourself the opportunity to be absolutely fresh and attentive on the day of the examination. This will help you control the nervousness that is natural, achieve the clear thought processes required, and feel confident that you have done all that is necessary to prepare and conquer this challenge. The day before the examination is to be one of pleasure. Treat yourself to what you enjoy the most.

Relax. You have prepared yourself well for the challenge of tomorrow. Allow yourself a good night's sleep, and wake up on the day of the examination knowing that you are absolutely ready to succeed. Look at your name with *R.N.* after it and the word *YES!*

THE DAY OF THE EXAMINATION

Wake up believing in yourself and that all you have accomplished is about to propel you to the professional level of registered nurse. Allow yourself plenty of time, eat a nutritious breakfast, and groom yourself for success. You are ready to meet the challenges of the day and overcome any obstacle that may face you. Today will soon be history, and tomorrow will bring you the envelope on which you read your name with the words *Registered Nurse* after it.

Be proud and confident of your achievements. You have worked hard to achieve your goal of becoming a registered nurse. If you believe in yourself and your goals, no one person or obstacle can move you off the pathway that leads to success, to the peak of the Pyramid.

Congratulations, and I wish you the very best in your career as a registered nurse.

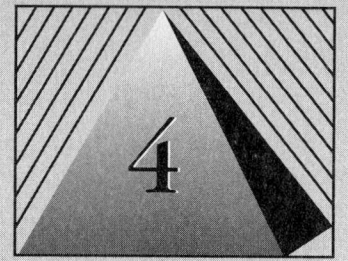

The NCLEX-RN Examination: From a Student's Perspective

KIMBERLY GREEN

Not so long ago, I was a nursing student worrying about the NCLEX-RN exam and thinking that this is the examination that will change the rest of my life. Yeah, that adds a little bit of stress to the whole situation of graduation and everything else that is going on in your life, but with preparation, confidence, and some luck, you will soon have your license and the letters *R.N.* at the end of your name.

Before I begin telling you about my experiences and how I prepared for this very important examination, I want to congratulate you on your outstanding achievements of success in your nursing program. I am sure that you spent many days studying and getting ready for your tests at school. I found that the same study patterns that I used while in school helped me to stay focused and disciplined while studying for the NCLEX-RN exam. But, as we know, all of that hard and dedicated work comes down to passing this one examination. Well, just hang in there. All it takes is equipping yourself with the information that you need to be successful with this examination, and guess what? You have all that knowledge from school. Now, it is time to tie up any loose ends in the preparation process.

First and foremost, I had some overwhelming thoughts and questions. I asked myself, where do I begin and what is the most important thing to study? Do not be afraid to present these questions to your teachers, friends, and other nurses to help determine which content areas to focus on. Second, I kept saying to myself, "Do not procrastinate!" It is so important to be familiar with the style of the test questions and to allot an appropriate amount of time to review all the important content areas. Third, I formulated a study plan and a timeline that I followed and adhered to until my testing day.

I started preparing for this examination while in school by correlating topics presented in class with chapters in *Saunders Comprehensive Review for the NCLEX-RN Examination* and by practicing questions from this book

and its CD-ROM. I also used the *Saunders Q&A Review for the NCLEX-RN Examination* and the CD-ROM accompanying this book to strengthen my knowledge base. This definitely helped me become familiar and comfortable with test questions, how to answer test questions, use of test-taking strategies, and other tools and strategies necessary for both learning in the classroom and for preparing for the NCLEX exam.

A few months before I graduated from nursing school, I decided that I needed a "study buddy" or two to prepare for the NCLEX-RN exam. A few of my fellow classmates and I developed a study time and met at the library to review content areas and practice test questions together. This was very helpful because it gave us the opportunity to share study ideas as well as reinforce important nursing content areas. We also shared our plans for registering for the examination and completing the forms that we needed to submit before we took the examination. This was a low-pressure, fun environment for starting my high stress task of preparing.

Once I graduated from nursing school, I decided that I needed 2 months to study for the examination. I began by focusing on using *Saunders Comprehensive Review for the NCLEX-RN Examination* and the *Saunders Q&A Review for the NCLEX-RN Examination* and primarily used the CD-ROMs during this time. I studied Monday through Friday only, leaving the weekends for relaxing and having fun, and I truly believe that the relaxation and fun time is a key component to success. I felt that I had a "vast task" ahead of me, and I did not want to become overwhelmed. That's why some time away from studying is so important.

During my study time, I spent at least 2 hours answering practice questions. When I answered a question incorrectly or if I encountered a question that contained content that I was unfamiliar with, I wrote the information down in my own special notebook that I called "My Study Notes." At the end of each study session

I reviewed any notes that I made and then went back to the *Saunders Comprehensive Review for the NCLEX-RN Examination* to review the content or, if necessary, my nursing course textbook.

Another preparation strategy that I decided would be helpful for me was to take a weeklong live review class for preparing for the examination. It was very helpful to me because the course focused on key content areas, practice test questions, and use of test-taking strategies. I would recommend this strategy or using an online review course because it will help you "tie up those loose ends."

The week before the examination date I took a drive to the testing facility to see how long it would take me to get there and to allow enough time for any obstacles, such as traffic, road construction, or ample parking that I may encounter. The night before the examination I ate a healthful dinner and reviewed "My Study Notes" for a short time before going to bed. On the morning of my examination, I ate a healthful, well-balanced breakfast and headed out to take the examination. During my entire drive to the testing facility I was worrying about whether or not I would pass, if I studied enough, and if I was ready. I really think that these thoughts and worries are normal and thoughts that everyone getting ready to take this examination has.

Before I left my house on the morning of the examination, I checked to be sure that I was bringing everything that I needed, such as my identification cards and my Authorization to Test form. I dressed in layers of clothing, as suggested, so that I would be able to adapt to the temperature in the testing room. I arrived to the testing center early, my palms were sweating, and I was fidgeting in my seat until my name was called. When I was brought into the testing room, I was seated at a computer cubical. There was only one other person when I began the examination. Other individuals came into the testing room after I started the examination, and some individuals left before I finished. At some points during the examination I became nervous and I had to stop and remind myself to deep breathe, and that really helped me to focus and continue. My computer did not turn off after answering 75 questions, and my heart began to race. But I maintained my stamina and finally, after 130 questions, my examination was complete. I felt very ambivalent as to whether or not I passed. I felt very unsure and could not gauge my performance, but I knew that this was a normal feeling. I decided to get my mind off of the examination, and I went to a movie with a friend.

I was told that I would receive my results via mail, but I was too anxious to wait. Each day I checked the state license Web site to see if my license number appeared next to my name. About one week after the examination, I popped up out of bed at 6 AM and ran downstairs to my computer. I quickly went to the state license Web site, entered in my name, and found my license number next to my name. I had passed! What a relief! I was dancing, yelling, and calling all my friends and family to spread the news. It was time to celebrate the hard work and achievement.

After everything was behind me and the stress of the examination was over, I realized that the studying and the examination were not as dreadful as I had anticipated. Just remember that it is extremely important to remain confident in yourself and your ability to pass this examination. This is the closing of one chapter in your life and the beginning of an exciting, rewarding new chapter, your career as a registered nurse. I look forward to working together with you as a colleague in the nursing profession and in the community. Again, congratulations on your achievements and good luck with the examination.

Test-Taking Strategies

I. PYRAMID TO SUCCESS (BOX 5-1)

II. HOW TO AVOID READING INTO THE QUESTION (BOX 5-2)

A. Pyramid Points

1. Read every word in the question and specifically determine what the question is asking.
2. Focus only on the information in the question and avoid asking yourself, "Well, what if …?"
3. Look for the key words in the question, such as *early signs* or *late signs*.
4. In multiple-choice questions, multiple-response questions, or questions that require you to number in order of priority, read every choice or option presented.
5. Use the process of elimination when choices or options are presented; reread the question and what the question is asking specifically to assist you in determining your final choice or choices.
6. With questions that require you to fill in the blank, focus on the information in the question and determine what the question is asking; if the question requires you to calculate a medication dose or intake and output amounts, recheck your work in calculating to verify the answer.
7. Remember, focus on the information in the question and specifically what the question is asking.

B. The parts of a question (Box 5-3)

1. The question will consist of a case situation, question stem, and the options (a fill in the blank question will not contain options).
2. The case situation provides you with the information about the client and the information that you need to consider in answering the question.
3. The question stem asks something specific about the case situation.
4. The options are all of the answers.
5. A multiple-choice question will have four options, and you must select one; read every option carefully, and always use the process of elimination.

BOX 5-1

Pyramid to Success

Read the question and every option thoroughly and carefully.

Ask yourself, "What is the question specifically asking?"

Be alert to key words and true and false response questions.

Eliminate the incorrect options.

Use all of your nursing knowledge, your clinical experiences, and your test-taking skills and strategies to answer the question.

BOX 5-2

Practice Question: Avoid Reading into the Question

A client with metastatic cancer is receiving a continuous intravenous infusion of morphine sulfate to alleviate pain. The nurse monitors the client for which *adverse or toxic effect* of the medication?

1. Dizziness
2. Sedation
3. Skeletal muscle flaccidity
4. Nausea

Answer: 3

Test-Taking Strategy: Read every word in the question and specifically determine what the question is asking. The question is asking about the adverse or toxic effect of morphine sulfate. Dizziness, sedation, and nausea are side effects of morphine sulfate that the client may experience but are not toxic effects. Remember, focus on the information in the question and what the question is asking.

BOX 5-3

Multiple Choice Question: Case Situation, Question Stem, and Options

Case situation: The nurse is monitoring a child for bleeding following surgery for removal of a brain tumor. The nurse checks the head dressing for the presence of blood and notes a colorless drainage on the back of the dressing. *Question stem:* Which of the following would be the most appropriate nursing intervention?
Options
1. Circle the area of drainage and continue to monitor.
2. Reinforce the dressing.
3. Notify the physician.
4. Document the findings and continue to monitor.

BOX 5-4

Common Key Words

Early or late
Best
First
Initial
Immediately
Most likely or least likely
Most appropriate or least appropriate

6. A multiple-response question will have several options, and you must select all options that apply to the situation in the question; read each option carefully, visualize the situation, and use your nursing knowledge to answer the question.
7. In a prioritizing (ordered response) question, you will be required to list in order of priority certain nursing interventions; visualize the situation, and use your nursing knowledge to answer the question.

III. LOOK FOR KEY WORDS (BOXES 5-4 AND 5-5)
A. Key words focus your attention on a specific or critical point to consider when answering the question.
B. Some key words may indicate that all of the options are correct, and that it will be necessary to prioritize in order to select the correct option.
C. As you read the question, look for the key words; key words will make a difference regarding how you will answer the question.

IV. THE ISSUE OF THE QUESTION (BOX 5-6)
A. The issue of the question is the specific subject content about which the question is asking.
B. Identifying the issue of the question will assist in eliminating the incorrect options and direct you to selecting the correct option.
C. The issue of the question can include the following:
   1. A medication or intravenous therapy
   2. A side effect of a medication

BOX 5-5

Practice Question: Look for the Key Words

A nurse is caring for a client who just returned from the recovery room after undergoing abdominal surgery. The nurse monitors the client for which *early sign* of hypovolemic shock?
1. Increased pulse rate
2. Increased depth of respiration
3. Lethargy
4. Decreased deep tendon reflexes
Answer: 1
Test-Taking Strategy: Note the key words *early sign*. Focusing on these key words and recalling that the earliest clinical signs of hypovolemic shock are cardiovascular changes will direct you to the correct option. Although increased depth of respirations, lethargy, and decreased or absent deep tendon reflexes occur in hypovolemic shock, these are not early signs. Rather they occur as the shock progresses. Remember to look for key words.

BOX 5-6

Practice Question: The Issue of the Question

Fat emulsion is prescribed for the client receiving total parenteral nutrition. The nurse is preparing to hang the fat emulsion and notes the *presence of fat globules* in the solution. The most appropriate nursing action is to
1. Shake the solution to dissolve the globules
2. Call the physician
3. Return the solution to the pharmacy
4. Place the solution in a bath of warm water until the globules dissolve
Answer: 3
Test-Taking Strategy: Focus on the issue, the presence of fat globules in the solution. Thinking about the significance of fat globules in the solution and the potential adverse effect of fat globules entering the client's bloodstream will direct you to the correct option.

   3. An adverse or toxic effect of a medication
   4. A treatment or procedure
   5. A complication of a health care problem, treatment, or procedure
   6. A specific nursing action

V. TRUE AND FALSE RESPONSE QUESTIONS (BOXES 5-7 AND 5-8)
A. True response questions use key words that ask you to select an option that is accurate regarding the information in the question.
B. False response questions use key words that ask you to select an option that is not accurate regarding the information in the question.
C. Read every word in the question and be especially alert in noting key words that ask you to select an

BOX 5-7

Practice Question: True Response

A client suspected of having meningitis is being scheduled for diagnostic tests. The nurse anticipates that which of the following diagnostic tests will *most likely* be prescribed to confirm the diagnosis?
1. Serum electrolytes
2. Electromyography
3. White blood cell count
4. Lumbar puncture

Answer: 4

Test-Taking Strategy: This question identifies an example of a true response question. Note the key words *most likely* and *confirm*. Focus on the diagnosis presented in the question and the associated pathophysiology to assist in directing you to option 4. Remember, meningitis is an acute or chronic inflammation of the meninges and the cerebrospinal fluid. The key diagnostic test used in meningitis is the lumbar puncture. A white blood cell count and serum electrolytes test also may be performed. Electromyography is not a key diagnostic test. Remember true response questions ask you to select an option that is accurate.

BOX 5-8

Practice Question: False Response

Cortisone (Cortone) is prescribed for a client with adrenal insufficiency, and the nurse provides instructions to the client regarding the medication. Which of the following statements if made by the client would indicate a *need for further instruction*?
1. "I will eat a good breakfast every day."
2. "I will avoid people with colds."
3. "I will limit my sodium intake."
4. "I will stop the medication when I feel better."

Answer: 4

Test-Taking Strategy: This question identifies an example of a false response question. Note the key words *need for further instruction*. These key words indicate that you should select an option that identifies an incorrect client statement. Glucocorticoids should not be abruptly discontinued to prevent acute adrenal insufficiency. You easily should be able to eliminate options 1, 2, and 3, remembering that the client should not stop these medications or in fact any medication without physician approval. Remember false response questions ask you to select an option that is not accurate regarding the information in the question.

option that is not accurate regarding the information in the question.

VI. QUESTIONS THAT REQUIRE PRIORITIZING

A. Questions in the examination may require you to use the skill of prioritizing nursing actions.
B. Look for the key words in the question that indicate the need to prioritize (Box 5-9).

BOX 5-9

Common Key Words That Indicate the Need to Prioritize

Best
Essential
First
Highest priority
Immediate
Initial
Most important
Next
Primary
Vital

C. Remember, when a question requires prioritization, all options may be correct, and you need to determine the correct order of action.
D. Guidelines to use include the ABCs airway, breathing, and circulation; Maslow's hierarchy of needs theory; and the steps of the nursing process.
E. The ABCs (Box 5-10)
   1. Use the ABCs—airway, breathing, and circulation—when selecting an answer or determining the order of priority.
   2. Remember the order of priority: airway, breathing, and circulation.
   3. Airway is always the first priority.
F. Maslow's hierarchy of needs theory (Box 5-11)
   1. Use Maslow's hierarchy of needs theory as a guide to prioritize.
   2. Physiological needs are the priority; therefore select an option or determine the order of priority by addressing physiological needs first.
   3. When a physiological need is not addressed in the question or noted in one of the options, continue to use Maslow's hierarchy of needs theory as a guide and look for the option that addresses safety.

BOX 5-10

Practice Question: Use of the ABCs

The client with a diagnosis of cancer is receiving morphine sulfate 10 mg subcutaneously every 3 to 4 hours for pain. When preparing the plan of care for the client, the nurse includes which *priority* action?
1. Monitor stools.
2. Monitor the urine output.
3. Encourage the client to cough and deep breath.
4. Encourage fluid intake.

Answer: 3

Test-Taking Strategy: Use the ABCs—airway, breathing, and circulation—as a guide to direct you to the correct option. Recall that morphine sulfate suppresses the cough reflex and the respiratory reflex. Although options 1, 2, and 4 are components of the plan of care, the correct option addresses airway. Remember use the ABCs airway, breathing, and circulation to prioritize.

BOX 5-11

Practice Question: Maslow's Hierarchy of Needs Theory

A nurse is reviewing the plan of care for a pregnant client with a diagnosis of sickle cell anemia. Which nursing diagnosis, if stated on the plan of care, would the nurse select as receiving the *highest priority*?
1. Anxiety
2. Ineffective coping
3. Disturbed body image
4. Deficient fluid volume
Answer: 4
Test-Taking Strategy: Note the key words *highest priority*. Use Maslow's hierarchy of needs theory to prioritize, remembering that physiological needs come first. Using this guideline will direct you to option 4. Deficient fluid volume is a physiological need and is the priority nursing diagnosis. Remember, physiological needs are the priority.

BOX 5-12

Assessment Key Words

Ascertain
Assess
Check
Determine
Find out
Identify
Monitor
Observe
Obtain information

BOX 5-13

Practice Question: The Nursing Process—Assessment

A nurse is teaching a client with coronary artery disease about dietary measures to follow. During the session, the client expresses frustration in learning the dietary regimen. The nurse would *initially*
1. Identify the cause of the frustration.
2. Continue with the dietary teaching.
3. Notify the physician.
4. Tell the client that the diet needs to be followed.
Answer: 1
Test-Taking Strategy: Use the steps of the nursing process. Assessment is the first step. Of the four options presented, the only assessment action is option 1. Options 2, 3, and 4 identify the implementation step of the nursing process. The initial action is to identify the cause of the frustration. Remember assessment is the first step of the nursing process.

BOX 5-14

Practice Question: The Nursing Process—Analysis

A nurse is reviewing the laboratory results of an infant suspected of having hypertrophic pyloric stenosis. Which of the following laboratory findings would the nurse most likely expect to note in this infant?
1. A blood pH of 7.50
2. A blood pH of 7.30
3. A blood bicarbonate of 22 mEq/L
4. A blood bicarbonate of 19 mEq/L
Answer: 1
Test-Taking Strategy: An understanding of the physiology associated with hypertrophic pyloric stenosis and that metabolic alkalosis is likely to occur as a result of vomiting is necessary. Next, the nurse must know which laboratory findings would be noted in this acid-base condition. Analysis of this data will direct you to the correct option. Remember analysis is the second step of the nursing process

G. Steps of the nursing process
  1. Use the steps of the nursing process to prioritize.
  2. The steps include assessment, analysis, planning, implementation, and evaluation and are followed in this order.
  3. Assessment
    a. Remember that assessment is the first step in the nursing process.
    b. When you are asked to select your first and initial nursing action, follow the steps of the nursing process to prioritize when selecting the correct option.
    c. Assessment questions address the process of gathering subjective and objective data relative to the client, confirming that data, and communicating and documenting the data
    d. Look for key words in the options that reflect assessment (Box 5-12).
    e. If an option contains the concept of assessment or the collection of client data, the best choice is to select that option (Box 5-13).
    f. If an assessment action is not one of the options, follow the steps of the nursing process as your guide to select your initial or first action.
    g. Possible exception to the guideline: If the question presents an emergency situation, read carefully; in an emergency situation, an intervention may be the priority.
  4. Analysis (Box 5-14)
    a. Analysis questions are the most difficult questions because they require understanding of the principles of physiological responses and require interpretation of the data based on assessment.
    b. Analysis questions require critical thinking and determining the rationale for therapeutic interventions that may be addressed in the question.

BOX 5-15

Practice Question: The Nursing Process—Planning

A nurse develops a plan of care for a client with a cataract. Which nursing diagnosis is the priority?
1. Fear related to loss of eyesight
2. Social Isolation related to decreased ability to mobilize in the community
3. Disturbed Sensory Perception (Visual) related to ocular lens opacity
4. Risk for Injury related to decreased vision

Answer: 3

Test-Taking Strategy: This question relates to planning nursing care and asks you to identify the priority nursing diagnosis. Use Maslow's hierarchy of needs theory to answer the question. Remembering that physiological needs are the priority will direct you to option 3. Although Risk for Injury is a potential rather than an actual problem, according to Maslow's hierarchy of needs theory, safety is the second priority. Fear and Social Isolation are psychosocial needs. Remember planning is the third step of the nursing process.

BOX 5-16

Practice Question: The Nursing Process—Implementation

A nurse is caring for a client with angina pectoris who begins to experience chest pain. The nurse administers a sublingual nitroglycerin (Nitrostat) tablet sublingually as prescribed, but the pain is unrelieved. The nurse should take which of the following actions *next*?
1. Contact the physician.
2. Call the client's family.
3. Administer another nitroglycerin tablet.
4. Reposition the client.

Answer: 3

Test-Taking Strategy: Implementation questions address the process of organizing and managing care. This question also requires that you prioritize the nursing actions. Note the key word *next*. Recalling that the nurse would administer three nitroglycerin tablets 5 minutes apart from each other to relieve chest pain will assist in directing you to option 3. Remember implementation is the fourth step of the nursing process.

c. Analysis questions may address the formulation of a nursing diagnosis and the communication and documentation of the results of the process of analysis.

5. Planning (Box 5-15)
  a. Planning questions require prioritizing nursing diagnoses, determining goals and outcome criteria for goals of care, developing the plan of care, and communicating and documenting the plan of care.
  b. Regarding nursing diagnoses, remember that actual client problems rather than potential or at-risk client problems will most likely be the priority.
  c. Remember that this is a nursing examination and the answer to the question most likely involves something that is included in the nursing care plan, rather than the medical plan.

6. Implementation (Box 5-16)
  a. Implementation questions address the process of organizing and managing care, counseling and teaching, providing care to achieve established goals, supervising and coordinating care, and communicating and documenting nursing interventions.
  b. This examination is about nursing, so focus on the nursing action rather than on the medical action, unless the question is asking you what prescription (medical order) is anticipated.
  c. The only client about whom you need to be concerned is the client in the question that you are answering; remember that this client is your only assigned client.
  d. Answer the question as if the situation were textbook and ideal and the nurse had all the time

and resources needed and readily available at the client's bedside.

7. Evaluation (Box 5-17)
  a. Evaluation questions focus on comparing the actual outcomes of care with the expected outcomes and focus on how the nurse should monitor or make a judgment concerning a client's response to therapy or to a nursing action.
  b. These questions address evaluating the client's ability to implement self-care, health care team members' ability to implement care, and the process of communicating and documenting evaluation findings.

BOX 5-17

Practice Question: The Nursing Process—Evaluation

A client with multiple sclerosis has been taking oxybutynin (Ditropan). The nurse *determines the degree of effectiveness* of the medication by asking the client about changes in the following:
1. Extent of muscle spasms
2. Level of fatigue
3. Bowel movements
4. Patterns of urination

Answer: 4

Test-Taking Strategy: This is an evaluation question. Note the key words *determines the degree of effectiveness*. Oxybutynin is an antispasmodic used to relieve symptoms of urinary urgency, frequency, nocturia, and incontinence in clients with uninhibited or reflex neurogenic bladder. Recalling that this medication is used to treat bladder dysfunction will direct you to option 4. Remember evaluation is the fifth step of the nursing process.

c. In an evaluation question, be alert to false response questions because they are used frequently in evaluation-type questions, and the question may ask for a client statement that indicates accurate or inaccurate information related to the issue of the question.

VII. CLIENT NEEDS
A. Safe, Effective Care Environment
   1. These questions address the nurse's role in providing and directing care that will ensure an environment that promotes protecting the client, family or significant other(s), and other health care personnel.
   2. Content addressed in these questions relates to the nursing role of coordinating and integrating cost-effective care, supervising and/or collaborating with members of the multidisciplinary health care team, and environmental safety.
   3. Be alert to safety needs addressed in a question, and remember the importance of handwashing, call bells, bed positioning, the appropriate use of side rails, and standard precautions.
B. Physiological Integrity
   1. These questions address the nurse's role in promoting physical health and well-being in the client by providing care and comfort, reducing client risk potential, and managing the client's health alterations.
   2. Content addressed in these questions relates to basic care and comfort, pharmacological and parenteral therapies, reducing the risk of the development of complications, and managing and providing care to clients with acute, chronic, or life-threatening conditions.
   3. Remember that physiological needs are a priority and are addressed first.
   4. Use the ABCs airway, breathing, and circulation; Maslow's hierarchy of needs theory; and the steps of the nursing process when selecting an option addressing physiological integrity.
C. Psychosocial Integrity
   1. These questions address the nurse's role in providing nursing care that supports and promotes the emotional, mental, and social well-being of the client and significant other(s).
   2. Content addressed in these questions relates to promoting the client's or significant other's ability to cope, adapt, or problem solve in situations such as illness or stressful events and to providing care to clients with maladaptive behavior or acute or chronic mental illness.
   3. In this Client Needs category you may be asked communication-type questions that relate to how you would respond to a client, a client's family member or significant other, or to other health care team members.

BOX 5-18

Practice Question: Communication

A mother says to the nurse, "I am afraid that my child might have another seizure." Which response by the nurse is most therapeutic?
1. "Why worry about something that you cannot control?"
2. "Most children will never experience a second seizure."
3. "Tell me what frightens you the most about seizures."
4. "Acetaminophen (Tylenol) can prevent another seizure from occurring."

Answer: 3

Test-Taking Strategy: Option 3 is the only option that addresses the client's fears. Option 1 blocks communication because it states that the mother should not worry. Options 2 and 4 are incorrect because the nurse is giving false assurance that a seizure will not reoccur or can be prevented in this child. Remember focus on feelings, concerns, anxieties, or fears.

---

   4. Use therapeutic communication techniques to answer communication questions because of their effectiveness in the communication process.
   5. Remember to select the answer that focuses on the client's, client's family member's, or significant other's feelings, concerns, anxieties, or fears (Box 5-18).
D. Health Promotion and Maintenance
   1. These questions address the nurse's role in providing and directing nursing care that prevents health problems, provides early detection of health problems, and provides and directs care that incorporates knowledge of expected growth and development principles.
   2. Content addressed in these questions relates to assisting the client and significant other(s) through the normal stages of growth and development and assisting the client and significant other(s) to develop health practices that promote wellness and to recognize alterations in health care status.
   3. Use the teaching/learning theory if the question addresses client education, remembering that client motivation and client readiness to learn is the first priority.
   4. Be alert to false response questions that address health promotion and maintenance and client education.

VIII. ELIMINATING SIMILAR OPTIONS (BOX 5-19)
A. When answering the question, use the process of elimination and look for similar options.
B. If any of the options include the same idea, then they are incorrect and can be eliminated.
C. Remember that there is only one correct option, and the answer to the question is the option that is different.

BOX 5-19

Practice Question: Eliminate Similar Options

A nurse is assigned to care for a group of clients. On review of the clients' medical records, the nurse determines that which client is at risk for excess fluid volume?
1. The client with an ileostomy
2. The client taking diuretics
3. The client who requires gastrointestinal suctioning
4. The client with renal failure

Answer: 4

Test-Taking Strategy: Focus on what the question is asking: the client at risk for excess fluid volume. Think about the pathophysiology associated with each condition identified in the options. The only client that retains fluid is the client with renal failure. The client with an ileostomy, the client taking diuretics, and the client requiring gastrointestinal suctioning all lose fluid. Remember eliminate similar options.

IX. ELIMINATE OPTIONS THAT CONTAIN ABSOLUTE WORDS (BOX 5-20)

A. As you read each option, look for absolute words.
B. Absolute words tend to make an option incorrect, and if you note an absolute word in an option, eliminate that option.
C. Some of these absolute words include *all*, *always*, *every*, *must*, *none*, *never*, and *only*.

X. LOOK FOR THE UMBRELLA OPTION (BOX 5-21)

A. When answering a question, if you note that more than one option appears to be correct, look for the umbrella option (also known as global option or comprehensive option).

BOX 5-20

Practice Question: Eliminate Options That Contain Absolute Words

A nurse is providing safety instructions to the mother of a child with hemophilia and tells the mother to do which of the following to promote a safe environment for the child?
1. Remove toys with sharp edges from the child's toy box.
2. Allow the child to play with toys only if a parent is present.
3. Place a helmet and elbow pads on the child every day.
4. Allow the child to play indoors only.

Answer: 1

Test-Taking Strategy: Eliminate options that contain absolute words. Options 2 and 4 contain the absolute word *only*. Option 3 contains the absolute word *every*. Remember that absolute words tend to make an option incorrect.

BOX 5-21

Practice Question: Look for the Umbrella Option

A nurse in the emergency room receives a telephone call from emergency medical services and is told that several victims who survived a plane crash and are suffering from cold exposure will be transported to the hospital. The initial nursing action of the emergency room nurse is which of the following?
1. Supply the trauma rooms with bottles of sterile water and normal saline.
2. Call the laundry department and ask the department to send as many warm blankets as possible to the emergency room.
3. Call the nursing supervisor to activate the agency disaster plan.
4. Call the intensive care unit to request that nurses be sent to the emergency room.

Answer: 3

Test-Taking Strategy: Option 3 is the umbrella option. Activating the agency disaster plan will ensure that the interventions in options 1, 2, and 4 will occur. Remember the umbrella option embraces the ideas of the other options within it.

B. The umbrella option is one that is a general statement and may contain the ideas of the other options within it.
C. The umbrella option will be the correct answer.

XI. USE THE GUIDELINES FOR DELEGATING AND ASSIGNMENT MAKING (BOX 5-22)

A. You may be asked a question that will require you to decide how you will delegate a task or assign clients to other health care providers.
B. Focus on the information in the question and what task or assignment is to be delegated.
C. Once you have determined what task or assignment is to be delegated, consider the client's needs and match the client's needs with the scope of practice of the health care providers identified in the question.
D. The nurse practice act and any practice limitations define which aspects of care can be delegated and which must be performed by the registered nurse.
E. Generally, noninvasive interventions such as skin care, range of motion exercises, ambulation, grooming, and hygiene measures can be assigned to a nursing assistant.
F. A licensed practical nurse can perform the tasks that a nursing assistant can perform and additionally can perform certain invasive tasks such as dressings, suctioning, urinary catheterization, and administering medications orally or by subcutaneous or intramuscular injections.
G. The registered nurse can perform the tasks that a licensed practical nurse can perform and is responsible for assessment and planning care, supervising

BOX 5-22

Practice Question: Use the Guidelines for Delegating and Assignment Making

A nurse is planning the client assignments for the day and has a licensed practical nurse (LPN) and a nursing assistant on the nursing team. Which client would the nurse most appropriately assign to the LPN?
1. A client with stable congestive heart failure who has early stage Alzheimer's disease
2. A client who was treated for dehydration and is weak and needs assistance with bathing
3. A client with emphysema who is receiving oxygen at 2 L by nasal cannula and becomes dyspneic on exertion
4. A client who is scheduled for an electrocardiogram and a chest x-ray

Answer: 3

Test-Taking Strategy: The nurse would most appropriately assign the client with emphysema to the LPN. This client has an airway problem and has the highest priority needs from the clients presented in the options. The clients described in option 1, 2, and 4 can be cared for appropriately by the nursing assistant. Remember to match the client's needs with the scope of practice of the health care provider.

care, initiating teaching, and administering medications intravenously.

XII. ANSWERING PHARMACOLOGY QUESTIONS (BOX 5-23)

A. If you are familiar with the medication, use nursing knowledge to answer the question.
B. Remember that the question will identify the generic name and the trade name of the medication.

BOX 5-23

Practice Question: Answering Pharmacology Questions

Orally administered levothyroxine (Synthroid) 50 μg daily is prescribed for a client with hypothyroidism. The nurse provides medication instructions to the client and tells the client to take the medication
1. Just after breakfast.
2. With a snack at 3 PM.
3. In the morning on an empty stomach.
4. With food.

Answer: 3

Test-Taking Strategy: Note that a medical diagnosis is presented in the question. This will assist you in determining that the medication is used to treat this condition. Additionally, most thyroid replacement medications contain "thy" in their names. Also use the strategy of eliminating similar options. Note that options 1, 2, and 4 are similar and indicate that the medication should be taken with food. Remember with pharmacology questions, focus on the information in the question and the classification of the medication.

C. If the question identifies a medical diagnosis, then try to make a relationship between the medication and the diagnosis; for example, you can determine that cyclophosphamide (Cytoxan) is an antineoplastic medication if the question refers to a client with breast cancer who is taking this medication.
D. Try to determine the classification of the medication being addressed to assist in answering the question; identifying the classification will assist in determining a medication action and side effects (diltiazem [Cardizem] is a cardiac medication).
E. Recognize the common side effects associated with each medication classification and then relate the appropriate nursing interventions to each side effect; for example, if a side effect is hypertension, then the associated nursing intervention would be to monitor the blood pressure.
F. Learn medications that belong to a classification by commonalities in their medication names; for example, medications that are xanthine bronchodilators end with "line" (theophylline).
G. Look at the medication name and use medical terminology to assist in determining the medication action; for example, *Lopressor* lowers (*lo*) the blood pressure (*pressor*).
H. If the question requires a medication calculation, remember that a calculator is available on the computer; talk yourself through each step to be sure the answer makes sense, and recheck the calculation before answering the question, particularly if the answer seems like an unusual dosage.
I. Pyramid Points to remember
   1. Generally, the client should not take an antacid with medication because the antacid will affect the absorption of the medication.
   2. Enteric-coated and sustained-release tablets should not be crushed; additionally, capsules should not be opened.
   3. The client should never adjust or change a medication dose or abruptly stop taking a medication.
   4. The nurse never adjusts or changes the client's medication dosage and never discontinues a medication.
   5. The client needs to avoid taking any over-the-counter medications or any other medications such as herbal preparations unless they are approved for use by the health care provider.
   6. The client needs to avoid alcohol and smoking.
   7. Medications are never administered if the order is difficult to read, is unclear, or identifies a medication dose that is not a normal one.

REFERENCES

Harkreader, H., & Hogan, M. A. (2004). *Fundamentals of nursing: Caring and clinical judgment* (2nd ed.). Philadelphia: W. B. Saunders.
Ignatavicius, D., & Workman, M. (2002). *Medical-surgical nursing: Critical thinking for collaborative care* (4th ed.). Philadelphia: W. B. Saunders.

Keltner, N., Schwecke, L., & Bostrom, C. (2003). *Psychiatric nursing* (4th ed.). St. Louis: Mosby.

Lewis, S., Heitkemper, M., & Dirksen, S. (2004). *Medical-surgical nursing: Assessment and management of clinical problems* (6th ed.). St. Louis: Mosby.

National Council of State Boards of Nursing (Eds.). (2003). *Test Plan for the National Council Licensure Examination for Registered Nurses* (effective date: April 2004). Chicago: Author.

Phipps, W., Monahan, F., Sands, J., Marek, J., & Neighbors, M. (2003). *Medical-surgical nursing: Health and illness perspectives* (7th ed.). St. Louis: Mosby.

Potter, P., & Perry, A. (2001). *Fundamentals of nursing* (5th ed.). St. Louis: Mosby.

Riley, J. (2004). *Communication in nursing* (5th ed.). St. Louis: Mosby.

Varcarolis, E. M. (2002). *Foundations of psychiatric mental health nursing* (4th ed.). Philadelphia: W. B. Saunders.

UNIT II

Issues in Nursing

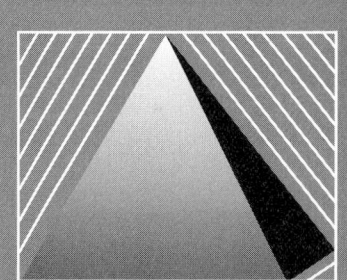

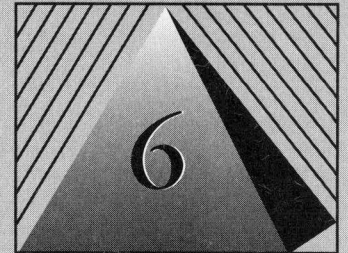

6 Cultural Diversity

PYRAMID TERMS

acculturation Process of learning norms, beliefs, and behavioral expectations of a group other than one's own group.

belief Something accepted as true by a culture.

cultural assimilation Process in which individuals from a minority group are absorbed by the dominant culture and take on the characteristics of the dominant culture.

cultural competence The acquisition of knowledge, understanding, and appreciation of a culture that facilitates the provision of culturally appropriate health care.

cultural diversity The differences among groups of people that result from ethnic, racial, and cultural variables.

cultural imposition The tendency to impose one's own beliefs, values, and patterns of behavior on individuals from another culture.

culture The dynamic network of knowledge, beliefs, patterns of behavior, ideas, attitudes, values, and norms that are unique to a particular group of people.

dominant culture The group whose values prevail within a society.

ethnic group A group of people within a culture who share an identity based on race, religion, color, national origin, or language.

ethnicity An individual's identification of self as part of an ethnic group.

ethnocentrism An assumption of cultural superiority and an inability to accept the ways of another culture.

minority group An ethnic, cultural, racial, or religious group that constitutes less than a numerical majority of the population.

race A grouping of people based on biological similarities. Members of a racial group have similar physical characteristics, such as blood group, facial features, and color of skin, hair, and eyes.

racism Discrimination directed toward individuals or groups who are perceived to be inferior because of biological differences; often accompanied by oppression.

stereotyping An expectation that all people within the same racial, ethnic, or cultural group act alike and share the same beliefs and attitudes.

subculture A group of people with characteristic patterns of behavior that distinguish the group from the larger culture or society.

values Principles and standards that have meaning and worth to an individual, family, group, community, or culture.

THE PYRAMID TO SUCCESS

Often nurses care for clients who come from ethnic, cultural, or religious backgrounds that are different from their own. Awareness of and sensitivity to the unique health and illness beliefs and practices are essential in the delivery of safe and effective care. Acknowledgment and acceptance of cultural differences with a nonjudgmental attitude are essential to providing culturally sensitive care. The belief underlying the NCLEX-RN exam test plan is that persons are unique individuals and define their own systems of daily living, which reflect their values, motives, and lifestyles. The Integrated Processes addressed in this chapter are Caring, Communication and Documentation, Nursing Process, and Teaching/Learning.

CLIENT NEEDS
Safe, Effective Care Environment

Advocacy
Client rights
Confidentiality
Continuity of care
Establishment of priorities
Ethical practice
Legal rights and responsibilities
Referrals
Resource management

Health Promotion and Maintenance

Aging process
Disease prevention
Family planning and family systems
Growth and development
Health and wellness
Health screening
Lifestyle choices

Psychosocial Integrity

Coping mechanisms
Cultural diversity
End of life
Family dynamics
Religious and spiritual influences on health
Support systems
Therapeutic communications
Therapeutic environment

Physiological Integrity

Alternative and complementary therapies
Blood and blood products
Illness management
Nonpharmacological comfort interventions
Nutrition and oral hydration (Boxes 6-1 and 6-2)
Palliative/comfort care
Therapeutic procedures

BOX 6-1
Dietary Preferences

AFRICAN-AMERICANS
Fried foods
Pork, greens, rice
Some pregnant African Americans engage in pica.

ASIAN AMERICANS
Soy sauce
Raw fish
Rice

AMERICANS OF EUROPEAN (WHITE) ORIGIN
Carbohydrates (potatoes)
Red meat

HISPANIC AMERICANS
Beans
Fried foods
Spicy foods
Tortillas
Carbonated beverages

AMERICAN INDIANS, ALEUTS, ESKIMOS
Blue cornmeal
Fish
Game
Fruits and berries
Navajos prefer meat and blue cornmeal and tend to avoid consumption of milk.

I. AFRICAN AMERICANS

A. Communication
1. Members are competent in standard English and in black English, a variation based on pronunciation, grammar, and vocabulary.
2. Head nodding does not necessarily mean agreement.
3. Direct eye contact may be interpreted as rudeness or aggressive behavior.
4. Nonverbal communication is important.
5. Personal questions asked on initial contact with a person may be viewed as intrusive.
B. Time orientation and personal space preferences
1. Time orientation varies according to age, socio-economics, and subgroups and may include past, present, or future orientation.
2. Members may be late for an appointment because relationships and events may be deemed more important than being on time.
3. Members are comfortable with close personal space when interacting with family and friends.
C. Social roles
1. Large extended family networks are important; the elderly are respected.

2. Many households are headed by single-parent woman.
3. Religious **beliefs** and church affiliation are sources of strength.
D. Health and illness
1. Religious beliefs profoundly affect ideas about health and illness.
2. Members believe illness can be prevented by nutritious meals, rest, and cleanliness.
E. Health risks
1. Sickle cell anemia
2. Hypertension
3. Heart disease
4. Cancer
5. Lactose intolerance
6. Diabetes mellitus
F. Interventions
1. Recognize the presence of many individual and subgroup variations.
2. Build a relationship based on trust.
3. Clarify the meaning of client's verbal and nonverbal behavior.
4. Be flexible and avoid rigidity in scheduling care.
5. Encourage family involvement.
6. Alternative modes of healing may include herbs, prayer, and laying on of hands.

BOX 6-2

Religions and Dietary Practices

SEVENTH DAY ADVENTIST (CHURCH OF GOD)
Alcohol, coffee, and tea are prohibited.
Some groups prohibit meat.

BUDDHISM
Alcohol and drug use is discouraged.
Some sects are vegetarian.

ROMAN CATHOLICISM
Avoid meat on Ash Wednesday and Good Friday.
Optional fasting during Lent season.
During Lent, discourage eating of meat on Friday.
Children and the ill are exempt from fasting.

CHURCH OF JESUS CHRIST OF LATTER-DAY SAINTS (MORMON)
Alcohol, coffee, and tea are prohibited.
Consumption of meat is limited.
First Sunday of the month is time for fasting.

HINDUISM
Beef and veal are prohibited.
Many individuals are vegetarians.
Consumption of meat is limited.
Fasting occurs on specific days of the week according to which god the person worships.
Children are not allowed to participate in fasting.
Fasting rituals vary from complete abstinence to consumption of only one meal per day.

ISLAM
Pork is prohibited.
Any meat product not ritually slaughtered is prohibited.
Alcohol or drugs are avoided.

During Ramadan (ninth month of Mohammedan year), fasting occurs during daytime.

JEHOVAH'S WITNESS
Any foods to which blood has been added are prohibited.
Can consume animal flesh that has been drained.

JUDAISM
Orthodox believers must adhere to dietary kosher laws.
Meats allowed include animals that are vegetable eaters, cloven-hoofed animals, and animals that are ritually slaughtered.
Fish that have scales and fins are allowed.
Any combination of meat and milk is prohibited.
During Yom Kippur, 24-hour fasting is observed.
Pregnant women and those who are seriously ill are exempt from fasting.
During Passover week, only unleavened bread is eaten.

PENTECOSTAL (ASSEMBLY OF GOD)
Alcohol is prohibited.
Members avoid consumption of anything to which blood has been added.
Some individuals avoid pork.

RUSSIAN ORTHODOX
Abstention from meat and dairy products on Wednesday, Friday, and during Lent is observed.
During Lent, all animal products, including dairy products, are forbidden.
Fasting occurs during Advent.
Exceptions from fasting include illness and pregnancy.

II. ASIAN AMERICANS
A. Communication
   1. Languages include Chinese, Japanese, Korean, Vietnamese, and English.
   2. Silence is valued.
   3. Eye contact may be considered inappropriate or disrespectful.
   4. Criticism or disagreement is not expressed verbally.
   5. Head nodding does not necessarily mean agreement.
   6. The word *no* may be interpreted as disrespect for others.
B. Time orientation and personal space preferences
   1. Time orientation reflects respect for the past but includes emphasis on the present and the future.
   2. Preference is for a formal personal space except with family and close friends.
   3. Usually members do not touch others during conversation.
   4. Touching is unacceptable with members of opposite sex.
   5. The head is considered to be sacred; therefore touching someone on the head is disrespectful.
C. Social roles
   1. Members are devoted to tradition.
   2. Large extended family networks are common.
   3. Loyalty to immediate and extended family and honor are valued.
   4. Family unit is structured and hierarchical.
   5. Men have the power and authority, and women are expected to be obedient.
   6. Education is viewed as important.
   7. Religions include Taoism (Buddhism), Islam, and Christianity.
   8. Social organizations are strong within the community.
D. Health and illness
   1. Health is a state of physical and spiritual harmony with nature and a balance between positive and negative energy forces (yin and yang).
   2. A healthy body is viewed as a gift from ancestors.

3. Illness is viewed as an imbalance between yin and yang.
4. Yin foods are cold, and yang foods are hot; one eats cold foods when one has a hot illness, and one eats hot foods when one has a cold illness.
5. Illness is attributed to prolonged sitting or lying or to overexertion.

E. Health risks
   1. Hypertension
   2. Heart disease
   3. Cancer
   4. Lactose intolerance
   5. Thalassemia

F. Interventions
   1. Avoid physical closeness and excessive touching; only touch a client's head when necessary, informing the client before doing so.
   2. Limit eye contact.
   3. Avoid gesturing with hands.
   4. If possible, a female client prefers a female health care provider.
   5. Clarify responses to questions and expectations of health care provider.
   6. Be flexible and avoid rigidity in scheduling care.
   7. Encourage family involvement.
   8. Alternative modes of healing may include herbs, acupuncture, restoration of balance with foods, massage, and offering of prayers and incense.

III. AMERICANS OF EUROPEAN (WHITE) ORIGIN

A. Communication
   1. Languages include national languages and English.
   2. Silence can be used to show respect or disrespect for another, depending on situation.
   3. Eye contact is viewed as indicating trustworthiness.

B. Time orientation and personal space preferences.
   1. Members are future oriented.
   2. Time is valued; members tend to be on time and to be impatient with people who are not on time.
   3. Members may be aloof and tend to avoid close physical contact.
   4. Handshakes may be used for formal greetings.

C. Social roles
   1. The nuclear family is the basic unit; the extended family is also important.
   2. The man is the dominant figure, but variation of gender roles exists within families/relationships.
   3. Religion includes Judeo-Christian beliefs.
   4. Community social organizations are important.

D. Health and illness
   1. Health is usually viewed as an absence of disease or illness.
   2. Members have a tendency to be stoical when expressing physical concerns.
   3. Members primarily rely on modern Western health care delivery system.

E. Health risks
   1. Cancer
   2. Heart disease
   3. Diabetes mellitus
   4. Injury

F. Interventions
   1. Monitor and assess client's body language.
   2. Respect client's personal space.

IV. HISPANIC AMERICANS

A. Communication
   1. Languages include Spanish and Portuguese.
   2. Members tend to be verbally expressive, yet confidentiality is important.
   3. Avoiding eye contact with a person in authority indicates respect and attentiveness.
   4. Direct confrontation is disrespectful, and the expression of negative feelings is impolite.
   5. Dramatic body language, such as gestures or facial expressions, is used to express emotion or pain.

B. Time orientation and personal space preferences
   1. Members are oriented more to present.
   2. Members may be late for an appointment because relationships and events are valued more than being on time.
   3. Members are comfortable with close proximity with family, friends, and acquaintances.
   4. Members are very tactile and use embraces and handshakes.
   5. Members value the physical presence of others.
   6. Politeness and modesty are essential.

C. Social roles
   1. The nuclear family is the basic unit; also, large extended family networks are common.
   2. The extended family is highly regarded.
   3. Needs of the family take precedence over individual family members' needs.
   4. Depending on age and **acculturation** factors, men are the decision makers and breadwinners and women are the caretakers and homemakers.
   5. Religions include Catholicism, evangelicalism, Jehovah's Witness, and Mormons.
   6. Members have strong church affiliations.
   7. Social organizations are strong within the community.

D. Health and illness
   1. Health may be a reward from God or a result of good luck.
   2. Health results from a state of balance between "hot and cold" forces and "wet and dry" forces.
   3. Illness may be viewed as a result of God's punishment for sins.
   4. Members may adhere to folk medicine traditions.

E. Health risks
   1. Lactose intolerance
   2. Diabetes mellitus
   3. Parasites

4. Hypertension
5. Heart disease
F. Interventions
   1. Allow time for the client to discuss treatment options with family members.
   2. Protect privacy.
   3. Offer to call clergy because of the significance of religious practices related to illnesses.
   4. Ask if it would be all right to touch a child before examining him or her.
   5. Be flexible regarding time of arrival for appointments, and avoid rigidity in scheduling care.
   6. Alternative modes of healing include herbs, consultation with lay healers, restoration of balance with hot or cold foods, prayer, and religious medals.

V. NATIVE AMERICANS

A. Communication
   1. Languages include English, Navajo, and other tribal languages.
   2. Silence indicates respect for the speaker.
   3. Members speak in a low tone of voice and expect others to be attentive.
   4. Eye contact is viewed as a sign of disrespect.
   5. Body language is important.
B. Time orientation and personal space preferences
   1. Oriented more to present.
   2. Personal space is important.
   3. Members will lightly touch another person's hand during greetings.
   4. Massage is used for the newborn infant to promote bonding between infant and mother.
   5. Some tribes may prohibit touching of a dead body.
C. Social roles
   1. Members are family oriented.
   2. Basic family unit is the extended family, which often includes persons from several households.
   3. In some tribes, grandparents are viewed as family leaders.
   4. Elders are honored.
   5. Children are taught to respect traditions.
   6. The father does all the work outside the home, and the mother assumes responsibility for domestic duties.
   7. Sacred myths and legends provide spiritual guidance.
   8. Religion and healing practices are integrated.
   9. Community social organizations are important.
D. Health and illness
   1. Health is a state of harmony between the person, the family, and the environment.
   2. Illness is caused by supernatural forces and disequilibrium between person and environment.
   3. Traditional health and illness beliefs may continue to be observed, including natural and religious folk medicine tradition.

E. Health risks
   1. Alcohol abuse
   2. Injury
   3. Heart disease
   4. Diabetes mellitus
   5. Tuberculosis
   6. Arthritis
   7. Lactose intolerance
   8. Gallbladder disease
   9. American Eskimos susceptible to glaucoma
F. Interventions
   1. Clarify communication.
   2. Understand that the client may be attentive even when eye contact is absent.
   3. Be attentive to own use of body language.
   4. Obtain input from members of extended family.
   5. Encourage client to personalize space in which health care is delivered; for example, encourage client to bring personal items or objects to the hospital.
   6. In the home, assess for the availability of running water, and modify infection control and hygiene practices as necessary.
   7. Alternative modes of healing include herbs, restoration of balance between the person and the universe, and consultation with traditional healers.

VI. END-OF-LIFE ISSUES (BOX 6-3)

A. Christian Science religion is unlikely to use medical means to prolong life.
B. Jewish faith generally opposes prolonging life after irreversible brain damage.
C. Eastern Orthodox religions, Muslims, Jehovah's Witnesses, and Orthodox Jews may prohibit, oppose, or discourage autopsy.
D. Jehovah's Witnesses and Muslims prohibit organ donation.
E. Buddhists in America encourage organ donation and consider it an act of mercy.
F. The Mormon, Eastern Orthodox, Islamic, and Jewish faiths discourage, oppose, or prohibit cremation.
G. Hindus prefer cremation, and cast the ashes in a holy river.
H. Hispanic and Latino groups
   1. The family generally makes decisions and may request to withhold the diagnosis or prognosis from the client.
   2. Extended family members often are involved in end-of-life care (pregnant women may be prohibited from caring for the dying or attending funerals).
   3. Several family members may be at the dying client's bedside.
   4. Vocal expression of grief and mourning is acceptable and expected.
   5. Members refuse procedures that alter the body such as organ donation or autopsy.
   6. Members prefer to die at home.

BOX 6-3

Religion and End-of-Life Care

CHRISTIANITY

Catholic and Orthodox religions
A priest anoints the sick.
Other sacraments before death include reconciliation and holy communion.

PROTESTANT
No last rites (anointing of the sick is accepted by some groups).
Prayers are given to offer comfort and support.

CHURCH OF JESUS CHRIST OF LATTER-DAY SAINTS (MORMONS)
May administer a sacrament if the client requests.

JEHOVAH WITNESS
Do not believe in sacraments.
Will be excommunicated if they receive a blood transfusion.

ISLAM
Second-degree male relatives such as cousins or uncles should be the contact person and determine whether the client and/or family should be given information about the client.
Client may choose to face Mecca (west or southwest in the United States).
The head should be elevated above the body.
Discussions about death usually are not welcomed.
Stopping medical treatment is against Allah's (Arabic word for God) will.

Grief may be expressed through slapping or hitting the body.
If possible, only a same-sex Muslim should handle the body after death; if not possible, non-Muslims should wear gloves so as not to touch the body.

JUDAISM
Prolongation of life is important (a client on life support must remain so until death).
A dying person should not be left alone (a rabbi's presence is desired).
Autopsy and cremation are forbidden.

HINDUISM
Rituals include tying a thread around the neck or wrist of the dying person, sprinkling the person with special water, or placing a leaf of basil on their tongue.
After death, the sacred threads are not removed and the body is not washed.

BUDDHISM
A shrine to Buddha may be placed in the client's room.
Time for meditation at the shrine is important and should be respected.
Clients may refuse medications that may alter their awareness (such as opioids).
After death, a monk may recite prayers for 1 hour (need not be done in the presence of the body).

I. African Americans
   1. Members discuss issues with the spouse or older family member (elders are held in high respect).
   2. Family is highly valued and is central to the care of the terminally ill.
   3. Open displays of emotion are common and accepted.
   4. Organ and blood donation usually are not allowed.
   5. Members prefer to die at home.
J. Chinese Americans
   1. Family members may make decisions about care and often do not tell the client the diagnosis or prognosis.
   2. Dying at home may be considered bad luck.
K. Native Americans
   1. Family meetings may be held to make decisions about end-of-life and the type of treatments that should be pursued.
   2. Some tribes avoid contact with the dying (may prefer to die in the hospital).

VII. COMPLEMENTARY AND ALTERNATIVE THERAPIES
A. Description
   1. Therapies are used in addition to conventional treatment to provide healing resources and focus on the mind-body connection.

   2. Included are high-risk therapies (some that are invasive) and low-risk therapies (those that are noninvasive).
   3. The National Center for Complementary and Alternative Medicine proposed a classification system that includes five categories of complementary and alternative types of therapy (Box 6-4).
B. Alternative medical systems
   1. Environmental medicine: Focuses on preventing the harmful effects of environmental toxins, and interventions include teaching, therapeutic diets, detoxification, immunotherapy, counseling, and use of environmentally safe products.
   2. Traditional Chinese medicine: Focuses on restoring and maintaining a balanced flow of vital energy, and interventions include acupressure, acupuncture, herbal therapies, diet, meditation, tai chi

BOX 6-4

Categories of Complementary and Alternative Therapies

Alternative medical systems
Mind-body interventions
Biological-based therapies
Manipulative and body-based interventions
Energy therapies

and qigong (exercise that focuses on breathing, visualization, and movement).

3. Ayurveda: Focuses on the balance of mind, body, and spirit, and interventions include diet, medicinal herbs, detoxification, breathing exercises, meditation, and yoga.

4. Homeopathy: Focuses on healing and interventions consist of small doses of specially prepared plant and mineral extracts that assist in the innate healing process of the body.

5. Naturopathy: Focuses on enhancing the natural healing responses of the body, and interventions include nutrition, herbology, hydrotherapy, homeopathy, acupuncture, physical therapies, and counseling and psychotherapy.

C. Mind-body interventions
1. Mind-body interventions focus on controlling physical functions through positive mental processes.
2. Interventions include biofeedback, hypnosis, relaxation therapy, meditation, music or art therapy, qigong, prayer and mental healing.

D. Biological-based therapies (Box 6-5)
1. Therapies includes natural and biological-derived products, interventions, and practices.
2. Interventions include aromatherapy, herbal therapies, macrobiotic diet, and orthomolecular therapy.

E. Manipulative and body-based interventions
1. Interventions involve manipulation and movement of the body by a therapist.
2. Interventions include acupressure, movement reeducation techniques, chiropractic therapy, and therapeutic massage.

BOX 6-5

Biological-Based Therapies

AROMATHERAPY
The use of topical or inhaled oils (plant extracts) that will promote and maintain health

HERBAL THERAPIES
The use of herbs derived from mostly plant sources that will maintain and restore balance and health

MACROBIOTIC DIET
Diet high in whole grain cereals, vegetables, beans and sea vegetables and vegetarian soups
Elimination of meat, animal fat, eggs, poultry, dairy products, sugars, and artificially produced food from the diet

ORTHOMOLECULAR THERAPY
Focus on nutritional balance, including the use of vitamins, essential amino acids, essential fats, and minerals

---

F. Energy therapies
1. Energy therapies focus on energy originating within the body or on energy from other sources.
2. Interventions include therapeutic touch and magnetic therapy.

VIII. HERBAL THERAPIES (BOX 6-6)
A. Herbal therapy is the use of herbs (plant or a plant part) for its therapeutic value on health.
B. Some herbs have been determined to be safe, yet some herbs, even in small amounts, can be toxic.

BOX 6-6

Commonly Used Herbs

Aloe: Antiinflammatory and antimicrobial effect; accelerates wound healing

Angelica: Antispasmodic and vasodilator; balances the effects of estrogen

Bilberry: Improves microcirculation in the eyes

Black cohosh: Produces estrogen-like effects

Cat's claw: Antioxidant; stimulates the immune system, lowers the blood pressure

Chamomile: Antispasmodic and antiinflammatory; produces a mild sedative effect

Dehydroepiandrosterone (DHEA): Converts to androgens and estrogen; slows the effects of aging and is used for erectile dysfunction

Echinacea: Stimulates the immune system

Evening primrose: Assists with the metabolism of fatty acid

Feverfew: Antiinflammatory; used for migraine headaches, arthritis, and fever

Garlic: Antioxidant; used to lower cholesterol levels

Ginger: Antiemetic; used for nausea and vomiting

Ginkgo biloba: Antioxidant; used to improve memory

Ginseng: Increases physical endurance and stamina; used for stress and fatigue

Glucosamine: An amino acid that assists in the synthesis of cartilage

Goldenseal: Antiinflammatory and antimicrobial that is used to stimulate the immune system; has an anticoagulant effect and may increase blood pressure

Kava: Antianxiety and skeletal muscle relaxant; produces a sedative effect

Melatonin: A hormone that regulates sleep; used for insomnia

Milk thistle: Antioxidant; stimulates the production of new liver cells, reduces liver inflammation, and is used for liver and gallbladder disease

St. John's wort: Antibacterial, antiviral, and antidepressant

Saw palmetto: Antiestrogen activity; used for urinary tract infections and benign prostatic hypertrophy

Valerian: Used to treat nervous disorders such as anxiety, restlessness, and insomnia

Zinc: Antiviral and stimulates the immune system

C. If the client is taking prescription medications, the client should consult with the health care provider regarding the use of herbs because serious herb-medication interactions can occur.

D. Client teaching points
1. Discuss herbal therapies with health care provider before use.
2. Contact the physician if any side effects of the herbal substance occur.
3. Contact the health care provider before stopping the use of a prescription medication.
4. Avoid using herbs to treat a serious medical condition such as heart disease.
5. Avoid taking herbs if pregnant or attempting to get pregnant or if nursing.
6. Do not give herbs to infants or young children.
7. Purchase herbal supplements only from a reputable manufacturer; the label should contain the scientific name of the herb, name and address of the manufacturer, batch or lot number, date of manufacture, and expiration date.
8. Adhere to the recommended dose; if herbal preparations are taken in high doses, they can be toxic.
9. Moisture, sunlight, and heat may alter the components of herbal preparations.
10. If surgery is planned, the herbal therapy may need to be discontinued 2 to 3 weeks before surgery.

IX. LOW-RISK THERAPIES

A. Low-risk therapies are those that have no adverse effects, and when implementing care can be used by the nurse.

B. Common low-risk therapies
1. Meditation
2. Relaxation techniques
3. Imagery
4. Music therapy
5. Massage
6. Touch
7. Laughter and humor
8. Spiritual measures such as prayer

X. NURSING CONSIDERATIONS

A. Principle: If health care recommendations, interventions, or treatments do not fit within the client's cultural **values**, they will not be followed.

B. Assessment skills: Be alert to cues regarding eye contact, personal space, time concepts, and understanding of the recommended plan of care.

C. Knowledge: Learn about the **cultures** of clients with whom you will be working; additionally, learn from your clients about their health care practices.

D. Flexibility: Allow for variation in accomplishing goals of health care; negotiate with the client until establishing a mutually agreeable plan.

E. Communication principles
1. Treat each client and those accompanying the client with respect.

2. Appreciate the differences/diversity of beliefs about health, illness, and treatment modalities.
3. Ask the client who has been consulted about the illness/condition and what treatments were recommended by the consultant.
4. Clarify perceptions of what the client has said or done and the perception about the client's expectations of the health care provider.
5. If language barriers pose a problem, seek an interpreter; avoid using family members as interpreters except as a last resort.

PRACTICE QUESTIONS

1. A nurse in an ambulatory care clinic is performing an admission assessment for an African American client scheduled for a cataract removal with an intraocular lens implant. Which of the following questions would be inappropriate for the nurse to ask on an initial assessment?
   1. "Do you have any difficulty breathing?"
   2. "Do you have a close family relationship?"
   3. "Do you ever experience chest pain?"
   4. "Do you frequently have episodes of headache?"

2. A nurse is providing discharge instructions to a Chinese client regarding prescribed dietary modifications. During the teaching session, the client continuously turns away from the nurse. Which nursing action is most appropriate?
   1. Continue with the instructions, verifying client understanding.
   2. Tell the client about the importance of the instructions for the maintenance of health care.
   3. Walk around the client so that the nurse continuously faces the client.
   4. Give the client a dietary booklet and return later to continue with the instructions.

3. A nurse is preparing a plan of care for a client whose religion is Jehovah's Witness. The client has been told that surgery is necessary. The nurse considers the client's religious preferences in developing the plan of care and documents that
   1. Surgery is prohibited in this religious group.
   2. The administration of blood and blood products is forbidden.
   3. Medication administration is not allowed.
   4. Faith healing is practiced primarily.

4. A nurse is preparing to deliver a food tray to a client whose religion is Jewish. The nurse checks the food on the tray and notes that the client has received a roast beef dinner with whole milk as a beverage. Which action will the nurse take?
   1. Deliver the food tray to the client.
   2. Call the dietary department and ask for a new meal tray.
   3. Replace the whole milk with fat-free milk.

4. Ask the dietary department to replace the roast beef with pork.

5. An ambulatory care nurse is discussing preoperative procedures with a Chinese American client who is scheduled for surgery the following week. During the discussion, the client continually smiles and nods the head. The nurse interprets this nonverbal behavior as
   1. The client understands the preoperative procedures.
   2. The client is agreeable to the required procedures.
   3. Reflecting a cultural value.
   4. An acceptance of the treatment.

6. A nurse educator is describing the yin and yang theory of the ancient Chinese philosophy of Tao to a group of nursing students. The nurse educator explains that foods are classified as hot and cold in this theory and are transformed into yin and yang energy when metabolized by the body. The nurse educator informs the students that a client who practices this belief
   1. Consumes cold foods when a "hot" illness is present.
   2. Consumes hot foods when a "hot" illness is present.
   3. Believes that yin foods are hot.
   4. Believes that yang foods are cold.

7. A client is diagnosed with cancer and is told that surgery followed by chemotherapy will be necessary. The client states to the nurse, "I have read a lot about complementary therapies. Do you think that I should try it?" The nurse responds by making which most appropriate statement?
   1. "No, because it will interact with the chemotherapy."
   2. "You need to ask your physician about it."
   3. "I would try anything that I could if I had cancer."
   4. "There are many different forms of complementary therapies. Let's talk about these therapies."

8. A nursing student is discussing cultural diversity issues in a clinical conference. The nursing instructor asks the student to describe ethnocentrism. Which of the following, if stated by the student, would indicate a lack of understanding of the issue of ethnocentrism?
   1. "It is a tendency to view one's own ways as best."
   2. "It is acting in a manner that is superior to other cultures."
   3. "It is believing that one's own ways are the only acceptable way."
   4. "It is imposing one's beliefs on individuals from another culture."

9. A home health nurse is visiting a client who does not speak English. The nurse attempts to obtain a translator to assist in communication but is unsuccessful in doing so. The nurse avoids which communication technique during the visit with the client?
   1. Communicating by writing medical terms
   2. Using simple words and avoiding medical terms
   3. Using simple words with simple actions while verbalizing them
   4. Discussing one topic at a time

10. A nurse is preparing to assist a Jewish client with eating lunch. A kosher meal is delivered to the client. Which nursing action is most appropriate in assisting the client with the meal?
    1. Carefully placing the food from the paper plates to glass plates
    2. Unwrapping the eating utensils for the client
    3. Replacing the plastic utensils with metal eating utensils
    4. Asking the client to unwrap the eating utensils and allowing the client to prepare the meal for eating

11. A nurse is planning the menu for a Chinese client with the hospital dietitian. In collaboration with the dietitian, the meal plan is designed to include which of the following foods that are generally included in the diet of this cultural group?
    1. Vegetables
    2. Milk
    3. A dessert high in sugar content
    4. Large portions of meat at every meal

12. A nurse is instructing a Native American client of the Navajo culture regarding the procedure for collecting a urine sample. The nurse observes that the client continuously stares at the floor during the instructional session. The nurse interprets this behavior as
    1. Rude.
    2. Lack of interest.
    3. Embarrassment.
    4. Indicative that the client is paying close attention.

13. An antihypertensive medication has been prescribed for a client with hypertension. The client tells the clinic nurse that she would like to take an herbal substance to help lower her blood pressure. The nurse most appropriately
    1. Tells the client that if she takes the herbal substance that she will need to have her blood pressure checked frequently.
    2. Advises the client to discuss the use of an herbal substance with the physician.
    3. Teaches the client how to take her blood pressure so that it can be monitored closely.
    4. Tells the client that herbal substances are not safe and should never be used.

14. A nurse educator is providing in-service education to the nursing staff regarding transcultural nursing care. A staff member asks the nurse educator to describe the concept of acculturation. The most appropriate response is which of the following?
    1. "It is a subjective perspective of the person's heritage and a sense of belonging to a group."
    2. "It is a group of individuals in a society that is culturally distinct and has a unique identity."
    3. "It is a group that shares some of the characteristics of the larger population group of which it is a part."

4. "It is a process of learning a different culture to adapt to a new or changing environment."

15. A nurse consults with a nutritionist regarding the dietary preferences of a European American client. Which of the following foods most likely would be requested by the client to be included in the diet?
   1. Red meat
   2. Rice
   3. Fried foods
   4. Raw fish

CRITICAL THINKING: FILL IN THE BLANK

A nurse is planning to instruct an African American client about nutrition to promote health and prevent disease. When developing the plan, the nurse is aware that a common dietary practice of African Americans is to eat what types of food that place them at risk for disease?

Answer: _____

ANSWERS

1. 2
Rationale: In the African American culture, asking personal questions on the initial contact or meeting is considered intrusive. African Americans are highly verbal and express feelings openly to family or friends, but what transpires within the family is viewed as private. Respiratory, cardiovascular, and neurological assessments include physiological assessments that are the priority assessments.
Test-Taking Strategy: Use Maslow's hierarchy of needs theory to answer the question. Note the key words "inappropriate" and "initial." Options 1, 3, and 4 address physiological needs. Option 2 addresses the psychosocial need. Review characteristics of the African American culture if you had difficulty with this question.
Level of Cognitive Ability: Application
Client Needs: Psychosocial Integrity
Integrated Process: Nursing Process—assessment
Content Area: Fundamental skills
Reference: Potter, P., & Perry, A. (2001). *Fundamentals of nursing* (5th ed., pp. 125, 146, 727). St. Louis: Mosby.

2. 1
Rationale: Most Chinese maintain a formal distance with others, which is a form of respect. Many Chinese are uncomfortable with face-to-face communications, especially when eye contact is direct. If the client turns away from the nurse during a conversation, the most appropriate action is to continue with the conversation. Walking around to the client so that the nurse faces the client is in direct conflict with the cultural practice. Telling the client about the importance of the instructions for the maintenance of health care may be viewed as degrading. The client may view returning later to continue with the explanation as a rude gesture.
Test-Taking Strategy: Use the process of elimination. Eliminate options 2 and 4 first because these actions are nontherapeutic. From the remaining options, option 1 is the most therapeutic. If you had difficulty with this question, review the communication practices of this cultural group.
Level of Cognitive Ability: Application
Client Needs: Psychosocial Integrity
Integrated Process: Nursing Process—implementation
Content Area: Fundamental skills
Reference: Potter, P., & Perry, A. (2001). *Fundamentals of nursing* (5th ed., p. 457). St. Louis: Mosby.

3. 2
Rationale: Among Jehovah's Witnesses, surgery is not prohibited, but the administration of blood and blood products is forbidden. Administration of medication is an acceptable practice except if the medication is derived from blood products. Faith healing is forbidden in this religious group.
Test-Taking Strategy: Use the process of elimination, recalling that the administration of blood and any associated blood products is forbidden. Review the characteristics of this religious group if you had difficulty with this question.
Level of Cognitive Ability: Application
Client Needs: Psychosocial Integrity
Integrated Process: Communication and Documentation
Content Area: Fundamental skills
Reference: Potter, P., & Perry, A. (2001). *Fundamentals of nursing* (5th ed., p. 437). St. Louis: Mosby.

4. 2
Rationale: In the Jewish religion the dairy-meat combination is not acceptable. Pork and pork products are not allowed in the traditional Jewish religion. The nurse would not deliver the food tray to the client and would ask the dietary department to deliver a new meal tray.
Test-Taking Strategy: Use the process of elimination, recalling that the dairy-meat combination is not acceptable in the Jewish religion. Review the dietary rules of this religious group if you had difficulty with this question.
Level of Cognitive Ability: Application
Client Needs: Psychosocial Integrity
Integrated Process: Nursing Process—implementation
Content Area: Fundamental skills
Reference: Potter, P., & Perry, A. (2001). *Fundamentals of nursing* (5th ed., p. 1347). St. Louis: Mosby.

5. 3
Rationale: Nodding or smiling by a Chinese American client may reflect only the cultural value of interpersonal harmony. This nonverbal behavior may not be an indication of agreement with the speaker, an acceptance of the treatment, or an understanding of the procedure.
Test-Taking Strategy: Use the process of elimination. Eliminate options 2 and 4 first because they are similar. From the remaining options, select option 3 because it is the most global option. In addition, option 1 is an incorrect interpretation of the client's nonverbal behavior. Review the cultural

characteristics of the Chinese American population if you had difficulty with this question.

Level of Cognitive Ability: Comprehension
Client Needs: Psychosocial Integrity
Integrated Process: Nursing Process—assessment
Content Area: Fundamental skills
Reference: Jarvis, C. (2000). *Physical examination & health assessment* (3rd ed., pp. 52, 76). Philadelphia: W. B. Saunders.

6. 1

Rationale: In the yin and yang theory, health is believed to exist when all aspects of the person are in perfect balance. Foods are classified as hot or cold in this theory and are transformed into yin and yang energy when metabolized by the body. Yin foods are cold, and yang foods are hot. Cold foods are eaten when one has a hot illness, and hot foods are eaten when one has a cold illness.

Test-Taking Strategy: Use the process of elimination and knowledge regarding the theory of yin and yang. If you are unfamiliar with this theory, review its elements.

Level of Cognitive Ability: Application
Client Needs: Psychosocial Integrity
Integrated Process: Teaching/Learning
Content Area: Fundamental skills
Reference: Potter, P., & Perry, A. (2001). *Fundamentals of nursing* (5th ed., p 981). St. Louis: Mosby.

7. 4

Rationale: Complementary (alternative) therapies include a wide variety of treatment modalities that are used in addition to conventional treatment to treat a disease or illness. These therapies complement conventional treatment but should be approved by the person's health care provider to ensure that the treatment does not interact with prescribed therapy. Although the physician should approve the use of a complementary therapy and although some of these therapies can interact with the prescribed treatment plan, the statements in options 1 and 2 are inappropriate. Likewise, option 3 is an inappropriate response to the client. Option 4 addresses the client's question and encourages discussion.

Test-Taking Strategy: Use therapeutic communication techniques. Eliminate options 1, 2, and 3 because they are nontherapeutic. Options 4 is the only option that addresses the client's question and encourages discussion. Review therapeutic communication techniques if you had difficulty with this question.

Level of Cognitive Ability: Application
Client Needs: Physiological Integrity
Integrated Process: Communication and Documentation
Content Area: Fundamental skills
References: Lewis, S., Heitkemper, M., & Dirksen, S. (2004). *Medical-surgical nursing: Assessment and management of clinical problems* (6th ed., p. 94). St. Louis: Mosby.
Potter, P., & Perry, A. (2001). *Fundamentals of nursing* (5th ed., p. 459). St. Louis: Mosby.

8. 4

Rationale: Ethnocentrism is a tendency to view one's own ways of life as the most desirable, acceptable, or best and to act in a superior manner toward another culture. Cultural imposition is the tendency to impose one's own beliefs, values, and patterns of behavior on individuals from another culture.

Test-Taking Strategy: Use the process of elimination and note the key words "indicate a lack of understanding" in the stem of the question. Also, note the similarity between options 1, 2, and 3. If you had difficulty with this question, review culturally related concepts.

Level of Cognitive Ability: Comprehension
Client Needs: Psychosocial Integrity
Integrated Process: Teaching/Learning
Content Area: Fundamental skills
Reference: Jarvis, C. (2000). *Physical examination & health assessment* (3rd ed., p. 46). Philadelphia: W. B. Saunders.

9. 1

Rationale: Communicating with the client by writing medical terms does not overcome the language barrier because the client likely will not be able to understand the written language or the medical terms. Options 2, 3, and 4 identify techniques that will assist in overcoming language barriers when an interpreter is not present.

Test-Taking Strategy: Note the key word "avoids" in the stem of the question. Use the process of elimination and attempt to visualize each of the methods identified in the options to assist in answering the question. Remember that the client may not be able to interpret medical terms or a written language that is different from his or her own. Review these communication techniques if you had difficulty with this question.

Level of Cognitive Ability: Application
Client Needs: Psychosocial Integrity
Integrated Process: Communication and Documentation
Content Area: Fundamental skills
Reference: Jarvis, C. (2000). *Physical examination & health assessment* (3rd ed., pp. 76-77). Philadelphia: W. B. Saunders.

10. 4

Rationale: Kosher meals arrive on paper plates and with plastic utensils sealed. Health care providers should not unwrap the utensils or transfer the foodstuffs to another serving dish. Although the nurse may want to be helpful in assisting the client with the meal, the only appropriate option for this client is option 4.

Test-Taking Strategy: Use the process of elimination and knowledge regarding the rituals associated with kosher meals. Options 1 and 3 are similar and can be eliminated first. To choose from the remaining options, one must be familiar with kosher rituals. If you had difficulty with this question, review the dietary practices of the Jewish culture.

Level of Cognitive Ability: Application
Client Needs: Psychosocial Integrity
Integrated Process: Nursing Process—implementation
Content Area: Fundamental skills
References: Jarvis, C. (2000). *Physical examination & health assessment* (3rd ed., p. 133). Philadelphia: W. B. Saunders.
Potter, P., & Perry, A. (2001). *Fundamentals of nursing* (5th ed., pp. 606-607). St. Louis: Mosby.

11. 1
Rationale: The Chinese diet is generally vegetarian, although meat may be served. Native Chinese generally do not drink milk or eat milk products because of a genetic tendency toward lactose intolerance. Most Chinese do not eat desserts high in sugar content, and their desserts are usually fruits.
Test-Taking Strategy: Use the process of elimination and knowledge regarding the food rituals related to the Chinese culture to answer this question. If you had difficulty with this question, review the characteristics of this culture.
Level of Cognitive Ability: Application
Client Needs: Psychosocial Integrity
Integrated Process: Nursing Process—planning
Content Area: Fundamental skills
Reference: Potter, P., & Perry, A. (2001). *Fundamentals of nursing* (5th ed., pp. 970, 1348). St. Louis: Mosby.

12. 4
Rationale: Native American clients often stare at the floor when a nurse is talking. This culturally appropriate behavior indicates that the listener is paying close attention to the speaker. In this culture, eye contact is considered a sign of disrespect. Options 1, 2, and 3 are inappropriate interpretations of the client's behavior.
Test-Taking Strategy: Use the process of elimination and knowledge regarding the culturally appropriate behaviors of Navajo clients. If you had difficulty with this question, review the characteristics of this culture.
Level of Cognitive Ability: Analysis
Client Needs: Psychosocial Integrity
Integrated Process: Nursing Process—analysis
Content Area: Fundamental skills
Reference: Jarvis, C. (2000). *Physical examination & health assessment* (3rd ed., p. 76). Philadelphia: W. B. Saunders.

13. 2
Rationale: Although herbal substances may have some beneficial effects, not all herbs are safe to use. Clients who are being treated with conventional medication therapy should be advised to avoid herbal substances with similar pharmacological effects because the combination may lead to an excessive reaction or to unknown interaction effects. Therefore the nurse would advise the client to discuss the use of the herbal substance with the physician.
Test-Taking Strategy: Use the process of elimination. Eliminate option 4 first because of the absolute word "never." Next eliminate options 1 and 3 because they are similar. Review the limitations associated with the use of herbal substances if you had difficulty with this question.
Level of Cognitive Ability: Application
Client Needs: Physiological Integrity
Integrated Process: Nursing Process—implementation
Content Area: Fundamental skills
References: Lewis, S., Heitkemper, M., & Dirksen, S. (2004). *Medical-surgical nursing: Assessment and management of clinical problems* (6th ed., p. 101). St. Louis: Mosby.
Skidmore-Roth, L. (2001). *Mosby's handbook of herbs & natural supplements* (p. 182). St. Louis: Mosby.

14. 4
Rationale: Acculturation is a process of learning a different culture to adapt to a new or changing environment. Option 1 describes ethnic identity. Option 2 describes an ethnic group. Option 3 describes a subculture.
Test-Taking Strategy: Knowledge regarding the descriptions and definitions of the foundational concepts related to culture is required to answer this question. Review these concepts if you are unfamiliar with them.
Level of Cognitive Ability: Comprehension
Client Needs: Psychosocial Integrity
Integrated Process: Teaching/Learning
Content Area: Fundamental skills
Reference: Jarvis, C. (2000). *Physical examination & health assessment* (3rd ed., p. 10). Philadelphia: W. B. Saunders.

15. 1
Rationale: European Americans prefer carbohydrates and red meat. African American food preferences include pork, greens, rice, and fried foods. Asian American food preferences include raw fish, rice, and soy sauce.
Test-Taking Strategy: Use the process of elimination and knowledge regarding the food practices and preferences related to the various cultures. Correlate carbohydrates and red meat with European Americans. This may assist in answering other questions similar to this one. If you had difficulty with this question, review the food preferences associated with the European American culture.
Level of Cognitive Ability: Comprehension
Client Needs: Psychosocial Integrity
Integrated Process: Nursing Process—planning
Content Area: Fundamental skills
References: Jarvis, C. (2000). *Physical examination & health assessment* (3rd ed.). Philadelphia: W. B. Saunders.
Williams, S. (2001). *Basic nutrition & diet therapy* (11th ed., p. 827). St. Louis: Mosby.

CRITICAL THINKING: FILL IN THE BLANK
Answer: Fried foods
Rationale: African American food preferences include primarily pork, greens, rice, and fried foods. Fried foods usually are prepared in lard. Consumption of foods from the fruit group is minimal. Eating foods that are fried places the African American client at risk for heart disease.
Test-Taking Strategy: Recalling that African Americans are at risk for hypertension and coronary artery disease will assist in identifying the types of food that these clients tend to eat. If you had difficulty with this question, review the food preferences associated with the African American culture.
Level of Cognitive Ability: Comprehension
Client Needs: Psychosocial Integrity
Integrated Process: Nursing Process—planning
Content Area: Fundamental skills
Reference: Williams, S. (2001). *Basic nutrition & diet therapy* (11th ed., p. 827). St Louis: Mosby.

REFERENCES

Jarvis, C. (2000). *Physical examination & health assessment* (3rd ed.). Philadelphia: W. B. Saunders.

Lewis, S., Heitkemper, M., & Dirksen, S. (2004). *Medical-surgical nursing: Assessment and management of clinical problems* (6th ed.). St. Louis: Mosby.

National Council of State Boards of Nursing (Eds.). (2003). *Test Plan for the National Council Licensure Examination for Registered Nurses* (effective date: April 2004). Chicago: Author.

Potter, P., & Perry, A. (2001). *Fundamentals of nursing* (5th ed.). St. Louis: Mosby.

Skidmore-Roth, L. (2001). *Mosby's handbook of herbs & natural supplements*. St. Louis: Mosby.

Williams, S. (2001). *Basic nutrition & diet therapy* (11th ed.) St Louis: Mosby.

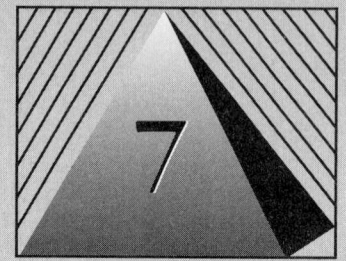

Ethical and Legal Issues

PYRAMID TERMS

advance directive Written document recognized by state law that provides directions concerning the provision of care when a person is unable to make his or her own treatment choices.

advocacy Acting on the behalf of the client and protecting the client's rights to make his or her own decisions.

consent Voluntary act by which a person agrees to allow someone else to do something.

ethics The distinction between right and wrong based on a body of knowledge, not just based on opinions.

informed consent A client's understanding of the reason for the proposed intervention, with its benefits and risks, and agreement with the treatment by signing a consent form.

law A system composed of general rules governing conduct and the procedures for resolving disputes when rules are not followed.

malpractice Failure to meet the standards of acceptable care, which results in harm to another person.

negligence Failure to provide care that a reasonable person ordinarily would use in a similar circumstance.

patient's bill of rights The rights and responsibilities of clients receiving care.

values Beliefs and attitudes that may influence behavior and the process of decision making.

▲ THE PYRAMID TO SUCCESS

Across all settings in the practice of nursing, nurses frequently are confronted with ethical and legal issues related to client care. The professional nurse has the responsibility to be aware of the ethical principles, laws, and guidelines related to providing safe and quality care to clients. In the Pyramid to Success, focus on ethical practices; the nurse practice act and client rights, particularly confidentiality and informed consent; advocacy, documentation, advance directives, and cultural, religious, and spiritual issues. The Integrated Processes addressed in this chapter are Caring, Communication and Documentation, Nursing Process, and Teaching/Learning.

CLIENT NEEDS
Safe, Effective Care Environment

Acting as an advocate
Advance directives
Client rights
Confidentiality
Continuous quality improvement
Establishing priorities
Ethical practice
Incident reports
Informed consent
Legal responsibilities
Resource management

Health Promotion and Maintenance

Developmental stages and transitions
Family systems
Lifestyle choices

Psychosocial Integrity

Abuse/neglect
Chemical dependency
Coping mechanisms
Cultural, spiritual, and religious issues
End of life
Grief and loss
Support systems

Physiological Integrity

Alterations in body systems
Palliative/comfort care
Unexpected responses to therapies

I. ETHICS

A. Description: The branch of philosophy that concerns the distinction between right and wrong based on a body of knowledge, not just based on opinions

B. Morality: Behavior in accordance with customs or tradition, usually reflecting personal or religious beliefs

C. Ethical principles: Codes that direct or govern nursing actions (Box 7-1)

D. **Values:** Beliefs and attitudes that may influence behavior and the process of decision making

E. **Values** clarification: Process of analyzing one's own values to understand better what is truly important

F. Ethical codes
   1. Ethical codes provide broad principles for determining and evaluating client care.
   2. These codes are not legally binding, but in most states, the board of nursing has authority to reprimand nurses for unprofessional conduct that results from violation of the ethical codes.
   3. Specific ethical codes follow:
      a. The Code for Nurses developed by the International Council of Nurses
      b. American Nurses Association Code of Ethics

G. Ethical dilemma
   1. An ethical dilemma occurs when there is a conflict between two or more ethical principles.
   2. No correct decision exists.
   3. The nurse must make a choice between two alternatives that are equally unsatisfactory.
   4. Such dilemmas may occur as a result of differences in cultural or religious beliefs.
   5. Ethical reasoning is the process of thinking through what one ought to do in an orderly and systematic manner to provide justification for actions based on principles.

H. Advocate
   1. An advocate is a person who speaks up for or acts on the behalf of the client, protects the client's right to make his or her own decisions, and upholds the principle of fidelity.
   2. An advocate represents the client's viewpoint to others.
   3. An advocate avoids letting personal **values** influence **advocacy** for the client.
   4. An advocate supports the client's decision even when it conflicts with his or her own preferences or choices.

I. **Ethics** committees
   1. **Ethics** committees take a multidisciplinary approach to facilitate dialogue regarding ethical dilemmas.
   2. These committees develop and establish policies and procedures for the prevention and resolution of dilemmas.

II. REGULATION OF NURSING PRACTICE

A. Nurse practice act
   1. A series of statutes have been enacted by each state legislature to regulate the practice of nursing in that state.
   2. Nurse practice acts set educational requirements for the nurse, distinguish between nursing practice and medical practice, and define the scope of nursing practice.
   3. Additional issues covered by nurse practice acts include licensure requirements for protection of the public, grounds for disciplinary action, rights of the nurse licensee if a disciplinary action is taken, and related topics.
   4. All nurses are responsible for knowing the provisions of the act for the state or province in which they work.

B. Standards of care
   1. Standards of care are guidelines by which the nurse should practice.
   2. The guidelines determine whether nurses have performed duties in an appropriate manner.
   3. If a nurse does not perform duties within accepted standards of care, the nurse places himself or herself in jeopardy of legal action.
   4. If a nurse is named as a defendant in a **malpractice** lawsuit and proceedings show that the nurse followed neither the accepted standards of care outlined by the state or province nursing practice act nor the policies of the employing institution, the nurses' legal liability is clear.

C. Employee guidelines
   1. Respondent superior: Employer will be held liable for any negligent acts of an employee if the alleged negligent act occurred during the employment

BOX 7-1

Ethical Principles

Autonomy	Respect for an individual's right to self-determination
Nonmaleficence	The obligation to do or cause no harm to another
Beneficence	The duty to do good to others and to maintain a balance between benefits and harms; paternalism is an undesirable outcome of beneficence, in which the health care provider decides what is best for the client and attempts to encourage the client to act against his or her own choices
Justice	The equitable distribution of potential benefits and tasks; determining the order in which client's should be cared for
Veracity	The obligation to tell the truth
Fidelity	The duty to do what one has promised

relationship and was within the scope of the employee's responsibilities.

2. Contracts
   a. Nurses are responsible for carrying out the terms of a contractual agreement with the employing agency and the client.
   b. The nurse employee relationship is governed by established employee handbooks and client care policies and procedures that create obligations, rights, and duties between those parties.

3. Institutional policies
   a. Written policies and procedures of the employing institution detail how nurses are to perform their duties.
   b. Policies and procedures are usually specific and are located in manuals in most health care facilities.
   c. Although policies are not laws, courts generally rule against nurses who violate policies.
   d. If the nurse practices nursing according to client care policies and procedures established by the employer, functions within the job responsibility, and provides care consistently in a nonnegligent manner, the nurse minimizes the potential for liability.

D. Hospital staffing
   1. Nurses should not walk out when staffing is inadequate because charges of abandonment can be made.
   2. Nurses in short staffing situations are obligated to make a report to the nursing administration.

E. Floating
   1. Floating is an acceptable, legal practice used by hospitals to solve their understaffing problems.
   2. Legally, a nurse cannot refuse to float unless a union contract guarantees that nurses can work only in a specified area or the nurse can prove lack of knowledge for the performance of assigned tasks.
   3. Nurses in a floating situation must not assume responsibility beyond their level of experience or qualification.
   4. Nurses who float should inform the supervisor of any lack of experience in caring for the type of clients on the new nursing unit.
   5. The nurse should request and be given orientation to the new unit.

F. Disciplinary action
   1. Boards of nursing may deny, revoke, or suspend any license to practice as a registered nurse, according to their statutory authority.
   2. Causes for disciplinary action are as follows:
      a. Unprofessional conduct
      b. Conduct that could affect the health and welfare of the public adversely
      c. Breach of client confidentiality
      d. Failure to use sufficient knowledge, skills, or nursing judgment

   e. Physically or verbally abusing a client
   f. Assuming duties without sufficient preparation
   g. Knowingly delegating to unlicensed personnel nursing care that places the client as risk for injury
   h. Failure to maintain an accurate record for each client
   i. Falsifying a client's record
   j. Leaving a nursing assignment without properly notifying appropriate personnel

III. LEGAL LIABILITY

A. Laws
   1. Nurses are governed by civil and criminal **law** in roles as providers of services, employees of institutions, and private citizens.
   2. A nurse has a personal and legal obligation to provide a standard of client care expected of a reasonably competent professional nurse.
   3. Professional nurses are held responsible (liable) for harm resulting from their negligent acts or their failure to act.

B. Types of laws (Box 7-2)

C. **Negligence** and **malpractice**
   1. **Negligence** is conduct that falls below the standard of care.
   2. **Negligence** can include acts of commission and acts of omission.
   3. If a nurse gives care that does not meet appropriate standards, the nurse may be held liable for **negligence**.

BOX 7-2

Types of Laws

CONTRACT LAW
Contract law is concerned with enforcement of agreements among private individuals.

CIVIL LAW
Civil law is concerned with relationships among persons and the protection of a person's rights.
Violation may cause harm to an individual or property, but no grave threat to society exists.

CRIMINAL LAW
Criminal law is concerned with relationships between individuals and governments and with acts that threaten society and its order; a crime is an offense against society that violates a law and is defined as a misdemeanor (less serious nature) or felony (serious nature).

TORT LAW
A tort is a civil wrong, other than a breach in contract, in which the law allows an injured person to seek damages from a person who caused the injury.

4. **Malpractice** is **negligence** on the part of a nurse.

5. **Malpractice** is determined if the nurse owed a duty to the client and did not carry out the duty, and the client was injured because the nurse failed to perform the duty.

6. Proof of liability
   a. Duty: At the time of injury, a duty existed between the plaintiff and the defendant.
   b. Breach of duty: The defendant breached duty of care to the plaintiff.
   c. Proximate cause: The breach of the duty was the legal cause of injury to the client.
   d. Damage or injury: The plaintiff experienced injury or damages or both and can be compensated by **law**.

D. Professional liability insurance
   1. Nurses need their own liability insurance for protection against **malpractice** lawsuits.
   2. Having their own insurance provides nurses protection as individuals and allows nurses to have an attorney present who has only the nurses' interests in mind.

E. Good Samaritan laws
   1. State legislatures pass Good Samaritan laws, which may vary from state to state.
   2. These laws encourage health care professionals to assist in emergency situations without fear of being sued for the care provided.
   3. These laws limit liability and offer legal immunity for persons helping in an emergency, providing they give reasonable care.
   4. Immunity from suit applies only when all conditions of the state **law** are met, such as the health care provider receives no compensation for the care provided and the care given is not intentionally negligent.

F. Controlled substances
   1. The nurse should adhere to facility policies and procedures concerning administration of controlled substances, which are governed by federal and state laws.
   2. Controlled substances must be kept locked securely, and only authorized personnel should have access to them.

IV. COLLECTIVE BARGAINING

A. Collective bargaining is a formalized decision-making process between representatives of management and representatives of labor to negotiate wages and conditions of employment.

B. When collective bargaining breaks down because the parties cannot reach an agreement, the employees usually call a strike.

C. Striking presents a moral dilemma to many nurses because nursing practice is a service to people.

V. LEGAL RISK AREAS

A. Assault
   1. Assault occurs when a person puts another person in fear of a harmful or offensive contact.
   2. The victim fears and believes that harm will result as a result of the threat.

B. Battery is an intentional touching of another's body without the other's **consent**.

C. Invasion of privacy includes violating confidentiality, intruding on private client or family matters, and sharing client information with unauthorized persons.

D. False imprisonment
   1. False imprisonment occurs when a client is not allowed to leave a health care facility when there is no legal justification to detain the client.
   2. False imprisonment occurs when restraining devices are used without an appropriate clinical need.
   3. A client can sign an Against Medical Advice form when the client refuses care and is competent to make decisions.
   4. The nurse should document circumstances in the medical record to avoid allegations by the client that cannot be defended.

E. Defamation is a false communication or a careless disregard for the truth that causes damage to someone's reputation, either in writing (libel) or verbally (slander).

F. Fraud results from a deliberate deception intended to produce unlawful gains.

VI. CLIENT RIGHTS

A. Description
   1. The client rights document, also called the **patient's bill of rights**, reflects acknowledgement of clients' right to participate in their health care with an emphasis on client autonomy.
   2. The document provides a list of the rights of the client and responsibilities that the hospital cannot violate (Box 7-3).
   3. The client's rights affect the relationship between the client and health care provider and between the client and health care delivery system and protect the client's ability to determine the level and type of care received.
   4. Several laws and standards pertain to client's rights (Box 7-4).

B. Rights for the mentally ill (Box 7-5)
   1. The Mental Health Systems Act created rights for the mentally ill.
   2. The Joint Commission on Accreditation of Healthcare Organizations developed policy statements on the rights of the mentally ill.
   3. Psychiatric facilities are required to have a client's bill of rights posted in a visible area.

BOX 7-3

Patient's Rights When Hospitalized

Right to considerate and respectful care

Right to be informed about illness, possible treatments, likely outcome, and to discuss this information with the physician

Right to know the names and roles of the persons who are involved in care

Right to consent or refuse a treatment

Right to have an advance directive

Right to privacy

Right to expect that medical records are confidential

Right to review the medical record and to have information explained

Right to expect that the hospital will provide necessary health services

Right to know if the hospital has relationships with outside parties that may influence treatment or care

Right to consent or refuse to take part in research

Right to be told of realistic care alternatives when hospital care is no longer appropriate

Right to know about hospital rules that affect treatment and about charges and payment methods

From Christensen, B., & Kockrow, E. (2003). *Foundations of Nursing* (4th ed., p.13). St. Louis: Mosby.

BOX 7-5

Rights for the Mentally Ill

Right to be treated with dignity and respect

Right to communicate with persons outside the hospital

Right to keep clothing and personal effects with them

Right to religious freedom

Right to be employed

Right to manage property

Right to execute wills

Right to enter into contractural agreements

Right to make purchases

Right to education

Right to habeas corpus (written request for release from the hospital)

Right to an independent psychiatric examination

Right to civil service status, including the right to vote

Right to retain licenses, privileges, or permits

Right to sue or be sued

Right to marry or divorce

Right to treatment in the least restrictive setting

Right not to be subject to unnecessary restraints

Right to privacy and confidentiality

Right to informed consent

Right to treatment and to refuse treatment

Right to refuse participation in experimental treatments or research

Adapted from Stuart, G., & Laraia, M. (2001). *Principles and practice of psychiatric nursing* (7th ed., p. 167). St. Louis: Mosby.

C. Organ donation and transplantation
   1. Client has the right to decide to become an organ donor and a right to refuse organ transplant as a treatment option.
   2. An individual who is at least 18 years of age may indicate a wish to become a donor on his or her driver's license (state specific) or in an **advance directive.**
   3. The Uniform Anatomical Gift Act provides a list of individuals who can provide **informed consent** for the donation of a deceased individual's organs.
   4. The United Network for Organ Sharing sets the criteria for organ donations.
   5. Some organs such as the heart, lungs, and liver can be obtained only from a person who was on mechanical ventilation and has suffered brain death, whereas other organs or tissues can be removed several hours after death.
   6. Donor must be free of infectious disease and cancer.
   7. Requests to the family for organ donation from a deceased family member usually are done by the physician or nurse specially trained for making such requests.
   8. Donation of organs does not delay funeral arrangements, no obvious evidence that the organs were removed from the body shows when the body is dressed, and the family incurs no cost for removal of the organs donated.
D. Religious beliefs: organ donation and transplantation
   1. Catholic Church: Organ donation and transplants are acceptable.
   2. Orthodox Church: Church discourages organ donation.
   3. Islam (Muslim) beliefs: Body parts may not be removed or donated for transplantation.
   4. Jehovah's Witness: An organ transplant may be accepted, but the organ must be cleansed with a nonblood solution before transplantation.

BOX 7-4

Laws and Standards

AMERICAN HOSPITAL ASSOCIATION
Issued a patients' bill of rights.

AMERICAN NURSES ASSOCIATION
Developed the Code for Nurses, which defines the nurse's responsibility for upholding the client's rights.

MENTAL HEALTH SYSTEMS ACT
Developed rights for the mentally ill client.

JOINT COMMISSION ON ACCREDITATION OF HEALTHCARE ORGANIZATIONS
Developed policy statements on the rights of the mentally ill.

5. Orthodox Judaism
   a. All body parts removed during autopsy must be buried with the body because it is believed that the entire body must be returned to the earth.
   b. Organ transplantation may be allowed with the rabbi's approval.

VII. INFORMED CONSENT

A. Description
   1. **Informed consent** is the client's approval (or that of the client's legal representative) to have his or her body touched by a specific individual.
   2. Consents, or releases, are legal documents that indicate the client's permission to perform surgery, perform a treatment, or give information to a third party.
   3. Types of consents (Box 7-6)
   4. **Informed consent** indicates the client's participation in the decision regarding health care.
   5. The client must be informed, in understandable terms, of the risks and benefits of the surgery or treatment, what the consequences are for not having the surgery or procedure performed, treatment options, and the name of the health care provider performing the surgery or procedure.
   6. A client's questions about the surgery or procedure must be answered before signing the **consent**.
   7. A **consent** must be signed freely by the client without threat or pressure and must be witnessed by an another adult.
   8. A client who has been medicated with sedating medications or any other medications that can affect the client's cognitive abilities should not be asked to sign a **consent**.
   9. Legally, the client must be mentally and emotionally competent to give **consent**.
   10. If a client is declared mentally or emotionally incompetent, the next of kin, appointed guardian (appointed by the court), or the durable power of attorney has legal authority to give **consent** (Box 7-7).
   11. A competent client over 18 years of age must sign the **consent**.
   12. In most states, when a nurse is involved in the **informed consent** process, the nurse is witnessing only the signature of the client on the **informed consent** form.
   13. An **informed consent** can be waived for urgent medical or surgical intervention as long as institutional policy so indicates.
   14. A client has the right to refuse information and waive the **informed consent** and undergo treatment, but this decision must be documented in the medical record.
   15. A client may withdraw **consent** at any time.

B. Minors
   1. A minor is a client under legal age as defined by state statute (usually under 18 years).
   2. A minor may not give legal **consent**, and **consent** must be obtained from a parent or the legal guardian.
   3. Parental or guardian **consent** should be obtained before treatment is initiated for a minor except in an emergency; in situations in which the **consent** of the minor is sufficient, such as treatment related to substance abuse, treatment of a sexually transmitted disease, human immunodeficiency virus testing and acquired immunodeficiency syndrome treatment, birth control services, pregnancy, or psychiatric services; emancipated minor; or if a court order or other legal authorization has been obtained.

BOX 7-6

Types of Consents

ADMISSION AGREEMENT
Admission agreements are obtained at the time of admission and identify the health care agency's responsibility to the client.

BLOOD TRANSFUSION CONSENT
A blood transfusion consent indicates that the client was informed of the benefits and risks of the transfusion.
Some clients hold religious beliefs that would prohibit receiving a blood transfusion, even in a life-threatening situation.

SURGICAL CONSENT
Surgical consent is obtained for all surgical or invasive procedures or diagnostic tests that are invasive.
The physician, surgeon, or anesthesiologist who performs the operative or other procedure is responsible for explaining the procedure, its risks, benefits, and possible alternative options.

RESEARCH CONSENT
The research consent obtains permission from the client regarding participation in a research study.
The consent informs the client about the possible risks, consequences, and benefits of the research.

SPECIAL CONSENTS
Special consents are required for the use of restraints, photographing the client, the disposal of body parts during surgery, donating organs after death, or performing an autopsy.

BOX 7-7

Mentally or Emotionally Incompetent Clients

Declared incompetent
Unconscious
Under the influence of alcohol or drugs
Chronic dementia or other mental deficiency

C. Emancipated minor
   1. An emancipated minor has established independence from the parents through marriage, pregnancy, service in the armed forces, or by a court order.
   2. An emancipated minor is considered legally capable of signing an **informed consent**.

▲ **VIII. HEALTH INSURANCE PORTABILITY AND ACCOUNTABILITY ACT (HIPAA)**
A. Description
   1. The Health Insurance Portability and Accountability Act describes how personal health information (PHI) may be used and how the client can obtain access to the information.
   2. Personal health information includes individually identifiable information that relates to the client's past, present, or future health; treatment; and payment for health care services.
   3. The act requires health care agencies to keep PHI private, provides information to the client about the legal responsibilities regarding privacy, and explains the client's rights with respect to PHI.
   4. The client has various rights as a consumer of health care under HIPAA, and any client requests may need to be placed in writing; a fee may be attached to certain client requests.
   5. The client may file a complaint if the client feels that privacy rights have been violated.
B. Client's rights
   1. To inspect and copy PHI
   2. To ask the health care agency to amend the PHI that is contained in a record if the PHI is inaccurate
   3. To request a list of disclosures made regarding the PHI as specified by HIPAA
   4. To request to restrict the way the health care agency uses or discloses PHI regarding treatment, payment, or health care operations unless information is needed to provide emergency treatment
   5. To request that the health care agency communicates with the client in a certain way or at a certain location; the request must specify how or where the client wishes to be contacted
   6. To request a paper copy of the HIPAA notice
C. Health care agency use and disclosure of PHI
   1. The health care agency obtains PHI in the course of providing or administering health insurance benefits for the client and may use or disclose PHI in administering benefits.
   2. Use or disclosure of PHI may be done for the following:
      a. Health care payment purposes
      b. Health care operations purposes
      c. Treatment purposes
      d. To provide information about health care services
      e. Data aggregation purposes to make health care benefit decisions

---

BOX 7-8

Uses or Disclosures of Personal Health Information

Compliance with legal proceedings or for limited law enforcement purposes

To a family member or significant other in a medical emergency

To a personal representative appointed by the client or designated by law

For research purposes in limited circumstances

To a coroner, medical examiner, or funeral director about a deceased person

To an organ procurement organization in limited circumstances

To avert a serious threat to the client's health or safety or the health or safety of others

To a governmental agency authorized to oversee the health care system or government programs

To the Department of Health and Human Services for the investigation of compliance with the Health Insurance Portability and Accountability Act or to fulfill another lawful request

To federal officials for lawful intelligence or national security purposes

To protect health authorities for public health purposes

To appropriate military authorities if a client is a member of the armed forces

In accordance with a valid authorization signed by the client

Adapted from Combined Life Insurance Company of New York. (2003). *HIPAA notice of privacy practices for personal health information.* (retrieved January, 2004). http://www.keio.edu/parents/hippa.html

   f. Administering health care benefits
   3. Additional uses or disclosures of PHI (Box 7-8)

IX. CLIENT PRIVACY ▲
A. Client's right to protection against unreasonable and unwarranted interference into private affairs
B. Violations (Box 7-9)

X. CONFIDENTIALITY ▲
A. Description
   1. Clients have a right to privacy in the health care system.
   2. A special relationship exists between the client and nurse, in which information discussed will not be shared with a third party who is not involved in the client's care directly.
B. Nurse's responsibility
   1. Nurses are bound to protect client confidentiality by most nurse practice acts, by ethical principles and standards, and by institutional and agency policies and procedures.
   2. Disclosure of confidential information exposes the nurse to liability for invasion of the client's privacy.
   3. The nurse needs to protect the client from indiscriminate disclosure of health care information that may cause harm (Box 7-10).

BOX 7-9

Invasion of Privacy

Taking photographs of the client
Release of medical information to an unauthorized person, such as a member of the press, family, friend, or neighbor of the client, without the client's permission
Use of the client's name or picture for the health care agency's sole advantage
Intrusion by the health care agency regarding the client's affairs
Publication of information about the client
Publication of embarrassing facts
Public disclosure of private information
Leaving the curtains or room door open while a treatment or procedure is being performed
Allowing individuals to observe a treatment or procedure without the client's consent
Leaving a confused or agitated client sitting in the nursing unit hallway
Interviewing a client in a room with only a curtain between clients or where conversation can be overheard
Accessing medical records when unauthorized to do so

C. Medical records
 1. Medical records are confidential.
 2. Client has the right to read the medical record and have copies of the record.
 3. Only staff directly involved in care have legitimate access to a client's record and may include physicians and nurses caring for the client, technicians, therapists, social workers, unit secretaries, client advocates, administrators (for statistical analysis, staffing, quality care review); others must ask permission from the client to review a record.
 4. The medical record is sent to hospital records or the health information department after hospital discharge.
D. Computerized medical records
 1. Health care employees should have access only to the client's records in the nursing unit or work area.

BOX 7-10

Maintenance of Confidentiality

Not discussing client issues with other clients or uninvolved staff in the client's care
Not sharing health care information with others without the client's consent (includes family members or friends of the client)
Keeping all information about a client private and not revealing it to someone not directly involved in care
Sharing client information only in private and secluded areas
Protecting the medical record from all unauthorized readers

 2. Confidentiality can be protected by the use of special computer access codes to limit what employees can find in computer systems.
 3. The use of a password or identification code is needed to enter and sign off a computer system.
 4. A password or identification code should never be shared with another person.
 5. Periodic changes in personal passwords should be done to prevent unauthorized computer access.
E. In research, any information provided by the client will not be reported in any manner that identifies the client and will not be made accessible to anyone outside the research team.

XI. LEGAL SAFEGUARDS
A. Risk management
 1. Risk management is a planned method to identify, analyze, and evaluate risks followed by a plan for reducing the frequency of accidents and injuries.
 2. Programs are based on a systematic reporting system for incidents or unusual occurrences.
B. Incident reports (Box 7-11)
 1. The report is used as a means of identifying risk situations and improving client care.
 2. Follow specific documentation guidelines.
 3. Fill out the report completely, accurately, and factually.
 4. The report form should not be copied or placed in the client's record.
 5. Make no reference to the incident report form in the client's record.
 6. The report is not a substitute for a complete entry in the client's record regarding the incident.
C. Safeguarding valuables
 1. Client's valuables should be given to a family member or secured for safekeeping in a stored and locked designated location, such as the agency's safe, and the location of the client's valuables is documented per agency policy.
 2. Many health care agencies require a client to sign a release to free the agency of the responsibility for lost valuables.
 3. A client's wedding band can be taped in place unless a risk exists for swelling of the hands or fingers.

BOX 7-11

Incidents

Accidental omission of ordered therapies
Circumstances that led to injury or a risk for client injury
Client falls
Medication administration errors
Needlestick injuries
Procedure-related or equipment-related accidents
A visitor having symptoms of an illness

BOX 7-12

Telephone Orders

Date and time the entry.
Repeat the order to the physician and record the order.
Sign the order; begin with "t.o." (telephone order), write the physician's name, and then sign the order.
If another nurse witnessed the order, that nurse's signature follows.
The physician needs to countersign the order within a time frame according to agency policy.

4. Religious items, such as medals or scapulas, may be pinned to the client's gown if allowed by agency policy.
D. Physicians' orders
   1. A nurse is obligated to carry out a physician's order except when the nurse believes an order to be inappropriate or inaccurate.
   2. A nurse carrying out an inaccurate order may be legally responsible for any harm suffered by the client.
   3. The nurse should clarify with the physician an unclear or inappropriate order or an order in question.
   4. If no resolution occurs regarding the order in question, the nurse should contact the nurse manager or supervisor.
   5. The nurse should follow these guidelines for telephone orders (Box 7-12).
   6. The nurse should ensure that all components of a medication order are documented (Box 7-13).
E. Documentation
   1. Documentation is legally required by accrediting agencies, state licensing laws, and state nurse and medical practice acts.
   2. The nurse should follow agency guidelines and procedures (Box 7-14).
F. Client/family teaching
   1. Provide complete instructions in a language that client or family can understand.
   2. Document client and family teaching, what was taught, evaluation of understanding, and who was present during the teaching.
   3. Inform client of what would happen if information shared during teaching is not followed.

BOX 7-13

Components of a Medication Order

Date and time the order was written
Medication name
Medication dosage
Route of administration
Frequency of administration
Physician or health care provider's signature

BOX 7-14

Documentation Guidelines

NARRATIVE
Use a black pen.
Date and time entries.
Provide objective, factual, and complete documentation.
Document care, medications, treatments, and procedures as soon as possible after completion.
Document client responses to interventions.
Document consent for or refusal of treatments.
Document calls made to other health care providers.
Do not document for others or change documentation for other individuals.
Sign and title each entry.
Use quotes as appropriate for subjective data.
Use correct spelling, grammar, and punctuation.
Avoid unacceptable abbreviations.
Avoid judgmental or evaluative statements such as "uncooperative client."
Do not leave blank spaces on documentation forms.
Follow agency policies when an error is made (draw one line through the error, initial, and date).
Follow agency guidelines regarding late entries.

COMPUTERIZED
Use only the user identification code, name, or password.
Never lend access identification to another.
Maintain privacy and confidentiality of documented information printed from the computer.

XII. LEGAL DOCUMENTS

A. **Advance directives**
   1. An **advance directive** is a written document (sometimes called a living will) recognized by state **law** that provides directions concerning the provision of care when a client is unable to make his or her own treatment choices.
   2. The directive also may include the naming of a relative or friend (health care proxy) who will make health care decisions in the event of the client's incapacitation.
B. Patient Self-Determination Act
   1. The Patient Self-Determination Act became a law in the United States in 1990 and was implemented in all health care institutions.
   2. Clients must be provided with information about their rights to identify written directions about the care that they wish to receive in the event that they become incapacitated and are unable to make health care decisions.
   3. On admission to a health care facility, the client is asked about the existence of an **advance directive**; if one exists, it must be documented and included as part of the medical record.
   4. If the client signs an **advance directive** at the time of admission, it must be documented in the client's medical record.

C. Living will
  1. An **advance directive** lists the medical treatment that a client chooses to omit or refuse if the client becomes unable to make decisions and is terminally ill.
  2. States have their own requirements for executing living wills, but generally two witnesses, neither of whom can be a relative or physician, are needed when the client signs the living will.
D. Durable powers of attorney is a legal document that appoints a person (health care proxy) chosen by the client to carry out the client's wishes as expressed in the **advance directive** or to make decisions on the client's behalf when the client can no longer make decisions.
▲ E. Do not resuscitate (DNR) orders
  1. The DNR is an order written by a physician when a client has indicated a desire to be allowed to die if the client stops breathing or the client's heart stops beating.
  2. The client or his or her legal representative must provide **informed consent** for the DNR status.
  3. The DNR order must be defined clearly so that other treatment, not refused by the client, will be continued.
  4. The DNR order must be reviewed regularly according to agency policy (usually every 3 days for hospitalized clients and every 60 days for clients in residential health facilities).
  5. All health care personnel must know whether a client has a DNR order.
  6. A nurse who attempts to resuscitate a client who has an order for DNR would be acting without the client's **consent** and committing battery.
  7. The nurse must follow specific agency guidelines regarding when and under what circumstances a verbal DNR order is acceptable.
F. The nurse's role
  1. Discussing **advance directives** with the client opens the communication channel to establish what is important to the client and what the client may view as promoting life versus prolonging dying.
  2. The nurse needs to ensure that the client was provided with information about the right to identify written directions about the care that the client wishes to receive.
  3. On admission to a health care facility, the nurse determines whether an **advance directive** exists and ensures that it is part of the medical record.
  4. The nurse ensures that the physician was notified of the presence of an **advance directive**.
  5. All health care workers need to follow the directions of an **advance directive** to be immune from liability.
  6. Some agencies have specific policies that prohibit a nurse from signing as a witness to a legal document such as a living will.
  7. If a nurse witnesses a legal document, the nurse must document the event and the factual circumstances surrounding the signing in the medical record.
  8. Documentation as a witness should include who was present, any significant comments by the client, and the nurse's observations of the client's conduct during this process.

XIII. REPORTING RESPONSIBILITIES ▲

A. Nurses are required to report certain communicable diseases or criminal activities such as abuse, gunshot or stab wounds, assaults, homicides, and suicides to the appropriate authorities.
B. The impaired nurse
  1. If a nurse suspects that a co-worker is abusing chemicals, the nurse must report the individual to nursing administration in a confidential manner with the goal of treatment being the priority issue.
  2. Nursing administration then notifies the board of nursing regarding the nurse's behavior.
C. Occupational Safety and Health Act
  1. The Occupational Safety and Health Act requires that an employer provide a safe workplace for employees according to regulations.
  2. Employees confidentially can report working conditions that violate regulations.
  3. An employee who reports unsafe working conditions cannot be retaliated against by the employer.
D. Sexual harassment
  1. Sexual harassment is prohibited by state and federal laws.
  2. Sexual harassment includes unwelcome conduct of a sexual nature.
  3. Follow agency policies and procedures to handle reporting of a concern or complaint.

PRACTICE QUESTIONS

1. A client arrives in the emergency room and is assessed by the nurse. The client is staggering, confused, and verbally abusive. The client complains of a headache from drinking alcohol and is asking for medication. The nurse explains to the client that the physician will need to perform an assessment before the administration of medication. When the client becomes verbally abusive, the nurse obtains leather restraints and threatens to place the client in the restraints. With which of the following can the client legally charge the nurse as a result of the nursing action?
  1. Assault
  2. Battery
  3. Negligence
  4. Invasion of privacy
2. The nurse calls the physician regarding a new medication order because the dosage prescribed is higher

than the recommended dosage. The nurse is unable to locate the physician and the medication is due to be administered. Which of the following actions would the nurse take?
1. Hold the medication until the physician can be contacted.
2. Administer the dose prescribed.
3. Administer the recommended dose until the physician can be located.
4. Contact the nursing supervisor.

3. A nursing graduate is employed as a staff nurse in a local hospital. During orientation, the new graduate asks the nurse educator about the need to obtain professional liability insurance. The most appropriate response by the nurse educator is
1. "The hospital's liability insurance will cover your actions."
2. "It is very expensive and not necessary."
3. "Nurses are encouraged to have their own malpractice insurance."
4. "The majority of suits are filed against physicians and the hospital."

4. The registered nurse arrives at work and is told to report (float) to the intensive care unit (ICU) for the day because the ICU is understaffed and needs additional nurses to care for the clients. The nurse has never worked in the ICU. Which of the following is the most appropriate nursing action?
1. Refuse to float to the ICU.
2. Call the hospital lawyer.
3. Call the nursing supervisor.
4. Report to the ICU and identify tasks that can be performed safely.

5. The nurse gives an inaccurate dose of a medication to a client. Following assessment of the client, the nurse completes an incident report. The nurse notifies the nursing supervisor of the medication error and calls the physician to report the occurrence. The nurse who administered the inaccurate medication dose understands that the
1. Error will result in suspension.
2. Incident report is a method of promoting quality care and risk management.
3. Incident will be reported to the board of nursing.
4. Incident will be documented in the personnel file.

6. A nurse who works on the night shift enters the medication room and finds a co-worker with a tourniquet wrapped around the upper arm. The co-worker is about to insert a needle, attached to a syringe containing a clear liquid, into the antecubital area. The most appropriate initial action by the nurse is which of the following?
1. Call the police.
2. Call security.
3. Lock the co-worker in the medication room until help is obtained.
4. Call the nursing supervisor.

7. A hospitalized client tells the nurse that a living will is being prepared and that the lawyer will be bringing the will to the hospital today for witness signatures. The client asks the nurse for assistance in obtaining a witness to the will. The most appropriate response to the client is which of the following?
1. "I will sign as a witness to your signature."
2. "You will need to find a witness on your own."
3. "I will call the nursing supervisor to seek assistance regarding your request."
4. "Whoever is available at the time will sign as a witness for you."

8. The nurse has made an error in documenting an assessment finding on a client and obtains the client's record to correct the error. The nurse corrects the error by
1. Trying to erase the error for space to write in the correct data.
2. Using whiteout to delete the error and writing in the correct data.
3. Drawing one line through the error, initialing and dating the line, and then documenting the correct information.
4. Documenting a late entry into the client's record.

9. The nurse employed in a hospital is waiting to receive a report from the laboratory via the facsimile machine. The facsimile machine activates and the nurse expects the report but instead receives a sexually oriented photograph. The most appropriate nursing action is to
1. Cut up the photograph and throw it away.
2. Call the laboratory and ask for the individual's name that sent the photograph.
3. Call the police.
4. Call the nursing supervisor and report the incident.

10. The nursing instructor provides a lecture to nursing students regarding the issue of client rights. The instructor asks a nursing student to identify a situation that represents an example of invasion of client privacy. Which of the following, if identified by the student, indicates an understanding of a violation of this client right?
1. Performing a procedure without consent.
2. Telling the client that he or she cannot leave the hospital.
3. Threatening to give a client a medication.
4. Observing care provided to the client without the client's permission.

11. The nursing staff is sitting in the lounge taking their morning break. A nursing assistant tells the group that she thinks that the unit secretary has acquired immunodeficiency syndrome. The nursing assistant proceeds to tell the nursing staff that the secretary probably contracted the disease from her husband, who is supposedly a drug addict. Which legal tort has the nursing assistant violated?
1. Slander

2. Libel

3. Assault

4. Negligence

12. The nurse hears a client calling out for help. The nurse hurries down the hallway to the client's room and finds a client lying on the floor. The nurse performs a thorough assessment and assists the client back to bed. The nurse notifies the physician of the incident and completes an incident report. Which of the following would the nurse document on the incident report?

   1. The client was found lying on the floor.

   2. The client climbed over the side rails.

   3. The client fell out of bed.

   4. The client became restless and tried to get out of bed.

13. A client is brought to the emergency room by the emergency medical services after being hit by a car. The name of the client is not known. The client has sustained a severe head injury, multiple fractures, and is unconscious. An emergency craniotomy is required. Regarding informed consent for the surgical procedure, which of the following is the best action?

   1. Call the police to identify the client and locate the family.

   2. Obtain a court order for the surgical procedure.

   3. Ask the emergency medical services team to sign the informed consent.

   4. Transport the victim to the operating room for surgery.

14. An 87-year-old woman is brought to the emergency room for treatment of a fractured arm. On physical assessment the nurse notes old and new ecchymotic areas on the client's chest and legs. The nurse asks the client how the bruises were sustained. The client, although reluctant, tells the nurse in confidence that her son frequently hits her if supper is not prepared on time when he arrives home from work. Which of the following is the most appropriate nursing response?

   1. "Oh really, I will discuss this situation with your son."

   2. "Do you have any friends that can help you out until you resolve these important issues with your son."

   3. "Let's talk about the ways you can manage your time to prevent this from happening."

   4. "This is a legal issue, and I need to let you know that I will need to report it."

15. The nurse is working in a long-term care facility and is administering medications to assigned clients. A client refuses to take the prescribed medication, and the nurse threatens the client and tells the client that if the medication is not taken orally, then restraints will be applied and the medication will be given by injection. This statement by the nurse constitutes which legal tort?

   1. Invasion of privacy

   2. Negligence

   3. Assault

   4. Battery

CRITICAL THINKING: FILL IN THE BLANK

The nurse is reviewing the physician's orders for a newly admitted client and notes that the physician has prescribed a medication dose that is twice the amount that the client reports taking before admission. The nurse verifies the medication amount taken before admission with the client. What is the next most appropriate nursing action?

Answer: _____

ANSWERS

1. Answer: **1**

Rationale: An assault occurs when a person puts another person in fear of a harmful or offensive contact. For this intentional tort to be actionable, the victim must be aware of the threat of harmful or offensive contact. Battery is the actual contact with one's body. Negligence involves actions below the standards of care. Invasion of privacy occurs with unreasonable intrusion into the individual's private affairs.

Test-Taking Strategy: Use the process of elimination. Note the key word *threatens* in the question. This key word easily should direct you to option 1. If you had difficulty with this question, review the descriptions associated with the terms in each option.

Level of Cognitive Ability: Comprehension

Client Needs: Safe, Effective Care Environment

Integrated Process: Nursing Process—implementation

Content Area: Fundamental skills

Reference: Brent, N. (2001). *Nurses and the law* (2nd ed., p. 114). Philadelphia: W. B. Saunders

2. Answer: **4**

Rationale: If the physician writes an order that requires clarification, the nurse's responsibility is to contact the physician for clarification. If there is no resolution regarding the order because the physician cannot be located or because the order remains as it was written after talking with the physician, the nurse then should contact the nurse manager or nursing supervisor for further clarification as to what the next step should be. Under no circumstances should the nurse proceed to carry out the order until obtaining clarification.

Test-Taking Strategy: Use the process of elimination and eliminate options 2 and 3 first because they are similar and unsafe actions. Holding the medication can result in client injury. The nurse needs to take action. Option 4 clearly identifies the required action in this situation. Review nursing responsibilities

related to physician's orders if you had difficulty with this question.
Level of Cognitive Ability: Application
Client Needs: Safe, Effective Care Environment
Integrated Process: Nursing Process—implementation
Content Area: Fundamental skills
Reference: Potter, P., & Perry, A. (2001) *Fundamentals of nursing* (5th ed., pp. 899, 902, 904). St. Louis: Mosby.

3. Answer: **3**
Rationale: Nurses need their own liability insurance for protection against malpractice law suits. Nurses erroneously assume that they are protected by an agency's professional liability policies. Usually when a nurse is sued, the employer also is sued for the nurse's actions or inactions. Even though this is the norm, nurses are encouraged to have their own malpractice insurance.
Test-Taking Strategy: Note that the issue of the question relates to "obtaining professional liability insurance." This issue easily should direct you to option 3. Review liability related to malpractice insurance if you had difficulty with this question.
Level of Cognitive Ability: Comprehension
Client Needs: Safe, Effective Care Environment
Integrated Process: Teaching/Learning
Content Area: Fundamental skills
Reference: Brent, N. (2001). *Nurses and the law* (2nd ed., p. 87). Philadelphia: W. B. Saunders.

4. Answer: **4**
Rationale: Floating is an acceptable legal practice used by hospitals to solve their understaffing problems. Legally, a nurse cannot refuse to float unless a union contract guarantees that nurses can work only in a specified area or the nurse can prove the lack of knowledge for the performance of assigned tasks. When encountering this situation, nurses should set priorities and identify potential areas of harm to the client.
Test-Taking Strategy: Use the process of elimination, noting the key words "most appropriate." This may indicate that more than one option may be correct. Options 1 and 2 can be eliminated first. From the remaining options, calling the nursing supervisor is premature. Option 4 is most appropriate. Review nursing responsibilities related to floating if you had difficulty with this question.
Level of Cognitive Ability: Application
Client Needs: Safe, Effective Care Environment
Integrated Process: Nursing Process—implementation
Content Area: Fundamental skills
Reference: Potter, P., & Perry, A. (2001). *Fundamentals of nursing* (5th ed., p. 435). St. Louis: Mosby.

5. Answer: **2**
Rationale: Documentation of unusual occurrences, incidents, and accidents and the nursing actions taken as a result of the occurrence is internal to the institution or agency and allows the nurse and administration to review the quality of care and determine any potential risks present. Based on the information provided in the question, the nurse's error will not result in suspension nor will it be documented in the personnel file. The error and the situation presented in

the question are not a reason for notifying the board of nursing.
Test-Taking Strategy: Focus on the information provided in the question. Use the process of elimination and knowledge regarding the purpose of incident reports to assist in eliminating options 1, 3, and 4. Note that the correct option is also the global option. If you had difficulty with this question, review the purpose of incident reports.
Level of Cognitive Ability: Comprehension
Client Needs: Safe, Effective Care Environment
Integrated Process: Nursing Process—implementation
Content Area: Fundamental skills
Reference: Potter, P., & Perry, A. (2001). *Fundamentals of nursing* (5th ed., pp. 440, 521). St. Louis: Mosby.

6. Answer: **4**
Rationale: Nurse practice acts require reporting impaired nurses. The board of nursing has jurisdiction over the practice of nursing and may develop plans for treatment and supervision of the impaired nurse. This incident needs to be reported to the nursing supervisor, who will then report to the board of nursing and other authorities, such as the police, as required. Option 3 is an inappropriate and unsafe action. The nurse may call security if a disturbance occurs, but no data in the question supports this need, and therefore this is not the initial action.
Test-Taking Strategy: Note the key words "initial action." Eliminate option 3 first because this is an inappropriate and unsafe action. Recall the lines of organizational structure to assist in directing you to option 4. If you had difficulty with this question, review the nurse's responsibilities when substance abuse is suspected or occurs in the workplace.
Level of Cognitive Ability: Application
Client Needs: Safe, Effective Care Environment
Integrated Process: Nursing Process—implementation
Content Area: Fundamental skills
Reference: Brent, N. (2001). *Nurses and the law* (2nd ed., p. 309). Philadelphia: W. B. Saunders.

7. Answer: **3**
Rationale: Living wills are required to be in writing and signed by the client. The client's signature either must be witnessed by specified individuals or notarized. Many states prohibit any employee, including a nurse of a facility where the client is receiving care, from being a witness. Option 2 is nontherapeutic and not a helpful response. The nurse should seek the assistance of the nursing supervisor.
Test-Taking Strategy: Note the key words "most appropriate." Options 1 and 4 are similar and should be eliminated first. Option 2 is eliminated because it is a nontherapeutic response. Review legal implications associated with wills if you had difficulty with this question.
Level of Cognitive Ability: Application
Client Needs: Safe, Effective Care Environment
Integrated Process: Communication and Documentation
Content Area: Fundamental skills
References: Potter, P., & Perry, A. (2001). *Fundamentals of nursing* (5th ed., p. 437). St. Louis: Mosby.
Brent, N. (2001). *Nurses and the law* (2nd ed., p. 217). Philadelphia: W. B. Saunders.

8. Answer: 3

Rationale: If the nurse makes an error in documenting in the client's record, the nurse should follow agency policies to correct the error. This includes drawing one line through the error, initialing and dating the line, and then documenting the correct information. Erasing data from the client's record and the use of whiteout are prohibited. A late entry is used to document additional information not remembered at the initial time of documentation.

Test-Taking Strategy: Use the process of elimination and principles related to documentation. Recalling that alterations to a client's record are to be avoided will assist in eliminating options 1 and 2. From the remaining options, focusing on the issue of the question and using knowledge regarding the principles related to documentation easily will direct you to option 3. Review these principles if you had difficulty with this question.
Level of Cognitive Ability: Application
Client Needs: Safe, Effective Care Environment
Integrated Process: Communication and Documentation
Content Area: Fundamental skills
Reference: Perry, A., & Potter, P. (2002). *Clinical nursing skills & techniques* (5th ed., p. 40). St. Louis: Mosby.

9. Answer: 4

Rationale: Sexual harassment in the workplace is prohibited by state and federal laws. Sexually suggestive jokes, touching, pressuring a co-worker for a date, and open displays of sexually oriented photographs or posters are examples of conduct that could be considered sexual harassment by another worker. If the nurse believes that he or she is being subjected to unwelcome sexual conduct, these concerns should be reported to the nursing supervisor immediately. Option 3 is unnecessary at this time. Options 1 and 2 are not the most appropriate actions.
Test-Taking Strategy: Note the key words "most appropriate." This may indicate that one or more than one of the options is partially or totally correct. Use the skills of prioritizing to select the correct option. Remember that using the organizational channels of communication is best. This will assist in directing you to option 4. Review nursing responsibilities when sexual harassment occurs in the workplace if you had difficulty with this question.
Level of Cognitive Ability: Application
Client Needs: Safe, Effective Care Environment
Integrated Process: Nursing Process—implementation
Content Area: Fundamental skills
References: Brent, N. (2001). *Nurses and the law* (2nd ed., p. 38). Philadelphia: W. B. Saunders.
Potter, P., & Perry, A. (2001). *Fundamentals of nursing* (5th ed., pp. 402, 404). St. Louis: Mosby.

10. Answer: 4

Rationale: Invasion of privacy takes place with unreasonable intrusion into an individual's private affairs. Telling the client that the client cannot leave the hospital constitutes false imprisonment. Threatening to give a client a medication constitutes assault. Performing a procedure without consent is an example of battery.
Test-Taking Strategy: The key words in the question are "invasion of client privacy." Focus on these key words to direct you

to option 4. If you had difficulty with this question, review those situations that include invasion of privacy.
Level of Cognitive Ability: Comprehension
Client Needs: Safe, Effective Care Environment
Integrated Process: Caring
Content Area: Fundamental skills
Reference: Potter, P., & Perry, A. (2001). *Fundamentals of nursing* (5th ed., p. 425). St. Louis: Mosby.

11. Answer: 1

Rationale: Defamation takes place when something untrue is said (slander) or written (libel) about a person, resulting in injury to that person's good name and reputation. An assault occurs when a person puts another person in fear of a harmful or an offensive contact. Negligence involves the actions of professionals that fall below the standard of care for a specific professional group.
Test-Taking Strategy: Use the process of elimination and eliminate options 3 and 4 first. Recalling that slander constitutes verbal defamation easily will direct you to option 1. If you had difficulty with this question, review the torts identified in each option.
Level of Cognitive Ability: Comprehension
Client Needs: Safe, Effective Care Environment
Integrated Process: Nursing Process—implementation
Content Area: Fundamental skills
Reference: Brent, N. (2001). *Nurses and the law* (2nd ed., p. 121). Philadelphia: W. B. Saunders.

12. Answer: 1

Rationale: The incident report should contain the client's name, age, and diagnosis. The report should contain a factual description of the incident, any injuries experienced by those involved, and the outcome of the situation. Option 1 is the only option that describes the facts as observed by the nurse. Options 2, 3, and 4 are interpretations of the situation and are not factual data as observed by the nurse.
Test-Taking Strategy: Use the process of elimination and read the information contained in the question to select the correct option. Remember to focus on factual information when documenting, and avoid including interpretations. Review documentation principles related to incident reports if you had difficulty with this question.
Level of Cognitive Ability: Application
Client Needs: Safe, Effective Care Environment
Integrated Process: Communication and Documentation
Content Area: Fundamental skills
Reference: Brent, N. (2001). *Nurses and the law* (2nd ed., pp. 95-96). Philadelphia: W. B. Saunders.

13. Answer: 4

Rationale: Generally, in only two instances is the informed consent of an adult client not needed. One instance is when an emergency is present and delaying treatment for the purpose of obtaining informed consent would result in injury or death to the client. The second instance is when the client waives the right to give informed consent. Option 2 will delay emergency treatment and option 3 is inappropriate. Although option 1 may be pursued, it is not the best action.

Test-Taking Strategy: Use the process of elimination. Recalling that when an emergency is present and a delay in treatment for the purpose of obtaining informed consent could result in injury or death easily will direct you to option 4. Review the issues surrounding informed consent, if you had difficulty with this question.
Level of Cognitive Ability: Application
Client Needs: Safe, Effective Care Environment
Integrated Process: Nursing Process—implementation
Content Area: Fundamental skills
Reference: Brent, N. (2001). *Nurses and the law* (2nd ed., pp. 41, 210, 213). Philadelphia: W. B. Saunders.

14. Answer: **4**
Rationale: Confidential issues are not to be discussed with nonmedical personnel or the person's family or friends without the person's permission. Clients should be assured that information is kept confidential, unless it places the nurse under a legal obligation. The nurse must report situations related to child or elderly abuse, gunshot wounds, and certain infectious diseases. Options 1, 2, and 3 do not address the legal implications of the situation and do not assure a safe environment for the client.
Test-Taking Strategy: Use the process of elimination and knowledge regarding the nursing responsibilities related to reporting obligations. Options 1, 2, and 3 should be eliminated because they are similar in that they do not protect the client from injury. Review the nursing responsibilities related to reporting obligations if you had difficulty with this question.
Level of Cognitive Ability: Application
Client Needs: Safe, Effective Care Environment
Integrated Process: Nursing Process—implementation
Content Area: Fundamental skills
Reference: Brent, N. (2001). *Nurses and the law* (2nd ed., p. 121). Philadelphia: W. B. Saunders.

15. Answer: **3**
Rationale: An assault occurs when a person puts another person in fear of a harmful or offensive contact. For this intentional tort to be actionable, the victim must be aware of the threat of harmful or offensive contact. Battery is the actual contact with one's body. Negligence involves actions below the standards of care. Invasion of privacy occurs with unreasonable intrusion into the individual's private affairs.
Test-Taking Strategy: Use the process of elimination and knowledge regarding the descriptions of the items in each option. Note the key word "threatens" in the question. This key word easily should direct you to option 3. If you had difficulty with this question, take time to review the descriptions associated with the terms in each option.
Level of Cognitive Ability: Comprehension
Client Needs: Safe, Effective Care Environment
Integrated Process: Nursing Process—implementation
Content Area: Fundamental skills
Reference: Brent, N. (2001). *Nurses and the law* (2nd ed., p. 114). Philadelphia: W. B. Saunders.

CRITICAL THINKING: FILL IN THE BLANK
Answer: Contact the physician
Rationale: If the nurse determines that a physician's order is unclear or if the nurse has a question about an order, the nurse should contact the physician before implementing the order. Under no circumstances should the nurse carry out the order unless the physician has clarified the order.
Test Taking Strategy: Use prioritizing skills to determine the next most appropriate nursing action. Noting that the nurse verifies with the client the medication amount taken before admission will guide you to determine that the nurse needs to contact the physician. Review guidelines related to physicians' orders if you had difficulty with this question.
Level of Cognitive Ability: Application
Client Needs: Safe, Effective Care Environment
Integrated Process: Nursing Process: implementation
Content Area: Fundamental skills
Reference: Potter, P., & Perry, A. (2001). *Fundamentals of nursing* (5th ed., p. 434). St. Louis: Mosby.

REFERENCES

Brent, N. (2001). *Nurses and the law* (2nd ed.). Philadelphia: W. B. Saunders.
Christensen, B., & Kockrow, E. (2003) *Foundations of nursing* (4th ed., p.13). St. Louis: Mosby.
Combined Life Insurance Company of New York. (2003). HIPAA notice of privacy practices for personal health information (retrieved January 2004). http://www.keio.edu/parents/hippa.html
Harkreader, H., & Hogan, M. A. (2004). *Fundamentals of nursing: caring and clinical judgment* (2nd ed.). Philadelphia: W. B. Saunders.
National Council of State Boards of Nursing (Eds). (2003). *Test Plan for the National Council Licensure Examination for registered nurses* (effective date: April 2004). Chicago: Author.

Perry, A., & Potter, P. (2002). *Clinical nursing skills & techniques* (5th ed.). St. Louis: Mosby.
Potter, P., & Perry, A. (2001). *Fundamentals of nursing* (5th ed.). St. Louis: Mosby.
Stuart, G., & Laraia, M. (2001). *Principles and practice of psychiatric nursing* (7th ed., p. 167). St. Louis: Mosby.
Yoder-Wise, P. (2003). *Leading and managing in nursing* (3rd ed.). St. Louis: Mosby.

Leadership, Delegating, and Prioritizing Client Care

PYRAMID TERMS

accountability A moral concept that involves acceptance by the professional nurse of the consequences of a decision or action.

authority Legitimate power or official right to act.

case management An interdisciplinary health care delivery system designed to promote appropriate use of hospital personnel and material resources to maximize hospital revenues while providing for optimal outcome of care.

change A dynamic process that leads to an alteration in behavior.

critical path Effective clinical management system for monitoring care and for reducing or controlling the length of hospital stay.

delegation Process of transferring a selected nursing task in a situation to an individual who is competent to perform that specific task.

empowerment An interpersonal process of enabling others to do for themselves.

leadership An interpersonal process that involves motivating and guiding others to achieve goals.

management The accomplishment of tasks by one's self or by directing others.

power The ability to do or act that results in the achievement of desired results.

prioritizing Deciding which needs or problems require immediate action and which ones could be delayed until a later time because they are not urgent.

responsibility The duty to act.

variances Actual deviations or detours from the critical paths.

◣ THE PYRAMID TO SUCCESS

The professional nurse is a leader and a manager. As described in the NCLEX-RN exam test plan, the professional nurse needs to provide integrated, cost-effective care to clients by coordinating, supervising, and collaborating with members of the multidisciplinary health care team. Pyramid Points focus on concepts of leadership and management, case management, resource management, the change process, the process of delegation, and prioritizing client care. The Integrated Processes addressed in this chapter include Caring, Communication and Documentation, Nursing Process, and Teaching/Learning.

CLIENT NEEDS
Safe, Effective Care Environment

Case management
Concepts of management
Consultation with members of the health care team
Cost-effective measures when providing nursing care
Delegation of client care
Establishing priorities of care
Identifying professional practice limitations
Performance improvement (quality assurance)
Resource management
Supervising the delivery of client care
Variance reports

Health Promotion and Maintenance

Client's ability to perform self-care
Disease prevention
Family systems
Health and wellness
Health promotion programs
Health screening

Psychosocial Integrity

Cultural, spiritual, and religious issues
Support systems
Therapeutic interactions

Physiological Integrity

Ensuring palliative/comfort care is provided to the client
Potential for alterations in body systems
Unexpected responses to therapy

I. HEALTH CARE DELIVERY

A. Managed care
1. Managed care is designed to control the cost of health services and promote a continuum of care through the development and use of integrated services.
2. Managed care uses a select group of providers who agree to a predetermined payment before delivering care.
3. Client care is outcome driven and is managed by a **case management** process.
4. Managed care emphasizes the promotion of health, client education and responsible self-care, early identification of disease, and the use of health care resources.

B. **Case management**
1. **Case management** is an organized system for delivering health care to an individual client or a group of clients throughout their illnesses.
2. **Case management** includes assessment and development of a plan of care, coordination of all services, referral, and follow-up.

C. Case manager
1. A professional nurse who assumes **responsibility** for coordinating the client's care from admission and following discharge is a case manager.
2. The case manager establishes a plan of care with the client, coordinates any consultations and referrals, and facilitates discharge.

D. **Critical path**
1. A multidisciplinary treatment plan that identifies the clinical interventions over a projected length of stay or a projected time frame for specific case types is a **critical path**.
2. All members of the health care team work with one plan to achieve the same client outcomes.
3. The goal of a **critical path** is to anticipate and recognize negative **variance** early so that appropriate action can be taken and better client outcomes can result.
4. **Variances**
   a. Actual deviations or detours from the **critical path** are variances.
   b. Positive **variance** occurs when a client achieves maximum benefit and is discharged earlier than anticipated on the **critical path**.
   c. Negative **variance** occurs when untoward events prevent a timely discharge and the length of hospital stay is longer than planned for a client on a specific **critical path**.
   d. **Variance** analysis occurs continually as the case manager and other caregivers monitor client outcomes against the **critical path**.
   e. Accurate monitoring of **critical path** with **variance** analysis can estimate the financial impact of client care.
   f. If the **variance** is predictable, negotiation with insurers for an additional length of hospital stay can maximize client care revenues.

E. CareMaps
1. CareMaps initially were developed at the New England Medical Center in Boston.
2. A CareMap is a model for a critical path.
3. The CareMap incorporates day-to-day expected client outcomes and those outcomes anticipated at discharge or at the end of a treatment phase.
4. The CareMap outlines clinical assessments, treatments and procedures, dietary interventions, activity and exercise therapies, client education, and discharge planning.

F. Nursing care plan
1. A nursing care plan is a written guideline and communication tool that identifies the client's pertinent assessment data, problems and nursing diagnoses, goals, interventions, and expected outcomes.
2. The plan enhances continuity of care by identifying specific nursing actions necessary to achieve the goals of care.
3. The client and family are involved in developing the plan of care, and the plan identifies short-term and long-term goals.
4. Client problems, goals, interventions, and expected outcomes are documented in the care plan, and the plan provides a framework for evaluation of the client's response to nursing actions.

II. FORMAL ORGANIZATIONS

A. The mission statement communicates in broad terms an organization's reason for existence, the geographical area the organization serves, and attitudes and beliefs and values within which the organization functions.
B. Goals and objectives are measurable activities specific to the development of designated services and programs of an organization.
C. The organizational chart depicts and communicates how activities are arranged, how **authority** relationships are defined, and how communication channels are established.
D. Procedures and protocols
1. Guidelines define appropriate courses of action.
2. Procedures define tasks.
3. Protocols signify the definitions of clinical processes.
E. Centralization is the making of decisions by a limited number of individuals at the top of the organization or by managers of a department or unit, and decisions are communicated thereafter to the employees.

F. Decentralization is the distribution of **authority** throughout the organization to allow for increased **responsibility** and **delegation** in decision making.

III. CONTINUOUS (TOTAL) QUALITY IMPROVEMENT

A. The total quality improvement program focuses on processes or systems that significantly contribute to effective client care outcomes.

B. When total quality improvement is a part of the philosophy of a health care agency, every staff member becomes involved in ways to improve care and outcomes.

C. The quality of a health care organization is defined in its mission statement and in the philosophy of the nursing department; these statements identify how nurses are to perform, identify the services that are made available to the client, and provide directions for professional standards and care guidelines that should guarantee excellent client outcomes.

D. The Joint Commission on Accreditation of Healthcare Organizations describes quality improvement as an approach to the continuous assessment and improvement of the methods of providing health care to meet the needs of others.

E. The quality improvement process is similar to the nursing process and involves a multidisciplinary process.

F. An outcome indicates whether the interventions are effective, whether the client has progressed, how well standards are met, and whether changes are necessary.

G. The evaluation of health care is a process used to determine the quality of care and service provided to clients.

H. The nurse has the **responsibility** to recognize trends in nursing practice, identify when recurrent problems occur, and initiate opportunities to improve the quality of care.

IV. NURSING DELIVERY SYSTEMS

A. Functional nursing
   1. Functional nursing involves a task approach to client care, with major tasks being delegated by the charge nurse to individual members of the team.
   2. The goals are concerned with work productivity at the lowest possible cost.
   3. Tasks generally are assigned to the lowest-skilled, paid workers who are available to do the work.

B. Team nursing
   1. The team generally is led by a registered nurse who is responsible for assessing, developing nursing diagnoses, planning, and evaluating each client's plan of care.
   2. Each staff member works fully within the realm of his or her educational and clinical expertise.
   3. Each staff member is accountable for client care and outcomes of care delivered in accordance with

the licensing and practice scope as determined by hospital policy and state law.
   4. Team nursing is characterized by a high degree of respect for and maturity of team members and a high degree of communication and collaboration between members.

C. Primary nursing
   1. Primary nursing focuses on client outcomes as opposed to nursing tasks.
   2. Primary nursing is concerned with keeping the nurse at the bedside, actively involved in client care, while planning goal-directed, individualized care.

V. PROFESSIONAL RESPONSIBILITIES

A. **Accountability**
   1. **Accountability** is the process that mandates that individuals are answerable for their actions and have an obligation (or duty) to act.
   2. **Accountability** involves assuming only the responsibilities that are within one's scope of practice and not assuming **responsibility** for activities in which competence has not been achieved.
   3. **Accountability** involves admitting mistakes rather than blaming others and evaluating the outcomes of one's own actions.
   4. **Accountability** includes a **responsibility** to the client to be competent, to render nursing services in accordance with standards of nursing practice, and to adhere to the professional ethics code.

B. **Leadership**
   1. **Leadership** is the interpersonal process that involves motivating and guiding others to achieve goals.
   2. **Leadership** is a method of modeling accountable behavior to others.

C. **Leadership** styles
   1. Autocratic **leadership**
      a. Leader is focused.
      b. Leader maintains strong control, makes the decisions, and solves all problems.
      c. Leader dominates the group and commands rather than makes suggestions or seeks input.
   2. Democratic **leadership**
      a. Democratic **leadership** also is called participative **leadership**.
      b. Democratic **leadership** is based on the belief that every group member should have input into the development of goals and problem solving.
      c. Leader acts primarily as a facilitator and a resource person.
      d. Leader is concerned for each member of the group.
      e. Democratic **leadership** is a more participative style and much less authoritarian than the autocratic **leadership** style.
   3. Laissez-faire **leadership**
      a. Leader assumes a passive, nondirective, and inactive approach.

b. **Leadership** responsibilities are assumed by the members of the group or are relinquished completely.

c. All decision making is left to the group, with the leader giving little if any guidance, support, or feedback.

d. Uncooperative behavior by the group may be permissible as a result of the leader's lack of limit setting and stated expectations.

4. Situational **leadership**

a. Situational **leadership** uses a combination of styles based on current circumstances and events.

b. **Leadership** styles are assumed according to the needs of the group and the tasks to be achieved.

D. **Leadership** qualities

1. Communication

a. Leaders listens actively to others.

b. Leader communicates in an assertive manner and speaks directly and honestly to others.

c. Leader differentiates between aggressive, passive, and assertive behavior to communicate appropriately in a given situation (Box 8-1).

2. Credibility

a. **Leadership** enhances a nurse's **accountability**.

b. Individuals who perform well are those who can influence others.

3. Critical thinking

a. An individual with an open-minded, questioning attitude is a critical thinker.

b. The ineffective leader is one who falls into routine ways of thinking without even being aware of what is happening.

4. Initiation of action

a. Leader initiates measures to solve problems.

b. Leader puts ideas into action and demonstrates flexibility.

c. If an approach is ineffective, the leader is not hesitant to try another approach.

5. Risk taking

a. Taking risks involves acting to solve problems.

b. Risk-taking activities are goal directed.

BOX 8-1

Types of Behavior

AGGRESSIVE BEHAVIOR
Occurs when an individual meets one's own needs regardless of the effect on others

PASSIVE BEHAVIOR
Occurs when one gives up one's own rights and does not have one's own needs met

ASSERTIVE BEHAVIOR
Occurs when an individual seeks to meet one's own needs while respecting the rights of others

---

BOX 8-2

Managerial Functions

Planning: Determining objectives and identifying methods that leads to the achievement of those objectives
Organizing: Using resources (human and material) to achieve predetermined outcomes
Directing: Guiding and motivating others to meet the expected outcomes
Controlling: Using performance standards as criteria for measuring success and taking corrective action
Decision making: Identifying a problem and deciding which alternative(s) can best achieve the objectives

---

6. Persuasiveness and influence

a. Leader motivates and inspires others to achieve goals.

b. Leader understands how to use **power** effectively and does not dominate but rather motivates others.

c. Persuasiveness can create enthusiasm, encourage collaboration, and increase cohesiveness among team members.

E. **Management** is the accomplishment of tasks by oneself or by directing others.

F. Managerial functions (Box 8-2)

G. Problem-solving process

1. Problem solving involves obtaining information and using it to reach an acceptable solution to a problem.

2. Steps of the problem solving process are similar to the steps of the nursing process (Table 8-1).

H. Types of managers

1. Frontline manager

a. Manager functions in a role closely identified with the actual delivery of client care.

b. Roles include charge nurse, team leader, and client care coordinator.

c. Manager coordinates the activity of all staff who provide client care and supervises team members.

2. Middle manager

a. Roles include unit manager or supervisor.

TABLE 8-1

Problem-Solving Process and Nursing Process

Problem-Solving Process	Nursing Process
Identifying a problem	Assessment
Collecting data about the problem	
Identifying the exact nature of the problem	Analysis
Determining a plan of action	Planning
Carrying out the plan	Implementation
Evaluating the plan	Evaluation

b. Responsibilities include managing staff, preparing budgets, preparing work schedules, writing and implementing policies that guide client care and unit operations, and maintaining the quality of client services.

3. Nurse executive
   a. A nurse executive is a top-level nurse manager and may be the director of nursing services or the vice president for client care services.
   b. The nurse executive supervises multiple departments and works closely with the administrative team of the organization.
   c. The nurse executive ensures that all client care provided by nurses is carried out in keeping with the objectives of the health care organization.

VI. POWER

A. **Power** is the ability to do or act and results in the achievement of desired results.

B. Powerful persons are able to modify behavior and influence others to **change**, even when others are resistant to **change**.

C. Effective nurse leaders use **power** to improve the delivery of care and to enhance the profession.

D. **Power** that is effective is **power** that is shared.

E. Types of **power** (Box 8-3)

VII. EMPOWERMENT

A. **Empowerment** is an interpersonal process of enabling others to do for themselves.

B. **Empowerment** occurs when individuals are better able to influence what happens to them.

C. **Empowerment** involves open communication, mutual goal setting, and decision making.

D. Nurses can **empower** clients through advocacy.

VIII. THE CHANGE PROCESS

A. **Change** is a dynamic process that leads to an alteration in behavior.

B. Types of **change**
   1. Planned **change**: a deliberate effort to improve a situation
   2. Unplanned **change**

BOX 8-3

Types of Power

Reward: Ability to provide incentives
Coercive: Ability to punish
Referent: Based on attraction
Expert: Based on having an expert knowledge base and skill level
Legitimate: Based on a position in society
Personal: Derived from a high degree of self-confidence
Informational: When one person provides explanations why another should behave in a certain way

---

BOX 8-4

Reasons for Resisting Change

CONFORMITY
One goes along with others to avoid conflict.

DISSIMILAR BELIEFS AND VALUES
Differences can impede positive change.

HABIT
Routine, set behaviors are often hard to change.

SECONDARY GAINS
Benefits or payoff are present and so desirable that there is no incentive to change.

THREATS TO SATISFY BASIC NEEDS
Change may be perceived as a threat to self-esteem, security, or survival.

FEAR
One fears failure or has fear of the unknown.

---

   a. **Change** that just happens
   b. **Change** that is unpredictable and may be imposed by others or by uncontrollable natural events

C. Resistance to **change** (Box 8-4)
   1. Resistance to **change** occurs when an individual rejects proposed new ideas without critically thinking about the proposal.
   2. **Change** requires energy.
   3. The **change** activity does not guarantee positive outcomes.

D. Overcoming barriers
   1. Create a flexible and adaptable environment.
   2. Encourage those involved to plan and set goals for **change**.
   3. Include all involved in the plan for **change**.
   4. Focus on the benefits of the **change** in relation to improvement of client care.
   5. Evaluate the process on an ongoing basis, keeping everyone informed of the progress.
   6. Provide positive feedback to all involved.
   7. Commit to the time it takes to **change**.

IX. CONFLICT

A. Conflict arises from a perception of incompatibility or difference in beliefs, attitudes, values, goals, priorities, or decisions.

B. Types of conflict
   1. Intrapersonal: Occurs within a person
   2. Interpersonal: Occurs between and among clients, nurses, and other staff members
   3. Organizational: Occurs when an employee confronts policies and procedures of the organization

▲ C. Modes of conflict resolution
1. Avoidance
   a. Person is unassertive and uncooperative.
   b. The individual neither pursues needs, goals, or concerns nor assists others to pursue theirs.
   c. Person postpones the issue.
2. Accommodation
   a. The individual neglects own needs, goals, or concerns (unassertive) while trying to satisfy those of others.
   b. The individual obeys and serves others and often feels resentment and disappointment because he or she "gets nothing in return."
3. Competion
   a. The individual pursues own needs and goals at the expense of others.
   b. Competition also may take the form of standing up for rights and defending important principles.
4. Compromise
   a. Person is assertive and cooperative.
   b. Individuals work creatively and openly to find the solution that most fully satisfies all important goals and concerns to be achieved.

▲ **X. ROLES OF HEALTH CARE TEAM MEMBERS**
A. Nurse roles are as follows:
   1. Promote health and disease prevention
   2. Provide comfort and care to clients
   3. Make decisions
   4. Act as a client advocate
   5. Lead and manage the nursing team
   6. Serve as a case manager
   7. Function as a rehabilitator
   8. Be a communicator
   9. Educate clients and health team members
   10. Act as a resource person
   11. Allocate resources in a cost-effective manner
B. Physician: The physician diagnoses and treats disease.
C. Physician assistant
   1. The physician assistant provides assistance to the physician.
   2. The physician assistant conducts physical examinations, performs diagnostic procedures, assists in the operating room and emergency room, and performs treatments.
D. Physical therapist: The therapist assists in examining, testing, and treating the physically disabled.
E. Occupational therapist: The therapist develops adaptive devices that help chronically ill or handicapped clients perform activities of daily living.
F. Respiratory therapist: The therapist delivers treatments designed to improve the client's ventilation and oxygenation status.
G. Nutritionist: The nutritionist assists in planning dietary measures to improve or maintain a client's nutritional status.
H. Continuing care nurse: This nurse coordinates discharge plans for the client.
I. Assistive personnel/nursing assistant: Assistants help the registered nurse with specified tasks and functions.
J. Pharmacist: The pharmacist formulates and dispenses medications.
K. Social worker: The social worker counsels clients and families.
L. Pastoral care: The cleric offers spiritual support and guidance to clients and families.
M. Secretarial staff: Members provide support to the health care team, organize and schedule diagnostic tests and procedure, and arrange for services needed by the client and family.

XI. HEALTH CARE TEAM COMMUNICATION ▲
A. Client care planning can be accomplished through referrals or consultations to other health care specialists and through client care conferences, which involve members from all health care disciplines
B. Reports
   1. Reports should be factual, accurate, current, complete, and organized.
   2. Reports should include essential background information, subjective data, objective data, any changes in the client's status, nursing diagnoses, treatments and procedures, medication administration, client teaching, discharge planning, family information, the client's response to treatments and procedures, and the client's priority needs.
   3. Change of shift report
      a. The report provides continuity of care among nurses who are caring for a client.
      b. The report may be written, given orally, by audiotape, or during client walking rounds at the client's bedside.
      c. The report describes the client's health status and informs the nurse on the next shift about the client's needs and priorities for care.
   4. Telephone reports
      a. Purposes
         i. To inform a physician of a client's change in status
         ii. To communicate information about a client's transfer to or from another unit or facility
         iii. To obtain results of laboratory or diagnostic tests
      b. The telephone report should be documented and should include when the call was made, who made the call, who was called, to whom information was given, what information was given, and what information was received
   5. Transfer reports
      a. Transfer reports provide continuity of care and may be given by telephone or in person (Box 8-5).
      b. The receiving nurse needs to be given an opportunity to ask questions about the client's status.

BOX 8-5
Transfer Reports
Client's name, age, physician, and diagnosis
Current health status and current plan of care
Client's needs and priorities for care
Any assessments or interventions that need to be done after transfer, such as laboratory tests, medication administration, or dressing changes
The need for any special equipment
Any additional considerations such as resuscitation status, precautionary considerations, or family issues

BOX 8-6
Discharge Teaching
How to administer prescribed medications
Side effects of medications that need to be reported to the physician
Prescribed dietary and activity measures
Complications of the medical condition that need to be reported to the physician
How to perform prescribed treatments
How to use any special equipment prescribed for the client
Schedule for any home care services that are planned
How to access available community resources
When to obtain follow-up care

XII. CONSULTATION WITH THE HEALTH CARE TEAM

A. Consultation is a process in which a specialist is sought to identify methods of care or treatment plans to meet the needs of a client.

B. Consultation is needed when the nurse encounters a problem that cannot be solved using nursing knowledge, skills, and available resources.

C. Consultation also is needed when the exact problem remains unclear; a consultant can objectively and more clearly assess and identify the exact nature of the problem.

XIII. DISCHARGE PLANNING

A. Discharge planning begins when the client is admitted to the hospital or health care facility.

B. Discharge planning is a multidisciplinary process that ensures that the client has a plan for continuing care after leaving the health care facility and assists in the client's transition from one environment to another.

C. All caregivers need to be involved in discharge planning, and referrals to other health care professionals or agencies may be needed; a physician's order may be needed for the referral, and the referral needs to be approved by the client's insurer.

D. The nurse should anticipate the client's discharge needs and make the referral as soon as possible (involve the client and family in the referral process).

E. The nurse needs to educate the client and family regarding care at home (Box 8-6).

XIV. PERFORMANCE IMPROVEMENT (QUALITY ASSURANCE)

A. Description
1. Performance improvement is a process of evaluating the outcome of care measured against predetermined standards.
2. Aspects of care that represent the predetermined standards are selected, criteria for achievement of the standards are identified, and the methods of monitoring are defined.
3. Compliance in achieving the predetermined standards is measured, and ways to improve compliance are sought if needed.

B. Retrospective audit is an evaluation method to inspect the medical record for documentation of compliance with the standards.

C. Concurrent audit is an evaluation method to inspect the nursing staffs compliance with predetermined standards and criteria while the nurses are providing care

D. The quality assurance staff, charge nurse, or nurse educator may perform the review; a peer review approach may be implemented in which all members of the nursing staff are involved.

XV. DELEGATION AND ASSIGNMENTS

A. **Delegation**
1. **Delegation** is a process of transferring a selected nursing task in a situation to an individual who is competent to perform that specific task.
2. **Delegation** involves achieving outcomes and sharing activities with other individuals who have the **authority** to accomplish the task.
3. The nurse practice act and any practice limitations define which aspects of care can be delegated and which must be performed by the registered nurse.
4. Even though a task may be delegated to someone, the nurse who delegates maintains **accountability** for the overall nursing care of the client.
5. Only the task, not the ultimate **accountability**, may be delegated to another.

B. Principles and guidelines of delegating (Box 8-7)

C. Assignments
1. Assignment is transferring **responsibility** and **accountability**.
2. Guidelines for client care assignments
   a. Always ensure client safety.
   b. Be aware of individual variations in work abilities.
   c. Determine which tasks can be delegated and to whom.
   d. Match the task to the delegatee based on the nurse practice act and appropriate position descriptions.

BOX 8-7

Principles and Guidelines of Delegating

Delegate the right task to the right delegatee: Be familiar with the experience of the delegatees, their scopes of practice, their job descriptions, agency policy and procedures, and the state nurse practice act.

Provide clear directions about the task and ensure that the delegatee understands the expectations.

Determine the degree of supervision that may be required.

Provide the delegatee with the authority to complete the task; provide a deadline for completion of the task.

Evaluate the outcome of care that has been delegated.

Provide feedback to the delegatee regarding their performance.

Generally noninvasive interventions such as skin care, range-of-motion exercises, ambulation, grooming, and hygiene measures can be assigned to a nursing assistant.

A licensed practical nurse can perform the tasks that a nursing assistant can perform and additionally can perform certain invasive tasks such as dressings, suctioning, urinary catheterization, and administration of medications orally, subcutaneously, and intramuscularly.

The registered nurse can perform the tasks that an licensed practical nurse can perform and is responsible for assessment and planning care, initiating teaching, and administering medications intravenously.

   e. Provide directions that are clear, concise, accurate, and complete.
   f. Validate the person's understanding of the directions.
   g. Communicate a feeling of confidence to the delegate, and provide feedback promptly after the task is performed.
   h. Maintain continuity of care as much as possible when assigning client care.

XVI. TIME MANAGEMENT
A. Description
   1. Time management is a technique designed to assist in completing tasks within a definite time period.
   2. Learning how, when, and where to use one's time and establishing personal goals and time frames is part of time management.
   3. Time management requires an ability to anticipate the day's activities, to combine activities when possible, and to not be interrupted by nonessential activities.
   4. Time management involves efficiency in completing tasks as quickly as possible and effectiveness in deciding on the most important task to do and doing it correctly.

B. Principles and guidelines
   1. Identify tasks, obligations, and activities, and write them down.
   2. Organize the workday; identify which tasks must be completed in specified time frames.
   3. Prioritize client needs according to importance.
   4. Anticipate the needs of the day, and provide time for unexpected and unplanned tasks that may arise.
   5. Focus on beginning the daily tasks working on the most important first while keeping goals in mind; look at the final goal for the day, which will help you break down tasks into manageable parts.
   6. Begin client rounds at the beginning of the shift, collecting data on each assigned client.
   7. Delegate tasks when appropriate.
   8. Keep a daily hour-by-hour log to assist in providing structure to the tasks that must be accomplished, and cross tasks off the list as you accomplish them.
   9. Use hospital resources wisely, anticipating resource needs, and gather the necessary supplies before beginning the task.
   10. Organize paperwork and continuously document task completion and necessary client data throughout the day.
   11. At the end of the day, evaluate the effectiveness of time management.

XVII. PRIORITIZING CARE
A. **Prioritizing** is deciding which needs or problems require immediate action and which ones could be delayed until a later time because they are not urgent.
B. Guidelines for **prioritizing** (Box 8-8)
C. Setting priorities for client teaching
   1. Determine client's immediate needs.
   2. Review the learning objectives established for the client.
   3. Determine what the client perceives as important.
   4. Assess the client's anxiety level and the time available to teach.
D. **Prioritizing** when caring for a group of clients
   1. Identify the problems of each client.
   2. Review nursing diagnoses.
   3. Determine which client problems are most urgent based on basic needs, the client's changing or unstable status, and complexity of the client's problem.
   4. Anticipate the time that it may take to care for the priority needs of the clients.
   5. Combine activities if possible to resolve more than one problem at a time.
   6. Involve the client in the care as much as possible.

XVIII. DISASTERS AND DISASTER PLANNING
A. Description
   1. A disaster is any human-made or natural event that causes destruction and devastation that cannot be alleviated without assistance (Box 8-9).

BOX 8-8

Guidelines for Prioritizing

The nurse and the client mutually rank the client's needs in order of importance based on the client's physical and psychological needs, safety, and the client's own needs and expectations; what the client sees as his or her priority needs may be different from what the nurse sees as the priority.

Priorities are classified as high, intermediate, or low.

Client needs that are life threatening or that could result in harm to the client if they are left untreated are high priorities.

Nonemergency and non–life-threatening client needs are intermediate priorities.

Client needs that are not related directly to the client's illness or prognosis are low priorities.

When providing care, the nurse needs to decide which needs or problems require immediate action and which ones could be delayed until a later time because they are not urgent.

The nurse considers client problems that involve actual or life-threatening concerns before potential health-threatening concerns.

When prioritizing care, the nurse must consider time constraints and available resources.

Problems identified as important by the client must be given high priority.

The nurse can use the ABCs—airway, breathing, and circulation—as a guide when determining priorities; client needs related to maintaining a patent airway are always the priority.

The nurse can use Maslow's hierarchy of needs theory as a guide to determine priorities and identify the levels of physiological needs; safety; love and belonging; self-esteem; and self-actualization (basic needs are met before moving to other needs in the hierarchy).

The nurse can use the steps of the nursing process as a guide to determine priorities; remember that assessment is the first step of the nursing process.

BOX 8-9

Types of Disasters

HUMAN-MADE DISASTERS
Dam failures resulting in flooding
Hazardous substance accidents such as pollution, chemical spills, or toxic gas leaks
Radiological accidents
Resource shortages such as food, water, and electricity
Structural collapse, fire, or explosions
Terrorist attacks such as bombing, riots, and bioterrorism
Transportation accidents

NATURAL DISASTERS
Blizzards
Communicable disease epidemics
Cyclones
Droughts
Earthquakes
Floods
Forest fires
Hailstorms
Hurricanes
Landslides
Mudslides
Tidal waves
Tornadoes
Volcanic eruptions

---

2. Regarding a health care agency, a disaster can be external or internal: external disasters include those that occur outside of the health care agency, and internal disasters includes those that occur inside the health care agency.
3. A disaster preparedness plan is a formal plan of action for coordinating the response of health care agency staff in the event of a disaster in the health care agency or surrounding community.

B. American Red Cross (ARC)
   1. The ARC has been given **authority** by the federal government to provide disaster relief.
   2. All ARC disaster relief assistance is free, and local offices are located across the United States.
   3. The ARC participates with the government in developing and testing community disaster plans.
   4. The ARC identifies and trains personnel for disaster response.
   5. The ARC works with businesses and labor organizations to identify resources and persons for disaster work.
   6. The ARC educates the public about ways to prepare for a disaster.
   7. The ARC operates shelters, provides assistance to meet immediate emergency needs, and provides disaster health services including mental support.
   8. The ARC handles inquires from family members.
   9. The ARC coordinates relief activities with other agencies.
   10. Nurses are involved directly with the ARC and assume functions such as managers, supervisors, and educators of first aid; they also participate in disaster preparedness and disaster relief programs and provide services such as disaster relief, blood collection drives, and immunization programs.

C. Phases of disaster management
   1. The Federal Emergency Management Agency (FEMA) identifies four disaster management phases: mitigation, preparedness, response, and recovery.
   2. Mitigation encompasses the following:
      a. Actions or measures that can prevent the occurrence of a disaster or reduce the damaging effects of a disaster
      b. Determination of the community hazards and community risks (actual and potential threats) before a disaster occurs

c. Awareness of available community resources and community health personnel to facilitate mobilization of activities and minimize chaos and confusion if a disaster occurs

d. Determination of the resources available for care to infants, the older client, the disabled, and those with chronic health problems

3. Preparedness encompasses the following:

a. Plans for rescue, evacuation, and caring for disaster victims

b. Plans for training disaster personnel and gathering resources, equipment, and other materials needed for dealing with the disaster

c. Identification of specific responsibilities for various disaster response personnel

d. Establishment of a community disaster plan and an effective public communication system

e. Setting up of an emergency medical system and a plan for activation

f. Checking the proper functioning of emergency equipment

g. Making anticipatory provisions and setting up a location for food, water, clothing, shelter, other supplies, and needed medicine

h. Checking of supplies regularly and replenishment of outdated supplies

i. Practice of community disaster plans (mock disaster drills)

4. Response

a. Response includes putting disaster planning services into action and the actions taken to save lives and prevent further damage.

b. Primary concerns include safety, physical health, and mental health of the victims and the members of the disaster response team.

5. Recovery

a. Recovery includes actions taken to return to a normal situation following the disaster.

b. Recovery includes preventing debilitating effects and restoring personal, economic, and environmental health and stability to the community.

D. Levels of disaster: FEMA identifies three levels of disaster, and the level determines the response from FEMA (Box 8-10).

1. Once a federal emergency has been declared, the federal response plan may take effect and activate emergency support functions.

2. The emergency support functions of the ARC include sheltering, feeding, performing emergency first aid, providing a disaster welfare information system, and coordinating bulk distribution of emergency relief supplies.

3. Disaster medical assistant teams, teams of specially trained personnel, can be activated and sent to a disaster site to provide triage and medical care to victims until they can be evacuated to a hospital.

BOX 8-10

Levels of Disaster

LEVEL III DISASTER
A minor disaster that involves a minimal level of damage but could result in a presidential declaration of an emergency

LEVEL II DISASTER
A moderate disaster that likely will result in a presidential declaration of an emergency, with moderate federal assistance

LEVEL I DISASTER
A massive disaster that involves significant damage and results in a presidential disaster declaration, with major federal involvement and full engagement of federal, regional, and national resources

---

BOX 8-11

Emergency Plans and Supplies

Plan a meeting place for family members.
Identify where to go if an evacuation is necessary.
Determine when and how to turn off water, gas, and electricity at main switches.
Locate the safe spots in the home for each type of disaster.
Replace water supply every 3 months and food supply every 6 months.
Include the following supplies:
A 3-day supply of water (1 gallon per person per day)
A 3-day supply of nonperishable food
Clothing and blankets
A first aid kit
Adequate supply of prescription medication
Battery-operated radio
Flashlight and batteries
Credit card, cash, or traveler's checks
An extra set of car keys and a full tank of gas in the car
Sanitation supplies for washing, toileting, and for disposing of trash
An extra pair of eyeglasses
Special items for infants, the older client, or the disabled
Items needed for a pet such as food, water, and a leash
Important documents in a waterproof case

E. Nurse's role in disaster planning

1. Personal and professional preparedness

a. Make personal and family preparations (Box 8-11).

b. Be aware of the disaster plan at the place of employment and in the community.

c. Maintain certification in disaster training and in cardiopulmonary resuscitation.

d. Participate in mock disaster drills.

e. Prepare professional emergency response items such as a copy of the nursing license, personal health care equipment such as a stethoscope, cash, warm clothing, record-keeping materials, and other nursing care supplies.

2. Disaster response
   a. In the heath care agency setting, if a disaster occurs, the agency disaster preparedness plan (emergency response plan) is activated immediately, and the nurse responds by following the directions identified in the plan.
   b. In the community setting, if the nurse is the first responder to a disaster, the nurse would care for the victims by attending to those with life-threatening problems first; once rescue workers arrive at the scene, immediate plans for triage should begin.

F. Triage
   1. In a disaster or war, triage is classifying victims according to the severity of the injury, urgency of treatment, and place for treatment.
   2. In an emergency department, triage is classifying clients according to their need for care and establishing priorities of care; the kind of illness, the severity of the problem, and the resources available govern the process.

G. Triage rating systems: Various rating systems categories are used in clinical settings, and the nurse must be familiar with the rating system in the health care agency in which he or she is employed (Box 8-12).

H. Emergency department triage system
   1. A commonly used rating system in an emergency department is a three-tier system that uses the categories of emergent, urgent, and nonurgent and also may identify these categories by color coding or numbers (Box 8-13).
   2. The nurse needs to be familiar with the triage system of the health care agency.

BOX 8-12

Triage Rating Systems

FIVE-TIER SYSTEM (MOST OFTEN USED IN MILITARY TRIAGE)
Victim is dead or will die.
Life threatening (emergent): Victim has life-threatening injuries, but they are readily correctable.
Urgent: Victim must be treated within 1 to 2 hours.
Delayed (nonurgent): Victim is noncritical or ambulatory; victim has no injury and no treatment is necessary.
No injury: No treatment is necessary.

FOUR-TIER SYSTEM
Immediate (emergent): Victim is seriously injured but has a reasonable chance for survival.
Delayed (nonurgent): Victim can wait for care after simple first aid.
Expectant: Victim is extremely critical and dying.
Minimal (nonurgent): Victim has no impairment of function and can treat self or be treated by a nonprofessional.

THREE-TIER SYSTEM (COMMONLY USED IN HEALTH CARE AGENCIES)
Life threatening (emergent): Victim has life-threatening injuries, but they are readily correctable.
Urgent: Victim must be treated within 1 to 2 hours.
Delayed (nonurgent): Victim has no injury, is noncritical, or is ambulatory.

TWO-TIER SYSTEM
Immediate: Category includes victims who have life-threatening injuries that are readily correctable on the scene (emergent) and victims who must be treated within 1 to 2 hours (urgent).
Delayed (nonurgent): Category includes victims who have no injuries or noncritical injuries, are ambulatory, are dying, or are dead.

Adapted from *Mosby's medical, nursing, & allied health dictionary* (6th ed., p. 1747). (2002). St. Louis: Mosby.

BOX 8-13

Emergency Department Triage System

EMERGENT (RED): PRIORITY 1 (HIGHEST)
This classification is given to clients who have life-threatening injuries and need immediate attention and continuous evaluation yet have a high probability for survival once stabilized.
Such clients include those with trauma, chest pain, severe respiratory distress or cardiac arrest, limb amputation, acute neurological deficits, and those who sustained chemical splashes to the eyes

URGENT (YELLOW): PRIORITY 2
This classification is given to clients who require treatment and whose injuries have complications that are not life threatening, provided they are treated within 1 to 2 hours; these clients require continuous evaluation every 30 to 60 minutes thereafter.
Such clients include those with a simple fracture, asthma without respiratory distress, fever, hypertension, abdominal pain, or the client with a renal stone.

NONURGENT (GREEN): PRIORITY 3
This classification is given to clients with local injuries who do not have immediate complications and who can wait several hours for medical treatment; these clients require evaluation every 1 to 2 hours thereafter.
Such clients include those with conditions such as a minor laceration, sprain, or cold symptoms.

3. When caring for the client who has died, the nurse needs to recognize the importance of family rituals and provide support to loved ones.

4. Organ donation procedures of the health care agency need to be addressed if appropriate.

▲ I. Client assessment in the emergency department

1. Primary assessment

a. The purpose of primary assessment is to identify any client problem that poses an immediate or potential threat to life.

b. The nurse gathers information primarily through objective data, and on finding any abnormalities, immediately initiates interventions.

c. The nurse uses the ABCs—airway, breathing, and circulation—as a guide in assessing the client's needs and also assesses the client who sustained a traumatic injury for signs of a head injury or cervical spine injury.

2. Secondary assessment

a. The nurse performs secondary assessment following the primary assessment and after treatment for any problems identified.

b. Secondary assessment identifies any other life-threatening problems that the client might be experiencing.

c. The nurse obtains subjective and objective data, including a history, general overview, vital sign measurements, neurological assessment, pain assessment, and a complete or focused physical assessment.

PRACTICE QUESTIONS

1. The nurse is reviewing the critical paths of the clients on the nursing unit. In performing a variance analysis, which of the following would indicate the need for further action and analysis?
   1. A client's family attending a diabetic teaching session
   2. Canceling physical therapy sessions on the weekend
   3. Normal vital signs and absence of wound infection in a postoperative client
   4. A client demonstrating accurate medication administration following teaching

2. A new nursing graduate is attending an agency orientation regarding the nursing model of practice implemented in the facility. The nurse is told that the nursing model is a team nursing approach. The nurse understands that planning care delivery will be based on which characteristic of this type of nursing model of practice?
   1. A task approach method is used to provide care to clients.
   2. A single registered nurse (RN) is responsible for providing nursing care to a group of clients.

3. Managed care concepts and tools are used in providing client care.
   4. Nursing personnel are led by an RN leader in providing care to a group of clients.

3. The nurse manager has implemented a change in the method of the nursing delivery system from functional to team nursing. A nursing assistant is resistant to the change and is not taking an active part in facilitating the process of change. Which of the following would be the best approach in dealing with the nursing assistant?
   1. Ignore the resistance.
   2. Exert coercion with the nursing assistant.
   3. Provide a positive reward system for the nursing assistant.
   4. Confront the nursing assistant to encourage verbalization of feelings regarding the change.

4. The registered nurse (RN) is planning the client assignments for the day. Which of the following is the most appropriate assignment for the nursing assistant?
   1. A client with difficulty swallowing food and fluids
   2. A client who requires urine specimen collections
   3. A client requiring a colostomy irrigation
   4. A client receiving continuous tube feedings

5. The registered nurse (RN) employed in a long-term care facility is planning assignments for the clients on a nursing unit. The RN needs to assign four clients and has a licensed practical (vocational) nurse and three nursing assistants on a nursing team. Which of the following clients would the nurse most appropriately assign to the licensed practical (vocational) nurse?
   1. The client who requires a bed bath
   2. An older client requiring frequent ambulation
   3. A client who requires a Fleet enema
   4. A client with an abdominal wound requiring wound irrigations and dressing changes every 3 hours

6. The registered nurse (RN) has received the assignment for the day shift. After making initial rounds and checking all of the assigned clients, which client will the RN plan to care for first?
   1. A client who is ambulatory
   2. A client with a fever who is diaphoretic and restless
   3. A client scheduled for physical therapy at 1 PM
   4. A postoperative client who has just received pain medication

7. The nurse is assigned to care for four clients. In planning client rounds, which client would the nurse assess first?
   1. A client receiving oxygen via nasal cannula who had difficulty breathing during the previous shift
   2. A postoperative client preparing for discharge
   3. A client scheduled for a chest x-ray
   4. A client requiring daily dressing changes

8. The nurse is giving a bed bath to an assigned client. A nursing assistant enters the client's room and tells

the nurse that another assigned client is in pain and needs pain medication. The most appropriate nursing action is which of the following?

1. Finish the bed bath and then administer the pain medication to the other client.
2. Cover the client, raise the side rails, tell the client that you will return shortly, and administer the pain medication to the other client.
3. Ask the nursing assistant to tell the client in pain that medication will be administered as soon as the bed bath is complete.
4. Ask the nursing assistant to find out when the last pain medication was given to the client.

9. The home health care nurse is planning client visits for the day. The nurse is assigned to admit a client who was discharged yesterday from the hospital following a diagnosis of pneumonia. The nurse also is scheduled to visit a client requiring twice daily abdominal dressing changes. The third client to be seen is a client whose spouse is performing daily dressing changes, and the nurse needs to supervise the spouse in performing the dressing change. The fourth client to be seen will be visited by a home health aide at 10 AM, and the nurse needs to orient the aide and provide supervision of client care. The nurse begins the visits at 9 AM. All clients live within a 5-mile radius. How would the nurse plan the order of the assignments for the day?

1. Client being visited by the home health aide, the client requiring admission, the client regarding supervision of the dressing change, client requiring twice daily dressing changes, client requiring the second twice daily dressing change
2. The client requiring admission, the client regarding supervision of the dressing change, client requiring twice daily dressing changes, client being visited by the home health aide, client requiring the second twice daily dressing change
3. Client being visited by the home health aide, client requiring twice daily dressing changes, the client requiring admission, the client regarding supervision of the dressing change, client requiring the second twice daily dressing change
4. Client requiring twice daily dressing changes, client being visited by the home health aide, the client regarding supervision of the dressing change, the client requiring admission, client requiring the second twice daily dressing change

10. A nurse employed in an emergency department is assigned to triage clients arriving to the emergency room for treatment on the evening shift. The nurse would assign highest priority to which of the following clients?

1. A client with chest pain who states that he just ate pizza that was made with a very spicy sauce
2. A client with a minor laceration on the index finger sustained while cutting an eggplant
3. A client complaining of muscle aches, a headache, and malaise
4. A client who twisted her ankle when she fell while rollerblading

CRITICAL THINKING: FILL IN THE BLANK

The nurse on the day shift is assigned to care for three clients. One client has a tracheostomy and is on a mechanical ventilator. Another client is scheduled for a cardiac catheterization at 10 AM, and the other client was newly diagnosed with diabetes mellitus and is scheduled for discharge to home. Following report from the night shift, which client will the nurse plan to assess first?

Answer: _____

ANSWERS

1. **2**

Rationale: Variances are actual deviations or detours from the critical paths. Variances can be positive or negative, avoidable or unavoidable, and can be caused by a variety of things. Positive variance occurs when the client achieves maximum benefit and is discharged earlier than anticipated. Negative variance occurs when untoward events prevent a timely discharge. Variance analysis occurs continually ito anticipate and recognize negative variance early so that appropriate action can be taken.

Test-Taking Strategy: Use the process of elimination noting the key words "indicate the need for further action and analysis." Options 1, 3, and 4 identify positive outcomes. Option 2 identifies a negative outcome. Review the purpose of variance analysis if you had difficulty with this question.

Level of Cognitive Ability: Analysis
Client Needs: Safe, Effective Care Environment
Integrated Process: Nursing Process—evaluation

Content Area: Leadership/Management
Reference: Potter, P., & Perry, A. (2001). *Fundamentals of nursing* (5th ed., p. 512). St. Louis: Mosby

2. **4**

Rationale: In team nursing, nursing personnel are led by an registered nurse leader in providing care to a group of clients. Option 1 identifies functional nursing. Option 2 identifies primary nursing. Option 3 identifies a component of case management.

Test-Taking Strategy: Note that the issue of the question relates to team nursing. Keep this issue in mind and use the process of elimination. Option 4 is the only option that identifies the concept of a team approach. Review the various types of nursing delivery systems if you had difficulty with this question.

Level of Cognitive Ability: Analysis
Client Needs: Safe, Effective Care Environment
Integrated Process: Nursing Process—planning
Content Area: Leadership/Management

Reference: Potter, P., & Perry, A. (2001). *Fundamentals of nursing* (5th ed., pp. 70-71, 353). St. Louis: Mosby.

3. 4

Rationale: Confrontation is an important strategy to meet resistance head-on. Face-to-face meetings to confront the issue at hand will allow verbalization of feelings, identification of problems and issues, and development of strategies to solve the problem. Option 1 will not address the problem. Option 2 may produce additional resistance. Option 3 may provide a temporary solution to the resistance but will not address the concern specifically.

Test-Taking Strategy: Use the process of elimination. Options 1 and 2 easily can be eliminated first. From the remaining options, select option 4 over option 3 because this option specifically addresses the issue and would provide problem-solving measures. If you had difficulty with this question, review the strategies associated with dealing with resistance to change.

Level of Cognitive Ability: Application
Client Needs: Safe, Effective Care Environment
Integrated Process: Nursing Process—implementation
Content Area: Leadership/Management
Reference: Potter, P., & Perry, A. (2001). *Fundamentals of nursing* (5th ed., p. 462). St. Louis: Mosby.

4. 2

Rationale: The nurse must determine the most appropriate assignment based on the skills of the staff member and the needs of the client. In this case, the most appropriate assignment for a nursing assistant would be to care for the client who requires urine specimen collections. The nursing assistant is skilled in this procedure. The client with difficulty swallowing food and fluids is at risk for aspiration. Colostomy irrigations and tube feedings are not performed by unlicensed personnel.

Test-Taking Strategy: Note the key words "most appropriate." Use the process of elimination, recalling the principles of delegation and supervision of the work of others. Remember that work that is delegated to others must be consistent with the individual's level of expertise and licensure or lack of licensure. Review the principles of delegation if you had difficulty with this question.

Level of Cognitive Ability: Application
Client Needs: Safe, Effective Care Environment
Integrated Process: Nursing Process—planning
Content Area: Delegating/Prioritizing
Reference: Potter, P., & Perry, A. (2001). *Fundamentals of nursing* (5th ed., p. 359). St. Louis: Mosby.

5. 4

Rationale: When delegating nursing assignments, the nurse needs to consider the skills and educational level of the nursing staff. Collecting a 24-hour urine sample, giving a bed bath and assisting with frequent ambulation, and administering enemas can be provided most appropriately by the nursing assistant. The licensed practical (vocational nurse) is skilled in wound irrigations and dressing changes and most appropriately would be assigned to the client who needs this care.

Test-Taking Strategy: Use the process of elimination and knowledge regarding the principles of delegation and assignment making. Recall that education and job position as described by the nurse practice act and employee guidelines needs to be considered when delegating activities and making assignments. Options 1, 2, and 3 easily can be eliminated because a nursing assistant can perform these tasks. If you had difficulty with this question, review the principles of delegation and assignment making.

Level of Cognitive Ability: Application
Client Needs: Safe, Effective Care Environment
Integrated Process: Nursing Process—planning
Content Area: Delegating/Prioritizing
Reference: Potter, P., & Perry, A. (2001). *Fundamentals of nursing* (5th ed., pp. 37-38, 383). St. Louis: Mosby.

6. 2

Rationale: The RN would plan to care for the client who has a fever and is diaphoretic and restless first because this client's needs are the priority. Waiting for pain medication to take effect before providing care to the postoperative client is best. The client who is ambulatory and the client scheduled for physical therapy later in the day do not have priority needs related to care.

Test-Taking Strategy: Use the process of elimination and principles related to prioritizing. Noting the key words "diaphoretic and restless" will assist in directing you to this option. Review the principles related to prioritizing if you had difficulty with this question.

Level of Cognitive Ability: Application
Client Needs: Safe, Effective Care Environment
Integrated Process: Nursing Process—planning
Content Area: Delegating/Prioritizing
Reference: Potter, P., & Perry, A. (2001). *Fundamentals of nursing* (5th ed., p. 280). St. Louis: Mosby.

7. 1

Rationale: Airway is always a high priority, and the nurse would attend to the client who has been experiencing an airway problem first. The clients described in options 2, 3, and 4 have needs that would be identified as intermediate priorities.

Test-Taking Strategy: Use Maslow's hierarchy of needs theory and the ABCs airway, breathing, and circulation to answer the question. Remember that airway is always the first priority. Review principles related to prioritizing if you had difficulty with this question.

Level of Cognitive Ability: Application
Client Needs: Safe, Effective Care Environment
Integrated Process: Nursing Process—planning
Content Area: Delegating/Prioritizing
Reference: Potter, P., & Perry, A. (2001). *Fundamentals of nursing* (5th ed., pp. 92, 327). St. Louis: Mosby.

8. 2

Rationale: The nurse is responsible for the care provided to the assigned clients. The most appropriate action is to provide safety to the client who is receiving the bed bath and prepare to administer the pain medication. Options 1 and 3 delay the administration of medication to the client in pain. Option 4 is not a responsibility of the nursing assistant.

Test-Taking Strategy: Use the process of elimination and principles related to priorities of care. Options 1 and 3 delay the administration of pain medication, and option 4 is not a responsibility of the nursing assistant. The most appropriate action is to plan to administer the medication. Review principles related to priorities of care if you had difficulty with this question.
Level of Cognitive Ability: Application
Client Needs: Safe, Effective Care Environment
Integrated Process: Nursing Process—implementation
Content Area: Delegating/Prioritizing
References: Jarvis, C. (2000). *Physical examination and health assessment* (3rd ed., p. 903). Philadelphia: W. B. Saunders. Potter, P., & Perry, A. (2001). *Fundamentals of nursing* (5th ed., p. 1028). St. Louis: Mosby.

9. **4**
Rationale: The nurse would plan to see the client requiring twice daily dressing changes first because the dressing changes should be spaced as far apart as possible. The nurse next would plan to see the client being visited by the home health aide and provide instructions and directions to the home health aide regarding care to the client. The nurse then would visit the client regarding supervision of the dressing change and would perform the admission last because that may take more time than the other clients. The nurse then would return to the client regarding the second twice daily dressing.
Test-Taking Strategy: Use the process of elimination, noting the needs of the client and the role of the nurse in caring for each of the clients. Noting that the client requiring twice daily dressing changes will need to be seen twice will assist in directing you to the correct option. This client should be seen first because dressing changes should be spaced as far apart as possible. If you had difficulty with this question, review the process of planning care and time management.
Level of Cognitive Ability: Application
Client Needs: Safe, Effective Care Environment
Integrated Process: Nursing Process—planning
Content Area: Delegating/Prioritizing
References: Jarvis, C. (2000). *Physical examination and health assessment* (3rd ed., p. 903). Philadelphia: W. B. Saunders. Lewis, S., Heitkemper, M., & Dirksen, S. (2004). *Medical-surgical nursing: Assessment and management of clinical problems* (6th ed., p. 1846). St. Louis: Mosby.

10. **1**
Rationale: In an emergency department, triage is classifying clients according to their need for care and includes establishing priorities of care. The kind of illness, the severity of the problem, and the resources available govern the process. Clients with trauma, chest pain, severe respiratory distress or cardiac arrest, limb amputation, acute neurological deficits, and those who sustained chemical splashes to the eyes are classified as emergent and are the number 1 priority. Clients with conditions such as a simple fracture, asthma without respiratory distress, fever, hypertension, abdominal pain, or the client with a renal stone have urgent needs and are classified as number 2 priority. Clients with conditions such as a minor laceration, sprain, or cold symptoms are classified as nonurgent and are the number 3 priority.
Test-Taking Strategy: Note the key words "highest priority." Use the ABCs—airway, breathing, and circulation—to direct you to option 1. A client experiencing chest pain is always classified as priority number 1 until a myocardial infarction has been ruled out. Review the triage classification system commonly used in a hospital emergency department if you had difficulty with this question.
Level of Cognitive Ability: Application
Client Needs: Safe, Effective Care Environment
Integrated Process: Nursing Process—implementation
Content Area: Delegating/Prioritizing
Reference: Lewis, S., Heitkemper, M., & Dirksen, S. (2004). *Medical-surgical nursing: Assessment and management of clinical problems* (6th ed., p. 1846). St. Louis: Mosby.

CRITICAL THINKING: FILL IN THE BLANK
Answer: The client that has a tracheostomy and is on a mechanical ventilator.
Rationale: Airway is always a high priority, and the nurse would assess the client who has a tracheostomy and is on a mechanical ventilator first. The nurse next would assess the client scheduled for the cardiac catheterization, followed by the client scheduled for discharge.
Test-Taking Strategy: Use Maslow's hierarchy of needs theory and the ABCs—airway, breathing, and circulation. Focus only on the data identified in the question. Remember that airway is always the first priority. Review principles related to prioritizing if you had difficulty with this question.
Level of Cognitive Ability: Application
Client Needs: Safe, Effective Care Environment
Integrated Process: Nursing Process—planning
Content Area: Delegating/Prioritizing
Reference: Jarvis, C. (2000). *Physical examination and health assessment* (3rd ed., p. 902). Philadelphia: W. B. Saunders.

REFERENCES

Harkreader, H., & Hogan, M. A. (2004). *Fundamentals of nursing: caring and clinical judgment.* (2nd ed.). Philadelphia: W. B. Saunders.

Jarvis, C. (2000). *Physical examination and health assessment* (3rd ed.). Philadelphia: W. B. Saunders.

Lewis, S., Heitkemper, M., & Dirksen, S. (2004). *Medical-surgical nursing: Assessment and management of clinical problems* (6th ed.). St. Louis: Mosby.

Mosby's medical, nursing, & allied health dictionary (6th ed.). (2002). St. Louis: Mosby.

National Council of State Boards of Nursing (Eds.). (2003). *Test Plan for the National Council Licensure Examination for Registered Nurses* (effective date: April 2004). Chicago: Author.

Potter, P., & Perry, A. (2001). *Fundamentals of nursing* (5th ed.). St. Louis: Mosby.

Stanhope, M., & Lancaster, J. (2002). *Foundations of community health nursing: Community-oriented practice.* St. Louis: Mosby.

Nursing Sciences

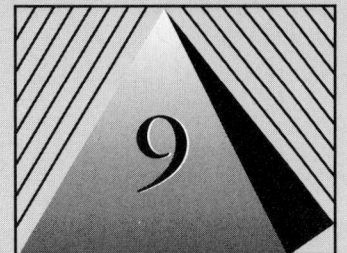

Fluids and Electrolytes

PYRAMID TERMS

fluid volume deficit Dehydration in which the fluid intake of the body is not sufficient to meet the fluid needs of the body.

fluid volume excess Fluid intake or fluid retention that exceeds the fluid needs of the body. Also called overhydration or fluid overload.

homeostasis The tendency of biological systems to maintain relatively constant conditions in the internal environment while continuously interacting with and adjusting to changes originating within or outside the system.

hypercalcemia A serum calcium level that exceeds 10 mg/dL

hyperkalemia A serum potassium level that exceeds 5.1 mEq/L

hypermagnesemia A serum magnesium level that exceeds 2.6 mg/dL.

hypernatremia A serum sodium level that exceeds 145 mEq/L

hyperphosphatemia A serum phosphorus level that exceeds 4.5 mg/dL

hypocalcemia A serum calcium level less than 8.6 mg/dL

hypokalemia A serum potassium level less than 3.5 mEq/L

hypomagnesemia A serum magnesium level less than 1.6 mg/dL.

hyponatremia A serum sodium level less than 135 mEq/L

hypophosphatemia A serum phosphorus level less than 2.7 mg/dL

▲ THE PYRAMID TO SUCCESS

Pyramid Points focus primarily on the assessment of a fluid and electrolyte imbalance, interventions, and evaluating the expected outcomes. Fluids and electrolytes constitute a content area that is sometimes complex and difficult to understand. The nurse must understand cell functions and properties and the concepts related to body fluids as outlined in this chapter. Review this content. Pyramid Points focus on the common fluid and electrolyte disturbances. As you review this content, focus on the Pyramid Points related to the causes, assessment findings, and related treatments. In any fluid or electrolyte imbalance, nursing interventions include monitoring the significant laboratory results and monitoring the client's cardiovascular, respiratory, gastrointestinal, neuromuscular, renal, and central nervous system status. Integrated Processes addressed in this chapter are Nursing Process, Caring, Communication and Documentation, and Teaching/Learning.

CLIENT NEEDS ▲
Safe, Effective Care Environment

Accident prevention and protection and safety of the client when an imbalance exists, particularly when changes in cardiovascular, respiratory, gastrointestinal, neuromuscular, renal, or central nervous systems occur, or when the client is at risk for complications such as seizures, respiratory depression, or dysrhythmias

Consultation with members of the health care team

Establishing priorities

Handling hazardous and infectious materials to prevent injury to health care personnel and others

Medical and surgical asepsis and prevention of infection in the client when samples for laboratory studies are obtained or when intravenous solutions are administered

Standard, transmission-based, and other precautions to prevent transmission of infection to self and others

Health Promotion and Maintenance

Health screening and the potential risk for a fluid and electrolyte imbalance

Education related to medication and diet management

Education related to the potential risk for a fluid and electrolyte imbalance, measures to prevent an imbalance, signs and symptoms of an imbalance, and actions to take if signs and symptoms develop

Psychosocial Integrity

Provision of support and continuously informing the client of the purposes for prescribed interventions

Provision of reassurance for the client who is experiencing a fluid or electrolyte imbalance

Physiological Integrity

Assistance in managing emergencies

Identification of clients who are at risk for a fluid or electrolyte imbalance

Identification of the expected and unexpected responses to therapeutic interventions and corresponding documentation

Monitoring for complications related to the imbalance

Monitoring of laboratory values

I. CONCEPTS OF FLUID AND ELECTROLYTE BALANCE

A. Electrolytes

1. Description: a substance that is dissolved in solution and some of its molecules split or dissociate into electrically charged atoms or ions (Box 9-1)
2. Measurement
   a. One uses the metric system to measure volumes of fluids: liters (L) or milliliters (mL).
   b. The unit of measure that expresses the combining activity of an electrolyte is the milliequivalent (mEq).
   c. One milliequivalent of any cation will always react chemically with one milliequivalent of an anion.
   d. Milliequivalents provide information about the number of anions or cations available to combine with other anions or cations.

B. Body fluid compartments

1. Description
   a. Fluid in each of the body compartments contains electrolytes.
   b. Each compartment has a particular composition of electrolytes, which differs from that of other compartments.
   c. To function normally, body cells must have fluids and electrolytes in the right compartments and in the right amounts.
   d. Whenever an electrolyte moves out of a cell, another electrolyte moves in to take its place.
   e. The numbers of cations and anions must be the same for **homeostasis** to exist.
   f. Compartments are separated by semipermeable membranes.
2. Intracellular compartment
   a. The intracellular compartment refers to all fluid inside the cells.
   b. Most of the body fluids are inside the cells.
3. The extracellular compartment is the fluid outside the cells.
4. The intravascular compartment is the fluid within blood vessels.
5. Interstitial fluids are fluids between the cells and blood vessels.

C. Third-spacing

1. Third-spacing is the accumulation and sequestration of trapped extracellular fluid in an actual or potential body space as a result of disease or injury.

BOX 9-1

Properties of Electrolytes and Their Components

ATOM

An atom is the smallest part of an element that still has the properties of the element.

The atom is composed of particles known as the proton (positive charge), neutron (neutral), and electron (negative charge).

Protons and neutrons are in the nucleus of the atom; therefore the nucleus is positively charged.

Electrons carry a negative charge and revolve around the nucleus.

As long as the number of electrons is the same as the number of protons, the atom has no net charge; that is, it is neither positive nor negative.

Atoms may gain, lose, or share electrons and then no longer are neutral.

MOLECULE

A molecule is two or more atoms that combine to form a substance.

ION

An ion is an atom that carries an electrical charge because it has gained or lost electrons.

Some ions carry a negative electrical charge, and some carry a positive charge.

CATION

A cation is an ion that carries a positive charge and has given away or lost electrons.

The result is fewer electrons than protons, and the result is a positive charge.

ANION

An anion is an ion that has gained electrons and therefore carries a negative charge.

When an ion has gained or taken on electrons, it assumes a negative charge and the result is a negatively charged ion.

2. The trapped fluid represents a volume loss and is unavailable for normal physiological processes.
3. Fluid may be trapped in body spaces such as the pericardial, pleural, peritoneal, or joint cavities; the bowel; or the abdomen; or within soft tissues after trauma or burns.
4. Assessing the intravascular fluid loss is difficult; the loss may not be reflected in weight changes or intake and output records and may not become apparent until after organ malfunction occurs.

D. Edema
1. Edema is an excess accumulation of fluid in the interstitial spaces.
2. Localized edema occurs as a result of traumatic injury from accidents or surgery, local inflammatory processes, or burns.
3. Generalized edema, also called anasarca, is an excessive accumulation of fluid in the interstitial space throughout the body as a result of a condition such as cardiac, renal, or liver failure.

E. Body fluid
1. Description
   a. Body fluid provides transportation of nutrients to the cells and carries waste products from the cells.
   b. Total body fluid amounts to about 60% of body weight.
   c. A loss of 10% of body fluid in the adult is serious.
   d. A loss of 20% of the body fluid in the adult is fatal.
2. Constituents of body fluids
   a. Body fluids consist of water and dissolved substances.
   b. The largest single fluid constituent of the body is water.
   c. Some substances, such as glucose, urea, and creatinine, do not dissociate in solution; that is, they do not separate from their complex forms into simpler substances when they are in solutions.
   d. Other substances do dissociate; for example, when sodium chloride is in a solution, it dissociates or separates into two parts or elements.

F. Body fluid transport
1. Diffusion
   a. Diffusion is the movement of particles in all directions through a solution.
   b. Diffusion is the process by which a solute (substance that is dissolved) may spread through a solution or solvent (solution in which the solute is dissolved).
   c. Diffusion of a solute will spread the molecules from an area of high concentration to an area of lower concentration.
   d. A permeable membrane will allow substances to pass through it without restriction.
   e. A selectively permeable membrane will allow some solutes to pass through without restriction but will prevent other solutes from passing freely.
   f. Diffusion occurs within fluid compartments and from one compartment to another, if the barrier between the compartments is permeable to the diffusing substances.
2. Osmosis
   a. Osmotic pressure is the force that draws the water from a less concentrated solution through a selectively permeable membrane into a more concentrated solution.
   b. If a membrane is permeable to water but not to all the solutes present, the membrane is a selective or semipermeable membrane.
   c. When the solvent or water moves across the membrane, the process is called osmosis.
   d. Osmosis is the diffusion of solvent molecules across a membrane in response to a concentration gradient, usually from a solution of lesser to one of greater solute concentration.
   e. When a more concentrated solution is on one side of a selectively permeable membrane and a less concentrated solution is on the other side, a pull called osmotic pressure draws the water through the membrane to the more concentrated side or the side with more solute.
3. Filtration
   a. Filtration is the movement of solutes and solvents by hydrostatic pressure.
   b. The movement is from an area of greater pressure to an area of lesser pressure.
4. Hydrostatic pressure
   a. Hydrostatic pressure is the force exerted by the weight of a solution.
   b. When a difference exists in the hydrostatic pressure on two sides of a membrane, water and diffusible solutes move out of the solution that has the higher hydrostatic pressure by the process of filtration.
   c. At the arterial end of the capillary, the hydrostatic pressure is greater than the osmotic pressure; therefore fluids and diffusible solutes move out of the capillary.
   d. At the venous end the osmotic pressure or pull is greater than the hydrostatic pressure, and fluids and some solutes move into the capillary.
   e. The excess fluid and solutes remaining in the interstitial spaces are returned to the intravascular compartment by the lymph channels.
5. Osmolality
   a. Osmolality refers to the number of osmotically active particles per kilogram of water.
   b. In the body, osmotic pressure is measured in milliosmoles.

c. The normal osmolality of plasma is 280 to 294 milliosmoles per kilogram (mOsm/kg).

G. Movement of body fluid
1. Description
   a. Cell membranes separate the interstitial fluid from the intravascular fluid.
   b. Cell membranes are selectively permeable; that is, the cell membrane and the capillary wall will allow water and some solutes free passage through them.
   c. Several forces affect the movement of water and solutes through the walls of cells and capillaries.
   d. The greater the number of particles in the concentrated solution, the more pull exists to move the water through the membrane.
   e. If the body loses more electrolytes than fluids, as can happen in diarrhea, then the extracellular fluid will contain fewer electrolytes or less solute than the intracellular fluid.
   f. Fluids and electrolytes must be kept in balance for health; when they remain out of balance, death can occur.
2. Isotonic solutions (Table 9-1)
   a. When the solutions on both sides of a selectively permeable membrane have established equilibrium or are equal in concentration, they are then isotonic.
   b. An example of an isotonic solution is 0.9% sodium chloride, which is referred to as isotonic saline solution or normal saline solution.
   c. Isotonic solutions are isotonic to human cells, and thus very little osmosis occurs.
   d. Other solutions that are isotonic are 5% dextrose in water, 5% dextrose in 0.225% saline, and lactated Ringer's solution.
3. Hypotonic solutions (Table 9-1)
   a. When a solution contains a lower concentration of salt or solute than other solutions, the solution is hypotonic.
   b. A hypotonic solution has less salt or more water than an isotonic solution.
   c. Distilled water and 0.45% normal saline are examples of hypotonic solutions.

d. Hypotonic solutions are hypotonic to the cells; therefore osmosis would continue in an attempt to bring about balance or equality.
4. Hypertonic solutions (Table 9-1)
   a. A solution that has a higher concentration of solutes than another solution is a hypertonic solution.
   b. Hypertonic solutions include 10% dextrose in water, 5% dextrose in 0.9% saline, 5% dextrose in 0.45% saline, and 5% dextrose in lactated Ringer's solution.
5. Osmotic pressure
   a. Osmotic pressure is the force that draws the solvent from a solution with more solvent activity through a selectively permeable membrane to a solution with less solvent activity.
   b. The amount of osmotic pressure is determined by the relative number of particles of solute on the side of greater concentration.
   c. When the solutions on each side of a selectively permeable membrane are equal in concentration, they are isotonic.
   d. A hypotonic solution has less solute than an isotonic solution, whereas a hypertonic solution contains more solute.
   e. If the selectively permeable membrane will allow the solvent to pass through but will not allow the solute through freely, the solvent will move to the side of greater solute concentration.
6. Active transport
   a. If an ion is to move through a membrane from an area of low concentration to an area of high concentration, an active transport system is necessary.
   b. An active transport system moves molecules or ions against concentration and osmotic pressure.
   c. Metabolic processes in the cell supply the energy for active transport.
   d. Substances that are transported actively through the cell membrane include ions of sodium, potassium, calcium, iron, and hydrogen, some of the sugars, and the amino acids.

H. Body fluid excretion (Box 9-2)
1. Description
   a. Fluids leave the body by several routes, including the skin, lungs, gastrointestinal tract, and kidneys.

TABLE 9-1

Tonicity of Intravenous Fluids

Solution	Tonicity
0.45% saline (½ NS)	Hypotonic
0.9% saline (NS)	Isotonic
5% dextrose in water (5% D/W)	Isotonic
5% dextrose in 0.225% saline (5% D/¼ NS)	Isotonic
Lactated Ringer's solution	Isotonic
5% dextrose in lactated Ringer's solution	Hypertonic
5% dextrose in 0.45% saline (5% D/½ NS)	Hypertonic
5% dextrose in 0.9% saline (5% D/NS)	Hypertonic
10% dextrose in water (10% D/W)	Hypertonic

BOX 9-2

Daily Body Fluid Excretion

Skin by diffusion: 400 mL
Skin by perspiration: 100 mL
Lungs: 350 mL
Feces: 150 mL
Kidneys: 1500 mL

b. The kidneys excrete the largest quantity of fluid.

c. As long as all organs are functioning normally, the body is able to maintain balance in its fluid content.

2. Skin

a. Water is lost through the skin by diffusion in the amount of about 400 mL per day and by perspiration.

b. The amount of water lost by perspiration varies according to the temperature of the environment and of the body, but the average amount of loss is 100 mL per day.

c. Water lost through the skin by diffusion is called insensible loss (the individual is unaware of losing that water).

3. Lungs

a. Water is lost from the lungs through expired air that is saturated with water vapor.

b. The amount of water lost from the lungs varies with the rate and the depth of respiration.

c. The average amount of water lost from the lungs is about 350 mL per day.

d. Water lost from the lungs is called insensible loss.

4. Gastrointestinal tract

a. Large quantities of water are secreted into the gastrointestinal tract, but almost all of this fluid is reabsorbed.

b. A large volume of electrolyte-containing liquids moves into the gastrointestinal tract and then returns again into the extracellular fluid.

c. The average amount of water lost in the feces is 150 mL per day, equal to the amount of water gained through the oxidation of foods.

d. Severe diarrhea results in the loss of large quantities of fluids and electrolytes.

5. Kidneys

a. The kidneys play a major role in regulating fluid and electrolyte balance.

b. Normal kidneys can adjust the amount of water and electrolytes leaving the body.

c. The quantity of fluid excreted by the kidneys is determined by the amount of water ingested and the amount of waste and solutes excreted.

d. The usual urine output is about 1500 mL per day; however, this varies greatly depending on fluid intake, amount of perspiration, and other factors.

I. Body fluid replacement

1. Description: Water enters the body through three sources: orally ingested liquids, water in foods, and water formed by oxidation of foods.

2. Amounts

a. The average total amount of water taken into the body by all three sources is 2500 mL per day.

b. About 10 mL of water is released by the metabolism of each 100 calories of fat, carbohydrates, or proteins.

3. Electrolytes

a. Electrolytes are present in foods and liquids.

b. With a normal diet an excess of essential electrolytes is taken in and the unused electrolytes are excreted.

J. Maintaining fluid and electrolyte balance

1. Description

a. **Homeostasis** is a term that indicates the relative stability of the internal environment.

b. Concentration and composition of body fluids must be nearly constant.

c. In a client, when one of the substances is deficient, either fluids or electrolytes, the substance must be replaced normally by the intake of food and water or by therapy such as intravenous solutions and medications.

d. When the client has an excess of fluid or electrolytes, therapy is directed toward assisting the body to eliminate the excess.

2. The kidneys play a major role in controlling all types of balance in fluid and electrolytes.

3. The adrenal glands, through the secretion of aldosterone, also aid in controlling extracellular fluid volume by regulating the amount of sodium reabsorbed by the kidneys.

4. Antidiuretic hormone from the pituitary gland regulates the osmotic pressure of extracellular fluid by regulating the amount of water reabsorbed by the kidney.

II. FLUID VOLUME DEFICIT

A. Description

1. Dehydration occurs when the fluid intake of the body is not sufficient to meet the fluid needs of the body.

2. The goal of treatment is to restore fluid volume, replace electrolytes as needed, and eliminate the cause of the **fluid volume deficit.**

B. Types of fluid volume deficits

1. Isotonic dehydration

a. Water and dissolved electrolytes are lost in equal proportions.

b. Known as hypovolemia, isotonic dehydration is the most common type of dehydration.

c. Isotonic dehydration results in decreased circulating blood volume and inadequate tissue perfusion.

2. Hypertonic dehydration

a. Water loss exceeds electrolyte loss.

b. The clinical problems that occur result from alterations in the concentrations of specific plasma electrolytes.

c. Fluid moves from the intracellular compartment into the plasma and interstitial fluid spaces, causing cellular dehydration and shrinkage.

3. Hypotonic dehydration

a. Electrolyte loss exceeds water loss.

b. The clinical problems that occur result from fluid shifts between compartments, causing a decrease in plasma volume.

c. Fluid moves from the plasma and interstitial fluid spaces into the cells, causing a plasma volume deficit and causing the cells to swell.

▲ C. Causes of **fluid volume deficits**

1. Isotonic dehydration
   a. Inadequate intake of fluids and solutes
   b. Fluid shifts between compartments
   c. Excessive losses of isotonic body fluids

2. Hypertonic dehydration: conditions that increase fluid loss, such as excessive perspiration, hyperventilation, ketoacidosis, prolonged fevers, diarrhea, early-stage renal failure, and diabetes insipidus

3. Hypotonic dehydration
   a. Chronic illness
   b. Excessive fluid replacement (hypotonic)
   c. Renal failure
   d. Chronic malnutrition

▲ D. Assessment

1. Cardiovascular
   a. Thready, increased pulse rate
   b. Decreased blood pressure and orthostatic (postural) hypotension
   c. Flat neck and hand veins in dependent positions
   d. Diminished peripheral pulses

2. Respiratory: increased rate and depth of respirations

3. Neuromuscular
   a. Decreased central nervous system activity, from lethargy to coma
   b. Fever

4. Renal
   a. Decreased urinary output
   b. Increased specific gravity

5. Integumentary
   a. Dry skin
   b. Poor turgor, tenting present
   c. Dry mouth

6. Gastrointestinal
   a. Decreased motility and diminished bowel sounds
   b. Constipation
   c. Thirst

7. Hypotonic dehydration: skeletal muscle weakness

8. Hypertonic dehydration
   a. Hyperactive deep tendon reflexes
   b. Pitting edema

E. Interventions

1. Monitor cardiovascular, respiratory, neuromuscular, renal, integumentary, and gastrointestinal status.

2. Prevent further fluid losses and increase fluid compartment volumes to normal ranges.

3. Provide oral rehydration therapy if possible and intravenous (IV) fluid replacement if the dehydration is severe.

4. Generally, isotonic dehydration is treated with isotonic fluid solutions; hypertonic dehydration with hypotonic fluid solutions; and hypotonic dehydration with hypertonic fluid solutions.

5. Administer medications as prescribed to correct the cause and treat any symptoms, such as antidiarrheal, antimicrobial, antiemetic, or antipyretic medications.

6. Administer oxygen as prescribed.

7. Monitor electrolyte values and prepare to administer medication to treat an imbalance if present.

III. FLUID VOLUME EXCESS

A. Description

1. Fluid intake or fluid retention exceeds the fluid needs of the body.

2. **Fluid volume excess** also is called overhydration or fluid overload.

3. The goal of treatment is to restore fluid balance, correct electrolyte imbalances if present, and eliminate or control the underlying cause of the overload.

B. Types

1. Isotonic overhydration
   a. Known as hypervolemia, isotonic overhydration results from excessive fluid in the extracellular fluid compartment.
   b. Only the extracellular fluid compartment is expanded, and fluid does not shift between the extracellular and intracellular compartments.
   c. Isotonic overhydration causes circulatory overload and interstitial edema; when severe or when it occurs in a client with poor cardiac function, congestive heart failure and pulmonary edema can result.

2. Hypertonic overhydration
   a. Occurrence of hypertonic overhydration is rare and is caused by an excessive sodium intake.
   b. Fluid is drawn from the intracellular fluid compartment; the extracellular fluid volume expands, and the intracellular fluid volume contracts.

3. Hypotonic overhydration
   a. Hypotonic overhydration is known as water intoxication.
   b. The excessive fluid moves into the intracellular space, and all body fluid compartments expand.
   c. Electrolyte imbalances occur as a result of dilution.

C. Causes

1. Isotonic overhydration
   a. Inadequately controlled IV therapy
   b. Renal failure
   c. Long-term corticosteroid therapy

2. Hypertonic overhydration
   a. Excessive sodium ingestion
   b. Rapid infusion of hypertonic saline
   c. Excessive sodium bicarbonate therapy

3. Hypotonic overhydration
   a. Early renal failure
   b. Congestive heart failure
   c. Syndrome of inappropriate antidiuretic hormone
   d. Inadequately controlled IV therapy
   e. Replacement of isotonic fluid loss with hypotonic fluids
   f. Irrigation of wounds and body cavities with hypotonic fluids

D. Assessment
   1. Cardiovascular
      a. Bounding, increased pulse rate
      b. Elevated blood pressure
      c. Distended neck and hand veins
      d. Elevated central venous pressure
   2. Respiratory
      a. Increased respiratory rate (shallow respirations)
      b. Dyspnea
      c. Moist crackles on auscultation
   3. Neuromuscular
      a. Altered level of consciousness
      b. Headache
      c. Visual disturbances
      d. Skeletal muscle weakness
      e. Paresthesias
   4. Integumentary
      a. Pitting edema in dependent areas
      b. Skin pale and cool to touch
   5. Increased motility in the gastrointestinal tract
   6. Isotonic overhydration
      a. Liver enlargement
      b. Ascites
   7. Hypotonic overhydration
      a. Polyuria
      b. Diarrhea
      c. Nonpitting edema
      d. Dysrhythmias
      e. Projectile vomiting
E. Interventions
   1. Monitor cardiovascular, respiratory, neuromuscular, renal, integumentary, and gastrointestinal status.
   2. Prevent further fluid overload, and restore normal fluid balance.
   3. Administer diuretics; osmotic diuretics typically are prescribed first to prevent severe electrolyte imbalances.
   4. Restrict fluid and sodium intake.
   5. Monitor intake and output and weight.
   6. Monitor electrolyte values, and prepare to administer medication to treat an imbalance if present.

IV. HYPONATREMIA
A. Description
   1. **Hyponatremia** is serum sodium level less than 135 mEq/L (Box 9-3).
   2. Sodium imbalances usually are associated with fluid volume imbalances.

BOX 9-3
Sodium

NORMAL VALUE
135 to 145 mEq/L

COMMON FOOD SOURCES
Bacon
Butter
Canned food
Cheese, such as American or cottage cheese
Frankfurters
Ketchup
Lunch meat
Milk
Mustard
Processed food
Snack food
Soy sauce
Table salt
White and whole-wheat bread

B. Causes
   1. Increased sodium excretion
      a. Excessive diaphoresis
      b. Diuretics
      c. Wound drainage, especially gastrointestinal
      d. Decreased secretion of aldosterone
      e. Renal disease
   2. Inadequate sodium intake
      a. Nothing by mouth
      b. Low-salt diet
   3. Dilution of serum sodium
      a. Excessive ingestion of hypotonic fluids or irrigation with hypotonic fluids
      b. Renal failure
      c. Freshwater drowning
      d. Syndrome of inappropriate antidiuretic hormone secretion
      e. Hyperglycemia
      f. Congestive heart failure
C. Assessment
   1. Cardiovascular
      a. Symptoms vary with changes in vascular volume
      b. Normovolemic: rapid pulse rate; normal blood pressure
      c. Hypovolemic: thready, weak, rapid pulse rate; hypotension; flat neck veins; normal or low central venous pressure
      d. Hypervolemic: rapid, bounding pulse; blood pressure normal or elevated; normal or elevated central venous pressure
   2. Respiratory: shallow, ineffective respiratory movements as a late manifestation related to skeletal muscle weakness
   3. Neuromuscular

a. Generalized skeletal muscle weakness that is worse in the extremities

b. Diminished deep tendon reflexes

4. Cerebral function

a. Headache

b. Personality changes

5. Gastrointestinal

a. Increased motility and hyperactive bowel sounds

b. Nausea

c. Abdominal cramping and diarrhea

6. Renal

a. Decreased specific gravity

b. Increased urinary output

D. Interventions

1. Monitor cardiovascular, respiratory, neuromuscular, cerebral, renal, and gastrointestinal status.

2. If **hyponatremia** is accompanied by a fluid deficit (hypovolemia), IV saline infusions are administered to restore sodium content and fluid volume.

3. If **hyponatremia** is accompanied by fluid excess (hypervolemia), osmotic diuretics are administered to promote the excretion of water rather than sodium.

4. If the cause is inappropriate or excessive secretion of antidiuretic hormone, medications that antagonize antidiuretic hormone, such as lithium and demeclocycline (Declomycin), may be administered.

5. Instruct client to increase oral sodium intake and inform the client about the foods to include in the diet (Box 9-3).

6. If the client is taking lithium, monitor lithium level because **hyponatremia** can cause diminished lithium excretion, resulting in toxicity.

V. HYPERNATREMIA

A. Description: **Hypernatremia** is a serum sodium level that exceeds 145 mEq/L (Box 9-3).

B. Causes

1. Decreased sodium excretion

a. Corticosteroids

b. Cushing's syndrome

c. Renal failure

d. Hyperaldosteronism

2. Increased sodium intake: excessive oral sodium ingestion or excessive administration of sodium-containing IV fluids

3. Decreased water intake: nothing by mouth

4. Increased water loss: increased rate of metabolism; fever; hyperventilation; infection; excessive diaphoresis; or watery diarrhea

C. Assessment

1. Cardiovascular: heart rate and blood pressure that respond to vascular volume status

2. Respiratory: pulmonary edema if hypervolemia is present

3. Neuromuscular

a. Early: spontaneous muscle twitches; irregular muscle contractions

b. Late: skeletal muscle weakness; deep tendon reflexes diminished or absent

4. Central nervous system

a. Altered cerebral function is the most common manifestation of **hypernatremia.**

b. Normovolemia or hypovolemia: agitation, confusion, seizures

c. Hypervolemia: lethargy, stupor, coma

5. Renal

a. Increased specific gravity

b. Decreased urinary output

6. Integumentary

a. Dry skin

b. Presence or absence of edema, depending on fluid volume changes

D. Interventions

1. Monitor cardiovascular, respiratory, neuromuscular, cerebral, renal, and integumentary status.

2. If the cause is fluid loss, prepare to administer IV infusions.

3. If the cause is inadequate renal excretion of sodium, prepare to administer diuretics that promote sodium loss.

4. Restrict sodium and fluid intake as prescribed (Box 9-3).

VI. HYPOKALEMIA

A. Description

1. **Hypokalemia** is a serum potassium level less than 3.5 mEq/L (Box 9-4).

2. Potassium deficit is potentially life threatening because every body system is affected.

B. Causes

1. Actual total body potassium loss

BOX 9-4

Potassium

NORMAL VALUE
3.5 mEq/L to 5.1 mEq/L

COMMON FOOD SOURCES
Avocado
Bananas
Cantaloupe
Carrots
Fish
Mushrooms
Oranges
Potatoes
Pork, beef, veal
Raisins
Spinach
Strawberries
Tomatoes

a. Excessive use of medications such as diuretics or corticosteroids

b. Increased secretion of aldosterone, such as in Cushing's syndrome

c. Vomiting; diarrhea

d. Wound drainage, particularly gastrointestinal

e. Prolonged nasogastric suction

f. Excessive diaphoresis

g. Renal disease impairing reabsorption of potassium

2. Inadequate potassium intake: nothing by mouth

3. Movement of potassium from the extracellular fluid to the intracellular fluid

a. Alkalosis

b. Hyperinsulinism

4. Dilution of serum potassium

a. Water intoxication

b. Intravenous therapy with potassium-poor solutions

C. Assessment

1. Cardiovascular

a. Thready, weak, irregular pulse

b. Peripheral pulses weak

c. Orthostatic hypotension

d. Electrocardiogram changes: ST depression; shallow, flat or inverted T wave; and prominent U wave (Table 9-2)

2. Respiratory

a. Shallow, ineffective respirations that result from profound weakness of the skeletal muscles of respiration

b. Diminished breath sounds

3. Neuromuscular

a. Anxiety, lethargy, confusion, coma

b. Skeletal muscle weakness; eventual flaccid paralysis

c. Loss of tactile discrimination

d. Deep tendon hyporeflexia

4. Gastrointestinal

a. Decreased motility, hypoactive to absent bowel sounds

b. Nausea, vomiting, constipation, abdominal distention

c. Paralytic ileus

5. Renal

a. Decreased specific gravity

b. Increased urinary output

D. Interventions

1. Monitor cardiovascular, respiratory, neuromuscular, gastrointestinal, and renal status, and place on a cardiac monitor.

2. Monitor electrolyte values.

3. Administer potassium supplements orally or intravenously as prescribed.

4. Oral potassium supplements

a. Oral potassium supplements may cause nausea and vomiting; they should not be taken on an empty stomach; if the client complains of abdominal pain, distention, nausea, vomiting, diarrhea, or gastrointestinal bleeding, the supplement may need to be discontinued.

b. Liquid potassium chloride has an unpleasant taste and should be taken with juice or another liquid.

5. Take the following precautions with intravenously administered potassium:

a. Potassium is never given by IV push or by the intramuscular or subcutaneous route.

b. A dilution of no more than 1 mEq/10 mL of solution is recommended.

c. After adding potassium to an IV solution, shake the bag and invert it to ensure that the potassium is distributed evenly throughout the IV solution.

d. The maximum recommended infusion rate is 5 to 10 mEq/hr, never to exceed 20 mEq/hr under any circumstances.

e. A client receiving more than 10 mEq/hr should be placed on a cardiac monitor and monitored for cardiac changes, and the infusion should be controlled by an infusion device.

f. Potassium infusion can cause phlebitis; therefore the nurse should assess the IV site frequently for signs of phlebitis or infiltration; if either of these occurs, the infusion is stopped immediately.

g. The nurse should assess renal function before administering potassium and monitor intake and output during administration.

6. Institute safety measures for the client experiencing muscle weakness.

7. If the client is taking a potassium-losing diuretic, it may be discontinued; a potassium-sparing diuretic may be prescribed.

8. Instruct client about foods that are high in potassium content (Box 9-4).

TABLE 9-2

Electrocardiographic Changes in Electrolyte Imbalances

Electrolyte Imbalance	Electrocardiographic Changes
Hypocalcemia	Prolonged ST interval
	Prolonged QT interval
Hypercalcemia	Shortened ST segment
	Widened T wave
Hypokalemia	ST depression
	Shallow, flat, or inverted T wave
	Prominent U wave
Hyperkalemia	Tall peaked T waves
	Flat P waves
	Widened QRS complex
	Prolonged PR interval
Hypomagnesemia	Tall T waves
	Depressed ST segment
Hypermagnesemia	Prolonged PR interval
	Widened QRS complexes

VII. HYPERKALEMIA

A. Description: **Hyperkalemia** is a serum potassium level that exceeds 5.1 mEq/L (Box 9-4).

B. Causes
1. Excessive potassium intake
   a. Overingestion of potassium-containing foods or medications such as potassium chloride or salt substitutes
   b. Rapid infusion of potassium-containing IV solutions
2. Decreased potassium excretion
   a. Potassium-sparing diuretics
   b. Renal failure
   c. Adrenal insufficiency, such as in Addison's disease
3. Movement of potassium from the intracellular fluid to the extracellular fluid
   a. Tissue damage
   b. Acidosis
   c. Hyperuricemia
   d. Hypercatabolism

C. Assessment
1. Cardiovascular
   a. Slow, weak, irregular heart rate
   b. Decreased blood pressure
   c. Electrocardiogram changes: tall peaked T waves; widened QRS complexes; prolonged PR intervals; and flat P waves (Table 9-2)
2. Respiratory: profound weakness of the skeletal muscles causes respiratory failure
3. Neuromuscular
   a. Early: muscle twitches, cramps, paresthesias (tingling and burning followed by numbness in the hands and feet and around the mouth)
   b. Late: profound weakness, ascending flaccid paralysis in the arms and legs (trunk, head, and respiratory muscles become affected when the serum potassium level reaches a lethal level)
4. Gastrointestinal
   a. Increased motility, hyperactive bowel sounds
   b. Diarrhea

D. Interventions
1. Monitor cardiovascular, respiratory, neuromuscular, renal, and gastrointestinal status; place client on a cardiac monitor.
2. Discontinue IV potassium (keep IV catheter patent), and hold oral potassium supplements.
3. Initiate a potassium-restricted diet.
4. Prepare to administer potassium-excreting diuretics if renal function is not impaired.
5. If renal function is impaired, prepare to administer sodium polystyrene sulfonate (Kayexalate), a cation exchange resin that promotes gastrointestinal sodium absorption and potassium excretion.
6. Prepare the client for dialysis if potassium levels are critically high.
7. Prepare for the IV administration of glucose with regular insulin to move excess potassium into the cells.
8. Monitor renal function.
9. When blood transfusions are prescribed for a client with a potassium imbalance, the client should receive fresh blood if possible; transfusions of stored blood may elevate the potassium level because the breakdown of older blood cells releases potassium.
10. Teach the client to avoid foods high in potassium (Box 9-4).
11. Instruct the client to avoid the use of salt substitutes or other potassium-containing substances.

VIII. HYPOCALCEMIA

A. Description: **Hypocalcemia** is a serum calcium level less than 8.6 mg/dL (Box 9-5).

B. Causes
1. Inhibition of calcium absorption from the gastrointestinal tract
   a. Inadequate oral intake of calcium
   b. Lactose intolerance
   c. Malabsorption syndromes such as celiac sprue or Crohn's disease
   d. Inadequate intake of vitamin D
   e. End-stage renal disease
2. Increased calcium excretion
   a. Renal failure, polyuric phase
   b. Diarrhea
   c. Steatorrhea
   d. Wound drainage, especially gastrointestinal
3. Conditions that decrease the ionized fraction of calcium
   a. Hyperproteinemia
   b. Alkalosis
   c. Medications such as calcium chelators or binders
   d. Acute pancreatitis
   e. **Hyperphosphatemia**
   f. Immobility
   g. Removal or destruction of the parathyroid glands

BOX 9-5

Calcium

NORMAL VALUE
8.6 to 10.0 mg/dL

COMMON FOOD SOURCES
Cheese
Collard greens
Milk and soy-milk
Rhubarb
Sardines
Spinach
Tofu
Yogurt, low-fat

C. Assessment
  1. Cardiovascular
     a. Decreased heart rate
     b. Hypotension
     c. Diminished peripheral pulses
     d. Electrocardiogram changes: prolonged ST interval; prolonged QT interval (Table 9-2)
  2. Respiratory: not directly affected; however, respiratory failure or arrest can result from decreased respiratory movement because of muscle tetany or seizures
  3. Neuromuscular
     a. Irritable skeletal muscles: twitches, cramps, tetany, seizures
     b. Painful muscle spasms in the calf or foot during periods of inactivity
     c. Paresthesias followed by numbness that may affect the lips, nose, and ears in addition to the limbs
     d. Positive Trousseau's and Chvostek's signs
     e. Hyperactive deep tendon reflexes
     f. Anxiety, irritability
  4. Gastrointestinal
     a. Increased gastric motility; hyperactive bowel sounds
     b. Abdominal cramping, diarrhea
D. Interventions
  1. Monitor cardiovascular, respiratory, neuromuscular, and gastrointestinal status; place client on a cardiac monitor.
  2. Administer calcium supplements orally or calcium intravenously.
  3. When administering calcium intravenously, warm injection to body temperature before administration; administer slowly; monitor for electrocardiogram changes; observe for infiltration; and monitor for **hypercalcemia.**
  4. Administer medications that increase calcium absorption.
     a. Aluminum hydroxide reduces serum phosphorus levels, causing the countereffect of increasing calcium levels.
     b. Vitamin D aids in the absorption of calcium from the intestinal tract.
  5. Provide a quiet environment to reduce environmental stimuli.
  6. Initiate seizure precautions.
  7. Move client carefully, and monitor for signs of a fracture.
  8. Keep 10% calcium gluconate available for treatment of acute calcium deficit.
  9. Instruct client to consume foods high in calcium (Box 9-5).

IX. HYPERCALCEMIA
A. Description: **Hypercalcemia** is a serum calcium level that exceeds 10 mg/dL (Box 9-5).

B. Causes
  1. Increased calcium absorption
     a. Excessive oral intake of calcium
     b. Excessive oral intake of vitamin D
  2. Decreased calcium excretion
     a. Renal failure
     b. Use of thiazide diuretics
  3. Increased bone resorption of calcium
     a. Hyperparathyroidism
     b. Hyperthyroidism
     c. Malignancy
     d. Immobility
     e. Use of glucocorticoids
  4. Hemoconcentration
     a. Dehydration
     b. Use of lithium
     c. Adrenal insufficiency
C. Assessment
  1. Cardiovascular
     a. Increased heart rate in early phase; bradycardia that can lead to cardiac arrest in late phases
     b. Increased blood pressure
     c. Bounding, full peripheral pulses
     d. Electrocardiogram changes: shortened ST segment; widened T wave (Table 9-2)
  2. Respiratory: ineffective respiratory movement as a result of profound skeletal muscle weakness
  3. Neuromuscular
     a. Profound muscle weakness
     b. Diminished or absent deep tendon reflexes
     c. Disorientation, lethargy, coma
  4. Renal
     a. Increased urinary output leading to dehydration
     b. Formation of renal calculi
  5. Gastrointestinal
     a. Decreased motility and hypoactive bowel sounds
     b. Anorexia, nausea, abdominal distention, constipation
D. Interventions
  1. Monitor cardiovascular, respiratory, neuromuscular, renal, and gastrointestinal status; place client on a cardiac monitor.
  2. Discontinue IV infusions of solutions containing calcium and oral medications containing calcium or vitamin D.
  3. Discontinue thiazide diuretics and replace with diuretics that enhance the excretion of calcium.
  4. Administer medications as prescribed that inhibit calcium resorption from the bone, such as phosphorus, calcitonin (Calcimar), biphosphonates (etidronate), and prostaglandin synthesis inhibitors (aspirin, nonsteroidal antiinflammatory drugs)
  5. Prepare the client with severe **hypercalcemia** for dialysis, if medications fail to reduce the serum calcium level.
  6. Move client carefully and monitor for signs of a fracture.

7. Monitor for flank or abdominal pain, and strain urine to check for the presence of urinary stones.
8. Instruct the client to avoid foods high in calcium (Box 9-5).

X. HYPOMAGNESEMIA

A. Description: **Hypomagnesemia** is a serum magnesium level less than 1.6 mg/dL (Box 9-6).
B. Causes
   1. Insufficient magnesium intake
      a. Malnutrition and starvation
      b. Vomiting or diarrhea
      c. Malabsorption syndrome
      d. Celiac disease
      e. Crohn's disease
   2. Increased magnesium secretion
      a. Medications such as diuretics
      b. Chronic alcoholism
   3. Intracellular movement of magnesium
      a. Hyperglycemia
      b. Insulin administration
      c. Sepsis
C. Assessment
   1. Cardiovascular
      a. Electrocardiogram changes: tall T waves; depressed ST segments (Table 9-2)
      b. Tachycardia
      c. Hypertension
   2. Gastrointestinal
      a. Decreased motility; decreased bowel sounds
      b. Anorexia, nausea, abdominal distention
   3. Respiratory: shallow respirations
   4. Neuromuscular
      a. Twitches; paresthesias
      b. Positive Trousseau's and Chvostek's signs

BOX 9-6

Magnesium

NORMAL VALUE
1.6 to 2.6 mg/dL

COMMON FOOD SOURCES
Avocado
Canned white tuna
Cauliflower
Cooked rolled oats
Green leafy vegetables such as spinach and broccoli
Low fat yogurt
Milk
Peanut butter
Peas
Pork, beef, chicken
Potatoes
Raisins

---

c. Hyperreflexia
d. Tetany; seizures
   5. Central nervous system
      a. Irritability
      b. Confusion
D. Interventions
   1. Monitor cardiovascular, gastrointestinal, respiratory, neuromuscular, and central nervous system status; place client on a cardiac monitor.
   2. Because **hypocalcemia** frequently accompanies **hypomagnesemia,** interventions also aim to restore normal serum calcium levels.
   3. Administer magnesium sulfate by the IV route in severe cases (intramuscular injections cause pain and tissue damage); monitor serum magnesium levels frequently.
   4. Initiate seizure precautions.
   5. Monitor for reduced deep tendon reflexes, suggesting **hypermagnesemia,** during administration of magnesium.
   6. Oral preparations of magnesium may cause diarrhea and increase magnesium loss.
   7. Instruct the client to increase the intake of foods that contain magnesium (Box 9-6).

XI. HYPERMAGNESEMIA

A. Description: **Hypermagnesemia** is a serum magnesium level that exceeds 2.6 mg/dL (Box 9-6).
B. Causes
   1. Increased magnesium intake
      a. Magnesium-containing antacids and laxatives
      b. Excessive administration of magnesium intravenously
   2. Decreased renal excretion of magnesium as a result of renal insufficiency
C. Assessment
   1. Cardiovascular
      a. Bradycardia, dysrhythmias
      b. Hypotension
      c. Electrocardiogram changes: prolonged PR interval; widened QRS complexes (Table 9-2)
   2. Respiratory: respiratory insufficiency when the skeletal muscles of respiration are involved
   3. Neuromuscular
      a. Diminished or absent deep tendon reflexes
      b. Skeletal muscle weakness
   4. Central nervous system: drowsiness and lethargy that progresses to coma
D. Interventions
   1. Monitor cardiovascular, respiratory, neuromuscular, and central nervous system status; place client on cardiac monitor.
   2. Diuretics are prescribed to increase renal excretion of magnesium.
   3. Intravenously administered calcium chloride or calcium gluconate may be prescribed to reverse the effects of magnesium on cardiac muscle.

4. Instruct the client to restrict dietary intake of magnesium-containing foods (Box 9-6).
5. Instruct the client to avoid the use of laxatives and antacids containing magnesium.

XII. HYPOPHOSPHATEMIA
A. Description
　1. **Hypophosphatemia** is a serum phosphorus level less than 2.7 mg/dL (Box 9-7).
　2. A decrease in the serum phosphorus level is accompanied by an increase in the serum calcium level.
B. Causes
　1. Insufficient phosphorus intake: malnutrition and starvation
　2. Increased phosphorus excretion
　　a. Hyperparathyroidism
　　b. Renal failure
　　c. Malignancy
　　d. Use of aluminum hydroxide-based or magnesium-based antacids
　3. Intracellular shift
　　a. Hyperglycemia
　　b. Respiratory alkalosis
C. Assessment
　1. Cardiovascular
　　a. Decreased contractility and cardiac output
　　b. Slowed peripheral pulses
　2. Respiratory: shallow respirations
　3. Neuromuscular
　　a. Weakness
　　b. Decreased deep tendon reflexes
　　c. Decreased bone density that can cause fractures and alterations in bone shape
　　d. Rhabdomyolysis
　4. Central nervous system
　　a. Irritability
　　b. Confusion
　　c. Seizures
　5. Hematological
　　a. Decreased platelet aggregation and increased bleeding
　　b. Immunosuppression

BOX 9-7

Phosphorus

NORMAL VALUE
2.7 to 4.5 mg/dL

COMMON FOOD SOURCES
Fish
Organ meats
Nuts
Pork, beef, chicken
Whole-grain breads and cereals

D. Interventions
　1. Monitor cardiovascular, respiratory, neuromuscular, central nervous system, and hematological status.
　2. Discontinue medications that contribute to **hypophosphatemia**.
　3. Administer phosphorus orally along with a vitamin D supplement.
　4. Administer phosphorus intravenously only when serum phosphorus levels fall below 1 mg/dL and when the client experiences critical clinical manifestations.
　5. Administer phosphorus intravenously slowly because of the risks associated with **hyperphosphatemia**.
　6. Assess renal system before administering phosphorus.
　7. Move client carefully, and monitor for signs of a fracture.
　8. Instruct client to increase intake of phosphorus-containing foods while decreasing the intake of calcium-containing foods (Boxes 9-5 and 9-7).

XIII. HYPERPHOSPHATEMIA
A. Description
　1. **Hyperphosphatemia** is a serum phosphorus level that exceeds 4.5 mg/dL (Box 9-7).
　2. Most body systems tolerate elevated serum phosphorus levels well.
　3. An increase in the serum phosphorus level is accompanied by a decrease in the serum calcium level.
　4. The problems that occur in **hyperphosphatemia** center on the **hypocalcemia** that results when serum phosphorus levels increase.
B. Causes
　1. Decreased renal excretion resulting from renal insufficiency
　2. Tumor lysis syndrome
　3. Increased intake of phosphorus, including dietary intake or overuse of phosphate-containing laxatives or enemas
　4. Hypoparathyroidism
C. Assessment: refer to assessment of **hypocalcemia**
D. Interventions
　1. Interventions entail the management of **hypocalcemia**.
　2. Administer phosphate-binding medications that increase fecal excretion of phosphorus by binding phosphorus from food in the gastrointestinal tract.
　3. Instruct client to avoid phosphate-containing medications, including laxatives and enemas.
　4. Instruct client to decrease the intake of food that is high is phosphorus (Box 1-7).
　5. Instruct client in how to take phosphate-binding medications, emphasizing that they should be taken with meals or immediately after meals.

PRACTICE QUESTIONS

1. A nurse is reading a physician's progress notes in the client's record and reads that the physician has documented "insensible fluid loss of approximately 800 mL daily." The nurse understands that this type of fluid loss can occur through
   1. The gastrointestinal tract.
   2. Urinary output.
   3. Wound drainage.
   4. The skin.

2. A nurse is assigned to care for a group of clients. On review of the clients' medical records, the nurse determines that which client is at risk for fluid volume deficit?
   1. A client with a colostomy
   2. A client receiving frequent wound irrigations
   3. A client with congestive heart failure
   4. A client with decreased kidney function

3. A nurse is caring for a client who has been taking diuretics on a long-term basis. The nurse suspects a fluid volume deficit. Which assessment finding would the nurse note in a client with this condition?
   1. Rales
   2. Increased blood pressure
   3. Decreased hematocrit
   4. Decreased central venous pressure (CVP)

4. A nurse is assigned to care for a group of clients. On review of the clients' medical records, the nurse determines that which client is at risk for a fluid volume excess?
   1. The client with renal failure
   2. The client with an ileostomy
   3. The client taking diuretics
   4. The client who requires gastrointestinal suctioning

5. The nurse is caring for a client with congestive heart failure. On assessment the nurse notes that the client is dyspneic and that rales are audible on auscultation. The nurse suspects fluid volume excess. What additional signs would the nurse expect to note in this client if fluid volume excess is present?
   1. A decreased central venous pressure (CVP)
   2. Flat neck and hand veins
   3. An increase in blood pressure
   4. Weight loss

6. A nurse is preparing to care for a client with a potassium deficit. The nurse reviews the client's record and determines that the client is at risk for developing the potassium deficit because the client
   1. Requires nasogastric suction.
   2. Has a history of renal disease.
   3. Has a history of Addison's disease.
   4. Is taking a potassium-sparing diuretic.

7. A nurse reviews a client's electrolyte laboratory report and notes that the potassium level is 3.2 mEq/L. Which of the following would the nurse note on the electrocardiogram as a result of the laboratory value?
   1. Elevated T waves
   2. Absent P waves
   3. Elevated ST segment
   4. U waves

8. A nurse prepares to administer potassium chloride intravenously as prescribed to a client with hypokalemia. Which of the following would not be a part of the nurse's plan regarding the preparation and administration of the potassium?
   1. Prepare the medication for bolus administration.
   2. Obtain a controlled IV infusion pump.
   3. Dilute in appropriate amount of normal saline.
   4. Monitor urine output during administration.

9. A nurse instructs a client at risk for hypokalemia about the foods high in potassium that should be included in the daily diet. The nurse determines that the client understands the food sources of potassium if the client states that the food item lowest in potassium is
   1. Spinach.
   2. Carrots.
   3. Avocado.
   4. Apples.

10. A nurse caring for a group of clients reviews the electrolyte laboratory results and notes a potassium level of 5.5 mEq/L on one client's laboratory reports. The nurse understands that which client is at most risk for the development of a potassium value at this level?
    1. The client who has sustained a traumatic burn
    2. The client with Cushing's syndrome
    3. The client with colitis
    4. The client who has been overusing laxatives

11. A nurse reviews the electrolyte results of an assigned client and notes that the potassium level is 5.4 mEq/L. Which of the following would the nurse expect to note on the electrocardiogram as a result of the laboratory value?
    1. Tall peaked T waves
    2. Prominent U wave
    3. ST depression
    4. Inverted T wave

12. A nurse caring for a group of clients reviews the electrolyte laboratory results and notes a sodium level of 130 mEq/L on one client's laboratory reports. The nurse understands that which client is at most risk for the development of a sodium value at this level?
    1. The client who is taking diuretics
    2. The client who is taking corticosteroids
    3. The client with renal failure
    4. The client with hyperaldosteronism

13. A nurse is caring for a client with acute congestive heart failure who is receiving high doses of a diuretic. On assessment the nurse notes that the client has flat neck veins, generalized muscle weakness, and diminished deep tendon reflexes. The nurse

suspects hyponatremia. What additional signs would the nurse expect to note in this client if hyponatremia were present?
1. Dry skin
2. Decreased urinary output
3. Increased specific gravity of the urine
4. Hyperactive bowel sounds

14. A nurse is caring for a client with a nasogastric tube. Nasogastric tube irrigations are prescribed to be performed once every shift. The client's serum electrolyte results indicate a potassium level of 4.5 mEq/L and a sodium level of 132 mEq/L. Based on these laboratory findings, the nurse selects which solution to use for the nasogastric tube irrigation?
1. Tap water
2. Distilled water
3. Sterile water
4. Normal saline

15. A nurse is reviewing laboratory results and notes that a client's serum sodium level is 150 mEq/L. The nurse reports the serum sodium level to the physician, and the physician prescribes dietary instructions based on the sodium level. Which food item does the nurse instruct the client to avoid?
1. Low-fat yogurt
2. Cauliflower
3. Processed oat cereals
4. Peas

16. A nurse is reviewing a client's laboratory reports and notes that the serum calcium level is 4.0 mg/dL. The nurse understands that which condition most likely caused this serum calcium level?
1. Prolonged bed rest
2. Excessive administration of vitamin D
3. Renal insufficiency
4. Hyperparathyroidism

17. A nurse is assessing a client with a suspected diagnosis of hypocalcemia. Which of the following clinical manifestations are not associated this diagnosis?

1. Hypoactive bowel sounds
2. Paresthesias
3. Hyperactive deep tendon reflexes
4. Positive Trousseau's sign

18. A nurse caring for a client with hypocalcemia would expect to note which of the following changes on the electrocardiogram?
1. Prominent U wave
2. Widened T wave
3. Shortened ST segment
4. Prolonged QT interval

19. A nurse caring for a client with severe malnutrition reviews the laboratory results and notes a magnesium level of 1.0 mg/dL. Which electrocardiogram change would the nurse expect to note based on the magnesium level?
1. Prominent U waves
2. Depressed ST segment
3. Widened QRS complexes
4. Prolonged PR interval

20. A nurse reviews the serum phosphorus level and notes that the client's level is 2.0 mg/dL. Which condition most likely caused this serum phosphorus level?
1. Alcoholism
2. Hypoparathyroidism
3. Tumor lysis syndrome
4. Renal insufficiency

CRITICAL THINKING: FILL IN THE BLANK

A nurse is caring for a client with a diagnosis of hyperthyroidism. Laboratory studies are performed, and the serum calcium level is 12.0 mg/dL. Is this calcium level high or low, and what is the normal serum calcium level?

Answer: _____

ANSWERS

1. 4

Rationale: Sensible losses are those of which the person is aware, such as through wound drainage, gastrointestinal tract losses, and urination. Insensible losses may occur without the person's awareness. Insensible losses occur daily through the skin and the lungs.

Test-Taking Strategy: Note that the issue of the question is fluid loss. Use the process of elimination, noting the similarity between options 1, 2, and 3. In options 1, 2 and 3, these types of losses can be measured for accurate output. Fluid loss through the skin cannot be measured accurately, only approximated. If you had difficulty with this question, review the difference between sensible and insensible fluid loss.

Level of Cognitive Ability: Comprehension
Client Needs: Physiological Integrity
Integrated Process: Communication and Documentation
Content Area: Fundamental skills
Reference: Ignatavicius, D., & Workman, M. (2002). *Medical surgical nursing: Critical thinking for collaborative care* (4th ed., pp. 140, 150, 156). Philadelphia: W. B. Saunders.

2. 1

Rationale: Causes of a fluid volume deficit include vomiting, diarrhea, conditions that cause increased respirations or increased urinary output, insufficient IV fluid replacement, draining fistulas, and the presence of an ileostomy or colostomy. A client with congestive heart failure or decreased

kidney function or a client receiving frequent wound irrigations is at risk for fluid volume excess.
Test-Taking Strategy: Read the question carefully, noting that it asks for the client at risk for a deficit. Read each option and think about the fluid imbalance that can occur in each. The clients presented in options 2, 3, and 4 retain fluid. The only condition that can cause a deficit is the condition noted in option 1. If you had difficulty with this question, review the causes of fluid volume deficit.
Level of Cognitive Ability: Analysis
Client Needs: Physiological Integrity
Integrated Process: Nursing Process—assessment
Content Area: Fundamental skills
Reference: Phipps, W., Monahan, F., Sands, J., Marek, J., & Neighbors, M. (2003). *Medical-surgical nursing: Health and illness perspectives* (7th ed., p. 245). St. Louis: Mosby.

3. 4
Rationale: Assessment findings in a client with a fluid volume deficit include increased respirations and heart rate, decreased central venous pressure (CVP), weight loss, poor skin turgor, dry mucous membranes, decreased urine volume, increased specific gravity of the urine, increased hematocrit, and altered level of consciousness. The normal CVP is between 4 and 11 mm H_2O. A client with dehydration has a low CVP. The assessment findings in options 1, 2, and 3 are seen in a client with fluid volume excess.
Test-Taking Strategy: Use the process of elimination and focus on the issue: fluid volume deficit. Eliminate options 1 and 2 first. Rales are noted in fluid volume excess, as is increased blood pressure. From the remaining options, recall that central venous pressure reflects the pressure under which blood is returned to the superior vena cava and right atrium. Therefore pressure (volume) would be decreased in a fluid volume deficit. If you had difficulty with this question, review the assessment findings noted in fluid volume deficit.
Level of Cognitive Ability: Analysis
Client Needs: Physiological Integrity
Integrated Process: Nursing Process—assessment
Content Area: Fundamental skills
Reference: Phipps, W., Monahan, F., Sands, J., Marek, J., & Neighbors, M. (2003). *Medical-surgical nursing: Health and illness perspectives* (7th ed., pp. 143, 294, 641). St. Louis: Mosby.

4. 1
Rationale: The causes of fluid volume excess include decreased kidney function, congestive heart failure, the use of hypotonic fluids to replace isotonic fluid losses, excessive irrigation of wounds and body cavities, and excessive ingestion of sodium. The client with an ileostomy, the client taking diuretics, and the client who requires gastrointestinal suctioning are at risk for fluid volume deficit.
Test-Taking Strategy: Use the process of elimination and focus on the issue: fluid volume excess. Read each option and think about the fluid imbalance that can occur in each. The clients presented in options 2, 3, and 4 lose fluid. The only condition that can cause an excess is the condition noted in option 1. If you had difficulty with this question, review the causes of fluid volume excess.
Level of Cognitive Ability: Analysis

Client Needs: Physiological Integrity
Integrated Process: Nursing Process—assessment
Content Area: Fundamental skills
Reference: Phipps, W., Monahan, F., Sands, J., Marek, J., & Neighbors, M. (2003). *Medical-surgical nursing: Health and illness perspectives* (7th ed., pp. 247-248). St. Louis: Mosby.

5. 3
Rationale: Assessment findings associated with fluid volume excess include cough, dyspnea, rales, tachypnea, tachycardia, an elevated blood pressure and a bounding pulse, an elevated CVP, weight gain, edema, neck and hand vein distention, altered level of consciousness, and a decreased hematocrit. Options 1, 2, and 4 identify signs noted in fluid volume deficit.
Test-Taking Strategy: Use the process of elimination and knowledge regarding the assessment findings in fluid volume excess. Note the similarities in options 1, 2, and 4. Each of these signs reflects a decrease. Option 3 reflects an increase. Remember that CVP reflects the pressure under which blood is returned to the superior vena cava and right atrium. Pressure (volume) would be elevated in fluid volume excess. If you had difficulty with this question, review the assessment findings noted in fluid volume excess.
Level of Cognitive Ability: Analysis
Client Needs: Physiological Integrity
Integrated Process: Nursing Process—assessment
Content Area: Fundamental skills
Reference: Phipps, W., Monahan, F., Sands, J., Marek, J., & Neighbors, M. (2003). *Medical-surgical nursing: Health and illness perspectives* (7th ed., p. 262). St. Louis: Mosby.

6. 1
Rationale: Potassium-rich gastrointestinal fluids are lost through gastrointestinal suction, placing the client at risk for hypokalemia. The client with renal disease or Addison's disease and the client taking a potassium-sparing diuretic are at risk for hyperkalemia.
Test-Taking Strategy: Use the process of elimination. Note that the issue is a potassium deficit. Option 1 is the only option that identifies a loss of body fluid. If you had difficulty with this question, review the causes of hypokalemia.
Level of Cognitive Ability: Analysis
Client Needs: Physiological Integrity
Integrated Process: Nursing Process:—assessment
Content Area: Fundamental skills
References: Phipps, W., Monahan, F., Sands, J., Marek, J., & Neighbors, M. (2003). *Medical-surgical nursing: Health and illness perspectives* (7th ed., pp. 237, 252-253). St. Louis: Mosby.
Potter, P., & Perry, A. (2001). *Fundamentals of nursing* (5th ed., pp. 1353, 1444). St. Louis: Mosby.

7. 4
Rationale: A serum potassium level less than 3.5 mEq/L indicates hypokalemia. Potassium deficit is a relatively common electrolyte imbalance and is potentially life threatening. Electrocardiogram changes include inverted T waves, ST segment depression, and prominent U waves.
Test-Taking Strategy: From the information in the question, you need to determine that the client is experiencing hypokalemia.

From this point, you must know the electrocardiogram changes that are expected when hypokalemia exists. If you had difficulty with this question, review the electrocardiogram changes that occur in hypokalemia.
Level of Cognitive Ability: Analysis
Client Needs: Physiological Integrity
Integrated Process: Nursing Process—analysis
Content Area: Fundamental skills
References: Lewis, S., Heitkemper, M., & Dirksen, S. (2004). *Medical-surgical nursing: Assessment and management of clinical problems* (6th ed., pp. 342-344). St. Louis: Mosby.
Phipps, W., Monahan, F., Sands, J., Marek, J., & Neighbors, M. (2003). *Medical-surgical nursing: Health and illness perspectives* (7th ed., p. 255). St. Louis: Mosby.

8. 1
Rationale: Potassium chloride administered intravenously must always be diluted in IV fluid and infused via a pump or controller. The usual concentration of IV potassium chloride is 20 to 40 mEq/L. Potassium chloride is never given by bolus (IV push). Giving potassium chloride by IV push can result in cardiac arrest. Dilution in normal saline is recommended, and dextrose solution is avoided because this type of solution increases intracellular potassium shifting. The IV bag containing the potassium chloride is always gently agitated before hanging. The IV site is monitored closely because potassium chloride is irritating to the veins and the risk of phlebitis exists. The nurse monitors urinary output during administration and contacts the physician if the urinary output is less than 30 mL/hr.
Test-Taking Strategy: Use the process of elimination and knowledge regarding the administration of potassium chloride intravenously. Noting the key word "not" in the stem of the question will direct you to option 1. Review the administration of potassium chloride if you had difficulty with this question.
Level of Cognitive Ability: Application
Client Needs: Physiological Integrity
Integrated Process: Nursing Process—planning
Content Area: Pharmacology
Reference: Hodgson, B., & Kizior, R. (2003). *Saunders nursing drug handbook 2003* (p. 910). Philadelphia: W. B. Saunders.

9. 4
Rationale:
A medium apple provides about 159 mg of potassium. Spinach (3½ oz) provides 470 mg. A large carrot provides 341 mg, and a medium avocado provides 1097 mg of potassium.
Test-Taking Strategy: Note the key words "lowest in potassium" in the stem of the question. Recalling the potassium content of the foods identified in the options will direct you to option 4. Review the foods that are high and low in potassium content if you had difficulty with this question.
Level of Cognitive Ability: Analysis
Client Needs: Health Promotion and Maintenance
Integrated Process: Nursing Process—evaluation
Content Area: Fundamental skills
Reference: Peckenpaugh, N. (2003). *Nutrition essentials and diet therapy* (9th ed., pp. 98, 116). Philadelphia: W. B. Saunders.

10. 1
Rationale: A serum potassium level greater than 5.1 mEq/L indicates hyperkalemia. Clients who experience cellular shifting of potassium in the early stages of massive cell destruction, such as in trauma, burns, or sepsis or with metabolic or respiratory acidosis, are at risk for hyperkalemia. The client with Cushing's syndrome or colitis and the client who has been overusing laxatives are at risk for hypokalemia.
Test-Taking Strategy: Use the process of elimination. Eliminate option 3 and 4 first because they are similar, both reflecting a gastrointestinal loss. From the remaining options, recalling that cell destruction causes potassium shifts will assist in directing you to the correct option. Remember that Cushing's syndrome presents a risk for hypokalemia and that Addison's disease presents a risk for hyperkalemia. If you had difficulty with this question, review the risk factors associated with hyperkalemia.
Level of Cognitive Ability: Analysis
Client Needs: Physiological Integrity
Integrated Process: Nursing Process—assessment
Content Area: Fundamental skills
References: Chernecky, C., & Berger, B. (2001). *Laboratory tests and diagnostic procedures* (3rd ed., p. 836). Philadelphia: W. B. Saunders.
Potter, P., & Perry, A. (2001). *Fundamentals of nursing* (5th ed., p. 1207). St. Louis: Mosby.

11. 1
Rationale: A serum potassium level greater than 5.4 mEq/L indicates hyperkalemia. Electrocardiogram changes include flat P waves, prolonged PR intervals, widened QRS complexes, and tall peaked T waves.
Test-Taking Strategy: From the information in the question, you need to determine that this condition is a hyperkalemic one. From this point, you must know the electrocardiogram changes that are expected when hyperkalemia exists. If you had difficulty with this question, review the normal serum potassium level and the electrocardiogram changes that occur in hyperkalemia.
Level of Cognitive Ability: Analysis
Client Needs: Physiological Integrity
Integrated Process: Nursing Process—analysis
Content Area: Fundamental skills
Reference: Lewis, S., Heitkemper, M., & Dirksen, S. (2004). *Medical-surgical nursing: Assessment and management of clinical problems* (6th ed., p. 343). St. Louis: Mosby.

12. 1
Rationale: Hyponatremia is evidenced by a serum sodium level of less than 135 mEq/L. Hyponatremia can occur in the client taking diuretics. The client taking corticosteroids and the client with renal failure or hyperaldosteronism are at risk for hypernatremia.
Test-Taking Strategy: Use the process of elimination. First determine that the client is experiencing hyponatremia. Next, you must know the causes of hyponatremia to direct you to option 1. Review the normal serum sodium level and the causes of hyponatremia if you had difficulty with this question.
Level of Cognitive Ability: Analysis
Client Needs: Physiological Integrity

Integrated Process: Nursing Process—assessment
Content Area: Fundamental skills
Reference: Ignatavicius, D., & Workman, M. (2002). *Medical surgical nursing: Critical thinking for collaborative care* (4th ed., p. 182). Philadelphia: W. B. Saunders.

13. **4**

Rationale: Hyperactive bowel sounds indicate hyponatremia. Options 1, 2, and 3 are signs of hypernatremia. In hyponatremia, increased urinary output and decreased specific gravity of the urine would be noted. Dry skin occurs in fluid volume deficit.

Test-Taking Strategy: Knowledge regarding the signs of hyponatremia is needed to answer the question. If you had difficulty with this, review the assessment signs associated with hyponatremia and hypernatremia.

Level of Cognitive Ability: Analysis
Client Needs: Physiological Integrity
Integrated Process: Nursing Process—assessment
Content Area: Fundamental skills
Reference: Potter, P., & Perry, A. (2001). *Fundamentals of nursing* (5th ed., p. 1201). St. Louis: Mosby.

14. **4**

Rationale: A potassium level of 4.5 mEq/L is within normal range. A sodium level of 132 mEq/L is low, indicating hyponatremia. In clients with hyponatremia, normal (isotonic) saline should be used rather than water for gastrointestinal irrigations.

Test-Taking Strategy: Use the process of elimination. Eliminate options 1, 2, and 3 because they are similar (sterile water, distilled water, and tap water). Also, recalling that the serum sodium level identified in the question indicates hyponatremia will direct you to option 4. If you had difficulty with this question, review the care of the client experiencing hyponatremia.

Level of Cognitive Ability: Application
Client Needs: Physiological Integrity
Integrated Process: Nursing Process—implementation
Content Area: Fundamental skills
Reference: Ignatavicius, D., & Workman, M. (2002). *Medical surgical nursing: Critical thinking for collaborative care* (4th ed., p. 182). Philadelphia: W. B. Saunders.

15. **3**

Rationale: The normal serum sodium level is 135 to 145 mEq/L. A serum sodium level of 150 mEq/L indicates hypernatremia. Based on this finding, the nurse would instruct the client to avoid foods high in sodium. Low-fat yogurt, cauliflower, and peas are good food sources of phosphorus. Processed foods are high in sodium content.

Test-Taking Strategy: First you must determine that the client has hypernatremia. Next, note the key word "avoid" in the stem of the question. Eliminate options 2 and 4 first because these are vegetables. From the remaining two options, note the word "processed" in option 3. Processed foods tend to be higher in sodium content. Review foods high in sodium content if you had difficulty with this question.

Level of Cognitive Ability: Application
Client Needs: Health Promotion and Maintenance

Integrated Process: Teaching/Learning
Content Area: Fundamental skills
Reference: Peckenpaugh, N. (2003). *Nutrition essentials and diet therapy* (9th ed., p. 156). Philadelphia: W. B. Saunders.

16. **1**

Rationale: The normal serum calcium level is 8.6 to 10.0 mg/dL. A client with a serum calcium level of 4.0 mg/dL is experiencing hypocalcemia. The excessive administration of vitamin D and hyperparathyroidism are causative factors associated with hypercalcemia. End-stage renal disease rather than renal insufficiency is a cause of hypocalcemia. Prolonged bed rest is a cause of hypocalcemia. Although immobilization initially can cause hypercalcemia, the long-term effect of prolonged bed rest is hypocalcemia.

Test-Taking Strategy: Note the key words "most likely." First, you must determine that the client is experiencing hypocalcemia. This should assist in eliminating option 2. Next, you must recall the causative factors associated with hypocalcemia to direct you to option 1. If you had difficulty with question, review the causative factors associated with hypocalcemia.

Level of Cognitive Ability: Analysis
Client Needs: Physiological Integrity
Integrated Process: Nursing Process—analysis
Content Area: Fundamental skills
Reference: Ignatavicius, D., & Workman, M. (2002). *Medical surgical nursing: Critical thinking for collaborative care* (4th ed., p. 186). Philadelphia: W. B. Saunders.

17. **1**

Rationale: Hypoactive bowel sounds are noted in hypercalcemia. Signs of hypocalcemia include paresthesias followed by numbness, hyperactive deep tendon reflexes, and a positive Trousseau's or Chvostek's sign. Additional signs of hypocalcemia include increased neuromuscular excitability, muscle cramps, twitching, tetany, seizures, irritability, and anxiety. Gastrointestinal symptoms include increased gastric motility, hyperactive bowel sounds, abdominal cramping, and diarrhea.

Test-Taking Strategy: Note the key word "not" in the stem of the question. Use the process of elimination, noting that options 2, 3, and 4 are similar in that they reflect a hyperactivity of the neuromuscular system. The option that is different is option 1. Review the assessment signs and symptoms noted in hypocalcemia if you had difficulty with this question.

Level of Cognitive Ability: Analysis
Client Needs: Physiological Integrity
Integrated Process: Nursing Process—assessment
Content Area: Fundamental skills
Reference: Ignatavicius, D., & Workman, M. (2002). *Medical surgical nursing: Critical thinking for collaborative care* (4th ed., p. 186). Philadelphia: W. B. Saunders.

18. **4**

Rationale: Electrocardiogram changes that occur in a client with hypocalcemia include a prolonged ST or QT interval. A shortened ST segment and a widened T wave occur with hypercalcemia. Prominent U waves occur with hypokalemia.

Test-Taking Strategy: Use knowledge regarding the electrocardiogram changes that occur in calcium imbalances to answer the question. Remember that hypocalcemia causes a prolonged

ST or QT interval. If you had difficulty with this question, review the electrocardiogram changes that occur in these conditions.
Level of Cognitive Ability: Analysis
Client Needs: Physiological Integrity
Integrated Process: Nursing Process—analysis
Content Area: Fundamental skills
Reference: Ignatavicius, D., & Workman, M. (2002). *Medical surgical nursing: Critical thinking for collaborative care* (4th ed., p. 186). Philadelphia: W. B. Saunders.

19. **2**
Rationale: The normal magnesium level is 1.6 to 2.6 mg/dL. A magnesium level of 1.0 mg/dL indicates hypomagnesemia. In hypomagnesemia, the nurse would note tall T waves and a depressed ST segment. Options 3 and 4 would be noted in a client experiencing hypermagnesemia. Prominent U waves occur with hypokalemia.
Test-Taking Strategy: First you must determine that the client is experiencing hypomagnesemia. Next, identify the electrocardiogram changes that occur in this condition. If you had difficulty with this question, review the normal magnesium level and the electrocardiogram changes that occur in hypomagnesemia and hypermagnesemia.
Level of Cognitive Ability: Analysis
Client Needs: Physiological Integrity
Integrated Process: Nursing Process—analysis
Content Area: Fundamental skills
Reference: Ignatavicius, D., & Workman, M. (2002). *Medical surgical nursing: Critical thinking for collaborative care* (4th ed., pp. 192-193). Philadelphia: W. B. Saunders.

20. **1**
Rationale: The normal serum phosphorus level is 2.7 to 4.5 mg/dL. The client is experiencing hypophosphatemia. Causative factors relate to malnutrition or starvation and the use of aluminum hydroxide-based or magnesium-based antacids. Malnutrition is associated with alcoholism. Hypoparathyroidism, renal insufficiency, and tumor lysis syndrome are causative factors of hyperphosphatemia.
Test-Taking Strategy: First you must determine that the client is experiencing hypophosphatemia. From this point, you must know the causes of hypophosphatemia. If you had difficulty with this question, review the causative factors associated with hypophosphatemia.
Level of Cognitive Ability: Analysis
Client Needs: Physiological Integrity
Integrated Process: Nursing Process—analysis
Content Area: Fundamental skills
References: Chernecky, C., & Berger, B. (2001). *Laboratory tests and diagnostic procedures* (3rd ed., p. 821). Philadelphia: W. B. Saunders.
Ignatavicius, D., & Workman, M. (2002). *Medical surgical nursing: Critical thinking for collaborative care* (4th ed., p. 193). Philadelphia: W. B. Saunders.

CRITICAL THINKING: FILL IN THE BLANK

Answer: The normal serum calcium level is 8.6 to 10.0 mg/dL; therefore a level of 12.0 mg/dL is high.
Rationale: The normal serum calcium level is 8.6 to 10.0 mg/dL. This client is experiencing hypercalcemia.
Test-Taking Strategy: You must know the normal serum calcium level to answer this question. If you are unfamiliar with this level, review and learn it.
Level of Cognitive Ability: Comprehension
Client Needs: Physiological Integrity
Integrated Process: Nursing Process—assessment
Content Area: Fundamental skills
Reference: Chernecky, C., & Berger, B. (2001). Laboratory tests and diagnostic procedures (3rd ed., p. 290). Philadelphia: W. B. Saunders.

REFERENCES

Chernecky, C., & Berger, B. (2001). *Laboratory tests and diagnostic procedures* (3rd ed.). Philadelphia: W. B. Saunders.

Hodgson, B., & Kizior, R. (2003). *Saunders nursing drug handbook 2003.* Philadelphia: W. B. Saunders.

Ignatavicius, D., & Workman, M. (2002). *Medical surgical nursing: Critical thinking for collaborative care* (4th ed.). Philadelphia: W. B. Saunders.

Lewis, S., Heitkemper, M., & Dirksen, S. (2004). *Medical-surgical nursing: Assessment and management of clinical problems* (6th ed.). St. Louis: Mosby.

National Council of State Boards of Nursing (Eds.). (2003). *Test Plan for the National Council Licensure for Registered Nurses* (effective date: April 2004). Chicago: Author.

Peckenpaugh, N. (2003). *Nutrition essentials and diet therapy* (9th ed.). Philadelphia: W. B. Saunders.

Phipps, W., Monahan, F., Sands, J., Marek, J., & Neighbors, M. (2003). *Medical-surgical nursing: health and illness perspectives* (7th ed.). St. Louis: Mosby.

Potter, P., & Perry, A. (2001). *Fundamentals of nursing* (5th ed.). St. Louis: Mosby.

Acid-Base Balance

PYRAMID TERMS

Allen's test   A test for collateral circulation to the hand by evaluation of the patency of the radial and ulnar arteries.

metabolic acidosis   A total concentration of buffer base that is lower than normal, with a relative increase in the hydrogen ion concentration, that results from loss of buffer bases or retention of too many acids without sufficient bases and occurs in conditions such as renal failure and diabetic ketoacidosis, from the production of lactic acid, and from the ingestion of toxins, such as aspirin.

metabolic alkalosis   A deficit or loss of hydrogen ions or acids or an excess of base (bicarbonate) that results from the accumulation of base or from a loss of acid without a comparable loss of base in the body fluids such as from conditions resulting in hypovolemia, the loss of gastric fluid, excessive bicarbonate intake, the massive transfusion of whole blood, and hyperaldosteronism.

respiratory acidosis   A total concentration of buffer base that is lower than normal, with a relative increase in hydrogen ion concentration; thus a greater number of hydrogen ions are circulating in the blood than the buffer system can absorb; caused by primary defects in the function of the lungs or by changes in normal respiratory patterns as a result of secondary problems. Any condition that causes an obstruction of the airway or depresses respiratory status can cause respiratory acidosis.

respiratory alkalosis   A deficit of carbonic acid or a decrease in hydrogen ion concentration that results from the accumulation of base or from a loss of acid without a comparable loss of base in the body fluids such as from conditions that cause overstimulation of the respiratory status.

▲ THE PYRAMID TO SUCCESS

Acid-base imbalance is a content area that sometimes is viewed as complex and difficult to understand. You must understand the description of each imbalance and then review the causes of each disorder, correlating the pathophysiology with each cause. From this point, note the assessment signs related to each disorder and the treatment associated with the clinical manifestations. Maintenance of a patent airway is a priority. The nurse also needs to monitor vital signs, cardiovascular status, neurological status, intake and output, laboratory values, and arterial blood gas values. Remember, safety and seizure precautions may need to be initiated. Integrated Processes addressed in this chapter are Nursing Process, Caring, Communication and Documentation, and Teaching/Learning.

CLIENT NEEDS
Safe, Effective Care Environment

Accident prevention
Establishment of priorities
Informed consent for invasive procedures
Medical and surgical asepsis
Provision of safety for the client during implementation of various treatments for the acid-base imbalance
Standard, transmission-based, and other precautions

Health Promotion and Maintenance

Client and family education about prevention, early detection, and treatment measures for health disorders
Disease prevention
Health and wellness
Identification of clients at risk for an acid-base imbalance
Techniques of physical assessment

Psychosocial Integrity

Emotional support of the client and family
Sensory/perceptual alterations
Support systems
Therapeutic interactions

Physiological Integrity

Administration and monitoring of medications, intravenous fluids, and other therapeutic interventions

Alterations in body systems

Basic care and comfort

Diagnostic tests

Expected effects of pharmacological and parenteral therapies

Laboratory values

Monitoring for changes in status and for complications

Obtaining an arterial blood gas specimen and analyzing the results

Provision of wound care when blood is obtained for an arterial blood gas study

Reducing the likelihood that an acid-base imbalance will occur

▲

I. HYDROGEN IONS, ACIDS, AND BASES

A. Hydrogen ions
  1. Vital to life
  2. Expressed as pH
  3. Circulate in the body in two forms:
     a. Volatile hydrogen of carbonic acid
     b. Nonvolatile form of hydrogen and organic acids
B. Acids
  1. Acids are produced as end products of metabolism.
  2. Acids contain hydrogen ions.
  3. Acids are hydrogen ion donors, which means that acids give up hydrogen ions to neutralize or decrease the strength of an acid or to form a weaker base.
  4. The strength of an acid is determined by the number of hydrogen ions it contains.
  5. The number of hydrogen ions in body fluid determines its acidity, alkalinity, or neutrality.
  6. The lungs excrete 13,000 to 30,000 mEq of volatile hydrogen per day in the form of carbonic acid as CO_2.
  7. The kidneys excrete 50 mEq of nonvolatile acids per day.
C. Bases
  1. Bases contain no hydrogen ions.
  2. Bases are hydrogen ion acceptors; they accept hydrogen ions from acids to neutralize or decrease the strength of a base or to form a weaker acid.

II. REGULATORY SYSTEMS FOR HYDROGEN ION CONCENTRATION IN THE BLOOD

A. Buffers
  1. Buffers are the fastest-acting regulatory system.
  2. Buffers provide immediate protection against changes in hydrogen ion concentration in the extracellular fluid.
  3. Buffers are reactors that function only to keep the pH within the narrow limits of stability when too much acid or base is released into the system.
  4. Buffers absorb or release hydrogen ions as needed.
  5. Buffers serve as a transport mechanism that carries excess hydrogen ions to the lungs.
  6. Once the primary buffer systems react, they are consumed, and this leaves the body less able to withstand further stress until they are replaced.
B. Primary buffer systems in extracellular fluid
  1. Hemoglobin system
     a. Red blood cells contain hemoglobin.
     b. System maintains acid-base balance by a process called chloride shift.
     c. Chloride shifts in and out of the cells in response to the level of O_2 in the blood.
     d. For each chloride ion that leaves a red blood cell, a bicarbonate ion enters.
     e. For each chloride ion that enters a red blood cell, a bicarbonate ion leaves.
  2. Plasma proteins system
     a. The system functions along with the liver to vary the amount of hydrogen ions in the chemical structure of protein.
     b. Plasma proteins have the ability to attract or release hydrogen ions.
  3. Carbonic acid/bicarbonate system ▲
     a. The system maintains a pH of 7.4 with a ratio of 20 parts bicarbonate to 1 part carbonic acid.
     b. This ratio (20:1) determines hydrogen ion concentration of body fluid.
     c. Carbonic acid concentration is controlled by the excretion of CO_2 by the lungs; the rate and depth of respiration change in response to changes in CO_2.
     d. The kidneys control the bicarbonate concentration and selectively retain or secrete bicarbonates in response to the body needs.
  4. Phosphate buffer system
     a. System is present in the cells and body fluids.
     b. System is especially active in the kidneys.
     c. System acts like bicarbonate and clears spare hydrogen ions.
C. Lungs
  1. The lungs are the second defense of the body and interact with the buffer system to maintain acid-base balance.
  2. In acidosis the pH decreases and the respiratory ▲ rate and depth increase in an attempt to exhale acids; the carbonic acid created by the neutralizing action of bicarbonate can be carried to the lungs, where it is reduced to CO_2 and water and exhaled; thus hydrogen ions are inactivated and excreted.
  3. In alkalosis the pH increases and the respiratory ▲ rate and depth decrease; the CO_2 is retained, and the carbonic acid builds to neutralize and decrease the strength of excess bicarbonate.
  4. The action of the lungs is reversible in controlling an excess or deficit.

5. The lungs can hold hydrogen ions until the deficit is corrected or can inactivate hydrogen ions, changing the ions to water molecules to be exhaled along with CO_2, thus correcting the excess.

6. The process of correcting a deficit or excess takes 10 to 30 seconds to complete.

7. The lungs are capable of inactivating only hydrogen ions carried by carbonic acid; excess hydrogen ions created by other problems must be excreted by the kidneys.

D. Kidneys

1. The ultimate correction of acid-base disturbances depends on the kidneys, even though the renal excretion of acids and alkali occurs more slowly.

2. Compensation requires a few hours to several days; however, the compensation is more thorough and selective than that of other regulators.

3. In acidosis the pH decreases and excess hydrogen ions are secreted into the tubules and combine with buffers for excretion in the urine.

4. In alkalosis the pH increases and bicarbonate ions move into the tubules, combine with sodium, and are excreted in the urine.

5. Selective regulation of bicarbonate occurs in the kidneys.
   a. The kidneys restore bicarbonate by the release of hydrogen ions and by holding bicarbonate ions.
   b. Extra hydrogen ions are excreted in the urine in the form of phosphoric acid.
   c. The alteration of certain amino acids in the renal tubules results in a diffusion of ammonia into the kidneys, and the ammonia combines with extra hydrogen ions and is excreted in the urine.

E. Potassium

1. Potassium plays an exchange role in maintaining acid-base balance.

2. The body changes the potassium level by drawing hydrogen ions into the cell or by pushing them out of the cell.

3. The potassium level changes to compensate for hydrogen ion level changes.
   a. In acidosis the body protects itself from the acid state by moving hydrogen ions into the cell; therefore potassium moves out to make room for hydrogen ions; the serum potassium level increases.
   b. In alkalosis the cells release hydrogen ions into the blood in an attempt to increase the acidity of the blood and combat alkalinity; the potassium moves into the cells, and the serum potassium level decreases.

III. RESPIRATORY ACIDOSIS

A. Description: The total concentration of buffer base is lower than normal, with a relative increase in hydrogen ion concentration; thus a greater number

---

BOX 10-1

Causes of Respiratory Acidosis

Asthma
Atelectasis
Brain trauma
Bronchiectasis
Bronchitis
Emphysema
Hypoventilation
Medications
Pulmonary edema

---

of hydrogen ions are circulating in the blood than can be absorbed by the buffer system.

B. Causes (Box 10-1)

1. **Respiratory acidosis** is caused by primary defects in the function of the lungs or changes in normal respiratory patterns.

2. Any condition that causes an obstruction of the airway or depresses respiratory status can cause **respiratory acidosis**.

3. Hypoventilation: Carbon dioxide is retained and the hydrogen ion concentration increases, leading to the acid state; carbonic acid is retained and the pH decreases.

4. Medications: Sedatives, narcotics, and anesthetics depress the respiratory center, leading to hypoventilation; carbon dioxide is retained and the hydrogen ion concentration increases.

5. Bronchitis: Inflammation causes airway obstruction, resulting in inadequate oxygenation.

6. Atelectasis: Excessive mucus collection, with the collapse of alveolar sacs caused by mucous plugs, infectious drainage, or anesthetic medications, results in decreased respirations.

7. Brain trauma: Excessive pressure on the respiratory center or medulla oblongata depresses respirations.

8. Emphysema: Loss of elasticity of alveolar sacs restricts air flow in and out, primarily out, leading to an increased CO_2 level.

9. Asthma: Spasms resulting from allergens, irritants, or emotions cause the smooth muscles of the bronchioles to constrict.

10. Pulmonary edema: Extracellular accumulation of fluid in acute congestive heart failure causes disturbances in alveolar diffusion and perfusion.

11. Bronchiectasis: Bronchi become dilated as a result of inflammation, and destructive changes and weakness in the walls of the bronchi occur.

C. Assessment

1. In an attempt to compensate, the respiratory rate and depth increase.

2. Headache

3. Restlessness

4. Mental status changes, such as drowsiness and confusion
5. Visual disturbances
6. Diaphoresis
7. Cyanosis as the hypoxia becomes more acute
8. Hyperkalemia
9. Rapid, irregular pulse
10. Dysrhythmias leading to ventricular fibrillation

D. Interventions
1. Monitor for signs of respiratory distress.
2. Administer oxygen as prescribed.
3. Place client in semi-Fowler position unless contraindicated.
4. Encourage and assist the client to turn, cough, and breathe deeply.
5. Prepare to administer respiratory treatments as prescribed.
6. Encourage hydration to thin secretions unless excess fluid intake is contraindicated.
7. Suction the client's airway if necessary.
8. Reduce restlessness by improving ventilation rather than by the administration of tranquilizers, sedatives, or narcotics because they further depress respirations.
9. Monitor electrolyte values, particularly the potassium level.
10. Administer antibiotics for respiratory infection or other medications as prescribed.

IV. RESPIRATORY ALKALOSIS

A. Description: A deficit of carbonic acid and a decrease in hydrogen ion concentration that results from the accumulation of base or from a loss of acid without a comparable loss of base in the body fluids
B. Causes (Box 10-2)
1. **Respiratory alkalosis** results from conditions that cause overstimulation of the respiratory system.
2. Hyperventilation: Rapid respirations cause the blowing off of CO_2, leading to a decrease in carbonic acid.
3. Hysteria: Hysteria often is neurogenic and related to a psychoneurosis; however, this condition leads to vigorous breathing and excessive exhaling of CO_2.
4. Overventilation by mechanical ventilators: The administration of O_2 and the depletion of CO_2

can occur from mechanical ventilation; the client may be hyperventilated.
5. Conditions that increase metabolism, such as fever, can cause **respiratory alkalosis**.
6. Pain: Overstimulation of the respiratory center in the brainstem results in a carbonic acid deficit.
7. Salicylates: Stimulation of the respiratory center causes hyperventilation.
8. Hypoxia: Respiratory stimulation results in a carbonic acid deficit.

C. Assessment
1. Initially the hyperventilation and respiratory stimulation will cause abnormal rapid respirations (tachypnea); in an attempt to compensate, respiratory rate and depth then decrease.
2. Headache
3. Light-headedness, vertigo
4. Mental status changes
5. Paresthesias, such as tingling of the fingers and toes
6. Hypokalemia, hypocalcemia
7. Tetany, convulsions

D. Interventions
1. Provide emotional support and reassurance to the client.
2. Encourage appropriate breathing patterns.
3. Assist with breathing techniques and breathing aids as prescribed.
   a. Voluntary holding of breath
   b. Use of rebreathing mask as prescribed
   c. Carbon dioxide breaths as prescribed
4. Provide cautious care with ventilator clients so that they are not forced to take breaths too deeply or rapidly.
5. Monitor electrolyte values, particularly potassium and calcium levels.
6. Administer medications as prescribed.
7. Prepare to administer calcium gluconate for tetany as prescribed.

V. METABOLIC ACIDOSIS

A. Description: A total concentration of buffer base that is lower than normal, with a relative increase in the hydrogen ion concentration, resulting from loss of too many bases and retention of too many acids without sufficient bases
B. Causes (Box 10-3)
1. Diabetes mellitus/diabetic ketoacidosis: An insufficient supply of insulin causes increased fat metabolism, leading to an excess accumulation of ketones or other acids; the bicarbonate then ends up being exhausted.
2. Renal insufficiency or failure results in the following:
   a. Increased waste products of protein metabolism are retained.
   b. Excessive acids build up, and bicarbonate is unable to maintain acid-base balance.

BOX 10-2

Causes of Respiratory Alkalosis

Fever
Hyperventilation
Hypoxia
Hysteria
Overventilation by mechanical ventilators
Pain

BOX 10-3

Causes of Metabolic Acidosis

Diabetes mellitus or diabetic ketoacidosis
Excessive ingestion of acetylsalicylic acid (aspirin)
High-fat diet
Insufficient metabolism of carbohydrates
Malnutrition
Renal insufficiency or renal failure
Severe diarrhea

3. Insufficient metabolism of carbohydrates: When an insufficient supply of O_2 is available for the proper burning of carbohydrates, glucose, and water, lactic acid increases and lactic acidosis results.
4. Excessive ingestion of acetylsalicylic acid (aspirin) causes an increase in the hydrogen ion concentration.
5. Severe diarrhea: Intestinal and pancreatic secretions are normally alkaline; therefore excessive loss of base leads to acidosis.
6. Malnutrition: Improper metabolism of nutrients causes fat catabolism, leading to an excess buildup of ketones and acids.
7. High-fat diet: A high intake of fat causes a much too rapid accumulation of the waste products of fat metabolism, leading to a buildup of ketones and acids.

C. Assessment
1. In an attempt to exhale the extra CO_2 and compensate for the acidosis, hyperpnea with Kussmaul's respiration occurs.
2. Headache
3. Nausea, vomiting, diarrhea
4. Fruity-smelling breath resulting from improper fat metabolism
5. Central nervous system depression: mental dullness, drowsiness, stupor, coma
6. Twitching, convulsions
7. Hyperkalemia

D. Interventions
1. Assess level of consciousness for central nervous system depression.
2. Monitor intake and output and assist with fluid and electrolyte replacement as prescribed.
3. Prepare to administer solutions intravenouly as prescribed to increase the buffer base.
4. Initiate safety and seizure precautions.
5. Monitor the serum potassium level closely; when acidosis is being treated, potassium will move back into the cell and the serum potassium level will drop.

E. Interventions in diabetes mellitus/diabetic ketoacidosis
1. Give insulin as prescribed to hasten the movement of serum glucose into the cell, thereby decreasing the concurrent ketosis.

2. When glucose is being properly metabolized, the body will stop converting fats to glucose.
3. Monitor for circulatory collapse caused by polyuria, which may result from the hyperglycemic state because polyuria or diuresis may lead to extracellular volume deficit.

F. Interventions in renal failure
1. In renal failure, dialysis may be used to remove protein and waste products, thereby lessening the acidosis state.
2. A diet low in protein and high in calories will decrease the amount of protein waste products; this in turn will lessen the acidosis.

VI. METABOLIC ALKALOSIS

A. Description: A deficit of carbonic acid and a decease in hydrogen ion concentration that results from the accumulation of base or from a loss of acid without a comparable loss of base in the body fluids

B. Causes (Box 10-4)
1. **Metabolic alkalosis** results from a malfunction of metabolism leading to an increased amount of available basic solution in the blood and a decrease in available acids in the blood.
2. Ingestion of excess sodium bicarbonate causes an increase in the amount of base in the blood.
3. Excessive vomiting or gastrointestinal suctioning leads to an excessive loss of acids.
4. Diuretics: The loss of hydrogen ions and chloride causes a compensatory increase in the bicarbonate in the blood.
5. Hyperaldosteronism: Increased renal tubular reabsorption of sodium occurs, with the resultant loss of hydrogen ions.
6. Massive transfusion of whole blood: The citrate anticoagulant used for the storage of blood is metabolized to bicarbonate.

C. Assessment
1. In an attempt to compensate, respiratory rate and depth decrease to conserve CO_2.
2. Nausea, vomiting, diarrhea
3. Restlessness
4. Numbness and tingling in the extremities
5. Twitching in the extremities
6. Hypokalemia
7. Hypocalcemia
8. Dysrhythmias: tachycardia

BOX 10-4

Causes of Metabolic Alkalosis

Diuretics
Excessive vomiting or gastrointestinal suctioning
Hyperaldosteronism
Ingestion of excess sodium bicarbonate
Massive transfusion of whole blood

D. Interventions
1. Monitor potassium and calcium serum blood levels.
2. Institute safety precautions.
3. Prepare to administer medications as prescribed to promote the kidney excretion of bicarbonate.
4. Prepare to replace potassium chloride as prescribed.

VII. ARTERIAL BLOOD GASES (BOX 10-5)

A. Collection of an arterial blood gas specimen
1. Obtain vital signs.
2. Determine whether the client has an arterial line in place.
3. Perform the **Allen's test** to determine the presence of collateral circulation (Box 10-6).
4. Assess factors that may affect the accuracy of the results, such as changes in the O_2 settings, suctioning within the last 20 minutes, and client activities.
5. Provide emotional support to the client.
6. Assist with the specimen draw by preparing a heparinized syringe.
7. Apply pressure immediately to the puncture site following the blood draw; maintain pressure for 5 minutes, or for 10 minutes if the client is taking anticoagulants.
8. Appropriately label the specimen and transport it on ice to the laboratory.
9. On the laboratory form, record the client's temperature and the type of supplemental oxygen that the client is receiving.
B. Respiratory imbalances
1. Remember, the respiratory function indicator is the P_{CO_2}.

BOX 10-5

Normal Blood Gas Values

pH	7.35-7.45
P_{CO_2}	35-45 mm Hg
HCO_3	22-27 mEq/L
P_{O_2}	80-100 mm Hg

BOX 10-6

Performing the Allen's Test

Apply direct pressure over the client's ulnar and radial arteries simultaneously.
While applying pressure, ask the client to open and close the hand repeatedly; the hand should blanch.
Release pressure from the ulnar artery while compressing the radial artery and assess the color of the extremity distal to the pressure point.
If pinkness fails to return within 6 seconds, the ulnar artery is insufficient, indicating that the radial artery should not be used for obtaining a blood specimen.

2. In a respiratory imbalance, you will find an opposite response between the pH and the P_{CO_2}; in other words, the pH will be up with a P_{CO_2} down (alkalosis), or the pH will be down with an elevated P_{CO_2} (acidosis).
3. Look at the pH and the P_{CO_2} to determine if the condition is a respiratory problem.
4. **Respiratory acidosis**: The pH is down; the P_{CO_2} is up.
5. **Respiratory alkalosis**: The pH is up; the P_{CO_2} is down.
C. Metabolic imbalances
1. Remember, the metabolic function indicator is the bicarbonate ion.
2. In a metabolic imbalance, you will find a corresponding response between the pH and the bicarbonate concentration; in other words, the pH will be up and the bicarbonate concentration will be up (alkalosis), or the pH will be down and the bicarbonate concentration will be down (acidosis).
3. Look at the pH and the bicarbonate concentration to determine whether the condition is a metabolic problem.
4. **Metabolic acidosis**: The pH is down; the bicarbonate concentration is down.
5. **Metabolic alkalosis**: The pH is up; the bicarbonate concentration is up.
D. Compensation
1. **Respiratory acidosis** and **respiratory alkalosis**
a. When compensation has occurred, the pH will be within normal limits.
b. The blood gas result reflects partial compensation if the bicarbonate concentration is abnormal.
c. The blood gas result reflects an uncompensated condition if the bicarbonate concentration is normal.
2. **Metabolic acidosis** and **metabolic alkalosis**
a. When compensation has occurred, the pH will be within normal limits.
b. The blood gas result reflects partial compensation if the P_{CO_2} is abnormal.
c. The blood gas result reflects an uncompensated condition if the P_{CO_2} is normal.
E. Steps for analyzing arterial blood gas results (Box 10-7)

PRACTICE QUESTIONS

1. A nurse plans care for a client with chronic obstructive pulmonary disease, knowing that the client is most likely to experience what type of acid-base imbalance?
   1. Respiratory acidosis
   2. Respiratory alkalosis
   3. Metabolic acidosis
   4. Metabolic alkalosis

BOX 10-7

Analyzing Arterial Blood Gas Results

If you can remember the following Pyramid Points and Pyramid Steps, you will be able to analyze any blood gas report.

PYRAMID POINTS
In acidosis the pH is down.
In alkalosis the pH is up.
The respiratory function indicator is the P_{CO_2}.
The metabolic function indicator is the bicarbonate ion.

PYRAMID STEPS
Pyramid Step 1
Look at the blood gas report. Look at the pH. Is the pH up or down? If the pH is up, it reflects alkalosis. If the pH is down, it reflects acidosis.
Pyramid Step 2
Look at the P_{CO_2}. Is the P_{CO_2} up or down? If the P_{CO_2} reflects an opposite response to the pH, then you know that the condition is a respiratory imbalance. If the P_{CO_2} does not reflect an opposite response to the pH, then move on to Pyramid Step 3.
Pyramid Step 3
Look at the bicarbonate concentration. Does the bicarbonate concentration reflect a corresponding response with the pH? If it does, then the condition is a metabolic imbalance.
Pyramid Step 4
Remember, compensation has occurred if the pH is in a normal range of 7.35 to 7.45. If the pH is not within normal range, look at the respiratory or metabolic function indicators.
Respiratory Imbalances
If the condition is a respiratory imbalance, look at the bicarbonate concentration to determine the state of compensation.
If the bicarbonate concentration is normal, then the condition is uncompensated. If the bicarbonate concentration is abnormal, then the condition is partial compensation.
Metabolic Imbalances
If the condition is a metabolic imbalance, look at the P_{CO_2} to determine the state of compensation.
If the P_{CO_2} is normal, then the condition is uncompensated. If the P_{CO_2} is abnormal, then the condition is partial compensation.

2. A nurse reviews the blood gas results of a client with Guillain-Barré syndrome. The nurse analyzes the results and determines that the client is experiencing respiratory acidosis. Which of the following validates the nurse's findings?
   1. pH 7.50, P_{CO_2} 52 mm Hg
   2. pH 7.35, P_{CO_2} 40 mm Hg
   3. pH 7.25, P_{CO_2} 50 mm Hg
   4. pH 7.50, P_{CO_2} 30 mm Hg

3. A nurse is caring for a client who is on a mechanical ventilator. Blood gas results indicate a pH of 7.50 and a P_{CO_2} of 30 mm Hg. The nurse has determined that the client is experiencing respiratory alkalosis. Which laboratory value would most likely be noted in this condition?
   1. Sodium level of 145 mEq/L
   2. Potassium level of 3.0 mEq/L
   3. Magnesium level of 2.0 mg/dL
   4. Phosphorus level of 4.0 mg/dL

4. A nurse reviews the arterial blood gas results of a client and notes the following: pH 7.45, P_{CO_2} of 30 mm Hg, and bicarbonate concentration of 22 mEq/L. The nurse analyzes these results as indicating
   1. Metabolic acidosis, compensated.
   2. Metabolic alkalosis, uncompensated.
   3. Respiratory alkalosis, compensated.
   4. Respiratory acidosis, uncompensated.

5. A client is scheduled for blood to be drawn from the radial artery for an arterial blood gas determination. Before the blood is drawn, an Allen's test is performed to determine the adequacy of the
   1. Popliteal circulation.
   2. Ulnar circulation.
   3. Femoral circulation.
   4. Carotid circulation.

6. A nurse is caring for a client with a nasogastric tube that is attached to low suction. The nurse monitors the client, knowing that the client is at risk for which acid-base disorder?
   1. Respiratory acidosis
   2. Respiratory alkalosis
   3. Metabolic acidosis
   4. Metabolic alkalosis

7. A nurse caring for a client with an ileostomy understands that the client is at most risk for developing which acid-base disorder?
   1. Respiratory acidosis
   2. Respiratory alkalosis
   3. Metabolic acidosis
   4. Metabolic alkalosis

8. A nurse is caring for a client with diabetic ketoacidosis and documents that the client is experiencing Kussmaul's respirations. Based on this documentation, which of the following did the nurse observe?
   1. Respirations that are abnormally deep, regular, and increased in rate
   2. Respirations that are regular but abnormally slow
   3. Respirations that are labored and increased in depth and rate
   4. Respirations that cease for several seconds

9. A nurse understands that the excessive use of oral antacids containing bicarbonate can result in which acid-base disturbance?
   1. Respiratory alkalosis

2. Respiratory acidosis
3. Metabolic acidosis
4. Metabolic alkalosis

10. A nurse is caring for a client with renal failure. Blood gas results indicate a pH of 7.30, a P_{CO_2} of 32 mm Hg, and a bicarbonate concentration of 20 mEq/L. The nurse has determined that the client is experiencing metabolic acidosis. Which of the following laboratory values would the nurse expect to note?
1. Sodium level of 145 mEq/L
2. Magnesium level of 2.0 mg/dL
3. Potassium level of 5.2 mEq/L
4. Phosphorus level of 4.0 mg/dL

CRITICAL THINKING: PRIORITIZING (ORDERED RESPONSE)

A nurse is preparing to obtain an arterial blood gas specimen from a client and plans to perform the Allen's test on the client. Number in order of priority the steps for performing the Allen's test. (Number 1 is the first step.)

___ Ask the client to open and close the hand repeatedly.
___ Apply pressure over the ulnar and radial arteries.
___ Assess the color of the extremity distal to the pressure point.
___ Release pressure from the ulnar artery.
___ Explain the procedure to the client.

ANSWERS

1. 1
Rationale: Respiratory acidosis is most often due to hypoventilation. Chronic respiratory acidosis is most commonly caused by chronic obstructive pulmonary disease. In end-stage disease, pathological changes lead to airway collapse, air trapping, and disturbance of ventilation-perfusion relationships. Options 2, 3, and 4 are incorrect options.
Test-Taking Strategy: Use the process of elimination. Note the key words "most likely." Remembering that hypoventilation results in respiratory acidosis will direct you to option 1. Review the causes of respiratory acidosis if you had difficulty with this question.
Level of Cognitive Ability: Analysis
Client Needs: Physiological Integrity
Integrated Process: Nursing Process—planning
Content Area: Fundamental skills
Reference: Phipps, W., Monahan, F., Sands, J., Marek, J., & Neighbors, M. (2003). *Medical-surgical nursing: Health and illness perspectives* (7th ed., p. 274). St. Louis: Mosby.

2. 3
Rationale: The normal pH is 7.35 to 7.45. The normal P_{CO_2} is 35 to 45 mm Hg. In respiratory acidosis the pH is down and the P_{CO_2} is up. Option 1 identifies an alkalotic condition. Option 2 identifies normal values. Option 4 identifies respiratory alkalosis.
Test-Taking Strategy: Use the process of elimination. Remember that in a respiratory imbalance you will find an opposite response between the pH and the P_{CO_2}. Also remember that the pH is down in an acidotic condition. Options 1 and 4 reflect an elevated pH, which indicates an alkalotic condition. Option 2 reflects a normal blood gas result. Option 3 is the only option that reflects an acidotic condition. Review blood gas analysis if you had difficulty with this question.
Level of Cognitive Ability: Analysis
Client Needs: Physiological Integrity
Integrated Process: Nursing Process—analysis
Content Area: Fundamental skills
Reference: Chernecky, C., & Berger, B. (2001). *Laboratory tests and diagnostic procedures* (3rd ed., p. 226). Philadelphia: W. B. Saunders.

3. 2
Rationale: Clinical manifestations of respiratory alkalosis include headache, tachypnea, paresthesias, tetany, vertigo, convulsions, hypokalemia, and hypocalcemia. Options 1, 3, and 4 identify normal laboratory values. Option 2 identifies the presence of hypokalemia.
Test-Taking Strategy: Use the process of elimination and knowledge regarding the clinical manifestations of respiratory alkalosis and normal laboratory values to answer the question. The only abnormal laboratory value is the potassium level, option 2. Review the clinical manifestations of respiratory alkalosis and normal laboratory values if you had difficulty with this question.
Level of Cognitive Ability: Analysis
Client Needs: Physiological Integrity
Integrated Process: Nursing Process—analysis
Content Area: Fundamental skills
Reference: Potter, P., & Perry, A. (2001). *Fundamentals of nursing* (5th ed., p. 1204). St. Louis: Mosby.

4. 3
Rationale: The normal pH is 7.35 to 7.45. In a respiratory condition, an opposite effect will be seen between the pH and the P_{CO_2}. In this situation, the pH is at the high end of the normal value and the P_{CO_2} is low. In an alkalotic condition, the pH is up. Therefore, the values identified in the question indicate a respiratory alkalosis. Compensation occurs when the pH returns to a normal value. Because the pH is in the normal range at the high end, compensation has occurred.
Test-Taking Strategy: Remember that in a respiratory imbalance you will find an opposite response between the pH and the P_{CO_2} as indicated in the question. Therefore you can eliminate options 1 and 2. Also remember that the pH is up in an alkalotic condition and compensation occurs as evidenced by a normal pH. Option 3 reflects a respiratory alkalotic condition and compensation and describes the blood gas values as indicated in the question. Review the steps related to reading blood gas values if you had difficulty with this question.
Level of Cognitive Ability: Analysis
Client Needs: Physiological Integrity
Integrated Process: Nursing Process—analysis
Content Area: Fundamental skills

References: Chernecky, C., & Berger, B. (2001). *Laboratory tests and diagnostic procedures* (3rd ed., p. 226). Philadelphia: W. B. Saunders.

Potter, P., & Perry, A. (2001). *Fundamentals of nursing* (5th ed., p. 1202). St. Louis: Mosby.

5. 2

Rationale: Before radial puncture for obtaining an arterial specimen for arterial blood gases, you should perform an Allen's test to determine adequate ulnar circulation. Failure to determine the presence of adequate collateral circulation could result is severe ischemic injury to the hand if damage to the radial artery occurs with arterial puncture. Options 1, 3, and 4 are incorrect options.

Test-Taking Strategy: Use the process of elimination and knowledge regarding the purpose and procedure for the Allen's test. Remember that the purpose of this test is to assess the adequacy of the ulnar circulation. Review the purpose and procedure of the Allen's test if you had difficulty with this question.

Level of Cognitive Ability: Comprehension
Client Needs: Physiological Integrity
Integrated Process: Nursing Process—assessment
Content Area: Fundamental skills
Reference: Potter, P., & Perry, A. (2001). *Fundamentals of nursing* (5th ed., p. 790). St. Louis: Mosby.

6. 4

Rationale: Loss of gastric fluid via nasogastric suction or vomiting causes metabolic alkalosis as a result of the loss of hydrochloric acid. Options 1, 2, and 3 are incorrect.

Test-Taking Strategy: Remembering that a client receiving nasogastric suction loses hydrochloric acid will direct you to the option identifying an alkalotic condition. Because the question addresses a situation other than a respiratory one, the acid-base disorder would be a metabolic condition. If you had difficulty with this question, review the causes of metabolic alkalosis.

Level of Cognitive Ability: Analysis
Client Needs: Physiological Integrity
Integrated Process: Nursing Process—analysis
Content Area: Fundamental skills
Reference: Ignatavicius, D., & Workman, M. (2002). *Medical-surgical nursing: Critical thinking for collaborative care* (4th ed., p. 230). Philadelphia: W. B. Saunders.

7. 3

Rationale: Intestinal secretions are high in bicarbonate and may be lost through enteric drainage tubes or an ileostomy or with diarrhea. These conditions result in metabolic acidosis. Options 1, 2, and 4 are incorrect because they do not occur in the client with an ileostomy.

Test-Taking Strategy: Use the process of elimination. Note that the client's condition described in the question is a gastrointestinal disorder. This will direct you toward a metabolic disorder. Remembering that intestinal fluids are primarily alkaline will assist you in selecting the correct option. When excess bicarbonate is lost, acidosis will result. If you had difficulty with this question, review the causes of metabolic acidosis.

Level of Cognitive Ability: Analysis
Client Needs: Physiological Integrity
Integrated Process: Nursing Process—analysis
Content Area: Fundamental skills
Reference: Phipps, W., Monahan, F., Sands, J., Marek, J., & Neighbors, M. (2003). *Medical-surgical nursing: Health and illness perspectives* (7th ed., p. 275). St. Louis: Mosby.

8. 1

Rationale: Kussmaul's respirations are abnormally deep, regular, and increased in rate. In bradypnea, respirations are regular but abnormally slow. In hyperpnea, respirations are labored and increased in depth and rate. Apnea is described as respirations that cease for several seconds.

Test-Taking Strategy: Use the process of elimination and knowledge of the description of Kussmaul's respirations. Recalling that this type of respiration occurs in diabetic ketoacidosis will direct you to option 1. Review the characteristics of this type of respiration if you had difficulty with this question.

Level of Cognitive Ability: Comprehension
Client Needs: Physiological Integrity
Integrated Process: Nursing Process—assessment
Content Area: Fundamental skills
Reference: Potter, P., & Perry, A. (2001). *Fundamentals of nursing* (5th ed., p. 703). St. Louis: Mosby.

9. 4

Rationale: Increases in base components occur as a result of oral or parenteral intake of bicarbonates, carbonates, acetates, citrates, or lactates. Excessive use of oral antacids containing bicarbonate can cause a metabolic alkalosis. Options 1, 2, and 3 are incorrect.

Test-Taking Strategy: Use the process of elimination. Eliminate options 1 and 2 first because a respiratory condition is not addressed in the question. From the remaining options, remembering that antacids contain bicarbonate and that an excess oral intake will increase bicarbonate will assist in directing you to option 4. Review the causes of metabolic alkalosis if you had difficulty with the question.

Level of Cognitive Ability: Comprehension
Client Needs: Physiological Integrity
Integrated Process: Nursing Process—assessment
Content Area: Fundamental skills
Reference: Ignatavicius, D., & Workman, M. (2002). *Medical-surgical nursing: Critical thinking for collaborative care* (4th ed., p. 230). Philadelphia: W. B. Saunders.

10. 3

Rationale: Clinical manifestations of metabolic acidosis include hyperpnea with Kussmaul's respirations; headache; nausea, vomiting, and diarrhea; fruity-smelling breath resulting from improper fat metabolism; central nervous system depression, including mental dullness, drowsiness, stupor, and coma; twitching; and convulsions. Hyperkalemia will occur.

Test-Taking Strategy: Use the process of elimination and knowledge regarding the clinical manifestations of metabolic acidosis and normal laboratory values to answer the question. The only abnormal laboratory value is the potassium level, option 3. Review the clinical manifestations of metabolic acidosis and normal laboratory values if you had difficulty with this question.

Level of Cognitive Ability: Analysis
Client Needs: Physiological Integrity
Integrated Process: Nursing Process—assessment
Content Area: Fundamental skills
References: Chernecky, C., & Berger, B. (2001). *Laboratory tests and diagnostic procedures* (3rd ed., p. 836). Philadelphia: W. B. Saunders.
Ignatavicius, D., & Workman, M. (2002). *Medical-surgical nursing: Critical thinking for collaborative care* (4th ed., p. 230). Philadelphia: W. B. Saunders.

CRITICAL THINKING: PRIORITIZING (ORDERED RESPONSE)

Answer: 32541
Rationale: The Allen's test is performed before obtaining an arterial blood specimen from the radial artery to determine the presence of collateral circulation and the adequacy of the ulnar artery. Failure to determine the presence of adequate collateral circulation could result in severe ischemic injury to the hand if damage to the radial artery occurs with arterial puncture. The nurse first would explain the procedure to the client. To perform the test, the nurse applies direct pressure over the client's ulnar and radial arteries simultaneously. While applying pressure, the nurse asks the client to open and close the hand repeatedly; the hand should blanch. The nurse then releases pressure from the ulnar artery while compressing the radial artery and assesses the color of the extremity distal to the pressure point. If pinkness fails to return within 6 seconds, the ulnar artery is insufficient, indicating that the radial artery should not be used for obtaining a blood specimen.

Test-Taking Strategy: Recalling that the procedure needs to be explained to the client will assist in determining the first action. Next, think about the purpose and reason for performing this test and visualize the procedure. This will assist in determining the steps for performing the Allen's test. Review this test if you had difficulty with this question.
Level of Cognitive Ability: Application
Client Needs: Physiological Integrity
Integrated Process: Nursing Process—assessment
Content Area: Fundamental skills
Reference: Potter, P., & Perry, A. (2001). *Fundamentals of nursing* (5th ed., p. 790). St. Louis: Mosby.

REFERENCES

Chernecky, C., & Berger, B. (2001). *Laboratory tests and diagnostic procedures* (3rd ed.). Philadelphia: W. B. Saunders.

Ignatavicius, D., & Workman, M. (2002). *Medical-surgical nursing: Critical thinking for collaborative care* (4th ed.). Philadelphia: W. B. Saunders.

National Council of State Boards of Nursing (Eds.). (2003). *Test Plan for the National Council Licensure Examination for Registered Nurses* (effective date: April 2004). Chicago: Author.

Phipps, W., Monahan, F., Sands, J., Marek, J., & Neighbors, M. (2003). *Medical-surgical nursing: health and illness perspectives* (7th ed.). St. Louis: Mosby.

Potter, P., & Perry, A. (2001). *Fundamentals of nursing* (5th ed.). St. Louis: Mosby.

Laboratory Values

PYRAMID TERMS

plasma The fluid ground substance; what remains after the cells have been removed from a sample of whole blood.

serum Blood plasma from which clotting agents have been removed.

venipuncture Puncture into a vein to obtain a blood specimen for testing; the antecubital veins are the veins of choice because of ease of access.

▲ THE PYRAMID TO SUCCESS

This chapter identifies the normal adult values for the most common laboratory tests. If you are familiar with the normal values, you will be able to determine whether an abnormality exists when a laboratory value is presented in a question. The questions on the NCLEX-RN exam related to laboratory values require you to identify whether the laboratory value is normal or abnormal, and then you are required to think critically about the effects of the laboratory value in terms of the client. Pyramid Points focus on knowledge of the normal values for the most common laboratory tests, therapeutic serum medication levels of commonly prescribed medications, and determination of the need to implement specific actions based on the findings. Remember that most blood samples should not be drawn during hemodialysis. When a question is presented on the NCLEX-RN examination regarding a specific laboratory value, note the disorder presented in the question and the associated body organ that is affected as a result of the disorder. This process will assist you in determining the correct answer. For example, if the question asks about the immune status of a client receiving chemotherapy, assessment of laboratory values will focus on the white blood cell count and the neutrophils. You will need to analyze these results as possibly being low and determine the specific client need, which in this case would be the risk for infection. In the client receiving

chemotherapy who has a low white blood cell count, your plan centers on the immune system and protecting that client from infection. Implementation focuses on preventive interventions related to infection, perhaps protective isolation measures. Evaluation may focus on maintenance of a normal temperature in the client. Integrated Processes addressed in this chapter are Nursing Process, Caring, Communication and Documentation, and Teaching/Learning. Box 11-1 lists the abbreviations found in laboratory values.

CLIENT NEEDS
Safe, Effective Care Environment

Informed consent for specific procedures
Verification of the identity of the client
Medical and surgical asepsis when obtaining a specimen
Principles of infection control
Standard, transmission-based, and other precautions
Procedures for handling hazardous and infectious materials

BOX 11-1

Pyramid Abbreviations

Abbreviation	Description
g/dL	grams per deciliter
mcg/dL	micrograms per deciliter
mg/dL	milligrams per deciliter
mEq/L	milliequivalents per liter
units/L	units per liter
mm/hr	millimeters per hour
IU/L	International Units per liter
mcg/mL	micrograms per milliliter
ng/mL	nanograms per milliliter
microunits/mL	microunits per milliliter
mL/kg	milliliters per kilogram

Health Promotion and Maintenance

Client preparation for the laboratory test
Posttest procedures
Signs and symptoms that indicate the need to notify the health care provider
Importance of follow-up laboratory studies
Community resources available for the follow-up

Psychosocial Integrity

Communication of the purpose of test to client
Provision of emotional support during testing
Communication with the client regarding laboratory results
Description of specific interventions or home care measures required based on the results

Physiological Integrity

Comfort interventions
Normal values for the most common laboratory tests
Therapeutic serum medication levels of commonly prescribed medications
Reporting of significant laboratory values
Determining the need to implement specific actions based on the laboratory results
Monitoring for clinical manifestations associated with an abnormal laboratory value
Monitoring for potential complications related to a test

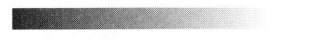

I. ELECTROLYTES (TABLE 11-1)
A. **Serum** sodium
　1. Description
　　a. Sodium is a major cation of extracellular fluid.
　　b. Sodium maintains osmotic pressures and acid-base balance and assists in transmission of nerve impulses.
　　c. Sodium is absorbed from the small intestine and excreted in the urine in amounts dependent on dietary intake.
　　d. Minimum daily requirement of sodium is about 15 mEq.
　2. Nursing consideration: Drawing blood samples proximal to intravenous (IV) infusion of sodium chloride will elevate results falsely.

TABLE 11-1

Normal Adult Electrolyte Values

Electrolyte	Value
Sodium	135-145 mEq/L
Potassium	3.5-5.1 mEq/L
Chloride	98-107 mEq/L
Bicarbonate (venous)	22-29 mEq/L

B. **Serum** potassium
　1. Description
　　a. Potassium is a major intracellular cation; it regulates cellular water balance, electrical conduction in muscle cells, and acid-base balance.
　　b. The body obtains potassium through dietary ingestion, and the kidneys preserve or excrete potassium depending on cellular need.
　　c. Potassium levels are used to evaluate cardiac function, renal function, gastrointestinal function, and the need for IV replacement therapy.
　2. Nursing considerations
　　a. Use of a tourniquet and clenching and unclenching the hand before venous sampling can increase the value.
　　b. Do not draw blood from a site where an IV infusion exists.
　　c. If the client is receiving potassium supplementation, note this on the laboratory form.
　　d. Clients with elevated white blood cell counts and platelet counts may have falsely elevated potassium levels.
C. **Serum** chloride
　1. Description
　　a. Chloride is a hydrochloric acid salt that is the most abundant body anion in the extracellular fluid.
　　b. Chloride functions to counterbalance cations, such as sodium, and acts as a buffer during oxygen and carbon dioxide exchange in red blood cells.
　　c. Chloride aids in digestion and maintaining osmotic pressure and water balance.
　2. Nursing considerations
　　a. Draw blood from an extremity that does not have normal saline infusing into it.
　　b. Do not allow the client to clench and unclench the hand before drawing blood.
　　c. Any condition accompanied by prolonged vomiting, diarrhea, or both will alter chloride levels.

II. COAGULATION STUDIES
A. Activated partial thromboplastin time (aPTT)
　1. Description
　　a. The aPTT evaluates how well the coagulation sequence is functioning by measuring the amount of time it takes for recalcified, citrated **plasma** to clot after partial thromboplastin is added to it.
　　b. The test screens for deficiencies and inhibitors of all factors except VII and XIII.
　　c. The aPTT most commonly is used to monitor heparin therapy and screen for coagulation disorders.
　2. Value: 20 to 36 seconds, depending on the type of activator used

3. Nursing considerations
   a. If the client is receiving intermittent heparin therapy, draw the blood sample 1 hour before the next scheduled dose.
   b. Do not draw samples from an arm into which heparin is infusing.
   c. Transport specimen to the laboratory immediately.
   d. The aPTT should be between 1.5 and 2.5 times normal when the client is receiving heparin therapy; if the value is prolonged, initiate bleeding precautions.

B. Prothrombin time (PT) and international normalized ratio (INR)
   1. Description
      a. Prothrombin is a vitamin K–dependent glycoprotein produced by the liver that is necessary for firm fibrin clot formation.
      b. Each laboratory establishes a normal value or control value based on the method used to perform the PT test.
      c. The PT measures the amount of time it takes for clot formation and is used to monitor response to warfarin sodium (Coumadin) therapy or to screen for dysfunction of the extrinsic system resulting from liver disease, vitamin K deficiency, or disseminated intravascular coagulation.
      d. A PT value within 2 seconds (plus or minus) of the control is considered normal.
      e. The INR standardized the PT ratio and is calculated in the laboratory setting by raising the observed PT ratio to the power of the International Sensitivity Index specific to the thromboplastin reagent used.
      f. The INR measures the effects of oral anticoagulants.
   2. Values
      a. PT: 9.6 to 11.8 seconds (male adult) and 9.5 to 11.3 seconds (female adult)
      b. INR: 2.0 to 3.0 for standard warfarin therapy
      c. INR: 3.0 to 4.5 for high-dose warfarin therapy
   3. Nursing considerations
      a. A baseline PT should be drawn before anticoagulation therapy is started; note the time of collection on laboratory form.
      b. Provide direct pressure to the **venipuncture** site for 3 to 5 minutes if a coagulation defect is present.
      c. Concurrent warfarin therapy with heparin therapy can lengthen the PT for up to 5 hours after dosing.
      d. Diets high in green leafy vegetables can increase the absorption of vitamin K, which shortens the PT.
      e. Orally administered anticoagulation therapy usually maintains the PT at 1.5 to 2 times the laboratory control value.

f. A PT greater than 30 seconds places the client at risk for hemorrhage.

C. Clotting time
   1. Description: The time required for the interaction of all factors involved in the clotting process
   2. Value: 8 to 15 minutes
   3. Nursing considerations
      a. The client should not receive heparin therapy for 3 hours before specimen collection because the heparin therapy will affect the results.
      b. The test result is prolonged by any anticoagulant therapy, test tube agitation, or high temperature changes that may affect the specimen.

D. Platelet count
   1. Description
      a. Platelets function in hemostatic plug formation, clot retraction, and coagulation factor activation.
      b. Platelets are produced by the bone marrow to function in hemostasis.
   2. Value: 150,000 to 400,000 cells/μL
   3. Nursing considerations
      a. Monitor the **venipuncture** site for bleeding in clients with known thrombocytopenia.
      b. High altitudes, chronic cold weather, and exercise increase platelet counts.
      c. Bleeding precautions should be instituted in clients with a low platelet count.

III. ERYTHROCYTE STUDIES

A. Erythrocyte sedimentation rate
   1. Description
      a. The rate at which erythrocytes settle out of anticoagulated blood in 1 hour
      b. Not diagnostic of any particular disease but indicative that a disease process is ongoing
   2. Value: 0 to 30 mm/hr, depending on age of client
   3. Nursing consideration: Fasting is not necessary, but a fatty meal may cause **plasma** alterations.

B. Hemoglobin and hematocrit
   1. Description
      a. Hemoglobin is the main component of erythrocytes and serves as the vehicle for the transportation of oxygen and carbon dioxide.
      b. Hemoglobin determinations are important in identifying anemia.
      c. Hematocrit represents red blood cell mass and is an important measurement in the identification of anemia or polycythemia (Table 11-2).
   2. Nursing consideration: Fasting is not required.

C. **Serum** iron
   1. Description
      a. Iron is found mostly in hemoglobin.
      b. Iron acts as a carrier of oxygen from the lungs to the tissues and indirectly aids in the return of carbon dioxide to the lungs.
      c. Iron aids in diagnosing anemias and hemolytic disorders.

TABLE 11-2

Normal Adult Hemoglobin and Hematocrit Levels

Blood Component	Normal Value
HEMOGLOBIN	
Male adult	14-16.5 g/dL
Female adult	12-15 g/dL
HEMATOCRIT	
Male adult	42%-52%
Female adult	35%-47%

2. Values
   a. Male adult: 65 to 175 mcg/dL
   b. Female adult: 50 to 170 mcg/dL
3. Nursing consideration: Level of iron will be increased if the client has ingested iron before the test.

D. Red blood cell count
   1. Description
      a. Red blood cells function in hemoglobin transport, which results in delivery of oxygen to the body tissues.
      b. Red blood cells are formed by red bone marrow, have a life span of 120 days, and are removed from the blood by the liver, spleen, and bone marrow.
      c. The red blood cell count aids in diagnosing anemias and blood dyscrasias.
      d. The red blood cell count evaluates the ability of the body to produce red blood cells in sufficient numbers.
   2. Values
      a. Female adult: 4 million to 5.5 million cells/μL
      b. Male adult: 4.5 million to 6.2 million cells/μL
   3. Nursing consideration: Fasting is not required.

IV. SERUM ENZYMES/CARDIAC MARKERS
   A. Creatine kinase (CK)
      1. Description
         a. Creatine kinase is an enzyme found in muscle and brain tissue that reflects tissue catabolism resulting from cell trauma.
         b. The test for CK is performed to detect myocardial or skeletal muscle damage or central nervous system damage; a normal CK value is 26 to 174 units/L.
         c. Isoenzymes include CK-MB (cardiac), CK-BB (brain), and CK-MM (muscles).
         d. Isoenzyme CK-MB is found mainly in cardiac muscle, CK-BB is found mainly in brain tissue, and CK-MM is found mainly is skeletal muscle.
      2. Values
         a. CK-MB: 0% to 5% of total

b. CK-MM: 95% to 100% of total
         c. CK-BB: 0%
      3. Nursing considerations
         a. If the test is to evaluate skeletal muscle, instruct the client to avoid strenuous physical activity for 24 hours before the test.
         b. Instruct the client to avoid ingestion of alcohol for 24 hours before the test.
         c. Invasive procedures and intramuscular injections may elevate CK levels falsely.
   B. Lactate dehydrogenase (LDH)
      1. Description
         a. The isoenzymes that are affected particularly with acute myocardial infarction are LDH_1 and LDH_2.
         b. The LDH level begins to rise about 24 hours after myocardial infarction and peaks in 48 to 72 hours; thereafter it returns to normal, usually within 7 to 14 days (Table 11-3).
         c. The presence of an LDH flip (when LDH_1 is higher than LDH_2) is helpful in diagnosing a myocardial infarction.
      2. Nursing considerations
         a. The LDH isoenzymes should be interpreted in view of the clinical findings.
         b. Testing should be repeated on 3 consecutive days.
   C. Troponins
      1. Description
         a. Troponin is a regulatory protein found in striated muscle (skeletal and myocardial).
         b. Increased amounts of troponins are released into the bloodstream when an infarction causes damage to the myocardium.
         c. Serial measurements are important to compare with a baseline test.
      2. Values
         a. Troponin I: Value usually is less than 0.6 ng/mL; greater than 1.5 ng/mL is consistent with a myocardial infarction.
         b. Troponin T: Greater than 0.1 to 0.2 ng/mL is consistent with a myocardial infarction.
      3. Nursing consideration: Client does not need to be fasting.

TABLE 11-3

Normal Adult Lactate Dehydrogenase

Serum Enzyme	Normal Value
Lactate dehydrogenase	140-280 units/L
Lactate dehydrogenase isoenzymes	
LDH_1	14%-26%
LDH_2	29%-39%
LDH_3	20%-26%
LDH_4	8%-16%
LDH_5	6%-16%

V. SERUM GASTROINTESTINAL STUDIES

A. Albumin
  1. Description
     a. Albumin is a main **plasma** protein of blood.
     b. Albumin maintains oncotic pressure and transports bilirubin, fatty acids, medications, hormones, and other substances that are insoluble in water.
  2. Value: 3.4 to 5 g/dL
  3. Nursing considerations: Draw from an extremity the does not have an IV infusion in it.
B. Alkaline phosphatase
  1. Description
     a. Alkaline phosphatase is an enzyme normally found in bone, liver, intestine, and placenta.
     b. The level rises during periods of bone growth, liver disease, and bile duct obstruction.
  2. Value: 4.5 to 13 King-Armstrong units/dL
  3. Nursing considerations
     a. The client may need to fast 12 hours before the test.
     b. Hepatotoxic medications administered within 12 hours before specimen collection can cause false values.
     c. Transport the specimen to laboratory immediately.
C. Ammonia
  1. Description
     a. Ammonia is a waste product from nitrogen breakdown during protein metabolism.
     b. Ammonia is metabolized by the liver and excreted by the kidneys as urea.
     c. Elevated levels resulting from hepatic dysfunction may lead to encephalopathy.
     d. Ammonia is not a reliable indicator of hepatic coma.
  2. Value: 35 to 65 mcg/dL
  3. Nursing considerations
     a. Instruct the client to fast, except for water, and to refrain from smoking for 8 to 10 hours before the test.
     b. Place the specimen in ice and transport to the laboratory immediately.
D. Amylase
  1. Description
     a. Amylase is an enzyme produced by the pancreas and salivary glands that aids in the digestion of complex carbohydrates and is excreted by the kidneys.
     b. In acute pancreatitis the amylase level is greatly increased; the level starts rising in 3 to 6 hours after the onset of pain, peaks at about 24 hours, and returns to normal in 2 to 3 days after the onset of pain.
  2. Value: 25 to 151 units/L
  3. Nursing considerations

a. On the laboratory form, list medications that the client has taken for the 24 hours before the test.
     b. Note that many medications may cause false-positive or false-negative results.
     c. Results are invalidated if the specimen was obtained less than 72 hours after cholecystography with radiopaque dyes.
E. Lipase
  1. Description
     a. Lipase is a pancreatic enzyme that changes fats and triglycerides into fatty acids and glycerol.
     b. Elevated lipase levels occur in pancreatic disorders; elevations may not occur until 24 to 36 hours after the onset of illness and may remain elevated for up to 14 days.
  2. Value: 10 to 140 units/L
  3. Nursing considerations: Endoscopic retrograde cholangiopancreatography may increase lipase activity.
F. Bilirubin
  1. Description
     a. Bilirubin is produced by the liver, spleen, and bone marrow and is also a by-product of hemoglobin breakdown.
     b. Total bilirubin levels can be broken down into direct bilirubin, which is excreted primarily via the intestinal tract, and indirect bilirubin, which circulates primarily in the bloodstream.
     c. Total bilirubin levels rise with any type of jaundice, whereas direct and indirect levels rise depending on the cause of the jaundice.
  2. Values
     a. Bilirubin, direct: 0 to 0.3 mg/dL
     b. Bilirubin, indirect: 0.1 to 1.0 mg/dL
     c. Bilirubin, total: less than 1.5 mg/dL
  3. Nursing considerations
     a. Instruct the client to eat a diet low in yellow foods, such as carrots, yams, yellow beans, and pumpkins, for 3 to 4 days before the blood is drawn.
     b. Instruct the client to fast for 4 hours before the blood is drawn.
     c. Note that results will be elevated with the ingestion of alcohol or the administration of morphine sulfate, theophylline, ascorbic acid (vitamin C), or acetylsalicylic acid (aspirin).
     d. Note that results are invalidated if the client has received a radioactive scan within 24 hours before the test.
G. Lipids
  1. Description
     a. Blood lipids consist primarily of cholesterol, triglycerides, and phospholipids.
     b. Lipid assessment includes total cholesterol, high-density lipoprotein, low-density lipoprotein, and triglycerides.

c. Cholesterol is present in all body tissues and is a major component of low-density lipoproteins, brain and nerve cells, cell membranes, and some gallbladder stones.

d. Triglycerides constitute a major part of very low-density lipoproteins and a small part of low-density lipoproteins.

e. Triglycerides are synthesized in the liver from fatty acids, protein, and glucose, and are obtained from the diet.

2. Values:
   a. Cholesterol: 140 to 199 mg/dL
   b. Low-density lipoproteins: less than 130 mg/dL
   c. High-density lipoproteins: 30 to 70 mg/dL
   d. Triglycerides: less than 200 mg/dL

3. Nursing considerations
   a. Oral contraceptives may increase the lipid level.
   b. Instruct the client to abstain from foods and fluid, except for water, for 12 to 14 hours and from alcohol for 24 hours before the test.
   c. Instruct the client that the evening meal before the test should be free of high-cholesterol foods.

H. Protein
   1. Description
      a. Protein reflects the total amount of albumin and globulins in the **serum**.
      b. Protein regulates osmotic pressure and comprises coagulation factors for hemostasis, enzymes, hormones, tissue growth and repair, and pH buffers.
   2. Value: 6.0 to 8.0 g/dL
   3. Nursing considerations
      a. Do not draw blood from an extremity with an IV infusion.
      b. Instruct the client to avoid a high-fat diet for 8 hours before the test.

I. Uric acid
   1. Description
      a. Uric acid is formed as the purines, adenine and guanine, and is metabolized continuously during the formation and degradation of DNA and RNA and from the metabolism of dietary purines.
      b. Elevated amounts of uric acid deposit in joints and soft tissue and cause gout.
      c. Conditions of fast cell turnover, as well as slowed renal excretion of uric acid, may cause hyperuricemia.
      d. Elevated amounts of urinary uric acid precipitate into urate stones in the kidneys.
   2. Values
      a. Male adult: 4.5 to 8 mg/dL
      b. Female adult: 2.5 to 6.2 mg/dL
   3. Nursing considerations
      a. Instruct the client to fast for 8 hours before the test.
      b. Aminophylline, caffeine, and vitamin C may cause falsely elevated results.

VI. GLUCOSE STUDIES

A. Fasting blood glucose
   1. Description
      a. Glucose is a monosaccharide found in fruits and is formed from the digestion of carbohydrates and the conversion of glycogen by the liver.
      b. Glucose is the main source of cellular energy for the body and is essential for brain and erythrocyte function.
      c. Fasting blood glucose levels are used to help diagnose diabetes mellitus and hypoglycemia (Table 11-4).
   2. Nursing considerations
      a. Instruct the client to fast for 8 to 12 hours before the test.
      b. Instruct a client with diabetes mellitus to withhold morning insulin or oral hypoglycemic medication until after the blood is drawn.

B. Glucose tolerance test (Table 11-4)
   1. Description
      a. The glucose tolerance test aids in the diagnosis of diabetes mellitus.
      b. If the glucose levels peak at higher than normal at 1 and 2 hours after injection or ingestion of glucose and are slower than normal to return to fasting levels, then diabetes mellitus is confirmed.
   2. Nursing considerations
      a. Instruct the client to eat a high-carbohydrate (200 to 300 g) diet for 3 days before the test.
      b. Instruct the client to avoid alcohol, coffee, and smoking for 36 hours before the test.
      c. Instruct the client to fast for 10 to 16 hours before the test.
      d. Instruct the client to avoid strenuous exercise for 8 hours before and after the test.
      e. Instruct the client with diabetes mellitus to withhold morning insulin or oral hypoglycemic medication.
      f. Instruct the client that the test will take 3 to 5 hours, requires intravenous or oral administration of glucose, and multiple blood samples.

TABLE 11-4

Normal Adult Glucose Values

Point of Measurement	Normal Value
Glucose, fasting	70-110 mg/dL
Glucose monitoring (capillary blood)	60-110 mg/dL
Glucose tolerance test, oral	
Baseline fasting	70-110 mg/dL
30-minute fasting	110-170 mg/dL
60-minute fasting	120-170 mg/dL
90-minute fasting	100-140 mg/dL
120-minute fasting	70-120 mg/dL
Glucose, 2-hour postprandial	<140 mg/dL

C. Glycosylated hemoglobin
   1. Description
      a. Glycosylated hemoglobin is blood glucose bound to hemoglobin.
      b. Hemoglobin A_{1c} (glycosylated hemoglobin A) is a reflection of how well blood glucose levels have been controlled for up to the prior 4 months.
      c. Hyperglycemia in diabetics is usually a cause of an increase in hemoglobin A_{1c}.
   2. Values
      a. Values are expressed as a percentage of the total hemoglobin.
      b. Diabetic with good control: 7.5% or less
      c. Diabetic with fair control: 7.6% to 8.9%
      d. Diabetic with poor control: 9% or greater
   3. Nursing consideration: Fasting is not required before the test.

VII. RENAL FUNCTION STUDIES
A. **Serum** creatinine
   1. Description
      a. Creatinine is a specific indicator of renal function.
      b. Increased levels of creatinine indicate a slowing of the glomerular filtration rate.
   2. Value: 0.6 to 1.3 mg/dL
   3. Nursing considerations: Instruct the client to avoid excessive exercise for 8 hours and excessive red meat intake for 24 hours before the test.
B. Blood urea nitrogen
   1. Description
      a. Urea nitrogen is the nitrogen portion of urea, a substance formed in the liver through an enzymatic protein breakdown process.
      b. Urea is normally freely filtered through the renal glomeruli, with a small amount reabsorbed in the tubules and the remainder excreted in the urine.
      c. Elevated levels indicate a slowing of the glomerular filtration rate.
   2. Value: 8 to 25 mg/dL
   3. Nursing considerations: Creatinine levels and urea nitrogen levels should be analyzed when renal function is evaluated.

VIII. ELEMENTS
A. Calcium
   1. Description
      a. Calcium is a cation that is absorbed into the bloodstream from dietary sources and functions in bone formation, nerve impulse transmission, and contraction of myocardial and skeletal muscles.
      b. Calcium aids in blood clotting by converting prothrombin to thrombin.
   2. Value: 8.6 to 10.0 mg/dL

   3. Nursing considerations
      a. Instruct the client to eat a diet with normal calcium levels (800 mg/day) for 3 days before the test.
      b. Instruct the client that fasting may be required for 8 hours before the test.
B. Magnesium
   1. Description
      a. Magnesium is used as an index to determine metabolic activity and renal function.
      b. Magnesium is needed in the blood-clotting mechanism, regulates neuromuscular activity, acts as a cofactor that modifies the activity of many enzymes, and has an effect on the metabolism of calcium.
   2. Value: 1.6 to 2.6 mg/dL
   3. Nursing considerations
      a. Prolonged use of magnesium products will cause increased levels.
      b. Long-term total parenteral nutrition therapy or excessive loss of body fluids may cause decreased levels.
C. Phosphorus
   1. Description
      a. Phosphorus is important in bone formation, energy storage and release, urinary acid-base buffering, and carbohydrate metabolism.
      b. Phosphorus is absorbed from food and is excreted by the kidneys.
      c. High concentrations of phosphorus are stored in bone and skeletal muscle.
   2. Value: 2.7 to 4.5 mg/dL
   3. Nursing considerations: Instruct the client to fast before the test.

IX. THYROID STUDIES
A. Description
   1. Thyroid studies are performed if a thyroid disorder is suspected.
   2. Thyroid studies are helpful to differentiate primary thyroid disease from secondary causes and from abnormalities in thyroxine-binding globulin levels.
B. Values
   1. Thyroid-stimulating hormone (also called thyrotropin): 0.2 to 5.4 microunits/mL
   2. Thyroxine: 5.0 to 12.0 mcg/dL
   3. Thyroxine, free: 0.8 to 2.4 ng/dL
   4. Triiodothyronine: 80 to 230 ng/dL
C. Nursing consideration: Test results may be invalid if client has undergone a radionuclide scan within 7 days before the test.

X. WHITE BLOOD CELL COUNT
A. Description
   1. White blood cells function in the immune defense system of the body

TABLE 11-5

Normal Adult White Blood Cell Differential Count

Cell Type	Percentage and Count
Neutrophils	56% or 1800-7800 cells/μL
Bands	3% or 0-700 cells/μL
Eosinophils	2.7% or 0-450 cells/μL
Basophils	0.3% or 0-200 cells/μL
Lymphocytes	34% or 1000-4800 cells/μL
Monocytes	4% or 0-800 cells/μL

2. The white blood cell count assesses each leukocyte distribution.

B. Value: 4500 to 11,000 cells/μL (Table 11-5)

C. Nursing considerations
   1. A "shift to the left" means that an increased number of immature neutrophils are in the peripheral blood.
   2. A low total white blood cell count with a left shift indicates a recovery from bone marrow depression or an infection of such intensity that the demand for neutrophils in the tissue is greater than the capacity of the bone marrow to release them into the circulation.
   3. A high total white blood cell count with a left shift indicates an increased release of neutrophils by the bone marrow in response to an overwhelming infection or inflammation.
   4. A "shift to the right" means that cells have more than the usual number of nuclear segments; found in liver disease, Down syndrome, or megaloblastic and pernicious anemia.

XI. HEPATITIS TESTS

A. Description
   1. Tests include radioimmunoassay, enzyme-linked immunosorbent assay (ELISA), and microparticle enzyme immunoassay.
   2. Serological tests for specific hepatitis virus markers assist in defining the specific type of hepatitis.

B. Values
   1. The presence of immunoglobulin M (IgM) antibody to hepatitis A virus and the total antibody to hepatitis A virus identify the disease.
   2. Detection of hepatitis B core antigen (HBcAg), envelope antigen (HBeAg), and surface antigen (HBsAg), or their corresponding antibodies, constitutes hepatitis B assessment.
   3. Hepatitis C is confirmed by the presence of antibodies to hepatitis C virus.
   4. Serological hepatitis D virus determination is made by detection of the hepatitis D antigen (HDAg) early in the course of the infection and by detection of anti–hepatitis D virus antibody in the later disease stages.

5. Specific serological tests for hepatitis E virus include detection of IgM and IgG antibodies to hepatitis E.
   6. Hepatitis G virus has been found in some blood donors, IV drug users, hemodialysis clients, and clients with hemophilia; however, hepatitis G virus does not appear to cause significant liver disease.

C. Nursing consideration: If the radioimmunoassay technique is being used, the injection of radionuclides within 1 week before the blood test may elevate results falsely.

XII. HUMAN IMMUNODEFICIENCY VIRUS (HIV) AND ACQUIRED IMMUNODEFICIENCY SYNDROME (AIDS) TESTING

A. Description
   1. The test detects HIV, which cause AIDS.
   2. Tests used to determine the presence of antibodies to HIV include ELISA, Western blot, and immunofluorescence assay (IFA).
   3. A single reactive ELISA test by itself cannot be used to diagnose HIV and should be repeated in duplicate with the same blood sample; if the result is repeatedly reactive, follow-up tests using Western blot or IFA should be done.
   4. A positive Western blot or IFA is considered confirmatory for HIV.
   5. A positive ELISA that fails to be confirmed by Western blot or IFA should not be considered negative, and repeat testing should take place in 3 to 6 months.

B. CD4$^+$ T cell counts
   1. This cell count monitors the progression of HIV.
   2. As the disease progresses, usually the number of CD4 T cell counts decrease, with a resultant decrease in immunity.
   3. Normal CD4 T cell count is between 500 and 1600 cells/μL.
   4. Generally the immune system remains healthy with CD4 T cell counts greater than 500 cells/μL.
   5. Immune system problems occur when the CD4 T cell count is between 200 and 499 cells/μL.
   6. Severe immune system problems occur when the CD4 T cell count is less than 200 cells/μL.

C. CD4 to CD8 ratio
   1. The ratio monitors the progression of the disease.
   2. The normal ratio is about 2:1.
   3. In HIV and AIDS, because of the low number of CD4 cells, this ratio is low.

D. Viral culture involves placing the infected client's blood cells in a culture medium and measuring the amount of reverse transcriptase activity over a specified period of time.

E. Viral load testing measures the presence of HIV viral genetic material (RNA) or another viral protein in the client's blood.

F. The p24 antigen assay quantifies the amount of HIV viral core protein in the client's **serum**.

G. Nursing considerations
  1. Maintain issues of confidentiality surrounding HIV and AIDS testing.
  2. Follow prescribed state regulations and protocols related to reporting positive test results.

XIII. URINE TESTS (TABLE 11-6)

XIV. THERAPEUTIC SERUM MEDICATION LEVELS (TABLE 11-7)

TABLE 11-6

Normal Adult Values: Urine Tests

Name of Test	Value
Chloride	110-250 mEq/24 hr
Magnesium	7.3-12.2 mg/dL per day
Potassium	25-125 mEq/24 hr
Protein	40-150 mg/24 hr
Sodium	40-220 mEq/24 hr
Uric acid	250-750 mg/24 hr
pH	4.5-7.8
Specific gravity	1.016 to 1.022

TABLE 11-7

Therapeutic Serum Medication Levels

Medication	Therapeutic Range
Acetaminophen (Tylenol)	10-20 mcg/mL
Amikacin (Amikin)	25-30 mcg/mL
Amitriptyline (Elavil)	120-150 ng/mL
Carbamazepine (Tegretol)	5-12 mcg/mL
Chloramphenicol (Chloromycetin)	10-20 mcg/mL
Desipramine (Norpramin)	150-300 ng/mL
Digitoxin (Crystodigin)	15-25 ng/mL
Digoxin (Lanoxin)	0.5-2.0 ng/mL
Disopyramide (Norpace)	2-5 mcg/mL
Ethosuximide (Zarontin)	40-100 mcg/mL
Gentamicin (Garamycin)	5-10 mcg/mL
Imipramine (Tofranil)	150-300 ng/mL
Lidocaine (Xylocaine)	1.5-5.0 mcg/mL
Lithium (Lithobid)	0.5-1.3 mEq/L
Magnesium sulfate	4-7 mg/dL
Nortriptyline (Aventyl)	50-150 ng/mL
Phenobarbital (Luminal)	10-30 mcg/mL
Phenytoin (Dilantin)	10-20 mcg/mL
Primidone (Mysoline)	5-20 mcg/mL
Procainamide (Pronestyl)	4-10 mcg/mL
Propranolol (Inderal)	50-100 ng/mL
Quinidine (Quinaglute, Cardioquin)	2-5 mcg/mL
Salicylate	100-250 mcg/mL
Theophylline (aminophylline; Theo-Dur)	10-20 mcg/mL
Tobramycin (Nebcin)	5-10 mcg/mL
Valproic acid (Depakene)	50-100 mcg/mL

PRACTICE QUESTIONS

1. A nurse is assigned to a 40 year-old client who has a diagnosis of chronic pancreatitis. The nurse reviews the laboratory result, anticipating a laboratory report that indicates a serum amylase level of
   1. 45 units/L.
   2. 100 units/L.
   3. 300 units/L.
   4. 500 units/L.

2. A client is suspected of having a myocardial infarction. A nurse assesses for elevations in which of the following isoenzyme values reported with the creatinine phosphokinase level?
   1. MM
   2. MB
   3. BB
   4. MK

3. An adult client has had laboratory work done as part of a routine physical examination. A nurse interprets that the client may have a mild degree of renal insufficiency if which of the following serum creatinine levels is found?
   1. 0.2 mg/dL
   2. 0.5 mg/dL
   3. 1.9 mg/dL
   4. 3.5 mg/dL

4. A client with a history of a seizure disorder who has been compliant with medication therapy is admitted to the hospital with seizure activity. Phenytoin (Dilantin) is administered to the client intravenously, and subsequently a serum phenytoin level is drawn. A nurse evaluates that the medication therapy has been most effective if the laboratory result is
   1. 3 mcg/mL.
   2. 8 mcg/mL.
   3. 16 mcg/mL.
   4. 24 mcg/mL.

5. A client who takes theophylline (Theo-Dur) for chronic obstructive pulmonary disease is seen in the urgent care center for respiratory distress. Just before therapy is initiated, a blood sample to determine the baseline theophylline level is drawn. Once the client is stabilized, a nurse begins discharge teaching. The nurse would be especially vigilant to include information about complying with medication therapy if the client's baseline result was
   1. 10 mcg/mL.
   2. 12 mcg/mL.
   3. 15 mcg/mL.
   4. 18 mcg/mL.

6. A nurse checks the laboratory result for a serum digoxin level that was drawn for a client earlier in the day and notes that the result is 2.4 ng/mL. Which of the following is the most important action on the part of the nurse?

1. Record the normal value on the client's flowsheet.
2. Administer the next dose of the medication as scheduled.
3. Check the client's last pulse rate.
4. Notify the physician.

7. A client is receiving a continuous intravenous infusion of heparin sodium to treat deep vein thrombosis. The client's activated partial thromboplastin time level is 65 seconds. The client's baseline before the initiation of therapy was 30 seconds. A nurse anticipates that which action is needed?
   1. Shutting off the heparin infusion.
   2. Decreasing the rate of the heparin infusion.
   3. Leaving the rate of the heparin infusion as is.
   4. Increasing the rate of the heparin infusion.

8. A client with atrial fibrillation who is receiving maintenance therapy of warfarin sodium (Coumadin) has a prothrombin time of 30 seconds. Based on the prothrombin time, a nurse anticipates which of the following orders?
   1. Holding the next dose of warfarin
   2. Administering the next dose of warfarin
   3. Increasing the next dose of warfarin
   4. Adding a dose of heparin

9. An adult client who has had preadmission testing before surgery has had blood drawn for serum electrolyte testing. A nurse would report which of the following abnormal values to the surgeon's office preoperatively?
   1. Sodium, 148 mEq/L
   2. Potassium, 3.8 mEq/L
   3. Chloride, 101 mEq/L
   4. Bicarbonate, 26 mEq/L

10. A client with a history of cardiac disease is due for a morning dose of furosemide (Lasix). A nurse plans to report which serum potassium level before administering the dose of furosemide?
    1. 3.8 mEq/L
    2. 3.2 mEq/L
    3. 4.8 mEq/L
    4. 4.2 mEq/L

11. An adult client with a history of gastrointestinal bleeding has a platelet count of 300,000 cells/μL. Which action by a nurse is most appropriate after reading this report?
    1. Report the abnormally low count.
    2. Report the abnormally high count.
    3. Place the client on bleeding precautions.
    4. Place the normal report in the client's medical record.

12. An adult client with hepatic cirrhosis has been following a diet with optimal amounts of protein because neither an excess nor a deficiency of protein has been helpful. The nurse evaluates the client's status as being most satisfactory if the total protein level is which of the following values, in the normal range?

1. 0.4 g/dL
2. 3.7 g/dL
3. 6.4 g/dL
4. 9.8 g/dL

13. A client is seen in the urgent care center for complaints of chest pain that began 3 days ago. Since that time the client has not been feeling well and fatigues easily. A nurse would suspect myocardial infarction at the time of chest pain if which of the following isoenzymes for lactate dehydrogenase came back positive?
    1. LDH_1
    2. LDH_3
    3. LDH_4
    4. LDH_5

14. An adult client was diagnosed with acute pancreatitis 9 days ago. A nurse interprets that the client is recovering from this episode if the serum lipase level drops to which of the following values, which is just underneath the upper limit of normal?
    1. 20 units/L
    2. 80 units/L
    3. 135 units/L
    4. 350 units/L

15. An adult female client has a hemoglobin level of 10.8 g/dL. A nurse interprets that this result is most likely due to which of the following conditions noted in the client's history?
    1. Chronic obstructive pulmonary disease
    2. Heart failure
    3. Dehydration
    4. Iron deficiency anemia

16. A client with diabetes mellitus has a glycosylated hemoglobin A_{1c} level of 9%. Based on this test result, a nurse plans to teach the client about the need to
    1. Avoid infection.
    2. Take in adequate fluids.
    3. Prevent hyperglycemia.
    4. Prevent hypoglycemia.

17. A nurse is caring for a client with a diagnosis of cancer who is immunosuppressed. A nurse would consider implementing neutropenic precautions if the client's white blood cell count was
    1. 2000 cells/μL.
    2. 5800 cells/μL.
    3. 8400 cells/μL.
    4. 11,500 cells/μL.

18. A 22-year-old adult has a cholesterol blood test done at a screening clinic sponsored by a local health club. A nurse volunteering at the screening teaches the client that diet and exercise should be used as health measures to keep the total cholesterol level below
    1. 140 mg/dL.
    2. 200 mg/dL.
    3. 250 mg/dL.
    4. 300 mg/dL.

19. A client has been admitted to the hospital for urinary tract infection and dehydration. A nurse evaluates that the client has received adequate volume replacement if the blood urea nitrogen level drops to
    1. 35 mg/dL.
    2. 29 mg/dL.
    3. 15 mg/dL.
    4. 3 mg/dL.

20. A client arrives in the emergency room complaining of chest pain that began 4 hours ago. A troponin T blood specimen is obtained, and the results indicate a level of 0.6 ng/mL. The nurse interprets that this result indicates
    1. A normal level.
    2. A level that indicates the presence of possible angina.
    3. A low value indicating possible gastritis.
    4. A level that indicates a myocardial infarction.

CRITICAL THINKING: MULTIPLE RESPONSE

Several laboratory tests are prescribed for a client, and the nurse reviews the results of the tests. Select the laboratory tests that are abnormal.

____ White blood cells, 3000 cells/μL

____ Neutrophils, 1000 cells/mL

____ Thyroid-stimulating hormone (thyrotropin), 0.4 microunit/mL

____ Phosphorus, 3.6 mg/dL

____ Magnesium, 1.0 mg/dL

____ Calcium, 7.0 mg/dL

____ Blood urea nitrogen, 10 mg/dL

____ Serum creatinine, 1.0 mg/dL

ANSWERS

1. **3**

Rationale: The normal serum amylase level is 25 to 151 IU/L. With chronic cases of pancreatitis the rise in serum amylase levels usually does not exceed 3 times the normal value. In acute pancreatitis the value may exceed 5 times the normal value. Options 1 and 2 are within normal limits. Option 4 is an extremely elevated level seen in acute pancreatitis.

Test-Taking Strategy: Use the process of elimination. Note the key word "chronic" in the question. You must understand the effects of chronic pancreatitis on the amylase level to answer this question. Review these effects if you had difficulty with this question.

Level of Cognitive Ability: Analysis
Client Needs: Physiological Integrity
Integrated Process: Nursing Process—analysis
Content Area: Adult health—gastrointestinal
Reference: Chernecky, C., & Berger, B. (2001). *Laboratory tests and diagnostic procedures* (3rd ed., p. 158). Philadelphia: W. B. Saunders.

2. **2**

Rationale: Creatine phosphokinase (CPK) is a cellular enzyme that can be fractionated into three isoenzymes. The MB band reflects CPK from cardiac muscle. This is the level that elevates with myocardial infarction. The MM band reflects CPK from skeletal muscle. The BB band reflects CPK from the brain. There is no MK band.

Test-Taking Strategy: To answer this question correctly, you must have specific knowledge of the isoenzymes that are produced with elevations in CPK. If necessary, review this important laboratory value for detecting myocardial infarction.

Level of Cognitive Ability: Comprehension
Client Needs: Physiological Integrity
Integrated Process: Nursing Process—assessment
Content Area: Adult health—cardiovascular

Reference: Chernecky, C., & Berger, B. (2001). *Laboratory tests and diagnostic procedures* (3rd ed., p. 397). Philadelphia: W. B. Saunders.

3. **3**

Rationale: The normal serum creatinine level for adults is 0.6 to 1.3 mg/dL. The client with a mild degree of renal insufficiency would have a slightly elevated level. A creatinine level of 0.2 mg/dL is low, and a level of 0.5 mg/dL is just below normal. A creatinine level of 3.5 mg/dL may be associated with acute or chronic renal failure.

Test-Taking Strategy: Note the key word "mild." This tells you that the correct option will be an abnormal value but perhaps not the most abnormal of all the options. Recall the normal value for this common laboratory test to direct you to option 3. Review the normal value for this laboratory test if you had difficulty with this question.

Level of Cognitive Ability: Analysis
Client Needs: Physiological Integrity
Integrated Process: Nursing Process—analysis
Content Area: Adult health—renal
Reference: Chernecky, C., & Berger, B. (2001). *Laboratory tests and diagnostic procedures* (3rd ed., p. 400). Philadelphia: W. B. Saunders.

4. **3**

Rationale: The therapeutic range for serum phenytoin (Dilantin) level is 10 to 20 mcg/mL. If the level is below the therapeutic range, the client may continue to experience seizure activity. If the level is too high, the client could experience phenytoin toxicity.

Test-Taking Strategy: Use the process of elimination. Recalling that the therapeutic range is 10 to 20 mcg/mL will direct you to option 3. Learn this therapeutic range if you had difficulty with this question.

Level of Cognitive Ability: Analysis
Client Needs: Physiological Integrity

Integrated Process: Nursing Process—evaluation
Content Area: Adult health—neurological
Reference: Hodgson, B., & Kizior, R. (2003). *Saunders nursing drug handbook 2003* (p. 892). Philadelphia: W. B. Saunders.

5. **1**
Rationale: The therapeutic range for the serum theophylline (or aminophylline) level is 10 to 20 mcg/mL. If the level is below the therapeutic range, the client may experience frequent exacerbations of the disorder. Although all of the options identify values within the therapeutic range, option 1 is the option that reflects a need for compliance with medication.
Test-Taking Strategy: Use the process of elimination. Note the key words "especially vigilant." Recalling the therapeutic level of theophylline will direct you to option 1. Review this therapeutic range if you had difficulty with this question.
Level of Cognitive Ability: Analysis
Client Needs: Physiological Integrity
Integrated Process: Teaching/Learning
Content Area: Adult health—respiratory
Reference: Chernecky, C., & Berger, B. (2001). *Laboratory tests and diagnostic procedures* (3rd ed., p. 974). Philadelphia: W. B. Saunders.

6. **4**
Rationale: The normal therapeutic range for digoxin is 0.5 to 2.0 ng/mL. A value of 2.4 ng/mL exceeds the therapeutic range and could be toxic to the client. The most important action is to notify the physician, who may give further orders about holding further doses of digoxin. Option 1 is incorrect because the value is not normal. The next dose should not be administered because the serum digoxin level exceeds the therapeutic range. Checking the client's last pulse rate is not incorrect but may have limited value in this situation. Depending on the time that has elapsed since the last assessment, a current assessment of the client's status may be more useful.
Test-Taking Strategy: Use the process of elimination and note the key words "most important action." To choose correctly, you must be familiar with the therapeutic range for this medication and note that the value of 2.4 ng/mL is a toxic one. If this question was difficult, review the information on this commonly used medication and measurement of its therapeutic serum level.
Level of Cognitive Ability: Application
Client Needs: Physiological Integrity
Integrated Process: Nursing Process—implementation
Content Area: Adult health—cardiovascular
References: Chernecky, C., & Berger, B. (2001). *Laboratory tests and diagnostic procedures* (3rd ed., p. 447). Philadelphia: W. B. Saunders.
Hodgson, B., & Kizior, R. (2003). *Saunders nursing drug handbook 2003* (p. 350). Philadelphia: W. B. Saunders.

7. **3**
Rationale: The normal activated partial thromboplastin time (aPTT) varies between 20 and 36 seconds, depending on the type of activator used in testing. The therapeutic dose of heparin for treatment of deep vein thrombosis is to keep the aPTT between 1.5 and 2.5 times normal. Thus the client's aPTT is within the therapeutic range, and the dose should remain unchanged.

Test-Taking Strategy: To answer this question accurately, you must be familiar with the normal aPTT level and the therapeutic level needed following institution of heparin therapy. Remember that the normal range is 20 to 36 seconds and that the aPTT should be between 1.5 and 2.5 times normal when the client is receiving heparin therapy. If this question was difficult, review this laboratory test and the expected level if the client is receiving heparin.
Level of Cognitive Ability: Analysis
Client Needs: Physiological Integrity
Integrated Process: Nursing Process—analysis
Content Area: Adult health—cardiovascular
Reference: Chernecky, C., & Berger, B. (2001). *Laboratory tests and diagnostic procedures* (3rd ed., pp. 795-796). Philadelphia: W. B. Saunders.

8. **1**
Rationale: The normal prothrombin time (PT) is 9.6 to 11.8 seconds (male adult) or 9.5 to 11.3 seconds (female adult). A therapeutic PT level is 1.5 to 2.0 times greater than the client's control level. Because the value of 30 seconds is high (and perhaps near the critical range), the nurse should anticipate that the client would not receive further doses at this time.
Test-Taking Strategy: Use the process of elimination, recalling that the normal PT is 9.6 to 11.8 seconds (male adult) or 9.5 to 11.3 seconds (female adult) and that a therapeutic PT level is 1.5 to 2.0 times greater than the client's control level. If this question was difficult, review this laboratory test and the expected level if the client is receiving warfarin sodium.
Level of Cognitive Ability: Analysis
Client Needs: Physiological Integrity
Integrated Process: Nursing Process—analysis
Content Area: Adult health—cardiovascular
Reference: Chernecky, C., & Berger, B. (2001). *Laboratory tests and diagnostic procedures* (3rd ed., pp. 865-867). Philadelphia: W. B. Saunders.

9. **1**
Rationale: The normal serum electrolyte ranges for adults are as follows: sodium, 135 to 145 mEq/L; potassium, 3.5 to 5.1 mEq/L; chloride, 98 to 107 mEq/L; and bicarbonate (venous), 22 to 29 mEq/L. The only abnormal value identified in the options is the serum sodium. The nurse reports any abnormal preoperative laboratory value to the surgeon's office.
Test-Taking Strategy: Use the process of elimination and knowledge of the normal serum electrolyte values to direct you to option 1. If this question was difficult, memorize these common laboratory values.
Level of Cognitive Ability: Application
Client Needs: Physiological Integrity
Integrated Process: Nursing Process—implementation
Content Area: Fundamental skills
Reference: Chernecky, C., & Berger, B. (2001). *Laboratory tests and diagnostic procedures* (3rd ed., p. 460). Philadelphia: W. B. Saunders.

10. **2**
Rationale: The normal serum potassium level in the adult is 3.5 to 5.1 mEq/L. Option 2 is the only value that falls below the therapeutic range. Administering furosemide to a client

with a low potassium level and a history of cardiac problems could precipitate ventricular dysrhythmias. Options 1, 3, and 4 are within the normal range.
Test-Taking Strategy: Use the process of elimination and knowledge of the normal serum potassium level to answer this question. This will assist you in identifying the value that is not within normal range. If this question was difficult, memorize this common laboratory value.
Level of Cognitive Ability: Comprehension
Client Needs: Physiological Integrity
Integrated Process: Nursing Process—planning
Content Area: Adult health—cardiovascular
Reference: Ignatavicius, D., & Workman, M. (2002). *Medical-surgical nursing: Critical thinking for collaborative care* (4th ed., p. 152). Philadelphia: W. B. Saunders.

11. 4
Rationale: A normal platelet count ranges from 150,000 to 400,000 cells/mL. The nurse should place the report containing the normal laboratory value in the client's medical record. A platelet count of 300,000 cells/μL is not an elevated count. The count also is not low; therefore bleeding precautions are not needed.
Test-Taking Strategy: Use the process of elimination. Remember that options that are similar are not likely to be correct. With this in mind, eliminate options 1 and 3 first. From the remaining options, you must be familiar with the normal range for this laboratory test. Because this is a common hematological study, the normal range is worth memorizing.
Level of Cognitive Ability: Application
Client Needs: Physiological Integrity
Integrated Process: Nursing Process—implementation
Content Area: Adult health—gastrointestinal
Reference: Chernecky, C., & Berger, B. (2001). *Laboratory tests and diagnostic procedures* (3rd ed., p. 827). Philadelphia: W. B. Saunders.

12. 3
Rationale: The normal range for total serum protein level in the adult client is 6.0 to 8.0 g/dL. The client with cirrhosis often has low total protein levels as a result of inadequate nutrition. Excess protein is not helpful, though, because a function of the liver is to metabolize protein. A diseased liver may not metabolize protein well. Options 1 and 2 identify low values, and option 4 identifies a high protein value.
Test-Taking Strategy: Use the process of elimination. Note the key words "normal range." Recalling the normal total protein level will direct you to option 3. Review this laboratory range if you had difficulty with this question.
Level of Cognitive Ability: Analysis
Client Needs: Physiological Integrity
Integrated Process: Nursing Process—evaluation
Content Area: Adult health—gastrointestinal
Reference: Chernecky, C., & Berger, B. (2001). *Laboratory tests and diagnostic procedures* (3rd ed., p. 859). Philadelphia: W. B. Saunders.

13. 1
Rationale: The particular isoenzymes that are affected after acute myocardial infarction are LDH_1 and LDH_2.

The lactate dehydrogenase (LDH) begins to elevate about 24 hours after myocardial infarction and peaks in 48 to 72 hours. Thereafter, it returns to normal, usually within 7 to 14 days.
Test-Taking Strategy: Use the process of elimination. Recalling that the levels of LDH_1 and LDH_2 are affected after an acute myocardial infarction will direct you to option 1. Review the LDH levels if you had difficulty with this question.
Level of Cognitive Ability: Analysis
Client Needs: Physiological Integrity
Integrated Process: Nursing Process—analysis
Content Area: Adult health—cardiovascular
Reference: Ignatavicius, D., & Workman, M. (2002). *Medical-surgical nursing: Critical thinking for collaborative care* (4th ed., p. 640). Philadelphia: W. B. Saunders.

14. 3
Rationale: The normal serum lipase level is 10 to 140 units/L. The client who is recovering from acute pancreatitis usually has elevated lipase levels for about 10 days after the onset of symptoms. This makes lipase a valuable test in monitoring the client's pancreatic function because serum amylase levels usually return to normal 3 days after the onset of symptoms. Option 3 is the only option that contains a value just underneath the upper limit of normal.
Test-Taking Strategy: Use the process of elimination and knowledge of the serum lipase level to answer this question. Noting the key words "just underneath the upper limit of normal" will assist in directing you to option 3. Review the range for this laboratory study if you had difficulty with this question.
Level of Cognitive Ability: Analysis
Client Needs: Physiological Integrity
Integrated Process: Nursing Process—evaluation
Content Area: Adult health—gastrointestinal
Reference: Malarkey, L., & McMorrow, M. (2000). *Nurse's manual of laboratory tests and diagnostic procedures* (2nd ed., pp. 508-509). Philadelphia: W. B. Saunders.

15. 4
Rationale: The normal hemoglobin level for an adult female client is 12 to 15 g/dL. Iron deficiency anemia can result in lower hemoglobin levels. Heart failure and chronic obstructive pulmonary disease may increase the hemoglobin level as a result of the need of the body for more oxygen-carrying capacity. Dehydration may increase the hemoglobin level by hemoconcentration.
Test-Taking Strategy: Use the process of elimination. Evaluate each of the options in terms of whether each is likely to raise or lower the hemoglobin level. Also note the relationship between "hemoglobin level" in the question and option 4. Review the normal hemoglobin level if you had difficulty with this question.
Level of Cognitive Ability: Analysis
Client Needs: Physiological Integrity
Integrated Process: Nursing Process—analysis
Content Area: Fundamental skills
Reference: Chernecky, C., & Berger, B. (2001). *Laboratory tests and diagnostic procedures* (3rd ed., p. 594). Philadelphia: W. B. Saunders.

16. 3

Rationale: In the glycosylated hemoglobin A_{1c}, 7.5% indicates good control, 7.6% to 8.9% indicates fair control, and 9% or higher indicates poor control. This test measures the amount of glucose that has become permanently bound to the red blood cells from circulating glucose. Elevations in blood glucose will cause elevations in the amount of glycosylation. Thus the test is useful in identifying clients who have periods of hyperglycemia that are undetected in other ways. Elevations indicate continued need for teaching related to prevention of hyperglycemic episodes.

Test-Taking Strategy: Use the process of elimination and knowledge regarding the values for this test and their significance to answer the question. If you had difficulty with this question or are unfamiliar with this test, review this content.

Level of Cognitive Ability: Application
Client Needs: Health Promotion and Maintenance
Integrated Process: Nursing Process—planning
Content Area: Adult health—endocrine
Reference: Chernecky, C., & Berger, B. (2001). *Laboratory tests and diagnostic procedures* (3rd ed., pp. 573-574). Philadelphia: W. B. Saunders.

17. 1

Rationale: The normal white blood cell count ranges from 4500 to 11,000 cell/μL. The client who is immunosuppressed has a decrease in the number of circulating white blood cells. The nurse implements neutropenic precautions when the client's values fall sufficiently below the normal level. The specific value for implementing neutropenic precautions usually is determined by agency policy. Options 2, 3, and 4 are normal values.

Test-Taking Strategy: Use the process of elimination. Recalling that the normal white blood cell count is 4500 to 11,000 cells/μL will direct you to option 1. Review this hematological test if you had difficulty with this question.

Level of Cognitive Ability: Analysis
Client Needs: Physiological Integrity
Integrated Process: Nursing Process—analysis
Content Area: Adult health—oncology
Reference: Phipps, W., Monahan, F., Sands, J., Marek, J., & Neighbors, M. (2003). *Medical-surgical nursing: Health and illness perspectives* (7th ed., pp. 807, 836). St. Louis: Mosby.

18. 2

Rationale: The nurse should counsel the client to keep the total cholesterol level under 200 mg/dL. This will aid in the prevention of atherosclerosis, which can lead to a number of cardiovascular disorders later in life. Options 3 and 4 are elevated values and place the client at risk for cardiovascular disease. Although option 1 is a low cholesterol level, option 2 identifies the realistic value to assist in preventing cardiovascular disease.

Test-Taking Strategy: Recalling that the cholesterol level ranges from 140 to 199 mg/dL and noting the issue of the question will direct you to option 2. Because of the importance of the health problems resulting from atherosclerosis and cardiovascular disease, review this laboratory test.

Level of Cognitive Ability: Application
Client Needs: Health Promotion and Maintenance
Integrated Process: Teaching/Learning
Content Area: Adult health—cardiovascular
Reference: Chernecky, C., & Berger, B. (2001). *Laboratory tests and diagnostic procedures* (3rd ed., p. 345). Philadelphia: W. B. Saunders.

19. 3

Rationale: The normal blood urea nitrogen level is 8 to 25 mg/dL. Values such as those in options 1 and 2 reflect continued dehydration. Option 4 reflects a lower than normal value, which may occur with fluid volume overload, among other conditions.

Test-Taking Strategy: Use the process of elimination and knowledge of the normal blood urea nitrogen level to answer the question. Option 3 is the only option that identifies a normal value. Review this laboratory test if you had difficulty with this question.

Level of Cognitive Ability: Analysis
Client Needs: Physiological Integrity
Integrated Process: Nursing Process—evaluation
Content Area: Adult health—renal
Reference: Phipps, W., Monahan, F., Sands, J., Marek, J., & Neighbors, M. (2003). *Medical-surgical nursing: Health and illness perspectives* (7th ed., pp. 1194-1195). St. Louis: Mosby.

20. 4

Rationale: Troponin is a regulatory protein found in striated muscle. The troponins function together in the contractile apparatus for striated muscle in skeletal muscle and in the myocardium. Increased amounts of troponins are released into the bloodstream when an infarction causes damage to the myocardium. A troponin T value that is greater than 0.1 to 0.2 ng/mL is consistent with a myocardial infarction. A normal troponin I level is less than 0.6 ng/mL.

Test-Taking Strategy: Note that the issue of the question relates to the troponin T. Knowledge that a level that is greater than 0.1 to 0.2 ng/mL is consistent with a myocardial infarction will direct you to option 4. Review this diagnostic test if you are unfamiliar with it.

Level of Cognitive Ability: Analysis
Client Needs: Physiological Integrity
Integrated Process: Nursing Process—analysis
Content Area: Adult health—cardiovascular
Reference: Malarkey, L., & McMorrow, M. (2000). *Nurse's manual of laboratory tests and diagnostic procedures* (2nd ed., p. 317). Philadelphia: W. B. Saunders.

CRITICAL THINKING: MULTIPLE RESPONSE

Answer:
White blood cells, 3000 cells/μL
Neutrophils, 1000 cells/μL
Magnesium, 1.0 mg/dL
Calcium, 7.0 mg/dL
Rationale: The normal values include the following: white blood cells, 4500 to 11,000 cells/μL; neutrophils, 56% or 1800 to 7800 cells/μL; thyroid-stimulating hormone, 0.2 to 5.4 microunits/mL; phosphorus, 2.7 to 4.5 mg/dL; magnesium, 1.6 to 2.6 mg/dL; calcium, 8.6 to 10.0 mg/dL; blood urea nitrogen, 5 to 20 mg/dl; and serum creatinine, 0.6 to 1.3 mg/dL.

Test-Taking Strategy: Note the word "abnormal" in the question. Knowledge of the normal laboratory values for these studies will assist in answering this question. Review these normal values if you had difficulty with this question.
Level of Cognitive Ability: Analysis
Client Needs: Physiological Integrity

Integrated Process: Nursing Process—assessment
Content Area: Fundamental skills
Reference: Lewis, S., Heitkemper, M., & Dirksen, S. (2004). Medical-surgical nursing: Assessment and management of clinical problems (6th ed., pp. 700, 1034, 1163, 1263-1264). St. Louis: Mosby.

REFERENCES

Chernecky, C., & Berger, B. (2001). *Laboratory tests and diagnostic procedures* (3rd ed.). Philadelphia: W. B. Saunders.

Hodgson, B., & Kizior, R. (2003). *Saunders nursing drug handbook 2003*. Philadelphia: W. B. Saunders.

Ignatavicius, D., & Workman, M. (2002). *Medical-surgical nursing: Critical thinking for collaborative care* (4th ed.). Philadelphia: W. B. Saunders.

Lewis, S., Heitkemper, M., & Dirksen, S. (2004). *Medical-surgical nursing: Assessment and management of clinical problems* (6th ed., pp. 700, 1034, 1163, 1263-1264). St. Louis: Mosby.

Malarkey, L., & McMorrow, M. (2000). *Nurse's manual of laboratory tests and diagnostic procedures* (2nd ed.). Philadelphia: W. B. Saunders.

National Council of State Boards of Nursing (Eds.). (2003). *Test Plan for the National Council Licensure Examination for Registered Nurses* (effective date: April 2004). Chicago: Author.

Phipps, W., Monahan, F., Sands, J., Marek, J., & Neighbors, M. (2003). *Medical-surgical nursing: Health and illness perspectives* (7th ed.). St. Louis: Mosby.

Nutrition

PYRAMID TERMS

absorption Passage of digested nutrients through the wall of the stomach or small intestine into the blood or lymph system.

digestion The breakdown of carbohydrates, fats, and proteins into monosaccharides, fatty acids, and amino acids.

enteral nutrition Administration of nutrition with liquefied foods into the gastrointestinal tract via a tube.

malnutrition Deficiency of the nutrients required for development and maintenance of the human body.

metabolism Ongoing chemical process within the body that converts digested nutrients into energy for the functioning of body cells.

nutrients Carbohydrates, fats or lipids, proteins, vitamins, minerals, and water that must be supplied in adequate amounts to provide energy, growth, development, and maintenance of the human body.

◢ THE PYRAMID TO SUCCESS

Nutrition is a basic need that must be met for all clients. Nurses must have the knowledge required to educate and care for healthy clients and for clients with nutritional needs or disorders requiring alterations in dietary measures. The NCLEX-RN examination addresses the dietary measures required for basic needs and for particular body system alterations. When presented with a question related to nutrition, consider the client's diagnosis and the particular requirement or restriction necessary for treatment of the disorder. Pyramid Points focus on the common types of therapeutic diets, nutrients contained in food items, and supplemental or enteral feedings. Integrated Processes addressed in this chapter include Nursing Process, Caring, Communication and Documentation, and Teaching/Learning.

CLIENT NEEDS ◢
Safe, Effective Care Environment

Consultation with members of the health care team
Dietary consultation and referral
Informed consent for invasive procedures
Medical and surgical asepsis
Standard, transmission-based, and other precautions

Health Promotion and Maintenance

Dietary teaching
Disease prevention
Health and wellness
Health promotion programs
Techniques of physical assessment

Psychosocial Integrity

Coping mechanisms
Cultural preferences related to nutritional patterns and lifestyle choices
Religious and spiritual influences on health

Physiological Integrity

Alteration in body systems
Elimination patterns
Monitoring of enteral feedings and the client's ability to tolerate feedings
Monitoring of laboratory values
Monitoring of fluid and electrolyte balance
Monitoring of nutritional intake and oral hydration

I. NUTRIENTS

A. Carbohydrates (Box 12-1)
1. Carbohydrates are the preferred source of energy.
2. Carbohydrates include sugars, starches, and cellulose and provide 4 cal/g.
3. Carbohydrates promote normal fat **metabolism**, spare protein, and enhance lower gastrointestinal function.
4. Major food sources of carbohydrates include milk, grains, fruits, and vegetables.
5. Inadequate carbohydrate intake affects **metabolism**.

B. Fats (Box 12-2)
1. Fats provide a concentrated source and a stored form of energy.
2. Fats protect internal organs and maintain body temperature.

BOX 12-1
Food Sources of Carbohydrates

CELLULOSE
Apples
Beans
Bran
Cabbage

FRUCTOSE
Fruits
Honey

GLUCOSE
Carrots
Corn
Dates
Grapes
Oranges

LACTOSE
Milk

STARCH
Barley
Beets, carrots, and peas
Corn
Oats
Potatoes and pasta
Rye
Wheat

SUCROSE
Apricots
Granulated table sugar
Honeydew and cantaloupe
Molasses
Peaches
Peas and corn
Plums

BOX 12-2
Food Sources of Fats

CHOLESTEROL
Animal products
Egg yolks
Liver and organ meats

MONOUNSATURATED FATS
Duck and goose
Eggs
Olive and peanut oils

POLYUNSATURATED FATS
Corn oil
Safflower oil
Sunflower oil

SATURATED FATS
Beef
Butter
Hard yellow cheeses
Luncheon meats

BOX 12-3
Food Sources of Protein

Bread and cereal products
Dairy products
Dried beans
Meats

3. Fats enhance **absorption** of the fat-soluble vitamins.
4. Fats provide 9 cal/g.
5. Inadequate fat intake leads to clinical manifestations of sensitivity to cold, skin lesions, increased risk of infection, and amenorrhea in women.
6. Diets high in fat can lead to obesity and increase the risk of cardiovascular disease and some cancers.

C. Proteins (Box 12-3)
1. Proteins are made from amino acids, are critical to all aspects of growth and development of body tissues, and provide 4 cal/g.
2. Proteins build and repair body tissues, regulate fluid balance, maintain acid-base balance, produce antibodies, provide energy, and produce enzymes and hormones.
3. Essential amino acids are required in the diet because the body cannot manufacture them.
4. High-quality proteins or complete proteins such as eggs, dairy products, meat, fish, and poultry contain adequate amounts of essential amino acids.
5. Foods that do not contain the essential amino acids in sufficient amounts are lower-quality or incomplete proteins.
6. Inadequate protein can cause protein energy **malnutrition** and severe wasting of fat and muscle tissue.

BOX 12-4

Food Sources of Vitamins

WATER SOLUBLE

Folic acid: Green, leafy vegetables; liver, beef, and fish; legumes; grapefruit and oranges
Niacin: Meats, poultry, fish, beans, peanuts, grains
Vitamin B_1 (thiamine): Pork and nuts, whole grain cereals, and legumes
Vitamin B_2 (riboflavin): Milk, lean meats, fish, grains
Vitamin B_6 (pyridoxine): Yeast, corn, meat, poultry, fish
Vitamin B_{12} (cobalamin): Meat, liver
Vitamin C (ascorbic acid): Citrus fruits, tomatoes, broccoli, cabbage

FAT SOLUBLE

Vitamin A: Liver, egg yolk, whole milk, green or orange vegetables, fruits
Vitamin D: Fortified milk, fish oils, cereals
Vitamin E: Vegetable oils; green, leafy vegetables; cereals; apricots, apples, and peaches
Vitamin K: Green, leafy vegetables; cauliflower and cabbage

D. Vitamins (Box 12-4)
1. Vitamins facilitate **metabolism** of proteins, fats, and carbohydrates; act as catalysts for metabolic functions; promote life and growth processes; and maintain and regulate body functions.
2. Fat-soluble vitamins A, D, E, and K can be stored in the body, so an excess can cause toxicity.
3. The B vitamins and vitamin C are water soluble, are not stored in the body, and can be excreted in the urine.
4. Vitamin K acts as a catalyst for facilitating blood-clotting factors, especially prothrombin.
5. Vitamin C functions in the production of collagen, a vital component in wound healing.
6. Vitamin A maintains eyesight and epithelial linings.

E. Minerals (Box 12-5)
1. Minerals are components of hormones, cells, tissues, and bones.
2. Minerals act as catalysts for chemical reactions and enhancers of cell function.
3. Almost all foods contain some form of minerals.
4. A deficiency of minerals can occur in chronically ill or hospitalized clients.

BOX 12-5

Food Sources of Minerals

CALCIUM	PHOSPHORUS	Cured pork
Broccoli	Fish	Frankfurters
Carrots	Nuts	Ketchup
Cheese	Organ meats	Lunch meat
Collard greens	Pork, beef, chicken	Milk
Green beans	Whole-grain breads and cereals	Mustard
Milk		Processed food
Rhubarb	**POTASSIUM**	Snack food
Spinach	Avocado	Soy sauce
Tofu	Bananas	Table salt
Yogurt, low-fat	Cantaloupe	White and whole-wheat bread
	Carrots	
CHLORIDE	Fish	**IRON**
Salt	Mushrooms	Breads and cereals
	Oranges	Dark green vegetables
MAGNESIUM	Pork, beef, veal	Egg yolk
Avocado	Potatoes	Liver
Canned white tuna	Raisins	Meats
Cauliflower	Spinach	
Cooked rolled oats	Strawberries	**ZINC**
Green leafy vegetables	Tomatoes	Eggs
Low-fat yogurt		Leafy vegetables
Milk	**SODIUM**	Meats
Peanut butter	American cheese	Protein-rich foods
Peas	Bacon	
Pork, beef, chicken	Butter	
Potatoes	Canned food	
Raisins	Cottage cheese	

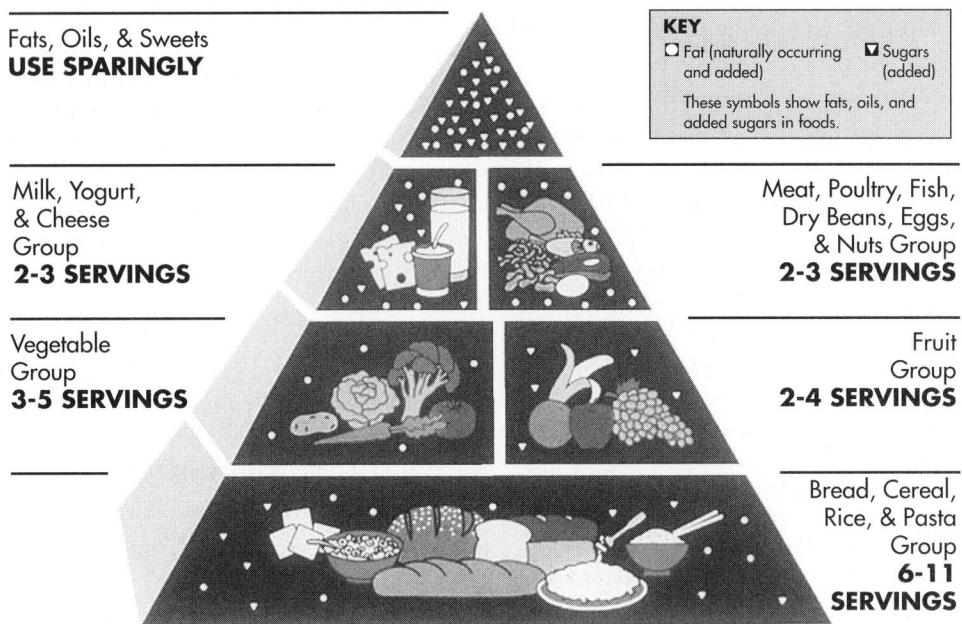

FIG. 12-1 U.S. Food Guide Pyramid. (From Potter, P., & Perry, A. [2001]. *Fundamentals of nursing* [5th ed.]. St. Louis: Mosby.)

II. FOOD GUIDE PYRAMID (FIG. 12-1)

A. The Food Guide Pyramid groups six broad families of foods with similar kinds of **nutrients** together.

B. Levels of the pyramid
1. Level one (base of the pyramid)
   a. This level is the bread, cereal, rice, and pasta group.
   b. Daily recommendation is 6 to 11 servings.
2. Level two
   a. This level is the vegetables and fruit group.
   b. Daily recommendation is 3 to 5 servings of vegetables and 2 to 4 servings of fruit.
3. Level three
   a. This level is the milk, yogurt, and cheese group and the meats, poultry, fish, dry beans, eggs, and nuts group.
   b. Daily recommendation is 2 to 3 servings for each group.
   c. The recommendation for the milk group depends on the various life stage of the individual.
4. Peak of the pyramid
   a. The peak is the fats, oils, and sweets group.
   b. Foods that are high in fats, sugar, or alcohol are to be eaten sparingly because they are kilocalorie-dense, nutrient-sparse foods.

III. THERAPEUTIC DIETS

A. Clear liquid diet
1. Indications
   a. A clear liquid diet serves a primary function of providing fluids and electrolytes to prevent dehydration.
   b. The diet is used as an initial feeding after complete bowel rest.
   c. The diet is used initially to feed a malnourished person or a person who has not had any oral intake for some time.
   d. The diet also is used for bowel preparation for surgery or tests.
   e. The diet is a postoperative diet.
   f. A clear liquid diet is used in cases of diarrhea.
2. Nursing considerations
   a. Clear liquid is deficient in energy and most **nutrients**.
   b. The body digests and absorbs clear liquids easily.
   c. Clear liquid contributes to little or no residue in the gastrointestinal tract.
   d. Clear liquid can be unappetizing and boring.
   e. Client should not stay on a clear liquid diet for more than a day or two.
   f. Clear liquid consists of foods that are relatively transparent to light and are clear and liquid at room and body temperature.
   g. Foods include items such as water, bouillon, clear broth, carbonated beverages, gelatin, hard candy, lemonade, popsicles, and regular or decaffeinated coffee or tea.
   h. The nurse should limit the amount of caffeine consumed by the client because caffeine can cause an upset stomach and sleeplessness.
   i. The client may have salt or sugar.
   j. Dairy products are not allowed.

B. Full liquid diet
1. Indication: A full liquid diet may be used as a second diet after clear liquids following surgery or for a client who is unable to chew or swallow.

2. Nursing considerations
   a. A full liquid diet is nutritionally deficient in energy and most **nutrients**.
   b. The diet includes clear and opaque liquid foods and those that liquefy at body temperature.
   c. Foods include all clear liquids and items such as plain ice cream, sherbet, breakfast drinks, milk, pudding and custard, soups that are strained, and strained vegetable juices.

C. Soft diet
  1. Indications
    a. A soft diet is used for clients with dental problems, clients with poor-fitting dentures, and clients who have difficulty chewing or swallowing.
    b. The diet is used for clients who have ulcerations of the mouth or gums, oral surgery, a broken jaw, plastic surgery of the head or neck, dysphasia, or for the client who had a stroke.
    c. The diet is therapeutic for clients with impaired **digestion** or **absorption** as a result of conditions such as ulcerative colitis and Crohn's disease.
  2. Nursing considerations
    a. Clients with mouth sores should be served foods at cooler temperatures.
    b. Clients who have difficulty chewing and swallowing because of a reduced flow of saliva can increase salivary flow by sucking on sour candy.
    c. Encourage the client to eat a variety of foods.
    d. Provide plenty of fluids with meals to ease chewing and swallowing of foods.
    e. Sucking fluids through a straw may be easier than drinking them from a cup or glass.
    f. All foods and seasonings are permitted; however, liquid, chopped, or pureed foods or regular foods with a soft consistency are best tolerated.
    g. Avoid foods than contain nuts or seeds, which easily can become trapped in the mouth and cause discomfort.
    h. Avoid raw fruits and vegetables, fried foods, and whole grains.

D. Bland diet
  1. Indication: A bland diet may be prescribed for the client with gastritis, ulcers, reflux esophagitis, or other gastrointestinal disorders, congestive heart failure, or myocardial infarction.
  2. Nursing considerations
    a. Bland foods are less likely to form gas than regular diets.
    b. Eliminate foods that stimulate gastric acid secretions.
    c. Eliminate foods that are irritating to the gastric mucosa.
    d. Foods to be avoided include alcohol; caffeine and caffeine-containing beverages such as cola, cocoa, coffee, and tea; fried foods; pepper and spicy foods.

E. Low-residue/low-fiber diet
  1. Indications
    a. The diet supplies foods that are least likely to form an obstruction when the intestinal tract is narrowed by inflammation or scarring or when gastrointestinal motility is slowed.
    b. The diet is used for inflammatory bowel disease, partial obstructions of the intestinal tract, enteritis, diarrhea, or other gastrointestinal disorders.
  2. Nursing considerations
    a. Foods high in carbohydrate are usually low in residue and include white bread, cereals, and pasta.
    b. Foods to be avoided are raw fruits (except bananas), vegetables, seeds, plant fiber, and whole grains.
    c. Dairy products are limited to two servings a day.

F. High-residue/high-fiber diet
  1. Indications
    a. The diet is used for clients who have constipation.
    b. The diet is used for irritable bowel syndrome when the primary symptom is alternating constipation and diarrhea and for asymptomatic diverticular disease.
    c. The diet helps regulate blood glucose in clients with diabetes mellitus.
    d. The diet helps control blood cholesterol in clients with heart disease.
  2. Nursing considerations
    a. The diet provides 20 to 25 g of dietary fiber daily.
    b. The diet adds volume and weight to the stool and speeds the movement of undigested materials through the intestine.
    c. The diet consists of fruits and vegetables and whole grain products.

G. Fat-controlled diet (Box 12-2)
  1. Indications
    a. The fat-controlled diet is indicated for atherosclerosis, diabetes mellitus, hyperlipidemia, hypertension, myocardial infarction, nephrotic syndrome, and renal failure.
    b. The diet reduces the risk of heart disease.
  2. Nursing consideration: Limit the total amount of fats and amounts of polyunsaturated, monounsaturated, and saturated fats and cholesterol.

H. High-calorie diet
  1. Indications: Persons with severe stress, burns, cancer, human immunodeficiency virus infections, acquired immunodeficiency syndrome, chronic obstructive pulmonary disease, respiratory failure, or any other type of debilitating disease require a high-calorie diet.
  2. Nursing considerations
    a. The high-calorie diet also should be high in protein because the purpose of the diet is to build or maintain lean body mass.

b. Add fats to foods whenever possible.

c. Add nuts and dried fruits such as raisins to desserts or cereals if the client can tolerate and eat these foods.

d. Add sugar to food, and provide high-calorie desserts.

e. Encourage snacks between meals, such as milk-shakes and instant breakfasts.

I. Sodium-restriction diet

1. Indications: Persons with hypertension, congestive heart failure, kidney diseases, cardiac diseases, and cirrhosis of the liver require a sodium-restriction diet.

2. Nursing considerations (Box 12-6)

a. This type of diet includes 2000 to 4000 mg of sodium daily (mild restriction), 1000 mg of sodium daily (moderate restriction), or 500 mg of sodium daily (strict and seldom prescribed).

b. Cereals allowed on a sodium-restricted diet include dried or instant cereals, puffed wheat, puffed rice, and shredded wheat.

J. Protein-restriction diet

1. Indications: Persons with acute renal failure, chronic renal disease, cirrhosis of the liver, and hepatic coma require a protein-restriction diet.

2. Nursing considerations

a. Provide enough protein to maintain nutritional status but not an amount that will allow the buildup of waste products from protein **metabolism** (40 to 60 g of protein daily).

b. The smaller the amount of protein allowed, the more important it becomes that all protein included in the diet be of high quality.

c. An adequate total energy intake from foods is critical for clients on protein-restricted diets (protein will be used for energy, rather than for protein synthesis).

d. Special low-protein products, such as pastas, bread, cookies, wafers, and gelatin made with wheat starch, can improve energy intake and add variety to the diet.

e. Carbohydrates in powdered or liquid forms also can provide additional energy.

f. Vegetables and fruits contain some protein, and for very low-protein diets, these foods must be calculated into the diet.

g. Foods are limited from the milk, meat, bread, and starch exchange.

K. High-protein diet

1. Indications: High-protein diets are for tissue building, burns, liver disease, and older clients.

2. Nursing considerations

a. High-protein diets correct protein loss or assist with tissue repair.

b. Increase foods such as meat, fish, fowl, and dairy products.

c. The client may need protein supplements.

L. Low-calcium diet

1. Indication: A low-calcium diet may be prescribed to prevent renal calculi in the client at risk for forming calculi composed of calcium.

2. Nursing considerations: Decrease the total intake of calcium to prevent further stone formation; avoid whole grains, milk and dairy products, and green, leafy vegetables.

M. High-calcium diet

1. Indications: Calcium is needed during bone growth and in adulthood to prevent osteoporosis.

2. Nursing considerations

a. Primary dietary sources of calcium are dairy products (refer to Chapter 9, Box 9-5, for food items high in calcium).

b. Clients experiencing lactose intolerance need to incorporate sources of calcium other than dairy products into their dietary patterns regularly.

N. Low-purine diet

1. Indication: The diet is used to treat gout.

2. Nursing considerations

a. Purine is a precursor for uric acid that forms stones and crystals.

b. The client needs to avoid consuming fish such as anchovies, herring, mackerel, sardines, and scallops.

c. The client needs to avoid consuming glandular meats, gravies, meat extracts, wild game, goose, and sweetbreads.

O. High-iron diet

1. Indication: The diet is used for clients with anemia.

2. Nursing considerations

a. The high-iron diet replaces iron deficit from inadequate intake or loss.

b. The diet includes organ meats, meat, egg yolks, whole wheat products, leafy vegetables, dried fruit, legumes.

P. Diet for diverticular disease

BOX 12-6

Sodium-Free Spices and Flavorings

Allspice
Almond extract
Bay leaves
Caraway seeds
Cinnamon
Curry powder
Garlic powder or garlic
Ginger
Lemon extract
Maple extract
Marjoram
Mustard powder
Nutmeg

1. Symptomatic diverticulitis: The client avoids fiber because a high-fiber diet is irritating to the bowel.
2. Asymptomatic diverticular disease: The client consumes a high-fiber diet to prevent constipation.
3. The client should maintain a liberal fluid intake of 2500 to 3000 mL/day, unless contraindicated.
4. The client should avoid seeds and nuts because they become trapped in the diverticula and cause irritation.
5. The client should avoid gas-forming foods (Box 12-7).

Q. Fluid restriction (Box 12-8)
1. Indications: Acute renal failure-oliguric phase, chronic renal disease, cirrhosis of the liver, congestive heart failure and other cardiac disorders, and hepatic coma require fluid restriction.
2. Nursing considerations: Usually this diet restricts those foods that are composed largely of water, such as carbonated beverages, coffee, juices, milk, tea, water, frozen yogurt, gelatin, ice cream, ice milk, Popsicles, sherbet, soup, cream, and liquid medications.

BOX 12-7

Gas-Forming Foods

Apples
Artichokes
Barley
Beans
Bran
Broccoli
Brussels sprouts
Cabbage
Celery
Cherries
Coconuts
Eggplant
Figs
Honey
Melons
Milk
Molasses
Nuts
Onions
Radishes
Soybeans
Wheat
Yeast

BOX 12-8

Measures to Relieve Thirst

Chew gum or suck hard candy.
Freeze fluids so they take longer to consume.
Add lemon juice to water to make it more refreshing.
Gargle with refrigerated mouthwash

R. Carbohydrate-controlled diet
1. Indications
a. The diet helps maintain normal glucose levels in clients with disorders that cause blood glucose levels to rise or fall abnormally.
b. The diet is used for client with diabetes mellitus, hypoglycemia, lactose intolerance, galactosemia, dumping syndrome, and obesity.
2. Nursing considerations: Exchange System for Meal Planning
a. The Exchange System for Meal Planning, developed by the American Dietetic Association and the American Diabetes Association, is a food guide used to control diabetes mellitus and manage weight.
b. The Exchange System groups foods according to the amounts of the carbohydrates, fats, and proteins they contain.
c. Major food groups include carbohydrate group, meat and meat substitute group, and fat group.

S. Miscellaneous diets: Refer to Chapter 9, Boxes 9-3, 9-4, 9-6, and 9-7, for foods high in sodium, potassium, magnesium, and phosphorus, respectively.

IV. VEGETARIAN DIETS
A. Types (Box 12-9)
B. Nursing considerations
1. Ensure that the client eats a sufficient amount of varied foods to meet normal nutrient and energy needs.
2. Protein intake can be increased by consumption of a variety of vegetable protein sources based on whole grains, legumes, seeds, nuts, and vegetables combined to provide all of the essential amino acids.
3. Adequate energy intakes are important to ensure that dietary protein is used for protein synthesis.

V. ENTERAL NUTRITION
A. Description: **Enteral nutrition** provides liquefied foods into the gastrointestinal tract via a tube.

BOX 12-9

Types of Vegetarian Diets

LACTO-OVO VEGETARIANS
Diet consists of plant foods with dairy products and eggs. Persons may consume fish and occasionally poultry.

LACTO-VEGETARIANS
Diet consists of plant foods and dairy products excluding eggs.

VEGANS
Persons follow a strict vegetarian diet and use no animal foods.
Food pattern consists entirely of plant foods.

B. Indications
   1. **Enteral nutrition** is necessary when the gastrointestinal tract is functional but oral intake is not feasible.
   2. **Enteral nutrition** is used for clients with swallowing problems, burns, major trauma, liver failure, or severe **malnutrition**.
C. Nursing considerations
   1. Clients with lactose intolerance need to be placed on lactose-free formulas.
   2. Refer to Chapter 21 for information regarding the administration of gastrointestinal tube feedings.

PRACTICE QUESTIONS

1. Spironolactone (Aldactone), a diuretic, is prescribed for a client with congestive heart failure. A nurse provides dietary instructions to the client and instructs the client to avoid foods that are high in which electrolyte?
   1. Calcium
   2. Potassium
   3. Magnesium
   4. Phosphorus

2. A client with hypertension has been told to maintain a diet low in sodium. A nurse who is teaching this client about foods that are allowed would plan to include which food item in a list provided to the client?
   1. Tomato soup
   2. Summer squash
   3. Instant oatmeal
   4. Boiled shrimp

3. A client has been diagnosed with gout. In developing a dietary plan for the client, a nurse plans to include which item on a list of foods to be avoided?
   1. Liver
   2. Chocolate
   3. Carrots
   4. Broccoli

4. A client who is recovering from gastric surgery has been advanced from a clear liquid diet to a full liquid diet. The client is looking forward to the diet change because he has been "bored" with the clear liquid diet. The nurse would most appropriately offer which full liquid item to the client?
   1. Gelatin
   2. Custard
   3. Tea
   4. Popsicle

5. A female adult client with diabetes mellitus has been instructed in the dietary exchange system. The client tells a nurse that she would like to eat 8 oz of nonfat yogurt with breakfast. The nurse determines that the client understands the principles of the exchange system if the client states that she will
   1. Not eat ice cream for 1 week.
   2. Omit 8 oz of skim milk at that meal.

   3. Omit salad dressing and butter for the day.
   4. Eat only half of a meat exchange at supper.

6. A nurse is planning to teach a client with heart disease about the necessity of following a low-fat diet. The nurse develops a list of high-fat foods to avoid. Which food item would the nurse plan to include in this list?
   1. Broccoli
   2. Oranges
   3. Cream cheese
   4. Broiled haddock

7. A client is recovering from abdominal surgery and has a large abdominal wound. A nurse encourages the client to eat which food item that is naturally high in vitamin C to promote wound healing?
   1. Chicken
   2. Bananas
   3. Oranges
   4. Milk

8. A nurse is caring for a client with cirrhosis of the liver. To minimize the effects of the disorder, the nurse teaches the client about foods that are high in thiamine. The nurse determines that the client has the best understanding of the dietary measures to follow if the client states an intention to increase the intake of
   1. Pork
   2. Milk
   3. Chicken
   4. Broccoli

9. A client who has developed atrial fibrillation that is not responding to medication therapy has been prescribed warfarin sodium (Coumadin). A nurse is doing discharge dietary teaching with the client. The nurse would plan to teach the client to avoid which of the following foods while taking this medication?
   1. Cherries
   2. Potatoes
   3. Spaghetti
   4. Broccoli

10. A client who recently has been started on enteral feedings begins to complain of abdominal cramping, followed by the passage of two liquid stools. A nurse notes that the client has abdominal distention as well. The nurse reviews the nutritional content on the label of the can of feeding to see if it has which of the following ingredients?
    1. Maltose
    2. Lactose
    3. Sucrose
    4. Fructose

CRITICAL THINKING: MULTIPLE RESPONSE

A postoperative client has been placed on a clear liquid diet. Select all of the items that the client is allowed to consume on this diet.

___ Broth

___ Gelatin

___ Pudding

___ Pureed vegetables

___ Coffee

___ Vegetable juice

ANSWERS

1. 2

Rationale: Spironolactone is a potassium-sparing diuretic, and the client should avoid foods high in potassium. If the client does not avoid foods high in potassium, the client could develop hyperkalemia. The client does not need to avoid foods that contain calcium, magnesium, or phosphorus while taking this medication.

Test-Taking Strategy: Recalling that spironolactone is a potassium-sparing diuretic will direct your thinking to the need for the client to avoid consuming foods high in potassium. If you had difficulty answering this question, review this medication and the client teaching points related to its administration.

Level of Cognitive Ability: Application
Client Needs: Physiological Integrity
Integrated Process: Teaching/Learning
Content Area: Adult health—cardiovascular
Reference: Hodgson, B., & Kizior, R. (2003). *Saunders nursing drug handbook 2003* (pp. 1029-1030). Philadelphia: W. B. Saunders.

2. 2

Rationale: Foods that are lower in sodium include fruits and vegetables (option 2), because they do not contain physiological saline. Highly processed or refined foods (options 1 and 3) are higher in sodium unless their food labels specifically state "low sodium." Saltwater fish and shellfish are high in sodium.

Test-Taking Strategy: Use the process of elimination. Begin to answer this question by eliminating option 4, recalling that saltwater fish and shellfish are high in sodium. Next, eliminate options 1 and 3 because they are processed foods. Review the foods that are high in sodium if you had difficulty with this question.

Level of Cognitive Ability: Application
Client Needs: Health Promotion and Maintenance
Integrated Process: Teaching/Learning
Content Area: Adult health—cardiovascular
Reference: Peckenpaugh, N. (2003). *Nutrition essentials and diet therapy* (9th ed., pp. 156; 241). Philadelphia: W. B. Saunders.

3. 1

Rationale: Liver should be omitted from the diet of a client who has gout because of its high purine content. The food items identified in the other options contain negligible amounts of purines and may be consumed freely by the client with gout.

Test-Taking Strategy: Use the process of elimination. Recalling that high-purine foods need to be avoided will direct you to option 1. Review foods high in purine if you had difficulty with this question.

Level of Cognitive Ability: Application
Client Needs: Health Promotion and Maintenance
Integrated Process: Teaching/Learning
Content Area: Adult health—musculoskeletal
Reference: Phipps, W., Monahan, F., Sands, J., Marek, J., & Neighbors, M. (2003). *Medical-surgical nursing: Health and illness perspectives* (7th ed., p. 1542). St. Louis: Mosby.

4. 2

Rationale: Full liquid food items include items such as plain ice cream, sherbet, breakfast drinks, milk, pudding and custard, soups that are strained, and strained vegetable juices. A clear liquid diet consists of foods that are relatively transparent. The food items in options 1, 3, and 4 are clear liquids.

Test-Taking Strategy: Focus on the issue, a full liquid item. Remember that a clear liquid diet consists of foods that are relatively transparent. This will assist you in eliminating options 1, 3, and 4. Review food items allowed on a clear liquid diet and a full liquid diet if you had difficulty with this question.

Level of Cognitive Ability: Application
Client Needs: Physiological Integrity
Integrated Process: Nursing Process—implementation
Content Area: Adult health—gastrointestinal
Reference: Peckenpaugh, N. (2003). *Nutrition essentials and diet therapy* (9th ed., pp. 154-155). Philadelphia: W. B. Saunders.

5. 2

Rationale: Yogurt belongs to the milk exchange. On the exchange system, foods are exchanged within that food group only. Salad dressing and butter belong to the fat exchange. Meats are a separate exchange. Ice cream is not recommended for use in the diabetic diet because it is high in fat and sugar. The exchange system is used within a meal, not between meals (options 3 and 4) or spread out over extended periods of time (option 1).

Test-Taking Strategy: Familiarity with the various foods in the diabetic diet and the exchange system is needed to answer this question. However, note the relationship between the words "with breakfast" in the question and "at that meal" in the correct option. Review foods and categories in the exchange system if you had difficulty with this question.

Level of Cognitive Ability: Analysis
Client Needs: Health Promotion and Maintenance
Integrated Process: Teaching/Learning
Content Area: Adult health—endocrine
Reference: Phipps, W., Monahan, F., Sands, J., Marek, J., & Neighbors, M. (2003). *Medical-surgical nursing: health and illness perspectives* (7th ed., pp. 949, 951). St. Louis: Mosby.

6. 3

Rationale: Fruits and vegetables tend to be lower in fat because they do not come from animal sources. Fish is also naturally lower in fat. Cream cheese is a high-fat food.

Test-Taking Strategy: Use the process of elimination and focus on the issue of the question, the high-fat food. Options 1 and 2 (vegetable and fruit) can be eliminated first. From the remaining options, remember that cheese is high in fat content. Review foods that are high in fat content if you had difficulty with this question.
Level of Cognitive Ability: Application
Client Needs: Health Promotion and Maintenance
Integrated Process: Teaching/Learning
Content Area: Adult health—cardiovascular
References: Peckenpaugh, N. (2003). *Nutrition essentials and diet therapy* (9th ed., p. 156). Philadelphia: W. B. Saunders. Phipps, W., Monahan, F., Sands, J., Marek, J., & Neighbors, M. (2003). *Medical-surgical nursing: Health and illness perspectives* (7th ed., pp. 666-668). St. Louis: Mosby.

7. 3
Rationale: Citrus fruits and juices are especially high in vitamin C. Bananas are high in potassium. Meats and dairy products are two food groups that are high in the B vitamins.
Test-Taking Strategy: Note the key words "naturally high" in the stem of the question. Use the process of elimination, recalling that citrus fruits and juices are high in vitamin C. Review the foods high in vitamin C if you are unfamiliar with them.
Level of Cognitive Ability: Application
Client Needs: Health Promotion and Maintenance
Integrated Process: Teaching/Learning
Content Area: Fundamental skills
Reference: Peckenpaugh, N. (2003). *Nutrition essentials and diet therapy* (9th ed., p. 96). Philadelphia: W. B. Saunders.

8. 1
Rationale: The client with cirrhosis needs to consume foods high in thiamine. Thiamine is present in a variety of foods of plant and animal origin. Pork products are especially rich in this vitamin. Other good food sources include nuts, whole grain cereals, and legumes. Milk contains vitamins A, D, and B_2. Poultry contains niacin. Broccoli contains vitamins C, E, and K and folic acid.
Test-Taking Strategy: Note the key words "best understanding" in the stem of the question. This may indicate that more than one option may be a food that contains thiamine. Remembering that pork products are especially rich in thiamine will direct you to option 1. Review food items high in thiamine if you had difficulty with this question.
Level of Cognitive Ability: Analysis
Client Needs: Health Promotion and Maintenance
Integrated Process: Teaching/Learning
Content Area: Adult health—gastrointestinal
References: Phipps, W., Monahan, F., Sands, J., Marek, J., & Neighbors, M. (2003). *Medical-surgical nursing: Health and illness perspectives* (7th ed., p. 1172). St. Louis: Mosby. Williams, S. (2001). *Basic nutrition & diet therapy* (11th ed., pp. 456-457). St. Louis: Mosby.

9. 4
Rationale: Anticoagulant medications work by antagonizing the action of vitamin K, which is needed for clotting. When a client is taking an anticoagulant, foods high in vitamin K often are omitted from the diet. Vitamin K is found in green,

leafy vegetables such as broccoli. The other options listed are foods that are lower in vitamin K.
Test-Taking Strategy: Knowledge about the relationship between warfarin sodium and vitamin K is needed to answer this question. Note the key word "avoid" in the stem of the question. This tells you that the correct option is a food that is high in vitamin K. Remember that green, leafy vegetables are high in vitamin K. If you had difficulty with this question, review the foods high in vitamin K.
Level of Cognitive Ability: Analysis
Client Needs: Physiological Integrity
Integrated Process: Teaching/Learning
Content Area: Pharmacology
Reference: Potter, P., & Perry, A. (2001). *Fundamentals of nursing* (5th ed., p. 1341). St. Louis: Mosby.

10. 2
Rationale: Several tube feeding formulas contain lactose. A client with an unreported history of lactose intolerance would develop symptoms such as these in response to nutritional therapy with these formulas. If the client is diagnosed as lactose intolerant, a lactose-free formula should be prescribed by the physician. This will resolve the client's symptoms and promote adequate nutrition for the client.
Test-Taking Strategy: The issue of the question is the ability to associate the symptoms experienced by the client with the symptoms of lactose intolerance. If you had difficulty with this question, review the symptoms of lactose intolerance and the nursing considerations related to enteral feedings.
Level of Cognitive Ability: Analysis
Client Needs: Physiological Integrity
Integrated Process: Nursing Process—assessment
Content Area: Fundamental skills
Reference: Williams, S. (2001). *Basic nutrition & diet therapy* (11th ed., p. 44). St. Louis: Mosby.

CRITICAL THINKING: MULTIPLE RESPONSE
Answer:
Broth
Gelatin
Coffee
Rationale: A clear liquid diet consists of foods that are relatively transparent to light and are clear and liquid at room and body temperature. These foods include items such as water, bouillon, clear broth, carbonated beverages, gelatin, hard candy, lemonade, popsicles, and regular or decaffeinated coffee or tea. The incorrect food items are items that are allowed on a full liquid diet.
Test-Taking Strategy: Focus on the issue, a clear liquid diet. Recalling that a clear liquid diet consists of foods that are relatively transparent to light and are clear will assist in answering the question. Review foods allowed on a clear and full liquid diet if you had difficulty with this question.
Level of Cognitive Ability: Application
Client Needs: Physiological Integrity
Integrated Process: Nursing Process—implementation
Content Area: Fundamental skills
Reference: Potter, P., & Perry, A. (2001). *Fundamentals of nursing* (5th ed., p. 1359). St. Louis: Mosby.

REFERENCES

Hodgson, B., & Kizior, R. (2003). *Saunders nursing drug handbook 2003*. Philadelphia: W. B. Saunders.

National Council of State Boards of Nursing (Eds.). (2003). *Test Plan for the National Council Licensure Examination for Registered Nurses* (effective date: April 2004). Chicago: Author.

Peckenpaugh, N. (2003). *Nutrition essentials and diet therapy* (9th ed.). Philadelphia: W. B. Saunders.

Phipps, W., Monahan, F., Sands, J., Marek, J., & Neighbors, M. (2003). *Medical-surgical nursing: Health and illness perspectives* (7th ed.). St. Louis: Mosby.

Potter, P., & Perry, A. (2001). *Fundamentals of nursing* (5th ed.). St. Louis: Mosby.

Williams, S. (2001). *Basic nutrition & diet therapy* (11th ed.). St. Louis: Mosby.

Total Parenteral Nutrition

PYRAMID TERMS

fat emulsion (lipids) Preparation administered during parenteral nutrition therapy to prevent fatty acid deficiency.

parenteral nutrition The administration of nutrition through a central or peripheral intravenous catheter.

peripheral parenteral nutrition (PPN) Parenteral nutrition administered through a peripheral vein in an extremity.

total parenteral nutrition (TPN) Parenteral nutrition administered through a central vein, such as the subclavian vein; also called hyperalimentation, central venous parenteral nutrition, or central parenteral nutrition.

▲ THE PYRAMID TO SUCCESS

The NCLEX-RN exam test plan addresses total parenteral nutrition (TPN) as related content in the Client Needs area of Physiological Integrity, Pharmacological and Parenteral Therapies. Pyramid Points focus on the administration of TPN and fat emulsions, nursing interventions, and the interventions required in monitoring for complications. Pyramid Points also focus on home care instructions for the client receiving TPN at home. Integrated Processes addressed in this chapter are Nursing Process, Communication and Documentation, Caring, and Teaching/Learning.

▲ CLIENT NEEDS
Safe, Effective Care Environment

Consultation with members of the health care team
Dietary consultation
Handling hazardous and infectious materials
Home health care referral
Informed consent for venous access and placement of the catheter

Medical and surgical asepsis to prevent infection
Standard, transmission-based, and other precautions

Health Promotion and Maintenance

Health and wellness related to nutrition
Client and family education regarding the administration of TPN at home
Client and family education regarding monitoring for complications

Psychosocial Integrity

Role changes related to the need to receive TPN
Support systems in the home to assist with the administration of TPN

Physiological Integrity

Nutritional needs
Providing comfort and assistance in the performance of activities of daily living
Rest and sleep
Central venous access device for administering TPN
Laboratory values
Monitoring for potential complications
Monitoring for expected effects

I. TOTAL PARENTERAL NUTRITION (TPN)
A. Description
   1. **Total parenteral nutrition** supplies necessary nutrients via the veins.
   2. **Total parenteral nutrition** supplies carbohydrates in the form of dextrose, fats in special emulsified form, proteins in the form of amino acids, vitamins, minerals, and water.

3. **Total parenteral nutrition** prevents subcutaneous fat and muscle protein from being catabolized by the body for energy.

B. Indications
1. Clients whose gastrointestinal tracts are severely dysfunctional or nonfunctional and are unable to process nutrients normally require **TPN**.
2. Clients who can take some oral nutrition, but not enough to meet the needs of the body require **TPN**.
3. Clients with multiple gastrointestinal surgeries, gastrointestinal trauma, severe intolerance to enteral feedings, or intestinal obstructions or who need to rest the bowel for healing require **TPN**.
4. Clients with acquired immunodeficiency syndrome, cancer, or malnutrition or clients receiving chemotherapy require **TPN**.

C. Components
1. Carbohydrates
   a. Carbohydrates are mainly in the form of glucose, with ranges from a 5% glucose solution for **peripheral parenteral nutrition** to a 50% to 70% glucose (hypertonic) solution for central **parenteral nutrition**.
   b. The strength of the glucose solution prescribed depends on the client's nutritional needs and on agency protocols.
   c. Carbohydrates provide 60% to 70% of caloric (energy) needs.
2. Amino acids provide 3% to 15% of the total calories.
3. **Lipids (fat emulsion)**
   a. **Lipids** provide up to 30% of caloric (energy) needs.
   b. **Lipids** provide nonprotein calories and prevent or correct fatty acid deficiency.
4. Vitamins
5. Minerals and trace elements
6. Water
7. Electrolytes
8. Insulin may be added to control the blood glucose level because of the high concentration of glucose solution in the **TPN**.
9. Heparin may be added to reduce the buildup of a fibrinous clot at the catheter tip.

II. INTRAVENOUS SITES (FIG. 13-1)
A. Central parenteral nutrition (CPN)
1. For central parenteral nutrition, **TPN** is administered through a central venous access when the client requires a larger concentration of carbohydrates (greater than 10% glucose).
2. The subclavian or internal jugular veins are used when **TPN** is a short-term intervention (less than 4 weeks).
3. When **TPN** is anticipated for an extended period (greater than 4 weeks), a more permanent catheter, such as a peripherally inserted central catheter line, a tunneled catheter, or an implanted vascular access device, is used.

B. **Peripheral parenteral nutrition (PPN)**
1. **Peripheral parenteral nutrition** is administered through a peripheral vein.
2. **Peripheral parenteral nutrition** is used for short periods (5 to 7 days) and when the client needs only small concentrations of carbohydrates, fats, and proteins.

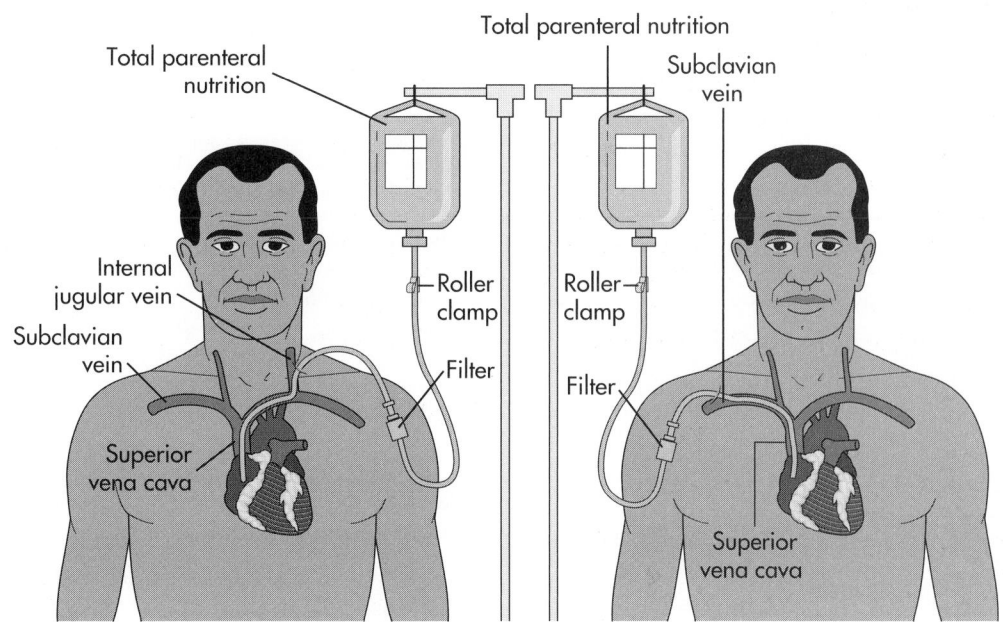

FIG. 13-1 Total parenteral nutrition. (From Leahy, J., & Kizilay, P. [1998]. *Foundations of nursing practice.* Philadelphia: W. B. Saunders.)

3. **Peripheral parenteral nutrition** is used to deliver isotonic or mildly hypertonic solutions; the delivery of highly hypertonic solutions into peripheral veins can cause sclerosis, phlebitis, or swelling.

III. LIPIDS (FAT EMULSION)

A. **Lipids** are given in an isotonic solution that can be administered through a peripheral vein.

B. **Lipids** are administered to prevent or correct fatty acid deficiency.

C. Most fat emulsions are prepared from soybean oil; the primary components are linoleic, oleic, palmitic, linolenic, and stearic acids.

D. Examine bottle for separation of emulsion into layers or fat globules or for the accumulation of froth; if observed, do not use and return the solution to the pharmacy.

E. Do not put additives into the **fat emulsion** solution.

F. Do not use an intravenous (IV) filter because particles in the **fat emulsion** are too large to pass through filters.

G. If the **fat emulsion** has been added to the **parenteral nutrition** solution, a 1.2-μm filter or a larger filter should be used to allow the **fat emulsion** to pass through.

H. Use vented IV tubing because the solution is supplied in a glass container for administration.

I. Infuse solution initially at 1 mL/min, monitor vital signs every 10 minutes, and observe for adverse reactions for the first 30 minutes of the infusion; if signs of an adverse reaction occur, stop the infusion and notify the physician (Box 13-1).

J. If no adverse reaction occurs, adjust flow to prescribed rate.

K. Monitor serum **lipids** 4 hours after discontinuing infusion.

L. Monitor liver function tests for evidence of impaired liver function indicating the inability of the liver to metabolize the **lipids**.

IV. FILTERS

A. **Total parenteral nutrition** and **peripheral parenteral nutrition** must be administered through tubing with an in-line filter to remove crystals from the solution.

B. A 0.22-μm filter is sufficient for administering solutions without lipid additives.

C. **Lipids** are administered through separate tubing attached below the filter of the main IV administration because particles in the **fat emulsion** are too large to pass through filters.

D. If the **parenteral nutrition** solution has **lipids** added to it, a 1.2-μm filter or a larger filter should be used.

V. COMPLICATIONS (BOX 13-2)

A. Description

1. Pneumothorax and air embolism are associated with central line placement; air embolism is also associated with tubing changes.

2. Other complications include infection (catheter related), fluid overload, and metabolic alterations such as hyperglycemia and hypoglycemia; these complications are usually due to the **parenteral nutrition** solution itself.

B. Pneumothorax (Box 13-3)

1. Monitor for signs of pneumothorax.

2. After insertion of the catheter, obtain a portable chest x-ray film to confirm correct catheter placement and to detect the presence of a pneumothorax; **parenteral nutrition** is not initiated until verification of correct catheter placement and the absence of pneumothorax.

3. After confirmation of catheter placement and the absence of pneumothorax, **parenteral nutrition** is initiated.

C. Air embolism (Box 13-4)

1. Instruct the client in Valsalva's maneuver for tubing and cap changes.

BOX 13-1

Signs of an Adverse Reaction to Lipids

Chest and back pain
Chills
Cyanosis
Diaphoresis
Dyspnea
Fever
Flushing
Headache
Nausea and vomiting
Pressure over the eyes
Thrombophlebitis
Vertigo

BOX 13-2

Complications of Total Parenteral Nutrition

Air embolism
Fluid overload
Hyperglycemia
Hypoglycemia
Infection
Pneumothorax

BOX 13-3

Signs of a Pneumothorax

Absence of breath sounds on affected side
Chest or shoulder pain
Sudden shortness of breath
Tachycardia

BOX 13-4

Signs of an Air Embolism

Apprehension
Chest pain
Dyspnea
Hypotension
Loud churning sound heard over the pericardium
Rapid and weak pulse
Respiratory distress

BOX 13-5

Signs of an Infection

Chills
Elevated white blood cell count
Erythema or drainage at the insertion site
Fever

BOX 13-6

Signs of Fluid Overload

Bounding pulse
Crackles on lung auscultation
Headache
Increased blood pressure
Jugular vein distension
Weight gain greater than desired

BOX 13-7

Signs of Hyperglycemia

Coma, when severe
Confusion
Diuresis
Elevated blood glucose level
Excessive thirst
Fatigue
Kussmaul's respirations
Restlessness
Weakness

BOX 13-8

Signs of Hypoglycemia

Anxiousness
Diaphoresis
Hunger
Low blood glucose level (usually less than 70 mg/dL)
Shakiness
Weakness

2. For tubing and cap changes, place the client in a head down position (if not contraindicated) with the head turned in the opposite direction of insertion site (increases intrathoracic venous pressure).
3. Check all catheter connections and secure (use tape per agency protocol) tubing connections.
4. If an air embolism is suspected, do the following:
   a. Clamp the intravenous catheter.
   b. Place the client in a left side-lying position with the head lower than the feet (to trap air in right side of the heart).
   c. Notify the physician.
   d. Administer oxygen as prescribed.
D. Infection (Box 13-5)
   1. Use strict aseptic technique; because the **TPN** solution has a high concentration of glucose, it is a medium for bacterial growth.
   2. Monitor temperature; in the event of fever, suspect sepsis.
   3. Assess the IV site for redness, swelling, tenderness, or drainage.
   4. Change **TPN** solution every 12 to 24 hours or according to agency protocol.
   5. Change IV tubing every 24 hours or according to agency protocol.
   6. Change dressing at the IV site every 48 hours or according to agency protocol.
   7. If signs of infection occur at the site, do the following:
      a. The IV line must be removed and restarted at a different site.
      b. Remove the tip of the IV catheter and send it to the laboratory for culture.
      c. Prepare the client for blood cultures.
E. Fluid overload (Box 13-6)
   1. Fluid overload occurs if the client receives the IV solution too rapidly.

2. **Total parenteral nutrition** is always delivered via an electronic infusion device.
3. Never increase the infusion rate to "catch up" if the IV infusion gets behind.
4. Monitor intake and output.
5. Weigh the client daily (ideal weight gain is 1 to 2 lb per week).
F. Hyperglycemia (Box 13-7)
   1. Assess the client for a history of glucose intolerance.
   2. Assess the client's medication history (corticosteroids may increase the blood glucose level).
   3. Begin infusion at a slow rate (usually 40 to 60 mL/hr) as prescribed.
   4. Monitor blood glucose levels every 4 to 6 hours or according to agency protocol.
   5. Administer regular insulin as prescribed.
G. Hypoglycemia (Box 13-8)
   1. Continue blood glucose monitoring.
   2. Gradually decrease the infusion when discontinuing **TPN**.
   3. When an infusion of hypertonic glucose is stopped, an infusion of 10% dextrose should be

instituted and maintained for 1 to 2 hours to prevent hypoglycemia.

4. Assess blood glucose level 1 hour after discontinuing **TPN**.

5. Prepare for the administration of glucose if hypoglycemia occurs.

▲ **VI. ADDITIONAL NURSING CONSIDERATIONS**

A. Always check the **TPN** solution with the physician's order to ensure that the prescribed components are contained in the solution.

B. To prevent infection and solution incompatibility, IV medications and blood are not given through the **TPN** line.

C. Monitor partial thromboplastin time and prothrombin time for clients receiving anticoagulants.

D. Monitor electrolytes, albumin, and liver and renal function studies.

E. In severely dehydrated clients, the albumin level may drop initially as the treatment restores hydration.

F. With severely malnourished clients, monitor for "refeeding syndrome" (a rapid drop in potassium, magnesium, and phosphate serum levels).

G. Abnormal liver function values may indicate intolerance to or an excess of fat emulsions or problems with metabolism with glucose and protein.

H. Abnormal renal function tests may indicate an excess of amino acids.

I. **Total parenteral nutrition** solutions should be stored under refrigeration and administered within 24 hours from the time that they were prepared (remove from refrigerator 0.5 to 1 hour before use).

BOX 13-9

Home Care Instructions

Teach caregiver how to administer and maintain total parenteral nutrition fluids.

Teach caregiver how to change a sterile dressing.

Obtain a daily weight at the same time of day in the same clothes.

Stress that a weight gain of more than 3 lb per week may indicate excessive fluid intake and should be reported.

Monitor the blood glucose level and report abnormalities immediately.

Check for signs and symptoms of infection, thrombosis, air embolism, and catheter displacement.

Instruct in the importance of reporting signs and symptoms of complications.

Symptoms of an air embolus should be taught to another person in the client's home.

For symptoms of thrombosis the client should report edema of the arm or at the catheter insertion site, neck pain, and jugular vein distention.

Leaking of fluid from the insertion site or pain or discomfort as the fluids are infused may indicate displacement of the catheter; this must be reported immediately.

J. **Total parenteral nutrition** solutions that are cloudy or darkened should not be used and should be returned to the pharmacy.

VII. HOME CARE INSTRUCTIONS (BOX 13-9) ▲

PRACTICE QUESTIONS

1. A client has been discharged to home on total parenteral nutrition (TPN). With each visit, a home care nurse assesses which of the following parameters most closely in monitoring this therapy?
   1. Temperature and weight
   2. Temperature and blood pressure
   3. Pulse and weight
   4. Pulse and blood pressure

2. A nurse is caring for a group of adult clients on an acute care medical-surgical nursing unit. The nurse understands that which of the following clients would be the least likely candidate for total parenteral nutrition (TPN)?
   1. A 66-year-old client with extensive burns
   2. A 42-year-old client who had an open cholecystectomy
   3. A 35-year-client with persistent nausea and vomiting from chemotherapy
   4. A 27-year-old client with severe exacerbation of regional enteritis (Crohn's disease)

3. A nurse is planning to hang the first bag of total parenteral nutrition (TPN) solution via the central line of an assigned client. The nurse plans to obtain which of the following most essential pieces of equipment before hanging the solution?
   1. Electronic infusion pump
   2. Blood glucose meter
   3. Urine test strips
   4. Noninvasive blood pressure monitor

4. A home care nurse is monitoring a client's response to total parenteral nutrition (TPN). The client's weight 1 week ago was 114 pounds. The nurse determines that the client is not gaining weight too rapidly if this morning's weight was
   1. 116 lb.
   2. 119 lb.
   3. 120 lb.
   4. 122 lb.

5. A nurse is assigned to a client receiving total parenteral nutrition (TPN) who had a blood glucose measurement done at 06:00. The nurse documents on the client's clinical worksheet for the day that the blood glucose level should be checked at which of the following times?
   1. 08:00
   2. 12:00
   3. 16:00
   4. 18:00

6. A client is receiving nutrition by means of total parenteral nutrition (TPN). A nurse monitors the client for

complications of the therapy and assesses the client for which of the following signs of hyperglycemia?
1. Nausea, vomiting, and oliguria
2. Sweating, chills, and abdominal pain
3. Fever, weak pulse, and thirst
4. Weakness, thirst, and increased urine output

7. At 8 AM a nurse checks the amount of solution left in a total parenteral nutrition (TPN) infusion bag for an assigned client. It is a 3000-mL bag with 1000 mL remaining. The solution is running at a rate of 100 mL/hr. The bag was hung the previous day at noon. The nurse plans to change the infusion bag and tubing today at
1. Noon.
2. 2 PM.
3. 4 PM.
4. 8 PM.

8. A nurse is changing the central line dressing of a client receiving total parenteral nutrition (TPN). The nurse notes that the catheter insertion site appears reddened. The nurse next assesses which of the following items?
1. Tightness of tubing connections
2. Client's temperature
3. Expiration date on the bag
4. Time of last dressing change

9. A nurse is preparing to hang a fat emulsion. The nurse notes that fat globules are visible at the top of the solution. The nurse takes which of the following actions?
1. Runs the bottle of solution under warm water.
2. Rolls the bottle of solution gently.
3. Shakes the bottle of solution vigorously.
4. Obtains a different bottle of solution.

10. A client is being weaned from total parenteral nutrition (TPN) and is expected to begin taking solid food today. The ongoing solution rate has been 100 mL/hr. A nurse anticipates that which of the following orders regarding the TPN solution will accompany the diet order?
1. Discontinue the TPN.
2. Continue current infusion rate orders for TPN.
3. Decrease TPN rate to 50 mL/hr.
4. Hang 1000 mL 0.9% normal saline.

11. A nurse is preparing to change the total parenteral nutrition (TPN) solution bag and tubing. The client's central venous line is located in the right subclavian vein. The nurse asks the client to do which of the following most essential items during the tubing change?
1. Take a deep breath, hold it, and bear down.
2. Exhale slowly and evenly.
3. Turn the head to the right.
4. Breathe normally.

12. A client with total parenteral nutrition (TPN) infusing has disconnected the tubing from the central line catheter. A nurse assesses the client and suspects an air embolism. The nurse should immediately place the client in which of the following positions?
1. On the left side with the head higher than the feet
2. On the left side with the head lower than the feet
3. On the right side with the head higher than the feet
4. On the right side with the head lower than the feet

13. A client receiving total parenteral nutrition (TPN) complains of a headache. A nurse notes that the client has an increased blood pressure, bounding pulse, jugular vein distention, and crackles bilaterally. The nurse interprets that the client is experiencing which complication of TPN therapy?
1. Hyperglycemia
2. Air embolism
3. Sepsis
4. Fluid overload

14. A client receiving total parenteral nutrition (TPN) suddenly spikes a fever. A nurse notifies the physician, and the physician initially orders that the solution and tubing be changed. The nurse should do which of the following with the discontinued materials?
1. Return them to the hospital pharmacy.
2. Send them to the laboratory for culture.
3. Save them for return to the manufacturer.
4. Discard them in the unit trash.

15. A nurse enters the room of a client receiving total parenteral nutrition (TPN) and discovers that the electronic infusion pump has been shut off. After checking the line for patency and restarting the infusion, the nurse assesses the client for which of the following signs and symptoms?
1. Weakness, thirst, and excessive urination
2. Fever and chills
3. Weakness, shakiness, diaphoresis, and complaints of hunger
4. Dyspnea and hypotension

16. A nurse is making initial rounds at the beginning of the shift. The total parenteral nutrition (TPN) bag of an assigned client is empty. Which of the following solutions readily available on the nursing unit should the nurse hang until another TPN solution is mixed and delivered to the nursing unit?
1. 5% dextrose in water
2. 5% dextrose in 0.9% sodium chloride
3. 5% dextrose in Ringer's lactate
4. 10% dextrose in water

17. At the beginning of a shift a nurse assesses a client receiving total parenteral nutrition (TPN) with fat emulsion piggybacked to the line. The nurse notes that the fat emulsion tubing has a 0.22-μm filter. Which of the following actions by the nurse is most appropriate?
1. Inspect the filter for clogging.
2. Replace with a tubing without a filter.

3. Leave the system alone.

4. Check the line for patency.

18. A nurse is monitoring the status of a client's fat emulsion infusion. The nurse notes that the infusion is 1 hour behind. Which of the following actions by the nurse is most appropriate?

    1. Adjust the infusion rate to run wide open until the solution is back on time.

    2. Ensure that the fat emulsion infusion rate is infusing at the prescribed rate.

    3. Increase the infusion rate to catch up over the next 2 hours.

    4. Adjust the infusion rate to catch up over the next hour.

19. A client receiving total parenteral nutrition (TPN) in the home setting has a weight gain of 5 lb in 1 week. The nurse next assesses the client to detect the presence of which of the following?

    1. Crackles on auscultation of the lungs

    2. Thirst

    3. Decreased blood pressure

    4. Polyuria

20. A nurse is caring for a restless client who is beginning nutritional therapy with total parenteral nutrition (TPN). The nurse should plan to ensure that which of the following is done to prevent the client from injury?

    1. Monitor blood glucose levels every 12 hours.

    2. Secure all connections in the TPN system.

    3. Monitor the temperature once daily.

    4. Calculate daily intake and output.

CRITICAL THINKING: PRIORITIZING (ORDERED RESPONSE)

A nurse is monitoring a client receiving total parenteral nutrition. The client suddenly develops respiratory distress, dyspnea, and chest pain, and the nurse suspects air embolism. Number the actions that the nurse would take in order of priority. (Number 1 is the first action.)

____ Contact the physician.

____ Clamp the intravenous catheter.

____ Administer oxygen.

____ Position the client in left Trendelenburg's position.

____ Take the client's vital signs.

ANSWERS

1. **1**

Rationale: The client receiving total parenteral nutrition (TPN) at home should have the temperature monitored as a means of detecting infection, which is a potential complication of this therapy. An infection also could result in sepsis because the catheter is in a blood vessel. The client's weight is monitored as a measure of the effectiveness of this nutritional therapy and to detect fluid overload. The pulse and blood pressure are important parameters to assess, but they do not relate specifically to the effects of TPN.

Test-Taking Strategy: Note the key words "TPN" and "most closely," which tell you that more than one or all of the options may be partially or totally correct. Remember also that when there are multiple parts to an option, all of the parts must be correct in order for that option to be correct. Recalling that infection and fluid overload are complications of TPN and that weight is monitored as a measure of the effectiveness of this nutritional therapy will direct you to option 1. Review these important assessments if you had difficulty with this question.

Level of Cognitive Ability: Application

Client Needs: Physiological Integrity

Integrated Process: Nursing Process—assessment

Content Area: Fundamental skills

References: Ignatavicius, D., & Workman, M. (2002). *Medical-surgical nursing: Critical thinking for collaborative care* (4th ed., pp. 1372-1373). Philadelphia: W. B. Saunders.

Peckenpaugh, N. (2003). *Nutrition essentials and diet therapy* (9th ed., p. 171). Philadelphia: W. B. Saunders.

2. **2**

Rationale: Total parenteral nutrition is indicated in clients whose gastrointestinal tracts are not functional or who cannot take in a diet enterally for extended periods of time. Examples of these conditions include those of the clients identified in options 1, 3, and 4. Other clients would be those who have had extensive surgery, have multiple fractures, are septic, or have advanced cancer or acquired immunodeficiency syndrome. The client with the open cholecystectomy is not a candidate because this client would resume a diet within a few days following surgery.

Test-Taking Strategy: Note the key words "TPN" and "least likely," which tell you that the correct option is the client who does not require this type of nutritional support. Use nursing knowledge of these various conditions and baseline knowledge of the purposes of TPN to make your selection. Review the indications for TPN if you had difficulty with this question.

Level of Cognitive Ability: Analysis

Client Needs: Physiological Integrity

Integrated Process: Nursing Process—assessment

Content Area: Fundamental skills

References: Ignatavicius, D., & Workman, M. (2002). *Medical-surgical nursing: Critical thinking for collaborative care* (4th ed., p. 1331). Philadelphia: W. B. Saunders.

Lewis, S., Heitkemper, M., & Dirksen, S. (2004). *Medical-surgical nursing: Assessment and management of clinical problems* (6th ed., p. 1145). St. Louis: Mosby.

3. **1**

Rationale: The nurse obtains an electronic infusion pump before hanging a TPN solution. Because of the high glucose content, use of an infusion pump is necessary to ensure that the solution does not infuse too rapidly or fall behind. Because the client's blood glucose is monitored every 4 to 6 hours during administration of TPN, a blood glucose meter also will be needed, but this is not the most essential item needed before hanging the solution. Urine test strips (to measure glucose) rarely are used because of the advent of blood glucose monitoring. A noninvasive blood pressure monitor is unnecessary for this procedure.

Test-Taking Strategy: Note the key words "most essential." They tell you that the correct option identifies the item that is needed to start the infusion. Use the process of elimination and knowledge of the procedure for initiating TPN to answer the question. Review these procedures if you had difficulty with this question.

Level of Cognitive Ability: Application
Client Needs: Physiological Integrity
Integrated Process: Nursing Process—planning
Content Area: Fundamental skills
Reference: Ignatavicius, D., & Workman, M. (2002). *Medical-surgical nursing: Critical thinking for collaborative care* (4th ed., p. 1372). Philadelphia: W. B. Saunders.

4. 1

Rationale: The client receiving TPN should not gain more than 3 lb per week, with optimal weight gain being 1 to 2 lb per week. The weight goal for the client on TPN is individual and depends on the client's metabolic needs and baseline weight (whether underweight, overweight, or at optimal weight). The correct option identifies a reasonable weight gain of 2 lb per week. Options 2, 3, and 4 indicate a weekly weight gain that is greater than expected.

Test-Taking Strategy: Use the process of elimination and recall that the optimal weekly weight gain for the client receiving TPN is 1 to 2 lb weekly. Review the expected outcomes of TPN if you had difficulty with this question.

Level of Cognitive Ability: Analysis
Client Needs: Physiological Integrity
Integrated Process: Nursing Process—evaluation
Content Area: Fundamental skills
References: Lehne, R. (2001). *Pharmacology for nursing care* (4th ed., p. 894.). Philadelphia: W. B. Saunders.
Perry, A., & Potter, P. (2002). *Clinical nursing skills and techniques* (5th ed., p. 693). St. Louis: Mosby.

5. 2

Rationale: The client's blood glucose level should be monitored every 4 to 6 hours during TPN. Depending on agency policy, this may be done every 8 hours instead. Monitoring the blood glucose level every 2 hours (option 1) is unnecessary. Monitoring every 10 or 12 hours (options 3 and 4) is insufficient.

Test-Taking Strategy: Use the process of elimination. Recalling that the client on TPN should have the blood glucose level monitored every 4 to 6 hours and knowledge of military time will direct you to the correct option. If you had difficulty with this question, review the nursing interventions related to the administration of TPN.

Level of Cognitive Ability: Application
Client Needs: Physiological Integrity
Integrated Process: Communication and Documentation
Content Area: Fundamental skills
References: Ignatavicius, D., & Workman, M. (2002). *Medical-surgical nursing: Critical thinking for collaborative care* (4th ed., p. 1372). Philadelphia: W. B. Saunders.

Lewis, S., Heitkemper, M., & Dirksen, S. (2004). *Medical-surgical nursing: Assessment and management of clinical problems* (6th ed., p. 989). St. Louis: Mosby.

6. 4

Rationale: The high glucose concentration in TPN places the client at risk for hyperglycemia. Signs of hyperglycemia include excessive thirst, fatigue, restlessness, confusion, weakness, Kussmaul's respirations, diuresis, and coma, when hyperglycemia is severe. If the client has these symptoms, the blood glucose level should be checked immediately. Options 1, 2, and 3 do not identify signs specific to hyperglycemia.

Test-Taking Strategy: Use the process of elimination. Remember that for an option to be correct, all of the parts of that option must be correct. Begin to answer this question by eliminating options 2 and 3 because chills and fever are indicative of infection. Choose option 4 over option 1 because the client with hyperglycemia has increased urine output rather than decreased urine output. Review the signs of hyperglycemia if you had difficulty with this question.

Level of Cognitive Ability: Comprehension
Client Needs: Physiological Integrity
Integrated Process: Nursing Process—assessment
Content Area: Fundamental skills
Reference: Ignatavicius, D., & Workman, M. (2002). *Medical-surgical nursing: Critical thinking for collaborative care* (4th ed., p. 1372). Philadelphia: W. B. Saunders.

7. 1

Rationale: Total parenteral nutrition solution should be changed every 24 hours because the TPN solution is a high-concentrate glucose and is a medium for bacterial growth. Infection control is also aided by use of aseptic technique with bag and tubing changes. Most agencies recommend that tubing be changed every 24 hours along with the bag, although some agencies recommend changing tubing every 48 to 72 hours. The nurse always should adhere to specific agency policies. Options 2, 3, and 4 identify insufficient time frames and present the risk for infection.

Test-Taking Strategy: Use the process of elimination. Recalling that the infusion bag should be changed every 24 hours will direct you to the correct option. Review the principles related to the prevention of infection in the client receiving TPN if you had difficulty with this question.

Level of Cognitive Ability: Application
Client Needs: Physiological Integrity
Integrated Process: Nursing Process—planning
Content Area: Fundamental skills
Reference: Ignatavicius, D., & Workman, M. (2002). *Medical-surgical nursing: Critical thinking for collaborative care* (4th ed., p. 1372). Philadelphia: W. B. Saunders.

8. 2

Rationale: Redness at the catheter insertion site is a possible indication of infection. The nurse would next assess for other signs of infection. Of the options given, the temperature is the next item to assess. The tightness of tubing connections should be assessed each time the TPN is checked; loose connections would result in leakage, not skin redness. The expiration date on the bag is a viable option, but that also should be checked at the time the solution is hung and with each shift change. The time of the last dressing change should be checked with each shift change.

Test-Taking Strategy: Note the key word "next." This question requires that you prioritize based on the information provided in the question. Also note the relationship between "site appears reddened" in the question and the word "temperature" in the correct option. Focusing on the issue of infection will direct you to option 2. Review the signs of infection in the client receiving TPN if you had difficulty with this question.

Level of Cognitive Ability: Application
Client Needs: Physiological Integrity
Integrated Process: Nursing Process—assessment
Content Area: Fundamental skills
Reference: Lewis, S., Heitkemper, M., & Dirksen, S. (2004). *Medical-surgical nursing: Assessment and management of clinical problems* (6th ed., p. 990). St. Louis: Mosby.

9. 4

Rationale: The nurse should examine the bottle of fat emulsion for separation of emulsion into layers or fat globules or for the accumulation of froth. The nurse should not hang a fat emulsion if any of these observations are made and should return the solution to the pharmacy. Options 1, 2, and 3 are inappropriate actions.

Test-Taking Strategy: Use the process of elimination. Remember that options that are similar are not likely to be correct. With this in mind, eliminate options 2 and 3 first. Select between the remaining options by recalling the significance of fat globules in the solution. Also, think about the potential adverse effect of fat globules entering the client's bloodstream. Review the procedure for administering fat emulsion if you had difficulty with this question.

Level of Cognitive Ability: Application
Client Needs: Physiological Integrity
Integrated Process: Nursing Process—implementation
Content Area: Fundamental skills
References: Lehne, R. (2001). *Pharmacology for nursing care* (4th ed., p. 894). Philadelphia: W. B. Saunders.
Lewis, S., Heitkemper, M., & Dirksen, S. (2004). *Medical-surgical nursing: Assessment and management of clinical problems* (6th ed., p. 989). St. Louis: Mosby.

10. 3

Rationale: When a client begins taking a diet after a period of receiving parenteral nutrition, the TPN is decreased gradually. Total parenteral nutrition that is discontinued abruptly can cause hypoglycemia. Clients often have anorexia after being without food for some time, and the digestive tract also is not used to producing the digestive enzymes that will be needed. Gradually decreasing the infusion rate allows the client to remain adequately nourished during the transition to a normal diet and prevents the occurrence of hypoglycemia. Even before clients are started on a solid diet, they are given clear liquids followed by full liquids to further ease the transition. A solution of normal saline will not provide the glucose needed during the transition of discontinuing the TPN and also could cause the client to experience hypoglycemia.

Test-Taking Strategy: Use the process of elimination and note the key word "weaned" in the question. Recalling the effects

of TPN and the complications that occur will direct you to option 3. If you had difficulty with this question, review the concepts related to discontinuing TPN solution.

Level of Cognitive Ability: Analysis
Client Needs: Physiological Integrity
Integrated Process: Nursing Process—analysis
Content Area: Fundamental skills
References: Kee, J., & Hayes, E. (2003). *Pharmacology: A nursing process approach* (4th ed., p. 228). Philadelphia: W. B. Saunders.
Lewis, S., Heitkemper, M., & Dirksen, S. (2004). *Medical-surgical nursing: Assessment and management of clinical problems* (6th ed., p. 990). St. Louis: Mosby.

11. 1

Rationale: The client should be asked to perform Valsalva's maneuver during tubing changes. This helps to avoid air embolism during tubing changes. The nurse asks the client to take a deep breath, hold it, and bear down. If the IV line is on the right, the client turns the head to the left. This position will increase intrathoracic pressure. Options 2 and 4 are inappropriate and could cause the potential for an air embolism during the tubing change.

Test-Taking Strategy: Note the key words "most essential." Use the process of elimination, recalling that air embolism is a complication that can occur during tubing changes. Review the procedure for TPN bag and tubing change if you had difficulty with this question.

Level of Cognitive Ability: Application
Client Needs: Physiological Integrity
Integrated Process: Nursing Process—implementation
Content Area: Fundamental skills
Reference: Ignatavicius, D., & Workman, M. (2002). *Medical-surgical nursing: Critical thinking for collaborative care* (4th ed., p. 2207). Philadelphia: W. B. Saunders

12. 2

Rationale: When air embolism is suspected, the client should be placed in a left side-lying position. The head should be lower than the feet. This position is used to try to minimize the effect of the air traveling as a bolus to the lungs by trapping it in the right side of the heart. Options 1, 3, and 4 are incorrect positions if an air embolism is suspected.

Test-Taking Strategy: Use the process of elimination and recall the concept that the goal is to trap air in the right side of the heart. If you had difficulty with this question, review the immediate interventions when air embolism is suspected.

Level of Cognitive Ability: Application
Client Needs: Physiological Integrity
Integrated Process: Nursing Process—implementation
Content Area: Fundamental skills
Reference: Perry, A., & Potter, P. (2002). *Clinical nursing skills and techniques* (5th ed., p. 687). St. Louis: Mosby.

13. 4

Rationale: The client's signs and symptoms are consistent with fluid overload. The increased intravascular volume increases the blood pressure, while the pulse rate increases as the heart tries to pump the extra fluid volume. The volume also causes neck vein distention and shifting of fluid into the alveoli, resulting in lung crackles. The signs and symptoms presented in the question do not indicate hyperglycemia, air embolism, or sepsis.

Test-Taking Strategy: Use the process of elimination, focusing on the signs and symptoms presented in the question. Recalling the signs of fluid overload will direct you to option 4. If you had difficulty with this question, review the signs of fluid overload.

Level of Cognitive Ability: Analysis
Client Needs: Physiological Integrity
Integrated Process: Nursing Process—analysis
Content Area: Fundamental skills
Reference: Lewis, S., Heitkemper, M., & Dirksen, S. (2004). *Medical-surgical nursing: Assessment and management of clinical problems* (6th ed., p. 990). St. Louis: Mosby.

14. **2**
Rationale: When the client who is receiving TPN spikes a temperature, a catheter-related infection should be suspected. The solution and tubing should be changed, and the discontinued materials should be cultured for infectious organisms. The other options are incorrect.

Test-Taking Strategy: Use the process of elimination. Identifying the issue of the question, infection, and correlating the elevated temperature with infection associated with the IV should direct you to option 2. Review the procedure when infection is suspected in the client receiving TPN if you had difficulty with this question.

Level of Cognitive Ability: Application
Client Needs: Physiological Integrity
Integrated Process: Nursing Process—implementation
Content Area: Fundamental skills
Reference: Lewis, S., Heitkemper, M., & Dirksen, S. (2004). *Medical-surgical nursing: Assessment and management of clinical problems* (6th ed., p. 989). St. Louis: Mosby.

15. **3**
Rationale: If the pump that is infusing TPN shuts off for a period of time, the nurse assesses the client for signs and symptoms of hypoglycemia. These signs include weakness, shakiness, headache, anxiety, diaphoresis, and complaints of hunger. The blood glucose level will be less than 70 mg/dL. The other signs and symptoms described are those of hyperglycemia (option 1), infection (option 2), and air embolism (option 4).

Test-Taking Strategy: Use the process of elimination and focus on the issue of the question that the infusion pump has been shut off. Recall that the client is at risk for hypoglycemia when the TPN is stopped or discontinued. Next, recalling the signs of hypoglycemia will direct you to option 3. Review the complications associated with TPN and the signs of the complications if you had difficulty with this question.

Level of Cognitive Ability: Analysis
Client Needs: Physiological Integrity
Integrated Process: Nursing Process—assessment
Content Area: Fundamental skills
References: Lewis, S., Heitkemper, M., & Dirksen, S. (2004). *Medical-surgical nursing: Assessment and management of clinical problems* (6th ed., p. 990). St. Louis: Mosby.
Phipps, W., Monahan, F., Sands, J., Marek, J., & Neighbors, M. (2003). *Medical-surgical nursing: Health and illness perspectives* (7th ed., p. 1060). St. Louis: Mosby.

16. **4**
Rationale: The solution containing the highest amount of glucose should be hung until the new TPN becomes available. Because TPN solutions contain high glucose concentrations, the 10% dextrose in water solution is the best of the choices presented. The solution selected should be one that minimizes the risk of hypoglycemia. Options 1, 2, and 3 will not be as effective in minimizing the risk of hypoglycemia.

Test-Taking Strategy: Use the process of elimination, recalling that this particular client is at risk for hypoglycemia. With this in mind, you would then select the solution that minimizes this risk to the client. Also, remember that options that are similar are not likely to be correct. Each of the incorrect options represents a solution commonly stocked on the nursing unit and contains 5% dextrose. Review the nursing actions to prevent hypoglycemia in the client receiving TPN if you had difficulty with this question.

Level of Cognitive Ability: Application
Client Needs: Physiological Integrity
Integrated Process: Nursing Process—implementation
Content Area: Fundamental skills
Reference: Phipps, W., Monahan, F., Sands, J., Marek, J., & Neighbors, M. (2003). *Medical-surgical nursing: Health and illness perspectives* (7th ed., p. 1059). St. Louis: Mosby.

17. **2**
Rationale: The most appropriate action by the nurse is to replace the tubing. A 0.22-μm filter is appropriate for the administration of TPN, but fat emulsion should be administered without a filter. If fat emulsion is mixed into the TPN solution, then a 1.2-μm filter or a larger filter should be used to allow the fat emulsion to pass through.

Test-Taking Strategy: Use the process of elimination, recalling that fat emulsion should be administered without a filter. If you had difficulty with this question, review the procedure for the administration of fat emulsion.

Level of Cognitive Ability: Application
Client Needs: Physiological Integrity
Integrated Process: Nursing Process—implementation
Content Area: Fundamental skills
References: Lewis, S., Heitkemper, M., & Dirksen, S. (2004). *Medical-surgical nursing: Assessment and management of clinical problems* (6th ed., p. 989). St. Louis: Mosby.
Phipps, W., Monahan, F., Sands, J., Marek, J., & Neighbors, M. (2003). *Medical-surgical nursing: Health and illness perspectives* (7th ed., p. 1059). St. Louis: Mosby.

18. **2**
Rationale: The nurse should not increase the rate of a fat emulsion to make up the difference if the infusion falls behind time. Doing so could place the client at risk for fat overload. The same principle applies to TPN; increasing the rate suddenly in this case could cause hyperglycemia and fluid overload.

Test-Taking Strategy: Note the key words "most appropriate." Remember also that options that are similar are not likely to be correct. This guides you to eliminate options 3 and 4 first. Choose option 2 over option 1, recalling that the nurse never increases the infusion rate or adjusts an infusion rate to run wide open if an infusion is behind. Review these safety principles if you had difficulty with this question.

Level of Cognitive Ability: Application
Client Needs: Physiological Integrity
Integrated Process: Nursing Process—implementation
Content Area: Fundamental skills
References: Lewis, S., Heitkemper, M., & Dirksen, S. (2004). *Medical-surgical nursing: Assessment and management of clinical problems* (6th ed., p. 989). St. Louis: Mosby.
Phipps, W., Monahan, F., Sands, J., Marek, J., & Neighbors, M. (2003). *Medical-surgical nursing: Health and illness perspectives* (7th ed., p. 1060). St. Louis: Mosby.

19. 1
Rationale: Optimal weight gain on TPN is 1 to 2 lb per week. The client who has a weight gain of 5 lb per week while receiving TPN is likely to have fluid retention that can result in fluid overload. Signs of fluid overload include a bounding pulse, jugular vein distention, headache, increased blood pressure, crackles on lung auscultation, and weight gain greater than desired. Options 2 and 4 are associated with hyperglycemia. Option 3 is likely to be noted in a fluid volume deficit.
Test-Taking Strategy: Focus on the issue of the question, a weight gain of 5 lb in 1 week. This should direct your thinking to the potential for fluid overload. With this in mind, use the process of elimination, selecting the option that identifies the signs of fluid overload. If you had difficulty with this question, review the signs and symptoms of the complications associated with the administration of TPN.
Level of Cognitive Ability: Analysis
Client Needs: Physiological Integrity
Integrated Process: Nursing Process—assessment
Content Area: Fundamental skills
Reference: Perry, A., & Potter, P. (2002). *Clinical nursing skills and techniques* (5th ed., p. 693). St. Louis: Mosby.

20. 2
Rationale: The nurse should plan to secure (tape is used per agency protocol) all connections in the tubing. This will help prevent the restless client from pulling the connections apart accidentally. The nurse should also monitor intake and output, but this does not relate specifically to a risk for injury as presented in the question. Also, options 1 and 3 do not relate to a risk for injury as presented in the question. In addition, the client's temperature and blood glucose levels are monitored

more frequently than the time frames identified in the options to detect signs of infection and hyperglycemia, respectively.
Test-Taking Strategy: Note the key words "restless," "ensure," "prevent," and "injury." Focus on the issue of the question, and use the process of elimination to direct you to option 2. Review the precautions related to TPN if you had difficulty with this question.
Level of Cognitive Ability: Application
Client Needs: Safe, Effective Care Environment
Integrated Process: Nursing Process—planning
Content Area: Fundamental skills
Reference: Ignatavicius, D., & Workman, M. (2002). *Medical-surgical nursing: Critical thinking for collaborative care* (4th ed., p. 207). Philadelphia: W. B. Saunders.

CRITICAL THINKING: PRIORITIZING (ORDERED RESPONSE)
Answer: 31425
Rationale: If air embolism is suspected, the nurse would first clamp the intravenous catheter to prevent the embolism from traveling through the heart to the pulmonary system. The nurse would next place the client in a left side-lying position with the head lower than the feet (to trap air in right side of the heart). The nurse would notify the physician and administer oxygen as prescribed. The nurse would monitor the client closely and take the client's vital signs.
Test-Taking Strategy: Think about the pathophysiology and effects of an air embolism. Recalling that a primary concern is that the embolism will travel to the pulmonary system will assist in determining that the catheter needs to be clamped first and that the client needs to be positioned to trap the air in the right side of the heart. Because this event is an emergency, the nurse notifies the physician next and the physician will provide an order for oxygen if necessary. The nurse monitors the client and takes the client's vital signs frequently.
Level of Cognitive Ability: Application
Client Needs: Physiological Integrity
Integrated Process: Nursing Process—implementation
Content Area: Fundamental skills
Reference: Perry, A., & Potter, P. (2002). *Clinical nursing skills and techniques* (5th ed., p. 687). St. Louis: Mosby.

REFERENCES

Ignatavicius, D., & Workman, M. (2002). *Medical-surgical nursing: Critical thinking for collaborative care* (4th ed.). Philadelphia: W. B. Saunders.

Kee, J., & Hayes, E. (2003). *Pharmacology: A nursing process approach* (4th ed.). Philadelphia: W. B. Saunders.

Lehne, R. (2001). *Pharmacology for nursing care* (4th ed.). Philadelphia: W. B. Saunders.

Lewis, S., Heitkemper, M., & Dirksen, S. (2004). *Medical-surgical nursing: Assessment and management of clinical problems* (6th ed.). St. Louis: Mosby.

National Council of State Boards of Nursing (Eds.). (2003). *Test Plan for the National Council Licensure Examination for Registered Nurses* (effective date: April 2004). Chicago: Author.

Peckenpaugh, N. (2003). *Nutrition essentials and diet therapy* (9th ed.). Philadelphia: W. B. Saunders.

Perry, A., & Potter, P. (2002). *Clinical nursing skills and techniques* (5th ed.). St. Louis: Mosby.

Phipps, W., Monahan, F., Sands, J., Marek, J., & Neighbors, M. (2003). *Medical-surgical nursing: Health and illness perspectives* (7th ed.). St. Louis: Mosby.

Potter, P., & Perry, A. (2001). *Fundamentals of nursing* (5th ed.). St. Louis: Mosby.

Intravenous Therapy

PYRAMID TERMS

air embolism Obstruction caused by a bolus of air that enters the vein through an inadequately primed intravenous line, from a loose connection, or during tubing change or removal of the intravenous line.

catheter embolism Obstruction that results from breakage of the tip of the catheter during intravenous line insertion or removal.

hypertonic Solutions that are more concentrated or have a higher osmolality than body fluids.

hypotonic Solutions that are more dilute or have a lower osmolality than body fluids.

infiltration Seepage of intravenous fluid out of the vein and into the surrounding interstitial spaces.

isotonic Solutions that have the same osmolality as body fluids.

phlebitis An inflammation of the vein that can result mechanical or chemical (medication) trauma or a local infection.

THE PYRAMID TO SUCCESS

Professional nurses are responsible for managing and providing care to clients receiving intravenous (IV) therapy. Pyramid Points focus on the safety measures required to initiate and maintain an IV line. Assessment of the client for allergies, including latex sensitivity, before initiation of an IV line is a critical nursing duty. Additional nursing responsibilities include monitoring for complications related to the IV line, and the initiation of measures required when an IV complication occurs. Pyramid Points focus on the signs and symptoms of infection, infiltration, phlebitis, circulatory overload, and air embolism, and the treatment measures associated with each. Integrated Processes addressed in this chapter include Nursing Process, Caring, Communication and Documentation, and Teaching/Learning.

CLIENT NEEDS
Safe, Effective Care Environment

Informed consent for invasive procedures
Establishment of priorities
Consultation with members of the health care team
Medical and surgical asepsis during handling of equipment and supplies
Error prevention in administering IV lines
Applying principles of infection control
Standard, transmission-based, and other precautions
Handling of hazardous or infectious materials

Health Promotion and Maintenance

Health and wellness
Lifestyle choices related to home care of an IV
Teaching the client and family about care to the IV
Evaluation of client's home environment for self-care modifications
Client's ability to perform self-care

Psychosocial Integrity

Assessment of coping mechanisms
Support systems in the home for caring for the IV line
Client's emotional response to treatment

Physiological Integrity

Intravenous therapy
Parenteral therapies
Central venous access devices
Expected effects of IV therapy
Monitoring laboratory values for fluid and electrolyte imbalances
Monitoring for complications of IV therapy
Immediate interventions if a complication occurs

I. INTRAVENOUS THERAPY

A. Purpose and uses
1. Intravenous therapy is used to sustain clients who are unable to take substances orally.
2. Intravenous therapy replaces water, electrolytes, and nutrients more rapidly than oral administration.
3. Intravenous therapy provides immediate access to the vascular system for the rapid delivery of specific solutions without the time required for gastrointestinal tract absorption.
4. Intravenous therapy provides a vascular route for the administration of medication or blood components.

B. Types of solutions (Table 14-1)
1. **Isotonic**
   a. Solutions have the same osmolality as body fluids.
   b. **Isotonic** solutions increase extracellular fluid volume.
   c. These solutions do not enter the cells because no osmotic force exists to shift the fluids.
2. **Hypotonic**
   a. Solutions are more dilute or have a lower osmolality than body fluids.
   b. **Hypotonic** solutions cause movement of water into cells by osmosis.
   c. These solutions should be administered slowly to prevent cellular edema.
3. **Hypertonic**
   a. Solutions are more concentrated or have a higher osmolality than body fluids.
   b. **Hypertonic** solutions concentrate extracellular fluid and cause movement of water from cells into the extracellular fluid by osmosis.

4. Crystalloids
   a. Solutions contain electrolytes.
   b. Crystalloids may be used for fluid volume replacement.
5. Colloids
   a. Colloids also are called plasma expanders.
   b. Colloids pull fluid from the interstitial compartment into the vascular compartment.
   c. Colloids are used to increase the vascular volume rapidly, such as in hemorrhage or severe hypovolemia.

II. INTRAVENOUS DEVICES

A. Intravenous cannulas
1. Steel needles or butterfly sets
   a. The set is a wing-tip needle with a metal cannula, plastic or rubber wings, and a plastic catheter or hub.
   b. The needle is 0.5 to 1.5 inches in length, with needle gauge sizes from 16 to 26.
   c. Intravenous cannulas are used when the infusion time will be short.
   d. **Infiltration** is more common with these devices.
   e. The butterfly infusion set commonly is used in children and the older client, whose veins are likely to be small or fragile.
2. Plastic cannulas
   a. Plastic cannulas may be an over-the-needle device or an in-needle catheter and are used primarily for short-term therapy.
   b. The over-the-needle device is preferred for rapid infusion and is more comfortable for the client.
   c. The in-needle catheter can cause **catheter embolism** if the tip of the cannula breaks.

B. Intravenous gauges
1. The smaller the gauge number, the larger the outside diameter of the cannula.
2. The size used depends on the solution to be administered and the diameter of the available vein.
3. Larger gauges allow a higher fluid rate than smaller ones and allow the administration of higher concentrations of solutions.
4. For rapid emergency fluid administration, blood products, or anesthetics, a large gauge is used, such as a 14-, 16-, 18-, or 19-gauge needle.
5. For peripheral fat infusions (lipids), a 20- or 21-gauge is used.
6. For standard IV fluid and clear liquid IV medications, a 22- or 24-gauge is used.
7. If the client has very small veins, a 24- to 25-gauge is used.

C. IV containers (Fig. 14-1)
1. Container may be glass or plastic.
2. Squeeze the plastic bag to ensure intactness and assess the glass bottle for any cracks before hanging.

TABLE 14-1

Types of Intravenous Solutions

Solution	Tonicity
0.9% saline (NS)	Isotonic
5% dextrose in water (D_5W)	Isotonic
5% dextrose in 0.225% saline (5% D/¼ NS)	Isotonic
Lactated Ringer's (RL) solution	Isotonic
0.45% saline (½ NS)	Hypotonic
0.225% saline (¼ NS)	Hypotonic
0.33% saline (⅓ NS)	Hypotonic
3% saline (3% NS)	Hypertonic
5% saline (5% NS)	Hypertonic
10% dextrose in water ($D_{10}W$)	Hypertonic
5% dextrose in 0.9% saline (5% D/NS)	Hypertonic
5% dextrose in 0.45% saline (5% D/½ NS)	Hypertonic
5% dextrose in lactated Ringer's solution	Hypertonic
Dextran	Colloid
Albumin	Colloid

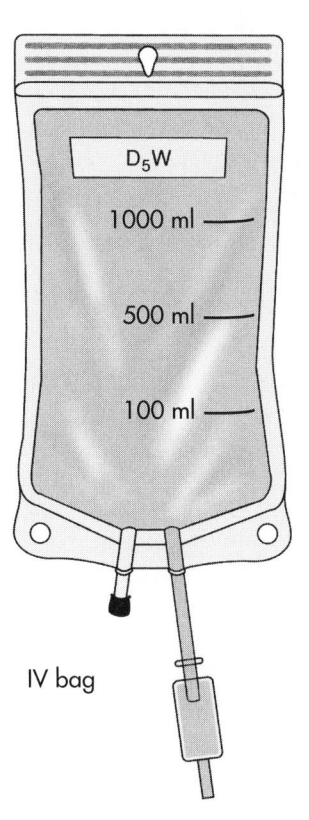

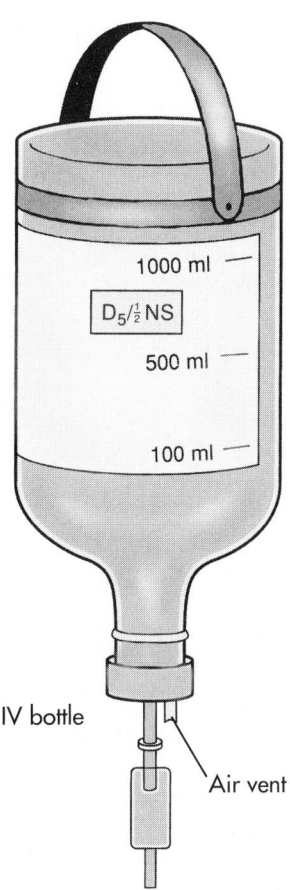

IV bag

IV bottle

Air vent

FIG. 14-1 Intravenous containers. (From Kee, J. L., & Marshall, S. M. [2004]. *Clinical calculations: With applications to general and specialty areas* [5th ed]. Philadelphia: W. B. Saunders.)

3. Do not write on the plastic IV bag with a marking pen because the ink may be absorbed through the plastic into the solution.
4. Use a label and a ballpoint pen for marking the bag, placing the label onto the bag.

D. Intravenous tubing (Fig. 14-2)
1. Intravenous tubing contains a spike end for the bag or bottle, a drop chamber, a roller clamp, a Y-site, and an adapter end for attachment to the needle.
2. Extension tubing is available for children, clients who are restless, or clients who have special mobility needs.
3. Shorter secondary tubing is used for piggyback solutions, connecting them to the injection sites nearest to the drip chamber (Fig. 14-3).
4. Special tubing is used for medication that absorbs into plastic.
5. Vented and nonvented tubing is available.
   a. A vent allows air to enter the IV container as the fluid leaves.
   b. A vented adapter can be used to add a vent to a nonvented IV tubing system.
   c. Use nonvented tubing for flexible containers.

d. Use vented tubing for glass or rigid plastic containers to allow air to enter and displace the fluid as it leaves; fluid will not flow from a rigid IV container unless it is vented.

E. Drip chambers (Fig. 14-4)
1. Microdrip chamber
   a. Normally the chamber has a short vertical metal piece where the drop forms.
   b. The chamber delivers about 60 drops/mL.
   c. Read the tubing package to determine how many drops per milliliter are delivered (drop factor).
   d. Microdrip chambers are used if fluid will be infused at a slow rate (less than 50 mL/hr).
   e. Microdrip chambers are used if the solution contains potent medication that needs to be titrated, such as in a critical care setting or in pediatrics.
2. Macrodrip chamber
   a. The chamber is used if the solution is thick or is to be infused rapidly.
   b. Drop factor varies from 10 to 20 drops/mL.
   c. Read the tubing package to determine how many drops per milliliter are delivered (drop factor).

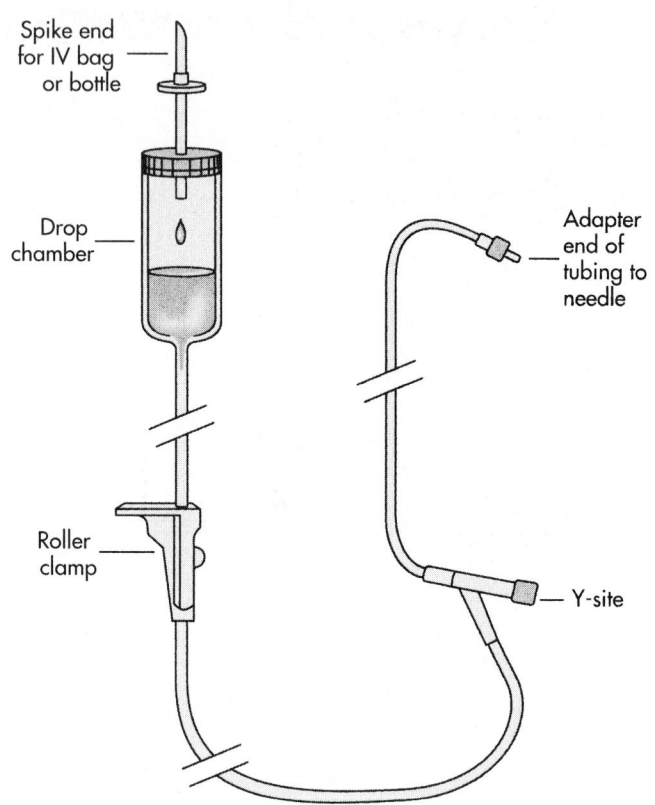

FIG. 14-2 Intravenous tubing. (From Kee, J. L., & Marshall, S. M. [2004]. *Clinical calculations: With applications to general and specialty areas* [5th ed]. Philadelphia: W. B. Saunders.)

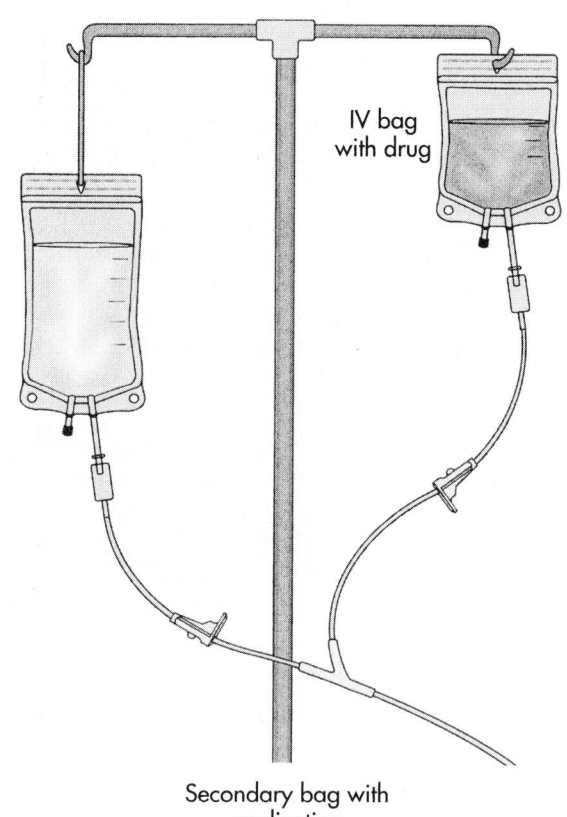

FIG. 14-3 Secondary bag with medication. (From Kee, J. L., & Marshall, S. M. [2004]. *Clinical calculations: With applications to general and specialty areas* [5th ed]. Philadelphia: W. B. Saunders.)

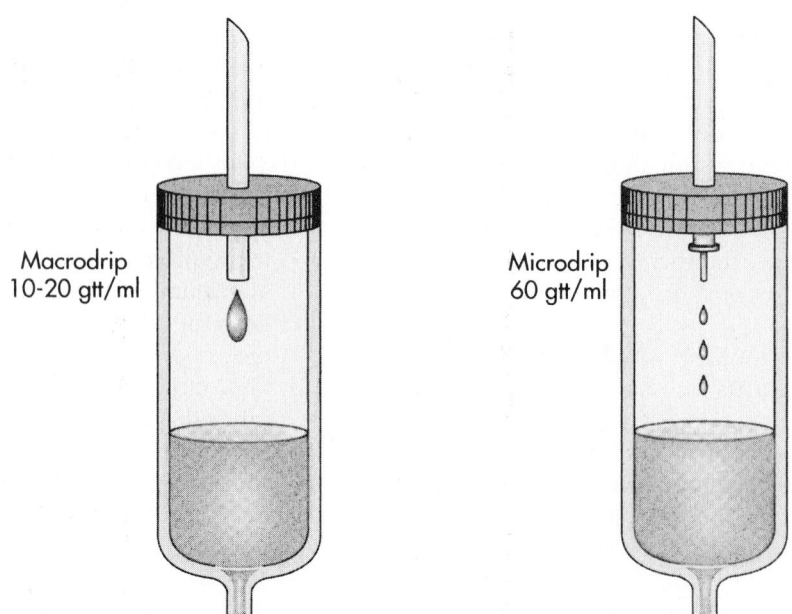

FIG. 14-4 Macrodrip and microdrip sizes. (From Kee, J. L., & Marshall, S. M. [2004]. *Clinical calculations: With applications to general and specialty areas* [5th ed]. Philadelphia: W. B. Saunders.)

F. Filters
1. Filters provide protection by preventing particles from entering the client's veins.
2. Filters are used in IV lines to trap small particles such as undissolved antibiotics or salt or medications that have precipitated in solution.
3. Assess the agency policy regarding the use of filters.
4. A 0.22-μm filter is used for most solutions, a 1.2-μm for solutions containing lipids or albumin, and a special filter for blood components.
5. Change filters every 24 to 72 hours (depending on agency policy) to prevent bacterial growth.
G. Needleless systems
1. Needleless systems include recessed needles, plastic cannulas, and one-way valves; these systems decrease the exposure to contaminated needles.
2. Do not administer total parenteral nutrition or blood products through a one-way valve.
H. Intermittent infusion sets (Fig. 14-5)
1. Intermittent infusion sets are used when intravascular accessibility is desired for intermittent administration of medications by IV push or IV piggyback.
2. An IV lock is attached for intermittent infusion devices.
3. Patency is maintained by periodic flushing with normal saline solution (sodium chloride and normal saline are interchangeable names).
4. When administering medication, flush with 1 to 2 mL (depending on agency policy) of normal saline to confirm placement of the IV cannula; administer the prescribed medication, and then flush the cannula again with 1 to 2 mL (depending on agency policy) of normal saline to maintain patency.

III. LATEX ALLERGY
A. Assess the client for an allergy to latex.
B. Intravenous supplies may contain latex including IV catheters, IV tubing, IV ports (particularly IV rubber injection ports), rubber stoppers on multidose vials, and adhesive tape.

BOX 14-1

Peripheral Intravenous: Sites to Avoid

Edematous extremity
An arm that is weak, traumatized, or paralyzed
The arm on the same side as a mastectomy
An arm that has an arteriovenous fistula or shunt for dialysis
An infected area

C. Latex-safe IV supplies need to be used on clients with a latex allergy.
D. A three-way stopcock, rather than a rubber injection port, needs to be used on plastic tubing.
E. Refer to Chapter 69 for additional information regarding latex allergy.

IV. SELECTION OF A PERIPHERAL IV SITE
A. Veins in the hand, forearm, and antecubital fossa are suitable sites.
B. Veins in the lower extremities are not suitable because of the risk of thrombus formation and possible pooling of medication in areas of decreased venous return (Box 14-1).
C. Veins in the scalp and feet may be suitable sites for infants.
D. The most frequently used sites are the veins of the forearm because the bones of the forearm act as a natural support and splint.
E. Assess the veins of both arms closely before selecting a site.
F. Start the IV infusion distally to provide the option of proceeding up the extremity if the vein is ruptured or **infiltration** occurs; if **infiltration** occurs from the antecubital vein, the lower veins usually cannot be used for further puncture sites.
G. Determine the client's dominant side, and select the opposite side for a venipuncture site.
H. Bending the elbow on the arm with an IV may easily obstruct the flow of solution, causing **infiltration** that could lead to thrombophlebitis.

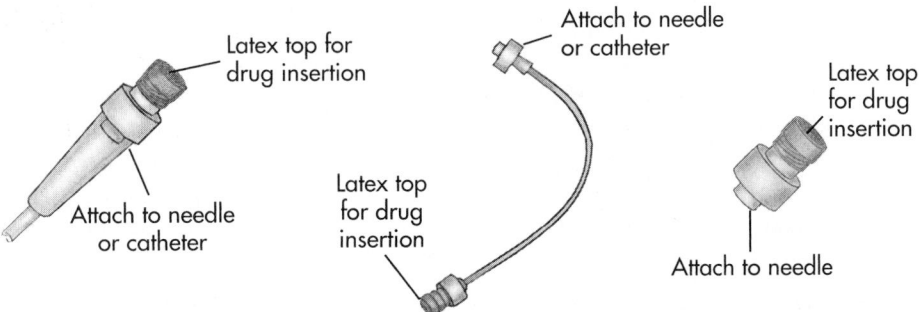

FIG. 14-5 Infusion devices. (From Kee, J. L., & Marshall, S. M. [2000]. *Clinical calculations: With applications to general and specialty areas* [4th ed]. Philadelphia: W. B. Saunders.)

I. Avoid checking the blood pressure on the arm receiving the IV infusion if possible.

J. Do not place restraints over the venipuncture site.

K. Use an armboard as needed when the venipuncture site is located in an area of flexion.

V. ADDITION OF MEDICATION TO AN IV LINE

A. Assess for compatibility of medication and solution.

B. When adding medication to the bag, mix the bag end-to-end several times before hanging it to disperse the medication.

C. Ensure that medication can be mixed in soft plastic because some medications absorb into the soft plastic and should be mixed only in glass.

VI. ADMINISTRATION OF IV SOLUTIONS

A. Check the IV solution against the physician's orders for the type, amount, percent of solution, and rate of flow.

B. Assess the health status and medical disorders of the client.

C. Identify client conditions that contraindicate use of a particular IV solution.

D. Wash hands thoroughly before inserting an IV line and before working with an IV line.

E. Use sterile technique when inserting an IV line and when changing the dressing over the IV site.

F. When inserting an IV line, clean the skin with an antimicrobial solution, using an inner to outer circular motion.

G. Prime the tubing to remove air from the system.

H. Change the venipuncture site every 48 to 72 hours, depending on agency policy.

I. Change the IV dressing every 72 hours, when the dressing is wet or contaminated, or as specified by the agency policy.

J. Change the IV tubing every 24 to 72 hours, depending on agency policy.

K. Label the tubing, dressing, and solution bags clearly, indicating the date and time when changed.

L. Do not let an IV bag or bottle of solution hang for more than 24 hours because of the potential for sepsis.

M. Do not allow the IV tubing to touch the floor because of the potential for bacterial contamination.

N. Before adding medications or solutions, swab access ports with 70% alcohol, another equally effective solution, or as specified by the agency policy.

VII. PRECAUTIONS FOR IV LINES

A. On insertion, an IV line can cause initial pain and discomfort for the client.

B. An IV puncture provides a route of entry for microorganisms into the body.

C. Medications enter the blood immediately, and any adverse reactions or allergic responses can occur immediately.

D. Fluid (circulatory) overload or electrolyte imbalances can occur from an excessive or too rapid infusion of IV fluids.

E. Incompatibilities between certain solutions and medications can occur.

F. Clients with respiratory, cardiac, renal, or liver diseases, older clients, and very young persons cannot tolerate an excessive fluid volume, and the risk of fluid overload exists with these clients.

G. A client with congestive heart failure usually is not given a solution containing saline because this type of fluid encourages the retention of water and would therefore exacerbate heart failure by increasing the fluid overload.

H. A client with diabetes mellitus usually does not receive dextrose (glucose) solutions.

I. Lactated Ringer's solution contains potassium and should not be administered to clients with renal failure.

VIII. COMPLICATIONS (TABLE 14-2)

A. Infection
1. Description
   a. Infection occurs from the entry of microorganisms into the body through the venipuncture site.
   b. Venipuncture interrupts the integrity of the skin, the first line of defense against infection.
   c. The longer the therapy continues, the greater the risk of infection.
   d. Infection can occur locally at the IV insertion site or systemically from the entry of microorganisms into the body.
2. At-risk clients
   a. Immunocompromised clients with diseases such as cancer or acquired immunodeficiency syndrome is at risk.
   b. Clients receiving treatments such as chemotherapy who have an altered or lowered white blood cell count are at risk.
   c. Older clients, because aging alters the effectiveness of the immune system, are at risk.
3. Prevention and interventions
   a. Assess client for predisposition to or risk for infection.
   b. Maintain strict asepsis when caring for the IV site.
   c. Monitor for signs of local infection, such as redness, swelling, and drainage at the IV site.
   d. Monitor for signs of systemic infection, such as chills, fever, malaise, headache, nausea, vomiting, backache, and tachycardia.
   e. Monitor white blood cell counts.
   f. Check fluid containers for cracks, leaks, cloudiness, or other evidence of contamination.
   g. Change tubing and site dressing every 24 to 72 hours according to agency policy.
   h. Use antimicrobial ointment at the IV site.

TABLE 14-2

Signs of Complications of Intravenous Therapy

Complication	Signs
Infection	Local: redness, swelling, and drainage at site
	Systemic: chills, fever, malaise, headache, nausea, vomiting, backache, tachycardia
Tissue damage	Skin color changes, sloughing of the skin, discomfort at site
Phlebitis	Heat, redness, tenderness at site
	Not swollen or hard
	Intravenous infusion sluggish
Thrombophlebitis	Hard and cordlike vein
	Heat, redness, tenderness at site
	Intravenous infusion sluggish
Infiltration	Edema, pain, and coolness at site
	May or may not have a blood return
Catheter embolism	Decrease in blood pressure
	Pain along vein
	Weak, rapid pulse
	Cyanosis of nail beds
	Loss of consciousness
Circulatory overload	Increased blood pressure
	Distended jugular veins
	Rapid breathing
	Dyspnea
	Moist cough and crackles
Electrolyte overload	Signs depend on the specific electrolyte imbalance
Hematoma	Ecchymosis, immediate swelling and leakage of blood at the site, and hard and painful lumps at the site
Air embolism	Tachycardia
	Dyspnea
	Hypotension
	Cyanosis
	Decreased level of consciousness

i. Label the IV site, bag or bottle, and tubing with the date and time to ensure that these are changed on time according to agency policy.

j. Ensure that the IV solution is not hanging for more than 24 hours.

k. If infection occurs, discontinue the IV, place a sterile cover on the venipuncture device for possible culture, and notify the physician.

l. Prepare to obtain blood cultures as prescribed if infection occurs.

m. Restart an IV in the opposite arm to differentiate sepsis (systemic infection) from local infection at the IV site.

n. Document the assessment of the finding related to infection.

B. Tissue damage
   1. Description
      a. Tissues most commonly damaged include the skin, veins, and the subcutaneous tissue.
      b. Tissue damage can be uncomfortable and can cause permanent negative effects.
   2. Prevention and interventions
      a. Use a careful and gentle approach when applying a tourniquet.
      b. Avoid tapping the skin over the vein when starting an IV.
      c. Monitor for ecchymosis when penetrating the skin with the cannula.
      d. Assess for any allergies to tape or dressing adhesives.
      e. Monitor for skin color changes, sloughing of the skin, or discomfort at the IV site.
      f. Notify the physician if tissue damage is suspected.
      g. Document the assessment of the tissue damage and its effects.

C. **Phlebitis** and thrombophlebitis
   1. Description
      a. **Phlebitis** is an inflammation of the vein that can occur from mechanical or chemical (medication) trauma or from a local infection.
      b. **Phlebitis** can cause the development of a clot (thrombophlebitis).
   2. Prevention and interventions
      a. Use an IV cannula smaller than the vein, and avoid using very small veins when administering irritating solutions.
      b. Avoid using the lower extremities as an access area for the IV.
      c. Avoid venipuncture over an area of flexion.
      d. Anchor the cannula and a loop of tubing securely with tape.
      e. Use an armboard or a splint as needed if the client is restless or active.
      f. Change the venipuncture site every 48 to 72 hours, depending on agency policy.
      g. If **phlebitis** occurs, remove the IV device immediately and restart it in the opposite extremity.
      h. Notify the physician if **phlebitis** is suspected, and apply warm, moist compresses as prescribed.
      i. If thrombophlebitis occurs, never irrigate the IV catheter; remove the IV, notify the physician, and restart the IV in the opposite extremity.
      j. Document the assessment of the **phlebitis** or thrombophlebitis and its effects.

D. **Infiltration**
   1. Description
      a. **Infiltration** is a form of tissue damage and also is called extravasation.
      b. **Infiltration** is seepage of the intravenous fluid out of the vein and into the surrounding interstitial spaces.
      c. **Infiltration** occurs when an access device has become dislodged or perforates the wall of the vein or when vein back pressure occurs because of a clot or venospasm.

2. Prevention and interventions
   a. Avoid venipuncture over an area of flexion.
   b. Anchor the cannula and a loop of tubing securely with tape.
   c. Use an armboard or a splint as needed if the client is restless or active.
   d. Assess the IV site for pain, edema, or coolness, comparing it with the opposite extremity.
   e. Monitor the IV rate for a decrease or a stop in flow.
   f. Evaluate the IV site for **infiltration** by occluding the vein proximal to the IV site; if the IV fluid continues to flow, the cannula is probably outside the vein (infiltrated); if the IV flow stops after occlusion of the vein, the IV device is still in the vein.
   g. Lower the IV fluid container below the IV site, and monitor for the appearance of blood in the IV tubing; if blood appears, the IV device is most likely in the vein.
   h. If **infiltration** has occurred, remove the IV device immediately.
   i. Do not rub an infiltrated area, which can cause the development of a hematoma.
   j. If **infiltration** has occurred, elevate the extremity and apply compresses (warm or cool, depending on the IV solution that was infusing and the physician's order) over the affected area.
   k. Document the assessment of the **infiltration**, its effects, and the action taken.

E. **Catheter embolism**
   1. Description: The tip of the catheter breaks off during IV insertion or removal, resulting in the possibility of an embolus.
   2. Prevention and interventions
      a. Monitor for signs of **catheter embolism**, including a decrease in blood pressure, pain along the vein, weak and rapid pulse, cyanosis of nail beds, and loss of consciousness.
      b. Remove the catheter carefully.
      c. Inspect the catheter when removed.
      d. If the catheter tip has broken off, place a tourniquet high on the limb of the IV site, notify the physician immediately, prepare to obtain an x-ray, and prepare the client for surgery to remove the catheter pieces if prescribed.

F. Circulatory overload
   1. Description
      a. Circulatory overload also is known as fluid overload.
      b. Circulatory overload results from the administration of fluids too rapidly or in a client at risk for fluid overload.
   2. Prevention and interventions
      a. Identify clients at risk for circulatory overload.
      b. Calculate and monitor the drip (flow) rate frequently.
      c. Use an infusion controller device, and frequently check the drip rate or pump setting, particularly in clients at risk for overload.
      d. Add a time strip to the IV bag or bottle.
      e. Monitor for signs of circulatory overload, including increased blood pressure, distended jugular veins, rapid breathing, dyspnea, moist cough, and crackles.
      f. If circulatory overload occurs, decrease the flow rate to a minimum at a keep vein open rate, elevate the head of the bed, keep the client warm, assess lung sounds and for edema, and notify the physician.
      g. Document the assessment and actions taken.

G. Electrolyte overload
   1. Description: An electrolyte imbalance is caused by too rapid or excessive infusion or by use of an inappropriate intravenous solution.
   2. Prevention and interventions
      a. Assess laboratory value reports.
      b. Verify the correct solution.
      c. Calculate and monitor the flow rate.
      d. Use an infusion controller device, and frequently check the flow rate or pump setting.
      e. Add a time strip to the IV bag or bottle.
      f. Place a medication sticker on the bag or bottle if a medication, such as potassium chloride, has been added to the IV solution.
      g. Monitor for signs of electrolyte imbalance, and notify the physician if they occur.

H. Hematoma
   1. Description: The collection of blood in the tissues after an unsuccessful venipuncture or after the venipuncture site is discontinued is a hematoma.
   2. Prevention and interventions
      a. When starting an IV, avoid piercing the posterior wall of the vein.
      b. Do not apply a tourniquet to the extremity immediately after an unsuccessful venipuncture.
      c. When discontinuing an IV, apply pressure to the site for at least 1 minute and elevate the extremity; apply pressure longer for clients with a bleeding disorder or who are taking anticoagulants.
      d. Monitor for ecchymosis, immediate swelling and leakage of blood at the site, and hard and painful lumps at the site.
      e. If a hematoma develops, elevate the extremity and apply pressure and ice as prescribed.

I. **Air embolism**
   1. Description: A bolus of air enters the vein through an inadequately primed IV line, from a loose connection, during tubing change, or during removal of the IV.
   2. Prevention and interventions
      a. Prime tubing with fluid before use, and monitor for any air bubbles in the tubing.
      b. Secure all connections

c. Replace the IV fluid before the bag or bottle is empty.

d. Monitor for signs of **air embolism**, including tachycardia, dyspnea, hypotension, cyanosis, and decreased level of consciousness; a loud churning sound heard over the pericardium that results from air in the right ventricle may be audible.

e. If **air embolism** is suspected, clamp the tubing, turn the client on the left side with the head of the bed lowered (Trendelenburg's position) to trap the air in the right atrium, and notify the physician.

IX. CENTRAL VENOUS CATHETERS (FIG. 14-6)

A. Description

1. Central venous catheters are used to deliver hyperosmolar solutions, to measure central venous pressure, or to infuse total parenteral nutrition or multiple IV infusions or medications.

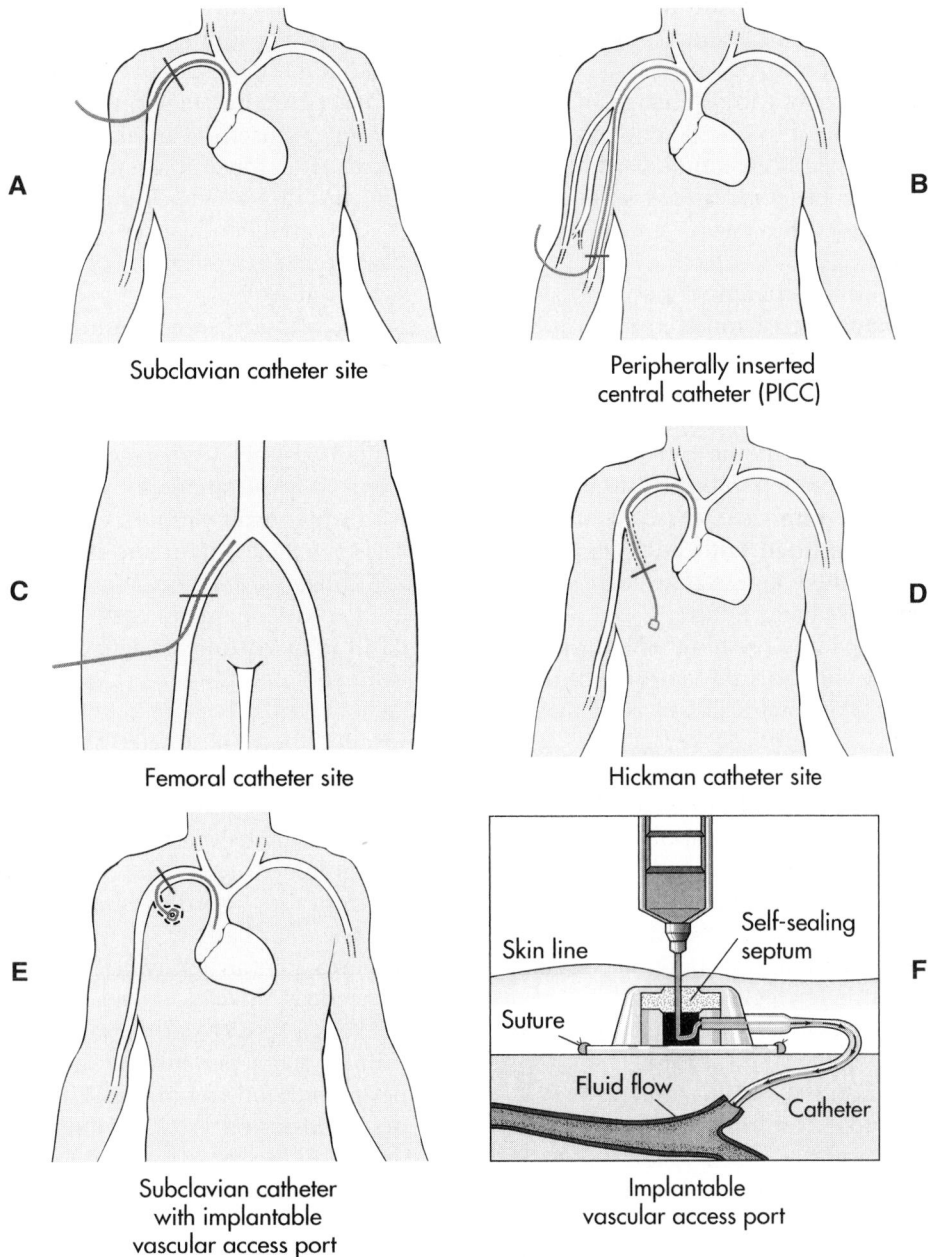

FIG. 14-6 Central venous access site(s). **A,** Subclavian catheter. **B,** Peripherally inserted central catheter. **C,** Femoral catheter. **D,** Hickman catheter. **E,** Subclavian catheter with implantable vascular access port. **F,** Implantable vascular access port. (From Kee, J. L., & Marshall, S. M. [2004]. *Clinical calculations: With applications to general and specialty areas* [5th ed]. Philadelphia: W. B. Saunders. **F** redrawn from Winters, B. [1984]. Implantable vascular access devices. *Oncology Nursing Forum, 11*[6], 25-30.)

▲ 2. Catheter position is determined by radiography after insertion.

3. The catheter may have a single, double, or triple lumen.

4. The catheter may be inserted peripherally and threaded through the basilic or cephalic vein into the superior vena cava, inserted centrally through the internal jugular or subclavian veins, or surgically tunneled through subcutaneous tissue into the cephalic vein.

5. With multilumen catheters, more than one medication can be administered at the same time without incompatibility problems, and only one insertion site requires care.

▲ 6. For central line insertion, tubing change, and line removal, place the client in Trendelenburg's position if not contraindicated, or supine position, and instruct the client to perform Valsalva's maneuver to increase pressure in the central veins when the IV system is open.

B. Tunneled central venous catheters

1. A more permanent type of catheter, such as the Hickman, Broviac, or Groshong catheter, is used for long-term IV therapy.

2. The catheter may be single lumen or multilumen.

3. The catheter is inserted in the operating room, and the catheter is threaded into the lower part of the vena cava at the entrance of the right atrium.

4. The catheter will be fitted with an intermittent infusion device to allow access as needed and to keep the system closed and intact.

▲ 5. Patency is maintained by flushing with a diluted heparin solution or normal saline solution depending on the type of catheter and as per agency policy.

C. Vascular access ports (implantable port)

1. Surgically implanted under the skin, ports such as a Port-a-Cath, Mediport, or Infusaport are used for long-term administration of repeated IV therapy.

▲ 2. For access, the port requires palpation and injection through the skin into the self-sealing port with a noncoring needle such as a Huber-point needle.

3. Patency is maintained by periodic flushing with a diluted heparin solution as prescribed and as per agency policy.

D. Peripherally inserted central catheter line

1. The catheter is used for long-term IV therapy, frequently in the home.

2. The basilic vein usually is used, but the median cubital and cephalic veins in the antecubital area also can be used.

3. The catheter is threaded so that the catheter tip may terminate in the subclavian vein or the superior vena cava.

4. A small amount of bleeding may occur at the time of insertion and may continue for 24 hours, but bleeding thereafter is not expected.

5. **Phlebitis** is a common complication.

6. Insertion is below the heart level; therefore **air embolism** is not common.

PRACTICE QUESTIONS

1. A nurse has an order to hang an IV bag of 1000 mL 5% dextrose in water with 20 mEq potassium chloride. The nurse should plan to do which of the following immediately after injecting the potassium chloride into the port of the intravenous (IV) bag?
   1. Attach the tubing to the client.
   2. Check the solution for yellowish discoloration.
   3. Rotate the bag gently.
   4. Place the time tape on the IV.

2. A nurse is inserting an intravenous line into a client's vein. After the initial stick the nurse continues to advance the catheter if the nurse notes that
   1. The catheter advances easily.
   2. Blood return shows in the backflash chamber of the catheter.
   3. The vein is distended under the needle.
   4. The client does not complain of discomfort.

3. A client is scheduled for insertion of a peripherally inserted central catheter (PICC). The nurse has explained the advantages of this catheter to the client. Which statement by the client indicates a need for further explanation?
   1. "There is less pain and discomfort."
   2. "This type of catheter is very reliable."
   3. "It is reasonable in cost."
   4. "It is specifically designed for short-term use."

4. A nurse is planning to provide a list of instructions to a client being discharged to home with a peripherally inserted central catheter (PICC). The nurse would avoid writing which of the following incorrect items on the instruction sheet?
   1. Keep activity level to a minimum while this catheter is in place.
   2. Keep the insertion site protected when in the shower or bath.
   3. Have a repair kit available in the home for use if needed.
   4. Wear a Medic-Alert tag or bracelet.

5. A nurse is assessing the IV dressing of a client with a peripheral intravenous infusion running. The date on the dressing is 7/25 (July 25). The nurse documents on the client's record that the dressing should be changed on which of the following dates?
   1. 7/26
   2. 7/28
   3. 7/30
   4. 8/1

6. A nurse is making initial rounds on the nursing unit to assess the condition of assigned clients. The nurse notes that a client's intravenous (IV) site is cool, pale, and swollen, and the solution is not infusing. The nurse

concludes that which of the following complications has been experienced by the client?
1. Thrombosis
2. Infection
3. Infiltration
4. Phlebitis

7. A client rings the call bell and complains of pain at the site of an intravenous (IV) infusion. A nurse assesses the site and determines that the client has developed phlebitis. The nurse avoids which action in the care of this client?
   1. Applies warm moist packs to the site.
   2. Starts a new IV line in a proximal portion of the same vein.
   3. Discontinues the IV catheter at that site.
   4. Notifies the physician.

8. A client had a 1000-mL bag of 5% dextrose in 0.9% sodium chloride hung at 15:00. A nurse making rounds at 15:45 finds the client to be complaining of a pounding headache and to be dyspneic, experiencing chills, apprehensive, and with an increased pulse rate. The intravenous (IV) bag has 400 mL remaining. The nurse should take which of the following actions first?
   1. Sit the client up in bed.
   2. Call the physician.
   3. Slow the IV infusion.
   4. Remove the IV catheter.

9. A nurse notes that the site of a client's peripheral intravenous (IV) catheter is reddened, warm, painful, and slightly edematous proximal to the insertion point of the IV catheter. After taking appropriate steps to care for the client, the nurse documents in the medical record that the client experienced
   1. Hypersensitivity to the IV solution.
   2. Allergic reaction to the IV catheter material.
   3. Infiltration of the IV line.
   4. Phlebitis of the vein.

10. A physician has written an order to discontinue an intravenous line. A nurse obtains which of the following supplies from the unit supply area for use in applying pressure to the site after removing the intravenous (IV) catheter?
    1. Adhesive bandage
    2. Sterile 2 × 2 gauze
    3. Alcohol swab
    4. Betadine swab

11. A client has just undergone insertion of a central venous catheter at the bedside. A nurse would be sure to check the results of which of the following before increasing the flow rate of the IV solution attached to the line from a keep vein open rate to 100 mL/hour?
    1. Serum electrolytes
    2. Serum osmolality
    3. Portable chest x-ray film
    4. Intake and output record

12. A nurse is preparing a continuous intravenous (IV) infusion at the medication cart. As the nurse goes to attach the distal end of the IV tubing to a needleless device, the tubing drops and hits the top of the medication cart. Which of the following is the appropriate action by the nurse?
    1. Wipe the distal end of the tubing with Betadine.
    2. Scrub the needleless device with an alcohol swab.
    3. Attach a new needleless device.
    4. Obtain new IV tubing.

13. A nurse is preparing to insert an intravenous (IV) angiocatheter into a client's inner forearm. Before cannulating the vein, the nurse cleanses the entry site by using which of the following motions?
    1. Scrubbing from the wrist toward the elbow
    2. Scrubbing from the elbow toward the wrist
    3. Using a circular motion from the center outward
    4. Using a circular motion inward toward the center

14. A client is hypovolemic, and plasma expanders are not available. A nurse anticipates that which of the following solutions available on the nursing unit will be prescribed by the physician?
    1. 5% dextrose in 0.45% sodium chloride
    2. 5% dextrose in water
    3. 0.9% sodium chloride
    4. 0.45% sodium chloride

15. A nurse hears an attending physician asking an intern to prescribe a hypotonic intravenous (IV) solution for a client. Which of the following IV solutions would the nurse expect the intern to prescribe?
    1. 0.45% saline (½ NS)
    2. 5% dextrose in water (D_5W)
    3. 10% dextrose in water ($D_{10}W$)
    4. 5% dextrose in 0.9% saline (D_5NS)

CRITICAL THINKING: FILL IN THE BLANK

A nurse is completing a time tape for a 1000-mL IV bag that is scheduled to infuse over 8 hours. The nurse has just placed the 11:00 AM marking at the 500-mL level. The nurse would place the mark for noon at which numerical level (mL) on the time tape?

Answer: _____

ANSWERS

1. 3

Rationale: After adding a medication to a bag of intravenous (IV) solution, the nurse should agitate or rotate the bag gently to mix the medication evenly in the solution. The nurse should then attach a completed medication label. The nurse then can place a time tape on the bag if this has not been done. The IV solution should have been checked for discoloration before the medication was added to the solution. The tubing is attached to the client last.

Test-Taking Strategy: Use the process of elimination. Note the key words "immediately after injecting." They imply a correct time sequence, and you need to prioritize. Visualize and think through the steps of adding medication to an IV bag, and make your choice accordingly. Review the procedure for adding potassium chloride to an IV bag if you had difficulty with this question.

Level of Cognitive Ability: Application
Client Needs: Physiological Integrity
Integrated Process: Nursing Process—implementation
Content Area: Pharmacology
Reference: Potter, P., & Perry, A. (2001). *Fundamentals of nursing* (5th ed., p. 953). St. Louis: Mosby.

2. 2

Rationale: The IV catheter has entered the lumen of the vein successfully when blood backflash shows in the IV catheter. The vein should have been distended by the tourniquet before the vein was cannulated. Client discomfort varies with the client, the site, and the nurse's insertion technique, and is not a reliable measure of catheter placement. The nurse should not advance the catheter until placement in the vein is verified by blood return.

Test-Taking Strategy: Use the process of elimination, focusing on the issue of the question: correct placement of an IV catheter. Noting the key words "blood return" in option 2 will direct you to this option. Review the steps for inserting an IV catheter if you had difficulty with this question.

Level of Cognitive Ability: Application
Client Needs: Physiological Integrity
Integrated Process: Nursing Process—implementation
Content Area: Fundamental skills
Reference: Potter, P., & Perry, A. (2001). *Fundamentals of nursing* (5th ed., p. 955). St. Louis: Mosby.

3. 4

*Rationale:*Peripherally inserted central catheters (PICCs) are intended to be used for clients needing long-term catheter placement. They are reasonable in cost because they do not need routine replacement, as do traditional peripheral IV catheters. The catheter is also reliable. The catheter is less likely to infiltrate and can be used for administration of a number of different types of medications.

Test-Taking Strategy: Use the process of elimination, noting the key words "need for further explanation." Noting the key words "short-term" in option 4 will assist in directing you to this option. Review the characteristics of a PICC if you had difficulty with this question.

Level of Cognitive Ability: Analysis
Client Needs: Physiological Integrity

Integrated Process: Teaching/Learning
Content Area: Fundamental skills
Reference: Phipps, W., Monahan, F., Sands, J., Marek, J., & Neighbors, M. (2003). *Medical-surgical nursing: Health and illness perspectives* (7th ed., p. 143). St. Louis: Mosby.

4. 1

Rationale: The client should be taught that only minor activity restrictions apply with this type of catheter. The client should protect the site during bathing and should carry or wear a Medic-Alert identification. The client should have a repair kit in the home for use as needed because the catheter is for long-term use.

Test-Taking Strategy: Use the process of elimination. Note the key word "avoid." Recalling that the PICC is for long-term use will assist in directing you to option 1. To keep activity to a minimum with such a catheter is unreasonable. Review home care instructions for a client with a PICC if you had difficulty with this question.

Level of Cognitive Ability: Application
Client Needs: Physiological Integrity
Integrated Process: Teaching/Learning
Content Area: Fundamental skills
Reference: Perry, A., & Potter, P. (2002). *Clinical nursing skills and techniques* (5th ed., p. 587). St. Louis: Mosby.

5. 2

Rationale: The IV site dressing should be changed every 48 to 72 hours, which is every 2 to 3 days. With an insertion date of 7/25, the due date for change, depending on agency policy, would be 7/27 or 7/28. It would be unnecessary, uncomfortable, and not cost-effective to change the site dressing daily (option 1). Changing the site dressing every 5 or 7 days (options 3 and 4) would place the client at higher risk for infection or other catheter complications.

Test-Taking Strategy: Use the process of elimination. Recalling that the IV site dressing should be changed every 48 to 72 hours will direct you to option 2. Review the standard accepted guidelines for intravenous site maintenance if you had difficulty with this question.

Level of Cognitive Ability: Application
Client Needs: Safe, Effective Care Environment
Integrated Process: Communication and Documentation
Content Area: Fundamental skills
Reference: Perry, A., & Potter, P. (2002). *Clinical nursing skills and techniques* (5th ed., p. 599). St. Louis: Mosby.

6. 3

Rationale: An infiltrated IV is one that has dislodged from the vein and is lying in subcutaneous tissue. Pallor, coolness, and swelling are the result of IV fluid being deposited in the subcutaneous tissue. When the pressure in the tissues exceeds the pressure in the tubing, the flow of the IV solution will stop. The corrective action is to remove the catheter and start a new IV line at another site. The other three options are likely to be accompanied by warmth at the site, not coolness.

Test-Taking Strategy: Use the process of elimination, focusing on the clinical manifestations identified in the question. Noting the key word "cool" in the question will direct you to

option 3. Review the signs of infiltration if you had difficulty with this question.
Level of Cognitive Ability: Analysis
Client Needs: Physiological Integrity
Integrated Process: Nursing Process—assessment
Content Area: Fundamental skills
Reference: Potter, P., & Perry, A. (2001). *Fundamentals of nursing* (5th ed. , p. 1233). St. Louis: Mosby.

7. **2**
Rationale: The nurse should discontinue the IV at the phlebitic site and apply warm moist compresses to the area to speed resolution of the inflammation. Because phlebitis has occurred, the nurse also notifies the physician about the IV complication. The nurse should restart the IV in a vein other than the one that has developed phlebitis.
Test-Taking Strategy: Use the process of elimination. Note the key word "avoid." This tells you that the correct option is an incorrect nursing action. Recalling that the nurse should restart the IV in a vein other than the one that has developed phlebitis will direct you to option 2. Review nursing interventions related to phlebitis if you had difficulty with this question.
Level of Cognitive Ability: Application
Client Needs: Physiological Integrity
Integrated Process: Nursing Process—implementation
Content Area: Fundamental skills
Reference: Potter, P., & Perry, A. (2001). *Fundamentals of nursing* (5th ed., p. 1235). St. Louis: Mosby.

8. **3**
Rationale: The client's symptoms are compatible with circulatory overload. This may be verified by noting that 600 mL has infused in the course of 45 minutes. The first action of the nurse is to slow the infusion. Other actions may follow in rapid sequence. The nurse may elevate the head of the bed to aid the client's breathing, if necessary. The nurse also notifies the physician immediately. The IV catheter does not need to be removed; it may be needed once the complication has been resolved.
Test-Taking Strategy: Use the process of elimination. Note the key word "first." This tells you that more than one or all of the options are likely to be correct actions, and the nurse needs to prioritize them according to a time sequence. You must be able to recognize the signs of circulatory overload. From this point, select the option that provides the intervention specific to circulatory overload. Review nursing actions related to this complication if you had difficulty with this question.
Level of Cognitive Ability: Application
Client Needs: Physiological Integrity
Integrated Process: Nursing Process—implementation
Content Area: Delegating/prioritizing
Reference: Potter, P., & Perry, A. (2001). *Fundamentals of nursing* (5th ed., p. 1245). St. Louis: Mosby.

9. **4**
Rationale: Phlebitis at an IV site can be distinguished by client discomfort at the site and by redness, warmth, and swelling proximal to the catheter. If phlebitis occurs, the nurse should discontinue the IV line and should insert a new IV line at a different site. Coolness at the site would be noted if the IV catheter was infiltrated. An allergic reaction produces a rash, redness, and itching. A major reaction, such as hypersensitivity, can cause dyspnea, a swollen tongue, and cyanosis.
Test-Taking Strategy: Use the process of elimination. Remember that options that are similar are not likely to be correct. In this situation, options 1 and 2 are similar and therefore are eliminated. Choose option 4 over option 3 after recalling the signs of common IV complications. Review the signs and symptoms of phlebitis if you had difficulty with this question.
Level of Cognitive Ability: Analysis
Client Needs: Physiological Integrity
Integrated Process: Communication and Documentation
Content Area: Fundamental skills
Reference: Potter, P., & Perry, A. (2001). *Fundamentals of nursing* (5th ed., p. 1235). St. Louis: Mosby.

10. **2**
Rationale: A dry sterile dressing such as a sterile 2 × 2 is used to apply pressure to the discontinued IV site. This material is absorbent, sterile, and nonirritating. A Betadine swab or an alcohol swab would irritate the opened puncture site and would not stop the blood flow. An adhesive bandage may be used to cover the site once hemostasis has occurred.
Test-Taking Strategy: Use the process of elimination. Note the key words "applying pressure." Visualize this procedure, thinking about each of the items identified in the options to direct you to option 2. Review this basic procedure if you had difficulty with this question.
Level of Cognitive Ability: Application
Client Needs: Physiological Integrity
Integrated Process: Nursing Process—implementation
Content Area: Fundamental skills
Reference: Potter, P., & Perry, A. (2001). *Fundamentals of nursing* (5th ed., p. 1240). St. Louis: Mosby.

11. **3**
Rationale: Before beginning administration of large volumes of IV solution, the nurse should assess whether the results of the chest radiograph reveal that the central catheter is in the proper place. This is necessary to prevent infusion of IV fluid into pulmonary or subcutaneous tissues. The other options represent items that are useful for the nurse to be aware of in the general care of this client, but they do not relate to this procedure.
Test-Taking Strategy: Use the process of elimination. Note the words "central venous catheter at the bedside." Recalling the potential complications associated with insertion of central venous catheters will direct you to option 3. Review the principles of care for a central venous catheter after insertion if you had difficulty with this question.
Level of Cognitive Ability: Application
Client Needs: Physiological Integrity
Integrated Process: Nursing Process—assessment
Content Area: Fundamental skills
References: Ignatavicius, D., & Workman, M. (2002). *Medical-surgical nursing: Critical thinking for collaborative care* (4th ed., p. 204). Philadelphia: W. B. Saunders.
Potter, P., & Perry, A. (2001). *Fundamentals of nursing* (5th ed., pp. 1370-1372). St. Louis: Mosby.

12. 4

Rationale: The nurse should obtain a new IV tubing because contamination has occurred and could cause systemic infection to the client. Wiping with Betadine is insufficient and would be contraindicated anyway because the tubing will be attached directly to an angiocatheter in the client's vein. The needleless device has not been contaminated and does not need replacement or cleansing.

Test-Taking Strategy: Use the process of elimination and knowledge of basic infection control measures and intravenous therapy concepts to answer this question. Clearly, only one option is correct. Remember that if an item is contaminated, discard it and obtain a new sterile item. Review aseptic technique if you had difficulty with this question.

Level of Cognitive Ability: Application

Client Needs: Safe, Effective Care Environment

Integrated Process: Nursing Process—implementation

Content Area: Fundamental skills

Reference: Perry, A., & Potter, P. (2002). *Clinical nursing skills and techniques* (5th ed., p. 601). St. Louis: Mosby.

13. 3

Rationale: The nurse cleans the skin by using a circular motion from inward to outward. This is the standard accepted aseptic technique to carry microorganisms away from the insertion site. The same technique is used to cleanse any area requiring surgical asepsis. Options 1, 2, and 4 are incorrect procedures.

Test-Taking Strategy: Use the process of elimination and basic principles of asepsis to answer the question. Knowledge of these principles allows you to choose correctly even without specific knowledge of IV insertion techniques. Review the basic principles of asepsis if you had difficulty with this question.

Level of Cognitive Ability: Application

Client Needs: Safe, Effective Care Environment

Integrated Process: Nursing Process—implementation

Content Area: Fundamental skills

Reference: Perry, A., & Potter, P. (2002). *Clinical nursing skills and techniques* (5th ed., p. 610). St. Louis: Mosby.

14. 1

Rationale: A solution of 5% dextrose in 0.45% sodium chloride is hypertonic. An advantage of hypertonic solutions is that they may be used to treat hypovolemia when plasma expanders are not readily available. Options 2 and 3 are isotonic solutions. Option 4 is a hypotonic solution.

Test-Taking Strategy: Use the process of elimination. Noting the key word "hypovolemic" will assist in directing you to option 1 if you are familiar with the IV solutions that are

hypertonic. If this question was difficult, review the nature and purposes of hypertonic, isotonic, and hypotonic IV solutions.

Level of Cognitive Ability: Analysis

Client Needs: Physiological Integrity

Integrated Process: Nursing Process—analysis

Content Area: Fundamental skills

Reference: Ignatavicius, D., & Workman, M. (2002). *Medical-surgical nursing: Critical thinking for collaborative care* (4th ed., pp. 140-143, 1226). Philadelphia: W. B. Saunders.

15. 1

Rationale: Hypotonic solutions contain a lower concentration of salt or more water than an isotonic solution. A solution of 0.45% saline (½ NS) is hypotonic. A solution of 5% dextrose in water (D_5W) is isotonic. Solutions of 10% dextrose in water ($D_{10}W$) and 5% dextrose in 0.9% saline (D_5NS) are hypertonic solutions. Distilled water is another example of a hypotonic solution.

Test-Taking Strategy: Use the process of elimination. Note the similarities in options 2, 3, and 4. All of these solutions contain dextrose. Option 1 is different from the other options. If you had difficulty with this question, review the tonicity of the various IV solutions.

Level of Cognitive Ability: Analysis

Client Needs: Physiological Integrity

Integrated Process: Nursing Process—planning

Content Area: Fundamental skills

Reference: Ignatavicius, D., & Workman, M. (2002). *Medical-surgical nursing: Critical thinking for collaborative care* (4th ed., pp. 140-143). Philadelphia: W. B. Saunders.

CRITICAL THINKING: FILL IN THE BLANK

Answer: 375 mL

Rationale: If the IV is scheduled to run over 8 hours, then the hourly rate is 125 mL per hour. Using 500 mL as the reference point, the next hourly marking would be at 375 mL, which is 125 mL less than 500.

Test-Taking Strategy: Use basic principles related to pharmacology math and IV administration to answer this question. If this question was difficult, review the concepts related to marking an IV solution by using a time tape.

Level of Cognitive Ability: Application

Client Needs: Physiological Integrity

Integrated Process: Nursing Process—implementation

Content Area: Fundamental skills

Reference: Perry, A., & Potter, P. (2002). *Clinical nursing skills and techniques* (5th ed., p. 590). St. Louis: Mosby.

REFERENCES

Ignatavicius, D., & Workman, M. (2002). *Medical-surgical nursing: Critical thinking for collaborative care* (4th ed.). Philadelphia: W. B. Saunders.

National Council of State Boards of Nursing (Eds.). (2003). *Test Plan for the National Council Licensure Examination for Registered Nurses* (effective date: April 2004). Chicago: Author.

Perry, A., & Potter, P. (2002). *Clinical nursing skills and techniques* (5th ed.). St. Louis: Mosby.

Phipps, W., Monahan, F., Sands, J., Marek, J., & Neighbors, M. (2003). *Medical-surgical nursing: health and illness perspectives* (7th ed.). Louis: Mosby.

Potter, P., & Perry, A. (2001). *Fundamentals of nursing* (5th ed.). St. Louis: Mosby.

Administration of Blood Products

PYRAMID TERMS

ABO   A type of antigen system. The ABO type of the donor should be compatible with the recipient's. Type A can match with types A or O; type B can match with types B or O; type O can match only with type O; type AB can match with A, B, or O.

autologous donation   A donation of the client's own blood before a scheduled procedure.

blood salvage   An autologous donation that involves suctioning blood from body cavities, joint spaces, or other closed body sites during a procedure.

circulatory overload   A complication resulting from the infusion of blood at a rate too rapid for the size, cardiac status, or clinical condition of the recipient.

compatibility   Matching of blood from two persons by two different types of antigen systems, ABO and Rh, present on the membrane surface of the red blood cells, so as to prevent a transfusion reaction.

crossmatching   The testing of the donor's blood and the recipient's blood for compatibility.

designated donor   A compatible donor who has been selected by the recipient.

fresh frozen plasma   A blood product administered to increase the level of clotting factors in clients with such a deficiency.

iron overload   A delayed transfusion complication that occurs in clients who are chronically dependent on blood transfusions, such as clients with anemia or thrombocytopenia.

platelets   A blood product administered to clients with low platelet counts and to thrombocytopenic clients who are bleeding actively or are scheduled for an invasive procedure.

red blood cells   A blood product used to replace erythrocytes lost as a result of trauma or surgical interventions or in clients with bone marrow suppression.

Rh factor   A person having the factor is Rh positive; a person lacking the factor is Rh negative.

septicemia   The presence of infective agents or their toxins in the bloodstream. Septicemia is a serious infection and must be treated promptly; otherwise, the infection leads to circulatory collapse, profound shock, and death.

transfusion reaction   A hemolytic reaction caused by blood type or Rh incompatibility. An allergic transfusion reaction most often occurs in clients with a history of allergy. A febrile transfusion reaction most commonly occurs in clients with antibodies directed against the transfused white blood cells. A bacterial transfusion reaction occurs after transfusion of contaminated blood products.

whole blood   Whole blood is composed of red blood cells, plasma, and plasma proteins and is administered primarily to treat hypovolemic shock resulting from hemorrhage.

THE PYRAMID TO SUCCESS

Pyramid Points focus on the safe administration of blood components, managing and providing care related to the procedure for administering blood components, and monitoring for complications. Focus is on the safe procedure for administering blood and on the signs and symptoms of transfusion reaction. Pyramid Points also focus on the immediate interventions if a transfusion reaction occurs, and evaluation and documentation of expected and unexpected effects of the therapy. Integrated Processes addressed in this chapter are Nursing Process, Caring, Communication and Documentation, and Teaching/Learning.

CLIENT NEEDS
Safe, Effective Care Environment

Client rights
Continuity of care and close supervision during transfusion
Establishment of priorities
Ethical practice and legal responsibilities
Handling of hazardous and infectious materials

Informed consent for the administration of blood products

Medical and surgical asepsis

Standard, transmission-based, and other precautions

Health Promotion and Maintenance

Client education about the signs of a transfusion reaction

Lifestyle choices related to receiving a blood transfusion

Psychosocial Integrity

Religious, spiritual, and cultural considerations related to blood administration

Therapeutic interactions with the client regarding the procedure for blood administration

Physiological Integrity

Documentation of the client's response to receiving the blood product

Management of medical emergencies if a transfusion reaction or other complication occurs

Monitoring for complications related to blood administration

Monitoring of laboratory values

Monitoring for expected effects

Safe administration of blood and blood products

Venous access devices for blood administration

I. TYPES OF BLOOD COMPONENTS

A. **Red blood cells**
   1. **Red blood cells** are a blood product used to replace erythrocytes.
   2. Packed **red blood cells** usually are supplied in 250-mL unit bags; however, they can be supplied in other amounts, such as 250- to 350- or 350- to 400-mL bags. Always check the unit for the volume of the blood component.
   3. Each unit increases the hemoglobin by 1 g/dL and hematocrit by 2% to 3%; the change in laboratory values takes 4 to 6 hours after completion of the blood transfusion.
   4. Evaluation of an effective response is based on the resolution of the symptoms of anemia and an increase in the erythrocyte count.
B. **Whole blood**
   1. **Whole blood** rarely is used; treatment with a specific blood component usually is prescribed.
   2. **Whole blood** is used to resolve hypovolemic shock resulting from hemorrhage.
   3. **Whole blood** contains **red blood cells**, plasma, and plasma proteins, and each unit normally contains 500 mL. Always check the bag for the volume of the blood component.

4. Evaluation of an effective response is based on the resolution of the symptoms of hypovolemia.
C. Platelets
   1. **Platelets** are used to treat thrombocytopenia and platelet dysfunctions.
   2. **Crossmatching** is not required but usually is done (platelet concentrates contain few **red blood cells**).
   3. The volume in a unit of **platelets** may vary from 50 to 70 mL per unit to 200 to 400 mL per unit. Always check the bag for the volume of the blood component.
   4. **Platelets** are administered immediately on receipt from the blood bank and are given rapidly, usually over 15 to 30 minutes.
   5. Evaluation of an effective response is based on improvement in the platelet count, and platelet counts normally are evaluated 1 hour and 18 to 24 hours after the transfusion.
D. **Fresh frozen plasma**
   1. **Fresh frozen plasma** may be used to provide clotting factors or volume expansion; it contains no platelets.
   2. **Fresh frozen plasma** is infused within 6 hours of thawing, while clotting factors are still viable, and is infused as rapidly as possible.
   3. **Rh compatibility** and **ABO** compatibility are required for the transfusion of plasma products.
   4. A unit usually contains 200 to 250 mL. Always check the bag for the volume of the blood component.
   5. Evaluation of an effective response is assessed by monitoring coagulation studies, particularly the prothrombin time and the partial thromboplastin time, and resolution of hypovolemia.
E. Albumin
   1. Albumin is prepared from plasma and can be stored for 5 years.
   2. Albumin is used to treat hypovolemic shock or hypoalbuminemia.
   3. Albumin 25g/100 mL is equal to 500 mL of plasma.
F. Cryoprecipitates
   1. Cryoprecipitates are prepared from **fresh frozen plasma** and can be stored for 1 year; once thawed, the product must be used.
   2. Cryoprecipitates are used to replace clotting factors, especially factor VIII and fibrinogen.

II. TYPES OF BLOOD DONATIONS

A. Autologous
   1. A donation of the client's own blood before a scheduled procedure is autologous; it reduces the risk of disease transmission and potential transfusion complications.
   2. **Autologous donation** is not an option for a client with leukemia or bacteremia.
   3. A donation can be made every 3 days as long as the hemoglobin remains within a safe range.

4. Donations should begin within 5 weeks of the transfusion date and end at least 3 days before the date of transfusion.

B. **Blood salvage**
   1. **Blood salvage** is an **autologous donation** that involves suctioning blood from body cavities, joint spaces, or other closed body sites.
   2. Blood may need to be "washed," a special process that removes tissue debris before reinfusion.

C. **Designated donor**
   1. Designated donation occurs when recipients select their own compatible donors.
   2. Donation does not reduce the risk of contracting infections transmitted by the blood; however, recipients feel more comfortable identifying their donors.

III. COMPATIBILITY

A. Client blood samples are drawn and labeled at the bedside when drawn; the client is asked to state his or her name, which is compared with the name on the client's identification band or bracelet.

B. The recipient's **ABO** type and **Rh** type are identified.

C. An antibody screen is done to determine the presence of antibodies other than anti-A and anti-B.

D. **Crossmatching** is done, in which donor **red blood cells** are combined with recipient's serum and Coombs' serum; crossmatch is compatible if no red blood cell agglutination occurs.

E. The universal red blood cell donor is O negative; the universal recipient is AB positive.

IV. INFUSION CONTROLLERS AND PUMPS

A. Infusion controllers and pumps may be used to administer blood products if they are designed to function with opaque solutions; however, the negative pressure exerted by the cassette of the machine can cause hemolysis of **red blood cells**.

B. Always consult manufacturer guidelines for the controller or pump.

C. Special manual pressure cuffs may be used to increase the flow rate but should not exceed 300 mm Hg.

D. Standard sphygmomanometer cuffs are not to be used to increase the flow rate because they do not exert uniform pressure against all parts of the bag.

V. BLOOD WARMERS

A. Blood warmers may be used to prevent hypothermia and adverse reactions when several units of blood are being administered.

B. Special warmers have been designed for this purpose, and only devices specifically tested and approved for this use can be used.

C. Do not warm blood products in a microwave or in hot water.

VI. PRECAUTIONS AND NURSING RESPONSIBILITIES (BOX 15-1)

VII. COMPLICATIONS (BOX 15-2)

A. Transfusion reactions
   1. Signs of an immediate **transfusion reaction**
      a. Chills and diaphoresis

BOX 15-1

Precautions and Nursing Responsibilities

GENERAL PRECAUTIONS

A large volume of refrigerated blood infused rapidly through a central catheter into the ventricle of the heart can cause cardiac dysrhythmias.

No solution other than normal saline should be added to blood components.

Medications are never added to blood components or piggybacked into a blood transfusion.

To avoid the risk of septicemia, infusions (1 unit) should not exceed 4 hours.

The blood administration set should be changed every 4 to 6 hours or according to institution policy to reduce the risk of septicemia.

Always check the blood bag for the date of expiration; components expire at midnight on the day marked on the bag unless otherwise specified.

Inspect the blood bag for leaks, abnormal color, clots, and bubbles.

Blood must be administered as soon as possible (within 20 to 30 minutes) from its being received at the blood bank, as this is the maximal allowable time out of monitored storage.

Never refrigerate blood in refrigerators other than those used in blood banks; if the blood is not administered within 20 to 30 minutes, return it to blood bank.

The recommended rate of infusion varies with the blood component being transfused and depends on the client's condition; generally, blood is infused as quickly as the client's condition allows.

Components containing few red blood cells and platelets may be infused rapidly, but caution should be taken to avoid circulatory overload.

The nurse should measure vital signs and assess lung sounds before the transfusion and again after the first 15 minutes and every hour until 1 hour after the transfusion is completed.

BLOOD BANK PRECAUTIONS

Blood will be released from the blood bank only to personnel as specified by agency policy.

The name and identification number of the intended recipient must be provided to the blood bank, and a documented permanent record of this information must be maintained.

Continued

BOX 15-1

Precautions and Nursing Responsibilities—cont'd

Blood should be transported from the blood bank to only one client at a time to prevent blood delivery to the wrong client.

CLIENT IDENTITY AND COMPATIBILITY

The most critical phase of the transfusion is confirming product compatibility and verifying client identity.

Two registered nurses need to check the physician's order, the client's identity, and the client's identification band or bracelet and number, verifying that the name and number are identical to those on the blood component tag.

At the bedside, the nurse asks the client to state his or her name, and the nurse compares the name with the name on the identification band or bracelet.

The nurse checks the blood bag tag, label, and blood requisition form to ensure that ABO and Rh types are compatible.

If the nurse notes any inconsistencies when verifying client identity and compatibility, the nurse notifies the blood bank immediately.

CLIENT ASSESSMENT

Assess for any cultural or religious beliefs regarding blood transfusions.

A Jehovah Witness cannot receive blood or blood products; this group believes that blood transfusions have eternal consequences.

Ensure that an informed consent has been obtained.

Determine whether the client has ever experienced any previous reactions to blood transfusions.

Check the client's vital signs; assess renal, circulatory, and respiratory status and the client's ability to tolerate intravenously administered fluids.

If the client's temperature is elevated, notify the physician before beginning the transfusion; a fever may be a cause for delaying the transfusion in addition to masking a possible symptom of an acute transfusion reaction.

ADMINISTRATION OF THE TRANSFUSION

Maintain standard, transmission-based, and other precautions as necessary.

Insert an intravenous (IV) line and infuse normal saline; maintain the infusion at a keep vein open rate.

An 18- or 19-gauge IV needle will be needed to achieve a maximum flow rate of blood products and prevent damage to red blood cells; if a smaller-gauge needle must be used, red blood cells may be diluted with normal saline.

A central catheter is an acceptable venous access option for blood transfusions.

Always check the bag for the volume of the blood component.

Blood products should be infused through administration sets designed specifically for blood; use a Y tubing or straight tubing blood administration set that contains a filter designed to trap fibrin clots and other debris that accumulate during blood storage.

Premedicate the client with acetaminophen (Tylenol) or diphenhydramine (Benadryl) as prescribed if the client has a history of adverse reactions; if prescribed, oral medications should be administered 30 minutes before the transfusion is started, and intravenously administered medications may be given immediately before the transfusion is started.

Instruct the client to report anything unusual immediately.

Determine the rate of infusion by physician order or, if not specified, by agency policy.

Begin the transfusion slowly under close supervision; if no reaction is noted within the first 15 minutes, the flow can be increased to the prescribed rate.

During the transfusion, monitor the client for signs and symptoms of a transfusion reaction; the first 15 minutes of the transfusion are the most critical, and the nurse must stay with client.

If a major ABO incompatibility exists or a severe allergic reaction occurs, the reaction is usually evident within the first 50 mL of the transfusion.

Document the client's tolerance to the administration of the blood product.

Monitor appropriate laboratory values and document effectiveness of treatment related to the specific type of blood product.

REACTIONS TO THE TRANSFUSION

If a transfusion reaction occurs, stop the transfusion, change the IV tubing down to the IV site, keep the IV line open with normal saline, notify the physician and blood bank, and return the blood bag and tubing to the blood bank.

Do not leave the client alone, and monitor the client for any life-threatening symptoms.

Obtain appropriate laboratory samples according to agency policies, such as blood and urine samples (free hemoglobin indicates that red blood cells were hemolyzed).

b. Muscle aches, back pain, or chest pain
c. Rashes, hives, itching, and swelling
d. Rapid, thready pulse
e. Dyspnea, cough, wheezing, or rales
f. Pallor and cyanosis
g. Apprehension
h. Tingling and numbness

i. Headache
j. Nausea, vomiting, abdominal cramping, and diarrhea
2. Signs of **transfusion reaction** in an unconscious client
   a. Weak pulse
   b. Fever

BOX 15-2

Complications of a Blood Transfusion

Transfusion reactions
Circulatory overload
Septicemia
Iron overload
Disease transmission
Hypocalcemia and citrate intoxication
Hyperkalemia

c. Tachycardia or bradycardia
d. Hypotension
e. Visible hemoglobinuria
f. Oliguria or anuria
3. Delayed transfusion reactions
   a. Reactions can occur days to years after a transfusion.
   b. Signs include fever, mild jaundice, and a decreased hematocrit level.
4. Interventions
   a. Stop the transfusion.
   b. Keep the intravenous line open with 0.9% normal saline.
   c. Notify the physician and blood bank.
   d. Remain with the client, observing signs and symptoms and monitoring vital signs as often as every 5 minutes.
   e. Prepare to administer emergency medications such as antihistamines, vasopressors, fluids, and corticosteroids as prescribed.
   f. Obtain a urine specimen for laboratory studies.
   g. Return blood bag, tubing, attached labels, and transfusion record to the blood bank.

B. **Circulatory overload**
1. Description: **Circulatory overload** is caused by infusion of blood at a rate too rapid for the client to tolerate.
2. Assessment
   a. Cough, dyspnea, chest pain, and rales on auscultation of the lungs
   b. Headache
   c. Hypertension
   d. Tachycardia and a bounding pulse
   e. Distended neck veins
3. Interventions
   a. Slow the rate of infusion.
   b. Place the client in an upright position, with the feet in a dependent position.
   c. Notify the physician.
   d. Administer oxygen, diuretics, and morphine sulfate as prescribed.
   e. Monitor for dysrhythmias.
   f. Phlebotomy also may be a method of prescribed treatment in a severe case.

C. **Septicemia**
1. Description: **Septicemia** occurs with the transfusion of blood that is contaminated with microorganisms.
2. Assessment
   a. Rapid onset of chills and a high fever
   b. Vomiting
   c. Diarrhea
   d. Hypotension
   e. Shock
3. Interventions
   a. Notify the physician.
   b. Obtain blood cultures and cultures of the blood bag.
   c. Administer oxygen, intravenous fluids, antibiotics, vasopressors, and corticosteroids as ordered.

D. **Iron overload**
1. Description: **Iron overload** is a delayed transfusion complication that occurs in clients who are chronically dependent on blood transfusions, such as clients with anemia or thrombocytopenia.
2. Assessment
   a. Vomiting
   b. Diarrhea
   c. Hypotension
   d. Altered hematological values
3. Interventions
   a. Deferoxamine (Desferal), administered intravenously or subcutaneously, removes accumulated iron via the kidneys.
   b. Urine turns red as iron is excreted after administration of deferoxamine; treatment is discontinued when serum iron levels return to normal.

E. Disease transmission
1. A disease commonly transmitted is hepatitis C, which is manifested by anorexia, nausea, vomiting, dark urine, and jaundice; the symptoms usually occur within 4 to 6 weeks after the transfusion.
2. Other infectious agents transmitted by blood transfusion include hepatitis B virus, human immunodeficiency virus, human herpesvirus type 6, Epstein-Barr virus, human T-cell leukemia, cytomegalovirus, and malaria.
3. Donor screening has greatly reduced the risk of transmission of infectious agents; additionally, antibody testing of donors for human immunodeficiency virus has greatly reduced the risk of transmission.

F. Hypocalcemia
1. Citrate in transfused blood binds with calcium and is excreted.
2. Assess serum calcium before and after transfusion.
3. Monitor for signs of hypocalcemia.
4. Slow the transfusion and notify the physician if signs of hypocalcemia occur.

G. Hyperkalemia
   1. Stored blood liberates potassium through hemolysis.
   2. The older the blood, the greater the risk of hyperkalemia; therefore clients at risk for hyperkalemia, such as those with renal insufficiency or renal failure, should receive fresh blood.
   3. Assess the date on the blood and the serum potassium level before and after the transfusion.
   4. Monitor the potassium level and for signs of hyperkalemia.
   5. Slow the transfusion and notify the physician if signs of hyperkalemia occur.

PRACTICE QUESTIONS

1. A nurse has just obtained a unit of blood from the blood bank to transfuse into a client as ordered. Before preparing the blood for transfusion, the nurse next looks for which of the following members of the health care team to assist in checking the unit of blood?
   1. Blood bank technician
   2. Registered nurse
   3. Medical student
   4. Phlebotomist

2. A nurse has obtained a unit of blood from the blood bank and has checked the blood bag properly with another nurse. Just before beginning the transfusion, the nurse assesses which of the following items?
   1. Vital signs
   2. Latest hematocrit level
   3. Skin color
   4. Urine output

3. A nurse has just received an order to transfuse a unit of packed red blood cells for an assigned client. In planning coverage for the client assignment, the nurse asks if another nurse will be available to check on the other assigned clients for how long when the unit of blood is hung?
   1. 5 minutes
   2. 15 minutes
   3. 30 minutes
   4. 45 minutes

4. A client has an order to receive a unit of packed red blood cells. A nurse would obtain which of the following intravenous (IV) solutions from the IV storage area to hang with the blood product at the client's bedside?
   1. 0.9% sodium chloride
   2. Lactated Ringer's
   3. 5% dextrose in 0.9% sodium chloride
   4. 5% dextrose in 0.45% sodium chloride

5. A nurse is assigned to care for a client who was just admitted to the hospital for the treatment of iron overload. The nurse reviews the physician's admission orders and anticipates that the physician will prescribe which medication to treat the iron overload?
   1. Granisetron (Kytril)
   2. Deferoxamine (Desferal)
   3. Ketoconazole (Nizoral)
   4. Terbinafine (Lamisil)

6. A client with severe blood loss resulting from multiple trauma requires rapid transfusion of several units of blood. A nurse asks another health team member to obtain which of the following devices for use during the transfusion procedure to help reduce the risk of cardiac dysrhythmias?
   1. Cardiac monitor
   2. Pulse oximetry
   3. Blood warming device
   4. Infusion controller

7. A nurse enters a client's room to assess the client, who began receiving a blood transfusion 45 minutes earlier. The client is flushed and dyspneic. On assessment the nurse auscultates the presence of crackles in the lung bases. The nurse determines that this client most likely is experiencing which of the following complications of blood transfusion therapy?
   1. Hypovolemia
   2. Transfusion reaction
   3. Fluid overload
   4. Bacteremia

8. A nurse determines that a client is having a transfusion reaction. As the nurse is stopping the unit of packed red blood cells that currently is infusing, the nurse plans to take which of the following actions next?
   1. Run normal saline at a keep vein open rate.
   2. Change the solution to 5% dextrose in water.
   3. Remove the IV line.
   4. Obtain a culture of the tip of the catheter device removed from the client.

9. A nurse has discontinued a unit of blood that was infusing into a client because the client has experienced a transfusion reaction. After documenting the incident appropriately, the nurse sends the blood bag to which of the following most appropriate areas?
   1. Infection Control Department
   2. Blood Bank
   3. Risk Management
   4. Environmental Services

10. A nurse has just received a unit of packed red blood cells from the blood bank for transfusion to an assigned client. The nurse is careful to select tubing especially made for blood products, knowing that this tubing is manufactured with
    1. A microdrip chamber.
    2. Tinted tubing to protect the blood from light.
    3. An air vent.
    4. An in-line filter.

11. Packed red blood cells have been prescribed for a client with a low hemoglobin and hematocrit.

A nurse measuring a client's temperature before hanging a blood transfusion finds it to be 100.6° F orally. The nurse does which of the following as the most appropriate nursing action?
1. Administer an antihistamine and begin the transfusion.
2. Administer two tablets of acetaminophen (Tylenol) and begin the transfusion.
3. Begin the transfusion as prescribed.
4. Delay hanging the blood and notify the physician.

12. A nurse has received an order to transfuse a client with a unit of packed red blood cells. Before explaining the procedure to the client, the nurse asks which initial question?
1. "Why do you think that you need the transfusion?"
2. "Do you know the complications and risks of a transfusion?"
3. "Have you ever had a transfusion before?"
4. "Have you ever gone into shock for any reason in the past?"

13. A nurse is signing for a unit of packed blood cells at the hospital blood bank. After putting the pen down, the nurse glances at the clock, which reads 1:00. The nurse calculates that the transfusion must be started by
1. 1:30.
2. 2:00.
3. 2:30.
4. 3:00.

14. A client has received a transfusion of platelets. The nurse evaluates that the client is benefiting most from this therapy if the client exhibits which of the following?
1. Decline of temperature to normal
2. Decreased oozing of blood from puncture sites and gums
3. Increased hemoglobin level
4. Increased hematocrit level

15. A nurse listening to morning report learns that an assigned client received a unit of granulocytes the previous evening. The nurse makes a note to assess the results of which of the following daily serum laboratory studies to assess the effectiveness of the transfusion?
1. White blood cell count
2. Erythrocyte count
3. Hemoglobin level
4. Hematocrit level

16. A client ordered to receive a transfusion has experienced a rash with pruritus during previous transfusions. The client asks the nurse whether it is safe to receive the transfusion. In formulating a response, the nurse incorporates the understanding that which of the following medications most likely will be ordered before the transfusion is begun?
1. Diphenhydramine (Benadryl)
2. Acetylsalicylic acid (ASA, aspirin)

3. Acetaminophen (Tylenol)
4. Ibuprofen (Motrin)

17. A nurse who is about to begin a blood transfusion knows that blood cells start to deteriorate after a certain period of time. The nurse checks which of the following items carefully before beginning the transfusion to ensure that this has not happened?
1. Blood identification number
2. Expiration date
3. Blood group and type
4. Presence of clots

18. A nurse overhears a physician stating that a client who is in hypovolemic shock requires plasma expansion. The nurse anticipates receiving an order to transfuse which of the following blood products to this client?
1. Cryoprecipitate
2. Packed red blood cells
3. Albumin
4. Platelets

19. A physician tells a client that the client needs a blood transfusion and that a blood sample must be drawn first for blood typing and crossmatching. After the physician leaves, the client asks the nurse, "What exactly is a blood type, anyway?" The nurse incorporates which of the following statements into a response?
1. "The blood type represents an antibody that normally circulates in the blood plasma."
2. "The blood type represents an antigen that normally circulates in the blood plasma."
3. "The blood type represents an antigen found on the surface of the red blood cells."
4. "The blood type represents an antibody found on the surface of the red blood cells."

20. A client requiring upcoming surgery is anxious about the possible need for blood transfusion during or after surgery. The nurse advises the client to do which of the following as the most effective way to eliminate the risk of cross-infection?
1. Take iron supplements before surgery to boost hemoglobin levels.
2. Request that any donated blood be screened twice by the blood bank.
3. Ask a friend or family member to donate blood ahead of time.
4. Give an autologous blood donation before the surgery.

CRITICAL THINKING: PRIORITIZING (ORDERED RESPONSE)

A unit of packed red blood cells has been prescribed for a client with low hemoglobin and hematocrit levels. The nurse notifies the blood bank of the order, and a blood specimen is drawn from the client for typing and crossmatching. The nurse receives a telephone call from the blood bank and is informed that the unit of blood is ready for administration. Number the actions in priority that the nurse would take to administer the blood. (Number 1 is the first priority.)

___ Verify the physician's order for the blood transfusion.

___ Ask a licensed nurse to assist in confirming blood compatibility and verifying client identity.

___ Ensure that an informed consent has been signed.

___ Insert an 18- or 19- gauge IV catheter into the client.

___ Obtain the unit of blood from the blood bank.

ANSWERS

1. 2

Rationale: Two registered nurses (RNs) or one RN and a licensed practical nurse (depending on agency policy) must check the label on the blood product together against the client's identification number, blood group, and complete name. This minimizes the risk of error in checking information on the blood bag and thereby minimizes the risk of harm or injury to the client. A blood bank technician will verify data with the nurse when the blood is obtained from the blood bank but will not verify information on the nursing unit or at the client's bedside. The other options are also incorrect.

Test-Taking Strategy: Use the process of elimination and specific knowledge of blood administration methods and techniques. Remember that two RNs or one RN and a licensed practical nurse (depending on agency policy) must check the blood product together. Review the procedures related to checking blood before administration if you had difficulty with this question.
Level of Cognitive Ability: Application
Client Needs: Physiological Integrity
Integrated Process: Nursing Process—planning
Content Area: Fundamental skills
Reference: Potter, P., & Perry, A. (2001). *Fundamentals of nursing* (5th ed., p. 1243). St. Louis: Mosby.

2. 1

Rationale: A change in vital signs during the transfusion may indicate that a transfusion reaction is occurring. This is why the nurse assesses vital signs before the procedure, every 15 minutes for the first half hour, and every half hour thereafter. The other options do not identify assessments that are required just before beginning a transfusion.

Test-Taking Strategy: Use the process of elimination. Note the key words "just before beginning the transfusion." This tells you that more than one of the options may be partially or totally correct and that the correct option needs to be assessed for possible comparison during the transfusion. Use the ABCs—airway, breathing, and circulation—to direct you to option 1. Review the nursing interventions for preparing to administer a blood transfusion if you had difficulty with this question.
Level of Cognitive Ability: Application
Client Needs: Physiological Integrity
Integrated Process: Nursing Process—assessment
Content Area: Fundamental skills
Reference: Potter, P., & Perry, A. (2001). *Fundamentals of nursing* (5th ed., pp. 1242-1243). St. Louis: Mosby.

3. 2

Rationale: The nurse must remain with the client for the first 15 minutes of a transfusion, which is the most frequent period during which a transfusion reaction may occur. This enables the nurse to detect a reaction and intervene quickly. The nurse engages in safe nursing practice by obtaining coverage for the other assigned clients during this time. Options 1, 3, and 4 are incorrect.

Test-Taking Strategy: Use the process of elimination and knowledge regarding blood transfusion procedures to answer this question. Remember, the client must be monitored directly for the first 15 minutes of the transfusion. Review the nursing responsibilities involved in beginning a blood transfusion if you had difficulty with this question.
Level of Cognitive Ability: Application
Client Needs: Physiological Integrity
Integrated Process: Nursing Process—planning
Content Area: Fundamental skills
Reference: Potter, P., & Perry, A. (2001). *Fundamentals of nursing* (5th ed., p.1243). St. Louis: Mosby.

4. 1

Rationale: Sodium chloride 0.9% (normal saline) is a standard isotonic solution that is used to precede and to follow infusion of blood products. Dextrose is not used because it could result in clumping and subsequent hemolysis of red blood cells. Lactated Ringer's is not the solution of choice with this procedure.

Test-Taking Strategy: Use the process of elimination and eliminate options 3 and 4 first because they are similar in that both solutions contain dextrose. From the remaining options, remember that normal saline is the solution that is compatible with red blood cells. If this question was difficult, review the procedures related to the administration of blood.
Level of Cognitive Ability: Application
Client Needs: Physiological Integrity
Integrated Process: Nursing Process—implementation
Content Area: Fundamental skills
Reference: Perry, A., & Potter, P. (2002). *Clinical nursing skills and techniques* (5th ed., p. 622). St. Louis: Mosby.

5. 2

Rationale: Deferoxamine (Desferal) is an antidote used to treat iron toxicity. Granisetron (Kytril) is an antiemetic. Ketoconazole (Nizoral) and terbinafine (Lamisil) are antifungal medications.

Test-Taking Strategy: Use the process of elimination and knowledge of the classifications of the medications identified in the options. Eliminate options 3 and 4 first because they are both antifungal medications. From the remaining options you must know that granisetron is an antiemetic and that deferoxamine is the medication used to treat iron toxicity. Review the medications identified in the options if you had difficulty with this question.

Level of Cognitive Ability: Analysis
Client Needs: Physiological Integrity
Integrated Process: Nursing Process—analysis
Content Area: Fundamental skills
Reference: Hodgson, B., & Kizior, R. (2003). *Saunders nursing drug handbook 2003* (pp. 315, 536, 630, 1063). Philadelphia: W. B. Saunders.

6. 3
Rationale: If several units of blood are to be administered, a blood warmer should be used. Rapid transfusion of cool blood places the client at risk for cardiac dysrhythmias. To prevent this occurrence, the nurse warms the blood as needed using a blood warming device. Electronic infusion devices are not helpful in this case because the infusion must be rapid, and infusion devices generally are used to control the flow rate. In addition, not all infusion devices are made to handle blood or blood products. Pulse oximetry and cardiac monitoring equipment is useful for the early assessment of complications but does not reduce the occurrence of cardiac dysrhythmias.
Test-Taking Strategy: Use the process of elimination. Note that the key words "rapid" and "reduce the risk." The words tell you that the infusions will infuse quickly and that the correct option is the one that will minimize the risk of cardiac dysrhythmias occurring. Eliminate option 1 and 2 first because these items are used to assess for rather than reduce the risk of complications. From the remaining options, use knowledge related to the complications of transfusion therapy and note the relationship between the words "several units of blood" in the question and "blood warming device" in the correct option. Review the concepts related to the use of a blood warmer if you had difficulty with this question.
Level of Cognitive Ability: Application
Client Needs: Physiological Integrity
Integrated Process: Nursing Process—planning
Content Area: Fundamental skills
References: Perry, A., & Potter, P. (2002). *Clinical nursing skills and techniques* (5th ed., p. 619). St. Louis: Mosby.
Potter, P., & Perry, A. (2001). *Fundamentals of nursing* (5th ed., p. 1243). St. Louis: Mosby.

7. 3
Rationale: With fluid overload the client has the presence of crackles in addition to dyspnea. An allergic reaction, which is one type of blood transfusion reaction, would produce symptoms such as flushing, dyspnea, itching, and a generalized rash. With bacteremia the client would have a fever, which is not part of the clinical picture presented. Hypovolemia is not a complication of a blood transfusion.
Test-Taking Strategy: Use the process of elimination, noting the key words "most likely." Read the question carefully and focus on the symptoms identified in the question. Eliminate option 1 first because it is not a complication of a blood transfusion. Next eliminate option 4 because no data in the question indicate that the client has an elevated temperature. From the remaining options, focusing on the key words "crackles in the lung bases" will direct you to option 3. Review the complications of blood transfusion therapy if you had difficulty with this question.

Level of Cognitive Ability: Analysis
Client Needs: Physiological Integrity
Integrated Process: Nursing Process—analysis
Content Area: Fundamental skills
Reference: Perry, A., & Potter, P. (2002). *Clinical nursing skills and techniques* (5th ed., pp. 624, 629). St. Louis: Mosby.

8. 1
Rationale: If the nurse suspects a transfusion reaction, the nurse stops the transfusion and infuses normal saline at a keep vein open rate pending further physician orders. This maintains a patent IV access line and aids in maintaining the client's intravascular volume. The nurse would not discontinue the IV line because then there would be no IV access route. Obtaining a culture of the tip of the catheter device removed from the client is incorrect. First, the catheter should not be removed. Second, cultures are performed when infection, not transfusion reaction, is suspected. Normal saline is the solution of choice over solutions containing dextrose because saline does not cause red blood cells to clump.
Test-Taking Strategy: Use the process of elimination, noting the key word "next." Knowing that the IV should not be removed or discontinued assists in eliminating options 3 and 4. Recalling that normal saline, not dextrose, is used when administering a unit of blood will direct you to option 1. Review care to the client when a transfusion reaction occurs if you had difficulty with this question.
Level of Cognitive Ability: Application
Client Needs: Physiological Integrity
Integrated Process: Nursing Process—planning
Content Area: Delegating/prioritizing
Reference: Potter, P., & Perry, A. (2001). *Fundamentals of nursing* (5th ed., p. 1243). St. Louis: Mosby.

9. 2
Rationale: The nurse returns the blood transfusion bag containing any remaining blood to the blood bank. This allows the blood bank to complete any follow-up testing procedures needed once a transfusion reaction has been documented. The other options are incorrect.
Test-Taking Strategy: Use the process of elimination and specific knowledge related to routine transfusion-related procedures to answer the question. Recalling that blood is issued from the blood bank will help you to eliminate each of the incorrect options. Review nursing responsibilities if a transfusion reaction occurs if you had difficulty with this question.
Level of Cognitive Ability: Application
Client Needs: Physiological Integrity
Integrated Process: Nursing Process—implementation
Content Area: Fundamental skills
Reference: Potter, P., & Perry, A. (2001). *Fundamentals of nursing* (5th ed., p. 1243). St. Louis: Mosby.

10. 4
Rationale: The tubing used for blood administration has an in-line filter. The filter helps ensure that any particles larger than the size of the filter are caught in the filter and are not infused into the client. The tubing should be macrodrip, not microdrip, to allow blood to flow freely through the drip chamber. An air vent is unnecessary because the blood bag is

not made of glass. Option 2 is incorrect, and in addition, blood does not need to be protected from light.
Test-Taking Strategy: Use the process of elimination. Read each option carefully and visualize the process of blood administration. Remember that tubing used for blood administration has an in-line filter. Review concepts related to tubing used for blood administration if you had difficulty with this question.
Level of Cognitive Ability: Application
Client Needs: Physiological Integrity
Integrated Process: Nursing Process—implementation
Content Area: Fundamental skills
Reference: Potter, P., & Perry, A. (2001). *Fundamentals of nursing* (5th ed., p. 1242). St. Louis: Mosby.

11. 4
Rationale: If the client has a temperature greater than 100° F, the unit of blood should not be hung until the physician is notified and has the opportunity to give further orders. The physician likely will prescribe that the blood be administered regardless of the temperature, but the decision is not within the nurse's scope of practice to make. The other options are incorrect.
Test-Taking Strategy: Use the process of elimination. Eliminate options 1, 2, and 3 because they all indicate beginning the transfusion. Review the nursing responsibilities before administering a blood transfusion if you had difficulty with this question.
Level of Cognitive Ability: Application
Client Needs: Physiological Integrity
Integrated Process: Nursing Process—implementation
Content Area: Fundamental skills
Reference: Phipps, W., Monahan, F., Sands, J., Marek, J., & Neighbors, M. (2003). *Medical-surgical nursing: Health and illness perspectives* (7th ed., p. 1643). St. Louis: Mosby.

12. 3
Rationale: Asking the client about personal experience with transfusion therapy provides a good starting point for client teaching about this procedure. Options 2 and 4 are not helpful because they may elicit a fearful response from the client. Although to determine whether the client knows the reason for the transfusion is important, option 1 is not an appropriate statement in terms of eliciting information from the client regarding an understanding of the need for the transfusion.
Test-Taking Strategy: Use the process of elimination. Note that the key words in the question are "initial question." This tells you that the correct option is the best starting point for discussion about the transfusion therapy. Options 2 and 4 have emotionally laden trigger words, including "risks" and "gone into shock," respectively, which make them incorrect. From the remaining options, focus on the key words and use therapeutic communication techniques to direct you to option 3. Review pretransfusion assessment procedures if you had difficulty with this question.
Level of Cognitive Ability: Application
Client Needs: Physiological Integrity
Integrated Process: Nursing Process—assessment
Content Area: Fundamental skills

Reference: Potter, P., & Perry, A. (2001). *Fundamentals of nursing* (5th ed., p. 1242). St. Louis: Mosby.

13. 1
Rationale: Blood must be hung as soon as possible (within 30 minutes) after obtaining it from the blood bank. After that time the blood temperature will be in excess of 50° F and could be unsafe for use. For this reason options 2, 3, and 4 are incorrect.
Test-Taking Strategy: Use the process of elimination. You must know that blood must be hung within 30 minutes after obtaining it from the blood bank to answer this question correctly. Review the standard procedures related to safe blood administration if you had difficulty with this question.
Level of Cognitive Ability: Application
Client Needs: Physiological Integrity
Integrated Process: Nursing Process—planning
Content Area: Fundamental skills
Reference: Perry, A., & Potter, P. (2002). *Clinical nursing skills and techniques* (5th ed., p. 625). St. Louis: Mosby.

14. 2
Rationale: Platelets are necessary for proper blood clotting. The client with insufficient platelets may exhibit frank bleeding or oozing of blood from puncture sites, wounds, and mucous membranes. A temperature would decline to normal after infusion of granulocytes if those cells were then instrumental in fighting infection in the body. Increased hemoglobin and hematocrit would occur when the client has received a transfusion of red blood cells.
Test-Taking Strategy: Use the process of elimination and knowledge regarding the potential uses and benefits of the various types of blood product transfusions. Eliminate options 3 and 4 first because they are similar. From the remaining options, recalling that platelets are necessary for proper blood clotting will direct you to option 2. If this question was difficult, review the types of blood products available for transfusion.
Level of Cognitive Ability: Analysis
Client Needs: Physiological Integrity
Integrated Process: Nursing Process—evaluation
Content Area: Fundamental skills
Reference: Ignatavicius, D., & Workman, M. (2002). *Medical-surgical nursing: Critical thinking for collaborative care* (4th ed., p. 821). Philadelphia: W. B. Saunders.

15. 1
Rationale: The client who has neutropenia may receive a transfusion of granulocytes, or white blood cells. These clients often have severe infections and are unresponsive to antibiotic therapy. The nurse notes the results of follow-up white blood cell counts to evaluate the effectiveness of therapy. The nurse also continues to monitor the client for signs and symptoms of infection. Erythrocyte count and hemoglobin and hematocrit levels are measured after transfusion of whole blood or packed red blood cells.
Test-Taking Strategy: Use the process of elimination. Recalling that granulocytes are a component of white blood cells will assist in directing you to option 1. In addition, note that options 2, 3, and 4 are similar in that these options all refer

to erythrocytes. Review the key points related to types of blood products if you had difficulty with this question.
Level of Cognitive Ability: Analysis
Client Needs: Physiological Integrity
Integrated Process: Nursing Process—evaluation
Content Area: Fundamental skills
Reference: Ignatavicius, D., & Workman, M. (2002). *Medical-surgical nursing: Critical thinking for collaborative care* (4th ed., p. 865). Philadelphia: W. B. Saunders.

16. **1**
Rationale: An urticarial reaction is characterized by a rash accompanied by pruritus. This type of transfusion reaction is prevented by pretreating the client with an antihistamine such as diphenhydramine. Acetaminophen and acetylsalicylic acid are analgesics, and ibuprofen is a nonsteroidal antiinflammatory drug.
Test-Taking Strategy: Use the process of elimination, recalling the classifications of the medications noted in each option. Recalling that diphenhydramine is an antihistamine will direct you to option 1. Review the measures implemented to prevent a transfusion reaction if you had difficulty with this question.
Level of Cognitive Ability: Analysis
Client Needs: Physiological Integrity
Integrated Process: Nursing Process—analysis
Content Area: Pharmacology
Reference: Hodgson, B., & Kizior, R. (2003). *Saunders nursing drug handbook 2003* (p. 356). Philadelphia: W. B. Saunders.

17. **2**
Rationale: The nurse notes the expiration date on the unit of blood to ensure that the blood is fresh. Blood cells begin to degenerate over time, so safe storage usually is limited to 35 days. Careful notation of the expiration date by the nurse is an essential part of the verification process before hanging a unit of blood. The nurse also notes the blood identification (unit) number, blood group and type, and client's name. The nurse also inspects the unit of blood for clots and returns the unit to the blood bank if clots are noted.
Test-Taking Strategy: Use the process of elimination and note that the key word in this question is "deteriorate." To answer this question correctly, you must know which part of the pre-transfusion verification procedure relates to the "freshness" of the unit of blood. Keeping this issue in mind should allow you to eliminate each of the incorrect options systematically. Review the procedure for checking blood if you had difficulty with this question.
Level of Cognitive Ability: Application
Client Needs: Physiological Integrity
Integrated Process: Nursing Process—implementation
Content Area: Fundamental skills
Reference: Phipps, W., Monahan, F., Sands, J., Marek, J., & Neighbors, M. (2003). *Medical-surgical nursing: Health and illness perspectives* (7th ed., p. 1646). St. Louis: Mosby.

18. **3**
Rationale: Albumin may be used as a plasma expander. Cryoprecipitate is useful in treating bleeding from hemophilia or disseminated intravascular coagulopathy because it is rich in clotting factors. Packed red blood cells replace erythrocytes and are not a plasma expander. Platelets are used when the client's platelet count is low.
Test-Taking Strategy: Use the process of elimination, noting the key words "requires plasma expansion." Recalling the composition of each of the blood components identified in the options will direct you to option 3. If you had difficulty with this question, review the various blood component therapies.
Level of Cognitive Ability: Analysis
Client Needs: Physiological Integrity
Integrated Process: Nursing Process—analysis
Content Area: Fundamental skills
Reference: Phipps, W., Monahan, F., Sands, J., Marek, J., & Neighbors, M. (2003). *Medical-surgical nursing: Health and illness perspectives* (7th ed., p. 298). St. Louis: Mosby.

19. **3**
Rationale: The major blood types are A, B, AB, and O. The blood type indicates an antigen that is found on the surface of the red blood cells. Acute hemolytic transfusion reaction (ABO incompatibility) can occur if a client receives blood that is not compatible with his or her blood type. Acute hemolytic reaction is the most serious adverse reaction to a blood transfusion.
Test-Taking Strategy: Use the process of elimination and specific knowledge related to the meaning of blood groups. If you had difficulty with this question, review these concepts.
Level of Cognitive Ability: Analysis
Client Needs: Physiological Integrity
Integrated Process: Nursing Process—analysis
Content Area: Fundamental skills
References: Phipps, W., Monahan, F., Sands, J., Marek, J., & Neighbors, M. (2003). *Medical-surgical nursing: Health and illness perspectives* (7th ed., p. 1642). St. Louis: Mosby.
Potter, P., & Perry, A. (2001). *Fundamentals of nursing* (5th ed., p. 1242). St. Louis: Mosby.

20. **4**
Rationale: Donating autologous blood to be reinfused as needed during or after surgery eliminates the risk of cross-infection from contaminated blood. The next most effective way is to ask a family member to donate blood before surgery. Blood banks do not provide extra screening on request. Preoperative iron supplements are helpful for iron deficiency anemia but are not most helpful in replacing blood lost during the surgery.
Test-Taking Strategy: Use the process of elimination. Note that the question contains the key words "most effective." This tells you that more than one or all of the options may be partially or totally correct. Recalling that an autologous transfusion is the collection of the client's own blood will direct you to option 4. Review the concepts related to disease transmission and blood donation procedures if you had difficulty with this question.
Level of Cognitive Ability: Application
Client Needs: Physiological Integrity
Integrated Process: Nursing Process—Implementation

Content Area: Fundamental skills
Reference: Potter, P., & Perry, A. (2001). *Fundamentals of nursing* (5th ed., p. 1242). St. Louis: Mosby.

CRITICAL THINKING: PRIORITIZING (ORDERED RESPONSE)

Answer: 15234
Rationale: The nurse would first verify the physician's order for the blood transfusion and ensure that the client has been informed about the procedure and has signed an informed consent. Once this has been done, the nurse would ensure that at least an 18- or 19-gauge intravenous needle is inserted into the client. Blood has a thicker and stickier consistency than intravenous solutions, and using an 18- or 19-gauge catheter ensures that the bore of the catheter is large enough to prevent damage to the blood cells. The blood is obtained from the blood bank next, once the nurse is assured that the client has been informed and has an adequate access for administering the blood. Once the blood has been obtained, two registered nurses or one registered and a licensed practical nurse (depending on agency policy) must together check the label on the blood product against the client's identification number, blood group, and complete name. This minimizes the risk of error in checking information on the blood bag and thereby minimizes the risk of harm or injury to the client. The nurse should measure vital signs and assess lung sounds before hanging the transfusion.

Test-Taking Strategy: Remember that a physician's order is needed for the treatments and procedures. This will direct you to the first nursing action. Recalling that the client needs to be informed about a procedure will assist in determining that the next action would be to ensure that the client has signed a consent form. Next remember that client preparation for the procedure is important. You would not obtain the blood from the blood bank unless the client was prepared; therefore the nurse would ensure that the client had an adequate intravenous access. Once blood is obtained, remember that verifying compatibility and client identity is critical. Review the procedure for administering blood if you had difficulty with this question.

Level of Cognitive Ability: Application
Client Needs: Physiological Integrity
Integrated Process: Nursing Process—implementation
Content Area: Delegating/prioritizing
Reference: Potter, P., & Perry, A. (2001). *Fundamentals of nursing* (5th ed., pp. 1242-1243). St. Louis: Mosby.

REFERENCES

Hodgson, B., & Kizior, R. (2003). *Saunders nursing drug handbook 2003.* Philadelphia: W. B. Saunders.

Ignatavicius, D., & Workman, M. (2002). *Medical-surgical nursing: Critical thinking for collaborative care* (4th ed.). Philadelphia: W. B. Saunders.

National Council of State Boards of Nursing (Eds.) (2003). *Test Plan for the National Council Licensure Examination for Registered Nurses* (effective date: April 2004). Chicago: Author.

Perry, A., & Potter, P. (2002). *Clinical nursing skills and techniques* (5th ed.). St. Louis: Mosby.

Phipps, W., Monahan, F., Sands, J., Marek, J., & Neighbors, M. (2003). *Medical-surgical nursing: Health and illness perspectives* (7th ed.). St. Louis: Mosby.

Potter, P., & Perry, A. (2001). *Fundamentals of nursing* (5th ed.). St. Louis: Mosby.

UNIT IV
Fundamental Skills

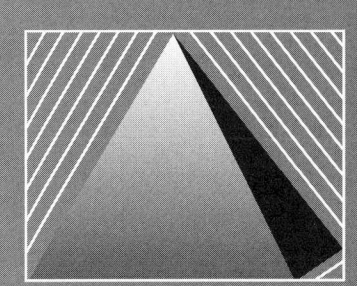

Provision of a Safe Environment

PYRAMID TERMS

chemical restraints Medications given to inhibit a specific behavior or movement.

nosocomial infections Infections acquired in the hospital or other health care facility that were not present or incubating at the time of the client's admission; also referred to as hospital-acquired infections.

physical restraints Devices that are applied to restrict a client's movement.

poison Any substance that impairs health or destroys life when ingested, inhaled, or otherwise absorbed by the body.

standard precautions Guidelines used by all health care providers with all clients to reduce the risk of infection for clients and caregivers.

transmission-based precautions Guidelines that are used in addition to standard precautions such as for specific syndromes that are highly suggestive of infections until a diagnosis is confirmed.

warfare agent Biological or chemical substances that can cause mass destruction and fatality.

▲ THE PYRAMID TO SUCCESS

Safety and Infection Control is a subcategory of the Client Needs component Safe, Effective Care Environment of the NCLEX-RN exam test plan. Pyramid Points focus on maintaining environmental safety, preventing accidents, the use of restraints, priority nursing actions in the event of a disaster, and biological and chemical warfare agents. Pyramid Points also focus on standard and transmission-based precautions and the measures required to handle hazardous or infectious materials. The Integrated Processes addressed in this chapter include Caring, Communication and Documentation, Nursing Process, and Teaching/Learning.

CLIENT NEEDS
Safe, Effective Care Environment

Establishment of priorities
Client rights and informed consent
Maintenance of precautions to prevent accidents
Standard, transmission-based, and other precautions
Handling of hazardous and infectious materials
Guidelines regarding the use of restraints
Disaster planning
Biological and chemical warfare agents

Health Promotion and Maintenance

Home safety assessment
Assisting clients and families to identify environmental hazards in the home
Client and family education regarding accident prevention
Client and family education to prevent the spread of infection
Client and family education regarding measures to be implemented in an emergency or disaster

Psychosocial Integrity

Cultural and religious lifestyles
Sensory/perceptual alterations
Support systems

Physiological Integrity

Provision of comfort and assistance to the client
Assisting the client with activities of daily living
Use of assistive devices to prevent injury

177

Management and provision of care to clients with infectious diseases

Priority nursing actions in an emergency or disaster

▲

I. ENVIRONMENTAL SAFETY

A. Fire safety (Box 16-1)
1. Keep open spaces free of clutter.
2. Clearly mark fire exits.
3. Know the locations of all fire alarms, exits, and extinguishers (Table 16-1; Box 16-2).
4. Know the telephone number for reporting fires.
5. Know the fire drill and evacuation plan of the agency.
6. Never use the elevator in the event of a fire.
▲ 7. Turn off oxygen and appliances in the vicinity of the fire.
8. In the event of a fire, if a client is on life support, maintain respiratory status manually with an Ambu-bag until the client is moved away from the threat of the fire and can be placed back on life support.
9. In the event of a fire, ambulatory clients can be directed to walk by themselves to a safe area and

in some cases may be able to assist in moving clients in wheelchairs.
10. Bedridden clients generally are moved from the scene of a fire by stretcher, their beds, or wheelchair.
11. If a client must be carried from the area of a fire, appropriate transfer techniques need to be used.
12. If fire department personnel are at the scene of the fire, they can help evacuate clients.

B. Electrical safety
1. Electrical equipment must be maintained in good working order and should be grounded.
2. Use a three-pronged electrical cord. ▲
3. In a three-pronged electrical cord, the third, longer prong of the cord is the ground; the other two prongs carry the power to the piece of electrical equipment.
4. Any electrical equipment that the client brings ▲ into the health care facility must be inspected for safety before use.
5. Check electrical cords and outlets for exposed, ▲ frayed, or damaged wires.
6. Avoid overloading any circuit.
7. Read warning labels on all equipment; never operate unfamiliar equipment.
8. Use safety extension cords only when absolutely necessary, and tape them to the floor with electrical tape.
9. Never run electrical wiring under carpets.
10. Never pull a plug by using the cord; always grasp the plug itself.
11. Never use electrical appliances near sinks, bathtubs, or other water sources.
12. Always disconnect a plug from the outlet before cleaning equipment or appliances.
13. If a client receives an electrical shock, turn off the ▲ electricity before touching the client.

C. Radiation safety
1. Know the protocols and guidelines of the health care agency.
2. Label potentially radioactive material.
3. To reduce exposure to radiation, do the following:
   a. Limit the time spent near the source.
   b. Make the distance from the source as great as possible.
   c. Use a shielding device such as a lead apron.
4. Monitor radiation exposure with a film badge.
5. Place the client who has a radiation implant in a private room.
6. Never touch dislodged radiation implants. ▲

D. Disposal of infectious wastes
1. Handle all infectious materials as a hazard.
2. Dispose of waste in designated areas only, using proper containers for disposal.
3. Ensure that infectious material is labeled properly.
4. Needles should not be recapped, bent, or broken. ▲

BOX 16-1

Priority Actions in the Event of a Fire

Remember the mnemonic RACE to set priorities in the event of a fire:

R, Rescue: Remove all clients from the vicinity of a fire.
A, Alarm: Activate the fire alarm; report a fire before attempting to extinguish it.
C, Confine: Close doors and windows when a fire is detected.
E, Extinguish: Extinguish the fire, using the appropriate fire extinguisher

---

TABLE 16-1

Types of Fire Extinguishers

Type	Class of Fire
A	Wood, cloth, upholstery, paper, rubbish, plastic
B	Flammable liquids or gases, grease, tar, and oil-based paint
C	Electrical equipment

BOX 16-2

Using a Fire Extinguisher

Remember the mnemonic PASS to use a fire extinguisher:
P: Pull the pin.
A: Aim at the base of the fire.
S: Squeeze the handles.
S: Sweep the fire from side to side.

BOX 16-3

Measures to Prevent Falls

Assess the client's risk for falling.
Assign the client at risk for falling to a room near the nurses' station.
Alert all personnel to the client's risk for falling.
Orient the client to physical surroundings.
Instruct the client to seek assistance when getting up.
Explain use of the call bell system.
Keep the bed in the low position with side rails up if required.
Lock all beds, wheelchairs, and stretchers.
Keep personal items within reach.
Eliminate clutter and obstacles in the client's room.
Provide adequate lighting.
Reduce bathroom hazards.
Maintain the client's toileting schedule throughout the day.

BOX 16-4

Documentation Points with the Use of a Restraint

Reason for restraint
Method of restraint
Date and time of application of restraint
Duration of use of restraint and client's response
Release from restraint with periodic exercise and circulatory, neurovascular, and skin assessment
Assessment of continued need for restraint
Evaluation of client's response

---

5. Dispose of all sharps immediately after use in closed, puncture-resistant disposal containers that are leak proof and labeled or color coded.

E. Falls (see Box 16-3 for measures to prevent falls)

F. Restraints

1. Restraints are protective devices used to limit the physical activity of a client or to immobilize a client or an extremity.

2. **Physical restraints** restrict client movement through the application of a device.

3. **Chemical restraints** are medications given to inhibit a specific behavior or movement.

4. Interventions

a. When restraints are necessary, the physician's orders should state the type of restraint, identify specific client behaviors for which restraints are to be used, and identify a limited time frame for use.

b. Physicians' orders for restraints should be renewed within a specific time frame according to the policy of the agency.

c. Restraints are not to be ordered "prn"; that is, as needed.

d. The reason for the restraints should be given to the client and the family, and their permission should be sought.

e. Restraints should not interfere with any treatments or affect the client's health problem.

f. Use a half-bow or safety knot to secure the device to the bedframe or chair, not to the side rails (provides for a quick release).

g. Ensure that enough slack is on the straps to allow some movement of the body part.

h. Assess skin integrity and neurovascular and circulatory status every 30 minutes and remove the restraint at least every 2 hours to permit muscle exercise and to promote circulation.

i. Continually assess the need for restraints (Box 16-4).

5. Alternatives to restraints

a. Orient the client and family to the surroundings.

b. Explain all procedures and treatments to client and family.

c. Encourage family and friends to stay with the client, and use sitters for clients who need supervision.

d. Assign confused and disoriented clients to rooms near the nurses' station.

e. Provide appropriate visual and auditory stimuli to the client, such as clocks, calendars, television, and a radio.

f. Place familiar items, such as family pictures, near the client's bedside.

g. Maintain toileting routines.

h. Eliminate bothersome treatments, such as tube feedings, as soon as possible.

i. Evaluate all medications that the client is receiving.

j. Use relaxation techniques with the client.

k. Institute exercise and ambulation schedules as the client's condition allows.

G. Poisons

1. Any substance that impairs health or destroys life when ingested, inhaled, or otherwise absorbed by the body is a **poison.**

2. Specific antidotes or treatments are available for only some types of poisons.

3. The capacity of body tissue to recover from a **poison** determines the reversibility of the effect.

4. **Poison** can impair the respiratory, circulatory, central nervous, hepatic, gastrointestinal, and renal systems of the body.

5. The toddler, the preschooler, and the young school-aged child must be protected from accidental poisoning.

6. In older adults, diminished eyesight and impaired memory may result in accidental ingestion of poisonous substances or an overdose of prescribed medications.

7. A **Poison** Control Center phone number should be visible on the telephone in homes with small

children; in all cases of expected poisoning, the number should be called immediately.

8. Interventions
   a. Remove any obvious materials from the mouth, eyes, or body area immediately.
   b. Identify the type and amount of substance ingested.
   c. Call the **Poison** Control Center before attempting an intervention.
   d. If the victim vomits or vomiting is induced, save the vomitus if requested to do so, and deliver it to the **Poison** Control Center.
   e. If instructed by the **Poison** Control Center to take the person to the emergency department, call an ambulance.
   f. Never induce vomiting following ingestion of lye, household cleaners, grease, or petroleum products.
   g. Never induce vomiting in an unconscious victim.

II. NOSOCOMIAL INFECTIONS (BOX 16-5)

A. **Nosocomial infections** also are referred to as hospital-acquired infections.
B. Such infections are infections acquired in a hospital or other health care facility that were not present or incubating at the time of a client's admission.
C. Illness impairs the normal defense mechanisms of the body.
D. The hospital environment provides exposure to a variety of virulent organisms that the client has not been exposed to in the past; therefore the client has not developed resistance to these organisms.
E. Infections can be transmitted by health care personnel who fail to practice proper handwashing procedures or fail to change gloves between client contacts.
F. Some health care agencies have dispensers containing an alcohol-based solution for hand rubs mounted at the entrance to each client's room.

III. STANDARD PRECAUTIONS

A. Description
   1. Nurses must practice **standard precautions** with all clients in any setting, regardless of the diagnosis or presumed infectiousness.
   2. **Standard precautions** promote handwashing and the use of gloves, masks, eye protection, and gowns, when appropriate, for client contact.
   3. These precautions apply to blood; all body fluids, secretions, and excretions except sweat, regardless

of whether they contain blood; nonintact skin; and mucous membranes.

B. Interventions
   1. Handle all blood and body fluids from all clients as if they were contaminated.
   2. Wash hands between client contacts; after contact with blood, body fluids, secretions, or excretions, and after contact with equipment or articles contaminated by them; and immediately after removing gloves.
   3. Wear gloves when touching blood, body fluids, secretions, excretions, nonintact skin, mucous membranes, or contaminated items; remove gloves and wash hands between client care contacts.
   4. Wear masks, eye protection, or face shields if client care activities may generate splashes or sprays of blood or body fluid.
   5. Wear gowns if soiling of clothing is likely from blood or body fluid; wash hands after removing a gown.
   6. Clean and reprocess client care equipment properly and discard single-use items.
   7. Place contaminated linen in leakproof bags and handle to prevent skin and mucous membrane exposure.
   8. Discard all sharp instruments and needles in a puncture-resistant container; dipose of needles uncapped or use a mechanical device for recapping the needle if necessary and available.
   9. Clean spills of blood or body fluids with a solution of bleach and water (diluted 1:10) or agency-approved disinfectant.
   10. A private room is unnecessary unless the client's hygiene is unacceptable; the nurse should consult with the infection-control professional.

IV. TRANSMISSION-BASED PRECAUTIONS

A. **Transmission-based precautions** include airborne, droplet, and contact precautions
B. Airborne precautions
   1. Diseases
      a. Measles
      b. Chickenpox (varicella)
      c. Disseminated varicella zoster
      d. Tuberculosis
   2. Barrier protection for airborne precautions
      a. Single room maintained under negative pressure; door kept closed except when someone is entering or exiting the room
      b. Negative airflow pressure in the room, with a minimum of 6 to 12 air exchanges per hour depending on the health care agency
      c. Use of ultraviolet germicide irradiation or high-efficiency particulate air filter in the room
      d. Mask or personal respiratory protection device
      e. Mask placed on the client when the client needs to leave the room; the client leaves the room only if necessary

---

BOX 16-5

Common Drug-Resistant Nosocomial Infections

Vancomycin-resistant enterococci
Methicillin-resistant *Staphylococcus aureus*
Multidrug-resistant tuberculosis

C. Droplet precautions
   1. Diseases
      a. Adenovirus
      b. Diphtheria (pharyngeal)
      c. Epiglottitis
      d. Influenza
      e. Meningitis
      f. Mumps
      g. Mycoplasmal pneumonia or meningococcal pneumonia
      h. Parvovirus B19
      i. Pertussis
      j. Pneumonia
      k. Rubella
      l. Scarlet fever
      m. Sepsis
      n. Streptococcal pharyngitis
   2. Barrier protection
      a. Private room or cohort client
      b. Use of a mask
      c. Mask placed on the client when the client is out of the room; the client leaves the room only if necessary
D. Contact precautions
   1. Diseases
      a. Colonization or infection with a multidrug-resistant organism
      b. Enteric infections such as *Clostridium difficile*
      c. Respiratory infections such as respiratory syncytial virus
      d. Wound infections
      e. Skin infections such as cutaneous diphtheria, herpes simplex, impetigo, pediculosis, scabies, staphylococcus, and varicella zoster
      f. Eye infection such as conjunctivitis
   2. Barrier protection
      a. Private room or cohort client
      b. Use of gloves and a gown when in contact with the client

V. DISASTERS
A. Know the disaster plan of the agency.
B. Internal disasters are those in which the agency is in danger.
C. External disasters occur in the community, and victims will be brought to the health care facility for care.
D. When the health care agency is notified of a disaster, the nurse would follow the guidelines specified in the disaster plan of the agency.
E. Refer to Chapter 8 for additional information on disaster planning.

VI. BIOLOGICAL WARFARE AGENTS
A. A **warfare agent** is a biological or chemical substance that can cause mass destruction and fatality.
B. Anthrax
   1. The disease is caused by *Bacillus anthracis* and can be contracted through the digestive system,

---

> **BOX 16-6**
>
> **Transmission and Symptoms of Anthrax**
>
> **SKIN**
> Spores enter the skin through cuts and abrasions and are contacted by handling contaminated animal skin products.
> Infection starts with an itchy bump like a mosquito bite that progresses to a small liquid-filled sac.
> The sac becomes a painless ulcer with an area of black, dead tissue in the middle.
> Toxins destroy surrounding tissue.
>
> **GASTROINTESTINAL**
> Infection occurs following the ingestion of contaminated, undercooked meat.
> Symptoms begin with nausea, loss of appetite, and vomiting.
> The disease progresses to severe abdominal pain, vomiting of blood, and severe diarrhea.
>
> **INHALATION**
> Infection is caused by the inhalation of bacterial spores, which multiply in the alveoli.
> The disease begins with the same symptoms as the flu, including fever, muscle aches, and fatigue.
> Symptoms suddenly become more severe with the development of breathing problems and shock.
> Toxins cause hemorrhage and destruction of lung tissue.

abrasions in the skin, or inhalation through the lungs.
   2. Anthrax is transmitted by direct contact with bacteria and spores; spores are dormant encapsulated bacteria that become active when they enter a living host (no person-to-person spread) (Box 16-6).
   3. The infection is carried to the lymph node, and then spreads to the rest of the body by way of the blood and lymph; high levels of toxins lead to shock and death.
   4. In the lungs, anthrax can cause buildup of fluid, tissue decay, and death (fatal if untreated).
   5. A blood test is available to detect anthrax (magnifies DNA from the blood sample and matches it to anthrax DNA).
   6. Anthrax is treated with ciprofloxacin (Cipro), doxycycline, or penicillin.
   7. Vaccine has limited availability.
C. Smallpox
   1. Smallpox is transmitted in air droplets and by handling of contaminated materials.
   2. Smallpox is highly contagious.
   3. Symptoms include fever, back pain, vomiting, malaise, and headache.
   4. Papules develop 2 days after symptoms develop and progress to pustular vesicles that are abundant on the face and extremities initially.
   5. A vaccine is available to those at risk for exposure to smallpox.

D. Botulism
1. Botulism is a serious paralytic illness caused by a nerve toxin that is produced by the bacterium *Clostridium botulinum* (the client can die within 24 hours).
2. Spore is found in the soil and can spread through the air or food (improperly canned food) or via a contaminated wound.
3. Botulism cannot be spread from person to person.
4. Symptoms include abdominal cramps, diarrhea, nausea and vomiting, double vision, blurred vision, drooping eyelids, difficulty swallowing or speaking, dry mouth, and muscle weakness.
5. Botulism can progress to paralysis of the arms, legs, trunk, or respiratory muscles (mechanical ventilation is necessary).
6. If diagnosed early, food-borne and wound botulism can be treated with an antitoxin that blocks the action of toxin circulating in the blood.
7. Other treatments include induction of vomiting, enemas, and penicillin.
8. No vaccine is available.

E. Plague
1. The plague is caused by *Yersinia pestis*, a bacteria found in rodents and fleas.
2. One contracts the plague by being bitten by a rodent or flea that is carrying the plague bacterium, by the ingestion of contaminated meat, or by handling an animal infected with the bacteria.
3. Transmission is by direct person-to-person spread.
4. Forms include bubonic (most common), pneumonic, and septicemic (most deadly).
5. The plague begins with a fever, chest pain, lymph node swelling, and a productive cough (hemoptysis).
6. The disease rapidly progresses to dyspnea, stridor, and cyanosis; death occurs from respiratory failure, shock, and bleeding.
7. Antibiotics are only effective if administered immediately; drugs of choice include streptomycin or gentamicin (Garamycin).
8. A vaccine is available.

F. Tularemia
1. Tularemia is an infectious disease of animals caused by the bacillus *Francisella tularensis* (also called deerfly fever or rabbit fever).
2. The disease is transmitted by ticks, deer flies, or contact with an infected animal.
3. Symptoms include fever, headache, an ulcerated skin lesion with localized lymph node enlargement, eye infections, gastrointestinal ulcerations, or pneumonia.
4. Treatment is with antibiotics.
5. Recovery produces lifelong immunity (a vaccine is available).

G. Hemorrhagic fever
1. Hemorrhagic fever is caused by several viruses including Marburg, Lassa, Junin, and Ebola.
2. The virus is carried by rodents and mosquitoes.
3. The disease can be transmitted by direct person-to-person spread via body fluids.
4. Symptoms include fever, headache, malaise, conjunctivitis, nausea, vomiting, hypotension, hemorrhage of tissues and organs, and organ failure.
5. No known specific treatment is available; treatment is symptomatic.

VII. CHEMICAL WARFARE AGENTS
A. Sarin
1. Sarin is a highly toxic nerve gas that can cause death within minutes of exposure.
2. Sarin enters the body through the eyes and skin and acts by paralyzing the respiratory muscles.
B. Phosgene is a colorless gas normally used in chemical manufacturing that if inhaled at high concentrations for a long enough period will lead to severe respiratory distress, pulmonary edema, and death.
C. Mustard gas is yellow to brown and has a garliclike odor that irritates the eyes and causes skin burns and blisters.
D. Ionizing radiation
1. Acute radiation exposure develops after a substantial exposure to radiation.
2. Exposure can occur from external radiation or internal absorption.
3. Symptoms depend on the amount of exposure to the radiation and range from nausea and vomiting, diarrhea, fever, electrolyte imbalances, and neurological and cardiovascular impairment to leukopenia, purpura, hemorrhage, and death.

PRACTICE QUESTIONS

1. A nurse enters a client's room and finds that the wastebasket is on fire. The nurse immediately assists the client out of the room. The next nursing action would be to
   1. Confine the fire by closing the room door.
   2. Activate the fire alarm.
   3. Call for help.
   4. Extinguish the fire.
2. A nurse enters the nursing lounge and discovers that a chair is on fire. She activates the alarm, closes the lounge door, and obtains the fire extinguisher to extinguish the fire. The nurse pulls the pin on the fire extinguisher. The next appropriate action in the use of the fire extinguisher is to
   1. Squeeze the handle on the extinguisher.
   2. Aim at the base of the fire.
   3. Sweep the fire from side to side with the extinguisher.
   4. Sweep the fire from top to bottom with the extinguisher.

3. A home care nurse performs a home safety assessment and discovers that a client is using a space heater to heat her apartment. Which of the following instructions would the nurse provide to the client regarding the use of the space heater?
   1. A space heater should not be used in an apartment.
   2. The space heater needs to be placed at least 3 feet from anything that can burn.
   3. The space heater should be placed in the hallway at night.
   4. The space heater should be kept at a low setting at all times.

4. A nurse is preparing to initiate an intravenous line containing a high dose of potassium chloride and plans to use an intravenous infusion pump. The nurse brings the pump to the bedside, prepares to plug the pump cord into the wall, and notes that no receptacle is available in the wall socket. Which of the following is the most appropriate nursing action?
   1. Use an extension cord from the nurses' lounge for the pump plug.
   2. Initiate the intravenous line without the use of a pump.
   3. Plug in the pump cord in the available plug above the room sink.
   4. Contact the electrical maintenance department for assistance.

5. A nurse obtains an order from a physician to restrain a client by using a jacket restraint. The nurse instructs a nursing assistant to apply the restraint to the client. Which of the following observations, if made by the nurse, would indicate inappropriate application of the restraint by the nursing assistant?
   1. A safety knot in the restraint straps
   2. Restraint straps that are safely secured to the side rails
   3. The jacket restraint secured such that two fingers can slide easily between the restraint and the client's skin
   4. Jacket restraint straps that do not tighten when force is applied against them

6. A nurse is giving report to a nursing assistant who will be caring for a client who has hand restraints. The nurse instructs the nursing assistant to assess the skin integrity of the restrained hands
   1. Every 30 minutes.
   2. Every 2 hours.
   3. Every 3 hours.
   4. Every 4 hours.

7. A nurse is planning care for a client with an internal radiation implant. Which of the following is an inappropriate component for the nurse to include in the plan of care?
   1. Placing the client in a semiprivate room at the end of the hallway
   2. Wearing gloves when emptying the client's bedpan
   3. Keeping all linens in the room until the implant is removed
   4. Wearing a lead apron when providing direct care to the client

8. A mother calls the home care nurse and tells the nurse that her 3-year-old child has just ingested liquid furniture polish. The home care nurse would direct the mother immediately to
   1. Induce vomiting.
   2. Bring the child to the emergency room.
   3. Call an ambulance.
   4. Call the Poison Control Center.

9. An emergency room nurse receives a telephone call and is informed that a tornado has hit a local residential area and that numerous casualties have occurred. The victims will be brought to the emergency room. The initial nursing action is which of the following?
   1. Prepare the triage rooms.
   2. Obtain additional supplies from the central supply department.
   3. Activate the agency disaster plan.
   4. Obtain additional nursing staff to assist in treating the casualties.

10. A nurse is caring for a client with a nosocomial infection caused by methicillin-resistant *Staphylococcus aureus*. Contact precautions are initiated. The nurse prepares to provide colostomy care to the client. The nurse obtains which of the following protective items required to perform this procedure?
    1. Gloves, gown, and goggles
    2. Gloves and goggles
    3. Gloves, gown, and shoe protectors
    4. Gloves and a gown

CRITICAL THINKING: FILL IN THE BLANK

A community health nurse is providing a teaching session about terrorism to members of the community and is discussing information regarding anthrax. The nurse tells those attending that anthrax can be transmitted by which route(s)?

Answer: _____

ANSWERS

1. 2
Rationale: The order of priority in the event of a fire is to rescue the clients who are in immediate danger. The next step is to activate the fire alarm. The fire then is confined by closing all doors, and last, the fire is extinguished.
Test-Taking Strategy: Remember the mnemonic RACE to prioritize in the event of a fire. R is rescue clients in immediate danger; A is alarm (sound the alarm); C is confine the fire by closing all doors; and E is extinguish or evacuate. If you had difficulty with this question, review the principles related to fire safety.
Level of Cognitive Ability: Application
Client Needs: Safe, Effective Care Environment
Integrated Process: Nursing Process—implementation
Content Area: Fundamental skills
Reference: Potter, P., & Perry, A. (2001). *Fundamentals of nursing* (5th ed., p. 1044). St. Louis: Mosby.

2. 2
Rationale: A fire can be extinguished by smothering it with a blanket or by the use of a fire extinguisher. To use the extinguisher, pull the pin first. You then should aim at the base of the fire. Squeeze the handle of the extinguisher, and extinguish the fire by sweeping from side to side to coat the area evenly.
Test-Taking Strategy: Remember the mnemonic PASS to prioritize in the use of a fire extinguisher. P is pull the pin; A is aim at the base of the fire; S is squeeze the handle; and S is sweep from side to side to coat the area evenly. If you had difficulty with this question, review the steps in the appropriate use of a fire extinguisher.
Level of Cognitive Ability: Application
Client Needs: Safe, Effective Care Environment
Integrated Process: Nursing Process—implementation
Content Area: Fundamental skills
Reference: Potter, P., & Perry, A. (2001). *Fundamentals of nursing* (5th ed., p. 1045). St. Louis: Mosby.

3. 2
Rationale: Space heaters need to be used appropriately because they present a great risk of fire. A space heater needs to be placed at least 3 feet from anything that can burn. Placing a heater in a hallway does not guarantee that it will be 3 feet from anything that can burn. A low setting does not reduce the risk of fire. A space heater can be used in an apartment if there is ample space and safety precautions are followed.
Test-Taking Strategy: Use the process of elimination, keeping in mind the issue related to fire safety. Note that option 2 is the only option that specifically defines a safety measure related to the use of a space heater. Review fire safety prevention measures in the home if you had difficulty with this question.
Level of Cognitive Ability: Application
Client Needs: Safe, Effective Care Environment
Integrated Process: Teaching/Learning
Content Area: Fundamental skills
Reference: Potter, P., & Perry, A. (2001). *Fundamentals of nursing* (5th ed., p. 1099). St. Louis: Mosby.

4. 4
Rationale: The nurse needs to use hospital resources for assistance. A regular extension cord should not be used because it poses the risk of fire. The use of electrical appliances near a sink also presents a hazard. An intravenous line that contains a high dose of potassium chloride should be administered by the use of a pump.
Test-Taking Strategy: Use the process of elimination. Noting the key words "high dose" in the question will assist in eliminating option 2. Recalling safety issues related to electrical hazards will assist in eliminating options 1 and 3. If you had difficulty with this question, review the interventions related to electrical safety.
Level of Cognitive Ability: Application
Client Needs: Safe, Effective Care Environment
Integrated Process: Nursing Process—implementation
Content Area: Fundamental skills
Reference: Potter, P., & Perry, A. (2001). *Fundamentals of nursing* (5th ed., p. 1046). St. Louis: Mosby.

5. 2
Rationale: A half-bow or safety knot should be used for applying a restraint because it does not tighten when force is applied against it and allows quick and easy removal of the restraint in the case of an emergency. The restraint straps are secured to the bed frame and never to the side rail to avoid accidental injury in the event that the side rail is released. The jacket restraint should be secure, and one to two fingers should slide easily between the restraint and the client's skin.
Test-Taking Strategy: Use the process of elimination. Note the key words "indicate inappropriate application." This indicates that you are looking for an option that identifies an inaccurate measure related to the application of restraints. Read each option carefully. The words "secured to the side rails" in option 2 should direct your attention as an inappropriate action. Review guidelines related to the application of restraints if you had difficulty with this question.
Level of Cognitive Ability: Analysis
Client Needs: Safe, Effective Care Environment
Integrated Process: Teaching/Learning
Content Area: Fundamental skills
Reference: Perry, A., & Potter, P. (2002). *Clinical nursing skills and techniques* (5th ed., p. 76). St. Louis: Mosby.

6. 1
Rationale: The nurse should instruct the nursing assistant to assess restraints and skin integrity every 30 minutes. Agency guidelines regarding the use of restraints should always be followed.
Test-Taking Strategy: Use the process of elimination. In this situation, to select the option that identifies the most frequent time frame is best. Review the guidelines related to the use of restraints if you had difficulty with this question.
Level of Cognitive Ability: Application
Client Needs: Safe, Effective Care Environment
Integrated Process: Teaching/Learning
Content Area: Fundamental skills
Reference: Potter, P., & Perry, A. (2001). *Fundamentals of nursing* (5th ed., p. 1043). St. Louis: Mosby.

7. 1
Rationale: A private room with a private bath is essential if a client has an internal radiation implant. This is necessary to prevent accidental exposure of other clients to radiation. Options 2, 3, and 4 are accurate interventions for a client with a radiation implant.
Test-Taking Strategy: Use the process of elimination. Note the key words "inappropriate component." Option 2 can be eliminated first because this is a component of standard precautions for all clients. Options 3 and 4 can be eliminated next because they directly relate to radiation safety. Review radiation safety principles if you had difficulty with this question.
Level of Cognitive Ability: Application
Client Needs: Safe, Effective Care Environment
Integrated Process: Nursing Process—planning
Content Area: Fundamental skills
Reference: Phipps, W., Monahan, F., Sands, J., Marek, J., & Neighbors, M. (2003). *Medical-surgical nursing: Health and illness perspectives* (7th ed., p. 334). St. Louis: Mosby.

8. 4
Rationale: If a poisoning occurs, the Poison Control Center should be contacted immediately. Vomiting should not be induced if the victim is unconscious or if the substance ingested is a strong corrosive or petroleum product. Bringing the child to the emergency room or calling an ambulance would not be the initial action because this would delay treatment. The Poison Control Center may advise the mother to bring the child to the emergency room, and if this is the case, the mother should call an ambulance.
Test-Taking Strategy: Use the process of elimination. Note the key word "immediately" in the stem of the question. Eliminate options 2 and 3 because these options will delay treatment. Recalling that vomiting should not be induced if a corrosive substance was ingested will assist in eliminating option 1. Review poison control measures if you had difficulty with this question.
Level of Cognitive Ability: Application
Client Needs: Safe, Effective Care Environment
Integrated Process: Nursing Process—implementation
Content Area: Fundamental skills
Reference: Potter, P., & Perry, A. (2001). *Fundamentals of nursing* (5th ed., pp. 1046-1047). St. Louis: Mosby.

9. 3
Rationale: In an external disaster, many victims may be brought to the emergency room for treatment. Although options 1, 2, and 4 may be components of preparing for the casualties, the initial nursing action must be to activate the disaster plan.
Test-Taking Strategy: Use the process of elimination to determine the priority action. Note the key word "initial" in the stem of the question. Note that option 3 is the global option. Review procedures related to management of a disaster if you had difficulty with this question.
Level of Cognitive Ability: Application
Client Needs: Safe, Effective Care Environment
Integrated Process: Nursing Process—implementation
Content Area: Fundamental skills
Reference: Clemen-Stone, S., McGuire, S., & Eigsti, D. (2002). *Comprehensive community health nursing: Family, aggregate & community practice* (6th ed., pp. 164-165). St. Louis: Mosby.

10. 1
Rationale: Goggles are worn to protect the mucous membranes of the eyes during interventions that may produce splashes of blood, body fluids, secretions, or excretions. In addition, contact precautions require the use of gloves, and a gown should be worn if direct client contact is anticipated. Shoe protectors are not necessary.
Test-Taking Strategy: Note the key words "contact precautions" and "colostomy." Use the process of elimination to determine the necessary items required in caring for this client. If you had difficulty with this question, review transmission-based precautions.
Level of Cognitive Ability: Application
Client Needs: Safe, Effective Care Environment
Integrated Process: Nursing Process—implementation
Content Area: Fundamental skills
Reference: Potter, P., & Perry, A. (2001). *Fundamentals of nursing* (5th ed., pp. 857-859). St. Louis: Mosby.

CRITICAL THINKING: FILL IN THE BLANK
Answer: Skin, gastrointestinal tract, or by inhalation
Rationale: Anthrax is caused by *Bacillus anthracis* and can be contracted through the digestive system, abrasions in the skin, or inhalation through the lungs.
Test-Taking Strategy: Knowledge regarding the methods of contracting anthrax is needed to answer this question. Recall the three modes of entry into the body. Review information related to this infection if you had difficulty with this question.
Level of Cognitive Ability: Application
Client Needs: Safe, Effective Care Environment
Integrated Process: Teaching/Learning
Content Area: Fundamental skills
Reference: Lewis, S., Heitkemper, M., & Dirksen, S. (2004). *Medical-surgical nursing: Assessment and management of clinical problems* (6th ed., p. 1863). St. Louis: Mosby.

REFERENCES

Clemen-Stone, S., McGuire, S., & Eigsti, D. (2002). *Comprehensive community health nursing: Family, aggregate & community practice* (6th ed). St. Louis: Mosby.

Lewis, S., Heitkemper, M., & Dirksen, S. (2004). *Medical-surgical nursing: Assessment and management of clinical problems* (6th ed.). St. Louis: Mosby.

National Council of State Boards of Nursing (Eds.). (2003). *Test Plan for the National Council Licensure Examination for Registered Nurses* (effective date: April 2004). Chicago: Author.

Perry, A., & Potter, P. (2002). *Clinical nursing skills and techniques* (5th ed.). St. Louis: Mosby.

Phipps, W., Monahan, F., Sands, J., Marek, J., & Neighbors, M. (2003). *Medical-surgical nursing: Health and illness perspectives* (7th ed.). St. Louis: Mosby.

Potter, P., & Perry, A. (2001). *Fundamentals of nursing* (5th ed.). St. Louis: Mosby.

Administration of Medication and Intravenous Solutions

PYRAMID TERMS

conversion The first step in the calculation of a medication problem.

generic name The common or chemical name of a medication, printed on the label in small letters, usually under the trade name.

milliequivalent An expression of the number of grams of a medication contained in 1 mL of a normal solution; abbreviated mEq.

parenteral Given by injection such as by intravenous, intramuscular, and subcutaneous routes.

percentage solutions The number of grams of a medication per 100 mL of solution.

ratio solutions The number of grams of a medication per total milliliters of solution.

reconstitution Dissolving a powder in a sterile diluent before use, usually in sterile water or normal saline.

trade name Also called the brand name; usually printed on the label in large, bold letters.

unit A measurement of a medication in terms of its action, not its physical weight.

◢ THE PYRAMID TO SUCCESS

When a medication or intravenous calculation question is presented, a nurse should always use the appropriate formula to solve the problem. The nurse should not use shortcuts to make these calculations. The problem and the answer should be expressed in the correct units of measure. Be careful with decimal points. Correct placement of the decimal point is important, or the answer will be incorrect. When solving a medication calculation problem, the nurse determines whether the answer is within reason and makes sense. In the clinical setting the nurse should always seek assistance if the nurse is unsure of the accuracy of a calculation.

On the NCLEX-RN examination, the fill in the blank questions may require that you calculate a medication dose or an intravenous flow rate. You will be provided with a computer on-screen calculator for these medication and intravenous problems. Even if you use the calculator to calculate dosages and flow rates, you must check the calculation before selecting an option or typing the answer. Follow the formula, place the decimal point in the correct place, and check the accuracy of the calculation. Remember, practice makes perfect.

The Integrated Processes addressed in this chapter are Caring, Nursing Process, Communication and Documentation, and Teaching/Learning.

CLIENT NEEDS
Safe, Effective Care Environment

Client rights
Error prevention
Handling of hazardous or infectious materials
Intravenous fluid and medication calculations
Medical and surgical asepsis
Medication calculations
Standard and other precautions

Health Promotion and Maintenance

Client teaching regarding prescribed medication(s) or intravenous (IV) therapy
Disease prevention
Lifestyle choices
Physical assessment of client

Psychosocial Integrity

Cultural, religious, and spiritual influences on health
Support systems
Therapeutic interactions
Use of coping mechanisms

Physiological Integrity

Actions of medications and IV therapy

Administration of medications and IV therapy

Adverse effects of and contraindications to medication or IV therapy

Alterations in body systems

Expected effects of pharmacological therapy

Laboratory values

Unexpected responses to therapy

I. MEDICATION ADMINISTRATION (BOX 17-1)

BOX 17-1

Medication Administration

Assess medication order.

Ask client about a history of allergies.

Assess client's current condition and the purpose for the medication or intravenous solution.

Determine client's understanding regarding the purpose of the prescribed medication or need for intravenous solution.

Teach client about the medication and about self-administration at home.

Identify and address concerns (social, cultural, religious) that the client may have about taking the medication.

Assess the need for conversion when preparing a dose of medication for administration to the client.

Assess the five rights: right medication, right dose, right client, right route, and right time.

Assess vital signs before administering medication.

Document the administration of the prescribed therapy and client's response to the therapy.

II. DRUG MEASUREMENT SYSTEMS

A. Metric system (Box 17-2)
1. The basic units of metric measures are meter, liter, and gram.
   a. Meter measures length.
   b. Liter measures volume.
   c. Gram measures mass.

B. Apothecary and household systems (Box 17-3)
1. The apothecary and household systems are the oldest of the medication measurement systems.
2. The three apothecary measures sometimes used are grain, dram, and ounce.
   a. Grain, dram, and ounce measure weight.
   b. Fluid dram and fluid ounce measure volume.

BOX 17-2

Metric System

ABBREVIATIONS

meter: m

liter: L

milliliter: mL

kilogram: kg

gram: g

milligram: mg

microgram: mcg

EQUIVALENTS

1 mcg = 0.000001 g

1 mg = 1000 mcg or 0.001 g

1 g = 1000 mg

1 kg = 1000 g

1 kg = 2.2 lb

1 mL = 0.001 L

BOX 17-3

Apothecary and Household Systems

ABBREVIATIONS	EQUIVALENTS
Apothecary (Weight)	1 gr = 60 mg
grain: gr	5 gr = 300 mg
dram: dr	15 gr = 1000 mg or 1 g
ounce: oz	$\frac{1}{150}$ gr = 0.4 mg
Household (Volume)	1 fl oz = 30 mL
drops: gtt	1 fl dr = 4 mL
minim: min	1 T = 15 mL or 3 tsp
fluid dram: fl dr	1 t or tsp = 5 mL
teaspoon: t or tsp	1 min = 1 gtt
tablespoon: T or tbs	15 min = 1 mL
fluid ounce: fl oz	60 min = 1 fl dr
pint: pt	8 fl dr = 1 fl oz
quart: qt	1 qt = 946 mL or 0.946 L
Household (Weight)	1 qt = 2 pt or 32 fl oz
pound: lb	1 pt = 16 fl oz
	16 oz = 1 lb
	2.2 lbs = 1 kg

c. The four household measures commonly used are tablespoon, teaspoon, minim, and drop.

C. Additional common drug measures
1. **Milliequivalent**
   a. **Milliequivalent** is abbreviated mEq.
   b. The **milliequivalent** is an expression of the number of grams of a medication contained in 1 mL of a normal solution.
   c. For example, the measure of serum potassium is given in milliequivalents.
2. **Unit**
   a. **Unit** measures a medication in terms of its action, not its physical weight.
   b. For example, penicillin, heparin sodium, insulin are measured in units.

III. CONVERSIONS

A. **Conversion** between metric units (Box 17-4)
1. The metric system is a decimal system; therefore conversions between the units in this system can be done by dividing or multiplying by 1000 or by moving the decimal point three places to the right or three places to the left.
2. In the metric system, to convert larger to smaller, multiply by 1000 or move the decimal point three places to the right.
3. In the metric system, to convert smaller to larger, divide by 1000 or move the decimal point three places to the left.

B. **Conversion** between apothecary, household, and metric systems
1. Metric, apothecary, and household measures are equivalent not equal measures.
2. **Conversion** to equivalent measures between systems is necessary when a medication order is written in one system but the medication label is stated in another.
3. Medications are not always ordered and prepared in the same system of measurement; therefore **conversion** of units from one system to another is necessary.

4. **Conversion** is the first step in the calculation of dosages.
5. Calculating equivalents between two systems may be done by using the method of ratio and proportion (Box 17-5).

IV. CELSIUS AND FAHRENHEIT TEMPERATURE (BOX 17-6)

A. To convert Fahrenheit to Celsius, subtract 32 and divide result by 1.8.
B. To convert Celsius to Fahrenheit, multiply by 1.8 and add 32.

V. MEDICATION LABELS

A. A medication label contains the **generic name** and the **trade name** of the medication.
B. Each medication has only one official name but may have several trade names, each for the exclusive use of the company that manufactures the medication.
C. Always check expiration dates on medication labels.

VI. MEDICATION ORDERS (BOX 17-7)

A. In a medication order, the name of the medication is written first, followed by the dosage, route, and frequency
B. If the nurse has any questions about or sees inconsistencies in the written order, the nurse must contact the person who wrote the order immediately and must verify the order.

BOX 17-5

Calculating Equivalents between Two Systems

Calculating equivalents between two systems may be done by using the method of ratio and proportion.

PROBLEM
The physician orders nitroglycerin, $\frac{1}{150}$ gr. The medication label reads 0.4 mg per tablet. The nurse prepares to administer how many tablets to the client?
Solution
gr 1: 60 mg = $\frac{1}{150}$ gr : x mg
60 × 1/150 = x
x = 0.4 mg (1 tablet)

BOX 17-4

Conversion between Metric Units

1. PROBLEM
Convert 2 g to milligrams.
Solution
Change a larger unit to a smaller unit.
2 g = 2000 mg (moving decimal three places to right)

2. PROBLEM
Convert 250 mL to liters.
Solution
Change a smaller unit to a larger unit.
250 mL = 0.25 L (moving decimal three places to left)

BOX 17-6

Celsius and Fahrenheit Temperature

FAHRENHEIT TO CELSIUS
To convert Fahrenheit to Celsius, subtract 32 and divide result by 1.8.
Formula: $C = \frac{(F - 32)}{1.8}$

CELSIUS TO FAHRENHEIT
To convert Celsius to Fahrenheit, multiply by 1.8 and add 32.
Formula: $F = (1.8 \times C) + 32$

Medication Orders

Name of client
Date and time when order is written
Name of medication to be given
Dosage of medication
Medication route
Time and frequency of administration
Signature of person writing the order

VII. ORAL MEDICATIONS

A. Scored tablets contain an indented mark to be used for possible breakage into partial dosages; when necessary, scored tablets (those marked for division) can be divided into halves or quarters.

B. Enteric-coated tablets and sustained-released capsules delay absorption until the medication reaches the small intestine; these medications should not be crushed.

C. Capsules contain a powered or oily medication in a gelatin cover.

D. Orally administered liquids are supplied in solution form and contain a specific amount of medication in a given amount of solution, as stated on the label.

E. The medicine cup
   1. The medicine cup has a capacity of 30 mL or 1 oz.
   2. The medicine cup is used for orally administered liquids.
   3. The medicine cup is calibrated to measure teaspoons, tablespoons, and fluid drams.
   4. To pour accurately, hold the medication cup at eye level, and then line up the measure that is needed and pour.

F. Volumes of less than 5 mL are measured by using a syringe with the needle removed.

G. A calibrated dropper is used for giving medicine to children or for adding small amounts of liquid to water or juice; calibrations are in milliliters, drops, or minims.

VIII. PARENTERAL MEDICATIONS

A. **Parenteral** always means an injection route, and **parenteral** medications are administered by intravenous, intramuscular (IM), or subcutaneous injection.

B. **Parenteral** medications are packaged in single-use ampules, in single- and multiple-use rubber-stoppered vials, and in premeasured syringes and cartridges.

C. The nurse should not administer more than 3 mL per intramuscular or 1 mL per subcutaneous injection site; larger volumes are difficult for an injection site to absorb and if prescribed, need to be verified.

D. Always question and verify excessively large or small volumes of medication.

E. The standard 3-mL syringe is used to measure most injectable medications and is calibrated in tenths (0.1) of a milliliter (Fig. 17-1).

F. The calibrations on a syringe are read from the top black ring on the syringe, not the middle section and not the bottom ring

G. Prefilled medication cartridge (Fig. 17-2)
   1. The medication cartridge slips into the cartridge holder, which provides a plunger for injection of the medication.
   2. The cartridge is designed to provide sufficient capacity to allow for the addition of a second medication when combined dosages are prescribed.
   3. The prefilled medication cartridge is to be used once and discarded; if a nurse is to give less than a full single dose provided, the nurse needs to discard the extra amount before giving the client the injection, following agency policies and procedures.

H. Standard medication doses for adults are to be rounded to the nearest tenth (0.1) of a milliliter and measured on the milliliter scale; for example, 1.25 mL is rounded to 1.3 mL.

I. When volumes larger than 3 mL are required, the nurse may use a 5-, 6-, 10-, or 12-mL syringe; these syringes are calibrated in fifths (Fig. 17-3).

J. Syringes larger than 12 mL are calibrated in 1-mL measures.

K. Tuberculin syringe (Fig. 17-4)
   1. The tuberculin syringe holds 1 mL and is used to measure small or critical amounts of medication, such as allergen extract, vaccine, or a child's medication.
   2. The syringe is calibrated in hundredths (0.01) of a milliliter, with each one tenth (0.1) marked on the metric scale.

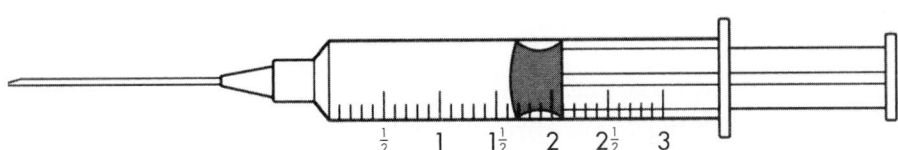

FIG. 17-1 Three-milliliter syringe. (From Kee, J., & Marshall, S. [2004]. *Clinical calculations: With applications to general and specialty areas* [5th ed.]. Philadelphia: W. B. Saunders.)

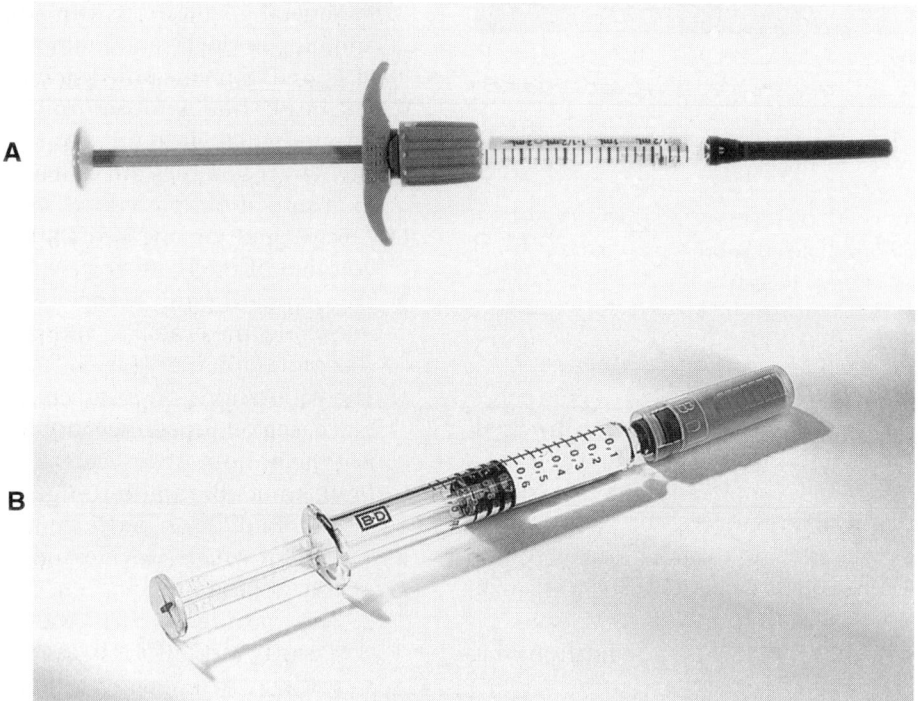

FIG. 17-2   **A,** Tubex syringe with cartridge. **B,** BD Hypak prefilled syringe. (From Kee, J., & Marshall, S. [2000]. *Clinical calculations: With applications to general and specialty areas* [4th ed.]. Philadelphia: W. B. Saunders. **A,** Courtesy Wyeth-Ayerst Laboratories, Philadelphia, PA; **B,** courtesy Becton, Dickinson, and Company, Franklin Lakes, NJ.)

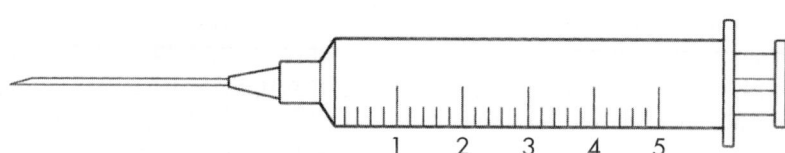

FIG. 17-3   Five-milliliter syringe. (From Kee, J., & Marshall, S. [2004]. *Clinical calculations: With applications to general and specialty areas* [5th ed.]. Philadelphia: W. B. Saunders.)

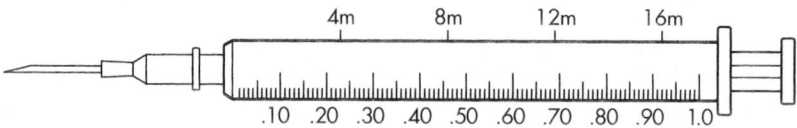

FIG. 17-4   Tuberculin syringe. (From Kee, J., & Marshall, S. [2004]. *Clinical calculations: With applications to general and specialty areas* [5th ed.]. Philadelphia: W. B. Saunders.)

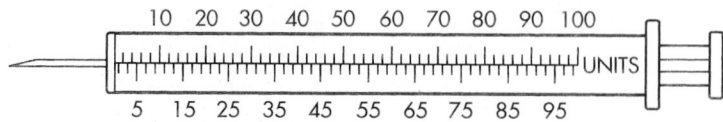

FIG. 17-5   Insulin syringe. (From Kee, J., & Marshall, S. [2004]. *Clinical calculations: With applications to general and specialty areas* [5th ed.]. Philadelphia: W. B. Saunders.)

L. Insulin syringe (Fig. 17-5)
  1. The standard 100-**unit** insulin syringe is used to measure 100 units of insulin only; the syringe is calibrated for 100 units, or 1 mL.
  2. Insulin should not be measured in any other type of syringe.
  3. When the insulin order states to combine regular and NPH insulin, remember "R.N.": draw *Regular* insulin first, and then draw the *NPH* insulin.
M. Safety needles contain shielding devices to reduce the incidence of needlestick injuries (Fig. 17-6).

IX. INJECTABLE MEDICATIONS IN POWDER FORM

A. Some medications become unstable when stored in solution form and are therefore packaged in powder form.
B. Powders must be dissolved with a sterile diluent before use; usually sterile water or normal saline is used. The dissolving procedure is called **reconstitution** (Box 17-8).

X. CALCULATING THE CORRECT DOSAGE (BOX 17-9)

A. When calculating dosages of oral medications, check the calculation and question an order if the calculation calls for more than three tablets.
B. When calculating dosages of **parenteral** medications, check the calculation and question an order if the amount to be given is too large a dose.
C. Regardless of the source of an error, if a nurse gives an incorrect dose, the nurse is legally responsible for the action.
D. Be sure that all measures are in the same system, and that all units are in the same size, converting when necessary; carefully consider what is the reasonable amount of the medication that should be administered.
E. Round standard injection doses to tenths and measure in a 3-mL syringe.
F. Round small, critical amounts, or children's doses to hundredths and measure in the 1-mL tuberculin syringe.

XI. CALCULATING DOSAGES EXPRESSED AS A RATIO OR PERCENT

A. **Percentage solutions**
  1. Express the number of grams of the medication per 100 mL of solution.
  2. For example, calcium gluconate 10% is 10 g of pure medication per 100 mL of solution.
B. **Ratio solutions**
  1. Express the number of grams of the medication per total milliliters of solution.
  2. For example, epinephrine 1:1000 is 1 g of pure medication per 1000 mL solution.

XII. INTRAVENOUS FLOW RATES (BOX 17-10)

A. Monitor IV flow rate every 30 minutes for adults and every 15 minutes for children.
B. If an IV is running behind schedule, collaborate with the physician to determine the client's ability to tolerate an increased flow rate, particularly clients

---

BOX 17-8

Reconstitution

In reconstituting the medication, locate the instructions on the label or in the vial package insert, and read and follow the directions carefully.

Instructions will state the volume of diluent to be used and the resulting volume of the reconstituted medication.

Often the powdered medication adds volume to the solution in addition to the amount of diluent added.

When reconstituting a multiple-dose vial, label the medication vial with the date and time of preparation, your initials, and the date of expiration.

Indicating the strength per volume on the label also is important.

The total volume of the prepared solution will exceed the volume of the diluent added.

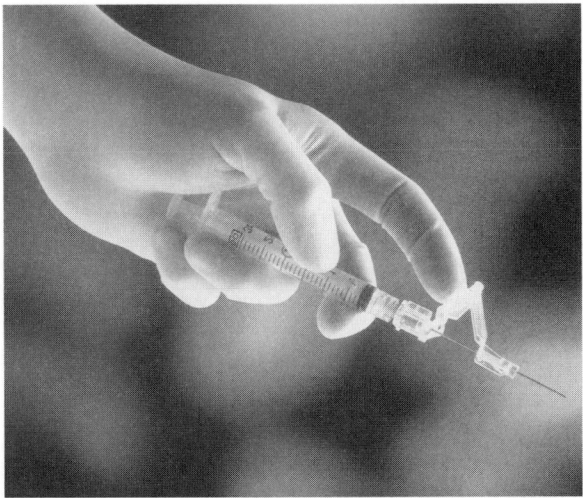

FIG. 17-6 SafetyGlyde needle. (From Kee, J., & Marshall, S. [2004]. *Clinical calculations: With applications to general and specialty areas* [5th ed.]. Philadelphia: W. B. Saunders. Courtesy Becton, Dickinson, and Company, Franklin Lakes, NJ.)

BOX 17-9

Formula for Calculating a Medication Dosage

$$\frac{D}{A} \times Q = X$$

D (desired) is the dosage that the physician ordered.

A (available) is the dosage strength as stated on the medication label.

Q (quantity) is the volume that the dosage strength is available in, such as tablets, capsules, or milliliters.

BOX 17-10

Formulas for Intravenous Calculations

FLOW RATES

$$\frac{\text{Total volume} \times \text{Drop factor}}{\text{Time in minutes}} = \text{Drops per minute}$$

INFUSION TIME

$$\frac{\text{Total volume to infuse}}{\text{Milliliters per hour being infused}} = \text{Infusion time}$$

NUMBER OF MILLILITERS PER HOUR

$$\frac{\text{Total volume in milliliters}}{\text{Number of hours}} = \text{Number of milliliters per hour}$$

with cardiac, pulmonary, renal, or neurological conditions.

C. The nurse should never increase the rate (speed up) of an IV infusion to catch up if the infusion is running behind schedule.

D. Whenever a prescribed IV rate is increased, the nurse should assess the client for increased heart rate, increased respirations, or increased lung congestion, which could indicate fluid overload.

E. Intravenously administered fluids are ordered most frequently based on milliliters per hour to be administered.

F. The volume per hour ordered is administered by setting the flow rate, which is counted in drops per minute.

G. Most flow rate calculations involve changing milliliters per hour into drops per minute.

H. Intravenous tubing
1. Intravenous tubing is calibrated in drops per milliliter, and this calibration is needed for calculating flow rates.
2. A standard or macrodrip set is used for routine adult IV administrations; depending on the manufacturer and type of tubing, the set will require 10, 15, or 20 gtt to equal 1 mL.
3. A minidrip or microdrip set is used when more exact measurements are needed, such as in intensive care units and pediatric units.
4. In a minidrip or microdrip set, 60 gtt is usually equal to 1 mL.
5. The calibration, in drops per milliliter, is written on the IV tubing package.

XIII. ELECTRONIC IV FLOW RATE REGULATORS

A. Controller
1. The controller works on the same principle of gravity as a regular IV drip, with the rate of flow being maintained by rapid compression and decompression of the IV tubing by the machine.
2. The desired flow rate is set on the controller in milliliters per hour.
3. Because controllers work by gravity, the height of the solution bag is critical; the bag must be maintained a minimum of 36 inches above the controller.

BOX 17-11

Infusions Ordered by Unit Dosage per Hour

Calculation of these problems can be done by a two-step process:
1. Determine the amount of medication per 1 mL.
2. Determine the infusion rate or milliliters per hour.

PROBLEM

Order: Continuous heparin sodium by IV at 1000 units per hour
Available: IV bag of 500 mL D₅W with 20,000 units of heparin sodium
How many milliliters per hour are required to administer the correct dose?

Solution

STEP 1: Calculate the units per milliliter.

$$\frac{\text{Known amount of medication in solution}}{\text{Total volume of diluent}} = \text{Amount of medication per milliliter}$$

$$\frac{20,000 \text{ units}}{500 \text{ mL}} = 40 \text{ units per 1 mL}$$

STEP 2: Calculate milliliters per hour.

$$\frac{\text{Dose per hour desired}}{\text{Concentration per milliliter}} = \text{Infusion rate or milliliter per hour}$$

$$\frac{1000 \text{ units}}{40 \text{ units}} = 25 \text{ mL per hour}$$

PROBLEM

Order: Continuous regular insulin by IV at 10 units per hour
Available: IV bag of 100 mL NS with 50 units regular insulin
How many milliliters per hour are required to administer the correct dose?

Solution

STEP 1: Calculate the units per milliliter.

$$\frac{\text{Known amount of medication in solution}}{\text{Total volume of diluent}} = \text{Amount of medication per milliliter}$$

$$\frac{50 \text{ units}}{100 \text{ mL}} = 0.5 \text{ units per milliliter}$$

STEP 2: Calculate milliliters per hour.

$$\frac{\text{Dose per hour desired}}{\text{Concentration per milliliter}} = \text{Infusion rate or milliliters per hour}$$

$$\frac{10 \text{ units}}{0.5 \text{ units/mL}} = 20 \text{ mL per hour}$$

4. The nurse should continue to assess the amount of IV solution in the IV container and monitor the controller to ensure proper functioning of the machine.

B. Pump

1. A pump is different from a controller in that it physically pumps fluids against resistance.
2. Gravity is not a factor in the use of a pump, and the height of the IV solution container is not a critical factor.
3. The flow rate on a pump is set in milliliters per hour.
4. The nurse should continue to assess the amount of IV solution in the IV container and monitor the pump to ensure proper functioning of the machine.

XIV. CALCULATION OF INFUSIONS ORDERED BY UNIT DOSAGE PER HOUR (BOX 17-11)

A. The most common medications that will be ordered by **unit** dosage per hour and run by continuous infusion are heparin sodium and regular insulin.

B. Calculation of these infusions can be done by a two-step process:

1. Determine the amount of medication per 1 mL.
2. Determine the infusion rate or milliliters per hour.

PRACTICE QUESTIONS

1. A physician orders 1000 mL of normal saline (NS) to infuse over 12 hours. The drop factor is 15 drops per 1 mL. A nurse prepares to set the flow rate at how many drops per minute?
   1. 15 drops per minute
   2. 17 drops per minute
   3. 21 drops per minute
   4. 23 drops per minute

2. A physician orders an intravenous (IV) dose of 400,000 units of penicillin G benzathine (Bicillin). The label on the 10-mL ampule sent from the pharmacy reads penicillin G benzathine (Bicillin), 300,000 units per milliliter. A nurse prepares how much medication to administer the correct dose?
   1. 1.3 mL
   2. 1.5 mL
   3. 10 mL
   4. 13 mL

3. A physician's order reads potassium chloride 30 mEq to be added to 1000 mL normal saline (NS) and to be administered over a 10-hour period. The label on the medication bottle reads 40 mEq per 20 mL. A nurse prepares how many milliliters of potassium chloride to administer the correct dose of medication?
   1. 10 mL
   2. 15 mL
   3. 20 mL
   4. 50 mL

4. A physician orders 3000 mL of 5% dextrose in water (D_5W) to infuse over a 24-hour period. The drop factor is 10 drops per 1 mL. A nurse sets the flow rate at how many drops per minute?
   1. 15 drops per minute
   2. 17 drops per minute
   3. 21 drops per minute
   4. 24 drops per minute

5. A physician's order reads clindamycin phosphate (Cleocin Phosphate) 0.3 g in 50 mL normal saline (NS) to be administered intravenously over 30 minutes. The medication label reads clindamycin phosphate (Cleocin Phosphate) 900 mg in 6 mL. A nurse prepares how many milliliters of the medication to administer the correct dose?
   1. 1 mL
   2. 2 mL
   3. 3 mL
   4. 5 mL

6. A physician's order reads phenytoin (Dilantin) 0.2 g PO bid. The medication label states 100-mg capsules. A nurse prepares how many capsule(s) to administer one dose?
   1. One capsule
   2. Two capsules
   3. Three capsules
   4. Four capsules

7. A physician orders 1000 mL of ½ normal saline (NS) to infuse over 8 hours. The drop factor is 15 drops per 1 mL. The nurse sets the flow rate at how many drops per minute?
   1. 20 drops per minute
   2. 22 drops per minute
   3. 28 drops per minute
   4. 31 drops per minute

8. A physician orders 2000 mL of 5% dextrose and ½ normal saline (NS) to infuse over 24 hours. The drop factor is 15 drops per 1 mL. A nurse sets the flow rate at how many drops per minute?
   1. 15 drops per minute
   2. 17 drops per minute
   3. 21 drops per minute
   4. 28 drops per minute

9. A physician orders heparin sodium (Liquaemin), 1300 units per hour by continuous intravenous (IV) infusion. The pharmacy prepares the medication and delivers an IV bag labeled heparin sodium (Liquaemin) 20,000 units per 250 mL D_5W. An infusion pump must be used to administer the medication. The nurse sets the infusion pump at how many milliliters per hour to deliver 1300 units per hour?
   1. 12 mL
   2. 16 mL
   3. 20 mL
   4. 22 mL

10. A physician's order reads cyanocobalamin (vitamin B_{12}) 1000 mcg IM. The medication label reads

cyanocobalamin (vitamin B$_{12}$) 0.5 mg/mL. A nurse prepares the medication and administers how many milliliters to the client?
1. 0.5 mL
2. 1 mL
3. 2 mL
4. 3 mL

11. A physician orders 3000 mL of D$_5$W to be administered over a 24-hour period. A nurse determines that how many milliliters per hour will be administered to the client?
1. 50 mL per hour
2. 75 mL per hour
3. 100 mL per hour
4. 125 mL per hour

12. Gentamicin sulfate (Garamycin), 80 mg in 100 mL normal saline (NS), is to be administered over 30 minutes. The drop factor is 10 drops per milliliter. A nurse sets the flow rate at how many drops per minute?
1. 18 drops
2. 23 drops
3. 33 drops
4. 43 drops

13. A physician's order reads levothyroxine (Synthroid), 150 mcg PO daily. The medication label reads Synthroid, 0.1 mg per tablet. A nurse administers how many tablet(s) to the client?
1. 1 tablet
2. 1.5 tablets
3. 2 tablets
4. 2.5 tablets

14. Cefuroxime axetil (Ceftin), 1 g in 50 mL normal saline (NS), is to be administered over 30 minutes. The drop factor is 15 drops per mL. A nurse sets the flow rate at how many drops per minute?
1. 15 drops
2. 25 drops
3. 20 drops
4. 22 drops

15. A physician orders 1000 mL D$_5$W to infuse at a rate of 125 mL per hour. A nurse determines that it will take how many hours for 1 L to infuse?
1. 8 hours
2. 10 hours
3. 12 hours
4. 15 hours

16. A physician orders 500 mL of normal saline (NS) to infuse over 5 hours. The drop factor is 10 drops per 1 mL. A nurse sets the flow rate at how many drops per minute?
1. 15 drops
2. 17 drops

3. 20 drops
4. 22 drops

17. A physician orders 1 unit of packed red blood cells to infuse over 4 hours. The unit of blood contains 250 mL. The drop factor is 10 drops per 1 mL. A nurse prepares to set the flow rate at how many drops per minute?
1. 10 drops
2. 15 drops
3. 17 drops
4. 20 drops

18. A physician orders 3000 mL of normal saline (NS) to infuse over 24 hours. The drop factor is 15 drops per 1 mL. The nurse prepares to set the flow rate at how many drops per minute?
1. 17 drops per minute
2. 20 drops per minute
3. 24 drops per minute
4. 31 drops per minute

19. A physician's order reads morphine sulfate, ⅛ gr IM stat. The medication ampule reads morphine sulfate, 10 mg per mL. A nurse prepares how many milliliters to administer the correct dose?
1. 0.5 mL
2. 0.75 mL
3. 0.85 mL
4. 1.5 mL

20. A physician orders regular insulin, 8 units per hour by continuous intravenous (IV) infusion. The pharmacy prepares the medication and then delivers an IV bag labeled 100 units of regular insulin in 100 mL normal saline (NS). An infusion pump must be used to administer the medication. The nurse sets the infusion pump at how many milliliters per hour to deliver 8 units per hour?
1. 1 mL
2. 4 mL
3. 8 mL
4. 10 mL

CRITICAL THINKING: FILL IN THE BLANK

The physician orders meperidine (Demerol) 60 mg and atropine sulfate ¹/₁₅₀ gr IM for a preoperative client. The medications are compatible and will be mixed into one syringe. The label on the meperidine bottle states 100 mg per mL. The label on the atropine sulfate bottle states 0.4 mg per mL. How many milliliters of meperidine and how many milliliters of atropine sulfate will be prepared for administration?

Answer: _____

ANSWERS

1. 3

Rationale: Use the intravenous (IV) flow rate formula.

Formula:

$$\frac{\text{Total volume} \times \text{Drop factor}}{\text{Time in minutes}} = \text{Drops per minute}$$

$$\frac{1000 \text{ mL} \times 15 \text{ gtt}}{720 \text{ minutes}} = \frac{15,000}{720} = 20.8, \text{ or } 21 \text{ drops per minute}$$

Test-Taking Strategy: Use the formula for calculating IV flow rates when answering the question. Be careful with the multiplication and division. Using the formula carefully will direct you to the correct option. Review IV infusion rates if you had difficulty with this question.

Level of Cognitive Ability: Application
Client Needs: Physiological Integrity
Integrated Process: Nursing Process—planning
Content Area: Fundamental skills
Reference: Potter, P., & Perry, A. (2001). *Fundamentals of nursing* (5th ed., p. 1229). St. Louis: Mosby.

2. 1

Rationale: Use the medication formula.

Formula:

$$\frac{\text{Desired}}{\text{Available}} \times x \text{ mL} = \text{Milliliters per dose}$$

$$\frac{400,000 \text{ units}}{300,000 \text{ units}} \times 1 \text{ mL} = \text{Milliliters per dose}$$

$$\frac{400,000}{300,000} = 1.3 \text{ mL}$$

Test-Taking Strategy: Follow the formula for the calculation of the correct dose. This problem does not require you to perform a conversion. Label each figure, including the answer. Recheck your work, and make sure that the answer makes sense. If you had difficulty with this question, review medication calculation problems.

Level of Cognitive Ability: Application
Client Needs: Physiological Integrity
Integrated Process: Nursing Process—planning
Content Area: Fundamental skills
Reference: Potter, P., & Perry, A. (2001). *Fundamentals of nursing* (5th ed., p. 898). St. Louis: Mosby.

3. 2

Rationale: Use the medication calculation formula.

Formula:

$$\frac{\text{Desired}}{\text{Available}} \times x \text{ mL} = \text{Milliliters per dose}$$

$$\frac{30 \text{ mEq}}{40 \text{ mEq}} \times 20 \text{ mL} = 15 \text{ mL}$$

Test-Taking Strategy: Follow the formula for the calculation of the correct dose. This problem does not require you to perform a conversion. Label each figure, including the answer. Recheck your work, and make sure that the answer makes sense. If you had difficulty with this question, review medication calculation problems.

Level of Cognitive Ability: Application
Client Needs: Physiological Integrity
Integrated Process: Nursing Process—planning
Content Area: Fundamental skills

Reference: Potter, P., & Perry, A. (2001). *Fundamentals of nursing* (5th ed., p. 898). St. Louis: Mosby.

4. 3

Rationale: Use the IV flow rate formula.

Formula:

$$\frac{\text{Total volume} \times \text{Drop factor}}{\text{Time in minutes}} = \text{Drops per minute}$$

$$\frac{3000 \text{ mL} \times 10 \text{ gtt}}{1440 \text{ minutes}} = \frac{30,000}{1440} = 20.8, \text{ or } 21 \text{ drops per minute}$$

Test-Taking Strategy: Use the formula for calculating IV flow rates when answering the question. Be careful with multiplication and division. Using the formula carefully will direct you to the correct option. Review IV infusion rates if you had difficulty with this question.

Level of Cognitive Ability: Application
Client Needs: Physiological Integrity
Integrated Process: Nursing Process—implementation
Content Area: Fundamental skills
Reference: Potter, P., & Perry, A. (2001). *Fundamentals of nursing* (5th ed., p. 1229). St. Louis: Mosby.

5. 2

Rationale: You must convert 0.3 g to milligrams. In the metric system, to convert larger to smaller, multiply by 1000 or move the decimal three places to the right. Therefore, 0.3 g = 300 mg. Following conversion from grams to milligrams, use the formula to calculate the correct dose.

Formula:

$$\frac{\text{Desired}}{\text{Available}} \times x \text{ mL} = \text{Milliliters per dose}$$

$$\frac{300 \text{ mg}}{900 \text{ mg}} \times 6 \text{ mL} = \frac{1800}{900} = 2 \text{ mL}$$

Test-Taking Strategy: In this medication calculation problem, first you must convert grams to milligrams. Next, follow the formula for the calculation of the correct dose. Recheck your work, and make sure that the answer makes sense. If you had difficulty with this question, review medication calculation problems.

Level of Cognitive Ability: Application
Client Needs: Physiological Integrity
Integrated Process: Nursing Process—planning
Content Area: Fundamental skills
Reference: Potter, P., & Perry, A. (2001). *Fundamentals of nursing* (5th ed., p. 898). St. Louis: Mosby.

6. 2

Rationale: You must convert 0.2 g to milligrams. In the metric system, to convert larger to smaller, multiply by 1000 or move the decimal three places to the right. Therefore, 0.2 g equals 200 mg. After conversion from grams to milligrams, use the formula to calculate the correct dose.

Formula:

$$\frac{\text{Desired}}{\text{Available}} \times \text{Capsules} = \text{Capsules per dose}$$

$$\frac{200 \text{ mg}}{100 \text{ mg}} \times 1 \text{ capsule} = 2 \text{ capsules}$$

Test-Taking Strategy: In this medication calculation problem, first you must convert grams to milligrams. Once you have done the conversion and reread the medication calculation problem, you will know that two capsules is the correct answer. Follow the formula for the calculation of the correct dose. Recheck your work, and make sure that the answer makes sense. If you had difficulty with this question, review medication calculation problems.

Level of Cognitive Ability: Application
Client Needs: Physiological Integrity
Integrated Process: Nursing Process—planning
Content Area: Fundamental skills
Reference: Potter, P., & Perry, A. (2001). *Fundamentals of nursing* (5th ed., p. 898). St. Louis: Mosby.

7. **4**
Rationale: Use the IV flow rate formula.
Formula:

$$\frac{\text{Total volume} \times \text{Drop factor}}{\text{Time in minutes}} = \text{Drops per minute}$$

$$\frac{1000 \text{ mL} \times 15 \text{ gtt}}{480 \text{ minutes}} = \frac{15,000}{480} = 31.2, \text{ or } 31 \text{ drops per minute}$$

Test-Taking Strategy: Use the formula for calculating IV flow rates when answering the question. Be careful with the multiplication and division. Using the formula carefully will direct you to the correct option. Review IV infusion rates if you had difficulty with this question.
Level of Cognitive Ability: Application
Client Needs: Physiological Integrity
Integrated Process: Nursing Process—implementation
Content Area: Fundamental skills
Reference: Potter, P., & Perry, A. (2001). *Fundamentals of nursing* (5th ed., p. 1229). St. Louis: Mosby.

8. **3**
Rationale: Use the IV flow rate formula.
Formula:

$$\frac{\text{Total volume} \times \text{Drop factor}}{\text{Time in minutes}} = \text{Drops per minute}$$

$$\frac{2000 \text{ mL} \times 15 \text{ gtt}}{1440 \text{ minutes}} = \frac{30,000}{1440} = 20.8, \text{ or } 21 \text{ drops per minute}$$

Test-Taking Strategy: Use the formula for calculating IV flow rates when answering the question. Be careful with the multiplication and division. Using the formula carefully will direct you to the correct option. Review IV infusion rates if you had difficulty with this question.
Level of Cognitive Ability: Application
Client Needs: Physiological Integrity
Integrated Process: Nursing Process—implementation
Content Area: Fundamental skills
Reference: Potter, P., & Perry, A. (2001). *Fundamentals of nursing* (5th ed., p. 1229). St. Louis: Mosby.

9. **2**
Rationale: Calculation of this problem requires a two-step process. First you need to determine the amount of heparin sodium in 1 mL. The next step is to determine the infusion rate, or milliliters per hour.
Step 1:

$$\frac{\text{Known amount of medication in solution}}{\text{Total volume of diluent}} =$$

Amount of medication per milliliter

$$\frac{20,000 \text{ units}}{250 \text{ mL}} = 80 \text{ units/mL}$$

Step 2:

$$\frac{\text{Dose per hour desired}}{\text{Concentration per milliliter}} =$$

Infusion rate or milliliters per hour

$$\frac{1300 \text{ units}}{80 \text{ units/mL}} = 16.25, \text{ or } 16 \text{ mL per hour}$$

Test-Taking Strategy: Read the question carefully, noting that two steps are required to solve this medication problem. If you had difficulty with this question, learn these steps now. These steps can be used for similar medication problems related to the administration of heparin sodium or regular insulin by IV infusion.
Level of Cognitive Ability: Application
Client Needs: Physiological Integrity
Integrated Process: Nursing Process—implementation
Content Area: Fundamental skills
Reference: Kee, J., & Marshall, S. (2000). *Clinical calculations: With applications to general and specialty areas* (4th ed., pp. 240-241). Philadelphia: W. B. Saunders.

10. **3**
Rationale: You must convert 1000 mcg to milligrams. In the metric system, to convert smaller to larger, divide by 1000 or move the decimal three places to the left. Therefore, 1000 mcg equals 1 mg. Next, use the formula to calculate the correct dose.
Formula:

$$\frac{\text{Desired}}{\text{Available}} \times \text{x mL} = \text{Milliliters per dose}$$

$$\frac{1 \text{ mg}}{0.5 \text{ mg}} \times 1\text{mL} = \frac{1}{0.5} = 2 \text{ mL}$$

Test-Taking Strategy: In this medication calculation problem, first you must convert micrograms to milligrams. Next, follow the formula for the calculation of the correct dose. Label each figure, including the answer. Recheck your work, and make sure that the answer makes sense. If you had difficulty with this question, review medication calculation problems.
Level of Cognitive Ability: Application
Client Needs: Physiological Integrity
Integrated Process: Nursing Process—implementation
Content Area: Fundamental skills
Reference: Potter, P., & Perry, A. (2001). *Fundamentals of nursing* (5th ed., p. 898). St. Louis: Mosby.

11. **4**
Rationale: Use the IV formula to determine milliliters per hour.
Formula:

$$\frac{\text{Total volume in milliliters}}{\text{Number of hours}} = \text{Number of milliliters per hour}$$

$$\frac{3000 \text{ mL}}{24 \text{ hours}} = 125 \text{ mL per hour}$$

Test-Taking Strategy: Read the question carefully, noting that the question is asking about milliliters per hour to be administered to the client. Use the formula for calculating milliliters per hour to direct you to the correct option. Review the IV formula for calculating milliliters per hour if you had difficulty with this question.
Level of Cognitive Ability: Comprehension
Client Needs: Physiological Integrity

Integrated Process: Nursing Process—planning
Content Area: Fundamental skills
Reference: Potter, P., & Perry, A. (2001). *Fundamentals of nursing* (5th ed., p. 1229). St. Louis: Mosby.

12. 3
Rationale: Use the IV flow rate formula.
Formula:

$$\frac{\text{Total volume} \times \text{Drop factor}}{\text{Time in minutes}} = \text{Drops per minute}$$

$$\frac{100 \text{ mL} \times 10 \text{ gtt}}{30 \text{ minutes}} = \frac{1000}{30} = 33.3, \text{ or } 33 \text{ drops per minute}$$

Test-Taking Strategy: Use the formula for calculating IV flow rates when answering the question. Be careful with the multiplication and division. Using the formula carefully will direct you to the correct option. Review IV infusion rates if you had difficulty with this question.
Level of Cognitive Ability: Application
Client Needs: Physiological Integrity
Integrated Process: Nursing Process—implementation
Content Area: Fundamental skills
Reference: Potter, P., & Perry, A. (2001). *Fundamentals of nursing* (5th ed., p. 1229). St. Louis: Mosby.

13. 2
Rationale: You must convert 150 mcg to milligrams. In the metric system, to convert smaller to larger, divide by 1000 or move the decimal three places to the left. Therefore 150 mcg equals 0.15 mg. Next, use the formula to calculate the correct dose.
Formula:

$$\frac{\text{Desired}}{\text{Available}} \times \text{Tablet} = \text{Tablets per dose}$$

$$\frac{0.15 \text{ mg}}{0.1 \text{ mg}} \times 1 \text{ tablet} = 1.5 \text{ tablets}$$

Test-Taking Strategy: In this medication calculation problem, first you must convert micrograms to milligrams. Next, follow the formula for the calculation of the correct dose. Label each figure, including the answer. Recheck your work, and make sure that the answer makes sense. If you had difficulty with this question, review medication calculation problems.
Level of Cognitive Ability: Application
Client Needs: Physiological Integrity
Integrated Process: Nursing Process—implementation
Content Area: Fundamental skills
Reference: Potter, P., & Perry, A. (2001). *Fundamentals of nursing* (5th ed., p. 898). St. Louis: Mosby.

14. 2
Rationale: Use the IV flow rate formula.
Formula:

$$\frac{\text{Total volume} \times \text{Drop factor}}{\text{Time in minutes}} = \text{Drops per minute}$$

$$\frac{50 \text{ mL} \times 15 \text{ gtt}}{30 \text{ minutes}} = \frac{750}{30} = 25 \text{ drops per minute}$$

Test-Taking Strategy: Use the formula for calculating IV flow rates when answering the question. Be careful with the multiplication and division. Using the formula carefully will direct you to the correct option. Review IV infusion rates if you had difficulty with this question.

Level of Cognitive Ability: Application
Client Needs: Physiological Integrity
Integrated Process: Nursing Process—implementation
Content Area: Fundamental skills
Reference: Potter, P., & Perry, A. (2001). *Fundamentals of nursing* (5th ed., p. 1229). St. Louis: Mosby.

15. 1
Rationale: You must determine that 1 L equals 1000 mL. Next, use the formula for determining infusion time in hours.
Formula:

$$\frac{\text{Total volume to infuse}}{\text{Milliliters per hour being infused}} = \text{Infusion time}$$

$$\frac{1000 \text{ mL}}{125 \text{ mL}} = 8 \text{ hours}$$

Test-Taking Strategy: Read the question carefully, noting that the question is asking about infusion time in hours. First, convert 1 L to milliliters. Next, use the formula for determining infusion time in hours. Review the IV formula for calculating infusion time if you had difficulty with this question.
Level of Cognitive Ability: Comprehension
Client Needs: Physiological Integrity
Integrated Process: Nursing Process—planning
Content Area: Fundamental skills
Reference: Potter, P., & Perry, A. (2001). *Fundamentals of nursing* (5th ed., p. 1229). St. Louis: Mosby.

16. 2
Rationale: Use the IV flow rate formula.
Formula:

$$\frac{\text{Total volume} \times \text{Drop factor}}{\text{Time in minutes}} = \text{Drops per minute}$$

$$\frac{500 \text{ mL} \times 10 \text{ gtt}}{300 \text{ minutes}} = \frac{5000}{300} = 16.6, \text{ or } 17 \text{ drops per minute}$$

Test-Taking Strategy: Use the formula for calculating IV flow rates when answering the question. Be careful with the multiplication and division. Using the formula carefully will direct you to the correct option. Review IV infusion rates if you had difficulty with this question.
Level of Cognitive Ability: Application
Client Needs: Physiological Integrity
Integrated Process: Nursing Process—implementation
Content Area: Fundamental skills
Reference: Potter, P., & Perry, A. (2001). *Fundamentals of nursing* (5th ed., p. 1229). St. Louis: Mosby.

17. 1
Rationale: Use the IV flow rate formula.
Formula:

$$\frac{\text{Total volume} \times \text{Drop factor}}{\text{Time in minutes}} = \text{Drops per minute}$$

$$\frac{250 \text{ mL} \times 10 \text{ gtt}}{240 \text{ minutes}} = \frac{2,500}{240} = 10.4, \text{ or } 10 \text{ drops per minute}$$

Test-Taking Strategy: Use the formula for calculating IV flow rates when answering the question. Be careful with the multiplication and division. Using the formula carefully will direct you to the correct option. Review IV infusion rates if you had difficulty with this question.
Level of Cognitive Ability: Application
Client Needs: Physiological Integrity
Integrated Process: Nursing Process—planning

Content Area: Fundamental skills
Reference: Potter, P., & Perry, A. (2001). *Fundamentals of nursing* (5th ed., p. 1229). St. Louis: Mosby.

18. **4**

Rationale: Use the IV flow rate formula.
Formula:

$$\frac{\text{Total volume} \times \text{Drop factor}}{\text{Time in minutes}} = \text{Drops per minute}$$

$$\frac{3000 \text{ mL} \times 15 \text{ gtt}}{1440 \text{ minutes}} = \frac{45,000}{1440} = 31.2, \text{ or } 31 \text{ drops per minute}$$

Test-Taking Strategy: Use the formula for calculating IV flow rates when answering the question. Be careful with the multiplication and division. Using the formula carefully will direct you to the correct option. Review IV infusion rates if you had difficulty with this question.
Level of Cognitive Ability: Application
Client Needs: Physiological Integrity
Integrated Process: Nursing Process—planning
Content Area: Fundamental skills
Reference: Potter, P., & Perry, A. (2001). *Fundamentals of nursing* (5th ed., p. 1229). St. Louis: Mosby.

19. **2**

Rationale: You must convert $\frac{1}{8}$ gr to milligrams. After converting grains to milligrams, use the formula to calculate the correct dose.
Conversion:
60 mg: 1 gr :: x mg : $\frac{1}{8}$ gr
1x = 1/8 × 60/1
x = 60/8 = 7.5 mg
Formula:

$$\frac{\text{Desired}}{\text{Available}} \times x \text{ mL} = \text{Milliliters per dose}$$

$$\frac{7.5 \text{ mg}}{10 \text{ mg}} \times 1 \text{ mL} = 0.75 \text{ mL}$$

Test-Taking Strategy: In this medication calculation problem, first you must convert grains to milligrams. Next, follow the formula for the calculation of the correct dose. Label each figure, including the answer. Recheck your work, and make sure that the answer makes sense. If you had difficulty with this question, review medication calculation problems.
Level of Cognitive Ability: Application
Client Needs: Physiological Integrity
Integrated Process: Nursing Process—planning
Content Area: Fundamental skills
Reference: Potter, P., & Perry, A. (2001). *Fundamentals of nursing* (5th ed., p. 898). St. Louis: Mosby.

20. **3**

Rationale: Calculation of this problem requires a two-step process. First you need to determine the amount of regular insulin in 1 mL. The next step is to determine the infusion rate, or milliliters per hour.
Formula:
Step 1

$$\frac{\text{Known amount of medication in solution}}{\text{Total volume of diluent}} =$$

Amount of medication per milliliter

$$\frac{100 \text{ units}}{100 \text{ mL}} = 1 \text{ unit/mL}$$

Step 2

$$\frac{\text{Dose per hour desired}}{\text{Concentration per milliliter}} =$$

Infusion rate or milliliters per hour

$$\frac{8 \text{ units}}{1 \text{ unit/mL}} = 8 \text{ mL per hour}$$

Test-Taking Strategy: Read the question carefully, noting that two steps are required to solve this medication problem. If you had difficulty with this question, learn these steps now. These steps can be used for similar medication problems related to the administration of heparin sodium or regular insulin by IV infusion.
Level of Cognitive Ability: Application
Client Needs: Physiological Integrity
Integrated Process: Nursing Process—implementation
Content Area: Fundamental skills
Reference: Kee, J., & Marshall, S. (2000). *Clinical calculations: With applications to general and specialty areas* (4th ed., pp. 240-241). Philadelphia: W. B. Saunders.

CRITICAL THINKING: FILL IN THE BLANK

Answer: Meperidine (Demerol), 0.6 mL; atropine sulfate, 1 mL
Rationale: Use the formula for calculating the milliliters of meperidine to be administered. Next, convert atropine sulfate $\frac{1}{150}$ gr to milligrams. After converting grains to milligrams, use the formula to calculate the correct dose.
Meperidine (Demerol)
Formula:

$$\frac{\text{Desired}}{\text{Available}} \times x \text{ mL} = \text{Milliliters per dose}$$

$$\frac{60 \text{ mg}}{100 \text{ mg}} \times 1 \text{ mL} = 0.6 \text{ mL}$$

Atropine Sulfate
Conversion:
60 mg : 1 gr :: x mg : $\frac{1}{150}$ gr
1x = 1/150 × 60/1
x = 60/150 = 0.4 mg
Formula:

$$\frac{\text{Desired}}{\text{Available}} \times x \text{ mL} = \text{Milliliters per dose}$$

$$\frac{0.4 \text{ mg}}{0.4 \text{ mg}} \times 1 \text{ mL} = 1 \text{ mL}$$

Test-Taking Strategy: This medication calculation requires determining the milliliters to be administered for two medications, meperidine (Demerol) and atropine sulfate. First, calculate the milliliters for the meperidine. To calculate the milliliters of atropine sulfate to be administered, first you must convert grains to milligrams. Next, follow the formula for the calculation of the correct dose. Label each figure, including the answer. Recheck your work, and make sure that the answer makes sense. If you had difficulty with this question, review medication calculation problems.
Level of Cognitive Ability: Application
Client Needs: Physiological Integrity
Integrated Process: Nursing Process—implementation
Content Area: Fundamental skills
Reference: Kee, J., & Marshall, S. (2000). *Clinical calculations: With applications to general and specialty areas* (4th ed., p. 158). Philadelphia: W. B. Saunders.

REFERENCES

Kee, J., & Marshall, S. (2000). *Clinical calculations: With applications to general and specialty areas* (4th ed.). Philadelphia: W. B. Saunders.

National Council of State Boards of Nursing (Eds.). (2003). *Test Plan for the National Council Licensure Examination for Registered Nurses* (effective date: April 2004). Chicago: Author.

Potter, P., & Perry, A. (2001). *Fundamentals of nursing* (5th ed.). St. Louis: Mosby.

Basic Life Support

PYRAMID TERMS

automated external defibrillator (AED) Machine that converts ventricular fibrillation into a perfusing rhythm and allows for early defibrillation by first responders.

basic life support (BLS) Provision of oxygen to the brain, heart, and other vital organs until help arrives.

cardiopulmonary resuscitation (CPR) An interchangeable term for basic life support.

head tilt–chin lift Preferred method to open a victim's airway.

Heimlich maneuver Method to relieve a foreign body airway obstruction.

jaw thrust maneuver Method used to open a victim's airway if a neck injury is suspected.

▲ THE PYRAMID TO SUCCESS

The Pyramid to Success focuses on the emergency measures related to performing basic life support measures. Focus on the points related to the breaths and compression ratio with one-person and two-person adult cardiopulmonary resuscitation (CPR) and CPR in the infant and the child. Pyramid Points focus on airway management in CPR and on performing the Heimlich maneuver to relieve a foreign body airway obstruction. Focus on the correct hand placements for cardiac compressions and on the differences between the adult, the child, and the infant. Remember, before initiating CPR, the initial action is to determine unresponsiveness. Remember the ABCDs—airway, breathing, circulation, and defibrillation or definitive treatment—when performing CPR. The Integrated Processes addressed in this chapter include Nursing Process, Caring, Communication and Documentation, and Teaching/Learning.

CLIENT NEEDS ▲
Safe, Effective Care Environment

Advanced directives regarding the client's documented requests
Advocacy regarding the client's wishes
Client rights
Establishing priorities
Ethical and legal responsibilities
Standard, transmission-based, and other precautions

Health Promotion and Maintenance

Health promotion programs
Teaching significant others to perform CPR and the Heimlich maneuver
Techniques of physical assessment

Psychosocial Integrity

Cultural diversity
End-of-life issues
Emotional support to significant others
Grief and loss
Religious and spiritual influences
Therapeutic communications

Physiological Integrity

Alterations in cardiopulmonary system
Handling of medical emergencies
Performing CPR or the Heimlich maneuver
Use of special equipment
Administration of emergency medications and intravenous solutions
Documentation of response to basic life support measures

I. BASIC LIFE SUPPORT (BLS) (BOX 18-1)

A. **Basic life support** is provision of oxygen to the brain, heart, and other vital organs until help arrives.

B. Basic life support also is known as **cardiopulmonary resuscitation**.

II. ADULT BLS

A. Description: An adult can be defined as a person who is 8 years of age or older.

B. Airway

1. Remember that assessment is the first step of the nursing process; assessing a victim of sudden illness or accident for unconsciousness is the initial action; assess for 5 to 10 seconds.

2. Gently shake the victim's shoulders and ask "Are you OK?"; be alert to the potential for a head or neck injury.

3. Activate emergency medical system (EMS): "phone first" for children 8 years of age or older and adults; "phone last" for children less than 8 years old.

4. Place the victim in a supine position on a firm, flat surface (logroll the victim, using spine precautions).

   a. One-person rescue: The rescuer is positioned on his or her knees, perpendicular to victim's sternum and facing the victim.

   b. Two-person rescue: One rescuer faces the victim, kneeling perpendicular to victim's head; the second rescuer moves to the opposite side and faces the victim, kneeling perpendicular to the victim's sternum.

   c. The rescuers apply gloves and face shields, if available.

5. Open the airway.

6. The **head tilt–chin lift** is the preferred method for opening the airway; if the victim has a neck injury, one uses the **jaw thrust maneuver** to open the airway.

7. Look for any foreign material, liquids, or solids in the victim's mouth; wipe out any foreign material with a hooked index or middle finger.

C. Breathing

1. Assess breathing and maintain an open airway.

2. The rescuer places his or her ear over the victim's nose and mouth and looks for the chest to rise and fall, listens for air moving in and out of the lungs, and feels for the flow of air.

3. For the breathing victim, do the following:

   a. Place victim on side if no cervical trauma is suspected; logroll victim onto side as a unit (without twisting) to help maintain an open airway and decrease the risk of aspiration.

   b. If trauma or injury is suspected, do not move the victim.

4. For the nonbreathing victim, do the following:

   a. Maintain the **head tilt–chin lift**; pinch the nostrils closed, and give two, slow full ventilations (breaths) of 2 seconds per breath (use a resuscitation bag or face shield if available, ensuring an adequate air seal); allow victim to exhale between breaths.

   b. Give 10 to 12 ventilations per minute.

   c. If unsuccessful at giving the breath or ventilation, reposition the victim's head and try again (improper chin and head position is the most common cause of difficulty in ventilating the victim).

   d. If still unsuccessful, check the victim's mouth for a foreign body or for loose dentures (remove dentures only if they interfere with the mouth seal), clear the airway, and try to ventilate again.

   e. Be alert to gastric distention when giving ventilations.

5. Mouth to nose: This method is recommended when ventilating through the victim's mouth is impossible, the mouth cannot be opened, the mouth is seriously injured, or a tight mouth-to-mouth seal is difficult to achieve.

6. Mouth to stoma: This method is used for the victim who has had a laryngectomy or has a temporary tracheostomy; to be effective, an adequate seal over the victim's mouth and nose is necessary.

D. Circulation

1. Assess circulation; always check for the absence of a pulse before beginning chest compressions on the victim.

2. Maintain an open airway and palpate for a carotid pulse for 5 to 10 seconds.

3. If there is a pulse, continue to give 10 to 12 ventilations per minute.

4. Recheck the pulse after 1 minute; if there is no pulse, start chest compressions.

E. Chest compressions

1. Hand placement

   a. Correct hand placement for chest compressions is crucial.

   b. Hand placement is on the lower half of the sternum.

   c. With the hand closest to the victim's feet, locate the lower margin of the rib cage.

   d. Move the fingertips along the margin to the notch where the ribs meet the sternum.

BOX 18-1

The ABCDs of Basic Life Support

A: Airway
B: Breathing
C: Circulation
D: Defibrillation or definitive treatment
Each step of the ABCDs of basic life support begins with assessment.

e. Place the middle finger on the notch and the index finger next to middle finger

f. Place the heel of the opposite hand next to the index finger, and place the other hand on top.

2. Complications of chest compressions
   a. Laceration of internal organs
   b. Punctured lungs
   c. Fractured ribs or sternum

III. ADULT ONE-PERSON BLS

A. The ratio is 15:2; that is, 15 compressions at a rate of 100 per minute and at a depth of 1.5 to 2 inches, and 2 ventilations at 2 seconds per breath.

B. Perform four complete cycles and then reassess the victim.

C. Check the carotid pulse after the first four cycles of **CPR** and every few minutes thereafter; if you feel no pulse, continue **CPR**.

IV. ADULT TWO-PERSON BLS

A. The ratio is 15:2, the same as adult one-person **BLS**.

B. One person is at the victim's side performing chest compressions; one person is at the victim's head, maintaining an open airway, monitoring the carotid pulse, and doing the rescue breathing.

C. When the second rescuer arrives at the scene, that rescuer must identify himself or herself and tell the first rescuer that he or she knows two-person **CPR**.

D. The second rescuer then activates the EMS, if this has not been done, and then returns to the scene to help.

E. The second rescuer can perform one-person **CPR** if the first rescuer is fatigued; or, the first rescuer finishes 15 compressions, gives 2 ventilations, moves to the head, opens the airway, and checks the carotid pulse.

F. If there is no pulse, the first rescuer announces "No pulse, continue **CPR**."

G. The second rescuer locates the landmark for chest compressions.

H. The two rescuers begin **CPR** at a ratio of 15 compressions to 2 ventilations.

I. At the end of 1 minute, the ventilator checks for a pulse and checks for breathing; if there is none, the ventilator says "No pulse, continue **CPR**."

J. When the compressor becomes tired, the compressor should change positions with minimal interruption of chest compressions.

K. The rescuer ventilating the victim assumes responsibility for monitoring for signs of circulation and breathing.

V. PEDIATRIC DIFFERENCES

A. Description
   1. A child can be defined as a person between 1 and 8 years of age.
   2. An infant can be defined as a person under 1 year of age.

B. Airway: Assess unresponsiveness.

C. Breathing
   1. Breathing victim: Keep the airway open.
   2. Nonbreathing victim
      a. Give two ventilations at 1 to 1½ seconds per breath.
      b. With the infant, provide ventilations by mouth to mouth and nose.
      c. With the larger child, provide ventilations by mouth to mouth.
      d. With the infant or the child, give 20 ventilations per minute.
      e. Activate the EMS as soon as possible.

D. Circulation
   1. Assess circulation.
   2. If the victim is older than 1 year, assess circulation via the carotid pulse.
   3. If the victim is younger than 1 year, assess circulation via the brachial pulse.
   4. The ratio is five compressions to one ventilation.
   5. Reassess every few minutes.
   6. For infant chest compressions, do the following:
      a. Locate the imaginary line between the nipples over the breastbone (sternum).
      b. Place the index finger of the hand farthest from the infant's head just under the intermammary line where it intersects the sternum.
      c. The area of compression is one fingerwidth below this intersection, at the location of the middle and ring fingers.
      d. Using two or three fingers, compress the breastbone ½ to 1 inch at least 100 times per minute.
      e. The two-thumb encircling hands technique is the preferred two-rescuer technique.
   7. For chest compressions for a child, do the following:
      a. The location for hand placement is the same as for an adult.
      b. Depress the chest 1 to 1½ inches at 100 times per minute with the heel of one hand.

VI. FOREIGN BODY AIRWAY OBSTRUCTION

A. Conscious adult
   1. Ask the victim, "Are you choking?" (the victim will not be able to speak or cough if he or she is choking).
   2. If the victim's airway is obstructed partially, a crowing sound is audible; encourage the victim to cough.
   3. Relieve the obstruction by the **Heimlich maneuver** (Box 18-2).
   4. Continue abdominal thrusts until the object is dislodged or the victim becomes unconscious.

B. Unconscious adult
   1. Assess unconsciousness.
   2. Call for help; activate the EMS as soon as possible.
   3. Perform tongue-jaw lift technique; fingersweep to remove the object.

BOX 18-2

Heimlich Maneuver

Stand behind the victim.
Place arms around the victim's waist.
Make a fist.
Place the thumb side of the fist just above the umbilicus (belly button) and well below the xiphoid process.
Perform five quick in and up thrusts (between the umbilicus and the xiphoid process).
Use chest thrusts for the obese or for the advanced pregnancy victim.

4. Open the airway.
5. Attempt ventilation.
6. Reposition the head if unsuccessful; reattempt ventilation.
7. Relieve the obstruction by the **Heimlich maneuver** with five thrusts; then fingersweep the mouth.
8. To perform the **Heimlich maneuver**, straddle the victim's thighs, place the heel of one hand on top of the other between umbilicus and xiphoid process, and give five thrusts in and up with the heel of the bottom hand.
9. Reattempt ventilation.
10. Repeat the sequence of tongue-jaw lift, fingersweep, breaths, and **Heimlich maneuver** until successful.
11. Be sure to assess the victim's pulse and respirations.
12. Perform **CPR** if required.

C. Choking child or infant
1. Choking is suspected in infants and children experiencing acute respiratory distress associated with coughing, gagging, or stridor (high-pitched noisy breathing).
2. Allow the victim to continue to cough if the cough is forceful.
3. If the cough is ineffective or the victim develops increased respiratory difficulty accompanied by a high-pitched noise while inhaling, help is needed.
4. For the conscious child, do the following:
   a. Assess for obstruction by asking the child, "Are you choking?"
   b. Relieve the obstruction by the **Heimlich maneuver** until the obstruction is dislodged or the child becomes unconscious.
5. For the unconscious child, do the following:
   a. Assess unconsciousness.
   b. Open the airway by the tongue-jaw lift.
   c. Check for breathing and look for a foreign object.
   d. Attempt ventilation.
   e. If unsuccessful, reposition the head; reattempt ventilation.
   f. Relieve the obstruction by using the **Heimlich maneuver**, giving five abdominal thrusts, and fingersweep the mouth only if the object is visible.

g. Assess the airway for a foreign object and reattempt ventilation.
h. Repeat the sequence.
i. Assess pulse and respirations and perform **CPR** if required.
6. For the conscious infant, do the following:
   a. Assess for obstruction and note breathing problems.
   b. Relieve the obstruction by five back blows and five chest thrusts.
   c. Straddle the infant over the arm, place the infant's head lower than the trunk, and support the head firmly, holding the jaw.
   d. Give five back blows with the heel of the hand between the shoulder blades.
   e. Turn the infant; place the head lower than the trunk.
   f. Give five chest thrusts at the same location as for chest compressions.
   g. Check for the object and remove if visible.
   h. Avoid blind fingersweeps in infants and small children because the object may be pushed back farther into the airway, causing further obstruction.
   i. Continue until the object is removed or the infant becomes unconscious.
7. For the unconscious infant, do the following:
   a. Assess unconsciousness by gentle taps.
   b. Open the airway by the tongue-jaw lift.
   c. Check for breathing and look for a foreign object.
   d. Attempt ventilation.
   e. Reposition the head if unsuccessful; reattempt ventilation.
   f. Relieve the obstruction by five back blows and five chest thrusts.
   g. Fingersweep the mouth only if the object is visible.
   h. Reattempt ventilation and repeat the sequence.
   i. Activate the EMS after 1 minute of unresponsiveness.
   j. Perform **CPR** if required.

VII. PREGNANT OR OBESE VICTIM
A. **Heimlich maneuver** and relieving a foreign body airway obstruction.
1. Place arms under the woman's axilla and across the chest.
2. Place the thumb side of a clenched fist against the middle of the sternum, and place the other hand over the fist.
3. Perform backward chest thrusts until the foreign body is expelled or until the woman becomes unconscious.
4. If she becomes unconscious, place her on her back; a wedge, such as a pillow or rolled blanket, should be placed under the right abdominal flank

BOX 18-3

Pyramid Points

Do not interrupt cardiopulmonary resuscitation (CPR) for more than 5 seconds.
STOP CPR ONLY IF THE FOLLOWING OCCURS:
Pulse and respiration return.
Emergency medical help arrives.
To administer the automated external defibrillator.
A physician declares the victim deceased.
Additional Pyramid Point: In a non–health care setting, another indication to stop CPR would be that the rescuer was exhausted and physically unable to continue to perform CPR.

and hip to displace the uterus to the left side of the abdomen.

5. If unable to ventilate, position the hands as for chest compressions and deliver chest thrusts firmly to remove the obstruction.

B. Defibrillation in the pregnant client: If defibrillation is needed, place the paddles one rib interspace higher than usual because the heart is displaced slightly by the enlarged uterus.

VIII. AUTOMATED EXTERNAL DEFIBRILLATOR (AED)

A. Description
  1. The **automated external defibrillator** is used to convert ventricular fibrillation into a perfusing rhythm.
  2. The **AED** differentiates nonventricular fibrillation rhythms and allows for early defibrillation by first responders.
  3. Use of an **AED** is not recommended on a child who is less than 8 years of age or a child who weighs less than 25 kg.
B. Interventions
  1. Attach **AED** leads to the victim.
  2. Turn on the **AED** and push the button to activate the analyzer.
  3. Follow instructions given for the **AED**, usually to "assess," "stand back," "shock," and "reassess."
  4. Evaluate for return of the pulse, and if the victim is pulseless, repeat defibrillation as directed up to 3 times; if defibrillation is still ineffective, perform **CPR** for 1 minute, and then deliver another series of three shocks (Box 18-3).

PRACTICE QUESTIONS

1. A nurse on the day shift walks into a client's room and finds the client unresponsive. The client is not breathing and does not have a pulse, and the nurse immediately calls out for help. The next nursing action is which of the following?
   1. Ventilate with a mouth-to-mask device.
   2. Start chest compressions.
   3. Give the client oxygen.
   4. Open the airway.
2. A nurse is performing cardiopulmonary resuscitation (CPR) on an adult client. When performing chest compressions, the nurse understands that correct hand placement is located over the
   1. Lower third of the sternum.
   2. Upper half of the sternum.
   3. Upper third of the sternum.
   4. Lower half of the sternum.
3. A nurse witnesses a neighbor's husband sustain a fall from the roof of his house. The nurse rushes to the victim and determines the need to open the airway. The nurse opens the airway in this victim by using which most appropriate method?
   1. Head tilt–chin lift
   2. Flexed position
   3. Modified head tilt–chin lift
   4. Jaw thrust maneuver
4. A nurse is preparing to attempt to relieve an airway obstruction on a 3-year-old conscious child. The nurse performs this maneuver by placing the hands between the
   1. Umbilicus and the groin.
   2. Groin and the abdomen.
   3. Umbilicus and the xiphoid process.
   4. Lower abdomen and the chest.
5. A nurse is performing BLS on a 7-year-old child. The nurse delivers how many breaths per minute to the child?
   1. 12
   2. 16
   3. 18
   4. 20
6. A nurse is performing cardiopulmonary resuscitation (CPR) on an infant. When performing chest compressions, the nurse understands that the compression rate is at least
   1. 60 times per minute.
   2. 80 times per minute.
   3. 100 times per minute.
   4. 160 times per minute.
7. A nursing instructor teaches a group of students about basic life support (BLS). The instructor asks a student to identify the most appropriate location to assess the pulse of an infant under 1 year of age. Which of the following, if stated by the student, would indicate that the student understands the appropriate assessment procedure?
   1. Brachial
   2. Carotid
   3. Popliteal
   4. Radial
8. A nurse is teaching cardiopulmonary resuscitation (CPR) to a group of community members. The nurse

asks a member of the group to describe the reason why blind fingersweeps are avoided in infants. The nurse determines that the person understands this reason if the person makes which statement?

1. "The object may be forced back farther into the throat."
2. "The mouth is too small to see the object."
3. "The object may have been swallowed."
4. "The infant may bite down on the finger"

9. A nurse is performing cardiopulmonary resuscitation (CPR) on an adult client. The nurse understands that when performing chest compressions, one should depress the sternum

1. ½ to ¾ inch.
2. ¾ to 1 inch.
3. 1½ to 2 inches.
4. 2½ to 3 inches.

10. A nursing instructor asks a nursing student to describe the procedure for performing the Heimlich maneuver on an unconscious pregnant woman at 8 months' gestation. The student describes the procedure correctly if the student states to

1. Perform abdominal thrusts until the object is dislodged.
2. Place the hands in the pelvis to perform the thrusts.
3. Place a rolled blanket under the right abdominal flank and hip area.
4. Perform left lateral abdominal thrusts until the object is dislodged.

CRITICAL THINKING: FILL IN THE BLANK

A nurse is using an automated external defibrillator (AED) on a victim who collapsed while shopping at a local mall. The nurse follows the instructions on the AED and repeats the defibrillation 3 times as directed. The defibrillation attempts are unsuccessful. What is the nurse's next action while waiting for emergency medical services to arrive?

Answer: _____

ANSWERS

1. **4**

Rationale: The next nursing action would be to open the airway. Ventilation cannot be initiated unless the airway is opened. One starts chest compressions after opening the airway and intiating ventilation. Oxygen may be helpful at some point, but the airway is opened first.

Test-Taking Strategy: Visualize the steps of basic life support (BLS) to answer the question. Recalling the ABCDs—airway, breathing, circulation, defibrillation or definitive treatment—will assist in directing you to option 4. Review the steps of BLS if you had difficulty with this question.

Level of Cognitive Ability: Application
Client Needs: Physiological Integrity
Integrated Process: Nursing Process—implementation
Content Area: Delegating/Prioritizing
Reference: Potter, P., & Perry, A. (2001). *Fundamentals of nursing* (5th ed., p. 1184). St. Louis: Mosby.

2. **4**

Rationale: Determine proper hand placement for chest compressions by locating the notch where the rib margin meets the sternum and placing the middle finger on this notch and the index finger next to it. Then place the heel of the opposite hand on the lower half of the sternum close to the index finger. Remove the first hand and place it on top of the hand on the sternum, and begin chest compressions. This location is the lower half of the sternum.

Test-Taking Strategy: Use the process of elimination. Eliminate options 2 and 3 first because these locations would be ineffective. From the remaining options, visualizing the procedure and considering the anatomical location of the heart will direct you to option 4. If you had difficulty with this question, review the landmarks for chest compressions.

Level of Cognitive Ability: Application
Client Needs: Physiological Integrity

Integrated Process: Nursing Process—implementation
Content Area: Adult health—cardiovascular
Reference: Potter, P., & Perry, A. (2001). *Fundamentals of nursing* (5th ed., pp. 1184-1187). St. Louis: Mosby.

3. **4**

Rationale: If a neck injury is suspected, the jaw thrust maneuver is used to open the airway. The head tilt–chin lift produces hyperextension of the neck and could cause complications if a neck injury is present. A flexed position is an inappropriate position for opening the airway.

Test-Taking Strategy: Use the process of elimination. Eliminate options 1 and 3 first because they are similar. Next, eliminate option 2 because this position would not open the airway. If you had difficulty with this question, review the appropriate methods to open an airway.

Level of Cognitive Ability: Application
Client Needs: Physiological Integrity
Integrated Process: Nursing Process—implementation
Content Area: Adult health—neurological
Reference: Potter, P., & Perry, A. (2001). *Fundamentals of nursing* (5th ed., p. 1185). St. Louis: Mosby.

4. **3**

Rationale: To perform the Heimlich maneuver on a child, the rescuer stands behind the victim and places the arms directly under the victim's axillas and around the victim. The rescuer places the thumb side of one fist against the victim's abdomen in the midline slightly above the umbilicus and well below the tip of the xiphoid process. The rescuer grasps the fist with the other hand and delivers up to five thrusts. One must take care not to touch the xiphoid process or the lower margins of the rib cage because force applied to these structures may damage internal organs.

Test-Taking Strategy: Use the process of elimination, noting the age of the child. Eliminate options 1 and 2 first because

they are similar. From the remaining options, considering the anatomical location and the effect of the maneuver in dislodging an obstruction will direct you to option 3. If you had difficulty with this question, review the correct hand placement for the Heimlich maneuver.
Level of Cognitive Ability: Application
Client Needs: Physiological Integrity
Integrated Process: Nursing Process—implementation
Content Area: Child health
Reference: Wong, D., Perry, S., & Hockenberry, M. (2002). *Maternal child nursing care* (2nd ed., p. 1229). St. Louis: Mosby.

5. **4**
*Rationale:*In a child between the ages of 1 and 8 years, 20 breaths per minute are delivered. Options 1, 2, and 3 are incorrect.
Test-Taking Strategy: Use the process of elimination and note the age of the child. Recalling the normal respiratory rate in a child at this age will assist in directing you to option 4. If you had difficulty with this question, review BLS for a child.
Level of Cognitive Ability: Application
Client Needs: Physiological Integrity
Integrated Process: Nursing Process—implementation
Content Area: Child health
Reference: Potter, P., & Perry, A. (2001). *Fundamentals of nursing* (5th ed., p. 1188). St. Louis: Mosby.

6. **3**
Rationale: In an infant the rate of chest compressions is at least 100 times per minute. Options 1 and 2 identify rates that are too low, and option 4 identifies a rate that is too high.
Test-Taking Strategy: Use the process of elimination, considering the normal heart rate of an infant. Eliminate options 1 and 2 because of the low rates identified in the options. Eliminate option 4 because this rate would be much too rapid for an infant. If you had difficulty with this question, review CPR for an infant.
Level of Cognitive Ability: Application
Client Needs: Physiological Integrity
Integrated Process: Nursing Process—implementation
Content Area: Child health
Reference: Potter, P., & Perry, A. (2001). *Fundamentals of nursing* (5th ed., p. 1188). St. Louis: Mosby.

7. **1**
Rationale: To assess a pulse in an infant (under 1 year of age), check the pulse at the brachial artery. The infant's relatively short, fat neck makes palpation of the carotid artery difficult. The popliteal and radial pulses are also difficult to palpate in an infant.
Test-Taking Strategy: Use the process of elimination and knowledge regarding circulatory assessment in an infant. Considering the body structure of an infant will assist in directing you to option 1. Review cardiac assessment and BLS for an infant if you had difficulty with this question.
Level of Cognitive Ability: Analysis
Client Needs: Physiological Integrity
Integrated Process: Teaching/Learning
Content Area: Child health

Reference: Potter, P., & Perry, A. (2001). *Fundamentals of nursing* (5th ed., p. 1188). St. Louis: Mosby.

8. **1**
Rationale: Blind fingersweeps are not recommended for infants and children because of the risk of forcing the object farther down into the airway. Options 2, 3, and 4 are not related directly to the issue of the question.
Test-Taking Strategy: Use the ABCDs—airway, breathing, circulation, and defibrillation or definitive treatment—to answer this question. Option 1 addresses the concern of airway patency. If you had difficulty with this question, review obstructed airway management for an infant or a child.
Level of Cognitive Ability: Analysis
Client Needs: Physiological Integrity
Integrated Process: Teaching/Learning
Content Area: Child health
References: American Heart Association. (1997-1999). Pediatric basic life support. In *Basic life support for health care providers* (pp. 6-11). Dallas: Author.
Wong, D., Hockenberry-Eaton, M. (2000). *Wong's essentials of pediatric nursing* (6th ed., p. 875). St. Louis: Mosby.

9. **3**
Rationale: When performing cardiopulmonary resuscitation (CPR) on an adult client, depress the sternum 1½ to 2 inches. Options 1 and 2 identify compression depths that would be ineffective in an adult. Option 4 identifies a depth that could cause injury to the client.
Test-Taking Strategy: Note the key word "adult" in the question. Consider the normal body structure of an adult to assist in answering the question. If you had difficulty with this question, review the procedure for performing adult BLS.
Level of Cognitive Ability: Application
Client Needs: Physiological Integrity
Integrated Process: Nursing Process—implementation
Content Area: Adult health—cardiovascular
Reference: Potter, P., & Perry, A. (2001). *Fundamentals of nursing* (5th ed., p. 1187). St. Louis: Mosby.

10. **3**
Rationale: To perform the Heimlich maneuver on a woman in an advanced stage of pregnancy, place the woman on her back. Place a wedge, such as a pillow or rolled blanket, under the right abdominal flank and hip to displace the uterus to the left side of the abdomen. Options 1, 2, and 4 are incorrect and can cause harm to the woman and the fetus.
Test-Taking Strategy: Use the process of elimination and note that the client is an unconscious pregnant woman at 8 months' gestation. Recall the concepts associated with hypotension and vena cava syndrome to assist in directing you to option 3. Review the principles associated with performing the Heimlich maneuver on a pregnant woman if you had difficulty with this question.
Level of Cognitive Ability: Analysis
Client Needs: Physiological Integrity
Integrated Process: Nursing Process—evaluation
Content Area: Maternity—antepartum
Reference: Lowdermilk, D., Perry, S., & Bobak, I. (2000). *Maternity & women's health care* (7th ed., p. 590). St. Louis: Mosby.

CRITICAL THINKING: FILL IN THE BLANK

Answer: Perform CPR.

Rationale: If the attempt at defibrillation is ineffective, the nurse performs CPR for 1 minute and then another series of three shocks is delivered.

Test-Taking Strategy: Focus on the key words "next action" and the issue, that defibrillation attempts have been unsuccessful. Also note that the nurse is waiting for emergency medical services to arrive. Use the ABCDs—airway, breathing, circulation, and defibrillation or definitive treatment—to direct your thinking to the need to perform CPR.

Level of Cognitive Ability: Application

Client Needs: Physiological Integrity

Integrated Process: Nursing Process—implementation

Content Area: Adult health—cardiovascular

Reference: Ignatavicius, D., & Workman, M. (2002). *Medical-surgical nursing: Critical thinking for collaborative care* (4th ed., p. 691). Philadelphia: W. B. Saunders.

REFERENCES

American Heart Association. (1997-1999). Pediatric basic life support. In *Basic life support for health care providers*. Dallas: Author.

American Heart Association. (2001). *Basic life support for health care providers*. Dallas: Author.

American Heart Association & International Liaison Committee on Resuscitation. (2000). *Guidelines 2000 for cardiopulmonary resuscitation and emergency cardiovascular care*. Dallas: Author.

Ignatavicius, D., & Workman, M. (2002). *Medical-surgical nursing: Critical thinking for collaborative care* (4th ed.). Philadelphia: W. B. Saunders.

Lowdermilk, D., Perry, S., & Bobak, I. (2000). *Maternity & women's health care* (7th ed.). St. Louis: Mosby.

National Council of State Boards of Nursing (Eds.). (2003). *Test Plan for the National Council Licensure Examination for Registered Nurses* (effective date: April 2004). Chicago: Author.

Potter, P., & Perry, A. (2001). *Fundamentals of nursing* (5th ed.). St. Louis: Mosby.

Wong, D., Hockenberry-Eaton, M. (2000). *Wong's essentials of pediatric nursing* (6th ed.). St. Louis: Mosby.

Wong, D., Perry, S., & Hockenberry, M. (2002). *Maternal child nursing care* (2nd ed.). St. Louis: Mosby.

Perioperative Nursing Care

PYRAMID TERMS

atelectasis A collapsed or airless state of the lung that may be the result of airway obstruction caused by accumulated secretions or failure of the client to deep breathe; a common postoperative complication that usually occurs 1 to 2 days after surgery.

extended postoperative stage The period of at least 1 to 4 days after surgery.

immediate postoperative stage The period of 1 to 4 hours after surgery.

intermediate postoperative stage The period of 4 to 24 hours after surgery.

wound dehiscence Separation of the wound edges.

wound evisceration Protrusion of internal organs through an incision.

▲ THE PYRAMID TO SUCCESS

Pyramid Points focus on teaching the client and family or significant other in the preoperative stage, preparing the client for the operative procedure, ensuring that prescribed preoperative tests and procedures such as x-ray films or laboratory studies have been performed, and ensuring that the results of the tests and procedures are within expected ranges and are documented. In the postoperative stage, Pyramid Points focus on monitoring for surgical complications and on the implementation of initial nursing measures if a complication arises. Pyramid Points also focus on preparing the client for discharge, teaching related to the prescribed treatments, and the mobilization of home care support services as needed. The Integrated Processes addressed in this chapter include Caring, Communication and Documentation, Nursing Process, and Teaching/Learning.

CLIENT NEEDS ▲

Safe, Effective Care Environment

Advance directives
Client rights
Establishing priorities
Informed consent for the surgical procedure
Informing the client of the surgical process
Prevention of a surgical infection
Provision of safety to the medicated client
Referral to home care and other support services
Surgical asepsis
Standard precautions

Health Promotion and Maintenance

Client and family teaching related to the prescribed discharge plan
Expected body image changes
Health and wellness teaching to prevent complications
Promotion of lifestyle choices
Techniques of physical assessment

Psychosocial Integrity

Assessment of psychosocial concerns
Assisting the client to develop coping methods
Promotion of an environment that will allow the client to express concerns
Support systems
Therapeutic interactions
Unexpected body image changes

Physiological Integrity

Initiating nursing interventions when surgical complications arise

Monitoring for surgical complications

Monitoring for unexpected responses to treatments and procedures

Monitoring for wound infection

Provision of basic care and comfort

Provision of respiratory therapy

Safe administration of intravenous (IV) fluids and blood products

Safe administration of preoperative and postoperative medications

I. PREOPERATIVE CARE

A. Obtaining informed consent
   1. The surgeon is responsible for obtaining the consent for surgery.
   2. No sedation should be administered to the client before the client signs the consent.
   3. Minors may need a parent or legal guardian to sign the consent form.
   4. Older clients may need a legal guardian to sign the consent form.
   5. The nurse may witness the client's signing of the consent form, but the nurse must be sure that the client has understood the surgeon's explanation of the surgery.
   6. The nurse needs to document the witnessing of the signing of the consent form, after the client acknowledges understanding the procedure.

B. Nutrition
   1. Review the physician's orders regarding the NPO status before surgery.
   2. Solid foods and liquids usually are withheld for 6 to 8 hours before general anesthesia and for 3 hours before surgery with local anesthesia to avoid aspiration.
   3. Prepare to initiate an IV line and administer IV fluids as prescribed.
   4. Prepare to administer total parenteral nutrition to clients who are malnourished, have protein or metabolic deficiencies, or cannot ingest foods.

C. Elimination
   1. If the client is to have intestinal or abdominal surgery, an enema or laxative or both may be prescribed the night before surgery.
   2. The client should void immediately before surgery.
   3. Prepare to insert a Foley catheter if ordered.
   4. If a Foley catheter is in place, it should be emptied immediately before surgery, and the nurse should document the amount and characteristics of the urine.

D. Surgical site
   1. Prepare to clean the surgical site with a mild antiseptic soap the night before surgery as prescribed.
   2. Prepare to shave the operative site as prescribed.

   3. Hair should be shaved only if it will interfere with the surgical procedure and only if prescribed.

E. Preoperative client teaching
   1. Inform the client about what to expect postoperatively.
   2. Inform the client to notify the nurse if the client experiences any pain postoperatively and that pain medication will be prescribed to be given as the client requests.
   3. Inform the client that requesting a narcotic after surgery will not make the client a drug addict.
   4. Demonstrate the use of a client-controlled analgesia pump if its use is prescribed.
   5. Instruct the client to use noninvasive pain relief techniques such as relaxation, distraction techniques, and guided imagery before the pain occurs and as soon as the pain is noticed.
   6. The nurse should instruct the client not to smoke for at least 24 hours before surgery.
   7. Instruct the client in deep breathing and coughing techniques, use of incentive spirometry, and the importance of performing the techniques postoperatively to prevent the development of pneumonia and **atelectasis** (Box 19-1; Fig. 19-1).
   8. Instruct the client in leg and foot exercises to prevent venous stasis of blood and to facilitate venous blood return (Box 19-1; Fig. 19-2).
   9. Instruct the client in how to splint an incision, turn, and reposition (Box 19-1; Fig. 19-3).
   10. Inform the client of any invasive devices that may be needed after surgery, such as a nasogastric tube, drain, Foley catheter, epidural catheter, or intravenous or subclavian lines.
   11. Instruct the client not to pull on any of the invasive devices, for they will be removed as soon as possible.

F. Psychosocial preparation
   1. Be alert to the client's level of anxiety.
   2. Answer any questions or concerns the client may have regarding surgery.
   3. Allow time for privacy for the client to prepare for surgery psychologically.
   4. Provide support and assistance as needed.

G. Preoperative checklist
   1. Ensure that the client is wearing an identification bracelet.
   2. Assess for allergies (refer to Chapter 69 for information on latex allergy).
   3. Review the preoperative checklist to be sure that each item is addressed before the client is transported to surgery.
   4. Ensure that informed consent forms were signed for the operative procedure, for any blood transfusions, for disposal of a limb, or for surgical sterilization procedures.
   5. Ensure that a history and physical examination were completed and documented in the client's record.

BOX 19-1

Client Teaching

DEEP BREATHING AND COUGHING EXERCISES

Instruct the client that a sitting position gives the best lung expansion for coughing and deep breathing exercises.

Instruct the client to breathe deeply 3 times, inhaling through the nostrils and exhaling slowly through pursed lips.

Instruct the client that the third breath should be held for 3 seconds; then the client should cough deeply 3 times.

The client should perform this exercise every 2 hours.

INCENTIVE SPIROMETRY

Instruct the client to assume a sitting or upright position.

Instruct the client to place the mouth tightly around the mouthpiece.

Instruct the client to inhale slowly to raise and maintain the flow rate indicator between the 600 and 900 marks.

Instruct the client to hold the breath for 5 seconds, and then to exhale through pursed lips.

Instruct the client to repeat this process 10 times every hour.

LEG AND FOOT EXERCISES

Gastrocnemius (calf) pumping: Instruct the client to move both ankles by pointing the toes up and then down.

Quadriceps (thigh) setting: Instruct the client to press the back of the knees against the bed, and then to relax the knees; this contracts and relaxes the thigh and calf muscles to prevent thrombus formation.

Foot circles: Instruct the client to rotate each foot in a circle.

Hip and knee movements: Instruct the client to flex the knee and thigh and to straighten the leg and hold the position for 5 seconds before lowering (not performed if the client is having abdominal surgery or if the client has a back problem).

SPLINTING OF THE INCISION

If the surgical incision is abdominal or thoracic, instruct the client to place a pillow, or one hand with the other hand on top, over the incisional area.

During deep breathing and coughing, the client presses gently against the incisional area to splint or support it.

---

6. Ensure that consultation requests were completed and documented in the client's record.
7. Ensure that prescribed laboratory results are documented in the client's record.
8. Ensure that the electrocardiogram and chest radiography reports are documented in the client's record.
9. Ensure that a blood type, screen, type and cross-match is performed and documented in the client's record.

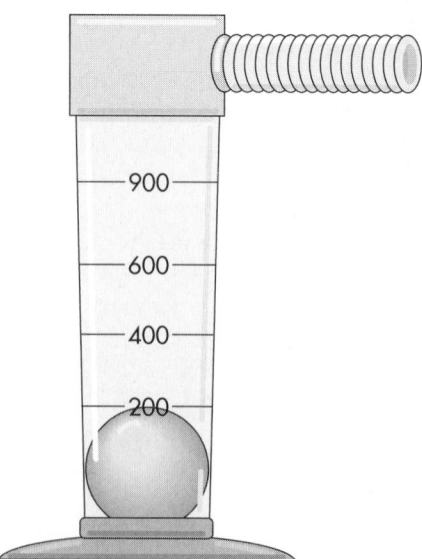

FIG. 19-1 Incentive spirometer. (From Phipps, W., Monahan, F., Sands, J., Marek, J., & Neighbors, M. [2003]. *Medical-surgical nursing: Health and illness perspectives* [7th ed.]. St. Louis: Mosby.)

Essential
Gastrocnemius (calf) pumping

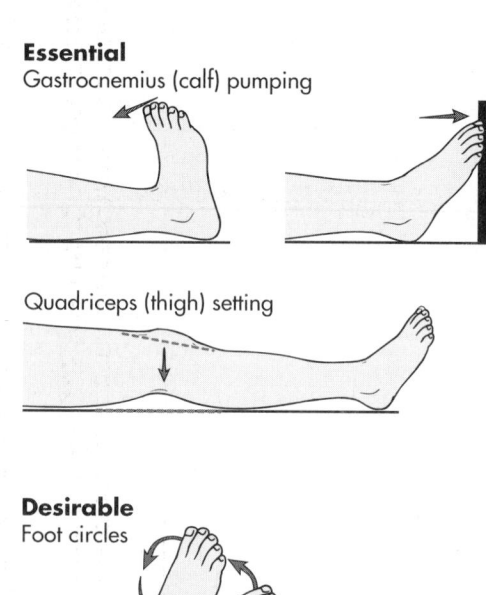

Quadriceps (thigh) setting

Desirable
Foot circles

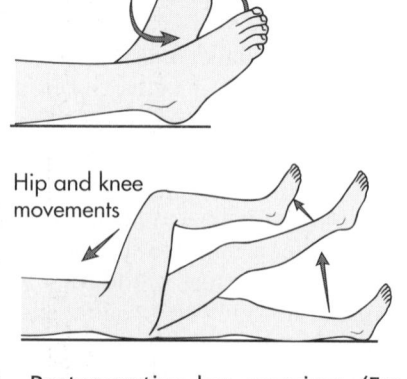

Hip and knee movements

FIG. 19-2 Postoperative leg exercises. (From Lewis, S., Heitkemper, M., & Dirksen, S. [2000]. *Medical-surgical nursing: Assessment and management of clinical problems* [5th ed.]. St. Louis: Mosby.)

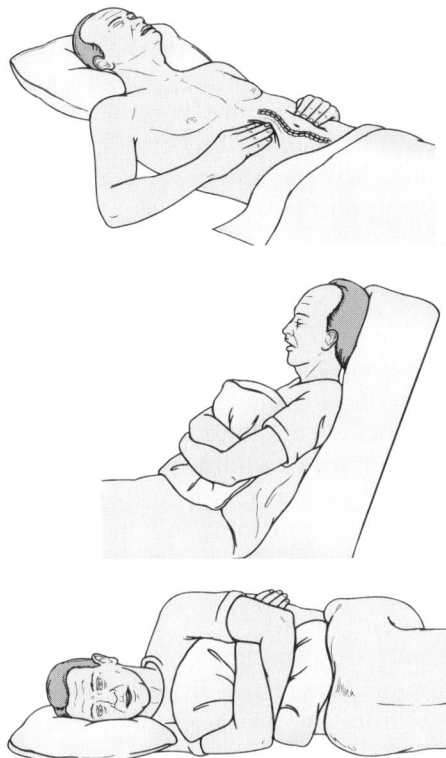

FIG. 19-3 Techniques for splinting a wound when coughing. (From Lewis, S., Heitkemper, M., & Dirksen, S. [2000]. *Medical-surgical nursing: Assessment and management of clinical problems* [5th ed.]. St. Louis: Mosby.)

10. Remove jewelry, makeup, dentures, hairpins, nail polish (depending on agency procedures), glasses, and prostheses.
11. Document that valuables were given to the client's family members or locked in the hospital safe.
12. Document the last time that the client ate or drank.
13. Document that the client voided before surgery.
14. Document that the prescribed preoperative medication was given (Box 19-2).
15. Monitor and document the client's vital signs.

H. Preoperative medications
1. Prepare to administer preoperative medications as prescribed or on call to the operating room immediately before surgery.
2. Instruct the client about the desired effects of the preoperative medication.
3. After administering the preoperative medications, keep the client in bed with the side rails up.
4. Place the call bell next to the client; instruct the client not to get out of bed and to call for assistance if needed.

I. Arrival in the operating room
1. When the client arrives in the operating room, the operating room nurse will verify the identification bracelet with the client's verbal response and will review the client's chart.
2. The operating room nurse will confirm the operative procedure and the operative site.

BOX 19-2

Substances That Can Affect the Client in Surgery

ANTIBIOTICS
Antibiotics potentiate the action of anesthetic agents.

ANTICHOLINERGICS
Medications with anticholinergic effects increase the potential for confusion.

ANTICOAGULANTS
Anticoagulants alter normal clotting factors and increase the risk of hemorrhaging.
Aspirin (acetylsalicylic acid) and nonsteroidal antiinflammatory medications are commonly used medications that can alter clotting mechanisms.
These medications should be discontinued at least 48 hours before surgery.

ANTICONVULSANTS
Long-term use of certain anticonvulsants can alter the metabolism of anesthetic agents.

ANTIDEPRESSANTS
Antidepressants may lower the blood pressure during anesthesia.

ANTIDYSRHYTHMICS
Antidysrhythmic medications reduce cardiac contractility and impair cardiac conduction during anesthesia.

ANTIHYPERTENSIVES
Antihypertensive medications can interact with anesthetic agents and cause bradycardia, hypotension, and impaired circulation.

CORTICOSTEROIDS
Corticosteroids cause adrenal atrophy and reduce the ability of the body to withstand stress.
Before and during surgery, dosages may be increased temporarily.

DIURETICS
Diuretics potentiate electrolyte imbalances after surgery.

HERBAL SUBSTANCES
Herbal substances can interact with anesthesia and cause a variety of adverse effects. These substances may need to be stopped at a specific time before surgery. During the preoperative period, the client needs to be asked if he or she is taking an herbal substance.

INSULIN
The need for insulin after surgery in a diabetic may be reduced because the client's nutritional intake is decreased or may be increased because of the stress response and intravenous administration of glucose solutions.

3. The client's chart will be checked for completeness, reviewed for informed consent forms, history and physical examination, and allergic reaction information.
4. Physicians' orders will be verified and implemented.
5. The IV line may be initiated at this time if prescribed.
6. The anesthesia team will administer the prescribed anesthesia.

II. POSTOPERATIVE CARE

A. **Immediate postoperative stage**
   1. Description: The period of 1 to 4 hours after surgery
   2. Respiratory system
      a. Monitor vital signs.
      b. Monitor airway patency and adequate ventilation because prolonged mechanical ventilation during anesthesia may affect postoperative lung function.
      c. Remember that extubated clients who are lethargic may not be able to maintain an airway.
      d. Monitor for secretions; if the client is unable to clear the airway by coughing, suction the secretions from the client's airway.
      e. Observe chest movement for symmetry and the use of accessory muscles.
      f. Monitor oxygen administration if prescribed.
      g. Monitor pulse oximetry.
      h. Encourage deep breathing and coughing exercises as soon as possible.
      i. Note the rate, depth, and quality of respirations; the respiratory rate should be greater than 10 and less than 30 breaths per minute.
      j. Assess breath sounds; stridor, wheezing, or crowing can indicate partial obstruction, bronchospasm, or laryngospasm; crackles or rhonchi may indicate pulmonary edema.
      k. Monitor for signs of **atelectasis**, pneumonia, or pulmonary embolism.
   3. Cardiovascular system
      a. Assess the skin and check capillary refill.
      b. Assess peripheral pulses.
      c. Assess for peripheral edema.
      d. Monitor for bleeding.
      e. Assess pulse for rate and rhythm; a bounding pulse may indicate hypertension, fluid overload, or excitement.
      f. Monitor for signs of hypertension and hypotension.
      g. Monitor for cardiac dysrhythmias.
      h. Assess for Homans' sign, particularly in clients positioned in lithotomy position during surgery.
   4. Musculoskeletal system
      a. Assess the client for movement of the extremities.
      b. Review physician's orders regarding client positioning or restrictions.
      c. Unless contraindicated, place client in a low Fowler's position after surgery to increase the size of the thorax for lung expansion.
      d. Avoid positioning the client in a supine position until pharyngeal reflexes have returned.
      e. If the client is comatose or semicomatose, position on the side and keep an oral airway in place.
   5. Neurological system
      a. Assess level of consciousness.
      b. Frequent periodic attempts to awaken the client should continue until the client awakens.
      c. Orient the client to environment.
      d. Speak in a soft tone; filter out extraneous noises in the environment.
      e. Maintain body temperature and prevent heat loss by providing the client with warm blankets and raising the room temperature as necessary.
   6. Temperature control
      a. Monitor temperature.
      b. Monitor for signs of hypothermia that may result from anesthesia, a cool operating room, or exposure of the skin and internal organs during surgery.
      c. Apply warm blankets and continue oxygen as prescribed if the client is shivering.
   7. Integumentary system
      a. Assess surgical site, drains, and wound dressings.
      b. Monitor for and document any drainage or bleeding from the surgical site.
      c. Assess skin for redness, abrasions, or breakdown that may have resulted from surgical positioning.
   8. Fluid and electrolyte balance
      a. Monitor IV administration as prescribed.
      b. Record intake and output.
      c. Monitor for signs of hypocalcemia, hyperglycemia, and metabolic or respiratory acidosis or alkalosis.
   9. Gastrointestinal system
      a. Monitor for nausea and vomiting.
      b. Maintain patency of nasogastric tube if present.
      c. Monitor for abdominal distention.
      d. Monitor for return of bowel sounds.
   10. Renal system
      a. Assess bladder for distention.
      b. Monitor color, quantity, and quality of urine output if a Foley catheter is present.
      c. Expect the client to void 6 to 8 hours after the surgical procedure, depending on the type of anesthesia administered.
   11. Pain management
      a. Assess for pain.
      b. Assess the type of anesthetic used and preoperative medication that the client received, and note whether the client received any

pain medications in the postanesthesia period.

   c. Inquire about the type and location of pain.
   d. Ask the client to rate the degree of pain on a scale of 1 to 10, with 10 being the most severe.
   e. Monitor for objective data related to pain, such as facial expressions, body gestures, increased pulse rate, increased blood pressure, and increased respirations.
   f. Inquire about the effectiveness of the last pain medication.
   g. Administer pain medication as prescribed.
   h. Ensure that a client with a client-controlled analgesia pump understands how to use it.
   i. If a narcotic has been prescribed, during the initial administration, assess the client every 30 minutes for respiratory rate and pain relief.
   j. Use noninvasive measures to relieve postoperative pain, including distraction, comfort measures, positioning, backrubs, and providing a quiet and restful environment.
   k. Document effectiveness of pain medication and noninvasive pain relief measures.

B. **Intermediate postoperative stage**
   1. Description: The period of 4 to 24 hours after surgery
   2. Respiratory system
      a. Monitor vital signs.
      b. Continue the same assessments as during the immediate stage.
      c. Monitor patency of airway, verifying that the lungs are clear on auscultation or describe sounds heard.
      d. Encourage deep breathing and coughing.
   3. Cardiovascular system
      a. Monitor circulatory status, such as peripheral pulses, capillary refill, and the absence of edema, numbness, and tingling.
      b. Encourage the use of antiembolism stockings, if prescribed, to promote venous return, strengthen muscle tone, and prevent pooling of secretions in the lungs.
   4. Musculoskeletal system
      a. Assess for range of motion in all extremities.
      b. Encourage ambulation; before ambulation, instruct the client to sit at the edge of the bed with the feet supported.
      c. If the client is unable to get out of bed, turn client every 1 to 2 hours.
   5. Neurological system
      a. Assess level of consciousness.
      b. Maintain orientation to the environment.
   6. Integumentary system
      a. Assess surgical site and drains.
      b. Monitor body temperature and wound for signs of infection.

   c. Maintain a dry, intact dressing.
   d. Reinforce wound with a sterile dressing if necessary, and notify the physician if bleeding occurs from the site.
   e. Change dressings as prescribed, noting the amount of bleeding or drainage, odor, and intactness of sutures or staples.
   f. Use an abdominal binder for obese and debilitated individuals to prevent dehiscense of the incision.
   g. Drains should be patent with minimal bleeding or drainage.
   h. Prepare to assist with the removal of drains (as prescribed by the physician) when the drainage amount becomes insignificant.
   7. Gastrointestinal system
      a. Monitor intake and output.
      b. Monitor for nausea and vomiting.
      c. Turn the client to a side-lying position if vomiting occurs and have suctioning equipment available and ready to use.
      d. Administer frequent mouth care.
      e. Maintain the NPO status until the gag reflex and peristalsis returns.
      f. Continue IV fluids as prescribed until the client can tolerate fluids.
      g. When oral fluids are permitted, start with ice chips and water.
      h. Ensure that the client advances to clear liquids and then to a regular diet as prescribed.
      i. Assess for bowel sounds in all four quadrants.
      j. Monitor the client for flatus and encourage ambulation.
   8. Renal system
      a. Monitor urinary output (should be greater than 30 mL per hour).
      b. If the client does not have a Foley catheter, the client is expected to void within 6 to 8 hours postoperatively; ensure that the amount is at least 200 mL.
   9. Pain management: Continue with assessments and interventions as during the immediate stage.

C. **Extended postoperative stage**
   1. Description: The period of at least 1 to 4 days postoperatively
   2. Interventions
      a. Continue to assess and observe the client's body systems during this stage.
      b. Monitor for signs of infection, such as redness, swelling, and tenderness at the surgical site; fever; and leukocytosis.
      c. Encourage active range of motion exercises every 2 hours.
      d. Continue to encourage ambulation to promote peristalsis and the passage of flatus.
      e. Increase ambulation every day to increase muscle strength.

f. Encourage the client to perform as many of activities of daily living as possible.

g. Instruct the client to eat foods that are high in protein and vitamin C content to promote wound healing.

III. PNEUMONIA AND ATELECTASIS (BOX 19-3; FIG. 19-4)

A. Description
1. Pneumonia: An inflammation of the alveoli caused by an infectious process that may develop 3 to 5 days postoperatively as a result of infection, aspiration, or immobility
2. **Atelectasis**: A collapse of the alveoli with retained mucous secretions; the most common postoperative

---

BOX 19-3

Postoperative Complications

Constipation
Hemorrhage
Hypoxia
Paralytic ileus
Pneumonia and atelectasis
Pulmonary embolism
Shock
Thrombophlebitis
Urinary retention
Wound dehiscence
Wound evisceration
Wound infection

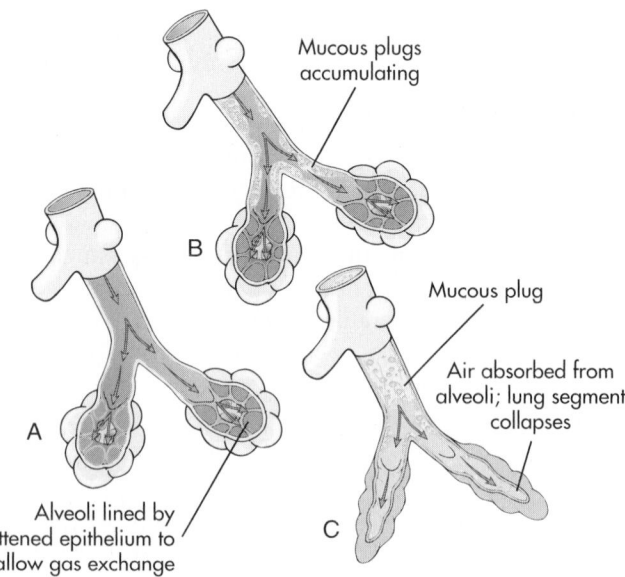

Mucous plugs accumulating

Mucous plug

Air absorbed from alveoli; lung segment collapses

Alveoli lined by flattened epithelium to allow gas exchange

FIG. 19-4   Postoperative atelectasis. **A,** Normal bronchiole and alveoli. **B,** Mucous plug in bronchiole. **C,** Collapse of alveoli caused by atelectasis following absorption of air. (From Lewis, S., Heitkemper, M., & Dirksen, S. [2000]. *Medical-surgical nursing: Assessment and management of clinical problems* [5th ed.]. St. Louis: Mosby.)

---

complication, usually occurring 1 to 2 days postoperatively

B. Assessment
1. Assess for factors that may increase the risk of pneumonia and **atelectasis**.
2. Assess for dyspnea and increased respiratory rate.
3. Assess for crackles over involved lung area.
4. Assess for elevated temperature.
5. Assess for productive cough and chest pain.

C. Interventions
1. Assess lung and breath sounds.
2. Reposition the client every 1 to 2 hours.
3. Encourage the client to deep breathe, cough, and use the incentive spirometer.
4. Provide chest physiotherapy and postural drainage as prescribed.
5. Use suction to clear secretions if the client is unable to cough.
6. Encourage fluid intake and early ambulation.

IV. HYPOXIA (BOX 19-3)

A. Description: An inadequate concentration of oxygen in arterial blood

B. Assessment
1. Restlessness
2. Dyspnea
3. Hypertension
4. Tachycardia
5. Diaphoresis
6. Cyanosis

C. Interventions
1. Monitor for signs of hypoxia.
2. Eliminate the cause of hypoxia.
3. Monitor lung sounds and pulse oximetry.
4. Administer oxygen as prescribed.
5. Encourage deep breathing and coughing and use of the incentive spirometer.
6. Turn and reposition the client.

V. PULMONARY EMBOLISM (BOX 19-3)

A. Description: An embolus blocking the pulmonary artery and disrupting blood flow to one or more lobes of the lung

B. Assessment
1. Dyspnea
2. Sudden sharp chest or upper abdominal pain
3. Cyanosis
4. Tachycardia
5. A drop in blood pressure

C. Interventions
1. Notify the physician immediately.
2. Monitor vital signs.
3. Administer oxygen and medications as prescribed.

VI. HEMORRHAGE (BOX 19-3)

A. Description: The loss of a large amount of blood externally or internally in a short time

B. Assessment
   1. Restlessness
   2. Weak and rapid pulse
   3. Hypotension
   4. Tachypnea
   5. Cool, clammy skin
   6. Reduced urine output
C. Interventions
   1. Provide pressure to the site of bleeding.
   2. Notify the physician immediately.
   3. Administer oxygen as prescribed.
   4. Administer IV fluids and blood as prescribed.
   5. Prepare client for surgical procedure if necessary.

▶ VII. SHOCK (BOX 19-3)
A. Description: Loss of circulatory fluid volume, which usually is caused by hemorrhage
B. Assessment: Similar to assessment findings in hemorrhage
C. Interventions
   1. If shock develops, elevate the legs.
   2. If the client had spinal anesthesia, do not elevate the legs any higher than placing them on the pillow; otherwise the diaphragm muscles could be impaired.
   3. Determine and treat the cause of shock.
   4. Administer oxygen as prescribed.
   5. Monitor level of consciousness.
   6. Monitor vital signs for increased pulse or decreased blood pressure.
   7. Monitor intake and output.
   8. Assess color, temperature, turgor, and moisture of skin and mucous membranes.
   9. Administer IV fluids, blood, and colloid solutions as prescribed.

VIII. THROMBOPHLEBITIS (BOX 19-3)
A. Description
   1. Thrombophlebitis is inflammation of a vein, often accompanied by clot formation.
   2. Veins in the legs are affected most commonly.
B. Assessment
   1. Vein inflammation
   2. Aching or cramping pain
   3. Vein feels hard and cordlike and is tender to touch
   4. Elevated temperature
▲ 5. Positive Homans' sign
C. Interventions
   1. Monitor legs for swelling, inflammation, pain, tenderness, venous distention, and cyanosis.
   2. Elevate the extremity 30 degrees without allowing any pressure on the popliteal area.
   3. Encourage the use of antiembolism stockings as prescribed; remove stockings twice a day to wash and inspect the legs.
   4. Use intermittent pulsatile compression device as prescribed (Fig. 19-5).

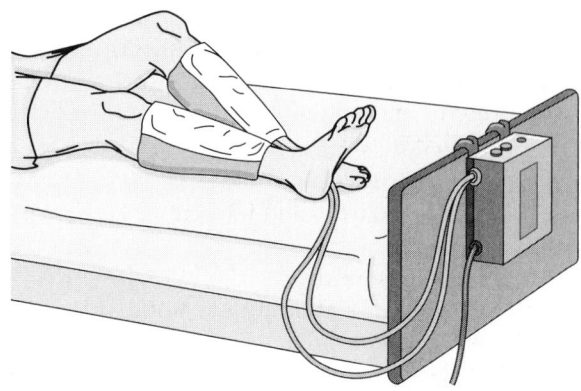

FIG. 19-5 Intermittent pulsatile compression device. (From Phipps, W., Monahan, F., Sands, J., Marek, J., & Neighbors, M. [2003]. *Medical-surgical nursing: Health and illness perspectives* [7th ed.]. St. Louis: Mosby.)

   5. Perform passive range of motion exercises every 2 hours if the client is confined to bed rest.
   6. Encourage early ambulation as prescribed.
   7. Do not allow the client to dangle the legs.
   8. Instruct the client not to sit in one position for an extended period of time.
   9. Administer heparin sodium or warfarin (Coumadin) as prescribed.

IX. URINARY RETENTION (BOX 19-3)
A. Description
   1. Urinary retention is involuntary accumulation of urine in the bladder as a result of loss of muscle tone.
   2. Urinary retention is caused by the effects of anesthetics or narcotic analgesics.
   3. Urinary retention appears 6 to 8 hours after surgery.
B. Assessment
   1. Inability to void
   2. Restlessness and diaphoresis
   3. Lower abdominal pain
   4. Distended bladder
   5. Hypertension
   6. On percussion, the bladder sounds like a drum
C. Interventions
   1. Monitor for voiding.
   2. Assess for distended bladder.
   3. Encourage ambulation when prescribed.
   4. Encourage fluid intake unless contraindicated.
   5. Assist the client to void by helping to stand.
   6. Provide privacy.
   7. Pour warm water over the perineum or allow the client to hear running water to promote voiding.
   8. Catheterize the client as prescribed after all noninvasive techniques have been attempted.

X. CONSTIPATION (BOX 19-3)
A. Description
   1. Constipation is an abnormal infrequent passage of stool.

2. When the client resumes a solid diet postoperatively, failure to pass stool within 48 hours is a cause for concern.

B. Assessment
1. Abdominal distention
2. Absence of bowel movements
3. Anorexia, headache, and nausea

C. Interventions
1. Assess bowel sounds.
2. Encourage fluid intake up to 3000 mL per day unless contraindicated.
3. Encourage early ambulation.
4. Encourage consumption of fiber foods unless contraindicated.
5. Administer stool softeners and laxatives as prescribed.
6. Provide privacy and adequate time for bowel elimination.

XI. PARALYTIC ILEUS (BOX 19-3)

A. Description
1. Paralytic ileus is failure of appropriate forward movement of bowel contents.
2. The condition may occur as a result of anesthetic medications or manipulation of the bowel during the surgical procedure.

B. Assessment
1. Nausea and vomiting immediately postoperatively
2. Abdominal distention
3. Absence of bowel sounds, bowel movement, or flatus

C. Interventions
1. Monitor intake and output.
2. Maintain NPO status until bowel sounds return.
3. Maintain patency of a nasogastric tube if in place.
4. Encourage ambulation.
5. Administer IV fluids or total parenteral nutrition as prescribed.
6. Administer medications as prescribed to increase gastrointestinal motility and secretions.
7. If ileus occurs, it is treated first nonsurgically by bowel decompression by insertion of an nasogastric tube attached to intermittent or constant suction.

XII. WOUND INFECTION (BOX 19-3)

A. Description
1. Infection is caused by poor aseptic technique or a contaminated wound before surgical exploration.
2. Infection usually occurs 3 to 6 days after surgery.
3. Purulent material may exit from the drains or separated wound edges.

B. Assessment
1. Fever and chills
2. Warm, tender, painful, and inflamed incision site
3. Edematous skin at incision and tight skin sutures
4. Elevated white blood cell count

C. Interventions
1. Monitor temperature.
2. Monitor incision site for approximation of suture line, edema, or bleeding, and signs of infection (REEDA: redness, erythema, ecchymosis, drainage, approximation of the wound edges).
3. Maintain patency of drains, and assess drainage amount, color, and consistency.
4. Keep drain and tubes away from incision line, and maintain asepsis.
5. Change dressing as prescribed.
6. Administer antibiotics as prescribed.

XIII. WOUND DEHISCENCE (BOX 19-3; FIG. 19-6)

A. Description
1. **Wound dehiscence** is separation of the wound edges at the suture line.
2. Dehiscence usually occurs 6 to 8 days after surgery.

B. Assessment
1. Increased drainage
2. Opened wound edges
3. Appearance of underlying tissues through the wound

C. Interventions
1. Place the client in low Fowler's position with knees bent to prevent abdominal tension on an abdominal suture line.
2. Cover the wound with a sterile normal saline dressing.
3. Notify the physician.
4. Prevent wound infection.

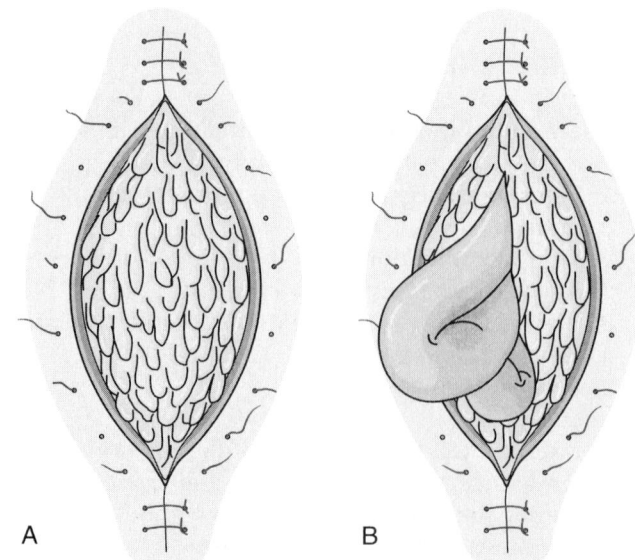

FIG. 19-6 **A,** Wound dehiscence. **B,** Wound evisceration. (From Phipps, W., Monahan, F., Sands, J., Marek, J., & Neighbors, M. [2003]. *Medical-surgical nursing: Health and illness perspectives* [7th ed.]. St. Louis: Mosby.)

BOX 19-4

Postoperative Discharge Teaching

Assess the client's readiness to learn, educational level, and desire to change or modify lifestyle.

Assess the need for resources needed for home care.

Demonstrate care to the incision and how to change the dressing.

Instruct the client to cover the incision with plastic if showering is allowed.

Be sure the client is provided with a 48-hour supply of dressings for home use.

Instruct the client on the importance of returning to the physician's office for follow-up.

Instruct the client that sutures usually are removed in the physician's office 7 to 10 days after surgery.

Inform the client that staples are removed 7 to 14 days after surgery and that the skin may become slightly reddened when they are ready to be removed.

Steri-Strips may be applied to provide extra support after the sutures are removed.

Instruct the client on the use of medications, their purpose, doses, administration, and side effects.

Instruct the client on diet and to drink 6 to 8 glasses of liquid a day.

Instruct the client on activity levels and to resume normal activities gradually.

Instruct the client to avoid lifting for 6 weeks if a major surgical procedure was performed.

Instruct the client with an abdominal incision not to lift anything weighing 10 lb or more and not to engage in any activities that involve pushing or pulling.

Clients usually can return to work in 6 to 8 weeks as prescribed by the physician.

Instruct the client on the signs and symptoms of complications and when to call a physician.

---

5. Administer antiemetics as prescribed to prevent vomiting and further strain on the abdominal incision.
6. Instruct the client to splint the abdominal incision when coughing.

XIV. WOUND EVISCERATION (BOX 19-3; FIG. 19-6)

A. Description
   1. **Wound evisceration** is protrusion of the internal organs through an incision.
   2. Evisceration is most common among obese clients, clients who have had abdominal surgery, or those who have poor wound-healing ability.
   3. Evisceration usually occurs 6 to 8 days after surgery.
   4. **Wound evisceration** is an emergency.

B. Assessment
   1. Discharge of serosanguinous fluid from a previously dry wound
   2. The appearance of loops of bowel or other abdominal contents through the wound
   3. Client reporting feeling a popping sensation after coughing or turning

C. Interventions
   1. Place the client in low Fowler's position with knees bent to prevent abdominal tension.
   2. Cover the wound with a sterile normal saline dressing.
   3. Notify the physician.
   4. Prevent wound infection through strict asepsis.
   5. Administer antiemetics as prescribed to prevent vomiting and further strain on the incision.
   6. Instruct the client to splint the incision when coughing.

XV. AMBULATORY SURGERY

A. Criteria for client discharge
   1. Client is alert and oriented.
   2. Client has voided.
   3. Client has no respiratory distress.
   4. Client is able to ambulate, swallow, and cough.
   5. Client has minimal pain.
   6. Client is not vomiting.
   7. Client has minimal, if any, bleeding from incision site.
   8. Client has a responsible adult available to drive the client home.
   9. The surgeon has signed a release form.

B. Discharge teaching (Box 19-4)
   1. Discharge teaching should be performed before the date of the scheduled procedure.
   2. Provide written instructions to the client and family regarding the specifics of care.
   3. Instruct the client and family about postoperative complications that can occur.
   4. Provide appropriate resources for home care support.
   5. Instruct the client not to drive for 24 hours after general anesthesia.
   6. Instruct the client to call the surgeon, ambulatory center, or emergency department if postoperative problems occur.
   7. Instruct the client to keep follow-up appointments with the surgeon.

PRACTICE QUESTIONS

1. A client with a perforated gastric ulcer is scheduled for emergency surgery. The client cannot sign the operative consent form because of sedation from narcotic analgesics that have been administered. The nurse should take which of the following most appropriate actions in the care of this client?
   1. Obtain a telephone consent from a family member and have the consent witnessed by two persons.

2. Obtain a court order for the surgery.
3. Send the client to surgery without the consent form being signed.
4. Have the hospital chaplain sign the informed consent immediately.

2. A preoperative client expresses anxiety to a nurse about upcoming surgery. Which response by the nurse is most likely to stimulate further discussion between the client and the nurse?
   1. "I will be happy to explain the entire surgical procedure to you."
   2. "Let me tell you about the care you'll receive after surgery and the amount of pain you can anticipate."
   3. "If it's any help, everyone is nervous before surgery."
   4. "Can you share with me what you've been told about your surgery?"

3. A nurse is conducting preoperative teaching with a client about the use of an incentive spirometer in the postoperative period. The nurse would include which piece of information in discussions with the client?
   1. Keep a loose seal between the lips and the mouthpiece.
   2. Inhale as rapidly as possible.
   3. After maximum inspiration, hold the breath for 15 seconds and exhale.
   4. The best results are achieved when the head of the bed is elevated 45 to 90 degrees.

4. A nurse has conducted preoperative teaching for a client scheduled for surgery in 1 week. The client has a history of arthritis and has been taking acetylsalicylic acid (aspirin). The nurse determines that the client needs additional teaching if the client states
   1. "I need to continue to take the aspirin as prescribed until the day of surgery."
   2. "Aspirin can cause bleeding after surgery."
   3. "Aspirin can cause my ability to clot blood to be abnormal."
   4. "I need to discontinue the aspirin 48 hours before the scheduled surgery."

5. A nurse is preparing a preoperative client for transfer to the operating room. The nurse should take which of the following actions in the care of this client at this time?
   1. Administer all the daily medications.
   2. Ensure that the client has voided.
   3. Verify that the client has not eaten for the last 24 hours.
   4. Practice postoperative breathing exercises.

6. A nurse in a surgical unit receives a postoperative client from the postanesthesia care unit. After the initial assessment of the client, the nurse plans to continue with postoperative assessment activities
   1. Every 5 minutes for the first half hour, every 15 minutes for 2 hours, every 30 minutes for 4 hours, and then every hour as needed.

2. Every 15 minutes for the first hour, every 30 minutes for 2 hours, every hour for 4 hours, and then every 4 hours as needed.
3. Every 30 minutes for the first hour, every hour for 2 hours, and then every 4 hours as needed.
4. Every hour for 2 hours, and then every 4 hours as needed.

7. A nurse receives a telephone call from the postanesthesia care unit stating that a client is being transferred to the surgical unit. The nurse plans to do which of the following first on arrival of the client?
   1. Assess the patency of the airway.
   2. Assess the vital signs to compare with preoperative measurements.
   3. Check the dressing to assess for bleeding.
   4. Check tubes or drains for patency.

8. A nurse has just reassessed the condition of a postoperative client who was admitted 1 hour ago to the surgical unit. The nurse plans to monitor which of the following parameters most carefully during the next hour?
   1. Serous drainage on the surgical dressing
   2. Blood pressure of 100/70 mm Hg
   3. Urinary output of 20 mL/hr
   4. Temperature of 37.6° C (99.6° F)

9. A postoperative client asks a nurse why it is so important to deep breathe and cough after surgery. In formulating a response the nurse incorporates the understanding that retained pulmonary secretions in a postoperative client can lead to
   1. Fluid imbalance.
   2. Carbon dioxide retention.
   3. Pulmonary edema.
   4. Pneumonia

10. A client is admitted to a surgical unit postoperatively with a wound drain in place. Which action would the nurse avoid in the care of the drain?
    1. Check the drain for patency.
    2. Curl the drain tightly and tape firmly to the body.
    3. Maintain aseptic technique when emptying the drain.
    4. Observe for bright red bloody drainage.

11. A nurse assesses a client's surgical incision for signs of infection. Which finding by the nurse would be interpreted as a normal finding at the surgical site?
    1. Red, hard skin
    2. Purulent drainage
    3. Serous drainage
    4. Warm, tender skin

12. When performing a surgical dressing change of a client's abdominal dressing, a nurse notes an increase in the amount of drainage and separation of the incision line. The underlying tissue is visible to the nurse. The nurse would do which of the following in the initial care of this wound?
    1. Leave the incision open to the air to dry the area.

2. Apply a sterile dressing soaked in povidone-iodine (Betadine).

3. Irrigate the wound and apply a sterile dry dressing.

4. Apply a sterile dressing soaked with normal saline.

13. A nurse is monitoring the status of a postoperative client. The nurse would become most concerned with which of the following signs that could indicate an evolving complication?

1. Blood pressure of 110/70 mm Hg and a pulse of 86 beats per minute

2. Increasing restlessness

3. Hypoactive bowel sounds in all four quadrants

4. A negative Homans' sign

14. A nurse is reviewing a physician's order sheet for a preoperative client that states that the client must be NPO after midnight. The nurse would telephone the physician to clarify whether which of the following medications should be given to the client and not withheld?

1. Conjugated estrogen (Premarin)

2. Prednisone (Deltasone)

3. Cyclobenzaprine (Flexeril)

4. Ferrous sulfate

15. A client who underwent preadmission testing had blood drawn for serum laboratory studies, including a complete blood count, electrolytes, coagulation studies, and a creatinine level. Which of the following laboratory results would be reported to the surgeon's office by the nurse, knowing that it could cause surgery to be postponed?

1. Platelets, 210,000 cells/µL

2. Serum creatinine, 0.8 mg/dL

3. Sodium, 141 mEq/L

4. Hemoglobin, 8.9 g/dL

16. A nurse is developing a plan of care for a preoperative client who has a latex allergy. Which of the following interventions would be included in the plan?

1. Apply a cloth barrier to the client's arm under a blood pressure cuff when taking the blood pressure.

2. Use medications that are from ampules with rubber stoppers.

3. Avoid using medications from glass ampules.

4. Avoid using IV tubing that is made of polyvinyl chloride.

17. A nurse is developing a plan of care for a client scheduled for surgery. The nurse would include which of the following activities in the nursing care plan for the client on the day of surgery?

1. Have the client void immediately before surgery.

2. Report immediately any slight increase in blood pressure or pulse.

3. Verify that the client has not eaten for the last 24 hours.

4. Avoid oral hygiene and rinsing with mouthwash.

18. A nurse is developing a list of home care instructions for a client being discharged after a laparoscopic cholecystectomy. Which of the following instructions would be least appropriate to include in the postoperative discharge plan of care?

1. Wound care

2. Activity restrictions

3. Follow-up care

4. Deep breathing exercises

19. A nurse is monitoring a postoperative client after abdominal surgery for signs of complications. The nurse assesses the client for the presence of Homans' sign and determines that this sign is positive if which of the following is noted?

1. Pain with dorsiflexion of the foot

2. Incisional pain

3. Absent bowel sounds

4. Crackles on auscultation of the lungs

20. An operating room nurse is positioning a client on the operating room table so as to prevent the client's extremities from dangling over the sides of the table. A nursing student who is observing for the day asks the nurse why this is so important. The nurse responds that this is done primarily to prevent

1. A drop in blood pressure.

2. Muscle fatigue in the extremities.

3. An increase in pulse rate.

4. Nerve and muscle damage.

CRITICAL THINKING: MULTIPLE RESPONSE

A client who had abdominal surgery complains of feeling as though "something gave way" in the incisional site. The nurse removes the dressing and notes the presence of a loop of bowel protruding through the incision. Select all nursing interventions that the nurse would take.

____ Place the client in a supine position without a pillow under the head.

____ Instruct the client to remain quiet.

____ Place a sterile saline dressing and ice packs over the wound.

____ Contact the surgeon.

____ Prepare the client for wound closure.

ANSWERS

1. 1

Rationale: Every effort must be made to obtain permission from a responsible family member to perform surgery if the client is unable to sign the consent form. A telephone consent must be witnessed by two persons who hear the family member's oral consent. The two witnesses then sign the consent with the name of the family member, noting that an oral consent was obtained. Consent is not informed if it is obtained from a client who is confused, unconscious, mentally incompetent, or under the influence of sedatives. In emergencies a client may be unable to sign and family members may not be available. In this situation a physician is permitted legally to perform surgery without consent. Options 2 and 4 are not appropriate. In addition, actions that delay treatment in an emergency are not appropriate.

Test-Taking Strategy: Use the process of elimination. Note the key words "most appropriate" in the question. Eliminate options 2 and 4 first. Option 2 will delay necessary surgery, and option 4 is inappropriate. Select option 1 over option 3 because it is the most appropriate of the options presented and it is legally acceptable to obtain a telephone permission from a family member if it is witnessed by two persons. Review the implications surrounding informed consent, if you had difficulty with this question.

Level of Cognitive Ability: Application
Client Needs: Safe, Effective Care Environment
Integrated Process: Nursing Process—implementation
Content Area: Fundamental skills
Reference: Potter, P., & Perry, A. (2001). *Fundamentals of nursing* (5th ed., p. 1677). St. Louis: Mosby.

2. 4

Rationale: Explanations should begin with the information that the client knows. By providing the client with individualized explanations of care and procedures, the nurse can assist the client in handling anxiety and fear for a smooth preoperative experience. Clients who are calm and emotionally prepared for surgery withstand anesthesia better and experience fewer postoperative complications. Options 1, 2, and 3 will produce anxiety in the client.

Test-Taking Strategy: Use the process of elimination. Note that the stem of the question contains the key words "most likely" and "stimulate further discussion." Use the steps of the nursing process and therapeutic communication techniques. Option 4 addresses assessment and is the only therapeutic response. If this question was difficult, review the fundamental principles of communication.

Level of Cognitive Ability: Application
Client Needs: Psychosocial Integrity
Integrated Process: Communication and Documentation
Content Area: Fundamental skills
Reference: Potter, P., & Perry, A. (2001). *Fundamentals of nursing* (5th ed., pp. 459-462). St. Louis: Mosby.

3. 4

Rationale: For optimal lung expansion with the incentive spirometer, the client should assume the semi-Fowler or high Fowler's position. The mouthpiece should be covered completely and tightly while the client inhales slowly with a constant flow through the unit. The breath should be held for 5 seconds before exhaling slowly.

Test-Taking Strategy: Use the process of elimination and knowledge of the procedure for using the incentive spirometer. Options 1, 2, and 3 are incorrect steps regarding incentive spirometer use. If you had difficulty with this question, review the correct procedure related to the use of an incentive spirometer.

Level of Cognitive Ability: Application
Client Needs: Physiological Integrity
Integrated Process: Teaching/Learning
Content Area: Fundamental skills
Reference: Perry, A., & Potter, P. (2002). *Clinical nursing skills and techniques* (5th ed., p. 328). St. Louis: Mosby.

4. 1

Rationale: Anticoagulants alter normal clotting factors and increase the risk of bleeding after surgery. Aspirin has properties that can alter the clotting mechanism and should be discontinued at least 48 hours before surgery.

Test-Taking Strategy: Use the process of elimination. Note the key words "the client needs additional teaching." Eliminate options 2 and 3 first because they are similar. From the remaining options, recalling that aspirin has properties that can alter the clotting mechanism will direct you to option 1. If you had difficulty with this question, review medications that affect the client preparing for surgery.

Level of Cognitive Ability: Analysis
Client Needs: Physiological Integrity
Integrated Process: Teaching/Learning
Content Area: Pharmacology
Reference: Potter, P., & Perry, A. (2001). *Fundamentals of nursing* (5th ed., p. 1668). St. Louis: Mosby.

5. 2

Rationale: The nurse should ensure that the client has voided, if a Foley catheter is not in place. The nurse does not administer all daily medications just before sending a client to the operating room. Rather the physician writes a specific order outlining which medications may be given with a sip of water. The client has nothing by mouth for 8 hours before surgery, not 24 hours. The time of transfer to the operating room is not the time to practice breathing exercises. This should have been accomplished earlier.

Test-Taking Strategy: Use the process of elimination. Note that the question contains the key words "at this time." This tells you that you must prioritize your answer according to a time line. With this in mind, eliminate options 1 and 3 first because they are incorrect. Choose correctly between the remaining two options by knowing that the client must empty the bladder or by knowing that the client is likely to be anxious at this time, making it inappropriate to practice breathing exercises. Review preoperative nursing interventions if you had difficulty with this question.

Level of Cognitive Ability: Application
Client Needs: Physiological Integrity
Integrated Process: Nursing Process—implementation
Content Area: Fundamental skills
Reference: Potter, P., & Perry, A. (2001). *Fundamentals of nursing* (5th ed., p. 1689). St. Louis: Mosby.

6. 2

Rationale: When the postoperative client arrives from the postanesthesia care unit, the nurse performs an initial assessment. Common time frames for continuing postoperative assessment activities are every 15 minutes the first hour, every 30 minutes for 2 hours, every hour for 4 hours, and then every 4 hours as needed. Options 3 and 4 identify time frames that are too infrequent and will not provide adequate assessment of the postoperative client. Option 1 identifies close time frames that are unnecessary.

Test-Taking Strategy: Use the process of elimination. Eliminate option 1 first because the time frames are so close. By the time that the nurse completed the assessment, the 5 minutes would have lapsed and the nurse would have to perform the assessment immediately again. This is unnecessary and unreasonable. Eliminate options 3 and 4 because they identify time frames that are too infrequent and will not provide adequate assessment of the postoperative client. Review postoperative assessment procedures if you had difficulty with this question.

Level of Cognitive Ability: Application
Client Needs: Physiological Integrity
Integrated Process: Nursing Process—planning
Content Area: Fundamental skills
Reference: Potter, P., & Perry, A. (2001). *Fundamentals of nursing* (5th ed., p. 1702). St. Louis: Mosby.

7. 1

Rationale: The first action of the nurse is to assess the patency of the airway and respiratory function. The nurse then takes vital signs followed by checking the dressing and the tubes or drains. If the airway is not patent, the nurse must take immediate measures for the survival of the client.

Test-Taking Strategy: Use the principles of prioritization when answering this question. Remember the ABCs—airway, breathing, and circulation. Ensuring airway patency is the first action to be taken; therefore option 1 is correct. Options 2, 3, and 4 are all nursing actions that should be performed after a patent airway has been established.

Level of Cognitive Ability: Application
Client Needs: Physiological Integrity
Integrated Process: Nursing Process—planning
Content Area: Delegating/Prioritizing
Reference: Potter, P., & Perry, A. (2001). *Fundamentals of nursing* (5th ed., p. 1704). St. Louis: Mosby.

8. 3

Rationale: Urine output should be maintained at a minimum of 30 mL/hr for an adult. An output of less than 30 mL for each of 2 consecutive hours should be reported to the physician. A temperature higher than 37.7° C (100° F) or lower than 36.1° C (97° F) and a falling systolic blood pressure under 90 mm Hg usually are considered reportable at once. The client's preoperative or baseline blood pressure is used to make informed postoperative comparisons. Moderate or light serous drainage from the surgical site is considered normal.

Test-Taking Strategy: To answer this question correctly, you must know the normal ranges for temperature, blood pressure, urinary output, and wound drainage. Through the process of elimination, you then can determine that the urinary output

is the only observation that is not within the normal range. Review these basic postoperative assessment findings if you had difficulty with this question.

Level of Cognitive Ability: Analysis
Client Needs: Physiological Integrity
Integrated Process: Nursing Process—planning
Content Area: Fundamental skills
Reference: Potter, P., & Perry, A. (2001). *Fundamentals of nursing* (5th ed., pp. 1707, 1397). St. Louis: Mosby.

9. 4

Rationale: The most common postoperative respiratory problems are atelectasis, pneumonia, and pulmonary emboli. Pneumonia is inflammation of lung tissue that causes productive cough, dyspnea, and crackles. Pulmonary edema usually results from failure of the left side of the heart and can be caused by medications or fluid overload. Carbon dioxide retention results from inability to exhale carbon dioxide in conditions such as chronic obstructive pulmonary disease. Fluid imbalance can be a deficit or excess related to fluid loss or overload.

Test-Taking Strategy: Use the process of elimination. Focus on the relationship between the words "deep breathe and cough" in the question and "pneumonia" in the correct option. Review the common postoperative complications if you had difficulty with this question.

Level of Cognitive Ability: Comprehension
Client Needs: Physiological Integrity
Integrated Process: Teaching/Learning
Content Area: Fundamental skills
Reference: Potter, P., & Perry, A. (2001). *Fundamentals of nursing* (5th ed., p. 1709). St. Louis: Mosby.

10. 2

Rationale: A postoperative drain should not be curled tightly or obstructed in any way. This could prevent the drain from functioning properly. The nurse should check the tube/drain for patency to provide an exit for the fluid/blood to promote healing. The nurse must use aseptic technique for emptying the drainage container or changing the dressing, to avoid contamination of the wound. Usually the drainage from the wound is pale, red, and watery. Active bleeding will be bright red.

Test-Taking Strategy: Use the process of elimination, noting the key word "avoid." Remember that surgical drains need to remain patent so that accumulated secretions can escape from the wound bed. If you had difficulty with this question, review nursing care for the client with a surgical drain.

Level of Cognitive Ability: Application
Client Needs: Physiological Integrity
Integrated Process: Nursing Process—implementation
Content Area: Fundamental skills
Reference: Potter, P., & Perry, A. (2001). *Fundamentals of nursing* (5th ed., p. 1712). St. Louis: Mosby.

11. 3

Rationale: Serous drainage is an expected finding at a surgical site. The other options indicate signs of wound infection. Signs and symptoms of infection include warm, red, and tender skin around the incision. Purulent material may exit from drains or from separated wound edges. Infection may be caused by poor aseptic technique and a contaminated wound before surgical exploration. Wound infection usually appears 3 to 6 days after surgery. The client also may have a fever and chills.

Test-Taking Strategy: Use the process of elimination, noting the key words "normal finding." Recalling the signs of a wound infection and noting these key words will direct you easily to option 3. Review the signs of a wound infection if you had difficulty with this question.

Level of Cognitive Ability: Analysis
Client Needs: Physiological Integrity
Integrated Process: Nursing Process—assessment
Content Area: Fundamental skills
Reference: Linton, A., & Maebius, N. (2003). *Introduction to medical-surgical nursing* (3rd ed., p. 230). Philadelphia: W. B. Saunders.

12. 4
Rationale: Wound dehiscence is the separation of wound edges at the suture line. Signs and symptoms include increased drainage and the appearance of underlying tissues. Dehiscence usually occurs 6 to 8 days after surgery. The client should be instructed to remain quiet and to avoid coughing or straining. The client should be positioned to prevent further stress on the wound. Sterile dressings soaked with sterile normal saline should be used to cover the wound. The nurse must notify the physician after applying this initial dressing to the wound.

Test-Taking Strategy: Use the process of elimination. Eliminate option 1 first because this action would dry the wound and also present a risk of infection to the underlying tissues. Eliminate options 2 and 3 next because a dry dressing and a dressing soaked with povidone-iodine will irritate the exposed body tissues. Review initial nursing care when dehiscence or evisceration occurs if you had difficulty with this question.

Level of Cognitive Ability: Application
Client Needs: Physiological Integrity
Integrated Process: Nursing Process—implementation
Content Area: Fundamental skills
Reference: Phipps, W., Monahan, F., Sands, J., Marek, J., & Neighbors, M. (2003). *Medical-surgical nursing: Health and illness perspectives* (7th ed., p. 452). St. Louis: Mosby.

13. 2
Rationale: Increasing restlessness is a sign that requires continuous and close monitoring because it could indicate a potential complication such as hemorrhage and shock. Hypoactive bowel sounds heard in all four quadrants are a normal occurrence, as is a negative Homans' sign. (A positive Homans' sign may indicate thrombophlebitis). A blood pressure of 110/70 mm Hg with a pulse of 86 beats per minute is within normal limits.

Test-Taking Strategy: Use the process of elimination, noting the key words "indicate an evolving complication." Eliminate each of the incorrect options because they are normal expected findings. If you had difficulty with this question, review the normal expected postoperative findings and the signs and symptoms of postoperative complications.

Level of Cognitive Ability: Analysis
Client Needs: Physiological Integrity
Integrated Process: Nursing Process—analysis
Content Area: Fundamental skills

Reference: Potter, P., & Perry, A. (2001). *Fundamentals of nursing* (5th ed., p. 1709). St. Louis: Mosby.

14. 2
Rationale: Prednisone is a corticosteroid. With prolonged use, corticosteroids cause adrenal atrophy, which reduces the ability of the body to withstand stress. When stress is severe, corticosteroids are essential to life. Before and during surgery, dosages may be increased temporarily. Cyclobenzaprine (Flexeril) is a skeletal muscle relaxant. Ferrous sulfate is an oral iron preparation used to treat iron deficiency anemia. Conjugated estrogen (Premarin) is an estrogen used for hormonal replacement therapy in postmenopausal women. The other three medications may be withheld before surgery without undue effects on the client.

Test-Taking Strategy: Use the process of elimination and knowledge about medications that may have special implications for the surgical client. Remember that when stress is severe, corticosteroids are essential to life. Review the effects of corticosteroids if you had difficulty with this question.

Level of Cognitive Ability: Analysis
Client Needs: Physiological Integrity
Integrated Process: Nursing Process—analysis
Content Area: Pharmacology
Reference: Potter, P., & Perry, A. (2001). *Fundamentals of nursing* (5th ed., p. 1668). St. Louis: Mosby.

15. 4
Rationale: Routine screening tests include a complete blood count, serum electrolyte analysis, coagulation studies, and serum creatinine tests. The complete blood count includes the hemoglobin analysis. All of these values are within normal range except the hemoglobin. If a client has a low hemoglobin level, the surgery likely could be postponed by the surgeon.

Test-Taking Strategy: Use the process of elimination and knowledge of the normal laboratory values. The only option that identifies an abnormal laboratory value is option 4. Review these laboratory values, if you had difficulty answering this question.

Level of Cognitive Ability: Analysis
Client Needs: Physiological Integrity
Integrated Process: Nursing Process—analysis
Content Area: Fundamental skills
Reference: Potter, P., & Perry, A. (2001). *Fundamentals of nursing* (5th ed., p. 1673). St. Louis: Mosby.

16. 1
Rationale: If a client has a latex allergy, a cloth barrier should be applied to the client's arm under a blood pressure cuff to prevent skin contact with the cuff. Medications from glass ampules are safe to use, and medications from ampules with rubber stoppers are unsafe to use. Latex-safe intravenous tubing made of polyvinyl chloride should be used for the client with a latex allergy.

Test-Taking Strategy: Use the process of elimination, focusing on the issue of the question, latex allergy. Recalling the causes of a latex allergy will direct you easily to option 1. Review nursing interventions for the client with a latex allergy if you had difficulty with this question.

Level of Cognitive Ability: Application

Client Needs: Safe, Effective Care Environment
Integrated Process: Nursing Process—planning
Content Area: Fundamental skills
Reference: Lewis, S., Heitkemper, M., & Dirksen, S. (2004). *Medical-surgical nursing: Assessment and management of clinical problems* (6th ed., p. 253). St. Louis: Mosby.

17. **1**
Rationale: The nurse would assist the client to void immediately before surgery so that the bladder will be empty. A slight increase in blood pressure and pulse is common during the preoperative period and is usually the result of anxiety. The client usually has a restriction of food and fluids for 8 hours before surgery instead of 24 hours. Oral hygiene is allowed, but the client should not swallow any water.
Test-Taking Strategy: Use the process of elimination, and read each option carefully. Eliminate option 2 because of the words "immediately" and "slight." Eliminate option 3, knowing that the client should be NPO for 8 hours before surgery. There is no useful reason for option 4; in fact, oral hygiene may make the client feel more comfortable. Review general preoperative care if you had difficulty with this question.
Level of Cognitive Ability: Application
Client Needs: Physiological Integrity
Integrated Process: Nursing Process—planning
Content Area: Fundamental skills
Reference: Potter, P., & Perry, A. (2001). *Fundamentals of nursing* (5th ed., p. 1689). St. Louis: Mosby.

18. **4**
Rationale: The type of planning and instruction required varies with each individual and the type of surgery. Specific instructions that the client needs to receive before discharge should include wound care, activity restrictions, dietary instructions, postoperative medication instructions, personal hygiene, and follow-up appointments. Deep breathing exercises are taught in the preoperative period.
Test-Taking Strategy: Use the process of elimination, noting the key words "least appropriate." Options 1, 2, and 3 are similar and refer to information that needs to be taught postoperatively. Option 4 refers to information that should be taught preoperatively. Review the client education points related to discharge teaching preoperatively and postoperatively if you had difficulty with this question.
Level of Cognitive Ability: Application
Client Needs: Health Promotion and Maintenance
Integrated Process: Teaching/Learning
Content Area: Fundamental skills
Reference: Potter, P., & Perry, A. (2001). *Fundamentals of nursing* (5th ed., p. 1679). St. Louis: Mosby.

19. **1**
Rationale: To elicit Homans' sign, the nurse would dorsiflex the client's foot and assesses the client for pain in the calf area. If pain is present, a positive Homans' sign is present, which is an indication of thrombophlebitis. Incisional pain is an expected occurrence after abdominal surgery. Absent bowel sounds may occur in the immediate postoperative period. Crackles on auscultation of the lungs may indicate a respiratory complication.

Test-Taking Strategy: Use the process of elimination and knowledge of the significance of a positive Homans' sign. Knowing that a positive Homans' sign indicates thrombophlebitis will direct you easily to option 1. Review this assessment technique if you had difficulty with this question.
Level of Cognitive Ability: Analysis
Client Needs: Physiological Integrity
Integrated Process: Nursing Process—assessment
Content Area: Fundamental skills
Reference: Linton, A., & Maebius, N. (2003). *Introduction to medical-surgical nursing* (3rd ed., p. 227). Philadelphia: W. B. Saunders.

20. **4**
Rationale: The client's extremities should not be allowed to dangle over the sides of the table because this may impair circulation to the local area or cause nerve and muscle damage. Part of the operating room nurse's role is to ensure that the safety needs of the client are met, which includes proper positioning.
Test-Taking Strategy: Use the process of elimination and knowledge regarding the basic principles related to positioning. Recalling that the client is anesthetized will direct you easily to option 4. Review the nurse's role during surgery if you had difficulty with this question.
Level of Cognitive Ability: Application
Client Needs: Physiological Integrity
Integrated Process: Teaching/Learning
Content Area: Fundamental skills
Reference: Potter, P., & Perry, A. (2001). *Fundamentals of nursing* (5th ed., p. 1699). St. Louis: Mosby.

CRITICAL THINKING: MULTIPLE RESPONSE
Answer:
Instruct the client to remain quiet.
Contact the surgeon.
Prepare the client for wound closure.
Rationale: Wound dehiscence is the separation of the wound edges. Wound evisceration is protrusion of the internal organs through an incision. If wound dehiscence or evisceration occurs, the surgeon is notified immediately. The client is placed in a low Fowler's position, kept quiet, and instructed not to cough. Protruding organs are covered with a warm, sterile saline dressing. The treatment for evisceration is immediate wound closure under local or general anesthesia.
Test-Taking Strategy: Focus on the information in the question to determine that the client is experiencing wound evisceration. Visualizing this occurrence will assist you in determining that the client would not be placed supine and that ice packs would not be placed on the incision. Review this surgical complication if you had difficulty with this question.
Level of Cognitive Ability: Application
Client Needs: Physiological Integrity
Integrated Process: Nursing Process—implementation
Content Area: Fundamental skills
Reference: Phipps, W., Monahan, F., Sands, J., Marek, J., & Neighbors, M. (2003). *Medical-surgical nursing: Health and illness perspectives* (7th ed., p. 452). St. Louis: Mosby.

REFERENCES

Lewis, S., Heitkemper, M., & Dirksen, S. (2004). *Medical-surgical nursing: Assessment and management of clinical problems* (6th ed.). St. Louis: Mosby.

Linton, A., & Maebius, N. (2003). *Introduction to medical-surgical nursing* (3rd ed.). Philadelphia: W. B. Saunders.

National Council of State Boards of Nursing (Eds.). (2003). *Test Plan for the National Council Licensure Examination for Registered Nurses* (effective date: April 2004). Chicago: Author.

Perry, A., & Potter, P. (2002). *Clinical nursing skills and techniques* (5th ed.). St. Louis: Mosby.

Phipps, W., Monahan, F., Sands, J., Marek, J., & Neighbors, M. (2003). *Medical-surgical nursing: Health and illness perspectives* (7th ed.). St. Louis: Mosby.

Potter, P., & Perry, A. (2001). *Fundamentals of nursing* (5th ed.). St. Louis: Mosby.

Positioning Clients

PYRAMID TERMS

Fowler's position The client is supine and the head of the bed is elevated to 45 to 60 degrees.

high Fowler's position The client is supine and the head of the bed is elevated to 90 degrees.

lateral (side-lying) position The client is lying on the side, and the head and shoulders are aligned with the hips and the spine and are parallel to the edge of the mattress. The head, neck, and upper arm are supported by a pillow. The lower shoulder is pulled forward slightly and, along with the elbow, flexed at 90 degrees. The legs are flexed or extended. A pillow is placed to support the back.

lithotomy position The client is lying on the back with the hips and knees flexed at right angles and the feet in stirrups.

prone position The client is lying on the abdomen with head turned to the side.

reverse Trendelenburg's position The bed is tilted so that the client's foot of the bed is down.

semi-Fowler position (low Fowler's) The client is supine and the head of the bed is elevated about 30 degrees.

Sims' position The client is lying on the side with the body turned prone at 45 degrees. The lower leg is extended, with the upper leg flexed at the hip and knee to a 45- to 90-degree angle.

supine position The client is lying on the back. The head and shoulders usually are elevated slightly with a small pillow. The arms and legs are extended, and the legs are slightly abducted.

Trendelenburg's position The bed is tilted so that the client's head of the bed is down. This position is contraindicated in clients with head injuries, increased intracranial pressure, spinal cord injuries, and certain respiratory disorders.

◢ THE PYRAMID TO SUCCESS

Nursing responsibility includes positioning clients in a safe and appropriate manner to provide safety and comfort. Knowledge regarding the client position required for a certain procedure or condition is expected.

The nurse has the responsibility to reduce the likelihood and prevent the development of complications related to an existing condition, prescribed treatment, or medical or surgical procedure. The nurse must review the physician's orders after treatments or procedures and take note of instructions regarding positioning and mobility (Figs. 20-1 to 20-3). The Integrated Processes

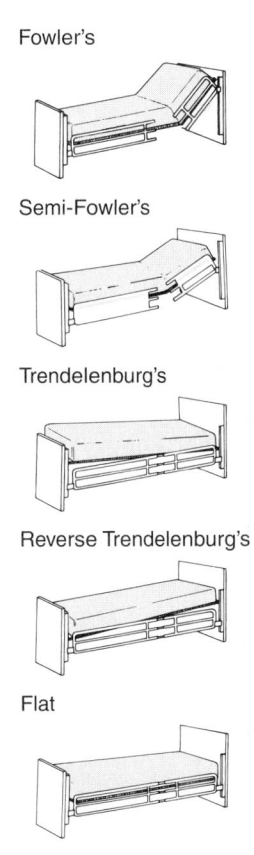

Fowler's

Semi-Fowler's

Trendelenburg's

Reverse Trendelenburg's

Flat

Fig. 20-1 Common bed positions. (From Potter, P., & Perry, A. [2001]. *Fundamentals of nursing* [5th ed.]. St. Louis: Mosby.)

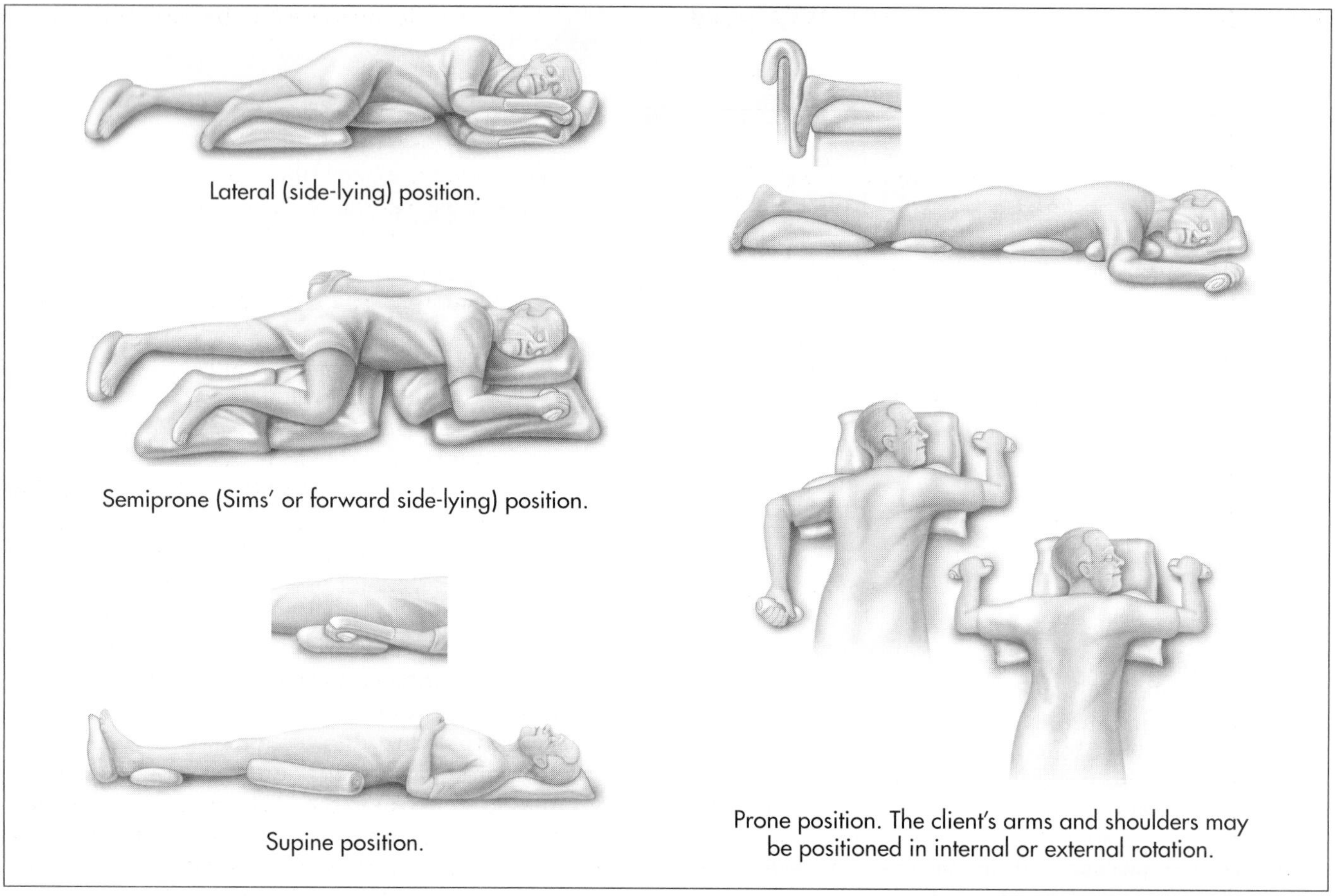

Lateral (side-lying) position.

Semiprone (Sims' or forward side-lying) position.

Supine position.

Prone position. The client's arms and shoulders may be positioned in internal or external rotation.

Fig. 20-2   Common client positions. (From Harkreader, H. [2000]. *Fundamentals of nursing: Caring and clinical judgment.* Philadelphia: W. B. Saunders.)

addressed in this chapter include Caring, Communication and Documentation, Nursing Process, and Teaching/Learning.

▲ CLIENT NEEDS
Safe, Effective Care Environment

Accident and injury prevention
Appropriate positioning
Environmental and personal safety
Establishing priorities
Protective measures
Safe use of equipment

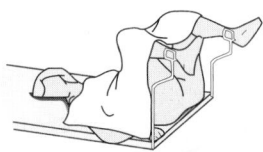

Fig. 20-3   Lithotomy position for examination. (From Potter, P., & Perry, A. [2001]. *Fundamentals of nursing* [5th ed.]. St. Louis: Mosby.)

Health Promotion and Maintenance

Information regarding the need for prescribed therapies
Techniques of physical assessment

Psychosocial Integrity

Assisting the client to use coping mechanisms
Keeping the family informed of client progress
Provision of support to the client
Therapeutic communications

Physiological Integrity

Comfort measures for rest and sleep
Immobility
Prevention of complications
Provision of nutrition and oral intake
Provision of personal hygiene as needed
Use of assistive devices

PROVISION OF SAFETY AND COMFORT

A. Integumentary system
1. Autograft: After surgery, the site is immobilized for 3 to 7 days to provide the time needed for the graft to adhere and attach to the wound bed.
2. Burns of the face and head: Elevate the head of the bed to prevent or reduce facial, head, and tracheal edema.
3. Circumferential burns of the extremities: Elevate the extremities above the level of the heart to prevent or reduce dependent edema.
4. Skin graft: Elevate and immobilize the graft site to prevent movement and shearing of the graft and disruption of tissue; avoid weight bearing.

B. Reproductive system
1. Mastectomy
   a. Position the client with the head of the bed elevated at least 30 degrees (**semi-Fowler position**), with the affected arm elevated on a pillow to promote lymphatic fluid return after the removal of axillary lymph nodes.
   b. Turn the client only to the back and unaffected side.
2. Perineal and vaginal procedures: Place the client in **lithotomy position**.

C. Endocrine system
1. Hypophysectomy: Elevate the head of the bed to prevent increased intracranial pressure.
2. Thyroidectomy
   a. Place client in the **semi-Fowler position** to reduce swelling and edema in the neck area.
   b. Sandbags or pillows may be used to support the client's head or neck.

D. Gastrointestinal system
1. Hemorrhoidectomy: Assist the client to a **lateral (side-lying) position** to prevent pain and bleeding.
2. Gastroesophageal reflux disease: **Reverse Trendelenburg's position** may be prescribed to promote gastric emptying and prevent esophageal reflux.
3. Liver biopsy
   a. During the procedure, do the following:
      (1) Position client **supine**, with the right side of the upper abdomen exposed.
      (2) The client's right arm is raised and extended over the left shoulder behind the head.
      (3) The liver is located on the right side, and this position provides for maximal exposure of the right intercostal space.
   b. After the procedure, do the following:
      (1) Assist the client into a right **lateral (side-lying) position**.
      (2) Place a small pillow or folded towel under the puncture site for at least 3 hours to provide pressure to the site and prevent bleeding.
4. Nasogastric tube
   a. Insertion
      (1) Position the client in **high Fowler's position** with the head tilted forward.
      (2) This position will assist to close the trachea and open the esophagus.
   b. Irrigations and tube feedings
      (1) Elevate the head of the bed 30 degrees (**semi-Fowler position**) to prevent aspiration.
      (2) Maintain head elevation for 1 hour after an intermittent feeding.
      (3) Head of the bed should remain elevated for continuous feedings.
5. Rectal enemas/irrigations: Place client in left **Sims' position** to allow the solution to flow by gravity in the natural direction of the colon.
6. Sengstaken-Blakemore and Minnesota tubes: Maintain elevation of the head of the bed to enhance lung expansion and reduce portal blood flow, permitting effective compression of the esophageal varices.

E. Respiratory system
1. Chronic obstructive pulmonary disease: In advanced disease, place client in a sitting position, leaning forward, with the client's arms over several pillows or an overbed table; this position will assist the client to breathe easier.
2. Laryngectomy (radical neck dissection): Place the client in **semi-Fowler** or **Fowler's position** to maintain a patent airway and minimize edema.
3. Bronchoscopy postprocedure: Place the client in a **semi-Fowler position** to prevent choking or aspiration resulting from an impaired ability to swallow.
4. Postural drainage: The lung segment to be drained should be in the uppermost position; **Trendelenburg's position** may be used.
5. Thoracentesis
   a. During the procedure, to facilitate removal of fluid from the chest wall, position the client sitting on the edge of the bed and leaning over the bedside table, with the feet supported on a stool, or lying in bed on the unaffected side with the head of the bed elevated about 45 degrees (**Fowler's position**).
   b. After the procedure, assist the client to a position of comfort.
6. Thoracotomy: Check physician's orders regarding positioning.

F. Cardiovascular system
1. Abdominal aneurysm resection
   a. After surgery, limit elevation of the head of the bed to 45 degrees (**Fowler's position**) to avoid flexion of the graft.
   b. The client may be turned from side to side.

2. Amputation of the lower extremity
   a. During the first 24 hours after amputation, elevate the foot of the bed (the stump is supported with pillows but not elevated because of the risk of flexion contractures) to reduce edema.
   b. Consult with the physician, and then put the client in a **prone position** twice a day for a 20- to 30-minute period to stretch muscles and prevent flexion contractures of the hip.
3. Arterial vascular grafting of an extremity
   a. To promote graft patency after the procedure, bed rest usually is maintained for about 24 hours, and the affected extremity is kept straight.
   b. Limit movement and avoid flexion of the hip and knee.
4. Cardiac catheterization
   a. If the femoral artery was used, the client is maintained on bed rest for 3 to 4 hours; the client may turn from side to side.
   b. The affected extremity is kept straight and the head is elevated no greater than 30 degrees until hemostasis is adequately achieved.
5. Congestive heart failure and pulmonary edema: Position the client upright, preferably with the legs dangling over the side of the bed, to decrease venous return and lung congestion.
6. Peripheral arterial disease
   a. Obtain the physician's order for positioning.
   b. Because swelling can prevent arterial blood flow, clients may be advised to elevate their feet at rest, but they should not raise their legs above the level of the heart because extreme elevation slows arterial blood flow; some clients may be advised to maintain a slightly dependent position to promote perfusion.
7. Deep vein thrombosis
   a. If the extremity is red, edematous, and painful, and traditional heparin sodium therapy is initiated, bed rest with leg elevation may be prescribed for the client.
   b. Clients receiving low-molecular-weight heparin usually can be out of bed after 24 hours if pain level permits.
8. Varicose veins: Leg elevation above heart level usually is prescribed; the client also is advised to minimize prolonged sitting or standing during daily activities.
9. Venous leg ulcers: Leg elevation usually is prescribed.

G. Sensory system
1. Cataract surgery: Postoperatively, elevate the head of the bed (**semi-Fowler** to **Fowler's position**) and position the client on the back or the nonoperative side to prevent the development of edema at the operative site.
2. Retinal detachment
   a. If the detachment is large, bed rest and bilateral eye patching may be prescribed to minimize eye movement and prevent extension of the detachment.
   b. Restrictions in activity and positioning following repair of the detachment depends on the physician's preference and the surgical procedure performed.
   c. If a gas bubble has been injected into the eye to flatten the retina and reinforce the repair, the client may have to be positioned so that the gas rises in the eye and presses against the repair (usually face down or angled toward the unoperative side).

H. Neurological system
1. Autonomic dysreflexia: Elevate the head of the bed to a **high Fowler's position** to assist with adequate ventilation and assist in the prevention of hypertensive stroke.
2. Cerebral aneurysm: Bed rest is maintained with the head of the bed elevated 30 to 45 degrees (**semi-Fowler** to **Fowler's position**) to prevent pressure on the aneurysm site.
3. Cerebral angiography
   a. Maintain bed rest for 12 to 24 hours as prescribed.
   b. The extremity into which the contrast medium was injected is kept straight and immobilized for about 8 hours.
4. Cerebrovascular accident
   a. In clients with hemorrhagic strokes, the head of the bed is elevated to 30 degrees to reduce intracranial pressure and to facilitate venous drainage.
   b. For clients with ischemic strokes, the head of the bed is kept flat.
   c. Maintain the head in a midline, neutral position to facilitate venous drainage from the head.
   d. Avoid extreme hip and neck flexion; extreme hip flexion may increase intrathoracic pressure, whereas extreme neck flexion prohibits venous drainage from the brain.
5. Craniotomy
   a. The client should *not* be positioned on the site that was operated on, especially if the bone flap has been removed, because the brain has no bony covering on the affected site.
   b. Elevate the head of the bed 30 to 45 degrees (**semi-Fowler** to **Fowler's position**) and maintain the head in a midline, neutral position to facilitate venous drainage from the head.
   c. Avoid extreme hip and neck flexion.
6. Laminectomy
   a. Logroll the client.
   b. When the client is out of bed, the client's back is kept straight (the client is placed in a

straight-backed chair) with the feet resting comfortably on the floor.

7. Increased intracranial pressure
   a. Elevate the head of the bed 30 to 45 degrees (**semi-Fowler** to **Fowler's position**) and maintain the head in a midline, neutral position to facilitate venous drainage from the head.
   b. Avoid extreme hip and neck flexion.
8. Lumbar puncture
   a. During the procedure, assist the client to the **lateral (side-lying) position**, with the back bowed at the edge of the examining table, the knees flexed up to the abdomen, and the head bent so that the chin is resting on the chest.
   b. After the procedure, place the client in the **supine position** for 4 to 12 hours as prescribed.
9. Myelogram postprocedure
   a. If water-soluble dye is used, the head of the bed should be elevated 30 to 60 degrees for about 12 hours to keep the dye from irritating the cerebral meninges.
   b. If an oil-based dye is used, a **supine position** is maintained for several hours after the dye is removed to prevent leakage of cerebrospinal fluid.
10. Spinal cord injury
    a. Immobilize the client on a spinal backboard, with the head in a neutral position, to prevent incomplete injury from becoming complete.
    b. Prevent head flexion, rotation, or extension; the head is immobilized with a firm, padded cervical collar.
    c. Logroll the client; no part of the body should be twisted or turned, nor should the client be allowed to assume a sitting position.

I. Musculoskeletal system
1. Total hip replacement
   a. Positioning depends on the surgical techniques used, the method of implantation, and the prosthesis.
   b. Avoid extreme internal and external rotation.
   c. Avoid adduction; side-lying on the operative side is not allowed (unless specifically prescribed by the physician).
   d. Maintain abduction when the client is in a supine position or positioned on the unoperative side.
   e. Place a pillow between the client's legs to maintain abduction; instruct the client not to cross the legs.
   f. Check the physician's orders regarding elevation of the head of the bed; flexion usually is limited to 60 degrees during the first postoperative week (usually 90 degress for 2 to 3 months thereafter).

PRACTICE QUESTIONS

1. A client has just returned to a nursing unit after an above-the-knee amputation of the right leg. A nurse places the client in which of the following most appropriate positions?
   1. Supine with the stump flat on the bed
   2. Supine with the stump supported with pillows
   3. Reverse Trendelenburg's
   4. Prone
2. A nurse is caring for a client with a severe burn. The client is scheduled for an autograft to be placed on the lower extremity. The nurse develops a postoperative plan of care for the client and includes which of the following in the plan?
   1. Maintain surgical extremity in a flat position.
   2. Keep surgical extremity covered with a blanket.
   3. Maintain the client in a prone position.
   4. Elevate and immobilize the grafted extremity.
3. A nurse is preparing to care for a client who has returned to the nursing unit following cardiac catheterization performed through the femoral artery. The nurse plans to place the client in which most appropriate client position/activity following the procedure?
   1. Bed rest with head elevation at 60 degrees
   2. Bed rest with head elevation no greater than 30 degrees
   3. Bed rest with bathroom privileges only
   4. Bed rest in high Fowler's position
4. A nurse is providing instructions to a client and the family regarding home care after right eye cataract removal. Which statement by the client would indicate an understanding of the instructions?
   1. "I will not sleep on my right side."
   2. "I will not sleep on my left side."
   3. "I will not sleep with my head elevated."
   4. "I will not wear my glasses until my physician says it is okay."
5. A nurse assists a physician in performing a liver biopsy. After the biopsy the nurse plans to place the client in which of the following positions?
   1. Supine
   2. Prone
   3. A left side-lying position with a small pillow or folded towel under the puncture site
   4. A right side-lying position with a small pillow or folded towel under the puncture site
6. A nurse is administering a cleansing enema to a client with a fecal impaction. Before administering the enema, the nurse places the client in which of the following positions?
   1. On the left side of the body, with the head of the bed elevated 45 degrees
   2. On the right side of the body, with the head of the bed elevated 45 degrees
   3. Left Sims' position
   4. Right Sims' position

7. A client is being prepared for a thoracentesis. A nurse assists the client to which of the following positions for the procedure?
   1. Lying in bed on the affected side
   2. Lying in bed on the unaffected side
   3. Prone with the head turned to the side and supported by a pillow
   4. Sims' position with the head of the bed flat

8. A nurse is preparing to insert a nasogastric tube into a client. The nurse places the client in which position for insertion?
   1. High Fowler's
   2. Supine with the head flat
   3. Right side
   4. Low Fowler's

9. A client is diagnosed with deep vein thrombophlebitis. A nurse develops a plan of care for the client and includes which client position/activity in the plan?
   1. Bed rest with the affected extremity in a dependent position
   2. Out-of-bed activities as desired
   3. Bed rest with the affected extremity kept flat
   4. Bed rest with elevation of the affected extremity

10. A nurse is preparing to care for a client who has had a supratentorial craniotomy. The nurse plans to place the client in which position?
    1. Prone
    2. Supine
    3. Semi-Fowler
    4. Side-lying

CRITICAL THINKING: FILL IN THE BLANK

A nurse is caring for a client with congestive heart failure. The client suddenly becomes anxious and restless, has a sudden onset of breathlessness, and becomes cyanotic. The nurse suspects pulmonary edema and immediately places the client in what position?

Answer: _____

ANSWERS

1. 2
Rationale: The stump is supported on pillows for the first 24 hours following surgery to promote venous return and decrease edema, which will increase mobility. After the first 24 hours the stump usually is placed flat on the bed to reduce hip contracture. Edema also is controlled by stump-wrapping techniques. Options 1, 3, and 4 are inappropriate positions for the client immediately after surgery.
Test-Taking Strategy: Use the process of elimination. A key issue in this question is that the client has just returned from surgery. Using basic principles related to immediate postoperative care will assist in directing you to option 2. If you had difficulty with this question, review postoperative positioning following amputation.
Level of Cognitive Ability: Application
Client Needs: Physiological Integrity
Integrated Process: Nursing Process—implementation
Content Area: Fundamental skills
Reference: Phipps, W., Monahan, F., Sands, J., Marek, J., & Neighbors, M. (2003). *Medical-surgical nursing: Health and illness perspectives* (7th ed., p. 779). St. Louis: Mosby.

2. 4
Rationale: Autografts placed over joints or on lower extremities are elevated and immobilized following surgery for 3 to 7 days, depending on the surgeon's preference. This period of immobilization allows the autograft time to adhere and attach to the wound bed, and the elevation minimizes edema. Keeping the client in a prone position and covering the extremity with a blanket can disrupt the graft site.
Test-Taking Strategy: Use the process of elimination. Options 2 and 3 can be eliminated first because a blanket and a prone position can disrupt a graft easily. From the remaining options, recall the principles related to gravity and edema to

assist in directing you to option 4. Review care to the client following an autograft if you had difficulty with this question.
Level of Cognitive Ability: Application
Client Needs: Physiological Integrity
Integrated Process: Nursing Process—planning
Content Area: Fundamental skills
Reference: Phipps, W., Monahan, F., Sands, J., Marek, J., & Neighbors, M. (2003). *Medical-surgical nursing: Health and illness perspectives* (7th ed., p. 2000). St. Louis: Mosby.

3. 2
Rationale: After cardiac catheterization the extremity into which the catheter was inserted is kept straight for 4 to 6 hours. If the femoral artery was used, bed rest is enforced for 3 to 4 hours. The client may turn from side to side. The affected leg is kept straight and the head is elevated no greater than 30 degrees until hemostasis is adequately achieved.
Test-Taking Strategy: Use the process of elimination. Knowing that the head of the bed should not be elevated more than 30 degrees will assist in eliminating options 1 and 4. Remembering that bathroom privileges are not allowed in the immediate postcatheterization period will assist in eliminating option 3. If you had difficulty with this question, review care after cardiac catheterization.
Level of Cognitive Ability: Application
Client Needs: Physiological Integrity
Integrated Process: Nursing Process—planning
Content Area: Fundamental skills
Reference: Ignatavicius, D., & Workman, M. (2002). *Medical-surgical nursing: Critical thinking for collaborative care* (4th ed., p. 644). Philadelphia: W. B. Saunders.

4. 1
Rationale: After cataract surgery the client should not sleep on the side of the body that was operated on. The client also

should be placed in a semi-Fowler position to assist in minimizing edema and intraocular pressure. During the day, the client may wear glasses or a protective shield; at night, the protective shield alone is sufficient.

Test-Taking Strategy: Use the process of elimination. Remember to instruct the client to remain off the operative side. This will assist you with answering questions related to cataract surgery. Review postoperative instructions for the client following cataract surgery if you had difficulty with this question.

Level of Cognitive Ability: Analysis
Client Needs: Health Promotion and Maintenance
Integrated Process: Teaching/Learning
Content Area: Fundamental skills
Reference: Ignatavicius, D., & Workman, M. (2002). *Medical-surgical nursing: Critical thinking for collaborative care* (4th ed., p. 1033). Philadelphia: W. B. Saunders.

5. 4
Rationale: After a liver biopsy the client is assisted to assume a right side-lying position with a small pillow or folded towel under the puncture site for 2 hours. This position compresses the liver against the chest wall at the biopsy site.

Test-Taking Strategy: Use the process of elimination and knowledge regarding the anatomy of the body to answer this question. Remember that the liver is on the right side of the body, and that the application of pressure on the right side will minimize the escape of blood or bile through the puncture site. Review care to the client following a liver biopsy if you had difficulty with this question.

Level of Cognitive Ability: Application
Client Needs: Physiological Integrity
Integrated Process: Nursing Process—planning
Content Area: Fundamental skills
Reference: Lewis, S., Heitkemper, M., & Dirksen, S. (2004). *Medical-surgical nursing: Assessment and management of clinical problems* (6th ed., p. 964). St. Louis: Mosby.

6. 3
Rationale: For administering an enema, the client is placed in a left Sims' position so that the enema solution can flow by gravity in the natural direction of the colon. The head of the bed is not elevated in the Sims' position.

Test-Taking Strategy: Use the process of elimination and knowledge regarding the anatomy of the bowel to answer the question. This will assist in eliminating options 2 and 4. Attempt to visualize the procedure for administering an enema and eliminate option 1 because the head of the bed should be flat during enema administration. Review the procedure for administering an enema if you had difficulty with this question.

Level of Cognitive Ability: Application
Client Needs: Physiological Integrity
Integrated Process: Nursing Process—implementation
Content Area: Fundamental skills
Reference: Potter, P., & Perry, A. (2001). *Fundamentals of nursing* (5th ed., p. 1463). St. Louis: Mosby.

7. 2
Rationale: To facilitate removal of fluid from the chest wall, the client is positioned sitting at the edge of the bed leaning over the bedside table with the feet supported on a stool or lying in bed on the unaffected side with the head of the bed elevated 30 to 45 degrees. The prone and Sims' positions are inappropriate positions for this procedure.

Test-Taking Strategy: Use the process of elimination. Eliminate option 1 first because if the client were lying on the affected side, it would be difficult to perform the procedure. Option 4 can be eliminated next because the Sims' position is used primarily for rectal enemas or irrigations. Next, visualize the prone position. In the prone position the client is lying on the abdomen, which is not an appropriate position for this procedure. Review the procedure for a thoracentesis if you had difficulty with this question.

Level of Cognitive Ability: Application
Client Needs: Physiological Integrity
Integrated Process: Nursing Process—implementation
Content Area: Fundamental skills
Reference: Perry, A., & Potter, P. (2002). *Clinical nursing skills and techniques* (5th ed., p. 1249). St. Louis: Mosby.

8. 1
Rationale: During insertion of a nasogastric tube, the client is placed in a sitting or high Fowler's position to reduce the risk of pulmonary aspiration if the client should vomit. Options 2, 3, and 4 will not facilitate insertion of the tube or prevent aspiration.

Test-Taking Strategy: Use the process of elimination. Recalling that a concern with insertion of a nasogastric tube is pulmonary aspiration will direct you to option 1. Review the procedure for inserting a nasogastric tube if you had difficulty with this question.

Level of Cognitive Ability: Application
Client Needs: Physiological Integrity
Integrated Process: Nursing Process—implementation
Content Area: Fundamental skills
Reference: Perry, A., & Potter, P. (2002). *Clinical nursing skills and techniques* (5th ed., p. 660). St. Louis: Mosby.

9. 4
Rationale: Elevation of the affected leg facilitates blood flow by the force of gravity and also decreases venous pressure, which in turn relieves edema and pain. Bed rest is indicated to prevent emboli and to prevent pressure fluctuations in the venous system that occurs with walking.

Test-Taking Strategy: Use the process of elimination. Focus on the client's diagnosis and think about the principles related to gravity flow and edema to answer the question. If you had difficulty with this question, review nursing care for clients with a venous disorder.

Level of Cognitive Ability: Application
Client Needs: Physiological Integrity
Integrated Process: Nursing Process—planning
Content Area: Fundamental skills
Reference: Ignatavicius, D., & Workman, M. (2002). *Medical-surgical nursing: Critical thinking for collaborative care* (4th ed., p. 763). Philadelphia: W. B. Saunders.

10. 3
Rationale: After supratentorial surgery (surgery above the tentorium of the brain), the client's head usually is elevated

30 degrees to promote venous outflow through the jugular veins. Options 1, 2, and 4 are incorrect positions after this surgery.
Test-Taking Strategy: Use the process of elimination and knowledge regarding supratentorial surgery and craniotomy to answer this question. A helpful strategy is to remember the following: *supra,* above the tentorium of the brain, head up. If you had difficulty with this question, review positioning after craniotomy surgery.
Level of Cognitive Ability: Application
Client Needs: Physiological Integrity
Integrated Process: Nursing Process—planning
Content Area: Fundamental skills
Reference: Ignatavicius, D., & Workman, M. (2002). *Medical-surgical nursing: Critical thinking for collaborative care* (4th ed., p. 1003). Philadelphia: W. B. Saunders.

CRITICAL THINKING: FILL IN THE BLANK
Answer: High Fowler's position
Rationale: Positioning the client upright (high Fowler's) with the legs dangling over the side of the bed has an immediate

effect of decreasing venous return and decreasing lung congestion.
Test-Taking Strategy: Think about the physiological occurrence in pulmonary edema. Recall that the lung congestion that occurs in this disorder results in severe hypoxemia. This will assist you in determining the optimal position for the client. Review care to the client that develops pulmonary edema if you had difficulty with this question.
Level of Cognitive Ability: Application
Client Needs: Physiological Integrity
Integrated Process: Nursing Process—implementation
Content Area: Fundamental skills
Reference: Ignatavicius, D., & Workman, M. (2002). *Medical-surgical nursing: Critical thinking for collaborative care* (4th ed., p. 710). Philadelphia: W. B. Saunders.

REFERENCES

Ignatavicius, D., & Workman, M. (2002). *Medical-surgical nursing: Critical thinking for collaborative care* (4th ed.). Philadelphia: W. B. Saunders.

Lewis, S., Heitkemper, M., & Dirksen, S. (2004). *Medical-surgical nursing: Assessment and management of clinical problems* (6th ed.). St. Louis: Mosby.

National Council of State Boards of Nursing (Eds.). (2003). *Test Plan for the National Council Licensure Examination for Registered Nurses* (effective date: April 2004). Chicago: Author.

Perry, A., & Potter, P. (2002). *Clinical nursing skills and techniques* (5th ed.). St. Louis: Mosby.

Phipps, W., Monahan, F., Sands, J., Marek, J., & Neighbors, M. (2003). *Medical-surgical nursing: Health and illness perspectives* (7th ed.). St. Louis: Mosby.

Care of a Client with a Tube

PYRAMID TERMS

chest tube Tube that returns negative pressure to the intrapleural space; used to remove abnormal accumulations of air and fluid from the pleural space.

endotracheal tube Tube used to maintain a patent airway; indicated when a client needs mechanical ventilation.

gastrointestinal intubation Insertion of a tube into the stomach or intestine.

intestinal tube Tube passed nasally and designed so that it enters the small intestine through the pyloric sphincter because of the weight of a small bag of mercury at the end of the tube; used to decompress the bowel or to remove intestinal contents.

Sengstaken-Blakemore tube Triple-lumen gastric tube with an inflatable esophageal balloon, an inflatable gastric balloon, and a gastric aspiration lumen; used as a treatment modality for a client with esophageal varices.

tracheostomy Artificial opening created into the trachea to establish an airway.

▲ THE PYRAMID TO SUCCESS

The Pyramid to Success focuses on the common types of tubes used in the clinical setting. The NCLEX-RN examination is likely to address content areas related to the appropriate care of certain tubes and the immediate interventions required if a complication arises. Focus on the specific assessment points related to the specific type of tube. Review procedures for inserting a particular tube, verifying correct placement, and administering medications or feedings, if appropriate. Pyramid Points also focus on interventions associated with complications ,or emergencies that may occur. The Integrated Processes addressed in this chapter include Caring, Communication and Documentation, Nursing Process, and Teaching/Learning.

CLIENT NEEDS
Safe, Effective Care Environment

Advance directives
Advocacy related to client's concerns
Client rights
Consultations with members of the health care team
Establishing priorities
Handling of infectious materials
Informed consent for invasive procedure
Medical and surgical asepsis
Standard precautions

Health Promotion and Maintenance

Client and family education regarding care at home
Disease prevention
Lifestyle changes
Techniques of physical assessment

Psychosocial Integrity

Home care services
Sensory/perceptual alterations
Situational role changes
Support systems
Therapeutic interactions
Unexpected body image changes

Physiological Integrity

Diagnostic tests to confirm accurate placement of tube
Emergency interventions for complications
Laboratory values
Measures to ensure basic care and comfort

233

Medication administration
Nutrition and oral hydration
Potential complications associated with the tube
Respiratory care

I. NASOGASTRIC TUBES

A. Description
  1. Short tubes used to intubate the stomach
  2. Tube inserted from nose to stomach
B. Types of tubes
  1. Levin (Fig. 21-1)
     a. Single-lumen nasogastric tube
     b. Used to remove gastric contents via intermittent suction or to provide tube feedings
  2. Salem sump (Fig. 21-1)
     a. A Salem sump is a double-lumen nasogastric tube with an air vent (pigtail) used for decompression with continuous suction.
     b. Air vent is not to be clamped and is to be kept above the level of the stomach.
     c. If leakage occurs through the air vent, instill 30 mL of air into the air vent and irrigate the main lumen with normal saline (NS).
C. Intubation procedures
  1. Place the client in high Fowler's position.
  2. Measure from tip of nose to earlobe to xiphoid process to determine the length of insertion, and mark with tape.
  3. Lubricate tube about 3 inches with a water-soluble jelly only oil-soluble is not used because of the risk of pneumonia if the tube accidentally slips into the bronchus.
  4. Instruct the client to bend the head forward, which closes the epiglottis and opens the esophagus.
  5. Insert into nostril and advance backward and through the nasopharynx.
  6. Have the client take a sip of water, and advance the tube as the client swallows.
  7. Do not force the tube.
  8. If the client experiences any respiratory distress (coughing or choking) during insertion, pull back on the tube and wait until the distress subsides.
  9. Advance until reaching the taped mark; tape tube in place when correct placement is confirmed.
  10. If feedings are prescribed, x-ray confirmation should be done before feedings are initiated.
  11. Following **gastrointestinal intubation**, the tube may be attached to continuous or intermittent suction, with a pressure not exceeding 25 mm Hg as prescribed by the physician.
D. Assessment of placement
  1. Note that the most reliable method to determine placement is by radiography, which should be performed after initial placement.

  2. Assess tube placement every 4 hours and before administering feedings or medications.
  3. Assess tube placement by aspirating gastric contents and measuring the pH, which should be 4 or less (pH values greater than 6 indicate intestinal placement).
  4. Inserting 5 to10 mL of air into the nasogastric tube and listening for the rush of air over the stomach with a stethoscope is an alternative method for assessing placement but is not as reliable as radiography or checking gastric pH.
E. Assessment of residual
  1. Check residual volumes every 4 hours, before each feeding, and before giving medications.
  2. Aspirate all stomach contents (residual) and measure amount.
  3. Reinstill residual feeding to prevent excessive fluid and electrolyte losses, unless the residual volume appears abnormal.
F. Irrigation
  1. Perform irrigation every 4 hours to check the patency of the tube.
  2. Assess placement before irrigating.
  3. Gently instill 30 to 50 mL of water or NS (depending on agency policy) with an irrigation syringe.
  4. Pull back on the syringe plunger to withdraw the fluid to check patency; repeat if tube remains sluggish.
G. Removal of an nasogastric tube: Ask the client to take a deep breath and hold; remove the tube slowly and evenly over the course of 3 to 6 seconds (coil the tube around the hand while removing it).

II. GASTROINTESTINAL TUBE FEEDINGS

A. Tubes
  1. Nasogastric: nose to stomach
  2. Nasoduodenal/nasojejunal: nose to duodenum or jejunum
  3. Gastrostomy: stomach
  4. Jejunostomy: jejunum
B. Types of administration
  1. Bolus
     a. A bolus resembles normal meal feeding patterns.
     b. Administration consists of 300 to 400 mL of formula given over a 30- to 60-minute period every 3 to 6 hours.
  2. Continuous
     a. Feeding is administered continually for 24 hours.
     b. An infusion pump regulates the flow.
  3. Cyclical
     a. Feeding is administered in the daytime or the nighttime for 8 to 16 hours.
     b. An infusion pump regulates the flow.
     c. Feedings at night allow for more freedom during the day.

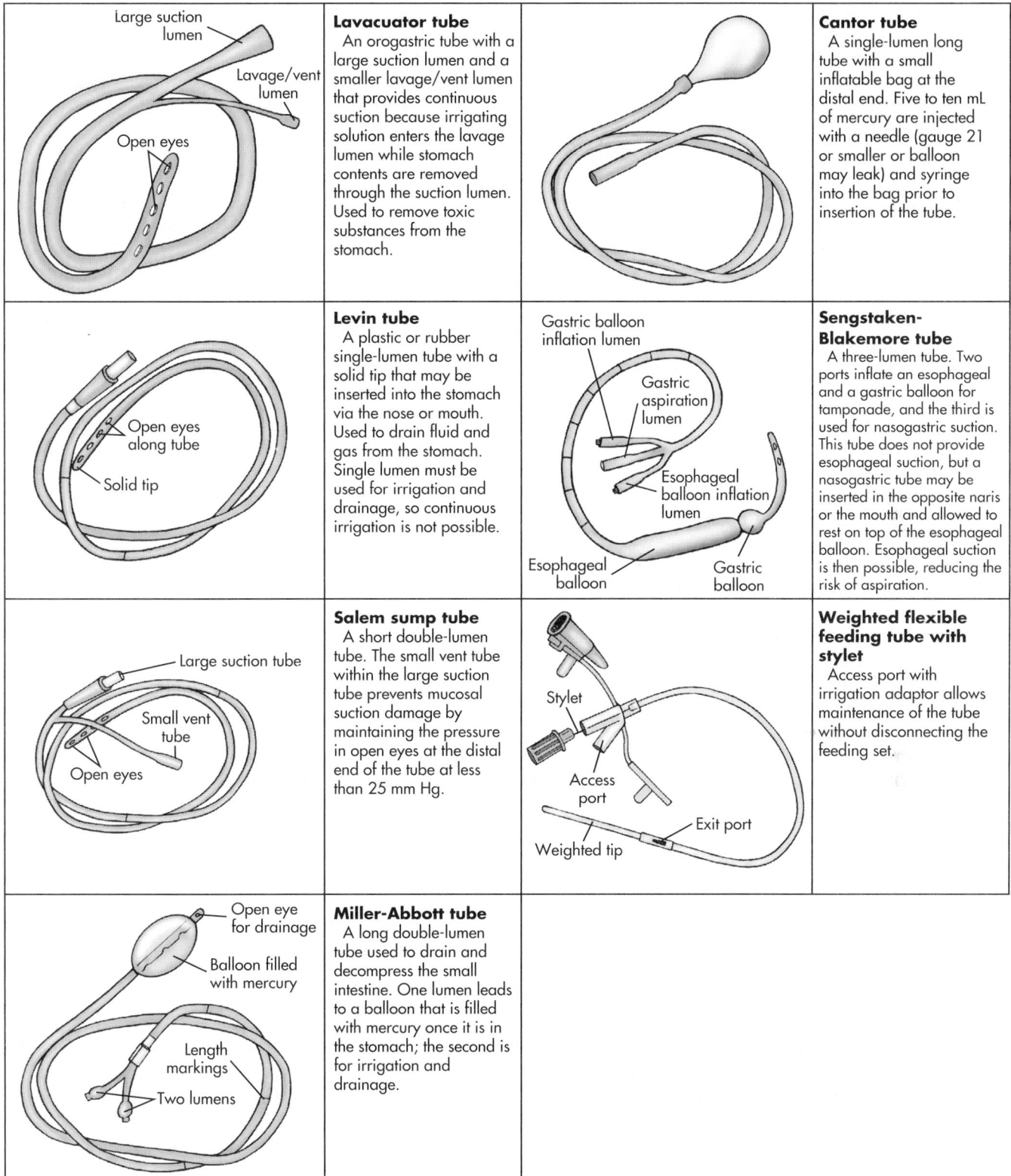

Lavacuator tube
An orogastric tube with a large suction lumen and a smaller lavage/vent lumen that provides continuous suction because irrigating solution enters the lavage lumen while stomach contents are removed through the suction lumen. Used to remove toxic substances from the stomach.

Cantor tube
A single-lumen long tube with a small inflatable bag at the distal end. Five to ten mL of mercury are injected with a needle (gauge 21 or smaller or balloon may leak) and syringe into the bag prior to insertion of the tube.

Levin tube
A plastic or rubber single-lumen tube with a solid tip that may be inserted into the stomach via the nose or mouth. Used to drain fluid and gas from the stomach. Single lumen must be used for irrigation and drainage, so continuous irrigation is not possible.

Sengstaken-Blakemore tube
A three-lumen tube. Two ports inflate an esophageal and a gastric balloon for tamponade, and the third is used for nasogastric suction. This tube does not provide esophageal suction, but a nasogastric tube may be inserted in the opposite naris or the mouth and allowed to rest on top of the esophageal balloon. Esophageal suction is then possible, reducing the risk of aspiration.

Salem sump tube
A short double-lumen tube. The small vent tube within the large suction tube prevents mucosal suction damage by maintaining the pressure in open eyes at the distal end of the tube at less than 25 mm Hg.

Weighted flexible feeding tube with stylet
Access port with irrigation adaptor allows maintenance of the tube without disconnecting the feeding set.

Miller-Abbott tube
A long double-lumen tube used to drain and decompress the small intestine. One lumen leads to a balloon that is filled with mercury once it is in the stomach; the second is for irrigation and drainage.

FIG. 21-1 Comparison of design and function of selected gastrointestinal tubes. (From Monahan, F., & Neighbors, M. [1998]. *Medical-surgical nursing* [2nd ed]. Philadelphia: W. B. Saunders.)

▲ C. Administration of feedings
   1. Position the client in high Fowler's and on the right side if comatose.
   2. Warm feeding to room temperature to prevent diarrhea and cramps.
   3. Aspirate all stomach contents (residual), measure the amount, and return the contents to the stomach to prevent electrolyte imbalances.
   4. Check physician's order and agency policy regarding residual amounts; usually if the residual is less than 100 mL, feeding is administered; large-volume aspirates indicate delayed gastric emptying and place the client at risk for aspiration.
   5. Assess tube placement by aspirating gastric contents and measuring the pH (should be 4 or less).
   6. Assess bowel sounds; hold feeding and notify the physician if bowel sounds are absent.
   7. Use a feeding pump for continuous or cyclic feedings.
   8. For bolus feeding, leave the client in a high Fowler's position for 30 minutes after feeding.
   9. For a continuous feeding, keep the client in a semi-Fowler position at all times.
▲ D. Precautions
   1. Change the feeding container and tubing every 24 hours.
   2. Do not hang more solution than will be required for a 4-hour period to prevent bacterial growth.
   3. Check the expiration date on the formula before administering.
   4. Shake the formula well before inserting into container.
   5. Always assess placement of the tube before feeding.
   6. Always assess bowel sounds; do not administer any feedings if bowel sounds are absent.
   7. Add a drop of methyline blue to the feeding, particularly with clients who have endotracheal or tracheal tubes; suspect a tracheoesophageal fistula when blue gastric contents appear in tracheal excretion, and if this is noted, notify the physician immediately.
   8. Administer feeding at prescribed rate or via gravity flow (intermittent, bolus feedings) with a 60-mL syringe with the plunger removed.
   9. Gently flush with 30 to 50 mL of water or normal saline (depending on agency policy) with the irrigation syringe after the feeding.
▲ E. Prevention of complications
   1. Diarrhea
      a. Use fiber-containing feedings.
      b. Administer feeding slowly and at room temperature.
   2. Aspiration
      a. Verify tube placement.
      b. Do not administer feeding if residual is greater than 100 mL (check physician's order and agency policy).
      c. Keep the head of the bed elevated.
      d. If aspiration occurs, suction as needed, assess respiratory rate, auscultate lung sounds, monitor temperature for aspiration pneumonia, and prepare to obtain chest radiograph.
   3. Clogged tube
      a. Use liquid forms of medication, if possible.
      b. Flush the tube with 30 to 50 mL of water or NS (depending on agency policy) before and after medication administration and before and after bolus feeding.
      c. Flush with water every 4 hours for continuous feeding.
   4. Vomiting
      a. Administer feedings slowly, and for bolus feedings, make the feeding last for 30 minutes.
      b. Measure abdominal girth.
      c. Do not allow feeding bag to empty.
      d. Do not allow air to enter the tubing.
      e. Administer feeding at room temperature.
      f. Elevate the head of the bed.
      g. Administer antiemetics as prescribed.
      h. If client vomits, place client in side-lying position.

III. MEDICATIONS VIA NASOGASTRIC OR GASTROSTOMY TUBE   ▲
A. Crush medications or use elixir forms of medications.
B. Ensure that the medication ordered can be crushed or that the capsule can be opened.
C. Dissolve crushed medication or capsule contents in 5 to 10 mL of water.
D. Check placement and residual before instilling medications.
E. Draw up the medication into a catheter tip syringe, clear excess air, and insert medication into the tube.
F. Flush with 30 to 50 mL of water or NS (depending on agency policy).
G. Clamp the tube for 30 to 60 minutes (depending on medication and agency policy).

IV. INTESTINAL TUBES
A. Description
   1. The **intestinal tube** is passed nasally into the small intestine.
   2. The tube may be used to decompress the bowel or to remove intestinal contents.
   3. The tube enters the small intestine through the pyloric sphincter because of the weight of a small bag of mercury at the end.
B. Types of tubes (Fig. 21-1)
   1. Cantor or Harris
   2. Miller-Abbott
C. Interventions   ▲
   1. Assess physician's orders and agency policy for advancement and removal of tube.
   2. Position client on the right side to facilitate passage of the mercury weights within the tube through

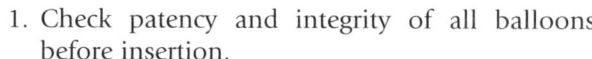

the pylorus of the stomach and into the small intestine.

3. Do not secure the tube to the face with tape until it has reached final placement (may take several hours) in the intestines.
4. Radiography is performed to verify desired placement.
5. Monitor drainage from the tube.
6. If the tube becomes blocked, notify the physician; a small amount of air injected into the lumen may be prescribed to clear the tube.
7. Assess the abdomen and measure abdominal girth.
8. To remove the tube, the mercury and air are removed from the balloon portion of the tube with a 5-mL syringe; the tube is removed gradually (6 inches every hour) as prescribed by the physician.
9. Dispose of the mercury in the appropriate manner as per agency policy.

V. ESOPHAGEAL AND GASTRIC TUBES
A. Description
   1. Used to apply pressure against esophageal veins to control bleeding
   2. Not used if the client has ulceration or necrosis of the esophagus or has had previous esophageal surgery
B. **Sengstaken-Blakemore tube** (Fig. 21-1)
   1. The **Sengstaken-Blakemore tube** is a triple-lumen gastric tube with an inflatable esophageal balloon, an inflatable gastric balloon, and a gastric aspiration lumen.
   2. The gastric balloon applies pressure at the cardio-esophageal junction to compress gastric varices directly and to decrease blood flow to esophageal varices; traction is applied to maintain the gastric balloon in place.
   3. The esophageal balloon directly compresses esophageal varices.
   4. If bleeding is not stopped with inflation of the gastric balloon, the esophageal balloon is inflated to 25 to 45 mm Hg.
   5. A radiograph of the upper abdomen and chest confirms placement.
   6. Gastric contents are aspirated by gastric lavage or intermittent suction via the gastric aspiration port.
   7. With the **Sengstaken-Blakemore tube**, a nasogastric tube also is inserted in the opposite naris to collect secretions that accumulate above the esophageal balloon.
C. Minnesota tube
   1. Four-lumen gastric tube
   2. A modified **Sengstaken-Blakemore tube** with an additional lumen for aspirating esophagopharyngeal secretions

D. Interventions
   1. Check patency and integrity of all balloons before insertion.
   2. Label each lumen.
   3. Place the client in the upright or Fowler's position for insertion.
   4. Immediately after insertion, prepare for radiography to verify placement.
   5. Maintain head elevation once the tube is in place.
   6. Double-clamp the balloon ports to prevent air leaks.
   7. Keep scissors at the bedside at all times; monitor for respiratory distress, and if it occurs, cut tubes to deflate balloons.
   8. To prevent ulceration or necrosis of the esophagus, release esophageal pressure as prescribed and per agency policy.
   9. Monitor for increased bloody drainage, which may indicate persistent bleeding.
   10. Monitor for signs of esophageal rupture, which includes a drop in blood pressure, increased heart rate, and back and upper abdominal pain; esophageal rupture is an emergency and must be reported to the physician immediately.

VI. LAVAGE TUBES
A. Description: Used to remove toxic substances from the stomach
B. Types of tubes
   1. Lavacuator
      a. The Lavacuator is an orogastric tube with a large suction lumen and a smaller lavage/vent lumen that provides continuous suction.
      b. Irrigation solution enters the lavage lumen while stomach contents are removed through the suction lumen.
   2. Ewald's: Reusable single-lumen large tube used for rapid one-time irrigation and evacuation

VII. URINARY AND RENAL TUBES
A. Routine urinary catheter care
   1. Use gloves and wash perineal area with warm soapy water.
   2. With nondominant hand, pull back the labia or foreskin to expose the meatus (in the adult male, return foreskin to its normal position).
   3. Cleanse along the catheter with soap and water.
   4. Anchor catheter to the thigh.
   5. Maintain catheter bag below the level of the bladder.
B. Ureteral and nephrostomy tubes
   1. Never clamp the tube.
   2. Maintain patency.
   3. Monitor output closely; urine output of less than 30 mL per hour or lack of output for more than 15 minutes should be reported to the physician immediately.

4. Irrigate only if prescribed by a physician, using strict aseptic technique; a maximum of 5 mL of sterile normal saline is instilled slowly and gently.

5. If patency cannot be established with prescribed irrigation, notify the physician immediately.

VIII. RESPIRATORY SYSTEM TUBES

A. Endotracheal tubes (Fig. 21-2)
1. Description
   a. The **endotracheal tube** is used to maintain a patent airway.
   b. Endotracheal tubes are indicated when the client needs mechanical ventilation.
   c. If the client requires an artificial airway for longer than 10 to 14 days, a **tracheostomy** may be created to avoid mucosal and vocal cord damage that can be caused by the **endotracheal tube**.
   d. The cuff (located at the distal end of the tube), when inflated, produces a seal between the trachea and the cuff to prevent aspiration and ensure delivery of a set tidal volume when mechanical ventilation is used; an inflated cuff also prevents air from passing to the vocal cords, nose, or mouth.
   e. The pilot balloon permits air to be inserted into the cuff, prevents air from escaping, and is used as a guideline for determining the presence or absence of air in the cuff.
   f. The universal adapter enables attachment of the tube to mechanical ventilation tubing or other types of oxygen delivery systems.
2. Orotracheal
   a. The orotracheal tube allows use of a larger-diameter tube and reduces the work of breathing.
   b. The orotracheal tube is indicated when the client has a nasal obstruction or a predisposition to epistaxis.

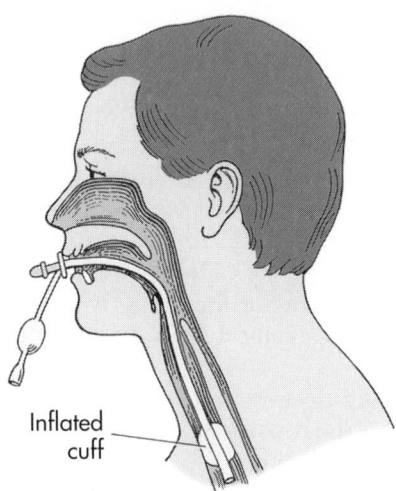

FIG. 21-2 Endotracheal tube with inflated cuff. (From Perry, A., & Potter, P. [2002]. *Clinical nursing skills and techniques* [5th ed.]. St. Louis: Mosby.)

c. The orotracheal tube is uncomfortable and can be manipulated by the tongue, causing airway obstruction; an oral airway may be needed to keep the client from biting on the tube.
3. Nasotracheal
   a. The nasotracheal tube is a smaller-sized tube and increases resistance and the client's work of breathing.
   b. The nasotracheal tube is discouraged in clients with bleeding disorders.
   c. The tube is more comfortable for the client, and the client is unable to manipulate the tube with the tongue.
4. Interventions
   a. Placement is confirmed by chest x-ray film (correct placement is 1 to 2 cm above the carina).
   b. Assess placement by auscultating both sides of chest while manually ventilating with a resuscitation (Ambu) bag (if breath sounds and chest wall movement are absent of the left side, the tube may be in the right main stem bronchus).
   c. Perform auscultation over the stomach to rule out esophageal intubation.
   d. If the tube is in the stomach, louder breath sounds will be heard over the stomach than over the chest, and abdominal distention will be present.
   e. Secure the tube with adhesive tape immediately after intubation.
   f. Monitor the position of the tube at the lip or nose.
   g. Monitor skin and mucous membranes.
   h. Suction the tube only when needed.
   i. The oral tube needs to be moved to the opposite side of the mouth daily to prevent pressure and necrosis of the lip and mouth area, prevent nerve damage, and facilitate inspection and cleaning of the mouth; moving the tube to the opposite side of the mouth should be done by two health care providers.
   j. Prevent dislodgment and pulling or tugging on the tube; suction, coughing, and speaking attempts by the client place extra stress on the tube and can cause dislodgment.
   k. Keep a resuscitation (Ambu) bag at the bedside at all times.
   l. Assess the pilot balloon to ensure that the cuff is inflated; maintain cuff inflation, which creates a seal and allows complete mechanical control of respiration.
   m. Monitor cuff pressures at least every 8 hours; they should not exceed 20 mm Hg.
5. Minimal leak technique
   a. Inflate the cuff until a seal is established.
   b. No harsh sound should be heard through a stethoscope placed over the trachea when the

client breathes in, but a slight air leak on peak inspiration is present and heard.

c. The client cannot make verbal sounds, and no air is felt coming out of the client's mouth.

6. Minimal occluding volume

   a. Provides an adequate seal in the trachea at the lowest possible cuff pressure.

   b. Use the same procedure as minimal leak technique, without an air leak.

7. Extubation

   a. Hyperoxygenate the client and suction the **endotracheal tube** and the oral cavity.

   b. Place the client in semi-Fowler position.

   c. Deflate the cuff; have the client inhale, and at peak inspiration, remove the tube, suctioning the airway through the tube while pulling it out.

   d. After removal, instruct the client to cough and deep breathe to assist in removing accumulated secretions in the throat.

   e. Apply oxygen therapy as prescribed.

   f. Monitor for respiratory difficulty; contact the physician if respiratory difficulty occurs.

   g. Inform the client that hoarseness or a sore throat is normal and that the client should limit talking if it occurs.

B. **Tracheostomy** (Fig. 21-3)

1. Description

   a. A tracheotomy is a surgical incision into the trachea for the purpose of establishing an airway.

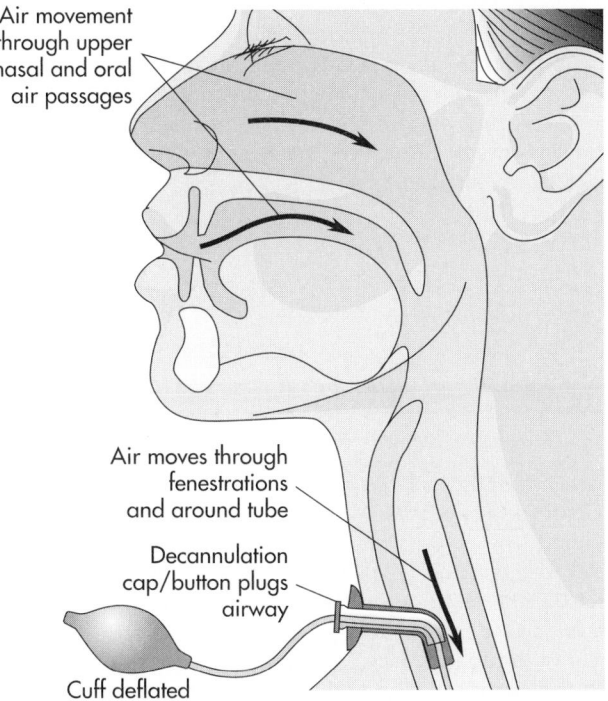

Air movement through upper nasal and oral air passages

Air moves through fenestrations and around tube

Decannulation cap/button plugs airway

Cuff deflated

FIG. 21-3   Breathing through a fenestrated tracheostomy tube with a cap in place and the cuff deflated. (From Ignatavicius, D., & Workman, M. [2002]. *Medical-surgical nursing: Critical thinking for collaborative care* [4th ed.]. Philadelphia: W. B. Saunders.)

   b. A **tracheostomy** is the stoma or opening that results from the tracheotomy (Box 21-1).

   c. The **tracheostomy** can be temporary or permanent.

2. Interventions

   a. Assess respirations and for bilateral breath sounds.

   b. Monitor arterial blood gases and pulse oximetry.

   c. Encourage coughing and deep breathing.

   d. Maintain a semi-Fowler to high Fowler's position.

   e. Monitor for bleeding, difficulty with breathing, absence of breath sounds, and crepitus, which are indications of hemorrhage, pneumothorax, and subcutaneous emphysema.

   f. Provide respiratory treatments as prescribed.

   g. Suction fluids as needed; hyperoxygenate the client before suctioning.

   h. If the client is allowed to eat, sit client up for meals and ensure that the cuff is inflated (if the tube is not capped) for meals and for 1 hour after meals.

   i. Monitor cuff pressures as prescribed.

   j. Assess the stoma and secretions for blood or purulent drainage.

   k. Follow the physician's orders and agency policy for cleaning the **tracheostomy** site and inner cannula; usually one-half strength hydrogen peroxide is used.

   l. Administer humidified oxygen as prescribed, for the normal humidification process is bypassed in a client with a **tracheostomy**.

   m. Obtain assistance in changing **tracheostomy** ties; after placing the new ties, cut and remove the old ties holding the **tracheostomy** in place.

   n. Never insert a decannulation plug into a **tracheostomy** tube until the cuff is deflated and the inner cannula is removed; prior insertion prevents airflow to the client.

   o. Keep a resuscitation (Ambu) bag, obturator, clamps, and a tracheotomy set at the bedside.

3. Complications of a **tracheostomy** (Box 21-2 and Table 21-1)

IX. CHEST TUBE DRAINAGE SYSTEM (FIG. 21-4)

A. Description

1. The **chest tube** drainage system returns negative pressure to the intrapleural space.

2. The system is used to remove abnormal accumulations of air and fluids from the pleural space.

B. Collection chamber

1. The collection chamber is located where the **chest tube** from the client connects to the system.

2. Drainage from the tube drains into and collects in a series of calibrated columns in this chamber.

BOX 21-1

Types of Tracheostomy Tubes

DOUBLE-LUMEN TUBE

The double-lumen tube has three major parts:

Outer cannula—fits into the stoma and keeps the airway open. The faceplate indicates the size and type of tube and has small holes on both sides for securing the tube with tracheostomy ties.

Inner cannula—fits snugly into the outer cannula and locks into place and provides the universal adaptor for use with the ventilator and other respiratory therapy equipment. Some may be removed, cleaned, and reused; others are disposable.

Obturator—a stylet with a smooth end used to facilitate the direction of the tube when inserting or changing a tracheostomy tube. The obturator is removed immediately after tube placement and is always kept with the client and at the bedside in case of accidental decannulation.

SINGLE-LUMEN TUBE

The single-lumen tube is a long tube used for clients with long or extra thick necks. The tube often is called a "bull neck trach" because of the long distance from the skin to the trachea or the longer length of the trachea in large persons. More intensive nursing care is required with this tube because there is no inner cannula to ensure a patent lumen.

CUFFED TUBE

A cuff, when inflated, seals the airway. The cuffed tube is used with mechanical ventilation, in preventing aspiration of oral or gastric secretions, or for tube feeding. A pilot balloon attached to the outside of the tube indicates the presence or absence of air in the cuff.

CUFFLESS TUBE

The cuffless tube is a plastic, silicone-like (Silastic), or metal tube, usually double lumen. The tube is used for long-term airway management in those clients who require

a tracheostomy, who can protect themselves from aspiration, and who do not require mechanical ventilation. Many persons can speak with this tube in place.

FENESTRATED TUBE

The fenestrated tube has a precut opening (fenestration) in the upper posterior wall of the outer cannula. The tube is used to wean the client from a tracheostomy by ensuring that the client can tolerate breathing through his or her natural airway before the entire tube is removed. This tube allows the client to speak.

CUFFED FENESTRATED TUBE

The cuffed fenestrated tube facilitates mechanical ventilation and speech and often is used for clients with spinal cord paralysis or neuromuscular disease who do not require ventilation all the time. When not on the ventilator, the client can have the cuff deflated and the tube capped for speech. A cuffed fenestrated tube is never used in weaning from a tracheostomy because the cuff, even fully deflated, may obstruct the airway partially.

METAL TRACHEOSTOMY TUBE

The metal tracheostomy tube is used for permanent tracheostomy, is a cuffless double-lumen tube, and can be cleaned and reused indefinitely. A special adaptor attaches a manual resuscitation bag. Popular types are the Jackson and Holinger tubes.

TALKING TRACHEOSTOMY TUBE

The talking tracheostomy tube provides a means of communication for the client who is using a ventilator on a long-term basis. An extra air channel allows air to flow up through the vocal cords so that the client can speak with the cuff inflated. The air can cause drying of the vocal cords from constant dry airflow.

From Ignatavicius, D., & Workman, M. (2002). *Medical-surgical nursing* (4th ed). Philadelphia: W. B. Saunders.

BOX 21-2

Complications of a Tracheostomy

TUBE OBSTRUCTION
Assessment
Difficulty in breathing
Noisy respirations
Difficulty in inserting the suction catheter
Thick, dry secretions
Unexplained peak pressures if client is on a mechanical ventilator
Prevention and Interventions
Assist the client to cough and deep breath.
Provide humidification and suctioning.
Clean the inner cannula regularly.

Physician repositions or replaces the tube if obstruction occurs as a result of cuff prolapse over the end of the tube.

TUBE DISLODGMENT
Prevention and Interventions
Secure the tube in place.
Minimize manipulation and traction on the tube.
Ensure that the client does not pull on the tube.
Ensure that a tracheostomy tube of the same type and size is at the client's bedside.

Continued

BOX 21-2

Complications of a Tracheostomy—cont'd

Be familiar with institutional policy regarding replacement of a tracheostomy tube as a nursing procedure.

During the first 72 hours following surgical placement of the tracheostomy:

The nurse manually ventilates the client by using a manual resuscitation (Ambu) bag while another nurse calls the resuscitation team for help.

After 72 hours following surgical placement of the tracheostomy:

Extend the client's neck and open the tissues of the stoma to secure the airway.

Grasp the retention sutures (if they are present) to spread the opening.

Use a tracheal dilator (curved clamp) to hold the stoma open.

Prepare to insert tracheostomy tube; place obturator into tracheostomy tube, replace the tube, and remove the obturator.

Maintain ventilation by resuscitation (Ambu) bag.

Assess airflow and bilateral breath sounds.

If unable to secure an airway, call the resuscitation team and the anesthesiologist.

TABLE 21-1

Complications of Tracheostomy

Complications and Description	Signs and Symptoms	Management	Prevention
Tracheomalacia: Constant pressure exerted by the cuff causes tracheal dilation and erosion.	An increased amount of air is required in the cuff to maintain the seal. A larger tracheostomy tube is required to prevent an air leak at the stoma. Food particles are seen in tracheal secretions. The client does not receive the set tidal volume on the ventilator.	No special management is needed unless bleeding occurs.	Use an uncuffed tube as soon as possible. Monitor cuff pressure and air volumes closely and detect changes.
Tracheal stenosis: Narrowed tracheal lumen is due to scar formation from irritation of tracheal mucosa by the cuff.	Stenosis usually is seen after the cuff is deflated or the tracheostomy tube is removed. The client has increased coughing, inability to expectorate secretions, or difficulty in breathing or talking.	Tracheal dilation or surgical intervention is used.	Prevent pulling of and traction on the tracheostomy tube. Properly secure the tube in the midline position. Maintain proper cuff pressure. Minimize oronasal intubation time.
Tracheoesophageal fistula (TEF): Excessive cuff pressure causes erosion of the posterior wall of the trachea. A hole is created between the trachea and the anterior esophagus. The client at highest risk also has a nasogastric tube present.	Similar to tracheomalacia: • Food particles are seen in tracheal secretions. • Increased air in cuff is needed to achieve a seal. • The client has increased coughing and choking while eating. • The client does not receive the set tidal volume on the ventilator.	Manually administer oxygen by mask to prevent hypoxemia. A small soft feeding tube is used instead of a nasogastric tube for tube feedings. A gastrostomy or jejunostomy may be performed. Monitor the client with a nasogastric tube closely; assess for TEF and aspiration.	Maintain cuff pressure. Monitor the amount of air needed for inflation and detect changes. Progress to a deflated cuff or cuffless tube as soon as possible.
Trachea-innominate artery fistula: A malpositioned tube causes its distal tip to push against the lateral wall of the tracheostomy. Continued pressure causes necrosis and erosion of the innominate artery. *This is a medical emergency.*	The tracheostomy tube pulsates in synchrony with the heartbeat. There is heavy bleeding from the stoma. This is a life-threatening complication.	Remove the tracheostomy tube immediately. Apply direct pressure to the innominate artery at the stoma site. Prepare the client for immediate surgical repair.	Use correct tube size and maintain tube in midline position. Prevent pulling or tugging on the tracheostomy tube. Immediately notify the physician of the pulsating tube.

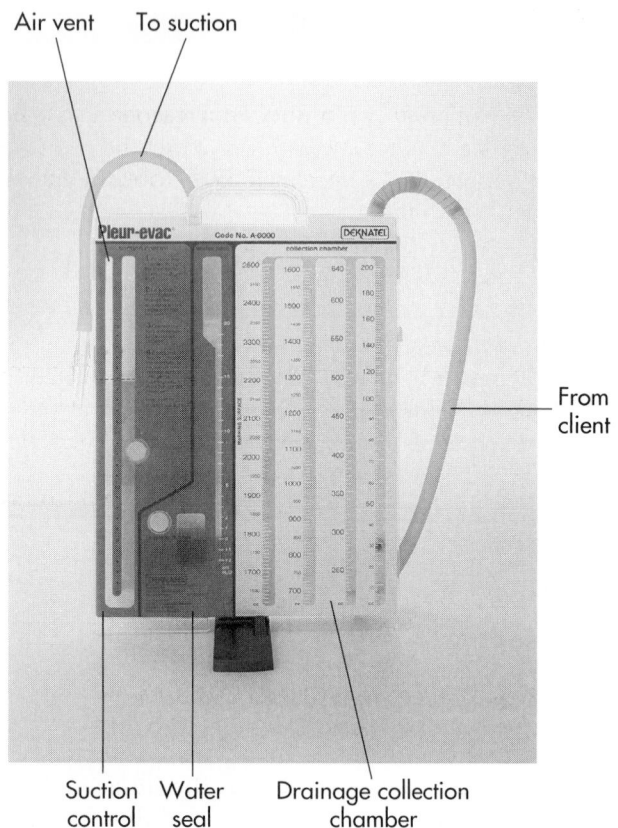

Air vent   To suction

From client

Suction control   Water seal   Drainage collection chamber

FIG. 21-4   The Pleur-Evac drainage system, a commercial three-bottle chest drainage device. (From Ignatavicius, D., & Workman, M. [2002]. *Medical-surgical nursing: Critical thinking for collaborative care* [4th ed.]. Philadelphia: W. B. Saunders.)

C. Water seal chamber
1. The tip of the tube is underwater, allowing fluid and air to drain from the pleural space and preventing air from entering the pleural space.
2. Water oscillates (moves up as the client inhales and moves down as the client exhales).
3. Bubbling indicates an air leak in the **chest tube** system.
D. Suction control chamber
1. The suction control chamber provides the suction, which can be controlled to provide negative pressure to the chest.
2. This chamber is filled with various levels of water to achieve the desired level of suction; without this control, lung tissue could be sucked into the **chest tube**.
3. Gentle bubbling in this chamber indicates that there is suction and does not indicate that air is escaping from the pleural space.
E. Dry suction system
1. Because this is a dry suction system, absence of bubbling is noted in the suction control chamber.
2. A knob on the collection device is used to set the prescribed amount of suction; then the wall

suction source dial is turned until a small orange floater valve appears in the window on the device (when the orange floater valve is in the window, the correct amount of suction is applied).
F. Interventions
1. Collection chamber
a. Monitor drainage; notify the physician if drainage is greater than 100 mL per hour or if drainage becomes bright red or increases suddenly.
b. Mark the **chest tube** drainage in the collection chamber at 1- to 4-hour intervals, using a piece of tape.
2. Water seal chamber
a. Monitor for fluctuation of the fluid level in the water seal chamber.
b. Fluctuation in the water seal chamber stops if the tube is obstructed, if a dependent loop exists, if the suction is not working properly, or if the lung has reexpanded.
c. If the client has a known pneumothorax, intermittent bubbling in the water seal chamber is expected as air is drained from the chest, but continuous bubbling indicates of an air leak in the system.
d. Notify the physician if there is continuous bubbling in the water seal chamber.
3. Suction control chamber: Gentle bubbling should be noted in the suction control chamber (vigorous bubbling indicates an air leak, and the physician should be notified).
4. An occlusive sterile dressing is maintained at the insertion site.
5. A chest radiograph assesses the position of the tube and determines whether the lung has reexpanded.
6. Assess respiratory status and auscultate lung sounds.
7. Monitor for signs of extended pneumothroax or hemothorax.
8. Keep the drainage system below the level of the chest and the tubes free of kinks, dependent loops, or other obstructions.
9. Ensure that all connections are secure.
10. Encourage coughing and deep breathing.
11. Change the client's position frequently to promote drainage and ventilation.
12. Do not strip or milk a **chest tube** unless specifically directed to do so by a physician and if the agency policy allows it.
13. Keep a clamp and a sterile occlusive dressing at the bedside at all times.
14. Never clamp a **chest tube** without a written order from the physician; also, determine agency policy for clamping a **chest tube**.
15. If the drainage system cracks or breaks, insert the **chest tube** into a bottle of sterile water,

remove the cracked or broken system, and replace it with a new system.

16. If the **chest tube** is pulled out of the chest accidentally, pinch the skin opening together, apply an occlusive sterile dressing, cover the dressing with overlapping pieces of 2-inch tape, and call the physician immediately.

17. When the **chest tube** is removed, the client is asked to take a deep breath and hold it, and the tube is removed; a dry sterile dressing, petroleum gauze dressing, or Telfa dressing (depending on the physician's preference) is taped in place after removal of the **chest tube**.

18. Depending on the physician's preference, when the **chest tube** is removed, the client may be asked to take a deep breath, exhale, and bear down (Valsalva's maneuver).

PRACTICE QUESTIONS

1. A nurse orientee is preparing to insert a nasogastric tube, and a nurse educator is observing the procedure. Which of the following supplies if obtained by the nurse orientee would indicate a need for further education regarding this procedure?
   1. Half-inch or one-inch tape
   2. Oil-soluble lubricant
   3. A glass of tap water with a straw
   4. A 50-mL catheter tip syringe

2. A registered nurse is observing a new orientee who is inserting a nasogastric tube in an adult client. The new orientee is determining the length of tube insertion. Which of the following observations indicates accurate measurement of the length of the tube to be inserted?
   1. The new orientee places the tube at the tip of the nose and measures by extending the tube to the earlobe and then down to the xiphoid process.
   2. The new orientee places the tube at the tip of the nose and measures by extending the tube to the earlobe and then down to the top of the sternum.
   3. The new orientee marks the tube at 10 inches.
   4. The new orientee marks the tube at 32 inches.

3. A nurse is inserting a nasogastric tube in an adult client. During the procedure, the client begins to cough and has difficulty breathing. Which of the following is the most appropriate nursing action?
   1. Remove the tube and reinsert when the respiratory distress subsides.
   2. Pull back on the tube and wait until the respiratory distress subsides.
   3. Quickly insert the tube.
   4. Notify the physician immediately.

4. A nurse is assessing for correct placement of a nasogastric tube. The nurse aspirates the stomach contents and checks the contents for pH. The nurse verifies correct tube placement if which pH value is noted?
   1. 7.5

2. 7.35
3. 7.0
4. 4.0

5. A nurse is preparing to remove a nasogastric tube from a client. The nurse would instruct the client to do which of the following just before the nurse removes the tube?
   1. To perform a Valsalva's maneuver
   2. To take and hold a deep breath
   3. To exhale
   4. To inhale and exhale quickly

6. A nurse is preparing to administer medication through a nasogastric tube that is connected to suction. To administer the medication accurately, the nurse would
   1. Aspirate the nasogastric tube after medication administration to maintain patency.
   2. Position the client supine to assist in medication absorption.
   3. Clamp the nasogastric tube for 30 minutes following administration of the medication.
   4. Change the suction setting to low intermittent suction for 30 minutes after medication administration.

7. A nurse assists a physician with the insertion of a Miller-Abbott tube. After insertion of the tube, the nurse would assist the client to which of the following positions?
   1. On the right side
   2. On the left side
   3. Prone
   4. Left lateral Sims'

8. A nurse is preparing to care for a client with esophageal varices who has just had a Sengstaken-Blakemore tube inserted. The nurse gathers supplies, knowing that which of the following items must be kept at the bedside at all times?
   1. An irrigation set
   2. A pair of scissors
   3. A Kelly clamp
   4. An obturator

9. A nurse is inserting an indwelling urinary catheter into the urethra of a male client. As the nurse inflates the balloon, the client complains of discomfort. The most appropriate nursing action is to
   1. Remove the syringe from the balloon; discomfort is normal and temporary.
   2. Aspirate the fluid, advance the catheter farther, and reinflate the balloon.
   3. Aspirate the fluid, withdraw the catheter slightly, and reinflate the balloon.
   4. Aspirate the fluid, remove the catheter and insert a new catheter.

10. A nurse is inserting an indwelling urinary catheter into a male client. As the catheter is inserted into the urethra, urine begins to flow into the tubing. At this point, the nurse

1. Immediately inflates the balloon.
2. Withdraws the catheter about 1 inch and inflates the balloon.
3. Inserts the catheter until resistance is met and inflates the balloon.
4. Inserts the catheter 2.5 to 5 cm and inflates the balloon.

11. A nurse has assisted a physician with the insertion of a chest tube. The nurse monitors the client and notes fluctuation of the fluid level in the water seal chamber after the tube is inserted. Based on this assessment, which of the following actions would be most appropriate?
    1. Inform the physician.
    2. Encourage the client to deep breathe.
    3. Continue to monitor, for this is an expected finding.
    4. Reinforce the occlusive dressing.

12. A nurse is caring for a client with a chest tube. The nurse turns the client to the side, and the chest tube accidentally disconnects. The initial nursing action is to
    1. Call the physician.
    2. Place the tube in a bottle of sterile water.
    3. Immediately replace the chest tube system.
    4. Place a sterile dressing over the disconnection site.

13. A nurse is assisting a physician with the removal of a chest tube. The nurse most appropriately instructs the client to
    1. Stay very still.
    2. Inhale and exhale quickly.
    3. Exhale slowly.
    4. Perform Valsalva's maneuver.

14. A nurse is changing the tapes on a tracheostomy tube. The client coughs and the tube is dislodged. The initial nursing action is to

1. Cover the tracheostomy site with a sterile dressing to prevent infection.
2. Call the physician to reinsert the tube.
3. Grasp the retention sutures to spread the opening.
4. Call the respiratory therapy department to reinsert the tracheotomy.

15. A nurse is caring for a client immediately after removal of the endotracheal tube following radical neck dissection. The nurse reports which of the following signs immediately if experienced by the client?
    1. Stridor
    2. Occasional pink-tinged sputum
    3. Respiratory rate of 24 breaths per minute
    4. A few basilar crackles on the right

CRITICAL THINKING: MULTIPLE RESPONSE

A nurse is assessing the functioning of a chest tube drainage system in a client who just returned from the recovery room following a thoracotomy with wedge resection. Select all expected assessment findings.

___ Excessive bubbling in the water seal chamber

___ Vigorous bubbling in the suction control chamber

___ Fluctuation of water in the tube in the water seal chamber during inhalation and exhalation

___ 50 mL of drainage in the drainage collection chamber

___ An occlusive dressing is in place over the chest tube insertion site

___ The drainage system is maintained below the client's chest

ANSWERS

1. 2

Rationale: Water-soluble lubricant is used to lubricate 3 to 4 inches of the tube at the insertion end. An oil lubricant is not used because if the tube accidentally goes into the bronchus, pneumonia can develop. Half-inch tape is used to secure the tube after correct placement is verified. A 50-mL catheter tip syringe is used to aspirate gastric contents to confirm placement. The client will be asked to take a sip of water through a straw to help with the passage of the tube.

Test-Taking Strategy: Use the process of elimination. Note the key words "indicate a need for further education." Attempt to visualize the procedure as you answer the question. Remember that water-soluble lubricant must be used to lubricate the tube. If you had difficulty with this question, review the procedure for inserting a nasogastric tube.

Level of Cognitive Ability: Analysis
Client Needs: Physiological Integrity
Integrated Process: Teaching/Learning

Content Area: Adult health—gastrointestinal
Reference: Potter, P., & Perry, A. (2001). *Fundamentals of nursing* (5th ed., p. 1474). St. Louis: Mosby.

2. 1

Rationale: Measuring the length of tube needed is done by placing the tube at the tip of the client's nose and extending the tube to the earlobe and then down to the xiphoid process. The average length for an adult is about 22 to 26 inches.

Test-Taking Strategy: Use the process of elimination. Attempt to visualize this procedure. Eliminate options 3 and 4 first because 10 inches is short and 32 inches is rather lengthy. Remember the abbreviation *NEX*, which stands for nose, earlobe, xiphoid process, to assist in answering questions similar to this one. Review the procedure for measuring the length of a nasogastric tube for insertion if you had difficulty with this question.

Level of Cognitive Ability: Analysis
Client Needs: Physiological Integrity

Integrated Process: Teaching/Learning
Content Area: Adult health—gastrointestinal
Reference: Potter, P., & Perry, A. (2001). *Fundamentals of nursing* (5th ed., p. 1475). St. Louis: Mosby.

3. 2
Rationale: During the insertion of a nasogastric tube, if the client experiences difficulty breathing or any respiratory distress, withdraw the tube slightly, stop the tube advancement, and wait until the distress subsides. Options 1 and 4 are unnecessary. Quickly inserting the tube is not an appropriate action because, in this situation, it may be likely that the tube has entered the bronchus.
Test-Taking Strategy: Use the process of elimination. Options 3 and 4 can be eliminated first. Visualizing the procedure and anticipating potential complications will assist in eliminating option 1 as an unnecessary action. Review the cautions related to inserting a nasogastric tube if you had difficulty with this question.
Level of Cognitive Ability: Application
Client Needs: Physiological Integrity
Integrated Process: Nursing Process—implementation
Content Area: Adult health—gastrointestinal
Reference: Potter, P., & Perry, A. (2001). *Fundamentals of nursing* (5th ed., p. 1476). St. Louis: Mosby.

4. 4
Rationale: If the nasogastric tube is in the stomach, the pH of the contents will be acidic. Gastric aspirates have acidic pH values and should be 4 or less. Option 1 indicates an alkaline pH. Option 2 indicates a neutral pH. Option 3 indicates a slightly acidic pH.
Test-Taking Strategy: Use the process of elimination and note the key word "verifies." Recalling that gastric contents are acidic will direct you to option 4. If you had difficulty with this question, review the procedure for assessing nasogastric tube placement.
Level of Cognitive Ability: Analysis
Client Needs: Physiological Integrity
Integrated Process: Nursing Process—analysis
Content Area: Adult health—gastrointestinal
Reference: Potter, P., & Perry, A. (2001). *Fundamentals of nursing* (5th ed., p. 1476). St. Louis: Mosby.

5. 2
Rationale: When the nurse removes a nasogastric tube, the client is instructed to take and hold a deep breath. This will close the epiglottis, and the airway will be obstructed temporarily during the tube removal. This allows for easy withdrawal through the esophagus into the nose. The nurse removes the tube with one smooth, continuous pull.
Test-Taking Strategy: Use the process of elimination and focus on the issue, removing a nasogastric tube. Visualize the procedure as a guide, considering what each action identified in the options would produce. Review the procedure for removing a nasogastric tube, if you had difficulty with this question.
Level of Cognitive Ability: Application
Client Needs: Physiological Integrity
Integrated Process: Nursing Process—implementation
Content Area: Adult health—gastrointestinal

Reference: Potter, P., & Perry, A. (2001). *Fundamentals of nursing* (5th ed., p. 1479). St. Louis: Mosby.

6. 3
Rationale: If a client has a nasogastric tube connected to suction, the nurse should wait up to 30 minutes before reconnecting the tube to the suction apparatus to allow adequate time for medication absorption. Aspirating the nasogastric tube will remove the medication just administered. Low intermittent suction also will remove the medication just administered. The client should not be placed in the supine position because of the risk for aspiration.
Test-Taking Strategy: Use the process of elimination. Eliminate options 1 and 4 first because these actions are similar and will produce the same effect. Recalling that the client should not be placed in a supine position will assist in eliminating option 2. If you had difficulty with this question, review the procedure for administering medications through a nasogastric tube.
Level of Cognitive Ability: Application
Client Needs: Physiological Integrity
Integrated Process: Nursing Process—implementation
Content Area: Adult health—gastrointestinal
Reference: Perry, A., & Potter, P. (2002). *Clinical nursing skills and techniques* (5th ed., p. 464). St. Louis: Mosby.

7. 1
Rationale: A Miller-Abbott tube is an intestinal tube that has a double lumen, one for a mercury balloon and the other for suction or drainage. After insertion, the tube is allowed to advance over several hours. The client is positioned on the right side to facilitate passage through the pylorus of the stomach and into the small intestine.
Test-Taking Strategy: Use the process of elimination. Eliminate options 2 and 4 because they are similar. From the remaining options, recalling the purpose of this tube and the anatomy of the body will assist in directing you to option 1. If you had difficulty with this question, review care to the client with a Miller-Abbott tube.
Level of Cognitive Ability: Application
Client Needs: Physiological Integrity
Integrated Process: Nursing Process—implementation
Content Area: Adult health—gastrointestinal
Reference: Lewis, S., Heitkemper, M., & Dirksen, S. (2004). *Medical-surgical nursing: Assessment and management of clinical problems* (6th ed., pp. 1080-1081). St. Louis: Mosby.

8. 2
Rationale: When the client has a Sengstaken-Blakemore tube, a pair of scissors must be kept at the client's bedside at all times. The client needs to be observed for sudden respiratory distress, which occurs if the gastric balloon ruptures and the entire tube moves upward. If this occurs, the nurse immediately cuts all balloon lumens and removes the tube. An obturator and a Kelly clamp are kept at the bedside of a client with a tracheostomy. An irrigation set may be kept at the bedside, but it is not the priority item.
Test-Taking Strategy: Use the process of elimination and knowledge regarding the structure, function, and placement of a Sengstaken-Blakemore tube to answer this question. Note the key word "must" in the stem of the question. This should

assist in eliminating options 1, 3, and 4. If you had difficulty with this question, review nursing care for a client with a Sengstaken-Blakemore tube.
Level of Cognitive Ability: Application
Client Needs: Physiological Integrity
Integrated Process: Nursing Process—planning
Content Area: Adult health—gastrointestinal
Reference: Ignatavicius, D., & Workman, M. (2002). *Medical-surgical nursing: Critical thinking for collaborative care* (4th ed., p. 1309). Philadelphia: W. B. Saunders.

9. 2
Rationale: If the balloon is malpositioned in the urethra, inflating the balloon could produce trauma, and pain will occur. If pain occurs, the fluid should be aspirated and the catheter inserted a little farther to provide sufficient space to inflate the balloon. The balloon of the catheter is behind the opening at the insertion tip. Inserting the catheter the extra distance will ensure that the balloon is inflated inside the bladder and not in the urethra. There is no need to remove the catheter and insert a new one. Pain when the balloon is inflated is not normal.
Test Taking Strategy: Use the process of elimination, noting the issue of the question, the client's complaint of discomfort. Attempt to visualize this procedure and the anatomy of the urinary system to answer this question. If you had difficulty with this question, review the procedure for inserting a urinary catheter.
Level of Cognitive Ability: Application
Client Needs: Physiological Integrity
Integrated Process: Nursing Process—implementation
Content Area: Adult health—renal
Reference: Perry, A., & Potter, P. (2002). *Clinical nursing skills and techniques* (5th ed., p. 712). St. Louis: Mosby.

10. 4
Rationale: The balloon of the catheter is behind the opening at the insertion tip. The catheter is inserted 2.5 to 5 cm after urine begins to flow to provide sufficient space to inflate the balloon. Inserting the catheter the extra distance will ensure that the balloon is inflated inside the bladder and not in the urethra. Inflating the balloon in the urethra could produce trauma.
Test-Taking Strategy: Knowledge of the proper procedure for inserting an indwelling urinary catheter will assist you in answering this question. Note the key words "urine begins to flow." Options 2 and 3 can be eliminated easily. Eliminate option 1 next because of the word "immediately." If you had difficulty with this question, review the procedure for bladder catheterization.
Level of Cognitive Ability: Application
Client Needs: Physiological Integrity
Integrated Process: Nursing Process—implementation
Content Area: Adult health—renal
Reference: Potter, P., & Perry, A. (2001). *Fundamentals of nursing* (5th ed., p. 1419). St. Louis: Mosby.

11. 3
Rationale: The presence of fluctuation of the fluid level in the water seal chamber indicates a patent drainage system.

With normal breathing the water level rises with inspiration and falls with expiration. Fluctuation stops if the tube is obstructed, if a dependent loop exists, if the suction is not working properly, or if the lung has reexpanded. Options 1, 2, and 4 are incorrect.
Test-Taking Strategy: Use the process of elimination, focusing on the issue, fluctuation of the fluid level in the water seal chamber. Recalling that this is an expected finding will direct you to the correct option. Review the expected and unexpected assessment findings in the care of a client with a chest tube if you had difficulty with this question.
Level of Cognitive Ability: Analysis
Client Needs: Physiological Integrity
Integrated Process: Nursing Process—implementation
Content Area: Adult health—respiratory
Reference: Potter, P., & Perry, A. (2001). *Fundamentals of nursing* (5th ed., p. 1174). St. Louis: Mosby.

12. 2
Rationale: If the chest drainage system is disconnected, the end of the tube is placed in a bottle of sterile water held below the level of the chest. The system is replaced if it breaks or cracks or if the collection chamber is full. Placing a sterile dressing over the disconnection site will not prevent complications resulting from the disconnection. The physician may need to be notified, but this is not the initial action.
Test-Taking Strategy: Use the process of elimination. Note the key word "initial" in the stem of the question. This indicates that a nursing action is required that will prevent a serious complication as a result of the disconnection. Eliminate options 1 and 3 because these actions delay required and immediate intervention. Knowledge of the complications that can occur from a disconnection will direct you easily to option 2. Review interventions related to the complications of a chest tube if you had difficulty with this question.
Level of Cognitive Ability: Application
Client Needs: Physiological Integrity
Integrated Process: Nursing Process—implementation
Content Area: Adult health—respiratory
Reference: Potter, P., & Perry, A. (2001). *Fundamentals of nursing* (5th ed., pp. 1175-1176). St. Louis: Mosby.

13. 4
Rationale: When the chest tube is removed, the client is asked to perform Valsalva's maneuver (take a deep breath, exhale, and bear down). The tube is quickly withdrawn, and an airtight dressing is taped in place. An alternative instruction is to ask the client to take a deep breath and hold the breath while the tube is removed. Options 1, 2, and 3 are incorrect client instructions.
Test-Taking Strategy: Use the process of elimination. Visualize the procedure and the client instructions as you select an option. If you had difficulty with this question, review the procedure for removal of a chest tube.
Level of Cognitive Ability: Application
Client Needs: Physiological Integrity
Integrated Process: Nursing Process—implementation
Content Area: Adult health—respiratory
References: Perry, A., & Potter, P. (2002). *Clinical nursing skills and techniques* (5th ed., p. 690). St. Louis: Mosby.

Potter, P., & Perry, A. (2001). *Fundamentals of nursing* (5th ed., p. 1440). St. Louis: Mosby.

14. 3

Rationale: If the tube is dislodged accidentally, the initial nursing action is to grasp the retention sutures and spread the opening. If agency policy permits, the nurse then attempts immediately to replace the tube. Covering the tracheostomy site will block the airway. Options 2 and 4 will delay treatment in this emergency situation.

Test-Taking Strategy: Use the process of elimination. Eliminate options 2 and 4 first because they are similar and will delay the immediate intervention needed. Eliminate option 1 because this action will block the airway. If you had difficulty with this question, review the intervention required if a tracheostomy tube dislodges.

Level of Cognitive Ability: Application
Client Needs: Physiological Integrity
Integrated Process: Nursing Process—implementation
Content Area: Adult health—respiratory
Reference: Lewis, S., Heitkemper, M., & Dirksen, S. (2004). *Medical-surgical nursing: Assessment and management of clinical problems* (6th ed., p. 582). St. Louis: Mosby.

15. 1

Rationale: The nurse reports stridor to the physician immediately. This is a high-pitched, coarse sound that is heard with the stethoscope over the trachea. Stridor indicates airway edema and places the client at risk for airway obstruction. Options 2, 3, and 4 are not signs that require immediate notification of the physician.

Test Taking Strategy: Use the process of elimination. Recall that the prime danger after removal of an artificial airway is the client's ability to maintain a patent airway and breathe independently. In comparing each of the options with this risk in mind, eliminate options 2, 3, and 4. Because stridor indicates laryngeal edema and possible airway obstruction, it is the symptom that must be reported immediately. Review care to the client following removal of an endotracheal tube if you had difficulty with this question.

Level of Cognitive Ability: Analysis
Client Needs: Physiological Integrity
Integrated Process: Nursing Process—implementation
Content Area: Adult health—respiratory

Reference: Lewis, S., Heitkemper, M., & Dirksen, S. (2004). *Medical-surgical nursing: Assessment and management of clinical problems* (6th ed., p. 1791). St. Louis: Mosby.

CRITICAL THINKING: MULTIPLE RESPONSE

Answer:
Fluctuation of water in the tube in the water seal chamber during inhalation and exhalation
50 mL of drainage in the drainage collection chamber
An occlusive dressing is in place over the chest tube insertion site
The drainage system is maintained below the client's chest

Rationale: The bubbling of water in the water seal chamber indicates air drainage from the client and usually is seen when intrathoracic pressure is greater than atmospheric pressure and may occur during exhalation, coughing, or sneezing. Excessive bubbling in the water seal chamber may indicate an air leak, an unexpected finding. Fluctuation of water in the tube in the water seal chamber during inhalation and exhalation is expected. An absence of fluctuation may indicate that the chest tube is obstructed or that the lung has reexpanded and that no more air is leaking into the pleural space.

Gentle (not vigorous) bubbling should be noted in the suction control chamber. A total of 50 mL of drainage is not excessive in a client returning to the nursing unit from the recovery room. Drainage that is more that 100 mL per hour is considered excessive and requires physician notification. The chest tube insertion site is covered with an occlusive (airtight) dressing to prevent air from entering the pleural space. Positioning the drainage system below the client's chest allows gravity to drain the pleural space.

Test-Taking Strategy: Thinking about the physiology associated with the functioning of a chest tube drainage system will assist in answering this question. The words "excessive bubbling" and "vigorous bubbling" will assist in eliminating these assessment findings. Review care to the client with a chest tube drainage system if you had difficulty with this question.

Level of Cognitive Ability: Analysis
Client Needs: Physiological Integrity
Integrated Process: Nursing Process—assessment
Content Area: Adult health—respiratory
Reference: Ignatavicius, D., & Workman, M. (2002). *Medical-surgical nursing: Critical thinking for collaborative care* (4th ed., pp. 564-568). Philadelphia: W. B. Saunders.

REFERENCES

Ignatavicius, D., & Workman, M. (2002). *Medical-surgical nursing: Critical thinking for collaborative care* (4th ed.). Philadelphia: W. B. Saunders.

Lewis, S., Heitkemper, M., & Dirksen, S. (2004). *Medical-surgical nursing: Assessment and management of clinical problems* (6th ed.). St. Louis: Mosby.

National Council of State Boards of Nursing (Eds.) (2003). *Test Plan for the National Council Licensure Examination for Registered Nurses* (effective date: April 2004). Chicago: Author.

Perry, A., & Potter, P. (2002). *Clinical nursing skills and techniques* (5th ed.). St. Louis: Mosby.

Phipps, W., Monahan, F., Sands, J., Marek, J., & Neighbors, M. (2003). *Medical-surgical nursing: Health and illness perspectives* (7th ed.). St. Louis: Mosby.

Potter, P., & Perry, A. (2001). *Fundamentals of nursing* (5th ed.). St. Louis: Mosby.

UNIT V

Maternity Nursing

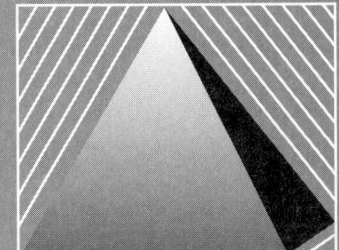

PYRAMID TERMS

amniotic fluid   Fluid that surrounds and protects the fetus and consisting of 800 to 1200 mL by the end of pregnancy. The fetus floats in the amniotic fluid, which serves as a cushion against injury from sudden blows or movements and helps maintain a constant body temperature for the fetus. The fetus voids into the amniotic fluid and also drinks and breathes the fluid.

ballottement   Rebounding of the fetus against the examiner's finger on palpation. When the examiner taps the cervix, the fetus floats upward in the amniotic fluid. The examiner feels a rebound when the fetus falls back.

Chadwick's sign   Bluish coloration of the mucous membranes of the cervix, vagina, and vulva that occurs at about 6 weeks of pregnancy and is a probable sign of pregnancy.

delivery is   Actual event of birth; the expulsion or extraction of the neonate.

fertilization   Uniting of the sperm and ovum, which occurs within 12 hours of ovulation and within 2 to 3 days of insemination, the average duration of viability for the ovum and sperm.

Goodell's sign   Softening of the cervix that occurs at the beginning of the second month of gestation and is a probable sign of pregnancy.

gravida   A pregnant woman; called gravida I (primagravida) during the first pregnancy, gravida II during the second, and so on.

Hegar's sign   Compressibility and softening of the lower uterine segment that occurs at about week 6 of gestation; a probable sign of pregnancy.

implantation   Attachment of the zygote to the uterine wall 6 to 8 days after ovulation.

infant   A baby born alive; also from 28 days of age until the first birthday.

labor   Coordinated sequence of involuntary uterine contractions resulting in effacement and dilation of cervix, followed by expulsion of the products of conception.

lochia   Discharge from the uterus that consists of blood from the vessels of the placental site and debris from the decidua; lasts for 2 to 3 weeks after delivery.

Nägele's rule   Determines the estimated date of confinement and works on the premise that the woman has a 28-day menstrual cycle. Add 7 days to the first day of the last menstrual period. Subtract 3 months and add 1 year. Alternatively, add 7 days to the last menstrual period and count forward 9 months.

neonate   A human offspring from the time of birth to the twenty-eighth day of life; also called newborn.

newborn   A human offspring from the time of birth to the twenty-eighth day of life; also called neonate.

parity   The number of pregnancies that have been carried to viability.

placenta   The organ that provides for the exchange of nutrients and waste products between the fetus and the mother, produces hormones to maintain pregnancy, and develops by the third month of gestation; also called afterbirth.

quickening   First perception of fetal movement, appearing usually in the sixteenth to eighteenth week of pregnancy.

▲ THE PYRAMID TO SUCCESS

The Pyramid to Success focuses on the physiological and psychosocial aspects related to the experience of pregnancy. Pyramid Points begin with instructing the pregnant client in measures that will promote a healthy environment for the mother and the fetus. Focus on the importance of antepartum follow-up, nutrition, and the interventions for common discomforts that occur during pregnancy. Review the purpose of the commonly prescribed diagnostic tests and procedures in the antepartum period. Focus on disorders that can occur during pregnancy, particularly pregnancy-induced hypertension and diabetes. Review the labor and delivery process and the immediate interventions for conditions in which the mother or fetal status is compromised, such as prolapsed cord or altered fetal heart rate. Review fetal effects from the mother with human immunodeficiency virus or acquired immunodeficiency syndrome or the substance-abusing mother. Focus on the normal expectations of the postpartum period and the complications that can occur. Pyramid Points also focus on the normal physical assessment findings in the neonate and the early identification of disorders in the neonate. Integrated Processes addressed in this unit include Nursing Process, Caring, Communication and Documentation, and Teaching/Learning.

▲ CLIENT NEEDS

Safe, Effective Care Environment

Confidentiality
Consultations with members of the health care team
Continuity of care
Establishing of priorities
Handling of infectious materials
Informed consent for procedures
Medical and surgical asepsis
Parent rights
Referrals
Standard, transmission-based, and other precautions during delivery of care

Health Promotion and Maintenance

Birthing and parenting issues
Concepts of wellness
Expected body image changes
Family planning and family systems
Growth and development and health care screening
Lifestyle choices
Reproduction and human sexuality
Teaching regarding antepartum, intrapartum, and postpartum care
Techniques of physical assessment

Psychosocial Integrity

Coping mechanisms
Cultural, religious, and spiritual influences regarding birth and motherhood
Situational role changes
Support systems
Therapeutic interactions

Physiological Integrity

Alterations in body systems
Commonly prescribed diagnostic tests and procedures
Interventions for unexpected events during pregnancy
Labor and delivery process
Normal expectations during pregnancy
Nutrition
Physiological changes that occur during pregnancy
Risk identification during pregnancy

REFERENCES

Herlihy, B., & Maebius, N. (2003). *The human body in health and illness* (2nd ed.). Philadelphia: W. B. Saunders.

Lowdermilk, D., & Perry, S. (2003). *Maternity nursing* (6th ed.). St. Louis: Mosby.

Matteson, P. (2001). *Women's health during the childbearing years: A community-based approach.* St. Louis: Mosby.

Murray, S., McKinney, E., & Gorrie, T. (2002). *Foundations of maternal-newborn nursing* (3rd ed.). Philadelphia: W. B. Saunders.

National Council of State Boards of Nursing (Eds.) (2003). *Test Plan for the National Council Licensure Examination for Registered Nurses* (effective date: April 2004). Chicago: Author.

Potter, P., & Perry, A. (2001). *Fundamentals of nursing* (5th ed.). St. Louis: Mosby.

Varcarolis, E. M. (2002). *Foundations of psychiatric mental health nursing* (4th ed.). Philadelphia: W. B. Saunders.

Wong, D., Hockenberry-Eaton, M. (2000). *Wong's essentials of pediatric nursing* (6th ed.). St. Louis: Mosby.

Wong, D., Perry, S., & Hockenberry, M. (2002). *Maternal child nursing care.* (2nd ed.). St. Louis: Mosby.

Female Reproductive System

I. REPRODUCTIVE STRUCTURES
A. Ovaries
1. Formation and expulsion of ova
2. Secretion of estrogen and progesterone

B. Fallopian tubes
1. Muscular tubes (oviducts) approximate to the ovaries and connected to the uterus
2. Tubes that propel the ova from the ovaries to the uterus

C. Uterus
1. A muscular, pear-shaped cavity in which the fetus develops
2. The cavity from which menstruation occurs

D. Cervix
1. The cervix is the internal os that opens into the body of the uterine cavity.
2. Cervical canal is located between the internal os and the external os.
3. External cervical os opens into the vagina.

E. Vagina
1. Mucous membrane-lined channel through the muscles of the pelvic floor
2. Known as the birth canal
3. Passage between the cervical os and the external environment
   a. Passageway for menstrual blood flow
   b. Passageway for fetus

II. MENSTRUAL CYCLE (BOX 22-1)
A. Ovarian hormones
1. Ovarian hormones include the follicle-stimulating hormone and luteinizing hormone.
2. The hormones are released by the anterior pituitary gland.
3. The hormones produce changes in the ovaries.
4. Secretion of ovarian hormones leads to changes in the endometrium.
5. The menstrual cycle, the regularly recurring physiological changes in the endometrium that culminate in its shedding, may vary in length, with the average length being about 28 days.

B. Ovarian changes
1. Preovulatory phase
2. Luteal phase

C. Uterine changes
1. Menstrual phase
2. Proliferative phase
3. Secretory phase

III. FEMALE PELVIS AND MEASUREMENTS
A. True pelvis
1. The true pelvis lies below the pelvic brim.
2. The true pelvis consists of the pelvic inlet, midpelvis, and pelvic outlet.

B. False pelvis
1. The false pelvis is the shallow portion above the pelvic brim.
2. The false pelvis supports the abdominal viscera.

C. Types of pelvis
1. Gynecoid
   a. Normal female pelvis
   b. Transversely rounded or blunt
   c. Most favorable for successful **labor** and birth
2. Anthropoid
   a. Oval shaped
   b. Adequate outlet, with a normal or moderately narrow pubic arch
3. Android
   a. Wedge-shaped or angulated
   b. Seen in males
   c. Not favorable for **labor**

BOX 22-1

Menstrual Cycle

OVARIAN CHANGES

Preovulatory Phase

The hypothalamus releases gonadotropin-releasing hormone through the portal system to the anterior pituitary system.

Secretion of follicle-stimulating hormone (FSH) by the anterior lobe of the pituitary gland stimulates growth of follicles.

Most follicles die, leaving one to mature into a large graafian follicle.

Estrogen produced by the follicle stimulates increased secretions of luteinizing hormone (LH) by the anterior lobe of the pituitary gland.

The follicle ruptures and releases an ovum into the peritoneal cavity.

Luteal Phase

The luteal phase begins with ovulation.

Body temperature drops and then rises by 0.5° to 1° F around the time of ovulation.

Corpus luteum is formed from follicle cells that remain in the ovary following ovulation.

Corpus luteum secretes estrogen and progesterone during the remaining 14 days of the cycle.

Corpus luteum degenerates if the ovum is not fertilized, and secretion of estrogen and progesterone declines.

The decline of estrogen and progesterone stimulates the anterior pituitary to secrete more FSH and LH, initiating a new reproductive cycle.

UTERINE CHANGES

Menstrual Phase

The menstrual phase consists of 4 to 6 days of bleeding as the endometrium breaks down because of the decreased amount of estrogen and progesterone.

The amount of FSH rises, enabling the beginning of a new cycle.

Proliferative Phase

The proliferative phase lasts about 9 days.

Estrogen stimulates proliferation and growth of the endometrium.

As estrogen increases, it suppresses secretion of FSH and increases secretion of LH.

Secretion of LH stimulates ovulation and the development of the corpus luteum.

Ovulation occurs between day 12 and day 16.

Estrogen is high and progesterone is low.

Secretory Phase

The secretory phase lasts about 12 days.

The secretory phase follows ovulation.

This phase is initiated in response to the increase in LH.

Graafian follicle is replaced by corpus luteum.

Corpus luteum secretes progesterone and estrogen.

Progesterone prepares the endometrium for pregnancy should a fertilized ovum be implanted.

---

    d. Narrow pelvic planes can cause slow descent and midpelvis arrest

  4. Platypelloid

    a. Flat with an oval inlet

    b. Wide transverse diameter but short anteroposterior diameter, making the outlet inadequate

D. Pelvic inlet diameters

  1. Anteroposterior diameters

    a. Diagonal conjugate: distance from the lower margin of the symphysis pubis to the sacral promontory

    b. True conjugate or conjugate vera: distance from the upper margin of the symphysis pubis to the sacral promontory

    c. Obstetric conjugate: the smallest front-to-back distance through which the fetal head must pass in moving through the pelvic inlet

  2. Transverse diameter: the largest of the pelvic inlet diameters; located at right angles to the true conjugate

  3. Oblique (diagonal) diameter: not clinically measurable

  4. Posterior sagittal diameter: Distance from the point where the anteroposterior and transverse diameters cross each other to the middle of the sacral promontory

E. Pelvic midplane diameters

  1. Transverse diameter (interspinous diameter)

  2. Midplane normally is the largest plane and the one of greatest diameter

F. Pelvic outlet diameters

  1. Transverse (intertuberous diameter)

  2. Outlet presents the smallest plane of the pelvic canal

IV. FERTILIZATION AND IMPLANTATION

A. Fertilization

  1. **Fertilization** occurs in the upper region of the fallopian tubes.

  2. **Fertilization** occurs within 12 hours of ovulation and within 2 to 3 days of insemination, the average durations of viability for the ovum and sperm.

  3. **Fertilization** takes place when sperm and ovum unite.

  4. Once fertilized, the membrane of the ovum undergoes changes that prevent the entry of other sperm.

5. Each reproductive cell carries 23 chromosomes.
6. Sperm carry an X and a Y chromosome; XY: male, XX: female.

▲ B. **Implantation**
1. Zygote is propelled toward the uterus.
2. Zygote implants 6 to 8 days after ovulation.
3. Blastocyst secretes chorionic gonadotropin to ensure that the corpus luteum remains viable and secretes estrogen and progesterone for the first 2 to 3 months of gestation.

V. FETAL DEVELOPMENT (BOX 22-2)
A. Preembryonic period: the first 2 weeks after conception
B. Embryonic period: beginning of the third week through the eighth week after conception
C. Fetal period: beginning of the ninth week after conception and ending with birth

VI. FETAL ENVIRONMENT
A. Amnion
1. The amnion encloses the amniotic cavity.

BOX 22-2

Fetal Development

EMBRYONIC PERIOD (WEEKS 3 TO 8)
Week 1
Blastocyst is free-floating.
Weeks 2 to 3
Embryo is 2 mm in length.
Groove forms along middle of back.
Blood circulation begins.
Heart is tubular.
Week 5
Embryo is 4 to 6 mm in length.
Embryo is 0.4 g.
Double heart chambers are visible.
Heart begins to beat.
Limb buds form.
Week 8
Embryo is 3 cm in length.
Embryo is 2 g.
Eyelids begin to fuse.
Circulatory system through umbilical cord is well established.
Every organ system is present.

FETAL PERIOD (WEEKS 9 TO BIRTH)
Week 12
Fetus is 8 cm in length.
Fetus is 45 g.
Face is well formed
Limbs are long and slender.
Kidneys begin to form urine.
Spontaneous movements occur.
Heartbeat is detected by Doppler transducer between 10 and 12 weeks.
Sex is visually recognizable.
Week 16
Active movements are present.
Fetal skin is transparent.
Lanugo hair begins to develop.
Skeletal ossification occurs.
Week 20
Fetus is 19 cm in length.
Fetus is 465 g.
Lanugo covers the entire body.
Fetus has nails.
Muscles are developed.

Enamel and dentin are depositing.
Heartbeat is detected by regular (nonelectronic) fetoscope.
Week 24
Fetus is 28 cm in length.
Fetus is 780 g.
Hair on head is well formed.
Skin is reddish and wrinkled.
Reflex hand grasp functions.
Vernix caseosa covers entire body.
Fetus has ability to hear.
Week 28
Fetus is 38 cm in length.
Fetus is 1200 g.
Limbs are well flexed.
Brain is developing rapidly.
Eyelids open and close.
Lungs are developed sufficiently to provide gas exchange (lecithin forming).
If born, neonate can breathe at this time.
Week 32
Fetus is 40 cm in length.
Fetus is 2000 g.
Bones are fully developed.
Subcutaneous fat has collected.
The L/S (lecithin/sphingomyelin) ratio is 1.2:1.
Week 36
The fetus is 42 to 48 cm length.
The fetus is 2500 g.
The skin is pink and the body is rounded.
The skin is less wrinkled.
Lanugo is disappearing.
The L/S ratio is greater than 2:1.
Week 40
The fetus is 48 to 52 cm in length.
The fetus is 3000 to 3600 g.
The skin is pinkish and smooth.
Lanugo is present on upper arms and shoulders.
Vernix caseosa decreases
Fingernails extend beyond fingertips.
Sole (plantar) creases run down to the heel.
The testes are in the scrotum.
The labia majoria are well developed.

2. The amnion is the inner membrane that forms about the second week of embryonic development.

3. The amnion forms a fluid-filled sac that surrounds the embryo and later the fetus.

B. Chorion

1. The chorion is the outer membrane.

2. The chorion becomes vascularized and forms the fetal part of the **placenta.**

► C. **Amniotic fluid**

1. The **amniotic fluid** consists of 800 to 1200 mL by the end of pregnancy.

2. The **amniotic fluid** surrounds, cushions, and protects the fetus and allows for fetal movement.

3. The **amniotic fluid** maintains the body temperature of the fetus.

4. The **amniotic fluid** consists largely of fetal urine and is therefore a measure of fetal kidney function.

5. The fetus drinks, swallows, and urinates the **amniotic fluid** and breathes the **amniotic fluid** into its lungs.

► D. **Placenta**

1. The **placenta** provides for exchange of nutrients and waste products between the fetus and mother.

2. The **placenta** develops by the third month.

3. The **placenta** depends on maternal circulation.

4. The **placenta** produces hormones to maintain pregnancy and assumes full responsibility for the production of these hormones by the twelfth week of gestation.

5. Large particles such as bacteria cannot pass through the **placenta.**

6. Nutrients, drugs, antibodies, and viruses can pass through the **placenta.**

7. In the third trimester, transfer of maternal immunoglobulin provides the fetus passive immunity to certain diseases for the first few months after birth.

8. By week 8, genetic testing can be done.

VII. FETAL CIRCULATION

A. Umbilical cord

1. The umbilical cord contains two arteries and one vein.

2. Arteries carry deoxygenated blood and waste products from the fetus.

3. The vein carries oxygenated blood and provides oxygen and nutrients to the fetus.

B. Fetal heart rate

1. The fetal heart rate depends on gestational age: 160 to 170 beats per minute in the first trimester but slows with fetal growth to 120 to 160 beats per minute near or at term.

2. The fetal heart rate is about twice the maternal heart rate.

C. Fetal circulation bypass

1. Fetal circulation bypass is present because of nonfunctioning lungs.

2. Bypasses must close following birth to allow blood to flow through the lungs and the liver.

3. Ductus arteriosus connects the pulmonary artery to the aorta, bypassing the lungs.

4. Ductus venosus connects the umbilical vein and the inferior vena cava, bypassing the liver.

5. Foramen ovale is the opening between right and left atriums of heart, bypassing the lungs.

PRACTICE QUESTIONS

1. A nurse is conducting a prenatal teaching class and is reviewing the functions of the female reproductive system. A client in the class asks the nurse about the function of the fallopian tubes. The nurse tells the client that

1. Estrogen and progesterone are secreted from the fallopian tubes.

2. The fallopian tubes are the passageway for the fetus.

3. The fetus develops in the fallopian tubes.

4. Fertilization occurs in the fallopian tubes.

2. A nursing instructor is reviewing the menstrual cycle with a nursing student who will be conducting a prenatal teaching session. The instructor asks the student to describe the follicle-stimulating hormone (FSH) and the luteinizing hormone (LH). The student accurately responds by stating that

1. FSH and LH are released from the anterior pituitary gland.

2. FSH and LH are secreted by the corpus luteum of the ovary.

3. FSH and LH are secreted by the adrenal glands.

4. FSH and LH stimulate the formation of milk during pregnancy.

3. A nurse employed in a prenatal clinic reviews a client's chart and notes that the physician documents that the client has a gynecoid pelvis. The nurse plans care for this client, knowing that this type of pelvis

1. Is not favorable for labor.

2. Has a narrow pubic arch.

3. Is a wide pelvis with a short diameter.

4. Is the most favorable for labor and birth.

4. A pregnant client asks a nurse about the purpose of the placenta. The nurse responds most appropriately by telling the client that the placenta

1. Prevents antibodies and viruses from passing to the fetus.

2. Cushions and protects the fetus.

3. Provides an exchange of nutrients and waste products between the mother and the fetus.

4. Maintains the body temperature of the fetus.

5. A nurse is describing the process of fetal circulation to a client during a prenatal visit. The nurse accurately tells the client that fetal circulation consists of

1. Two umbilical veins and one umbilical artery.

2. Two umbilical arteries and one umbilical vein.

3. Arteries carrying oxygenated blood to the fetus.

4. Veins carrying deoxygenated blood to the fetus.

6. A nursing student is assigned to a client in labor. A nursing instructor asks the student to describe fetal circulation, specifically the ductus venosus. The nursing instructor determines that the student understands fetal circulation if the student states that the ductus venosus

1. Connects the pulmonary artery to the aorta.

2. Is an opening between the right and left atriums.

3. Connects the umbilical artery to the inferior vena cava.

4. Connects the umbilical vein to the inferior vena cava.

7. A nurse is caring for a client during the prenatal period. The client tells that nurse that she wants to know the sex of the fetus as soon as it can be determined. The nurse responds to the client, knowing that the sex of the fetus can be visually recognizable as early as week

1. 4.

2. 6.

3. 8.

4. 12.

8. A nurse prepares to assess a fetal heartbeat. The nurse uses a fetoscope, knowing that the fetal heartbeat first can be heard with a regular (nonelectronic) fetoscope at gestational week

1. 5.

2. 10.

3. 16.

4. 20.

9. During a prenatal visit at 38 weeks, a nurse assesses the fetal heart rate. The nurse determines that the fetal heart rate is normal if which of the following is noted?

1. 80 beats per minute

2. 100 beats per minute

3. 150 beats per minute

4. 180 beats per minute

10. A pregnant adolescent client asks the nurse about the menstrual cycle. The nurse describes the cycle and tells the adolescent that its normal duration is about

1. 14 days.

2. 28 days.

3. 30 days.

4. 45 days.

CRITICAL THINKING: FILL IN THE BLANK

A client who has just been told that she is pregnant asks a clinic nurse when the fetus's heart will be developed and beating. The nurse tells the client that the fetal heart is beating at what gestational week?

Answer: _____

ANSWERS

1. **4**

Rationale: Each fallopian tube is a hollow, muscular tube that transports a mature oocyte for final maturation and fertilization. Fertilization typically occurs near the boundary between the ampulla and isthmus of the tube. Estrogen is a hormone produced by the ovarian follicles, corpus luteum, adrenal cortex, and placenta during pregnancy. Progesterone is a hormone secreted by the corpus luteum of the ovary, adrenal glands, and placenta during pregnancy. The vagina is the passageway for the fetus, and the fetus develops in the uterus.

Test-Taking Strategy: Use the process of elimination and knowledge of the anatomy and physiology of the female reproductive system. Remember that fertilization occurs in the fallopian tubes. If you had difficulty with this question, review anatomy and physiology of the reproductive system.

Level of Cognitive Ability: Comprehension

Client Needs: Physiological Integrity

Integrated Process: Teaching/Learning

Content Area: Maternity—antepartum

Reference: Murray, S., McKinney, E., & Gorrie, T. (2002). *Foundations of maternal-newborn nursing* (3rd ed., p. 64). Philadelphia: W. B. Saunders.

2. **1**

Rationale: Follicle-stimulating hormone and LH, when stimulated by gonadotropin-releasing hormone from the hypothalamus, are released from the anterior pituitary gland to stimulate follicular growth and development, growth of the graafian follicle, and the production of progesterone. Options 2, 3, and 4 are incorrect.

Test-Taking Strategy: Use the process of elimination, recalling that FSH and LH are released from the anterior pituitary gland. If you had difficulty with this question, review the menstrual cycle.

Level of Cognitive Ability: Analysis

Client Needs: Physiological Integrity

Integrated Process: Nursing Process—evaluation

Content Area: Maternity—antepartum

Reference: Wong, D., Perry, S., & Hockenberry, M. (2002). *Maternal child nursing care* (2nd ed., p. 56). St. Louis: Mosby.

3. **4**

Rationale: A gynecoid pelvis is a normal female pelvis and is the most favorable for successful labor and birth. An android pelvis (resembling a male pelvis) would not be favorable for labor because of the narrow pelvic planes. An anthropoid pelvis has an outlet that is adequate, with a normal or moderately narrow pubic arch. The platypelloid pelvis (flat pelvis) has a wide transverse diameter, but the anteroposterior diameter is short, making the outlet inadequate.

Test-Taking Strategy: Use the process of elimination. Recalling that the gynecoid pelvis is the normal female pelvis will direct you to the correct option. Review pelvic types if you had difficulty with this question.

Level of Cognitive Ability: Comprehension
Client Needs: Physiological Integrity
Integrated Process: Nursing Process—planning
Content Area: Maternity—antepartum
References: Lowdermilk, D., & Perry, S. (2003). *Maternity nursing* (6th ed., p. 262). St. Louis: Mosby.
Wong, D., Perry, S., & Hockenberry, M. (2002). *Maternal child nursing care* (2nd ed., p. 318). St. Louis: Mosby.

4. **3**
Rationale: The placenta provides an exchange of nutrients and waste products between the mother and the fetus. The amniotic fluid surrounds, cushions, and protects the fetus and maintains the body temperature of the fetus. Nutrients, drugs, antibodies, and viruses can pass through the placenta.
Test-Taking Strategy: Use the process of elimination and recall that the placenta provides nutrients. If you had difficulty with this question, review the structure and function of the placenta and amniotic fluid.
Level of Cognitive Ability: Comprehension
Client Needs: Physiological Integrity
Integrated Process: Teaching/Learning
Content Area: Maternity—antepartum
Reference: Murray, S., McKinney, E., & Gorrie, T. (2002). *Foundations of maternal-newborn nursing* (3rd ed., p. 114). Philadelphia: W. B. Saunders.

5. **2**
Rationale: Blood pumped by the embryo's heart leaves the embryo through two umbilical arteries. Once oxygenated, the blood then is returned by one umbilical vein. Arteries carry deoxygenated blood and waste products from the fetus, and veins carry oxygenated blood and provide oxygen and nutrients to the fetus.
Test-Taking Strategy: Use the process of elimination and recall that three umbilical vessels are within an umbilical cord (two arteries and one vein). If you had difficulty with this question, review fetal circulation.
Level of Cognitive Ability: Comprehension
Client Needs: Physiological Integrity
Integrated Process: Teaching/Learning
Content Area: Maternity—antepartum
Reference: Murray, S., McKinney, E., & Gorrie, T. (2002). *Foundations of maternal-newborn nursing* (3rd ed., p. 114). Philadelphia: W. B. Saunders.

6. **4**
Rationale: The ductus venosus connects the umbilical vein to the inferior vena cava. Options 1, 2, and 3 are incorrect. The foramen ovale is a temporary opening between the right and left atriums. The ductus arteriosus joins the aorta and the pulmonary artery.
Test-Taking Strategy: Use the process of elimination and knowledge regarding fetal circulation to answer this question. Remember that the ductus venosus connects the umbilical vein to the inferior vena cava. Review fetal circulation if you had difficulty with this question.
Level of Cognitive Ability: Analysis
Client Needs: Physiological Integrity
Integrated Process: Nursing Process—evaluation

Content Area: Maternity—intrapartum
Reference: Murray, S., McKinney, E., & Gorrie, T. (2002). *Foundations of maternal-newborn nursing* (3rd ed., p. 114). Philadelphia: W. B. Saunders.

7. **4**
Rationale: By the end of the twelfth week, the external genitalia of the fetus have developed to such a degree that the sex of the fetus can be determined visually. Options 1, 2, and 3 are incorrect.
Test-Taking Strategy: Use knowledge regarding fetal development to answer this question. Remember that the sex of the fetus can be recognizable visually by gestational week 12. If you had difficulty with this question, review fetal development.
Level of Cognitive Ability: Comprehension
Client Needs: Physiological Integrity
Integrated Process: Teaching/Learning
Content Area: Maternity—antepartum
Reference: Murray, S., McKinney, E., & Gorrie, T. (2002). *Foundations of maternal-newborn nursing* (3rd ed., p. 56). Philadelphia: W. B. Saunders.

8. **4**
Rationale: The fetal heartbeat first can be heard with a regular (nonelectronic) fetoscope at 18 to 20 weeks of gestation. If a Doppler transducer device is used, the fetal heartbeat can be detected as early as 10 to 12 weeks of gestation. Options 1, 2, and 3 are incorrect.
Test-Taking Strategy: Note the key word "fetoscope" in the question. Recalling fetal development and the use of a fetoscope will direct you to option 4. If you had difficulty with this question, review fetal heart assessment.
Level of Cognitive Ability: Comprehension
Client Needs: Physiological Integrity
Integrated Process: Nursing Process—implementation
Content Area: Maternity—antepartum
Reference: Murray, S., McKinney, E., & Gorrie, T. (2002). *Foundations of maternal-newborn nursing* (3rd ed., p. 104). Philadelphia: W. B. Saunders.

9. **3**
Rationale: The fetal heart rate depends on gestational age and ranges from 160 to 170 beats per minute in the first trimester but slows with fetal growth to 120 to 160 beats per minute near or at term. At or near term, if the fetal heart rate is less than 120 or more than 160 beats per minute with the uterus at rest, the fetus may be in distress. Options 1 and 2 indicate bradycardia. Option 4 indicates tachycardia.
Test-Taking Strategy: Use the process of elimination and note that the client is at 38 weeks of gestation. Remember that the normal fetal heart rate at or near term is 120 to 160 beats per minute. Review fetal heart rate if you had difficulty with this question.
Level of Cognitive Ability: Comprehension
Client Needs: Physiological Integrity
Integrated Process: Nursing Process—assessment
Content Area: Maternity—antepartum
Reference: Murray, S., McKinney, E., & Gorrie, T. (2002). *Foundations of maternal-newborn nursing* (3rd ed., p. 978). Philadelphia: W. B. Saunders.

10. 2

Rationale: The normal duration of the menstrual cycle is about 28 days, although it may range from 20 to 45 days. Significant deviations from the 28-day cycle are associated with reduced fertility. The first day of the menstrual period is counted as day 1 of the woman's cycle.

Test-Taking Strategy: Use the process of elimination and note the key words "normal duration" in the question. Recalling the duration of the menstrual cycle will assist in eliminating options 1, 3, and 4. If you had difficulty with this question, review the menstrual cycle.

Level of Cognitive Ability: Application
Client Needs: Physiological Integrity
Integrated Process: Teaching/Learning
Content Area: Maternity—antepartum
Reference: Lowdermilk, D., & Perry, S. (2003). *Maternity nursing* (6th ed., p. 62). St. Louis: Mosby.

CRITICAL THINKING: FILL IN THE BLANK

Answer: Week 5
Rationale: By gestational week 5, double heart chambers are visible and the heart begins to beat.

Test-Taking Strategy: Recalling the weekly development of the fetus will assist in answering this question. Review fetal development in relation to the fetal heartbeat if you had difficulty with this question.

Level of Cognitive Ability: Application
Client Needs: Physiological Integrity
Integrated Process: Teaching/Learning
Content Area: Maternity—antepartum
Reference: Murray, S., McKinney, E., & Gorrie, T. (2002). *Foundations of maternal-newborn nursing* (3rd ed., p. 106). Philadelphia: W. B. Saunders.

REFERENCES

Herlihy, B., & Maebius, N. (2003). *The human body in health and illness* (2nd ed.). Philadelphia: W. B. Saunders.

Lowdermilk, D., & Perry, S. (2003). *Maternity nursing* (6th ed.). St. Louis: Mosby.

Murray, S., McKinney, E., & Gorrie, T. (2002). *Foundations of maternal-newborn nursing* (3rd ed.). Philadelphia: W. B. Saunders.

Wong, D., Perry, S., & Hockenberry, M. (2002). *Maternal child nursing care* (2nd ed.). St. Louis: Mosby.

Obstetrical Assessment

I. GESTATION
A. Time until the estimated date of confinement or estimated date of delivery
B. About 280 days
C. **Nägele's rule** for estimating the date of confinement (Box 23-1)
   1. For **Nägele's rule** to be accurate requires that the woman have a regular 28-day menstrual cycle.
   2. Add 7 days to the first day of the last menstrual period, subtract 3 months, and then add 1 year to that date, alternatively, add 7 days to the date of the last menstrual period and count forward 9 months.

II. GRAVIDITY AND PARITY
A. Gravidity
   1. **Gravida** refers to a pregnant woman.
   2. Gravidity refers to the number of pregnancies.
   3. Nulligravida is a woman who has never been pregnant.
   4. Primigravida is a woman who is pregnant for the first time.
   5. Multigravida is a woman in at least her second pregnancy.
B. **Parity**
   1. **Parity** is the number of births (not the number of fetuses; e.g., twins) past 20 weeks' gestation, whether the fetus was born alive or not.

   2. Nullipara is a woman who has not had a birth at more than 20 weeks of gestation.
   3. Primipara is a woman who has had one birth that occurs after the twentieth week of gestation.
   4. Multipara is a woman who has had two or more pregnancies resulting in viable offspring.
C. Use of GTPAL: Pregnancy outcomes can be described with the acronym GTPAL (Box 23-2).
   1. G is gravidity, the number of pregnancies
   2. T is term births, the number born at term (40 weeks)
   3. P is preterm births, the number born before 40 weeks' gestation
   4. A is abortions/miscarriages, the number of abortions/miscarriages (included in gravida if before 20 weeks' gestation; included in parity if past 20 weeks' gestation)
   5. L is live births, the number of live births or living children

---

BOX 23-1

Nägele's Rule for Estimating the Date of Confinement

First day of last menstrual period: September 11, 2006
Add 7 days: September 18, 2006
Subtract 3 months: June 18, 2006
Add 1 year: June 18, 2007
Estimated date of confinement: June 18, 2007

BOX 23-2

GTPAL

G, gravidity
T, term births
P, preterm births
A, abortions/miscarriages
L, live births
Example: A woman is pregnant for the fourth time. She had one elective abortion in the first trimester, a daughter who was born at 40 weeks' gestation, and a son who was born at 36 weeks' gestation. Therefore she is gravida (G) 4, parity 2, and term (T) 1 (the daughter born at 40 weeks'); preterm (P) 1 (the son born at 36 weeks'); abortion (A) 1 (the abortion is counted in the gravida but is not included in the para because it occurred before 20 weeks); live births (L) 2.
GTPAL = 4, 1, 1, 1, 2

III. PREGNANCY SIGNS

A. Presumptive signs
1. Amenorrhea
2. Nausea and vomiting
3. Increased size and increased feeling of fullness in breasts
4. Pronounced nipples
5. Urinary frequency
6. **Quickening:** The first perception of fetal movement may occur as early as the fourteenth to sixteenth week of gestation.
7. Fatigue
8. Discoloration of the vaginal mucosa

B. Probable signs
1. Uterine enlargement
2. **Hegar's sign:** softening and thinning of the lower uterine segment that occurs about week 6
3. **Goodell's sign:** softening of the cervix that occurs at the beginning of the second month
4. **Chadwick's sign:** bluish coloration of the mucous membranes of cervix, vagina, and vulva that occurs about week 6
5. **Ballottement:** rebounding of the fetus against the examiner's fingers on palpation
6. Braxton Hicks contractions
7. Positive pregnancy test measuring for human chorionic gonadotropin

C. Positive signs
1. Fetal heart rate detected by electronic device (Doppler transducer) at 10 to 12 weeks and by nonelectronic device (fetoscope) at 20 weeks of gestation
2. Active fetal movements palpable by examiner
3. Outline of fetus via radiography or ultrasound

IV. FUNDAL HEIGHT (BOX 23-3)

A. Fundal height is measured to evaluate the fetus's gestational age.
B. During the second and third trimesters (weeks 18 to 30), fundal height in centimeters approximately equals the fetus's age in weeks plus or minus 2 cm.
C. At 16 weeks, the fundus can be found halfway between the symphysis pubis and the umbilicus.
D. At 20 to 22 weeks, the fundus is at the umbilicus.
E. At 36 weeks, the fundus is at the xiphoid process.

BOX 23-3

Measuring Fundal Height

1. Place the client in the supine position.
2. Place the end of the tape measure at the level of the symphysis pubis.
3. Stretch the tape to the top of the uterine fundus.
4. Note and record the measurement.

V. MATERNAL RISK FACTORS

A. German measles (rubella)
1. The risk of maternal and fetal or congenital infection is related to the trimester of placental infection.
2. Maternal infection during the first 8 weeks of gestation carries the highest rate of maternal and fetal infection.

B. Sexually transmitted diseases
1. Syphilis
   a. Infection may cross the **placenta**.
   b. Infection usually leads to spontaneous abortions.
   c. Infection increases the incidence of mental subnormality and physical deformities.
2. Genital herpes
   a. Infection may cross the **placenta**.
   b. Fetus is contaminated after membranes rupture or with vaginal **delivery**.
3. Gonorrhea
   a. Fetus is contaminated at the time of **delivery**.
   b. Maternal infection may result in postpartum infection of the **neonate**.
   c. Risks to the **neonate** include ophthalmia neonatorum, pneumonia, and sepsis.

C. Human immunodeficiency virus
1. The virus is transmitted through blood, blood products, and other bodily fluids, such as urine, semen, and vaginal fluid.
2. Repeated exposure to the virus during pregnancy through unsafe sex practices or intravenous drug use can increase the risk of transmission to the fetus.

D. Substance abuse
1. Many substances cross the **placenta**; therefore no drugs, including over-the-counter medications, should be taken unless prescribed by physician.
2. Substances commonly abused include alcohol, cocaine, crack, marijuana, amphetamines, barbiturates, and heroin.
3. Substance abuse threatens normal fetal growth and successful term completion of the pregnancy.
4. Substance abuse places the pregnancy at risk for fetal growth retardation, abruptio placentae, and fetal bradycardia.
5. Physical signs of drug abuse may include dilated or contracted pupils, fatigue, track (needle) marks, skin abscesses, inflamed nasal mucosa, and inappropriate behavior by the mother.
6. Consumption of alcohol during pregnancy may lead to fetal alcohol syndrome and can cause jitteriness, physical abnormalities, congenital anomalies, and growth deficits.
7. Smoking leads to low birth weights, a higher incidence of birth defects, and stillbirths.

E. Adolescent pregnancy
1. Factors that result in adolescent pregnancy include the early onset of menarche, changing sexual behaviors in this age group, problems with family

development, poverty, and the lack of knowledge of reproduction and birth control.

2. The major concerns related to adolescent pregnancy include poor nutritional status, emotional and behavioral difficulties, lack of support systems, increased risk of stillbirth, low-birth-weight **newborn** infants, fetal mortality, cephalopelvic disproportion, and the increased risk of maternal complications such as hypertension, anemia, prolonged **labor**, and infections.

PRACTICE QUESTIONS

1. A client arrives at a prenatal clinic for the first prenatal assessment. The client tells a nurse that the first day of her last menstrual period was September 19, 2005. Using Nägele's rule, the nurse determines the estimated date of confinement as
   1. July 26, 2006.
   2. June 12, 2007.
   3. June 26, 2006.
   4. July 12, 2007.

2. A nurse is collecting data during an admission assessment of a client who is pregnant with twins. The client has a healthy 5-year-old child that was delivered at 38 weeks and tells the nurse that she does not have a history of any type of abortion or fetal demise. The nurse would document the GTPAL for this client as
   1. G = 3, T = 2, P = 0, A = 0, L = 1
   2. G = 2, T = 0, P = 1, A = 0, L = 1
   3. G = 1, T = 1, P = 1, A = 0, L = 1
   4. G = 2, T = 0, P = 0, A = 0, L = 1

3. A nurse is performing an assessment of a primipara who is being evaluated in a clinic during her second trimester of pregnancy. Which of the following indicates an abnormal physical finding necessitating further testing?
   1. Consistent increase in fundal height
   2. Fetal heart rate of 180 beats per minute
   3. Braxton Hicks contractions
   4. Quickening

4. A nurse is providing instructions to a pregnant client with genital herpes about the measures that need to be implemented to protect the fetus. The nurse tells the client that
   1. Daily administration of acyclovir (Zovirax) is necessary during the entire pregnancy.
   2. Total abstinence from sexual intercourse is necessary during the entire pregnancy.
   3. Sitz baths need to be taken every 4 hours while awake if vaginal lesions are present.
   4. A cesarean section will be necessary if vaginal lesions are present at the time of labor.

5. A nurse is performing an assessment of a pregnant client who is at 28 weeks of gestation. The nurse measures the fundal height in centimeters and expects the findings to be which of the following?

   1. 22 cm
   2. 30 cm
   3. 36 cm
   4. 40 cm

6. A pregnant client is seen in a health care clinic for a regular prenatal visit. The client tells the nurse that she is experiencing irregular contractions, and the nurse determines that she is experiencing Braxton Hicks contractions. Based on this finding, which nursing action is most appropriate?
   1. Instruct the client to maintain bed rest for the remainder of the pregnancy.
   2. Inform the client that these are common and may occur throughout the pregnancy.
   3. Contact the physician.
   4. Call the maternity unit and inform them that the client will be admitted in a prelabor condition.

7. A nurse is reviewing the record of a client who has just been told that a pregnancy test is positive. The physician has documented the presence of Goodell's sign. The nurse determines that this sign indicates
   1. A softening of the cervix.
   2. A soft blowing sound that corresponds to the maternal pulse during auscultation of the uterus.
   3. The presence of human chorionic gonadotropin in the urine.
   4. The presence of fetal movement.

8. A nursing instructor asks a nursing student who is preparing to assist with the assessment of a pregnant client to describe the process of quickening. Which of the following statements if made by the student indicates an understanding of this term?
   1. "It is the irregular, painless contractions that occur throughout pregnancy."
   2. "It is the soft blowing sound that can be heard when the uterus is auscultated."
   3. "It is the fetal movement that is felt by the mother."
   4. "It is the thinning of the lower uterine segment."

9. A nurse midwife is performing an assessment of a pregnant client and is assessing the client for the presence of ballottement. Which of the following would the nurse implement to test for the presence of ballottement?
   1. Auscultating for fetal heart sounds
   2. Palpating the abdomen for fetal movement
   3. Assessing the cervix for thinning
   4. Initiating a gentle upward tap on the cervix

10. A pregnant client asks the nurse in the clinic when she will be able to start feeling the fetus move. The nurse responds by telling the mother that fetal movements will be noted between
    1. 6 and 8 weeks of gestation.
    2. 8 and 10 weeks of gestation.
    3. 10 and 12 weeks of gestation.
    4. 14 and 16 weeks of gestation.

CRITICAL THINKING: MULTIPLE RESPONSE

A nurse is assisting in performing an assessment on a client who suspects that she is pregnant and is checking the client for probable signs of pregnancy. Select all probable signs of pregnancy.

____ Uterine enlargement

____ Fetal heart rate detected by a nonelectronic device

____ Outline of fetus via radiography or ultrasound

____ Chadwick's sign

____ Braxton Hicks contractions

____ Ballottement

ANSWERS

1. 3

Rationale: Accurate use of Nägele's rule requires that the woman have a regular 28-day menstrual cycle. Add 7 days to the first day of the last menstrual period, subtract 3 months, and then add 1 year to that date. First day of the last menstrual period: September 19, 2005; add 7 days: September 26, 2005; subtract 3 months: June 26, 2005; add 1 year: June 26, 2006.

Test-Taking Strategy: Use knowledge regarding the use of Nägele's rule to answer this question. Read all of the options carefully, noting the dates and years in the options, before selecting an answer. Review Nägele's rule if you had difficulty with this question.

Level of Cognitive Ability: Analysis

Client Needs: Health Promotion and Maintenance

Integrated Process: Nursing Process—assessment

Content Area: Maternity—antepartum

Reference: Lowdermilk, D., & Perry, A. (2003). *Maternity nursing* (6th ed., p. 188). St. Louis: Mosby.

2. 2

Rationale: Pregnancy outcomes can be described with the acronym GTPAL. G is gravidity, the number of pregnancies. T is term births, the number born at term (40 weeks). P is preterm births, the number born before 40 weeks' gestation. A is abortions/miscarriages, the number of abortions/miscarriages (included in gravida if before 20 weeks' gestation; included in parity if past 20 weeks' gestation). L is live births, the number of live births or living children. Therefore a woman who is pregnant with twins and has a child has a gravida of 2. Because the child was delivered at 38 weeks, the number of preterm births is 1, and the number of term births is 0. The number of abortions is 0, and the number of live births is 1.

Test-Taking Strategy: Knowledge and understanding of the acronym GTPAL will direct you to option 2. If you had difficulty answering this question, review this method of describing pregnancy outcomes.

Level of Cognitive Ability: Application

Client Needs: Health Promotion and Maintenance

Integrated Process: Nursing Process—assessment

Content Area: Maternity—antepartum

Reference: Wong, D., Perry, S., & Hockenberry, M. (2002). *Maternal child nursing care* (2nd ed., p. 168). St. Louis: Mosby.

3. 2

Rationale: The normal range of the fetal heart rate depends on gestational age. The heart rate is usually 160 to 170 beats per minute in the first trimester and slows with fetal growth.

Near and at term, the fetal heart rate ranges from 120 to 160 beats per minute. Options 1, 3, and 4 are normal expected findings.

Test-Taking Strategy: Note the key words "indicates an abnormal physical finding" and note that the client is in the second trimester of pregnancy. Recalling the normal fetal heart rate will direct you to option 2. Review normal assessment findings in pregnancy if you had difficulty with this question.

Level of Cognitive Ability: Analysis

Client Needs: Physiological Integrity

Integrated Process: Nursing Process—assessment

Content Area: Maternity—antepartum

Reference: Wong, D., Perry, S., & Hockenberry, M. (2002). *Maternal child nursing care* (2nd ed., p. 353). St. Louis: Mosby.

4. 4

Rationale: For women with active lesions, either recurrent or primary at the time of labor, delivery should be by cesarean section to prevent the fetus from being in contact with the genital herpes. The safety of acyclovir has not been established during pregnancy, and it should be used only when a life-threatening infection is present. Clients should be advised to abstain from sexual contact while the lesions are present. If this is an initial infection, clients should continue to abstain until they become culture negative, because prolonged viral shedding may occur in such cases. Keeping the genital area clean and dry will promote healing.

Test-Taking Strategy: Use the process of elimination. Eliminate options 1 and 2 first because of the absolute word "entire" in these options. From the remaining options, recalling that the lesions should be kept clean and dry to promote healing will assist in eliminating option 3. If you had difficulty with this question, review the content related to genital herpes as a maternal risk factor.

Level of Cognitive Ability: Application

Client Needs: Health Promotion and Maintenance

Integrated Process: Teaching/Learning

Content Area: Maternity—antepartum

Reference: Murray, S., McKinney, E., & Gorrie, T. (2002). *Foundations of maternal-newborn nursing* (3rd ed., p. 725). Philadelphia: W. B. Saunders.

5. 2

Rationale: During the second and third trimesters (weeks 18 to 30), fundal height in centimeters approximately equals the fetus's age in weeks plus or minus 2 cm. At 16 weeks the fundus can be located halfway between the symphysis pubis and the umbilicus. At 20 to 22 weeks the fundus is at the umbilicus, and at 36 weeks the fundus is at the xiphoid process.

Test-Taking Strategy: Use the process of elimination. Remember that during the second and third trimesters (weeks 18 to 30), fundal height in centimeters approximately equals the fetus's age in weeks plus or minus 2 cm. If you are unfamiliar with this assessment technique, review this content area.

Level of Cognitive Ability: Analysis

Client Needs: Health Promotion and Maintenance

Integrated Process: Nursing Process—assessment

Content Area: Maternity—antepartum

Reference: Wong, D., Perry, S., & Hockenberry, M. (2002). *Maternal child nursing care* (2nd ed., p. 195). St. Louis: Mosby.

6. 2

Rationale: Braxton Hicks contractions are irregular, painless contractions that may occur intermittently throughout pregnancy. Because Braxton Hicks contractions may occur and are normal in some pregnant women during pregnancy, options 1, 3, and 4 are unnecessary and inappropriate actions.

Test-Taking Strategy: Use the process of elimination. Options 3 and 4 are similar and can be eliminated first. From the remaining options, knowing that Braxton Hicks contractions are common and can occur throughout pregnancy will assist in directing you to option 2. Review the physiology associated with Braxton Hicks contractions if you had difficulty with this question.

Level of Cognitive Ability: Application

Client Needs: Health Promotion and Maintenance

Integrated Process: Teaching/Learning

Content Area: Maternity—antepartum

Reference: Lowdermilk, D., & Perry, A. (2003). *Maternity nursing* (6th ed., p. 172) St. Louis: Mosby.

7. 1

Rationale: In the early weeks of pregnancy the cervix becomes softer as a result of increased vascularity and hyperplasia, which causes Goodell's sign. Cervical softening is noted by the examiner during pelvic examination. A soft blowing sound that corresponds to the maternal pulse may be auscultated over the uterus and is due to blood circulation through the placenta. Human chorionic gonadotropin is noted in maternal urine in a positive urine pregnancy test. Goodell's sign does not indicate the presence of fetal movement.

Test-Taking Strategy: Use the process of elimination and knowledge regarding the physiological findings in Goodell's sign to answer this question. Remember that Goodell's sign refers to a softening of the cervix. If you had difficulty with this question, review the changes in the cervix that occur during pregnancy.

Level of Cognitive Ability: Analysis

Client Needs: Health Promotion and Maintenance

Integrated Process: Nursing Process—analysis

Content Area: Maternity—antepartum

Reference: Lowdermilk, D., & Perry, A. (2003). *Maternity nursing* (6th ed., p. 172) St. Louis: Mosby.

8. 3

Rationale: Quickening is fetal movement and may occur as early as the sixteenth to eighteenth week of gestation, and the expectant mother first notices subtle fetal movements that gradually increase in intensity. A soft blowing sound that corresponds to the maternal pulse may be auscultated over the uterus, and this is known as uterine souffle. This sound is due to the blood circulation to the placenta and corresponds to the maternal pulse. Braxton Hicks contractions are irregular, painless contractions that may occur throughout pregnancy. A thinning of the lower uterine segment occurs about the sixth week of pregnancy and is called Hegar's sign.

Test-Taking Strategy: Use the process of elimination and knowledge regarding the term "quickening" to answer this question. Remember that quickening is fetal movement. If you are unfamiliar with this sign associated with pregnancy, review this content area.

Level of Cognitive Ability: Analysis

Client Needs: Health Promotion and Maintenance

Integrated Process: Teaching/Learning

Content Area: Maternity—antepartum

Reference: Lowdermilk, D., & Perry, A. (2003). *Maternity nursing* (6th ed., p. 172). St. Louis: Mosby.

9. 4

Rationale: Ballottement is a technique of palpating a floating structure by bouncing it gently and feeling it rebound. In the technique used to palpate the fetus, the examiner places a finger in the vagina and taps gently upward, causing the fetus to rise. The fetus then sinks, and the examiner feels a gentle tap on the finger. Options 1, 2, and 3 are incorrect.

Test-Taking Strategy: Use the process of elimination. Recalling that ballottement is a technique of palpating a floating structure by bouncing it gently and feeling it rebound will direct you to option 4. Review this assessment technique if you had difficulty with this question.

Level of Cognitive Ability: Application

Client Needs: Health Promotion and Maintenance

Integrated Process: Nursing Process—implementation

Content Area: Maternity—antepartum

Reference: Lowdermilk, D., & Perry, A. (2003). *Maternity nursing* (6th ed., p. 172) St. Louis: Mosby.

10. 4

Rationale: Quickening is fetal movement and may occur as early as the fourteenth to sixteenth week of gestation. The expectant mother first notices subtle fetal movements during this time, which gradually increase in intensity. Options 1, 2, and 3 are incorrect.

Test-Taking Strategy: Use the process of elimination and knowledge regarding the occurrence of quickening. In this situation, selecting the option that indicates the greatest length of gestational time is best. Review the process of quickening if you had difficulty with this question.

Level of Cognitive Ability: Application

Client Needs: Health Promotion and Maintenance

Integrated Process: Teaching/Learning

Content Area: Maternity—antepartum

Reference: Lowdermilk, D., & Perry, A. (2003). *Maternity nursing* (6th ed., p. 172). St. Louis: Mosby.

CRITICAL THINKING: MULTIPLE RESPONSE

Answer:

Uterine enlargement

Chadwick's sign

Braxton Hicks contractions

Ballottement

Rationale: The probable signs of pregnancy include uterine enlargement, Hegar's sign (softening and thinning of the lower uterine segment that occurs about week 6), Goodell's sign (softening of the cervix that occurs at the beginning of the second month), Chadwick's sign (bluish coloration of the mucous membranes of the cervix, vagina, and vulva that occurs about week 6), ballottement (rebounding of the fetus against the examiner's fingers on palpation), Braxton Hicks contractions, and a positive pregnancy test measuring for human chorionic gonadotropin. Positive signs of pregnancy include fetal heart rate detected by electronic device (Doppler transducer) at 10 to 12 weeks and by nonelectronic device (fetoscope) at 20 weeks of gestation, active fetal movements palpable by examiner, and an outline of the fetus via radiography or ultrasound.

Test-Taking Strategy: Focusing on the issue, probable signs of pregnancy, will assist in answering this question. Remember that detection of the fetal heart rate and an outline of the fetus via radiography or ultrasound are positive signs of pregnancy. Review the probable signs of pregnancy if you had difficulty with this question.

Level of Cognitive Ability: Analysis

Client Needs: Health Promotion and Maintenance

Integrated Process: Nursing Process—assessment

Content Area: Maternity—antepartum

Reference: Murray, S., McKinney, E., & Gorrie, T. (2002). *Foundations of maternal-newborn nursing* (3rd ed., p. 132). Philadelphia: W. B. Saunders.

REFERENCES

Lowdermilk, D., & Perry, A. (2003). *Maternity nursing* (6th ed.). St. Louis: Mosby.

Murray, S., McKinney, E., & Gorrie, T. (2002). *Foundations of maternal-newborn nursing* (3rd ed.). Philadelphia: W. B. Saunders.

Wong, D., Perry, S., & Hockenberry, M. (2002). *Maternal child nursing care* (2nd ed.). St. Louis: Mosby.

Prenatal Period

I. PHYSIOLOGICAL MATERNAL CHANGES

A. Cardiovascular system
1. Circulating blood volume increases, plasma increases, and total red blood cell volume increases (total volume increases by 40% to 50%).
2. Physiological anemia occurs as the plasma increase exceeds the increase in red blood cell production.
3. Iron requirements are increased.
4. Heart size increases and is elevated upward and to the left because of displacement of the diaphragm as the uterus enlarges.
5. Pulse may increase about 10 beats per minute.
6. Blood pressure may decline in the second trimester.
7. Retention of sodium and water may occur.

B. Respiratory system
1. Oxygen consumption increases by 15% to 20%.
2. Diaphragm is elevated because of the enlarged uterus.
3. Respiratory rate remains unchanged.
4. A woman may experience shortness of breath.

C. Gastrointestinal system
1. Nausea and vomiting may occur as a result of the secretion of human chorionic gonadotropin and subsides by the third month.
2. Poor appetite may occur because of the decreased gastric motility.
3. Alterations in taste and smell may occur.
4. Constipation may occur as a result of decreased gastrointestinal motility or pressure of the uterus.
5. Flatulence and heartburn may occur because of decreased gastrointestinal motility and slow emptying of the stomach.
6. Hemorrhoids may occur as a result of increased venous pressure.
7. Gum tissue may become swollen and easily bleed.
8. Ptyalism (excessive secretion of saliva) may occur.

D. Renal system
1. Frequency of urination occurs in the first and third trimesters as a result of pressure of the enlarging uterus on the bladder.
2. Decreased bladder tone may occur and is caused by hormonal changes.
3. Decreased bladder capacity is experienced.
4. Renal threshold for glucose may be reduced.

E. Endocrine system
1. Basal metabolic rate rises.
2. Anterior lobe of the pituitary gland enlarges.
3. Thyroid enlarges slightly, and thyroid activity increases.
4. Parathyroid increases in size.
5. Aldosterone levels gradually increase.

F. Reproductive system
1. Uterus
   a. Uterus enlarges, increasing in mass from 60 g to 1000 g.
   b. Size and number of blood vessels and lymphatics increase.
   c. Irregular contractions occur.
2. Cervix
   a. The cervix becomes shorter, more elastic, and larger in diameter.
   b. Endocervical glands secrete a thick mucus plug, which is expelled from the canal when dilation begins.
   c. Increased vascularization causes a softening and blue-purple discoloration known as **Chadwick's sign**, which occurs at about 6 weeks of gestational age.
3. Ovaries
   a. The maturation of new follicles is blocked.
   b. The ovaries cease ovum production.

4. Vagina
   a. Hypertrophy and thickening of the muscle occurs.
   b. Increase in vaginal secretions is experienced, and secretions are usually thick, white, and acidic.
5. Breasts
   a. Breast size increases.
   b. Nipples become more pronounced.
   c. Areola becomes darker in color.
   d. Superficial veins become prominent.
   e. Hypertrophy of the Montgomery's follicles occurs.
   f. Colostrum may appear from the breast.
G. Skin
1. Pigmentation increases.
2. A dark streak down the midline of the abdomen may appear (linea nigra).
3. Chloasma (mask of pregnancy), a blotchy brownish hyperpigmentation, may occur over the forehead, cheeks, and nose.
4. Reddish-purple stretch marks (striae) may occur on the abdomen, breasts, thighs, and upper arms.
5. Vascular spider nevi may occur on the neck, chest, face, arms, and legs.
6. Rate of hair growth may decrease.
H. Skeletal system
1. Center of gravity changes.
2. Postural changes occur as the increased weight of the uterus causes a forward pull of the bony pelvis.
I. Metabolism
1. Metabolic function increases.
2. Body weight increases.
3. Water retention is increased, which can contribute to weight gain.

II. PSYCHOLOGICAL MATERNAL CHANGES
A. Ambivalence
1. Ambivalence occurs early in pregnancy, even when the pregnancy is planned.
2. Mother may experience dependence-independence conflict and ambivalence related to role changes.
3. Father may experience ambivalence related to the new role he is assuming, the increased financial responsibilities, and sharing the wife's attention with the child.
B. Acceptance: Factors that may be related to acceptance of the pregnancy are the woman's readiness for the experience and her identification with the motherhood role.
C. Emotional lability
1. Emotional lability may be manifested by frequency in the change of emotional states or extremes in emotional states.
2. These emotional changes are common, and the mother may feel that these changes are abnormal.

D. Body image changes
1. The changes in a woman's perception of her image during pregnancy occurs gradually and may be positive or negative.
2. The physical changes and symptoms that the woman experiences during pregnancy contribute to her body image.
E. Relationship with the fetus
1. The woman may daydream to prepare for motherhood and think about the maternal qualities she would like to possess.
2. The woman first accepts the biological fact that she is pregnant.
3. The woman next accepts the growing fetus as distinct from herself and a person to nuture.
4. Finally, the woman prepares realistically for the birth and parenting of the child.

III. DISCOMFORTS OF PREGNANCY
A. Nausea and vomiting
1. Nausea and vomiting occur in the first trimester.
2. Nausea and vomiting are due to elevated levels of human chorionic gonadotropin and changes in carbohydrate metabolism.
3. Interventions
   a. Eating dry crackers before arising
   b. Avoiding brushing teeth immediately after arising
   c. Eating small, frequent, low-fat meals during the day
   d. Drinking liquids between meals rather than at meals
   e. Avoiding fried foods and spicy foods
   f. Acupressure (some types may require a prescription)
   g. Herbal remedies, only if approved by a physician or nurse-midwife
B. Syncope
1. Syncope usually occurs in the first trimester; supine hypotension occurs particularly in the second and third trimester.
2. Syncope may be triggered hormonally or caused by the increased blood volume, anemia, fatigue, sudden position changes, or lying supine.
3. Interventions
   a. Sitting with the feet elevated
   b. Changing positions slowly
   c. Changing the position to the lateral recumbent to relieve the pressure of the uterus on the inferior vena cava
C. Urinary urgency and frequency
1. Usually in the first and third trimesters
2. Due to pressure of the uterus on the bladder
3. Interventions
   a. Drinking 2 qt of fluid during the day
   b. Limiting fluid intake in the evening
   c. Voiding at regular intervals

d. Sleeping on the side at night

e. Wearing perineal pads if necessary

f. Performing Kegel exercises

D. Breast tenderness

1. Tenderness can occur from the first through the third trimesters.

2. Tenderness is due to increased levels of estrogen and progesterone.

3. Interventions

a. Encouraging wearing a supportive bra

b. Avoiding the use of soap on the nipples and areola area to prevent drying

E. Increased vaginal discharge

1. Increased discharge can occur from the first through the third trimesters.

2. Increased discharge is due to hyperplasia of vaginal mucosa and increased mucus production.

3. Interventions

a. Proper cleansing and hygiene

b. Wearing cotton underwear

c. Avoiding douching

d. Advising the client to consult the physician or nurse-midwife if infection is suspected

F. Nasal stuffiness

1. Nasal stuffiness occurs during the first through the third trimesters.

2. Nasal stuffiness results from increased estrogen, which causes swelling of the nasal tissues and dryness.

3. Interventions

a. Encouraging the use of a humidifier

b. Avoiding the use of nasal sprays or anti-histamines

G. Fatigue

1. Fatigue occurs usually in the first and third trimesters.

2. Fatigue usually results from hormonal changes.

3. Interventions

a. Arranging frequent rest periods throughout the day

b. Using correct body mechanics

c. Obtaining regular exercise

d. Performing muscle relaxation and strengthening exercises for the legs and hip joints

e. Avoiding eating and drinking foods containing stimulants throughout pregnancy

H. Heartburn

1. Heartburn occurs in the second and the third trimesters.

2. Heartburn results from increased progesterone levels, decreased gastrointestinal motility and esophageal reflux, and displacement of the stomach by the enlarging uterus.

3. Interventions

a. Eating small, frequent meals

b. Sitting upright for 30 minutes following a meal

c. Drinking milk between meals

d. Avoiding fatty and spicy food

e. Performing tailor-sitting exercises

f. Taking antacids only if recommended by the physician or nurse-midwife

I. Ankle edema

1. Edema usually occurs in the second and the third trimesters.

2. Edema results from vasodilation, venous stasis, and increased venous pressure below the uterus.

3. Interventions

a. Elevating the legs at least twice a day

b. Sleeping on the left side

c. Wearing supportive stockings

d. Avoiding sitting or standing in one position for long periods of time

J. Varicose veins

1. Varicose veins usually occur in the second and the third trimesters.

2. Varicose veins result from weakening walls of the veins or valves and venous congestion.

3. Interventions

a. Wearing support hose

b. Elevating the feet when sitting

c. Lying with the feet and hips elevated

d. Avoiding long periods of standing or sitting

e. Moving about while standing to improve circulation

f. Avoiding leg crossing

g. Avoiding constricting articles of clothing

K. Headaches

1. Headaches usually occur in the second and third trimesters.

2. Headaches result from changes in blood volume and vascular tone.

3. Interventions

a. Changing position slowly

b. Applying a cool cloth to the forehead

c. Eating a small snack

d. Using acetaminophen (Tylenol) only if prescribed by the physician or nurse-midwife

L. Hemorrhoids

1. Hemorrhoids usually occur in the second and third trimesters.

2. Hemorrhoids result from increased venous pressure and constipation.

3. Interventions

a. Soaking in a warm sitz bath

b. Sitting on a soft pillow

c. Eating high-fiber foods and avoiding constipation

d. Drinking sufficient fluids

e. Increasing exercise, such as walking

f. Applying ointments, suppositories, or compresses as prescribed by the physician or nurse-midwife

M. Constipation
1. Constipation usually occurs in the second and third trimesters.
2. Constipation results from decreased intestinal motility, the displacement of the intestines, and taking of iron supplements.
3. Interventions
   a. Eating high-fiber foods
   b. Drinking sufficient fluids
   c. Exercising regularly
   d. Avoiding laxatives or enemas without first consulting with the physician or nurse-midwife

N. Backache
1. Backache usually occurs in the second and third trimesters.
2. Backache results from an exaggerated lumbosacral curve resulting from the enlarged uterus.
3. Interventions
   a. Encouraging rest
   b. Using correct body mechanics and improving posture
   c. Wearing low-heeled shoes
   d. Performing pelvic rocking and abdominal breathing exercises
   e. Sleeping on a firm mattress

O. Leg cramps
1. Leg cramps usually occur in the second and third trimesters.
2. Leg cramps result from an altered calcium-phosphorus balance and pressure of the uterus on nerves or from fatigue.
3. Interventions
   a. Getting regular exercise, especially walking
   b. Dorsiflexing the foot of the affected leg
   c. Increasing calcium intake

P. Shortness of breath and dyspnea
1. Dyspnea can occur in the second and third trimesters.
2. Dyspnea results from pressure on the diaphragm.
3. Interventions
   a. Allowing frequent rest periods
   b. Sleeping with the head elevated or on the side
   c. Avoiding overexertion
   d. Performing tailor sitting exercises

IV. LABORATORY TESTS (BOX 24-1)

A. Blood type and Rh factor
1. ABO typing is performed to determine the woman's blood type.

2. Rh typing is done to determine the presence or absence of Rh antigen (Rh positive or Rh negative).
3. If the client is Rh negative and has a negative antibody screen, the client will need repeat antibody screens and should receive Rh immune globulin at 28 weeks' gestation.

B. Rubella titer
1. If the client has a negative titer, indicating susceptibility to the rubella virus, the client should receive the appropriate immunization postpartum.
2. The client must be using effective birth control at the time of the immunization and must be counseled not to become pregnant for 3 months following immunization and to avoid contact with anyone who is immunocompromised.
3. If the rubella vaccine is administered at the same time as Rh immune globulin, it may not be effective.

C. Hemoglobin and hematocrit levels
1. Hemoglobin and hematocrit levels will drop during gestation as a result of increased plasma volume.
2. An increase in the hematocrit level may indicate the development of pregnancy-induced hypertension.
3. A decrease in the hemoglobin level to less than 10 g/dL or in the hematocrit level less than 30 g/dL indicates anemia.

D. Papanicolaou's smear is done during the initial prenatal examination to screen for cervical neoplasia.

E. Sexually transmitted diseases (Table 24-1)

F. Sickle cell screening
1. Screening is indicated for clients at risk for sickle cell disease.

BOX 24-1

Usual Schedule for Prenatal Visits

Every 4 weeks for first 28 to 32 weeks
Every 2 weeks from 32 to 36 weeks
Every week from 36 to 40 weeks

TABLE 24-1

Monitoring for Sexually Transmitted Diseases

Disease	Laboratory Test
Gonorrhea	A culture is done during the initial prenatal examination to screen for gonorrhea.
	The culture may be repeated during the third trimester in high-risk clients.
Syphilis	A culture is done during the initial prenatal examination to screen for syphilis.
	The culture may be repeated during the third trimester in high-risk clients.
Herpes virus	A culture is indicated for clients with a positive history or those with active lesions.
	The test is performed to determine the route of delivery.
	Weekly cultures may be done at week 35 or 36 of pregnancy until delivery.
Chlamydia	A culture is indicated if the client is in a high-risk group or if infants from previous pregnancies have developed neonatal conjunctivitis or pneumonia.

2. A positive test may indicate a need for further screening.

▶ G. Tuberculin skin test
1. The health care provider may prefer to perform this skin test after **delivery**.
2. A positive skin test indicates the need for a chest radiograph (using an abdominal lead shield) to rule out active disease; in a pregnant client, a chest radiograph will not be performed until after 20 weeks of gestation (after fetal organs are formed).
3. Converters to positive may be referred for treatment with medication following **delivery**.

▶ H. Hepatitis B surface antigens
1. Testing for hepatitis antigens is recommended for all women because of the prevalence of the disease in the general population.
2. Vaccination for hepatitis B antigen may be specifically indicated for the following:
   a. Health care workers
   b. Clients born in Asia, Africa, Haiti, or the Pacific islands
   c. Clients with previously undiagnosed jaundice or chronic liver disease
   d. Intravenous drug abusers
   e. Clients with tattoos
   f. Clients with histories of blood transfusions
   g. Clients with histories of multiple episodes of sexually transmitted diseases
   h. Clients who have been rejected previously as blood donors
   i. Clients with histories of dialysis or renal transplantation
   j. Clients from households having hepatitis B–infected members or hemodialysis clients

I. Urinalysis and urine culture
1. A urine specimen for glucose and protein determinations should be obtained at every prenatal visit.
2. Glycosuria is a common result of decreased renal threshold that occurs during pregnancy.
3. If glycosuria persists, it may indicate diabetes.
4. White blood cells in the urine may indicate infection.
5. Ketonuria may result from insufficient food intake or vomiting.
6. Levels of 2+ to 4+ protein in the urine may indicate infection or pregnancy-induced hypertension.

▶ V. DIAGNOSTIC TESTS
▶ A. Ultrasonography
1. Ultrasonography outlines and identifies fetal and maternal structures.
2. Ultrasonography assists to confirm gestational age and estimated date of **delivery**.
3. Ultrasonography may be done abdominally or transvaginally during pregnancy.

4. Interventions
   a. If the abdominal ultrasound is being performed, the woman may need to drink water to fill the bladder before the procedure to obtain a better image of the fetus.
   b. If the transvaginal ultrasound is being performed, a lubricated probe is inserted into the vagina.
   c. Inform the client that the test presents no known risks to the client or the fetus.

B. Alpha-fetoprotein screening
1. Screening assesses the quantity of fetal serum proteins; elevated levels of protein are associated with open neural tube and abdominal wall defects.
2. Screenings can detect spina bifida and Down syndrome.
3. Interventions
   a. Explain that the level is determined by a single maternal blood sample drawn at 15 to 18 weeks' gestation.
   b. If the level is elevated and the gestation is less than 18 weeks, a second sample is drawn.
   c. An ultrasound is performed for elevated levels to rule out fetal abnormalities or multiple gestation.

C. Chorionic villus sampling
1. The physician aspirates a small sample of chorionic villus tissue at 8 to 12 weeks' gestation.
2. Test is performed for the purpose of detecting genetic abnormalities.
3. Interventions
   a. Obtain informed consent.
   b. Instruct the client to drink water to fill the bladder before the procedure to aid in positioning the uterus for catheter insertion.
   c. Instruct the client to report bleeding, infection, or leakage of fluid at insertion site after the procedure.
   d. Rh-negative women may be given $Rh_0(D)$ immune globulin (RhoGAM) because chorionic villus sampling increases the risk of Rh sensitization.

D. Kick counts (fetal movement counting)
1. Mother sits quietly or lies down on the left side and counts fetal kicks for a period of time as instructed.
2. Instruct the client to notify the physician or nurse-midwife if there are fewer than 10 kicks in a 12-hour period or as instructed by the physician or nurse-midwife.

E. Amniocentesis
1. Aspiration of **amniotic fluid**; may be done from 13 to 14 weeks of pregnancy.
2. Amniocentesis is performed to determine genetic disorders, metabolic defects, and fetal lung maturity.

3. Risks
   a. Maternal hemorrhage
   b. Infection
   c. Rh isoimmunization
   d. Abruptio placentae
   e. **Amniotic fluid** emboli
   f. Premature rupture of the membranes
4. Interventions
   a. Obtain informed consent.
   b. Instruct the client to empty the bladder before the procedure.
   c. Prepare the client for ultrasonography, which is performed to locate the **placenta**.
   d. Obtain baseline vital signs and fetal heart rate, and monitor every 15 minutes.
   e. Position the client supine.
   f. Instruct the client that if chills, fever, leakage of fluid at the needle insertion site, decreased fetal movement, or uterine contractions occur, she is to notify the physician or nurse-midwife.
F. Fern test
   1. The fern test is a microscopic slide test to determine the presence of **amniotic fluid** leakage.
   2. By use of sterile technique, a specimen is obtained from the external os of the cervix and vaginal pool and is examined on a slide under a microscope.
   3. A fernlike pattern occurring from the salts of **amniotic fluid** indicates the presence of **amniotic fluid**.
   4. Interventions
      a. Position the client in the dorsal lithotomy position.
      b. Instruct the client to cough to cause the fluid to leak from the uterus if the membranes are ruptured.

G. Nitrazine test
   1. A Nitrazine test strip is used to detect the presence of **amniotic fluid** in vaginal secretions.
   2. Vaginal secretions have a pH of 4.5 to 5.5 and do not affect the yellow Nitrazine strip or swab.
   3. **Amniotic fluid** has a pH of 7.0 to 7.5 and turns the yellow Nitrazine blue.
   4. Interventions
      a. Position the client in dorsal lithotomy position.
      b. Touch the test tape to the fluid.
      c. Assess the test tape for a blue-green, blue-gray, or deep blue color, which indicates that the membranes are probably ruptured.
H. Nonstress test (Box 24-2)
I. Contraction stress test (Box 24-3)

VI. NUTRITION
A. General guidelines
   1. The average expected weight gain during pregnancy is 25 to 35 lb for women with a normal prepregnancy weight.
   2. An increase of about 300 calories per day is needed during pregnancy.
   3. Calorie needs are greater in the last two trimesters than in the first.
   4. An increase of about 500 calories per day is needed during lactation.
   5. Encourage a diet high in folic acid with folic acid supplements.
   6. A diet rich in folic acid is necessary for all women of childbearing age to prevent neural tube defect in the fetus during the first trimester of pregnancy.
   7. An intake of at least 8 to 10 (8-oz) glasses of fluid each day, of which 4 to 6 glasses are water, is needed.

BOX 24-2

Nonstress Test

DESCRIPTION
The test is performed to assess placental function and oxygenation.
The test determines fetal well-being.
The test evaluates fetal heart rate (FHR) in response to fetal movement.

INTERVENTIONS
An external ultrasound transducer and the tocodynamometer are applied to the mother, and a tracing of at least 20 minutes' duration is obtained so that the FHR and the uterine activity can be observed.
Obtain baseline blood pressure and monitor blood pressure frequently.
Position mother in the left lateral position to avoid vena cava compression.
The mother may be asked to press a button every time she feels fetal movement; the monitor records a mark at each point of fetal movement, which is used as a reference point to assess FHR response.

RESULTS
Reactive Nonstress Test (Normal/Negative)
"Reactive" indicates a healthy fetus.
The result requires two or more FHR accelerations of at least 15 beats per minute, lasting at least 15 seconds from the beginning of the acceleration to the end, in association with fetal movement, during a 20-minute period.
Nonreactive Nonstress Test (Abnormal)
No accelerations or accelerations of less than 15 beats per minute or lasting less than 15 seconds in duration occur during a 40-minute observation.
Unsatisfactory
The result cannot be interpreted because of the poor quality of the FHR tracing.

BOX 24-3

Contraction Stress Test

DESCRIPTION

The test assesses placental oxygenation and function.

The test determines fetal ability to tolerate labor and determines fetal well-being.

The fetus is exposed to the stressor of contractions to assess the adequacy of placental perfusion under simulated labor conditions.

The test is performed if the nonstress test is abnormal.

INTERVENTIONS

The external fetal monitor is applied to the mother, and a 20- to 30-minute baseline strip is recorded.

The uterus is stimulated to contract by the administration of a dilute dose of oxytocin (Pitocin) or by having the mother use nipple stimulation until three palpable contractions with a duration of 40 seconds or more in a 10-minute period have been achieved.

Frequent maternal blood pressure readings are done, and the mother is monitored closely while increasing doses of oxytocin are given.

RESULTS

Negative Contraction Stress Test (Normal)

A negative result is represented by no late or variable decelerations of the fetal heart rate.

Positive Contraction Stress Test (Abnormal)

A positive result is represented by late or variable decelerations of the fetal heart rate with 50% or more of the contractions in the absence of hyperstimulation of the uterus.

Equivocal

An equivocal result contains decelerations but with less than 50% of the contractions, or the uterine activity shows a hyperstimulated uterus.

Unsatisfactory

An unsatisfactory result means that adequate uterine contractions cannot be achieved, or the fetal heart rate tracing is not of sufficient quality for adequate interpretation.

---

8. Sodium is not restricted unless specifically prescribed by the physician or nurse-midwife.

B. Vegetarianism (Box 24-4)

1. Ensure that the client eats a sufficient amount of varied foods to meet normal nutrient and energy needs.
2. Protein consumption can be increased by consumption of a variety of vegetable protein sources based on whole grains, legumes, seeds, nuts, and vegetables combined to provide all of the essential amino acids.
3. Adequate food intake is important to ensure that dietary protein is used for protein synthesis.

C. Lactose intolerance

1. Lactose consumed by an individual with an intolerance can cause abdominal distention, discomfort, nausea, vomiting, cramps, and loose stools.

BOX 24-4

Types of Vegetarian Diets

LACTO-OVO VEGETARIANS

Adherents consume plant foods with dairy products and eggs.

Adherents may consume fish and occasionally poultry.

LACTO-VEGETARIANS

Adherents consume plant foods and dairy products excluding eggs.

VEGANS

Vegans follow a strict vegetarian diet and use no animal foods.

The food pattern consists entirely of plant foods.

---

2. Clients experiencing lactose intolerance need to incorporate sources of calcium other than dairy products into their dietary patterns regularly.
3. Milk may be tolerated in cooked form, such as in custards or fermented dairy products.
4. Cheese and yogurt sometimes are tolerated.
5. Lactase, an enzyme, may be prescribed and is taken before ingesting milk or milk products.
6. Lactase-treated milk or lactose-free products are also available commercially.

D. Pica

1. Pica is the eating of nonfood substances such as dirt, clay, starch, and freezer frost.
2. The cause is unknown; cultural values, such as beliefs regarding the effect of a material on the mother or fetus, may make pica a common practice.
3. Iron deficiency anemia may occur as a result of pica.

E. Cultural considerations: Refer to Chapter 6 for information on cultural considerations in nutrition.

PRACTICE QUESTIONS

1. A physician has prescribed transvaginal ultrasonography for a woman in the first trimester of pregnancy and the woman asks the nurse about the procedure. The nurse accurately provides which of the following information to the client?

   1. The procedure takes about 2 hours.
   2. Transmission gel is spread over the abdomen, and a transducer will be moved over the abdomen to obtain the picture.

3. It will be necessary to drink 1 to 2 qt of water before the examination.
4. The transvaginal probe encased in a disposable cover and coated with a gel is inserted into the vagina.

2. A clinic nurse has instructed a pregnant client in measures to prevent varicose veins during pregnancy. Which statement by the client indicates a need for further instructions?
   1. "I should wear support hose."
   2. "I should be wearing flat nonslip shoes that have an arch support."
   3. "I should wear panty hose."
   4. "I should wear knee-high hose as long as I don't leave them on longer than 8 hours."

3. A pregnant client calls a clinic and tells a nurse that she is experiencing leg cramps and is awakened by the cramps at night. To provide relief from the leg cramps, the nurse tells the client to
   1. Dorsiflex the foot while extending the knee when the cramps occur.
   2. Dorsiflex the foot while flexing the knee when the cramps occur.
   3. Plantar flex the foot while flexing the knee when the cramps occur.
   4. Plantar flex the foot while extending the knee when the cramps occur.

4. A clinic nurse is providing instructions to a pregnant client regarding measures that will assist in alleviating heartburn. Which statement by the client indicates an understanding of these measures?
   1. "I should lie down for an hour after eating."
   2. "I should avoid between-meal snacks."
   3. "I should substitute spices for cooking rather than using salt."
   4. "I should avoid eating gas-producing foods and fatty foods."

5. A nurse in a health care clinic is instructing a pregnant woman in how to perform "kick counts." Which statement by the woman indicates a need for further instructions?
   1. "I should place my hands on the largest part of my abdomen and concentrate on the fetal movements to count the kicks."
   2. "I will record the number of movements or kicks."
   3. "I need to lie flat on my back to perform the procedure."
   4. "A count of fewer than 10 kicks in a 12-hour period indicates the need to contact the physician."

6. A clinic nurse is instructing a pregnant client regarding dietary measures to promote a healthy pregnancy. The nurse instructs the client to have an adequate intake of fluid daily. Which statement by the mother indicates an understanding of the daily fluid requirement?
   1. "I should drink at least 8 to 10 glasses of fluid each day, of which 4 to 6 glasses are water."

   2. "I should drink 12 glasses of fruit juices or milk every day."
   3. "I should drink 8 to 10 glasses of fluid a day, and I can count all of the diet soft drinks that I consume."
   4. "I should drink 12 glasses of fluid a day, and I can include the coffee or tea that I drink in the count."

7. A nurse is instructing a pregnant client regarding measures to increase sources of iron in the diet. The nurse tells the client to consume which food that contains the highest source of dietary iron?
   1. Milk
   2. Dark green, leafy vegetables
   3. Potatoes
   4. Cantaloupe

8. A nurse is providing instructions regarding treatment for hemorrhoids to a client who is in the second trimester of pregnancy. Which statement by the client indicates a need for further instruction?
   1. "I can apply ice packs to the hemorrhoids to reduce the swelling."
   2. " I should apply heat packs to the hemorrhoids to help the hemorrhoids shrink."
   3. "I should avoid straining during bowel movements."
   4. "I can gently replace the hemorrhoids into the rectum."

9. A nurse is providing instructions to a client in the first trimester of pregnancy regarding measures to assist in reducing breast tenderness. The nurse tells the client to
   1. Avoid wearing a bra.
   2. Wash the nipples and areola area daily with soap, and massage the breasts with lotion.
   3. Wear tight-fitting blouses or dresses to provide support.
   4. Wash the breasts with warm water and keep them dry.

10. A nonstress test is prescribed for a pregnant client, and the client asks the nurse about the procedure. The nurse tells the client that
    1. The test is an invasive procedure and requires that an informed consent be signed.
    2. The test will take about 2 hours and will require close monitoring for 2 hours after the procedure is completed.
    3. An ultrasound transducer that records fetal heart activity is secured over the abdomen where the fetal heart is heard most clearly.
    4. The fetus is challenged or stressed by uterine contractions to obtain the necessary information.

11. A nurse has assisted in performing a nonstress test on a pregnant client and is reviewing the documentation related to the results of the test. The nurse notes that the physician has documented the test results as reactive. The nurse interprets that this result indicates

1. Normal findings.
2. Abnormal findings.
3. The need for further evaluation.
4. That the findings on the monitor were difficult to interpret.

12. A nonstress test is performed on a client who is pregnant, and the results of the test indicate non-reactive findings. The physician prescribes a contraction stress test, the test is performed, and the nurse notes that the physician has documented the results as negative. The nurse interprets this finding as indicating
    1. A high risk for fetal demise.
    2. A normal test result.
    3. The need for a cesarean delivery.
    4. An abnormal test result.

13. A nurse is reviewing a nutritional plan of care with a pregnant client and is identifying the food items that are highest in folic acid. The nurse determines that the client understands which foods supply the highest amounts of folic acid if the client states that she will include which of the following in the daily diet?
    1. A banana
    2. Leafy, green vegetable
    3. Milk
    4. Yogurt

14. A pregnant client tells a nurse that she has been craving "unusual foods." The nurse gathers additional assessment data from the client and discovers that the client has been ingesting daily amounts of white clay dirt from her backyard. Laboratory studies are performed on the client. The nurse reviews the laboratory results and determines that which of the following indicates a physiological consequence of this client's practice?
    1. Hematocrit, 38%
    2. Hemoglobin, 9.1 g/dL
    3. Glucose, 86 mg/dL
    4. White blood cell count, 12,400/mm^3

15. A pregnant client who is at 30 weeks' gestation comes to a clinic for a routine visit, and the nurse performs an assessment on the client. Which observation made by the nurse during the assessment indicates a need for teaching?
    1. The client is wearing sneakers.
    2. The client is wearing flat shoes with rubber soles.
    3. The client is wearing pants with an elastic waistband.
    4. The client is wearing knee-high hose.

16. A nurse is developing a plan of care for a pregnant client who is complaining of intermittent episodes of constipation. The nurse includes in the plan of care measures to prevent the episodes of constipation and plans to tell the client to
    1. Take a mild stool softener daily in the evening.
    2. Drink 6 glasses of water per day.

3. Consume a low-roughage diet.
4. Use a Fleet enema when the episodes occur.

17. A pregnant client visits a clinic for a scheduled prenatal appointment. On assessment the client tells the nurse that she frequently has a backache, and the nurse provides instructions to the client regarding measures that will assist in relieving the backache. Which statement by the client indicates a need for further instructions regarding the measures to relieve the backache?
    1. "I need to try to maintain good posture."
    2. "I should do more exercises to strengthen my back muscles."
    3. "I should sleep on a firm mattress."
    4. "I should wear low-heeled shoes."

18. A nurse is providing instructions to a pregnant client who is scheduled for an amniocentesis. The nurse tells the client that
    1. A fever is expected following the procedure because of the trauma to the abdomen.
    2. Strict bed rest is required following the procedure.
    3. An informed consent will need to be signed before the procedure.
    4. Hospitalization is necessary for 24 hours following the procedure.

19. A pregnant client in the first trimester calls a nurse at a health care clinic and reports that she has noticed a thin, colorless, vaginal drainage. The nurse most appropriately tells the mother
    1. To come to the clinic immediately.
    2. To report to the emergency room at the maternity center immediately.
    3. That the vaginal discharge may be bothersome but is a normal occurrence.
    4. To use tampons if the discharge is bothersome but to be sure to change the tampons every 2 hours.

20. A pregnant client asks a nurse about the types of exercises that are allowable during the pregnancy. The nurse would instruct the client that the safest exercise to engage in is which of the following?
    1. Bicycling with the legs in the air
    2. Swimming
    3. Scuba diving
    4. Low-weight gymnastics

CRITICAL THINKING: FILL IN THE BLANK

A pregnant client has blood drawn for a rubella titer, and the results show a negative titer, indicating susceptibility to the rubella virus. The client is told that she will receive a rubella virus vaccine in the postpartum period following delivery. The nurse instructs the client that pregnancy needs to be avoided for what time period after receiving the vaccine?

Answer: _____

ANSWERS

1. 4

Rationale: Transvaginal ultrasonography allows clear visibility of the uterus, gestational sac, embryo, and deep pelvic structures such as the ovaries and fallopian tubes. The woman is placed in a lithotomy position and a transvaginal probe, encased in a disposable cover and coated with a gel that provides for lubrication and promotes conductivity, is inserted into the vagina. The woman may feel more comfortable if she is allowed to insert the probe. The procedure takes about 10 to 15 minutes. Options 2 and 3 identify components of the abdominal ultrasound.

Test-Taking Strategy: Use the process of elimination. Note the key words "transvaginal ultrasonography." Also note the relationship of the name of the test and the description in the correct option. If you had difficulty with this question, review the procedure for transvaginal ultrasonography.

Level of Cognitive Ability: Application
Client Needs: Physiological Integrity
Integrated Process: Teaching/Learning
Content Area: Maternity—Antepartum
Reference: Murray, S., McKinney, E., & Gorrie, T. (2002). *Foundations of maternal-newborn nursing* (3rd ed., p. 220). Philadelphia: W. B. Saunders.

2. 4

Rationale: Varicose veins often develop in the lower extremities during pregnancy. Any constrictive clothing, such as knee-high hose, impedes venous return from the lower legs and places the client at risk for developing varicosities. The client should be encouraged to wear support hose or panty hose. Flat nonslip shoes with proper support are important to assist the pregnant woman to maintain proper posture and balance and minimize falls.

Test-Taking Strategy: Use the process of elimination. Note the key words "a need for further instructions." Focus on the issue of the question as it relates to preventing varicose veins. Recall that anything that constricts the lower vessels and impedes venous return from the lower legs will place the client at risk for varicosities. If you had difficulty with this question, review measures to prevent varicose veins.

Level of Cognitive Ability: Analysis
Client Needs: Health Promotion and Maintenance
Integrated Process: Nursing Process—evaluation
Content Area: Maternity—antepartum
Reference: Murray, S., McKinney, E., & Gorrie, T. (2002). *Foundations of maternal-newborn nursing* (3rd ed., p. 149). Philadelphia: W. B. Saunders.

3. 1

Rationale: Leg cramps occur when the pregnant woman stretches the leg and plantar flexes the foot. Dorsiflexion of the foot while extending the knee stretches the affected muscle, prevents the muscle from contracting, and stops the cramping. Options 2, 3, and 4 are not measures that will provide relief from the leg cramps.

Test-Taking Strategy: Use the process of elimination. Focus on the issue of the question, to provide relief from the leg cramps. Attempt to visualize each of the descriptions in the options to assist in directing you to option 1. If you had difficulty with this question, review measures that assist in alleviating muscle cramps.

Level of Cognitive Ability: Application
Client Needs: Health Promotion and Maintenance
Integrated Process: Teaching/Learning
Content Area: Maternity—antepartum
Reference: Matteson, P. (2001). *Women's health during the childbearing years: A community-based approach* (p. 455). St. Louis: Mosby.

4. 4

Rationale: Lying down is likely to lead to reflux of stomach contents, especially immediately following a meal. The client should be instructed to avoid spices along with salt because spices will trigger heartburn. Salt will produce edema. The client should be encouraged to eat between-meal snacks and should be instructed that to control heartburn, eating smaller, more frequent portions is preferred over eating three large meals. The client also should limit or avoid gas-producing and fatty foods.

Test-Taking Strategy: Use the process of elimination and note the key words "indicates an understanding." Recalling that the client needs to limit or avoid gas-producing and fatty foods will assist in directing you to option 4. Review the measures that will alleviate heartburn in the pregnant client if you had difficulty with this question.

Level of Cognitive Ability: Analysis
Client Needs: Health Promotion and Maintenance
Integrated Process: Nursing Process—evaluation
Content Area: Maternity–antepartum
Reference: Williams, S. (2001). *Basic nutrition & diet therapy* (11th ed., p. 277). St Louis: Mosby.

5. 3

Rationale: The woman should sit or lie quietly on her side to perform kick counts. Lying flat on the back is not necessary to perform this procedure, can cause discomfort, and presents a risk of vena cava (hypotensive) syndrome. The woman is instructed to place her hands on the largest part of the abdomen and concentrates on the fetal movements. The woman records the number of movements felt during a specified time period. The client needs to notify the physician or nurse-midwife if there are fewer than 10 kicks in a 12-hour period or as instructed by the physician or nurse-midwife.

Test-Taking Strategy: Use the process of elimination, noting the key words "a need for further instructions." If you are unfamiliar with this procedure, recalling that the risk of vena cava (hypotensive) syndrome exists when the client lies on her back will direct you to option 3. Review the procedure for kick counts if you had difficulty with this question.

Level of Cognitive Ability: Analysis
Client Needs: Health Promotion and Maintenance
Integrated Process: Nursing Process—evaluation
Content Area: Maternity—antepartum
Reference: Lowdermilk, D., & Perry, S. (2003). *Maternity nursing* (6th ed., p. 660). St. Louis: Mosby.

6. 1

Rationale: The nurse should instruct the client to have an adequate fluid intake daily to assist in digestion and in the management of constipation. The pregnant woman should consume at least 8 to 10 (8-oz) glasses of fluid each day, of which 4 to 6 glasses are water. Because of their sodium content, diet soft drinks should be consumed in moderation. Caffeinated beverages have a diuretic effect, which may be counterproductive to increasing fluid intake.

Test-Taking Strategy: Use the process of elimination. Recalling that diet soft drinks and caffeine-containing products should be avoided will assist in eliminating options 3 and 4. From the remaining options, recalling that water needs to be included in the daily fluid intake will assist in directing you to option 1. If you had difficulty with this question, review client instructions regarding water and fluid intake during pregnancy.

Level of Cognitive Ability: Analysis
Client Needs: Health Promotion and Maintenance
Integrated Process: Nursing Process—evaluation
Content Area: Maternity—antepartum
References: Lowdermilk, D., & Perry, S. (2003). *Maternity nursing* (6th ed., p. 240). St. Louis: Mosby.
Williams, S. (2001). *Basic nutrition & diet therapy* (11th ed., p. 297). St Louis: Mosby.

7. **2**

Rationale: Dietary sources of iron include lean meats, liver, shellfish, dark green leafy vegetables, legumes, whole grains, and enriched grains, cereals, and molasses. Milk is high in calcium and also contains phosphorus. Cantaloupe and potatoes are high in vitamin C.

Test-Taking Strategy: Use the process of elimination and knowledge of the dietary sources of iron to assist in answering the question. Remember that dark green, leafy vegetables are high in iron. If you had difficulty with this question, review food items high in iron.

Level of Cognitive Ability: Application
Client Needs: Health Promotion and Maintenance
Integrated Process: Teaching/Learning
Content Area: Maternity—antepartum
References: Lowdermilk, D., & Perry, S. (2003). *Maternity nursing* (6th ed., p. 249). St. Louis: Mosby.
Williams, S. (2001). *Basic nutrition & diet therapy* (11th ed., p. 201). St Louis: Mosby.

8. **2**

Rationale: Measures that provide relief from hemorrhoids include avoiding constipation and straining during bowel movements; applying ice packs to reduce the hemorrhoidal swelling; gently replacing the hemorrhoids into the rectum; using stool softeners, ointments, or sprays as prescribed; and assuming certain positions to relieve pressure on the hemorrhoids. Heat packs will increase the blood flow to the area and worsen the discomfort from hemorrhoids.

Test-Taking Strategy: Use the process of elimination, noting the key words "need for further instruction." Recalling the principles regarding heat and cold will assist in directing you to option 2. If you had difficulty with this question, review the measures for the treatment of hemorrhoids.

Level of Cognitive Ability: Analysis
Client Needs: Health Promotion and Maintenance
Integrated Process: Teaching/Learning

Content Area: Maternity—antepartum
Reference: Murray, S., McKinney, E., & Gorrie, T. (2002). *Foundations of maternal-newborn nursing* (3rd ed., p. 149). Philadelphia: W. B. Saunders.

9. **4**

Rationale: The pregnant woman should be instructed to wash the breasts with warm water and keep them dry. The woman should be instructed to avoid using soap on the nipples and areola area to prevent the drying of tissues. Wearing a supportive bra with wide adjustable straps can decrease breast tenderness. Tight-fitting blouses or dresses will cause discomfort. The woman is instructed to wear soft-textured clothing to decrease nipple tenderness and to use breast pads inside the bra to prevent leakage if colostrum is a problem.

Test-Taking Strategy: Use the process of elimination. Focusing on the issue of the question, reducing breast tenderness, and visualizing each of the measures identified in the options will direct you to option 4. If you had difficulty with this question, review treatment measures for the client with breast tenderness.

Level of Cognitive Ability: Application
Client Needs: Health Promotion and Maintenance
Integrated Process: Teaching/Learning
Content Area: Maternity—antepartum
Reference: Matteson, P. (2001). *Women's health during the childbearing years: A community-based approach* (p. 376). St. Louis: Mosby.

10. **3**

Rationale: The nonstress test takes about 20 to 30 minutes. The test is termed *nonstress* because it consists of monitoring only; the fetus is not challenged or stressed by uterine contractions to obtain the necessary data. The test is noninvasive, and an ultrasound transducer that records fetal heart activity is secured over the maternal abdomen where the fetal heart is heard most clearly. A tocotransducer that detects uterine activity and fetal movement also is secured to the maternal abdomen. Fetal heart activity and movements are recorded.

Test-Taking Strategy: Use the process of elimination. Focus on the name of the test and the procedure for this test to eliminate options 1, 2, and 4. If you are unfamiliar with this test or had difficulty answering this question, review this procedure.

Level of Cognitive Ability: Application
Client Needs: Physiological Integrity
Integrated Process: Teaching/Learning
Content Area: Maternity—antepartum
Reference: Murray, S., McKinney, E., & Gorrie, T. (2002). *Foundations of maternal-newborn nursing* (3rd ed., p. 230). Philadelphia: W. B. Saunders.

11. **1**

Rationale: A reactive nonstress test is a normal result. To be considered reactive, the baseline fetal heart rate must be within normal range (120 to 160 beats per minute) with good long-term variability. In addition, two or more fetal heart rate accelerations of at least 15 beats per minute must occur, each with a duration of at least 15 seconds, in a 20-minute interval.

Test-Taking Strategy: Use the process of elimination. Eliminate options 2, 3, and 4 because they are similar. If you

had difficulty with this question and are unfamiliar with the interpretation of the results of a nonstress test, review this content.
Level of Cognitive Ability: Analysis
Client Needs: Physiological Integrity
Integrated Process: Nursing Process—analysis
Content Area: Maternity—antepartum
Reference: Murray, S., McKinney, E., & Gorrie, T. (2002). *Foundations of maternal-newborn nursing* (3rd ed., p. 231). Philadelphia: W. B. Saunders.

12. **2**
Rationale: Contraction stress test results may be interpreted as negative (normal), positive (abnormal), or equivocal. A negative test result indicates that no late decelerations occurred in the fetal heart rate, although the fetus was stressed by three contractions of at least 40 seconds' duration in a 10-minute period.
Test-Taking Strategy: Use the process of elimination, noting that options 1, 3, and 4 are similar in that they indicate an abnormal test result finding. If you had difficulty with this question and are unfamiliar with the interpretation of the results of a contraction stress test, review this content.
Level of Cognitive Ability: Analysis
Client Needs: Physiological Integrity
Integrated Process: Nursing Process—analysis
Content Area: Maternity—antepartum
Reference: Murray, S., McKinney, E., & Gorrie, T. (2002). *Foundations of maternal-newborn nursing* (3rd ed., p. 233). Philadelphia: W. B. Saunders.

13. **2**
Rationale: Leafy, green vegetables are rich in folate (folic acid). Bananas provide potassium; milk and yogurt supply calcium.
Test-Taking Strategy: Use the process of elimination. Eliminate options 3 and 4 first because they are similar. From the remaining options, recalling that leafy, green vegetables are high in folic acid will direct you to option 2. Review these foods if you had difficulty with this question.
Level of Cognitive Ability: Analysis
Client Needs: Physiological Integrity
Integrated Process: Teaching/Learning
Content Area: Maternity—antepartum
Reference: Williams, S. (2001). *Basic nutrition & diet therapy* (11th ed., p. 163). St Louis: Mosby.

14. **2**
Rationale: Pica cravings often lead to iron deficiency anemia, resulting in a lowered hemoglobin. The laboratory values in options 1, 3, and 4 are within normal limits for the pregnant woman.
Test-Taking Strategy: Use the process of elimination, recalling that pica results in anemia. This will assist in eliminating options 3 and 4. From the remaining options, recall the normal laboratory values in a pregnant client to assist in directing you to option 2. Review the physiological effects of pica and the normal laboratory values in a pregnant client, if you had difficulty with this question.
Level of Cognitive Ability: Analysis
Client Needs: Physiological Integrity

Integrated Process: Nursing Process—analysis
Content Area: Maternity—antepartum
Reference: Williams, S. (2001). *Basic nutrition & diet therapy* (11th ed., p. 280). St Louis: Mosby.

15. **4**
Rationale: Varicose veins often develop in the lower extremities during pregnancy. Any constricting clothing such as knee-high hose impede venous return from the lower legs and thus place the client at higher risk for developing varicosities. Clients should be encouraged to wear panty hose or support hose. Flat, nonslip shoes with proper support are important to assist the pregnant woman to maintain proper posture and balance and minimize the risk for falls. Pants with an elastic waistband are comfortable and are not constricting.
Test-Taking Strategy: Use the process of elimination, noting the key words "indicates a need for teaching." Remembering that the pregnant client is at risk for developing varicosities and recalling the measures to prevent their occurrence will direct you to option 4. Review the measures that will assist in preventing varicosities, if you had difficulty with this question.
Level of Cognitive Ability: Analysis
Client Needs: Physiological Integrity
Integrated Process: Nursing Process—assessment
Content Area: Maternity—antepartum
References: Matteson, P. (2001). *Women's health during the childbearing years: A community-based approach* (p. 429). St. Louis: Mosby.
Murray, S., McKinney, E., & Gorrie, T. (2002). *Foundations of maternal-newborn nursing* (3rd ed., p. 149). Philadelphia: W. B. Saunders.

16. **2**
Rationale: The nurse should instruct the client to drink 6 glasses of water per day and to consume a diet that includes roughage to prevent the constipation. The client should not take stool softeners, laxatives, mineral oil, other medications, or enemas without first consulting with the physician or nurse-midwife.
Test-Taking Strategy: Use the process of elimination and recall the basic principles related to the prevention of constipation. Also remember that the client is a pregnant client. Review measures to prevent constipation in the pregnant client if you had difficulty with this question.
Level of Cognitive Ability: Application
Client Needs: Health Promotion and Maintenance
Integrated Process: Teaching/Learning
Content Area: Maternity—antepartum
Reference: Matteson, P. (2001). *Women's health during the childbearing years: A community-based approach* (p. 428). St. Louis: Mosby.

17. **2**
Rationale: Some of the measures that will assist in relieving a backache include maintaining good posture and body mechanics, resting and avoiding fatigue, wearing low-heeled shoes, and sleeping on a firm mattress. The back discomfort that occurs in a pregnant client is often due to the exaggerated lumbar and cervicothoracic curves caused by a change in the

center of gravity resulting from the enlarged uterus. Performing more exercises to strengthen the back muscles could be harmful to a pregnant client.

Test-Taking Strategy: Use the process of elimination, focusing on the key words "need for further instructions." Recalling the principles related to relieving a backache will assist in directing you to the correct option. Review these measures if you had difficulty with this question.

Level of Cognitive Ability: Analysis
Client Needs: Health Promotion and Maintenance
Integrated Process: Teaching/Learning
Content Area: Maternity—antepartum
References: Matteson, P. (2001). *Women's health during the childbearing years: A community-based approach* (p. 381). St. Louis: Mosby.
Murray, S., McKinney, E., & Gorrie, T. (2002). *Foundations of maternal-newborn nursing* (3rd ed., p. 148). Philadelphia: W. B. Saunders.

18. 3

Rationale: Because amniocentesis is an invasive procedure, informed consent will need to be obtained before the procedure. After the procedure the client is instructed to rest but may resume light activity after the cramping subsides. The client is instructed to keep the puncture site clean and to report any complications such as vaginal discharge, severe, persistent cramping, or the onset of fever. Amniocentesis is an outpatient procedure and may be done in a physician's private office or in a special prenatal testing unit. Hospitalization is not necessary following the procedure.

Test-Taking Strategy: Use the process of elimination. Simply recalling that this procedure is invasive will direct you to option 3. If you had difficulty with this question, review the procedure related to amniocentesis.

Level of Cognitive Ability: Application
Client Needs: Physiological Integrity
Integrated Process: Teaching/Learning
Content Area: Maternity—antepartum
Reference: Chernecky, C., & Berger, B. (2001). *Laboratory tests and diagnostic procedures* (3rd ed., p. 153). Philadelphia: W. B. Saunders.

19. 3

Rationale: Leukorrhea begins during the first trimester. Many women notice a thin, colorless, or yellow vaginal discharge throughout pregnancy. Some clients become distressed about this condition. This occurrence does not require that the client report to the health care clinic or the emergency room immediately. If vaginal discharge is profuse, the woman may use panty liners but should not wear tampons because of the risk of infection. If the woman uses panty liners, she should change them frequently.

Test-Taking Strategy: Use the process of elimination. Eliminate options 1 and 2 first because they are similar. From the remaining options, recalling that this manifestation is a normal physiological occurrence or that tampons should be avoided will assist in directing you to the correct option. Review the normal occurrences related to vaginal discharge in a pregnant woman, if you had difficulty with this question.

Level of Cognitive Ability: Application
Client Needs: Health Promotion and Maintenance
Integrated Process: Nursing Process—implementation
Content Area: Maternity—antepartum
References: Lowdermilk, D., & Perry, S. (2003). *Maternity nursing* (6th ed., p. 173). St. Louis: Mosby.
Wong, D., Perry, S., & Hockenberry, M. (2002). *Maternal child nursing care* (2nd ed., p. 172). St. Louis: Mosby.

20. 2

Rationale: Non–weight-bearing exercises are preferable to weight-bearing exercises during pregnancy. Exercises to avoid are shoulder standing and bicycling with the legs in the air because the knee-chest position should be avoided. Competitive or high-risk sports such as scuba diving, water skiing, downhill skiing, horseback riding, basketball, volleyball, and gymnastics should be avoided. Non–weight-bearing exercises such as swimming are allowable.

Test-Taking Strategy: Use the process of elimination. Identify those activities or exercises that could cause or produce an injury to the fetus. This should direct you easily to option 2. If you had difficulty with this question, review the teaching points related to exercising for a client who is pregnant.

Level of Cognitive Ability: Application
Client Needs: Health Promotion and Maintenance
Integrated Process: Teaching/Learning
Content Area: Maternity—antepartum
References: Lowdermilk, D., & Perry, S. (2003). *Maternity nursing* (6th ed., p. 73). St. Louis: Mosby.
Wong, D., Perry, S., & Hockenberry, M. (2002). *Maternal child nursing care* (2nd ed., p. 38). St. Louis: Mosby.

CRITICAL THINKING: FILL IN THE BLANK

Answer: The client is counseled not to become pregnant for 3 months following immunization.

Rationale: The client must be using effective birth control at the time of the immunization. The client is counseled not to become pregnant for 3 months following immunization because of a possible risk to the fetus from the live virus vaccine.

Test-Taking Strategy: Focus on the issue, specific information about becoming pregnant. Recalling that the rubella vaccine is a live virus vaccine will assist in answering this question. Review client instructions following this immunization if you had difficulty with this question.

Level of Cognitive Ability: Application
Client Needs: Health Promotion and Maintenance
Integrated Process: Teaching/Learning
Content Area: Maternity—postpartum
Reference: Lowdermilk, D., & Perry, S. (2003). *Maternity nursing* (6th ed., p. 399). St. Louis: Mosby.

REFERENCES

Chernecky, C., & Berger, B. (2001). *Laboratory tests and diagnostic procedures* (3rd ed.). Philadelphia: W. B. Saunders.

Lowdermilk, D., & Perry, S. (2003). *Maternity nursing* (6th ed.). St. Louis: Mosby.

Matteson, P. (2001). *Women's health during the childbearing years: A community-based approach.* St. Louis: Mosby.

Murray, S., McKinney, E., & Gorrie, T. (2002). *Foundations of maternal-newborn nursing* (3rd ed.). Philadelphia: W. B. Saunders.

Williams, S. (2001). *Basic nutrition & diet therapy* (11th ed.). St Louis: Mosby.

Wong, D., Perry, S., & Hockenberry, M. (2002). *Maternal child nursing care* (2nd ed.). St. Louis: Mosby.

Risk Conditions Related to Pregnancy

I. ABORTION

Description: A pregnancy that ends before 20 weeks' gestation, spontaneously or electively

A. Types (Box 25-1)

B. Assessment
1. Spontaneous vaginal bleeding occurs.
2. Passage of clots or tissue through the vagina occurs.
3. Low uterine cramping or contractions occur.
4. Hemorrhage and shock can occur.

C. Interventions
1. Maintain bed rest.
2. Monitor vital signs.
3. Monitor cramping and bleeding.
4. Count perineal pads to evaluate blood loss, and save expelled tissues and clots.
5. Maintain intravenous fluids as prescribed; monitor for signs of shock.
6. Prepare client for dilatation and curettage as prescribed for incomplete abortion.

BOX 25-1

Types of Abortions

Spontaneous: pregnancy ends because of natural causes
Induced: therapeutic or elective reasons for terminating the pregnancy
Threatened: developing spontaneous abortion
Inevitable: threatened loss that cannot be prevented
Incomplete: loss of some products of conception and retention of others
Complete: loss of all products of conception
Missed: retention of products of conception in utero after fetal death
Habitual: spontaneous abortions in three or more successive pregnancies

---

7. Rh immune globulin is given to appropriate $Rh_0(D)$-negative woman.

II. ACQUIRED IMMUNODEFICIENCY SYNDROME

A. Description
1. The human immunodeficiency virus (HIV) is a causative factor in the development of acquired immunodeficiency syndrome.
2. Women infected with HIV first may demonstrate symptoms at the time of pregnancy or possibly develop life-threatening infections because normal pregnancy involves some suppression of the maternal immune system.
3. Zidovudine (AZT) is recommended for the prevention of maternal-fetal HIV transmission and is administered orally beginning after 14 weeks' gestation, intravenously during **labor**, and in the form of syrup to the **neonate** after birth for 6 weeks.

B. Transmission
1. Sexual exposure to genital secretions of an infected person
2. Parenteral exposure to infected blood and tissue
3. Perinatal exposure of an **infant** to infected maternal secretions through birth or breast-feeding

C. Risks to the mother: The mother with HIV is managed as high risk because she is vulnerable to infections.

D. Diagnosis
1. Tests used to determine the presence of antibodies to HIV include enzyme-linked immunosorbent assay (ELISA), Western blot, and immunofluorescence assay (IFA).
2. A single reactive ELISA test by itself cannot be used to diagnose HIV and should be repeated in duplicate with the same blood sample; if the result is repeatedly reactive, follow-up tests using Western blot or IFA should be done.
3. A positive Western blot or IFA is considered confirmatory for HIV.

4. A positive ELISA that fails to be confirmed by Western blot or IFA should not be considered negative, and repeat testing should take place in 3 to 6 months.

5. Refer to Chapter 11 for additional laboratory tests.

E. Assessment (Box 25-2)

F. Interventions

1. Prenatal period
   a. Prevent opportunistic infections.
   b. Avoid procedures that increase the risk of perinatal transmission, such as amniocentesis and fetal scalp sampling.

2. Intrapartum period
   a. If the fetus has not been exposed to HIV in utero, the highest risk exists during **delivery** through the birth canal.
   b. Avoid the use of scalp electrodes.
   c. Avoid episiotomy to decrease the amount of maternal blood in and around the birth canal.
   d. Avoid the administration of oxytocin (Pitocin) because contractions induced by oxytocin can be strong, causing vaginal tears or necessitating an episiotomy.
   e. Place heavy absorbent pads under the mother's hips to absorb **amniotic fluid** and maternal blood.
   f. Minimize the neonate's exposure to maternal blood and body fluids; promptly remove the **neonate** from the mother's blood following delivery.
   g. Suction fluids from the **neonate** promptly.
   h. Prepare to administer zidovudine intravenously as prescribed to the mother during **labor** and **delivery**.

3. Postpartum period
   a. Monitor for signs of infection.
   b. Place the mother in protective isolation if the mother is immunosuppressed.
   c. Restrict breast-feeding.
   d. Instruct the mother to monitor for signs of infection and report any signs if they occur.

G. The **neonate** and HIV

1. Description
   a. Neonates born to HIV-positive clients may test positive because the mother's positive antibodies may persist for as long as 18 months after birth; all neonates acquire maternal antibody to HIV infection, but not all acquire infection.
   b. The use of antiviral medication, reduction of **neonate** exposure to maternal blood and body fluids, and early identification of HIV in pregnancy reduce the risk of transmission to the **neonate**.

2. Interventions
   a. Bathe the **neonate** carefully before any invasive procedure, such as the administration of vitamin K, heel sticks, or venipunctures; clean the umbilical cord stump meticulously every day until healed.
   b. **Neonate** can room with mother.
   c. Prepare to administer zidovudine to the **newborn** infant as prescribed for the first 6 weeks of life.
   d. All HIV-exposed **newborn** infants should be treated with medication to prevent infection by *Pneumocystis carinii*.
   e. Note that an HIV culture is recommended at age 1 month and after 4 months of age; infants at risk for HIV infection should be seen by the physician at birth, 1 week, 2 weeks, 1 month, 2 months, and 4 months of life.
   f. Infants at risk for HIV infection need to receive all recommended immunizations at the regular schedule; no live immunizations should be administered.
   g. The **neonate** may be asymptomatic for the first several years of life and needs to be monitored for early signs of immunodeficiency

III. ANEMIA

A. Description

1. Anemia is a condition that can develop as a result of iron deficiency.
2. Anemia predisposes the client to postpartum infection and hemorrhage.

BOX 25-2

Stages of Acquired Immunodeficiency Syndrome

STAGE 1
Fever
Myalgia
Lymphadenopathy
Headache

STAGE 2
Infection is active but asymptomatic and may remain so for years.
Person may experience an outbreak of herpes zoster (shingles).
Person may experience a transient thrombocytopenia.

STAGE 3
Person is symptomatic.
Immune dysfunction is evident.
All body systems can show signs of immune dysfunction.
Integumentary and gynecological problems are common.

STAGE 4
Advanced human immunodeficiency virus infection.
Person is vulnerable to common bacterial infections.
Development of opportunistic infections occurs.
Serious immune compromise occurs.

B. Assessment
   1. Fatigue
   2. Headache
   3. Pallor
   4. Tachycardia
   5. Hemoglobin value usually less than 10 g/dL; hematocrit value usually less than 30 g/dL.
C. Interventions
   1. Monitor hemoglobin and hematocrit levels every 2 weeks.
   2. Administer and instruct the client about iron and folic acid supplements.
   3. Instruct the client to take iron with a source of vitamin C and to avoid taking iron with tea.
   4. Instruct the client to eat foods high in iron, folic acid, and protein.
   5. Teach the client to monitor for signs and symptoms of infection.
   6. Prepare to administer parenteral iron; may be prescribed for severe anemia.
   7. Prepare to administer transfusions if prescribed for severe anemia.
   8. Prepare for the administration of oxytoxic medications in the postpartum period to prevent hemorrhage.

▲ IV. CARDIAC DISEASE

A. Description
   1. The mother with cardiac disease may be unable physiologically to cope with the added plasma volume and the increased cardiac output.
   2. Blood volume is at a maximum during the last weeks of the second trimester.
B. Assessment
   1. Signs and symptoms of cardiac decompensation, particularly during the second trimester
   2. Cough
   3. Dyspnea and fatigue
   4. Palpitations and tachycardia
   5. Peripheral edema
   6. Anginal-type pain
   7. Signs of pulmonary edema
   8. Signs of respiratory infection
C. Interventions
   1. Monitor vital signs, fetal heart rate , and condition of the fetus.
   2. Plan activities and stress the need for sufficient rest.
   3. Encourage adequate nutrition to prevent anemia.
   4. Maintain bed rest for the client as prescribed during the last weeks of pregnancy.
   5. During **labor**, do the following:
      a. Monitor vital signs frequently.
      b. Place the client on a cardiac monitor and on an external fetal monitor.
      c. Maintain bed rest, with mother lying on her side with her head and shoulders elevated.

d. Administer oxygen as prescribed.
e. Monitor for signs of heart failure.

V. CHORIOAMNIONITIS

A. Description
   1. Chorioamnionitis is a bacterial infection of the amniotic cavity, which can result from premature rupture of the membrane, vaginitis, amniocentesis, or intrauterine procedures.
   2. Chorioamnionitis causes the development of postpartum endometritis.
B. Assessment
   1. Uterine tenderness and contractions
   2. Elevated temperature
   3. Maternal or fetal tachycardia
   4. Foul odor to **amniotic fluid**
   5. Leukocytosis
C. Interventions
   1. Monitor maternal vital signs and fetal heart rate.
   2. Monitor for uterine tenderness, contractions, and fetal activity.
   3. Monitor results of blood culture.
   4. Prepare for amniocentesis to obtain amniotic fluid for Gram stain and leukocyte count.
   5. Administer antibiotics as prescribed after cultures are obtained.
   6. Administer oxytoxic medications as prescribed to increase uterine tone.
   7. Obtain neonatal cultures after **delivery**.

VI. CHRONIC HYPERTENSION

A. Description
   1. Hypertension that occurs before pregnancy, is diagnosed before the twentieth week of gestation, or is diagnosed for the first time during pregnancy and persists beyond the forty-second day postpartum is chronic.
   2. The condition predisposes the client to pregnancy-induced hypertension (PIH).
   3. The condition can cause abruptio placentae and intrauterine growth retardation.
B. Assessment
   1. Headaches
   2. Visual changes
   3. Elevated blood pressure (usually 140/90 mm Hg or greater)
   4. Delayed fetal growth
   5. Oligohydramnios
C. Interventions
   1. Monitor blood pressure.
   2. Monitor fetal activity and fetal growth.
   3. Encourage frequent rest periods, instructing the client to lie in the left lateral position.
   4. Administer antihypertensive medications as prescribed for diastolic pressures greater than 100 mm Hg.
   5. Monitor intake and output.

6. Evaluate renal function through prescribed studies such as blood urea nitrogen, serum creatinine, and 24-hour urine levels for creatinine clearance and protein.

VII. DIABETES MELLITUS

A. Description
1. Pregnancy places demands on carbohydrate metabolism and causes insulin requirements to change.
2. Premature **delivery** is more frequent.
3. The **newborn infant** of a diabetic mother may be large in size but will have functions related to gestational age rather than size.
4. The **newborn infant** of a diabetic mother is subject to hypoglycemia, hyperbilirubinemia, respiratory distress syndrome, hypocalcemia, and congenital anomalies.
5. Stillborn and neonatal mortality rates are higher in pregnancies of women with diabetes.

B. Type 1 diabetes mellitus
1. Maternal glucose crosses the **placenta** but insulin does not.
2. The fetus produces its own insulin and pulls glucose from the mother, which predisposes the mother to hypoglycemic reactions.
3. During the first trimester, maternal insulin needs decrease.
4. During the second and third trimesters, increases in placental hormones cause an insulin-resistant state, requiring an increase in the client's insulin dose.
5. After placental **delivery**, placental hormone levels drop abruptly and insulin requirements decrease.

C. Gestational diabetes mellitus
1. Gestational diabetes occurs in pregnancy (during the second or third trimester) in clients not previously diagnosed as diabetic and occurs when the pancreas cannot respond to the demand for more insulin.
2. Pregnant women should be screened for gestational diabetes between 24 and 28 weeks of pregnancy.
3. An oral glucose tolerance test will be performed to confirm gestational diabetes mellitus.
4. Oral hypoglycemic agents are never used during pregnancy.
5. Gestational diabetes frequently can be treated by diet alone; however, some clients may need insulin.
6. Most women with gestational diabetes convert to normal after **delivery**; however, these individuals have an increased risk of developing diabetes mellitus in their lifetimes.

D. Predisposing conditions to gestational diabetes
1. Over age 35
2. Obesity
3. Multiple gestation
4. Family history of diabetes mellitus

E. Assessment
1. Excessive thirst
2. Hunger
3. Weight loss
4. Blurred vision
5. Frequent urination
6. Recurrent urinary tract infections and vaginal yeast infections
7. Glycosuria and ketonuria
8. Signs of PIH
9. Polyhydramnios
10. Large fetus for gestational age

F. Interventions
1. Include diet, insulin (if diet cannot control blood glucose levels), exercise, and blood glucose determinations to maintain blood glucose levels between 65 to 130 mg/dL.
2. Observe for signs of hyperglycemia, glycosuria and ketonuria, and hypoglycemia.
3. Monitor weight.
4. Increase calorie intake as prescribed, with adequate insulin therapy so that glucose will move into the cells.
5. Assess for signs of maternal complications such as preeclampsia (hypertension, proteinuria, and edema).
6. Monitor for signs of infection.
7. Instruct the client to report burning and pain on urination, vaginal discharge or itching, or any other signs of infection to the health care provider.
8. Assess fetal status and monitor for signs of fetal compromise.

G. Interventions during **labor**
1. Monitor fetal status continuously for signs of distress and, if noted, prepare the client for immediate cesarean section.
2. Carefully regulate insulin and provide glucose intravenously as prescribed because **labor** depletes glycogen.

H. Interventions during the postpartum period
1. Observe client closely for a hypoglycemic reaction because a precipitous drop in insulin requirements normally occurs (the client may not require insulin for the first 24 hours).
2. Reregulate insulin needs as prescribed after the first day, according to blood glucose testing.
3. Assess dietary needs based on blood glucose and insulin requirements.
4. Monitor for signs of infection or postpartum hemorrhage.

VIII. DISSEMINATED INTRAVASCULAR COAGULATION (DIC)

A. Description
1. Disseminated intravascular coagulation is a condition in the mother's body that results in an

exaggerated clotting process that increases the formation of clots in microcirculation.

2. Thromboplastin from placental tissue and clots enter the bloodstream through open vessels at the placental site and initiate an exaggeration of the normal clotting process.

3. The rapid and extensive formation of clots causes the platelets and clotting factors to be depleted; this results in bleeding and the potential vascular occlusion of organs from thromboembolus formation.

B. Predisposing conditions (Box 25-3)

C. Assessment
   1. Uncontrolled bleeding
   2. Bruising, purpura, petechiae, and ecchymosis
   3. Presence of occult blood
   4. Hematuria, hematemesis, or vaginal bleeding
   5. Signs of shock
   6. Decreased fibrinogen level, platelet count, and hematocrit level
   7. Increased prothrombin time and partial thromboplastin time, clotting time, and fibrin degradation products

D. Interventions
   1. Remove the underlying cause.
   2. Monitor vital signs; assess for bleeding and signs of shock.
   3. Prepare for oxygen therapy, volume replacement, blood component therapy, and possibly heparin therapy.
   4. Monitor for complications associated with fluid and blood replacement and heparin therapy.
   5. Monitor urine output and maintain at 30 mL per hour (renal failure is a complication of DIC).

IX. ECTOPIC PREGNANCY

A. Description: A pregnancy that occurs in an other than uterine site, with **implantation** usually occurring in fallopian tubes

B. Assessment
   1. Missed period
   2. Abdominal pain
   3. Vaginal spotting to bleeding that is dark red or brown
   4. Rupture: increased pain, referred shoulder pain, signs of shock

---

BOX 25-3

Predisposing Conditions for Disseminated Intravascular Coagulation

Abruptio placentae
Intrauterine fetal death
Amniotic fluid embolism
Pregnancy-induced hypertension
Liver disease
Sepsis

C. Interventions
   1. Obtain assessment data and vital signs.
   2. Monitor bleeding and initiate measures to prevent rupture and shock.
   3. Methotrexate (a folic acid antagonist) may be prescribed to inhibit cell division in the developing embryo.
   4. Prepare the client for laparotomy and removal of the pregnancy and tube, if necessary, or repair of the tube.
   5. Administer antibiotics; Rh immune globulin is given to appropriate $Rh_0(D)$-negative women.

X. ENDOMETRITIS

A. Description
   1. Endometritis is an infection of the lining of the uterus following **delivery** that is caused by bacteria that invade the uterus at the placental site.
   2. The infection may spread and involve the entire endometrium and cause peritonitis, pelvic thrombophlebitis, or cellulitis.

B. Assessment
   1. Chills and fever
   2. Increased pulse
   3. Decreased appetite
   4. Headache
   5. Backache
   6. Prolonged, severe afterpains
   7. Tender, large uterus
   8. Foul odor to **lochia** or reddish-brown **lochia**
   9. Ileus
   10. Elevated white blood cell count with a left shift and immature formed cells

C. Interventions
   1. Monitor vital signs.
   2. Position client in Fowler's position to facilitate drainage of **lochia**.
   3. Provide a private room for the mother.
   4. Inform the mother that isolation of the **newborn infant** from the mother is not necessary.
   5. Instruct the mother in proper handwashing techniques.
   6. Initiate wound and skin precautions as necessary.
   7. Monitor intake and output and encourage fluids.
   8. Administer antibiotics intravenously as prescribed.
   9. Administer comfort measures such as back rubs and position changes and pain medications as prescribed.
   10. Administer oxytoxic medications as prescribed to improve uterine tone.

XI. FETAL DEATH IN UTERO

A. Description
   1. The death of a fetus after the twentieth week of gestation and before birth
   2. The client can develop DIC if the dead fetus is retained in the uterus for 3 to 4 weeks or more.

B. Assessment
1. Absence of fetal movement
2. Absence of fetal heart tones
3. Maternal weight loss
4. Lack of fetal growth or decrease in fundal height
5. Lack of cardiac activity and other characteristics suggestive of fetal death noted on the ultrasound
C. Interventions
1. Prepare for the **delivery** of the fetus.
2. Support the client's decision about **labor**, birth, and the postpartum period.
3. Facilitate the grieving process.
4. Allow the parents to hold the **infant** after birth.
5. Allow the parents to name the **infant**.
6. Accept behaviors such as anger and hostility from the parents.
7. Refer parents to an appropriate support group.

▲ XII. HEPATITIS B
A. Description
1. The risk of prematurity, low birth weight, and neonatal death increases if the mother has hepatitis B infection.
2. Hepatitis is transmitted through blood, saliva, vaginal secretions, semen, breast milk, and across the placental barrier.
B. Interventions
1. Minimize the risk for intrapartum ascending infections (limit the number of vaginal examinations).
2. Remove maternal blood from the **neonate** immediately after birth.
3. Suction the fluids from the **neonate** immediately after birth.
4. Bathe the **neonate** before any invasive procedures.
5. Clean and dry the face and eyes of the **neonate** before instilling eye prophylaxis.
6. Infection of the **neonate** can be prevented by the administration of hepatitis B immune globulin and hepatitis B vaccine soon after birth.
7. Discourage the mother from kissing the **neonate** until the **neonate** has received the vaccine.
8. Support breast-feeding after neonatal treatment; breast-feeding is not contraindicated if the **neonate** has been vaccinated.
9. Inform the mother that the hepatitis B vaccine will be administered to the **neonate** and that the second dose is administered at 1 month and that the third dose is administered at 6 months.

XIII. HEMATOMA
A. Description
1. Hematoma occurs following the escape of blood into the tissues of the reproductive sac after the **delivery**.
2. Predisposing conditions include operative **delivery** with forceps or injury to a blood vessel.

BOX 25-4

Hematoma: Assessment Findings

Abnormal, severe pain
Pressure in perineal area
Palpable, sensitive tumor in perineal area, with discolored skin
Inability to void
Decreased hemoglobin and hematocrit levels
Signs of shock, such as pallor, tachycardia, and hypotension, if significant blood loss has occurred

---

B. Assessment (Box 25-4)
C. Interventions
1. Monitor vital signs.
2. Monitor client for abnormal pain, especially when forceps **delivery** has occurred.
3. Apply ice to the hematoma site.
4. Administer analgesics as prescribed.
5. Monitor intake and output.
6. Encourage fluids and voiding; prepare for urinary catheterization if client is unable to void.
7. Administer blood replacements as prescribed.
8. Monitor for signs of infection, such as increased temperature, pulse rate, and white blood cell count.
9. Administer antibiotics as prescribed because infection is common following hematoma formation.
10. Prepare for incision and evacuation of the hematoma if necessary.

XIV. HYDATIDIFORM MOLE
A. Description
1. The hydatidiform mole is a developmental anomaly of the **placenta** that changes chorionic villi into a mass of clear vesicles.
2. The mole presents as an edematous grapelike cluster that may be nonmalignant or may develop into choriocarcinoma.
B. Assessment
1. Fetal heart rate not detectable
2. Vaginal bleeding, which usually occurs by week 12, of a bright red or dark brown color; may be slight, profuse, or intermittent
3. Symptoms of PIH, such as an elevated blood pressure, edema, and proteinuria, which may be present before week 20
4. Fundal height greater than expected for date
5. Elevated human chorionic gonadotropin levels
6. Ultrasound showing a characteristic snowstorm pattern
C. Interventions
1. Prepare mother for uterine evacuation (before evacuation, diagnostic tests are done to detect metastatic disease).

2. Evacuation of the mole is done by vacuum aspiration; oxytocin is administered after evacuation to contract the uterus.

3. Tissue is sent to the laboratory for evaluation, and follow-up is important to detect changes suggestive of malignancy.

4. Monitor for postprocedure hemorrhage and infection.

5. Human chorionic gonadotropin levels are monitored every 1 to 2 weeks until normal prepregnancy levels are attained; then the levels are checked every 1 to 2 months for 1 year.

6. Instruct parents regarding birth control measures so that pregnancy can be prevented during the 1-year follow-up.

XV. HYPEREMESIS GRAVIDARUM

A. Description: Intractable nausea and vomiting that persist beyond the first trimester and cause disturbances in nutrition, electrolytes, and fluid balance

B. Assessment
1. Nausea most pronounced on arising; possibly occurring at other times during the day
2. Persistent vomiting
3. Weight loss
4. Signs of dehydration
5. Electrolyte imbalances

C. Interventions
1. Initiate measures to alleviate nausea, including medication therapy; if unsuccessful and weight loss and electrolyte imbalances occur, intravenously administered fluid and electrolyte replacement or total parenteral nutrition may be necessary.
2. Monitor vital signs, intake and output, weight, and calorie count.
3. Monitor laboratory data and for signs of dehydration and electrolyte imbalances.
4. Monitor urine for ketones.
5. Monitor fetal heart rate, fetal activity, and fetal growth.
6. Encourage intake of small portions of food (low fat, easily digestible carbohydrates, such as cereals, rice, and pasta).
7. Liquids should be taken between meals to avoid distending the stomach and triggering vomiting.
8. Encourage the client to sit upright after meals.

XVI. INCOMPETENT CERVIX

A. Description
1. Incompetent cervix is premature dilation of the cervix, which occurs most often in the fourth or fifth month of pregnancy.
2. Incompetent cervix is associated with cervical trauma as a result of previous surgery or birth.
3. Treatment is surgical.

B. Assessment
1. Vaginal bleeding

2. Fetal membranes visible through the cervix

C. Interventions
1. Provide bedrest, hydration, and tocolysis as prescribed to inhibit uterine contractions.
2. Prepare for cervical cerclage (at 10 to 14 weeks gestation) in which a band of fascia or nonabsorbable ribbon is placed around the cervix beneath the mucosa to constrict the internal os of the cervix.
3. Following cervical cerclage, the woman is told to refrain from intercourse and avoid prolonged standing and heavy lifting.
4. The cervical cerclage is removed at 37 weeks' gestation or left in place and a cesarean birth is performed; if removed, cerclage must be repeated with each successive pregnancy.
5. Following the procedure, monitor for contractions, rupture of the membranes, and signs of infection.
6. Instruct the woman to report any postprocedure vaginal bleeding or increased uterine contractions immediately to the health care provider.

XVII. INFECTIONS

A. Toxoplasmosis
1. Toxoplasmosis is caused by infection with the intracellular protozoan parasite *Toxoplasma gondii*.
2. Toxoplasmosis produces a rash and symptoms of acute, flulike infection in the mother.
3. Toxoplasmosis is transmitted to the mother through raw meat or handling of cat litter of infected cats.
4. Organism is transmitted to the fetus across the **placenta**.
5. Toxoplasmosis can cause spontaneous abortion.

B. Rubella (German measles)
1. Rubella is teratogenic in the first trimester.
2. Organism is transmitted to the fetus across the **placenta**.
3. Rubella causes congenital defects of the eyes, heart, ears, and brain.
4. If not immune (titer of 1:8 or less), the mother should be vaccinated in the postpartum period; she must wait at least 3 months before becoming pregnant.

C. Cytomegalovirus
1. Cytomegalovirus produces mononucleosis-like symptoms in the mother.
2. Organism is transmitted across the placenta to the fetus, or the fetus may be infected through the birth canal.
3. The mother may be asymptomatic at birth; cytomegalovirus causes fetal death, mental retardation, blindness, deafness, or seizures.
4. Antiviral therapy may be prescribed.

D. Genital herpes
1. Herpes affects the external genitalia, vagina, and cervix.

2. Herpes causes draining, painful vesicles.

3. Virus usually is transmitted to the fetus during birth through the infected vagina or via an ascending infection after rupture of the membranes.

4. No vaginal examinations are done in the presence of active vaginal herpetic lesions.

5. Herpes can cause death or severe neurological impairment in the **newborn.**

6. **Delivery** of the fetus is usually by cesarean section if active lesions are present in the vagina; **delivery** may be performed vaginally if the lesions are in the anal, perineal, or inner thigh area (strict precautions are necessary to protect the fetus during **delivery**).

7. Maintain contact precautions.

XVIII. MULTIPLE GESTATION
A. Description
   1. Multiple gestation results from double ovulation (fraternal or dizygotic) or a splitting of the fertilized egg (identical or monozygotic).
   2. Complications include spontaneous abortion, anemia, congenital anomalies, hyperemesis gravidarum, intrauterine growth retardation, PIH, polyhydramnios, postpartum hemorrhage, premature rupture of membranes, and preterm **labor** and **delivery**.
B. Assessment
   1. Excessive fetal activity
   2. Uterus large for gestational age
   3. Palpation of three or four large parts in the uterus
   4. Auscultation of more than one fetal heart rate
   5. Excessive weight gain
C. Interventions
   1. Monitor vital signs.
   2. Monitor fetal heart rates, fetal activity, and fetal growth.
   3. Monitor for cervical changes.
   4. Prepare client for ultrasound as prescribed.
   5. Monitor for anemia; administer supplemental vitamins as prescribed.
   6. Monitor for preterm **labor**, and treat preterm **labor** promptly.
   7. Prepare for cesarean section for abnormal presentations.
   8. Prepare to administer oxytoxic medications after **delivery** to prevent postpartum hemorrhage from uterine overdistention.

XIX. PREGNANCY-INDUCED HYPERTENSION
A. Description
   1. Pregnancy-induced hypertension is an acute hypertensive state that develops after the twentieth week of gestation.
   2. The condition can be mild or severe and can progress to seizures (eclampsia) (Box 25-5).
   3. The classic signs of preeclampsia are hypertension, generalized edema, and proteinuria.

BOX 25-5

Signs of Worsening Pregnancy-Induced Hypertension or Impending Seizures

Blood pressure 160/110 mm Hg or higher
Epigastric pain
Decreased urinary output
Visual changes
Headache
Excessive proteinuria

B. Predisposing conditions
   1. Primigravida
   2. Women under 19 years of age or over 40 years
   3. Chronic renal disease
   4. Chronic hypertension
   5. Diabetes mellitus
   6. Rh incompatibility
   7. History of or family history of PIH
C. Complications of PIH
   1. Abruptio placentae
   2. Disseminated intravascular coagulation
   3. Thrombocytopenia
   4. Placental insufficiency
   5. Intrauterine fetal death
D. Mild preeclampsia
   1. Assessment
      a. Elevated blood pressure (usually 15 to 30 mm Hg above baseline)
      b. Weight gain of 1 lb or more per week in the last trimester
      c. Mild, generalized edema
      d. Proteinuria of 1+ to 2+
   2. Interventions
      a. Provide bed rest and place the client in left lateral position.
      b. Monitor blood pressure and weight.
      c. Monitor neurological status because changes can indicate cerebral hypoxia or impending seizure.
      d. Monitor deep tendon reflexes and for the presence of clonus, because hyperreflexia indicates increased central nervous system irritability (Box 25-6).
      e. Provide adequate fluids.
      f. Monitor intake and output; a urinary output of 30 mL per hour indicates adequate renal perfusion.
      g. Increase dietary protein and carbohydrates with no added salt.
      h. Administer medications as prescribed to lower the blood pressure; blood pressure should not be lowered drastically because placental perfusion can be compromised.
E. Severe preeclampsia
   1. Assessment

BOX 25-6

Assessment of Reflexes

BICEPS

Position your thumb over the client's biceps tendon, supporting the client's elbow with the palm of the hand.
Strike a downward blow over the thumb with the percussion hammer.
Normal response: Flexion of the arm at the elbow

PATELLAR

Position the client with legs dangling over the edge of the examining table or lying on the back with the legs slightly flexed.
Strike the patellar tendon just below the kneecap with the percussion hammer.
Normal response: Extension or kicking out of leg

CLONUS

Position the client with the legs dangling over the edge of the examining table.
Support the leg with one hand and sharply dorsiflex the client's foot with the other hand.

Maintain the dorsiflexed position for a few seconds and then release the foot.
Normal response (negative clonus response):
Foot will remain steady in the dorsiflexed position.
No rhythmic oscillations or jerking of the foot will be felt.
When released, the foot will drop to a plantar flexed position with no oscillations.
Abnormal response (positive clonus response):
Rhythmic oscillations occur when the foot is dorsiflexed.
Similar oscillations will be noted when the foot drops to the plantar flexed position.

GRADING THE RESPONSE
0, Reflex absent
1+, Reflex present but hypoactive
2+, Normal reflex
3+, Hyperactive reflex
4+, Hyperactive reflex with clonus present

---

a. Severe hypertension (systolic blood pressure of at least 160 mmHg or a diastolic blood pressure of at least 110 mmHg)
b. Massive, generalized edema and weight gain
c. Proteinuria greater than 3+ to 4+
d. Oliguria, less than 400 to 500 mL urine output in 24 hours
e. Cerebral or visual disturbances such as altered level of consciousness
f. Headache or blurred vision
g. Epigastric pain, nausea, and vomiting
h. Hepatic, pulmonary, or cardiac involvement
i. Thrombocytopenia
j. HELLP syndrome: a laboratory diagnosis for severe preeclampsia characterized by hemolysis (H), elevated liver enzymes (EL), and low platelets (LP)
2. Interventions
   a. Maintain bedrest.
   b. Administer magnesium sulfate (use a controlled infusion device) as prescribed to prevent seizures; may be continued for 24 to 48 hours postpartum.
   c. Monitor for signs of magnesium toxicity, including flushing, sweating, hypotension, depressed deep tendon reflexes, and central nervous system depression including respiratory depression; keep antidote (calcium gluconate) at the client's bedside.
   d. Administer antihypertensives as prescribed.
   e. Prepare for the induction of **labor**.
F. Eclampsia
   1. Assessment: Characterized by generalized seizures (Box 25-7)

2. Interventions
   a. Maintain a patent airway and administer oxygen.
   b. Protect the client from injury.
   c. Monitor fetal heart rate and contractions.
   d. Administer medications to control the seizures (magnesium sulfate may be prescribed).
   e. Prepare for delivery of the fetus after stabilization of the client.

XX. PYELONEPHRITIS

A. Description
   1. Pyelonephritis results from bacterial infections that extend upward from the bladder through the blood vessels and lymphatics.
   2. Pyelonephritis frequently follows untreated urinary tract infections and is associated with increased incidence of anemia, low birth weight, PIH, premature **labor** and **delivery**, and premature rupture of the membranes.

BOX 25-7

Eclampsia

Seizure typically begins with twitching around the mouth.
The body then becomes rigid in a state of tonic muscular contractions that last 15 to 20 seconds.
The facial muscles and then all body muscles alternatively contract and relax in rapid succession (clonic phase that may last about 1 minute).
Respiration is halted during the seizure because the diaphragm tends to remain fixed (breathing resumes shortly after the seizure).

B. Assessment
1. Flank pain
2. Burning or painful urination
3. Increased frequency of urination
4. Chills, malaise, nausea
5. Increased temperature, pulse rate, and fetal heart rate
6. Vomiting
7. Uterine contractions
8. Elevated white blood cell count

C. Interventions
1. Monitor vital signs.
2. Monitor fetal heart rate and for contractions.
3. Encourage fluids; monitor intake and output.
4. Monitor renal function.
5. Administer antibiotics as prescribed.
6. Administer antipyretics such as acetaminophen (Tylenol) as prescribed.
7. Obtain urine cultures every 2 to 4 weeks after resolution of infection.

XXI. SEXUALLY TRANSMITTED DISEASES

A. Chlamydia
1. Description
   a. Chlamydia is a sexually transmitted pathogen associated with an increased risk for premature births, stillbirths, neonatal conjunctivitis, and **newborn** chlamydial pneumonia.
   b. In the nonpregnant state, chlamydia can cause salpingitis, pelvic abscesses, chronic pelvic pain, and infertility.
   c. Diagnostic test is a culture for *Chlamydia trachomatis.*
2. Assessment
   a. Usually asymptomatic
   b. Bleeding between periods or after coitus
   c. Mucoid or purulent cervical discharge
   d. Dysuria
   e. In the **newborn**, conjunctivitis and pneumonia
3. Interventions
   a. Screen the client to determine whether the client is high risk; instruct the client in the importance of rescreening because reinfection can occur as the client nears term.
   b. Instruct the client about the prescribed medication for treatment.
   c. Instruct the client about medication for the **neonate** if prescribed.
   d. Administer appropriate eye prophylaxis to the **neonate**.
   e. Monitor **neonate** for signs and symptoms of pneumonia, if at risk.
   f. Ensure that the sexual partner is treated.

B. Syphilis
1. Description
   a. Syphilis is a chronic infectious disease caused by the organism *Treponema pallidum.*
   b. Transmission is by physical contact with syphilitic lesions, which usually are found on the skin, the mucous membranes of the mouth, or on the genitals.
   c. The infection may cause abortion or premature **labor** and is passed to the fetus after the fourth month of pregnancy as congenital syphilis.
2. Assessment (Box 25-8)
3. Interventions
   a. Obtain a serum test for syphilis on the first prenatal visit; prepare to repeat the test at 36 weeks' gestation because the disease may be acquired after the initial visit.
   b. If the test result is positive, treatment is necessary with an antibiotic, such as penicillin.
   c. Instruct the client that treatment of her partner is necessary, if infection is present.

C. Gonorrhea
1. Description
   a. Infection, caused by *Neisseria gonorrhoeae,* causes inflammation of the mucous membranes of the genital and urinary tracts.
   b. Transmission of the organism is by sexual intercourse.
   c. Infection may be transmitted to the newborn's eyes during **delivery**, causing blindness (ophthalmia neonatorum).
2. Assessment
   a. Female: Usually asymptomatic; vaginal discharge, urinary frequency, and pain possible
   b. Male: Fever, painful urination, pelvic pain, epididymitis with pain, tenderness, and swelling

---

BOX 25-8

Stages of Syphilis

PRIMARY STAGE
Most infectious stage
Appearance of ulcerative, painless lesions produced by spirochetes at the point of entry into the body

SECONDARY STAGE
Highly infectious stage
Appearance of lesions about 3 weeks after the primary stage anywhere on the skin and mucous membranes
Generalized lymphadenopathy

TERTIARY STAGE
Entrance of spirochetes into the internal organs, causing permanent damage; symptoms occurring 10 to 30 years following the untreated primary lesion
Invasion of the central nervous system, causing meningitis, ataxia, general paresis, and progressive mental deterioration
Deleterious effects on the aortic valve and aorta

3. Interventions
   a. Obtain culture for gonorrhea on the first prenatal visit; prepare to repeat culture because infection may occur during pregnancy.
   b. Administer antibiotics prophylactically to the eyes of the **newborn infant**.
   c. Instruct the client that treatment of her partner is necessary if infection is present.

D. Condylomata acuminata (venereal warts)
   1. Description
      a. Venereal warts are caused by human papillomavirus; infection affects the cervix, urethra, anus, penis, and scrotum.
      b. Venereal warts are transmitted through sexual contact.
   2. Assessment
      a. Infection produces small to large wartlike growths on genitals.
      b. Cervical cell changes may be noted because human papillomavirus is associated with cervical malignancies.
   3. Interventions
      a. Lesions are removed by the use of cytotoxic agents, cryotherapy, electrocautery, and laser.
      b. Encourage yearly Papanicolaou's smear.
      c. Avoid sexual contact until the lesions are healed (condoms reduce transmission).

▶ **XXII. TUBERCULOSIS**
   A. Description
      1. Tuberculosis is a highly communicable disease caused by *Mycobacterium tuberculosis*.
      2. Tuberculosis is transmitted by the airborne route.
      3. A multidrug-resistant strain of tuberculosis can exist as a result of improper compliance or noncompliance with treatment programs and the development of mutations in the tubercle bacilli.
   B. Transmission
      1. Transplacental transmission is rare.
      2. Transmission can occur during birth through aspiration of infected **amniotic fluid**.
      3. **Neonate** can become infected from contact with infected individuals.
   C. Risk to mother: Active disease during pregnancy has been associated with an increase in hypertensive disorders of pregnancy.
   D. Diagnosis
      1. If a chest radiograph is required for the mother, it is done only after 20 weeks of gestation, and a lead shield for the abdomen is required.
      2. Tuberculin skin testing is safe during pregnancy.
   E. Assessment
      1. Maternal
         a. Possibly asymptomatic
         b. Fever and chills
         c. Night sweats
         d. Weight loss

         e. Fatigue
         f. Cough, hemoptysis, or green or yellow sputum
         g. Dyspnea
         h. Pleural pain
      2. **Neonate**
         a. Fever
         b. Lethargy
         c. Poor feeding
         d. Failure to thrive
         e. Respiratory distress
         f. Hepatosplenomegaly
         g. Meningitis
         h. Possible disease spread to all major organs
   F. Interventions
      1. Pregnant client
         a. Administration of isoniazid (INH), pyrazinamide, and rifampin (Rifadin) daily for 9 months; ethambutol (Myambutol) is added if medication resistance is probable.
         b. Pyridoxine (vitamin B_6) should be administered with isoniazid to pregnant women to prevent fetal neurotoxicity caused by the isoniazid.
         c. Promote breast-feeding only if the mother is noninfectious.
      2. **Newborn infant**
         a. Management focuses on preventing disease and treating early infection.
         b. The infant is skin tested at birth and may be placed on isoniazid therapy; the skin test is repeated in 3 to 4 months and isoniazid may be stopped if the skin test results remain negative.
         c. If the skin test result is positive, the infant should receive isoniazid for at least 6 months.
         d. If the mother's sputum is free of organisms, the infant does not need to be isolated from the mother while in the hospital.

XXIII. URINARY TRACT INFECTION
   A. Description: A urinary tract infection can occur during pregnancy; if untreated, the client can develop pyelonephritis.
   B. Predisposing conditions
      1. History of urinary tract infections
      2. Sickle cell trait
      3. Poor hygiene
      4. Anemia
      5. Diabetes mellitus
      6. Pregnancy
   C. Assessment
      1. Possibly asymptomatic during pregnancy
      2. Burning and pain on urination
      3. Increased frequency of urination
      4. Lower abdominal pain and costovertebral angle tenderness
      5. Fever
      6. Proteinuria, hematuria, bacteriuria, and white blood cells in urine

D. Interventions
1. Monitor vital signs.
2. Monitor fetal heart rate.
3. Increase fluid intake.
4. Monitor intake and output.
5. Monitor urine for consistency and odor.
6. Monitor for signs and symptoms of pyelonephritis (dip test urine with each prenatal visit).
7. Obtain urine for culture and sensitivity.
8. Provide heat to lower abdomen or back.
9. Administer antibiotics as prescribed.
10. Instruct the client to complete the course of antibiotics if prescribed.
11. Instruct the client regarding the need to repeat the culture after treatment is completed.

PRACTICE QUESTIONS

1. A pregnant client in the last trimester has been admitted to the hospital with a diagnosis of severe preeclampsia. A nurse monitors for complications associated with the diagnosis and assesses the client for
   1. Any bleeding, such as in the gums, petechiae, and purpura.
   2. Enlargement of the breasts.
   3. Periods of fetal movement followed by quiet periods.
   4. Complaints of feeling hot when the room is cool.
2. A nurse in a maternity unit is reviewing the records of the clients on the unit. Which of the clients would the nurse identify as being at most risk for developing disseminated intravascular coagulation (DIC)?
   1. A gravida IV who delivered 8 hours ago and has lost 500 mL of blood
   2. A gravida II who has just been diagnosed with dead fetus syndrome
   3. A primigravida with mild preeclampsia
   4. A primigravida who delivered a 10-lb baby 3 hours ago
3. A client in the first trimester of pregnancy arrives at a health care clinic and reports that she has been experiencing vaginal bleeding. A threatened abortion is suspected, and a nurse instructs the client regarding management of care. Which statement if made by the client indicates a need for further education?
   1. "I will maintain strict bed rest throughout the remainder of the pregnancy."
   2. "I will avoid sexual intercourse until the bleeding has stopped, and for 2 weeks following the last evidence of bleeding."
   3. "I will count the number of perineal pads used on a daily basis and note the amount and color of blood on the pad."
   4. "I will watch for the evidence of the passage of tissue."
4. A prenatal nurse is providing instructions to a group of pregnant clients regarding measures to prevent toxoplasmosis. Which statement if made by one of the clients indicates a need for further instructions?
   1. "I need to cook meat thoroughly."
   2. "I need to avoid touching mucous membranes of the mouth or eyes while handling raw meat."
   3. "I need to drink unpasteurized milk only."
   4. "I need to avoid contact with materials that are possibly contaminated with cat feces."
5. A pregnant woman reports to a health care clinic, complaining of loss of appetite, weight loss, and fatigue. Following assessment of the woman, tuberculosis is suspected. A sputum culture is obtained and identifies Mycobacterium tuberculosis. The nurse provides instructions to the mother regarding therapeutic management of the tuberculosis. The nurse tells the client that
   1. Medication will not be started until after delivery of the fetus.
   2. Isoniazid (INH) plus rifampin (Rifadin) will be required for a total of 9 months.
   3. The newborn infant will need to receive medication therapy immediately following birth.
   4. Therapeutic abortion is required.
6. A clinic nurse has provided home care instructions to a client with a history of cardiac disease who has just been told that she is pregnant. Which statement if made by the client indicates a need for further education?
   1. "During the pregnancy, I need to avoid contact with other individuals as much as possible to prevent infection."
   2. "I need to avoid excessive weight gain to prevent increased demands on my heart."
   3. "It is best that I rest on my left side to promote blood return to the heart."
   4. "I need to try to avoid stressful situations because stress increases the workload on the heart."
7. A nurse is providing instructions to a maternity client with a history of cardiac disease regarding appropriate dietary measures. Which statement if made by the client indicates an understanding of the measures to take?
   1. "I need to increase my fluid intake and intake of high-fiber foods."
   2. "I need to maintain a low-calorie diet to prevent any weight gain."
   3. "I need to lower my blood volume by limiting my fluids."
   4. "I do not need to be concerned about sodium intake during pregnancy."
8. A clinic nurse is performing a psychosocial assessment of a client who has been told that she is pregnant. Which of the following assessment findings would indicate to the nurse that the client is at high risk for contracting human immunodeficiency virus (HIV)?
   1. A history of intravenous drug use
   2. A history of one sexual partner for the past 10 years

3. No history of any sexually transmitted diseases

4. A significant other who is heterosexual

9. A nurse in a maternity unit is providing emotional support to a client and her husband who are preparing to be discharged from the hospital after the birth of a dead fetus. Which statement if made by the client indicates a component of the normal grieving process?

1. "We would really like to attend a support group."

2. "We're okay, and we are going to try to have another baby immediately."

3. "We never want to have a baby again."

4. "We are going to try to adopt a child immediately."

10. A nurse assists a pregnant client with cardiac disease to identify resources to help her care for her 18-month-old child during the last trimester of pregnancy. The nurse encourages the pregnant client to use these resources primarily to

1. Help the mother prepare for labor and delivery.

2. Reduce excessive maternal stress and fatigue.

3. Prepare the 18-month-old child for maternal separation during hospitalization.

4. Avoid exposure to potential pathogens and resulting infections.

11. A nurse evaluates a hepatitis B–positive client's ability to safely bottle-feed her infant during postpartum hospitalization. Which maternal action best exemplifies the client's knowledge of potential disease transmission to the infant?

1. The client tests the temperature of the formula before initiating feeding.

2. The client holds the infant properly during feeding and burping.

3. The client washes and dries her hands before and following self-care of the perineum and asks for a pair of gloves before feeding.

4. The client requests that the window be closed before feeding.

12. A nurse is providing instructions to a pregnant client with human immunodeficiency virus (HIV) regarding care to the newborn infant following delivery. The client asks the nurse about the feeding options that are available. Which statement will the nurse provide to the client regarding feeding the newborn infant?

1. "You will be able to breast-feed for 6 months and then will need to switch to bottle-feeding."

2. "You will be able to breast-feed for 9 months and then will need to switch to bottle-feeding."

3. "You will need to feed the newborn infant by nasogastric tube feeding."

4. "You will need to bottle-feed the newborn infant."

13. During the intrapartum period, a nurse is caring for a laboring client with sickle cell disease. The nurse ensures that the client receives appropriate intravenous fluid intake and oxygen consumption primarily to

1. Stimulate the labor process.

2. Avoid the necessity of a cesarean delivery.

3. Prevent dehydration and hypoxemia.

4. Eliminate the need for analgesic administration.

14. A home care nurse visits a pregnant client who has a diagnosis of mild preeclampsia and who is being monitored for pregnancy induced hypertension (PIH). Which assessment finding indicates a worsening of the preeclampsia and the need to notify the physician?

1. Blood pressure reading is at the prenatal baseline

2. Urinary output has increased

3. The client complains of a headache and blurred vision

4. Dependent edema has resolved

15. A client with a 38-week twin gestation is admitted to a birthing center in early labor. One of the fetuses is a breech presentation. Of the following interventions, which will the nurse list as the lowest priority in planning the nursing care of this client?

1. Attach electronic fetal monitoring.

2. Prepare the client for a possible cesarean section.

3. Measure fundal height.

4. Visually examine the perineum and vaginal opening.

16. A stillborn infant was delivered in the birthing suite a few hours ago. After the birth the family has remained together, holding and touching the baby. Which statement by the nurse would further assist the family in their initial period of grief?

1. "Don't worry, there is nothing you could do to prevent this from happening."

2. "We need to take the baby from you now so that you can get some sleep."

3. "What have you named your lovely baby?"

4. "We will see to it that you have an early discharge so that you don't have to be reminded of this experience."

17. A nurse implements a teaching plan for a pregnant client who is newly diagnosed with gestational diabetes mellitus. Which statement if made by the client indicates a need for further education?

1. "I need to stay on the diabetic diet."

2. "I will perform glucose monitoring at home."

3. "I need to avoid exercise because of the negative effects on insulin production."

4. "I need to be aware of any infections and report signs of infection immediately to my health care provider."

18. A primigravida is receiving magnesium sulfate for the treatment of pregnancy induced hypertension (PIH). The nurse who is caring for the client is performing assessments every 30 minutes. Which assessment finding would be of most concern to the nurse?

1. Urinary output of 20 mL since the previous assessment

2. Deep tendon reflexes of 2+

3. Respiratory rate of 10 breaths per minute

4. Fetal heart rate of 120 beats per minute

19. A nurse is caring for a pregnant client with preeclampsia. The nurse prepares a plan of care for the client and documents in the plan that if the client progresses from preeclampsia to eclampsia, the nurse's first action is to
    1. Administer magnesium sulfate intravenously
    2. Assess the blood pressure and fetal heart rate.
    3. Clear and maintain an open airway.
    4. Administer oxygen by face mask.
20. A client has just had surgery to deliver a nonviable fetus resulting from abruptio placenta. As a result of the abruptio placenta, the client develops disseminated intravascular coagulation (DIC) and is told about the complication. The client begins to cry and screams, "God, just let me die now!" Which nursing diagnosis should direct care for this client?

1. Hopelessness related to loss of baby and personal health
2. Deficient knowledge related to disease process
3. Situational low self-esteem related to being ill
4. Grieving related to loss of the baby

CRITICAL THINKING: FILL IN THE BLANK

A home care nurse is monitoring a pregnant client with pregnancy induced hypertension (PIH) who is at risk for preeclampsia. At each home care visit, the nurse assesses the client for which three classic signs of preeclampsia?

Answer: _____

ANSWERS

1. **1**

Rationale: Severe preeclampsia can trigger disseminated intravascular coagulation (DIC) because of the widespread damage to vascular integrity. Bleeding is an early sign of DIC and should be reported to the health care provider if noted on assessment. Options 2, 3, and 4 are normal occurrences in the last trimester of pregnancy.

Test-Taking Strategy: Use the process of elimination and knowledge regarding the normal physiological occurrences in pregnancy to answer the question. Eliminate options 2, 3, and 4 because they are normal occurrences in the last trimester of pregnancy. Review the assessment findings in DIC if you had difficulty with this question.

Level of Cognitive Ability: Analysis
Client Needs: Physiological Integrity
Integrated Process: Nursing Process—assessment
Content Area: Maternity—antepartum
References: Murray, S., McKinney, E., & Gorrie, T. (2002). *Foundations of maternal-newborn nursing* (3rd ed., p. 680). Philadelphia: W. B. Saunders.
Wong, D., Perry, S., & Hockenberry, M. (2002). *Maternal child nursing care* (2nd ed., p. 284). St. Louis: Mosby.

2. **2**

Rationale: Dead fetus syndrome is considered a risk factor for DIC. Hemorrhage is a risk factor with DIC; however, a loss of 500 mL is not considered hemorrhage. Severe preeclampsia is considered a risk factor for DIC; a mild case is not. Delivering a large baby is not considered a risk factor for DIC.

Test-Taking Strategy: Use the process of elimination and knowledge regarding the risk factors associated with DIC to answer this question. Recalling that dead fetus syndrome is a risk factor for DIC will assist in directing you to option 2. If you had difficulty answering this question, review these risk factors.

Level of Cognitive Ability: Analysis
Client Needs: Physiological Integrity
Integrated Process: Nursing Process—analysis
Content Area: Maternity—intrapartum
Reference: Lowdermilk, D., & Perry, S. (2003). *Maternity nursing* (6th ed., p. 701). St. Louis: Mosby.

3. **1**

Rationale: Strict bed rest throughout the remainder of the pregnancy is not required. The woman is advised to curtail sexual activities until bleeding has ceased, and for 2 weeks following the last evidence of bleeding or as recommended by the physician or other health care provider. The woman is instructed to count the number of perineal pads used daily and to note the quantity and color of blood on the pad. The woman also should watch for the evidence of the passage of tissue.

Test-Taking Strategy: Use the process of elimination to assist in answering the question. Note the key words "need for further education" in the stem of the question. Noting the word "strict" in option 1 will assist in directing you to this option. Review therapeutic management for a threatened abortion, if you had difficulty with this question.

Level of Cognitive Ability: Analysis
Client Needs: Health Promotion and Maintenance
Integrated Process: Teaching/Learning
Content Area: Maternity—antepartum
Reference: Murray, S., McKinney, E., & Gorrie, T. (2002). *Foundations of maternal-newborn nursing* (3rd ed., p. 663). Philadelphia: W. B. Saunders.

4. **3**

Rationale: All pregnant women should be advised to do the following to prevent the development of toxoplasmosis. Women should be instructed to cook meats thoroughly, particularly pork, beef, and lamb; avoid touching mucous membranes of the mouth or eyes while handling raw meat; thoroughly wash all kitchen surfaces that come in contact with uncooked meat; wash the hands thoroughly after handling raw meat; avoid uncooked eggs and unpasteurized milk; wash fruits and vegetables before consumption; and avoid contact with materials that possibly are contaminated with cat feces, such as cat litter boxes, sand boxes, or garden soil.

Test-Taking Strategy: Note the key words "need for further instructions." Also, note the absolute term "only" in option 3. If you are unfamiliar with the measures to prevent toxoplasmosis, review this content.

Level of Cognitive Ability: Analysis
Client Needs: Health Promotion and Maintenance

Integrated Process: Teaching/Learning
Content Area: Maternity—antepartum
Reference: Murray, S., McKinney, E., & Gorrie, T. (2002). *Foundations of maternal-newborn nursing* (3rd ed., p. 729). Philadelphia: W. B. Saunders.

5. 2
Rationale: More than one medication may be used to prevent growth of resistant organisms in the pregnant woman with tuberculosis. Treatment must continue for a prolonged period of time. The preferred treatment for the pregnant woman is isoniazid plus rifampin daily for a total of 9 months. Ethambutol is added initially if medication resistance is suspected. Pyridoxine (vitamin B_6) often is administered with isoniazid to prevent fetal neurotoxicity. The infant will be tested at birth and may be started on preventive isoniazid therapy. Skin testing should be repeated at 3 months on the infant, and isoniazid may be stopped if the skin test result remains negative. If the skin test result converts to positive, a full course of isoniazid would be given.
Test-Taking Strategy: Knowledge regarding the therapeutic management for the mother with tuberculosis and for the newborn infant is required to answer this question. If you had difficulty with this question, review treatment measures for the mother with tuberculosis.
Level of Cognitive Ability: Application
Client Needs: Physiological Integrity
Integrated Process: Teaching/Learning
Content Area: Maternity—antepartum
Reference: Murray, S., McKinney, E., & Gorrie, T. (2002). *Foundations of maternal-newborn nursing* (3rd ed., p. 730). Philadelphia: W. B. Saunders.

6. 1
Rationale: To avoid infections, visitors with active infections should not be allowed to visit the client; otherwise restrictions are not required. Stress causes increased heart workload, and the client should be instructed to avoid stress. Too much weight gain can place further demands on the heart. Resting should be on the left side to promote blood return.
Test-Taking Strategy: Use the process of elimination. Note the key words "cardiac disease" and "need for further education" in the question. Using principles related to the therapeutic management of cardiac disease in general will assist in directing you to option 1. If you had difficulty with this question, review the measures for the pregnant client with cardiac disease.
Level of Cognitive Ability: Analysis
Client Needs: Health Promotion and Maintenance
Integrated Process: Teaching/Learning
Content Area: Maternity—antepartum
Reference: Murray, S., McKinney, E., & Gorrie, T. (2002). *Foundations of maternal-newborn nursing* (3rd ed., p. 716). Philadelphia: W. B. Saunders.

7. 1
Rationale: Constipation can cause the client to use Valsalva's maneuver. This maneuver can cause blood to rush to the heart and overload the cardiac system. Therefore high-fiber foods are important. A low-calorie diet is not recommended during pregnancy. Diets low in fluid can cause a decrease in blood

volume that can deprive the fetus of nutrients. Therefore adequate fluid intake and high-fiber foods are important. Sodium should be restricted by some degree as prescribed by the physician because this will cause an overload to the circulating blood volume and contribute to cardiac complications.
Test-Taking Strategy: Use the process of elimination. Think about the physiology of the cardiac system, the maternal and fetus needs, and the factors that increase the workload on the heart to answer the question. If you had difficulty with this question, review nursing measures for the pregnant client with cardiac disease.
Level of Cognitive Ability: Analysis
Client Needs: Health Promotion and Maintenance
Integrated Process: Teaching/Learning
Content Area: Maternity—antepartum
Reference: Williams, S. (2001). *Basic nutrition & diet therapy* (11th ed., pp. 57, 478, 481). St Louis: Mosby.

8. 1
Rationale: Human immunodeficiency virus (HIV) is transmitted by intimate sexual contact and the exchange of body fluids, exposure to infected blood, and transmission from an infected woman to her fetus. Women who fall into the high-risk category for HIV infection include those with persistent and recurrent sexually transmitted diseases, those with a history of multiple sexual partners, and those who have used intravenous drugs. A heterosexual partner, particularly a partner who has had only one sexual partner in 10 years, does not have a high risk for contracting HIV.
Test-Taking Strategy: Use the process of elimination, recalling that exchange of blood and body fluids places the client at high risk for HIV infection. This will assist in directing you to the correct option. If you had difficulty with this question, review the risk factors for HIV.
Level of Cognitive Ability: Analysis
Client Needs: Psychosocial Integrity
Integrated Process: Nursing Process—assessment
*Content Area:*Maternity—antepartum
References: Matteson, P. (2001). *Women's health during the childbearing years: A community-based approach* (p. 266). St. Louis: Mosby.
Wong, D., Perry, S., & Hockenberry, M. (2002). *Maternal child nursing care* (2nd ed., p. 268). St. Louis: Mosby.

9. 1
Rationale: A support group can help the parents work through their pain by nonjudgmental sharing of feelings. Option 1 identifies a statement that would indicate positive, normal grieving. Although the other options may indicate reactions of the client and significant other, they are not specifically a part of the normal grieving process.
Test-Taking Strategy: Use the process of elimination. Read all of the options carefully before selecting an answer and focus on the issue of the question, the normal grieving process. Note the similarity between options 2, 3, and 4 in that they relate to childbearing. If you had difficulty with this question, review the components of the normal grieving process.
Level of Cognitive Ability: Analysis
Client Needs: Psychosocial Integrity
Integrated Process: Caring

Content Area: Maternity—postpartum
Reference: Murray, S., McKinney, E., & Gorrie, T. (2002). *Foundations of maternal-newborn nursing* (3rd ed., p. 650). Philadelphia: W. B. Saunders.

10. 2
Rationale: A variety of factors can cause increased emotional stress during pregnancy, resulting in further cardiac complications. The client with known cardiac disease is at greater risk for such complications. The use of resources will assist the client to avoid emotional stress, thus reducing additional cardiac compromise during the last trimester. These resources are not intended to minimize potential risk of maternal infection or prepare the client and family for the subsequent labor, delivery, and hospitalization.
Test-Taking Strategy: Focus on the issue of the question, noting the client's diagnosis. Also note the key word "primarily" in the stem of the question. Use Maslow's hierarchy of needs theory and focus on the client's condition to assist in directing you to option 2. Review considerations in caring for the pregnant client with cardiac disease if you had difficulty with this question.
Level of Cognitive Ability: Application
Client Needs: Health Promotion and Maintenance
Integrated Process: Nursing Process—implementation
Content Area: Maternity—antepartum
Reference: Murray, S., McKinney, E., & Gorrie, T. (2002). *Foundations of maternal-newborn nursing* (3rd ed., p. 717). Philadelphia: W. B. Saunders.

11. 3
Rationale: Hepatitis B virus is highly contagious when transmitted by direct contact with blood and body fluids of infected persons. The rationale for identifying childbearing women with this disease is to provide adequate protection of the fetus and the newborn infant, to minimize transmission to other human beings, and to reduce further maternal morbidity for the mother. Option 3 provides the best evaluation of maternal understanding of disease transmission. Options 1 and 2 are appropriate feeding techniques for bottle-feeding but do not minimize disease transmission for hepatitis B. Option 4 will not affect disease transmission.
Test-Taking Strategy: Focus on the issue of the question, "disease transmission to the infant." This focus and the process of elimination will easily direct you to option 3. Review measures to prevent transmission of hepatitis if you had difficulty with this question.
Level of Cognitive Ability: Analysis
Client Needs: Safe, Effective Care Environment
Integrated Process: Nursing Process—evaluation
Content Area: Maternity—postpartum
Reference: Murray, S., McKinney, E., & Gorrie, T. (2002). *Foundations of maternal-newborn nursing* (3rd ed., p. 728). Philadelphia: W. B. Saunders.

12. 4
Rationale: Perinatal transmission of HIV can occur during the antepartal period, during labor and birth, or in the postpartum period if the mother is breast-feeding. Women who carry HIV are advised not to breast-feed. There is no physiological reason why the newborn infant needs to be fed by nasogastric tube.
Test-Taking Strategy: Use the process of elimination and knowledge regarding the transmission of HIV to assist in answering the question. Eliminate options 1 and 2 first because these options are similar in that they both address breast-feeding. From the remaining options, select option 4, knowing that it is not necessary to feed the infant by nasogastric tube. Review feeding options for the newborn infant of an HIV client if you had difficulty with this question.
Level of Cognitive Ability: Application
Client Needs: Physiological Integrity
Integrated Process: Teaching/Learning
Content Area: Maternity—postpartum
Reference: Murray, S., McKinney, E., & Gorrie, T. (2002). *Foundations of maternal-newborn nursing* (3rd ed., p. 728). Philadelphia: W. B. Saunders.

13. 3
Rationale: A variety of conditions, including dehydration, hypoxemia, infection, and exertion, can stimulate the sickling process during the intrapartum period. Maintaining adequate intravenous fluid intake and the administration of oxygen via face mask will help to ensure a safe environment for maternal and fetal health during labor. These measures will not stimulate the labor process, avoid the need for a cesarean delivery, or eliminate the need for analgesic administration.
Test-Taking Strategy: Note the relationship between "appropriate intravenous fluid intake and oxygen consumption" in the question and "prevent dehydration and hypoxemia" in the correct option. This relationship and knowledge regarding the care measures for sickle cell anemia will direct you easily to option 3. Review these care measures if you had difficulty with this question.
Level of Cognitive Ability: Application
Client Needs: Physiological Integrity
Integrated Process: Nursing Process—implementation
Content Area: Maternity—intrapartum
Reference: Murray, S., McKinney, E., & Gorrie, T. (2002). *Foundations of maternal-newborn nursing* (3rd ed., p. 719). Philadelphia: W. B. Saunders.

14. 3
Rationale: If the client complains of a headache and blurred vision, the physician should be notified because these are signs of worsening preeclampsia. Options 1, 2, and 4 are normal signs.
Test-Taking Strategy: Use the process of elimination, noting the key word "worsening" in the stem of the question. Eliminate options 1, 2, and 4 because these options indicate normal findings. Review the signs that indicate a worsening of preeclampsia, if you had difficulty with this question.
Level of Cognitive Ability: Analysis
Client Needs: Physiological Integrity
Integrated Process: Nursing Process—assessment
Content Area: Maternity—antepartum
Reference: Lowdermilk, D., & Perry, S. (2003). *Maternity nursing* (6th ed., pp. 606-607). St. Louis: Mosby.

15. 3

Rationale: Option 3 is a low priority because fundal height should be measured at each antepartal clinic visit, not in the intrapartum period. Options 1, 2, and 4 are high priorities. Intrapartal management and assessment require careful attention to maternal and fetal status. The fetuses should be monitored by dual electronic fetal monitoring, and any signs of distress need to be reported to the physician or health care provider. A cesarean section may be necessary if a fetus is breech. The nurse should examine the perineum and vaginal opening visually for signs of the cord, which sometimes will prolapse through the cervix.

Test-Taking Strategy: Use the process of elimination and note the key words "lowest priority." Also note that the client is in early labor. With this in mind, think about the nursing interventions associated with early labor. Review care to the pregnant client with a twin pregnancy and a breech presentation if you had difficulty with this question.

Level of Cognitive Ability: Application
Client Needs: Physiological Integrity
Integrated Process: Nursing Process—planning
Content Area: Maternity—intrapartum
Reference: Murray, S., McKinney, E., & Gorrie, T. (2002). *Foundations of maternal-newborn nursing* (3rd ed., p. 742). Philadelphia: W. B. Saunders.

16. 3

Rationale: Nurses should be able to explore measures that assist the family to create memories of the newborn infant so that the existence of the child is confirmed and the parents can complete the grieving process. Option 3 provides this support and demonstrates a caring and empathetic response. Options 1, 2, and 4 are blocks to communication and devalue the parents' feelings.

Test-Taking Strategy: Use the process of elimination and therapeutic communication techniques to answer the question. Option 3 is the only option that reflects use of therapeutic communication techniques. Review these techniques and the nursing strategies in caring for parents who experience perinatal death if you had difficulty with this question.

Level of Cognitive Ability: Application
Client Needs: Psychosocial Integrity
Integrated Process: Caring
Content Area: Maternity—postpartum
Reference: Murray, S., McKinney, E., & Gorrie, T. (2002). *Foundations of maternal-newborn nursing* (3rd ed., p. 649). Philadelphia: W. B. Saunders.

17. 3

Rationale: Exercise is safe for the client with gestational diabetes mellitus and is helpful in lowering the blood glucose level. Dietary modifications are the mainstay of treatment, and the client is placed on a standard diabetic diet. Many women are taught to perform blood glucose monitoring. If the woman is not performing the blood glucose monitoring at home, then it will be performed at the clinic or health care provider's office. Signs of infection need to be reported to the health care provider.

Test-Taking Strategy: Use the process of elimination, noting the key words "need for further education." Noting these key words and the absolute term "avoid" in option 3 will assist in answering the question. If you had difficulty with this question, review the teaching points for a client with gestational diabetes mellitus.

Level of Cognitive Ability: Analysis
Client Needs: Health Promotion and Maintenance
Integrated Process: Teaching/Learning
Content Area: Maternity—antepartum
References: Lowdermilk, D., & Perry, S. (2003). *Maternity nursing* (6th ed., p. 581). St. Louis: Mosby.
Murray, S., McKinney, E., & Gorrie, T. (2002). *Foundations of maternal-newborn nursing* (3rd ed., p. 706). Philadelphia: W. B. Saunders.

18. 3

Rationale: Magnesium sulfate depresses the respiratory rate. If the respiratory rate is less than 12 breaths per minute, the physician or other health care provider needs to be notified, and continuation of the medication needs to be reassessed. A urinary output of 20 mL in a 30-minute period is adequate; less that 30 mL in 1 hour needs to be reported. Deep tendon reflexes of 2+ are normal. The fetal heart rate is within normal limits for a resting fetus.

Test-Taking Strategy: Use the process of elimination. Note the key words "most concern" in the stem of the question. Knowledge of the normal and abnormal assessment findings will direct you easily to option 3. Review care to the client receiving magnesium sulfate if you had difficulty with this question.

Level of Cognitive Ability: Analysis
Client Needs: Physiological Integrity
Integrated Process: Nursing Process—analysis
Content Area: Maternity—antepartum
Reference: Hodgson, B., & Kizior, R. (2004). *Saunders nursing drug handbook 2004* (p. 624). Philadelphia: W. B. Saunders.

19. 3

Rationale: The immediate care during a seizure (eclampsia) is to ensure a patent airway. Options 1, 2, and 4 are actions that follow or will be implemented after the seizure has ceased.

Test-Taking Strategy: Note the key words "first action" in the stem of the question. Use the ABCs—airway, breathing, and circulation—to answer the question. Remember that the airway is always the first priority. Review care to the client with eclampsia if you had difficulty with this question.

Level of Cognitive Ability: Application
Client Needs: Physiological Integrity
Integrated Process: Nursing Process—implementation
Content Area: Delegating/Prioritizing
Reference: Wong, D., Perry, S., & Hockenberry, M. (2002). *Maternal child nursing care* (2nd ed., p. 287). St. Louis: Mosby.

20. 1

Rationale: By seeing no way out of the situation except for death, the client meets the criteria for hopelessness. A person who lacks hope feels that life is too much to handle. Option 2 is a possible nursing diagnosis later, but not enough data support it at this point. The data given do not support the nursing diagnosis of situational low self-esteem. Option 4 is a possible nursing diagnosis at a later time; however, at this

time the diagnosis of hopelessness should take precedence.
Test-Taking Strategy: Use the process of elimination. When answering a question regarding a nursing diagnosis, focus on the issue of the question and only on the data in the question. No data support options 2, 3, or 4.
Level of Cognitive Ability: Analysis
Client Needs: Psychosocial Integrity
Integrated Process: Nursing Process—analysis
Content Area: Maternity—postpartum
References: Lowdermilk, D., & Perry, S. (2003). *Maternity nursing* (6th ed., p. 634). St. Louis: Mosby.
Wong, D., Perry, S., & Hockenberry, M. (2002). *Maternal child nursing care* (2nd ed., p. 305). St. Louis: Mosby.

CRITICAL THINKING: FILL IN THE BLANK
Answer: Hypertension, generalized edema, and proteinuria
Rationale: The three classic signs of preeclampsia are hypertension, generalized edema, and proteinuria.
Test-Taking Strategy: You must know the classic signs of preeclampsia to answer this question. If you had difficulty with this question, review preeclampsia and learn these signs.
Level of Cognitive Ability: Application
Client Needs: Physiological Integrity
Integrated Process: Nursing Process—assessment
Content Area: Maternity—antepartum
Reference: Wong, D., Perry, S., & Hockenberry, M. (2002). *Maternal child nursing care* (2nd ed., p. 277). St. Louis: Mosby.

REFERENCES

Hodgson, B., & Kizior, R. (2004). *Saunders nursing drug handbook 2004.* Philadelphia: W. B. Saunders.

Lowdermilk, D., & Perry, S. (2003). *Maternity nursing* (6th ed.). St. Louis: Mosby.

Murray, S., McKinney, E., & Gorrie, T. (2002). *Foundations of maternal-newborn nursing* (3rd ed.). Philadelphia: W. B. Saunders.

Williams, S. (2001). *Basic nutrition & diet therapy* (11th ed.). St Louis: Mosby.

Wong, D., Perry, S., & Hockenberry, M. (2002). *Maternal child nursing care* (2nd ed.). St. Louis: Mosby.

Labor and Delivery

26

I. THE PROCESS OF LABOR—FOUR *P*'S

A. Terms
1. **Labor**: coordinated sequence of involuntary uterine contractions
2. **Delivery**: actual event of birth
B. Four major factors (four *P*'s) interact during normal childbirth; the four *P*'s are interrelated and depend on each other for a safe delivery (Box 26-1).
C. Powers: uterine contractions
1. The forces acting to expel the fetus
2. Effacement: shortening and thinning of the cervix during the first stage of labor
3. Dilation: enlargement of cervical os and cervical canal during first stage
4. Pushing efforts of mother during second stage
D. Passageway: the mother's rigid bony pelvis and the soft tissues of the cervix, pelvic floor, vagina, and introitus
E. Passenger: the fetus
F. Psyche: The mother may experience anxiety or fear.
G. Attitude
1. Attitude is the relationship of the fetal body parts to one another.
2. Normal intrauterine attitude is flexion, in which the fetal back is rounded, the head is forward on the chest, and the arms and legs are folded in against the body.

BOX 26-1

Four *P*'s

Powers
Passageway
Passenger
Psyche

H. Lie
1. Relationship of the spine of the fetus to the spine of the mother
2. Longitudinal or vertical
   a. Fetal spine is parallel to the mother's spine.
   b. Fetus is in cephalic or breech presentation.
3. Transverse or horizontal
   a. Fetal spine is at a right angle, or perpendicular, to the mother's spine.
   b. Presenting part is the shoulder.
   c. **Delivery** by cesarean section is necessary.
4. Oblique
   a. Fetal spine is at a slight angle from a true horizontal lie.
   b. **Delivery** is by cesarean section if uncorrectable.
I. Presentation
1. Presenting part: portion of the fetus that enters the pelvis first
2. Cephalic
   a. Cephalic is the most common presentation.
   b. Fetal head presents first.
3. Breech
   a. Buttocks present first.
   b. **Delivery** by cesarean section may be required, although vaginal birth is often possible.
4. Shoulder
   a. Fetus is in a transverse lie, or the arm, back, abdomen, or side could present.
   b. If the fetus does not spontaneously rotate or if it is not possible to turn the fetus manually, a cesarean section may be performed.
J. Position: relationship of assigned area of the presenting part or landmark to the maternal pelvis (Box 26-2)
K. Station
1. The measurement of the progress of descent in centimeters above or below the midplane from the presenting part to the ischial spine
2. Station 0: at ischial spine

3. Minus station: above ischial spine
4. Plus station: below ischial spine

II. MECHANISMS OF LABOR (BOX 26-3)

A. Assessment
  1. Lightening or dropping: Fetus descends into the pelvis about 2 weeks before **delivery** for a primipara; the fetus may engage into the pelvis after **labor** commences for a multipara.
  2. Braxton Hicks contractions increase.
  3. Show is visible.
  4. The vaginal mucosa is congested and vaginal mucus increases.
  5. Brownish or blood-tinged cervical mucus is passed.
  6. Cervix ripens, becomes soft, partly effaced, and may begin to dilate.
  7. Mother has a sudden burst of energy.
  8. Loss of 1 to 3 lb from water loss results from fluid shifts produced by the changes in progesterone and estrogen levels.
  9. Spontaneous rupture of membranes occurs.
B. True **labor** (Box 26-4)
  1. Contractions increase in duration and intensity.
  2. Cervical dilation and effacement are progressive.
C. False labor (Box 26-4)
  1. Exaggeration of normal contractions occurs.
  2. **Labor** does not produce dilation, effacement, or descent.
  3. Contractions are irregular without progression.
  4. Walking has no effect on contractions and often relieves false **labor**.

BOX 26-2

Fetal Positions

ROA: Right occiput anterior
LOA: Left occiput anterior
ROP: Right occiput posterior
LOP: Left occiput posterior
ROT: Right occiput transverse
LOT: Left occiput transverse
RMA: Right mentum anterior
LMA: Left mentum anterior
RMP: Right mentum posterior
LSA: Left sacrum anterior
LSP: Left sacrum posterior

BOX 26-4

True Labor and False Labor

TRUE LABOR
Contractions increase in duration and intensity.
Cervical dilation and effacement are progressive.

FALSE LABOR
False labor does not produce dilation, effacement, or descent.
Contractions are irregular without progression.
Walking has no effect on contractions and often relieves false labor.
Example: If a woman has been sleeping and wakes up with contractions, if she gets up and moves around and her contractions become stronger and closer together, this is true labor. If the contractions go away, this is false labor.

BOX 26-3

Mechanisms of Labor

ENGAGEMENT
Engagement is the mechanism by which the fetus nestles into the pelvis.
Engagement also is termed *lightening* or *dropping*.

DESCENT
Descent is the process that the fetal head undergoes as it begins its journey through the pelvis.
Descent is a continuous process from the time of engagement until birth and is assessed by the measurement called station.

FLEXION
Flexion is a process of the fetal head's nodding forward toward the fetal chest.

INTERNAL ROTATION
Internal rotation of the fetus occurs most commonly from the occiput transverse position, assumed at engagement into the pelvis, to the occiput anterior position while continuously descending.

EXTENSION
Extension enables the head to emerge when the fetus is in a cephalic position.
Extension begins after the head crowns.
Extension is complete when the head passes under the symphysis pubis and occiput and the anterior fontanel, brow, face, and chin pass over the sacrum and coccyx and are over the perineum.

RESTITUTION
Restitution is realignment of the fetal head with the body after the head emerges.

EXTERNAL ROTATION
The shoulders externally rotate after the head emerges and restitution occurs so that the shoulders are in the anteroposterior diameter of the pelvis.

EXPULSION
Expulsion is the birth of the entire body.

III. LEOPOLD'S MANEUVERS

A. Description: method to determine position, presentation, and engagement

B. Preparation
1. Ask the mother to empty the bladder.
2. Warm hands and apply them to the mother's abdomen with firm and gentle pressure.

C. First maneuver
1. The first maneuver determines which part of the fetus is in the fundus.
2. Place palms on each side of the upper abdomen and palpate around the fundus.
3. If the head is in the fundus, one would feel a hard, round, movable object.
4. The buttocks will feel soft and have an irregular shape and are more difficult to move.

D. Second maneuver
1. Move hands downward over each side of the abdomen, applying firm, even pressure.
2. The fetus's back, which is a smooth, hard surface, should be felt on one side of the abdomen.
3. Irregular knobs and lumps, which may be the hands, feet, elbows, and knees, will be felt on the opposite side of the abdomen.

E. Third maneuver
1. The third maneuver confirms fetal position.
2. Place hand above the symphysis pubis.
3. Bring thumb and fingers together and grasp the part of fetus between them (may be the head or the buttocks).

F. Fourth maneuver
1. The fourth maneuver is used in the late stage of pregnancy to determine how far the fetus has descended into the pelvic inlet.
2. Place hands on the sides of the lower abdomen close to the midline.
3. Slide hands downward and press inward.
4. If you have determined that the buttocks are in the fundus, then feel for the head.
5. If you cannot feel the head, it probably has descended.

IV. BREATHING TECHNIQUES (BOX 26-5)

A. Provide a focus during contractions, interfering with pain sensory transmission.
B. Begin with simple breathing patterns and progress to more complex ones as needed.
C. Promote relaxation and oxygenation.

V. FETAL MONITORING

A. Description
1. The fetal monitor displays the fetal heart rate (FHR).
2. The device monitors uterine activity.
3. The monitor assesses frequency, duration, and intensity of contractions.
4. The monitor assesses FHR in relation to maternal contractions.
5. Baseline FHR is measured between contractions; the normal FHR at term is 120 to 160 beats per minute.

B. External fetal monitoring
1. External fetal monitoring is noninvasive and is performed using a tocotransducer or Doppler ultrasonic transducer.
2. Perform Leopold's maneuvers to determine on which side the fetal back is located, and place the ultrasound transducer over this area (fasten with a belt).
3. Place the tocotransducer over the fundus of the uterus where contractions feel the strongest (fasten with a belt).

BOX 26-5

Breathing Techniques

FIRST-STAGE BREATHING

Cleansing Breath
Each contraction begins and ends with a deep inspiration and expiration.

Slow-Paced Breathing
Slow, paced breathing promotes relaxation.
Slow-paced breathing is used as long as possible during labor.

Modified-Paced Breathing
Modified-paced breathing is used when slow-paced breathing is no longer effective.
Breathing is shallow and fast.

Pattern-Paced Breathing
Pattern-paced breathing sometimes is called pant-blow.
After a certain number of breaths (modified-paced breathing), the woman exhales with a slight emphasis or blow, and then begins the modified-paced breathing again.

Breathing to Prevent Pushing
The woman blows repeatedly using short puffs when the urge to push is strong.

SECOND STAGE BREATHING

Traditional Pushing
The woman takes one or more cleansing breaths at the beginning of a contraction and then holds her breath, pushing as hard as she can for as long as possible.
She then quickly exhales, takes another breath, and pushes again, repeating the process until the contraction is over.

Other Pushing Methods
Exhalation of small amounts of air through an open glottis during pushing is another breathing method.
The woman may push in short bursts only when the urge is strong instead of using prolonged expulsive efforts.

4. Allow the client to assume a comfortable position, avoiding vena cava compression.

C. Internal fetal monitoring
1. Internal fetal monitoring is invasive and requires rupturing of the membranes and attaching an electrode to the presenting part of the fetus.
2. Mother must be dilated 2 to 3 cm to perform internal monitoring.

D. Periodic patterns in the FHR
1. Fetal bradycardia and tachycardia
   a. Bradycardia: The FHR is less than 120 beats per minute for 10 minutes or more.
   b. Tachycardia: The FHR is greater than 160 beats per minute for 10 minutes or more.
   c. Change position of the mother and administer oxygen.
   d. Notify the physician.
2. Variability (Box 26-6)
   a. Fluctuations in the baseline FHR may include irregular fluctuations of 2 cycles per minute or greater.
   b. Decreased variability can result from fetal hypoxemia, acidosis, or certain medications.
   c. A temporary decrease in variability can occur when the fetus is in a sleep state (sleep states do not usually last longer than 30 minutes).
3. Accelerations
   a. Accelerations are brief, temporary increases in the FHR of at least 15 beats greater than the baseline and lasting at least 15 seconds.
   b. Accelerations usually are a reassuring sign, reflecting a responsive, nonacidotic fetus.
   c. Accelerations usually occur with fetal movement.
   d. Acclerations may be nonperiodic (having no relation to contractions) or periodic.
   e. Accelerations may occur with uterine contractions, vaginal examinations, or mild cord compression, or when the fetus is in a breech presentation.
4. Early decelerations
   a. Early decelerations are decreases in FHR below baseline; the rate at the lowest point of the deceleration usually remains greater than 100 beats per minute.
   b. Early decelerations occur during contractions as the fetal head is pressed against the woman's pelvis or soft tissues, such as the cervix, and return to the baseline FHR by the end of the contraction.
   c. Tracing shows a uniform shape and mirror image of uterine contractions.
   d. Early decelerations are not associated with fetal compromise and require no intervention.
5. Late decelerations
   a. Later deceleratins are nonreassuring patterns that reflect impaired placental exchange or uteroplacental insufficiency.
   b. The patterns look similar to early decelerations but begin well after the contraction begins and return to baseline after the contraction ends.
   c. The degree of fall in the heart rate from baseline is not related to the amount of uteroplacental insufficiency.
   d. Interventions include improving placental blood flow and fetal oxygenation.
6. Variable decelerations
   a. Variable decelerations are caused by conditions that restrict flow through the umbilical cord.
   b. Variable decelerations do not have the uniform appearance of early and late decelerations.
   c. Their shape, duration, and degree of fall below baseline heart rate are variable; they fall and rise abruptly with the onset and relief of cord compression.
   d. Variable decelerations also may be nonperiodic, occurring at times unrelated to contractions.
   e. One considers baseline rate and variability when evaluating variable decelerations.
   f. Variable decelerations are significant when the FHR repeatedly decreases to less than 70 beats per minutes and persists at that level for at least 60 seconds before returning to the baseline.
7. Hypertonic uterine activity
   a. Assessment of uterine activity includes frequency, duration, intensity of the contractions, and uterine resting tone.
   b. The uterus should relax between contractions for 60 seconds or longer.
   c. Uterine contraction intensity is about 50 to 75 mm Hg (with the intrauterine uterine catheter) during **labor** and may reach 110 mm Hg with pushing during the second stage.
   d. The average resting tone is 5 to 15 mm Hg.
   e. In hypertonic uterine activity the uterine resting tone between contractions is high, reducing uterine blood flow and decreasing fetal oxygen supply.
8. Interventions for nonreassuring patterns (Box 26-7)
   a. Identify the cause (assess for cord prolapse).
   b. Discontinue oxytocin (Pitocin) if infusing as prescribed.

BOX 26-6

Variability

Absent variability: undetected variability
Minimal variability: greater than undetected but not more than 5 beats per minute
Moderate variability: fetal heart rate fluctuations from 6 to 25 beats per minute
Marked variability: fetal heart rate fluctuations greater than 25 beats per minute

BOX 26-7

Nonreassuring Patterns

Tachycardia
Bradycardia
Decreased or absent variability
Late decelerations
Variable decelerations falling to less than 70 beats per
   minute for longer than 60 seconds
Prolonged decelerations
Hypertonic uterine activity

---

   c. Change the mother's position (avoid the supine position for patterns associated with cord compression).

   d. Administer oxygen by face mask at 8 to 10 L per minute.

   e. Increase intravenous (IV) fluids as prescribed.

   f. Notify the physician or nurse midwife as soon as possible.

   g. Prepare to initiate continuous electronic fetal monitoring with internal devices if not contraindicated.

   h. Prepare to obtain a fetal scalp pH monitor to determine a blood pH value.

   i. Prepare for cesarean **delivery** if necessary.

▲ VI. STAGES OF LABOR

A. Stage 1 latent phase
   1. Assessment
     a. Cervical dilation is 1 to 4 cm.
     b. Uterine contractions occur every 15 to 30 minutes and are 15 to 30 seconds in duration and of mild intensity.
     c. Mother is talkative and eager to be in **labor**.
   2. Interventions
     a. Encourage mother and partner to participate in care.
     b. Assist with comfort measures, changes of position, and ambulation.
     c. Keep mother and partner informed of progress.
     d. Offer fluids and ice chips.
     e. Encourage voiding every 1 to 2 hours.

B. Stage 1 active phase
   1. Assessment
     a. Cervical dilation is 4 to 7 cm.
     b. Uterine contractions occur every 3 to 5 minutes and are 30 to 60 seconds in duration and of moderate intensity.
     c. Mother may experience feelings of helplessness.
     d. Mother becomes restless and anxious as contractions become stronger.
   2. Interventions
     a. Encourage maintenance of effective breathing patterns.
     b. Provide a quiet environment.
     c. Keep mother and partner informed of progress.

     d. Promote comfort with backrubs, sacral pressure, pillow support, and position changes.
     e. Instruct partner in effleurage.
     f. Offer fluids and ice chips and ointment for dry lips.
     g. Encourage voiding every 1 to 2 hours.

C. Stage 1 transition phase
   1. Assessment
     a. Cervical dilation is 8 to 10 cm.
     b. Uterine contractions occur every 2 to 3 minutes and are 45 to 90 seconds in duration and of strong intensity.
     c. Mother becomes tired, is restless and irritable, and feels out of control.
   2. Interventions
     a. Encourage rest between contractions.
     b. Wake mother at beginning of contraction so she can begin breathing pattern.
     c. Keep mother and partner informed of progress.
     d. Provide privacy.
     e. Offer fluids and ice chips and ointment for dry lips.
     f. Encourage voiding every 1 to 2 hours.

D. Interventions throughout stage I.
   1. Monitor maternal vital signs.
   2. Monitor FHR via ultrasound Doppler, fetoscope, or electronic fetal monitor.
   3. Assess FHR before, during, and after a contraction, noting that the normal FHR is 120 to 160 beats per minute.
   4. Monitor uterine contractions by palpation or monitor, determining frequency, duration, and intensity.
   5. Assess status of cervical dilation and effacement.
   6. Assess fetal station presentation and position by Leopold's maneuvers.
   7. Assist with pelvic examination and prepare for a Nitrazine test and a fern test.
   8. Assess the color of the **amniotic fluid** if the membranes have ruptured because meconium-stained fluid can indicate fetal distress.

E. Stage 2
   1. Assessment
     a. Cervical dilation is complete.
     b. Progress of **labor** is measured by descent of fetal head through the birth canal (change in fetal station).
     c. Uterine contractions occur every 2 to 3 minutes, lasting 60 to 75 seconds, and the intensity is strong.
     d. Increase in bloody show occurs.
     e. Mother feels urge to bear down; assist mother in pushing efforts.
   2. Interventions
     a. Perform assessments every 5 minutes.
     b. Monitor maternal vital signs.
     c. Monitor FHR via ultrasound Doppler, fetoscope, or electronic fetal monitor.

d. Assess FHR before, during, and after a contraction, noting that normal fetal heart rate is 120 to 160 beats per minute.

e. Monitor uterine contractions by palpation or monitor, determining frequency, duration, and intensity.

f. Provide mother with encouragement and praise and provide for rest between contractions.

g. Keep mother and partner informed of progress.

h. Maintain privacy.

i. Provide ice chips and ointment for dry lips.

j. Assist mother into a position that promotes comfort and assists pushing efforts, such as lithotomy, semisitting, kneeling, side-lying, or squatting.

k. Monitor for signs of approaching birth, such as perineal bulging or visualization of the fetal head.

l. Prepare for birth.

F. Stage 3

1. Assessment

a. Contractions occur until the **placenta** is born.

b. Placental separation and expulsion occur.

c. Birth of **placenta** occurs 5 to 30 minutes after birth of the baby.

d. Schultze mechanism: Center portion of **placenta** separates first, and its shiny fetal surface emerges from the vagina.

e. Duncan mechanism: Margin of **placenta** separates, and the dull, red, rough maternal surface emerges from the vagina first.

2. Interventions

a. Assess maternal vital signs.

b. Assess uterine status.

c. Provide parents with an explanation regarding birth of the **placenta**.

d. Following birth of the **placenta**, uterine fundus remains firm and is located 2 fingerbreadths below the umbilicus.

e. Examine **placenta** for cotyledons and membranes to verify that it is intact.

f. Assess mother for shivering and provide warmth.

g. Promote parental-neonatal attachment.

G. Stage 4

1. Description: the period of time from 1 to 4 hours after **delivery**

2. Assessment

a. Blood pressure returns to prelabor level.

b. Pulse is slightly lower than during **labor**.

c. Fundus remains contracted, in the midline, 1 to 2 fingerbreadths below the umbilicus.

d. **Lochia** is moderate or scant and is red.

3. Interventions

a. Perform maternal assessments every 15 minutes for 1 hour, every 30 minutes for 1 hour, and hourly for 2 hours.

b. Provide warm blankets.

c. Apply ice packs to the perineum.

d. Massage the uterus if needed and teach the mother to massage the uterus.

e. Provide breast-feeding support as needed.

f. Refer to Chapter 30 for information on caring for the **newborn**.

VII. ANESTHESIA

A. Local anesthesia

1. Local anesthesia is used for blocking pain during episiotomy.

2. Local anesthesia is administered just before the birth of the baby.

3. The anesthetic has no effect on the fetus.

B. Pudendal block

1. A pudendal block is administered just before the birth of the baby.

2. Injection site is at the pudendal nerve through a transvaginal route.

3. Anesthetic blocks the perineal area for episiotomy.

4. Effect lasts about 30 minutes.

5. Anesthetic has no effect on contractions or the fetus.

C. Lumbar epidural block

1. Injection site is in epidural space at L3 to L4.

2. The block is administered after labor is established or just before a scheduled cesarean birth.

3. The anesthetic relieves pain from contractions and numbs the vagina and perineum.

4. The block may cause hypotension.

5. The anesthetic does not cause headache because the dura mater is not penetrated.

6. Assess maternal blood pressure.

7. Maintain the mother in side-lying position or place a rolled blanket beneath the right hip to displace the uterus from the vena cava.

8. Administer IV fluids as prescribed.

9. Increase fluids as prescribed if hypotension occurs.

D. Subarachnoid (spinal) block

1. Injection site is in the spinal subarachnoid space at L3 to L5.

2. The block is administered just before birth.

3. The anesthetic relieves uterine and perineal pain and numbs the vagina, perineum, and lower extremities.

4. The anesthetic may cause maternal hypotension.

5. The anesthetic may cause postpartum headache.

6. The mother must lie flat for 8 to 12 hours following spinal injection.

7. Administer IV fluids as prescribed.

E. General anesthesia

1. General anesthesia may be used for some surgical interventions.

2. The mother is not awake.

3. General anesthesia presents a danger of respiratory depression and vomiting.

TABLE 26-1

Factors of the Bishop Score

Score	0	1	2	3
Dilation of cervix	0	1-2 cm	3-4 cm	>5 cm
Effacement of cervix	0%-30%	40%-50%	60%-70%	>80%
Consistency of cervix	Firm	Medium	Soft	
Position of cervix	Posterior	Midposition	Anterior	
Station of presenting part	−3	−2	−1	+1, +2

VIII. OBSTETRICAL PROCEDURES

A. Bishop score (Table 26-1)
  1. The Bishop score is used to determine maternal readiness for **labor**.
  2. The Bishop score evaluates cervical status and fetal position.
  3. The Bishop score is indicated before the induction of **labor**.
  4. The five factors are assigned a score of 0 to 3, and the total score is calculated.
  5. A score of 6 or more indicates a readiness for **labor** induction.

B. Induction
  1. A deliberate initiation of uterine contractions that stimulates **labor**.
  2. Elective induction may be accomplished by oxytocin (Pitocin) infusion.
  3. Obtain baseline tracing of uterine contractions and FHR.
  4. Increase IV dosage of oxytocin as prescribed only after assessing contractions, FHR, and maternal blood pressure and pulse.
  5. Do not increase rate of oxytocin once the desired contraction pattern is obtained (contraction frequency of 2 to 3 minutes and lasting 60 seconds).
  6. Discontinue oxytocin as prescribed if contraction frequency is less than 2 minutes or duration is more than 90 seconds, or if fetal distress is noted.

C. Amniotomy
  1. Artificial rupture of membranes is performed by the physician to stimulate **labor**.
  2. Amniotomy is performed if the fetus is at 0 or a plus station.
  3. Amniotomy increases risk of prolapsed cord and infection.
  4. Monitor FHR before and after amniotomy.
  5. Record time of amniotomy, FHR, and characteristics of the fluid.
  6. Meconium-stained **amniotic fluid** may be associated with fetal distress.
  7. Bloody **amniotic fluid** may indicate abruptio placentae or fetal trauma.
  8. An unpleasant odor to **amniotic fluid** is associated with infection.
  9. Polyhydramnios is associated with maternal diabetes and certain congenital disorders.
  10. Oligohydramnios is associated with intrauterine growth retriction and congenital disorders.
  11. Expect more variable decelerations after rupture of the membranes as a result of possible cord compression during contractions.
  12. Limit client activity if prescribed.

D. External version
  1. External version is manipulation of the fetus from an abnormal position into a normal presentation.
  2. External version is indicated for an abnormal presentation that exists after the thirty-fourth week.
  3. Monitor vital signs.
  4. If the mother is Rh-negative, ensure that Rh immune globulin was given at 28 weeks' gestation.
  5. Prepare for nonstress test to evaluate fetal well-being.
  6. Intravenous fluids and tocolytic therapy may be administered to relax the uterus and permit easier manipulation of fetus.
  7. Ultrasound is used during the procedure to evaluate fetal position and placental placement and guide direction of the fetus.
  8. Abdominal wall is manipulated to direct fetus into a cephalic presentation if possible.
  9. Monitor blood pressure to identify vena cava compression.
  10. Monitor for unusual pain.
  11. After the procedure, do the following:
    a. Perform nonstress test to evaluate fetal well-being.
    b. Monitor for uterine activity, bleeding, ruptured membranes, and decreased fetal activity.
    c. With Rh-negative clients, perform Kleihauer-Betke test as prescribed to detect the presence and amount of fetal blood in the maternal circulation and to identify clients who need additional Rh immune globulin.

E. Episiotomy
  1. An episiotomy is an incision made into the perineum to enlarge the vaginal outlet and facilitate **delivery**.
  2. Check episiotomy site.
  3. Institute measures to relieve pain.
  4. Provide ice packs during the first 24 hours.
  5. Instruct the client in the use of sitz baths.
  6. Apply analgesic spray or ointment as prescribed.

7. Provide perineal care using clean technique.
8. Instruct the client in the proper care of the incision.
9. Instruct the client to dry the perineal area from front to back and to blot the area rather than wipe it.
10. Instruct the client to shower rather than bathe in a tub.
11. Apply a peripad without touching the inside surface of the pad.
12. Report any bleeding or discharge to the physician.

▲ F. Forceps **delivery**
  1. Two double-crossed, spoonlike articulated blades are used to assist in the **delivery** of the fetal head.
  2. Reassure the mother and explain the need for forceps.
  3. Monitor mother and fetus during **delivery**.
  4. Check **neonate** and mother after **delivery** for any possible injury.
  5. Assist with repair of any lacerations.

▲ G. Vacuum extraction
  1. A caplike suction device is applied to the fetal head to facilitate extraction.
  2. Suction is used to assist in **delivery** of the fetal head.
  3. Traction is applied during uterine contractions until descent of the fetal head is achieved.
  4. The suction device should not be kept in place any longer than 25 minutes.
  5. Monitor FHR every 5 minutes if external fetal monitoring is not used.
  6. Assess **newborn infant** at birth and throughout postpartum period for signs of cerebral trauma.
  7. Monitor for developing cephalohematoma.
  8. Caput succedaneum is normal and will resolve in 24 hours.

▲ H. Cesarean **delivery**
  1. Cesarean section is **delivery** of the fetus usually through a transabdominal, low-segment incision of the uterus.
  2. Preoperative
    a. If planned, prepare the mother and partner.
    b. If an emergency, quickly explain the need and procedure to the mother and partner.
    c. Obtain informed consent.
    d. Make sure that the preoperative diagnostic tests are done, including the Rh factor.
    e. Prepare to insert an IV line and a Foley catheter.
    f. Prepare the abdomen as prescribed.
    g. Monitor the mother and fetus continuously for signs of **labor**.
    h. Provide emotional support.
    i. Administer preoperative medications as prescribed.
  3. Postoperative
    a. Monitor vital signs.
    b. Provide pain relief.
    c. Encourage turning, coughing, and deep breathing.
    d. Encourage ambulation.
    e. Monitor for signs of infection and bleeding.
    f. Burning and pain on urination may indicate a bladder infection.
    g. A tender uterus and foul-smelling **lochia** may indicate endometritis.
    h. A productive cough or chills may indicate pneumonia.
    i. A positive Homans' sign, pain, or edema of an extremity may indicate thrombophlebitis.

PRACTICE QUESTIONS

1. A nurse is caring for a client in labor. The nurse determines that the client is beginning the second stage of labor when which of the following assessments is noted?
   1. The client begins to expel clear vaginal fluid.
   2. The contractions are regular.
   3. The membranes have ruptured.
   4. The cervix is dilated completely.

2. A nurse in the labor room is caring for a client in the active stage of labor. The nurse is assessing the fetal patterns and notes a late deceleration on the monitor strip. The most appropriate nursing action is to
   1. Place the mother in a supine position.
   2. Document the findings and continue to monitor the fetal patterns.
   3. Administer oxygen via face mask.
   4. Increase the rate of the oxytocin (Pitocin) IV infusion.

3. A nurse is performing an assessment of a client who is scheduled for a cesarean delivery. Which assessment finding would indicate a need to contact the physician?
   1. Fetal heart rate of 180 beats per minute.
   2. White blood cell count of 12,000 cells/mm³
   3. Maternal pulse rate of 85 beats per minute.
   4. Hemoglobin of 11.0 g/dL

4. A client in labor is transported to the delivery room and is prepared for a cesarean delivery. The client is transferred to the delivery room table, and the nurse places the client in the
   1. Trendelenburg's position with the legs in stirrups.
   2. Semi-Fowler position with a pillow under the knees.
   3. Prone position with the legs separated and elevated.
   4. Supine position with a wedge under the right hip.

5. A nurse has provided discharge instructions to a client who delivered a healthy newborn infant by cesarean delivery. Which statement if made by the client indicates a need for further instructions?
   1. "I will notify the physician if I develop a fever."
   2. "I will lift nothing heavier than the newborn infant for at least 2 weeks."

3. "I will begin abdominal exercises immediately."

4. "I will turn on my side and push up with my arms to get out of bed."

6. A nurse is caring for a client in labor and prepares to auscultate the fetal heart rate by using a Doppler ultrasound device. The nurse most accurately determines that the fetal heart sounds are heard by

1. Noting if the heart rate is greater than 140 beats per minute.

2. Placing the diaphragm of the Doppler on the mother's abdomen.

3. Performing Leopold's maneuvers first to determine the location of the fetal heart.

4. Palpating the maternal radial pulse while listening to the fetal heart rate.

7. A nurse is caring for a client in labor who is receiving oxytocin (Pitocin) by intravenous infusion to stimulate uterine contractions. Which assessment finding would indicate to the nurse that the infusion needs to be discontinued?

1. Three contractions occurring within a 10-minute period.

2. A fetal heart rate of 90 beats per minute.

3. Adequate resting tone of the uterus palpated between contractions.

4. Increased urinary output.

8. A nurse is preparing to care for a client in labor. The physician has prescribed an intravenous infusion of oxytocin (Pitocin). The nurse ensures that which of the following is implemented before initiating the infusion?

1. Placing the client on complete bed rest

2. Continuous electronic fetal monitoring

3. An intravenous infusion of antibiotics

4. Placing a code cart at the client's bedside

9. A nurse is monitoring a client in active labor and notes that the client is having contractions every 3 minutes that last 45 seconds. The nurse notes that the fetal heart rate between contractions is 100 beats per minute. Which of the following nursing actions is most appropriate?

1. Encourage the client's coach to continue to encourage breathing techniques.

2. Encourage the client to continue pushing with each contraction.

3. Continue monitoring the fetal heart rate.

4. Notify the physician or nurse-midwife.

10. A nurse is caring for a client in labor and is monitoring the fetal heart rate patterns. The nurse notes the presence of episodic accelerations on the electronic fetal monitor tracing. Which of the following actions is most appropriate?

1. Document the findings and tell the mother that the monitor indicates fetal well-being.

2. Take the mother's vital signs and tell the mother that bed rest is required to conserve oxygen.

3. Notify the physician or nurse-midwife of the findings.

4. Reposition the mother and check the monitor for changes in the fetal tracing.

11. A nurse is admitting a pregnant client to the labor room and attaches an external electronic fetal monitor to the client's abdomen. After attachment of the electronic fetal monitor, the initial nursing assessment is which of the following?

1. Identifying the types of accelerations

2. Assessing the baseline fetal heart rate

3. Determining the frequency of the contractions

4. Determining the intensity of the contractions

12. A nurse is reviewing the record of a client in the labor room and notes that the nurse midwife has documented that the fetus is at −1 station. The nurse determines that the fetal presenting part is

1. 1 cm above the ischial spine.

2. 1 fingerbreadth below the symphysis pubis.

3. 1 inch below the coccyx.

4. 1 inch below the iliac crest.

13. A pregnant client is admitted to the labor room. An assessment is performed, and the nurse notes that the client's hemoglobin and hematocrit levels are low, indicating anemia. The nurse determines that the client is at risk for which of the following?

1. Anxiety

2. Low self-esteem

3. Hemorrhage

4. Postpartum infection

14. A nurse assists in the vaginal delivery of a newborn infant. After the delivery, the nurse observes the umbilical cord lengthen and a spurt of blood from the vagina. The nurse documents these observations as signs of

1. Hematoma

2. Placenta previa

3. Uterine atony

4. Placental separation

15. A client arrives at a birthing center in active labor. Her membranes are still intact, and the nurse-midwife prepares to perform an amniotomy. A nurse who is assisting the nurse-midwife explains to the client that after this procedure, she will most likely have

1. Less pressure on her cervix.

2. Increased efficiency of contractions.

3. Decreased number of contractions.

4. The need for increased maternal blood pressure monitoring.

16. A nurse is monitoring a client in labor. The nurse suspects umbilical cord compression if which of the following is noted on the external monitor tracing during a contraction?

1. Early decelerations

2. Variable decelerations

3. Late decelerations

4. Short-term variability

17. A nurse explains the purpose of effleurage to a client in early labor. The nurse tells the client that effleurage is
    1. A form of biofeedback to enhance bearing down efforts during delivery.
    2. Light stroking of the abdomen to facilitate relaxation during labor and provide tactile stimulation to the fetus.
    3. The application of pressure to the sacrum to relieve a backache.
    4. Performed to stimulate uterine activity by contracting a specific muscle group while other parts of the body rest.
18. A client in labor has been pushing effectively for 1 hour. A nurse determines that the client's primary physiological need at this time is to
    1. Change positions frequently.
    2. Ambulate.
    3. Consume oral food and fluids.
    4. Rest between contractions.
19. A client in labor is dilated 10 cm. At this time during labor, the nurse would plan to assess and document the fetal heart rate at least
    1. Before each contraction.
    2. Every 15 minutes.
    3. Every 30 minutes.
    4. Hourly.
20. A nurse is caring for a client in the second stage of labor. The client is experiencing uterine contractions every 2 minutes and cries out in pain with each contraction. The nurse recognizes this behavior as
    1. Exhaustion.
    2. Fear of losing control.
    3. Involuntary grunting.
    4. Valsalva's maneuver.

CRITICAL THINKING: PRIORITIZING (ORDERED RESPONSE)

A nurse is monitoring a client in labor who is receiving oxytocin (Pitocin) and notes that the client is experiencing hypertonic uterine contractions. List in order of priority the actions that the nurse takes. (Number 1 is the first action.)

___ Stop the oxytocin infusion.

___ Perform a vaginal examination.

___ Reposition the client.

___ Check the client's blood pressure and heart rate.

___ Administer oxygen by face mask at 8 to 10 L/min.

ANSWERS
1. **4**
Rationale: The second stage of labor begins when the cervix is dilated completely and ends with birth of the neonate. Options 1, 2, and 3 are not specific assessment findings of the second stage of labor.
Test-Taking Strategy: Use the process of elimination. Eliminate options 1 and 3 first because they are similar. From the remaining options, recalling that regular contractions occur before the second stage of labor will direct you easily to option 4. Review the stages of labor if you had difficulty with this question.
Level of Cognitive Ability: Analysis
Client Needs: Physiological Integrity
Integrated Process: Nursing Process—assessment
Content Area: Maternity—intrapartum
Reference: Wong, D., Perry, S., & Hockenberry, M. (2002). *Maternal child nursing care* (2nd ed., p. 324). St. Louis: Mosby.

2. **3**
Rationale: Late decelerations are due to uteroplacental insufficiency as the result of decreased blood flow and oxygen to the fetus during the uterine contractions. This causes hypoxemia; therefore oxygen is necessary. The supine position is avoided because it decreases uterine blood flow to the fetus. The client should be turned onto her side to displace pressure of the gravid uterus on the inferior vena cava. An intravenous oxytocin infusion is discontinued when a late deceleration is noted. The oxytoxin would cause further hypoxemia because of increased uteroplacental insufficiency resulting from stimulation of

contractions by this medication. Option 2 would delay necessary treatment.
Test-Taking Strategy: Use the ABCs—airway, breathing, and circulation—and knowledge related to the significance of a late deceleration to answer this question. Review content related to late deceleration if you had difficulty with this question.
Level of Cognitive Ability: Application
Client Needs: Physiological Integrity
Integrated Process: Nursing Process—implementation
Content Area: Maternity—intrapartum
Reference: Lowdermilk, D., & Perry, S. (2003). *Maternity nursing* (6th ed., p. 309). St. Louis: Mosby.

3. **1**
Rationale: A normal fetal heart rate is 120 to 160 beats per minute. A count of 180 beats per minute could indicate fetal distress and would warrant physician notification. White blood cells counts in a normal pregnancy begin to rise in the second trimester and peak in the third trimester, with a normal range of 11,000 to 15,000 cells/mm³, up to 18,000 cells/mm³. During the immediate postpartum period, the count may be as high as 25,000 to 30,000 cells/mm³ as a result of increased leukocytosis during delivery. By full term, a normal maternal hemoglobin range is 11 to 13 g/dL as a result of the hemodilution caused by an increase in plasma volume during pregnancy. The maternal pulse rate during pregnancy increases 10 to 15 beats per minute over prepregnancy readings to facilitate increased cardiac output, oxygen transport, and kidney filtration.
Test-Taking Strategy: Use the process of elimination, noting the key words "indicate a need to contact the physician."

Knowledge regarding the normal and abnormal findings in the pregnant client and the fetus will direct you to option 1. If you are unfamiliar with these normal and abnormal findings, review this content.

Level of Cognitive Ability: Analysis
Client Needs: Physiological Integrity
Integrated Process: Nursing Process—analysis
Content Area: Maternity—intrapartum
Reference: Matteson, P. (2001). *Women's health during the childbearing years: A community-based approach* (p. 534). St. Louis: Mosby.

4. 4

Rationale: Vena cava and descending aorta compression by the pregnant uterus impedes blood return from the lower trunk and extremities. This leads to decreasing cardiac return, cardiac output, and blood flow to the uterus and subsequently the fetus. The best position to prevent this would be side-lying with the uterus displaced off the abdominal vessels. Positioning for abdominal surgery necessitates a supine position; however, a wedge placed under the right hip provides displacement of the uterus. Trendelenburg's positioning places pressure from the pregnant uterus on the diaphragm and lungs, decreasing respiratory capacity and oxygenation. A semi-Fowler or prone position is not practical for this type of abdominal surgery.

Test-Taking Strategy: Knowledge regarding vena cava syndrome and the appropriate position to prevent this syndrome is required to answer this question. Use the process of elimination, visualizing each of the positions identified in the options and considering the effect that the position may have on the mother and the fetus. If you had difficulty with this question, review care of the mother requiring cesarean delivery.

Level of Cognitive Ability: Application
Client Needs: Physiological Integrity
Integrated Process: Nursing Process—implementation
Content Area: Maternity—intrapartum
Reference: Lowdermilk, D., & Perry, S. (2003). *Maternity nursing* (6th ed., p. 678). St. Louis: Mosby.

5. 3

Rationale: Abdominal exercises should not start immediately following abdominal surgery, and the client should wait at least 3 to 4 weeks postoperatively to allow for healing of the incision. Options 1, 2, and 4 are appropriate instructions for the client following a cesarean delivery.

Test-Taking Strategy: Use the process of elimination. Note the key words "indicates a need for further instructions." Keep in mind that the client had a cesarean delivery and noting the absolute term "immediately" in option 3 will assist in directing you to this option. Review home care instructions for the client following cesarean delivery if you had difficulty with this question.

Level of Cognitive Ability: Analysis
Client Needs: Health Promotion and Maintenance
Integrated Process: Teaching/Learning
Content Area: Maternity—intrapartum
Reference: Lowdermilk, D., & Perry, S. (2003). *Maternity nursing* (6th ed., p. 682). St. Louis: Mosby.

6. 4

Rationale: The nurse simultaneously should palpate the maternal radial or carotid pulse and auscultate the fetal heart rate (FHR) to differentiate the two. If the fetal and maternal heart rates are similar, the nurse may mistake the maternal heart rate for the FHR. Noting if the heart rate is greater than 140 beats per minute or placing the diaphragm of the Doppler on the mother's abdomen will not ensure accuracy in obtaining the FHR. Leopold's maneuvers may help the examiner locate the position of the fetus but will not ensure a distinction between the two rates.

Test-Taking Strategy: Use the process of elimination and focus on the key words "most accurately determines." Option 4 is the only option that identifies an action that will directly distinguish the maternal heart rate from the FHR. Review FHR monitoring if you had difficulty with this question.

Level of Cognitive Ability: Analysis
Client Needs: Physiological Integrity
Integrated Process: Nursing Process—implementation
Content Area: Maternity—intrapartum
Reference: Lowdermilk, D., & Perry, S. (2003). *Maternity nursing* (6th ed., p. 203). St. Louis: Mosby.

7. 2

Rationale: A normal fetal heart rate is 120 to 160 beats per minute. Bradycardia or late or variable decelerations indicate fetal distress and the need to discontinue the oxytocin. The goal of labor augmentation is to achieve three good-quality contractions (appropriate intensity and duration) in a 10-minute period. The uterus should return to resting tone between contractions, and there should be no evidence of fetal distress. Increased urinary output is unrelated to the use of oxytocin.

Test-Taking Strategy: Use the process of elimination and note the key words "infusion needs to be discontinued." Eliminate option 4 first because it is unrelated to the use of oxytocin. Next eliminate option 3 because of the key words "adequate resting tone." From the remaining options, knowing that the normal fetal heart rate is 120 to 160 beats per minute will direct you easily to option 2. Review monitoring the client receiving an oxytocin infusion if you had difficulty with this question.

Level of Cognitive Ability: Analysis
Client Needs: Physiological Integrity
Integrated Process: Nursing Process—assessment
Content Area: Maternity—intrapartum
Reference: Murray, S., McKinney, E., & Gorrie, T. (2002). *Foundations of maternal-newborn nursing* (3rd ed., p. 402). Philadelphia: W. B. Saunders.

8. 2

Rationale: Continuous electronic fetal monitoring should be implemented during an intravenous infusion of oxytocin. No data in the question indicate the need for complete bed rest or the need for antibiotics. Placing a code cart at the bedside of a client receiving an oxytocin infusion is not necessary.

Test-Taking Strategy: Use the process of elimination and the ABCs—airway, breathing, and circulation—to assist in answering the question. Option 2 is the only option that addresses oxygenation and circulation. If you had difficulty

with this question, review the nursing considerations related to the administration of oxytocin.
Level of Cognitive Ability: Application
Client Needs: Physiological Integrity
Integrated Process: Nursing Process—planning
Content Area: Maternity—intrapartum
Reference: Murray, S., McKinney, E., & Gorrie, T. (2002). *Foundations of maternal-newborn nursing* (3rd ed., p. 401). Philadelphia: W. B. Saunders.

9. 4
Rationale: A normal fetal heart rate is 120 to 160 beats per minute. Fetal bardycardia between contractions may indicate the need for immediate medical management, and the physician or nurse midwife needs to be notified. Options 1, 2, and 3 are not appropriate nursing actions in this situation.
Test-Taking Strategy: Use the process of elimination. Knowledge that the normal fetal heart rate is 120 to 160 beats per minute will assist you to easily recognize that fetal bradycardia is present. If you had difficulty with this question, review the expected and unexpected findings during the labor process.
Level of Cognitive Ability: Application
Client Needs: Physiological Integrity
Integrated Process: Nursing Process—implementation
Content Area: Maternity—intrapartum
Reference: Murray, S., McKinney, E., & Gorrie, T. (2002). *Foundations of maternal-newborn nursing* (3rd ed., p. 402). Philadelphia: W. B. Saunders.

10. 1
Rationale: Accelerations are transient increases in the fetal heart rate that often accompany contractions or are caused by fetal movement. Episodic accelerations are thought to be a sign of fetal well-being and adequate oxygen reserve. Options 2, 3, and 4 are inaccurate nursing actions and are unnecessary.
Test-Taking Strategy: Use the process of elimination. Note that options 2, 3, and 4 are similar in that they indicate the need for further intervention. Knowing that accelerations indicate fetal well-being will direct you easily to option 1. Review the significance of episodic accelerations if you had difficulty with this question.
Level of Cognitive Ability: Application
Client Needs: Physiological Integrity
Integrated Process: Nursing Process—implementation
Content Area: Maternity—intrapartum
Reference: Lowdermilk, D., & Perry, S. (2003). *Maternity nursing* (6th ed., p. 306). St. Louis: Mosby.

11. 2
Rationale: Assessing the baseline fetal heart rate is important so that abnormal variations of the baseline rate will be identified if they occur. The intensity of contractions is assessed by an internal fetal monitor, not an external fetal monitor. Options 1 and 3 are important to assess, but not as the first priority. Fetal heart rate is evaluated by assessing baseline and periodic changes. Periodic changes occur in response to the intermittent stress of uterine contractions and the baseline beat-to-beat variability of the fetal heart rate.

Test-Taking Strategy: Use the process of elimination. Note the key word "initial" in the stem of the question. Use the ABCs—airway, breathing, and circulation. Fetal heart rate reflects the ABCs. Review the concepts related to external fetal monitoring if you had difficulty with this question.
Level of Cognitive Ability: Application
Client Needs: Physiological Integrity
Integrated Process: Nursing Process—assessment
Content Area: Maternity—intrapartum
Reference: Lowdermilk, D., & Perry, S. (2003). *Maternity nursing* (6th ed., p. 303). St. Louis: Mosby.

12. 1
Rationale: Station is the relationship of the presenting part to an imaginary line drawn between the ischial spines, is measured in centimeters, and is noted as a negative number above the line and a positive number below the line. At −1 station, the fetal presenting part is 1 cm above the ischial spines.
Test-Taking Strategy: Use the process of elimination. Knowledge that station is measured in centimeters and uses the ischial spines as a reference point will assist in answering this question. Note that options 2, 3, and 4 are similar in the use of "below," which would be represented by a positive measurement in determining station. Review stations of the presenting part if you had difficulty with this question.
Level of Cognitive Ability: Analysis
Client Needs: Physiological Integrity
Integrated Process: Nursing Process—analysis
Content Area: Maternity—intrapartum
Reference: Lowdermilk, D., & Perry, S. (2003). *Maternity nursing* (6th ed., p. 260). St. Louis: Mosby.

13. 4
Rationale: Anemic women have a greater likelihood of cardiac decompensation during labor, postpartum infection, and poor wound healing. Anemia does not specifically present a risk for hemorrhage. Anxiety and low self-esteem are unrelated to physiological integrity.
Test-Taking Strategy: Use the process of elimination and Maslow's hierarchy of needs theory. Eliminate options 1 and 2 first because they are not physiological needs. From the remaining options, focusing on the issue will direct you to option 4. Review the risks associated with anemia in pregnancy if you had difficulty with this question.
Level of Cognitive Ability: Analysis
Client Needs: Physiological Integrity
Integrated Process: Nursing Process—analysis
Content Area: Maternity—intrapartum
Reference: Lowdermilk, D., & Perry, S. (2003). *Maternity nursing* (6th ed., p. 592). St. Louis: Mosby.

14. 4
Rationale: As the placenta separates, it settles downward into the lower uterine segment. The umbilical cord lengthens, and a sudden trickle or spurt of blood appears. Options 1, 2, and 3 are incorrect interpretations.
Test-Taking Strategy: Use the process of elimination. Options 1, 2, and 3 are similar in that they identify complications of pregnancy. Option 4 indicates a normal finding following

delivery of the newborn infant vaginally. Review this stage of labor if you had difficulty with this question.
Level of Cognitive Ability: Comprehension
Client Needs: Physiological Integrity
Integrated Process: Communication and Documentation
Content Area: Maternity—intrapartum
References: Lowdermilk, D., & Perry, S. (2003). *Maternity nursing* (6th ed., p. 685). St. Louis: Mosby.
Murray, S., McKinney, E., & Gorrie, T. (2002). *Foundations of maternal-newborn nursing* (3rd ed., p. 764). Philadelphia: W. B. Saunders.

15. 2
Rationale: Amniotomy (artificial rupture of the membranes) can be used to induce labor when the condition of the cervix is favorable (ripe) or to augment labor if the progress begins to slow. Rupturing of membranes allows the fetal head to contact the cervix more directly and may increase the efficiency of contractions. Increased monitoring of maternal blood pressure is not necessary following this procedure. The fetal heart rate, however, needs to be monitored frequently.
Test-Taking Strategy: Use the process of elimination. Recalling that amniotomy is performed to augment labor if the progress begins to slow will direct you easily to option 2. Review the purpose of amniotomy if you had difficulty with this question.
Level of Cognitive Ability: Application
Client Needs: Physiological Integrity
Integrated Process: Nursing Process—implementation
Content Area: Maternity—intrapartum
Reference: Lowdermilk, D., & Perry, S. (2003). *Maternity nursing* (6th ed., p. 669). St. Louis: Mosby.

16. 2
Rationale: Variable decelerations occur if the umbilical cord becomes compressed, thus reducing blood flow between the placenta and the fetus. Early decelerations result from pressure on the fetal head during a contraction. Late decelerations are an ominous pattern in labor because it suggests uteroplacental insufficiency during a contraction. Short-term variability refers to the beat-to-beat range in the fetal heart rate.
Test-Taking Strategy: Use the process of elimination, focusing on the key issue, umbilical cord compression. Recalling that variable decelerations occur if the umbilical cord becomes compressed will direct you easily to option 2. Review the findings in umbilical cord compression if you had difficulty with this question.
Level of Cognitive Ability: Analysis
Client Needs: Physiological Integrity
Integrated Process: Nursing Process—assessment
Content Area: Maternity—intrapartum
Reference: Lowdermilk, D., & Perry, S. (2003). *Maternity nursing* (6th ed., p. 307). St. Louis: Mosby.

17. 2
Rationale: Effleurage is a specific type of cutaneous stimulation involving light stroking of the abdomen and is used before transition to promote relaxation and relieve mild to moderate pain. Effleurage provides tactile stimulation to the fetus. Options 1, 3, and 4 are inaccurate descriptions of effleurage.

Test-Taking Strategy: Use the process of elimination. Focus on the key words "in early labor" to eliminate option 1. Eliminate option 3 because not all clients in labor experience backache. Eliminate option 4 because it focuses on stimulation of uterine activity rather than relaxation. Review the components of effleurage if you had difficulty with this question.
Level of Cognitive Ability: Comprehension
Client Needs: Psychosocial Integrity
Integrated Process: Teaching/Learning
Content Area: Maternity—intrapartum
Reference: Lowdermilk, D., & Perry, S. (2003). *Maternity nursing* (6th ed., p. 280). St. Louis: Mosby.

18. 4
Rationale: The birth process expends a great deal of energy. Encouraging rest between contractions conserves maternal energy, facilitating voluntary pushing efforts with contractions. Uteroplacental perfusion also is enhanced, which promotes fetal tolerance of the stress of labor. Changing positions frequently is not the primary physiological need. Ambulation is encouraged during early labor. Ice chips should be provided. Food and fluids likely are to be withheld at this time.
Test-Taking Strategy: Use the process of elimination. Focusing on the key words "pushing effectively" will assist in directing you to option 4. Review care to the client in the transition stage of labor if you had difficulty with this question.
Level of Cognitive Ability: Analysis
Client Needs: Physiological Integrity
Integrated Process: Nursing Process—analysis
Content Area: Maternity—intrapartum
References: Lowdermilk, D., & Perry, S. (2003). *Maternity nursing* (6th ed., p. 327). St. Louis: Mosby.
Matteson, P. (2001). *Women's health during the childbearing years: A community-based approach* (p. 550). St. Louis: Mosby.

19. 2
Rationale: The second stage of labor begins when the cervix is dilated completely (10 cm). Maternal pulse, blood pressure, and fetal heart rate are assessed every 5 to 15 minutes; some agency protocols recommend assessment after each contraction. Options 3 and 4 represent lengthy time intervals for assessment in this stage of labor.
Test-Taking Strategy: Use the process of elimination and focus on the data in the question, dilated 10 cm. Noting the key words "at least" will assist in directing you to the option that identifies the most frequent time frame. Review care of the client in the second stage of labor if you had difficulty with this question.
Level of Cognitive Ability: Application
Client Needs: Physiological Integrity
Integrated Process: Nursing Process—planning
Content Area: Maternity—intrapartum
Reference: Lowdermilk, D., & Perry, S. (2003). *Maternity nursing* (6th ed., p. 332). St. Louis: Mosby.

20. 2
Rationale: Pains, helplessness, panicking, and fear of losing control are possible behaviors in the second stage of labor. Options 1, 3, and 4 are not indicative of the description provided in the question.

Test-Taking Strategy: Use the process of elimination, focusing on the information provided in the question. Recalling that during the second stage of labor the woman may feel out of control will direct you to option 2. Review maternal behavioral responses during the second stage of labor if you had difficulty with this question.
Level of Cognitive Ability: Analysis
Client Needs: Psychosocial Integrity
Integrated Process: Nursing Process—assessment
Content Area: Maternity—intrapartum
References: Lowdermilk, D., & Perry, S. (2003). *Maternity nursing* (6th ed., p. 353). St. Louis: Mosby.
Murray, S., McKinney, E., & Gorrie, T. (2002). *Foundations of maternal-newborn nursing* (3rd ed., p. 279). Philadelphia: W. B. Saunders.

CRITICAL THINKING: PRIORITIZING (ORDERED RESPONSE)

Answer: 14253
Rationale: If uterine hypertonicity occurs, the nurse immediately would intervene to reduce uterine activity and increase fetal oxygenation. The nurse would stop the oxytocin infusion and increase the rate of the nonadditive solution, position the woman in a side-lying position, and administer oxygen by snug face mask at 8 to 10 L/min. The nurse then would attempt to determine the cause of the uterine hypertonicity and perform a vaginal examination to check for a prolapsed cord. The nurse would check maternal blood pressure for the presence of hypertension or hypotension.
Test-Taking Strategy: Noting that the client is experiencing uterine hypertonicity will assist in determining that the first action would be to stop the oxytocin infusion. The mother's position would be changed next because this action would immediately provide oxygen to the fetus. Because fetal oxygenation is a concern, oxygen would be administered next. The nurse then would determine the cause of the uterine hypertonicity by performing a vaginal examination and checking the client's blood pressure.
Level of Cognitive Ability: Application
Client Needs: Physiological Integrity
Integrated Process: Nursing Process—implementation
Content Area: Maternity—intrapartum
Reference: Murray, S., McKinney, E., & Gorrie, T. (2002). *Foundations of maternal-newborn nursing* (3rd ed., pp. 352, 401). Philadelphia: W. B. Saunders.

REFERENCES

Lowdermilk, D., & Perry, S. (2003). *Maternity nursing* (6th ed.). St. Louis: Mosby.

Matteson, P. (2001). *Women's health during the childbearing years: A community-based approach.* St. Louis: Mosby.

Murray, S., McKinney, E., & Gorrie, T. (2002). *Foundations of maternal-newborn nursing* (3rd ed.). Philadelphia: W. B. Saunders.

Wong, D., Perry, S., & Hockenberry, M. (2002). *Maternal child nursing care* (2nd ed.). St. Louis: Mosby.

Problems with Labor and Delivery

I. DYSTOCIA

A. Description
   1. Dystocia is difficult **labor** that is prolonged or more painful.
   2. Dystocia occurs because of problems caused by uterine contractions, the fetus, or the bones and tissues of the maternal pelvis.
   3. Contractions may be hypotonic or hypertonic.
   4. Fetus may be excessively large, malpositioned, or in an abnormal presentation.
   5. Dystocia can result in maternal dehydration, infection, fetal injury, or death.

B. Assessment
   1. Excessive abdominal pain
   2. Abnormal contraction pattern
   3. Fetal distress
   4. Maternal or fetal tachycardia
   5. Lack of progress in **labor**

C. Interventions
   1. Assess fetal heart rate; monitor for fetal distress.
   2. Monitor uterine contractions.
   3. Monitor maternal temperature and heart rate.
   4. Assist with pelvic examination, measurements, ultrasounds, and other procedures.
   5. Administer prophylactic antibiotics as prescribed to prevent infection.
   6. Administer intravenous (IV) fluids as prescribed.
   7. Monitor intake and output.
   8. Assess for dehydration.
   9. Instruct the mother in breathing techniques and relaxation exercises.
   10. Perform fetal monitoring if oxytocin (Pitocin) is prescribed.
   11. Monitor color of **amniotic fluid**.
   12. Provide rest and comfort as with a normal **delivery**, such as backrubs and position changes.
   13. Assess mother's fatigue and pain, and administer sedatives and pain medications as prescribed.
   14. Assess for prolapse of the cord after rupture of the membranes.

II. PROLAPSED CORD

A. Description: The umbilical cord is displaced, between the presenting part and the amnion or protruding through the cervix, causing compression of the cord and compromising fetal circulation.

B. Assessment
   1. Mother has a feeling that something is coming through the vagina.
   2. Umbilical cord is visible or palpable.
   3. The fetal heart rate is irregular and slow.
   4. Fetal heart monitor will show variable deceleration or bradycardia after rupture of the membranes.
   5. If fetal hypoxia is severe, violent fetal activity may occur and then cease.

C. Interventions (Box 27-1)

BOX 27-1

Interventions: Cord Prolapse

Relieve cord pressure immediately.
Reposition mother; turn her side to side or elevate her hips to shift the fetal presenting part toward her diaphragm.
Elevate fetal presenting part that is lying on the cord by applying finger pressure with a sterile gloved hand.
Do not attempt to push the cord into the uterus.
Monitor the fetal heart rate.
Assess fetus for hypoxia.
Administer oxygen by face mask to the mother as prescribed.
Prepare for emergency cesarean birth.

III. PRECIPITOUS LABOR AND DELIVERY

A. Description: **labor** lasting less than 3 hours

B. Interventions

1. Stay with the mother at all times.
2. Provide emotional support and keep the mother calm.
3. Encourage the mother to pant between contractions.
4. Prepare for rupturing membranes when the head crowns if they are not already ruptured.
5. Do not try to keep fetus from being delivered.
6. If delivery is necessary before the arrival of the health care provider, do the following:
   a. Apply gentle pressure to fetal head upward toward the vagina to prevent damage to the fetal head and vaginal lacerations.
   b. Support the infant's body during delivery.
   c. Deliver the infant between contractions, checking for the cord around the neck.
   d. Use restitution to deliver the posterior shoulder.
   e. Use gentle downward pressure to move the anterior shoulder under the pubic symphysis.
   f. Clear the infant's mouth.
   g. Dry and cover the infant to keep the body warm.
   h. Allow the **placenta** to separate naturally.
   i. Place the **infant** on the mother's abdomen or breast to induce uterine contractions.

IV. PRETERM LABOR

A. Description

1. Preterm **labor** occurs after the twentieth week but before the thirty-seventh week.
2. Contractions occur more frequent than every 10 minutes, last 30 seconds or longer, and persist.
3. Preterm labor may be associated with infection.

B. Assessment

1. Uterine contractions (painful or painless)
2. Abdominal cramping (may be accompanied by diarrhea)
3. Low back pain
4. Pelvic pressure or heaviness
5. Change in the character and amount of usual discharge; may be thicker or thinner, bloody, brown or colorless, and may be odorous
6. Rupture of amniotic membranes

C. Interventions

1. Focus on stopping the labor: identify and treat infection, restrict activity, and ensure hydration.
2. Maintain bed rest and a lateral position.
3. Monitor fetal status.
4. Administer fluids.
5. Administer medications as prescribed (Box 27-2).

V. RUPTURE OF UTERUS

A. Description

1. Complete or incomplete separation of the uterine tissue as a result of a tear in the wall of the uterus from the stress of **labor**

BOX 27-2

Medications Used in Preterm Labor

Ritodrine (Yutopar)
Magnesium sulfate
Terbutaline (Brethine)
Nifedipine (Procardia)
Indomethacin (Indocin)

---

2. Complete: a direct communication between the uterine and peritoneal cavities
3. Incomplete: a rupture into the peritoneum covering the uterus but not into the peritoneal cavity
4. Manifestations vary with the degree of rupture.

B. Assessment

1. Abdominal pain or tenderness
2. Chest pain
3. Contractions may stop or fail to progress
4. Rigid abdomen
5. Absent fetal heart rate
6. Signs of maternal shock
7. Fetus palpated outside the uterus (complete rupture)

C. Interventions

1. Monitor for and treat signs of shock (administer oxygen, IV fluids, and blood products).
2. Prepare client for cesarean section or hysterotomy with hysterectomy.
3. Provide emotional support for the client and partner.

VI. PLACENTA PREVIA

A. Description

1. Placenta previa is an improperly implanted **placenta** in the lower uterine segment near or over the internal cervical os.
2. Total: The internal os is covered entirely by the **placenta** when the cervix is dilated fully.
3. Partial: The internal os in covered incompletely.
4. Marginal: Only an edge of the **placenta** extends to the internal os but may extend onto the os during dilation of the cervix during **labor**.
5. Low-lying placenta: The placenta is implanted in the lower uterine segment but does not reach the os.
6. Management depends on the classification of the previa and gestational age of the fetus.

B. Assessment

1. Sudden onset of painless, bright red vaginal bleeding occurs in the last half of pregnancy.
2. Uterus is soft, relaxed, and nontender.
3. Fundal height may be greater than expected for gestational age.

C. Interventions

1. Monitor maternal vital signs, fetal heart rate, and fetal activity.
2. Prepare for ultrasound to confirm diagnosis.

3. Vaginal examinations or any other actions that would stimulate uterine activity is avoided.
4. Maintain bed rest in a left lateral position.
5. Monitor amount of bleeding (treat signs of shock).
6. Administer IV fluids, blood products, or tocolytic medications as prescribed.
7. If bleeding is heavy, a cesarean section may be performed.
8. Prepare to administer Rh immune globulin if the mother is Rh-negative and has not been given the injection at 28 weeks' gestation.

VII. ABRUPTIO PLACENTAE
A. Description: premature separation of the placenta from the uterine wall after the twentieth week of gestation and before the fetus is delivered
B. Assessment
1. Painful vaginal bleeding (dark red)
2. Uterine tenderness
3. Uterine rigidity
4. Severe abdominal pain
5. Signs of fetal distress
6. Signs of maternal shock if bleeding is excessive
C. Interventions
1. Monitor maternal vital signs and fetal heart rate.
2. Assess for excessive vaginal bleeding, abdominal pain, and increase in fundal height.
3. Maintain bed rest; administer oxygen, IV fluids, and blood products as prescribed.
4. Monitor and report any uterine activity.
5. Prepare for the **delivery** of the fetus as quickly as possible, with vaginal **delivery** preferable if the fetus is healthy and stable and the presenting part is in the pelvis; emergency cesarean section is performed if the fetus is alive but shows signs of distress.
6. Monitor for signs of disseminated intravascular coagulation in the postpartum period.
7. Prepare to administer Rh immune globulin.

VIII. UTERINE INVERSION
A. Description
1. Uterus completely or partly turns inside out.
2. Usually occurs during **delivery** or after **delivery** of the **placenta**.
B. Assessment
1. A depression in the fundal area of the uterus is noted.
2. Interior of the uterus may be seen through the cervix or protruding through the vagina.
3. Woman has severe pain.
4. Hemorrhage is evident.
5. Woman shows signs of shock.
C. Interventions
1. Monitor for hemorrhage and signs of shock and treat shock.

2. Prepare the client for a return of the uterus to the correct position via the vagina; if unsuccessful, laparotomy with replacement is done.

IX. AMNIOTIC FLUID EMBOLISM
A. Description
1. **Amniotic fluid** embolism is the escape of amniotic fluid into the maternal circulation.
2. The debris containing **amniotic fluid** deposits in the pulmonary arterioles and is usually fatal to the mother.
B. Assessment
1. Abrupt onset of respiratory distress and chest pain
2. Cyanosis
3. Seizures
4. Heart failure and pulmonary edema
5. Fetal bradycardia and distress if delivery has not occurred at the time of the embolism
C. Interventions
1. Institute emergency measures to maintain life.
2. Administer oxygen at 8 to 10 L/min by face mask or resuscitation bag delivering 100% oxygen.
3. Prepare for intubation and mechanical ventilation.
4. Position the woman on her side.
5. Administer IV fluids, blood products, and medications to correct coagulation failure.
6. Monitor fetal status.
7. Prepare for emergency delivery once the woman is stabilized.
8. Provide emotional support to the woman, partner, and family.

X. SUPINE HYPOTENSIVE SYNDROME
A. Description
1. Supine hypotensive syndrome occurs when the venous return to the heart is impaired by the weight of the uterus.
2. The syndrome results in partial occlusion of the vena cava and descending aorta and in reduced cardiac return, cardiac output, and blood pressure.
B. Assessment
1. Faintness, light-headedness, dizziness
2. Hypotension
3. Fetal distress
C. Interventions
1. Position the client in a lateral recumbent position to shift the weight of the fetus off the inferior vena cava.
2. Monitor vital signs and fetal heart rate.

XI. FETAL DISTRESS
A. Assessment
1. Fetal heart rate less than 120 or greater than 160 beats per minute
2. Meconium-stained **amniotic fluid**
3. Fetal hyperactivity

4. Progressive decrease in baseline variability
5. Severe variable decelerations
6. Late decelerations

B. Interventions

1. Place the mother in a lateral position; elevate her legs.
2. Administer oxygen at 8 to 10 L/min via face mask.
3. Discontinue oxytocin (Pitocin) if infusing.
4. Monitor maternal and fetal status.
5. Prepare for emergency cesarean section.

PRACTICE QUESTIONS

1. A nurse in a labor room is monitoring a client with dysfunctional labor for signs of fetal or maternal compromise. Which of the following assessment findings would alert the nurse to a compromise?
   1. Persistent nonreassuring fetal heart rate
   2. Maternal fatigue
   3. Progressive changes in the cervix
   4. Coordinated uterine contractions

2. A nurse is assigned to care for a client with hypotonic uterine dysfunction and signs of a slowing labor. The nurse is reviewing the physician's orders and would expect to note which of the following prescribed treatments for this condition?
   1. Medication that will provide sedation
   2. Increased hydration
   3. Oxytocin (Pitocin) infusion
   4. Administration of a tocolytic medication

3. A nurse in a labor room is preparing to care for a client with hypertonic uterine dysfunction. The nurse is told that the client is experiencing uncoordinated contractions that are erratic in their frequency, duration, and intensity. The priority nursing intervention in caring for the client is to
   1. Monitor the oxytocin (Pitocin) infusion closely.
   2. Provide pain relief measures.
   3. Prepare the client for an amniotomy.
   4. Promote ambulation every 30 minutes.

4. A nurse is providing emergency measures to a client in labor who has been diagnosed with a prolapsed cord. The mother becomes anxious and frightened and says to the nurse, "Why are all of these people in here? Is my baby going to be all right?" Which of the following nursing diagnoses would be most appropriate for this client at this time?
   1. Fear
   2. Powerlessness
   3. Ineffective Coping
   4. Fatigue

5. A nurse has developed a plan of care for a client experiencing dystocia and includes several nursing interventions in the plan of care. The nurse prioritizes the plan of care and selects which of the following nursing interventions as the highest priority?

1. Keeping the significant other informed of the progress of the labor
2. Providing comfort measures
3. Monitoring the fetal heart rate
4. Changing the client's position frequently

6. A maternity nurse is preparing to care for a pregnant client in labor who will be delivering twins. The nurse monitors the fetal heart rates by placing the external fetal monitor
   1. Over the fetus that is most anterior to the mother's abdomen.
   2. Over the fetus that is most posterior to the mother's abdomen.
   3. So that each fetal heart rate is monitored separately.
   4. So that one fetus is monitored for a 15-minute period followed by a 15-minute fetal monitoring period for the second fetus.

7. A nurse is preparing a plan of care for a client who just delivered a dead fetus. The most appropriate initial intervention in planning to meet the emotional needs of the client and her spouse is which of the following?
   1. Encourage the client to talk about the dead fetus.
   2. Allow the client and the spouse to hold the baby.
   3. Allow family members to name the baby.
   4. Assess the client and the spouse's perception of the event.

8. A nurse in the postpartum unit is caring for a client who has just delivered a newborn infant following a pregnancy with a placenta previa. The nurse reviews the plan of care and prepares to monitor the client for which of the following risks associated with placenta previa?
   1. Disseminated intravascular coagulation
   2. Chronic hypertension
   3. Infection
   4. Hemorrhage

9. A nurse in a delivery room is assisting with the delivery of a newborn infant. After the delivery of the newborn, the nurse assists in delivering the placenta. Which observation would indicate that the placenta has separated from the uterine wall and is ready for delivery?
   1. The umbilical cord shortens in length and changes in color.
   2. A soft and boggy uterus
   3. Maternal complaints of severe uterine cramping
   4. Changes in the shape of the uterus

10. A nurse in a labor room is performing a vaginal assessment on a pregnant client in labor. The nurse notes the presence of the umbilical cord protruding from the vagina. Which of the following would be the initial nursing action?
   1. Place the client in Trendelenburg's position.

2. Call the delivery room to notify the staff that the client will be transported immediately.

3. Gently push the cord into the vagina.

4. Find the closest telephone and stat page the physician.

11. A maternity nurse is caring for a client with abruptio placenta and is monitoring the client for disseminated intravascular coagulopathy. Which assessment finding is least likely to be associated with disseminated intravascular coagulation?

1. Swelling of the calf of one leg
2. Prolonged clotting times
3. Decreased platelet count
4. Petechiae, oozing from injection sites, and hematuria

12. A nurse is assessing a pregnant client in the second trimester of pregnancy who was admitted to the maternity unit with a suspected diagnosis of abruptio placentae. Which of the following assessment findings would the nurse expect to note if this condition is present?

1. Absence of abdominal pain
2. A soft abdomen
3. Uterine tenderness
4. Painless, bright red vaginal bleeding

13. A maternity nurse is preparing for the admission of a client in the third trimester of pregnancy who is experiencing vaginal bleeding and has a suspected diagnosis of placenta previa. The nurse reviews the physician's orders and would question which order?

1. Prepare the client for an ultrasound.
2. Obtain equipment for external electronic fetal heart rate monitoring.
3. Obtain equipment for a manual pelvic examination.
4. Prepare to draw a hemoglobin and hematocrit blood sample.

14. An ultrasound is performed on a client at term gestation who is experiencing moderate vaginal bleeding. The results of the ultrasound indicate that abruptio placentae is present. Based on these findings, the nurse would prepare the client for

1. Complete bed rest for the remainder of the pregnancy.
2. Delivery of the fetus.
3. Strict monitoring of intake and output.
4. The need for weekly monitoring of coagulation studies until the time of delivery.

15. A nurse in a labor room is assisting with the vaginal delivery of a newborn infant. The nurse would monitor the client closely for the risk of uterine rupture if which of the following occurred?

1. Hypotonic contractions
2. Forceps delivery
3. Schultz presentation
4. Weak bearing down efforts

16. A clinic nurse is performing a prenatal assessment on a pregnant client. The nurse would implement teaching related to the risk of abruptio placentae if which of the following information was obtained on assessment?

1. The client has a history of hypertension.
2. The client performs moderate exercise on a regular daily schedule.
3. The client is 28 years of age.
4. This is the second pregnancy.

17. A nurse is performing an initial assessment on a client who has just been told that a pregnancy test is positive. Which assessment finding would indicate that the client is at risk for preterm labor?

1. The client is a 35-year-old primigravida.
2. The client is a 20-year-old primigravida of average weight and height.
3. The client's hemoglobin level is 13.5 g/dL.
4. The client has a history of cardiac disease.

18. A nurse is monitoring a client who is in the active stage of labor. The client has been experiencing contractions that are short, irregular, and weak. The nurse documents that the client is experiencing which type of labor dystocia?

1. Hypotonic
2. Precipitous
3. Hypertonic
4. Preterm labor

19. A nurse is caring for a client who is experiencing a precipitous birth. The nurse is waiting for the physician to arrive. When the infant's head crowns, the nurse would instruct the client to

1. Bear down.
2. Push with each contraction.
3. Breathe rapidly (pant).
4. Hold her breath.

20. After a precipitous delivery, a nurse notes that the new mother is passive and only touches her newborn infant briefly with her fingertips. The nurse would do which of the following to help the woman process what has happened?

1. Encourage the mother to breast-feed soon after birth.
2. Tell the mother that it is important to hold the newborn infant.
3. Document a complete account of the mother's reaction on the birth record.
4. Support the mother in her reaction to the newborn infant.

CRITICAL THINKING: MULTIPLE RESPONSE

A nurse is performing an assessment on a client diagnosed with placenta previa. Select all assessment findings that the nurse would expect to note?

____ Bright red vaginal bleeding

____ Uterine rigidity

____ Soft, relaxed, nontender uterus

____ Uterine tenderness

____ Severe abdominal pain

____ Fundal height may be greater than expected for gestational age

ANSWERS

1. 1
Rationale: Signs of a fetal or maternal compromise include a persistent nonreassuring fetal heart rate, fetal acidosis, and the passage of meconium. Maternal exhaustion and infection can occur if the labor is prolonged but do not indicate fetal or maternal compromise. Progressive changes in the cervix and coordinated uterine contractions are a reassuring pattern in labor.
Test-Taking Strategy: Focus on the issue of the question, signs of fetal or maternal compromise. Use the process of elimination, noting that options 2, 3, and 4 are normal expectations during labor. Review the assessment findings that indicate fetal or maternal compromise if you had difficulty with this question.
Level of Cognitive Ability: Analysis
Client Needs: Physiological Integrity
Integrated Process: Nursing Process—assessment
Content Area: Maternity—intrapartum
Reference: Murray, S., McKinney, E., & Gorrie, T. (2002). *Foundations of maternal-newborn nursing* (3rd ed., p. 737). Philadelphia: W. B. Saunders.

2. 3
Rationale: Therapeutic management for hypotonic uterine dysfunction includes oxytocin augmentation and amniotomy to stimulate a labor that slows. A cesarean birth will be performed if no progress in labor occurs. Options 1, 2, and 4 identify therapeutic measures for a client with hypertonic dysfunction.
Test-Taking Strategy: Focus on the key word "hypotonic" to assist in answering the question. Use the process of elimination and identify the option that will assist to stimulate labor. This should direct you easily to option 3. If you had difficulty with this question, review the therapeutic management for hypotonic uterine dysfunction.
Level of Cognitive Ability: Analysis
Client Needs: Physiological Integrity
Integrated Process: Nursing Process—analysis
Content Area: Maternity—intrapartum
Reference: Murray, S., McKinney, E., & Gorrie, T. (2002). *Foundations of maternal-newborn nursing* (3rd ed., p. 738). Philadelphia: W. B. Saunders.

3. 2
Rationale: Management of hypertonic labor depends on the cause. Relief of pain is the primary intervention to promote a normal labor pattern. An amniotomy and an oxytocin infusion are not treatment measures for hypertonic dysfunction; however, these treatments may be used in clients with hypotonic dysfunction. The client with hypertonic uterine dysfunction would not be encouraged to ambulate every 30 minutes but would be encouraged to rest.
Test-Taking Strategy: Use the process of elimination, focusing on the key word "hypertonic." This key word and knowledge of the therapeutic management for this condition will assist in directing you to option 2. Options 1, 3, and 4 are therapeutic measures for hypotonic dysfunction. If you had difficulty with this question, review the therapeutic management for hypertonic uterine dysfunction.
Level of Cognitive Ability: Application
Client Needs: Physiological Integrity
Integrated Process: Nursing Process—implementation
Content Area: Maternity—intrapartum
Reference: Murray, S., McKinney, E., & Gorrie, T. (2002). *Foundations of maternal-newborn nursing* (3rd ed., p. 739). Philadelphia: W. B. Saunders.

4. 1
Rationale: The mother is anxious and frightened, and the most appropriate nursing diagnosis for the client at this time is Fear. No data in the question support a nursing diagnosis of Powerlessness, Ineffective Coping, or Fatigue, although these nursing diagnoses may be considered for this client at some point during the hospitalization experience.
Test-Taking Strategy: When answering questions related to nursing diagnosis, focus specifically on the data provided in the question. Note the relationship between the words "frightened" in the question and "Fear" in the correct option. Review maternal psychosocial responses when a prolapsed cord occurs if you had difficulty with this question.
Level of Cognitive Ability: Analysis
Client Needs: Psychosocial Integrity
Integrated Process: Nursing Process—analysis
Content Area: Maternity—intrapartum
References: Lowdermilk, D., & Perry, S. (2003). *Maternity nursing* (6th ed., p. 687). St. Louis: Mosby.
Murray, S., McKinney, E., & Gorrie, T. (2002). *Foundations of maternal-newborn nursing* (3rd ed., p. 766). Philadelphia: W. B. Saunders.

5. 3
Rationale: The priority is to monitor the fetal heart rate. Although providing comfort measures, changing the client's position frequently, and keeping the significant other informed of the progress of the labor are components of the plan of care, the fetal status would be the priority.
Test-Taking Strategy: Note the key words "highest priority." Use Maslow's hierarchy of needs theory and the ABCs—airway, breathing, and circulation—to assist in answering the question. Review priority nursing interventions for the client with dystocia if you had difficulty with this question.

Level of Cognitive Ability: Application
Client Needs: Physiological Integrity
Integrated Process: Nursing Process—planning
Content Area: Maternity—intrapartum
Reference: Wong, D., Perry, S., & Hockenberry, M. (2002). *Maternal child nursing care* (2nd ed., p. 419). St. Louis: Mosby.

6. 3
Rationale: In a client with a multifetal pregnancy, each fetal heart rate is monitored separately. Options 1, 2, and 4 are incorrect because these actions would provide information regarding the status of only one fetus at one time.
Test-Taking Strategy: Use the process of elimination. Note that options 1, 2, and 4 are similar in that they relate to monitoring only one fetus at one time. Review care of the client with a multifetal pregnancy if you had difficulty with this question.
Level of Cognitive Ability: Application
Client Needs: Physiological Integrity
Integrated Process: Nursing Process—implementation
Content Area: Maternity—intrapartum
Reference: Matteson, P. (2001). *Women's health during the childbearing years: A community-based approach* (p. 765). St. Louis: Mosby.

7. 4
Rationale: The most appropriate initial intervention in planning to meet the emotional needs of the client and her spouse is to assess their perception of the event. Although options 1, 2, and 3 are likely to be components of the plan of care, the initial intervention in planning is to assess the perception of the event.
Test-Taking Strategy: Note the key word "initial" in the stem of the question. Use the process of elimination and the steps of the nursing process to assist in answering the question. Remember that assessment is the first step in the nursing process. Review nursing interventions when fetal demise occurs if you had difficulty with this question.
Level of Cognitive Ability: Application
Client Needs: Psychosocial Integrity
Integrated Process: Caring
Content Area: Maternity—postpartum
Reference: Matteson, P. (2001). *Women's health during the childbearing years: A community-based approach* (p. 458). St. Louis: Mosby.

8. 4
Rationale: Because the placenta is implanted in the lower uterine segment, which does not contain the same intertwining musculature as the fundus of the uterus, this site is more prone to bleeding. Options 1, 2, and 3 are not risks that are related specifically to placenta previa.
Test-Taking Strategy: Use the process of elimination, focusing on the issue of the question, placenta previa. Recalling that bleeding is a primary concern in this client will direct you easily to option 4. Review the complications associated with placenta previa if you had difficulty with this question.
Level of Cognitive Ability: Analysis
Client Needs: Physiological Integrity
Integrated Process: Nursing Process—assessment
Content Area: Maternity—postpartum

Reference: Murray, S., McKinney, E., & Gorrie, T. (2002). *Foundations of maternal-newborn nursing* (3rd ed., p. 672). Philadelphia: W. B. Saunders.

9. 4
Rationale: Signs of placental separation include lengthening of the umbilical cord, a sudden gush of dark blood from the introitus, a firmly contracted uterus, and the uterus changing from a discoid to a globular shape. The client may experience vaginal fullness, but not severe uterine cramping.
Test-Taking Strategy: Use the process of elimination, reading each option carefully. Recalling that the placenta is attached to the uterine wall will assist in directing you to option 4. Review the findings associated with placental separation if you had difficulty with this question.
Level of Cognitive Ability: Analysis
Client Needs: Physiological Integrity
Integrated Process: Nursing Process—assessment
Content Area: Maternity—intrapartum
Reference: Lowdermilk, D., & Perry, S. (2003). *Maternity nursing* (6th ed., p. 366). St. Louis: Mosby.

10. 1
Rationale: When cord prolapse occurs, prompt actions are taken to relieve cord compression and increase fetal oxygenation. The mother should be positioned with the hips higher than the head to shift the fetal presenting part toward the diaphragm. The nurse should push the call light to summon help, and other staff members should call the physician and notify the delivery room. If the cord is protruding from the vagina, no attempt should be made to replace it because to do so could traumatize it and further reduce blood flow. The examiner, however, may place a gloved hand into the vagina and hold the presenting part off of the umbilical cord. Oxygen at 8 to 10 L/min by face mask is administered to the mother to increase fetal oxygenation.
Test-Taking Strategy: Use the process of elimination, noting the key words "umbilical cord protruding from the vagina." Options 2 and 4 can be eliminated first because these actions delay necessary and immediate treatment. Knowledge that the cord should not be pushed back into the vagina will easily direct you to option 1. Review priority nursing measures for prolapsed cord if you had difficulty with this question.
Level of Cognitive Ability: Application
Client Needs: Physiological Integrity
Integrated Process: Nursing Process—implementation
Content Area: Maternity—intrapartum
Reference: Lowdermilk, D., & Perry, S. (2003). *Maternity nursing* (6th ed., p. 685). St. Louis: Mosby.

11. 1
Rationale: Disseminated intravascular coagulation (DIC) is a state of diffuse clotting in which clotting factors are consumed, leading to widespread bleeding. Platelets are decreased because they are consumed by the process; coagulation studies show no clot formation (and are thus normal to prolonged); and fibrin plugs may clog the microvasculature diffusely, rather than in an isolated area. The presence of petechiae, oozing from injection sites, and hematuria are signs associated with DIC.

Swelling and pain in the calf of one leg are more likely to be associated with thrombophlebitis.

Test-Taking Strategy: Use the process of elimination. Note the key words "least likely" in the stem of the question. Knowledge that DIC is a widespread problem rather than a localized one will direct you easily to option 1. Review the signs related to DIC if you had difficulty with this question.

Level of Cognitive Ability: Analysis
Client Needs: Physiological Integrity
Integrated Process: Nursing Process—assessment
Content Area: Maternity—intrapartum
References: Lowdermilk, D., & Perry, S. (2003). *Maternity nursing* (6th ed., pp. 637-638). St. Louis: Mosby.
Wong, D., Perry, S., & Hockenberry, M. (2002). *Maternal child nursing care* (2nd ed., p. 1370). St. Louis: Mosby.

12. 3
Rationale: Painless, bright red vaginal bleeding in the second or third trimester of pregnancy is a sign of placenta previa. In abruptio placentae, acute abdominal pain is present. Uterine tenderness accompanies placental abruption, especially with a central abruption and trapped blood behind the placenta. The abdomen will feel hard and boardlike on palpation as the blood penetrates the myometrium and causes uterine irritability. Observation of the fetal monitoring often reveals increased uterine resting tone, caused by failure of the uterus to relax in an attempt to constrict blood vessels and control bleeding.

Test-Taking Strategy: Use the process of elimination. Remember that the difference between placenta previa and abruptio placentae involves the presence of uterine pain and tenderness with an abruption, as opposed to painless bleeding with a previa. Review the signs of abruptio placentae if you had difficulty with this question.

Level of Cognitive Ability: Analysis
Client Needs: Physiological Integrity
Integrated Process: Nursing Process—assessment
Content Area: Maternity—intrapartum
References: Lowdermilk, D., & Perry, S. (2003). *Maternity nursing* (6th ed., p. 633). St. Louis: Mosby.
Wong, D., Perry, S., & Hockenberry, M. (2002). *Maternal child nursing care* (2nd ed., p. 301). St. Louis: Mosby.

13. 3
Rationale: Manual pelvic examinations are contraindicated when vaginal bleeding is apparent in the third trimester until a diagnosis is made and placental previa is ruled out. Digital examination of the cervix can lead to maternal and fetal hemorrhage. A diagnosis of placenta previa is made by ultrasound. The hemoglobin and hematocrit levels are monitored, and external electronic fetal heart rate monitoring is initiated. Electronic fetal monitoring (external) is crucial in evaluating the status of the fetus who is at risk for severe hypoxia.

Test-Taking Strategy: Use the process of elimination and knowledge of the pathophysiology associated with placenta previa. Note the key words "would question which order" in the stem of the question. Also, note that option 3 is the only procedure that is invasive to the pregnancy and endangers the physiological safety of the client and the fetus. Review care of

the client with placenta previa if you had difficulty with this question.

Level of Cognitive Ability: Application
Client Needs: Physiological Integrity
Integrated Process: Nursing Process—implementation
Content Area: Maternity—intrapartum
Reference: Wong, D., Perry, S., & Hockenberry, M. (2002). *Maternal child nursing care* (2nd ed., p. 301). St. Louis: Mosby.

14. 2
Rationale: The goal of management in abruptio placentae is to control the hemorrhage and deliver the fetus as soon as possible. Delivery is the treatment of choice if the fetus is at term gestation or if the bleeding is moderate to severe and the mother or fetus is in jeopardy. Because delivery of the fetus is necessary, options 1, 3, and 4 are incorrect regarding management of the client with abruptio placentae.

Test-Taking Strategy: Use the process of elimination and knowledge regarding the management of abruptio placentae to answer the question. Note the key words "term gestation" and "moderate vaginal bleeding." Knowing that the goal is to deliver the fetus will direct you easily to option 2. If you had difficulty with this question or are unfamiliar with the management of abruptio placentae, review this content.

Level of Cognitive Ability: Application
Client Needs: Physiological Integrity
Integrated Process: Nursing Process—planning
Content Area: Maternity—intrapartum
Reference: Wong, D., Perry, S., & Hockenberry, M. (2002). *Maternal child nursing care* (2nd ed., p. 303). St. Louis: Mosby.

15. 2
Rationale: Excessive fundal pressure, forceps delivery, violent bearing down efforts, tumultuous labor, and shoulder dystocia can place a woman at risk for traumatic uterine rupture. Hypotonic contractions and weak bearing down efforts do not alone add to the risk of rupture because they do not add to the stress on the uterine wall. Schultz presentation is the expulsion of the placenta with the fetal side presenting first and is not associated with uterine rupture.

Test-Taking Strategy: Use the process of elimination. Read each option carefully, and select the option that provides an additional source of pressure to the uterus and would be most likely to add to the risk of rupturing or "tearing" the uterus. Option 2 is the only option that would provide an additional source of pressure to the uterus. Review the risks associated with uterine rupture if you had difficulty with this question.

Level of Cognitive Ability: Analysis
Client Needs: Physiological Integrity
Integrated Process: Nursing Process—assessment
Content Area: Maternity—intrapartum
Reference: Lowdermilk, D., & Perry, S. (2003). *Maternity nursing* (6th ed., p. 687). St. Louis: Mosby.

16. 1
Rationale: Abruptio placentae is associated with conditions characterized by poor uteroplacental circulation, such as hypertension, smoking, and alcohol or cocaine abuse. The condition also is associated with physical and mechanical

factors such as overdistention of the uterus that occurs with multiple gestation or polyhydramnios. In addition, a short umbilical cord, physical trauma, and increased maternal age and parity are risk factors.
Test-Taking Strategy: Use the process of elimination, focusing on the risk factors associated with abruptio placentae. Eliminate options 2, 3, and 4 because they are not situations that would present a risk for this condition. Review the risk factors associated with abruptio placentae if you had difficulty with this question.
Level of Cognitive Ability: Analysis
Client Needs: Health Promotion and Maintenance
Integrated Process: Nursing Process—assessment
Content Area: Maternity—antepartum
Reference: Lowdermilk, D., & Perry, S. (2003). *Maternity nursing* (6th ed., p. 633). St. Louis: Mosby.

17. 4
Rationale: Several factors are associated with preterm labor. These include a history of medical conditions, present and past obstetric problems, social and environmental factors, and demographic factors such as race and age. Other risk factors include a multifetal pregnancy, which contributes to overdistention of the uterus; anemia, which decreases oxygen supply to the uterus; and age less than 18 years or first pregnancy over the age of 40.
Test-Taking Strategy: Use the process of elimination and note that option 4 is the only option that identifies an abnormal condition. Options 1, 2, and 3 are average and normal findings. Review the risk factors for preterm labor if you had difficulty with this question.
Level of Cognitive Ability: Analysis
Client Needs: Physiological Integrity
Integrated Process: Nursing Process—assessment
Content Area: Maternity—antepartum
Reference: Murray, S., McKinney, E., & Gorrie, T. (2002). *Foundations of maternal-newborn nursing* (3rd ed., p. 750). Philadelphia: W. B. Saunders.

18. 1
Rationale: Hypotonic labor contractions are short, irregular, and weak and usually occur during the active phase of labor. Hypertonic dysfunction usually occurs during the latent phase of labor. Precipitous labor is that which lasts in its entirety for 3 hours or less. Preterm labor is the onset of labor after 20 weeks of gestation and before the thirty-seventh week of gestation.
Test-Taking Strategy: Use the process of elimination. Note the relationship between the words "short, irregular, and weak" in the question and "hypotonic" in the correct option. If you are unfamiliar with dysfunctional labor (dystocia), review this content.
Level of Cognitive Ability: Application
Client Needs: Physiological Integrity
Integrated Process: Communication and Documentation
Content Area: Maternity—intrapartum
Reference: Murray, S., McKinney, E., & Gorrie, T. (2002). *Foundations of maternal-newborn nursing* (3rd ed., p. 738). Philadelphia: W. B. Saunders.

19. 3
Rationale: During a precipitous birth, when the infant's head crowns, the nurse instructs the client to breathe rapidly to decrease the urge to push. The client is not instructed to push or bear down. Holding the breath decreases the amount of oxygen to the mother and to the fetus.
Test-Taking Strategy: Use the process of elimination, focusing on the key words "precipitous birth." Option 4 can be eliminated first because this action decreases the amount of oxygen to the mother and to the fetus. Next, eliminate options 1 and 2 because they are similar. Review the nursing interventions in the care of a client experiencing a precipitous birth if you had difficulty with this question.
Level of Cognitive Ability: Application
Client Needs: Physiological Integrity
Integrated Process: Nursing Process—implementation
Content Area: Maternity—intrapartum
Reference: Murray, S., McKinney, E., & Gorrie, T. (2002). *Foundations of maternal-newborn nursing* (3rd ed., p. 746). Philadelphia: W. B. Saunders.

20. 4
Rationale: Women who have experienced precipitous labor and delivery often describe feelings of disbelief that their labor progressed so rapidly. To assist the woman to process what has happened, the best option is to support the mother in her reaction to the newborn infant. Options 1, 2, and 3 do not acknowledge the mother's feelings.
Test-Taking Strategy: Use therapeutic communication techniques. Option 4 is the only option that acknowledges the mother's feelings. If you had difficulty with this question, review these techniques and care to the mother following a precipitous birth.
Level of Cognitive Ability: Application
Client Needs: Psychosocial Integrity
Integrated Process: Caring
Content Area: Maternity—postpartum
References: Lowdermilk, D., & Perry, S. (2003). *Maternity nursing* (6th ed., p. 666). St. Louis: Mosby.
Matteson, P. (2001). *Women's health during the childbearing years: A community-based approach.* (p. 775). St. Louis: Mosby.

CRITICAL THINKING: MULTIPLE RESPONSE
Answer:
Bright red vaginal bleeding
Soft, relaxed, nontender uterus
Fundal height may be greater than expected for gestational age.
Rationale: Painless, bright red vaginal bleeding in the second or third trimester of pregnancy is a sign of placenta previa. The client will have a soft, relaxed, nontender uterus, and fundal height may be greater than expected for gestational age. In abruptio placentae, acute abdominal pain is present. Uterine tenderness accompanies placental abruption. Additionally, in abruptio placentae the abdomen will feel hard and boardlike on palpation as the blood penetrates the myometrium and causes uterine irritability.
Test-Taking Strategy: Remember that the difference between placenta previa and abruptio placentae involves the presence of uterine pain and tenderness with an abruption as opposed

to painless bleeding with placenta previa. Review the signs of placenta previa and abruptio placentae if you had difficulty with this question.
Level of Cognitive Ability: Analysis
Client Needs: Physiological Integrity

Integrated Process: Nursing Process—assessment
Content Area: Maternity—intrapartum
Reference: Murray, S., McKinney, E., & Gorrie, T. (2002). *Foundations of maternal-newborn nursing* (3rd ed., p. 353). Philadelphia: W. B. Saunders.

REFERENCES

Lowdermilk, D., & Perry, S. (2003). *Maternity nursing* (6th ed.). St. Louis: Mosby.

Matteson, P. (2001). *Women's health during the childbearing years: A community-based approach.* St. Louis: Mosby.

Murray, S., McKinney, E., & Gorrie, T. (2002). *Foundations of maternal-newborn nursing* (3rd ed.). Philadelphia: W. B. Saunders.

Wong, D., Perry, S., & Hockenberry, M. (2002). *Maternal child nursing care* (2nd ed.). St. Louis: Mosby.

The Postpartum Period

I. POSTPARTUM

A. Description: period when the reproductive tract returns to the normal, nonpregnant state

B. The postpartum period starts immediately after **delivery** and is completed usually by week 6 following **delivery**.

II. PHYSIOLOGICAL MATERNAL CHANGES

A. Involution
1. Description
   a. Involution is the rapid decrease in the size of the uterus as it returns to the nonpregnant state.
   b. Clients who breast-feed may experience a more rapid involution.
2. Assessment
   a. Weight of the uterus decreases from 2 lb to 2 oz in 6 weeks.
   b. Endometrium regenerates.
   c. Fundus steadily descends into the pelvis.
   d. Fundal height decreases about 1 fingerbreadth (1 cm) per day.
   e. By 10 days postpartum, the uterus cannot be palpated abdominally.
   f. Note that a flaccid fundus indicates uterine atony and should be massaged until firm; a tender fundus indicates an infection.

B. **Lochia**
1. Description: discharge from the uterus that consists of blood from the vessels of the placental site and debris from the decidua
2. Assessment
   a. Rubra is bright red discharge that occurs from **delivery** day to day 3.
   b. Serosa is brownish pink discharge that occurs from days 4 to 10.
   c. Alba is white discharge that occurs from days 10 to 14.
   d. The discharge should smell like normal menstrual flow.
   e. Discharge decreases daily in amount.
   f. Discharge may increase with ambulation.
   g. Weigh the perineal pad before and after use and identify the amount of time between pad changes to determine most accurately the amount of lochial flow.

C. Cervix: Cervical involution occurs, and after 1 week the muscle begins to regenerate.

D. Vagina: Vaginal distention decreases, although muscle tone is never restored completely to the pregravid state.

E. Ovarian function and menstruation
1. Ovarian function depends on the rapidity with which the pituitary function is restored.
2. Menstrual flow resumes within 8 weeks in non–breast-feeding mothers.
3. Menstrual flow usually resumes within 3 to 4 months in breast-feeding mothers.
4. Breast-feeding mothers may experience amenorrhea during the entire period of lactation.
5. Women may ovulate without menstruating, so breast-feeding should not be considered a form of birth control.

F. Breasts
1. Breasts continue to secrete colostrum.
2. A decrease in estrogen and progesterone levels after **delivery** stimulates increased prolactin levels, which promote breast milk production.
3. Breasts become distended with milk on the third day.

4. Engorgement occurs in 48 to 72 hours in non–breast-feeding mothers.
5. Breast-feeding will relieve engorgement.

G. Urinary tract
1. Woman may have urinary retention as a result of loss of elasticity and tone, loss of sensation in the bladder from trauma, medications, anesthesia, and lack of privacy.
2. Diuresis usually begins within the first 12 hours after **delivery**.

H. Gastrointestinal tract
1. Women are usually hungry after **delivery**.
2. Constipation can occur.
3. Hemorrhoids are common.

I. Vital signs
1. Temperature may be elevated during the first 24 hours because of dehydration.
2. Bradycardia is common during the first week, with a range of 50 to 70 beats per minute.
3. Blood pressure remains unchanged.

III. POSTPARTUM INTERVENTIONS

A. Assessment
1. Monitor vital signs.
2. Assess pain level.
3. Assess height, consistency, and location of the fundus.
4. Monitor color, amount, and odor of **lochia**.
5. Assess breasts for engorgement.
6. Monitor perineum for swelling or discoloration.
7. Monitor episiotomy for healing.
8. Assess incisions or dressings of cesarean birth client.
9. Monitor bowel status.
10. Monitor intake and output.
11. Encourage frequent voiding.
12. Encourage ambulation.
13. Administer $Rh_0(D)$ immune globulin (RhoGam) as prescribed within 72 hours postpartum to the Rh-negative client who has given birth to an Rh-positive **neonate**.
14. Assess bonding with the newborn infant.
15. Assess emotional status.

B. Client teaching
1. Initiate counseling of the client in discharge instructions.
2. Demonstrate **newborn** care skills as necessary.
3. Provide the opportunity for the mother to bathe the **newborn infant**.
4. Instruct in feeding technique.
5. Instruct the mother to avoid heavy lifting for at least 3 weeks.
6. Instruct the mother to plan at least one rest period per day.
7. Instruct the mother that contraception should begin after **delivery** or with the initiation of intercourse (intercourse should be postponed at least until the **lochia** ceases).
8. Instruct the mother in the importance of follow-up, which should be scheduled at 4 to 6 weeks.
9. Instruct the mother to report any signs of chills, fever, increased **lochia**, or depressed feelings to the physician immediately.

IV. POSTPARTUM DISCOMFORTS

A. After-birth pains
1. After-birth pains occur as a result of contractions of the uterus.
2. After-birth pains are more common in multiparas, breast-feeding mothers, clients treated with oxytocin (Pitocin), and clients who had an overdistended uterus during pregnancy, such as with carrying twins.

B. Perineal discomfort
1. Apply ice packs to the perineum during the first 24 hours to reduce swelling.
2. After the first 24 hours, apply warmth by sitz baths.

C. Episiotomy
1. Instruct the client to administer perineal care after each voiding.
2. Encourage the use of an analgesic spray as prescribed.
3. Administer analgesics as prescribed if comfort measures are unsuccessful.

D. Breast discomfort from engorgement
1. Encourage wearing of a support bra at all times, even while the client is sleeping.
2. Encourage the use of ice packs between feedings if the client is breast-feeding.
3. Encourage the use of warm soaks or a warm shower before feeding for the breast-feeding mother.
4. Administer analgesics as prescribed if comfort measures are unsuccessful.

E. Postpartum blues (Box 28-1)
1. The postpartum blues is a condition caused by physiological and emotional stress.
2. The mother may feel upset and depressed at times.
3. Verbalization should be encouraged.
4. Postpartum blues may progress to postpartum depression if unresolved.

V. NUTRITIONAL COUNSELING

A. Discuss caloric intake with breast-feeding and non–breast-feeding mothers.
B. Nutritional needs depend on prepregnancy weight, ideal weight for height, and whether the mother is breast-feeding.
C. If the mother is breast-feeding, calorie needs increase by 200 to 500 calories per day, and the mother may require increased fluids and the continuance of prenatal vitamins and minerals.

BOX 28-1

Rubin's Postpartum Phases of Regeneration

TAKING-IN PHASE: FIRST 3 DAYS

Mother focuses on her own primary needs, such as sleep and food.

For the nurse to listen and to help the mother interpret the events of delivery to make them more meaningful is important.

This phase is not an optimum time to teach the mother about baby care.

TAKING HOLD PHASE: DAYS 3 TO 10

The woman is more in control of independence.

The woman begins to assume the tasks of mothering.

This phase is an optimum time to teach the mother about baby care.

LETTING-GO PHASE

Mother may feel deep loss over separation of the baby from part of the body and may grieve over the loss.

Mother may be caught in a dependent/independent role, wanting to feel safe and secure yet wanting to make decisions.

Teenage mothers need special consideration because of the conflict taking place within them as part of adolescence.

BOX 28-2

Breast-feeding Procedure for Mother

Wash hands and assume a comfortable position.

Start with the breast with which the last feeding ended.

Brush the newborn infant's lower lip with nipple.

Tickle the lips to have the infant open the mouth wide.

Guide the nipple and surrounding areola into the infant's mouth.

After the baby has nursed, release suction by depressing the infant's chin or inserting a clean finger into the infant's mouth.

Burp the infant after the first breast.

Repeat the procedure on the second breast until the infant stops nursing.

Burp the infant again.

Instruct the mother to listen for audible sucking and swallowing.

VI. BREAST-FEEDING

A. Interventions

1. Put the baby to breast as soon as the mother's and baby's conditions are stable (on **delivery** table if possible).

2. Stay with the mother each time she nurses until she feels secure or confident with the baby and her feelings.

3. Assess L.A.T.C.H. (L, latch achieved by infant; A, audible swallowing; T, type of nipple; C, comfort of mother; H, help given to mother with nursing).

4. Uterine cramping may occur the first day after **delivery** while the mother is nursing, when oxytocin stimulation causes the uterus to contract.

5. Use general hygiene and wash the breasts once daily.

6. If engorgement occurs, breast-feed frequently, apply warm packs before feeding, apply ice packs between feedings, and massage the breasts.

7. Do not use soap on the breasts, for it tends to remove natural oils, which increases the chance of cracked nipples.

8. If cracked nipples develop, expose the nipples to air for 10 to 20 minutes after feeding, rotate the position of the baby for each feeding, and be sure that the baby is latched on to the areola, not just the nipple.

9. Bra should be well fitted and supporting.

10. Breasts may leak between feedings or during coitus; place breast pad in bra.

11. Calories should be increased by 200 to 500 per day, and the diet should include additional fluids; prenatal vitamins should be taken as prescribed.

12. Baby's stools will be light yellow, seedy, watery, and frequent.

13. Medications should be avoided unless prescribed.

14. Gas-producing foods and caffeine should be avoided.

15. Hormonal contraceptives may cause a decrease in the milk supply and are best avoided during the first 6 weeks after birth.

16. Oral contraceptives containing estrogen are not recommended for breast-feeding mothers; progestin-only birth control pills are less likely to interfere with the milk supply.

17. Baby will develop his or her own feeding schedule.

B. Breast-feeding procedure for mother (Box 28-2)

C. Engorgement

1. Breast-feed frequently.

2. Apply warm packs before feeding.

3. Apply ice packs between feedings.

D. Cracked nipples

1. Expose nipples to air for 10 to 20 minutes after feeding.

2. Rotate the position of the baby for each feeding.

3. Be sure that the baby is latched on to the areola, not just the nipple.

PRACTICE QUESTIONS

1. A postpartum nurse is preparing to care for a woman who has just delivered a healthy newborn infant. In the immediate postpartum period the nurse plans to take the woman's vital signs

   1. Every 30 minutes during the first hour and then every hour for the next 2 hours.

   2. Every 15 minutes during the first hour and then every 30 minutes for the next 2 hours.

3. Every hour for the first 2 hours and then every 4 hours.
4. Every 5 minutes for the first 30 minutes and then every hour for the next 4 hours.

2. A postpartum nurse is taking the vital signs of a woman who delivered a healthy newborn infant 4 hours ago. The nurse notes that the mother's temperature is 100.2° F. Which of the following actions would be most appropriate?
   1. Retake the temperature in 15 minutes.
   2. Notify the physician.
   3. Document the findings.
   4. Increase hydration by encouraging oral fluids.

3. A nurse is assessing a client who is 6 hours postpartum after delivering a full-term healthy newborn infant. The client complains to the nurse of feelings of faintness and dizziness. Which of the following nursing actions would be most appropriate?
   1. Obtain hemoglobin and hematocrit levels.
   2. Instruct the mother to request help when getting out of bed.
   3. Elevate the mother's legs.
   4. Inform the nursery room nurse to avoid bringing the newborn infant to the mother until the feelings of light-headedness and dizziness have subsided.

4. A nurse is preparing to perform a fundal assessment on a postpartum client. The initial nursing action in performing this assessment is which of the following?
   1. Ask the client to turn on her side.
   2. Ask the client to lie flat on her back with the knees and legs flat and straight.
   3. Ask the mother to urinate and empty her bladder.
   4. Massage the fundus gently before determining the level of the fundus.

5. A nurse is assessing the lochia discharge on a 1 day postpartum woman. The nurse notes that the lochia is red and has a foul-smelling odor. The nurse determines that this assessment finding is
   1. Normal.
   2. Indicates the presence of infection.
   3. Indicates the need for increasing oral fluids.
   4. Indicates the need for increasing ambulation.

6. When performing a postpartum assessment on a client, a nurse notes the presence of clots in the lochia. The nurse examines the clots and notes that they are larger than 1 cm. Which of the following nursing actions is most appropriate?
   1. Document the findings.
   2. Notify the physician.
   3. Reassess the client in 2 hours.
   4. Encourage increased oral intake of fluids.

7. A nurse in a postpartum unit is instructing a mother regarding lochia and the amount of expected lochia drainage. The nurse instructs the mother that the normal amount of lochia may vary but should never exceed the need for
   1. One peripad a day.
   2. Two peripads a day.
   3. Three peripads a day.
   4. Eight peripads a day.

8. A nurse is performing a postpartum assessment on a client who is preparing to breast-feed. Which of the following breast assessment findings would the nurse determine to be the most effective for breast-feeding?
   1. Flat nipples.
   2. Inverted nipples.
   3. Erectile nipples.
   4. Nipples that are level with the skin surface.

9. A postpartum nurse is providing instructions to a woman after delivery of a healthy newborn infant. The nurse instructs the mother that she should expect normal bowel elimination to return
   1. On the day of delivery.
   2. 3 days postpartum.
   3. 7 days postpartum.
   4. Within 2 weeks postpartum.

10. A nursing student is preparing to perform a cardiovascular assessment on a postpartum woman. A nursing instructor asks the student about the procedure to elicit Homans' sign. Which response by the nursing student would indicate an understanding of this assessment technique?
    1. "I will ask the woman to raise the legs up to the waist and then to lower the legs slowly."
    2. "I will ask the woman to extend her legs flat on the bed, and I will grasp the foot and gently dorsiflex it forward."
    3. "I will ask the woman to extend the legs flat on the bed, and I will grasp the foot and sharply extend it backward."
    4. "I will ask the woman to raise the legs and to try to lower them against pressure from my hand."

CRITICAL THINKING: FILL IN THE BLANK

A postpartum nurse is monitoring the amount of lochial flow in a client following delivery. The nurse implements which procedure to determine most accurately the amount of lochial flow?

Answer: _____

ANSWERS

1. **2**

Rationale: During the immediate postpartum period, the nurse takes vital signs every 15 minutes in the first hour after birth, every 30 minutes for the next 2 hours, and every hour for the next 2 to 6 hours. The nurse monitors vital signs thereafter every 4 hours for 24 hours and every 8 to 12 hours for the remainder of the hospital stay.

Test-Taking Strategy: Use the process of elimination, noting that the nurse is caring for the client in the immediate postpartum period. Read each option carefully. Taking vital signs every 5 minutes is not necessary unless an alteration in physiological integrity has occurred during the labor period. Options 1 and 3 can be eliminated next because the time frames are not frequent enough to monitor the immediate postpartum status. If you had difficulty with this question, review postpartum assessment procedures.

Level of Cognitive Ability: Application
Client Needs: Physiological Integrity
Integrated Process: Nursing Process—planning
Content Area: Maternity—postpartum
Reference: Murray, S., McKinney, E., & Gorrie, T. (2002). *Foundations of maternal-newborn nursing* (3rd ed., p. 438). Philadelphia: W. B. Saunders.

2. **4**

Rationale: The mother's temperature may be taken every 4 hours while she is awake. Temperatures up to 100.4° F (38° C) in the first 24 hours after birth often are related to the dehydrating effects of labor. The most appropriate action is to increase hydration by encouraging oral fluids, which should bring the temperature to a normal reading. Although the nurse also would document the findings, the most appropriate action would be to increase the hydration. Contacting the physician is not necessary. Taking the temperature in another 15 minutes is not the most appropriate action.

Test-Taking Strategy: Use the process of elimination and knowledge regarding the physiological findings in the immediate postpartum period to assist in answering this question. Note the key words "most appropriate" in the stem of the question. Recalling that a temperature elevation often is related to the dehydrating effects of labor will direct you to the correct option. Review normal postpartum assessment findings if you had difficulty with this question.

Level of Cognitive Ability: Application
Client Needs: Physiological Integrity
Integrated Process: Nursing Process—implementation
Content Area: Maternity—postpartum
Reference: Murray, S., McKinney, E., & Gorrie, T. (2002). *Foundations of maternal-newborn nursing* (3rd ed., p. 440). Philadelphia: W. B. Saunders.

3. **2**

Rationale: Orthostatic hypotension may be evident during the first 8 hours after birth. Feelings of faintness or dizziness are signs that caution the nurse to beware for the client's safety. The nurse should advise the mother to get help the first few times the mother gets out of bed. Option 1 requires a physician's order. Option 3 is not the most appropriate or helpful action. Option 4 is unnecessary.

Test-Taking Strategy: Use the process of elimination and focus on the issue of the question, client safety. Option 4 is inappropriate and should be eliminated first. Elevating the client's legs is not an appropriate nursing intervention. From the remaining options recall that safety is a primary issue. This should assist in directing you to the correct option. If you had difficulty with this question, review postpartum nursing interventions.

Level of Cognitive Ability: Application
Client Needs: Safe, Effective Care Environment
Integrated Process: Nursing Process—implementation
Content Area: Maternity—postpartum
Reference: Murray, S., McKinney, E., & Gorrie, T. (2002). *Foundations of maternal-newborn nursing* (3rd ed., pp. 438-439). Philadelphia: W. B. Saunders.

4. **3**

Rationale: Before starting the fundal assessment, the nurse should ask the mother to empty her bladder so that an accurate assessment can be done. When the nurse is performing fundal assessment, the nurse asks the woman to lie flat on her back with the knees flexed. Massaging the fundus is not appropriate unless the fundus is boggy or soft, and then it should be massaged gently until firm.

Test-Taking Strategy: Use the process of elimination. Note the key words "initial nursing action" in the stem of the question. Attempt to visualize the procedure when answering the question. This should direct you easily to option 3. If you had difficulty with this question, review fundal assessment in the postpartum period.

Level of Cognitive Ability: Application
Client Needs: Physiological Integrity
Integrated Process: Nursing Process—implementation
Content Area: Maternity—postpartum
Reference: Murray, S., McKinney, E., & Gorrie, T. (2002). *Foundations of maternal-newborn nursing* (3rd ed., p. 441). Philadelphia: W. B. Saunders.

5. **2**

Rationale: Lochia, the discharge present after birth, is red for the first 1 to 3 days and gradually decreases in amount. Normal lochia has a fleshy odor. Foul-smelling or purulent lochia usually indicates infection, and these findings are not normal. Encouraging the woman to drink fluids or increase ambulation is not an accurate nursing intervention.

Test-Taking Strategy: Use the process of elimination, noting the key words "foul-smelling." This should direct you easily to option 2. If you had difficulty with this question, review normal assessment findings of lochia in the postpartum woman.

Level of Cognitive Ability: Analysis
Client Needs: Physiological Integrity
Integrated Process: Nursing Process—analysis
Content Area: Maternity—postpartum
References: Matteson, P. (2001). *Women's health during the childbearing years: A community-based approach* (p. 597). St. Louis: Mosby.
Wong, D., Perry, S., & Hockenberry, M. (2002). *Maternal child nursing care* (2nd ed., p. 447). St. Louis: Mosby.

6. **2**

Rationale: Normally one may find a few small clots in the first 1 to 2 days after birth from pooling of the blood in the vagina. Clots larger than 1 cm are considered abnormal. The cause of these clots, such as uterine atony or retained placental fragments, needs to be determined and treated to prevent further blood loss. Although the findings would be documented, the most appropriate action is to notify the physician. Reassessing the client in 2 hours would delay necessary treatment. Increasing oral intake of fluids would not be an appropriate action in this situation.

Test-Taking Strategy: Use the process of elimination, focusing on the key words "larger than 1 cm." Knowledge regarding the presence of clots in the postpartum period and their significance will direct you to option 2. If you had difficulty with this question, review normal postpartum findings in the woman.

Level of Cognitive Ability: Application
Client Needs: Physiological Integrity
Integrated Process: Nursing Process—implementation
Content Area: Maternity—postpartum
Reference: Lowdermilk, D., & Perry, S. (2003). *Maternity nursing* (6th ed., p. 394). St. Louis: Mosby.

7. **4**

Rationale: The normal amount of lochia may vary with the individual but should never exceed 4 to 8 peripads a day. The average number of peripads used is 6 per day.

Test-Taking Strategy: Use the process of elimination and knowledge regarding the normal amount of lochia drainage in the postpartum period to answer the question. Noting the key words "should never exceed" will assist in directing you to option 4. If you had difficulty with this question, review postpartum assessment.

Level of Cognitive Ability: Application
Client Needs: Health Promotion and Maintenance
Integrated Process: Teaching/Learning
Content Area: Maternity—postpartum
Reference: Lowdermilk, D., & Perry, S. (2003). *Maternity nursing* (6th ed., p. 394). St. Louis: Mosby.

8. **3**

Rationale: For the breast-feeding woman, the nurse should note the presence of an erectile nipple that the infant can latch on to easily. The nurse also should observe and palpate for nipple soreness, breast tenderness, engorgement, mastitis, the presence of colostrum, and the presence of leaking milk. A flat or inverted nipple is more difficult for the infant to grasp and may require interventions for breast-feeding to be successful. Nipples that are level with the skin surface are the same as flat nipples.

Test-Taking Strategy: Use the process of elimination, noting the issue of the question, breast-feeding and assessment of the breasts. Eliminate options 1 and 4 first because they are similar. From the remaining options, thinking about the process of breast-feeding will direct you easily to option 3. If you had difficulty with this question, review preparing the postpartum client for breast-feeding.

Level of Cognitive Ability: Analysis
Client Needs: Physiological Integrity

Integrated Process: Nursing Process—evaluation
Content Area: Maternity—postpartum
Reference: Wong, D., Perry, S., & Hockenberry, M. (2002). *Maternal child nursing care* (2nd ed., p. 199). St. Louis: Mosby.

9. **2**

Rationale: After birth, the nurse should auscultate the woman's abdomen in all four quadrants to determine the return of bowel sounds. Normal bowel elimination usually returns 2 to 3 days postpartum. Surgery, anesthesia, and the use of narcotics and pain control agents also contribute to the longer period of altered bowel functions. Options 1, 3, and 4 are incorrect.

Test-Taking Strategy: Use the process of elimination and general principles related to postpartum care to assist in answering this question. Eliminate options 3 and 4 first because of the length of time stated in these options. From the remaining options, eliminate option 1 because it would seem unreasonable that bowel function would return that quickly in the postpartum woman. Review normal gastrointestinal functions in the postpartum client if you had difficulty with this question.

Level of Cognitive Ability: Application
Client Needs: Physiological Integrity
Integrated Process: Teaching/Learning
Content Area: Maternity—postpartum
Reference: Wong, D., Perry, S., & Hockenberry, M. (2002). *Maternal child nursing care* (2nd ed., p. 499). St. Louis: Mosby.

10. **2**

Rationale: To elicit Homans' sign, the nurse asks the woman to extend her legs flat on the bed. The nurse grasps the foot and dorsiflexes it forward. If this causes any discomfort or resistance, the nurse should notify the physician or midwife that Homans' sign is present. Options 1, 3, and 4 are incorrect descriptions of this assessment technique.

Test-Taking Strategy: Knowledge regarding the assessment technique to elicit Homans' sign is required to answer this question. Use the process of elimination and visualize this technique to assist in directing you to option 2. If you had difficulty with this question, review the technique to elicit Homans' sign.

Level of Cognitive Ability: Analysis
Client Needs: Health Promotion and Maintenance
Integrated Process: Teaching/Learning
Content Area: Maternity—postpartum
Reference: Murray, S., McKinney, E., & Gorrie, T. (2002). *Foundations of maternal-newborn nursing* (3rd ed., p. 445). Philadelphia: W. B. Saunders.

CRITICAL THINKING: FILL IN THE BLANK

Answer: Weighing the perineal pad before and after use and identifying the amount of time between pad changes

Rationale: The most accurate method for determining the amount of lochial flow is to weigh the perineal pads before and after use. Once these two weights are noted, the amount of lochial flow can be determined accurately. Each gram increase in the weight is roughly equivalent to 1 milliliter of blood loss. To obtain an accurate estimate of lochial flow, the time factor must be incorporated into the analysis.

Test Taking Strategy: Note the key words "to determine most accurately the amount." Recalling the need to weigh the perineal pads and to identify the time factor between pad changes will assist you in answering the question. Review postpartum assessment measures if you had difficulty with this question.

Level of Cognitive Ability: Application
Client Needs: Physiological Integrity
Integrated Process: Nursing Process—implementation
Content Area: Maternity—postpartum
Reference: Lowdermilk, D., & Perry, S. (2003). *Maternity nursing* (6th ed., p. 394). St. Louis: Mosby.

REFERENCES

Lowdermilk, D., & Perry, S. (2003). *Maternity nursing* (6th ed.). St. Louis: Mosby.

Matteson, P. (2001). *Women's health during the childbearing years: A community-based approach.* St. Louis: Mosby.

Murray, S., McKinney, E., & Gorrie, T. (2002). *Foundations of maternal-newborn nursing* (3rd ed.). Philadelphia: W. B. Saunders.

Riordan, J., Bibb, D., Miller, M., Rawlins, T. (2001). Predicting breast-feeding duration using the LATCH breastfeeding assessment tool. *Journal of Human Lactation, 17*(1), 20-23.

Wong, D., Perry, S., & Hockenberry, M. (2002). *Maternal child nursing care* (2nd ed.). St. Louis: Mosby.

Postpartum Complications

I. CYSTITIS
A. Description: an infection of the bladder
B. Assessment
   1. Burning and pain on urination
   2. Lower abdominal pain
   3. Increased frequency of urination
   4. Costovertebral angle tenderness
   5. Fever
   6. Proteinuria, hematuria, bacteriuria, white blood cells in the urine
C. Interventions
   1. Palpate bladder for distention.
   2. Palpate fundus.
   3. Obtain urine specimen for culture and sensitivity if prescribed.
   4. Institute measures to assist the client to void.
   5. Encourage frequent and complete emptying of the bladder.
   6. Force fluids to 3000 mL per day.
   7. Administer antibiotics as prescribed after the urine culture is obtained.
   8. Instruct the client in the methods of prevention and treatment of cystitis.

II. HEMATOMA
A. Description
   1. Hematoma is a localized collection of blood into the tissues of the reproductive sac after the **delivery**.
   2. Predisposing conditions include operative **delivery** with forceps and injury to a blood vessel.
   3. Hematoma can be a life-threatening condition.
B. Assessment
   1. Abnormal severe pain
   2. Pressure in the perineal area
   3. Sensitive, bulging mass in the perineal area with discolored skin

4. Inability to void
5. Decreased hemoglobin and hematocrit levels
6. Signs of shock, such as pallor, tachycardia, and hypotension, if significant blood loss has occurred
C. Interventions
   1. Monitor vital signs.
   2. Monitor client for abnormal pain, especially when forceps **delivery** has occurred.
   3. Place ice at the hematoma site.
   4. Administer analgesics as prescribed.
   5. Monitor intake and output.
   6. Encourage fluids and voiding.
   7. Prepare for urinary catheterization if the client is unable to void.
   8. Administer blood products as prescribed.
   9. Monitor for signs of infection, such as increased temperature, pulse rate, and white blood cell count.
   10. Administer antibiotics as prescribed because infection is common following hematoma formation.
   11. Prepare for incision and evacuation of hematoma if necessary.

III. HEMORRHAGE
A. Description: bleeding of 500 mL or more following **delivery**
B. Assessment
   1. Early
      a. Hemorrhage occurs during the first 24 hours after **delivery**.
      b. Hemorrhage is caused by uterine atony, lacerations, or inversion of the uterus.
   2. Late
      a. Hemorrhage occurs after the first 24 hours following **delivery**.
      b. Hemorrhage is caused by retained placental fragments.

C. Interventions
  1. Massage fundus, with care not to overmassage.
  2. Notify physician or health care provider if hemorrhage occurs.
  3. Monitor vital signs and fundus every 5 to 15 minutes.
  4. Remain with the client.
  5. Assess and estimate blood loss by pad count.
  6. Assess level of consciousness.
  7. Administer fluids and monitor intake and output.
  8. Monitor hemoglobin and hematocrit levels.
  9. Maintain asepsis because hemorrhage predisposes to infection.
  10. Prepare for the administration of oxytocin (Pitocin) if prescribed.
  11. Prepare for the administration of blood transfusions if prescribed.

IV. INFECTION

A. Description: any infection of the reproductive organs that occurs within 28 days of **delivery** or abortion
B. Assessment
  1. Fever
  2. Chills
  3. Anorexia
  4. Pelvic discomfort or pain
  5. Vaginal discharge
  6. Elevated white blood cell count
C. Interventions
  1. Monitor vital signs and temperature every 2 to 4 hours.
  2. Make the mother as comfortable as possible; position the mother for comfort and to promote drainage.
  3. Keep the mother warmed if chilled.
  4. Isolate the baby from the mother only if the mother can infect the baby.
  5. Provide nutritious, high-calorie, protein diet.
  6. Encourage fluids to 3000 to 4000 mL per day, if not contraindicated.
  7. Encourage frequent voiding and monitor intake and output.
  8. Monitor culture results if cultures were prescribed.
  9. Administer antibiotics according to organism, as prescribed.

V. MASTITIS

A. Description
  1. Mastitis is inflammation of the breast as a result of infection.
  2. Mastitis primarily occurs in breast-feeding mothers 2 to 3 weeks after **delivery** but may occur at any time during lactation.
B. Assessment
  1. Localized heat and swelling

  2. Pain
  3. Elevated temperature
  4. Complaints of flulike symptoms
C. Interventions
  1. Instruct the mother in good hand-washing and breast hygiene techniques.
  2. Promote comfort.
  3. Apply heat or cold to site as prescribed.
  4. Maintain lactation in breast-feeding mothers.
  5. Encourage manual expression of breast milk or use of breast pump every 4 hours.
  6. Encourage mother to support breasts by wearing a supportive bra.
  7. Administer analgesics as prescribed.
  8. Administer antibiotics as prescribed.

VI. PULMONARY EMBOLISM

A. Description: the passage of thrombus, often originating in one of the uterine or other pelvic veins, into the lungs, where it disrupts the circulation of the blood
B. Assessment
  1. Dyspnea, tachypnea, and tachycardia
  2. Cough and rales
  3. Hemoptysis
  4. Pleuritic chest pain
  5. Feeling of impending doom
C. Interventions
  1. Administer oxygen as prescribed.
  2. Position client with the head of the bed elevated to promote comfort.
  3. Monitor vital signs frequently.
  4. Frequently assess respiratory rate and breath sounds.
  5. Monitor for signs of respiratory distress and for signs of increasing hypoxemia.
  6. Administer intravenous fluids as prescribed.
  7. Administer anticoagulants as prescribed.
  8. Prepare to assist physician to administer streptokinase (Streptase) to dissolve the clot if prescribed.

VII. SUBINVOLUTION

A. Description: incomplete involution or failure of the uterus to return to its normal size and condition
B. Assessment
  1. Uterine pain on palpation.
  2. Uterus is larger than expected.
  3. Greater than normal vaginal bleeding.
C. Interventions
  1. Assess vital signs.
  2. Assess uterus and fundus.
  3. Monitor for vaginal bleeding.
  4. Elevate the legs to promote venous return.
  5. Encourage frequent voiding.
  6. Monitor hemoglobin and hematocrit.
  7. Prepare to administer methylergonovine maleate (Methergine) as prescribed.

BOX 29-1

Assessment of the Types of Thrombophlebitis

SUPERFICIAL
Tenderness and pain in the affected lower extremity
Warm and pinkish red color over thrombus area
Palpable thrombus that feels bumpy and hard

FEMORAL
Chills and fever
Malaise
Pain, stiffness, and swelling of the affected leg
Shiny, white skin over the affected area
Positive Homans' sign
Diminished peripheral pulses

PELVIC
Severe chills
Dramatic body temperature changes
Occurrence of pulmonary embolism may be the first sign

BOX 29-2

Client Education for Thrombophlebitis

SUPERFICIAL
Avoid pressure behind the knees.
Avoid prolonged sitting.
Avoid constrictive clothing.
Avoid crossing the legs.
Never massage the leg.
Know how to apply support hose if prescribed.
Understand the importance of anticoagulant therapy if prescribed.
Understand the importance of follow-up with the health care provider.

VIII. THROMBOPHLEBITIS

A. Description
   1. Thrombophlebitis is a condition in which a clot forms in a vessel wall as a result of the inflammation of the vessel wall.
   2. A partial obstruction of the vessel can occur.
   3. Increased blood-clotting factors in the postpartum period place the client at risk.

B. Types
   1. Superficial thrombophlebitis
   2. Femoral thrombophlebitis
   3. Pelvic thrombophlebitis

C. Assessment (Box 29-1)

D. Interventions
   1. Assess the lower extremities for edema, tenderness, varices, and increased skin temperature.
   2. Evaluate the legs for Homans' sign by extending the legs with the knees slightly flexed and dorsiflexing the foot.
   3. Maintain bed rest.
   4. Elevate the affected leg.
   5. Apply a bed cradle and keep bedclothes off affected leg.
   6. Never massage the leg.
   7. Monitor for manifestations of pulmonary embolism.
   8. Superficial thrombophlebitis
      a. Provide bed rest.
      b. Apply hot packs to the affected site as prescribed.
      c. Apply elastic stockings.
      d. Administer analgesics as prescribed.
   9. Femoral thrombophlebitis
      a. Provide bed rest.
      b. Elevate affected leg.
      c. Apply moist heat continuously to affected area if prescribed to alleviate discomfort.
      d. Administer analgesics as prescribed.
      e. Administer antibiotics if prescribed.
      f. Prepare to administer heparin sodium intravenously to prevent further thrombus formation if prescribed.
   10. Pelvic thrombophlebitis
      a. Provide bed rest.
      b. Administer analgesics as prescribed.
      c. Administer antibiotics if prescribed.
      d. Prepare to administer heparin sodium intravenously.

E. Client education (Box 29-2)

PRACTICE QUESTIONS

1. A nurse is caring for a postpartum woman who has received epidural anesthesia and is monitoring the woman for the presence of a vulvar hematoma. Which of the following assessment findings would best indicate the presence of a hematoma?
   1. Complaints of a tearing sensation
   2. Complaints of intense pain
   3. Changes in vital signs
   4. Signs of heavy bruising

2. A nurse is developing a plan of care for a postpartum woman with a small vulvar hematoma. The nurse includes which specific intervention in the plan during the first 12 hours following delivery for this client?
   1. Assess vital signs every 4 hours.
   2. Inform health care provider of assessment findings.
   3. Measure fundal height every 4 hours.
   4. Prepare an ice pack for application to the area.

3. A new mother received epidural anesthesia during labor and had a forceps delivery after pushing for 2 hours. At 6 hours postpartum, her systolic blood pressure has dropped 20 points, her diastolic blood pressure has dropped 10 points, and her pulse is 120 beats per minute. The client is anxious and restless. On further assessment, a vulvar hematoma

is verified. After notifying the health care provider, the nurse immediately plans to
1. Monitor fundal height.
2. Apply perineal pressure.
3. Prepare the client for surgery.
4. Reassure the client.

4. After surgical evacuation and repair of a paravaginal hematoma, the mother is discharged 3 days postpartum. A nurse knows that the new mother needs further discharge instructions when the new mother states
   1. "Because I am so sore, I will nurse the baby while lying on my side."
   2. "I will probably need my mother to help me with housekeeping."
   3. "My husband and I will not have intercourse until the stitches are healed."
   4. "The only medications I will take are prenatal vitamins and stool softeners."

5. A nurse is monitoring a new mother in the postpartum period for signs of hemorrhage. Which of the following signs, if noted in the mother, would be an early sign of excessive blood loss?
   1. A temperature of 100.4° F.
   2. An increase in the pulse rate from 88 to 102 beats per minute.
   3. An increase in the respiratory rate from 18 to 22 breaths per minute.
   4. A blood pressure change from 130/88 to 124/80 mm Hg.

6. A nurse is preparing to assess the uterine fundus of a client in the immediate postpartum period. When the nurse locates the fundus, she notes that the uterus feels soft and boggy. Which of the following nursing interventions would be most appropriate initially?
   1. Massage the fundus until it is firm.
   2. Elevate the mother's legs.
   3. Push on the uterus to assist in expressing clots.
   4. Encourage the mother to void.

7. A postpartum nurse is assessing a mother who delivered a healthy newborn infant by cesarean section. The nurse is assessing for signs and symptoms of superficial venous thrombosis. Which of the following signs or symptoms would the nurse note if superficial venous thrombosis were present?
   1. Paleness of the calf area
   2. Enlarged, hardened veins
   3. Coolness of the calf area
   4. Palpable dorsalis pedis pulses

8. A nurse is developing a plan of care for a postpartum client who was diagnosed with superficial venous thrombosis. Which of the following interventions would be a component of the plan of care?
   1. Elevation of the affected extremity
   2. Ambulation 4 to 6 times daily
   3. Application of ice packs to the affected area
   4. Administration of the prescribed anticoagulants

9. A client in a postpartum unit complains of sudden sharp chest pain. The nurse notes that the client is tachycardic and the respiratory rate is elevated. The nurse suspects a pulmonary embolism. The initial nursing action would be which of the following?
   1. Assess the client's blood pressure.
   2. Initiate an intravenous line.
   3. Administer oxygen at 8 to 10 L/min by face mask.
   4. Prepare to administer morphine sulfate.

10. A nurse is providing instructions to a mother who has been diagnosed with mastitis. Which of the following statements if made by the mother indicates a need for further education?
    1. "I need to take antibiotics, and I should begin to feel better in 24 to 48 hours."
    2. "I can use analgesics to assist in alleviating some of the discomfort."
    3. "I need to wear a supportive bra to relieve the discomfort."
    4. "I need to stop breast-feeding until this condition resolves."

11. A nurse is monitoring a postpartum client in the fourth stage of labor. Which of the following findings, if noted by the nurse, would indicate a complication related to a laceration of the birth canal?
    1. The presence of dark red lochia
    2. The saturation of more than one peripad per hour
    3. Palpation of the uterus as a firm contracted ball
    4. Palpation of the fundus at the level of the umbilicus

12. A nurse is developing a plan of care for a new mother recovering from a cesarean delivery. To prevent thrombophlebitis, the nurse plans to encourage the woman to
    1. Ambulate frequently.
    2. Apply warm moist packs to the legs.
    3. Remain on bed rest.
    4. Elevate the legs.

13. A postpartum client is being treated for deep venous thrombophlebitis. A nurse understands that the client's response to treatment will be evaluated by regularly assessing the client for
    1. Dysuria, ecchymosis, and vertigo.
    2. Epistaxis, hematuria, and dysuria.
    3. Hematuria, ecchymosis, and epistaxis.
    4. Hematuria, ecchymosis, and vertigo.

14. A nurse suspects that a postpartum client with femoral thrombophlebitis has developed a pulmonary embolism. The immediate nursing action would be to
    1. Administer oxygen by face mask as prescribed at 8 to 10 L/min.
    2. Elevate the head of the bed to 30 to 45 degrees.
    3. Initiate an intravenous line if one is not already in place.
    4. Monitor vital signs.

15. A nurse performs an assessment on a client who is 4 hours postpartum. The nurse notes that the client has cool, clammy skin and is restless and excessively thirsty. The nurse prepares immediately to
    1. Assess for hypovolemia and notify the health care provider.
    2. Begin hourly pad counts and reassure the client.
    3. Begin fundal massage and start oxygen by mask.
    4. Elevate the head of the bed and assess vital signs.

16. A nurse is assessing a client in the fourth stage of labor and notes that the fundus is firm but that bleeding is excessive. The initial nursing action would be which of the following?
    1. Massage the fundus.
    2. Place the mother in Trendelenburg's position.
    3. Notify the physician.
    4. Record the findings.

17. A new mother is seen in a health care clinic 2 weeks after giving birth to a healthy newborn infant. The mother is complaining that she feels as though she has the flu and complains of fatigue and aching muscles. On further assessment the nurse notes a localized area of redness on the left breast, and the mother is diagnosed with mastitis. The mother asks the nurse about the condition. The most appropriate nursing response is which of the following?
    1. "The infection can occur at any time during breast-feeding."
    2. "The infection is most common for women who have breast-fed in the past."
    3. "The infection usually involves both breasts."
    4. "The infection usually is caused by wearing a supportive bra."

18. A nurse is providing instructions to a mother who is breast-feeding her newborn infant regarding measures to prevent postpartum mastitis. Which of the following if stated by the mother would indicate a need for further instructions?
    1. "I should change the breast pads frequently."
    2. "I should wash the nipples daily with soap and water."
    3. "I should wash my hands well before breast-feeding."
    4. "I should breast-feed every 2 to 3 hours."

19. A home care nurse visits a client who delivered a healthy newborn infant via vaginal delivery. An episiotomy was performed, and the woman has developed a wound infection at the episiotomy site. The nurse provides instructions to the mother regarding care related to the infection. Which of the following statements if made by the mother would indicate a need for further instructions?
    1. "I need to take the antibiotics as prescribed."
    2. "I need to apply warm compresses to provide comfort."
    3. "I need to take warm sitz baths to promote healing."
    4. "I need to isolate the infant for 48 hours after the initiation of the antibiotics."

20. A nurse is caring for a postpartum client with a diagnosis of deep vein thrombosis who is receiving a continuous intravenous infusion of heparin sodium. Which of the following laboratory results will the nurse specifically review to determine if an effective and appropriate dose of the heparin is being delivered?
    1. Prothrombin time
    2. International normalized ratio
    3. Activated partial thromboplastin time
    4. Platelet count

CRITICAL THINKING: MULTIPLE RESPONSE

A nurse is preparing a list of self-care instructions for a postpartum client who was diagnosed with mastitis. Select all instructions that would be included on the list.

___ Take the prescribed antibiotics until the soreness subsides.

___ Wear a supportive bra.

___ Avoid decompression of the breasts by breast-feeding or breast pump.

___ Rest during the acute phase.

___ Continue to breast-feed if the breasts are not too sore.

ANSWERS

1. **3**

Rationale: Because the woman has had epidural anesthesia and is anesthetized, she cannot feel pain, pressure, or a tearing sensation. Changes in vital signs indicate hypovolemia in the anesthetized postpartum woman with vulvar hematoma. Option 4 (heavy bruising) may be visualized, but vital sign changes indicate hematoma caused by blood collection in the perineal tissues.

Test-Taking Strategy: Use the process of elimination, noting the key words "epidural anesthesia." With this in mind, eliminate options 1 and 2. From the remaining options, use the ABCs—airway, breathing, and circulation—to direct you to option 3. Review the signs of a vulvar hematoma in a woman who had epidural anesthesia if you had difficulty with this question.

Level of Cognitive Ability: Analysis
Client Needs: Physiological Integrity
Integrated Process: Nursing Process—assessment
Content Area: Maternity—postpartum
References: Matteson, P. (2001). *Women's health during the childbearing years: A community-based approach* (p. 816). St. Louis: Mosby.

Murray, S., McKinney, E., & Gorrie, T. (2002). *Foundations of maternal-newborn nursing* (3rd ed., p. 778). Philadelphia: W. B. Saunders.

2. 4

Rationale: Application of ice will reduce swelling caused by hematoma formation in the vulvar area. Options 1, 2, and 3 are not interventions that are specific to the plan of care for a client with a small vulvar hematoma.

Test-Taking Strategy: Use the process of elimination, noting the key words "small" and "specific intervention" in the question. This focus will assist in directing you to option 4. Review nursing care of the client with a hematoma if you had difficulty with this question.

Level of Cognitive Ability: Application
Client Needs: Physiological Integrity
Integrated Process: Nursing Process—planning
Content Area: Maternity—postpartum
Reference: Wong, D., Perry, S., & Hockenberry, M. (2002). *Maternal child nursing care* (2nd ed., p. 1054). St. Louis: Mosby.

3. 3

Rationale: The use of an epidural, prolonged second-stage labor, and forceps delivery are predisposing factors for hematoma formation, and a collection of up to 500 mL of blood can occur in the vaginal area. Although the other options may be implemented, the immediate action would be to prepare the client for surgery to stop the bleeding.

Test-Taking Strategy: Use the process of elimination and note the key word "immediately." Focus on the clinical manifestations identified in the question to direct you to option 3. Review nursing content related to vulvar hematomas if you had difficulty with this question.

Level of Cognitive Ability: Application
Client Needs: Physiological Integrity
Integrated Process: Nursing Process—planning
Content Area: Maternity—postpartum
Reference: Murray, S., McKinney, E., & Gorrie, T. (2002). *Foundations of maternal-newborn nursing* (3rd ed., pp. 779-781). Philadelphia: W. B. Saunders.

4. 4

Rationale: The postoperative client will need an antibiotic because she is at increased risk for infection as a result of the break in skin integrity and collection of blood at the hematoma site. Options 1, 2, and 3 indicate that the mother understands the home care measures following surgical evacuation and repair of a paravaginal hematoma.

Test-Taking Strategy: Use the process of elimination, noting the key words "needs further discharge instructions." Recalling that the client is at increased risk for infection because of the break in skin integrity and collection of blood at the hematoma site will direct you easily to option 4. Review treatment plans associated with hematoma if you had difficulty with this question.

Level of Cognitive Ability: Analysis
Client Needs: Health Promotion and Maintenance
*Integrated Process:*Teaching/Learning
Content Area: Maternity—postpartum
Reference: Matteson, P. (2001). *Women's health during the childbearing years: A community-based approach* (p. 819). St. Louis: Mosby.

5. 2

Rationale: During the fourth stage of labor, the maternal blood pressure, pulse, and respiration should be checked every 15 minutes during the first hour. A rising pulse is an early sign of excessive blood loss because the heart pumps faster to compensate for reduced blood volume. The blood pressure will fall as the blood volume diminishes, but a decreased blood pressure would not be the earliest sign of hemorrhage. A slight rise in temperature is normal. The respiratory rate is increased slightly.

Test-Taking Strategy: Use the process of elimination, noting the key word "early" in the stem of the question. Think about the physiological occurrences of shock and the expected findings in the postpartum period. This should assist in directing you to option 2. Review signs of early hemorrhage if you had difficulty with this question.

Level of Cognitive Ability: Analysis
Client Needs: Physiological Integrity
Integrated Process: Nursing Process—analysis
Content Area: Maternity—postpartum
Reference: Murray, S., McKinney, E., & Gorrie, T. (2002). *Foundations of maternal-newborn nursing* (3rd ed., pp. 438-440). Philadelphia: W. B. Saunders.

6. 1

Rationale: If the uterus is not contracted firmly, the first intervention is to massage the fundus until it is firm and to express clots that may have accumulated in the uterus. Pushing on an uncontracted uterus can invert the uterus and cause massive hemorrhage. Elevating the client's legs and encouraging the client to void will not assist in managing uterine atony. If the uterus does not remain contracted as a result of the uterine massage, the problem may be a distended bladder and the nurse should assist the mother to urinate, but this would not be the initial action.

Test-Taking Strategy: Use the process of elimination. Note the key word "initially" in the stem of the question. Focus on the issue of the question and knowledge regarding the therapeutic management for uterine atony to assist in directing you to the correct option. If you had difficulty with this question, review therapeutic management for the client with uterine atony.

Level of Cognitive Ability: Application
Client Needs: Physiological Integrity
Integrated Process: Nursing Process—implementation
Content Area: Maternity—postpartum
Reference: Murray, S., McKinney, E., & Gorrie, T. (2002). *Foundations of maternal-newborn nursing* (3rd ed., p. 775). Philadelphia: W. B. Saunders.

7. 2

Rationale: Thrombosis of superficial veins usually is accompanied by signs and symptoms of inflammation. These include swelling of the involved extremity and redness, tenderness, and warmth. It also may be possible to palpate the enlarged, hard vein. Clients sometimes experience pain when they walk.

Test-Taking Strategy: Use the process of elimination, eliminating option 4 first because this is a normal and expected finding. Next eliminate options 1 and 3 because they are similar. If you had difficulty with this question, review the clinical manifestations associated with venous thrombosis.

Level of Cognitive Ability: Analysis
Client Needs: Physiological Integrity
Integrated Process: Nursing Process—assessment
Content Area: Maternity—postpartum
Reference: Murray, S., McKinney, E., & Gorrie, T. (2002). *Foundations of maternal-newborn nursing* (3rd ed., p. 785). Philadelphia: W. B. Saunders.

8. **1**
Rationale: Thrombosis that is limited to the superficial veins of the saphenous system is treated with analgesics, rest, and elastic support stockings. Elevation of the affected lower extremity to improve venous return also may be recommended. Warm packs may be applied to the affected area to promote healing. There is no need for anticoagulants or antiinflammatory agents unless the condition persists. After 5 to 7 days of bed rest, and when symptoms disappear, the woman may ambulate gradually.
Test-Taking Strategy: Use the process of elimination, focusing on the diagnosis of superficial venous thrombosis. Recalling that anticoagulants are not used in this disorder will assist in eliminating option 4. From the remaining options, eliminate options 2 and 3 recalling that rest and warmth is prescribed to treat this complication. Review therapeutic management of superficial venous thrombosis if you had difficulty with this question.
Level of Cognitive Ability: Application
Client Needs: Physiological Integrity
Integrated Process: Nursing Process—planning
Content Area: Maternity—postpartum
Reference: Murray, S., McKinney, E., & Gorrie, T. (2002). *Foundations of maternal-newborn nursing* (3rd ed., p. 785). Philadelphia: W. B. Saunders.

9. **3**
Rationale: If pulmonary embolism is suspected, oxygen should be administered at 8 to 10 L/min by face mask. Oxygen is used to decrease hypoxia. The woman also is kept on bed rest with the head of the bed slightly elevated to reduce dyspnea. Morphine may be prescribed for the client, but this action would not be the initial nursing action. An intravenous line also will be required, and vital signs need to be monitored, but these actions would follow the administration of the oxygen.
Test-Taking Strategy: Use the process of elimination, noting the key words "initial" in the stem of the question. Use the ABCs—airway, breathing, and circulation—to assist in directing you to option 3. If you had difficulty with this question, review therapeutic management of the client with pulmonary embolism.
Level of Cognitive Ability: Application
Client Needs: Physiological Integrity
Integrated Process: Nursing Process—implementation
Content Area: Maternity—postpartum
Reference: Murray, S., McKinney, E., & Gorrie, T. (2002). *Foundations of maternal-newborn nursing* (3rd ed., p. 788). Philadelphia: W. B. Saunders.

10. **4**
Rationale: In most cases, the mother can continue to breast-feed with both breasts. If the affected breast is too sore, the mother can pump the breast gently. Regular emptying of the breast is important to prevent abscess formation. Antibiotic therapy assists in resolving the mastitis within 24 to 48 hours. Additional supportive measures include ice packs, breast supports, and analgesics.
Test-Taking Strategy: Use the process of elimination, noting the key words "need for further education." Knowledge regarding the therapeutic management associated with mastitis will assist in eliminating options 1, 2, and 3. Review measures for the client with mastitis if you had difficulty with this question.
Level of Cognitive Ability: Analysis
Client Needs: Physiological Integrity
Integrated Process: Teaching/Learning
Content Area: Maternity—postpartum
Reference: Murray, S., McKinney, E., & Gorrie, T. (2002). *Foundations of maternal-newborn nursing* (3rd ed., p. 792). Philadelphia: W. B. Saunders.

11. **2**
Rationale: In the first 24 hours after birth, the uterus will feel like a firmly contracted ball roughly the size of a large grapefruit. One easily can locate the uterus at the level of the umbilicus. Lochia should be dark red and moderate in amount. Saturation of more than one peripad per hour is considered excessive even in the early postpartum period.
Test-Taking Strategy: Use the process of elimination, focusing on the issue of the question. Eliminate those options that indicate normal physiological findings in the fourth stage of labor. Noting the key word "saturation" in option 2 will assist in directing you to this option. Review the normal findings in the fourth stage of labor if you had difficulty with this question.
Level of Cognitive Ability: Analysis
Client Needs: Physiological Integrity
Integrated Process: Nursing Process—assessment
Content Area: Maternity—postpartum
Reference: Lowdermilk, D., & Perry, S. (2003). *Maternity nursing* (6th ed., p. 394). St. Louis: Mosby.

12. **1**
Rationale: Stasis is believed to be a predisposing factor in the development of thrombophlebitis. Because cesarean delivery is also a risk factor for thrombophlebitis, new mothers should ambulate early and frequently to promote circulation and prevent stasis. Options 2, 3, and 4 are interventions for the client diagnosed with thrombophlebitis.
Test-Taking Strategy: Use the process of elimination, noting the key words "prevent thrombophlebitis." Eliminate options 2, 3, and 4 because they are similar and are interventions for the client who has been diagnosed with thrombophlebitis. Review content related to the prevention of thrombophlebitis in the postoperative period if you had difficulty with this question.
Level of Cognitive Ability: Application
Client Needs: Health Promotion and Maintenance
Integrated Process: Teaching/Learning
Content Area: Maternity—postpartum
References: Lowdermilk, D., & Perry, S. (2003). *Maternity nursing* (6th ed., p. 703). St. Louis: Mosby.
Murray, S., McKinney, E., & Gorrie, T. (2002). *Foundations of maternal-newborn nursing* (3rd ed., p. 785). Philadelphia: W. B. Saunders.

13. 3

Rationale: The treatment for deep venous thrombophlebitis is anticoagulant therapy. The nurse assesses for bleeding, which is an adverse effect of anticoagulants. This includes hematuria, ecchymosis, and epistaxis. Dysuria and vertigo (options 1, 2, and 4) are not associated specifically with bleeding.

Test-Taking Strategy: Use the process of elimination. Recall that deep venous thrombophlebitis is treated with anticoagulant therapy and that bleeding is an adverse effect. Eliminate options 1, 2, and 4 because dysuria and vertigo are not associated specifically with bleeding. Review the treatment for deep venous thrombophlebitis and the adverse effects of treatment if you had difficulty with this question.

Level of Cognitive Ability: Analysis
Client Needs: Physiological Integrity
Integrated Process: Nursing Process—evaluation
Content Area: Maternity—postpartum
References: Hodgson, B., & Kizior, R. (2003). *Saunders nursing drug handbook 2003* (p. 543). Philadelphia: W. B. Saunders.
Lowdermilk, D., & Perry, S. (2003). *Maternity nursing* (6th ed., pp. 702-703). St. Louis: Mosby.

14. 1

Rationale: Because pulmonary circulation is compromised in the presence of an embolus, cardiorespiratory support is initiated by oxygen administration. Although options 2, 3, and 4 may be implemented, they are not the immediate nursing action.

Test-Taking Strategy: Use the process of elimination, noting the key words "immediate nursing action." This question requires that you prioritize your actions. Use the ABCs—airway, breathing, and circulation—to direct you to option 1. Review immediate interventions for the client who has developed a pulmonary embolism if you had difficulty with this question.

Level of Cognitive Ability: Application
Client Needs: Physiological Integrity
Integrated Process: Nursing Process—implementation
Content Area: Maternity—postpartum
Reference: Wong, D., Perry, S., & Hockenberry, M. (2002). *Maternal child nursing care* (2nd ed., p. 503). St. Louis: Mosby.

15. 1

Rationale: Symptoms of hypovolemia include cool, clammy, pale skin, sensations of anxiety or impending doom, restlessness, and thirst. When these symptoms are present, the nurse should further assess for hypovolemia and notify the health care provider. Option 2 will delay necessary treatment. The question gives no indication of the cause of the hypovolemia or that the client is hemorrhaging and that fundal massage is needed. The head of the bed is not elevated in a hypovolemic condition.

Test-Taking Strategy: Use the process of elimination and focus on the data provided in the question. Note the key word "immediately." Use the steps of the nursing process to select the correct option. Option 1 is the only option that addresses assessment. Review the interventions for the client experiencing hypovolemia if you had difficulty with this question.

Level of Cognitive Ability: Application
Client Needs: Physiological Integrity
Integrated Process: Nursing Process—planning

Content Area: Maternity—postpartum
References: Lowdermilk, D., & Perry, S. (2003). *Maternity nursing* (6th ed., p. 394). St. Louis: Mosby.
Wong, D., Perry, S., & Hockenberry, M. (2002). *Maternal child nursing care* (2nd ed., p. 503). St. Louis: Mosby.

16. 3

Rationale: If bleeding is excessive, the cause may be laceration of the cervix or birth canal. Massaging the fundus if it is firm will not assist in controlling the bleeding. Trendelenburg's position is to be avoided because it may interfere with cardiac function. Although the nurse would record the findings, the initial nursing action would be to contact the physician.

Test-Taking Strategy: Read the question carefully, noting the issue of the question and the clinical manifestations identified in the question. Use the process of elimination and eliminate option 1 first, because if the uterus is firm, it would not be necessary to perform fundal massage. Knowing that Trendelenburg's position is not advised will assist in eliminating this option. From the remaining options, noting the key words "bleeding is excessive" will assist in directing you to option 3. Review the interventions related to a client who is hemorrhaging if you had difficulty with this question.

Level of Cognitive Ability: Application
Client Needs: Physiological Integrity
Integrated Process: Nursing Process—implementation
Content Area: Maternity—postpartum
References: Matteson, P. (2001). *Women's health during the childbearing years: A community-based approach* (p. 557). St. Louis: Mosby.
Murray, S., McKinney, E., & Gorrie, T. (2002). *Foundations of maternal-newborn nursing* (3rd ed., p. 781). Philadelphia: W. B. Saunders.

17. 1

Rationale: Mastitis is an infection of the lactating breasts and occurs most often during the second and third weeks after birth, although it may develop at any time during breastfeeding. Mastitis is more common in mothers nursing for the first time and usually affects one breast. A supportive bra will not cause mastitis; however, constriction of the breasts from a bra that is too tight may interfere with emptying of all the ducts and may lead to infection.

Test-Taking Strategy: Use the process of elimination. Focus on the diagnosis presented in the question to assist in directing you to the correct option. If you are unfamiliar with the cause and characteristics associated with mastitis, review this content.

Level of Cognitive Ability: Application
Client Needs: Health Promotion and Maintenance
Integrated Process: Teaching/Learning
Content Area: Maternity—postpartum
References: Lowdermilk, D., & Perry, S. (2003). *Maternity nursing* (6th ed., p. 535). St. Louis: Mosby.
Murray, S., McKinney, E., & Gorrie, T. (2002). *Foundations of maternal-newborn nursing* (3rd ed., p. 792). Philadelphia: W. B. Saunders.

18. 2

Rationale: Mastitis generally is caused by an organism that enters through an injured area of the nipples such as a crack or blister. Measures to prevent the development of mastitis include changing nursing pads when they are wet and avoiding continuous pressure on the breasts. Soap is drying and could lead to cracking of the nipples, and the mother should be instructed to avoid the use of soap on the nipples during breast-feeding. The mother is taught about the importance of hand washing and that she should breast-feed every 2 to 3 hours.

Test-Taking Strategy: Use the process of elimination. Note the key words "a need for further instructions" in the stem of the question. Recalling that the use of soap is drying to the skin, could cause cracking, and thus provide an entry point for organisms will direct you easily to option 2. Review these measures if you had difficulty with this question.

Level of Cognitive Ability: Analysis
Client Needs: Health Promotion and Maintenance
Integrated Process: Teaching/Learning
Content Area: Maternity—postpartum
Reference: Murray, S., McKinney, E., & Gorrie, T. (2002). *Foundations of maternal-newborn nursing* (3rd ed., pp. 582, 792). Philadelphia: W. B. Saunders.

19. **4**
Rationale: Broad-spectrum antibiotics will be prescribed for the mother, and the mother should be instructed to take the antibiotics as prescribed. Analgesics are often necessary, and warm compresses or sitz baths may be used to provide comfort in the area. The infant is not isolated routinely from the mother with a wound infection, but the mother must be taught how to protect the infant from contact with contaminated articles.

Test-Taking Strategy: Use the process of elimination, noting the key words "need for further instructions." Eliminate options 2 and 3 first because they are similar. Knowing that the infant does not need to be isolated from the mother will assist in directing you to the correct option. Review care to the client with a wound infection from an episiotomy site if you had difficulty with this question.

Level of Cognitive Ability: Analysis
Client Needs: Health Promotion and Maintenance
Integrated Process: Teaching/Learning
Content Area: Maternity—postpartum
Reference: Murray, S., McKinney, E., & Gorrie, T. (2002). *Foundations of maternal-newborn nursing* (3rd ed., p. 791). Philadelphia: W. B. Saunders.

20. **3**
Rationale: Anticoagulation therapy may be used to prevent the extension of thrombus by delaying the clotting time of the blood. Activated partial thromboplastin time should be

monitored, and a heparin dose should be adjusted to maintain a therapeutic level of 1.5 to 2.5 times the control. The prothrombin time and the international normalized ratio are used to monitor coagulation time when warfarin (Coumadin) is used. The platelet count cannot be used to determine an adequate dosage for the heparin infusion.

Test-Taking Strategy: Knowledge regarding the administration of heparin and the laboratory tests specific to monitoring for an appropriate and effective dose is required to answer this question. Remember that the activated partial thromboplastin time is used to monitor the effectiveness of a heparin infusion. If you are unfamiliar with the administration of heparin and the specific laboratory tests that are monitored, review this content.

Level of Cognitive Ability: Analysis
Client Needs: Physiological Integrity
Integrated Process: Nursing Process—analysis
Content Area: Maternity—postpartum
Reference: Lowdermilk, D., & Perry, S. (2003). *Maternity nursing* (6th ed., p. 703). St. Louis: Mosby.

CRITICAL THINKING: MULTIPLE RESPONSE

Answer:
Wear a supportive bra.
Rest during the acute phase.
Continue to breast-feed if the breasts are not too sore.
Rationale: Mastitis is an infection of the lactating breast. Client instructions include resting during the acute phase, maintaining a fluid intake of at least 3000 mL per day, and taking analgesics to relieve discomfort. Antibiotics may be prescribed and are taken until the complete prescribed course is finished. They are not stopped when the soreness subsides. Additional supportive measures include the use of moist heat or ice packs and wearing a supportive bra. Continued decompression of the breast by breast-feeding or breast pump is important to empty the breast and prevent the formation of an abscess.

Test-Taking Strategy: Think about the pathophysiology associated with mastitis. Recalling that supportive measures include rest, moist heat or ice packs, antibiotics, analgesics, breast support, and decompression of the breasts will assist in answering the question. Review the measures to treat mastitis if you had difficulty with this question.

Level of Cognitive Ability: Application
Client Needs: Physiological Integrity
Integrated Process: Teaching/Learning
Content Area: Maternity—postpartum
Reference: Gorrie, T., McKinney, E., & Murray, S. (1998). *Foundations of maternal-newborn nursing* (2nd ed., p. 792). Philadelphia: W. B. Saunders.

REFERENCES

Gorrie, T., McKinney, E., & Murray, S. (1998). *Foundations of maternal-newborn nursing* (2nd ed., p. 792). Philadelphia: W. B. Saunders.

Hodgson, B., & Kizior, R. (2003). *Saunders nursing drug handbook 2003*. Philadelphia: W. B. Saunders.

Lowdermilk, D., & Perry, S. (2003). *Maternity nursing* (6th ed.). St. Louis: Mosby.

Matteson, P. (2001). *Women's health during the childbearing years: A community-based approach*. St. Louis: Mosby.

Murray, S., McKinney, E., & Gorrie, T. (2002). *Foundations of maternal-newborn nursing* (3rd ed.). Philadelphia: W. B. Saunders.

Wong, D., Perry, S., & Hockenberry, M. (2002). *Maternal child nursing care* (2nd ed.). St. Louis: Mosby.

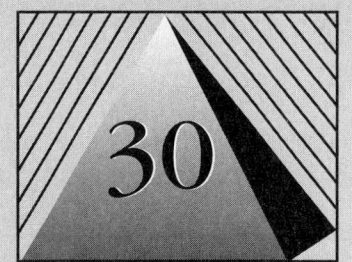

Care of the Newborn

I. INITIAL CARE OF THE NEWBORN

A. Assessment
1. Observe or assist with initiation of respirations.
2. Assess Apgar score.
3. Note characteristics of cry.
4. Monitor for nasal flaring, grunting, retractions, and abnormal respirations.
5. Obtain vital signs.
6. Observe **newborn** for signs of hypothermia or hyperthermia.
7. Assess for gross anomalies.

B. Interventions
1. Suction mouth, then nares, with bulb syringe.
2. Dry **newborn** and stimulate crying by rubbing.
3. Maintain temperature stability; wrap **newborn** in warm blankets and place a stockinette cap on newborn's head.
4. Keep **newborn** with mother to facilitate bonding.
5. Place **newborn** at mother's breast if breast-feeding is planned, or place on mother's abdomen.
6. Place **newborn** in warmer.
7. Position **newborn** on side or abdomen or in modified Trendelenburg's position to facilitate drainage of mucus.

8. Ensure newborn's proper identification.
9. Footprint **newborn** and fingerprint mother on identification sheet per agency policies and procedures.
10. Place matching identification bracelets on mother and **newborn**.

C. Apgar scoring system
1. Perform and record the Apgar score at 1 minute and at 5 minutes.
2. Assess each of five items to be scored, and assign value of 0 (very poor) to 2 (excellent) for each item.
3. Add the points to determine the newborn's total score.
4. Five vital indicators (Table 30-1)
5. Interventions: Apgar score (Table 30-2)

II. INITIAL PHYSICAL EXAMINATION

A. General guidelines
1. Keep **newborn** warm during the examination.
2. Begin with general observations and then perform assessments that are least disturbing to the **newborn** first.
3. Initiate nursing interventions for abnormal findings.
4. Document all abnormal findings.

TABLE 30-1

Five Vital Indicators of Apgar Scoring

Indicator	0 Points	1 Point	2 Points
Heart rate	Absent	Less than 100 beats per minute	More than 100 beats per minute
Respiratory rate	Absent	Slow, irregular, weak cry	Good, vigorous cry
Muscle tone	Flaccid, limp	Minimal flexion of extremities	Good flexion, active motion
Reflex irritability	No response	Minimal response (grimace) to suction or gentle slap on soles	Responds promptly with a cry or active movement
Skin color	Pallor or cyanosis	Body skin normal, extremities blue	Body and extremity skin color normal

TABLE 30-2

Apgar Score Interventions

Score	Intervention
8 to 10	No intervention is required except to support the infant's spontaneous efforts.
4 to 7	Gently stimulate. Rub infant's back. Administer oxygen to infant.
0 to 3	Infant requires resuscitation.

B. Vital signs
   1. Heart rate: 100 to 170 beats per minute (apical); assess for a full minute because of irregularities after birth
   2. Respirations: 30 to 80 breaths per minute; assess for a full minute
   3. Axillary temperature: 96.8° to 99° F
   4. Blood pressure: 73/55 mm Hg
C. Body measurements
   1. Length: 45 to 55 cm (18 to 22 inches)
   2. Weight: 2500 to 4300 g (5.5 to 9.5 lb)
   3. Head circumference: 33 to 35.5 cm (13 to 14 inches)
   4. Chest circumference: 30 to 33 cm (12 to 13 inches) and should be equal to or 2 to 3 cm less than the head circumference
D. Head
   1. Head should be 25% of the body length (cephalocaudal development).
   2. Bones of the skull are not fused.
   3. Sutures are palpable (connective tissue between the skull bones).
   4. Fontanels are unossified membranous tissue at the junction of the sutures (Table 30-3).
   5. Molding is asymmetry of the head resulting from pressure in the birth canal; molding disappears in about 72 hours.
   6. Masses from birth trauma
      a. Caput succedaneum is edema of the soft tissue over bone (crosses over suture line); it subsides within a few days.

TABLE 30-3

Fontanels

Fontanel	Characteristics	Closure
Anterior	Soft, flat, diamond shaped, 3 to 4 cm wide by 2 to 3 cm long	Between 12 and 18 months of age
Posterior	Triangular, 0.5 to 1 cm wide Located between occipital and parietal bones	Between birth and 2 to 3 months of age

      b. Cephalhematoma is swelling caused by bleeding into an area between the bone and its periosteum (does not cross over suture line); it usually is absorbed within 6 weeks with no treatment.
   7. Head lag
      a. Common when pulling **newborn** to a sitting position
      b. When prone, **newborn** should be able to lift the head slightly and turn the head from side to side
E. Eyes
   1. Slate gray (light skin) or brown-gray (dark skin)
   2. Symmetrical and clear
   3. Pupils equal, round, react to light by accommodation
   4. Blink reflex present
   5. Eyes cross because of weak extraocular muscles
   6. Ability to track and fixate momentarily
   7. Red reflex present
   8. Eyelids often edematous as a result of pressure during the birth process and the effects of eye medication
F. Ears
   1. Symmetrical
   2. Firm cartilage with recoil
   3. Pinna on or above line drawn from canthus of eye
   4. Low-set ears are associated with Down syndrome
G. Nose
   1. Flat, broad, in center of face
   2. Obligatory nose breathing
   3. Occasional sneezing to remove obstructions
H. Mouth
   1. Pink, moist gums
   2. Soft and hard palates intact
   3. Epstein's pearls (small, white cysts) that may be present on hard palate
   4. Uvula in midline
   5. Freely moving tongue that is symmetrical and has short frenulum
   6. Sucking and crying movements symmetrical
   7. Able to swallow
   8. Gag reflex present
I. Neck
   1. Short and thick
   2. Head held in midline
   3. Trachea on midline
   4. Good range of motion and ability to flex and extend
J. Chest
   1. Circular appearance because anteroposterior and lateral diameters are about equal
   2. Diaphragmatic respirations
   3. Bronchial sounds heard on auscultation
   4. Nipples prominent and often edematous
   5. Milky secretion (witch's milk) common
   6. Breast tissue present

7. Clavicles need to be palpated to assess for fractures

K. Skin
1. Pinkish red (light-skinned **newborn**) to pinkish brown or pinkish yellow (dark-skinned **newborn**)
2. Vernix caseosa
3. Lanugo
4. Milia
5. Dry, peeling skin
6. Dark red color common in premature newborns
7. Cyanosis common with hypothermia, infection, and hypoglycemia, and with cardiac, respiratory, or neurological abnormalities
8. Acrocyanosis (peripheral cyanosis) normal in the first few hours after birth and if the infant becomes cold and results from poor perfusion of blood to the periphery of the body
9. Assessment for ecchymosis and petechiae resulting from the trauma of birth
10. Assessment of skin turgor over the abdomen to determine hydration status
11. Observation for forceps marks
12. Harlequin sign
   a. Deep pink or red color develops over one side of the newborn's body while the other side remains pale or of normal color.
   b. Harlequin sign may indicate shunting of blood with a cardiac problem or may indicate sepsis.
13. Birthmarks (Table 30-4)

L. Abdomen
1. Umbilical cord
   a. The umbilical cord should have three vessels, two arteries and one vein; if fewer than three vessels are noted, notify the physician.
   b. Small, thin cord may be associated with poor fetal growth.
   c. Assess for intact cord, and ensure that the cord clamp is secured.
   d. Cord should be clamped for at least the first 24 hours after birth; clamp can be removed when the cord is dried and occluded.
   e. Note any bleeding or drainage from the cord.
   f. Triple dye or alcohol may be applied for initial cord care because it minimizes microorganism growth and promotes drying; use a cotton-tipped applicator to paint the dye, one time, on the cord and on 1 inch of surrounding skin.
   g. Application of alcohol to the cord should be done with each diaper change and at least 2 or 3 times a day to minimize microorganism growth and promote drying.
   h. If symptoms of infection such as moistness, oozing, discharge, and a reddened base occur, antibiotic treatment is prescribed.
2. Gastrointestinal
   a. Monitor cord for meconium staining.

TABLE 30-4

Birthmarks

Birthmark	Characteristics
Telangiectatic nevi (stork bites)	Pale pink or red, flat, dilated capillaries
	On eyelids, nose, lower occipital bone, and nape of neck
	Easily blanch
	More noticeable during crying periods
	Disappear by age 2 years
Nevus flammeus (port-wine stain)	Capillary angioma directly below epidermis
	Nonelevated, sharply demarcated, red to purple, dense areas of capillaries
	Commonly appearing on face
	No fading with time
	May require surgery in the future
Nevus vasculosus (strawberry mark)	Capillary hemangioma
	Raised, clearly delineated, dark red, with a rough surface
	Common in head region
	Disappears by age 7 to 9 years
Mongolian spots	Bluish black pigmentation
	On lumbar dorsal area and buttocks
	Gradual fading during first and second years of life
	Common in Asian and dark-skinned races

   b. Assess for umbilical hernia.
   c. Note for abdominal depression associated with diaphragmatic hernia.
   d. Assess for abdominal distention associated with obstruction, mass, or sepsis.
   e. Monitor bowel sounds, which should occur within 1 to 2 hours after birth.
3. Anus
   a. Ensure that anal opening is patent.
   b. First-stool meconium should pass within first 24 hours.

M. Genitals
1. Female
   a. Labia are edematous; clitoris is enlarged.
   b. Smegma may be present (thick, white mucus discharge).
   c. Pseudomenstruation is possible (blood-tinged mucus).
   d. Hymen tag may be visible.
   e. First voiding should occur within 24 hours.
2. Male
   a. Prepuce (foreskin) covers glans penis.
   b. Scrotum is edematous.
   c. Verify meatus at tip of penis.
   d. Testes descended but may retract with cold.

e. Assess for hernia or hydrocele.

f. First voiding should occur within 24 hours.

N. Spine
1. Straight
2. Posture flexed
3. Supportive of head momentarily when prone
4. Arms and legs flexed
5. Chin flexed on upper chest
6. Well-coordinated, sporadic movements
7. A degree of hypotonicity or hypertonicity indicative of central nervous system damage

O. Extremities
1. Flexed
2. Full range of motion; symmetrical movements
3. Fists clenched
4. Ten fingers and 10 toes, all separate
5. Legs bowed
6. Major gluteal folds even
7. Creases on soles of feet
8. Assessment for fractures (especially clavicle) or dislocations (hip)
9. Assessment for hip dysplasia; when thighs are rotated outward, no clicks should be heard
10. Pulses palpable (radial, brachial, femoral)
11. Slight tremors common but could be a sign of hypoglycemia or drug withdrawal

III. BODY SYSTEMS ASSESSMENT

A. Cardiovascular system
1. Keep **newborn** warm.
2. Take apical heart rate for 1 full minute.
3. Listen for murmurs.
4. Palpate pulses.
5. Assess for cyanosis; blanch skin on trunk and extremities to assess circulation.
6. Observe for cardiac distress when **newborn** is feeding.

B. Respiratory system
1. Position **newborn** on side.
2. Suction airway as necessary: use a bulb syringe for upper airway suctioning (compress bulb before insertion) and a French catheter for deeper suctioning.
3. Observe for respiratory distress and hypoxemia.
   a. Nasal flaring
   b. Increasingly severe retractions
   c. Grunting
   d. Cyanosis
   e. Bradycardia and periods of apnea lasting longer than 15 seconds
4. Administer oxygen via hood if necessary and as prescribed.

C. Hepatic system
1. Normal or physiological jaundice appears after the first 24 hours in full-term neonates and after the first 48 hours in premature neonates; jaundice occurring before this time (pathological jaundice) may indicate early hemolysis of red blood cells and must be reported to the physician.
2. Physiological jaundice peaks about the fifth day of life (indirect bilirubin levels: 6 to 7 mg/dL).
3. Monitor serum bilirubin levels.
4. Feed early to stimulate intestinal activity and to keep the bilirubin level low.
5. Prevent chilling, because hypothermia can cause acidosis that interferes with bilirubin conjugation and excretion.
6. Liver stores iron passed from the mother for 5 to 6 months.
7. Glycogen storage occurs in the liver.
8. **Neonate** is at risk for hemorrhagic disorders; coagulation factors synthesized in the liver depend on vitamin K, which is not synthesized until intestinal bacteria are present.
9. Handle **neonate** carefully and monitor for any bruising or bleeding episodes.
10. Watch for meconium stool and subsequent stools.
11. Administer one dose of vitamin K (AquaMEPHYTON), 0.5 to 1.0 mg intramuscularly as prescribed, to the **neonate** in the lateral aspect of the middle third of the vastus lateralis muscle to prevent hemorrhagic disorders.
12. Assess newborn's hemoglobin and blood glucose levels.

D. Renal system
1. The immature kidneys are unable to concentrate urine.
2. A weight loss of 5% to 15% during the first week of life occurs as a result of voiding and limited intake.
3. Weigh **newborn** daily.
4. Monitor intake and output; weigh diapers if necessary.
5. Measure specific gravity of urine if necessary.
6. Assess for signs of dehydration (dry mucous membranes, sunken eyeballs, poor skin turgor, sunken fontanels).

E. Immune system
1. Newborn receives passive immunity via the **placenta** (immunoglobulin G).
2. Newborn receives passive immunity from colostrum (immunoglobulin A).
3. Elevations in immunoglobulin M indicate infection in utero.
4. Use aseptic technique when caring for the **newborn**.
5. Observe standard precautions when handling the **newborn**.
6. Ensure meticulous hand washing.
7. Ensure that an infection-free staff cares for the **newborn**.
8. Monitor newborn's temperature.
9. Observe for any cracks or openings in the skin.

10. Administer eye medication within 1 hour after birth to prevent ophthalmia neonatorum.
    a. Eye prophylaxis may be delayed until an hour or so after birth to facilitate eye contact and parent-infant attachment and bonding.
    b. Erythromycin (0.5%) and tetracycline (1%) ophthalmic ointment or drops are bacteriostatic and bactericidal and provide prophylaxis against *Neisseria gonorrhoeae* and *Chlamydia trachomatis*.
    c. Silver nitrate (1%) solution may be prescribed, but its use is minimal because it does not protect against chlamydial infection and can cause chemical conjunctivitis.
11. Provide cord care.
    a. Umbilical clamp can be removed after 24 hours.
    b. Teach mother how to perform cord care.
    c. Keep the cord clean and dry; wash with soap and water at least 2 or 3 times a day.
    d. Keep diaper from covering cord; fold diaper below cord.
    e. Assess cord for odor, swelling, or discharge.
    f. The **newborn** is cleaned via a sponge bath until the cord falls off (within 2 weeks).
12. Provide circumcision care.
    a. Apply petroleum jelly gauze to the penis except when a Plastibell is used.
    b. Remove petroleum jelly gauze, if applied, after first voiding following circumcision.
    c. Observe for swelling, infection, or bleeding from the circumcision site.
    d. Teach mother care of circumcision site.
    e. Cleanse the penis after each voiding by squeezing warm water over the penis.
    f. A milky covering over the glans penis is normal and should not be disrupted.
    g. Monitor for urinary retention.

F. Metabolic system and gastrointestinal system
1. Newborns are able to digest simple carbohydrates but are unable to digest fats because of the lack of lipase.
2. Proteins may be broken down only partially, so they may serve as antigens and provoke an allergic reaction.
3. The **newborn** has a small stomach capacity (about 90 mL) with rapid intestinal peristalsis (bowel emptying time is 2.5 to 3 hours).
4. Breast-feeding usually can begin immediately after birth; bottle-fed newborns may be offered a few milliliters of sterile water or 5% dextrose 1 to 4 hours after birth before a feeding with formula.
5. Observe feeding reflexes, such as rooting, sucking, and swallowing.
6. Assist mother with breast-feeding or formula feeding.
7. Burp **newborn** during and after feeding.
8. Assess for regurgitation or vomiting.

9. Position **newborn** on right side after feeding.
10. Observe for normal stool and the passage of meconium.
    a. Meconium stool, which is greenish black with a thick, sticky, tarlike consistency, usually is passed within the first 24 hours of life.
    b. Transitional stool, the second type of stool excreted by the **newborn**, is greenish brown and of looser consistency than meconium.
    c. Seedy, yellow stools are noted in breast-fed newborns; pale yellow to light brown stools in formula-fed newborns.
11. Perform **newborn** screening test (includes the test for phenylketonuria) before discharge after sufficient protein intake occurs; the **newborn** should be on formula or breast milk for 24 hours before screening.

G. Neurological system
1. **Newborn** head size is proportionally larger than that of an adult because of cephalocaudal development.
2. Myelinization of nerve fibers is incomplete, so primitive reflexes are present.
3. Fontanels are open to allow for brain growth.
4. Assess for an abnormal head size and a bulging or depressed anterior fontanel.
5. Measure and graph head circumference in relation to chest circumference and length.
6. Assess newborn's movements, noting symmetry, posture, and abnormal movements.
7. Observe for jitteriness, marked tremors, and seizures.
8. Test newborn's reflexes.
9. Assess for lethargy.
10. Assess pitch of cry.

H. Thermal regulatory system
1. Newborns do not shiver to produce heat.
2. Newborns have brown fat deposits, which produce heat.
3. Heat is dissipated through vasodilation.
4. Prevent heat loss resulting from evaporation by keeping **newborn** dry and well-wrapped with a blanket.
5. Prevent heat loss resulting from radiation by keeping **newborn** away from cold objects and outside walls.
6. Prevent heat loss resulting from convection by shielding the **newborn** from drafts.
7. Prevent heat loss resulting from conduction by performing all treatments on a warm, padded surface.
8. Keep temperature in room warm.
9. Take newborn's axillary temperature every hour for the first 4 hours of life, every 4 hours for the remainder of the first 24 hours, and then every shift.

I. Reflexes
1. Sucking and rooting

a. Touch the newborn's lip, cheek, or corner of the mouth with a nipple.

b. **Newborn** turns head toward the nipple, opens the mouth, takes hold of the nipple, and sucks.

c. Rooting reflex usually disappears after 3 to 4 months but may persist for up to 1 year.

2. Swallowing reflex

a. Swallowing reflex occurs spontaneously after sucking and obtaining fluids.

b. **Newborn** swallows in coordination with sucking without gagging, coughing, or vomiting.

3. Tonic neck or fencing

a. While the **newborn** is falling asleep or sleeping, gently and quickly turn the head to one side.

b. As the **newborn** faces the left side, the left arm and leg extend outward while the right arm and leg flex.

c. When the head is turned to the right side, the right arm and leg extend outward while the left arm and leg flex.

d. Response usually disappears within 3 to 4 months.

4. Palmar-plantar grasp

a. Place a finger in the palm of the newborn's hand and then place a finger at the base of the toes.

b. The newborn's fingers curl around the examiner's fingers, and the newborn's toes curl downward.

c. Palmar response lessens within 3 to 4 months.

d. Plantar response lessens within 8 months.

5. Moro's reflex

a. Hold the **newborn** in a semisitting position and then allow the head and trunk to fall backward to at least a 30-degree angle.

b. The **newborn** symmetrically abducts and extends the arms.

c. The **newborn** fans the fingers out and forms a C with the thumb and the forefinger.

d. The **newborn** adducts the arms to an embracing position and returns to a relaxed flexion state.

e. Moro's reflex is present at birth; a complete response may occur up to 8 weeks.

f. A body jerk motion occurs from 8 to 18 weeks.

g. No response may be noted by 6 months as long as neurological maturation has not been delayed.

h. A persistent response lasting more than 6 months may indicate the occurrence of brain damage during pregnancy.

6. Startle reflex

a. The response is best elicited if the **newborn** is a least 24 hours old.

b. The examiner makes a loud noise or claps hands to elicit the response.

c. The newborn's arms adduct while the elbows flex.

d. The hands stay clenched.

e. The reflex should disappear within 4 months.

7. Pull-to-sit

a. Pull the **newborn** up from the wrist while the **newborn** is in the supine position.

b. The head will lag until the **newborn** is in an upright position, and then the head will be level with the chest and shoulders momentarily before falling forward.

c. The head will then lift for a few minutes.

d. The response depends on the newborn's general muscle tone and condition and on maturity level.

8. Babinski's sign: plantar

a. Beginning at the heel of the foot, gently stroke upward along the lateral aspect of the sole, and then move the finger along the ball of the foot.

b. The newborn's toes hyperextend while the big toe dorsiflexes.

c. Reflex disappears after the **newborn** is 1 year old.

d. Absence of this reflex indicates the need for a neurological examination.

9. Stepping or walking

a. Hold the **newborn** in a vertical position, allowing one foot to touch a table surface.

b. The **newborn** simulates walking, alternately flexing and extending the feet.

c. The reflex is usually present for 3 to 4 months.

10. Crawling

a. Place the **newborn** on the abdomen

b. The **newborn** begins making crawling movements with the arms and legs.

c. The reflex usually disappears after about 6 weeks.

IV. PARENT TEACHING

A. Formula feeding

1. Teach sterilization techniques if the water supply is located in areas where the purification process of the water is questionable.

2. Remind the mother not to heat the bottle of formula in a microwave oven.

3. Inform the mother that formula is a sufficient diet for the first 4 to 6 months.

4. Assess the mother's ability to burp the **newborn**.

B. Breast-feeding

1. Assess the newborn's ability to attach to the mother's breast and suck.

2. Teach the mother about engorgement.

3. Teach the mother how to pump her breasts and how to store breast milk properly.

4. Inform the mother that breast milk is a sufficient and superior diet for the first 4 to 6 months.

5. Give the mother the phone numbers of the local organizations that offer support to breast-feeding mothers.

C. Bathing
1. Bathe the **newborn** in a warm room before feeding.
2. Have all equipment for bathing available.
3. Use a mild soap (not on the face).
4. Proceed from the cleanest area to the dirtiest.
5. Clean eyes from the inner canthus outward.
6. Special care should be taken to clean under the folds of the neck, underarms, groin, and genitals.
7. Make bath time enjoyable for the **newborn** and the mother.
D. Clothing
1. Assess diaper and clothing needs for the **newborn** with the mother.
2. Instruct the mother that the newborn's head should be covered in cold weather to prevent heat loss.
3. Instruct the mother to layer the newborn's clothing in cooler weather.
E. Cord care: Refer to cord care under Body Systems Assessment.
F. Circumcision: Refer to circumcision care under Body Systems Assessment.
G. Uncircumcised **newborn**
1. Inform the mother that the foreskin and glans are two similar layers of cells that separate from each other and that the separation process normally is complete between 3 and 5 years of age.
2. Instruct the mother not to pull back the foreskin but to allow for the natural separation to occur.
3. Inform the mother that as the process of separation occurs, sterile sloughed cells build up between the layers of the foreskin and the glans, and that when retraction occurs, daily gentle washing of the glans with soap and water is sufficient to maintain adequate cleanliness.

V. PRETERM NEWBORN
A. Description
1. A preterm **neonate** is one born before 37 weeks of gestation.
2. The primary concern relates to immaturity of all body systems.
B. Assessment
1. Respirations are irregular with periods of apnea.
2. Body temperature is below normal.
3. **Newborn** has poor suck and swallow reflexes.
4. Bowel sounds are diminished.
5. Urinary output is increased or decreased.
6. Extremities are thin, with minimal creasing on soles and palms.
7. **Newborn** extends extremities and does not maintain flexion.
8. Lanugo, on skin and in the hair on the newborn's head, is present in woolly patches.
9. Skin is thin, with visible blood vessels and minimal subcutaneous fat pads.
10. Skin may appear jaundiced.

11. Testes are undescended in boys.
12. Labia are narrow in girls.
C. Interventions
1. Monitor vital signs every 2 to 4 hours.
2. Maintain cardiopulmonary functions.
3. Administer oxygen and humidification as prescribed.
4. Monitor intake and output and electrolyte balance.
5. Monitor daily weight.
6. Maintain **newborn** in a warming device.
7. Position every 1 to 2 hours, and handle **newborn** carefully.
8. Avoid exposure to infections.
9. Provide **newborn** with appropriate stimulation, such as touch.

VI. POSTTERM NEWBORN
A. Description: a **neonate** born after 42 weeks of gestation
B. Assessment
1. Hypoglycemia
2. Parchmentlike skin (dry and cracked) without lanugo
3. Fingernails long and extended over ends of fingers
4. Profuse scalp hair
5. Long and thin body
6. Wasting of fat and muscle in extremities
7. Meconium staining possibly present on nails and umbilical cord
C. Interventions
1. Provide normal **newborn** care.
2. Monitor for hypoglycemia.
3. Maintain newborn's temperature.
4. Monitor for meconium aspiration.

VII. SMALL FOR GESTATIONAL AGE
A. Description: a **neonate** who is plotted at or below the 10th percentile on the intrauterine growth curve
B. Assessment
1. Fetal distress
2. Gestational age and physical maturity
3. Lowered or elevated body temperature
4. Physical abnormalities
5. Hypoglycemia
6. Signs of polycythemia
   a. Ruddy appearance
   b. Cyanosis
   c. Jaundice
7. Signs of infection
8. Signs of aspiration of meconium
C. Interventions
1. Maintain airway.
2. Maintain body temperature.
3. Observe for signs of respiratory distress.
4. Monitor for infection and initiate measures to prevent sepsis.

5. Monitor blood glucose levels and for signs of hypoglycemia.
6. Initiate early feedings and monitor for signs of aspiration.
7. Provide stimulation, such as touch and cuddling.

VIII. LARGE FOR GESTATIONAL AGE

A. Description: a **neonate** who is plotted at or above the 90th percentile on the intrauterine growth curve
B. Assessment
 1. Gestational age
 2. Birth trauma or injury
 3. Respiratory distress
 4. Hypoglycemia
C. Interventions
 1. Monitor vital signs.
 2. Monitor blood glucose levels and for signs of hypoglycemia.
 3. Initiate early feedings.
 4. Monitor for infection and initiate measures to prevent sepsis.
 5. Provide stimulation, such as touch and cuddling.

IX. RESPIRATORY DISTRESS SYNDROME

A. Description: a serious lung disorder caused by immaturity and inability to produce surfactant, resulting in hypoxia and acidosis
B. Assessment
 1. Tachypnea
 2. Flaring nares
 3. Expiratory grunting
 4. Retractions
 5. Decreased breath sounds
 6. Apnea
 7. Pallor and cyanosis
 8. Hypothermia
 9. Poor muscle tone
C. Interventions
 1. Monitor color, respiratory rate, and degree of effort in breathing.
 2. Support respirations as prescribed.
 3. Monitor arterial blood gases and oxygen saturation levels (arterial blood gases from umbilical artery).
 4. Monitor arterial blood gases so that oxygen administered to the **newborn** is at the lowest possible concentration necessary to maintain adequate arterial oxygenation.
 5. Schedule any premature **newborn** who required oxygen support for an eye examination before discharge to assess for retinal damage.
 6. Suction every 2 hours or more often as necessary.
 7. Position **newborn** on side or back, with neck slightly extended.
 8. Prepare to administer surfactant replacement therapy (instilled into the endotracheal tube).
 9. Administer respiratory therapy (percussion and vibration) as prescribed; use padded small plastic cup or small oxygen mask for percussion; use padded electric toothbrush for vibration.
 10. Provide nutrition.
 11. Support bonding.
 12. Prepare parents for short- to long-term period of oxygen dependency if necessary.
 13. Encourage mother to pump breasts for future breast-feeding if she so desires.
 14. Encourage as much parental participation in newborn's care as condition allows.

X. HYPERBILIRUBINEMIA

A. Description
 1. At any serum bilirubin level, the appearance of jaundice during the first day of life indicates a pathological process.
 2. Evaluation is indicated when serum levels are more than 12 mg/dL in the term **newborn**.
 3. Therapy is aimed at preventing kernicterus, which results in permanent neurological damage resulting from the deposition of bilirubin in the brain cells.
B. Assessment
 1. Jaundice
 2. Elevated serum bilirubin levels
 3. Enlarged liver
 4. Poor muscle tone
 5. Lethargy
 6. Poor sucking reflex
C. Interventions
 1. Monitor for the presence of jaundice.
    a. Examine the newborn's skin color in natural light.
    b. Press finger over a bony prominence or tip of the newborn's nose to press out capillary blood from the tissues.
    c. Note that jaundice starts at the head first, spreads to the chest, then the abdomen, and then the arms and legs, followed by the hands and feet, which are the last to be jaundiced.
 2. Keep **newborn** well hydrated to maintain blood volume.
 3. Facilitate early, frequent feeding to hasten passage of meconium and encourage excretion of bilirubin.
 4. Report to the physician any signs of jaundice in the first 24 hours and any abnormal signs and symptoms.
 5. Prepare for phototherapy, and monitor the **newborn** closely during the treatment.
D. Phototherapy
 1. Description
    a. Phototherapy is use of intense florescent lights to reduce serum bilirubin levels in the **newborn**.
    b. Injury from treatment, such as eye damage, dehydration, or sensory deprivation, can occur.
 2. Interventions
    a. Expose as much of the newborn's skin as possible.

b. Cover the genital area, and monitor genital area for skin irritation or breakdown.

c. Cover the newborn's eyes with eye shields or patches; make sure eyelids are closed when shields or patches are applied.

d. Remove the shields or patches at least once per shift to inspect the eyes for infection or irritation and to allow eye contact.

e. Measure the quantity of light every 8 hours.

f. Monitor skin temperature closely.

g. Increase fluids to compensate for water loss.

h. Expect loose green stools and green urine.

i. Monitor the newborn's skin color with the florescent light turned off, every 4 to 8 hours.

j. Monitor the skin for bronze baby syndrome, a grayish brown discoloration of the skin.

k. Reposition **newborn** every 2 hours.

l. Provide stimulation.

m. After treatment, continue monitoring for signs of hyperbilirubinemia, as rebound elevations are normal after therapy is discontinued.

XI. ERYTHROBLASTOSIS FETALIS

A. Description
1. Erythroblastosis fetalis is destruction of red blood cells that results from an antigen-antibody reaction.
2. The disorder is characterized by hemolytic anemia or hyperbilirubinemia.
3. Exchange of fetal and maternal blood takes place primarily when the **placenta** separates at birth.
4. Rh antigens from the baby's blood enter the maternal bloodstream.
5. The mother produces anti-Rh antibodies against the fetal blood cells.
6. Antibodies are harmless to the mother but attach to the erythrocytes in the fetus and cause hemolysis.
7. Sensitization is rare with the first pregnancy.
8. ABO incompatibility is usually less severe.

B. Assessment
1. Anemia
2. Jaundice that develops rapidly after birth and before 24 hours
3. Edema

C. Interventions
1. Administer $Rh_0(D)$ immune globulin to the mother during the first 72 hours after **delivery** if the Rh-negative mother delivers an Rh-positive fetus but remains unsensitized.
2. Assist with exchange transfusion after birth or intrauterine transfusion as prescribed.
3. The baby's blood is replaced with Rh-negative blood to stop the destruction of the baby's red blood cells; the Rh-negative blood is replaced with the baby's own blood gradually.
4. Reassure the mother that the **newborn** will suffer no untoward effects from the condition.

XII. SEPSIS

A. Description: generalized infection resulting from the presence of bacteria in the blood

B. Assessment
1. Pallor
2. Tachypnea, tachycardia
3. Poor feeding
4. Abdominal distention
5. Temperature instability

C. Interventions
1. Assess for periods of apnea or irregular respirations.
2. If apnea is present, stimulate by gently rubbing chest or foot.
3. Administer oxygen as prescribed.
4. Monitor vital signs.
5. Maintain warmth in an Isolette.
6. Provide isolation as necessary.
7. Assess for a fever.
8. Monitor intake and output and obtain daily weight.
9. Monitor for diarrhea.
10. Assess feeding and sucking reflex, which may be poor.
11. Assess for jaundice.
12. Assess for irritability and lethargy.
13. Administer antibiotics as prescribed and observe carefully for toxicity because a newborn's liver and kidneys are immature.

XIII. TORCH SYNDROME

A. Description
1. Torch syndrome refers to infections of the fetus or **newborn**.
2. The syndrome is caused by one of the following:
   a. *T*oxoplasmosis
   b. *O*ther viruses
   c. *R*ubella
   d. *C*ytomegalovirus
   e. *H*erpes

B. Infections (Table 30-5)

XIV. SYPHILIS

A. Description
1. Syphilis is a sexually transmitted disease.
2. Congenital syphilis can result in premature **delivery**, skin lesions, abnormal skeletal development.
3. The organism *Treponema pallidum*, a spirochete, is able to cross the **placenta** throughout pregnancy and infect the fetus, usually after 18 weeks' gestation.
4. Risks include preterm birth, stillbirth, and low birth weight.
5. Congenital effects are irreversible and may include central nervous system damage and hearing loss.

B. Assessment
1. Hepatosplenomegaly
2. Joint swelling

TABLE 30-5

Infections Included in TORCH Syndrome

Infection	Characteristics
Toxoplasmosis	Disease is caused by a protozoan infection. Disease produces no serious effects in the mother. Organism can be transmitted to the fetus. Infection can result in severe physical and developmental abnormalities. Common carriers include cat feces and raw beef.
Other infections	Such as syphilis
Rubella	Rubella is a systemic viral infection. Rubella causes congenital rubella syndrome, which includes congenital heart disease, cataracts, growth retardation, and pneumonia if the mother becomes infected within the first trimester. Deafness and some learning disabilities can occur if the mother becomes infected during the first trimester.
Cytomegalovirus	Cytomegalovirus is a viral infection that persists in the body indefinitely, with periods of reactivation without symptoms. The virus can infect the fetus or infant during delivery or after birth through breast milk, blood transfusions, or contact with infected secretions. Infection may cause microcephaly, blindness, deafness, and mental and motor retardation.
Herpes simplex	Sexually transmitted disease is caused by a virus. The virus has periods of reactivation. Neonate commonly is infected during delivery by direct contact with lesions in the genital tract. Virus can cause neurological impairment or death.

3. Palmar rash
4. Anemia
5. Jaundice
6. Snuffles
7. Ascites
8. Pneumonitis
9. Cerebrospinal fluid changes

C. Interventions
1. Monitor **newborn** for signs of syphilis.
2. Monitor for palmar rash and snuffles.
3. Prepare **newborn** for serological testing if prescribed.
4. Administer antibiotic therapy as prescribed.
5. Use standard precautions and drainage/secretion (contact) precautions with suspected congenital syphilis.
6. Wear gloves when handling **neonate** until 24 hours of antibiotic therapy has been administered.
7. Provide psychological support to the mother, and provide instructions regarding follow-up care to the **newborn**.

▶ **XV. THE ADDICTED NEWBORN**
A. Description: **newborn** who has become passively addicted to drugs that have passed through the **placenta**
B. Addicting drugs
1. Heroin
   a. **Newborn** may appear normal at birth with a low birth weight.
   b. Withdrawal occurs within 12 to 24 hours and may last 5 to 7 days.

2. Methadone
   a. Withdrawal occurs within 1 to 2 days to 1 week or more, is most evident at 48 to 72 hours, and may last 6 days to 8 weeks.
   b. **Newborn** appears very ill.
   c. **Newborn** may develop jaundice as a result of prematurity.
3. Cocaine
   a. Cocaine addiction causes decreased interactive behavior.
   b. Feeding problems are present.
   c. Irregular sleep patterns and diarrhea occur.

C. Assessment
1. Irritability
2. Tremors
3. Hyperactivity and hypertonicity
4. Respiratory distress
5. Vomiting
6. High-pitched cry
7. Sneezing
8. Fever
9. Diarrhea
10. Excessive sweating
11. Poor feeding
12. Extreme sucking of fists
13. Convulsions

D. Interventions
1. Monitor respiratory and cardiac status frequently.
2. Monitor temperature and vital signs.
3. Hold **newborn** firm and close to the body during feeding and when giving care.
4. Initiate seizure precautions (pad sides of crib).

5. Provide small frequent feedings and allow a longer period for feeding.
6. Monitor intake and output.
7. Administer intravenous hydration if prescribed.
8. Protect neonate's skin from injury that can be caused by the constant rubbing from hyperactive jitters.
9. Swaddle **newborn**.
10. Place **newborn** in a quiet room and reduce stimulation.
11. Allow mother to ventilate feelings of anxiety and guilt.
12. Refer mother for treatment of substance abuse problem.

▲ XVI. FETAL ALCOHOL SYNDROME

A. Description
  1. Fetal alcohol syndrome is caused by maternal alcohol use during pregnancy.
  2. The syndrome is the most serious cause of teratogenesis.
  3. The syndrome causes mental and physical retardation.

B. Assessment
  1. Facial changes
    a. Short palpebral fissures
    b. Hypoplastic philtrum
    c. Short, upturned nose
    d. Flat midface
    e. Thin upper lip
    f. Low nasal bridge
  2. Abnormal palmar creases
  3. Respiratory distress (apnea, cyanosis)
  4. Congenital heart disorders
  5. Irritability, hypersensitivity to stimuli
  6. Tremors
  7. Poor feeding
  8. Seizures

C. Interventions
  1. Monitor for respiratory distress.
  2. Position **newborn** on side to facilitate drainage of secretions.
  3. Keep resuscitation equipment at the bedside.
  4. Monitor for hypoglycemia.
  5. Assess suck and swallow reflex.
  6. Administer small feedings and burp well.
  7. Suction as necessary.
  8. Monitor intake and output.
  9. Monitor weight and head circumference.
  10. Decrease environmental stimuli.

▲ XVII. NEWBORN WITH ACQUIRED IMMUNODEFICIENCY SYNDROME

A. Description
  1. The fetus of a human immunodeficiency virus (HIV) antibody–positive woman should be monitored closely throughout the pregnancy.
  2. Serial ultrasound screenings should be done during pregnancy to identify intrauterine growth restriction.
  3. Weekly nonstress testing after 32 weeks of gestation and biophysical profiles may be necessary during pregnancy.
  4. Neonates born to HIV-positive clients may test positive because the mother's positive antibodies may persist in the **newborn** for as long as 18 months after birth.
  5. The use of antiviral medication, the reduction of **neonate** exposure to maternal blood and body fluids, and the early identification of HIV in pregnancy reduce the risk of transmission to the **newborn**.
  6. All neonates born to HIV-positive mothers acquire maternal antibody to HIV infection, but not all acquire the infection.
  7. The **neonate** may be asymptomatic for the first several years of life.

B. Transmission
  1. Across placental barrier
  2. During **labor** and **delivery**
  3. Breast milk

C. Assessment
  1. Possibly no outward signs for the first several months of life
  2. Signs of immune deficiency
  3. Hepatomegaly
  4. Splenomegaly
  5. Lymphadenopathy
  6. Impairment in growth and development

D. Interventions
  1. Cleanse newborn's skin carefully before any invasive procedure, such as the administration of vitamin K, heel sticks, or venipunctures.
  2. Circumcisions are not done on newborns with HIV-positive mothers until the newborn's status is determined.
  3. **Newborn** can room with mother.
  4. All HIV-exposed newborns should be treated with medication to prevent infection by *Pneumocystis carinii*.
  5. Zidovudine (AZT) may be administered as prescribed for the first 6 weeks of life.
  6. Monitor for early signs of immune deficiency, such as enlarged spleen or liver, lymphadenopathy, and impairment in growth and development.
  7. Newborns at risk for HIV infection should be seen by the physician at birth and at 1 week, 2 weeks, 1 month, and 2 months of life.
  8. Inform the mother that an HIV culture is recommended at age 1 month and after 4 months of age.

E. Immunizations
  1. Newborns at risk for HIV infection need to receive all recommended immunizations at the regular schedule.

2. Immunizations with live vaccines, such as measles-mumps-rubella, should not be done until the newborn's, infant's, or child's status is confirmed.

3. If a child is infected, live vaccine will not be given.

XVIII. NEWBORN OF A DIABETIC MOTHER

A. Description
   1. **Neonate** born to an insulin-dependent mother or gestational diabetic mother
   2. High incidences of hypoglycemia, hyperbilirubinemia, respiratory distress syndrome, hypocalcemia, and congenital anomalies

B. Assessment
   1. Excessive size and weight as a result of excess fat and glycogen in tissues
   2. Edema or puffiness in the face and cheeks
   3. Signs of hypoglycemia, such as twitching, difficulty in feeding, lethargy, apnea, seizures, and cyanosis
   4. Hyperbilirubinemia
   5. Signs of respiratory distress, such as tachypnea, cyanosis, retractions, grunting, and nasal flaring

C. Interventions
   1. Monitor for signs of respiratory distress.
   2. Monitor bilirubin and blood glucose levels.
   3. Monitor weight.
   4. Feed the infant soon after birth with glucose in water, breast milk, or formula as prescribed.
   5. Administer glucose intravenously to treat hypoglycemia if necessary and as prescribed.
   6. Monitor for edema.
   7. Monitor for apnea, tremors, and seizures.

XIX. HYPOGLYCEMIA

A. Description
   1. Hypoglycemia is an abnormally low level of glucose in the blood (less than 30 mg/dL in the first 72 hours or less than 45 mg/dL after the first 3 days of life).
   2. Normal blood glucose level is 40 to 60 mg/dL in a 1-day-old **neonate** and 50 to 90 mg/dL in a **neonate** older than 1 day.

B. Assessment
   1. Increased respiratory rate
   2. Twitching, nervousness, or tremors
   3. Unstable temperature
   4. Cyanosis

C. Interventions
   1. Prevent low blood glucose through early feedings.
   2. Administer glucose orally or intravenously as prescribed.
   3. Monitor blood glucose levels as prescribed.
   4. Monitor for feeding problems.
   5. Monitor for apneic periods.
   6. Assess for shrill or intermittent cries.
   7. Evaluate lethargy and poor muscle tone.

PRACTICE QUESTIONS

1. A nurse instructs a mother in how to bathe a newborn infant. The nurse tells the mother to
   1. Start with the dirtiest area first.
   2. Begin with the eyes and face.
   3. Begin with the feet and work upward.
   4. Only wash the diaper area because this is the only part of the infant that gets soiled.

2. A nurse in a delivery room is assisting with the delivery of a newborn infant. After the delivery, the nurse prepares to prevent heat loss in the newborn infant resulting from evaporation by
   1. Warming the crib pad.
   2. Turning on the overhead radiant warmer.
   3. Closing the doors to the room.
   4. Drying the infant with a warm blanket.

3. A nurse is providing instructions to a new mother regarding cord care for a newborn infant. Which statement if made by the mother indicates a need for further education?
   1. "I should cleanse the cord 2 or 3 times a day."
   2. "The cord will fall off in 1 to 2 weeks."
   3. "Alcohol may be used to clean the cord."
   4. "I need to fold the diaper above the cord to prevent infection."

4. The mother of a newborn infant calls a clinic and reports to a nurse that when cleansing the umbilical cord, the mother noticed that the cord was moist and that discharge was present. The most appropriate nursing instruction to the mother is which of the following?
   1. To increase the number of times that the cord is cleansed per day
   2. To monitor the cord for another 24 to 48 hours and to call the clinic if the discharge continues
   3. To bring the infant to the clinic
   4. That this is a normal occurrence

5. A nurse is assessing a newborn infant following circumcision and notes that the circumcised area is red with a small amount of bloody drainage. Which of the following nursing actions would be most appropriate?
   1. Document the findings.
   2. Contact the physician.
   3. Circle the amount of bloody drainage on the dressing and reassess in 30 minutes.
   4. Reinforce the dressing.

6. A nurse has provided instructions to a mother of a male newborn infant who is not circumcised about measures to clean the penis. Which statement if made by the mother indicates an understanding of how to clean the newborn infant's penis?
   1. "I need to retract the foreskin and clean the penis every time I give my infant a bath."
   2. "I should gently retract the foreskin as far as it will go on the penis and then pull the skin back over the penis after cleaning."

3. "I should retract the foreskin and clean the penis every time I change the diaper."

4. "I need to avoid pulling back the foreskin to clean the penis because this may cause adhesions."

7. A nurse in a newborn nursery is monitoring a preterm newborn infant for respiratory distress syndrome. Which assessment signs if noted in the newborn infant would alert the nurse to the possibility of this syndrome?
   1. Hypotension and bradycardia
   2. Tachypnea and retractions
   3. Acrocyanosis and grunting
   4. The presence of a barrel chest with acrocyanosis

8. A nurse is assessing the reflexes of a newborn infant. In eliciting the Moro's reflex, the nurse would perform which of the following?
   1. Stimulate the perioral cavity of the newborn infant with a finger.
   2. Clap the hand or slap on the newborn infant's mattress.
   3. Stimulate the pads of the newborn infant's hands by firm pressure.
   4. Stimulate the newborn infant's ball of the foot by firm pressure.

9. A nurse in a newborn nursery is performing an assessment of a newborn infant. The nurse is preparing to measure the head circumference of the infant. The nurse would most appropriately
   1. Wrap the tape measure around the infant's head and measure just above the eyebrows.
   2. Place the tape measure under the infant's head at the base of the skull and wrap around to the front just above the eyes.
   3. Place the tape measure under the infant's head, wrap around the occiput, and measure just above the eyes.
   4. Place the tape measure at the back of the infant's head, wrap around across the ears, and measure across the infant's mouth.

10. A postpartum nurse is providing instructions to the mother of a newborn infant with hyperbilirubinemia who is being breast-fed. The nurse provides which most appropriate instruction to the mother?
    1. Switch to bottle-feeding the baby for 2 weeks.
    2. Stop the breast-feedings and switch to bottle-feeding permanently.
    3. Feed the newborn infant less frequently.
    4. Continue to breast-feed every 2 to 4 hours.

11. A nurse in the newborn nursery is caring for a neonate. On assessment the infant is exhibiting signs of cyanosis, tachypnea, nasal flaring, and grunting. Respiratory distress syndrome is diagnosed, and the physician prescribes surfactant replacement therapy. The nurse would prepare to administer this therapy by
    1. Subcutaneous injection.
    2. Intravenous injection.
    3. Instillation of the preparation into the lungs through an endotracheal tube.
    4. Intramuscular injection.

12. A nurse is assessing a newborn infant who was born to a mother who is addicted to drugs. Which of the following assessment findings would the nurse expect to note during the assessment of this newborn?
    1. Sleepiness
    2. Cuddles when being held
    3. Lethargy
    4. Incessant crying

13. A nurse is preparing to administer an injection of vitamin K to a newborn. In preparing to administer the injection, the nurse would select which of the following injection sites?
    1. The lateral aspect of the middle third of the vastus lateralis muscle
    2. The medial aspect of the upper third of the vastus lateralis muscle
    3. The lower aspect of the rectus femoris muscle
    4. The gluteal muscle

14. A 4-day-old newborn infant is receiving phototherapy at home for a bilirubin level of 14 mg/dL. The nurse should plan to include which of the following in the plan of care during the home visit to the mother of the newborn infant?
    1. Having minimal contact with the newborn infant to prevent stimulation
    2. Advising the mother to limit newborn infant oral intake during phototherapy
    3. Applying lotions to exposed newborn infant's skin
    4. Assessing skin integrity and fluid and electrolyte status of the newborn infant

15. A nurse notes hypotonia, irritability, and a poor sucking reflex in a full-term newborn infant on admission to the nursery. The nurse suspects fetal alcohol syndrome and is aware that which additional sign would be consistent with fetal alcohol syndrome?
    1. Head circumference appropriate for gestational age
    2. Birth weight of 6 lb 14 oz
    3. Length of 19 inches
    4. Abnormal palmar creases

16. A nurse is preparing a plan of care for a newborn infant with fetal alcohol syndrome. The nurse would include which of the following priority interventions in the plan of care?
    1. Monitor the newborn infant's response to feedings and weight gain pattern.
    2. Encourage frequent handling of the newborn infant by staff and parents.
    3. Maintain the newborn infant in a brightly lighted area of the nursery.
    4. Allow the newborn infant to establish own sleep/rest pattern.

17. A nurse administers erythromycin ointment (0.5%) to the eyes of a newborn infant. The mother asks the nurse why this is performed. The nurse explains to the mother that this is routinely done to
    1. Minimize the spread of microorganisms to the newborn infant from invasive procedures during labor.
    2. Protect the newborn infant's eyes from possible infections acquired while hospitalized.
    3. Prevent ophthalmia neonatorum from occurring after delivery in a newborn infant born to a woman with an untreated gonococcal infection.
    4. Prevent cataracts in the newborn infant born to a woman who is rubella susceptible.

18. A nurse prepares to administer a vitamin K injection to a newborn infant. The mother asks the nurse why her newborn infant needs the injection. The best response by the nurse would be
    1. "Your infant needs vitamin K to develop immunity."
    2. "The vitamin K will protect your infant from being jaundiced."
    3. "Newborn infants are deficient in vitamin K, and this injection prevents your infant from abnormal bleeding."
    4. "Newborn infants have sterile bowels, and vitamin K promotes the growth of bacteria in the bowel."

19. A nurse develops a plan of care for a human immunodeficiency virus–infected mother and her newborn infant. The nurse includes which intervention in the plan of care?
    1. Instruct the breast-feeding mother regarding the treatment of the nipples with nystatin ointment.
    2. Monitor the newborn infant's vital signs routinely.
    3. Maintain standard precautions at all times while caring for the newborn.
    4. Initiate referral to evaluate for blindness, deafness, learning, or behavioral problems.

20. A nurse in a newborn nursery receives a telephone call to prepare for the admission of a 43-week-gestation newborn infant with Apgar scores of 1 and 4. In planning for admission of this infant, the nurse's highest priority should be to
    1. Connect the resuscitation bag to the oxygen outlet.
    2. Turn on the apnea and cardiorespiratory monitors.
    3. Set up the intravenous line with 5% dextrose in water.
    4. Set the radiant warmer control temperature at 36.5° C (97.6° F).

CRITICAL THINKING: FILL IN THE BLANK

A nurse is caring for a post-term, small for gestational age newborn infant immediately after admission to the nursery. The priority nursing action would be to monitor the results of what serum laboratory study?

Answer: _____

ANSWERS

1. **2**

Rationale: Bathing should start at the eyes and face, usually the cleanest area. Next, the external ear and the areas behind the ears are cleansed. The infant's neck should be washed because formula, lint, or breast milk will often accumulate in the folds of the neck. Hands and arms then are washed. The infants legs are washed, and the diaper area is washed last.
Test-Taking Strategy: Use the process of elimination. Remember the basic techniques of bathing a client to assist in answering this question. Always start with the cleanest area of the body first and proceed to the dirtiest area. Use techniques related to washing an adult to assist in answering this question. If you had difficulty with this question, review home care measures related to the care of the newborn infant.
Level of Cognitive Ability: Application
Client Needs: Physiological Integrity
Integrated Process: Teaching/Learning
Content Area: Maternity—postpartum
Reference: Wong, D., Perry, S., & Hockenberry, M. (2002). *Maternal child nursing care* (2nd ed., p. 586). St. Louis: Mosby.

2. **4**

Rationale: Evaporation of moisture from a wet body dissipates heat along with the moisture. Keeping the newborn infant dry by drying the wet newborn infant at birth will prevent hypothermia via evaporation. Hypothermia caused by conduction occurs when the newborn infant is on a cold surface, such as a cold pad or mattress, and heat from the newborn infant's body is transferred to the colder object. Warming the crib pad will assist in preventing hypothermia by conduction. Convection occurs as air moves across the newborn infant's skin from an open door and heat is transferred to the air. Radiation occurs when heat from the newborn infant radiates to a colder surface.
Test-Taking Strategy: Use the process of elimination. Note the key word "evaporation" in the question to assist in selecting the correct option. Knowledge that evaporation of moisture from a wet body dissipates heat along with the moisture will assist in directing you to option 4. Review these heat loss concepts if you had difficulty with this question.
Level of Cognitive Ability: Application
Client Needs: Physiological Integrity
Integrated Process: Nursing Process—planning
Content Area: Maternity—postpartum
References: Lowdermilk, D., & Perry, S. (2003). *Maternity nursing* (6th ed.). St. Louis: Mosby.
Wong, D., Perry, S., & Hockenberry, M. (2002). *Maternal child nursing care* (2nd ed., p. 527). St. Louis: Mosby.

3. 4

Rationale: The cord should be kept clean and dry to decrease bacterial growth. The diaper should be folded below the cord to keep urine away from the cord. The cord should be cleansed 2 or 3 times a day with alcohol or other prescribed agents. Cord care is required until the cord dries up and falls off between 7 and 14 days.

Test-Taking Strategy: Use the process of elimination. Read each option carefully and attempt to visualize the descriptions in each of the options. Also note the key words "need for further education" in the stem of the question. Knowing that option 4 suggests folding the diaper above the cord should assist in directing you to this option because the cord can become saturated and contaminated with urine with this method of diapering. Review concepts related to cord care if you had difficulty with this question.

Level of Cognitive Ability: Analysis
Client Needs: Health Promotion and Maintenance
Integrated Process: Teaching/Learning
Content Area: Maternity—postpartum
Reference: Murray, S., McKinney, E., & Gorrie, T. (2002). *Foundations of maternal-newborn nursing* (3rd ed., p. 558). Philadelphia: W. B. Saunders.

4. 3

Rationale: Symptoms of infection are moistness, oozing, discharge, and a reddened base around the cord. If symptoms of infection occur, the mother should be instructed to notify a health care provider. If these symptoms occur, antibiotics are necessary. Options 1, 2, and 4 are inappropriate nursing interventions for the description given in the question.

Test-Taking Strategy: Use the process of elimination. Focus on the clinical manifestations provided in the question to assist in directing you to the correct option. Noting the key word "discharge" in the question will assist in directing you to the option that indicates that the newborn needs to be seen by the health care provider. Review interventions related to cord care, if you had difficulty with this question.

Level of Cognitive Ability: Application
Client Needs: Physiological Integrity
Integrated Process: Nursing Process—implementation
Content Area: Maternity—postpartum
Reference: Murray, S., McKinney, E., & Gorrie, T. (2002). *Foundations of maternal-newborn nursing* (3rd ed., p. 568). Philadelphia: W. B. Saunders.

5. 1

Rationale: The penis is normally red during the healing process. A yellow exudate may be noted in 24 hours, and this is part of normal healing. The nurse would expect that the area would be red with a small amount of bloody drainage. If the bleeding is excessive, the nurse would apply gentle pressure with a sterile gauze. If bleeding is not controlled, then the blood vessel may need to be ligated, and the nurse would notify the physician. Because the findings identified in the question are normal, the nurse would document the assessment.

Test-Taking Strategy: Use the process of elimination. Note the key words "small amount of bloody drainage." This should assist in directing you to the option that this is a normal occurrence following circumcision. If you had difficulty with

this question, review the expected findings following this procedure.

Level of Cognitive Ability: Application
Client Needs: Physiological Integrity
Integrated Process: Nursing Process—implementation
Content Area: Maternity—postpartum
Reference: Lowdermilk, D., Perry, S., & Bobak, I. (2000). *Maternity & women's health care* (7th ed., p. 748). St. Louis: Mosby.

6. 4

Rationale: In male newborn infants the prepuce is continuous with the epidermis of the glans and is not retractable. If retraction is forced, this may cause adhesions to develop. The mother should be told to allow separation to occur naturally, which usually occurs between 3 years and puberty. Most foreskins are retractable by 3 years of age and should be pushed back gently at this time for cleaning. Options 1, 2, and 3 identify an action that addresses retraction of the foreskin.

Test-Taking Strategy: Use the process of elimination. Note that options 1, 2, and 3 are similar in that they all identify retracting the foreskin. Option 4 is the option that is different. If you had difficulty with this question, review teaching points related to cleaning the penis of a newborn male infant who is uncircumcised.

Level of Cognitive Ability: Analysis
Client Needs: Health Promotion and Maintenance
Integrated Process: Teaching/Learning
Content Area: Maternity—postpartum
Reference: Murray, S., McKinney, E., & Gorrie, T. (2002). *Foundations of maternal-newborn nursing* (3rd ed., p. 530). Philadelphia: W. B. Saunders.

7. 2

Rationale: The newborn infant with respiratory distress syndrome may present with clinical signs of cyanosis, tachypnea or apnea, nasal flaring, chest wall retractions, or audible grunts. Acrocyanosis is the bluish discoloration of the hands and feet, is associated with immature peripheral circulation, and is not uncommon in the first few hours of life. Options 1, 3, and 4 do not indicate clinical signs of respiratory distress syndrome.

Test-Taking Strategy: Use the process of elimination. Recalling that acrocyanosis may be a normal sign in a newborn infant will assist in eliminating options 3 and 4. From the remaining options, you must be familiar with the signs of respiratory distress syndrome. Also, note the relationship between the diagnosis and the signs noted in option 2. If you had difficulty with this question, review the signs of respiratory distress syndrome.

Level of Cognitive Ability: Analysis
Client Needs: Physiological Integrity
Integrated Process: Nursing Process—assessment
Content Area: Maternity—postpartum
Reference: Murray, S., McKinney, E., & Gorrie, T. (2002). *Foundations of maternal-newborn nursing* (3rd ed., p. 831). Philadelphia: W. B. Saunders.

8. 2

Rationale: The Moro's reflex is elicited by a loud noise such as a hand clap or a slap on the mattress to startle the newborn infant. Symmetrical extension and abduction of the arms are seen; fingers fan out and form a C with the thumb and forefinger; slight tremor may be noted; and the arms are adducted in an embracing motion and then return to a relaxed flexion state. Legs may follow a similar pattern of response. This reflex disappears at 6 months of age. The rooting reflex is elicited by stimulating the perioral area with the finger. The palmar grasp reflex is elicited by stimulating the palm of the hand by firm pressure, and the plantar grasp reflex is elicited by stimulating the ball of the foot by firm pressure.

Test-Taking Strategy: Use the process of elimination. Options 3 and 4 are similar and should be eliminated first. Focusing on the issue of the question, the Moro's reflex, will assist in directing you to option 2. Review assessment of neonatal reflexes if you had difficulty with this question.

Level of Cognitive Ability: Application
Client Needs: Health Promotion and Maintenance
Integrated Process: Nursing Process—assessment
Content Area: Maternity—postpartum
Reference: Lowdermilk, D., & Perry, S. (2003). *Maternity nursing* (6th ed., p. 453). St. Louis: Mosby.

9. 3
Rationale: To measure head circumference, the nurse should place the tape measure under the infant's head, wrap the tape around the occiput, and measure just above the eyebrows so that the largest area of the occiput is included. Options 1, 2, and 4 are incorrect methods to measure the head circumference.

Test-Taking Strategy: Use the process of elimination. Attempt to visualize each of the descriptions in the options. Remembering that the largest area of the occiput is included in the measurement will assist in directing you to option 3. If you had difficulty with this question, review measuring head circumference in a newborn infant.

Level of Cognitive Ability: Application
Client Needs: Health Promotion and Maintenance
Integrated Process: Nursing Process—implementation
Content Area: Maternity—postpartum
Reference: Wong, D., Perry, S., & Hockenberry, M. (2002). *Maternal child nursing care* (2nd ed., p. 790). St. Louis: Mosby.

10. 4
Rationale: Breast-feeding should be initiated within 2 hours after birth and every 2 to 4 hours thereafter. The infant should not be fed less frequently. Switching to bottle-feeding for 2 weeks or stopping breast-feeding permanently is not necessary.

Test-Taking Strategy: Use the process of elimination. Note the similarities between options 1 and 2. These options discourage the continuation of breast-feeding and are therefore similar. From the remaining options, recalling the pathophysiology associated with hyperbilirubinemia will assist you in eliminating option 3. Review client instructions related to hyperbilirubinemia in the newborn infant if you had difficulty with this question.

Level of Cognitive Ability: Application
Client Needs: Physiological Integrity
Integrated Process: Teaching/Learning
Content Area: Maternity—postpartum

References: Lowdermilk, D., & Perry, S. (2003). *Maternity nursing* (6th ed., p. 499). St. Louis: Mosby.
Wong, D., Perry, S., & Hockenberry, M. (2002). *Maternal child nursing care* (2nd ed., p. 598). St. Louis: Mosby.

11. 3
Rationale: The aim of therapy in respiratory distress syndrome is to support the disease until the disease runs its course with the subsequent development of surfactant. The infant may benefit from surfactant replacement therapy. In surfactant replacement, an exogenous surfactant preparation is instilled into the lungs through an endotracheal tube. Options 1, 2, and 4 identify incorrect methods of administering surfactant.

Test Taking Strategy: Knowledge regarding surfactant replacement therapy is required to answer this question. If you are unfamiliar with the administration of this therapy, review this procedure.

Level of Cognitive Ability: Application
Client Needs: Physiological Integrity
Integrated Process: Nursing Process—planning
Content Area: Maternity—postpartum
Reference: Murray, S., McKinney, E., & Gorrie, T. (2002). *Foundations of maternal- newborn nursing* (3rd ed., p. 832). Philadelphia: W. B. Saunders.

12. 4
Rationale: A newborn infant born to a woman using drugs is irritable. The infant is overloaded easily by sensory stimulation. The infant may cry incessantly and be difficult to console. The infant would hyperextend and posture rather than cuddle when being held.

Test-Taking Strategy: Use the process of elimination. Note that options 1 and 3 are similar in that they indicate hypoactivity of the newborn. From the remaining options, recalling the pathophysiology associated with a newborn infant born to a drug-addicted mother will assist you in eliminating option 2. Review assessment findings in the newborn infant born to a drug-addicted mother if you had difficulty with this question.

Level of Cognitive Ability: Analysis
Client Needs: Physiological Integrity
Integrated Process: Nursing Process—assessment
Content Area: Maternity—postpartum
Reference: Murray, S., McKinney, E., & Gorrie, T. (2002). *Foundations of maternal-newborn nursing* (3rd ed., p. 857). Philadelphia: W. B. Saunders.

13. 1
Rationale: The preferred injection site for vitamin K in the newborn infant is the lateral aspect of the middle third of the vastus lateralis muscle in the infant's thigh. This muscle is the preferred injection site because it is free of major blood vessels and nerves and is large enough to absorb the medication.

Test-Taking Strategy: Use the process of elimination and knowledge regarding the preferred injection site for a newborn infant. If you had difficulty with this question, review the procedure for administering vitamin K to the newborn infant.

Level of Cognitive Ability: Application
Client Needs: Physiological Integrity
Integrated Process: Nursing Process—planning
Content Area: Maternity—postpartum

References: Lowdermilk, D., & Perry, S. (2003). *Maternity nursing* (6th ed., p. 496). St. Louis: Mosby.
Murray, S., McKinney, E., & Gorrie, T. (2002). *Foundations of maternal-newborn nursing* (3rd ed., p. 547). Philadelphia: W. B. Saunders.

14. **4**
Rationale: Assessing skin integrity and fluid and electrolyte status of the newborn infant is an essential component of phototherapy. Contact with the newborn infant is important. Lotions are not used to minimize skin breakdown and to ensure the therapeutic effect of light exposure in subcutaneous tissue. Adequate oral fluids are essential to prevent dehydration because diarrhea is a common side effect of therapy. In addition, safe care for the newborn infant during phototherapy requires shielding the eyes with a soft eye shield to prevent retinal damage, keeping the newborn's skin exposed except for a diaper, and changing position frequently.
Test-Taking Strategy: Use the process of elimination and knowledge regarding phototherapy. Note that option 4 addresses the first step of the nursing process, assessment. If you had difficulty with this question, review care to the newborn infant receiving phototherapy.
Level of Cognitive Ability: Application
Clients Needs: Physiological Integrity
Integrated Process: Teaching/Learning
Content Area: Maternity—postpartum
Reference: Murray, S., McKinney, E., & Gorrie, T. (2002). *Foundations of maternal-newborn nursing* (3rd ed., p. 847). Philadelphia: W. B. Saunders.

15. **4**
Rationale: Features of newborn infants diagnosed with fetal alcohol syndrome include craniofacial abnormalities, intrauterine growth retardation, cardiac abnormalities, abnormal palmar creases, and respiratory distress. Options 1, 2, and 3 are normal assessment findings in the full-term newborn infant.
Test-Taking Strategy: Use the process of elimination and knowledge regarding normal assessment findings in the full-term newborn infant to answer this question. Note that options 1, 2, and 3 are similar and represent normal assessment findings in the full-term newborn infant. If you had difficulty with this question, review the content related to normal newborn infant assessment findings and fetal alcohol syndrome.
Level of Cognitive Ability: Analysis
Client Needs: Physiological Integrity
Integrated Process: Nursing Process—assessment
Content Area: Maternity—postpartum
References: Lowdermilk, D., & Perry, S. (2003). *Maternity nursing* (6th ed., p. 758). St. Louis: Mosby.
Murray, S., McKinney, E., & Gorrie, T. (2002). *Foundations of maternal-newborn nursing* (3rd ed., p. 638). Philadelphia: W. B. Saunders.

16. **1**
Rationale: A primary nursing goal for the newborn infant diagnosed with fetal alcohol syndrome is to establish nutritional balance following delivery. These newborn infants may exhibit hyperirritability, vomiting, diarrhea, or an uncoordinated sucking and swallowing ability. A quiet environment with minimal stimuli and handling will help establish appropriate sleep/rest cycles in the newborn infant as well. Options 2, 3, and 4 are inappropriate interventions.
Test-Taking Strategy: Use the process of elimination. Recalling that these newborn infants may exhibit hyperirritability, vomiting, diarrhea, or an uncoordinated sucking and swallowing ability will direct you easily to option 1. Review care to the newborn infant with fetal alcohol syndrome if you had difficulty with this question.
Level of Cognitive Ability: Application
Client Needs: Physiological Integrity
Integrated Process: Nursing Process—planning
Content Area: Maternity—postpartum
Reference: Wong, D., Perry, S., & Hockenberry, M. (2002). *Maternal child nursing care* (2nd ed., p. 649). St. Louis: Mosby.

17. **3**
Rationale: Erythromycin ophthalmic ointment (Ilotycin ophthalmic) 0.5% is used as a prophylactic treatment for ophthalmia neonatorum, which is caused by the bacterium *Neisseria gonorrhoeae.* Preventive treatment of gonorrhea is required by law. Options 1, 2, and 4 are not the purposes for administering this medication to the newborn infant.
Test-Taking Strategy: Use the process of elimination and knowledge of the purpose of administering erythromycin ophthalmic ointment to the newborn infant. If you had difficulty with this question, review initial care to the newborn infant.
Level of Cognitive Ability: Application
Client Needs: Health Promotion and Maintenance
Integrated Process: Teaching/Learning
Content Area: Maternity—postpartum
Reference: Murray, S., McKinney, E., & Gorrie, T. (2002). *Foundations of maternal-newborn nursing* (3rd ed., p. 546). Philadelphia: W. B. Saunders.

18. **3**
Rationale: Vitamin K is necessary for the body to synthesize coagulation factors. Vitamin K is administered to the newborn infant to prevent abnormal bleeding. Vitamin K promotes liver formation of the clotting factors II, VII, IX, and X. Newborn infants are vitamin K deficient because the bowel does not have the bacteria necessary for synthesizing fat-soluble vitamin K. The normal flora in the intestinal tract produces vitamin K. The newborn infant's bowel does not support the normal production of vitamin K until bacteria adequately colonize it. The bowel becomes colonized by bacteria as food is ingested. Vitamin K does not promote the development of immunity or prevent the infant from becoming jaundiced.
Test-Taking Strategy: Use the process of elimination. Note the key word "best." Because jaundice and immunity are not related to the action of vitamin K, eliminate options 1 and 2. From the remaining options, recall the action of vitamin K to direct you to option 3. If you had difficulty with this question, review the purpose of vitamin K injection.
Level of Cognitive Ability: Application
Client Needs: Physiological Integrity
Integrated Process: Teaching/Learning

Content Area: Maternity—postpartum
Reference: Murray, S., McKinney, E., & Gorrie, T. (2002). *Foundations of maternal-newborn nursing* (3rd ed., p. 546). Philadelphia: W. B. Saunders.

19. 3
Rationale: The newborn infant born of a mother infected with human immunodeficiency virus (HIV) must be cared for with strict attention to standard precautions. This prevents the transmission of HIV from the newborn infant, if infected, to others, and prevents transmission of other infectious agents to the possibly immunocompromised newborn infant. Mothers infected with HIV should not breast-feed. Options 2 and 4 are not associated specifically with the care of a potentially HIV-infected newborn infant.
Test-Taking Strategy: Use the process of elimination and knowledge regarding care of a newborn infant born to an HIV-infected woman. Eliminate options 2 and 4 first because they are not associated specifically with the care of a potentially HIV-infected newborn infant. Recalling that HIV-infected mothers should not breast-feed will direct you easily to option 3. Review care of an infant born to an HIV-infected woman if you had difficulty with this question.
Level of Cognitive Ability: Application
Client Needs: Safe, Effective Care Environment
Integrated Process: Nursing Process—planning
Content Area: Maternity—postpartum
Reference: Murray, S., McKinney, E., & Gorrie, T. (2002). *Foundations of maternal-newborn nursing* (3rd ed., p. 728). Philadelphia: W. B. Saunders.

20. 1
Rationale: The highest priority on admission to the nursery for a newborn with low Apgar scores is airway, which would involve preparing respiratory resuscitation equipment. The remaining options are also important, although they are of lower priority. The newborn infant will be placed on a cardiorespiratory monitor. Setting up an intravenous line with 5% dextrose in water would provide circulatory support. The radiant warmer will provide an external heat source, which is necessary to prevent further respiratory distress.
Test-Taking Strategy: Use the process of elimination and note the key words "highest priority." This question asks you to prioritize care on the basis of information about a newborn infant's condition. Use the ABCs—airway, breathing, and circulation. A method of planning for airway support is to have the resuscitation bag connected to an oxygen source. Review care to the newborn infant with low Apgar scores if you had difficulty with this question.
Level of Cognitive Ability: Application
Client Needs: Physiological Integrity
Integrated Process: Nursing Process—planning
Content Area: Maternity—postpartum
Reference: Matteson, P. (2001). *Women's health during the childbearing years: A community-based approach.* (p. 655). St. Louis: Mosby.

CRITICAL THINKING: FILL IN THE BLANK
Answer: Blood glucose levels
Rationale: The most common metabolic complication in the small for gestational age newborn infant is hypoglycemia, which can produce central nervous system abnormalities and mental retardation if not corrected immediately.
Test-Taking Strategy: Recalling that the most common metabolic complication in the small for gestational age newborn infant is hypoglycemia will assist in answering the question. Review the small for gestational age newborn content if you had difficulty with this question.
Level of Cognitive Ability: Analysis
Client Needs: Physiological Integrity
Integrated Process: Nursing Process—assessment
Content Area: Maternity—postpartum
Reference: Lowdermilk, D., & Perry, S. (2003). *Maternity nursing* (6th ed., p. 743). St. Louis: Mosby.

REFERENCES

Lowdermilk, D., & Perry, S. (2003). *Maternity nursing* (6th ed.). St. Louis: Mosby.

Lowdermilk, D., Perry, S., & Bobak, I. (2000). *Maternity & women's health care* (7th ed.). St. Louis: Mosby.

Lowdermilk, D., & Perry, S. (2004). *Maternity & women's health care* (8th ed.). St. Louis: Mosby.

Matteson, P. (2001). *Women's health during the childbearing years: A community-based approach.* St. Louis: Mosby.

Murray, S., McKinney, E., & Gorrie, T. (2002). *Foundations of maternal-newborn nursing* (3rd ed.). Philadelphia: W. B. Saunders.

Wong, D., & Hockenberry, M. (2003). *Nursing care of infants and children* (7th ed.). St. Louis: Mosby.

Wong, D., Perry, S., & Hockenberry, M. (2002). *Maternal child nursing care* (2nd ed.). St. Louis: Mosby.

Maternity and Newborn Medications

I. OXYTOCIC MEDICATION: OXYTOCIN (PITOCIN)

A. Description
1. Oxytocin stimulates the smooth muscle of the uterus and induces contraction of the myocardium.
2. Oxytocin promotes milk letdown.
3. Routes of administration include intranasal, intramuscular, and intravenous (IV).
4. Minimal cervical change usually is noted until the active phase of **labor** is achieved.

B. Uses
1. Induce or augment **labor**.
2. Control postpartum bleeding.
3. Promote milk letdown and facilitate breast-feeding (intranasal route).
4. Induce or complete an abortion.

C. Adverse reactions and contraindications
1. Adverse reactions are rare but may include allergies, dysrhythmias, changes in blood pressure, uterine rupture, and water intoxication; intranasal administration may cause nasal vasoconstriction.
2. Oxytocin may produce uterine hypertonicity resulting in fetal or maternal injury.
3. High doses may cause hypotension, with rebound hypertension.
4. Postpartum hemorrhage can occur because the uterus may become atonic when the medication wears off.
5. Oxytocin should not be used in a client who cannot deliver vaginally or in a client with hypertonic uterine contractions.

D. Interventions
1. Monitor maternal vital signs (every 15 minutes), especially the blood pressure and heart rate, weight, intake and output, level of consciousness, and lung sounds.
2. Monitor frequency, duration, force of contractions, and resting uterine tone every 15 minutes.
3. Monitor fetal heart rate every 15 minutes, and notify the health care provider if significant changes occur; an internal fetal scalp electrode should be used if possible.
4. Administered by IV infusion via an infusion monitoring device (Y-setup or stopcock is used with normal saline in the primary line); carefully monitor dose being administered.
5. Do not leave the client unattended while the oxytocin is infusing.
6. Administer oxygen if prescribed.
7. Monitor for hypertonic contractions.
8. Stop the medication if uterine hyperstimulation or a nonreassuring fetal heart rate occurs; turn the client on her side, increase the IV rate of the normal saline, and administer oxygen via facemask.
9. Notify the health care provider if uterine hyperstimulation or a nonreassuring fetal heart rate occurs.
10. Monitor for signs of water intoxication.
11. Have emergency equipment available.
12. Document the dose of the medication and the time the medication was started, increased, maintained, and discontinued.
13. Keep the family informed of the client's progress.

II. ERGOT ALKALOIDS (BOX 31-1)

A. Description
1. Ergot alkaloids directly stimulate uterine muscle and increase the force and frequency of contractions.

BOX 31-1

Ergot Alkaloids

Ergonovine (Ergotrate)
Methylergonovine (Methergine)

---

2. The medications produce a firm tetanic contraction of the uterus.

3. The medications produce arterial vasoconstriction and can cause vasospasm of the coronary arteries.

4. Ergot alkaloids are not administered before the **delivery** of the **placenta**.

5. The medications may be administered by the oral or intramuscular route; for IV use in an emergency, either medication may be administered undiluted.

B. Uses
  1. Postpartum hemorrhage
  2. Postabortal hemorrhage resulting from atony or involution

C. Adverse reactions and contraindications
  1. Ergot alkaloids can cause nausea.
  2. The medications can cause uterine cramping.
  3. The medications can cause bradycardia, dysrhythmias, myocardial infarction, and severe hypertension.
  4. High doses are associated with peripheral vasospasm or vasoconstriction, angina, miosis, confusion, respiratory depression, seizures, or unconsciousness; uterine tetany can occur.
  5. The medications are contraindicated during pregnancy.
  6. The medications are contraindicated in clients with significant cardiovascular disease, peripheral vascular disease, or hypertension.

D. Interventions
  1. Monitor maternal vital signs, weight, intake and output, level of consciousness, and lung sounds.
  2. Monitor the blood pressure closely; the medication produces vasoconstriction, and if a rise in blood pressure is noted, withhold the medication and notify the health care provider.
  3. Monitor uterine contractions (frequency, strength, and duration).
  4. Assess for chest pain, headache, shortness of breath, itching, pale or cold hands or feet, nausea, diarrhea, or dizziness.
  5. Notify the health care provider if chest pain occurs.
  6. Assess the extremities for color, warmth, movement, and pain.
  7. Assess vaginal bleeding.
  8. Administer analgesics as prescribed; they may be required because the medication produces painful uterine contractions.

III. UTERINE RELAXANTS (BOX 31-2)

A. Description
  1. Uterine relaxants produce uterine relaxation.

2. Ritodrine is the medication of choice to control premature **labor**.

3. Ritodrine may be used orally or intravenously.

4. Ritodrine usually is administered intravenously when premature **labor** begins; when contractions have been controlled for 12 to 24 hours, the client may be started on orally administered ritodrine and the IV infusion may be discontinued.

5. Contractions may resume when the client is on oral therapy.

B. Uses
  1. Ritrodrine is used to halt spontaneous **labor** when it appears after the twentieth week of pregnancy and before the thirty-sixth week.
  2. Terbutaline, primarily used to control bronchospasm, is an alternative medication for the control of premature **labor**.

C. Adverse reactions and contraindications
  1. Ritodrine
    a. Ritodrine can cause heart palpitations, tachycardia, nausea and vomiting, trembling, flushing, and headache.
    b. Ritodrine can cause fetal tachycardia.
    c. High doses can cause cardiovascular symptoms and pulmonary edema.
    d. Ritodrine is contraindicated in clients with preexisting cardiac disease.
  2. Terbutaline
    a. Hypokalemia, pulmonary edema, and hypoglycemia may occur if given during **labor**.
    b. Hypoglycemia may be found in **neonate**.

D. Interventions
  1. Monitor vital signs, uterine contractions, and fetal heart rate every 5 minutes when initiating therapy, every 15 to 30 minutes when the client is stable, and every 4 hours when the client is taking oral maintenance doses.
  2. An infusion monitoring device is used when the medications are administered by the IV route.
  3. Monitor for pulmonary edema; assess lung sounds for rales.
  4. Monitor potassium and glucose levels.
  5. Instruct the client to contact the health care provider if four to six contractions per hour occur.

IV. PROSTAGLANDINS (BOX 31-3)

A. Description
  1. Prostaglandins are potent stimulators of the myometrium.
  2. Dinoprostone is administered as a gel or suppository directly into the vagina.

BOX 31-2

Uterine Relaxants

Ritodrine (Yutopar)
Terbutaline (Bricanyl)

BOX 31-3

Prostaglandins

Carboprost (Hemabate)
Dinoprostone (Cervidil)

3. Carboprost can be administered by deep intramuscular injection.

B. Uses
1. Prostaglandins are abortifacients.
2. Prostaglandins can induce abortion during the second trimester, when the uterus is resistant to oxytocin.
3. Dinoprostone also is used to soften and promote dilation of the cervix to facilitate vaginal **delivery**.

C. Adverse reactions and contraindications
1. Significant gastrointestinal side effects, including diarrhea, nausea, vomiting, and stomach cramps
2. Fever, chills, and flushing
3. Anaphylaxis, dysrhythmias, bronchoconstriction, chest pain, hypertension, and peripheral vasoconstriction
4. Contraindicated in clients with significant cardiovascular disease or those with a history of asthma or pulmonary disease
5. Uterine cramping and tetany caused by high doses

D. Interventions
1. Monitor maternal vital signs, especially the blood pressure and heart rate, weight, intake and output, level of consciousness, and lung sounds.
2. Monitor frequency, duration, force of uterine contractions, and resting uterine tone frequently; palpate the fundus.
3. Monitor vaginal bleeding.
4. Remain with the client for 30 minutes after administration to monitor for anaphylaxis; signs include shortness of breath or difficulty breathing, tachycardia, hives, tightness in the chest, or swelling of the face.
5. Maintain client in a supine position for 30 minutes following administration of the medication.
6. Keep side rails up; have a suction machine at the bedside.
7. Administer antidiarrheal and antiemetic medications as prescribed.

V. MAGNESIUM SULFATE

A. Description
1. Magnesium sulfate is a central nervous system depressant and anticonvulsant.
2. The medication causes smooth muscle relaxation.
3. The antidote is calcium gluconate.

B. Uses
1. Prevent and control seizures in preeclamptic and eclamptic clients
2. Treat preterm **labor**

C. Adverse reactions and contraindications
1. Magnesium sulfate can cause reduced respiratory rate, decreased reflexes, flushing, hypotension, and decreased heart rate.
2. Continuous IV infusion increases the risk of magnesium toxicity in the **neonate**.
3. Intravenous administration should not be used for 2 hours preceding **delivery**.

4. Magnesium sulfate is continued for the first 12 to 24 hours postpartum if it is used for preeclampsia.
5. High doses can cause loss of deep tendon reflexes, heart block, respiratory paralysis, and cardiac arrest.
6. The medication is contraindicated in the client with heart block, myocardial damage, or renal failure.
7. The medication is used with caution in the client with severe renal impairment.

D. Interventions
1. Monitor maternal vital signs, especially respirations, every 30 to 60 minutes.
2. Call the health care provider if respirations are less than 12, indicating respiratory depression.
3. Assess renal function and electrocardiogram for cardiac function.
4. Monitor magnesium levels, for the target range is 4 to 7 mEq/L; if a rise in the magnesium level occurs, notify the health care provider.
5. Administered by IV infusion via an infusion monitoring device; carefully monitor dose being administered.
6. Keep calcium gluconate on hand in case of a magnesium sulfate overdose, because calcium gluconate antagonizes the effect of magnesium sulfate.
7. Monitor deep tendon reflexes hourly for signs of developing toxicity.
8. Test patellar reflex or knee jerk reflex before administering repeat parenteral doses (used as an indicator of central nervous system depression; suppressed reflex may be a sign of impending respiratory arrest).
9. Patellar reflex must be present and respiratory rate must be greater than 16 breaths per minute before each parenteral dose.
10. Monitor intake and output hourly; output should be maintained at 30 mL per hour because the medication is eliminated through the kidneys.

VI. MEPERIDINE HYDROCHLORIDE (DEMEROL)

A. Description
1. Narcotic analgesic
2. Administered by intramuscular or IV route
3. Antidote: naloxone (Narcan)

B. Use: to relieve moderate to severe pain associated with **labor**

C. Adverse reactions and contraindications
1. Meperidine can cause dizziness, nausea, vomiting, sedation, decreased blood pressure, decreased respirations, diaphoresis, flushed face, decreased urination.
2. Meperidine may be administered with promethazine (Phenergan) to prevent nausea.
3. High dosages may result in respiratory depression, skeletal muscle flaccidity, cold, clammy skin, cyanosis, extreme somnolence progressing to convulsions, stupor, and coma.

4. Meperidine is used cautiously in clients delivering preterm infants.
5. Meperidine is not administered in early **labor** because it may slow the **labor** process.
6. Meperidine is not administered in advanced **labor** (within 1 hour of **delivery**) if the **neonate** is to be delivered before the medication is removed adequately from the fetal circulation (may cause respiratory depression).
7. Regular use of opiates during pregnancy may produce withdrawal symptoms in the **neonate** (irritability, excessive crying, tremors, hyperactive reflexes, fever, vomiting, diarrhea, yawning, sneezing, and seizures).

D. Interventions
1. Monitor vital signs, particularly respiratory status; if respirations are 12 per minute or fewer, withhold medication and contact the health care provider.
2. Monitor for blood pressure changes (hypotension); maintain in a recumbent position.
3. Have antidote available.

▲ VII. Rh$_0$(D) IMMUNE GLOBULIN (RhoGAM)
A. Description
1. Prevention of anti-Rh(D) antibody formation is most successful if the medication is administered twice: at 28 weeks of gestation and again within 72 hours after **delivery**.
2. The immune globulin also should be administered within 72 hours after potential or actual exposure to Rh-positive blood; must be given with each subsequent exposure or potential exposure to Rh-positive blood.
3. The immune globulin is of no benefit once the client has developed a positive antibody titer to the Rh antigen.
B. Use: to prevent isoimmunization in Rh-negative clients who are exposed or potentially exposed to Rh-positive red blood cells by transfusion, termination of pregnancy, amniocentesis, chorionic villus sampling (CVS), abdominal trauma, or bleeding during pregnancy or the birth process
▲ C. Adverse reactions and contraindications
1. Elevated temperature
2. Tenderness at the injection site
3. Contraindicated for Rh-positive women
4. Contraindicated in clients with a history of systemic allergic reactions to preparations containing human immunoglobulins
5. Not administered to a **newborn infant**
D. Interventions
1. Administer to mother by intramuscular injection at 28 weeks' gestation and within 72 hours after **delivery**.
2. Never administer by the IV route.
3. Monitor for temperature elevation.
4. Monitor injection site for tenderness.

VIII. BETAMETHASONE (CELESTONE)
A. Description
1. Betamethasone is a corticosteroid.
2. Betamethasone increases production of surfactant.
B. Use: for client in preterm **labor** between 28 and 32 weeks whose **labor** can be inhibited for 48 hours without jeopardizing the mother or fetus.
C. Adverse reactions and contraindications
1. Decreases mother's resistance to infection
2. Breast-feeding contraindicated during medication administration
D. Interventions
1. Monitor maternal vital signs.
2. Monitor mother for signs of infection.
3. Monitor white blood cell count.

IX. LUNG SURFACTANTS (BOX 31-4) ▲
A. Description
1. Lung surfactants replenish surfactant and restore surface activity to the lungs.
2. Lung surfactants are administered by the intratracheal route.
B. Use: to prevent or treat respiratory distress syndrome (hyaline membrane disease) in premature infants
C. Adverse reactions and contraindications
1. Side effects include transient bradycardia and oxygen desaturation.
2. Surfactants are administered with caution in those at risk for circulatory overload.
D. Interventions ▲
1. Instill surfactant through catheter inserted into infant's endotracheal tube; avoid suctioning for at least 2 hours after administration.
2. Monitor for bradycardia and decreased oxygen saturation during administration.
3. Assess lung sounds for rales and moist breath sounds.

X. EYE PROPHYLAXIS FOR THE NEONATE ▲
A. Description
1. Erythromycin (0.5% Ilotycin) and tetracycline (1%) ophthalmic ointment or drops are bacteriostatic and bactericidal and provide prophylaxis against *Neisseria gonorrhoeae* and *Chlamydia trachomatis*.
2. Silver nitrate (1%) solution may be prescribed, but its use is minimal because it does not protect against chlamydial infection and can cause chemical conjunctivitis.
3. Preventive treatment of gonorrhea is required by law.

BOX 31-4

Lung Surfactants

Beractant (Survanta)
Colfosceril palmitate (Exosurf)

B. Use: as a prophylactic measure to protect against *Neisseria gonorrhoeae* and *Chlamydia trachomatis*
C. Adverse reaction: Silver nitrate (1%) solution can cause chemical conjunctivitis.
D. Interventions
   1. Cleanse the neonate's eyes before instilling drops or ointment.
   2. Instill into each of the neonate's conjunctival sacs within 1 hour after **delivery**; eye prophylaxis may be delayed until an hour or so after birth to facilitate eye contact and parent-infant attachment and bonding.
   3. Do not flush the eyes after instillation.

XI. VITAMIN K (AquaMEPHYTON)

A. Description
   1. Vitamin K is necessary for aiding in the production of active prothrombin.
   2. Newborns are deficient in vitamin K for the first 5 to 8 days of life because of the lack of intestinal flora that is necessary to absorb vitamin K.
B. Use: for prophylaxis and to treat hemorrhagic disease of the **newborn**
C. Adverse reaction: Vitamin K can cause hyperbilirubinemia in the **newborn**.
D. Interventions
   1. Protect the medication from light.
   2. Administer during the early neonatal period.
   3. Administer in the vastus lateralis muscle of the thigh.
   4. Monitor for bruising at the injection site and for bleeding from the cord.
   5. Monitor for jaundice and monitor bilirubin level because the medication can cause hyperbilirubinemia in the **newborn**.

PRACTICE QUESTIONS

1. Epidural analgesia is administered to a woman for pain relief following a cesarean birth. The nurse assigned to care for the woman ensures that which medication is readily available if respiratory depression occurs?
   1. Betamethasone (Celestone)
   2. Morphine sulfate
   3. Meperidine hydrochloride (Demerol)
   4. Naloxone (Narcan)
2. Rh$_0$(D) immune globulin (RhoGAM) is prescribed for a woman following delivery of a newborn infant and the nurse provides information to the woman about the purpose of the medication. The nurse determines that the woman understands the purpose of the medication if the woman states that it will protect her next baby from which of the following?
   1. Being affected by Rh incompatibility
   2. Having Rh-positive blood
   3. Developing a rubella infection
   4. Developing physiological jaundice

3. Methylergonovine (Methergine) is prescribed for a woman to treat postpartum hemorrhage. Before administration of methylergonovine, the priority nursing assessment is to check the
   1. Amount of lochia.
   2. Blood pressure.
   3. Deep tendon reflexes.
   4. Uterine tone.
4. A nurse is preparing to administer beractant (Survanta) to a premature infant who has respiratory distress syndrome (hyaline membrane disease). The nurse plans to administer the medication by which of the following routes?
   1. Subcutaneous
   2. Intratracheal
   3. Intramuscular
   4. Intradermal
5. A nurse is caring for a client who is receiving oxytocin (Pitocin) to induce labor. The nurse discontinues the oxytocin infusion if which of the following is noted on assessment of the client?
   1. Drowsiness
   2. Fatigue
   3. Early decelerations of the fetal heart rate
   4. Uterine hyperstimulation
6. A pregnant client is receiving magnesium sulfate for the management of preeclampsia. A nurse determines that the client is experiencing toxicity from the medication if which of the following is noted on assessment?
   1. Presence of deep tendon reflexes
   2. Serum magnesium level of 6 mEq/L
   3. Proteinuria of +3
   4. Respirations of 10 per minute
7. A woman with preeclampsia is receiving magnesium sulfate. The nurse assigned to care for the client determines that the magnesium sulfate therapy is effective if
   1. Ankle clonus is noted.
   2. The blood pressure decreases.
   3. Seizures do not occur.
   4. Scotomas are present.
8. Methylergonovine (Methergine) is prescribed for a client with postpartum hemorrhage. Before administering the medication, a nurse contacts the health care provider who prescribed the medication if which of the following conditions is documented in the client's medical history?
   1. Peripheral vascular disease
   2. Hypothyroidism
   3. Hypotension
   4. Diabetes mellitus
9. Vitamin K (AquaMEPHYTON) is prescribed for a neonate. A nurse prepares the medication and selects which muscle site to administer the medication?
   1. Deltoid
   2. Triceps

3. Vastus lateralis
4. Biceps

10. A nursing instructor asks a nursing student to describe the procedure for administering erythromycin (0.5% Ilotycin) ointment to the eyes of a neonate. The instructor determines that the student needs to research this procedure further if the student states
   1. "I will cleanse the neonate's eyes before instilling ointment."
   2. "I will flush the eyes after instilling the ointment."
   3. "I will instill the eye ointment into each of the neonate's conjunctival sacs within 1 hour after birth."

4. "Administration of the eye ointment may be delayed until an hour or so after birth so that eye contact and parent-infant attachment and bonding can occur."

CRITICAL THINKING: FILL IN THE BLANK

A nurse is caring for a pregnant client with severe preeclampsia who is receiving magnesium sulfate intravenously. The nurse ensures that what medication, the antidote to magnesium sulfate, is in the client's room?

Answer: _____

ANSWERS

1. 4
Rationale: Narcotics are used for epidural analgesia. An adverse reaction of epidural analgesia is a delayed respiratory depression. Naloxone (Narcan) is a narcotic antagonist, which reverses the effects of narcotics and is given for respiratory depression. Morphine sulfate and meperidine hydrochloride are narcotics. Betamethasone is a corticosteroid administered to enhance fetal lung maturity.
Test-Taking Strategy: Use the process of elimination, focusing on the issue of the question, the antidote for respiratory depression. Eliminate options 2 and 3 first, knowing that these medications are narcotics. Next eliminate option 1, knowing that this medication is a corticosteroid. Review the purpose and actions of these medications if you had difficulty with this question.
Level of Cognitive Ability: Application
Client Needs: Physiological Integrity
Integrated Process: Nursing Process—planning
Content Area: Maternity—postpartum
Reference: Kee, J., & Hayes, E. (2003). *Pharmacology: A nursing process approach* (4th ed., p. 866). Philadelphia: W. B. Saunders.

2. 1
Rationale: Rh incompatibility can occur when an Rh-negative mother becomes sensitized to the Rh antigen. Sensitization may develop when an Rh-negative woman becomes pregnant with a fetus who is Rh positive. During pregnancy and at delivery, some of the baby's Rh-positive blood can enter the maternal circulation, causing the woman's immune system to form antibodies against Rh-positive blood. Administration of $Rh_0(D)$ immune globulin prevents the woman from developing antibodies against Rh-positive blood by providing passive antibody protection against the Rh antigen.
Test-Taking Strategy: Use the process of elimination. Options 3 and 4 can be eliminated first. From the remaining options, note the relationship between the name of the medication, $Rh_0(D)$ immune globulin, and the word "incompatibility" in the correct option. Review the purpose of this medication if you had difficulty with this question.
Level of Cognitive Ability: Analysis
Client Needs: Physiological Integrity
Integrated Process: Teaching/Learning
Content Area: Maternity—postpartum

Reference: Hodgson, B., & Kizior, R. (2003). *Saunders nursing drug handbook 2003.* (p. 972). Philadelphia: W. B. Saunders.

3. 2
Rationale: Methylergonovine, an ergot alkaloid, is an agent that is used to prevent or control postpartum hemorrhage by contracting the uterus. Methylergonovine causes continuous uterine contractions and may elevate blood pressure. A priority assessment before the administration of the medication is to check the blood pressure. The physician should be notified if hypertension is present. Although options 1, 3, and 4 may be components of the postpartum assessment, option 2, blood pressure, is related specifically to the administration of this medication.
Test-Taking Strategy: Use the process of elimination. Eliminate options 1 and 4 first because they are similar and related to one another. From the remaining options, use the ABCs—airway, breathing, and circulation. Blood pressure is a method of assessing circulation. Review the adverse effects of this medication if you had difficulty with this question.
Level of Cognitive Ability: Analysis
Client Needs: Physiological Integrity
Integrated Process: Nursing Process—assessment
Content Area: Maternity—postpartum
Reference: Kee, J., & Hayes, E. (2003). *Pharmacology: A nursing process approach* (4th ed., p. 785). Philadelphia: W. B. Saunders.

4. 2
Rationale: Respiratory distress is common in premature neonates and may be due to lung immaturity as a result of surfactant deficiency. The mainstay of treatment is the administration of exogenous surfactant, which is administered by the intratracheal route. Options 1, 3, and 4 are not routes of administration for this medication.
Test-Taking Strategy: Use the process of elimination. Note the relationship between the diagnosis "respiratory distress syndrome" and the correct option, "intratracheal." Review this medication if you had difficulty with this question.
Level of Cognitive Ability: Application
Client Needs: Physiological Integrity
Integrated Process: Nursing Process—planning
Content Area: Maternity—postpartum
Reference: Hodgson, B., & Kizior, R. (2004). *Saunders nursing drug handbook 2004* (p. 103). Philadelphia: W. B. Saunders.

5. 4

Rationale: Oxytocin stimulates uterine contractions and is one of the common pharmacological methods to induce labor. An adverse reaction associated with administration of the medication is hyperstimulation of uterine contractions. Therefore oxytocin infusion must be stopped when any signs of uterine hyperstimulation are present. Drowsiness and fatigue may be due to the labor experience. Early decelerations of the fetal heart rate are a reassuring sign and do not indicate fetal distress.

Test-Taking Strategy: Use the process of elimination, focusing on the issue, an adverse reaction to oxytocin. Options 1 and 2 can be eliminated first. From the remaining options, recalling that early decelerations of the fetal heart rate are a reassuring sign will direct you to option 4. Review the nursing responsibilities associated with this medication if you had difficulty with this question.

Level of Cognitive Ability: Application
Client Needs: Physiological Integrity
Integrated Process: Nursing Process—implementation
Content Area: Maternity—intrapartum
References: Hodgson, B., & Kizior, R. (2004). *Saunders nursing drug handbook 2004* (p. 770). Philadelphia: W. B. Saunders. Kee, J., & Hayes, E. (2003). *Pharmacology: A nursing process approach* (4th ed., p. 782). Philadelphia: W. B. Saunders.

6. 4

Rationale: Magnesium toxicity can occur from magnesium sulfate therapy. Signs of magnesium sulfate toxicity relate to central nervous system depressant effects of the medication and include respiratory depression, loss of deep tendon reflexes, and a sudden drop in fetal heart rate and maternal heart rate and blood pressure. Therapeutic serum levels of magnesium are 4 to 7 mEq/L. Proteinuria of +3 is likely to be noted in a client with preeclampsia.

Test-Taking Strategy: Use the process of elimination and eliminate option 1 first because it is a normal finding. Next eliminate option 2, knowing that the therapeutic serum level of magnesium is between 4 and 7 mEq/L. From the remaining options, recalling that proteinuria of +3 would be noted in a client with preeclampsia will direct you to the correct option. Review the adverse effects of magnesium sulfate if you had difficulty with this question.

Level of Cognitive Ability: Analysis
Client Needs: Physiological Integrity
Integrated Process: Nursing Process—assessment
Content Area: Maternity—intrapartum
Reference: Hodgson, B., & Kizior, R. (2004). *Saunders nursing drug handbook 2004* (p. 624). Philadelphia: W. B. Saunders.

7. 3

Rationale: For a client with preeclampsia, the goal of care is directed at preventing eclampsia (seizures). Magnesium sulfate is an anticonvulsant, not an antihypertensive agent. Although a decrease in blood pressure may be noted initially, this effect is usually transient. Ankle clonus indicates hyperreflexia and may precede the onset of eclampsia. Scotomas are areas of complete or partial blindness. Visual disturbances, such as scotomas, often precede an eclamptic seizure.

Test-Taking Strategy: Use the process of elimination. Knowing that magnesium sulfate is an anticonvulsant will direct you to

option 3. Review this medication if you had difficulty with this question.

Level of Cognitive Ability: Analysis
Client Needs: Physiological Integrity
Integrated Process: Nursing Process—evaluation
Content Area: Maternity—intrapartum
Reference: Lehne, R. (2001). *Pharmacology for nursing care* (4th ed., pp. 208, 486). Philadelphia: W. B. Saunders.

8. 1

Rationale: Methylergonovine is an ergot alkaloid used for postpartum hemorrhage. Ergot alkaloids are avoided in clients with significant cardiovascular disease, peripheral disease, hypertension, eclampsia, or preeclampsia. These conditions are worsened by the vasoconstrictive effects of the ergot alkaloids. Options 2, 3, and 4 are not contraindications related to the use of ergot alkaloids.

Test-Taking Strategy: Use the process of elimination. Recalling that ergot alkaloids produce vasoconstriction will direct you to option 1. Review the effects of this medication and the associated contraindications if you had difficulty with this question.

Level of Cognitive Ability: Application
Client Needs: Physiological Integrity
Integrated Process: Nursing Process—implementation
Content Area: Maternity—postpartum
Reference: Hodgson, B., & Kizior, R. (2004). *Saunders nursing drug handbook 2004* (p. 654). Philadelphia: W. B. Saunders.

9. 3

Rationale: Newborns are deficient in vitamin K for the first 5 to 8 days of life because of the lack of intestinal flora that is necessary to absorb vitamin K. Vitamin K is administered to the neonate to aid in the production of active prothrombin and to prevent hemorrhagic disease. Vitamin K is administered in the vastus lateralis muscle. Options 1, 2, and 4 are incorrect administration sites.

Test-Taking Strategy: Use the process of elimination. Visualize the procedure for administering an injection to a neonate to assist in directing you to option 3. Review this procedure if you had difficulty with this question.

Level of Cognitive Ability: Application
Client Needs: Physiological Integrity
Integrated Process: Nursing Process—implementation
Content Area: Maternity—postpartum
Reference: Murray, S., McKinney, E., & Gorrie, T. (2002). *Foundations of maternal-newborn nursing* (3rd ed., p. 547). Philadelphia: W. B. Saunders.

10. 2

Rationale: Eye prophylaxis protects the neonate against *Neisseria gonorrhoeae* and *Chlamydia trachomatis*. The eyes are not flushed after instillation of the medication because the flush will wash away the administered medication. Options 1, 3, and 4 are correct statements regarding the procedure for administering eye medication to the neonate.

Test-Taking Strategy: Use the process of elimination, noting the key words "needs to research further." Eliminate options 3 and 4 first because they are similar. From the remaining options, visualize the effect of each. This will direct you to

option 2. Review the procedure for administering eye medication to the neonate if you had difficulty with this question.
Level of Cognitive Ability: Analysis
Client Needs: Safe, Effective Care Environment
Integrated Process: Teaching/Learning
Content Area: Maternity—postpartum
Reference: Murray, S., McKinney, E., & Gorrie, T. (2002). *Foundations of maternal-newborn nursing* (3rd ed., p. 552). Philadelphia: W. B. Saunders.

CRITICAL THINKING: FILL IN THE BLANK
Answer: Calcium gluconate
Rationale: Calcium gluconate is the medication that acts as an antidote to magnesium sulfate and should be placed in the room of the client receiving magnesium sulfate intravenously.
Test-Taking Strategy: You must know the antidote for magnesium sulfate to answer this question. If you are unfamiliar with the guidelines for the administration of this medication, review this content.
Level of Cognitive Ability: Application
Client Needs: Physiological Integrity
Integrated Process: Nursing Process—implementation
Content Area: Maternity—intrapartum
Reference: Gutierrez, K., & Queener, S. (2003). *Pharmacology for nursing practice* (p. 1031). St. Louis: Mosby.

REFERENCES

Gutierrez, K., & Queener, S. (2003). *Pharmacology for nursing practice.* St. Louis: Mosby.

Hodgson, B., & Kizior, R. (2003). *Saunders nursing drug handbook 2003.* Philadelphia: W. B. Saunders.

Hodgson, B., & Kizior, R. (2004). *Saunders nursing drug handbook 2004.* Philadelphia: W. B. Saunders.

Kee, J., & Hayes, E. (2003). *Pharmacology: A nursing process approach* (4th ed.). Philadelphia: W. B. Saunders.

Lehne, R. (2001). *Pharmacology for nursing care* (4th ed.). Philadelphia: W. B. Saunders.

Murray, S., McKinney, E., & Gorrie, T. (2002). *Foundations of maternal-newborn nursing* (3rd ed.). Philadelphia: W. B. Saunders.

Growth and Development across the Life Span

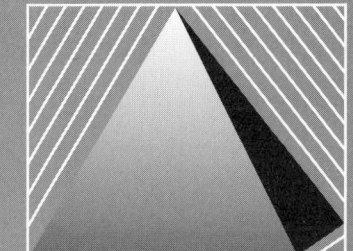

PYRAMID TERMS

abuse   The willful infliction of pain, injury, or mental anguish; unreasonable confinement or willful deprivation of services, including medical care. Abuse can include failure to prevent injury, verbal assaults, the demand to perform demeaning tasks, theft, or mismanagement of personal belongings.

accommodation   The ability to change a schema (an individual's cognitive structure or framework of thought) to introduce new ideas, objects, or experiences.

aging   The biopsychosocial process of change occurring between birth and death.

assimilation   The ability to incorporate new ideas, objects, and experiences into the framework of one's thoughts.

conscious   All experiences that are within an individual's awareness and that the individual is able to control.

dementia   Organic syndrome identified by gradual and progressive deterioration in intellectual functioning. Long- and short-term memory loss occurs with impairment in judgment, abstract thinking, problem-solving ability, and behavior, resulting in a self-care deficit. The most common type of dementia is Alzheimer's disease.

depression   A functional disorder of mood that is not linked with aging. The depression may be precipitated by losses related to aging. Depression can be manifested by cognitive impairment or may be the cause of a decline in mental status. Depression can be identified by feelings of sadness, hopelessness, and worthlessness, and a decreased interest in activities.

ego   One's "sense of self"; provides functions such as problem solving, mobilization of defense mechanisms, reality testing, and the capability of functioning independently; the mediator between the id and the superego.

exploitation   Illegal or improper use of the individual's resources.

gerontology   The study of the process of aging.

id   Source of all primitive drives and instincts; thought of as the reservoir of all psychic energy.

neglect   The lack of providing services necessary for physical or mental health.

schema   An individual's cognitive structure or framework of thought.

schemata   Categories that an individual forms in his or her mind to organize and understand the world.

self-neglect   The choice to avoid medical care or other services that could improve optimal function. Unless declared legally incompetent, an individual has the right to refuse care.

subconscious   Often called the preconscious; includes experiences, thoughts, feelings, or desires that might not be in immediate awareness but can be recalled to consciousness; helps repress unpleasant thoughts or feelings.

superego   The moral component of personality, including internalization of the values, ideals, and moral standards of society.

unconscious   Memories, feelings, thoughts, or wishes that are repressed and that are not available to the conscious mind.

◢ THE PYRAMID TO SUCCESS

Normal growth and development proceed in an orderly, systematic, and predictable pattern, which provides a basis for identifying and assessing an individual's abilities. Understanding the path of growth and development across the life span assists the nurse in identifying appropriate and expected human behavior. The Pyramid to Success focuses on Sigmund Freud's theory of psychosexual development, Jean Piaget's theory of cognitive development, Erik Erikson's psychosocial theory, and Lawrence Kohlberg's theory of moral development. Growth and development concepts focus on the aging process and on physical characteristics, nutritional behaviors, skills, play, and specific safety measures relevant to a particular age group that will ensure a safe and hazard-free environment. When a question is presented on the NCLEX-RN examination, if an age is identified in the question, note the age and think about the associated growth and developmental concepts. The Integrated Processes addressed in this unit include Nursing Process, Caring, Communication and Documentation, and Teaching/Learning.

◢ CLIENT NEEDS
Safe, Effective Care Environment

Accident prevention
Advocacy
Client rights
Confidentiality
Consultation with members of the health care team
Establishing priorities
Ethical practice
Legal responsibilities
Referrals
Respect for client and family needs based on their preferences

Health Promotion and Maintenance

Aging process
Client and family education
Developmental stages and transition
Expected body image changes
Family planning and family systems
Growth and development
Health and wellness
Health care beliefs and preferences
Lifestyle choices

Psychosocial Integrity

Abuse and neglect
Adjustment to potential deterioration in physical and mental health and well-being in the older client
Changes and adjustment in role function in the older client (threat to independent functioning)
Coping mechanisms
Grief and loss issues with the older client
Loss of quantity and quality of relationships with the older client
Sensory/perceptual alterations
Support systems
Use of resources for the client and family

Physiological Integrity

Alterations in body systems and the related risks from the aging process
Basic care and comfort needs
Health care preferences
Interventions compatible with the client's age, cultural, religious, and health care beliefs, education level, and language.
Practices or restrictions related to procedures and treatments
Provision of care using a nonjudgmental approach
Safe medication administration

REFERENCES

Ebersole, P., & Hess, P. (2001). *Geriatric nursing & healthy aging.* St. Louis: Mosby.
Ignatavicius, D., & Workman, M. (2002). *Medical-surgical nursing: Critical thinking for collaborative care* (4th ed.). Philadelphia: W. B. Saunders.
Leuckenotte, A. (2000). *Gerontologic nursing* (2nd ed.). St. Louis: Mosby.
Lewis, S., Heitkemper, M., & Dirksen, S. (2004). *Medical-surgical nursing: Assessment and management of clinical problems* (6th ed.). St. Louis: Mosby.
Lowdermilk, D., & Perry, S. (2003). *Maternity nursing* (6th ed.). St. Louis: Mosby.
National Council of State Boards of Nursing (Eds.). (2003). *Test Plan for the National Council Licensure Examination for Registered Nurses* (effective date: April 2004). Chicago: Author.
Phipps, W., Monahan, F., Sands, J., Marek, J., & Neighbors, M. (2003). *Medical-surgical nursing: health and illness perspectives* (7th ed.). St. Louis: Mosby.
Potter, P., & Perry, A. (2001). *Fundamentals of nursing* (5th ed.). St. Louis: Mosby.
Varcarolis, E. M. (2002). *Foundations of psychiatric mental health nursing* (4th ed.). Philadelphia: W. B. Saunders.
Wong, D., & Hockenberry, M. (2003). *Nursing care of infants and children* (7th ed.). St. Louis: Mosby.
Wong, D., & Hockenberry-Eaton, M. (2000). *Wong's essentials of pediatric nursing* (6th ed.). St. Louis: Mosby.
Wong, D., Perry, S., & Hockenberry, M. (2002). *Maternal child nursing care* (2nd ed.). St. Louis: Mosby.

Theories of Growth and Development

I. PSYCHOSOCIAL DEVELOPMENT AND ERIK ERIKSON

A. The theory

1. Erikson's theory of psychosocial development describes the human life cycle as a series of eight **ego** developmental stages from birth to death.

2. Each stage presents a psychosocial crisis, the goal of which is to integrate physical, maturation, and societal demands.

3. The theory focuses on psychosocial tasks that are accomplished throughout the life cycle.

4. The **ego** is separate and liberated from the **id**, developing across the course of the complete life cycle.

5. **Ego** development is influenced by family, social, and developmental factors.

B. Psychosocial development

1. Psychosocial development is a lifelong series of conflicts affected by social and cultural factors.

2. Each conflict must be resolved for the child or adult to progress emotionally.

3. Unsuccessful resolution leaves the individual emotionally handicapped.

C. Stages of psychosocial development (Table 32-1)

II. COGNITIVE DEVELOPMENT AND JEAN PIAGET

A. The theory

1. Piaget's theory of cognitive development defines cognitive acts as ways in which the mind organizes and adapts to its environment.

TABLE 32-1

Erik Erikson's Stages of Psychosocial Development

Age	Psychosocial Crisis	Task
Infancy (Birth to 18 months)	Trust vs. Mistrust	Attachment to the mother

Resolution of Crisis
Trust in persons; faith and hope about the environment and the future
Unsuccessful Resolution of Crisis
General difficulties relating to persons effectively; suspicion; trust-fear conflict, fear of the future

Age	Psychosocial Crisis	Task
Early childhood (18 months to 3 years)	Autonomy vs. Shame and Doubt	Gaining some basic control over self and environment

Resolution of Crisis
Sense of self-control and adequacy; will power
Unsuccessful Resolution of Crisis
Independence-fear conflict; severe feelings of self-doubt

Continued

TABLE 32-1

Erik Erikson's Stages of Psychosocial Development—cont'd

Age	Psychosocial Crisis	Task
Late childhood (3-6 years)	Initiative vs. Guilt	Becoming purposeful and directive

Resolution of Crisis
Ability to initiate one's own activities; sense of purpose
Unsuccessful Resolution of Crisis
Aggression-fear conflict; sense of inadequacy or guilt

Age	Psychosocial Crisis	Task
School age (6-12 years)	Industry vs. Inferiority	Developing social, physical, and school skills

Resolution of Crisis
Competence; ability to learn and work
Unsuccessful Resolution of Crisis
Sense of inferiority; difficulty learning and working

Age	Psychosocial Crisis	Task
Adolescence (12-20 years)	Identity vs. Role Confusion	Developing sense of identity

Resolution of Crisis
Sense of personal identity
Unsuccessful Resolution of Crisis
Confusion about who one is; identity submerged in relationships or group memberships

Age	Psychosocial Crisis	Task
Early adulthood (20-35 years)	Intimacy vs. Isolation	Establishing intimate bonds of love and friendship

Resolution of Crisis
Ability to love deeply and commit oneself
Unsuccessful Resolution of Crisis
Emotional isolation, egocentricity

Age	Psychosocial Crisis	Task
Middle adulthood (35-65 years)	Generativity vs. Stagnation	Fulfilling life goals that involve family, career, and society

Resolution of Crisis
Ability to give and care for others
Unsuccessful Resolution of Crisis
Self-absorption; inability to grow as a person

Age	Psychosocial Crisis	Task
Later (65 years to death)	Integrity vs. Despair	Looking back over one's life and accepting its meaning

Resolution of Crisis
Sense of integrity and fulfillment
Unsuccessful Resolution of Crisis
Dissatisfaction with life

Modified from Varcarolis, E. (2002). *Foundations of psychiatric mental health nursing* (4th ed., p. 30). Philadelphia: W. B. Saunders.

2. **Schema** refers to an individual's cognitive structure or framework of thought.
3. **Schemata**
   a. **Schemata** are categories that an individual forms in his or her mind to organize and understand the world.
   b. A young child has only a few **schemata** with which to understand the world, and gradually these are increased.
   c. Adults use a wide variety of **schemata** to understand the world.

4. **Assimilation**
   a. **Assimilation** is the ability to incorporate new ideas, objects, and experiences into the framework of one's thoughts.
   b. The growing child will perceive and give meaning to new information according to what is already known and understood.
5. **Accommodation**
   a. **Accommodation** is the ability to change a **schema** to introduce new ideas, objects, or experiences.

b. Accommodation changes the mental structure so that new experiences can be added.

B. Stages of cognitive development

1. Sensorimotor stage
   a. Birth to 2 years
   b. Development proceeds from reflex activity to imagining and solving problems through the senses and movement.

2. Preoperational stage
   a. 2 to 7 years
   b. The child learns to think in terms of past, present, and future.
   c. The child moves from knowing the world through sensation and movement to prelogical thinking and finding solutions to problems.

3. Concrete operational
   a. 7 to 11 years
   b. The child is able to classify, order, and sort facts.

   c. The child moves from prelogical thought to solving concrete problems through logic.

4. Formal operations
   a. 11 years to adulthood
   b. The person is able to think abstractly and logically.
   c. Logical thinking is expanded to include solving abstract and concrete problems.

III. MORAL DEVELOPMENT AND LAWRENCE KOHLBERG

A. Moral development
   1. Moral development is a complicated process involving the acceptance of the values and rules of society in a way that shapes behavior.
   2. Moral development is classified in a series of levels and behaviors.

B. Levels of moral development (Box 32-1)

BOX 32-1

Moral Development and Lawrence Kohlberg

LEVEL ONE: PRECONVENTIONAL

Stage 0 (Birth to 2 years)

The infant has no awareness of right or wrong.

Stage 1 (2-3 years)

At this stage children cannot reason as mature members of society.

Children view the world in a selfish way, with no real understanding of right or wrong.

The child obeys rules and demonstrates acceptable behavior to avoid punishment, to avoid displeasing those who are in power, and because the child fears punishment from a superior force as a parent.

A toddler typically is at the first substage of the preconventional stage, involving punishment and obedience orientation, in which the toddler makes judgments based on avoiding punishment or obtaining a reward.

Physical punishment and withholding privileges tend to give the toddler a negative view of morals.

Withdrawing love and affection as punishment leads to feelings of guilt in the toddler.

Appropriate discipline includes providing simple explanations why certain behaviors are unacceptable, praising appropriate behavior, and using distractions when the toddler is headed for an unsafe action.

Stage 2 (4-7 years)

The child conforms to rules to obtain rewards or have favors returned.

The child's moral standards are those of others, and the child's observes them to either avoid punishment or obtain rewards.

A preschooler is in the preconventional stage of moral development.

In this stage, conscience emerges and the emphasis is on external control.

LEVEL TWO: CONVENTIONAL

The child conforms to rules to please others.

The child has increased awareness of others' feelings.

A concern for social order begins to emerge.

A child views good behavior as that which those in authority will approve.

If the behavior is not acceptable, the child feels guilty.

Stage 3 (7-10 years)

Conformity occurs to avoid disapproval or dislike by others.

This stage involves living up to what is expected by individuals close to you or what individuals generally expect of others in their roles as son, brother, friend, and so on.

Being good is important and is interpreted as having good motives and showing concern about others.

Being good also means maintaining mutual relationships, such as trust, loyalty, respect, and gratitude.

Stage 4 (10-12 years)

The child has more concern with society as a whole.

Emphasis is on obeying laws to maintain social order.

Moral reasoning develops as the child shifts the focus of living to society.

The school-aged child is at the conventional level of the role conformity stage and has an increased desire to please others.

The child observes and to some extent internalizes the standards of others.

The child wants to be considered "good" by those individuals whose opinions matter to the child.

LEVEL THREE: POSTCONVENTIONAL

The individual focuses on individual rights and principles of conscience.

The focus is a concern regarding what is best for all.

Continued

BOX 32-1

Moral Development and Lawrence Kohlberg—cont'd

Stage 5
The person is aware that others hold a variety of values and opinions and that most values and rules are relative to the group.
The adolescent in this stage gives and takes and does not expect to get something without paying for it.
Stage 6
Conformity is based on universal principles of justice and occurs to avoid self-condemnation.
This stage involves following self-chosen ethical principles.

The development of the postconventional level of morality occurs in the adolescent at about age 13 years, marked by the development of an individual conscience and a defined set of moral values.
The adolescent can now acknowledge a conflict between two socially accepted standards and try to decide between them.
Control of conduct is now internal in standards observed and in reasoning about right and wrong.

IV. PSYCHOSEXUAL DEVELOPMENT AND SIGMUND FREUD

A. Components of the theory (Box 32-2)
  1. Levels of awareness
  2. Agencies of the mind (**id, ego, superego**)
  3. Concept of anxiety and defense mechanisms
  4. Psychosexual stages of development
B. Levels of awareness
  1. **Conscious** level of awareness
    a. The **conscious** mind is logical and is regulated by the Reality Principle.
    b. Consciousness includes all experiences that are within an individual's awareness and that the individual is able to control.
    c. Consciousness includes all information that is remembered easily and is immediately available to an individual.
  2. Preconscious level of awareness
    a. The preconscious is called the **subconscious.**
    b. The preconscious includes experiences, thoughts, feelings, or desires that might not be in immediate awareness but can be recalled to consciousness.
    c. The **subconscious** can help repress unpleasant thoughts or feelings and can examine and censor certain wishes and thinking.
  3. **Unconscious** level of awareness
    a. The **unconscious** is not logical and is governed by the Pleasure Principle, which refers to seeking immediate tension reduction.
    b. Memories, feelings, thoughts, or wishes are repressed and are not available to the conscious mind.

    c. These repressed memories, thoughts, or feelings, if made prematurely **conscious**, can cause anxiety.
C. Agencies of the mind
  1. **Id, ego,** and **superego**
    a. The **id, ego,** and **superego** are the three systems of personality.
    b. These psychological processes follow different operating principles.
    c. In a mature and well-adjusted personality, they work together as a team under the leadership of the **ego.**
  2. The **id**
    a. The **id** is the source of all drives.
    b. The **id** is present at birth.
    c. The **id** includes genetic inheritance, reflexes, capacities to respond, instincts, basic drives, needs, and wishes that motivate an individual.
    d. The **id** operates according to the Pleasure Principle.
    e. The **id** does not tolerate uncomfortable states and seeks to discharge the tension and return to a more comfortable, constant level of energy.
    f. The **id** acts immediately in an impulsive, irrational way and pays no attention to the consequences of its actions and therefore often behaves in ways harmful to self and others.
    g. The primary process is a psychological activity in which the **id** attempts to reduce tension.
    h. The primary process can include hallucinating or forming an image of the object that will satisfy its needs and remove the tension.
    i. The primary process by itself is not capable of reducing tension; therefore, a secondary psychological process must develop if the individual is to survive; when this occurs, the structure of the second system of the personality, the **ego,** begins to take form.
  3. The **ego**
    a. The functions of the **ego** include reality testing and problem solving.
    b. The **ego** begins its development during the fourth or fifth month of life.

BOX 32-2

Psychosexual Development and Sigmund Freud: Components of the Theory

Levels of awareness
Agencies of the mind (id, ego, superego)
Concept of anxiety and defense mechanisms
Psychosexual stages of development

c. The **ego** emerges out of the **id** and acts as an intermediary between the **id** and the external world.

d. The **ego** emerges because the needs, wishes, and demands of the **id** require appropriate exchanges with the outside world of reality.

e. The **ego** distinguishes between things in the mind and things in the external world.

f. Reality testing is a function of the **ego**, and the **ego** uses realistic thinking.

g. The **ego** follows the Reality Principle and operates by means of the secondary process; that is, realistic thinking.

h. The aim of the Reality Principle is to satisfy the id's impulses in the external world with an object that is suitable; the Reality Principle determines whether an experience is true or false and whether it has external existence.

i. The **ego** devises a plan and tests the plan by some kind of action to see if it will work.

4. The **superego**

a. The **superego** is a necessary part of socialization that develops during the phallic stage of 3 to 6 years of age.

b. The **superego** develops from the interactions with one's parents during the extended period of childhood dependency.

c. The **superego** includes the internalization of the values, ideals, and moral standards of society.

d. The child internalizes the moral standards of parents and society.

e. The **superego** consists of the conscience and the **ego** ideal.

f. The conscience refers to the capacity for self-evaluation and criticism.

g. When moral codes are violated, the conscience punishes the individual by instilling guilt.

h. What parents approve of and what they reward the child for doing become incorporated as the **ego** ideal by the mechanism of introjection.

i. The **superego** strives for perfection rather than pleasure and represents the ideal rather than the real.

j. Living up to one's **ego** ideal results in the individual feeling proud and increases self-esteem.

D. Anxiety and defense mechanisms

1. The **ego** develops defenses or defense mechanisms to fight off anxiety.

2. Defense mechanisms operate on an **unconscious** level, except for suppression, so the individual is not aware of their operation.

3. Defense mechanisms deny, falsify, or distort reality to make it less threatening.

4. An individual cannot survive without defense mechanisms; however, if they become too extreme in distorting reality, then interference in healthy adjustment and personal growth may occur.

E. Psychosexual stages of development (Box 32-3)

1. Human development proceeds through a series of stages from infancy to adulthood.

2. Each stage is characterized by the inborn tendency of all individuals to reduce tension and seek pleasure.

BOX 32-3

Freud's Psychosexual Stages of Development

ORAL STAGE (BIRTH TO 1 YEAR)
During this stage, the infant is concerned with self-gratification.
The infant is all id, operating on the Pleasure Principle and striving for immediate gratification of needs.
When the infant experiences gratification of basic needs, a sense of trust and security begins.
The ego begins to emerge as the infant begins to see self as separate from the mother; this marks the beginning of the development of a sense of self.

ANAL STAGE (1-3 YEARS)
Toilet training occurs during this period, and the child gains pleasure from the elimination of the feces and from their retention.
The conflict of this stage is between those demands from society and the parents and the sensations of pleasure associated with the anus.
The child begins to gain a sense of control over instinctive drives and learns to delay immediate gratification to gain a future goal.

PHALLIC STAGE (3-6 YEARS)
The child experiences pleasurable and conflicting feelings associated with the genital organs.
The pleasures of masturbation and the fantasy life of children set the stage for the Oedipus complex.
The child's unconscious sexual attraction to and wish to possess the parent of the opposite sex, the hostility and desire to remove the parent of the same sex, and the subsequent guilt for these wishes is the conflict the child faces.
The conflict is resolved when the child identifies with the parent of the same sex.
The emergence of the superego is the solution to and the result of these intense impulses.

LATENCY STAGE (6-12 YEARS)
The latency stage is a tapering off of conscious biological and sexual urges.
The sexual impulses are channeled and elevated into a more culturally accepted level of activity.

Continued

Freud's Psychosexual Stages of Development—cont'd

Growth of ego functions and the ability to care about and relate to others outside the home is the task of this stage of development.

GENITAL STAGE (12 YEARS AND BEYOND)
The genital stage emerges at adolescence with the onset of puberty when the genital organs mature.

The individual gains gratification from his or her own body.
During this stage, the individual develops satisfying sexual and emotional relationships with members of the opposite sex.
The individual plans life goals and gains a strong sense of personal identity.

3. Each stage is associated with a particular conflict that must be resolved before the child can move successfully to the next stage.

4. Experiences during the early stages determine an individual's adjustment patterns and the personality traits that the individual has as an adult.

PRACTICE QUESTIONS

1. A maternity nurse is providing instructions to a new mother regarding the psychosocial development of the newborn infant. Using Erikson's psychosocial development theory, the nurse would instruct the mother to
   1. Allow the newborn infant to signal a need.
   2. Anticipate all of the needs of the newborn infant.
   3. Avoid the newborn infant during the first 10 minutes of crying.
   4. Attend to the newborn infant immediately when crying.

2. A mother of a 3-year-old tells a clinic nurse that the child is rebelling constantly and having temper tantrums. The nurse most appropriately tells the mother to
   1. Punish the child every time the child says "no," to change the behavior.
   2. Allow the behavior because this is normal at this age period.
   3. Set limits on the child's behavior.
   4. Ignore the child when this behavior occurs.

3. A home health nurse visits a 70-year-old woman weekly. At each visit the client reminisces about past life experiences in a positive way. The home health nurse interprets this behavior as
   1. A normal psychosocial response.
   2. Requiring a psychiatric consultation.
   3. A mental status alteration.
   4. A sensory deficit requiring social activities.

4. The mother of an 8-year-old child tells the clinic nurse that she is concerned about the child because the child seems to be more attentive to friends than anything else. The most appropriate nursing response would be which of the following?
   1. "You need to be concerned."
   2. "You need to monitor the child's behavior closely."

   3. "At this age, the child is developing his own personality."
   4. "You need to provide more praise to the child to stop this behavior."

5. The mother of a 4-year-old child calls the clinic nurse and expresses concern because the child has been masturbating. The most appropriate response by the nurse is which of the following?
   1. "The child is very young to begin this behavior and should be brought to the clinic."
   2. "This is not normal behavior, and the child should be seen by the physician."
   3. "This is a normal behavior at this age."
   4. "Children usually begin this behavior at age 8 years."

6. A nursing instructor asks a nursing student to present a clinical conference to peers regarding Freud's psychosexual stages of development, specifically the anal stage. The student plans the conference, knowing that which of the following most appropriately relates to this stage of development?
   1. This stage is associated with toilet training.
   2. This stage is associated with pleasurable and conflicting feelings about the genital organs.
   3. This stage is characterized by a tapering off of conscious biological and sexual urges.
   4. This stage is characterized by the gratification of self.

7. A mother of a 5-year-old child tells the nurse that the child scolds the floor or a table if the child hurts herself on the object. According to Piaget's theory of cognitive development, this behavior is identified as
   1. Object permanence.
   2. Egocentric speech.
   3. Animism.
   4. Global organization.

8. A nursing instructor asks a nursing student to describe the formal operations stage of Piaget's cognitive developmental theory. The most appropriate response by the nursing student is
   1. "The child has the ability to think abstractly."
   2. "The child develops logical thought patterns."
   3. "The child has difficulty separating fantasy from reality."
   4. "The child begins to understand the environment."

9. A clinic nurse is preparing to discuss the concepts of moral development with a mother. The nurse

understands that according to Kohlberg's theory of moral development, in the preconventional level, moral development is thought to be motivated by which of the following?

1. The parents' behavior
2. Peer pressure
3. Social pressures
4. Punishment and reward

10. A nurse educator is preparing to conduct a session to the nursing staff regarding the theories of growth and development. The nurse educator plans to discuss Kohlberg's theory of moral development and understands that which of the following is not a component of the theory?
    1. Moral development progresses in relationship to cognitive development.
    2. Individuals move through all six stages in a sequential fashion.
    3. The theory provides a framework for understanding how individuals determine a moral code to guide their behavior.

4. A person's ability to make moral judgments develops over a period of time.

CRITICAL THINKING: PRIORITIZING (ORDERED RESPONSE)

Freud's psychosocial stages of human development proceed through a series of stages from infancy to adulthood. List the stages in order, as they proceed from infancy to adulthood. (Number 1 would indicate the stage that occurs at infancy.)

____ Latency stage

____ Anal stage

____ Oral stage

____ Phallic stage

____ Genital stage

ANSWERS

1. 1
Rationale: According to Erikson, the caregiver should not try to anticipate the newborn infant's needs at all times but must allow the newborn infant to signal needs. If a newborn infant is not allowed to signal a need, the newborn will not learn how to control the environment. Erikson believed that a delayed or prolonged response to a newborn infant's signal would inhibit the development of trust and lead to mistrust of others.
Test-Taking Strategy: Use the process of elimination. Eliminate options 2, 3, and 4 because of the absolute words "all," "avoid," and "immediately" in these options. Review Erikson's stages of psychosocial development if you had difficulty with this question.
Level of Cognitive Ability: Application
Client Needs: Psychosocial Integrity
Integrated Process: Teaching/Learning
Content Area: Child health
Reference: McKinney, E., Ashwill, J., Murray, S., James, S., Gorrie, T., Droske, S. (2000). *Maternal-child nursing* (pp. 60-61, 89). Philadelphia: W. B. Saunders.

2. 3
Rationale: According to Erikson, the child focuses on independence between ages 1 and 3 years. Gaining independence often means that the child has to rebel against the parents' wishes. Saying things like "no" or "mine" and having temper tantrums are common during this period of development. Being consistent and setting limits on the child's behavior are necessary elements.
Test-Taking Strategy: Use the process of elimination. Options 2 and 4 can be eliminated first because they are similar. Next, eliminate option 1 because this action is likely to produce a negative response during this normal developmental pattern. Review psychosocial development of the toddler according

to the Erikson, if you had difficulty with this question.
Level of Cognitive Ability: Application
Client Needs: Psychosocial Integrity
Integrated Process: Teaching/Learning
Content Area: Child health
Reference: James, S., Ashwill, J., & Droske, S. (2002). *Nursing care of children: Principles & practice* (2nd ed., pp. 70-71, 174). Philadelphia: W. B. Saunders.

3. 1
Rationale: According the Erikson, late adulthood is the period of old age. The adult reminisces about past life experiences, viewing them in a positive way. The adult needs to feel good about accomplishments, see successes in life, and feel that he or she has made a contribution to society.
Test-Taking Strategy: Use the process of elimination. Note the similarity in options 2, 3, and 4 in that all of these options indicate an abnormal response. Review Erikson's theory of psychosocial development of late adulthood if you had difficulty with this question.
Level of Cognitive Ability: Analysis
Client Needs: Psychosocial Integrity
Integrated Process: Nursing Process—analysis
Content Area: Fundamental skills
Reference: Wong, D., Perry, S., & Hockenberry, M. (2002). *Maternal child nursing care* (2nd ed., pp. 743, 973). St. Louis: Mosby.

4. 3
Rationale: According to Erikson, during school age years (ages 6 to 12 years), the child begins to move toward peers and friends and away from the parents for support. The child also begins to develop special interests that reflect his or her own developing personality instead of the parents.
Test-Taking Strategy: Use the process of elimination and knowledge of Erikson's psychosocial development theory

related to middle childhood. Options 1 and 2 can be eliminated easily first. Eliminate option 4 next because although praising the child for accomplishments is important at this age, the behavior that the child is exhibiting is normal. Review psychosocial development related to this age group according to Erikson if you had difficulty with this question.
Level of Cognitive Ability: Application
Client Needs: Psychosocial Integrity
Integrated Process: Caring
Content Area: Child health
Reference: McKinney, E., Ashwill, J., Murray, S., James, S., Gorrie, T., Droske, S. (2000). *Maternal-child nursing* (p. 161). Philadelphia: W. B. Saunders.

5. 3
Rationale: According to Freud's psychosexual stages of development, between the ages of 3 and 6, the child is in the phallic stage. At this time the child devotes much energy to examining his or her genitalia, masturbating, and expressing interest in sexual concerns.
Test-Taking Strategy: Use the process of elimination. Eliminate options 1 and 2 first because they are similar. Focus on the issue of the question and note the words "age 8 years" in option 4 to assist in eliminating this option. If you had difficulty with this question, review Freud's psychosocial stages of development.
Level of Cognitive Ability: Application
Client Needs: Psychosocial Integrity
Integrated Process: Caring
Content Area: Child health
Reference: McKinney, E., Ashwill, J., Murray, S., James, S., Gorrie, T., Droske, S. (2000). *Maternal-child nursing.* (pp. 113-114). Philadelphia: W. B. Saunders.

6. 1
Rationale: Generally, toilet training occurs during this period. According to Freud, the child gains pleasure from the elimination of feces and from their retention. Option 2 relates to the phallic stage. Option 3 relates to the latency period. Option 4 relates to the oral stage.
Test-Taking Strategy: Use the process of elimination. Note the relationship between the words "anal" in the question and "toilet training" in the correct option. If you had difficulty with this question, review Freud's psychosocial stages of development.
Level of Cognitive Ability: Comprehension
Client Needs: Psychosocial Integrity
Integrated Process: Nursing Process—planning
Content Area: Child health
Reference: Wong, D., Perry, S., & Hockenberry, M. (2002). *Maternal child nursing care* (2nd ed., pp. 742, 888-889). St. Louis: Mosby.

7. 3
Rationale: Animism means that all inanimate objects are given living meaning. Object permanence, the realization that something out of sight still exists, occurs in the later stages of the sensorimotor stage of development. Egocentric speech occurs when the child talks just for fun and cannot see another's point of view. Global organization means that if any

part of an object or situation changes, the whole thing has changed. Options 2 and 4 occur during the preoperational stage.
Test-Taking Strategy: Use the process of elimination. Note the relationship between the behavior identified in the question and option 3. If you had difficulty with this question, review the concepts of Piaget's theory of cognitive development.
Level of Cognitive Ability: Comprehension
Client Needs: Psychosocial Integrity
Integrated Process: Nursing Process—assessment
Content Area: Child health
Reference: McKinney, E., Ashwill, J., Murray, S., James, S., Gorrie, T., Droske, S. (2000). *Maternal-child nursing* (pp. 110-111). Philadelphia: W. B. Saunders.

8. 1
Rationale: In the formal operations stage the child has the ability the think abstractly and logically. Option 2 identifies the concrete operations stage. Option 3 identifies the preoperational stage. Option 4 identifies the sensorimotor stage.
Test-Taking Strategy: Use the process of elimination and knowledge regarding the characteristics of Piaget's cognitive developmental theory to answer this question. If you had difficulty with this question, review these concepts.
Level of Cognitive Ability: Comprehension
Client Needs: Psychosocial Integrity
Integrated Process: Teaching/Learning
Content Area: Child health
Reference: Wong, D., Perry, S., & Hockenberry, M. (2002). *Maternal child nursing care* (2nd ed., p. 974). St. Louis: Mosby.

9. 4
Rationale: In the preconventional stage, morals are thought to be motivated by punishment and reward. If the child is obedient and is not punished, then the child is being moral. The child sees actions as good or bad. If the child's actions are good, the child is praised. If the child's actions are bad, the child is punished.
Test-Taking Strategy: Use the process of elimination. Eliminate options 2 and 3 because they are similar. Knowledge that the preconventional stage occurs between birth and 7 years will assist in directing you to option 4. If you had difficulty with this question, review Kohlberg's theory of moral development.
Level of Cognitive Ability: Comprehension
Client Needs: Psychosocial Integrity
Integrated Process: Nursing Process—planning
Content Area: Child health
Reference: McKinney, E., Ashwill, J., Murray, S., James, S., Gorrie, T., Droske, S. (2000). *Maternal-child nursing* (pp. 59, 138). Philadelphia: W. B. Saunders.

10. 2
Rationale: Kohlberg's theory states that individuals move through the six stages of development in a sequential fashion but that not everyone reaches stages 5 and 6 in his or her development of personal morality. Options 1, 3, and 4 are correct statements regarding Kohlberg's theory.
Test-Taking Strategy: Use the process of elimination. Note the key word "not" in the stem of the question. Also, note the

absolute word "all" in option 2. If you had difficulty with this question, review Kohlberg's theory.
Level of Cognitive Ability: Comprehension
Client Needs: Psychosocial Integrity
Integrated Process: Nursing Process—planning
Content Area: Fundamental skills
Reference: Wong, D., Perry, S., & Hockenberry, M. (2002). *Maternal child nursing care* (2nd ed., p. 104). St. Louis: Mosby.

CRITICAL THINKING: PRIORITIZING (ORDERED RESPONSE)

Answer: 42135
Rationale: According to Freud, human development proceeds through a series of stages from infancy to adulthood. Each stage is characterized by the inborn tendency of all individuals to reduce tension and seek pleasure and is associated with a particular conflict that must be resolved before the child can move successfully to the next stage. Experiences during the early stages determine an individual's adjustment patterns and the personality traits that the individual has as an adult. The oral stage occurs in infancy from birth to 1 year of age; the anal stage, 1 to 3 years of age; the phallic stage, 3 to 6 years of age; latency stage, 6 to 12 years of age; and the genital stage, 12 years and beyond.
Test-Taking Strategy: Knowledge regarding Freud's psychosocial stages of development is needed to answer this question. Review these stages if you had difficulty with this question.
Level of Cognitive Ability: Comprehension
Client Needs: Psychosocial Integrity
Integrated Process: Nursing Process—implementation
Content Area: Child health
Reference: Wong, D., Perry, S., & Hockenberry, M. (2002). *Maternal child nursing care* (2nd ed., pp. 742-743). St. Louis: Mosby.

REFERENCES

James, S., Ashwill, J., & Droske, S. (2002). *Nursing care of children: Principles & practice* (2nd ed.). Philadelphia: W. B. Saunders.

McKinney, E., Ashwill, J., Murray, S., James, S., Gorrie, T., Droske, S. (2000). *Maternal-child nursing.* Philadelphia: W. B. Saunders.

Varcarolis, E. (2002). *Foundations of psychiatric mental health nursing* (4th ed.). Philadelphia: W. B. Saunders.

Wong, D., Perry, S., & Hockenberry, M. (2002). *Maternal child nursing care* (2nd ed.). St. Louis: Mosby.

Developmental Stages

▲ I. THE HOSPITALIZED INFANT AND TODDLER

A. **Separation** anxiety
1. Protest
   a. Crying, screaming, searching for a parent; avoidance and rejection of contact with strangers
   b. Verbal attacks on others
   c. Physical fighting; kicking, fighting, hitting, pinching
2. Despair
   a. Withdrawn, depressed, uninterested in the environment
   b. Loss of newly learned skills
3. Detachment
   a. Detachment is uncommon and occurs only after lengthy separations from the parent.
   b. Superficially, the toddler appears to have adjusted to the loss.
   c. During this phase, the toddler again becomes more interested in the environment, plays with others, and seems to form new relationships; this behavior is a form of resignation and is not a sign of contentment.
   d. The toddler detaches from the parents in an effort to escape the emotional pain of desiring the parent's presence.
   e. The toddler copes by forming shallow relationships with others, becoming increasingly self-centered, and attaching primary importance to material objects.
   f. This is the most serious phase because reversal of the potential adverse effects is less likely to occur once detachment is established; in most situations, the temporary separation imposed by hospitalization does not cause such prolonged parental absence that the toddler enters into detachment.

B. Fear of injury and pain: Affected by previous experiences, separation from parents, and preparation for the experience

C. Loss of control
1. Hospitalization with its own set of rituals and routines can disrupt the life of a toddler severely.
2. The lack of control often is exhibited in behaviors related to feeding, toileting, playing, and bedtime.
3. The toddler may demonstrate **regression**.

D. Interventions
1. Provide swaddling and soft talking to the infant.
2. Provide opportunities for sucking and oral stimulation for the infant using a pacifier if the infant is not to receive anything by mouth.
3. Provide stimulation if appropriate for the infant, using objects of contrasting colors and textures.
4. Provide routines and rituals as close as possible to what the toddler is used to at home.
5. Provide choices as much as possible to the toddler, to provide some control.
6. Approach the toddler with a positive attitude.
7. Allow the toddler to express feelings of protest.
8. Encourage the toddler to talk about parents or others in their lives.
9. Accept regressive behavior without ridiculing the toddler.
10. Provide the toddler with favorite and comforting objects.
11. Allow the toddler as much mobility as possible.
12. Anticipate temper tantrums from the toddler, and maintain a safe environment for physical acting out.
13. Employ pain-reduction techniques as appropriate.

II. THE HOSPITALIZED PRESCHOOLER

A. Separation anxiety
1. Separation anxiety is generally less obvious and less serious than in the toddler.
2. As stress increases, the preschooler's ability to separate from the parents decreases.
3. Protest
   a. Protest is less direct and aggressive than in the toddler.
   b. The preschooler may displace feelings onto others.
4. Despair
   a. The preschooler reacts in a manner similar to the toddler.
   b. The preschooler is quietly withdrawn, depressed, uninterested in the environment.
   c. The child exhibits loss of newly learned skills.
   d. The preschooler becomes generally uncooperative, refusing to eat or take medication.
   e. The preschooler repeatedly asks when the parents will be visiting.
5. Detachment: Similar to the toddler
B. Fear of injury and pain
1. The preschooler has a general lack of understanding of body integrity.
2. The child fears invasive procedures and mutilation.
3. The child imagines things to be much worse than they are.
4. Preschoolers believe that they are ill because of something they did or thought.
C. Loss of control
1. The preschooler likes familiar routines and rituals and may show **regression** if not allowed to maintain some control.
2. The child has attained a good deal of independence and self-care at home and may expect that to continue in the hospital.
D. Interventions
1. Provide a safe and secure environment.
2. Take time for communication.
3. Allow the preschooler to express anger.
4. Acknowledge fears and anxieties.
5. Accept regressive behavior; assist the preschooler in moving from regressive to appropriate behaviors according to age.
6. Encourage rooming-in or leave favorite toy.
7. Allow mobility and provide play and diversional activities.
8. Place the preschooler with other children of the same age if possible.
9. Encourage the preschooler to be independent.
10. Explain procedures simply on the preschooler's level.
11. Avoid intrusive procedures when possible.
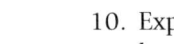
12. Allow wearing of underpants.

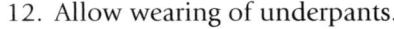

III. THE HOSPITALIZED SCHOOL-AGED CHILD

A. Separation anxiety
1. The school-aged child is accustomed to periods of separation from the parents, but as stressors are added, the separation becomes more difficult.
2. The child is more concerned with missing school and the fear that their friends will forget them.
3. Usually the stage of behavior of protest, despair, and detachment does not occur with school-aged children.
B. Fear of injury and pain
1. The school-aged child fears bodily injury and pain.
2. The child fears illness itself, disability, death, and intrusive procedures in genital areas.
3. The child is uncomfortable with any type of sexual examination.
4. The child groans or whines, holds rigidly still, and communicates about pain.
C. Loss of control
1. The child is usually highly social, independent, and involved with activities.
2. The child seeks information and asks relevant questions about tests and procedures and the illness.
3. The child associates his or her actions with the cause of the illness.
4. The child may feel helpless and dependent if physical limitations occur.
D. Interventions
1. Encourage rooming-in.
2. Focus on the school-aged child's abilities and needs.
3. Encourage the school-aged child to become involved with his or her own care.
4. Accept **regression** but encourage independence.
5. Provide choices to the school-aged child.
6. Allow expression of feelings verbally and nonverbally.
7. Acknowledge fears and concerns and allow for discussion.
8. Explain all procedures, using body diagrams or outlines.
9. Provide privacy.
10. Avoid intrusive procedures if possible.
11. Allow the school-aged child to wear underpants.
12. Involve the school-aged child in activities appropriate to developmental level and illness.
13. Encourage the school-aged child to contact friends.
14. Provide for educational needs.
15. Use appropriate interventions to relieve pain.

IV. THE HOSPITALIZED ADOLESCENT

A. Separation anxiety
1. Adolescents are not sure whether they want their parents with them when they are hospitalized.
2. Separation from friends is a source of anxiety.

3. Adolescents become upset if friends go on with their lives, excluding them.

B. Fear of injury and pain
   1. Adolescents fear being different from others and their peers.
   2. Adolescents may give the impression that they are not afraid even though they are terrified.
   3. Adolescents become guarded when any areas related to sexual development are examined.

C. Loss of control
   1. Behaviors exhibited include anger, withdrawal, and uncooperativeness.
   2. Adolescents seek help and then reject it.

D. Interventions
   1. Encourage questions about appearance and effects of the illness on the future.
   2. Explore feelings about the hospital and the significance the illness might have for relationships.
   3. Encourage adolescents to wear own clothes and perform normal grooming.
   4. Allow favorite foods to be brought in to the hospital if possible.
   5. Provide privacy.
   6. Use body diagrams to prepare for procedures.
   7. Introduce to other adolescents in the nursing unit.
   8. Encourage maintaining contact with peer groups.
   9. Provide for educational needs.
   10. Identify formation of future plans.
   11. Help develop positive coping mechanisms.

V. COMMUNICATION APPROACHES

A. General guidelines
   1. Allow the child to feel comfortable with the nurse.
   2. Communicate through the use of objects.
   3. Allow the child to express fears and concerns.
   4. Speak clearly and in a quiet, unhurried voice.
   5. Offer choices when possible.
   6. Be honest with the child.
   7. Set limits with the child as appropriate.

B. Infant
   1. Infants respond to nonverbal communication behaviors of adults, such as holding, rocking, patting, and touching.
   2. Use a slow approach and allow the infant to get to know the nurse.
   3. Use a calm, soft, soothing voice.
   4. Be responsive to cries.
   5. Talk and read to infants.
   6. Allow security objects such as blankets and pacifiers if the infant has them.

C. Toddler
   1. Approach the toddler cautiously.
   2. Remember that toddlers accept verbal communications of others literally.
   3. Learn the toddler's words for common items and use them in conversations.

4. Use short, concrete terms.
5. Prepare the toddler for procedures immediately before the event.
6. Repeat explanations and descriptions.
7. Use play for demonstrations.
8. Use visual aids such as picture books, puppets, and dolls.
9. Allow the toddler to handle the equipment or instruments; explain what the equipment or instrument does and how it feels.
10. Encourage the use of comfort objects.

D. Preschooler
   1. Seek opportunities to offer choices.
   2. Speak in simple sentences.
   3. Be concise and limit the length of explanations.
   4. Allow asking questions.
   5. Describe procedures as they are about to be performed.
   6. Use play to explain procedures and activities.
   7. Allow handling the equipment or instruments, which will ease fear and help to answer questions.

E. School-aged child
   1. Establish limits.
   2. Provide reassurance to help in alleviating fears and anxieties.
   3. Engage in conversations that encourage thinking.
   4. Use medical play techniques.
   5. Use photographs, books, dolls, and videos to explain procedures.
   6. Explain in clear terms.
   7. Allow time for composure and privacy.

F. Adolescent
   1. Remember that the adolescent may be preoccupied with body image.
   2. Encourage and support independence.
   3. Provide privacy.
   4. Use photographs, books, and videos to explain procedures.
   5. Engage in conversations about adolescents' interests.
   6. Avoid becoming too abstract, too detailed, and too technical.
   7. Avoid responding to less than desirable social behaviors by prying, confrontation, or judgmental attitudes.

VI. DEVELOPMENTAL CHARACTERISTICS

A. Infant
   1. Physical
      a. Height increases by ¾ inch per month.
      b. Weight is doubled at 5 to 6 months and tripled at 12 months.
      c. At birth, head circumference is 2 to 3 cm greater than chest circumference.
      d. By 1 to 2 years of age, head circumference and chest circumference are equal.
      e. Anterior fontanel (soft and flat in a normal infant) closes at 12 to 18 months.

f. Posterior fontanel (soft and flat in a normal infant) closes by 2 to 3 months.

g. Infant has 10 upper and 10 lower deciduous teeth by 2½ years of age.

h. Lower central incisors are present by 6 to 8 months.

i. Infant sleeps most of the time.

2. Vital signs (Box 33-1)

3. Nutrition

a. The infant may breast-feed or bottle-feed, depending on the mother's choice.

b. Iron stores from birth are depleted by 4 months.

c. Human milk is the best food for infants under 6 months of age.

d. Infants should remain on human milk or iron-fortified formula for the first year of life.

e. Whole milk should not be introduced to infants until after 1 year of age.

f. Skim and low-fat milk should not be given because the essential fatty acids are inadequate and the solute concentration of protein and electrolytes is too high.

g. Fluoride supplementation may be needed at about 6 months of age, depending on the infant's intake of fluoridated tap water.

h. Solid foods are introduced at 5 to 6 months of age; introduce solid foods one at a time, usually at intervals of 4 to 5 days, to identify food allergens.

i. Sequence of introduction of solid foods is as follows: rice cereal; fruits and vegetables, starting with yellow and then green; meats; and then egg yolks, avoiding egg whites (introduce egg white toward the end of the first year); cheese may be used as a substitute for meat and as a finger food.

j. Avoid solid foods that place the infant at risk for choking, such as nuts, foods with seeds, raisins, popcorn, grapes, pieces of a hot dog.

k. Avoid microwaving baby bottles and baby food.

l. Never mix food or medications with formula.

m. Avoid adding honey to formula, water, or other fluid to prevent botulism.

n. Offer fruit juice from a cup (12-13 months) rather than a bottle to prevent nursing (bottle-mouth) caries.

4. Skills (Box 33-2)

5. Play

a. Solitary

b. Birth to 3 months: verbal, visual, and tactile stimuli

c. 4 to 6 months: initiation of actions and recognition of new experiences

d. 6 to 12 months: awareness of self, imitation, repetition of pleasurable actions

e. Enjoyment of soft stuffed animals, crib mobiles with contrasting colors, squeeze toys, rattles, musical toys, water toys during the bath, large picture books, and push toys after he or she begins to walk

6. Safety

a. Parents must baby-proof the home.

b. Infants who weigh up to 20 lb should be restrained in a car seat (convertible restraint) in a semireclined, rear-facing position.

c. Rear-facing infant seats (convertible restraint) are not placed in the front seats of cars equipped with an air bag on the passenger side; the child could be injured seriously if the air bag is released because rear-facing infant seats extend closer to the dashboard.

d. Guard infant when on bed or changing table.

e. Use gates to protect infant from stairs.

f. Never vigorously shake an infant.

g. Be sure that bath water is not hot; do not leave unattended in bath.

h. Do not hold infant while drinking or working near hot liquids.

i. Cool vaporizers should be used instead of steam to prevent burn injuries.

j. Avoid offering food that is round and similar to the size of the airway to prevent choking.

k. Be sure toys have no small pieces.

l. Hanging toys or mobiles over the crib should be well out of reach to prevent strangulation.

m. Avoid placing large toys in the crib because an older infant may use them as steps to climb.

n. Cribs should be positioned away from curtains and blind cords.

o. Cover electrical outlets.

p. Remove hazardous objects from low, reachable places.

q. Remove chemicals, medications, poisons, and plants from infant's reach.

r. Keep the poison control number available.

s. Keep syrup of ipecac available; in the event of a poisoning, the poison control center is

---

BOX 33-1

Vital Signs: Newborn and 1-Year-Old Infant

NEWBORN
Temperature: axillary, 97.7° to 99.5° F
Apical rate: 120-160 beats per minute (100 sleeping, 180 crying)
Respirations: 30-60 (average 40) breaths per minute
Blood pressure: 73/55 mm Hg

1-YEAR-OLD INFANT
Temperature: axillary, 97° to 99° F
Apical rate: 90 to 130 beats per minute
Respirations: 20 to 40 breaths per minute
Blood pressure: 90/56 mm Hg

BOX 33-2

Infant Skills

2-3 MONTHS
Smiles
Turns head side to side
Cries
Follows objects
Holds head in midline

4-5 MONTHS
Grasps objects
Switches objects from hands
Rolls over for the first time
Enjoys social interaction
Begins to show memory
Aware of unfamiliar surroundings

6-7 MONTHS
Creeps
Sits with support
Imitates
Exhibits fear of strangers
Holds arms out
Frequent mood swings
Waves bye-bye

8-9 MONTHS
Sits steadily unsupported
Crawls
May stand while holding on
Begins to stand without help

10-11 MONTHS
Can change from prone to sitting position
Walks while holding onto furniture
Stands securely
Entertains self for periods of time

12-13 MONTHS
Walks with one hand held
Can take a few steps without falling
Can drink from a cup

14-15 MONTHS
Walks alone
Can crawl upstairs
Shows emotions such as anger and affection
Will explore away from mother in familiar surroundings

---

contacted immediately and will provide the mother with initial treatment instructions.

B. Toddler
1. Physical
   a. Height and weight increase in a steplike fashion, reflecting growth spurts and lags.
   b. Head circumference increases about 1 inch between ages 1 and 2; thereafter, head circumference increases about ½ inch per year until age 5.
   c. Anterior fontanel closes between ages 12 to 18 months.
   d. Weight gain is slower than in infancy; by age 2, the average weight is 22-27 lb.
   e. Normal height changes include a growth of about 3 inches per year; the average height of the toddler is 34 inches at age 2 years.
   f. Lordosis (pot belly) is evident.
   g. The toddler should see a dentist soon after the first teeth erupt, usually around 1 year of age; flouride supplements may be necessary if the water is not fluoridated.
   h. A toddler should never be allowed to fall asleep with a bottle containing milk, juice, soda pop, or sweetened water because of the risk of nursing (bottle-mouth) caries.
   i. Typically the toddler sleeps through the night and has one daytime nap and discontinues the daytime nap at about age 3.
   j. A consistent bedtime ritual helps prepare the toddler for sleep.
   k. Security objects at bedtime may assist in sleep.

2. Vital signs (Box 33-3)
3. Nutrition
   a. Most toddlers prefer to feed themselves.
   b. The toddler generally does best by eating several small nutritious meals each day rather than three large meals.
   c. Offer a limited number of foods at any one time.
   d. Offer finger foods and avoid concentrated sweets and empty calories.
   e. The toddler is at risk for aspiration of small foods that are not chewed easily, such as nuts, foods with seeds, raisins, popcorn, grapes, and pieces of a hot dog.
   f. Physiological anorexia is normal because of the alternating periods of fast and slow growth.
   g. Sit the toddler in a high chair at the family table for meals.
   h. Allow sufficient time to eat, but remove food when toddler begins to play with it.
   i. The toddler drinks well from a cup held with both hands.
   j. Avoid using food as a reward or punishment.

BOX 33-3

The Toddler's Vital Signs

Temperature: axillary, 97.5° to 98.6° F
Apical rate: 80 to 120 beats per minute
Respirations: 20 to 30 breaths per minute
Blood pressure: average, 92/55 mm Hg

4. Skills
   a. The toddler begins to walk with one hand held by age 12 to 13 months.
   b. The toddler runs by age 2 years and walks backward and hops on one foot by age 3 years.
   c. The toddler usually cannot alternate feet when climbing stairs.
   d. The toddler begins to master fine-motor skills for building, undressing, and drawing lines.
   e. The young toddler often uses "no" even when the toddler means "yes" to assert independence.
   f. The toddler begins to use short sentences and has a vocabulary of about 300 words by age 2.
   g. The toddler tends to ask many "why" questions.
5. Bowel and bladder control
   a. Signs that a toddler is ready for toilet training (Box 33-4)
   b. Bowel control develops before bladder control.
   c. By age 3, the toddler achieves fairly good bowel and bladder control.
   d. The toddler may stay dry during the day but may need a diaper at night until about age 4.
6. Play
   a. The major socializing mechanism is parallel play, and therapeutic play can begin at this age.
   b. The toddler has a short attention span, causing the toddler to change toys often.
   c. The toddler explores body parts of self and others.
   d. Typical toys include push/pull toys, blocks, sand, finger paints and bubbles, large balls, crayons, trucks and dolls, containers, Play-Doh, toy telephones, cloth books, and wooden puzzles.
7. Safety
   a. Toddlers are eager to explore the world around them.
   b. The toddler should be supervised at play.
   c. The toddler can be placed in an upright forward-facing position in a car seat (convertible restraint); the transition point for switching to a forward-facing position is defined by the manufacturer of the car seat but is generally at a body weight of at least 9 kg (20 lb) and 1 year of age.
   d. Convertible restraints (car safety seats) are used until the child weighs at least 40 lb.
   e. Lock car doors.
   f. Use back burners on the stove to prepare a meal, and turn pot handles inward and toward the middle of the stove.
   g. Keep dangling cords from small appliances away from the toddler.
   h. Place inaccessible locks on windows and doors, and keep furniture away from windows.
   i. Secure screens on all windows.
   j. Place gates at stairways.
   k. Do not allow the toddler to sleep or play in an upper bunk bed.
   l. Never leave the toddler alone near a bathtub, pail of water, swimming pool, or any other body of water.
   m. Keep toilet lids closed.
   n. Keep all medicines, poisons, household plants, and toxic products high and locked out of reach.
   o. Keep the poison control number available.
   p. Keep syrup of ipecac available; in the event of a poisoning, the poison control center should be contacted immediately and will provide the mother with initial treatment instructions.
C. Preschooler
   1. Physical
      a. The preschooler grows 2½ to 3 inches per year.
      b. Average height is 37 inches at age 3; 40½ inches at age 4; and 43 inches at age 5.
      c. The preschooler gains approximately 5 lb per year; average weight of 35-40 lb at age 5.
      d. The preschooler requires about 12 hours of sleep each day.
      e. A security object and a night-light assist with sleeping.
      f. At the beginning of the preschool period, the eruption of the deciduous (primary) teeth is complete.
      g. Regular dental care is essential, and the preschooler requires assistance with brushing and flossing of teeth; fluoride supplements may be necessary if the water is not fluoridated.
   2. Vital signs (Box 33-5)
   3. Nutrition
      a. The preschooler exhibits food fads and strong taste preferences.

BOX 33-4

Signs of Readiness for Toilet Training

Child is able to stay dry for 2 hours.
Child is waking up dry from a nap.
Child is able to sit, squat, and walk.
Child is able to remove clothing.
Child recognizes urge to defecate or urinate.
Child expresses willingness to please parent.
Child is able to sit on toilet for 5 to 10 minutes without fussing or getting off.

BOX 33-5

The Preschooler's Vital Signs

Temperature: axillary, 97.5° to 98.6° F
Apical rate: 70 to 110 beats per minute
Respirations: 16 to 22 breaths per minute
Blood pressure: average, 95/57 mm Hg

b. By 5 years old, the child tends to focus on social aspects of eating, table conversations, manners, and willingness to try new foods.

4. Skills
   a. The preschooler has good posture.
   b. The child develops fine-motor coordination.
   c. The child can hop, skip, and run more smoothly.
   d. Athletic abilities begin to develop.
   e. The preschooler demonstrates increased skills in balancing.
   f. The child alternates feet when climbing stairs.
   g. The child can tie shoelaces.
   h. The child may talk continuously and ask many "why" questions.
   i. Vocabulary increases to about 900 words by age 3 and 2100 words by age 5.
   j. By age 3 the preschooler usually talks in three- or four-word sentences and speaks in short phrases.
   k. By age 4 the preschooler speaks five- or six-word sentences and by age 5 speaks in longer sentences that contain all parts of speech.
   l. The child can be understood readily by others and can understand clearly what others are saying.

5. Bowel and bladder control
   a. By age 4 the preschooler has daytime control of bowel and bladder but may experience bed-wetting accidents at night.
   b. By age 5 the preschooler achieves bowel and bladder control, although accidents may occur in stressful situations.

6. Play
   a. The preschooler is cooperative.
   b. The preschooler has imaginary playmates.
   c. The child likes to build and create things, and play is simple and imaginative.
   d. The child understands sharing and is able to interact with peers.
   e. The child requires regular socialization with mates of similar age.
   f. Play activities include a large space for running and jumping.
   g. The preschooler likes dress-up clothes, paints, paper, and crayons for creative expressions.
   h. Swimming and sports aid with growth development.
   i. Puzzles and toys aid with fine-motor development.

7. Safety
   a. Preschoolers are active and inquisitive.
   b. Because of their magical thinking, they may believe that daring feats seen in cartoons are possible and they may attempt them.
   c. The preschooler can learn simple safety practices because they can follow simple verbal directions and their attention span is lengthened.

d. Once the child has outgrown the convertible restraint car safety seat (weight more than 40 lb), the preschooler should be placed and restrained in a booster seat (until the preschooler weighs at least 60 lb, is 8 years old, or his or her head is higher than the vehicle back seat).
e. A universal child safety seat system for automobiles provides a uniform anchorage in the rear seat of the vehicle for child safety seats; seat belts are not needed to anchor child safety seats.
f. Teach the preschooler basic safety rules to ensure safety when playing in a playground near swings and ladders.
g. Teach the preschooler never to play with matches or lighters.
h. The preschooler should be taught what to do in the event of a fire or if clothes catch fire; fire drills should be practiced with preschooler.
i. Guns should be stored unloaded and secured under lock and key; the preschooler should be taught to leave an area immediately if a gun is visible and to tell an adult.
j. The preschooler should be taught never to point a toy gun at another person.
k. Teach the preschooler that if another person touches his or her body in an inappropriate way to tell an adult.
l. Teach the preschooler to avoid speaking to strangers and never to accept a ride, toys, or gifts from a stranger.
m. Teach the preschooler his or her full name, address, parents' names, and telephone number.
n. Teach the preschooler how to dial 911 in an emergency situation.
o. Keep the poison control number available.
p. Keep syrup of ipecac available; in the event of a poisoning, the poison control center should be contacted immediately and will provide the mother with initial treatment instructions.

D. School-aged child
   1. Physical
      a. Girls usually grow faster than boys.
      b. Growth is about 2 inches per year between ages 6 and 12.
      c. Height ranges from 45 inches at age 6 to 59 inches at age 12.
      d. School-aged children gain weight at 4½ to 6½ lb per year.
      e. Average weight is 46 lb at age 6 and 88 lb at age 12.
      f. The first permanent (secondary) teeth erupt around age 6, and deciduous teeth are lost gradually.
      g. Regular dentist visits are necessary, and the school-aged child needs to be supervised with

    brushing and flossing teeth; fluoride supplements may be necessary if the water is not fluoridated.

  h. For school-aged children with primary and permanent dentition, the best toothbrush is one with soft nylon bristles and an overall length of about 6 inches.

  i. Sleep requirements range from 10 to 12 hours a night.

2. Vital signs (Box 33-6)

3. Nutrition

  a. School-aged children have increased growth needs.

  b. Children require a balanced diet from foods in the Food Guide Pyramid.

  c. Children still may be picky eaters but are willing to try new foods.

4. Skills

  a. School-aged children exhibit refinement of fine-motor skills.

  b. Development of gross-motor skills continues.

  c. Strength and endurance increases.

5. Play

  a. Play is more competitive.

  b. Rules and rituals are important aspects of play and games.

  c. The school-aged child enjoys drawing, collecting items, dolls, pets, guessing games, board games, listening to the radio, TV, reading, and videos and computer games.

  d. The child participates in team sports.

  e. The child may participate in secret clubs, gang activities, and scout organizations.

6. Safety

  a. The school-aged child experiences less fear in play activities and frequently imitates real life by using tools and household items.

  b. Car safety belts should be worn low on the hips; the shoulder belt is used only if it does not cross over the child's neck and face.

  c. Major causes of injuries include bicycles, skateboards, and team sports as the child increases in motor abilities and independence.

  d. Children should always wear a helmet when riding a bike or using inline skates or skateboards.

  e. Teach the school-aged child water safety rules.

  f. Instruct the school-aged child to avoid teasing or playing roughly with animals.

  g. Teach the school-aged child never to play with matches or lighters.

  h. The school-aged child should be taught what to do in the event of a fire or if clothes catch fire; fire drills should be practiced with the school-aged child.

  i. Guns should be stored unloaded and secured under lock and key; the school-aged child should be taught to leave an area immediately if a gun is visible and to tell an adult.

  j. Teach the school-aged child that if another person touches his or her body in an inappropriate way to tell an adult.

  k. Teach the school-aged child to avoid speaking to strangers and never to accept a ride, toys, or gifts from a stranger.

  l. Teach the school-aged child traffic safety rules.

  m. Teach the school-aged child how to dial 911 in an emergency situation.

  n. Keep the poison control number available.

  o. Keep syrup of ipecac available; in the event of a poisoning, the poison control center should be contacted immediately and will provide the mother with initial treatment instructions.

E. Adolescent

1. Physical

  a. Puberty is the maturational, hormonal, and growth process that occurs when the reproductive organs begin to function and the secondary sex characteristics develop.

  b. Body mass increases to adult size.

  c. Sebaceous and sweat glands become active and fully functional.

  d. Body hair distribution occurs.

  e. Increase in height, weight, breast development, and pelvic girth occurs in girls.

  f. Menstrual periods occur about $2\frac{1}{2}$ years after the onset of puberty.

  g. In boys, an increase in height, weight, muscle mass, and penis and testicle size occurs.

  h. Voice deepens in boys.

  i. Normal weight gain during puberty: Girls gain 15 to 55 lb and boys gain 15 to 65 lb.

  j. Careful brushing and care of the teeth are important, and many adolescents need to wear braces.

  k. Sleep patterns include a tendency to stay up late; therefore in an attempt to catch up on missed sleep, adolescents sleep late whenever possible; an overall average of 8 hours per night is recommended.

2. Vital signs (Box 33-7)

3. Nutrition

  a. Teaching about the Food Guide Pyramid is important.

  b. Adolescents typically eat whenever they have a break in activities.

   c. Calcium, zinc, iron, folic acid, and protein are especially important nutritional needs.

   d. Adolescents tend to snack on empty calories.

   e. Body image is important.

4. Skills

   a. Gross- and fine-motor skills are well developed.

   b. Strength and endurance increase.

5. Play

   a. Games and athletics are the most common forms of play.

   b. Competition and strict rules are important.

   c. Adolescents enjoy activities such as sports, videos, movies, reading, parties, dancing, hobbies, computer games, music, and experimenting such as with makeup and hairstyles.

   d. Friends are important, and adolescents like to gather in small groups.

6. Safety

   a. Adolescents are risk takers.

   b. Adolescents have a natural urge to experiment and to be independent.

   c. Instruct adolescents in the dangers related to drugs and alcohol.

   d. Help adolescents to recognize that they have choices when difficult or potentially dangerous situations arise.

   e. Advocate the use of seat belts.

   f. Instruct adolescents in the consequences of injuries that motor vehicle accidents can cause.

   g. Instruct adolescents in water safety and emphasize that they should enter the water feet first as opposed to diving, especially when the depth of the water is unknown.

   h. Instruct adolescents about the dangers associated with guns, violence, and gangs.

   i. Instruct adolescents about the complications associated with body piercing, tattooing, and suntanning.

   j. Discuss issues such as date rape, sexual relationships, and the transmission of sexually transmitted diseases.

F. Early adulthood

1. Description: period between the late teens and the mid- to late thirties

2. Physical changes

   a. Person has completed physical growth by the age of 20.

   b. Person is active.

   c. Severe illnesses are less common than in older age groups.

   d. Person tends to ignore physical symptoms and postpone seeking health care.

   e. Lifestyle habits such as smoking, stress, lack of exercise, poor personal hygiene, and family history of disease increase the risk of future illness.

3. Cognitive changes

   a. Person has rational thinking habits.

   b. Conceptual, problem-solving, and motor skills increase.

   c. Person identifies preferred occupational areas.

4. Psychosocial changes

   a. Person separates from the families of origin.

   b. Person gives much attention to occupational and social pursuits to improve socioeconomic status.

   c. Person makes decisions regarding career, marriage, and parenthood.

   d. Person needs to adapt to new situations.

5. Sexuality

   a. Person has the emotional maturity to develop mature sexual relationships.

   b. Person is at risk for sexually transmitted diseases.

G. Middle adulthood

1. Description: period between the mid- to late thirties and the mid-sixties

2. Physical changes

   a. Phyical changes occur between 40 and 65 years of age.

   b. Individual becomes aware that changes in reproductive and physical abilities signify the beginning of another stage in life.

   c. Menopause occurs in women and climacteric occurs in men.

   d. Physiological changes often have an impact on self-concept and body image.

   e. Physiological concerns include stress, level of wellness, and the formation of positive health habits.

3. Cognitive changes

   a. Person may be interested in learning new skills.

   b. Person may become involved in educational or vocational programs for entering the job market or for changing careers.

4. Psychosocial changes

   a. Changes may include expected events, such as children moving away from home (postparental family stage), or unexpected events such as death of a close friend.

   b. Time and financial demands decrease as children move away from home and the couple faces redefining their relationship.

   c. Adults may become grandparents.

   d. Adults are achieving generativity.

5. Sexuality

   a. Many couples renew their relationships and find increased marital and sexual satisfaction.

b. The onset of menopause and climacteric may affect sexual health.

c. Stress, health, and medications can affect sexuality.

PRACTICE QUESTIONS

1. The parents of a 2-year-old arrive at a hospital to visit their child. The child is in the playroom when the parents arrive. When the parents enter the playroom, the child does not readily approach the parents. The nurse interprets this behavior as indicating that
   1. The child is withdrawn.
   2. The child is self-centered.
   3. The child has adjusted to the hospitalized setting.
   4. This is a normal pattern.

2. A mother arrives at a clinic with her toddler and tells a nurse that she has a difficult time getting the child to go to bed at night. Which of the following is most appropriate for the nurse to suggest to the mother?
   1. Inform the child of bedtime a few minutes before it is time for bed.
   2. Allow the child to have temper tantrums.
   3. Allow the child to set bedtime limits.
   4. Avoid a nap during the day.

3. A mother of a 3-year-old asks a clinic nurse about appropriate and safe toys for the child. The nurse tells the mother that the most appropriate toy for a 3-year-old is which of the following?
   1. A farm set
   2. A golf set
   3. A jack set with marbles
   4. A wagon

4. A clinic nurse provides information to the mother of a toddler regarding toilet training. Which statement if made by the mother indicates a need for further information regarding the toilet training?
   1. "The child will not be ready to toilet train until the age of about 18 to 24 months."
   2. "Bladder control usually is achieved before bowel control."
   3. "The child should not be forced to sit on the potty for long periods."
   4. "The ability of the child to remove clothing is a sign of physical readiness."

5. The mother of a 3-year-old is concerned because her child still is insisting on a bottle at nap time and at bedtime. Which of the following is the most appropriate suggestion to the mother?
   1. Do not allow the child to have the bottle.
   2. Allow the bottle during naps but not at bedtime.
   3. Allow the bottle if it contains juice.
   4. Allow the bottle if it contains water.

6. A nurse assesses the vital signs of a 12-month-old infant with a respiratory infection. The respiratory rate is 35 breaths per minute. Based on this finding, which action is most appropriate?
   1. Notify the physician.
   2. Administer oxygen.
   3. Reassess the respiratory rate in 15 minutes.
   4. Document the findings.

7. A nurse prepares to take the blood pressure of a school-aged child. To obtain an accurate measurement, the nurse ensures that the blood pressure cuff covers
   1. One half of the distance between the antecubital fossa and the shoulder.
   2. One third of the distance between the antecubital fossa and the shoulder.
   3. Two thirds of the distance between the antecubital fossa and the shoulder.
   4. One quarter of the distance between the antecubital fossa and the shoulder.

8. A nurse provides instructions to the parents of an infant regarding car travel and safety seats. Which of the following is the most appropriate information related to the safety of the infant?
   1. Restrain in a car seat in the front seat in a semi-reclined, rear-facing position.
   2. Restrain in a car seat in the front seat in a semi-reclined, forward-facing position.
   3. Restrain in a car seat in the back seat in a semireclined, rear-facing position.
   4. Restrain in a car seat in the back seat in a semireclined, forward-facing position.

9. A nurse is monitoring a 3-month-old infant for signs of increased intracranial pressure. On palpation of the fontanels, the nurse notes that the anterior fontanel is soft and flat. Based on this finding, which nursing action is most appropriate?
   1. Elevate the head of the bed to 90 degrees.
   2. Notify the physician.
   3. Increase oral fluids.
   4. Document the finding.

10. A nurse is evaluating the developmental level of a 2-year-old. Which of the following does the nurse expect to observe in this child?
    1. Uses a fork to eat.
    2. Uses a cup to drink.
    3. Uses a knife for cutting food.
    4. Pours own milk into a cup.

11. A nurse is preparing to care for a 5-year-old who has been placed in traction following a fracture of the femur. The nurse plans care, knowing that which of the following is the most appropriate activity for this child?
    1. Large picture books
    2. A radio
    3. Crayons and a coloring book
    4. A sports video

12. The mother of a 16-year-old tells a nurse that she is concerned because the child sleeps about 8 hours every night and until noontime every weekend.

The most appropriate nursing response is which of the following?
1. "The child probably is anemic and should eat more foods containing iron."
2. "Adolescents need that amount of sleep every night."
3. "The child should not be staying up so late at night."
4. "If the child eats properly, that should not be happening."

13. A 4-year old child diagnosed with leukemia is hospitalized for chemotherapy. The child is fearful of the hospitalization. Which nursing intervention would be most appropriate to alleviate the child's fears?
1. Advise the family to visit only during the scheduled visiting hours.
2. Encourage play with other children of the same age.
3. Provide a private room, allowing the child to bring the favorite toys from home.
4. Encourage the child's parents to stay with the child.

14. A 16-year-old is admitted to the hospital for acute appendicitis, and an appendectomy is performed. Which of the following nursing interventions is most appropriate to facilitate normal growth and development?
1. Allow the family to bring in the child's favorite computer games.
2. Encourage the parents to room-in with the child.
3. Encourage the child to rest and read.
4. Allow the child to participate in activities with other individuals in the same age group when the condition permits.

15. A nurse prepares to administer digoxin (Lanoxin) to a 3-year-old child with a diagnosis of congestive heart failure. The nurse notes that the apical rate is 110 beats per minute. Based on this finding, which nursing action is most appropriate?
1. Administer the digoxin.
2. Recheck the apical rate in 15 minutes.
3. Notify the physician.
4. Hold the medication.

16. A 2-year-old child is treated in the emergency room for a burn to the chest and abdomen. The child sustained the burn by grabbing a cup of hot coffee that was left on the kitchen counter. The nurse reviews safety principles with the parents before discharge. Which statement, if made by the parents, indicates an understanding of the measures to provide safety in the home?
1. "I guess my children need to understand what the word *hot* means."

2. "We will install a safety gate as soon as we get home so the children cannot get into the kitchen."
3. "We will be sure that the children stay in their rooms when we work in the kitchen."
4. "We will be sure not to leave hot liquids unattended."

17. A clinic nurse provides instructions to a parent of a toddler experiencing physiological anorexia. Which statement if made by the parent indicates a need for further instructions?
1. "I will not force-feed my child."
2. "I will limit the juice intake to less than 12 ounces per day."
3. "I will feed my child if she will not eat."
4. "At mealtime, I will offer less than my child may eat and let my child ask for more."

18. A mother of a 4-year-old expresses concern because her hospitalized child has begun thumb sucking. The mother states that this behavior began 2 days after hospital admission. The most appropriate nursing response is which of the following?
1. "A 4-year-old is too old for this type of behavior."
2. "Your child is acting like a baby."
3. "The doctor will need to notified."
4. "It is best to ignore the behavior."

19. A clinic nurse assesses the communication patterns of a 5-month-old infant. The nurse determines that the infant is demonstrating the highest level of developmental achievement expected if the infant:
1. Uses simple words such as "mama."
2. Uses monosyllabic babbling.
3. Links syllables together.
4. Coos when comforted.

20. The mother of a toddler asks a nurse when it is safe to place the car safety seat in a face-forward position. The best nursing response is which of the following?
1. When the toddler weighs 20 lb.
2. The seat should not be placed in a face-forward position unless there are safety locks in the car.
3. The seat should never be placed in a face-forward position because of the risk of the child unbuckling the harness.
4. When the weight of the toddler is greater than 40 lb.

CRITICAL THINKING: FILL IN THE BLANK

The mother of a preschooler asks a clinic nurse when it will be safe to allow the child to use the car seat belts, rather than the booster seat, for traveling in the car. The nurse provides the mother with what information?

Answer: _____

ANSWERS

1. 4

Rationale: The phases through which young children progress when separated from their parents include protest, despair, and denial or detachment. In the stage of protest, when the parents return, the child readily goes to them. In the stage of despair, the child may not approach them readily or may cling to a parent. In denial or detachment, when the parents return, the child becomes cheerful, interested in the environment and new persons (seemingly unaware of the lost parents), friendly with the staff, and interested in developing superficial relationships. Options 1, 2, and 3 are incorrect interpretations of the child's behavior.

Test-Taking Strategy: Use the process of elimination and knowledge regarding the phases of separation anxiety to answer the question. In addition, focusing on the data in the question will assist in eliminating options 1, 2, and 3. Review the concepts related to the hospitalized toddler and separation anxiety if you had difficulty with this question.

Level of Cognitive Ability: Analysis
Client Needs: Psychosocial Integrity
Integrated Process: Nursing Process—analysis
Content Area: Child health
References: James, S., Ashwill, J., & Droske, S. (2002). *Nursing care of children: Principles & practice* (2nd ed., p. 310). Philadelphia: W. B. Saunders.
McKinney, E., Ashwill, J., Murray, S., James, S., Gorrie, T., Droske, S. (2000). *Maternal-child nursing* (p. 113). Philadelphia: W. B. Saunders.

2. 1

Rationale: Toddlers often resist going to bed. Bedtime protests may be reduced by establishing a consistent before-bedtime routine and enforcing consistent limits regarding the child's bedtime behavior. Informing the child of bedtime a few minutes before it is time for bed is the most appropriate option. Firm, consistent limits are needed for temper tantrums or when toddlers try stalling tactics. Most toddlers take an afternoon nap and until their second birthday also may require a morning nap.

Test-Taking Strategy: Use the process of elimination. Note the key words "most appropriate." Eliminate options 2, 3, and 4 by using concepts related to growth and development. Remember that preparing the toddler for an event will minimize resistive behavior. Review concepts related to sleep patterns and the toddler if you had difficulty with this question.

Level of Cognitive Ability: Application
Client Needs: Physiological Integrity
Integrated Process: Teaching/Learning
Content Area: Child health
Reference: McKinney, E., Ashwill, J., Murray, S., James, S., Gorrie, T., Droske, S. (2000). *Maternal-child nursing* (p. 120). Philadelphia: W. B. Saunders.

3. 4

Rationale: Toys for the toddler must be strong, safe, and too large to swallow or place in the ear or nose. Toddlers need supervision at all times. Push/pull toys, large balls, large crayons, trucks, and dolls are some of the appropriate toys. A farm set, a golf set, and jacks with marbles may contain items that the child could swallow.

Test-Taking Strategy: Use the process of elimination and focus on the issue, the appropriate toy for a 3-year-old. Options 1, 2, and 3 can be eliminated easily because they contain items that the child could swallow. Remember that large and strong toys are safest for the toddler. Review the principles related to play activities and the toddler if you had difficulty with this question.

Level of Cognitive Ability: Application
Client Needs: Safe, Effective Care Environment
Integrated Process: Teaching/Learning
Content Area: Child health
Reference: James, S., Ashwill, J., & Droske, S. (2002). *Nursing care of children: Principles & practice* (2nd ed., p. 163). Philadelphia: W. B. Saunders.

4. 2

Rationale: Bowel control usually is achieved before bladder control. The physical ability to control the anal and urethral sphincters is achieved sometime after the child is walking, probably between the ages of 18 and 24 months. The child should not be forced to sit for long periods. The ability to remove clothing is one of the physical signs of readiness.

Test-Taking Strategy: Use the process of elimination and knowledge of the concepts related to readiness for toilet training. Note the key words "indicates a need for further information." Look for the option that indicates that the nurse needs to provide additional information to the mother regarding the toilet training. Review the concepts related to readiness for toilet training if you had difficulty with this question.

Level of Cognitive Ability: Analysis
Client Needs: Physiological Integrity
Integrated Process: Nursing Process—evaluation
Content Area: Child health
Reference: James, S., Ashwill, J., & Droske, S. (2002). *Nursing care of children: Principles & practice* (2nd ed., p. 174). Philadelphia: W. B. Saunders.

5. 4

Rationale: A toddler should never be allowed to fall asleep with a bottle containing milk, juice, soda pop, or sweetened water because of the risk of nursing (bottle-mouth) caries. If a bottle is allowed at nap time or bedtime, it should contain only water.

Test-Taking Strategy: Use the process of elimination and note the key words "most appropriate." Eliminate options 1 and 2 first because they are similar. From the remaining options, recalling that nursing (bottle-mouth) caries is a concern in a child will assist in directing you to option 4. Review dental health principles related to children if you had difficulty with this question.

Level of Cognitive Ability: Application
Client Needs: Health Promotion and Maintenance
Integrated Process: Teaching/Learning
Content Area: Child health
Reference: James, S., Ashwill, J., & Droske, S. (2002). *Nursing care of children: Principles & practice* (2nd ed., p. 143). Philadelphia: W. B. Saunders.

6. 4

Rationale: The normal respiratory rate in a 12-month-old infant is 20 to 40 breaths per minute. The normal apical rate is 90 to 130 beats per minute, and the average blood pressure is 90/56 mm Hg. The nurse would document the findings.

Test-Taking Strategy: Knowledge regarding the normal vital signs of an infant is required to answer this question. If you had difficulty with this question, review these normal parameters.

Level of Cognitive Ability: Application
Client Needs: Physiological Integrity
Integrated Process: Nursing Process—implementation
Content Area: Child health
Reference: McKinney, E., Ashwill, J., Murray, S., James, S., Gorrie, T., Droske, S. (2000). *Maternal-child nursing* (p. 831). Philadelphia: W. B. Saunders.

7. **3**

Rationale: The size of the blood pressure cuff is important. Cuffs that are too small will cause falsely elevated values, and those that are too large will cause inaccurate low values. The cuff should cover two thirds of the distance between the antecubital fossa and the shoulder.

Test-Taking Strategy: Use the process of elimination. Attempt to visualize the placement measurements described in each of the options. This will assist in directing you to option 3. If you had difficulty with this question, review the procedure for taking a blood pressure in a child.

Level of Cognitive Ability: Comprehension
Client Needs: Health Promotion and Maintenance
Integrated Process: Nursing Process—implementation
Content Area: Child health
Reference: James, S., Ashwill, J., & Droske, S. (2002). *Nursing care of children: Principles & practice* (2nd ed., p. 235). Philadelphia: W. B. Saunders.

8. **3**

Rationale: Infants who weigh up to 20 lb should be restrained in a car seat (convertible restraint) in a semireclined, rear-facing position in the back seat of the car. Options 1, 2, and 4 are incorrect.

Test-Taking Strategy: Visualize each of the descriptions in the options, with a focus of safety in mind. Eliminate options 1 and 2 because of the words "front seat." Next, eliminate option 4 because of the words "forward-facing." If you had difficulty with this question, review the car safety measures for the infant.

Level of Cognitive Ability: Application
Client Needs: Safe, Effective Care Environment
Integrated Process: Teaching/Learning
Content Area: Child health
Reference: James, S., Ashwill, J., & Droske, S. (2002). *Nursing care of children: Principles & practice* (2nd ed., p. 122). Philadelphia: W. B. Saunders.

9. **4**

Rationale: The anterior fontanel is diamond shaped and located on the top of the head. The fontanel should be soft and flat in a normal infant, and it normally closes by 12 to 18 months of age. The nurse would document the finding because it is normal.

Test-Taking Strategy: Use the process of elimination. Note the key words "soft and flat." This should provide you with the clue that this is a normal finding. A bulging or tense fontanel

may result from crying or increased intracranial pressure. If you had difficulty with this question, review normal assessment findings in an infant.

Level of Cognitive Ability: Application
Client Needs: Physiological Integrity
Integrated Process: Nursing Process—implementation
Content Area: Child health
Reference: James, S., Ashwill, J., & Droske, S. (2002). *Nursing care of children: Principles & practice* (2nd ed., p. 240). Philadelphia: W. B. Saunders.

10. **2**

Rationale: By age 2 years, the child can use a cup and can use a spoon correctly but with some spilling. By ages 3 to 4, the child begins to use a fork. By the end of the preschool period, the child should be able to pour milk into a cup and begin to use a knife for cutting.

Test-Taking Strategy: Note the age of the child and use the process of elimination. Option 3 can be eliminated easily. Next, think about the fine-motor skills that need to be developed in selecting the correct option. With this in mind, eliminate options 1 and 4. If you had difficulty with this question, review the developmental skills of a 2-year-old.

Level of Cognitive Ability: Analysis
Client Needs: Health Promotion and Maintenance
Integrated Process: Nursing Process—assessment
Content Area: Child health
Reference: Wong, D., Perry, S., & Hockenberry, M. (2002). *Maternal child nursing care* (2nd ed., p. 420). St. Louis: Mosby.

11. **3**

Rationale: In the preschooler, play is simple and imaginative and includes activities such as crayons and coloring books, puppets, felt and magnetic boards, and Play-Doh. Large picture books are most appropriate for the infant. A radio and a sports video are most appropriate for the adolescent.

Test-Taking Strategy: Use the process of elimination. Note the age of the child, and think about the age-related activity that would be most appropriate. Eliminate options 3 and 4, knowing that they are most appropriate for the adolescent. From the remaining options, the word "large" in option 1 should provide you with the clue that this activity would be more appropriate for a child younger than age 5. If you had difficulty with this question, review the appropriate activities for a preschooler.

Level of Cognitive Ability: Application
Client Needs: Psychosocial Integrity
Integrated Process: Nursing Process—planning
Content Area: Child health
References: McKinney, E., Ashwill, J., Murray, S., James, S., Gorrie, T., Droske, S. (2000). *Maternal-child nursing* (pp. 912-913). Philadelphia: W. B. Saunders.
Wong, D., Perry, S., & Hockenberry, M. (2002). *Maternal child nursing care* (2nd ed., p. 1106). St. Louis: Mosby.

12. **2**

Rationale: The adolescent needs about 8 hours of sleep per night. During this age, with an increase in social activities, school commitments, and possibly work activities, it is important that the adolescent receive enough sleep at night.

Options 1, 3, and 4 are inaccurate and inappropriate nursing responses.

Test-Taking Strategy: Use the process of elimination and focus on the issue of the question. Note the key words "most appropriate." The question gives no indication that a physiological alteration is present; therefore eliminate option 1. From the remaining options, use therapeutic communication techniques to direct you to option 2. Review adolescent sleep patterns if you had difficulty with this question.

Level of Cognitive Ability: Application

Client Needs: Health Promotion and Maintenance

Integrated Process: Communication and Documentation

Content Area: Child health

Reference: McKinney, E., Ashwill, J., Murray, S., James, S., Gorrie, T., Droske, S. (2000). *Maternal-child nursing* (p. 166). Philadelphia: W. B. Saunders.

13. 4

Rationale: Although the preschooler already may be spending some time away from parents at a day care center or preschool, illness adds a stressor that makes separation more difficult. The child may ask repeatedly when parents will be coming for a visit or may be wanting constantly to call the parents. Options 1 and 3 will increase stress related to separation anxiety. Option 2 is unrelated to the issue of the question and, in addition, may not be appropriate for a child at risk for immunocompromise and infection.

Test-Taking Strategy: Note that the issue relates to the child's fear. Use the process of elimination. Options 1 and 3 will increase anxiety and fear further and should be eliminated. Bearing the issue of the question in mind and considering the child's diagnosis will assist you in eliminating option 2. Review interventions to prevent or minimize separation anxiety if you had difficulty with this question.

Level of Cognitive Ability: Application

Client Needs: Psychosocial Integrity

Integrated Process: Caring

Content Area: Child health

Reference: Wong, D., Perry, S., & Hockenberry, M. (2002). *Maternal child nursing care* (2nd ed., p. 1082). St. Louis: Mosby.

14. 4

Rationale: Adolescents often are not sure whether they want their parents with them when they are hospitalized. Because of the importance of the peer group, separation from friends is a source of anxiety. Ideally, the members of the peer group will support their ill friend. Options 1, 2, and 3 isolate the child from the peer group.

Test-Taking Strategy: Consider the psychosocial needs of the adolescent when answering the question. Options 1, 2, and 3 are similar in that they isolate the child from his or her own peer group. If you had difficulty with this question, review the psychosocial needs of the adolescent.

Level of Cognitive Ability: Application

Client Needs: Psychosocial Integrity

Integrated Process: Caring

Content Area: Child health

Reference: Wong, D., & Hockenberry-Eaton, M. (2001). *Wong's essentials of pediatric nursing* (6th ed., p. 709). St. Louis: Mosby.

15. 1

Rationale: The normal apical heart rate for a 3-year-old is 80 to 120 beats per minute. Because the apical rate is within the normal range, options 2, 3, and 4 are inappropriate.

Test-Taking Strategy: Use the process of elimination and knowledge of the normal apical heart rate for a 3-year-old to answer the question. Recalling that a heart rate of 110 beats per minute is within the normal range will direct you to option 1. Review the normal vital signs for a 3-year-old if you had difficulty with this question.

Level of Cognitive Ability: Application

Client Needs: Physiological Integrity

Integrated Process: Nursing Process—implementation

Content Area: Child health

Reference: McKinney, E., Ashwill, J., Murray, S., James, S., Gorrie, T., Droske, S. (2000). *Maternal-child nursing* (p. 831). Philadelphia: W. B. Saunders.

16. 4

Rationale: Toddlers, with their increased mobility and development of motor skills, can reach hot water or hot objects placed on counters and stoves and can reach open fires or stove burners above their eye level. The nurse should encourage parents to remain in the kitchen when preparing a meal, to use the back burners on the stove, and to turn pot handles inward and toward the middle of the stove. Hot liquids should never be left unattended, and the toddler should always be supervised. The statements in options 1, 2, and 3 do not indicate an understanding of the principles of safety.

Test-Taking Strategy: Use the process of elimination, noting the key words "indicates an understanding." Option 1 can be eliminated easily. Options 2 and 3 are similar in that they isolate the child from the environment. Option 4 is the only option that reflects an understanding of safety principles by the parents. Review these safety principles if you had difficulty with this question.

Level of Cognitive Ability: Analysis

Client Needs: Safe, Effective Care Environment

Integrated Process: Nursing Process—evaluation

Content Area: Child health

Reference: McKinney, E., Ashwill, J., Murray, S., James, S., Gorrie, T., Droske, S. (2000). *Maternal-child nursing* (p. 122). Philadelphia: W. B. Saunders.

17. 3

Rationale: A toddler has the skills required to feed himself or herself. The parent needs to be instructed not to feed children who can feed themselves and not to force-feed a child. To increase nutritious intake at mealtime, juice intake needs to be limited to less than 12 oz per day. At mealtime, the best option is to offer less than the toddler may eat and let the child ask for more food.

Test-Taking Strategy: Note the key words "a need for further instructions." Bearing in mind that the goal is to provide a nutritious intake should assist in directing you to option 3. In addition, feeding a child if he or she will not eat will impair independence. Review interventions that will promote nutrition in the toddler if you had difficulty with this question.

Level of Cognitive Ability: Analysis

Client Needs: Physiological Integrity

Integrated Process: Nursing Process—evaluation
Content Area: Child health
References: James, S., Ashwill, J., & Droske, S. (2002). *Nursing care of children: Principles & practice* (2nd ed., p. 165). Philadelphia: W. B. Saunders.
Wong, D., & Hockenberry-Eaton, M. (2001). *Wong's essentials of pediatric nursing* (6th ed., p. 424). St. Louis: Mosby.

18. **4**
Rationale: In the hospitalized preschooler, the best option is to accept regression if it occurs. Regression is most often due to the stress of the hospitalization. Parents may be overly concerned about regression and should be told that their child may continue the behavior at home. When regression does occur, the best approach is to ignore it while praising existing patterns of appropriate behavior. Calling the physician is not necessary. Options 1 and 2 are inappropriate.
Test-Taking Strategy: Use the process of elimination. Note the key words "most appropriate." Options 1 and 2 are clearly inappropriate and are eliminated first. Option 3 may cause increased concern in the mother. If you had difficulty with this question, review the psychosocial issues related to the hospitalized preschool child.
Level of Cognitive Ability: Application
Client Needs: Psychosocial Integrity
Integrated Process: Communication and Documentation
Content Area: Child health
References: Wong, D., & Hockenberry-Eaton, M. (2001). *Wong's essentials of pediatric nursing* (6th ed., p. 345). St. Louis: Mosby.
Wong, D., Perry, S., & Hockenberry, M. (2002). *Maternal child nursing care* (2nd ed., p. 844). St. Louis: Mosby.

19. **2**
Rationale: Using monosyllabic babbling occurs between 3 and 6 months of age. Using simple words such as "mama" occurs between 9 and 12 months of age. Linking syllables together when communicating occurs between 6 and 9 months of age. Cooing begins at birth and continues until 2 months of age.
Test-Taking Strategy: Use the process of elimination and knowledge of language and communication developmental milestones to answer the question. Focus on the age of the infant to assist in directing you to the correct option. Review the patterns of infant communication if you had difficulty with this question.
Level of Cognitive Ability: Analysis
Client Needs: Health Promotion and Maintenance

Integrated Process: Nursing Process—assessment
Content Area: Child health
References: James, S., Ashwill, J., & Droske, S. (2002). *Nursing care of children: Principles & practice* (2nd ed., p. 141). Philadelphia: W. B. Saunders.
Wong, D., Perry, S., & Hockenberry, M. (2002). *Maternal child nursing care* (2nd ed., p. 834). St. Louis: Mosby.

20. **1**
Rationale: The transition point for switching to the forward-facing position is defined by the manufacturer of the convertible car safety seat but is generally at a body weight of 9 kg (20 lb) and 1 year of age. Convertible car safety seats are used until the child weighs at least 40 lb. Options 2, 3, and 4 are incorrect.
Test-Taking Strategy: Use the process of elimination and focus on the issue of the question. Eliminate options 2 and 3 first because of the absolute words "not" and "never." From the remaining options, use knowledge regarding car safety and the toddler to answer the question. Review these safety principles if you had difficulty with this question.
Level of Cognitive Ability: Application
Client Needs: Safe, Effective Care Environment
Integrated Process: Teaching/Learning
Content Area: Child health
Reference: Wong, D., & Hockenberry-Eaton, M. (2001). *Wong's essentials of pediatric nursing* (6th ed., p. 374). St. Louis: Mosby.

CRITICAL THINKING: FILL IN THE BLANK
Answer: The preschooler is restrained in a booster seat until the preschooler weighs at least 60 lb, is 8 years old, or his or her head is higher than the vehicle back seat.
Rationale: At this developmental level the child's head is high enough to allow a car seat belt to be correctly positioned over the child's chest and pelvis.
Test-Taking Strategy: Focus on the issue of the question and the developmental level of the child, the preschooler, to answer the question. Review the principles and guidelines related to car safety if you had difficulty with this question.
Level of Cognitive Ability: Application
Client Needs: Safe, Effective Care Environment
Integrated Process: Teaching/Learning
Content Area: Child health
Reference: Wong, D., & Hockenberry-Eaton, M. (2001). *Wong's essentials of pediatric nursing* (6th ed., p. 430). St. Louis: Mosby.

REFERENCES

James, S., Ashwill, J., & Droske, S. (2002). *Nursing care of children: Principles & practice* (2nd ed.). Philadelphia: W. B. Saunders.

McKinney, E., Ashwill, J., Murray, S., James, S., Gorrie, T., Droske, S. (2000). *Maternal-child nursing.* Philadelphia: W. B. Saunders.

Murray, S., McKinney, E., & Gorrie, T. (2002). *Foundations of maternal-newborn nursing* (3rd ed.). Philadelphia: W. B. Saunders.

Wong, D., & Hockenberry-Eaton, M. (2001). *Wong's essentials of pediatric nursing* (6th ed.). St. Louis: Mosby.

Wong, D., Perry, S., & Hockenberry, M. (2002). *Maternal child nursing care* (2nd ed.). St. Louis: Mosby.

Care of the Older Client

I. PHYSIOLOGICAL CHANGES

A. Integumentary system
   1. Loss of pigment in hair and skin
   2. Wrinkling of the skin
   3. Thinning of the epidermis and easy bruising and tearing of the skin
   4. Decreased skin turgor, elasticity, and subcutaneous fat
   5. Increased nail thickness and decreased nail growth
   6. Decreased perspiration
   7. Dry, itchy, scaly skin
   8. Seborrheic dermatitis and keratosis formation

B. Neurological system
   1. Slowed reflexes
   2. Slight tremors and difficulty with fine motor movement
   3. Loss of balance
   4. Experience an increased incidence of awakening after sleep onset
   5. Increased susceptibility to hypothermia and hyperthermia
   6. Short-term memory decline possible
   7. Long-term memory usually maintained

C. Musculoskeletal system
   1. Decreased muscle mass and strength and atrophy of muscles
   2. Decreased mobility, range of motion, flexibility, coordination, and stability
   3. Change of gait, with shortened step and wider base
   4. Posture and stature changes causing a decrease in height
   5. Increased brittleness of the bones
   6. Deterioration of joint capsule components
   7. Kyphosis of the dorsal spine

D. Cardiovascular system
   1. Diminished energy and endurance with lowered tolerance to exercise
   2. Decreased compliance of the heart muscle, with heart valves becoming thicker and more rigid
   3. Decreased cardiac output and decreased efficiency of blood return to the heart
   4. Decreased resting heart rate
   5. Weak peripheral pulses
   6. Increased blood pressure but susceptibility to postural hypotension

E. Respiratory system
   1. Decreased stretch and compliance of the chest wall
   2. Decreased strength and function of respiratory muscles
   3. Decreased size and number of alveoli
   4. Increased rate of respirations, generally 16 to 25 breaths per minute
   5. Decreased depth of respirations and oxygen intake
   6. Decreased ability to cough and expectorate sputum

F. Hematological system
   1. Hemoglobin and hematocrit average levels toward the low end of normal
   2. Prone to increased blood clotting

G. Immune system
   1. Tendency of lymphocyte counts to be low
   2. Decreased resistance to infection and disease

H. Gastrointestinal system
   1. Decreased need for calories
   2. Decreased appetite, thirst, and oral intake
   3. Decreased lean body weight
   4. Digestive disturbances
   5. Decreased stomach-emptying time
   6. Decreased absorption of carbohydrates, proteins, fats, and vitamins

7. Increased tendency toward constipation
8. Increased susceptibility for dehydration
9. Tooth loss
10. Difficulty in chewing and swallowing food
I. Endocrine system
1. Decreased secretion of hormones, with specific changes related to each hormone function
2. Decreased metabolic rate
3. Decreased glucose tolerance with resistance to insulin in peripheral tissues
J. Renal system
1. Decreased kidney size, function, and ability to concentrate urine
2. Decreased glomerular filtration rate
3. Decreased capacity of the bladder
4. Increased residual urine and increased incidence of infection and incontinence
5. Impaired medication excretion
K. Reproductive system
1. Decreased testosterone production and decreased size of testes
2. Changes in the prostate gland leading to urinary problems
3. Decreased secretion of hormones with the cessation of menses
4. Vaginal changes, including decreased muscle tone and lubrication
5. Impotence or sexual dysfunction for both sexes; sexual function varies and depends on general physical condition and mental health status and medications
L. Special senses
1. Decreased visual acuity
2. Decreased accommodation in eyes requiring increased adjustment time to changes in light
3. Decreased peripheral vision and increased sensitivity to glare
4. Presbyopia and cataract formation
5. Possible loss of hearing ability; low pitched tones are heard more easily
6. Inability to discern taste of food
7. Decreased sense of smell
8. Changes in touch sensation
9. Decreased pain awareness

II. PSYCHOSOCIAL CONCERNS
A. Adjustment to deterioration in physical and mental health and well-being
B. Threat to independent functioning and fear of becoming a burden to loved ones
C. Adjustment to retirement and loss of income
D. Loss of skills and competencies developed early in life
E. Coping with changes in role function and social life
F. Diminished quantity and quality of relationships and coping with loss
G. Dependence on governmental and social systems

BOX 34-1

Mental Health Concerns

Depression
Grief
Isolation
Suicide

H. Access to social support systems
I. Costs of health care and medications

III. MENTAL HEALTH CONCERNS (BOX 34-1)
A. Isolation: Client is alone and desires contact with others but is unable to make that contact.
B. Grief: Client reacts to the perception of loss, including physical, psychological, social, and spiritual aspects.
C. **Depression:** The increased dependency that older adults may experience can lead to hopelessness, helplessness, a lowered sense of self-control, and decreased self-esteem and self-worth; these changes can interfere with daily functioning and lead to depression.
D. Suicide: All suicide threats from an older client should be taken seriously.

IV. PAIN
A. Description
1. Pain can occur from numerous causes and most often occurs from degenerative changes in the musculoskeletal system.
2. The failure to alleviate pain in the older client can lead to functional limitations affecting their ability to function independently.
B. Assessment
1. Agitation
2. Moaning
3. Crying
4. Restlessness
5. Verbal reporting of pain
C. Interventions
1. Monitor the client for signs of pain.
2. Identify the pattern of pain.
3. Identify the precipitating factor(s) for the pain.
4. Monitor the impact of the pain on activities of daily living.
5. Provide pain relief through measures such as distraction, relaxation, massage, and biofeedback.
6. Administer pain medication as prescribed, and instruct the client in its use.
7. Evaluate the effects of pain-reducing measures.

V. MEDICATIONS
A. Major problems with prescriptive medications include adverse affects, medication interactions, medication errors, noncompliance, and the cost.
B. Determine the use of over-the-counter medications.

C. Keep the use of medications to a minimum.

D. Medication dosages normally are prescribed at one third to one half of the normal adult doses.

E. Closely monitor client for adverse effects and response to therapy because of the increased risk for medication toxicity.

F. Note that a common sign of an adverse reaction in the older client in an acute change in mental status.

G. Assess for medication interactions in client taking multiple medications.

H. Advise the client to use one pharmacy and notify the consulting physicians of the medications taken.

I. Administration of medications

1. Place the client in a sitting position when administering medication.

2. Check for mouth dryness because medication may stick and dissolve in mouth.

3. Administer liquid preparations if the client has difficulty swallowing tablets.

4. Crush tablets if necessary and give with textured food (nectar, applesauce) if not contraindicated.

5. Do not crush enteric-coated tablets and do not open capsules.

6. If administering a suppository, do not insert suppository immediately after removing from the refrigerator.

7. A suppository may take longer to dissolve because of decreased body core temperature.

8. When administering parenteral medication, monitor the site because it may ooze medication or bleed because of decreased tissue elasticity.

9. Do not use an immobile limb for administering parenteral medication.

10. Monitor client compliance with taking prescribed medications.

11. Monitor client for safety in correctly taking medications.

12. Use a medication cassette to facilitate proper administration of medication.

VI. ABUSE TO THE OLDER ADULT

A. **Abuse** involves physical, emotional, or sexual **abuse** and also can involve **neglect** or economic **exploitation**.

B. Individuals at most risk include those who are dependent because of their immobility or altered mental status.

C. Factors that contribute to **abuse** and **neglect** include long-standing family violence, caregiver stress, and the individual's increasing dependence on others.

D. Victims may attempt to dismiss injuries as accidental, and abusers may prevent victims from receiving proper medical care to avoid discovery.

E. Victims often are isolated socially by their abusers.

F. For additional information on abuse to the older client, refer to Chapter 75.

PRACTICE QUESTIONS

1. The nurse is providing instructions to a nursing assistant regarding care to an older client with hearing loss. The nurse tells the assistant that clients with a hearing loss
   1. Are often distracted.
   2. Respond to low-pitched tones.
   3. Have middle-ear changes.
   4. Develop moist cerumen production.

2. An older male client is admitted to the hospital with a diagnosis of malnutrition. Which of the following laboratory data indicates that the client is experiencing a protein deficiency?
   1. Creatinine, 0.6 mg/dL
   2. Transferrin, 90 mg/dL
   3. Calcium, 10 mg/dL
   4. Sodium, 138 mEq/L

3. The nurse is providing an educational session to new employees, and the topic is abuse to the older client. The nurse tells the employees that which client is most characteristic of a victim of abuse?
   1. A 90-year-old woman with advanced Parkinson's disease.
   2. A 68-year-old man with newly diagnosed cataracts.
   3. A 70-year-old woman with early diagnosed Lyme's disease.
   4. A 75-year-old man with moderate hypertension.

4. An older female client confides to the visiting nurse that she is afraid she will fall while going to the bathroom at night. Which suggestion, if made by the nurse, indicates that the nurse understands the visual changes affecting the older client?
   1. "Use a bell to call your daughter if you need to get up."
   2. "Keep a red light on in the bathroom at night."
   3. "Use a commode in your bedroom at night."
   4. "Limit your fluid intake during the day."

5. The nurse is caring for an agitated older client with Alzheimer's disease. Which nursing intervention most likely would calm the client?
   1. Playing a radio
   2. Turning the lights out
   3. Putting an arm around the client's waist
   4. Encouraging group participation

6. The nurse who volunteers at a senior citizens center is planning activities for the members who attend the center. Which activity would best promote health and maintenance for these senior citizens?
   1. Gardening every day for an hour
   2. Cycling 3 times a week for 20 minutes
   3. Sculpting once a week for 40 minutes
   4. Walking 3 to 5 times a week for 30 minutes

7. The nurse is working with older clients in a long-term care facility. Which of the following activities performed by the nurse fosters reminiscence among these clients?

1. Displaying calendars and clocks
2. Encouraging client participation in pottery class
3. Setting up pet therapy sessions
4. Having storytelling hours

8. The home care nurse is performing an environmental assessment in the home of an older client. Which of the following, if observed by the nurse, requires immediate attention?
   1. An operable smoke detector
   2. A prefilled medication cassette
   3. Unsecured scatter rugs
   4. Clear exit passageways

9. The nurse is teaching an older client about measures to prevent constipation. Which statement, if made by the client, indicates that further teaching about bowel elimination is necessary?
   1. "I drink six to eight glasses of water per day."
   2. "I walk 1 to 2 miles per day."
   3. "I need to decrease fiber in my diet."
   4. "I have a bowel movement every other day."

10. The nurse educator is providing an information session to nursing assistants regarding caring for the older adult. The nurse educator tells the nursing assistants that which of the following situations portrays ageism?
    1. Accepting differences among older adults
    2. Allowing older adults to make decisions
    3. Informing the older adult of their rights
    4. Advising older adults to forego aggressive treatment

11. The nurse is providing medication instructions to an older client who is taking digoxin (Lanoxin) daily. The nurse bears in mind that which age-related body changes could place the client at risk for digoxin toxicity?
    1. Decreased cough efficiency and decreased vital capacity
    2. Decreased lean body mass and decreased glomerular filtration rate
    3. Decreased salivation and decreased gastrointestinal motility
    4. Decreased muscle strength and loss of bone density

12. The nurse employed in a long-term care facility is caring for an older male client. Which of the following nursing actions would contribute to encouraging autonomy in the client?
    1. Scheduling his barber appointments
    2. Allowing him to choose social activities
    3. Decorating his room
    4. Planning his meals

13. The nurse assigned to care for an older client places an extra blanket in the client's room. The nurse understands that the older client is less able to regulate hot and cold bodily changes because of alterations in the activity of the
    1. Parotid glands.
    2. Thymus gland.
    3. Pineal gland.
    4. Sweat glands.

14. The home care nurse is visiting an older female client whose husband died 6 months ago. Which behavior, by the client, indicates ineffective coping?
    1. Visiting her husband's grave once a month
    2. Participating in a senior citizens program
    3. Looking at old snapshots of her family
    4. Neglecting her personal grooming

15. The nurse is preparing to communicate with an older client who is hearing impaired. The most appropriate initial nursing action is to
    1. Stand in front of the client.
    2. Exaggerate lip movements.
    3. Obtain a sign language interpreter.
    4. Pantomime and write the client notes.

16. The nurse is performing an assessment on an older client who is having difficulty sleeping at night. Which statement, if made by the client, indicates that teaching concerning improving sleep is necessary?
    1. "I drink hot chocolate before bedtime."
    2. "I have stopped smoking cigars."
    3. "I swim 3 times a week."
    4. "I read for 40 minutes before bedtime."

17. The visiting nurse observes that the older male client is confined by his daughter-in-law to his room. When the nurse suggests he walk to the den and join the family, he says, "I'm in everyone's way; my daughter-in-law needs for me to stay here." The most important action for the nurse to take is to
    1. Suggest to the client and daughter-in-law that they consider a nursing home for the client.
    2. Suggest appropriate resources to the client and daughter-in-law such as respite care and senior citizens.
    3. Say nothing, for it is best for the nurse to remain neutral and wait to be asked for help.
    4. Say to the daughter-in-law, "Confining your father-in-law to his room is inhuman."

18. The nurse is performing an assessment on an older adult client. Which assessment data would indicate a potential complication associated with the skin of this client?
    1. Wrinkling
    2. Thinning and loss of elasticity in the skin
    3. Deepening of expression lines
    4. Crusting

19. The home care nurse provides medication instructions to an older hypertensive client who is taking lisinopril (Prinivil, Zestril) 20 mg PO daily. Which statement, if made by the client, indicates that further teaching is necessary?
    1. "I take the pill after breakfast each day."
    2. "I need to change my position slowly."

3. "If I get a bad headache, I should call my doctor immediately."
4. "I can skip a dose once a week."
20. The nurse is caring for an older client who is on bedrest. The nurse plans which intervention to prevent respiratory complications?
1. Monitoring vital signs every shift.
2. Decreasing oral fluid intake.
3. Changing the client's position every 2 hours.
4. Instructing the client to bear down every hour and hold the breath.

CRITICAL THINKING: MULTIPLE RESPONSE

Select all of the normal age-related physiological changes.

___ Decline in visual acuity

___ Decreased respiratory rate

___ Increased heart rate

___ Increased susceptibility to urinary tract infections

___ Decline in long-term memory

___ Increased incidence of awakening after sleep onset

ANSWERS
1. 2
Rationale: Presbycusis refers to the age-related irreversible degenerative changes of the inner ear leading to decreased hearing ability. As a result of these changes, the older client has a decreased response to high-frequency sounds. Low-pitched tones of voice are heard more easily and interpreted by the older client. Options 1, 3, and 4 are not accurate.
Test-Taking Strategy: Use the process of elimination. Recalling that the client with a hearing loss responds to low-pitched tones will direct you to option 2. If you had difficulty with this question, review the characteristics associated with presbycusis and hearing loss.
Level of Cognitive Ability: Application
Client Needs: Physiological Integrity
Integrated Process: Teaching/Learning
Content Area: Adult health—ear
Reference: Lueckenotte, A. (2000). *Gerontologic nursing* (2nd ed., p. 711). St. Louis: Mosby.

2. 2
Rationale: Serum transferrin is an iron-transport protein that can be measured directly or calculated as an indirect measurement of total iron-binding capacity. Transferrin is a more sensitive indicator of protein status than albumin. When serum transferrin is less than 100 mg/dL, the level of protein depletion is severe. Options 1, 3, and 4 identify normal laboratory values.
Test-Taking Strategy: Use the process of elimination. Note the key word "protein." The only option that refers to the analysis of protein is option 2. Additionally, eliminate options 1, 3, and 4 because these are normal laboratory values. Review these laboratory values if you had difficulty with this question.
Level of Cognitive Ability: Analysis
Client Needs: Physiological Integrity
Integrated Process: Nursing Process—analysis
Content Area: Fundamental skills
References: Lueckenotte, A. (2000). *Gerontologic nursing* (2nd ed., p. 409). St. Louis: Mosby.
O'Neill, P. (2002). *Caring for the older adult* (p. 916). Philadelphia: W. B. Saunders.

3. 1
Rationale: Elder abuse is widespread and occurs among all subgroups of the population. Elder abuse includes physical and psychological abuse, misuse of property, and violation of rights. The typical abuse victim is a woman of advanced age with few social contacts and at least one physical or mental impairment that limits the ability to perform activities of daily living. In addition, the client usually lives alone or with the abuser and depends on the abuser for care.
Test-Taking Strategy: Use the process of elimination. Read each option carefully and identify the client that is most defenseless as the result of the disease process. If you had difficulty with this question, review content related to elder abuse.
Level of Cognitive Ability: Application
Clients Needs: Psychosocial Integrity
Integrated Process: Teaching/Learning
Content Area: Mental health
Reference: O'Neill, P. (2002). *Caring for the older adult* (p. 255). Philadelphia: W. B. Saunders.

4. 2
Rationale: Because it takes longer to adapt to changes from dark to light and vice versa, older persons are at a greater risk of falls and injuries. Any place where a sudden change from dark to light or from light to dark occurs can be dangerous. Getting up during the night is a hazardous situation for an older client. Eyes adapt to the dark by using the rod receptors, which are sensitive to short blue-green wavelengths. Red wavelengths are longer and are perceived by the cones. Thus a red light in the bathroom at night will allow for vision to function in the dark adequately without the need for adaptation.
Test-Taking Strategy: Use the process of elimination focusing on the issue. Eliminate options 1 and 3 because they do not meet the client's need for independence. Additionally, no data in the question indicates that the client lives with the daughter. Option 4 is incorrect because the older client needs to be encouraged to drink at least 2 L of fluid a day to prevent dehydration. Review the physiological changes in the eye that occurs with aging if you had difficulty with this question.
Level of Cognitive Ability: Application
Clients Needs: Physiological Integrity
Integrated Process: Nursing Process—implementation
Content Area: Adult health—eye
Reference: Ebersole, P., & Hess, P. (2001). *Geriatric nursing & healthy aging* (p. 475). St. Louis: Mosby.

5. 3
Rationale: Nursing interventions for the client with Alzheimer's disease who is angry, frustrated, or hostile include decreasing

environmental stimuli, approaching the client calmly and with assurance, not demanding anything from the client, and distracting the client. For the nurse to reach out, touch, hold a hand, put an arm around the waist, or in some way maintain physical contact is important. Playing a radio may increase stimuli, and turning the lights out may produce more agitation. The client with Alzheimer's disease would not be a candidate for group work if the client is agitated.

Test-Taking Strategy: Note the key words "most likely". Use the process of elimination, recalling the need to decrease environmental stimuli and avoid further agitation. These concepts will direct you to option 3. Review care to the client with Alzheimer's disease if you had difficulty with this question.

Level of Cognitive Ability: Application
Clients Needs: Psychosocial Integrity
Integrated Process: Caring
Content Area: Mental health
Reference: Lueckenotte, A. (2000). *Gerontologic nursing* (2nd ed., pp. 631, 636). St. Louis: Mosby.

6. 4
Rationale: Exercise and activity are essential for health promotion and maintenance in the older adult and to achieve an optimal level of functioning. About half of the physical deterioration of the older client is caused by disuse rather than by the aging process or disease. One of the best exercises for an older adult is walking, progressing to 30 minute sessions 3 to 5 times each week. Swimming and dancing are also beneficial.

Test-Taking Strategy: Use the process of elimination noting the key word "best." Options 1, 2, and 3, although possible, are not the best activities. Remember, walking is one of the best forms of exercise. Review this content if you had difficulty with this question.

Level of Cognitive Ability: Application
Clients Needs: Health Promotion and Maintenance
Integrated Process: Nursing Process—planning
Content Area: Fundamental skills
Reference: Lueckenotte, A. (2000). *Gerontologic nursing* (2nd ed., p. 25). St. Louis: Mosby.

7. 4
Rationale: Clients who like to retell stories or past events need to be provided the opportunity to do so. This phenomenon is called life review or reminiscence. In a sense, reminiscence is a way for the older client to relive and restructure life experiences and is a part of achieving ego identity. Option 1 indicates reality orientation techniques. Options 2 and 3 indicate socialization and physical activity.

Test-Taking Strategy: Use the process of elimination. Focusing on the key word "reminiscence" and recalling the definition of this word will direct you to option 4. Review this form of activity if you had difficulty with this question.

Level of Cognitive Ability: Application
Clients Needs: Psychosocial Integrity
Integrated Process: Caring
Content Area: Mental health
Reference: Lueckenotte, A. (2000). *Gerontologic nursing* (2nd ed., p. 263). St. Louis: Mosby.

8. 3
Rationale: Trauma to the older client in the home may be caused by a variety of factors. Some of these factors include an unsteady gait, the presence of unsecured scatter rugs, cluttered passageways, inoperable smoke detectors, or a history of previous falls.

Test-Taking Strategy: Use the process of elimination. Note the key words "requires immediate attention." Focusing on the issue and looking for the item that identifies an unsafe condition will direct you to option 3. Review the components of an environmental assessment if you had difficulty with this question.

Level of Cognitive Ability: Analysis
Clients Needs: Safe, Effective Care Environment
Integrated Process: Nursing Process—assessment
Content Area: Fundamental skills
Reference: Lueckenotte, A. (2000). *Gerontologic nursing* (2nd ed., p. 245). St. Louis: Mosby.

9. 3
Rationale: Adequate dietary fiber is an important factor in aiding bowel function. Dietary fiber increases fecal weight and water content and accelerates the transit of fecal mass through the gastrointestinal tract. The retention of water by the fiber has the ability to soften stools and promote regularity. Fluid intake and exercise also facilitate bowel elimination.

Test-Taking Strategy: Note the key words "further teaching about bowel elimination is necessary." Use the process of elimination and basic principles related to preventing constipation. If you had difficulty with this question, review these basic principles.

Level of Cognitive Ability: Analysis
Clients Needs: Physiological Integrity
Integrated Process: Teaching/Learning
Content Area: Fundamental skills
References: Lueckenotte, A. (2000). *Gerontologic nursing* (2nd ed., p. 294). St. Louis: Mosby.
O'Neill, P. (2002). *Caring for the older adult* (p. 98). Philadelphia: W. B. Saunders.

10. 4
Rationale: Ageism is a form of prejudice in which older adults are stereotyped by characteristics found in only a few members of their group. Fundamental to ageism is the view that older persons are different from "me" and will remain different from "me." Therefore they are portrayed as not experiencing the same desires, needs, and concerns. Options 1, 2, and 3 identify supportive roles that the nurse engages in when dealing with the older adult. Option 4 suggests that the older adult is not worthy of aggressive treatment and demonstrates ageism.

Test-Taking Strategy: Use the process of elimination and focus on the issue, ageism. Recalling the definition of ageism will direct you to option 4. Review this concept if you had difficulty with this question.

Level of Cognitive Ability: Comprehension
Clients Needs: Health Promotion and Maintenance
Integrated Process: Caring
Content Area: Fundamental skills

References: Lueckenotte, A. (2000). *Gerontologic nursing* (2nd ed., p. 14). St. Louis: Mosby.
O'Neill, P. (2002). *Caring for the older adult* (p. 8). Philadelphia: W. B. Saunders.

11. 2
Rationale: The older client is at risk for medication toxicity because of decreased lean body mass and age-associated decreased glomerular filtration rate. Although options 1, 3, and 4 identify age-related changes that occur in the older client, they are not associated specifically with this risk.
Test-Taking Strategy: Use the process of elimination and focus on the issue, age-related body changes that could place the client at risk for medication toxicity. Note that option 2 is the only option that addresses renal excretion. If you had difficulty with this question, review the physiological changes associated with aging.
Level of Cognitive Ability: Analysis
Clients Needs: Physiological Integrity
Integrated Process: Teaching/Learning
Content Area: Fundamental skills
References: Lueckenotte, A. (2000). *Gerontologic nursing* (2nd ed., p. 389). St. Louis: Mosby.
O'Neill, P. (2002). *Caring for the older adult* (p. 112). Philadelphia: W. B. Saunders.

12. 2
Rationale: Autonomy is the personal freedom to direct one's own life as long as it does not impinge on the rights of others. An autonomous person is capable of rational thought. This individual can identify problems, search for alternatives, and select solutions that allow continued personal freedom as long as the rights and property of others are not harmed. Loss of autonomy and therefore independence, is a real fear among older clients. Option 2 is the only option that allows the client to be a decision maker.
Test-Taking Strategy: Use the process of elimination focusing on the issue, encouraging autonomy. Recalling the definition of autonomy will direct you to the correct option. Remember, giving the client choices is essential to promote independence. Review the concept of autonomy if you had difficulty with this question.
Level of Cognitive Ability: Application
Clients Needs: Safe, Effective Care Environment
Integrated Process: Caring
Content Area: Fundamental skills
Reference: O'Neill, P. (2002). *Caring for the older adult* (p. 250). Philadelphia: W. B. Saunders.

13. 4
Rationale: Functions of the skin include protection, sensory reception, homeostasis, and temperature regulation. The skin helps regulate the body temperature in two ways: by dilation and constriction of blood vessels and by the activity of the sweat glands. As aging progresses, alterations in sweat gland activity make the glands less effective in temperature regulation, so the aging person is less able to regulate hot and cold bodily changes. The parotid glands are responsible for the drainage of saliva, which plays an important role in digestion.

The pineal gland is a major site of melatonin biosynthesis. The thymus gland plays an immunological role throughout life.
Test-Taking Strategy: Use the process of elimination and focus on the issue, temperature regulation. Recalling the function of the skin and that the sweat glands control temperature regulation will direct you to the correct option. Review the age-related changes that occur in the older client if you had difficulty with this question.
Level of Cognitive Ability: Comprehension
Clients Needs: Physiological Integrity
Integrated Process: Nursing Process—implementation
Content Area: Fundamental skills
References: Ebersole, P., & Hess, P. (2001). *Geriatric nursing & healthy aging* (p. 236). St. Louis: Mosby.
Lueckenotte, A. (2000). *Gerontologic nursing* (2nd ed., p. 202). St. Louis: Mosby.

14. 4
Rationale: Coping mechanisms are behaviors used to decreased stress and anxiety. In response to a death, ineffective coping is manifested by an extreme behavior that in some instances may be harmful to the individual physically or psychologically. Option 4 is indicative of a behavior that identifies an ineffective coping behavior in the grieving process.
Test-Taking Strategy: Use the process of elimination and note the issue, an ineffective coping behavior. Eliminate options 1, 2, and 3 because they are similar and are positive activities that the individual is engaging in to get on with her life. Review coping mechanisms in response to grief and loss if you had difficulty with this question.
Level of Cognitive Ability: Analysis
Clients Needs: Psychosocial Integrity
Integrated Process: Nursing Process—assessment
Content Area: Mental Health
References: Ebersole, P., & Hess, P. (2001). *Geriatric nursing & healthy aging* (p. 556). St. Louis: Mosby.
Lueckenotte, A. (2000). *Gerontologic nursing* (2nd ed., p. 371). St. Louis: Mosby.

15. 1
Rationale: The nurse would ensure that the hearing impaired client can see the nurse when speaking by providing adequate lighting and by standing in front of the client. The nurse should enunciate words clearly but not exaggerate lip movements. If the client is profoundly hearing impaired and uses signing, the nurse should obtain a sign language interpreter. If a client cannot understand by reading lips, the nurse should try using gestures, pantomiming, or writing notes.
Test-Taking Strategy: Note the key words "initial nursing action." To communicate effectively with a hearing impaired client, the nurse first makes sure that the client can see her or him. If you had difficulty with this question, review the nursing interventions for the hearing impaired.
Level of Cognitive Ability: Application
Clients Needs: Health Promotion and Maintenance
Integrated Process: Nursing Process—implementation
Content Area: Fundamental skills
Reference: Lueckenotte, A. (2000). *Gerontologic nursing* (2nd ed., p. 713). St. Louis: Mosby.

16. 1

Rationale: Many nonpharmacological sleep aids can be used to influence sleep. The client should avoid caffeinated beverages and stimulants such as tea, cola, and chocolate, and foods with tyrosine such as cheddar cheese. The client should exercise regularly, for exercise enhances sleep by burning off tension that accumulates during the day. A 20- to 30-minute walk, swim, or bicycle ride 3 times a week is helpful. The client should sleep on a bed with a firm mattress. Smoking and alcohol should be avoided. The client should avoid large meals, peanuts, beans, fruit and raw vegetables that produce gas, and snacks high in fat that are difficult to digest.

Test-Taking Strategy: Focus on the issue, that teaching is necessary. Options 2, 3, and 4 are positive statements indicating that the client understands the methods of improving sleep. Review the factors that can interfere with sleep if you had difficulty with this question.

Level of Cognitive Ability: Analysis
Clients Needs: Physiological Integrity
Integrated Process: Teaching/Learning
Content Area: Fundamental skills
References: Ebersole, P., & Hess, P. (2001). *Geriatric nursing & healthy aging* (p. 215). St. Louis: Mosby.
Lueckenotte, A. (2000). *Gerontologic nursing* (2nd ed., pp. 40, 208). St. Louis: Mosby.

17. 2

Rationale: Assisting clients and families to become knowledgeable of community support systems that are available is a role and responsibility of the nurse. Option 1 suggests to commit the client to a nursing home and is a premature action on the nurse's part. Although the data provided tell the nurse that this client requires nursing care, the nurse does not know the extent of nursing care. Observing that the client has begun to be confined to his room makes it necessary for the nurse to intervene legally and ethically, so option 3 is not appropriate and is passive in terms of advocacy. Option 4 is incorrect and judgmental.

Test-Taking Strategy: Use the process of elimination. Note the key words "most important action." Using principles related to the ethical and legal responsibility of the nurse and knowledge of the nurse's role will direct you to option 2. Review these principles if you had difficulty with this question.

Level of Cognitive Ability: Application
Client Needs: Health Promotion and Maintenance
Integrated Process: Nursing Process—implementation
Content Area: Fundamental skills
Reference: Lueckenotte, A. (2000). *Gerontologic nursing* (2nd ed., p. 776.). St. Louis: Mosby.

18. 4

Rationale: The normal physiological changes that occur in the skin of older adults includes thinning of the skin, loss of elasticity, deepening of expression lines, and wrinkling. Crusting noted on the skin would indicate a potential complication.

Test-Taking Strategy: Use the process of elimination and note the key words "potential complication." Think about the normal physiological changes that occur in the aging process to direct you to option 4. Review these age-related skin changes if you had difficulty with this question.

Level of Cognitive Ability: Analysis
Client Needs: Physiological Integrity
Integrated Process: Nursing Process—assessment
Content Area: Fundamental skills
References: Lueckenotte, A. (2000). *Gerontologic nursing* (2nd ed., p. 656). St. Louis: Mosby.
O'Neill, P. (2002). *Caring for the older adult* (p. 69). Philadelphia: W. B. Saunders.

19. 4

Rationale: Lisinopril is an antihypertensive, angiotensin-converting enzyme inhibitor. The usual dosage range is 20 to 40 mg daily. Adverse effects include headache, dizziness, fatigue, orthostatic hypotension, tachycardia, and angioedema. Specific client teaching points include taking one pill a day, not stopping the medication without consulting the physician, and monitoring for side effects and adverse reactions. The client should notify the physician if side effects occur.

Test-Taking Strategy: Use the process of elimination. Note the key words "further teaching is necessary." Basic principles related to the administration of prescribed medications will direct you to option 4. If you had difficulty with this question, review teaching points related to medication administration.

Level of Cognitive Ability: Analysis
Clients Needs: Physiological Integrity
Integrated Process: Teaching/Learning
Content Area: Pharmacology
References: Hodgson, B., & Kizior, R. (2003). *Saunders nursing drug handbook 2003* (p. 670). Philadelphia: W. B. Saunders.
Lueckenotte, A. (2000). *Gerontologic nursing* (2nd ed., p. 456). St. Louis: Mosby.

20. 3

Rationale: Frequent position change helps to mobilize lung secretions and prevent pooling. This is the only intervention identified in the options that will prevent respiratory complications. The nurse should assess the client's vital signs every 4 hours to identify an elevated temperature that may suggest infection. The nurse would encourage fluid intake to thin secretions and thus enable the client to expectorate more easily. The nurse must encourage coughing and deep breathing to mobilize lung secretions. The client should be instructed to avoid Valsalva's maneuver or any activity involving holding the breath.

Test-Taking Strategy: Use the process of elimination. Note the key words "prevent respiratory complications." Changing the position of the immobilized client every 2 hours will help prevent pooling of lung secretions. The other options do not assist the client to improve ventilatory efforts or prevent respiratory complications. Review nursing interventions to prevent respiratory complications in the client who is immobilized if you had difficulty with this question.

Level of Cognitive Ability: Application
Clients Needs: Physiological Integrity
Integrated Process: Nursing Process—planning
Content Area: Fundamental skills
Reference: O'Neill, P. (2002). *Caring for the older adult* (p. 177). Philadelphia: W. B. Saunders.

CRITICAL THINKING: MULTIPLE RESPONSE

Answer:
Decline in visual acuity
Increased susceptibility to urinary tract infections
Increased incidence of awakening after sleep onset
Rationale: Anatomical changes to the eye affect the individual's visual ability, leading to potential problems with activities of daily living. Light adaptation and visual fields are reduced. Respiratory rates are generally higher in older adults, ranging from 16 to 25 breaths per minute. Heart rate decreases and heart valves thicken. Age-related changes that affect the urinary tract increase an older client's susceptibility to urinary tract infections. Short-term memory may decline with age, but long-term memory usually is maintained. Change in sleep patterns is a consistent, age-related change. Older persons experience an increased incidence of awakening after sleep onset.
Test-Taking Strategy: Knowledge regarding the normal age-related changes is needed to answer this question. Read each characteristic carefully and think about the physiological changes that occur with aging to select the correct items. Review the normal age-related changes if you had difficulty with this question.
Level of Cognitive Ability: Analysis
Client Needs: Health Promotion and Maintenance
Integrated Process: Nursing Process—assessment
Content Area: Fundamental skills
Reference: Lueckenotte, A. (2000). *Gerontologic nursing* (2nd ed., pp. 448, 486, 586, 617, 696). St. Louis: Mosby.

REFERENCES

Ebersole, P., & Hess, P. (2001). *Geriatric nursing & healthy aging.* St. Louis: Mosby.

Hodgson, B., & Kizior, R. (2004). *Saunders nursing drug handbook 2004.* Philadelphia: W. B. Saunders.

Lueckenotte, A. (2000). *Gerontologic nursing* (2nd ed.), St. Louis: Mosby.

O'Neill, P. (2002). *Caring for the older adult.* Philadelphia: W. B. Saunders.

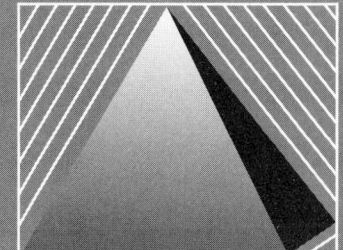
PYRAMID TERMS

abuse Nonaccidental physical injury or the nonaccidental act of omission by a parent or person responsible for the care of a child.

active immunity The protection, which can last months, years, or even a lifetime, that forms in response to exposure to antigens in nature or vaccines.

atresia Congenital absence or closure of a body orifice.

attenuated vaccines Vaccines derived from microorganisms or viruses the virulence of which has been weakened as a result of passage through another host.

cephalocaudal Characterized by growth and development that proceeds from head to toe.

chronological age Age in years.

developmental age Age based on functional behavior and ability to adapt to the environment. It does not necessarily correspond to chronological age.

encopresis Fecal incontinence after age 4.

functional age The age equivalent at which a child actually is able to perform specific self-care or related tasks.

growth Measurable physical and physiological changes that occur over time.

hereditary The transmission of genetic characteristics from parent to offspring.

inactivated vaccines Vaccines that contain killed microorganisms.

intelligence What an individual can do relative to learning, thinking, and problem solving.

learning Behavior changes that occur as a result of maturation and experience with the environment.

nasal flaring A serious sign of air hunger; a widening of the nares to enable an infant or child to take in more oxygen.

passive immunity Antibody transfer from a person with active immunity to a person who does not have that antibody.

puberty The period of time during which the adolescent experiences a growth spurt, develops secondary sex characteristics, and achieves reproductive maturity.

regression Behavior that is more appropriate to an earlier stage of development and often is used to cope with stress or anxiety.

regurgitation An abnormal backward flow of body fluid.

retraction An abnormal movement of the chest wall during inspiration.

shunt Movement of blood or body fluid through an abnormal anatomical or surgically created opening.

stenosis The narrowing or constriction of an opening.

stridor A shrill harsh sound heard during inspiration or expiration or both that is produced by the flow of air through a narrowed segment of the respiratory tract.

wheezing High-pitched musical whistles heard with or without a stethoscope.

PYRAMID TO SUCCESS

Pyramid Points focus on growth and development, safety and the age-appropriate measures to ensure a safe and hazard-free environment for the child, and on acute disorders that can occur in children. Focus on specific feeding techniques, positioning techniques, and interventions that will provide and maintain adequate airway, breathing, and circulation patterns in the child. On the NCLEX-RN examination, be alert to the age of the child, if the age is presented in a question. The Integrated Processes addressed in this unit include Nursing Process, Caring, Communication and Documentation, and Teaching/Learning.

CLIENT NEEDS

Safe, Effective Care Environment

Accident prevention
Confidentiality
Continuity of care
Environmental and personal safety related to the developmental age of the child
Establishing of priorities
Informed consent regarding minors
Parent and child rights
Protection of the child and other contacts to prevent illness
Protective measures
Spread and control of infectious agents, particularly regarding communicable diseases

Health Promotion and Maintenance

Developmental stages
Disease prevention
Family systems
Health promotion programs
Immunizations and communicable diseases
Instructions to the child and parents regarding care at home

Psychosocial Integrity

Child abuse and neglect
Communication
Cultural, religious, and spiritual differences
End-of-life issues
Family and support systems
Grief and loss
Play

Physiological Integrity

Age-appropriate normal body structure and function
Comfort measures
Elimination
Illness management
Infectious diseases
Intrusive procedures
Medical emergencies
Medication administration
Nutrition
Potential for alterations in body systems
Responses to therapies
Rest and sleep
Surgical procedures and health alterations

REFERENCES

James, S., Ashwill, J., & Droske, S. (2002). *Nursing care of children: Principles & practice* (2nd ed.). Philadelphia: W. B. Saunders.

McKinney, E., Ashwill, J., Murray, S., James, S., Gorrie, T., & Droske, S. (2000). *Maternal-child nursing.* Philadelphia: W. B. Saunders.

National Council of State Boards of Nursing (Eds.). (2003). *Test Plan for the National Council Licensure Examination for Registered Nurses* (effective date: April 2004). Chicago: Author.

Perry, A., & Potter, P. (2002). *Clinical nursing skills and techniques* (5th ed.). St. Louis: Mosby.

Potter, P., & Perry, A. (2001). *Fundamentals of nursing* (5th ed.). St. Louis: Mosby.

Stuart, G., & Laraia, M. (2001). *Principles and practice of psychiatric nursing* (7th ed.). St. Louis: Mosby.

Varcarolis, Elizabeth M. (2002). *Foundations of psychiatric mental health nursing* (4th ed.). Philadelphia: W. B. Saunders.

Wong, D., Hockenberry-Eaton, M. (2000). *Wong's essentials of pediatric nursing* (6th ed.). St. Louis: Mosby.

Wong, D., Perry, S., & Hockenberry, M. (2002). *Maternal child nursing care* (2nd ed.). St. Louis: Mosby.

Neurological, Cognitive, and Psychosocial Disorders

I. HEAD INJURY

A. Description
   1. Head injury is the pathological result of any mechanical force to the skull, scalp, meninges, or brain.
   2. Manifestations depend on the type of injury and the subsequent amount of increased intracranial pressure (ICP).

B. Assessment (ICP)
   1. Early signs
      a. Headache
      b. Visual disturbances, diplopia
      c. Nausea and vomiting
      d. Dizziness or vertigo
      e. Slight change in vital signs
      f. Change in pupillary response and equality
      g. Sunsetting eyes
      h. Slight change in level of consciousness
      i. Infant: bulging fontanel; wide sutures, increased head circumference; dilated scalp veins; high-pitched cry
   2. Late signs
      a. Significant decrease in level of consciousness
      b. Cushing's triad: increased systolic blood pressure and widened pulse pressure, bradycardia, and irregular respirations
      c. Decorticate posturing: adduction of the arms at the shoulders, the arms being flexed on the chest with the wrists flexed and the hands fisted, and the lower extremities being extended and adducted; seen with severe dysfunction of the cerebral cortex (Fig. 35-1)
      d. Decerebrate posturing: rigid extension and pronation of the arms and the legs; a sign of dysfunction at the level of the midbrain (Fig. 35-1)
      e. Fixed and dilated pupils

C. Interventions
   1. Monitor the airway.
   2. Assess injuries; immobilize the neck if a cervical injury is suspected.
   3. Monitor vital signs and neurological function.
   4. Monitor for decreased responsiveness to pain (a significant sign of altered level of consciousness).
   5. Initiate seizure precautions.
   6. Maintain a nothing-by-mouth status or provide clear liquids if prescribed, until it is determined that vomiting will not occur.
   7. Administer oxygen and intravenous fluids as prescribed.
   8. Monitor intravenous fluids carefully to avoid aggravating any cerebral edema and to minimize the possibility of overhydration.
   9. Elevate the head of the bed 15 to 30 degrees if not contraindicated.
   10. Position the client so that the head is maintained midline to facilitate venous drainage and avoid jugular vein compression; turning side to side is contraindicated because of the risk of jugular vein compression.
   11. Assess wound dressings for the presence of drainage and monitor for nose or ear drainage, which could indicate leakage of cerebrospinal fluid (CSF); drainage that is positive indicates leakage of CSF from a skull fracture.
   12. Administer tepid sponge baths or place on a hypothermia blanket if hyperthermia occurs.
   13. Suctioning through the nares is contraindicated because of the high risk of a secondary infection and the probability of the catheter entering the brain through a fracture.
   14. Administer acetaminophen (Tylenol) for headache, anticonvulsants for seizures, antibiotics if a laceration is present, and tetanus toxoid as appropriate.

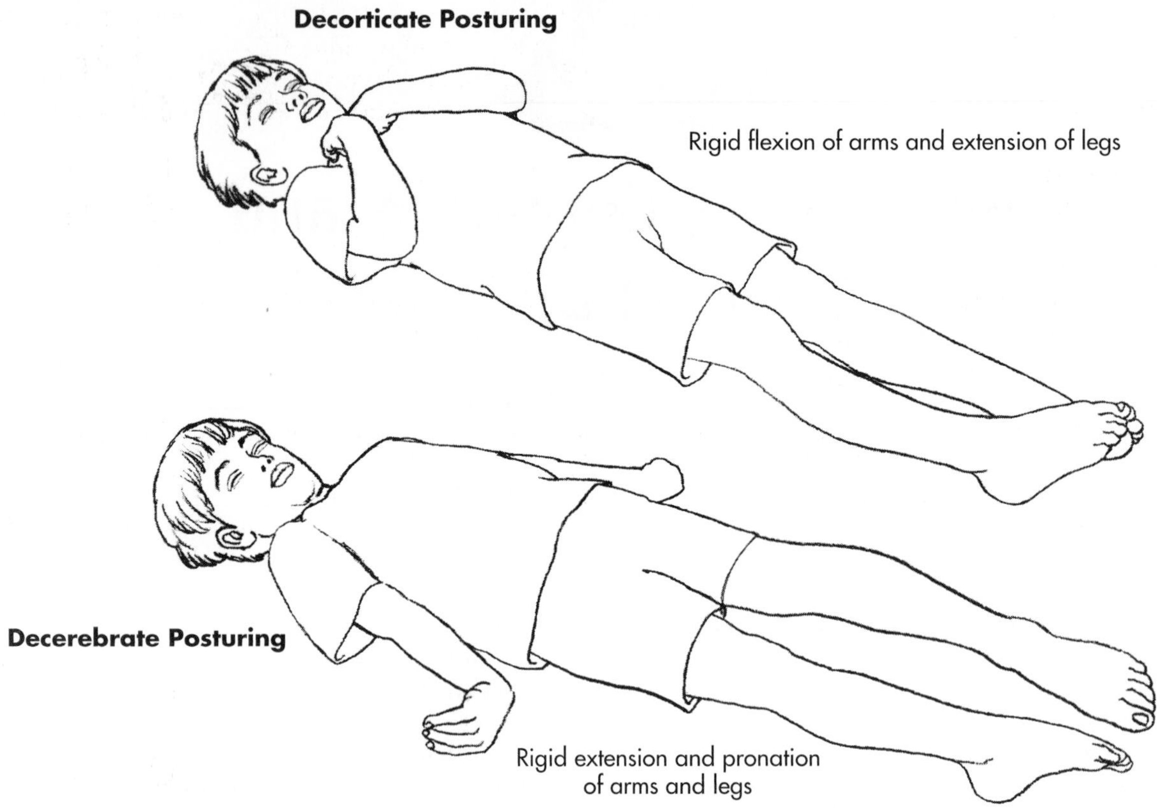

Decorticate Posturing

Rigid flexion of arms and extension of legs

Decerebrate Posturing

Rigid extension and pronation
of arms and legs

FIG 35-1 Decorticate and decerebrate posturing. (From James, S., Ashwill, J., & Droske, S. [2002]. *Nursing care of children: Principles & practice* [2nd ed.]. Philadelphia: W. B. Saunders.)

BOX 35-1

Signs of Brainstem Involvement

Deep, rapid, or intermittent and gasping respirations
Wide fluctuations or noticeable slowing of the pulse
Widening pulse pressure or extreme fluctuations in blood pressure

---

15. Sedating medications are withheld during the acute phase of the injury.
16. Monitor for signs of brainstem involvement (Box 35-1).
17. Epidural hematoma: Monitor for asymmetric pupils (one dilated, unreactive pupil in a comatose child is a neurosurgical emergency that may require evacuation of the hematoma).

II. HYDROCEPHALUS

A. Description
   1. Hydrocephalus is an imbalance of CSF absorption or production caused by malformations, tumors, hemorrhage, infections, or trauma.
   2. Hydrocephalus results in head enlargement and increased ICP.
B. Types (Box 35-2)

BOX 35-2

Types of Hydrocephalus

COMMUNICATING
Hydrocephalus occurs as a result of impaired absorption within the subarachnoid space.
Interference of the cerebrospinal fluid within the ventricular system does not occur.

NONCOMMUNICATING
Obstruction of cerebrospinal flow within the ventricular system occurs.

C. Assessment
   1. Infant
      a. Increased head circumference
      b. Thin, widely separated bones of the head that produce a cracked-pot sound (Macewen's sign) on percussion
      c. Anterior fontanel tense, bulging, and non-pulsating
      d. Dilated scalp veins
      e. Frontal bossing
      f. Sunsetting eyes
   2. Child
      a. Behavior changes such as irritability and lethargy

b. Headache on awakening
c. Nausea and vomiting
d. Ataxia
e. Nystagmus
3. Late signs: a high, shrill cry and seizure activities
D. Surgical interventions
1. The goal of surgical treatment is to prevent further CSF accumulation by bypassing the blockage and draining the fluid from the ventricles to a location where it may be reabsorbed.
2. In a ventriculoperitoneal **shunt,** the CSF drains into the peritoneal cavity from the lateral ventricle (Fig. 35-2).
3. In an atrioventricular **shunt,** CSF drains into the right atrium of the heart from the lateral ventricle, bypassing the obstruction (used in older children and in children with pathological conditions of the abdomen).
E. Interventions postoperatively
1. Monitor vital signs and neurological signs.
2. Position client on the unoperated side to prevent pressure on the **shunt** valve.
3. Keep the child flat as prescribed to avoid rapid reduction of intracranial fluid.
4. Observe for increased ICP; if increased ICP occurs, elevate the head of the bed to 15 to 30 degrees to enhance gravity flow through the **shunt.**
5. Monitor for signs of infection and assess dressings for drainage.
6. Measure head circumference.
7. Monitor intake and output.
8. Provide comfort measures; administer medications as prescribed, which may include diuretics, antibiotics, or anticonvulsants.

9. Instruct parents in how to recognize **shunt** infection or malfunction.
10. In a toddler, headache and a lack of appetite are the earliest common signs of **shunt** malfunction.

III. SPINA BIFIDA
A. Description
1. Spina bifida is a central nervous system defect that occurs as a result of neural tube failure to close during embryonic development.
2. Associated deficits include sensory motor disturbance, dislocated hips, clubfoot, and hydrocephalus.
3. Defect closure usually is done during infancy.
B. Types
1. Spina bifida occulta
a. Posterior vertebral arches fail to close in the lumbosacral area.
b. Spinal cord remains intact and usually is not visible.
c. Meninges are not exposed on the skin surface.
d. Neurological deficits are not usually present.
2. Spina bifida cystica
a. Protrusion of the spinal cord and/or its meninges occurs.
b. Defect results in incomplete closure of the vertebral and neural tubes, resulting in a saclike protrusion in the lumbar or sacral area, with varying degrees of nervous tissue involvement.
c. Defect can include meningocele, myelomeningocele, lipomeningocele, and lipomeningomyelocele.

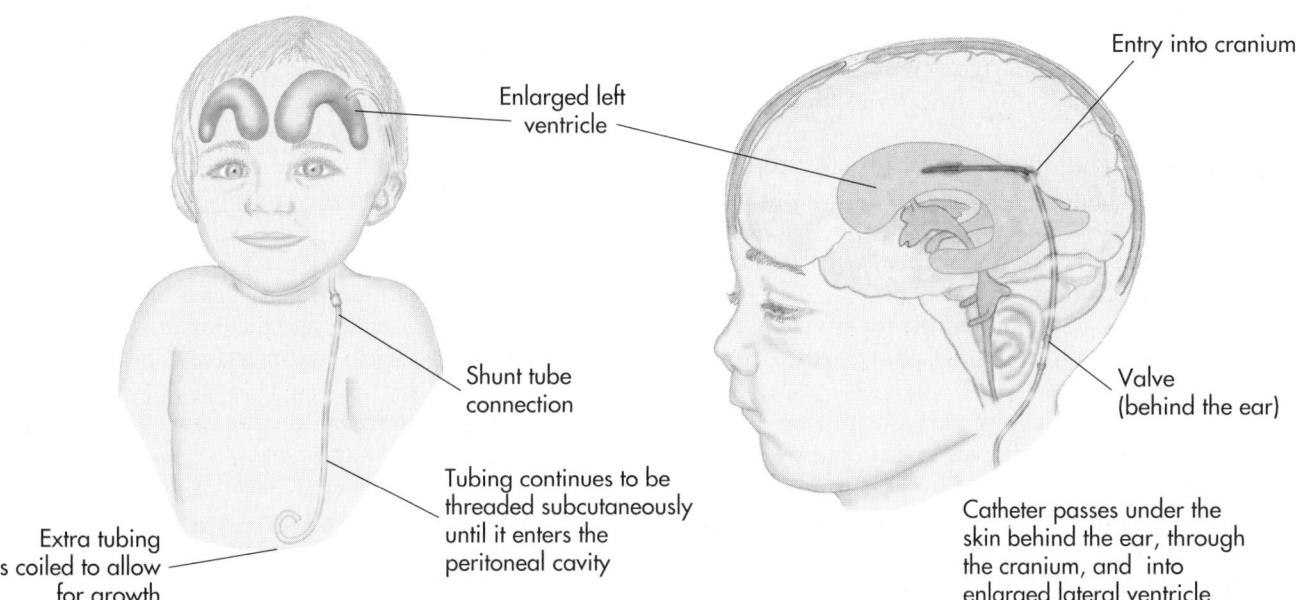

Enlarged left ventricle

Shunt tube connection

Extra tubing is coiled to allow for growth

Tubing continues to be threaded subcutaneously until it enters the peritoneal cavity

Entry into cranium

Valve (behind the ear)

Catheter passes under the skin behind the ear, through the cranium, and into enlarged lateral ventricle

FIG 35-2 Ventriculoperitoneal shunt. (From James, S., Ashwill, J., & Droske, S. [2002]. *Nursing care of children: Principles & practice* [2nd ed.]. Philadelphia: W. B. Saunders.)

3. Meningocele
   a. Protrusion involves meninges and a saclike cyst that contains CSF in the midline of the back, usually in the lumbosacral area.
   b. Spinal cord is not involved.
   c. Neurological deficits are usually not present.
4. Myelomeningocele
   a. Protrusion of meninges, CSF, nerve roots, and a portion of the spinal cord occurs.
   b. The sac (defect) is covered by a thin membrane that is prone to leakage or rupture.
   c. Neurological deficits are evident.
C. Assessment
   1. Depends on the spinal cord involvement
   2. Visible spinal defect
   3. Flaccid paralysis of the legs
   4. Altered bladder and bowel function
   5. Hip and joint deformities
D. Interventions
   1. Evaluate the sac and measure the lesion.
   2. Perform neurological assessment.
   3. Monitor for increased ICP, which might indicate developing hydrocephalus.
   4. Measure head circumference; assess the anterior fontanel for fullness.
   5. Protect the sac; cover with a sterile, moist (normal saline), nonadherent dressing to maintain the moisture of the sac and contents, and change the dressing every 2 to 4 hours as prescribed.
   6. Place in a prone position to minimize tension on the sac and the risk of trauma; the head is turned to one side for feeding.
   7. Change the dressing covering the sac whenever it becomes soiled because of the risk of infection; diapering may be contraindicated until the defect has been repaired.
   8. Use aseptic technique to prevent infection.
   9. Assess the sac for redness, clear or purulent drainage, abrasions, irritation, and signs of infection.
   10. Early signs of infection include elevated temperature (axillary), irritability, lethargy, and nuchal rigidity.
   11. Assess for physical impairments such as hip and joint deformities.
   12. Prepare the child and family for surgery.
   13. Administer antibiotics as prescribed to prevent infection.
   14. Administer anticholinergics to improve urinary continence and laxatives to achieve bowel continence in the child, and antispasmodics to control bladder spasms.

IV. REYE'S SYNDROME
A. Description
   1. Reye's syndrome is acute encephalopathy that follows a viral illness and is characterized pathologically by cerebral edema and fatty changes in the liver.
   2. The exact cause is not clear.
   3. Administration of aspirin is not recommended for children with varicella or influenza because of its association with Reye's syndrome.
   4. Acetaminophen (Tylenol) is considered the medication of choice for pediatric clients.
   5. The goal of treatment is to maintain effective cerebral perfusion and control increasing ICP.
B. Assessment
   1. History of systemic viral illness 4 to 7 days before the onset of symptoms
   2. Malaise
   3. Nausea and vomiting
   4. Progressive neurological deterioration
C. Interventions
   1. Assess neurological status.
   2. Monitor for altered level of consciousness and signs of increased ICP.
   3. Monitor intake and output.
   4. Provide rest and decrease stimulation in the environment.
   5. Monitor for signs of bleeding and signs of impaired coagulation, such as a prolonged bleeding time.
   6. Monitor liver function studies.

V. MENINGITIS
A. Description
   1. Meningitis is an infectious process of the central nervous system caused by bacteria and viruses that may be acquired as a primary disease or as a result of complications of neurosurgery, trauma, infection of the sinus or ears, or systemic infections.
   2. Diagnosis is made by testing CSF obtained by lumbar puncture, which shows increased pressure, cloudy CSF, high protein, and low glucose.
   3. Meningococcal meningitis occurs in epidemic form and is the only type readily transmitted by droplet infection from nasopharyngeal secretions.
   4. Viral meningitis is associated with viruses such as mumps, paramyxovirus, herpesvirus, and enterovirus.
B. Assessment
   1. Signs and symptoms vary, depending on the type, the age of the child, and the duration of the preceding illness; there is no one classic sign or symptom.
   2. Fever, chills
   3. Vomiting, diarrhea
   4. Poor feeding or anorexia
   5. Nuchal rigidity
   6. Poor or high-pitched cry
   7. Altered level of consciousness, such as lethargy or irritability
   8. Bulging anterior fontanel in the infant
   9. Kernig's sign and Brudzinski's sign in children and adolescents

10. Muscle or joint pain
11. Petechial or purpuric rashes (meningococcal infection)

C. Interventions
1. Provide isolation and maintain it for at least 24 hours after antibiotics are initiated.
2. Administer antibiotics as prescribed.
3. Perform neurological and cardiovascular assessment.
4. Assess for personality changes and irritability.
5. Monitor intake and output.
6. Assess nutritional status.
7. Determine close contacts of the child with meningitis because the contacts will need prophylactic treatment.

VI. SEIZURE DISORDERS
A. Description
1. Sudden, transient alterations in brain function resulting from excessive levels of electrical activity in the brain
2. Classified as partial or generalized, or unclassified, depending on the area of the brain involved
B. Assessment
1. Obtain information from the parents about the time of onset, precipitating events, and behavior before and after the seizure.
2. Determine the child's history related to seizures.
C. Seizure precautions (Box 35-3)
D. Interventions (Box 35-4)

VII. CEREBRAL PALSY
A. Description
1. Cerebral palsy is a disorder characterized by impaired movement and posture resulting from an abnormality in the extrapyramidal or pyramidal motor system.
2. The most common clinical type is spastic cerebral palsy, which represents an upper motor neuron type of muscle weakness.
B. Assessment
1. Extreme irritability and crying
2. Feeding difficulties
3. Stiff and rigid arms or legs

BOX 35-3

Seizure Precautions

Raise the side rails when the child is sleeping or resting.
Pad the side rails and other hard objects.
Place a waterproof mattress or pad on the bed or crib.
Instruct the child to wear or carry medical identification.
Instruct the child in precautions to take during potentially hazardous activities.
Instruct the child to swim with a companion.
Instruct the child to use a protective helmet and padding during bicycle riding, skateboarding, inline skating.
Alert caregivers to the need for any special precautions.

BOX 35-4

Emergency Treatment for Seizures

Ensure airway patency.
Time the seizure episode.
If the child is standing or sitting, ease the child down to the floor, placing the child in a side-lying position.
Place a pillow or folded blanket under the child's head; if no bedding is available, place your own hands under the child's head or place the child's head in your own lap.
Loosen restrictive clothing.
Remove eyeglasses from the child if present.
Clear area of any hazards or hard objects.
Allow seizure to proceed and end without interference.
If vomiting occurs, turn child to one side as a unit.
Do not restrain the child, place anything in the child's mouth, or give any food or liquids to the child.
Prepare to administer medications as prescribed.
Remain with the child until the child fully recovers.
Observe for incontinence, which may have occurred during the seizure.
Document the occurrence.

---

4. Delayed gross development
5. Abnormal motor performance
6. Alterations of muscle tone
7. Abnormal posturing, such as opisthotonic (exaggerated arching of the back)
8. Persistence of primitive infantile reflexes
C. Interventions
1. The goal of management is early recognition and intervention to maximize the child's abilities.
2. A multidisciplinary team approach is implemented to meet the many needs of the child.
3. Therapeutic management includes physical therapy, occupational therapy, speech therapy, education, and recreation.
4. Assess the child's developmental level and **intelligence.**
5. Encourage early intervention and participation in school programs.
6. Prepare for using mobilizing devices to help prevent or reduce deformities.
7. Encourage communication and interaction with the child on his or her developmental level rather than **chronological age** level.
8. Provide a safe environment such as by removing sharp objects, using a protective helmet if the child falls frequently, and implementing seizure precautions if necessary.
9. Provide safe, appropriate toys for age and developmental level.
10. Position the child upright after meals.
11. Administer medications as prescribed to decrease spasticity.
12. Surgical interventions are reserved for the child who does not respond to more conservative

measures or for the child whose spasticity causes progressive deformity.

VIII. MENTAL RETARDATION
A. Description
   1. In mental retardation, the child manifests sub-average intellectual functioning along with deficits in adaptive skills.
   2. Down syndrome is a congenital condition that results in moderate to severe retardation and has been linked to an extra group G chromosome, chromosome 21 (trisomy 21).
B. Assessment
   1. Deficits in cognitive skills and level of adaptive functioning
   2. Delays in fine- and gross-motor skills
   3. Speech delays
   4. Decreased spontaneous activity
   5. Nonresponsiveness
   6. Irritability
   7. Poor eye contact during feeding
C. Interventions
   1. Medical strategies are focused at correcting structural deformities and treating associated behaviors.
   2. Implement community and educational services using a multidisciplinary approach.
   3. Promote care skills as much as possible.
   4. Assist with communication and socialization skills.
   5. Facilitate appropriate playtime.
   6. Initiate safety precautions as necessary.
   7. Assist the family with decisions regarding care.
   8. Provide information regarding support services and community agencies.

IX. AUTISM
A. Description
   1. Autism is a severe mental disorder beginning in infancy or toddlerhood.
   2. The disorder is apparent to the parents before the child is 3 years old.
   3. Autism is characterized by impairment in reciprocal social interaction and in verbal and nonverbal communication.
   4. The cause is unknown and the prognosis may be poor.
   5. Diagnosis is established based on symptoms and through the use of specialized autism assessment tools.
   6. The disorder also is called infantile autism.
B. Assessment
   1. The child experiences a disturbance in the rate and appearance of physical, social, and language skills.
   2. The child expriences abnormal responses of body sensations.
   3. The child has abnormal ways of relating to persons, objects, and events; the child is self-absorbed and unable to relate to others.

4. The child has no delusions, hallucinations, or incoherence, and the facies is intelligent and responsive.
5. The child may play happily alone for hours but have temper tantrums if interrupted.
6. Language disturbance often includes repetition of previously heard speech and reversal of the pronouns "I" and "you."
7. If the child can talk, he or she uses speech not for communication but to repeat words or phrases meaninglessly.
8. The child may develop an unusual attachment to a significant object and display frequent rocking, spinning, twirling, or other bizarre behaviors.
C. Interventions
   1. Determine the child's routines, habits, and preferences and maintain consistency as much as possible.
   2. Determine the specific ways in which the child communicates.
   3. Facilitate communication through the use of picture boards.
   4. Evaluate the child for safety.
   5. Implement safety precautions as necessary for self-injurious behaviors such as head banging.
   6. Monitor for stress and anxiety.
   7. Avoid placing demands on the child.
   8. Initiate referrals to special programs as required.
   9. Provide support to parents.

X. ATTENTION-DEFICIT HYPERACTIVITY DISORDER
A. Description
   1. Attention-deficit hyperactivity disorder is a developmental disorder characterized by developmentally inappropriate degrees of inattention, overactivity, and impulsivity.
   2. The disorder is one of the most common reasons for referral of children to mental health services.
   3. Childhood problems include lowered intellectual development, some minor physical abnormalities, sleeping disturbances, behavioral or emotional disorders, and difficulty in social relationships.
   4. Diagnosis is established based on self-reports, parent and teacher reports, and psychological assessments.
B. Assessment
   1. Fidgets with hands or feet or squirms in the seat
   2. Easily distracted with external or internal stimuli
   3. Difficulty with following through on instructions
   4. Poor attention span
   5. Shifting from one uncompleted activity to another
   6. Talking excessively
   7. Interrupting or intruding on others
   8. Engaging in physically dangerous activities without considering the possible consequences

C. Interventions
1. Provide environmental and physical safety measures.
2. Enhance capabilities and self-esteem.
3. Encourage support groups for parents.
4. Administer prescribed medication; some commonly prescribed medications include methylphenidate hydrochloride (Ritalin), pemoline (Cylert), and dextroamphetamine sulfate (Dexedrine).
5. Instruct the child and parents regarding medication administration.
6. Inform the child and parents that positive effects of the medication may be seen within 1 to 2 weeks if taken as prescribed.

XI. TOURETTE'S DISORDER
A. Description: Tourette's disorder appears between ages 2 and 15 and is characterized by recurrent involuntary and rapid movements affecting various parts of the body, accompanied by vocal noises such as barks, grunts, or profanities.
B. Interventions
1. Establish a trusting one-to-one relationship.
2. Protect the child from harm by providing a helmet or protective padding.
3. Allow the child to have a favorite toy or other object.
4. Provide positive reinforcement for appropriate behaviors.
5. Maintain eye contact.
6. Assess suicide potential.
7. Remove dangerous objects from the environment.
8. Set limits on socially inappropriate or manipulative behaviors.
9. Encourage the child to confront tension and frustration before they emerge as inappropriate behaviors.
10. Provide noncompetitive group situations.

XII. CHILD ABUSE
A. Description: Child abuse involves emotional or physical abuse or neglect, as well as sexual exploitation or molestation by caretakers or other individuals.
B. Assessment
1. Physical abuse
   a. Unexplained bruises, burns, or fractures
   b. Bald spots on the scalp
   c. Apprehensive child
   d. Extreme aggressiveness or withdrawal
   e. Fear of parents
   f. Lack of crying when approached by a stranger
2. Physical neglect
   a. Inadequate weight gain
   b. Poor hygiene
   c. Consistent hunger
   d. Inconsistent school attendance
   e. Constant fatigue

   f. Reports of lack of child supervision
   g. Delinquency
3. Emotional abuse
   a. Speech disorders
   b. Habit disorders such as sucking, biting, and rocking
   c. Psychoneurotic reactions
   d. Learning disorders
   e. Suicide attempts
4. Sexual abuse
   a. Difficulty walking or sitting
   b. Torn, stained, or bloody underclothing
   c. Pain, swelling, or itching of the genitals
   d. Bruises, bleeding, or lacerations in the genital or anal area
   e. Unwillingness to change clothes or unwillingness to participate in gym activities
   f. Poor peer relations
5. Shaken baby syndrome
   a. Can cause intracranial hemorrhage leading to cerebral edema and death.
   b. Full bulging fontanelles and a head circumference greater than expected would be noted.
C. Interventions
1. Support the child during a thorough physical assessment.
2. Assess injuries.
3. Report case of suspected abuse.
4. Place the child in an environment that is safe, thereby preventing further injury.
5. Document in an objective manner information related to the suspected abuse.
6. Assess parents' strengths and weaknesses, normal coping mechanisms, and presence or absence of support systems.
7. Assist the family in identifying stressors, support systems, and resources.
8. Refer the family to appropriate support groups.

PRACTICE QUESTIONS

1. A nurse is performing an admission assessment on a 6-month-old infant with a diagnosis of hydrocephalus. The nurse assesses for the major sign associated with hydrocephalus when the nurse
   1. Tests the urine for protein.
   2. Takes the apical pulse.
   3. Palpates the anterior fontanel.
   4. Takes the blood pressure.
2. A nurse has provided discharge instructions to the parents of an infant who had a ventriculoperitoneal shunt procedure performed for the treatment of hydrocephalus. Which statement if made by the parents indicates an accurate understanding of the presence of a shunt complication?
   1. "If my infant has a high-pitched cry, I should call the doctor."

2. "I should position my infant on the side with the shunt when sleeping."

3. "My infant will pass urine more often now that the shunt is in place."

4. "I should call my doctor if my infant refuses baby food."

3. A nurse is performing an admission assessment on a newborn infant with a diagnosis of spina bifida (meningomyelocele). The nurse assesses for a major symptom associated with this type of spina bifida when the nurse

   1. Checks the capillary refill of the nailbeds of the upper extremities.
   2. Tests the urine for blood.
   3. Palpates the abdomen for masses.
   4. Checks for responses to painful stimuli from the torso downward.

4. A mother arrives at an emergency room with her 5-year-old child. The mother states that the child fell off a bunk bed. A head injury is suspected, and a nurse is assessing the child continuously for signs of increased intracranial pressure (ICP). Which of the following would indicate a late sign of increased ICP in this child?

   1. Bulging fontanel
   2. Dilated scalp veins
   3. Nausea
   4. Widened pulse pressure

5. A nurse is caring for a newborn infant with spina bifida (meningomyelocele type) who is scheduled for surgical closure of the sac. In the preoperative period the priority nursing action would be to monitor the

   1. Blood pressure.
   2. Moisture of the normal saline dressing covering the sac.
   3. Specific gravity of the urine.
   4. Anterior fontanel for depression.

6. A child is diagnosed with Reye's syndrome. A nurse develops a nursing care plan for the child and includes which intervention in the plan?

   1. Providing a quiet atmosphere with dimmed lighting
   2. Assessing hearing loss
   3. Monitoring urine output
   4. Changing body position every 2 hours

7. A physician prescribes home health nurse visits for a child discharged home with Reye's syndrome. During a home visit, a nurse instructs the parents about the residual effects of Reye's syndrome. Which statement if made by the parents would indicate a need for further instruction?

   1. "We need to decrease the stimuli at home to prevent intracranial pressure."
   2. "We need to give frequent, small, nutritious meals to decrease the amount of vomiting."
   3. "We need to have the child nap during the day to provide rest."
   4. "We need to check for jaundiced skin and eyes every day."

8. A nurse develops a plan of care for a child at risk for generalized tonic-clonic seizures. In the plan of care, the nurse initiates seizure precautions and documents that which items need to be placed at the child's bedside?

   1. Suctioning equipment and an airway
   2. Oxygen with a tracheotomy set
   3. Emergency cart
   4. Airway and a tracheotomy set

9. A nurse is caring for a child recently diagnosed with cerebral palsy. The parents of the child ask the nurse about the disorder. The nurse bases her response on the understanding that cerebral palsy is

   1. A chronic disability characterized by impaired muscle movement and posture.
   2. An infectious disease of the central nervous system.
   3. An inflammation of the brain as a result of a viral illness.
   4. A congenital condition that results in moderate to severe retardation.

10. A nurse is developing a plan of care for a child with cerebral palsy. The nurse includes interventions in the plan of care, understanding that a primary goal is to

   1. Eliminate the cause of the disorder.
   2. Prevent the occurrence of emotional disturbances.
   3. Maximize the child's assets and minimize the limitations caused by the disorder.
   4. Cure the disorder.

11. A nurse is caring for a child diagnosed with Down syndrome. In describing the disorder to the parents, the nurse bases the explanation on the fact that Down syndrome is a condition characterized by

   1. Above-average intellectual functioning with deficits in adaptive behavior.
   2. Average intellectual functioning and the absence of deficits in adaptive behavior.
   3. Moderate to severe retardation, congenital nature, and linkage to an extra chromosome 21, group G.
   4. Subaverage intellectual functioning with the absence of deficits in adaptive behavior.

12. A nurse is assigned to care for an 8-year-old child with a diagnosis of a basilar skull fracture. The nurse reviews the physician's orders and contacts the physician to question which order?

   1. Clear liquid intake
   2. Maintain a patent intravenous line
   3. Daily weight
   4. Suction as needed

13. A lumbar puncture is performed on a child suspected of having bacterial meningitis. Cerebrospinal fluid (CSF) is obtained for analysis. A nurse reviews the results of the CSF analysis and determines that which of the following results would verify the diagnosis?

   1. Cloudy CSF, decreased protein, and decreased glucose

2. Cloudy CSF, elevated protein, and decreased glucose

3. Clear CSF, elevated protein, and decreased glucose

4. Clear CSF, decreased pressure, and elevated protein

14. A nurse is planning care for a child with acute bacterial meningitis. Based on the mode of transmission of this infection, which of the following would be included in the plan of care?

    1. No precautions are required as long as antibiotics have been started.
    2. Maintain enteric precautions.
    3. Maintain respiratory isolation precautions for at least 24 hours after the initiation of antibiotics.
    4. Maintain neutropenic precautions.

15. A clinic nurse is observing a child diagnosed with autistic disorder. The nurse would expect to observe which characteristic of this disorder?

    1. Normal responses to sensory stimuli
    2. Normal social play
    3. Lack of social interaction
    4. Normal verbal but abnormal nonverbal communication

16. An emergency room nurse is performing an assessment on a child suspected of being sexually abused. Which assessment data obtained by the nurse most likely would support this suspicion?

    1. Poor hygiene
    2. Bald spots on the scalp
    3. Fear of the parents
    4. Difficulty walking

17. A nurse performs an admission assessment on a child and suspects physical abuse. Based on this suspicion, the primary legal nursing responsibility is which of the following?

    1. Document the child's physical assessment findings accurately and thoroughly.
    2. Report the case in which the abuse is suspected to the local authorities.
    3. Refer the family to the appropriate support groups.
    4. Assist the family in identifying resources and support systems.

18. A maternity nurse employed in a newborn nursery receives a telephone call from the delivery room and is told that a newborn with spina bifida (meningomyelocele type) will be transported to the nursery. The maternity nurse prepares for the arrival of the newborn and places which of the following priority items at the newborn's bedside?

    1. A blood pressure cuff
    2. A rectal thermometer
    3. A specific gravity urinometer
    4. A bottle of sterile normal saline

19. A nurse is performing an assessment of a 7-year-old child who is suspected of having episodes of absence seizures. Which of the following assessment questions to the mother will assist in providing information that will identify the symptoms associated with this type of seizure?

    1. "Does the child have a blank expression during these episodes?"
    2. "Does the muscle twitching occur on one side of the body?"
    3. "Does twitching occur in the face and neck?"
    4. "Does the muscle twitching occur on both sides of the body?"

20. A nurse is reviewing the record of a child with increased intracranial pressure and notes that the child has exhibited signs of decerebrate posturing. On assessment of the child, the nurse would expect to note which of the following if this type of posturing was present?

    1. Abnormal flexion of the upper extremities and extension of the lower extremities
    2. Rigid extension and pronation of the arms and legs
    3. Rigid pronation of all extremities
    4. Flaccid paralysis of all extremities

CRITICAL THINKING: MULTIPLE RESPONSE

A nurse is developing a plan of care for a child who is at risk for seizures. Select all interventions that apply if the child has a seizure.

____ Place the child in a prone position.

____ Restrain the child.

____ Time the seizure.

____ Insert a padded tongue blade in the child's mouth.

____ Stay with the child.

____ Move furniture away from the child.

ANSWERS

1. 3

Rationale: In infants with hydrocephalus the head grows at an abnormal rate, and the first sign of the disorder may be bulging fontanels without head enlargement. A bulging, tense, and nonpulsatile anterior fontanel indicates an increase in cerebrospinal fluid collection in the cerebral ventricle. A method of assessing fluid collection in the cranial cavity is to palpate the anterior fontanel. Proteinuria, apical pulse, and blood pressure changes are not specific to hydrocephalus.

Test-Taking Strategy: Use the process of elimination and the principles associated with excessive fluid buildup in the cranial cavity when answering the question. In addition, correlate "hydrocephalus" in the question with "anterior fontanel" in option 3. If you had difficulty with this question, review the signs associated with hydrocephalus.

Level of Cognitive Ability: Analysis
Client Needs: Physiological Integrity
Integrated Process: Nursing Process—assessment
Content Area: Child health
Reference: James, S., Ashwill, J., & Droske, S. (2002). *Nursing care of children: Principles & practice* (2nd ed., p. 961). Philadelphia: W. B. Saunders.

2. 1

Rationale: If the shunt is broken or malfunctioning, the fluid from the ventricle part of the brain will not be diverted to the peritoneal cavity. The cerebrospinal fluid will build up in the cranial area. The result is intracranial pressure, which then causes a high-pitched cry in the infant. The infant should not have pressure placed on the shunt side. Skin breakdown and possible compressions to the apparatus could result. This type of shunt affects the gastrointestinal system, not the genitourinary system. Option 4 is only a concern if the infant becomes malnourished or dehydrated, which then could raise the body temperature. Otherwise, the infant's refusing baby food has no direct relationship to the shunt functioning.

Test-Taking Strategy: Use the process of elimination, noting the key words "presence of a shunt complication." Recalling that shunt malfunction is a complication, and that if it occurs, the infant will exhibit signs of increased intracranial pressure, will direct you to the correct option. Remember that a high-pitched cry in an infant indicates a concern or problem. If you had difficulty with this question, review the assessment findings that indicate a complication with a shunt.

Level of Cognitive Ability: Analysis
Client Needs: Health Promotion and Maintenance
Integrated Process: Teaching/Learning
Content Area: Child health
Reference: James, S., Ashwill, J., & Droske, S. (2002). *Nursing care of children: Principles & practice* (2nd ed., p. 960). Philadelphia: W. B. Saunders.

3. 4

Rationale: Newborn infants with spina bifida (meningomyelocele type) demonstrate lack of innervation from below the site of the sac that contains the meninges and spinal cord and excess cerebrospinal fluid. They therefore show diminished or no responses to painful stimuli in these areas below the sac. Options 1, 2, and 3 are incorrect because the area above the sac is not affected. The capillary refill is normal. The urine will not have blood present. If the kidneys are affected, proteinuria could be present but generally is not noted in the newborn period. No abdominal masses are present besides the sac on the back area, externally protruding from the vertebral deformity.

Test-Taking Strategy: Use the process of elimination, recalling that diminished or absent innervation occurs in the area below the sac. If you had difficulty with this question, review the symptoms associated with meningomyelocele.

Level of Cognitive Ability: Analysis
Client Needs: Physiological Integrity
Integrated Process: Nursing Process—assessment
Content Area: Child health
References: James, S., Ashwill, J., & Droske, S. (2002). *Nursing care of children: Principles & practice* (2nd ed., p. 108). Philadelphia: W. B. Saunders.
Wong, D., Hockenberry-Eaton, M. (2000). *Wong's essentials of pediatric nursing* (6th ed., p. 211). St. Louis: Mosby.

4. 4

Rationale: Late signs of increased intracranial pressure (ICP) include a significant decrease in level of consciousness, Cushing's triad (increased systolic blood pressure and widened pulse pressure, bradycardia, and irregular respirations), and fixed and dilated pupils. A bulging fontanel and dilated scalp veins are early signs of increased ICP and would be noted in an infant, not a 5-year-old child. Nausea is an early sign of increased ICP.

Test-Taking Strategy: Use the process of elimination. Note the age of the child and the key word "late." Options 1 and 2 can be eliminated first because these signs would be noted in an infant, not a 5-year-old child. Focusing on the key word "late" will direct you to option 4. If you had difficulty with this question, review the early and late signs of increased ICP in an infant and in a child.

Level of Cognitive Ability: Analysis
Client Needs: Physiological Integrity
Integrated Process: Nursing Process—assessment
Content Area: Child health
Reference: James, S., Ashwill, J., & Droske, S. (2002). *Nursing care of children: Principles & practice* (2nd ed., p. 297). Philadelphia: W. B. Saunders.

5. 2

Rationale: The infant usually is placed in an incubator or a radiant warmer so that temperature can be maintained without clothing or covers that might irritate the delicate lesion. A sterile normal saline dressing is placed over the sac to maintain moisture of the sac and its contents and to prevent tearing or breakdown of the skin integrity at the site. Any opening in the sac greatly increases the risk of infection of the central nervous system. When an overhead warmer is used, the dressings over the defect require more frequent moistening because of the drying effect of the radiant heat. Blood pressure is difficult to assess during the newborn period and is not the best indicator of infection. Urine concentration is not well developed in the newborn stage of development. Depression of the anterior fontanel is a sign of dehydration. In spina bifida, monitoring for an increase in intracranial pressure is the priority, and it would be identified by the presence of a bulging anterior fontanel, among other signs.

Test-Taking Strategy: Note the key words "preoperative period" and "priority nursing action." Use the process of elimination, recalling the importance of the care of the sac in the preoperative period. Eliminate options 1 and 3 first. Although blood pressure and specific gravity are common preoperative assessments, they are not reliable indicators of the status of a newborn. Knowledge that an increase in intracranial pressure is a concern will assist in eliminating option 4. Review preoperative care for the infant with a meningomyelocele if you had difficulty with this question.

Level of Cognitive Ability: Application
Client Needs: Physiological Integrity
Integrated Process: Nursing Process—implementation
Content Area: Child health
Reference: Wong, D., Hockenberry-Eaton, M. (2000). *Wong's essentials of pediatric nursing* (6th ed., p. 1257). St. Louis: Mosby.

6. **1**
Rationale: In Reye's syndrome, supportive care is directed toward monitoring and managing cerebral edema. Decreasing stimuli in the environment by providing a quiet environment with dimmed lighting would decrease the stress on the cerebral tissue and neuron responses. Hearing loss and urine output are not affected. Changing the body position every 2 hours would not affect the cerebral edema directly. The child should be in a head-elevated position to decrease the progression of the cerebral edema and promote drainage of cerebrospinal fluid.

Test-Taking Strategy: Use the process of elimination. Knowledge that cerebral edema is a concern for the child with Reye's syndrome will direct you easily to option 1. If you had difficulty with this question, review the appropriate plan of nursing care for the child with Reye's syndrome.

Level of Cognitive Ability: Application
Client Needs: Physiological Integrity
Integrated Process: Nursing Process—planning
Content Area: Child health
Reference: Wong, D., Perry, S., & Hockenberry, M. (2002). *Maternal child nursing care* (2nd ed., p. 1457). St. Louis: Mosby.

7. **2**
Rationale: The vomiting that occurs in Reye's syndrome is caused by cerebral edema and is a symptom of increased intracranial pressure. Small, frequent meals will not affect the amount of vomiting, and if vomiting occurs, the parents should contact the health care provider. Options 1, 3, and 4 are correct. Decreasing stimuli and providing rest decrease stress on the brain tissue. Checking for jaundice will assist in identifying the presence of liver dysfunction that occurs in Reye's syndrome.

Test-Taking Strategy: Use the process of elimination, noting the key words "indicate a need for further instruction." Options 1 and 3 can be eliminated first because they are similar. Next eliminate option 4, knowing that liver dysfunction is a concern in the child with Reye's syndrome. Review home care instructions for the child with Reye's syndrome if you had difficulty with this question.

Level of Cognitive Ability: Analysis
Client Needs: Health Promotion and Maintenance

Integrated Process: Teaching/Learning
Content Area: Child health
Reference: Wong, D., Hockenberry-Eaton, M. (2000). *Wong's essentials of pediatric nursing* (6th ed., p. 1082). St. Louis: Mosby.

8. **1**
Rationale: Generalized tonic-clonic seizures cause rigidity of all body muscles, followed by intense jerking movements. Because airway obstruction and increased oral secretions can occur during and after the seizure, an airway and suctioning equipment are placed at the bedside. A tracheotomy is not performed during a seizure. An emergency cart would not be left at the bedside but would be available in the treatment room or nearby on the nursing unit.

Test-Taking Strategy: Use the process of elimination. Note the key words "need to be placed at the child's bedside." Remember that when an option contains two parts, both parts of the option must be correct in order for the option to be the correct one. Eliminate options 2 and 4 first, knowing that a tracheotomy is not performed. From the remaining options, focusing on the primary concern during seizure activity will direct you to option 1. If you had difficulty with this question, review the plan of care associated with seizure precautions.

Level of Cognitive Ability: Application
Client Needs: Physiological Integrity
Integrated Process: Nursing Process—planning
Content Area: Child health
Reference: Wong, D., Perry, S., & Hockenberry, M. (2002). *Maternal child nursing care* (2nd ed., p. 1485). St. Louis: Mosby.

9. **1**
Rationale: Cerebral palsy is a chronic disability characterized by impaired movement and posture resulting from an abnormality in the extrapyramidal or pyramidal motor system. Meningitis is an infectious process of the central nervous system. Encephalitis is an inflammation of the brain that occurs as a result of viral illness or central nervous system infection. Down syndrome is an example of a congenital condition that results in moderate to severe retardation.

Test-Taking Strategy: Use the process of elimination. Eliminate options 2 and 3 first, noting that they are similar. Next, note the relationship between "palsy" in the question and "impaired muscle movement" in option 1. If you had difficulty with this question, review the characteristics associated with cerebral palsy.

Level of Cognitive Ability: Comprehension
Client Needs: Physiological Integrity
Integrated Process: Nursing Process—implementation
Content Area: Child health
Reference: James, S., Ashwill, J., & Droske, S. (2002). *Nursing care of children: Principles & practice* (2nd ed., p. 962). Philadelphia: W B. Saunders.

10. **3**
Rationale: The goals of managing the child with cerebral palsy are early recognition and intervention to maximize the child's abilities. The cause of the disorder cannot be eliminated. Minimizing the occurrence of emotional disturbances is best if possible, but not to prevent them because expression of emotions is healthy for the child. The disorder is not curable.

Test-Taking Strategy: Use the process of elimination. Eliminate options 1 and 4 first because they are similar. Next, eliminate option 2 because emotional disturbances cannot be prevented. Also, option 3 is the most global option. Review the therapeutic management of the child with cerebral palsy if you had difficulty with this question.
Level of Cognitive Ability: Application
Client Needs: Health Promotion and Maintenance
Integrated Process: Nursing Process—planning
Content Area: Child health
Reference: James, S., Ashwill, J., & Droske, S. (2002). *Nursing care of children: Principles & practice* (2nd ed., p. 963). Philadelphia: W. B. Saunders.

11. **3**
Rationale: Down syndrome is a form of mental retardation and is a congenital condition that results in moderate to severe mental retardation. A high percentage of cases are attributable to an extra chromosome (group G); hence the name trisomy 21. Options 1, 2, and 4 are incorrect characteristics of this syndrome.
Test-Taking Strategy: Use the process of elimination. Eliminate options 1 and 2 first because average or above average intelligence is not associated with this disorder. Eliminate option 4 because deficits in adaptive behavior do occur with Down syndrome. Knowing that Down syndrome is associated with an extra chromosome will assist in directing you to the correct option. If you had difficulty with this question, review the characteristics associated with Down syndrome.
Level of Cognitive Ability: Comprehension
Client Needs: Physiological Integrity
Integrated Process: Nursing Process—implementation
Content Area: Child health
Reference: Wong, D., Perry, S., & Hockenberry, M. (2002). *Maternal child nursing care* (2nd ed., p. 1041). St. Louis: Mosby.

12. **4**
Rationale: Nasotracheal suctioning is contraindicated in a child with a basilar skull fracture. Because of the nature of the injury, there is a high risk of secondary infection and the probability of the catheter entering the brain through the fracture. The child is maintained on a nothing-by-mouth status or restricted to clear liquids until it is determined that vomiting will not occur. An intravenous line is maintained to administer fluids or medications if necessary. Fluid balance is monitored closely by daily weight, intake and output measurement, and serum osmolality to detect early signs of water retention, excessive dehydration, and states of hypertonicity or hypotonicity.
Test-Taking Strategy: Use the process of elimination. Eliminate options 1, 2, and 3 because they are similar in that they address the issue of fluids. Remember that nasotracheal suctioning is contraindicated in a child with a skull fracture. If you had difficulty with this question, review the care of a child with this type of a skull fracture.
Level of Cognitive Ability: Analysis
Client Needs: Physiological Integrity
Integrated Process: Nursing Process—implementation
Content Area: Child health
Reference: Wong, D., Hockenberry-Eaton, M. (2000). *Wong's essentials of pediatric nursing* (6th ed., p. 1071). St. Louis: Mosby.

13. **2**
Rationale: A diagnosis of meningitis is made by testing cerebrospinal fluid obtained by lumbar puncture. In the case of bacterial meningitis, findings usually include an elevated pressure, turbid or cloudy cerebrospinal fluid, elevated leukocytes, elevated protein, and decreased glucose levels.
Test-Taking Strategy: Use the process of elimination and knowledge regarding the diagnostic findings in meningitis. Eliminate options 3 and 4 first because clear cerebrospinal is not likely to be found if an infectious process such as meningitis. From this point, knowledge that an elevated protein level indicates a possible diagnosis of meningitis is helpful to answer the question. If you had difficulty with this question, review this diagnostic test.
Level of Cognitive Ability: Analysis
Client Needs: Physiological Integrity
Integrated Process: Nursing Process—analysis
Content Area: Child health
References: James, S., Ashwill, J., & Droske, S. (2002). *Nursing care of children: Principles & practice* (2nd ed., p. 944). Philadelphia: W. B. Saunders.
Wong, D., Hockenberry-Eaton, M. (2000). *Wong's essentials of pediatric nursing* (6th ed., p. 1093). St. Louis: Mosby.

14. **3**
Rationale: A major priority of nursing care for a child suspected of having meningitis is to administer the prescribed antibiotic as soon as it is ordered. The child also is placed on respiratory isolation for at least 24 hours while culture results are obtained and the antibiotic is having an effect. Enteric precautions and neutropenic precautions are not associated with the mode of transmission of meningitis. Enteric precautions are instituted when the mode of transmission is through the gastrointestinal tract. Neutropenic precautions are instituted when a child has a low neutrophil count.
Test-Taking Strategy: Use the process of elimination and knowledge regarding the mode of transmission of meningitis. Eliminate options 2 and 4 first because both enteric and neutropenic precautions are unrelated to the mode of transmission. Knowledge that it takes about 24 hours for antibiotics to reach a therapeutic blood level will assist in directing you to option 3. If you had difficulty with this question, review the mode of transmission of meningitis.
Level of Cognitive Ability: Application
Client Needs: Safe, Effective Care Environment
Integrated Process: Nursing Process—planning
Content Area: Child health
Reference: Wong, D., Hockenberry-Eaton, M. (2000). *Wong's essentials of pediatric nursing* (6th ed., p. 1093). St. Louis: Mosby.

15. **3**
Rationale: Autistic disorder is a complex childhood disorder that involves abnormalities in behavior, social interactions, and communication. Autistic children are unable to relate to persons or to respond to social and emotional cues. Characteristically, these children engage in repetitive behaviors, including head banging, twirling in circles, biting themselves, and flapping their hands or arms. Abnormal communication patterns include verbal and nonverbal communication.

Test-Taking Strategy: Use the process of elimination. Note that options 1, 2, and 4 are similar in that they address a normal response. If you had difficulty with this question, review the characteristics associated with autistic disorder.
Level of Cognitive Ability: Analysis
Client Needs: Psychosocial Integrity
Integrated Process: Nursing Process—assessment
Content Area: Child health
Reference: Wong, D., Hockenberry-Eaton, M. (2000). *Wong's essentials of pediatric nursing* (6th ed., p. 408). St. Louis: Mosby.

16. **4**
Rationale: The most likely assessment findings in sexual abuse include difficulty walking or sitting; torn, stained, or bloody underclothing; pain, swelling, or itching of the genitals; and bruises, bleeding, or lacerations in the genital or anal area. Poor hygiene may indicate physical neglect. Bald spots on the scalp and fear of the parents most likely are associated with physical abuse.
Test-Taking Strategy: Use the process of elimination, noting the key words "sexually abused." The only option that specifically addresses an assessment finding related to sexual abuse is option 4. If you had difficulty with this question, review the assessment findings in a child suspected of being abused.
Level of Cognitive Ability: Analysis
Client Needs: Physiological Integrity
Integrated Process: Nursing Process—assessment
Content Area: Child health
References: James, S., Ashwill, J., & Droske, S. (2002). *Nursing care of children: Principles & practice* (2nd ed., p. 1006). Philadelphia: W. B. Saunders.
Wong, D., Hockenberry-Eaton, M. (2000). *Wong's essentials of pediatric nursing* (6th ed., p. 1093). St. Louis: Mosby.

17. **2**
Rationale: The primary legal nursing responsibility when child abuse is suspected is to report the case. All states and provinces in North America have laws for mandatory reporting of child maltreatment. One should report suspected child abuse to the local authorities. Although documentation of assessment findings, assisting the family, and referring the family to appropriate resources and support groups are important, the primary legal responsibility is to report the suspected case.
Test-Taking Strategy: Use the process of elimination, noting the key words "primary" and "legal." In addition to the many implications associated with child abuse, abuse is a crime. With this in mind, option 2, reporting the case of abuse, is the primary responsibility. If you had difficulty with this question, review the responsibilities of the nurse when child abuse is suspected.
Level of Cognitive Ability: Application
Client Needs: Psychosocial Integrity
Integrated Process: Nursing Process—implementation
Content Area: Child health
Reference: Wong, D., Hockenberry-Eaton, M. (2000). *Wong's essentials of pediatric nursing* (6th ed., p. 489). St. Louis: Mosby.

18. **4**
Rationale: The newborn with spina bifida is at risk for infection before the closure of the sac. A sterile normal saline dressing is placed over the sac to maintain moisture of the sac and its contents. This prevents tearing or breakdown of the skin integrity at the site. Blood pressure may be difficult to assess during the newborn period and is not the best indicator of infection. Urine concentration is not well developed in the newborn stage of development. A thermometer will be needed to assess temperature, but in this newborn the priority is to maintain sterile normal saline dressings over the sac.
Test-Taking Strategy: Knowledge of the characteristics of spina bifida, the care involved, and the potential complications is needed to correctly answer this question. Eliminate options 1 and 3 first as unlikely needed items. Recalling that this newborn will have a sac and is at risk for infection will direct you easily to the correct option. Review care to the newborn with spina bifida if you had difficulty with this question.
Level of Cognitive Ability: Application
Client Needs: Physiological Integrity
Integrated Process: Nursing Process—planning
Content Area: Child health
Reference: Wong, D., Hockenberry-Eaton, M. (2000). *Wong's essentials of pediatric nursing* (6th ed., p. 1257). St. Louis: Mosby.

19. **1**
Rationale: Formerly called petit mal seizures, absence seizures are brief episodes of altered awareness. No muscle activity occurs except eyelid fluttering or twitching. The child has a blank facial expression. These seizures last only 5 to 10 seconds, but they may occur one after another several times a day. Myoclonic seizures are brief random contractions of a muscle group that can occur on one or both sides of the body. Simple partial seizures consist of twitching of an extremity, face, or neck, or the sensation of twitching or numbness in an extremity or face or neck.
Test-Taking Strategy: Knowledge of the characteristics of the various types of seizures is required to answer this question. Focusing on the type of seizure identified in the question, "absence" seizures, may assist in directing you to option 1. Review the characteristics of the various types of seizures if you had difficulty with this question.
Level of Cognitive Ability: Analysis
Client Needs: Physiological Integrity
Integrated Process: Nursing Process—assessment
Content Area: Child health
Reference: Wong, D., Perry, S., & Hockenberry, M. (2002). *Maternal child nursing care* (2nd ed., p. 1455). St. Louis: Mosby.

20. **2**
Rationale: Decerebrate posturing is characterized by the rigid extension and pronation of the arms and legs. Option 1 describes decorticate posturing. Options 3 and 4 are incorrect.
Test-Taking Strategy: Knowledge of the clinical manifestations associated with decerebrate posturing is required to answer this question. Review the characteristics of posturing if you had difficulty with this question.
Level of Cognitive Ability: Analysis
Client Needs: Physiological Integrity
Integrated Process: Nursing Process—assessment
Content Area: Child health
Reference: Wong, D., Perry, S., & Hockenberry, M. (2002). *Maternal child nursing care* (2nd ed., p. 1425). St. Louis: Mosby.

CRITICAL THINKING: MULTIPLE RESPONSE

Answer:

Time the seizure

Stay with the child

Move furniture away from the child

Rationale: During a seizure, the child is placed on his or her side in a lateral position. Positioning on the side will prevent aspiration because saliva will drain out the corner of the child's mouth. The child is not restrained because this could cause injury to the child. The nurse would loosen clothing around the child's neck and ensure a patent airway. Nothing is placed into the child's mouth during a seizure because this action may cause injury to the child's mouth, gums, or teeth.

The nurse would stay with the child to reduce the risk of injury and allow for observation and timing of the seizure.

Test-Taking Strategy: Visualize this clinical situation. Recalling that airway patency and safety is the priority will assist in determining the appropriate interventions. Review care to the child experiencing a seizure if you had difficulty with this question.

Level of Cognitive Ability: Application

Client Needs: Physiological Integrity

Integrated Process: Nursing Process—implementation

Content Area: Child health

Reference: James, S., Ashwill, J., & Droske, S. (2002). *Nursing care of children: Principles & practice* (2nd ed., p. 973). Philadelphia: W. B. Saunders.

REFERENCES

James, S., Ashwill, J., & Droske, S. (2002). *Nursing care of children: Principles & practice* (2nd ed.). Philadelphia: W. B. Saunders.

Wong, D., Hockenberry-Eaton, M. (2000). *Wong's essentials of pediatric nursing* (6th ed.). St. Louis: Mosby.

Wong, D., Perry, S., & Hockenberry, M. (2002). *Maternal child nursing care* (2nd ed.). St. Louis: Mosby.

Eye, Ear, and Throat Disorders

I. STRABISMUS

A. Description
1. Called "squint" or "lazy eye"
2. A condition in which the eyes are not aligned because of lack of coordination of the extraocular muscles
3. Most often results from muscle imbalance or paralysis of extraocular muscles but also may result from conditions such as a brain tumor, myasthenia gravis, or infection
4. Normal in the young infant but should not be present after about age 4 months

B. Assessment
1. Amblyopia if not treated early
2. Permanent loss of vision if not treated early
3. Loss of binocular vision
4. Impairment of depth perception
5. Frequent headaches
6. Squinting or tilting of the head to see

C. Interventions
1. Corrective lenses may be indicated.
2. Instruct the parents regarding patching (occlusion therapy) of the "good" eye to strengthen the weak eye.
3. Inform the parents that the injection of botulinum toxin wears off in about 2 months, and if successful, correction will occur.
4. Prepare for surgery to realign the weak muscles as prescribed if nonsurgical interventions are unsuccessful; performed before the age of 2 years
5. Instruct the parents in the need for follow-up visits.

II. CONJUNCTIVITIS

A. Description
1. Conjunctivitis also is known as "pinkeye."
2. Conjunctivitis is inflammation of the conjunctiva.
3. Conjunctivitis usually is caused by allergy, infection, or trauma.
4. Bacterial or viral conjunctivitis is extremely contagious.
5. Chlamydial conjunctivitis is rare in older children and if diagnosed in a child who is not sexually active, the child should be assessed for possible sexual **abuse**.

B. Assessment
1. Itching, burning, or scratchy eyelids
2. Redness
3. Edema
4. Discharge

C. Interventions
1. Instruct in infection control measures such as good hand washing and not sharing towels and washcloths.
2. Administer antibiotic or antiviral eye drops or ointment as prescribed if infection is present.
3. Administer antihistamines as prescribed if an allergy is present.
4. Instruct the child and parents in the administration of the prescribed medications.
5. Instruct the parents that the child should be kept home from school or day care until antibiotic eye drops have been administered for 24 hours.
6. Instruct in the use of cool compresses to lessen irritation and in wearing dark glasses for photophobia.
7. Instruct the child to avoid rubbing the eye to prevent injury.
8. Instruct the child who is wearing contact lenses to discontinue wearing them and to obtain new lenses to eliminate the chance of reinfection.
9. Instruct the adolescent that eye makeup should be discarded and replaced.

III. OTITIS MEDIA
A. Description
   1. Otitis media is infection of the middle ear occurring as a result of a blocked eustachian tube, which prevents normal drainage.
   2. Otitis media is a common complication of an acute respiratory infection.
   3. Infants and children are more prone to otitis media because their eustachian tubes are shorter, wider, and straighter.
B. Assessment
   1. Fever
   2. Irritability and restlessness
   3. Loss of appetite
   4. Rolling of head from side to side
   5. Pulling on or rubbing the ear
   6. Earache or pain
   7. Signs of hearing loss
   8. Purulent ear drainage
   9. Red, opaque, bulging, or retracting tympanic membrane
C. Interventions
   1. Encourage fluid intake.
   2. Teach the parents to feed infants in upright position.
   3. Instruct the child to avoid chewing during the acute period because chewing increases pain.
   4. Provide local heat and have the child lie with the affected ear down.
   5. Instruct the parents in the appropriate procedure to clean drainage from the ear with sterile cotton swabs.
   6. Instruct the parents in the administration of analgesics or antipyretics such as acetaminophen (Tylenol) to decrease fever and pain.
   7. Instruct the parents in the administration of the prescribed antibiotics, emphasizing that the 10- to 14-day period is necessary to eradicate infective organisms.
   8. Instruct the parents that screening for hearing loss may be necessary.
   9. Instruct the parents about the procedure for administering ear medications (Box 36-1).
D. Myringotomy
   1. Description: insertion of tympanoplasty tubes into the middle ear to equalize pressure and keep the ear aerated

---

BOX 36-1

Administration of Ear Medications

In a child younger than age 3, pull the pinna down and back.
In a child older than 3 years, pull the pinna up and back.

---

   2. Interventions postoperatively
      a. Instruct the parents and child to keep the ears dry.
      b. The client should wear earplugs during bathing, shampooing, and swimming.
      c. Diving and submerging under water are not allowed.

IV. TONSILLECTOMY AND ADENOIDECTOMY
A. Description
   1. Tonsillitis refers to inflammation and infection of the tonsils.
   2. Adenoiditis refers to inflammation and infection of the adenoids.
B. Assessment
   1. Persistent or recurrent sore throat
   2. Enlarged, bright red tonsils that may be covered with white exudate
   3. Difficulty in swallowing
   4. Mouth breathing and an unpleasant mouth odor
   5. Fever
   6. Cough
   7. Enlarged adenoids may cause nasal quality of speech, mouth breathing, hearing difficulty, snoring, or obstructive sleep apnea.
C. Interventions preoperatively
   1. Assess for signs of active infection.
   2. Assess bleeding and clotting studies because the throat is vascular.
   3. Prepare the child for a sore throat postoperatively, and inform the child that he or she will need to drink liquids.
   4. Assess for any loose teeth to decrease the risk of aspiration during surgery.
D. Interventions postoperatively
   1. Position client prone or side-lying to facilitate drainage.
   2. Have suction equipment available, but do not suction unless there is an airway obstruction.
   3. Monitor for signs of hemorrhage (frequent swallowing may indicate hemorrhage); if hemorrhage occurs, turn the child to the side and notify the physician.
   4. Discourage coughing or clearing the throat.
   5. Provide clear, cool, noncitrus and noncarbonated fluids.
   6. Avoid milk products initially because they will coat the throat.
   7. Avoid red liquids, which will simulate the appearance of blood if the child vomits.
   8. Do not give the child any straws, forks, or sharp objects that can be put in the mouth.
   9. Administer acetaminophen (Tylenol) for sore throat as prescribed.
   10. Instruct the parents to notify the physician if bleeding, persistent earache, or fever occurs.
   11. Instruct the parents to keep the child away from crowds until healing has occurred.

PRACTICE QUESTIONS

1. A day care nurse is observing a 2-year-old child. The nurse suspects that the child may have strabismus. Which of the following observations made by the nurse might indicate this condition?
   1. The child consistently tilts the head to see.
   2. The child consistently turns the head to see.
   3. The child does not respond when spoken to.
   4. The child has difficulty hearing.

2. A physician has told the mother of a newborn infant diagnosed with strabismus that surgery will be necessary to realign the weakened eye muscles. The mother asks the nurse when the surgery might be performed. The most appropriate response is to tell the mother that surgery will be performed
   1. Immediately.
   2. Shortly before the child starts school.
   3. Before the child is 2 years old.
   4. Before the child begins to read.

3. The mother of a 6-year-old child arrives at a clinic because the child has been experiencing scratchy, red, and swollen eyes. The nurse notes a discharge from the eyes and sends a culture to the laboratory for analysis. Chlamydial conjunctivitis is diagnosed. Based on this diagnosis, the nurse determines that which of the following would require further investigation?
   1. The presence of an allergy
   2. Possible trauma
   3. Possible sexual abuse
   4. The presence of a respiratory infection

4. A nurse prepares a teaching plan for a mother of a child diagnosed with bacterial conjunctivitis. Which of the following, if stated by the mother, would indicate a need for further education?
   1. "I need to wash my hands frequently."
   2. "I need to clean the eye as prescribed."
   3. "I need to give the eye drops as prescribed."
   4. "It is okay to share towels and washcloths."

5. The mother of a child who had a myringotomy with insertion of tympanostomy tubes calls the nurse and tells the nurse that the tubes have fallen out. Which of the following is the most appropriate response to the mother?
   1. "Replace the tubes immediately so that the created opening does not close."
   2. "This is an emergency and requires immediate intervention. Bring the child to the emergency room."
   3. "This is not an emergency. I will speak to the physician and call you right back."
   4. "Place the tubes in hydrogen peroxide for 1 hour before replacing them in the child's ears."

6. Antibiotics are prescribed for a child after a myringotomy with insertion of tympanostomy tubes. The nurse provides discharge instructions to the parents regarding the administration of the antibiotics.

Which of the following statements, if made by the parents, indicates that they understood the instructions?
   1. "Administer the antibiotics if the child has a fever."
   2. "Administer the antibiotics until the child feels better."
   3. "Administer the antibiotics until they are gone."
   4. "Begin to taper the antibiotics after 3 days of a full course."

7. The mother of a child who underwent a myringotomy with insertion of tympanostomy tubes calls a nurse and reports that the child is complaining of discomfort. Which of the following is the most appropriate response?
   1. "Give the child children's aspirin for the discomfort."
   2. "Give the child acetaminophen (Tylenol) for the discomfort."
   3. "You need to speak to the physician because the child should not be having any discomfort."
   4. "I will speak to the physician so that a narcotic can be prescribed."

8. A nurse provides discharge instructions to the mother of a child after a myringotomy with insertion of tympanostomy tubes. The nurse determines that the mother needs additional instructions if the mother states
   1. To be sure to give her child soft tissues to blow his nose.
   2. To place earplugs with petroleum jelly in the ears during baths and showers.
   3. That swimming in deep water is prohibited.
   4. That swimming in lake water needs to be avoided.

9. A nurse is reviewing the laboratory results for a child scheduled for tonsillectomy. The nurse determines that which of the following laboratory values is most significant to review?
   1. Prothrombin time
   2. Sedimentation rate
   3. Blood urea nitrogen
   4. Creatinine

10. A child is scheduled for a tonsillectomy. A nurse plans care, knowing that which of the following would present the highest risk of aspiration during surgery?
   1. Difficulty in swallowing
   2. The presence of loose teeth
   3. Bleeding during surgery
   4. Exudate in the throat area

11. A nurse is preparing to care for a child after a tonsillectomy. The nurse documents on the plan of care to place the child in which most appropriate position?
   1. Supine
   2. Trendelenburg's
   3. Side-lying
   4. High Fowler's

12. After a tonsillectomy, a nurse reviews the physician's postoperative orders. Which of the following physician's orders does the nurse question?
   1. Clear, cool liquids when awake
   2. No milk or milk products
   3. Monitor for bleeding
   4. Suction every 2 hours

13. A nurse is caring for a child after a tonsillectomy. The nurse monitors the child, knowing that which of the following may indicate that the child is bleeding?
   1. A decreased pulse rate
   2. An elevation in blood pressure
   3. Complaints of discomfort
   4. Frequent swallowing

14. After tonsillectomy, a child begins to vomit bright red blood. The most appropriate initial nursing action would be to
   1. Administer the prescribed antiemetic.
   2. Turn the child to the side.
   3. Notify the physician.
   4. Maintain a nothing-by-mouth status.

15. A child is scheduled for a tonsillectomy in a day-stay surgical unit. On the day following surgery, the mother calls the surgical unit and expresses concern because the child has a bad mouth odor. Which of the following responses is most appropriate?
   1. "The child probably has an infection."
   2. "You need to contact the physician immediately."
   3. "Bad mouth odor is normal and may be relieved by drinking more liquids."
   4. "Have the child gargle with mouthwash every 4 hours."

CRITICAL THINKING: FILL IN THE BLANK

A nurse is providing instructions to the mother of a 2-year-old-child regarding the correct procedure for administering ear drops. To straighten the auditory canal, the nurse tells the mother to pull on the pinna of the ear in which manner?

Answer: _____

ANSWERS

1. 1
Rationale: The nurse may suspect strabismus in a child when the child complains of frequent headaches, squints, or tilts the head to see. Options 2, 3, and 4 are not indicative of this condition.
Test-Taking Strategy: Use the process of elimination. Eliminate options 3 and 4 first because they are similar. From the remaining options, recalling that the child may tilt the head to see will direct you to option 1. Review the signs of strabismus if you had difficulty with this question.
Level of Cognitive Ability: Analysis
Client Needs: Physiological Integrity
Integrated Process: Nursing Process—assessment
Content Area: Child health
Reference: Wong, D., Hockenberry-Eaton, M. (2000). *Wong's essentials of pediatric nursing* (6th ed., p. 640). St. Louis: Mosby.

2. 3
Rationale: In a child diagnosed with strabismus, surgery may be indicated to realign the weakened muscles. Surgery most often is indicated when amblyopia (decreased vision in the deviated eye) is present. The surgery should be performed before the child is 2 years old. Options 1, 2, and 4 are incorrect.
Test-Taking Strategy: Use the process of elimination. Option 1 can be eliminated easily. Options 2 and 4 can be eliminated next because they address a similar time frame. If you had difficulty with this question, review the treatment for strabismus.
Level of Cognitive Ability: Application
Client Needs: Physiological Integrity
Integrated Process: Nursing Process—implementation
Content Area: Child health

Reference: McKinney, E., Ashwill, J., Murray, S., James, S., Gorrie, T., & Droske, S. (2000). *Maternal-child nursing* (p. 1563). Philadelphia: W. B. Saunders.

3. 3
Rationale: A diagnosis of chlamydial conjunctivitis in a child who is not sexually active should signal the health care provider to assess the child for possible sexual abuse. Allergy, infection, and trauma can cause conjunctivitis, but the causative organism is not likely to be chlamydia.
Test-Taking Strategy: Use the process of elimination. Note the age of the child and the organism that is identified in the question. This may assist in directing you to option 3. Options 1, 2, and 4 can be recognized as the common causes of conjunctivitis. These options are similar in that they relate to a physiological problem. Review content related to chlamydial conjunctivitis if you had difficulty with this question.
Level of Cognitive Ability: Analysis
Client Needs: Psychosocial Integrity
Integrated Process: Nursing Process—assessment
Content Area: Child health
Reference: McKinney, E., Ashwill, J., Murray, S., James, S., Gorrie, T., & Droske, S. (2000). *Maternal-child nursing* (p. 1055). Philadelphia: W. B. Saunders.

4. 4
Rationale: Bacterial conjunctivitis is highly contagious, and the nurse should teach infection control measures. These include good hand washing and not sharing towels and washcloths. Options 2 and 3 are correct treatment measures.
Test-Taking Strategy: Use the process of elimination. Note the key words "need for further education." Options 1, 2, and 3 can be eliminated easily by recalling that bacterial conjunctivitis is

highly contagious. If you had difficulty with this question, review infection control measures for bacterial conjunctivitis.
Level of Cognitive Ability: Analysis
Client Needs: Safe, Effective Care Environment
Integrated Process: Teaching/Learning
Content Area: Child health
Reference: Wong, D., Hockenberry-Eaton, M. (2000). *Wong's essentials of pediatric nursing* (6th ed., p. 486). St. Louis: Mosby.

5. 3
Rationale: The size and appearance of the tympanostomy tubes should be described to the parents after surgery. They should be reassured that if the tubes fall out, it is not an emergency, but that the physician should be notified.
Test-Taking Strategy: Use the process of elimination. Option 2 should be eliminated first because this will cause concern in the parent. Next, eliminate options 1 and 4 because they are similar and relate to replacing the tubes. Review parent instructions following this procedure, if you had difficulty with this question.
Level of Cognitive Ability: Application
Client Needs: Physiological Integrity
Integrated Process: Nursing Process—implementation
Content Area: Child health
References: McKinney, E., Ashwill, J., Murray, S., James, S., Gorrie, T., & Droske, S. (2000). *Maternal-child nursing* (p. 1204). Philadelphia; W .B. Saunders.
Wong, D., Hockenberry-Eaton, M. (2000). *Wong's essentials of pediatric nursing* (6th ed., p. 837). St. Louis: Mosby.

6. 3
Rationale: The nurse must instruct parents regarding the administration of antibiotics. Antibiotics need to be taken as prescribed, and the full course needs to be completed. Options 1, 2, and 4 are incorrect. Antibiotics are not tapered but are administered until they are used up.
Test-Taking Strategy: Use the process of elimination and recall that antibiotics must be taken for the full course, regardless of whether the child is feeling better. Note the key words "understood the instructions." Review concepts related to the administration of antibiotics if you had difficulty with this question.
Level of Cognitive Ability: Analysis
Client Needs: Physiological Integrity
Integrated Process: Teaching/Learning
Content Area: Child health
Reference: McKinney, E., Ashwill, J., Murray, S., James, S., Gorrie, T., & Droske, S. (2000). *Maternal-child nursing* (p. 1203). Philadelphia: W. B. Saunders.

7. 2
Rationale: After myringotomy with insertion of tympanostomy tubes, the child may experience some discomfort. Tylenol can be given to relieve the discomfort. A narcotic is not necessary, and aspirin should not be administered to a child.
Test-Taking Strategy: Use the process of elimination. Options 1 and 4 can be eliminated easily. It seems reasonable that the child may have some discomfort following this surgical procedure; therefore eliminate option 3. If you had difficulty with this question, review postoperative care following this procedure.

Level of Cognitive Ability: Application
Client Needs: Physiological Integrity
Integrated Process: Nursing Process—implementation
Content Area: Child health
Reference: McKinney, E., Ashwill, J., Murray, S., James, S., Gorrie, T., & Droske, S. (2000). *Maternal-child nursing* (p. 1203). Philadelphia: W. B. Saunders.

8. 1
Rationale: Parents need to be instructed that the child should not blow his or her nose for 7 to 10 days. Bath and lake water are potential sources of bacterial contamination. Diving and swimming in deep water are prohibited. The child's ears need to be kept dry. Options 2, 3, and 4 are appropriate instructions.
Test-Taking Strategy: Use the process of elimination. Note the key words "needs additional instructions" in the stem of the question. Options 2, 3, and 4 are similar; all relate to the concept of keeping the ears dry. Option 1 may cause disruption of the surgical site. Review parent discharge instructions following this procedure if you had difficulty with this question.
Level of Cognitive Ability: Analysis
Client Needs: Health Promotion and Maintenance
Integrated Process: Teaching/Learning
Content Area: Child health
Reference: James, S., Ashwill, J., & Droske, S. (2002). *Nursing care of children: Principles & practice* (2nd ed., p. 634). Philadelphia: W. B. Saunders.

9. 1
Rationale: Because the tonsillar area is so vascular, postoperative bleeding is a concern. The prothrombin time, partial thromboplastin time, platelet count, hemoglobin and hematocrit, white blood cell count, and urinalysis are performed preoperatively. The prothrombin time results would identify a potential for bleeding. The blood urea nitrogen, creatinine, and sedimentation rate would not determine the potential for bleeding.
Test-Taking Strategy: Focus on the issue of the question. The issue of the question relates to the potential for bleeding. Options 3 and 4 can be eliminated because they relate to kidney function. Similarly, option 2 can be eliminated because it is unrelated to the issue of the question. Review preoperative care to the child scheduled for tonsillectomy if you had difficulty with this question.
Level of Cognitive Ability: Analysis
Client Needs: Physiological Integrity
Integrated Process: Nursing Process—assessment
Content Area: Child health
Reference: James, S., Ashwill, J., & Droske, S. (2002). *Nursing care of children: Principles & practice* (2nd ed., p. 636). Philadelphia: W. B. Saunders, p. 636.

10. 2
Rationale: In the preoperative period, the child should be observed for the presence of loose teeth to decrease the risk of aspiration during surgery. Options 1 and 4 are incorrect because these are characteristics that may indicate the need for the surgery. Bleeding during surgery will be controlled via packing and suction as needed.

Test-Taking Strategy: Use the process of elimination, noting that the child is scheduled for surgery. The issue of the question relates to aspiration, and note the key words "highest risk" in the stem of the question. Options 1 and 4 can be eliminated easily because these are characteristics that may indicate the need for the surgery. Recall that the tonsillar area is vascular; bleeding during surgery is expected and would be controlled. Therefore eliminate option 3. Review preoperative assessment procedures related to tonsillectomy if you had difficulty with this question.
Level of Cognitive Ability: Analysis
Client Needs: Physiological Integrity
Integrated Process: Nursing Process—planning
Content Area: Child health
Reference: McKinney, E., Ashwill, J., Murray, S., James, S., Gorrie, T., & Droske, S. (2000). *Maternal-child nursing* (p. 1206). Philadelphia: W. B. Saunders.

11. **3**
Rationale: The child should be placed in a prone or side-lying position following tonsillectomy to facilitate drainage. Options 1, 2, and 4 will not achieve this goal.
Test-Taking Strategy: Use the process of elimination. Visualize each of the positions described in the options. Keeping in mind that the goal is to facilitate drainage will direct you easily to option 3. Review positioning procedures following tonsillectomy if you had difficulty with this question.
Level of Cognitive Ability: Application
Client Needs: Physiological Integrity
Integrated Process: Communication and Documentation
Content Area: Child health
Reference: McKinney, E., Ashwill, J., Murray, S., James, S., Gorrie, T., & Droske, S. (2000). *Maternal-child nursing* (p. 1207). Philadelphia: W. B. Saunders.

12. **4**
Rationale: After tonsillectomy, suction equipment should be available, but suctioning is not performed unless there is an airway obstruction because of the risk of trauma to the oropharynx. Clear, cool liquids are encouraged. Milk and milk products are avoided initially because they coat the throat, cause the child to clear the throat, and increase the risk of bleeding. Option 3 is an important nursing intervention following any type of surgery.
Test-Taking Strategy: Use the process of elimination. Option 3 can be eliminated first because this is a nursing action, not a medical order. From the remaining options, consider the anatomical location of the surgery. This should direct you easily to option 4. Review postoperative care following tonsillectomy if you had difficulty with this question.
Level of Cognitive Ability: Analysis
Client Needs: Physiological Integrity
Integrated Process: Nursing Process—implementation
Content Area: Child health
Reference: McKinney, E., Ashwill, J., Murray, S., James, S., Gorrie, T., & Droske, S. (2000). *Maternal-child nursing* (p. 1206). Philadelphia: W. B. Saunders.

13. **4**
Rationale: Frequent swallowing, restlessness, a fast and thready pulse, and vomiting bright red blood are signs of bleeding. An elevated blood pressure and complaints of discomfort are not indications of bleeding.
Test-Taking Strategy: Use the concepts related to the signs of shock to assist in answering the question. These concepts should assist in eliminating options 1 and 2. From the remaining options, knowing that discomfort does not indicate bleeding will direct you to option 4. Review the signs of bleeding after tonsillectomy if you had difficulty with this question.
Level of Cognitive Ability: Analysis
Client Needs: Physiological Integrity
Integrated Process: Nursing Process—assessment
Content Area: Child health
References: McKinney, E., Ashwill, J., Murray, S., James, S., Gorrie, T., & Droske, S. (2000). *Maternal-child nursing* (p. 1207). Philadelphia: W. B. Saunders.
Wong, D., Hockenberry-Eaton, M. (2000). *Wong's essentials of pediatric nursing* (6th ed., p. 834). St. Louis: Mosby.

14. **2**
Rationale: After tonsillectomy, if bleeding occurs, the nurse turns the child to the side and then notifies the physician. A nothing-by-mouth status would be maintained, and an antiemetic may be prescribed; however, the initial nursing action would be to turn the child to the side.
Test-Taking Strategy: Use the process of elimination. Note the key word "initial" in the stem of the question. Although all of the options may be appropriate, to maintain physiological integrity, the initial action is to turn the child to the side. Review care of the postoperative child who vomits if you had difficulty with this question.
Level of Cognitive Ability: Application
Client Needs: Physiological Integrity
Integrated Process: Nursing Process—implementation
Content Area: Child health
Reference: McKinney, E., Ashwill, J., Murray, S., James, S., Gorrie, T., & Droske, S. (2000). *Maternal-child nursing* (p. 1207). Philadelphia: W. B. Saunders.

15. **3**
Rationale: Bad mouth odor is normal following tonsillectomy and may be relieved by drinking more liquids. Options 1, 2, and 4 are incorrect. In addition, mouthwash gargles (option 4) will irritate the throat.
Test-Taking Strategy: Use the process of elimination. Eliminate option 4 first, knowing that mouthwash gargles will irritate the surgical site. Options 1 and 2 are similar and will cause additional concern in the mother. Review postoperative expectations following tonsillectomy if you had difficulty with this question.
Level of Cognitive Ability: Application
Client Needs: Health Promotion and Maintenance
Integrated Process: Nursing Process—implementation
Content Area: Child health

Reference: McKinney, E., Ashwill, J., Murray, S., James, S., Gorrie, T., & Droske, S. (2000). *Maternal-child nursing* (p. 1207). Philadelphia: W. B. Saunders.

CRITICAL THINKING: FILL IN THE BLANK

Answer: For children younger than age 3, the nurse instructs the parent that the auditory canal is straightened by pulling the pinna down and back.

Rationale: If ear drops are prescribed, instruct the parent that the auditory canal is straightened by pulling the pinna down and back in children younger than age 3 and by pulling the pinna up and back for a child older than 3 years.

Test-Taking Strategy: Focus on the age of the child and recall the anatomy of the ear and the principles related to the administration of ear drops in a child to answer the question. Review these age-related principles if you had difficulty with this question.

Level of Cognitive Ability: Application

Client Needs: Health Promotion and Maintenance

Integrated Process: Teaching/Learning

Content Area: Child health

Reference: McKinney, E., Ashwill, J., Murray, S., James, S., Gorrie, T., & Droske, S. (2000). *Maternal-child nursing* (p. 1003). Philadelphia: W. B. Saunders.

REFERENCES

James, S., Ashwill, J., & Droske, S. (2002). *Nursing care of children: Principles & practice* (2nd ed.). Philadelphia: W. B. Saunders.

McKinney, E., Ashwill, J., Murray, S., James, S., Gorrie, T., & Droske, S. (2000). *Maternal-child nursing*. Philadelphia: W. B. Saunders.

Wong, D., Hockenberry-Eaton, M. (2000). *Wong's essentials of pediatric nursing* (6th ed.). St. Louis: Mosby.

Wong, D., Perry, S., & Hockenberry, M. (2002). *Maternal child nursing care* (2nd ed.). St. Louis: Mosby.

Respiratory Disorders

I. EPIGLOTTITIS

A. Description
1. Epiglottitis is a bacterial form of croup.
2. Epiglottitis is an inflammation of the epiglottis, which may be caused by *Haemophilus influenzae* type B or *Streptococcus pneumoniae.*
3. Epiglottitis occurs most frequently between 2 to 5 years of age.
4. The onset is abrupt, and the condition occurs most often in the winter.
5. Epiglottitis is considered an emergency situation.

B. Assessment
1. High fever
2. Sore, red, and inflamed throat
3. Absence of spontaneous cough
4. Drooling
5. Difficulty in swallowing
6. Muffled voice
7. Inspiratory **stridor**
8. Agitation
9. Tripod positioning; while supporting the body with the hands, the child thrusts the chin forward and opens the mouth in an attempt to widen the airway.

C. Interventions
1. Maintain a patent airway.
2. Assess respiratory status and breath sounds, noting **nasal flaring,** the use of accessory muscles, and the presence of **stridor**.
3. Assess temperature by the axillary route, not the oral route.
4. To prevent spasm of the epiglottis and airway occlusion, *no* attempts should be made to visualize the posterior pharynx or to obtain a throat culture.
5. Prepare the child for lateral neck films to confirm the diagnosis.
6. Maintain nothing-by-mouth status.
7. Do not leave the child unattended.
8. Do not force the child to lie down.
9. Do not restrain the child.
10. Administer fluids and antibiotics intravenously as prescribed.
11. Administer analgesics and antipyretics (acetaminophen [Tylenol]) to reduce fever and throat pain as prescribed.
12. Provide cool-mist oxygen therapy as prescribed.
13. Provide high humidification to cool the airway and decrease swelling.
14. Have resuscitation equipment available, and prepare for endotracheal intubation or tracheotomy for severe respiratory distress.
15. Ensure that the child is up-to-date with immunization schedule including *Haemophilus influenzae* type b (Hib) conjugate vaccine.

II. LARYNGOTRACHEOBRONCHITIS

A. Description
1. Inflammation of the larynx, trachea, and bronchi
2. Most common type of croup and may be viral or bacterial
3. Gradual onset that may be preceded by an upper respiratory infection

B. Assessment
1. Fever, low-grade to high
2. Irritability and restlessness
3. Hoarse voice
4. Seal bark and brassy cough
5. Inspiratory **stridor** and suprasternal **retraction**
6. Use of accessory muscles for breathing
7. Crackles and **wheezing** on lung auscultation
8. Anorexia, nausea, and vomiting
9. Signs of anoxia and carbon dioxide retention
10. Cyanosis

C. Interventions
1. Maintain a patent airway.
2. Assess respiratory status, monitoring for **nasal flaring**, sternal **retraction**, and inspiratory **stridor**.
3. Monitor for pallor or cyanosis.
4. Elevate the head of the bed and provide bed rest.
5. Provide humidified oxygen via cool-mist tent for the hospitalized child.
6. Instruct the parents to use a cool-air vaporizer or humidifier at home; other measures include having the child breathe in the cool night air or the air from an open freezer or taking the child to a cool basement or garage.
7. Provide and encourage fluid intake; intravenous fluids may be prescribed to maintain hydration status if the child is unable to take fluids orally.
8. Administer acetaminophen (Tylenol) as prescribed to reduce fever.
9. Avoid cough syrups and cold medicines, which may dry and thicken secretions.
10. Administer bronchodilators if prescribed to relax smooth muscle and relieve **stridor**.
11. Administer corticosteroids if prescribed for the antiinflammatory effect.
12. Administer nebulized epinephrine (racemic epinephrine) as prescribed for children with severe disease, **stridor** at rest, retractions, or difficulty breathing.
13. Administer antibiotics as prescribed, noting that they are not indicated unless a bacterial infection is present.
14. Have resuscitation equipment available.

III. BRONCHITIS
A. Description: infection of the major bronchi that may be referred to as tracheobronchitis
B. Assessment
1. Fever
2. Dry, hacking, and nonproductive cough that is worse at night and becomes productive in 2 to 3 days
C. Interventions
1. Monitor for respiratory distress.
2. Provide cool, humidified air.
3. Monitor for signs of dehydration, such as a sunken fontanel, poor skin turgor, and decreased and concentrated urinary output.
4. Increased fluid intake.
5. Administer acetaminophen (Tylenol) for fever as prescribed.

IV. BRONCHIOLITIS/RESPIRATORY SYNCYTIAL VIRUS (RSV)
A. Description
1. Bronchiolitis is an inflammation of the bronchioles that causes a thick production of mucus that occludes bronchiole tubes and small bronchi.

2. Respiratory syncytial virus is a common cause of bronchiolitis
3. Respiratory syncytial virus, although not airborne, is highly communicable and is usually transferred by the hands.

B. Assessment
1. Upper respiratory infection symptoms such as rhinorrhea and low-grade fever
2. Lethargy, poor feeding, and irritability in infants
3. Tachypnea
4. Increased difficulty in breathing
5. **Nasal flaring** and retractions
6. Expiratory wheeze and grunt
7. Diminished breath sounds
C. Interventions
1. Maintain a patent airway.
2. Position the child at a 30- to 40-degree angle with the neck slightly extended to maintain an open airway and decrease pressure on the diaphragm.
3. Provide cool, humidified oxygen.
4. Encourage fluids; fluid administered intravenously may be necessary until the acute stage has passed.
5. Assess for signs of dehydration.
D. The child with RSV
1. Isolate the child in a single room or place in a room with another child with RSV.
2. Maintain good hand-washing procedures.
3. Ensure that nurses caring for these children do not care for other high-risk children.
4. Wear gowns when soiling of clothing may occur during care.
5. Administer ribavirin (Virazole), an antiviral respiratory medication, if prescribed (Box 37-1).
6. Prepare for the administration of respiratory syncytial virus immune globulin (RSV-IGIV or RespiGam or palivizumab [Synagis]) (Box 37-2).

BOX 37-1

Administration of Ribavirin (Virazole)

Administer ribavirin via aerosol by hood, tent, mask, or through ventilator tubing.
Pregnant health care providers should not care for a child receiving ribavirin.
The nurse wearing contact lenses should wear goggles when coming in contact with ribavirin because the mist may dissolve soft lenses.

BOX 37-2

Respiratory Syncytial Virus Immune Globulin

The immune globulin is used prophylactically to prevent respiratory syncytial virus infection in high-risk infants.
The immune globulin is not administered to infants or children with congenital heart disease or with cyanotic congenital heart disease.

BOX 37-3

Types of Pneumonia

Viral pneumonia
Primary atypical pneumonia (*Mycoplasma pneumoniae*)
Bacterial pneumonia
Aspiration pneumonia

V. PNEUMONIA
A. Description (Box 37-3)
   1. Pneumonia is inflammation of the alveoli caused by a virus, mycoplasmal agents, bacteria, or the aspiration of foreign substances.
   2. The causative agent usually is introduced into the lungs through inhalation or from the bloodstream.
   3. Viral pneumonia occurs more frequently than bacterial and often is associated with a viral upper respiratory infection.
   4. Primary atypical pneumonia (*Mycoplasma pneumoniae*) is the most common cause of pneumonia in children between the ages of 5 and 12 years; it occurs primarily in the fall and winter months and is more prevalent in crowded living conditions.
   5. Bacterial pneumonia is often a serious infection; hospitalization is indicated when pleural effusion or empyema accompanies the disease and is mandatory for children with staphylococcal pneumonia.
   6. Aspiration pneumonia occurs when food, secretions, liquids, or other materials enter the lung and cause inflammation and a chemical pneumonitis; classic symptoms include an increasing cough or fever with foul-smelling sputum, deteriorating results on chest x-rays, and other signs of airway involvement.
B. Viral pneumonia
   1. Assessment
      a. Mild fever, slight cough, and malaise, to high fever, severe cough, and prostration
      b. Nonproductive or productive cough of small amounts of whitish sputum
      c. Wheezes or fine crackles
   2. Interventions
      a. Administer oxygen with cool mist as prescribed.
      b. Increase fluid intake.
      c. Administer antipyretics for fever as prescribed.
      d. Administer chest physiotherapy and postural drainage as prescribed.
      e. Antimicrobial therapy is reserved for children in whom the presence of infection is demonstrated by cultures.
C. Primary atypical pneumonia
   1. Assessment
      a. Fever, chills, anorexia, headache, malaise, and muscle pain

      b. Rhinitis, sore throat, and dry, hacking cough
      c. Nonproductive cough initially; then production of seromucoid sputum that becomes mucopurulent or blood streaked
   2. Interventions: symptomatic
D. Bacterial pneumonia
   1. Assessment
      a. Acute onset, fever, toxic appearance
      b. Infant: irritability, lethargy, poor feeding; abrupt fever (may be accompanied by seizures); respiratory distress (air hunger, tachypnea, and circumoral cyanosis)
      c. Older child: headache, chills, abdominal pain, chest pain, meningeal symptoms (meningism)
      d. Hacking, nonproductive cough
      e. Diminished breath sounds or scattered crackles
      f. As the infection resolves, coarse crackles and **wheezing** are heard and the cough becomes productive with purulent sputum.
   2. Interventions
      a. Antimicrobial therapy is initiated as soon as the diagnosis is suspected.
      b. Administer oxygen (via hood, mist tent, or nasal cannula) for respiratory distress as prescribed.
      c. Place the child in a mist tent as prescribed; cool humidification moistens the airways and assists in temperature reduction.
      d. Suction mucus from the infant to maintain a patent airway if the infant is unable to handle secretions.
      e. Administer chest physiotherapy and postural drainage every 4 hours as prescribed.
      f. Promote bed rest to conserve energy.
      g. Encourage the child to lie on the affected side (if pneumonia is unilateral) to splint the chest and reduce the discomfort caused by pleural rubbing.
      h. Provide liberal fluid intake (administer cautiously to prevent aspiration); intravenously administered fluids may be necessary.
      i. Administer antipyretics for fever as prescribed; monitor temperature frequently because of the risk for febrile seizures.
      j. Institute isolation precautions with pneumococcal or staphylococcal pneumonia (according to agency policy).
      k. Administer antitussives as prescribed before rest times and meals if the cough is disturbing.
      l. Continuous closed chest drainage may be instituted if purulent fluid is present (usually noted in staphylococcus infections).
      m. Fluid accumulation in the pleural cavity may be removed by thoracentesis; thoracentesis also provides a means for obtaining fluid for culture and for instilling antibiotics directly into the pleural cavity.

VI. TUBERCULOSIS

A. Description

1. Tuberculosis is a contagious disease caused by *Mycobacterium tuberculosis*, an acid-fast bacillus.
2. Multidrug-resistant strains of *M. tuberculosis* occur because of client or family noncompliance with therapeutic regimens.
3. The route of transmission of *M. tuberculosis* is through inhalation of droplets from an individual with active tuberculosis.
4. Most children are infected by a family member or by another individual with whom they have frequent contact, such as a babysitter.

B. Assessment

1. Client may be asymptomatic or develop symptoms such as malaise, fever, cough, weight loss, anorexia, and lymphadenopathy.
2. Specific symptoms related to the site of infection, such as the lungs, brain, or bone, may be present.

C. Mantoux test (Box 37-4)

1. The test will produce a positive reaction 2 to 10 weeks after the initial infection.
2. The test determines whether the child has been infected and has developed a sensitivity to the protein of the tubercle bacillus; a positive reaction does not confirm the presence of active disease.
3. Once the child reacts positively, the child will always react positively; a positive reaction in a previously negative test indicates that the child has been infected since the last test.
4. Tuberculosis testing should not be done at the same time as measles immunization; viral interference from the measles vaccine may cause a false-negative reaction.

D. Sputum culture

1. A definitive diagnosis is made by demonstrating the presence of mycobacteria in a culture.
2. Because an infant or young child often swallows sputum rather than expectorates, gastric washings (aspiration of lavaged contents from the fasting stomach) may be done to obtain a specimen;

BOX 37-4

Mantoux Test Results

Induration measuring 15 mm or greater is considered to be a positive reaction in children 4 years of age or older who do not have any risk factors.
Induration measuring 10 mm or greater is considered to be a positive reaction in children younger than 4 years of age and in those with chronic illness or at high risk for exposure to tuberculosis.
Induration measuring 5 mm or greater is considered to be positive for the highest risk groups, such as children with immunosuppressive conditions or human immunodeficiency virus.

---

specimen is obtained in the early morning before breakfast.

E. Interventions

1. Medications
   a. Include isoniazid (INH), rifampin (Rifadin), and pyrazinamide
   b. A 9-month course of isoniazid may be prescribed to prevent a latent infection from progressing to clinically active tuberculosis and to prevent initial infection in children in high-risk situations; a 12-month course may be prescribed for the child infected with human immunodeficiency virus.
   c. Recommendation for the child with clinically active tuberculosis may include administration of isoniazid, rifampin, and pyrazinamide daily for 2 months and then isoniazid and rifampin twice weekly for 4 months.
2. Place children with infectious disease on airborne precautions until medications have been initiated, sputum cultures demonstrate a diminished number of organisms, and cough is improving.
3. Wear a mask if the child is coughing and does not reliably cover his or her mouth.
4. Maintain airborne precautions with family members until they are demonstrated not to have infectious tuberculosis.
5. Stress the importance of adequate rest and adequate diet.
6. Instruct the child and family in measures to prevent transmission of tuberculosis.

VII. ASTHMA

A. Description

1. Asthma is a chronic inflammatory disease of the airways.
2. Asthma commonly is caused by physical and chemical irritants such as foods, pollens, dust mites, cockroaches, smoke, animal dander, temperature changes, respiratory infection, activity, and stress.
3. The allergic reaction in the airways can cause an immediate reaction, with obstruction occurring, and it can precipitate a late bronchial obstructive reaction several hours after the initial exposure.
4. A common symptom is coughing in the absence of respiratory infection, especially at night.
5. Status asthmaticus
   a. Child displays respiratory distress despite vigorous treatment measures.
   b. Status asthmaticus is a medical emergency that can result in respiratory failure and death if left untreated.

B. Assessment

1. Client has episodes of **wheezing**, breathlessness, dyspnea, chest tightness, and cough, particularly at night and/or in the early morning.

2. Client has itching localized at the front of the neck or over the upper part of the back.
3. Exacerbations are episodes of progressively worsening shortness of breath, cough, **wheezing**, chest tightness, decreases in expiratory airflow because of bronchospasm, mucosal edema, and mucus plugging; air is trapped behind occluded or narrow airways, and hypoxemia can occur.
4. Asthmatic episode
   a. The episode begins with irritability, restlessness, headache, feeling tired, or chest tightness.
   b. Respiratory symptoms include a hacking, irritable, nonproductive cough caused by bronchial edema.
   c. Accumulated secretions stimulate the cough, and the cough becomes rattling and productive of frothy, clear, gelatinous sputum.
   d. Child may be pale or flushed, and the lips may have a deep, dark red color that may progress to cyanosis observed in the nailbeds and skin, especially around the mouth.
   e. Restlessness, apprehension, and diaphoresis occur.
   f. Younger children assume the tripod sitting position; older children sit upright with the shoulders in a hunched-over position, with the hands on the bed or a chair, and arms braced to facilitate the use of accessory muscles of breathing (child refuses to lie down).
   g. Child speaks in short, broken phrases.
   h. Child experiences retractions.
   i. Hyperresonance on percussion of the chest is noted.
   j. Breath sounds are coarse and loud, with crackles and coarse rhonchi and inspiratory and expiratory **wheezing**; expiration is prolonged.
5. Exercise-induced bronchospasm: cough, shortness of breath, chest pain or tightness, **wheezing**, and endurance problems during exercise.
6. Severe spasm or obstruction: breath sounds and crackles may become inaudible, and the cough is ineffective (represents a lack of air movement).
7. Ventilatory failure and asphyxia: shortness of breath, with air movement in the chest restricted to the point of absent breath sounds accompanied by a sudden rise in the respiratory rate.
C. Interventions: acute episode (Box 37-5)
D. Medications
1. Quick-relief (rescue medications): to treat symptoms and exacerbations (Box 37-6)
2. Long-term control (preventer medications): to achieve and maintain control of inflammation (Box 37-7)
3. Nebulizer, metered-dose inhaler or peak expiratory flow meters
   a. These devices deliver many of the medications used to treat asthma.

BOX 37-5

Interventions in the Event of an Acute Asthma Attack

Assess airway patency.
Administer humidified oxygen by nasal prongs or face mask.
Administer quick-relief (rescue) medications.
Continuously monitor respiratory status, pulse oximetry, and color; be alert to decreased wheezing or a silent chest, which may signal the inability to move air.
Initiate an intravenous line, and prepare to correct dehydration, acidosis, or electrolyte imbalances.
Prepare the child for a chest radiograph.
Prepare to obtain samples for determining arterial blood gases and serum electrolytes.

BOX 37-6

Quick-Relief (Rescue Medications)

Short-acting B_2-agonists
Anticholinergics (for relief of acute bronchospasm)
Systemic corticosteroids (for its antiinflammatory action to treat reversible airflow obstruction)

BOX 37-7

Long-term Control (Preventer Medications)

Corticosteroids
Antiallergic medications
Nonsteroidal antiinflammatory drugs
Long-acting B_2-agonists
Leukotriene modifiers to prevent bronchospasm and inflammatory cell infiltration
Long-acting bronchodilators
Nebulizer, metered-dose inhaler, or peak expiratory flow meters

---

   b. If the child has difficulty using the metered-dose inhaler, medication can be administered by nebulization (medication is mixed with saline and then nebulized with compressed air by a machine).
E. Chest physiotherapy
1. Chest physiotherapy includes breathing exercises and physical training.
2. Chest physiotherapy is not recommended during an acute exacerbation.
F. Allergen control
1. Prevention and reduction of exposure to airborne and environmental allergens
2. Skin testing to identify allergens; immunotherapy (hyposensitization) is not recommended for allergens that can be eliminated effectively
G. Home care measures
1. Instruct the client in measures to eliminate allergens.

2. Avoid extremes of environmental temperature; in cold temperatures, instruct the child to breathe through the nose, not the mouth, and to cover the nose and mouth with a scarf.
3. Avoid exposure to individuals with a viral respiratory infection.
4. Instruct the child in how to recognize early symptoms of an asthma attack.
5. Instruct the child in the administration of medications as prescribed.
6. Instruct the child in the use of a nebulizer, metered-dose inhaler, or peak expiratory flow meter.
7. Instruct the child about the importance of home monitoring of peak expiratory flow rate; decrease in rate may indicate impending infection or exacerbation.
8. Instruct the child in the cleaning of devices used for inhaled medications (oral candidiasis can occur with the use of aerosolized steroids).
9. Encourage adequate rest, sleep, and a well-balanced diet.
10. Instruct the child in the importance of adequate fluid intake to liquefy secretions.
11. Assist in developing an exercise program.
12. Instruct the child in the procedure for respiratory treatments and exercises as prescribed.
13. Encourage the child to cough effectively.
14. Encourage the parents to keep immunizations up to date; annual influenza vaccinations are recommended.
15. Inform other health care providers and school personnel of the asthma condition.
16. Allow the child to take control of self-care measures based on age appropriateness.

VIII. CYSTIC FIBROSIS

A. Description
1. Cystic fibrosis is a chronic multisystem disorder (autosomal recessive trait disorder) characterized by exocrine gland dysfunction.
2. The mucus produced by the exocrine glands is abnormally thick, causing obstruction of the small passageways of the affected organs.
3. The most common symptoms are pancreatic enzyme deficiency caused by duct blockage, progressive chronic lung disease associated with infection, and sweat gland dysfunction resulting in increased sodium and chloride sweat concentrations.
4. An increase in sodium and chloride in sweat and saliva forms the basis for the most reliable diagnostic test, the sweat chloride test.
B. Respiratory system
1. Symptoms are produced by the stagnation of mucus in the airway, leading to bacterial colonization and destruction of lung tissue.

2. Emphysema and atelectasis occur as the airways become increasingly obstructed.
3. Chronic hypoxemia causes contraction and hypertrophy of the muscle fibers in pulmonary arteries and arterioles, leading to pulmonary hypertension and eventual cor pulmonale.
4. Pneumothorax from ruptured bullae and hemoptysis from erosion of the bronchial wall through an artery occur as the disease progresses.
5. Other respiratory symptoms include the following:
   a. **Wheezing** and dry nonproductive cough
   b. Dyspnea
   c. Cyanosis
   d. Clubbing of the fingers and toes
   e. Repeated episodes of bronchitis and pneumonia
C. Gastrointestinal system
1. Meconium ileus in the neonate
2. Intestinal obstruction (distal intestinal obstructive syndrome) caused by thick intestinal secretions; signs include pain, abdominal distention, nausea, and vomiting
3. Steatorrhea (frothy, foul-smelling stools)
4. Deficiency of the fat-soluble vitamins A, D, E, and K, which causes easy bruising and anemia
5. Malnutrition and failure to thrive; demonstration of hypoalbuminemia from diminished absorption of protein, resulting in generalized edema
6. Rectal prolapse that can result from the large, bulky stools, and lack of the supportive fat pads around the rectum
D. Integumentary system
1. Abnormally high concentrations of sodium and chloride in sweat
2. Parents reporting that the infant tastes "salty" when kissed
3. Dehydration and electrolyte imbalances, especially during hyperthermic conditions
E. Reproductive system
1. Cystic fibrosis can delay **puberty** in girls.
2. Fertility can be inhibited by highly viscous cervical secretions, which act as a plug and block sperm entry.
3. Males are usually sterile, caused by the blockage of the vas deferens by abnormal secretions or by failure of normal development of duct structures.
F. Diagnostic tests
1. Quantitative sweat chloride test (Box 37-8)
2. Chest x-ray film reveals atelectasis and obstructive emphysema.
3. Pulmonary function tests provide evidence of abnormal small airway function.
4. Stool/fat and/or enzyme analysis: A 72-hour stool sample is collected to check the fat and/or enzyme (trypsin) content (food intake is recorded during the collection).
G. Interventions
1. Respiratory system

BOX 37-8

Quantitative Sweat Chloride Test

The production of sweat is stimulated (pilocarpine iontophoresis), the sweat is collected, and the sweat electrolytes are measured (a minimum of 50 mg of sweat is needed).

Normally, sweat chloride concentration is less than 40 mEq/L.

A chloride concentration greater than 60 mEq/L is a positive test result.

Chloride concentrations of 40 to 60 mEq/L are highly suggestive of cystic fibrosis and require a repeat test.

---

    a. Goals of treatment include preventing and treating pulmonary infection by improving aeration, removing secretions, and administering antimicrobial medications.

    b. Chest physiotherapy (percussion and postural drainage) on awakening and in the evening (more frequently during pulmonary infection).

    c. Chest physiotherapy should not be performed before or immediately after a meal.

    d. Bronchodilator medication by aerosol opens the bronchi for easier expectoration (administered before the chest physiotherapy when the child has reactive airway disease or is **wheezing**).

    e. Use of a Flutter Mucus Clearance Device (a small, handheld plastic pipe with a stainless steel ball on the inside) that facilitates removal of mucus; store away from small children because if the device separates, the steel ball poses a choking hazard.

    f. Use of a ThAIRapy vest device that provides high-frequency chest wall oscillation to help loosen secretions.

    g. Administration of recombinant human deoxyribonuclease (DNase), known generically as dornase alfa (Pulmozyme), which decreases the viscosity of mucus.

    h. Instruct the parents not to give cough suppressants, for they will inhibit expectoration of secretions and promote infection.

    i. Teach the child forced expiratory technique (huffing) to mobilize secretions.

    j. Develop a physical exercise program with the aim of establishing a good habitual breathing pattern.

    k. Administer antibiotics as prescribed, which may be prescribed prophylactically or when pulmonary symptoms develop.

    l. Aerosolized antibiotics may be prescribed and are administered after chest physiotherapy is performed, or antibiotics may be prescribed and administered intravenously at home through a central venous access device.

    m. Administer oxygen as prescribed during acute episodes; monitor closely for oxygen narcosis.

    n. Monitor for hemoptysis; greater than 300 mL in 24 hours for the older child (less for a younger child) needs to be treated immediately.

    o. Hemoptysis may be controlled by bed rest, cough suppressants, antibiotics, and vitamin K; if hemoptysis persists, the site of bleeding may be cauterized or embolized.

    p. Lung transplantation is a final therapeutic option for the child with end-stage disorder.

  2. Gastrointestinal system

    a. The goal of treatment for pancreatic insufficiency is to replace pancreatic enzymes; administered with meals and snacks (or within 30 minutes of eating meals and snacks) to ensure that digestive enzymes are mixed with food in the duodenum.

    b. The amount of pancreatic enzymes administered is adjusted to achieve normal **growth** and a decrease in the number of stools to two or three per day.

    c. Enteric-coated pancreatic enzymes should not be crushed or chewed.

    d. Pancreatic enzymes should not be given if the child is to receive nothing by mouth.

    e. Encourage a well-balanced, high-protein, high-calorie diet; multivitamins and vitamins A, D, E, and K are also administered.

    f. Assess weight and monitor for failure to thrive.

    g. Monitor for constipation and intestinal obstruction.

    h. Ensure adequate salt intake during extremely hot weather or if the child has a fever; include fluids such as Gatorade or Exceed, which provide an adequate supply of electrolytes.

H. Home care

  1. Instruct the parents about the prescribed treatment measures and their importance.

  2. Instruct the parents to be sure immunizations are up to date.

  3. Inform the parents that the child should be vaccinated yearly for influenza. Pneumococcus vaccine may also be prescribed.

  4. Inform the parents about the Cystic Fibrosis Foundation.

IX. SUDDEN INFANT DEATH SYNDROME

A. Description

  1. Unexpected death of an apparently healthy infant under age 1 year for which a thorough autopsy fails to demonstrate an adequate cause of death

  2. Unknown cause that may be related to a brainstem abnormality in the neurological regulation of cardiorespiratory control

  3. Time of year: Most frequently during winter months

  4. Time of death: Usually during sleep

  5. Age: Most frequently from 2 months to 4 months of life

6. Sex and race
    a. Incidence higher in males
    b. Incidence higher in Native Americans, African-Americans, and Hispanics
7. Sleep risk habits
    a. Prone position
    b. Use of soft bedding
    c. Overheating (thermal stress)
    d. Possibly sleeping with an adult
B. Appearance when found
    1. Child is apneic, blue, and lifeless.
    2. Frothy blood-tinged fluid is in the nose and mouth.
    3. Child may be found in any position but typically is found in a disheveled bed, with blankets over the head, and huddled in a corner.
    4. Child may be clutching bedding.
    5. Diaper may be wet and full of stool.
▲ C. Prevention
    1. Infants should be placed in the supine position for sleep.
    2. Soft moldable mattresses and bedding, such as pillows or quilts, should not be used under the infant for bedding.
    3. Stuffed animals should be removed from the crib while the infant is sleeping.
    4. Discourage bed sharing (sleeping with an adult).
    5. Avoid overheating during sleep.

PRACTICE QUESTIONS

1. A student nurse is caring for a 2-year-old child diagnosed with croup. A nursing instructor asks the student about the clinical manifestations associated with croup. Which statement by the student indicates a need for further research?
    1. "Symptoms usually worsen at night and are better during the day."
    2. "Symptoms usually worsen during the day and are relieved during sleep."
    3. "The cough is harsh and brassy."
    4. "Inspiratory stridor and a low-grade fever may be present."
2. A hospitalized 2-year-old child with croup is receiving corticosteroid therapy. The mother asks a nurse why the physician did not prescribe antibiotics. The most appropriate response is
    1. "The child is too young to receive antibiotics."
    2. "The child still has the maternal antibodies from birth and does not need antibiotics."
    3. "Antibiotics are not indicated unless a bacterial infection is present."
    4. "The child may be allergic to antibiotics."
3. A child with croup is placed in a cool mist tent. The mother becomes concerned because the child is frightened, consistently crying, and trying to climb

out of the tent. The most appropriate nursing action would be to
    1. Call the physician and obtain an order for a mild sedative.
    2. Tell the mother that the child must stay in the tent.
    3. Place a toy in the tent to make the child feel more comfortable.
    4. Let the mother hold the child and direct a cool mist over the child's face.
4. A nurse caring for an infant with bronchiolitis is assessing for signs of dehydration. The nurse assesses which of the following, knowing that it is the most reliable method of determining fluid loss?
    1. Intake and output
    2. Fontanels
    3. Mucous membranes
    4. Weight
5. An emergency room nurse is caring for a child diagnosed with epiglottitis. Assessing the child, the nurse monitors for which indication that the child may be experiencing airway obstruction?
    1. The child is leaning backward, supporting himself with the hands and arms.
    2. The child has a low-grade fever and complains of a sore throat.
    3. The child is leaning forward with the chin thrust out.
    4. The child exhibits nasal flaring and bradycardia.
6. A nurse is caring for an infant with bronchiolitis. Diagnostic tests have confirmed respiratory syncytial virus. Based on this finding, which of the following would be the most appropriate nursing action?
    1. Move the infant to a room with another child with RSV.
    2. Leave the infant in the present room because RSV is not contagious.
    3. Inform the staff that they must wear a mask when caring for the child.
    4. Initiate strict enteric precautions.
7. Ribavirin (Virazole) is prescribed for a hospitalized child with respiratory syncytial virus. The nurse prepares to administer this medication via which of the following routes?
    1. Subcutaneous
    2. Intramuscular
    3. Oxygen tent
    4. Oral
8. A 10-year-old child with asthma is treated for acute exacerbation in the emergency room. A nurse reports which of the following, knowing that it indicates a worsening of the condition?
    1. Increased wheezing
    2. Decreased wheezing
    3. Warm, dry skin
    4. A pulse rate of 90 beats per minute
9. The mother of an 8-year-old child being treated for right lower lobe pneumonia at home calls the clinic nurse. The mother tells the nurse that the child

complains of discomfort on the right side and that the acetaminophen (Tylenol) is not effective. The nurse most appropriately tells the mother to
1. Increase the dose of the acetaminophen.
2. Increase the frequency of the acetaminophen.
3. Encourage the child to lie on the right side.
4. Encourage the child to lie on the left side.

10. The charge nurse of a newborn nursery is providing a teaching session to new employees regarding sudden infant death syndrome (SIDS). The charge nurse tells the new employees that SIDS usually occurs during sleep and
    1. Most frequently occurs from 2 months to 4 months of life.
    2. Most frequently occurs during the summer months.
    3. Most frequently occurs in a toddler.
    4. Most frequently occurs in girls.

11. A new mother expresses concern to a nurse regarding sudden infant death syndrome. She asks the nurse how to position her new infant for sleep. The nurse most appropriately tells the mother that the infant should be placed on his
    1. Back rather than on the stomach.
    2. Side or prone.
    3. Stomach with the face turned.
    4. Back or prone.

12. A sweat test is performed on a child with a suspected diagnosis of cystic fibrosis. The nurse reviews the test results and determines that which of the following is a positive result for cystic fibrosis?
    1. Chloride level of 20 mEq/L
    2. Chloride level of 30 mEq/L
    3. Chloride level of 40 mEq/L
    4. Chloride level of 70 mEq/L

13. A clinic nurse is providing instructions to a mother of a child with cystic fibrosis regarding the immunization schedule for the child. Which statement would the nurse make to the mother?
    1. "The immunization schedule will need to be altered."
    2. "The child will receive all of the immunizations except for the polio series."

3. "The child will receive the recommended basic series of immunizations along with a yearly pneumococcus and influenza vaccination."
4. "The child should not receive any hepatitis vaccines."

14. A clinic nurse reads the results of a Mantoux test on a 3-year-old child. The results indicate an area of induration measuring 10 mm. The nurse would interpret these results as
    1. Negative
    2. Positive
    3. Inconclusive
    4. Definitive and requiring a repeat test

15. Isoniazid (INH) is prescribed for a 2-year-old child with human immunodeficiency virus infection who has a positive Mantoux test. The mother of the child asks the nurse how long the child will need to take the medication. The nurse tells the mother that the medication will need to be taken for
    1. 4 months.
    2. 6 months.
    3. 9 months.
    4. 12 months.

CRITICAL THINKING: MULTIPLE RESPONSE

A nurse is preparing for the admission of an infant with a diagnosis of bronchiolitis caused by the respiratory syncytial virus. Select all interventions that would be included in the plan of care.

____ Place the infant in a private room.

____ Position the infant side-lying with the head lower than the chest.

____ Place the infant in a room near the nurse's station.

____ Place the child in a tent that delivers warm humidified air.

____ Wear a mask at all times when in contact with the infant

ANSWERS
1. **2**
Rationale: Croup often begins at night and may be preceded by several days of upper respiratory infection symptoms. Croup is characterized by a sudden onset of a harsh, brassy cough, sore throat, and inspiratory stridor. Symptoms usually worsen at night and are better in the day. Croup usually is accompanied by a low-grade fever, but occasionally the temperature may be as high as 104° F.
Test-Taking Strategy: Use the process of elimination. Note the key words "need for further research." Eliminate option 4 first

because of the word "may." Knowledge of the manifestations associated with this illness will assist in eliminating options 1 and 3. If you had difficulty with this question, review this disorder.
Level of Cognitive Ability: Analysis
Client Needs: Physiological Integrity
Integrated Process: Teaching/Learning
Content Area: Child health
Reference: James, S., Ashwill, J., & Droske, S. (2002). *Nursing care of children: Principles & practice* (2nd ed., p. 638). Philadelphia: W. B. Saunders.

2. 3

Rationale: Antibiotics are not indicated in the treatment of croup unless a bacterial infection is present. Options 1, 2, and 4 are incorrect. In addition, no supporting data in the question indicate that the child may be allergic to antibiotics.

Test-Taking Strategy: Use the process of elimination. Eliminate option 4 because no supporting data are in the question regarding the potential for allergies. Noting the age of the child will assist in eliminating options 1 and 2. In addition, recalling the general principles related to the use of antibiotics will direct you to the correct option. Review the indications for the use of antibiotics if you had difficulty with this question.

Level of Cognitive Ability: Application
Client Needs: Health Promotion and Maintenance
Integrated Process: Teaching/Learning
Content Area: Child health
Reference: James, S., Ashwill, J., & Droske, S. (2002). *Nursing care of children: Principles & practice* (2nd ed., p. 639). Philadelphia: W. B. Saunders.

3. 4

Rationale: If the use of a tent or hood is causing distress, treatment may be more effective if the child is held by the parent and a cool mist is directed toward the child's face. A mild sedative would not be administered to the child. Crying will aggravate laryngospasm and increase hypoxia, which may cause airway obstruction. Options 2 and 3 will not alleviate the child's fear.

Test-Taking Strategy: Focus on the issue of the question. Options 1, 2, and 3 will not alleviate the child's fear and are similar in that they do not address the fear. Option 4 is the option that addresses the issue of the question. Review care to the child in a mist tent if you had difficulty with this question.

Level of Cognitive Ability: Application
Client Needs: Psychosocial Integrity
Integrated Process: Caring
Content Area: Child health
Reference: James, S., Ashwill, J., & Droske, S. (2002). *Nursing care of children: Principles & practice* (2nd ed., p. 641). Philadelphia: W. B. Saunders.

4. 4

Rationale: Weight is the most reliable method of measurement of body fluid loss or gain. One kilogram of weight change represents 1 L of fluid loss or gain. Although options 1, 2, and 3 identify components of the assessment for dehydration, these are not the most reliable determinants.

Test-Taking Strategy: Use the process of elimination. Note the key words "most reliable." Options 2 and 3 can be easily eliminated first. From the remaining options, recall that it would be difficult to obtain an accurate output on an infant. This concept should direct you easily toward option 4. Review assessment of dehydration if you had difficulty with this question.

Level of Cognitive Ability: Analysis
Client Needs: Physiological Integrity
Integrated Process: Nursing Process—assessment
Content Area: Child health
Reference: James, S., Ashwill, J., & Droske, S. (2002). *Nursing care of children: Principles & practice* (2nd ed., p. 646). Philadelphia: W. B. Saunders.

5. 3

Rationale: Clinical manifestations suggestive of airway obstruction include tripod positioning (leaning forward while supported by arms, chin thrust out, mouth open), nasal flaring, tachycardia, a high fever, and a sore throat.

Test-Taking Strategy: Use the process of elimination. Eliminate option 4 first because tachycardia rather than bradycardia will occur in a child experiencing respiratory distress. Eliminate option 2 next, knowing that a high fever occurs with epiglottitis. From the remaining options, visualize the descriptions in each and determine which position would best assist a child experiencing respiratory distress. Review the indications of airway obstruction if you had difficulty with this question.

Level of Cognitive Ability: Analysis
Client Needs: Physiological Integrity
Integrated Process: Nursing Process—assessment
Content Area: Child health
Reference: James, S., Ashwill, J., & Droske, S. (2002). *Nursing care of children: Principles & practice* (2nd ed., p. 644). Philadelphia: W. B. Saunders.

6. 1

Rationale: Respiratory syncytial virus (RSV) is a highly communicable disorder and is not transmitted via the airborne route. The virus usually is transferred by the hands, and meticulous hand washing is necessary to decrease the spread of organisms. The infant with RSV is isolated in a single room or placed in a room with another child with RSV. Enteric precautions are not necessary; however, the nurse should wear a gown when soiling of clothing may occur.

Test-Taking Strategy: Use the process of elimination. Recall the method of the transmission and that the infant with RSV is isolated in a single room or placed in a room with another child with RSV. Review the care of the infant with RSV if you had difficulty with this question.

Level of Cognitive Ability: Application
Client Needs: Safe, Effective Care Environment
Integrated Process: Nursing Process—implementation
Content Area: Child health
Reference: Wong, D., Perry, S., & Hockenberry, M. (2002). *Maternal child nursing care* (2nd ed., p. 1205). St. Louis: Mosby.

7. 3

Rationale: Ribavirin (Virazole) is an antiviral respiratory medication used mainly in hospitalized children with severe RSV. Administration is via hood, face mask, or oxygen tent. Ribavirin is not administered subcutaneously, intramuscularly, or orally.

Test-Taking Strategy: Use the process of eliminating. Recalling that this medication is aerosolized will direct you to option 3. If you are unfamiliar with this medication, review its method of administration.

Level of Cognitive Ability: Application
Client Needs: Physiological Integrity
Integrated Process: Nursing Process—planning
Content Area: Child health
Reference: Wong, D., Hockenberry-Eaton, M. (2000). *Wong's essentials of pediatric nursing* (6th ed., p. 842). St. Louis: Mosby.

8. 2

Rationale: Decreased wheezing in a child with asthma may be interpreted incorrectly as a positive sign when in fact it may signal an inability to move air. A "silent chest" is an ominous sign during an asthma episode. With treatment, increased wheezing actually may signal that the child's condition is improving. The normal pulse rate in a 10-year-old is 70 to 110 beats per minute. Warm, dry skin indicates an improvement in condition, for the child is normally diaphoretic during exacerbation.

Test-Taking Strategy: Use the process of elimination. Note the key word "worsening" in the stem of the question. Options 3 and 4 can be eliminated easily. From the remaining options, recall that a "silent chest" is an ominous sign during an asthma episode. Review these clinical manifestations if you had difficulty with this question.

Level of Cognitive Ability: Application
Client Needs: Physiological Integrity
Integrated Process: Nursing Process—implementation
Content Area: Child health
References: Wong, D., Hockenberry-Eaton, M. (2000). *Wong's essentials of pediatric nursing* (6th ed., p. 853). St. Louis: Mosby. Wong, D., Perry, S., & Hockenberry, M. (2002). *Maternal child nursing care* (2nd ed., p. 1213). St. Louis: Mosby.

9. 3

Rationale: Splinting of the affected side by lying on that side may decrease discomfort. To advise the mother to increase the dose or frequency of the acetaminophen is inappropriate. Lying on the left side will not be helpful in alleviating discomfort.

Test-Taking Strategy: Use the process of elimination. Options 1 and 2 can be eliminated easily. Recalling the principles related to splinting an incision in the postoperative client will assist in directing you to option 3 because these principles can be applied in this situation. Review care to the child with pneumonia if you had difficulty with this question.

Level of Cognitive Ability: Application
Client Needs: Physiological Integrity
Integrated Process: Nursing Process—implementation
Content Area: Child health
Reference: Wong, D., Hockenberry-Eaton, M. (2000). *Wong's essentials of pediatric nursing* (6th ed., p. 845). St. Louis: Mosby.

10. 1

Rationale: Sudden infant death syndrome (SIDS) usually occurs during sleep and during the winter months and most frequently occurs between the second and fourth months of life. The syndrome is more common in boys.

Test-Taking Strategy: Use the process of elimination and knowledge regarding the characteristics, etiology, and incidence of SIDS. Review this information if you are unfamiliar with it.

Level of Cognitive Ability: Application
Client Needs: Health Promotion and Maintenance
Integrated Process: Teaching/Learning
Content Area: Child health
Reference: Wong, D., Hockenberry-Eaton, M. (2000). *Wong's essentials of pediatric nursing* (6th ed., pp. 404-405). St. Louis: Mosby.

11. 1

Rationale: Nurses should encourage parents to place the infant on the back (supine) for sleep. The infant may have the ability to turn to a prone position from the side-lying position. Infants in the prone position (on the stomach) may be unable to move their heads to the side, thus increasing the risk of suffocation and lethal rebreathing.

Test-Taking Strategy: Use the process of elimination. Eliminate options 2, 3, and 4 because they are similar. Remember that the infant needs to be placed on his or her back. Review positioning of the healthy infant for sleep if you had difficulty with this question.

Level of Cognitive Ability: Application
Client Needs: Safe, Effective Care Environment
Integrated Process: Teaching/Learning
Content Area: Child health
Reference: Wong, D., Hockenberry-Eaton, M. (2000). *Wong's essentials of pediatric nursing* (6th ed., p. 405). St. Louis: Mosby.

12. 4

Rationale: In a sweat test, sweating is stimulated on the child's forearm with pilocarpine, the sample is collected on absorbent material, and the amounts of sodium and chloride are measured. A sample of at least 50 mg of sweat is required for accurate results. A chloride level greater than 60 mEq/L is considered to be a positive test result. A chloride level of 40 mEq/L suggests cystic fibrosis and requires a repeat test.

Test-Taking Strategy: Use the process of elimination. Note the key words "positive result." Use knowledge regarding this diagnostic test, and in this situation select the option that indicates the highest value. Review this diagnostic test if you are unfamiliar with it.

Level of Cognitive Ability: Analysis
Client Needs: Physiological Integrity
Integrated Process: Nursing Process—analysis
Content Area: Child health
Reference: Wong, D., Hockenberry-Eaton, M. (2000). *Wong's essentials of pediatric nursing* (6th ed., p. 864). St. Louis: Mosby.

13. 3

Rationale: Adequately protecting children with cystic fibrosis from communicable diseases by immunization is essential. In addition to the basic series of immunizations, a yearly influenza and possibly a pneumococcus vaccine also are recommended for children with cystic fibrosis.

Test-Taking Strategy: Use the process of elimination. Eliminate options 1, 2, and 4 because they are similar. Recalling the importance of protection from communicable diseases, particularly in children with a disorder such as cystic fibrosis, will assist in directing you to option 3. Review the immunization schedule for the child with cystic fibrosis if you had difficulty with this question.

Level of Cognitive Ability: Application
Client Needs: Health Promotion and Maintenance
Integrated Process: Teaching/Learning
Content Area: Child health
Reference: James, S., Ashwill, J., & Droske, S. (2002). *Nursing care of children: Principles & practice* (2nd ed., p. 680). Philadelphia: W. B. Saunders.

14. **2**

Rationale: Induration measuring 10 mm or greater is considered to be a positive result in children younger than 4 years of age and in those with chronic illness or at high risk for environmental exposure to tuberculosis. A reaction of 5 mm or greater is considered to be a positive result for the highest risk groups, such as the child with an immunosuppressive condition or the child with human immunodeficiency virus. A reaction of 15 mm or greater is positive in children 4 years of age or older without any risk factors.

Test-Taking Strategy: Use the process of elimination. Options 3 and 4 are similar and can be eliminated first. From the remaining options, note the child's age to assist in directing you to option 2. If you had difficulty with this question, review the analysis of a Mantoux test in children.

Level of Cognitive Ability: Analysis
Client Needs: Physiological Integrity
Integrated Process: Nursing Process—analysis
Content Area: Child health
Reference: James, S., Ashwill, J., & Droske, S. (2002). *Nursing care of children: Principles & practice* (2nd ed., pp. 626, 681). Philadelphia: W. B. Saunders.

15. **4**

Rationale: For children with human immunodeficiency virus infection, a minimum of 12 months of treatment with isoniazid is recommended.

Test-Taking Strategy: Focus on the child's diagnosis. Noting that the child has human immunodeficiency virus infection will direct you to option 4, the longest length of treatment time. Review the treatment plans for tuberculosis in children if you had difficulty with this question.

Level of Cognitive Ability: Application
Client Needs: Health Promotion and Maintenance
Integrated Process: Nursing Process—implementation
Content Area: Child health

Reference: James, S., Ashwill, J., & Droske, S. (2002). *Nursing care of children: Principles & practice* (2nd ed., p. 682). Philadelphia: W. B. Saunders.

CRITICAL THINKING: MULTIPLE RESPONSE

Answer:
Place the infant in a private room.
Place the infant in a room near the nurse's station.
Rationale: The infant with RSV should be isolated in a private room or in a room with another infant with RSV infection. The infant should be placed in a room near the nurse's station for easy observation. The infant should be positioned with the head and chest at a 30- to 40-degree angle and the neck slightly extended to maintain an open airway and decrease pressure on the diaphragm. Cool humidified oxygen is delivered to relieve dyspnea, hypoxemia, and insensible water loss from tachypnea. Contact precautions (wearing gloves and a gown) reduces nosocomial transmission of RSV.

Test-Taking Strategy: Recalling the mode of transmission of RSV will assist in determining that the infant needs to be placed in a private room or in a room with another infant with RSV infection and that contact precautions need to be maintained. Recalling the need to maintain a patent airway (edema and the accumulation of mucus obstruct the bronchioles) will assist in determining that the infant need to be observed closely, that the infant's head should be elevated, and that the infant should receive cool humidified oxygen. Review care to the child with bronchiolitis and RSV if you had difficulty with this question.

Level of Cognitive Ability: Application
Client Needs: Physiological Integrity
Integrated Process: Nursing Process—planning
Content Area: Child health
Reference: James, S., Ashwill, J., & Droske, S. (2002). *Nursing care of children: Principles & practice* (2nd ed., pp. 647-648). Philadelphia: W. B. Saunders.

REFERENCES

American Lung Association. www.lungusa.org.
American SIDS Institute. www.sids.org.
Asthma and Allergy Foundation of America. www.aafa.org.
Cystic Fibrosis Foundation. www.CFF.org.
Hodgson, B., & Kizior, R. (2004). *Saunders nursing drug handbook 2004.* Philadelphia: W. B. Saunders.
James, S., Ashwill, J., & Droske, S. (2002). *Nursing care of children: Principles & practice* (2nd ed.). Philadelphia: W. B. Saunders.

Perry, A., & Potter, P. (2002). *Clinical nursing skills and techniques* (5th ed.). St. Louis: Mosby.
Wong, D., Hockenberry-Eaton, M. (2000). *Wong's essentials of pediatric nursing* (6th ed.). St. Louis: Mosby.
Wong, D., Perry, S., & Hockenberry, M. (2002). *Maternal child nursing care* (2nd ed.). St. Louis: Mosby.

Cardiovascular Disorders

I. CONGESTIVE HEART FAILURE (CHF)

A. Description
1. Congestive heart failure is the inability of the heart to pump sufficiently to meet the metabolic needs of the body.
2. In infants and children, inadequate cardiac output most commonly is caused by congenital heart defects that produce an excessive volume or pressure load on the myocardium.
3. In infants and children, a combination of left-sided and right-sided heart failure is usually present.
4. The goals of treatment are to improve cardiac function, remove accumulated fluid and sodium, decrease cardiac demands, improve tissue oxygenation, and decrease oxygen consumption.

B. Assessment of early signs
1. Tachycardia, especially during rest and slight exertion
2. Tachypnea
3. Profuse scalp sweating, especially in infants
4. Fatigue and irritability
5. Sudden weight gain
6. Respiratory distress

C. Interventions
1. Monitor vital signs closely and for the early signs of CHF.
2. Monitor for respiratory distress (count respirations for 1 minute).
3. Monitor apical pulse (count pulse for 1 minute) and monitor for dysrhythmias.
4. Monitor temperature for hyperthermia and for other signs of infection, particularly respiratory infection.
5. Monitor intake and output; weigh diapers.
6. Monitor daily weight to assess for fluid retention; a weight gain of 0.5 kg (1 lb) in 1 day is due to the accumulation of fluid.

7. Monitor for facial or peripheral edema, auscultate lung sounds, and report abnormal findings.
8. Elevate the head of the bed (semi-Fowler position).
9. Maintain a neutral thermal environment to prevent cold stress in infants.
10. Provide rest; decrease environmental stimuli.
11. Administer cool, humidified oxygen as prescribed; use an oxygen hood for young infants and a nasal cannula or face tent for older infants and children.
12. Organize nursing activities to allow for uninterrupted sleep.
13. Maintain adequate nutritional status.
14. Feed when hungry and soon after awakening (crying exhausts the limited energy supply), accommodating the infant's sleep and wake patterns; the infant should be well rested before feeding.
15. Provide small, frequent feedings, which will be less tiring.
16. Administer sedation as prescribed during the acute stage to promote rest.
17. Administer digoxin (Lanoxin) as prescribed; monitor digoxin levels and for signs of digoxin toxicity, especially bradycardia and vomiting.
18. Assess apical heart rate for 1 minute before administering digoxin.
19. Check with physician regarding parameters for withholding digoxin; generally, digoxin is withheld if the pulse is fewer than 90 to 110 beats per minute in infants and young children or fewer than 70 beats per minute in older children.
20. Note that infants rarely receive more than 1 mL (50 mcg, or 0.05 mg) of digoxin (Lanoxin) in one dose.
21. Administer angiotensin-converting enzyme inhibitors as prescribed; captopril (Capoten) or enalapril (Vasotec) commonly is prescribed.

22. Monitor child for hypotension, renal dysfunction, and cough when angiotensin-converting enzyme inhibitors are administered.
23. Administer diuretics as prescribed; monitor for hypokalemia with furosemide (Lasix) and with the thiazide diuretics.
24. Administer potassium supplements and provide dietary sources of potassium as prescribed.
25. Monitor serum electrolytes, particularly the potassium level.
26. Restrict fluid as prescribed in the acute stage; monitor for dehydration.
27. Check with the physician regarding sodium restriction; note that most infant formulas have slightly more sodium than does breast milk.
28. Instruct the parents regarding the description of the diagnosis and administration of medications (Box 38-1).
29. Instruct the parents in cardiopulmonary resuscitation.

II. DEFECTS WITH INCREASED PULMONARY BLOOD FLOW (BOX 38-2)

A. Description
1. Intracardiac communications along the septum or an abnormal connection between the great arteries allows blood to flow from the high-pressure left side of the heart to the low-pressure right side of the heart.
2. The infant typically demonstrates signs and symptoms of CHF.

B. Atrial septal defect (ASD)
1. Atrial septal defect is an abnormal opening between the atria that causes an increased flow of oxygenated blood into the right side of the heart.
2. Right atrial and ventricular enlargement occurs.
3. Infant may be asymptomatic or may develop CHF.
4. Types
   a. ASD 1 (ostium primum): Opening is at the lower end of the septum
   b. ASD 2 (ostium secundum): Opening is near the center of the septum
   c. ASD 3 (sinus venosus defect): Opening is near the junction of the superior vena cava and the right atrium
5. Nonsurgical treatment: The defect may be closed by using devices during a cardiac catheterization.
6. Surgical treatment: Open repair with cardiopulmonary bypass usually is performed before school age.

C. Ventricular septal defect (VSD)
1. A VSD is an abnormal opening between the right and left ventricles.
2. Many VSDs close spontaneously during the first year of life in children having small or moderate defects.
3. A characteristic murmur is present; CHF is common.
4. Nonsurgical treatment: Device closure during cardiac catheterization may be possible.
5. Surgical treatment: Open repair is done with cardiopulmonary bypass.

D. Atrioventricular canal defect
1. The defect results from incomplete fusion of the endocardial cushions.
2. The defect is the most common cardiac defect in Down syndrome.
3. A characteristic murmur is present.
4. The infant usually has mild to moderate CHF; cyanosis increases with crying.
5. Surgical treatment can include pulmonary artery banding for infants with severe symptoms (palliative) or complete repair via cardiopulmonary bypass.

E. Patent ductus arteriosus
1. Patent ductus arteriosus is failure of the fetal ductus arteriosus (artery connecting the aorta and the pulmonary artery) to close within the first weeks of life.
2. A characteristic machinery-like murmur is present; the infant is asymptomatic or may show signs of CHF.
3. A widened pulse pressure and bounding pulses are present.

BOX 38-1

Home Care Instructions for Administering Digoxin

Administer as prescribed.
Administer 1 hour before or 2 hours after feedings.
Use a calendar to mark off the dose administered.
Do not mix the medication with foods or fluid.
If a dose is missed and more than 4 hours has elapsed, withhold the dose and give the next dose at the scheduled time; if less than 4 hours has elapsed, administer the missed dose.
If the child vomits, do not administer a second dose.
If more than two consecutive doses have been missed, notify the physician; do not increase or double the dose for missed doses.
If the child has teeth, give water after the medication; if possible, brush the teeth to prevent tooth decay from the sweetened liquid.
If the child becomes ill, notify the physician.
Keep the medication in a locked cabinet.
Call the poison control center immediately if accidental overdose occurs.

BOX 38-2

Defects with Increased Pulmonary Blood Flow

Atrial septal defect
Ventricular septal defect
Atrioventricular canal defect
Patent ductus arteriosus

4. Medical management: Indomethacin (Indocin), a prostaglandin inhibitor, may be administered to close a patent ductus in premature infants and some newborns

5. Management: Coils may be used to occlude the patent ductus arteriosus via a cardiac catheterization procedure or the defect may require surgical management.

III. OBSTRUCTIVE DEFECTS (BOX 38-3)

A. Description

1. Blood exiting the heart meets an area of anatomic narrowing (**stenosis**), causing obstruction to blood flow.
2. The location of narrowing is usually near the valve of the obstructive defect.
3. Infants and children exhibit signs of CHF.
4. Children with mild obstruction may be asymptomatic.

B. Coarctation of the aorta

1. Coarctation of the aorta is localized narrowing near the insertion of the ductus arteriosus.
2. Collateral circulation develops during fetal life to maintain flow from the ascending to the descending aorta.
3. Signs of CHF occur in infants.
4. High blood pressure and bounding pulses in the arms, weak or absent femoral pulses, and cool lower extremities may be present.
5. Children may experience headaches, dizziness, fainting, and epistaxis resulting from hypertension.
6. Nonsurgical treatment is balloon angioplasty in children; restenosis can occur.
7. Surgical management
   a. Mechanical ventilation and inotropic support are often necessary before surgery.
   b. Resection of the coarcted portion with end-to-end anastomosis of the aorta or enlargement of the constricted section using a graft of prosthetic material or a portion of the left subclavian artery is possible.
   c. Because the defect is outside the heart, cardiopulmonary bypass is not required and a thoracotomy incision is used.

C. Aortic **stenosis**

1. Aortic stenosis is narrowing or stricture of the aortic valve, causing resistance to blood flow in the left ventricle, decreased cardiac output, left

ventricular hypertrophy, and pulmonary vascular congestion.

2. Types
   a. Valvular **stenosis** is the most common type and usually is caused by malformed cusps, resulting in a bicuspid rather than a tricuspid valve, or fusion of the cusps.
   b. Subvalvular **stenosis** is a stricture caused by a fibrous ring below a normal valve.
   c. Supravalvular **stenosis** occurs rarely.
3. A characteristic murmur is present.
4. Infants with severe defects demonstrate signs of decreased cardiac output with faint pulses, hypotension, tachycardia, and poor feeding.
5. Children show signs of exercise intolerance, chest pain, and dizziness when standing for long periods of time.
6. Nonsurgical treatment for valvular aortic **stenosis** is balloon angioplasty done during cardiac catheterization to dilate the narrowed valve.
7. Surgical treatment for valvular aortic **stenosis** is aortic valvotomy under inflow occlusion (palliative); a valve replacement may be required at a second procedure.
8. Surgical treatment for subvalvular aortic **stenosis** may involve incising a membrane if one exists or cutting the fibromuscular ring; a patch may be required.

D. Pulmonary **stenosis**

1. Pulmonary stenosis is narrowing at the entrance to the pulmonary artery.
2. Resistance to blood flow causes right ventricular hypertrophy and decreased pulmonary blood flow; the right ventricle may be hypoplastic.
3. Pulmonary **atresia** is the extreme form of pulmonary stenosis in that there is total fusion of the commissures and no blood flows to the lungs.
4. A characteristic murmur is present.
5. The infant or child may be asymptomatic; mild cyanosis or CHF occurs.
6. Newborns with severe narrowing will be cyanotic.
7. If pulmonary stenosis is severe, CHF occurs.
8. Nonsurgical treatment is balloon angioplasty done during cardiac catheterization to dilate the narrowed valve.
9. Surgical treatment
   a. In infants, transventricular (closed) valvotomy procedure.
   b. In children, pulmonary valvotomy with cardiopulmonary bypass.

IV. DEFECTS WITH DECREASED PULMONARY BLOOD FLOW (BOX 38-4)

A. Description

1. Obstructed pulmonary blood flow and an anatomic defect (ASD or VSD) between the right and left sides of the heart are present.

BOX 38-3

Obstructive Defects

Coarctation of the aorta
Aortic stenosis
Pulmonary stenosis

Defects with Decreased Pulmonary Blood Flow

Tetralogy of Fallot
Tricuspid atresia

2. Pressure on the right side of the heart increases, exceeding pressure on the left side, which allows desaturated blood to **shunt** right to left, causing desaturation in the left side of the heart and in the systemic circulation.
3. Typically hypoxemia and cyanosis appear.
B. Tetralogy of Fallot
1. The tetralogy of Fallot includes four defects: VSD, pulomary stenosis, overriding aorta, and right ventricular hypertrophy.
2. If pulmonary vascular resistance is higher than systemic resistance, the **shunt** is from right to left; if systemic resistance is higher than pulmonary resistance, the **shunt** is left to right.
3. Infants
   a. The infant may be acutely cyanotic at birth or may have mild cyanosis that progresses over the first year of life as the pulmonic **stenosis** worsens.
   b. A characteristic murmur is present.
   c. Acute episodes of cyanosis and hypoxia (hypercyanotic spells), called blue spells or tet spells, occur when the infant's oxygen requirements exceed the blood supply (usually during crying or after feeding).
4. Children: With increasing cyanosis, squatting, clubbing of the fingers, and poor **growth** may occur.
5. Surgical treatment: palliative **shunt**.
   a. The **shunt** increases pulmonary blood flow and increases oxygen saturation in infants who cannot undergo primary repair.
   b. **Shunt** provides blood flow to the pulmonary arteries from the left or right subclavian artery.
6. Surgical treatment: complete repair
   a. Complete repair usually is performed in the first year of life.
   b. Complete repair involves closure of the VSD and resection of the **stenosis**, with a pericardial patch to enlarge the right ventricular outflow tract.
   c. The repair requires a median sternotomy and cardiopulmonary bypass.
C. Tricuspid **atresia**
1. Tricuspid **atresia** is failure of the tricuspid valve to develop.
2. No communication exists from the right atrium to the right ventricle.
3. Blood flows through an ASD or a patent foramen ovale to the left side of the heart and through a VSD to the right ventricle and out to the lungs.
4. The defect often is associated with pulmonic **stenosis** and transposition of the great arteries.

5. The defect results in complete mixing of unoxygenated and oxygenated blood in the left side of the heart, resulting in systemic desaturation, pulmonary obstruction, and decreased pulmonary blood flow.
6. Cyanosis, tachycardia, and dyspnea are seen in the newborn.
7. Older children exhibit signs of chronic hypoxemia and clubbing.
8. Surgical treatment
   a. If the ASD is small, atrial septostomy is performed during cardiac catheterization; otherwise surgery is needed.
   b. For the neonate whose pulmonary blood flow depends on the patency of the ductus arteriosus, a continuous infusion of prostaglandin E_1 is initiated until surgery.

V. MIXED DEFECTS (BOX 38-5)
A. Description
1. Fully saturated systemic blood flow mixes with the desaturated blood flow, causing a desaturation of the systemic blood flow.
2. Pulmonary congestion occurs and cardiac output decreases.
3. Signs of CHF are present; symptoms depend on the degree of desaturation.
B. The defects involve transposition of the great arteries or transposition of the great vessels.
1. The pulmonary artery leaves the left ventricle, and the aorta exits from the right ventricle.
2. No communication exists between the systemic and pulmonary circulation.
3. Infants with minimal communication are severely cyanotic and depressed at birth.
4. Infants with large septal defects or a patent ductus arteriosus may be less severely cyanotic but may have symptoms of CHF.
5. Cardiomegaly is evident a few weeks after birth.
6. Nonsurgical treatment
   a. Prostaglandin E_1 may be initiated to increase blood mixing temporarily if systemic and pulmonary mixing is inadequate.
   b. Balloon atrial septostomy during cardiac catheterization may be performed to increase mixing and maintain cardiac output over a longer period.

Mixed Defects

Transposition of the great arteries or transposition of the great vessels
Total anomalous pulmonary venous connection
Truncus arteriosus
Hypoplastic left heart syndrome

7. Surgical treatment: The arterial switch procedure reestablishes normal circulation with the left ventricle acting as the systemic pump; the procedure involves transection and anastomosis of the great arteries, and the coronary arteries are switched from the proximal aorta to the proximal pulmonary artery, creating a new aorta.

C. Total anomalous pulmonary venous connection
1. The defect is a failure of the pulmonary veins to join the left atrium.
2. The defect results in mixed blood being returned to the right atrium and shunted from the right to the left through an ASD.
3. The right side of the heart hypertrophies, whereas the left side of the heart may remain small.
4. Congestive heart failure develops.
5. Cyanosis worsens with pulmonary vein obstruction; once obstruction occurs, the infant's condition deteriorates rapidly.
6. Surgical treatment
   a. Corrective repair is performed in early infancy.
   b. The pulmonary vein is anastomosed to the left atrium, the ASD is closed, and the anomalous pulmonary venous connection is ligated.

D. Truncus arteriosus
1. Truncus arteriosus is failure of normal septation and division of the embryonic bulbar trunk into the pulmonary artery and the aorta, resulting in a single vessel that overrides both ventricles.
2. Blood from both ventricles mixes in the common great artery, causing desaturation and hypoxemia.
3. A characteristic murmur is present.
4. The infant exhibits moderate to severe CHF and variable cyanosis, poor **growth**, and activity intolerance.
5. Surgical treatment: Corrective surgical repair is performed in the first few months of life.

E. Hypoplastic left heart syndrome
1. Underdevelopment of the left side of the heart occurs, resulting in a hypoplastic left ventricle and aortic **atresia**.
2. Mild cyanosis and signs of CHF occur until the ductus arteriosus closes; then progressive deterioration with cyanosis and decreased cardiac output occurs, leading to cardiovascular collapse.
3. The defect is fatal in the first few months of life without intervention.
4. Surgical treatment
   a. Surgical treatment is necessary; transplantation in the newborn period may be considered.
   b. In the preoperative period, the neonate requires mechanical ventilation and a continuous infusion of prostaglandin E_1 to maintain ductal patency, ensuring adequate systemic blood flow.

▲ VI. INTERVENTIONS: CARDIOVASCULAR DEFECTS
A. Monitor for signs of a defect in the infant or child.
B. Monitor vital signs closely.

C. Monitor respiratory status for the presence of **nasal flaring** and use of accessory muscles, and notify the physician if any changes occur.
D. Auscultate breath sounds for crackles, rhonchi, or rales.
E. If respiratory effort is increased, place the child in reverse Trendelenburg's position (elevate head and upper body) to decrease the work of breathing.
F. Administer humidified oxygen as prescribed.
G. Provide endotracheal tube and ventilator care if necessary and as prescribed, and restrain the hands of an intubated child.
H. Monitor for hypercyanotic spells (Box 38-6) ▲
I. Assess for signs of CHF, such as fluid retention in the eyes, hands, feet, and chest.
J. Assess peripheral pulses.
K. Monitor intake and output, and notify the physician if a decrease in urine output occurs.
L. Assess urine output, weighing diapers as necessary.
M. Obtain daily weight.
N. Maintain fluid restriction if prescribed.
O. Provide adequate nutrition (high calorie requirements) as prescribed.
P. Administer medications as prescribed.
Q. Keep child as stress free as possible; plan interventions to allow maximal rest for the child.
R. Prepare parents and child, if appropriate, for surgery.
S. Allow parents and child to verbalize feelings and concerns regarding disorder.
T. Familiarize parents and child with hospital procedures and equipment.

VII. CARDIAC SURGERY
A. Interventions postoperatively
1. Monitor vital signs frequently.
2. Monitor temperature and notify the physician if a fever occurs.
3. Monitor for signs of sepsis, such as fever, chills, diaphoresis, lethargy, and altered levels of consciousness.
4. Maintain aseptic technique.
5. Monitor lines, tubes, or catheters that are in place and remove promptly as prescribed when no longer needed, to prevent infection.
6. Assess for signs of discomfort, such as irritability, changes in heart rate, respiratory rate, and blood pressure, and the inability to sleep.
7. Administer pain medications as prescribed, noting effectiveness.

BOX 38-6

Treatment for Hypercyanotic Spells

Place the infant in a knee-chest position.
Administer 100% oxygen by face mask.
Administer morphine sulfate as prescribed.
Administer fluids intravenously as prescribed.

BOX 38-7

Home Care after Cardiac Surgery

Omit play outside for several weeks.
Avoid activities in which the child could fall, such as bike riding, for 2 to 4 weeks.
Avoid crowds for 2 weeks after discharge.
Follow a no-added-salt diet if prescribed.
Do not add any new foods to the infant's eating schedule.
Do not place creams, lotions, or powders on the incision until completely healed.
The child may return to school the third week after discharge, starting with half days.
No physical education for 2 months.
Instruct the parents to discipline the child normally.
Instruct the parents about the importance of the 2-week follow-up.
Avoid immunizations, invasive procedures, and dental visits for 2 months.
Advise the parents regarding the importance of a dental visit every 6 months after age 3 and to inform the dentist of the cardiac problem so that antibiotics can be prescribed if necessary.
Instruct the parents to call the physician when coughing, tachypnea, cyanosis, vomiting, diarrhea, anorexia, pain, fever, or any swelling, redness, or drainage occurs at the site of the incision.

8. Administer antibiotics and antipyretics as prescribed.
9. Encourage rest periods.
10. Facilitate parent-child contact as soon as possible.
B. Postoperative home care (Box 38-7)

VIII. RHEUMATIC FEVER
A. Description
1. Rheumatic fever is an inflammatory autoimmune disease that affects the connective tissues of the heart, joints, subcutaneous tissues, and blood vessels of the central nervous system.
2. The most serious complication is rheumatic heart disease, which affects the cardiac valves.
3. Rheumatic fever presents 2 to 6 weeks following an untreated or partially treated group A β-hemolytic streptococcal infection of the upper respiratory tract.
4. Jones criteria are used to determine the diagnosis.
B. Assessment (Fig. 38-1)
1. Fever: low-grade fever that spikes in the late afternoon
2. Elevated antistreptolysin O titer
3. Elevated sedimentation rate
4. Elevated C-reactive protein
5. Aschoff's bodies (lesions): found in the heart, blood vessels, brain, and serous surfaces of the joints and pleura

C. Interventions
1. Assess vital signs.
2. Assess for the clinical manifestations.
3. Control joint pain and inflammation with massage and alternating hot and cold applications as prescribed.
4. Provide bed rest during acute febrile phase.
5. Limit physical exercise in the child with carditis.
6. Administer antibiotics (penicillin) as prescribed.
7. Administer salicylates and antiinflammatory agents as prescribed (should not be instituted before the diagnosis is confirmed, because these medications mask the polyarthritis).
8. Initiate seizure precautions if the child is experiencing chorea.
9. Instruct the parents about the importance of follow-up and the need for antibiotic prophylaxis for dental work, infection, and invasive procedures.
10. Advise the child to inform the parents if anyone in school develops a streptococcal throat infection.

IX. KAWASAKI DISEASE
A. Description
1. Kawasaki disease is known as mucocutaneous lymph node syndrome and is an acute systemic inflammatory illness.
2. The cause is unknown but may be associated with an infection from an organism or toxin.
3. Cardiac involvement is the most serious complication; aneurysms can develop.
B. Assessment
1. Acute stage
a. Fever
b. Conjunctival hyperemia
c. Red throat
d. Swollen hands, rash, and enlargement of the cervical lymph nodes
2. Subacute stage
a. Cracking lips and fissures
b. Desquamation of the skin on the tips of the fingers and toes
c. Joint pain
d. Cardiac manifestations
e. Thrombocytosis
3. Convalescent stage: Child appears normal but signs of inflammation may be present.
C. Interventions
1. Monitor temperature frequently.
2. Assess heart sounds and rhythm.
3. Assess extremities for edema, redness, and desquamation.
4. Examine eyes for conjunctivitis.
5. Monitor mucous membranes for inflammation.
6. Monitor dietary and fluid intake.
7. Administer soft foods and liquids that are neither too hot nor too cold.

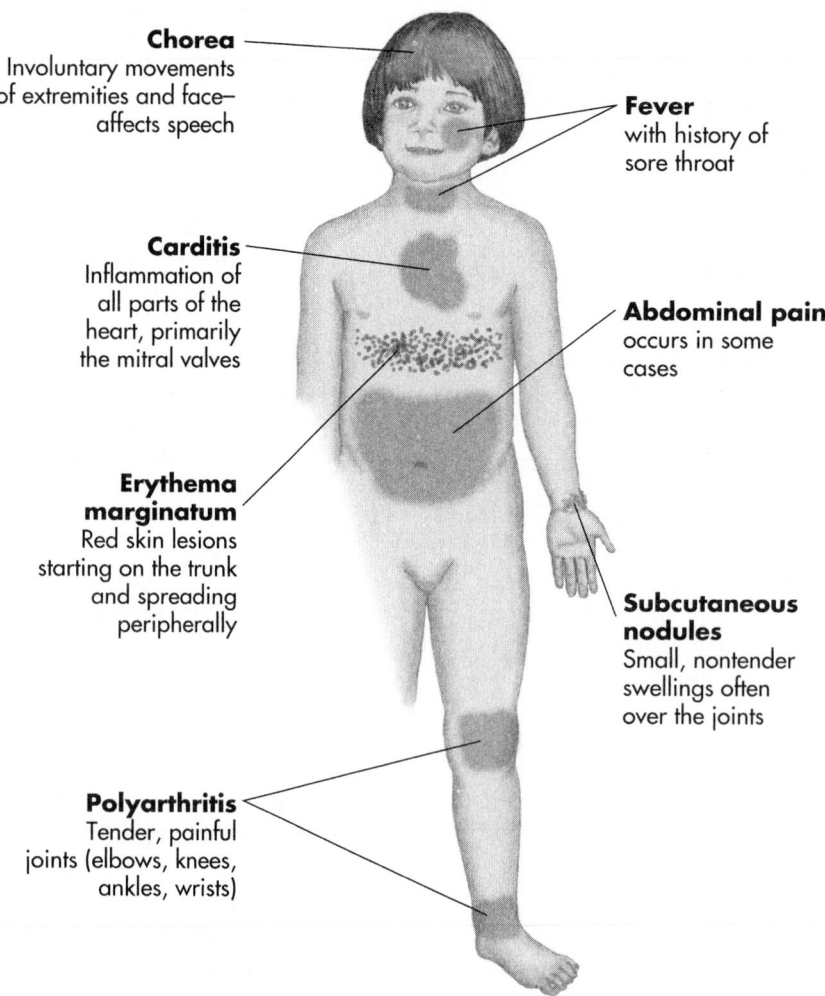

Chorea
Involuntary movements of extremities and face–affects speech

Fever
with history of sore throat

Carditis
Inflammation of all parts of the heart, primarily the mitral valves

Abdominal pain
occurs in some cases

Erythema marginatum
Red skin lesions starting on the trunk and spreading peripherally

Subcutaneous nodules
Small, nontender swellings often over the joints

Polyarthritis
Tender, painful joints (elbows, knees, ankles, wrists)

FIG 38-1 Clinical manifestations of rheumatic fever. (From James, S., Ashwill, J., & Droske, S. [2002]. *Nursing care of children: Principles & practice* [2nd ed.]. Philadelphia: W. B. Saunders.)

8. Weigh client daily.
9. Provide passive range-of-motion exercises to facilitate joint movement.
10. Administer acetylsalicylic acid (aspirin) as prescribed for its antipyretic and antiplatelet effect.
11. Administer immune globulin intravenously as prescribed to reduce the duration of fever and the incidence of coronary artery lesions and aneurysms.
12. Instruct the parents in the administration of prescribed medications, the need to monitor for bleeding, and the need for follow-up to monitor for cardiac complications.

PRACTICE QUESTIONS

1. A nurse caring for an infant with congenital heart disease is monitoring the infant closely for signs of congestive heart failure (CHF). The nurse assesses the infant closely for which early sign of CHF?
   1. Cough
   2. Tachycardia
   3. Slow and shallow breathing
   4. Pallor
2. A physician has prescribed oxygen as needed for an infant with congestive heart failure. In which situation would the nurse plan to administer the oxygen to the infant?
   1. During feeding
   2. When the mother is holding the infant
   3. When changing the infant's diapers
   4. When drawing blood for electrolyte values
3. An infant with congestive heart failure is receiving diuretic therapy, and a nurse is closely monitoring the intake and output. The nurse uses which most appropriate method to assess the urine output?

1. Inserting a Foley catheter
2. Weighing the diapers
3. Comparing intake with output
4. Measuring the amount of water added to formula
4. A nurse is monitoring the daily weight of an infant with congestive heart failure. Which of the following alerts the nurse to suspect fluid accumulation and the need to call the physician?
   1. Bradypnea
   2. Diaphoresis
   3. Decreased blood pressure
   4. A weight gain of 1 lb in 1 day
5. A nurse provides home care instructions to the parents of a child with congestive heart failure regarding the procedure for the administration of digoxin (Lanoxin). Which statement if made by a parent indicates the need for further instructions?
   1. "If the child vomits after medication administration, I will repeat the dose."
   2. "I will take the child's pulse before administering the medication."
   3. "I will not mix the medication with food."
   4. "If more than one dose is missed, I will call the physician."
6. A nurse is assigned to care for an infant with a diagnosis of tricuspid atresia. The nurse plans care, knowing that in this disorder
   1. No communication exists between the systemic and pulmonary circulation.
   2. Frequent episodes of hypercyanotic spells occur.
   3. No communication exists from the right atrium to the right ventricle.
   4. A single vessel overrides both ventricles.
7. Prostaglandin E_1 is prescribed for a child with transposition of the great arteries. The mother of the child is a registered nurse and asks the nurse why the child needs the medication. The most appropriate response would be to tell the mother that the medication
   1. Maintains an adequate hormonal level.
   2. Maintains the position of the great arteries.
   3. Provides adequate oxygen saturation and maintains cardiac output.
   4. Prevents tet spells.
8. A clinic nurse reviews the record of a child just seen by a physician. The physician has documented a diagnosis of suspected aortic stenosis. The nurse expects to note documentation of which of the following clinical manifestations specifically found in this disorder?
   1. Hyperactivity
   2. Exercise intolerance
   3. Pallor
   4. Gastrointestinal disturbances
9. A nurse has provided home care instructions to the mother of a child who is being discharged following cardiac surgery. Which statement made by the mother indicates a need for further instructions?

1. "Large crowds of people need to be avoided for at least 2 weeks following surgery."
2. "I can apply lotion or powder to the incision if it is itchy."
3. "A balance of rest and exercise is important."
4. "Activities in which the child could fall need to be avoided for 2 to 4 weeks."
10. A nurse receives a telephone call from the admitting office and is told that a child with rheumatic fever will be arriving in the nursing unit for admission. On admission, the nurse prepares to ask the mother which question to elicit assessment information specific to the development of rheumatic fever?
    1. "Did the child have a sore throat or an unexplained fever within the last 2 months?"
    2. "Has the child had any nausea or vomiting?"
    3. "Has the child complained of headaches?"
    4. "Has the child complained of back pain?"
11. Acetylsalicylic acid (aspirin) is prescribed for a child with rheumatic fever. A nurse would question this order if there were documented evidence that the child had which of the following?
    1. A viral infection
    2. Joint pain
    3. Facial edema
    4. Arthralgia
12. A nurse is caring for a child with a suspected diagnosis of rheumatic fever. The nurse reviews the laboratory results, knowing that which laboratory study would assist in confirming the diagnosis of rheumatic fever?
    1. White blood cell count
    2. Red blood cell count
    3. Immunoglobulin
    4. Antistreptolysin O titer
13. The nurse is caring for a child with a diagnosis of Kawasaki disease. The mother of the child asks the nurse about the disorder. The nurse tells the mother that
    1. It is an acquired cell-mediated immunodeficiency disorder.
    2. It is an inflammatory autoimmune disease that affects the connective tissue of the heart, joints, and subcutaneous tissues.
    3. It is a chronic multisystem autoimmune disease characterized by the inflammation of connective tissue.
    4. Is also called mucocutaneous lymph node syndrome and is a febrile generalized vasculitis of unknown origin.
14. A nurse is preparing for the admission of a child with a diagnosis of acute-stage Kawasaki disease. On assessment of the child, the nurse expects to note which clinical manifestation of the acute stage of the disease?
    1. Conjunctival hyperemia
    2. Cracked lips

3. Desquamation of the skin
4. A normal appearance
15. A nurse is reviewing the physician's orders for a child who was just admitted to the hospital with a diagnosis of Kawasaki disease. The nurse expects to note an order for which of the following as part of the treatment plan?
   1. Morphine sulfate
   2. Immune globulin
   3. Heparin infusion
   4. Digoxin (Lanoxin)

CRITICAL THINKING: FILL IN THE BLANK

A nurse is caring for an infant with a diagnosis of tetralogy of Fallot. The infant suddenly becomes cyanotic, and the nurse recognizes that the infant is experiencing a hypercyanotic spell. The nurse immediately places the infant in what position?

Answer: _____

ANSWERS

1. 2
Rationale: The early signs of congestive heart failure (CHF) include tachycardia, tachypnea, profuse scalp sweating, fatigue and irritability, sudden weight gain, and respiratory distress. A cough may occur in CHF as a result of mucosal swelling and irritation but is not an early sign. Pallor may be noted in the infant with CHF but is also not an early sign.
Test-Taking Strategy: Use the process of elimination and note the key word "early." Think about the physiology and the effects on the heart when fluid overload occurs. These concepts will assist in directing you to option 2. If you had difficulty with this question, review the early signs of CHF in an infant.
Level of Cognitive Ability: Analysis
Client Needs: Physiological Integrity
Integrated Process: Nursing Process—assessment
Content Area: Child health
Reference: Wong, D., Hockenberry-Eaton, M. (2000). *Wong's essentials of pediatric nursing* (6th ed., p. 952). St. Louis: Mosby.

2. 4
Rationale: Crying exhausts the limited energy supply, increases the workload of the heart, and increases the oxygen demands. Oxygen administration may be prescribed for stressful periods, especially during bouts of crying or invasive procedures. Options 1, 2, and 3 are not likely to produce crying in the infant.
Test-Taking Strategy: Use the process of elimination. Recall the situations that would place stress and an increased workload on the heart. This concept should direct you easily to option 4. Drawing blood is an invasive procedure, which would likely cause the child to cry. Review care to the child with CHF if you had difficulty with this question.
Level of Cognitive Ability: Analysis
Client Needs: Physiological Integrity
Integrated Process: Nursing Process—planning
Content Area: Child health
References: Wong, D., Hockenberry-Eaton, M. (2000). *Wong's essentials of pediatric nursing* (6th ed., p. 952). St. Louis: Mosby. Wong, D., Perry, S., & Hockenberry, M. (2002). *Maternal child nursing care* (2nd ed., p. 1326). St. Louis: Mosby.

3. 2
Rationale: The most appropriate method for assessing urine output in an infant receiving diuretic therapy is to weigh the diapers. Comparing intake with output would not provide an accurate measure of urine output. Measuring the amount of water added to formula is unrelated to the amount of output. Although Foley catheter drainage is most accurate in determining output, it is not the most appropriate method in an infant and places the infant at risk for infection.
Test-Taking Strategy: Use the process of elimination. Eliminate options 3 and 4 first because they will not provide an indication of urine output. From the remaining options, note the words "most appropriate" in the stem of the question. These words will direct you to option 2. Review care to the infant receiving diuretic therapy if you had difficulty with this question.
Level of Cognitive Ability: Application
Client Needs: Physiological Integrity
Integrated Process: Nursing Process—assessment
Content Area: Child health
Reference: James, S., Ashwill, J., & Droske, S. (2002). *Nursing care of children: Principles & practice* (2nd ed., p. 700). Philadelphia: W. B. Saunders.

4. 4
Rationale: A weight gain of 0.5 kg (1 lb) in 1 day is due to the accumulation of fluid. The nurse should assess urine output, assess for evidence of facial or peripheral edema, auscultate lung sounds, and report the weight gain to the physician. Tachypnea and an increased blood pressure would occur with fluid accumulation. Diaphoresis is a sign of CHF but is not specific to fluid accumulation, and usually occurs with exertional activities.
Test-Taking Strategy: Use the process of elimination and focus on the issue, fluid accumulation. Note the relationship between "fluid accumulation" in the question and "weight gain" in the correct option. Review the indications of fluid accumulation in an infant with CHF if you had difficulty with this question.
Level of Cognitive Ability: Analysis
Client Needs: Physiological Integrity
Integrated Process: Nursing Process—analysis
Content Area: Child health
Reference: James, S., Ashwill, J., & Droske, S. (2002). *Nursing care of children: Principles & practice* (2nd ed., p. 700). Philadelphia: W. B. Saunders.

5. 1
Rationale: The parents need to be instructed that if the child vomits after the digoxin is administered, they are not to repeat the dose. Options 2, 3, and 4 are accurate instructions

regarding the administration of this medication. In addition, the parents should be instructed that if a dose is missed and is not identified until 4 hours later, the dose should not be administered.

Test-Taking Strategy: Use the process of elimination. Note the key words "need for further instructions." General knowledge regarding digoxin administration will assist in eliminating option 2. Principles related to administering medications to children will assist in eliminating option 3. From the remaining options, select option 1 over option 4 because if the child vomits, it would be difficult to determine whether the medication also was vomited or was absorbed by the body. Review home care instructions regarding the administration of digoxin if you had difficulty with this question.

Level of Cognitive Ability: Analysis
Client Needs: Health Promotion and Maintenance
Integrated Process: Teaching/Learning
Content Area: Child health
Reference: Wong, D., Hockenberry-Eaton, M. (2000). *Wong's essentials of pediatric nursing* (6th ed., p. 953). St. Louis: Mosby.

6. **3**

Rationale: In tricuspid atresia, no communication exists from the right atrium to the right ventricle. Option 1 describes transposition of the great arteries. Frequent episodes of hypercyanotic spells occur in tetralogy of Fallot. Option 4 describes truncus arteriosus.

Test-Taking Strategy: Use the process of elimination. Note the relationship between "tricuspid atresia" and the description in option 3. Recalling that the tricuspid valve is located between the right atrium and the right ventricle will direct you to this option. Review the characteristics of tricuspid atresia if you had difficulty with this question.

Level of Cognitive Ability: Comprehension
Client Needs: Physiological Integrity
Integrated Process: Nursing Process—planning
Content Area: Child health
Reference: Wong, D., Hockenberry-Eaton, M. (2000). *Wong's essentials of pediatric nursing* (6th ed., p. 945). St. Louis: Mosby.

7. **3**

Rationale: A child with transposition of the great arteries may receive prostaglandin E_1 temporarily to increase blood mixing if systemic and pulmonary mixing is inadequate to maintain adequate cardiac output. Options 1, 2, and 4 are incorrect. In addition, tet spells occur in tetralogy of Fallot.

Test-Taking Strategy: Use the ABCs—airway, breathing, and circulation—to answer the question. Option 3 addresses circulation. Review the purpose of this medication in this condition if you had difficulty with this question.

Level of Cognitive Ability: Application
Client Needs: Physiological Integrity
Integrated Process: Nursing Process—implementation
Content Area: Child health
Reference: Wong, D., Hockenberry-Eaton, M. (2000). *Wong's essentials of pediatric nursing* (6th ed., p. 945). St. Louis: Mosby.

8. **2**

Rationale: The child with aortic stenosis shows signs of exercise intolerance, chest pain, and dizziness when standing for long periods of time. Pallor may be noted but is not specific to this type of disorder alone. Options 1 and 4 are not related to this disorder.

Test-Taking Strategy: Use the process of elimination, focusing on the disorder. Options 1 and 4 can be easily eliminated first because they are not associated with a cardiac disorder. From the remaining options, noting the word "specifically" in the stem of the question will direct you to option 2. Review the manifestations associated with aortic stenosis if you had difficulty with this question.

Level of Cognitive Ability: Analysis
Client Needs: Physiological Integrity
Integrated Process: Communication and Documentation
Content Area: Child health
Reference: Wong, D., Hockenberry-Eaton, M. (2000). *Wong's essentials of pediatric nursing* (6th ed., p. 942). St. Louis: Mosby.

9. **2**

Rationale: The mother should be instructed that lotions and powders should not be applied to the incision site. Options 1, 3, and 4 are accurate instructions regarding home care after cardiac surgery.

Test-Taking Strategy: Use the process of elimination. Note the key words "indicates a need for further instructions" in the stem of the question. Using general principles related to postoperative incisional site care will direct you to option 2. Review home care instructions following cardiac surgery if you had difficulty with this question.

Level of Cognitive Ability: Analysis
Client Needs: Health Promotion and Maintenance
Integrated Process: Teaching/Learning
Content Area: Child health
Reference: James, S., Ashwill, J., & Droske, S. (2002). *Nursing care of children: Principles & practice* (2nd ed., p. 721). Philadelphia: W. B. Saunders.

10. **1**

Rationale: Rheumatic fever characteristically presents 2 to 6 weeks after an untreated or partially treated group A β-hemolytic streptococcal infection of the upper respiratory tract. Initially, the nurse determines whether the child had a sore throat or an unexplained fever within the past 2 months. Options 2, 3, and 4 are unrelated to rheumatic fever.

Test-Taking Strategy: Use the process of elimination. Note the similarity between rheumatic "fever" in the question and the word "fever" in the correct option. If you had difficulty with this question, review the etiology related to rheumatic fever.

Level of Cognitive Ability: Analysis
Client Needs: Physiological Integrity
Integrated Process: Nursing Process—assessment
Content Area: Child health
Reference: James, S., Ashwill, J., & Droske, S. (2002). *Nursing care of children: Principles & practice* (2nd ed., p. 726). Philadelphia: W. B. Saunders.

11. **1**

Rationale: Antiinflammatory agents including aspirin may be prescribed for the child with rheumatic fever. Aspirin should not be given to a child who has chickenpox or other viral infections such as the flu. Options 2 and 4 are

clinical manifestations of rheumatic fever. Facial edema may be associated with the development of a cardiac complication.
Test-Taking Strategy: Use the process of elimination. Options 2 and 4 can be eliminated because they are similar. Knowledge that facial edema may indicate a cardiac complication will assist in eliminating this option. Review the contraindications related to the use of aspirin if you had difficulty with this question.
Level of Cognitive Ability: Analysis
Client Needs: Physiological Integrity
Integrated Process: Nursing Process—implementation
Content Area: Child health
References: Hodgson, B., & Kizior, R. (2003). *Saunders nursing drug handbook 2003* (p. 83). Philadelphia: W. B. Saunders.
McKinney, E., Ashwill, J., Murray, S., James, S., Gorrie, T., & Droske, S. (2000). *Maternal-child nursing* (p. 1275). Philadelphia: W. B. Saunders.

12. 4
Rationale: A diagnosis of rheumatic fever is confirmed by the presence of two major manifestations or one major and two minor manifestations from the Jones criteria. In addition, evidence of a recent streptococcal infection is confirmed by a positive antistreptolysin O titer, streptozyme assay, or an anti-DNase B assay. Options 1, 2, and 3 will not assist in confirming the diagnosis of rheumatic fever.
Test-Taking Strategy: Use the process of elimination. Recalling that rheumatic fever characteristically is associated with streptococcal infection will direct you easily to option 4. If you had difficulty with this question, review the Jones criteria.
Level of Cognitive Ability: Analysis
Client Needs: Physiological Integrity
Integrated Process: Nursing Process—assessment
Content Area: Child health
Reference: McKinney, E., Ashwill, J., Murray, S., James, S., Gorrie, T., & Droske, S. (2000). *Maternal-child nursing* (p. 1275). Philadelphia: W. B. Saunders.

13. 4
Rationale: Kawasaki disease, also called mucocutaneous lymph node syndrome, is a febrile generalized vasculitis of unknown origin. Option 1 describes human immunodeficiency virus infection. Option 2 describes rheumatic fever. Option 3 describes systemic lupus erythematosus.
Test-Taking Strategy: Knowledge regarding the description of Kawasaki disease is required to answer this question. Review this disorder if you are unfamiliar with it.
Level of Cognitive Ability: Comprehension
Client Needs: Physiological Integrity
Integrated Process: Nursing Process—implementation
Content Area: Child health
Reference: James, S., Ashwill, J., & Droske, S. (2002). *Nursing care of children: Principles & practice* (2nd ed., p. 727). Philadelphia: W. B. Saunders.

14. 1
Rationale: In the acute stage the child has a fever, conjunctival hyperemia, a red throat, swollen hands, a rash, and enlargement of the cervical lymph nodes. In the subacute stage, cracking lips and fissures, desquamation of the skin on the tips of the fingers and toes, joint pain, cardiac manifestations, and thrombocytosis occur. In the convalescent stage the child appears normal, but signs of inflammation may be present.
Test-Taking Strategy: Use the process of elimination. Noting the key words "acute stage" in the question will assist in directing you to option 1. Review the clinical manifestations associated with each stage of Kawasaki disease if you had difficulty with this question.
Level of Cognitive Ability: Analysis
Client Needs: Physiological Integrity
Integrated Process: Nursing Process—assessment
Content Area: Child health
Reference: James, S., Ashwill, J., & Droske, S. (2002). *Nursing care of children: Principles & practice* (2nd ed., p. 727). Philadelphia: W. B. Saunders.

15. 2
Rationale: Immune globulin is administered intravenously to the child with Kawasaki disease to decrease the incidence of coronary artery lesions and aneurysms and to decrease fever and inflammation. Options 1, 3, and 4 are not components of the treatment plan for this disease.
Test-Taking Strategy: Use the process of elimination. Remember that the pharmacological treatment for this disease is acetylsalicylic acid (aspirin) and intravenously administered immune globulin. If you had difficulty with this question, review the treatment plan for the child with Kawasaki disease.
Level of Cognitive Ability: Analysis
Client Needs: Physiological Integrity
Integrated Process: Nursing Process—analysis
Content Area: Child health
Reference: Wong, D., Hockenberry-Eaton, M. (2000). *Wong's essentials of pediatric nursing* (6th ed., p. 975). St. Louis: Mosby.

CRITICAL THINKING: FILL IN THE BLANK
Answer: The nurse places the infant in a knee-chest position.
Rationale: If a hypercyanotic spell occurs, the nurse immediately places the infant in a knee-chest position. This position improves systemic arterial oxygen saturation.
Test-Taking Strategy: Focus on the issue of the question, a hypercyanotic spell. Think about the position that will improve oxygenation. Review the interventions if a hypercyanotic spell occurs in an infant, if you had difficulty with this question.
Level of Cognitive Ability: Application
Client Needs: Physiological Integrity
Integrated Process: Nursing Process—implementation
Content Area: Child health
Reference: James, S., Ashwill, J., & Droske, S. (2002). *Nursing care of children: Principles & practice* (2nd ed., p. 711). Philadelphia: W. B. Saunders.

REFERENCES

Hodgson, B., & Kizior, R. (2003). *Saunders nursing drug handbook 2003*. Philadelphia: W. B. Saunders.

James, S., Ashwill, J., & Droske, S. (2002). *Nursing care of children: Principles & practice* (2nd ed.). Philadelphia: W. B. Saunders.

McKinney, E., Ashwill, J., Murray, S., James, S., Gorrie, T., & Droske, S. (2000). *Maternal-child nursing*. Philadelphia: W. B. Saunders.

Wong, D., Hockenberry-Eaton, M. (2000). *Wong's essentials of pediatric nursing* (6th ed.). St. Louis: Mosby.

Wong, D., Perry, S., & Hockenberry, M. (2002). *Maternal child nursing care* (2nd ed.). St. Louis: Mosby.

Gastrointestinal Disorders

I. VOMITING

A. Description

1. The major concerns when a child is vomiting are the risk of dehydration, the loss of fluid and electrolytes, and the development of metabolic alkalosis.
2. Additional concerns include aspiration, atelectasis, and the development of pneumonia.

B. Assessment

1. Signs of aspiration
2. Character of vomitus
3. Pain and abdominal cramping
4. Dehydration
5. Fluid and electrolyte imbalances
6. Metabolic alkalosis

C. Interventions

1. Maintain a patent airway.
2. Position the child on side to prevent aspiration.
3. Monitor vital signs.
4. Monitor the character, amount, and frequency of vomiting.
5. Assess the force of the vomiting, for projectile vomiting indicates pyloric **stenosis** or increased intracranial pressure.
6. Monitor intake and output and for signs of dehydration.
7. Monitor electrolyte levels.
8. Provide oral rehydration therapy as tolerated and as prescribed; start feeding slowly, with small amounts of fluid at frequent intervals.
9. Assess for diarrhea or abdominal pain.
10. Advise the parents to inform the physician when signs of dehydration, blood in vomitus, forceful vomiting, or abdominal pain is present.

II. DIARRHEA

A. Description: The major concerns when a child is having diarrhea are the risk of dehydration, the loss of fluid and electrolytes, and the development of metabolic acidosis.

B. Assessment

1. Character of stools
2. Pain and abdominal cramping
3. Dehydration
4. Fluid and electrolyte imbalances
5. Metabolic acidosis

C. Interventions

1. Monitor vital signs.
2. Monitor the character, amount, and frequency of diarrhea.
3. Monitor skin integrity.
4. Monitor intake and output and for signs of dehydration.
5. Monitor electrolyte levels.
6. For mild to moderate dehydration, provide oral rehydration therapy; avoid carbonated beverages and those containing high amounts of sugar.
7. For severe dehydration, maintain NPO status to place the bowel at rest and provide fluid and electrolyte replacement by the intravenous (IV) route as prescribed; if potassium is prescribed for IV administration, ensure that the child has voided before administering.
8. Reintroduce a normal diet once rehydration is achieved.
9. Provide enteric isolation as required.
10. Instruct the parents in good hand-washing technique.

III. CLEFT LIP AND CLEFT PALATE (FIG. 39-1)

A. Description

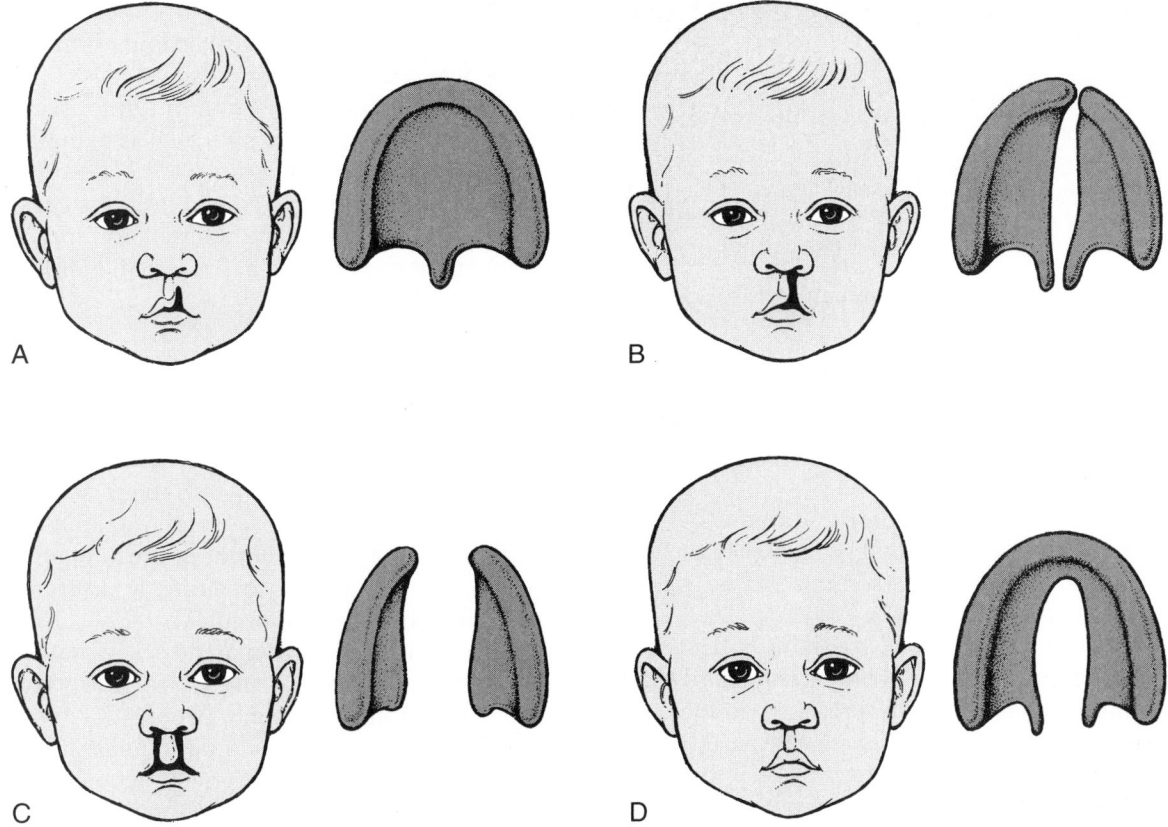

FIG. 39-1 Variations in clefts of lip and palate at birth. **A,** Notch in vermilion border. **B,** Unilateral cleft lip and palate. **C,** Bilateral cleft lip and palate. **D,** Cleft palate. (From Hockenberry, M. J. [2005]. *Wong's essentials of pediatric nursing* [7th ed.]. St. Louis: Mosby.)

1. Cleft lip or cleft palate is a congenital anomaly that occurs as a result of failure of soft tissue or bony structure to fuse during embryonic development.
2. The defects involve abnormal openings in the lip or palate that may occur unilaterally or bilaterally and are readily apparent at birth.
3. Causes include genetic, **hereditary,** and environmental factors; exposure to radiation or rubella virus; chromosome abnormalities; and teratogenic factors.
4. Closure of cleft lip defect precedes that of the palate and is performed usually during the first weeks of life.
5. Cleft palate repair is performed sometime between 12 and 18 months of age to allow for the palatal changes that take place with normal **growth**; a cleft palate is closed before the child develops faulty speech habits.

B. Assessment
1. Cleft lip can range from a slight notch to a complete separation from the floor of the nose.
2. Cleft palate can include nasal distortion, midline or bilateral cleft, and variable extension from the uvula and soft and hard palate.

C. Interventions
1. Assess the ability to suck, swallow, handle normal secretions, and breathe without distress.

2. Assess fluid and calorie intake daily and monitor weight.
3. Modify feeding techniques; plan to use specialized feeding techniques, obturators, and special nipples and feeders.
4. Hold the child in an upright position and direct the formula to the side and back of the mouth to prevent aspiration; feed small amounts gradually and burp frequently.
5. Position on side after feeding.
6. Keep suction equipment and bulb syringe at bedside.
7. Encourage breast-feeding if appropriate.
8. Teach the parents special feeding or suctioning techniques.
9. Teach the parents the ESSR (enlarge, stimulate sucking, swallow, rest) method of feeding (Box 39-1).
10. Encourage the parents to describe their feelings related to the deformity.

D. Interventions postoperatively
1. Cleft lip repair
   a. A lip protector device may be taped securely to the cheeks to prevent trauma to the suture line.
   b. Position the child on the side lateral to the repair or on the back; avoid the prone position

to prevent rubbing of the surgical site on the mattress.

   c. After feeding, cleanse the suture line of formula or serosanguineous drainage with a cotton-tipped swab dipped in saline; apply antibiotic ointment if prescribed.

2. Cleft palate repair
   a. Child is allowed to lie on the abdomen.
   b. Feedings are resumed by bottle, breast, or cup.
   c. Oral packing may be secured to the palate (removed in 2 to 3 days).
   d. Do not allow the child to brush his or her teeth.
   e. Instruct the parents to avoid offering hard food items to the child, such as toast or cookies.

3. Soft elbow or jacket restraints may be used (check agency policies and procedures) to keep the child from touching the repair site; remove restraints at least every 2 hours to assess skin integrity and allow for exercising the arms.

4. Avoid contact with sharp objects near the surgical site.

5. Avoid the use of oral suction or placing objects in the mouth such as a tongue depressor, thermometer, straws, spoons, forks, or pacifiers.

6. Provide analgesics for pain.
7. Instruct the parents in feeding techniques and in the care of the surgical site.
8. Instruct the parents to monitor for signs of infection at the surgical site, such as redness, swelling, or drainage.
9. Encourage the parents to hold the child.
10. Initiate appropriate referrals for speech impairment or language-based **learning** difficulties.

IV. ESOPHAGEAL ATRESIA AND TRACHEOESOPHAGEAL FISTULA (FIG. 39-2)

A. Description
1. The esophagus terminates before it reaches the stomach or a fistula is present that forms an unnatural connection with the trachea.
2. The condition causes oral intake to enter the lungs or a large amount of air to enter the stomach, and choking, coughing, and severe abdominal distention can occur.
3. Aspiration pneumonia and severe respiratory distress will develop, and death will occur without surgical intervention.
4. Treatment includes maintenance of a patent airway, prevention of pneumonia, gastric or blind pouch decompression, supportive therapy, and surgical repair.

B. Assessment
1. Frothy saliva in the mouth and nose and drooling
2. The "3 Cs"—coughing and choking during feedings and unexplained cyanosis
3. **Regurgitation** and vomiting
4. Abdominal distention

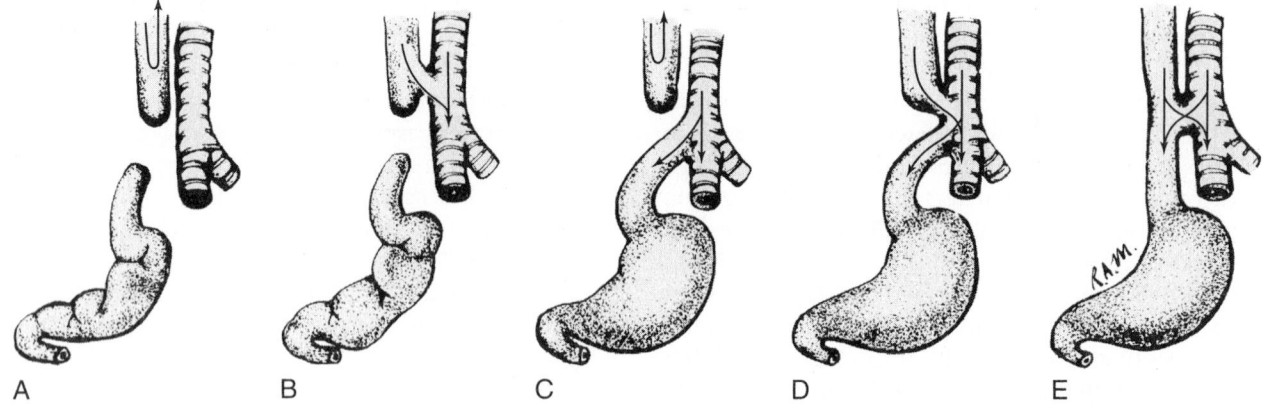

A   B   C   D   E

FIG. 39-2   Congenital atresia of esophagus and tracheoesophageal fistula. **A,** Upper and lower segments of esophagus end in blind sac (occurring in 5% to 8% of such infants). **B,** Upper segment of esophagus ends in atresia and connects to trachea by fistulous tract (occurring rarely). **C,** Upper segment of esophagus ends in blind pouch; lower segment connects with trachea by small fistulous tract (occurring in 80% to 95% of such infants). **D,** Both segments of esophagus connect by fistulous tracts to trachea (occurring in less than 1% of such infants). Infant may aspirate with first feeding. **E,** Esophagus is continuous but connects by fistulous tract to trachea; known as H-type. (From Wong, D., Perry, S., & Hockenberry, M. [2002]. *Maternal child nursing care* [2nd ed.]. St. Louis: Mosby.)

5. Inability to pass a small-gauge (such as a No. 5 French) orogastric feeding tube via the mouth into the stomach.

C. Interventions preoperatively

1. Infant may be placed in an incubator or radiant warmer in which humidified oxygen is administered (intubation and mechanical ventilation may be necessary if respiratory distress occurs).
2. Maintain an NPO status.
3. Maintain IV fluids as prescribed.
4. Suction accumulated secretions from the mouth and pharynx.
5. A double-lumen catheter is placed into the upper esophageal pouch and attached to intermittent or continuous low suction to keep the pouch empty of secretions; it is irrigated with normal saline as prescribed to prevent clogging.
6. Maintain in an upright position to facilitate drainage and to prevent aspiration of gastric secretions.
7. A gastrostomy tube may be placed and is left open so that air entering the stomach through the fistula can escape, minimizing the danger of **regurgitation**.
8. Administer broad-spectrum antibiotics as prescribed because of the high risk for aspiration pneumonia.

D. Interventions postoperatively

1. Monitor respiratory status.
2. Maintain IV fluids, antibiotics, and parenteral nutrition as prescribed.
3. Monitor intake and output and weight daily.
4. Inspect surgical site.
5. Provide care to the chest tube if in place.
6. Assess for signs of pain.
7. Assess for dehydration and possible fluid overload.
8. Monitor for anastomotic leaks as evidenced by purulent chest drainage, increased temperature, and an increased white blood cell count.
9. The double-lumen catheter is attached to low suction.
10. If a gastrostomy tube is present, it is attached to gravity drainage until the infant can tolerate feedings (usually the fifth to seventh day postoperatively).
11. Before oral feedings and removal of the chest tube, a barium swallow is performed to verify the integrity of the esophageal anastomosis.
12. Before feeding, the gastrostomy tube is elevated and secured above the level of the stomach to allow gastric secretions to pass to the duodenum and swallowed air to escape through the open gastrostomy tube.
13. Feedings through the gastrostomy tube may be prescribed until the anastomosis is healed.
14. Oral feedings are begun with sterile water, followed by frequent small feedings of formula.

15. The gastrostomy tube may be removed before discharge or may be maintained for supplemental feedings at home.
16. If the infant is awaiting esophageal replacement, a cervical esophagostomy may be performed.
17. Assess cervical esophagostomy site for redness, breakdown, or exudate (continued discharge or saliva can cause skin breakdown); remove drainage frequently and apply a protective ointment, a barrier dressing, and/or a collection device.
18. If the infant is awaiting esophageal replacement, nonnutritive sucking is provided by a pacifier; infants who remain NPO for extended periods and have not received oral stimulation frequently may have difficulty eating by mouth after surgery and develop oral hypersensitivity and food aversion.
19. Instruct the parents in the techniques of suctioning, gastrostomy tube care and feedings, and skin site care as appropriate.
20. Instruct parents to identify behaviors that indicate the need for suctioning, signs of respiratory distress, and signs of a constricted esophagus (poor feeding, dysphagia, drooling, or regurgitated undigested food).

V. GASTROESOPHAGEAL REFLUX

A. Description

1. Gastroesophageal reflux is backflow of gastric contents into the esophagus as a result of relaxation or incompetence of the lower esophageal or cardiac sphincter.
2. Complications include esophagitis, esophageal strictures, aspiration of gastric contents, and aspiration pneumonia.
3. Most infants with gastroesophageal reflux have a mild problem that improves in about 1 year and requires only medical therapy.
4. Treatment (Box 39-2)

B. Assessment

1. Passive **regurgitation** or emesis
2. Poor weight gain
3. Hematemesis and melena
4. Irritability
5. Heartburn (in older children)
6. Anemia from blood loss

C. Interventions

1. Assess amount and characteristics of emesis.

BOX 39-2

Treatment for Gastroesophageal Reflux

Diet
Positioning
Medications
Surgery: performed when severe complications occur

2. Assess the relation of vomiting to the times of feedings and infant activity.
3. Monitor breath sounds before and after feedings.
4. Place suction equipment at the bedside.
5. Monitor intake and output.
6. Monitor for signs and symptoms of dehydration.
7. Maintain IV fluids as prescribed.

▲ D. Positioning: Place child in the flat prone position or the head-elevated prone position following feedings and at night.

E. Diet
1. Provide small, frequent feedings to decrease the amount of **regurgitation**; nasogastric tube feedings are indicated if severe **regurgitation** and poor **growth** are present.
2. For infants, thicken formula by adding 1 tablespoon of rice cereal per 6 oz of formula and crosscut the nipple; monitor for coughing during feeding.
3. Breast-feeding may continue, and the mother may provide more frequent feeding times or express milk for thickening with rice cereal.
▲ 4. Burp the infant frequently when feeding and handle the infant minimally after feedings.
5. For toddlers, feed solids first, followed by liquids.
6. The parents are instructed to avoid feeding the child fatty foods, chocolate, tomato products, carbonated liquids, fruit juices, citrus products, and spicy foods.
7. Avoid vigorous play after feeding and avoid feeding just before bedtime.

F. Medications
1. Administer antacids and histamine receptor antagonists as prescribed to reduce the amount of acid present in gastric secretions and to prevent esophagitis.
2. Administer prokinetic agents to accelerate gastric emptying and decrease reflux.
3. Administer acetaminophen (Tylenol) as prescribed to relieve reflux pain.

G. Surgery
1. If surgery is prescribed, it will require a procedure known as fundoplication, in which a wrap to the stomach fundus is made around the distal esophagus (restores the competence of the lower esophageal sphincter).
2. A gastrostomy may be performed at the same time as the fundoplication for decompression of the stomach postoperatively.
3. Fundoplication may be combined with pyloroplasty in children with gastroesophageal reflux who also have delayed gastric emptying.
4. Postoperative care is similar to that for other types of abdominal surgery.
5. Instruct parents in the potential postoperative problems, such as bloating symptoms or discomfort after consuming large, solid meals.

VI. HYPERTROPHIC PYLORIC STENOSIS (FIG. 39-3)

A. Description
1. Hypertrophy of the circular muscles of the pylorus causes narrowing of the pyloric canal between the stomach and the duodenum.
2. The stenosis usually develops in the first few weeks of life, causing projectile vomiting, dehydration, metabolic alkalosis, and failure to thrive.

B. Assessment
1. Vomiting that progresses from mild **regurgitation** to forceful and projectile and usually occurs after a feeding.
2. Vomitus contains gastric contents such as milk or formula, may contain mucus, may be blood tinged, and does not usually contain bile.
3. The child exhibits hunger and irritability.
4. Peristaltic waves are visible from left to right across the epigastrium during or immediately following a feeding.
5. Olive-shaped mass is in the epigastrium just right of the umbilicus.

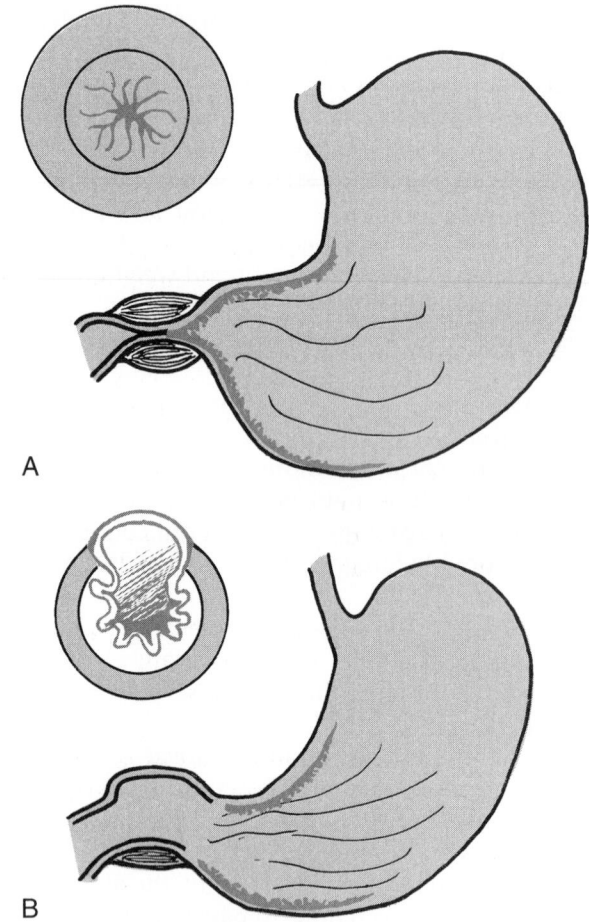

A

B

FIG. 39-3 Hypertrophic pyloric stenosis. **A,** Enlarged muscular area nearly obliterates pyloric channel. **B,** Longitudinal surgical division of muscle down to submucosa establishes adequate passageway. (From Hockenberry, M. J. [2005]. *Wong's essentials of pediatric nursing* [7th ed.]. St. Louis: Mosby.)

6. Dehydration and malnutrition can occur.
7. Electrolyte imbalances can occur.
8. Metabolic alkalosis can occur.
C. Interventions
 1. Monitor vital signs.
 2. Monitor intake and output and weight.
 3. Monitor for signs of dehydration and electrolyte imbalances.
 4. Prepare the child and parents for pyloromyotomy if prescribed.
D. Pyloromyotomy
 1. Description: An incision through the muscle fibers of the pylorus that may be performed by laparoscopy
 2. Interventions preoperatively
  a. Monitor hydration status by daily weights, intake and output, and urine for specific gravity.
  b. Correct fluid and electrolyte imbalances; administer fluids intravenously as prescribed for rehydration.
  c. Maintain NPO status.
  d. Monitor the number and character of stools.
  e. Maintain patency of the nasogastric tube placed for stomach decompression.
 3. Interventions postoperatively.
  a. Monitor intake and output.
  b. Maintain IV fluids until the infant is taking and retaining adequate amounts by mouth.
  c. Begin small, frequent feedings of glucose, water, or electrolyte solution 4 to 6 hours postoperatively as prescribed; advance the diet to formula 24 hours postoperatively as prescribed.
  d. Gradually increase amount and interval between feedings until a full feeding schedule is reinstated, usually by 48 hours postoperatively.
  e. Feed the infant slowly, burping frequently; handle the infant minimally after feedings.
  f. Monitor for abdominal distention.
  g. Monitor the surgical wound and for signs of infection.
  h. Instruct the parents about wound care and feeding.

VII. LACTOSE INTOLERANCE

A. Description: Inability to tolerate lactose as a result of an absence or deficiency of lactase, an enzyme found in the secretions of the small intestine that is required for the digestion of lactose
B. Assessment (Box 39-3)
C. Interventions
 1. Eliminate the offending dairy product or administer an enzyme replacement.
 2. Provide information to parents about enzyme tablets (Lactaid, Lactrase, Dairy Ease) that predigest the lactose in milk or supplement the body's own lactase.

BOX 39-3

Assessment Findings: Lactose Intolerance

Symptoms occurring after the ingestion of milk products
Abdominal distention
Crampy, abdominal pain
Diarrhea
Excessive flatus

---

 3. In infants, soy-based formulas can be substituted for cow's milk formula or human milk.
 4. Provide calcium and vitamin D supplements to prevent deficiency.
 5. Limit milk consumption to one glass at a time.
 6. If the child consumes milk, the child should drink it with other foods rather than alone.
 7. Encourage consumption of hard cheese, cottage cheese, or yogurt (contains inactive lactase enzyme) instead of drinking milk.
 8. Encourage consumption of small amounts of dairy foods daily to help colonic bacteria adapt to ingested lactose.
 9. Instruct parents about the importance of calcium and vitamin D supplements.
 10. Instruct parents about the foods that contain lactose, including hidden sources.

VIII. CELIAC DISEASE

A. Description
 1. Celiac disease also is known as gluten enteropathy or tropical sprue.
 2. Intolerance to gluten, the protein component of wheat, barley, rye, and oats, is characteristic.
 3. Celiac disease results in the accumulation of the amino acid glutamine, which is toxic to intestinal mucosal cells.
 4. Intestinal villi atrophy occurs, which affects absorption of ingested nutrients.
 5. Symptoms of the disorder occur most often between the ages of 1 and 5 years; there is usually an interval of several months between the introduction of gluten in the diet and the onset of symptoms.
 6. Strict dietary avoidance of gluten minimizes the risk of developing malignant lymphoma of the small intestine and other gastrointestinal malignancies.
B. Assessment
 1. Acute or insidious diarrhea; stools are watery and pale with an offensive odor
 2. Anorexia
 3. Abdominal pain and distention
 4. Muscle wasting, particularly in the buttocks and extremities
 5. Vomiting
 6. Anemia
 7. Irritability

▲ C. Celiac crisis (Box 39-4)
▲ D. Interventions
▲   1. Gluten-free diet and substituting corn, rice, and millet as grain sources
▲   2. Lifelong elimination of gluten sources such as wheat, rye, oats, and barley
   3. Mineral and vitamin supplements, including iron, folic acid, and fat-soluble supplements A, D, E, and K
   4. Teaching the parents about a gluten-free diet and to read food labels carefully for hidden sources of gluten (Box 39-5)
   5. Instructing the parents in the measures to prevent celiac crisis
   6. Informing the parents about the Celiac Sprue Association/United States of America

IX. APPENDICITIS

A. Description
   1. Appendicitis is inflammation of the appendix.
   2. When the appendix becomes inflamed or infected, perforation may occur within a matter of hours, leading to peritonitis and sepsis.
   3. Treatment is surgical removal of the appendix before perforation occurs.
B. Assessment
   1. Pain in periumbilical area that descends to the right lower quadrant
▲   2. Abdominal pain that is most intense at McBurney's point
   3. Referred pain indicating the presence of peritoneal irritation

   4. Rebound tenderness and abdominal rigidity
   5. Elevated white blood cell count
   6. Side-lying position with abdominal guarding (legs flexed)
   7. Difficulty walking and pain in the right hip
   8. Low-grade fever
   9. Anorexia, nausea, and vomiting after the pain develops
   10. Diarrhea
C. Peritonitis   ▲
   1. Description: Results from a perforated appendix
      a. Increased fever
      b. Sudden relief of pain after the perforation and then a subsequent increase in pain accompanied by right guarding of the abdomen
      c. Progressive abdominal distention
      d. Tachycardia and tachypnea
      e. Pallor
      f. Chills
      g. Restlessness and irritability
   2. Assessment
D. Appendectomy
   1. Description: Surgical removal of the appendix
   2. Interventions preoperatively
      a. Maintain NPO status.
      b. Administer fluids and electrolytes intravenously as prescribed to prevent dehydration and correct electrolyte imbalances.
      c. Monitor for signs of ruptured appendix and peritonitis.
      d. Administer antibiotics as prescribed.
      e. Monitor for changes in the level of pain.
      f. Monitor bowel sounds.
      g. Position in right side-lying or low to semi-Fowler
         position to promote comfort.
      h. Apply ice packs to the abdomen for 20 to 30 minutes every hour if prescribed.
      i. Avoid the application of heat to the abdomen.
      j. Avoid laxatives or enemas.
   3. Interventions postoperatively
      a. Monitor temperature for signs of infection.
      b. Maintain NPO status until bowel function has returned; advance diet gradually as tolerated and as prescribed when bowel sounds return.
      c. Assess incision for signs of infection, such as redness, swelling, drainage, and pain.
      d. If perforation of the appendix had occurred, expect a drain (Penrose drain) to be inserted or the incision may be left open to heal from the inside out.
      e. Expect that drainage from the drain may be profuse for the first 12 hours.
      f. Position the client in right side-lying or low to   ▲
         semi-Fowler position with legs flexed to facilitate drainage.
      g. Change the dressing as prescribed, and record type and amount of drainage.

BOX 39-4

Celiac Crisis

Crisis is precipitated by infection, fasting, and ingestion of gluten.
Crisis can lead to electrolyte imbalance, rapid dehydration, and severe acidosis.
Crisis causes profuse watery diarrhea and vomiting.

BOX 39-5

Basics of a Gluten-Free Diet

FOODS ALLOWED
Meat such as beef, pork, and poultry and fish, eggs, milk and dairy products, vegetables, fruits, grains, rice, corn, gluten-free wheat flour, puffed rice, cornflakes, cornmeal, and precooked gluten-free cereals

FOODS PROHIBITED
Commercially prepared ice cream; malted milk; prepared puddings; grains, including anything made from wheat, rye, oats, or barley, such as breads, rolls, cookies, cakes, crackers, cereal, spaghetti, macaroni noodles, beer, and ale

h. Perform wound irrigations if prescribed.
i. Maintain nasogastric tube suction and patency of tube if present.
j. Administer antibiotics and analgesics as prescribed.

X. HIRSCHSPRUNG'S DISEASE (FIG. 39-4)

A. Description
   1. Hirschsprung's disease is a congenital anomaly also known as congenital aganglionosis or megacolon.
   2. The disease occurs as the result of an absence of ganglion cells in the rectum and upward in the colon.
   3. The disease results in mechanical obstruction from inadequate motility in an intestinal segment.
   4. The disease may be a familial congenital defect or may be associated with other anomalies, such as Down syndrome and genital urinary abnormalities.
   5. A rectal biopsy demonstrates histologic evidence of the absence of ganglionic cells.
   6. The most serious complication is enterocolitis; signs include fever, severe prostration, gastrointestinal bleeding, and explosive watery diarrhea.
   7. Treatment for mild or moderate disease is based on relieving the chronic constipation with stool softeners and rectal irrigations; however, most children require surgery.
   8. Treatment for moderate to severe disease involves a two-step surgical procedure.
   9. Initially, in the neonatal period, a temporary colostomy is created to relieve obstruction and allow the normally innervated, dilated bowel to return to its normal size.

   10. A complete surgical repair is performed when the child weighs about 9 kg (20 pounds) via a pull-through procedure to excise portions of the bowel; at this time, the colostomy is closed.

B. Assessment
   1. Newborn infants
      a. Failure to pass meconium stool
      b. Refusal to suck
      c. Abdominal distention
      d. Bile-stained vomitus
   2. Children
      a. Failure to gain weight and delayed **growth**
      b. Abdominal distention
      c. Vomiting
      d. Constipation alternating with diarrhea
      e. Ribbonlike and foul-smelling stools

C. Interventions: medical management
   1. Dietary management
   2. Stool softeners
   3. Daily rectal irrigations with normal saline to promote adequate elimination and prevent obstruction

D. Surgical management: preoperative interventions
   1. Assess bowel function and administer bowel preparation as prescribed.
   2. Maintain NPO status.
   3. Monitor hydration and fluid and electrolyte status; provide fluids intravenously as prescribed for hydration.
   4. Administer antibiotics as prescribed to clear the bowel of bacteria.
   5. Monitor intake and output and weight.
   6. Measure abdominal girth.
   7. Avoid taking the temperature rectally.
   8. Monitor for respiratory distress associated with abdominal distention.

E. Interventions postoperatively
   1. Monitor vital signs, avoiding taking the temperature rectally.
   2. Measure abdominal girth.
   3. Assess surgical site for redness, swelling, and drainage.
   4. Assess the stoma if present for bleeding or skin breakdown (stoma should be pink and moist).
   5. Assess anal area for the presence of stool, redness, or discharge.
   6. Maintain NPO status until bowel sounds return or flatus is passed; bowel sounds usually return within 48 to 72 hours.
   7. Maintain the nasogastric tube to allow intermittent suction until peristalsis returns.
   8. Maintain IV fluids until the child tolerates appropriate oral intake; begin the diet with clear liquids, advancing to regular as tolerated and as prescribed.
   9. Assess for dehydration and fluid overload.
   10. Monitor intake and output and weight.

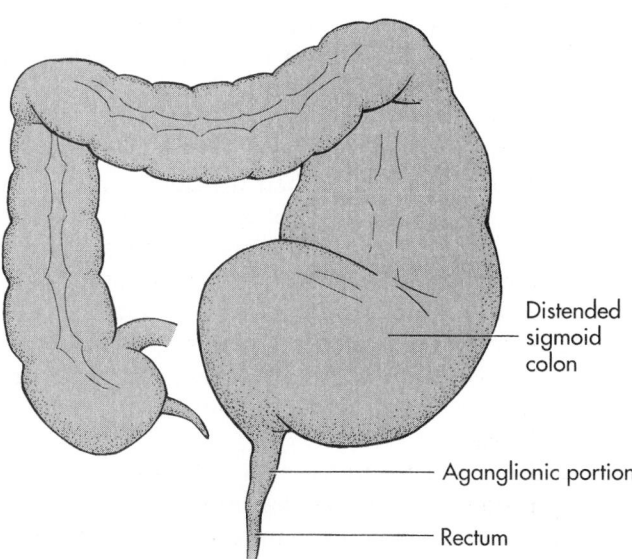

Distended
sigmoid
colon

Aganglionic portion

Rectum

FIG. 39-4   Hirschsprung's disease. (From Wong, D., Perry, S., & Hockenberry, M. [2002]. *Maternal child nursing care* [2nd ed.]. St. Louis: Mosby.)

11. Assess for pain and provide comfort measures as required.
12. Provide the parents with instructions regarding colostomy care and skin care.
13. Teach the parents about the appropriate diet and the need for adequate fluid intake.

XI. INTUSSUSCEPTION (FIG. 39-5)

A. Description
   1. Intussusception is telescoping of one portion of the bowel into another portion.
   2. The condition results in an obstruction to the passage of intestinal contents.

B. Assessment
   1. Colicky abdominal pain that causes the child to scream and draw the knees to the abdomen
   2. Vomiting of gastric contents
   3. Bile-stained fecal emesis
   4. Currant jelly–like stools containing blood and mucus
   5. Hypoactive or hyperactive bowel sounds
   6. Tender distended abdomen, possibly with a palpable sausage-shaped mass in the upper right quadrant

C. Interventions
   1. Monitor for signs of perforation and shock as evidenced by fever, increased heart rate, changes in level of consciousness or blood pressure, and respiratory distress, and report immediately.
   2. Prepare for hydrostatic reduction if prescribed (not performed if signs of perforation or shock occur).

   a. Antibiotics, IV fluids, and decompression via nasogastric tube may be prescribed.
   b. Monitor for the passage of normal, brown stool, which indicates that the intussusception has reduced itself.
   3. After hydrostatic reduction, do the following:
   a. Monitor for the return of normal bowel sounds, for the passage of barium, and the characteristics of stool.
   b. Administer clear fluids and advance the diet gradually as prescribed.
   4. If surgery is required, postoperative care is similar to that following any abdominal surgery.

XII. ABDOMINAL WALL DEFECTS

A. Omphalocele
   1. Omphalocele is a herniation of the abdominal contents through the umbilical ring (hernia of the umbilical cord), usually with an intact peritoneal sac.
   2. The protrusion is covered by a translucent sac that may contain bowel or other abdominal organs.
   3. Rupture of the sac results in evisceration of the abdominal contents.
   4. Immediately after birth, the sac is covered with sterile gauze soaked in normal saline to prevent drying of abdominal contents; a layer of plastic wrap is placed over the gauze to provide additional protection against moisture loss.
   5. Monitor vital signs every 2 to 4 hours, particularly temperature because the infant can lose heat through the sac.
   6. Preoperatively: Maintain NPO status, administer IV fluids as prescribed to maintain hydration and electrolyte balance, monitor for signs of infection, and handle the infant carefully to prevent rupture of the sac.
   7. Postoperatively: Control pain, prevent infection, maintain fluid and electrolyte balance, and ensure adequate nutrition.

B. Gastroschisis
   1. Gastroschisis occurs when the herniation of the intestine is lateral to the umbilical ring.
   2. No membrane covers the exposed bowel.
   3. The exposed bowel is covered loosely in saline-soaked pads, and the abdomen is wrapped in a plastic drape; wrapping around the exposed bowel is contraindicated because if the exposed bowel expands, wrapping could cause pressure and necrosis.
   4. Preoperatively: Care is similar to that for omphalocele; surgery is performed within several hours after birth because no membrane is covering the sac.
   5. Postoperatively: Most infants have a prolonged ileus and require mechanical ventilation and parenteral nutrition; otherwise, care is similar to that for omphalocele.

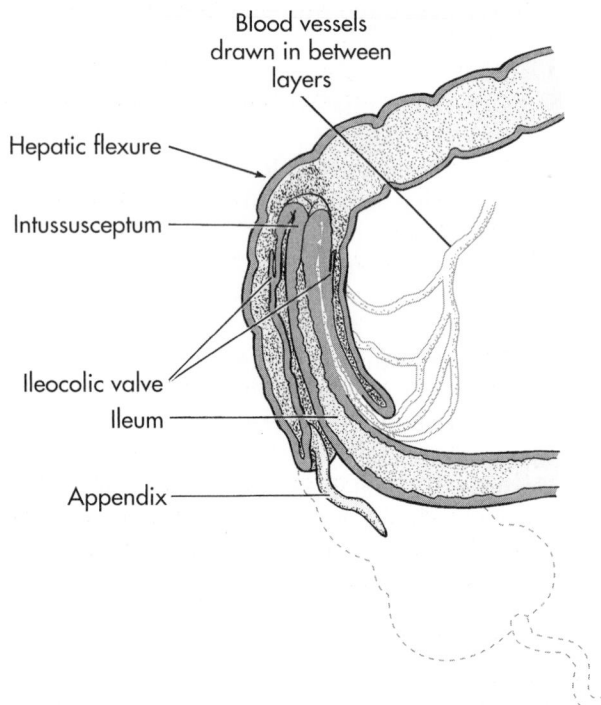

FIG. 39-5   Ileocolic intussusception. (From Hockenberry, M. J. [2005]. *Wong's essentials of pediatric nursing* [7th ed.]. St. Louis: Mosby.)

Blood vessels drawn in between layers

Hepatic flexure

Intussusceptum

Ileocolic valve

Ileum

Appendix

XIII. UMBILICAL HERNIA, INGUINAL HERNIA, OR HYDROCELE

A. Description
1. A hernia is a protrusion of the bowel through an abnormal opening in the abdominal wall.
2. In children, a hernia most commonly occurs at the umbilicus and through the inguinal canal.
3. A hydrocele is the presence of abdominal fluid in the scrotal sac.

B. Assessment
1. Umbilical hernia: soft swelling or protrusion around the umbilicus that is usually reducible with the finger
2. Inguinal hernia
   a. Painless inguinal swelling that is reducible
   b. Swelling that may disappear during periods of rest and is most noticeable when the infant cries or coughs
3. Incarcerated hernia
   a. When the descended portion of bowel becomes tightly caught in the hernial sac, compromising blood supply
   b. A medical emergency requiring surgical repair
   c. Irritability
   d. Tenderness at site
   e. Anorexia; possible vomiting
   f. Abdominal distention
   g. Difficulty defecating
   h. May lead to complete intestinal obstruction and gangrene
4. Noncommunicating hydrocele
   a. Residual peritoneal fluid is trapped with no communication to the peritoneal cavity.
   b. The hydrocele usually disappears by age 1 year.
5. Communicating hydrocele
   a. The hydrocele is associated with a hernia that remains open from the scrotum to the abdominal cavity.
   b. Assessment includes a bulge in the inguinal area or the scrotum that increases with crying or straining and decreases when the child is at rest.

C. Interventions postoperatively (hernia)
1. Monitor vital signs.
2. Assess for wound infection.
3. Monitor for redness or drainage.
4. Monitor intake and output and hydration status.
5. Advance the diet as tolerated.
6. Administer analgesics as prescribed.

D. Interventions postoperatively (hydrocele)
1. Provide ice bags and a scrotal support to relieve pain and swelling.
2. Instruct the child and parents to avoid tub bathing until the incision heals.
3. Instruct the child and parents that the child should avoid strenuous physical activities.

XIV. CONSTIPATION AND ENCOPRESIS

A. Description
1. Constipation is the infrequent and difficult passage of dry, hard stools.
2. **Encopresis** is fecal incontinence, and children often complain that soiling is involuntary and occurs without warning.
3. If the child does not have a neurological or anatomical disorder, **encopresis** is usually the result of fecal impaction and an enlarged rectum caused by chronic constipation.

B. Assessment
1. Constipation
   a. Abdominal pain and cramping without distention
   b. Palpable movable fecal masses
   c. Normal or decreased bowel sounds
   d. Malaise and headache
   e. Anorexia, nausea, and vomiting
2. **Encopresis**
   a. Evidence of soiling of clothing
   b. Scratching or rubbing of anal area
   c. Fecal odor
   d. Social withdrawal

C. Interventions
1. Simple constipation may resolve by using only dietary changes or methods to change the habit of retention.
2. Severe **encopresis** may require that interventions be continued over a period of 3 to 6 months.
3. Overcoming withholding
   a. Administer enemas as prescribed until the impaction is cleared.
   b. Monitor for hypernatremia or hyperphosphatemia when administering repeated enemas.
   c. Administer stool softener or laxative as prescribed.
   d. Administer mineral oil, 30 to 75 mL bid, as prescribed; administer chilled or mixed with cold drinks to disguise the taste.
4. Dietary changes
   a. Increase water and fiber intake.
   b. Decrease sugar and milk intake.
   c. Administer fat-soluble vitamins during the use of mineral oil because the oil can interfere with vitamin absorption in the small intestine.
5. Changing the retention habit: Have the child sit on the toilet for 5 to 10 minutes approximately 20 to 30 minutes after breakfast and dinner to assist with defecation.

XV. IRRITABLE BOWEL SYNDROME

A. Description
1. Irritable bowel syndrome results from increased motility that can lead to spasm and pain.
2. The diagnosis is based on the elimination of pathologic conditions.

3. The syndrome is a self-limiting, intermittent problem with no definitive treatment.
4. Stress and emotional factors may contribute to its occurrence.

B. Assessment
1. Diffuse abdominal pain unrelated to meals or activity.
2. Alternating constipation and diarrhea with the presence of undigested food and mucus in the stool.

C. Interventions
1. Reassure that the problem is self-limiting and intermittent and will resolve; medication may be prescribed.
2. Encourage the maintenance of a healthy, well-balanced, moderate-fiber diet.
3. Encourage health promotion activities such as exercise and school activities.
4. Inform the parents of psychosocial resources if required.

XVI. IMPERFORATE ANUS

A. Description: Incomplete development or absence of the anus in its normal position in the perineum
B. Assessment (Box 39-6)
C. Interventions
1. Determine patency of the anus.
2. Monitor for the presence of stool in the urine and vagina and report immediately.
D. Interventions postoperatively
1. Monitor the skin for signs of infection.
2. Position side-lying with legs flexed or in a prone position to keep the hips elevated to reduce edema and pressure on the surgical site.
3. Keep the anal surgical incision clean and dry, and monitor for redness, swelling, or drainage.
4. Maintain NPO status and nasogastric tube if in place.
5. Maintain IV fluids until gastrointestinal motility returns.
6. Provide colostomy care if present as prescribed.
7. A fresh colostomy stoma will be red and edematous, but this should decrease with time.
8. Instruct the parents to perform anal dilation if prescribed to achieve and maintain bowel patency.
9. Instruct the parents to use only dilators supplied by the physician and a water-soluble lubricant and to insert the dilator no more than 1 to 2 cm into the anus to prevent damage to the mucosa.

BOX 39-6

Assessment Findings: Imperforate Anus

Failure to pass meconium stool
Absence or stenosis of the anal rectal canal
Presence of an anal membrane
External fistula to the perineum or genitourinary system

XVII. HEPATITIS

A. This section contains specific information regarding hepatitis as it relates to infants and children; refer to Chapters 25 and 55 for additional information on hepatitis
B. Description: An acute or chronic inflammation of the liver that may be caused by a virus, a medication reaction, or another disease process
C. Hepatitis A (HAV)
1. Highest incidence of HAV infection occurs among preschool or school-aged children under 15 years of age.
2. Many affected children are asymptomatic, but mild nausea, vomiting, and diarrhea may occur.
3. Infected children who are asymptomatic still can spread HAV to others.
D. Hepatitis B (HBV)
1. Most HBV in children is acquired perinatally.
2. Newborn infants are at risk if the mother is infected with HBV or was a carrier of HBV during pregnancy.
3. Possible routes of maternal-fetal (infant) transmission include leakage of the virus across the placenta late in pregnancy or during labor; ingestion of amniotic fluid or maternal blood; and breast-feeding, especially if the mother has cracked nipples.
4. The severity in the infant varies from no liver disease to fulminant (severe, acute course) or chronic, active disease.
5. In children and adolescents, HBV occurs in specific high-risk groups, including children with hemophilia or other disorders who have received multiple blood transfusions, children or adolescents involved in drug abuse, institutionalized children, and preschool children in endemic areas, and if involvement with heterosexual activity or sexual activity with homosexual males occurs.
6. Infection with HBV can cause a carrier state and lead to eventual cirrhosis or hepatocellular carcinoma in adulthood.
E. Hepatitis C (HCV)
1. Transmission is primarily by the parenteral route.
2. Some children may be asymptomatic, but HCV often becomes a chronic condition and can cause cirrhosis and hepatocellular carcinoma.
F. Hepatitis D
1. Infection occurs in children already infected with HBV.
2. Acute and chronic forms tend to be more severe than HBV and can lead to cirrhosis.
G. Hepatitis E
1. Infection is uncommon in children.
2. Infection is not a chronic condition, does not cause chronic liver disease, and has no carrier state.
H. Hepatitis G
1. Hepatitis G virus is blood borne and is similar to HCV.

BOX 39-7

Assessment Findings: Hepatitis

PRODROMAL OR ANICTERIC PHASE
Lasts 5 to 7 days
Absence of jaundice
Anorexia, malaise, lethargy, easy fatigability
Fever (especially in adolescents)
Nausea and vomiting
Epigastric or right upper quadrant abdominal pain
Arthralgia and skin rashes (more likely with hepatitis B
  virus)
Hepatomegaly

ICTERIC PHASE
Jaundice, which is best assessed in the sclera, nail beds,
  and mucous membranes
Dark urine and pale stools
Pruritus

---

2. High-risk groups include transfusion recipients, IV drug users, and individuals infected with HCV.
3. Individuals are often asymptomatic, and most infections are chronic.

I. Assessment (Box 39-7)

J. Diagnostic evaluation: Refer to Chapter 11 for laboratory studies used to diagnose hepatitis.

K. Prevention
  1. Proper hand washing and standard precautions can prevent the spread of viral hepatitis.
  2. Prophylactic use of standard immune globulin to prevent HAV in situations of preexposure (such as anticipated travel to areas where HAV is prevalent) or within 2 weeks of exposure.
  3. Hepatitis B immune globulin is effective in preventing infection following one-time exposures, such as accidental needle punctures or other contact of contaminated material with mucous membranes, and should be given to newborns whose mothers are HbsAg-positive and should be given within 72 hours of exposure.
  4. Hepatitis A vaccine is recommended for children ages 2 to 18 years who reside in communities with high endemic rates and for preexposure prophylaxis.
  5. Hepatitis B vaccine: Refer to Chapter 47 for immunization schedule.

L. Interventions
  1. Strict hand washing is required.
  2. Hospitalization is required in the event of coagulopathy or fulminant hepatitis.
  3. Standard precautions are followed during hospitalization.
  4. Hospitalized child usually is not isolated in a separate room unless he or she is fecally incontinent and items are likely to become contaminated with feces.

5. Children are discouraged from sharing toys.
6. Instruct child and parents in good hand-washing techniques.
7. Instruct the parents to disinfect diaper-changing surfaces thoroughly with a solution of $\frac{1}{4}$ cup bleach in a gallon of water.
8. Maintain comfort and provide adequate rest and sleep.
9. Provide a low-fat, balanced diet.
10. Provide enteric precautions for at least 1 week after the onset of jaundice with HAV.
11. Inform the parents that because hepatitis A is not infectious 1 week after the onset of jaundice, the child may return to school at that time if he or she feels well enough.
12. Inform the parents that jaundice may get worse before it resolves.
13. Caution parents about administering any medications to the child (liver is unable to detoxify and excrete medications).
14. Instruct the parents in the signs indicating a worsening of the child's condition, such as changes in the neurological status, bleeding, and fluid retention.

XVIII. INGESTION OF POISONS

A. Lead poisoning
  1. Description: Excessive accumulation of lead in the blood
  2. Causes
    a. The pathway for exposure may be food, air, or water.
    b. Dust and soil contaminated with lead may be a source of exposure.
    c. Lead enters the child's body through ingestion or inhalation or through placental transmission to an unborn child when the mother is exposed; the most common route is ingestion from hand-to-mouth behavior from contaminated objects or from eating loose paint chips.
    d. When lead enters the body, it affects the erythrocytes, bones and teeth, and organs and tissues, including the brain and nervous system; the most serious consequences are the effects on the central nervous system.
  3. Universal screening
    a. Screening is recommended in high-risk areas at the age of 1 to 2 years; children at high risk should be screened earlier.
    b. Any child between the ages of 3 and 6 years who has not been screened should be tested.
  4. Targeted screening
    a. Targeted screening is acceptable in low-risk areas.
    b. At the age of 1 to 2 years (or a child between the ages of 3 and 6 years who has not been screened) may be targeted for screening if determined to be at risk.

TABLE 39-1

Blood Lead Level Test

Level	Intervention
Less than 10 mcg/dL	Reassess or rescreen in 1 year or sooner if exposure status changes.
10 to 14 mcg/dL	Provide family lead education, follow-up testing, and social service referral if necessary.
15 to 19 mcg/dL	Provide family lead education, follow-up testing, and social service referral if necessary; on follow-up testing, initiate actions for blood lead level of 20 to 44 mcg/dL.
20 to 44 mcg/dL	A blood lead level greater than 20 mcg/dL is considered acute; provide coordination of care, clinical management, including treatment, environmental investigation, and lead-hazard control (the child must not remain in a lead-hazardous environment if resolution is necessary).
70 mcg/dL or greater	Medical treatment is provided immediately, including coordination of care, clinical management, environmental investigation, and lead-hazard control.

5. Blood lead level test: Used for screening and diagnosis (Table 39-1)
6. Erythrocyte protoporphyrin test
   a. An indicator of anemia
   b. Normal value for a child is 35 mcg/100 mL of whole blood or less
7. Chelation therapy
   a. Chelation therapy removes lead from the circulating blood and from some organs and tissues.
   b. Therapy does not counteract any effects of the lead.
   c. Medications include dimercaprol (BAL in oil), calcium disodium edetate (CaNa$_2$EDTA), succimer (Chemet).
   d. Dimercaprol (BAL) is contraindicated in children with an allergy to peanuts because the medication is prepared in a peanut oil solution.
   e. Ensure adequate urinary output before administering medications.
   f. Provide adequate hydration and monitor kidney function for nephrotoxicity when medication is given because the medication is excreted via the kidneys.
   g. Follow-up lead levels to monitor progress are essential.
   h. Provide instructions to parents about safety from lead hazards, medication administration, and the need for follow-up.

   i. Confirm that the child will be discharged to home without lead hazards.
B. Acetaminophen (Tylenol)
   1. Description
      a. Seriousness of ingestion is determined by the amount ingested and the length of time before intervention.
      b. Toxic dose is 150 mg/kg or greater in children.
   2. Assessment
      a. First 2 to 4 hours: malaise, nausea, vomiting, sweating, pallor, weakness
      b. Latent period: 24 to 36 hours; child improves
      c. Hepatic involvement: may last up to 7 days and may be permanent; right upper quadrant pain, jaundice, confusion, stupor, elevated liver enzymes and bilirubin, prolonged prothrombin time
   3. Interventions
      a. Administer antidote: *N*-acetylcysteine
      b. Dilute antidote in juice or soda because of its offensive odor.
      c. Loading dose is followed by maintenance doses.
C. Acetylsalicylic acid (aspirin)
   1. Description
      a. Overdose may be caused by acute ingestion or chronic ingestion.
      b. Acute: Severe toxicity occurs with 300 to 500 mg/kg.
      c. Chronic: Ingestion of more than 100 mg/kg per day for 2 days or more, which can be more serious than acute ingestion.
   2. Assessment
      a. Gastrointestinal effects: nausea, vomiting, and thirst from dehydration
      b. Central nervous system effects: hyperpnea, confusion, tinnitus, convulsions, coma, respiratory failure, circulatory collapse
      c. Renal effects: oliguria
      d. Hematopoietic effects: bleeding tendencies
      e. Metabolic effects: diaphoresis, fever, hyponatremia, hypokalemia, dehydration, hypoglycemia
   3. Interventions
      a. Vomiting may be induced with syrup of ipecac or gastric lavage is performed.
      b. Administer activated charcoal to decrease absorption of salicylate (important in early acetylsalicylic acid toxicity).
      c. Administer IV fluids, sodium bicarbonate, electrolytes, or volume expanders as prescribed.
      d. Administer vitamin K for bleeding tendencies as prescribed.
      e. Administer glucose for hypoglycemia as prescribed.
      f. Prepare the child for dialysis as prescribed if the child is unresponsive to the therapy.

PRACTICE QUESTIONS

1. A 3-year-old child is hospitalized because of persistent vomiting. A nurse monitors the child closely for
   1. Diarrhea.
   2. Metabolic acidosis.
   3. Metabolic alkalosis.
   4. Hyperactive bowel sounds.
2. A nurse is monitoring for signs of dehydration in a 1-year-old child who has been hospitalized for diarrhea. The nurse prepares to take the child's temperature and avoids which method of measurement?
   1. Tympanic
   2. Axillary
   3. Rectal
   4. Electronic
3. A home care nurse provides instructions to the mother of an infant with cleft palate regarding feeding. Which statement if made by the mother indicates a need for further instructions?
   1. "I will use a nipple with a small hole to prevent choking."
   2. "I will stimulate sucking by rubbing the nipple on the lower lip."
   3. "I will allow the infant time to swallow."
   4. "I will allow the infant to rest frequently to provide time for swallowing what has been placed in the mouth."
4. An infant has just returned to the nursing unit following a surgical repair of a cleft lip located on the right side of the lip. The nurse places the infant in which most appropriate position?
   1. On the right side
   2. On the left side
   3. Prone
   4. Supine
5. A clinic nurse reviews the record of an infant seen in the clinic. The nurse notes that a diagnosis of esophageal atresia with tracheoesophageal fistula is suspected. The nurse expects to note which most likely sign of this condition documented in the record?
   1. Severe projectile vomiting
   2. Coughing at nighttime
   3. Choking with feedings
   4. Incessant crying
6. A nurse prepares a teaching plan for the parents of an infant with gastroesophageal reflux regarding proper positioning to manage reflux. The nurse documents that the infant should be maintained in which position following feedings and at night?
   1. 30-degree angle when supine
   2. 60-degree angle when supine
   3. Head-elevated prone position
   4. 20-degree angle when supine
7. A nurse provides feeding instructions to a mother of an infant diagnosed with gastroesophageal reflux.

To assist in reducing the episodes of emesis, the nurse tells the mother to
   1. Thin the feedings by adding water to the formula.
   2. Thicken the feedings by adding rice cereal to the formula.
   3. Provide less frequent, larger feedings.
   4. Burp the infant less frequently during feedings.
8. A nurse admits a child to the hospital with a diagnosis of pyloric stenosis. On admission assessment, which data would the nurse expect to obtain when asking the mother about the child's symptoms?
   1. Vomiting large amounts of bile
   2. Watery diarrhea
   3. Increased urine output
   4. Projectile vomiting
9. A home care nurse instructs the mother about dietary measures for a 5-year-old child with lactose intolerance. The nurse tells the mother that is necessary to provide which dietary supplement in the child's diet?
   1. Zinc
   2. Protein
   3. Calcium
   4. Fats
10. A nurse provides home care instructions to the parents of a child with celiac disease. The nurse teaches the parents to include which of the following food items in the child's diet?
    1. Rice
    2. Rye toast
    3. Oatmeal
    4. Wheat bread
11. A clinic nurse reviews the record of a 3-week-old infant and notes that the physician has documented a diagnosis of suspected Hirschsprung's disease. The nurse reviews the assessment findings documented in the record, knowing that which symptom most likely led the mother to seek health care for the infant?
    1. Diarrhea
    2. Projectile vomiting
    3. Regurgitation of feedings
    4. Foul-smelling ribbonlike stools
12. A nurse is caring for a newborn infant with a suspected diagnosis of imperforate anus. The nurse monitors the infant, knowing that which of the following is a clinical manifestation associated with this disorder?
    1. Sausage-shaped mass palpated in the upper right abdominal quadrant
    2. Bile-stained fecal emesis
    3. Failure to pass meconium stool in the first 24 hours after birth
    4. The passage of currant jelly–like stools
13. A nurse is preparing to care for a child with a diagnosis of intussusception. The nurse reviews the child's record and expects to note which symptom of this disorder documented?

1. Bright red blood and mucus in the stools
2. Profuse projectile vomiting
3. Watery diarrhea
4. Ribbonlike stools

14. A child is receiving succimer (Chemet) for the treatment of lead poisoning. A nurse monitors which of the following most important laboratory results?
   1. Potassium level
   2. Blood urea nitrogen
   3. Red blood cell count
   4. White blood cell count

15. An emergency room nurse is caring for a child brought to the emergency room after the ingestion of about one half bottle of acetylsalicylic acid (aspirin). The nurse anticipates that the most likely initial treatment will be

1. The administration of syrup of ipecac.
2. The administration of sodium bicarbonate.
3. The administration of vitamin K.
4. Dialysis.

CRITICAL THINKING: FILL IN THE BLANK

A nurse is caring for a child who is scheduled for an appendectomy. The nurse reviews the physician's preoperative orders and notes the following: initiate an IV line, maintain an NPO status, administer a Fleet enema, and administer preoperative medication on call to the operating room. Which order written by the physician would the nurse question?

Answer: _____

ANSWERS

1. **3**

Rationale: Vomiting will cause the loss of hydrochloric acid and subsequent metabolic alkalosis. Metabolic acidosis would occur in a child experiencing diarrhea because of the loss of bicarbonate. Diarrhea may not accompany vomiting. Hyperactive bowel sounds are not necessarily associated with vomiting.

Test-Taking Strategy: Use the process of elimination. Recalling that gastric fluids are acidic and that the loss of these fluids will lead to alkalosis will assist in answering the question. No data in the question support options 1 and 4. Review the manifestations that occur with vomiting if you had difficulty with this question.

Level of Cognitive Ability: Analysis
Client Needs: Physiological Integrity
Integrated Process: Nursing Process—assessment
Content Area: Child health
Reference: James, S., Ashwill, J., & Droske, S. (2002). *Nursing care of children: Principles & practice* (2nd ed., p. 526). Philadelphia: W. B. Saunders.

2. **3**

Rationale: Rectal temperature measurements should be avoided if diarrhea is present. Use of a rectal thermometer can stimulate peristalsis and cause more diarrhea. Axillary and tympanic measurements of temperature would be acceptable. Most measurements are done via electronic devices.

Test-Taking Strategy: Use the process of elimination. Note the key word "avoids." Eliminate option 4 first because most methods of temperature measurement are done through an electronic device. Note the diagnosis stated in the question. This should direct you easily to option 3. Review care of the child with diarrhea if you had difficulty with this question.

Level of Cognitive Ability: Analysis
Client Needs: Physiological Integrity
Integrated Process: Nursing Process—implementation
Content Area: Child health
Reference: James, S., Ashwill, J., & Droske, S. (2002). *Nursing care of children: Principles & practice* (2nd ed., p. 522). Philadelphia: W. B. Saunders.

3. **1**

Rationale: The mother is taught the ESSR method of feeding the child with a cleft palate: *enlarge* the nipple, *stimulate* the sucking reflex, *swallow*, and *rest* to allow the infant to finish swallowing what has been placed in the mouth.

Test-Taking Strategy: Use the process of elimination. Note the key words "need for further instructions." Eliminate options 3 and 4 first because they are similar. Use basic principles regarding the methods to stimulate sucking to eliminate option 2. Review teaching guidelines for the child with cleft lip or palate if you had difficulty with this question.

Level of Cognitive Ability: Analysis
Client Needs: Health Promotion and Maintenance
Integrated Process: Teaching/Learning
Content Area: Child health
References: James, S., Ashwill, J., & Droske, S. (2002). *Nursing care of children: Principles & practice* (2nd ed., p. 535). Philadelphia: W. B. Saunders.
Wong, D., Hockenberry-Eaton, M. (2000). *Wong's essentials of pediatric nursing* (6th ed., p. 913). St. Louis: Mosby.

4. **2**

Rationale: After cleft lip repair the infant should be positioned supine or on the side lateral to the repair to prevent the contact of the suture lines with the bed linens. Placing the infant on the left side rather than supine immediately after surgery is best to prevent the risk of aspiration if the infant vomits.

Test-Taking Strategy: Use the process of elimination. Note the key words "just returned" and "most appropriate." Consider the anatomical location of the surgical site and the key words "right side" in the question. You should be directed easily to the correct option by using these concepts. Review postoperative positioning techniques if you had difficulty with this question.

Level of Cognitive Ability: Application
Client Needs: Physiological Integrity
Integrated Process: Nursing Process—implementation
Content Area: Child health
References: James, S., Ashwill, J., & Droske, S. (2002). *Nursing care of children: Principles & practice* (2nd ed., p. 538). Philadelphia: W. B. Saunders.

Wong, D., Hockenberry-Eaton, M. (2000). *Wong's essentials of pediatric nursing* (6th ed., pp. 91-96). St. Louis: Mosby.

5. 3
Rationale: Any child who exhibits the "3 C's"—coughing and choking with feedings and unexplained cyanosis—should be suspected of tracheoesophageal fistula. Options 1, 2, and 4 are not specifically associated with tracheoesophageal fistula.
Test-Taking Strategy: Use the process of elimination, focusing on the diagnosis. Recalling the "3 C's" associated with this disorder will assist in directing you to the correct option. Review the clinical manifestations associated with this disorder if you had difficulty with this question
Level of Cognitive Ability: Analysis
Client Needs: Physiological Integrity
Integrated Process: Nursing Process—assessment
Content Area: Child health
Reference: Wong, D., Hockenberry-Eaton, M. (2000). *Wong's essentials of pediatric nursing* (6th ed., p. 918). St. Louis: Mosby.

6. 3
Rationale: The infant should be placed in the flat prone position or the head-elevated prone position following feedings and at night. The supine position is not recommended because aspiration could occur if the infant vomits.
Test-Taking Strategy: Use the process of elimination. Visualize each of the positions, and think about the effect of the position in the infant with gastroesophageal reflux. Also note that options 1, 2, and 4 are similar. Review positioning for gastroesophageal reflux if you had difficulty with this question.
Level of Cognitive Ability: Application
Client Needs: Physiological Integrity
Integrated Process: Communication and Documentation
Content Area: Child health
Reference: Wong, D., Hockenberry-Eaton, M. (2000). *Wong's essentials of pediatric nursing* (6th ed., p. 896). St. Louis: Mosby.

7. 2
Rationale: Small, more frequent feedings with frequent burping often are prescribed in the treatment of gastroesophageal reflux. Feedings thickened with rice cereal may reduce episodes of emesis. If thickened formula is used, crosscutting of the nipple may be required.
Test-Taking Strategy: Use the process of elimination and basic principles related to feeding an infant to assist in eliminating options 3 and 4. Noting the key words "reducing the episodes of emesis" will assist in directing you to select option 2 over option 1. Review therapeutic interventions associated with this disorder if you had difficulty with this question.
Level of Cognitive Ability: Application
Client Needs: Physiological Integrity
Integrated Process: Teaching/Learning
Content Area: Child health
Reference: Wong, D., Hockenberry-Eaton, M. (2000). *Wong's essentials of pediatric nursing* (6th ed., p. 896). St. Louis: Mosby.

8. 4
Rationale: Clinical manifestations of pyloric stenosis include projectile vomiting, irritability, hunger and crying, constipation, and signs of dehydration, including a decrease in urine output.

Test-Taking Strategy: Use the process of elimination. Considering the anatomical location of this disorder and its potential effects will assist in eliminating options 2 and 3. Recalling that a major clinical manifestation is projectile vomiting will assist in directing you to option 4. Review these clinical manifestations if you had difficulty with this question.
Level of Cognitive Ability: Analysis
Client Needs: Physiological Integrity
Integrated Process: Nursing Process—assessment
Content Area: Child health
Reference: Wong, D., Hockenberry-Eaton, M. (2000). *Wong's essentials of pediatric nursing* (6th ed., p. 912). St. Louis: Mosby.

9. 3
Rationale: Lactose intolerance is the inability to tolerate lactose, the sugar found in dairy products. Removing milk from the diet can provide adequate relief from symptoms. Additional dietary changes may be required to provide adequate sources of calcium and, in the infant, protein and calories.
Test-Taking Strategy: Use the process of elimination. Knowledge that lactose is the sugar found in dairy products will easily direct you to option 3, since dairy products contain high levels of calcium. Review the dietary management for lactose intolerance if you had difficulty with this question.
Level of Cognitive Ability: Application
Client Needs: Physiological Integrity
Integrated Process: Teaching/Learning
Content Area: Child health
Reference: Wong, D., Hockenberry-Eaton, M. (2000). *Wong's essentials of pediatric nursing* (6th ed., p. 399). St. Louis: Mosby.

10. 1
Rationale: Dietary management is the mainstay of treatment in celiac disease. All wheat, rye, barley, and oats should be eliminated from the diet and replaced with corn, rice, or millet. Vitamin supplements—especially the fat-soluble vitamins, iron, and folic acid—may be needed in the early period of treatment to correct deficiencies. Dietary restrictions are likely to be lifelong, although small amounts of grains may be tolerated after ulcerations have healed.
Test-Taking Strategy: Use the process of elimination. Recalling that corn, rice, and millet are substitute food replacements in this disease will direct you easily to option 1. Review the dietary management in this disorder if you had difficulty with this question.
Level of Cognitive Ability: Application
Client Needs: Health Promotion and Maintenance
Integrated Process: Teaching/Learning
Content Area: Child health
Reference: Wong, D., Hockenberry-Eaton, M. (2000). *Wong's essentials of pediatric nursing* (6th ed., p. 927). St. Louis: Mosby.

11. 4
Rationale: Chronic constipation beginning in the first month of life and resulting in pelletlike or ribbon stools that are foul smelling is a clinical manifestation of this disorder. Delayed passage or absence of meconium stool in the neonatal period is the cardinal sign. Bowel obstruction, especially in the neonatal period, abdominal pain and distension, and

failure to thrive are also clinical manifestations. Options 1, 2, and 3 are not associated specifically with this disorder.
Test-Taking Strategy: Use the process of elimination and knowledge regarding the pathophysiology associated with Hirschsprung's disease to direct you to option 4. If you are unfamiliar with this disorder, review the assessment findings associated with it.
Level of Cognitive Ability: Analysis
Client Needs: Physiological Integrity
Integrated Process: Communication and Documentation
Content Area: Child health
Reference: Wong, D., Hockenberry-Eaton, M. (2000). *Wong's essentials of pediatric nursing* (6th ed., p. 894). St. Louis: Mosby.

12. **3**
Rationale: During the newborn assessment, this defect should be identified easily on sight. However, a rectal thermometer or tube may be necessary to determine patency if meconium is not passed in the first 24 hours after birth. Other assessment findings include absence or stenosis of the anal rectal canal, presence of an anal membrane, and an external fistula to the perineum. Options 1, 2, and 4 are findings noted in intussusception.
Test-Taking Strategy: Use the process of elimination and the definition of the word "imperforate" to assist in answering this question. This should direct you to option 3. Review the assessment findings associated with this disorder if you had difficulty with this question.
Level of Cognitive Ability: Analysis
Client Needs: Physiological Integrity
Integrated Process: Nursing Process—assessment
Content Area: Child health
Reference: Wong, D., Hockenberry-Eaton, M. (2000). *Wong's essentials of pediatric nursing* (6th ed., p. 926). St. Louis: Mosby.

13. **1**
Rationale: The child with intussusception classically has severe abdominal pain that is crampy and intermittent, causing the child to draw in the knees to the chest. Vomiting may be present but is not projectile. Bright red blood and mucus are passed through the rectum and commonly are described as currant-jelly stools. Watery diarrhea and ribbonlike stools are not manifestations of this disorder.
Test-Taking Strategy: Use the process of elimination. Recalling that a classic manifestation is currant-jelly stools will assist in directing you to option 1. Review this disorder if you had difficulty with this question.
Level of Cognitive Ability: Analysis
Client Needs: Physiological Integrity
Integrated Process: Communication and Documentation
Content Area: Child health
Reference: Wong, D., Hockenberry-Eaton, M. (2000). *Wong's essentials of pediatric nursing* (6th ed., p. 923). St. Louis: Mosby.

14. **2**
Rationale: Renal function is monitored closely during the administration of chelation therapy because the medications

are excreted via the kidneys. Although it is important to monitor the red blood cell count for the presence of anemia in a child with lead poisoning, this laboratory result is not specific to chelation therapy. Options 1 and 4 are unrelated to the administration of chelation therapy.
Test-Taking Strategy: Use the process of elimination. Recalling that the medications used in chelation therapy are excreted via the kidneys will direct you to option 2. Review this treatment for lead poisoning if you had difficulty with this question.
Level of Cognitive Ability: Analysis
Client Needs: Physiological Integrity
Integrated Process: Nursing Process—assessment
Content Area: Child health
Reference: Wong, D., Hockenberry-Eaton, M. (2000). *Wong's essentials of pediatric nursing* (6th ed., p. 481). St. Louis: Mosby.

15. **1**
Rationale: Initial treatment of salicylate overdose includes inducing vomiting with syrup of ipecac or gastric lavage. Activated charcoal may be administered to decrease absorption. Fluids and sodium bicarbonate may be administered intravenously to enhance excretion but would not be the initial treatment. Dialysis is used in extreme cases if the child is unresponsive to therapy. Vitamin K is the antidote for warfarin sodium (Coumadin) overdose.
Test-Taking Strategy: Use the process of elimination and knowledge regarding the treatment for aspirin overdose to answer this question. Note the key word "initial" in the stem of the question. This key word will assist in directing you to option 1. Review the treatment for this common overdose in children if you had difficulty with this question.
Level of Cognitive Ability: Analysis
Client Needs: Physiological Integrity
Integrated Process: Nursing Process—planning
Content Area: Child health
Reference: Wong, D., Hockenberry-Eaton, M. (2000). *Wong's essentials of pediatric nursing* (6th ed., p. 476). St. Louis: Mosby.

CRITICAL THINKING: FILL IN THE BLANK

Answer: Administer a Fleet enema.
Rationale: In the preoperative period, enemas or laxatives should not be administered. Intravenous fluids would be started, and the child would not receive anything by mouth. Prescribed preoperative medications most likely would be administered on call to the operating room.
Test-Taking Strategy: Consider the anatomical location and the concern of rupture in this disorder. Administering a Fleet enema would place the child at risk for a perforated appendix. Review preoperative care in the child with appendicitis if you had difficulty with this question.
Level of Cognitive Ability: Analysis
Client Needs: Physiological Integrity
Integrated Process: Nursing Process—analysis
Content Area: Child health
Reference: Wong, D., Hockenberry-Eaton, M. (2000). *Wong's essentials of pediatric nursing* (6th ed., p. 899). St. Louis: Mosby.

REFERENCES

Celiac Sprue Association/United States of America: e-mail Celiacusa@aol.com

James, S., Ashwill, J., & Droske, S. (2002). *Nursing care of children: Principles & practice* (2nd ed.). Philadelphia: W. B. Saunders.

Hodgson, B., & Kizior, R. (2003). *Saunders nursing drug handbook 2003*. Philadelphia: W. B. Saunders.

Wong, D., Hockenberry-Eaton, M. (2000). *Wong's essentials of pediatric nursing* (6th ed.). St. Louis: Mosby.

Wong, D., Perry, S., & Hockenberry, M. (2002). *Maternal child nursing care* (2nd ed.). St. Louis: Mosby.

Metabolic and Endocrine Disorders

I. FEVER

A. Description
1. Fever is an abnormal body temperature elevation.
2. A child's temperature can vary depending on activity, emotional stress, the type of clothing the child is wearing, and the temperature of the environment.
3. Assessment findings associated with the fever provide important indications of the seriousness of the fever.

B. Assessment
1. Temperature elevation
2. Flushed skin
3. Diaphoresis
4. Chills
5. Restlessness or lethargy

C. Interventions
1. Monitor vital signs.
2. Administer a sponge bath with lukewarm water for 20 to 30 minutes.
3. Administer antipyretics such as acetaminophen (Tylenol) as prescribed.
4. Do not administer aspirin (acetylsalicylic acid) because of the risk of Reye's syndrome.
5. Retake the temperature 30 to 60 minutes after the antipyretic is administered.
6. Provide adequate fluid intake as tolerated and as prescribed.
7. Monitor for dehydration and fluid and electrolyte imbalance.
8. Instruct the parents in how to take the temperature, how to medicate their child safely, and when it is necessary to call the physician.

II. DEHYDRATION (BOX 40-1)

A. Description
1. Dehydration is a common fluid and electrolyte imbalance in infants and children.
2. Infants and children are more vulnerable to fluid volume deficit because a greater amount of their body water is in the extracellular fluid compartment.
3. In infants and children, the organs that conserve water are immature, placing them at risk for fluid volume deficit.
4. The causes can include decreased fluid intake, diaphoresis, vomiting, diarrhea, diabetic ketoacidosis, and extensive burns or other serious injuries.

B. Assessment
1. Tachycardia
2. Dry skin and mucous membranes
3. Sunken eyeballs and fontanels
4. Decreased urine output and increased urine specific gravity

---

BOX 40-1

Types of Dehydration

ISOTONIC DEHYDRATION
Electrolyte and water deficits occur in approximately balanced proportions.

HYPERTONIC DEHYDRATION
Water loss exceeds electrolyte loss.

HYPOTONIC DEHYDRATION
Electrolyte loss exceeds water loss.

---

5. Changes in level of consciousness and responses to stimuli
6. Signs of circulatory failure, such as coolness and mottling of the extremities
7. Loss of skin elasticity and turgor
8. Delayed capillary filling time
9. Weight loss
10. Decreased blood pressure
11. Thirst
12. Absence of tears

C. Interventions
1. Monitor vital signs.
2. Monitor for signs of dehydration.
3. Monitor weight and monitor for changes, including fluid gains and losses.
4. Monitor intake and output and urine for specific gravity.
5. Monitor level of consciousness.
6. Monitor skin turgor and mucous membranes for dryness.
7. Provide oral rehydration therapy with solutions, as prescribed, if the child is able to take fluids orally.
8. Administer fluids and electrolyte replacements intravenously, as prescribed, if the child is unable to take sufficient fluids orally.
9. Introduce a regular diet as prescribed when the child is rehydrated.
10. Provide instructions to the parents about the types and amounts of fluid to encourage, the signs of dehydration, and the indications of the need to notify the physician.

III. PHENYLKETONURIA

A. Description
1. Phenylketonuria is a genetic disorder that results in central nervous system damage from toxic levels of phenylalanine in the blood.
2. Phenylketonuria is an autosomal recessive disorder.
3. Phenylketonuria is characterized by blood phenylalanine levels greater than 8 mg/dL (normal level is less than 2 mg/dL 2 to 5 days after birth).
4. All 50 states require routine screening of all newborn infants for phenylketonuria.

B. Assessment
1. In all children
   a. Digestive problems and vomiting
   b. Seizures
   c. Musty odor of the urine
   d. Mental retardation
2. In older children
   a. Eczema
   b. Hypertonia
   c. Hypopigmentation of the hair, skin, and irises
   d. Hyperactive behavior

C. Interventions
1. Screening of newborn infants for phenylketonuria: the infant should have begun formula or breast milk feeding before specimen collection.
2. If initial screening is positive, a repeat test is performed and further diagnostic evaluation is required to verify the diagnosis.
3. Rescreen infants by 14 days of age if the initial screening was done before 48 hours of age.
4. If phenylketonuria is diagnosed, do the following:
   a. Restrict phenylalanine intake; high-protein foods (meats and dairy products) and aspartame are avoided because they contain large amounts of phenylalanine.
   b. Monitor physical, neurological, and intellectual development.
   c. Stress the importance of follow-up treatment.
   d. Encourage the parents to express feelings about the diagnosis and the risk of phenylketonuria in future children.

IV. TYPE 1 DIABETES MELLITUS

A. Description
1. Type 1 diabetes mellitus also is known as insulin-dependent diabetes mellitus; the majority of children with diabetes mellitus have type 1.
2. Type 1 diabetes mellitus is caused by the partial or complete lack of secretory capacity of the beta cells of the pancreas, resulting in insulin deficiency.
3. Complete insulin deficiency requires the use of exogenous insulin to promote appropriate glucose use and to prevent complications related to elevated blood glucose levels, such as hyperglycemia, diabetic ketoacidosis, and death.
4. Diagnosis is based on the presence of classic symptoms and an elevated blood glucose level (normal blood glucose level is 70 to 110 mg/dL).

B. Assessment
1. Polyuria, polydipsia, polyphagia
2. Hyperglycemia
3. Weight loss
4. Unexplained fatigue or lethargy
5. Headaches
6. Stomachaches
7. Occasional enuresis in a previously toilet-trained child
8. Vaginitis in adolescent girls (caused by *Candida*, which thrives in hyperglycemic tissues)
9. Fruity odor to breath
10. Dehydration
11. Blurred vision
12. Slow wound healing
13. Changes in level of consciousness

C. Long-term effects
1. Failure to grow at a normal rate
2. Delayed maturation

3. Recurrent infections
4. Neuropathy
5. Cardiovascular disease
6. Retinal microvascular disease
7. Renal microvascular disease

D. Complications
1. Hypoglycemia
2. Hyperglycemia
3. Diabetic ketoacidosis
4. Coma
5. Hypokalemia
6. Hyperkalemia
7. Microvascular changes
8. Cardiovascular changes

E. Diet
1. Total number of calories is individualized based on the child's age and growth expectations.
2. As prescribed by the physician, the child may be instructed to follow the food exchange from the American Diabetic Association diet or the dietary guidelines for Americans (Food Guide Pyramid) issued by the U.S. Departments of Agriculture and Health and Human Services.
3. Dietary intake should include three meals per day, eaten at consistent intervals, plus a midafternoon carbohydrate snack and a bedtime snack high in protein; a consistent intake of carbohydrates at each meal and snack is needed.
4. Instruct the child and the parents that the child should carry candy with him or her at all times to treat hypoglycemia if it occurs.
5. Incorporate the diet into individual child's needs, likes and dislikes, lifestyle, and cultural and socioeconomic patterns.
6. Allow the child to participate in making food choices to provide a sense of control.

F. Exercise
1. Instruct the child in dietary adjustments when exercising.
2. Extra food needs to be consumed for increased activity, usually 10 to 15 g of carbohydrates for every 30 to 45 minutes of activity.
3. Instruct the child to monitor blood glucose before exercising.
4. Plan with the child an appropriate exercise regimen, incorporating the developmental stage.

G. Insulin
1. Diluted insulin may be required for some infants to provide small enough doses to avoid hypoglycemia; diluted insulin should be labeled clearly to avoid dosage errors.
2. Laboratory evaluation of glycosylated hemoglobin should be performed every 3 months.
3. Illness, infection, and stress increase the need for insulin, and insulin should not be withheld during illness, infection, or stress, because hyperglycemia and ketoacidosis can result.

4. When the child is not receiving anything by mouth for a special procedure, verify with the physician the need to withhold the morning insulin, and when food, fluids, and insulin are to be resumed.
5. Instruct the child and parents in the administration of the insulin.
6. Instruct the child and parents to recognize symptoms of hypoglycemia and hyperglycemia.
7. Instruct the parents in the administration of glucagon intramuscularly or subcutaneously if the child has a hypoglycemic reaction and is unable to consume sugar-containing items orally.
8. Instruct the child and parents to always have a spare bottle of insulin available.
9. Advise the parents to obtain a Medic-Alert bracelet indicating the type and daily insulin dosage prescribed for the child.

H. Blood glucose monitoring
1. Results provide information needed to maintain good glycemic control.
2. Blood glucose monitoring is more accurate than urine testing.
3. Monitoring requires that the child prick himself or herself several times a day as prescribed.
4. Instruct the child and parents in the proper procedure for obtaining the blood glucose level.
5. Inform the child and parents that the procedure must be done precisely to obtain accurate results.
6. Stress the importance of hand washing before and after performing the procedure to prevent infection.
7. Stress the importance of following the manufacturer's instructions for the blood glucose monitoring device.
8. Instruct the child and parents to calibrate the monitor as instructed by the manufacturer.
9. Instruct the child and parents to check the expiration date on the test strips used for the blood glucose monitoring.
10. Instruct the child and parents that if the blood glucose results do not seem reasonable, reread the instructions, reassess technique, check the expiration date of the test strips, and perform the procedure again to verify results.

I. Urine testing
1. Instruct the parents and child in the procedure for testing urine for ketones and glucose.
2. Teach the child that the second voided urine specimen is most accurate.
3. The presence of ketones may indicate impending ketoacidosis.
4. Urine glucose testing is not recommended as the only means of monitoring control in the child taking insulin because it is a less reliable indicator compared with blood glucose monitoring.

J. Hypoglycemia
1. Description
   a. Hypoglycemia is a blood glucose level less than 70 mg/dL.
   b. Hypoglycemia results from too much insulin, not enough food, or excessive activity.
2. Interventions (Box 40-2 and 40-3)
K. Hyperglycemia
1. Description: elevated blood glucose level greater than 200 mg/dL
2. Interventions (Box 40-4)
3. Sick day rules (Box 40-5)
L. Diabetic ketoacidosis
1. Description
   a. Diabetic ketoacidosis is a complication of diabetes mellitus that develops when a severe insulin deficiency occurs.
   b. Diabetic ketoacidosis is a life-threatening condition.
   c. Hyperglycemia that progresses to metabolic acidosis occurs.
   d. Diabetic ketoacidosis develops over a period of several hours to days.
   e. The blood glucose level is greater than 300 mg/dL, and urine and serum ketone tests are positive.
2. Interventions
   a. Restore circulating volume and protect against cerebral, coronary, or renal hypoperfusion.
   b. Correct dehydration with intravenous (IV) infusions of 0.9% or 0.45% saline as prescribed.
   c. Correct hyperglycemia with IV regular insulin administration as prescribed.
   d. Monitor vital signs, urine output, and mental status closely.
   e. Correct acidosis and electrolyte imbalances.
   f. Administer oxygen as prescribed.
   g. Monitor blood glucose level frequently.
   h. Monitor potassium level closely because when the child receives insulin to lower the blood glucose level, the serum potassium will change; if the potassium level drops, potassium replacement may be required.
   i. Monitor the child closely for signs of fluid overload.
   j. Intravenously administered dextrose is added as prescribed when the blood glucose reaches an appropriate level.
   k. Treat the cause of hyperglycemia.

BOX 40-2

Interventions for Hypoglycemia

If able, the nurse should confirm hypoglycemia with a blood glucose reading.

Administer glucose immediately; the rapid-releasing sugar is followed by a complex carbohydrate and protein such as a slice of bread or a peanut butter cracker.

Give an extra snack if the next meal is not planned for more than 30 minutes or if activity is planned.

If the child becomes unconscious, squeeze cake frosting or glucose paste onto the gums and retest the blood glucose level if the child does not improve within 15 to 20 minutes; if the reading remains low, administer additional sugar.

If the child remains unconscious, administration of glucagon may be necessary.

In the hospital setting, prepare to administer dextrose intravenously.

BOX 40-3

Food items to Treat Hypoglycemia

½ cup of orange juice or a sugar-sweetened carbonated beverage
1 small box of raisins
3 to 4 hard candies
Sugar cubes
Life Savers
1 candy bar
1 tsp honey
2 or 3 glucose tablets

BOX 40-4

Interventions for Hyperglycemia

Instruct the parents to notify the physician when the following occur:
Blood glucose results are greater than the targeted range (usually 200 mg/dL).
Moderate or high ketonuria is present.
The child is unable to take food or fluids.
Illness persists.

BOX 40-5

Sick Day Rules for the Diabetic Child

Always give insulin even if the child does not have an appetite, or contact the physician for specific instructions.
Test blood glucose levels at least every 4 hours.
Test for urinary ketones with each voiding.
Notify the physician if moderate or large amounts of urinary ketones are present.
Follow the child's usual meal plan.
Encourage calorie-free liquids to aid in clearing ketones.
Encourage rest, especially if urinary ketones are present.
Notify the physician if vomiting, fruity odor to the breath, deep rapid respirations, decreasing level of consciousness, or persistent hyperglycemia occurs.

PRACTICE QUESTIONS

1. A nurse asks a nursing assistant to gather supplies in preparation to administer a tepid bath to a child with a fever. The nurse determines that the nursing assistant needs instructions about the procedure for administering a tepid bath if the nursing assistant obtained which item?
   1. Washcloths and towels
   2. A bottle of alcohol
   3. Toys
   4. Lightweight pajamas

2. A nursing student is assigned to admit to the hospital a child who has been experiencing vomiting and diarrhea. A physician establishes a diagnosis of gastroenteritis and isotonic dehydration. A nursing instructor asks the student to describe isotonic dehydration. The nursing student responds accurately by telling the instructor that isotonic dehydration
   1. Occurs when water and electrolytes are lost in about the same proportions as they exist in the body.
   2. Occurs when the loss of electrolytes is greater than the loss of water.
   3. Occurs when the loss of water is greater than the loss of electrolytes.
   4. Causes the serum sodium level to rise above 150 mEq/L.

3. A clinic nurse is assessing a child for dehydration. The nurse determines that the child is moderately dehydrated if which symptom is noted on assessment?
   1. Flat fontanels
   2. Moist mucous membranes
   3. Pale skin color
   4. Oliguria

4. A physician orders intravenously administered potassium for a child with hypertonic dehydration. A nurse performs which priority assessment before administering the potassium?
   1. Taking the temperature
   2. Taking the blood pressure
   3. Obtaining a weight
   4. Checking the amount of urine output

5. A pediatric nurse educator provides a teaching session to the nursing staff regarding phenylketonuria. The nurse educator tells the nursing staff that
   1. Phenylketonuria is an autosomal dominant disorder.
   2. Treatment includes dietary restriction of tyramine.
   3. All 50 states require routine screening of all newborn infants for phenylketonuria.
   4. Phenylketonuria primarily affects the gastrointestinal system.

6. A mother brings her 3-week-old infant to a clinic for a phenylketonuria rescreening blood test. The test indicates a serum phenylalanine level of 1 mg/dL. The nurse interprets this result as
   1. Inconclusive.
   2. Requiring rescreening at age 6 weeks.
   3. Positive.
   4. Negative.

7. A school-aged child with type 1 diabetes mellitus has soccer practice three afternoons a week. The school nurse provides instructions regarding how to prevent hypoglycemia during practice. The school nurse tells the child to
   1. Take one half of the amount of prescribed insulin on practice days
   2. Eat twice the amount normally eaten at lunchtime.
   3. Take the prescribed insulin at noontime rather than in the morning.
   4. Eat 6 graham crackers or drink a cup of orange juice before soccer practice.

8. A home care nurse is teaching an adolescent with type 1 diabetes mellitus about insulin administration and rotation sites. Which statement, if made by the adolescent, would indicate effective teaching?
   1. "I need to use a location in one major site for the morning injection and another location in the same major site for the evening injection for 2 to 3 weeks before changing major sites."
   2. "I need to use a different site for each insulin injection."
   3. "I need to use the same site for 1 month before rotating to another site."
   4. "I should use only my stomach and my thighs for injections."

9. The mother of a 6-year-old who has type 1 diabetes mellitus calls a clinic nurse and tells the nurse that the child has been sick. The mother reports that she checked the child's urine and it was positive for ketones. The nurse instructs the mother to
   1. Come to the clinic immediately.
   2. Hold the next dose of insulin.
   3. Administer an additional dose of regular insulin.
   4. Encourage the child to drink calorie-free liquids.

10. A child with type 1 diabetes mellitus is brought to an emergency room by the mother, who states that the child has been complaining of abdominal pain and has a fruity odor of the breath. Diabetic ketoacidosis is diagnosed. Anticipating the plan of care, the nurse prepares to administer
    1. 5% dextrose IV infusion.
    2. Normal saline IV infusion.
    3. NPH insulin IV infusion.
    4. Potassium IV infusion.

CRITICAL THINKING: MULTIPLE RESPONSE

Select all interventions for a child with type 1 diabetes mellitus who has a blood glucose level of 60 mg/dL.

___ Give the child a teaspoon of honey.

___ Prepare to administer glucagon subcutaneously if unconsciousness occurs.

___ Encourage the child to ambulate.

___ Administer regular insulin.

___ Provide electrolyte replacement therapy intravenously.

ANSWERS

1. 2

Rationale: Alcohol should not be used for bathing the child with a fever because it can cause rapid cooling, peripheral vasoconstriction, and chilling, thus elevating the temperature further. Washcloths can be used to squeeze water over the child's body. Towels are used to dry the child. Toys, especially water toys, can be used to provide distraction during the bath. Lightweight clothing should be placed on the child after the child is dried.

Test-Taking Strategy: Use the process of elimination, noting the key words "needs instructions." Options 1 and 4 can be eliminated easily. From the remaining options, recall the harmful effects of alcohol and the effect of potentially elevating the temperature with its use. Review the procedure for administering a tepid bath if you had difficulty with this question.

Level of Cognitive Ability: Analysis
Client Needs: Physiological Integrity
Integrated Process: Teaching/Learning
Content Area: Child health
References: James, S., Ashwill, J., & Droske, S. (2002). *Nursing care of children: Principles & practice* (2nd ed., p. 369). Philadelphia: W. B. Saunders
Wong, D., Hockenberry-Eaton, M. (2000). *Wong's essentials of pediatric nursing* (6th ed., p. 763). St. Louis: Mosby.

2. 1

Rationale: Isotonic dehydration occurs when water and electrolytes are lost in about the same proportions as they exist in the body. In this type of dehydration the serum sodium levels remain normal (135 to 145 mEq/L). Option 2 describes hypotonic dehydration; in this type the serum sodium level is less than 130 mEq/L. Options 3 and 4 describe hypertonic dehydration.

Test-Taking Strategy: Use the process of elimination. Thinking about the terms "hypotonic" and "hypertonic" and relating these terms to "losses" or "excesses" may assist in eliminating options 2, 3, and 4. Review these types of dehydration if you had difficulty with this question.

Level of Cognitive Ability: Comprehension
Client Needs: Physiological Integrity
Integrated Process: Teaching/Learning
Content Area: Child health
Reference: Wong, D., Hockenberry-Eaton, M. (2000). *Wong's essentials of pediatric nursing* (6th ed., p. 881). St. Louis: Mosby.

3. 4

Rationale: In moderate dehydration the fontanels would be slightly sunken, the mucous membranes would be dry, and the skin color would be dusky. In moderate dehydration, oliguria would be present.

Test-Taking Strategy: Use the process of elimination. Note the key words "moderately dehydrated." From the options presented, option 4 is the clinical manifestation of greatest concern. Review the manifestations related to mild, moderate, and severe dehydration if you had difficulty with this question.

Level of Cognitive Ability: Analysis
Client Needs: Physiological Integrity
Integrated Process: Nursing Process—assessment
Content Area: Child health
Reference: Wong, D., Hockenberry-Eaton, M. (2000). *Wong's essentials of pediatric nursing* (6th ed., p. 882). St. Louis: Mosby.

4. 4

Rationale: The priority assessment before administering potassium intravenously would be to assess the status of the urine output. Potassium should never be administered in the presence of oliguria or anuria. If the urine output is less than 1 to 2 mL/kg per hour, potassium should not be administered. Although options 1, 2, and 3 are appropriate assessments for the child with dehydration, these assessments are not related specifically to the intravenous (IV) administration of potassium.

Test-Taking Strategy: Use the process of elimination. Recalling that the kidneys play a key role in the excretion and reabsorption of potassium will direct you easily to option 4. Review this important medication if you had difficulty with this question.

Level of Cognitive Ability: Analysis
Client Needs: Physiological Integrity
Integrated Process: Nursing Process—assessment
Content Area: Child health
Reference: McKinney, E., Ashwill, J., Murray, S., James, S., Gorrie, T., & Droske, S. (2000). *Maternal-child nursing* (p. 1095). Philadelphia: W. B. Saunders.

5. 3

Rationale: Phenylketonuria is an autosomal recessive disorder. Treatment includes dietary restriction of phenylalanine intake. Phenylketonuria is a genetic disorder that results in central nervous system damage from toxic levels of phenylalanine in the blood. Option 3 is accurate.

Test-Taking Strategy: Use the process of elimination. Recalling that phenylketonuria is a recessive disorder will assist you in eliminating option 1. Reading option 2 carefully will direct you to eliminate this option because phenylalanine, not tyramine, is restricted. Recalling that phenylketonuria affects the central nervous system will direct you to option 3.

Review the characteristics associated with this disorder if you had difficulty with this question.
Level of Cognitive Ability: Application
Client Needs: Physiological Integrity
Integrated Process: Teaching/Learning
Content Area: Child health
Reference: James, S., Ashwill, J., & Droske, S. (2002). *Nursing care of children: Principles & practice* (2nd ed., p. 907). Philadelphia: W. B. Saunders.

6. **4**
Rationale: Phenylketonuria is characterized by blood phenylalanine levels greater than 8 mg/dL. A normal level is less than 2 mg/dL. A result of 1 mg/dL is a negative test result.
Test-Taking Strategy: Use the process of elimination. Eliminate options 1 and 2 first because they are similar. Note that the level identified in the question is a low level. This should assist in directing you to option 4. Review this important screening test if you had difficulty with this question.
Level of Cognitive Ability: Analysis
Client Needs: Physiological Integrity
Integrated Process: Nursing Process—analysis
Content Area: Child health
Reference: James, S., Ashwill, J., & Droske, S. (2002). *Nursing care of children: Principles & practice* (2nd ed., p. 907). Philadelphia: W. B. Saunders.

7. **4**
Rationale: An extra snack of 15 to 30 g of carbohydrates eaten before activities such as soccer practice will prevent hypoglycemia. Six graham crackers or a cup of orange juice will provide 15 to 30 g of carbohydrates. The child or parents should not be instructed to adjust the amount or time of insulin administration. Meal amounts should not be doubled.
Test-Taking Strategy: Use the process of elimination. Options 1 and 3 can be eliminated first because insulin doses and times should not be adjusted. From the remaining options, recalling the manifestations and treatment associated with hypoglycemia will direct you to option 4. Review treatment to prevent hypoglycemia if you had difficulty with this question.
Level of Cognitive Ability: Application
Client Needs: Health Promotion and Maintenance
Integrated Process: Teaching/Learning
Content Area: Child health
Reference: James, S., Ashwill, J., & Droske, S. (2002). *Nursing care of children: Principles & practice* (2nd ed., p. 927). Philadelphia: W. B. Saunders.

8. **1**
Rationale: To help decrease variations in absorption from day to day, the adolescent should use one major site for injections for 2 to 3 weeks before changing major sites. The injections are rotated to different locations within that major site. Options 2, 3, and 4 are incorrect.
Test-Taking Strategy: Use the process of elimination. Eliminate option 4 first because of the word "only." From the remaining options, recalling the physiology associated with absorption of insulin will direct you to option 1. If you had difficulty with this question, review insulin administration.
Level of Cognitive Ability: Analysis

Client Needs: Health Promotion and Maintenance
Integrated Process: Teaching/Learning
Content Area: Child health
Reference: Wong, D., Hockenberry-Eaton, M. (2000). *Wong's essentials of pediatric nursing* (6th ed., p. 1138). St. Louis: Mosby.

9. **4**
Rationale: When the child is sick, the mother should test for urinary ketones with each voiding. If ketones are present, liquids are essential to aid in clearing the ketones. The child should be encouraged to drink calorie-free liquids. Bringing the child to the clinic immediately is not necessary. Insulin doses should not be adjusted or changed.
Test-Taking Strategy: Use the process of elimination. Eliminate options 2 and 3 first because insulin doses should not be adjusted or changed. From the remaining options, note the words "positive for ketones." Recalling that liquids are essential to aid in clearing the ketones will direct you to the correct option. Review home care instructions for the sick diabetic child if you had difficulty with this question.
Level of Cognitive Ability: Application
Client Needs: Physiological Integrity
Integrated Process: Nursing Process—implementation
Content Area: Child health
Reference: James, S., Ashwill, J., & Droske, S. (2002). *Nursing care of children: Principles & practice* (2nd ed., p. 936). Philadelphia: W. B. Saunders.

10. **2**
Rationale: Rehydration is the initial step in resolving diabetic ketoacidosis. Normal saline is the initial IV rehydration fluid. NPH insulin is never administered by the IV route. Dextrose solutions are added to the treatment when the blood glucose level reaches an acceptable level. Intravenously administered potassium may be required, depending on the potassium level, but would not be part of the initial treatment.
Test-Taking Strategy: Use the process of elimination. Eliminate option 1, knowing that dextrose would not be administered in a hyperglycemic state. Eliminate option 3 next, knowing that NPH insulin is never administered by the IV route. Knowledge that hydration is the initial treatment in diabetic ketoacidosis will direct you easily to option 2. Review the treatment for this important condition if you had difficulty with this question.
Level of Cognitive Ability: Analysis
Client Needs: Physiological Integrity
Integrated Process: Nursing Process—planning
Content Area: Child health
Reference: James, S., Ashwill, J., & Droske, S. (2002). *Nursing care of children: Principles & practice* (2nd ed., pp. 934-935). Philadelphia: W. B. Saunders.

CRITICAL THINKING: MULTIPLE RESPONSE
Answer:
Give the child a teaspoon of honey.
Prepare to administer glucagon subcutaneously if unconsciousness occurs.
Rationale: Hypoglycemia is defined as a blood glucose level less than 70 mg/dL. Hypoglycemia occurs as a result of too much insulin, not enough food, or excessive activity. If able, the nurse should confirm hypoglycemia with a blood

glucose reading. Glucose is administered orally immediately; the rapid-releasing sugar is followed by a complex carbohydrate and protein, such as a slice of bread or a peanut butter cracker.

An extra snack is given if the next meal is not planned for more than 30 minutes or if activity is planned. If the child becomes unconscious, cake frosting or glucose paste is squeezed onto the gums and the blood glucose level is retested if the child does not improve within 15 to 20 minutes; if the reading remains low, additional sugar is administered. If the child remains unconscious, administration of glucagons may be necessary, and the nurse should be prepared for this intervention. In the hospital setting the nurse should be prepared to administer dextrose intravenously. Encouraging the child to ambulate and administering regular insulin will result in a lowered blood glucose level. Providing electrolyte replacement therapy intravenously is an intervention to treat diabetic ketoacidosis.

Test-Taking Strategy: Focus on the information in the question. Recalling that a blood glucose level of 60 mg/dL indicates hypoglycemia will assist in determining the correct interventions. Review the interventions for hypoglycemia if you had difficulty with this question.

Level of Cognitive Ability: Application

Client Needs: Physiological Integrity

Integrated Process: Nursing Process—implementation

Content Area: Child health

Reference: James, S., Ashwill, J., & Droske, S. (2002). *Nursing care of children: Principles & practice* (2nd ed., p. 925). Philadelphia: W. B. Saunders.

REFERENCES

Chernecky, C., & Berger, B. (2001). *Laboratory tests and diagnostic procedures* (3rd ed.). Philadelphia: W. B. Saunders.

James, S., Ashwill, J., & Droske, S. (2002). *Nursing care of children: Principles & practice* (2nd ed.). Philadelphia: W. B. Saunders.

McKinney, E., Ashwill, J., Murray, S., James, S., Gorrie, T., & Droske, S. (2000). *Maternal-child nursing*. Philadelphia: W. B. Saunders.

Wong, D., Hockenberry-Eaton, M. (2000). *Wong's essentials of pediatric nursing* (6th ed.). St. Louis: Mosby.

Wong, D., Perry, S., & Hockenberry, M. (2002). *Maternal child nursing care* (2nd ed.). St. Louis: Mosby.

Renal and Urinary Disorders

I. GLOMERULONEPHRITIS

A. Description
1. Glomerulonephritis is a term that includes a variety of disorders, most of which are caused by an immunological reaction.
2. The disorder results in proliferative and inflammatory changes within the glomerular structure.
3. Destruction, inflammation, and sclerosis of the glomeruli of both kidneys occur.
4. Inflammation of the glomeruli results from an antigen-antibody reaction produced by an infection elsewhere in the body.
5. Loss of kidney function develops.

B. Causes
1. Immunological diseases
2. Autoimmune diseases
3. Streptococcal infection, group A β-hemolytic
4. History of pharyngitis or tonsillitis 2 to 3 weeks before symptoms

C. Types (Box 41-1)

D. Complications
1. Renal failure
2. Hypertensive encephalopathy
3. Pulmonary edema
4. Heart failure

BOX 41-1

Types of Glomerulonephritis

Acute: Occurs 2 to 3 weeks after a streptococcal infection
Chronic: Can occur after the acute phase or slowly over time

E. Assessment
1. Periorbital and facial edema that is more prominent in the morning
2. Anorexia
3. Decreased urinary output
4. Cloudy, smoky, brown-colored urine
5. Pallor, irritability, lethargy
6. In the older child, headaches, abdominal or flank pain, dysuria
7. Hypertension
8. Proteinuria that produces a persistent and excessive foam in the urine
9. Azotemia
10. Increased blood urea nitrogen and creatinine levels
11. Increased antistreptolysin O titer (used to diagnose disorders caused by streptococcal infections)

F. Interventions
1. Monitor vital signs, weight, intake and output, and the characteristics of urine.
2. Limit activity; provide safety measures.
3. Nutrition
   a. Restrictions depend on the stage and severity of the disease, especially the extent of the edema.
   b. In uncomplicated cases, a regular diet is permitted but sodium is restricted to a no added salt to foods diet.
   c. Moderate sodium restriction is prescribed for the child with hypertension or edema.
   d. Foods high in potassium are restricted during periods of oliguria.
   e. Protein is restricted if the child has severe azotemia resulting from prolonged oliguria.
4. Monitor for complications (renal failure, hypertensive encephalopathy, pulmonary edema, and heart failure).

472

5. Administer diuretics (if significant edema and fluid overload are present), antihypertensives (for hypertension), and antibiotics (to the child with evidence of persistent streptococcal infections) as prescribed.
6. Initiate seizure precautions and administer anticonvulsants as prescribed for seizures associated with hypertensive encephalopathy.
7. Instruct the parents to report signs of bloody urine, headache, or edema.
8. Instruct the parents that the child needs to obtain treatment for infections, specifically sore throats and upper respiratory infections.

II. NEPHROTIC SYNDROME

A. Description
1. Nephrotic syndrome is a kidney disorder characterized by massive proteinuria, hypoalbuminemia, and edema.
2. The primary objective of therapeutic management is to reduce the excretion of urinary protein and maintain protein-free urine.

B. Assessment (Box 41-2)

C. Interventions
1. Monitor vital signs, intake and output, and daily weights.
2. Monitor urine for specific gravity and albumin.
3. Monitor for edema.
4. Nutrition: A regular diet without added salt is prescribed if the child is in remission; sodium is restricted during periods of massive edema.
5. Corticosteroid therapy is prescribed as soon as the diagnosis has been determined (monitor child closely for signs of infection).
6. Immunosuppressant therapy may be prescribed to reduce the relapse rate and induce long-term remission; therapy may be administered along with the corticosteroid.
7. Diuretics may be prescribed to reduce edema.
8. Plasma expanders such as salt-poor human albumin may be prescribed for the severely edematous child.
9. Instruct the parents about testing the urine for albumin, medication administration, side effects of medications, and general care of the child.

BOX 41-2

Assessment Findings in Nephrotic Syndrome

Child gains weight.
Periorbital and facial edema is most prominent in the morning.
Leg, ankle, labial or scrotal edema occurs.
Urine output decreases; urine is dark and frothy.
Abdominal swelling occurs.
Blood pressure is normal or slightly decreased.

---

10. Instruct the parents regarding the signs of infection and the need to avoid contact with other children who may be infectious.

III. ENURESIS

A. Description
1. Enuresis refers to a condition in which the child is unable to control bladder function even though the child has reached an age at which control of voiding is expected.
2. By age 5, most children are aware of bladder fullness and are able to control voiding.

B. Primary nocturnal enuresis
1. Primary nocturnal enuresis is bed-wetting in a child who has never been dry for extended periods.
2. The condition is common in children, and most children eventually will outgrow bed-wetting without therapeutic intervention.
3. The child is not able to sense a full bladder and does not awaken to void.
4. The child may have delayed maturation of the central nervous system.

C. Secondary or acquired enuresis
1. The onset of wetting occurs after a period of established urinary continence.
2. Secondary enuresis may occur during nighttime sleep (nocturnal), only during the waking hours (diurnal), or during both times of the day.
3. The child may complain of dysuria, urgency, or frequency.
4. The child should be assessed for urinary tract infections.

D. Assessment
1. Assess voiding pattern
2. History of bed-wetting with no extended period of dryness in a child older than age 5 years

E. Interventions
1. Obtain urinalysis and urine culture as prescribed to rule out infection or existing disorder.
2. Assist the family with identifying a treatment plan that will best fit their needs.
3. Limit fluid intake at night, and encourage the child to void just before going to bed.
4. Involve the child in caring for the wet sheets and changing the bed to assist the child to take ownership of the problem.
5. Provide reward systems as appropriate for the child.
6. Incorporate behavioral conditioning techniques.
7. Encourage follow-up to determine the effectiveness of the treatment.

IV. CRYPTORCHIDISM

A. Description: Cryptorchidism occurs when one or both testes fail to descend through the inguinal canal into the scrotal sac.

▶ B. Assessment: Testes are not palpable or easily guided into the scrotum.

C. Interventions

1. Monitor during the first 12 months of life to determine whether spontaneous descent occurs.
2. After age 1, medical or surgical treatment may be instituted.
3. Human chorionic gonadotropin, a pituitary hormone that stimulates the production of testosterone, may be prescribed.
4. Surgical correction, if needed, is done by orchiopexy before the child's second birthday (preferably between 1 and 2 years of age) if the testes do not descend spontaneously.
5. Monitor for bleeding and infection postoperatively.
6. Instruct the parents in postoperative home care measures, including preventing infection, pain control, and activity restrictions.
7. Provide an opportunity for parental counseling if the parents are concerned about the future fertility of the child.

V. EPISPADIAS AND HYPOSPADIAS (FIG. 41-1)

A. Description: Congenital defects involving abnormal placement of the urethral orifice of the penis

▶ B. Assessment

1. Epispadias: Urethral orifice is located on the dorsal surface of the penis; the condition often occurs with exstrophy of the bladder.
2. Hypospadias: Urethral orifice is located below the glans penis along the ventral surface.

C. Surgical interventions

1. Surgery is done before the age of toilet training, preferably between 16 and 18 months of age.
2. The child should not be circumcised because the foreskin may be used in surgical reconstruction.

▶ D. Interventions postoperatively

1. The child will have a pressure dressing and may have some type of urinary diversion or a urinary stent (used to maintain patency of the urethral opening) while healing of the meatus occurs.
2. Monitor vital signs.
3. Encourage fluid intake to maintain adequate urine output and to maintain patency of the stent.
4. Monitor intake and output and the urine for cloudiness or a foul odor.
5. Notify the physician if there is no urinary drainage for 1 hour because this may indicate kinks in the system or obstruction by sediment.
6. Provide pain medication (acetaminophen [Tylenol]) or medication to relieve bladder spasms (anticholinergic) as prescribed.
7. Administer antibiotics as prescribed.
8. Instruct the parents in the care of the urinary diversion or stent if present.
9. Instruct the parents to avoid giving the child a tub bath until the stent, if present, is removed.

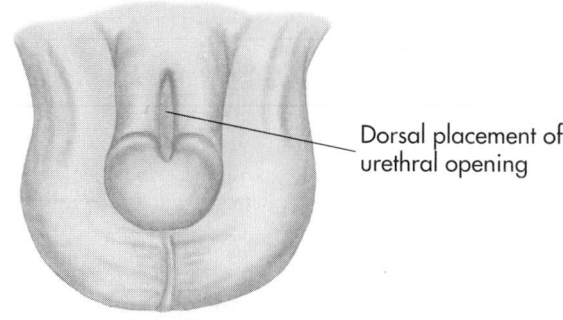

Epispadias

Dorsal placement of urethral opening

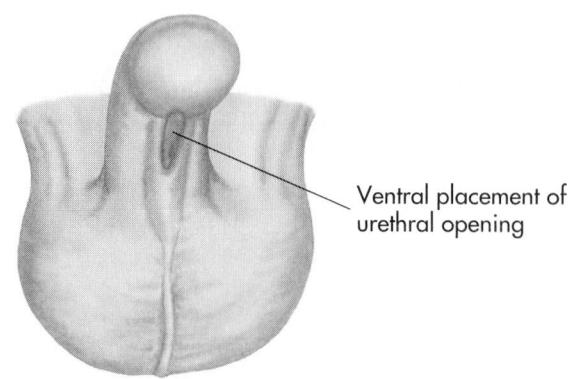

Hypospadias

Ventral placement of urethral opening

FIG. 41-1 Epispadias and hypospadias are genital anomalies in which the urethral opening is above or below its normal location on the glans of the penis. (From James, S., Ashwill, J., & Droske, S. [2002]. *Nursing care of children: Principles & practice* [2nd ed.]. Philadelphia: W. B. Saunders.)

10. Instruct the parents about fluid intake, medication administration, the signs and symptoms of infection, and the need for physician follow-up for dressing removal about 4 days after surgery.

VI. BLADDER EXSTROPHY

A. Description

1. Bladder exstrophy is a congenital anomaly characterized by extrusion of the urinary bladder to the outside of the body through a defect in the lower abdominal wall.
2. The cause is unknown.
3. Treatment requires surgical management and occurs in a series of staged reconstructions.
4. Initial surgery for closure of the abdominal defect should occur within the first few days of life.
5. The goal of subsequent operations is to reconstruct the bladder and genitalia and enable the child to achieve urinary continence.

B. Assessment

1. Exposed bladder mucosa
2. Widened symphysis pubis
3. Defects of the external genitalia

C. Interventions
1. Monitor urinary output.
2. Monitor for signs of urinary tract or wound infection.
3. Maintain the integrity of the exposed bladder mucosa.
4. Prevent the bladder tissue from drying, while allowing the drainage of urine, until surgical closure is performed.
   a. The bladder is covered with sterile, nonadherent clear plastic wrap or a sterile thin film dressing without adhesive.
   b. Petroleum jelly is avoided because it tends to dry out, adhere to the bladder mucosa, and damage the delicate tissues when the dressing is removed.
5. Monitor laboratory values and urinalysis to assess for renal function.
6. Administer antibiotics as prescribed
7. Provide emotional support to the parents, and encourage verbalization of their fears and concerns.

PRACTICE QUESTIONS

1. A nurse interviews the parents of a child recently diagnosed with glomerulonephritis. The nurse understands that which information collected during the assessment most often is associated with the diagnosis of glomerulonephritis?
   1. Streptococcal throat infection 2 weeks before diagnosis
   2. Child fell off a bike onto the handlebars
   3. Nausea and vomiting for the last 24 hours
   4. Urticaria and itching for 1 week before diagnosis
2. A nurse is assigned to care for a child suspected of having glomerulonephritis. The nurse reviews the child's record and notes that which finding is associated with the diagnosis of glomerulonephritis?
   1. Low blood urea nitrogen
   2. Hypotension
   3. Low urinary specific gravity
   4. Red-brown urine
3. A nurse is developing a plan of care for a 7-year-old child diagnosed with acute glomerulonephritis. The nurse includes which priority intervention in the plan of care?
   1. Encourage limited activity and provide safety measures.
   2. Catheterize the child to monitor intake and output strictly.
   3. Force oral fluids to prevent hypovolemic shock.
   4. Encourage classmates to visit and to keep the child informed of school events.
4. A nurse is performing an admission assessment on a 2-year-old child who has been diagnosed with nephrotic syndrome. The nurse knows that the most common characteristic associated with nephrotic syndrome is

1. Generalized edema.
2. Frank bright red blood in the urine.
3. Increased urinary output.
4. Hypertension.
5. A nurse is preparing a 2-year-old child with suspected nephrotic syndrome for diagnostic tests to confirm the diagnosis. The mother asks the nurse if the child will ever look thin again. The nurse most appropriately responds by telling the mother
   1. "Wearing loose-fitting clothing should help conceal the extra weight."
   2. "In most cases, medication and diet will control the fluid retention."
   3. "Do you feel guilty because you didn't notice the weight gain?"
   4. "When children are little, it's expected they'll look a little chubby."
6. A 7-year-old child is seen in a clinic, and the primary health care provider documents a diagnosis of primary nocturnal enuresis. The mother asks a nurse about the diagnosis. The nurse plans to respond, knowing that primary nocturnal enuresis
   1. Requires surgical intervention to improve the problem.
   2. Is caused by a psychiatric problem.
   3. Is common and most children will outgrow the bedwetting problem without therapeutic intervention.
   4. Does not respond to treatment.
7. A child with cryptorchidism is being discharged following orchiopexy, which was performed on an outpatient basis. A nurse informs the parents that which care measure should take priority in the plan of care at home?
   1. Administering anticholinergics
   2. Measuring intake and output
   3. Applying cold, wet compresses to the surgical site
   4. Preventing infection at the surgical site
8. A nurse has provided discharge instructions to the mother of a 2-year-old child who has had an orchiopexy to correct cyptorchidism. Which of the following statements, if made by the mother of the child, indicates that further teaching is necessary?
   1. "I'll check his temperature."
   2. "I'll let him decide when to return to his play activities."
   3. "I'll give him medication so he'll be comfortable."
   4. "I'll check his voiding to be sure there's no problem."
9. A nurse collects a urine specimen preoperatively from a child with epispadias who is scheduled for surgical repair. When the nurse is analyzing the results of the urinalysis, which of the following would the nurse most likely expect to note?
   1. Hematuria
   2. Proteinuria
   3. Bacteriuria
   4. Glucosuria

10. A 1-year-old child with hypospadias is scheduled for surgery to correct this condition. The nurse prepares a nursing care plan for this child and understands that this surgery is taking place at a time when
    1. Fears of separation are great.
    2. Sibling rivalry will cause regression to occur.
    3. Embarrassment about voiding irregularities is common.
    4. Concern over size and function of the penis is present.

11. An 18-month-old child is being discharged following surgical repair of hypospadias. Which postoperative nursing care measure should the nurse stress to the parents as they prepare to take this child home?
    1. Encourage toilet training to ensure that flow of urine is normal.
    2. Restrict fluid intake to reduce urinary output for the first few days.
    3. Avoid tub baths until the stent has been removed.
    4. Leave the diapers off to allow the site to heal.

12. A nurse is reviewing a treatment plan with the parents of a newborn infant with hypospadias. Which statement by the parents indicates their understanding of the plan?
    1. "Circumcision has been delayed to save tissue for surgical repair."
    2. "Catheterization will be necessary when the infant does not void."
    3. "Caution should be used when straddling the infant on a hip."
    4. "Vital signs should be taken daily to check for bladder infection."

13. The parents of a newborn infant have been told that their child was born with bladder exstrophy. The parents ask the nurse about this condition. The nurse plans to base the response on knowledge that this condition is
    1. Caused by the use of medications taken by the mother during pregnancy.
    2. A hereditary disorder that occurs in every other generation.
    3. A condition in which the urinary bladder is abnormally located in the pelvic cavity.
    4. An extrusion of the urinary bladder to the outside of the body through a defect in the lower abdominal wall.

14. After performing an assessment of an infant with bladder exstrophy, a nurse prepares a plan of care. The nurse identifies which of the following nursing diagnoses as the priority for the infant?
    1. Total urinary incontinence
    2. Impaired tissue integrity
    3. Deficient knowledge (parental)
    4. Risk for infection

15. A nurse is caring for an infant with a diagnosis of bladder exstrophy. To protect the exposed bladder tissue, the nurse plans to
    1. Cover the bladder with petroleum jelly gauze.
    2. Keep the bladder tissue dry by covering it with dry sterile gauze.
    3. Cover the bladder with a nonadhering plastic wrap.
    4. Apply sterile distilled water dressings over the bladder mucosa.

CRITICAL THINKING: FILL IN THE BLANK

A nurse is performing an assessment on a child admitted to the hospital with a probable diagnosis of nephrotic syndrome. The nurse reviews the physician's orders and notes that the physician has ordered a urinalysis. The nurse obtains the specimen and would expect to observe what characteristics in the urine if nephrotic syndrome is present?

Answer: _____

ANSWERS

1. **1**
Rationale: Group A β-hemolytic streptococcal infection is a cause of glomerulonephritis. Often the child becomes ill with streptococcal infection of the upper respiratory tract and then develops symptoms of acute poststreptococcal glomerulonephritis after an interval of 1 to 2 weeks. The assessment data in options 2, 3, and 4 are unrelated to a diagnosis of glomerulonephritis.
Test-Taking Strategy: Use the process of elimination. Option 2 relates to a kidney injury, not an infectious process. From the remaining options, recalling that a streptococcal infection 1 to 2 weeks before the development of glomerulonephritis is the classic assessment finding will assist in directing you to option 1. If you had difficulty with this question, review the causes of glomerulonephritis.

Level of Cognitive Ability: Analysis
Client Needs: Physiological Integrity
Integrated Process: Nursing Process—assessment
Content Area: Child health
Reference: Wong, D., Hockenberry-Eaton, M. (2000). *Wong's essentials of pediatric nursing* (6th ed., p. 1046). St. Louis: Mosby.

2. **4**
Rationale: Gross hematuria, resulting in dark, smoky, cola-colored or red-brown urine, is a classic symptom of glomerulonephritis. Hypertension is also common. Blood urea nitrogen levels may be elevated. A moderately elevated to high urinary specific gravity is associated with glomerulonephritis.
Test-Taking Strategy: Use the process of elimination. Eliminate options 2 and 3 first because hypertension and a high specific gravity are most likely to occur in this kidney disorder.

Knowledge that blood urea nitrogen levels elevate will assist in directing you to option 4. If you had difficulty with this question, review the clinical manifestations associated with glomerulonephritis.
Level of Cognitive Ability: Analysis
Client Needs: Physiological Integrity
Integrated Process: Nursing Process—analysis
Content Area: Child health
Reference: Wong, D., Hockenberry-Eaton, M. (2000). *Wong's essentials of pediatric nursing* (6th ed., p. 1046). St. Louis: Mosby.

3. **1**
Rationale: Activity is limited, and most children, because of fatigue, voluntarily restrict their activities during the active phase of the disease. Catheterization may cause a risk of infection. Fluids should not be forced. Visitors should be limited to allow for adequate rest.
Test-Taking Strategy: Use the process of elimination. Eliminate option 4 because rest is the priority over socialization. Eliminate option 2 next. Although monitoring intake and output is essential, the risk of infection could occur with catheterization. From the remaining options, eliminate option 3 because of the words "force oral fluids." Review the appropriate nursing interventions for the child with glomerulonephritis if you had difficulty with this question.
Level of Cognitive Ability: Application
Client Needs: Physiological Integrity
Integrated Process: Nursing Process—planning
Content Area: Child health
Reference: Wong, D., Hockenberry-Eaton, M. (2000). *Wong's essentials of pediatric nursing* (6th ed., p. 1048). St. Louis: Mosby.

4. **1**
Rationale: Nephrotic syndrome is defined as massive proteinuria, hypoalbuminemia, hyperlipemia, and edema. Other manifestations include the following: the child gains weight, periorbital and facial edema that is most prominent in the morning, leg, ankle, labial or scrotal edema, decreased urine output and urine that is dark and frothy, abdominal swelling, and a blood pressure that is normal or slightly decreased.
Test-Taking Strategy: Recall the pathophysiology associated with nephrotic syndrome. Associate edema with nephrotic syndrome to help you if you encounter a question similar to this one. If you had difficulty with this question, review the characteristics of nephrotic syndrome.
Level of Cognitive Ability: Analysis
Client Needs: Physiological Integrity
Integrated Process: Nursing Process—assessment
Content Area: Child health
Reference: Wong, D., Hockenberry-Eaton, M. (2000). *Wong's essentials of pediatric nursing* (6th ed., p. 1043). St. Louis: Mosby.

5. **2**
Rationale: The nurse must give the mother information that addresses the issue that is the parent's concern. Most children experience remission with treatment. Options 1 and 3 are nontherapeutic and may add to the mother's guilt. Option 4 does not acknowledge the concern and is a stereotypical response.
Test-Taking Strategy: Use therapeutic communication techniques, and focus on the mother's concern. Options 1, 3, and 4

do not address the mother's concern and are inappropriate and nontherapeutic responses. Remember, always address the mother's feelings and concerns.
Level of Cognitive Ability: Application
Client Needs: Psychosocial Integrity
Integrated Process: Communication and Documentation
Content Area: Child health
Reference: James, S., Ashwill, J., & Droske, S. (2002). *Nursing care of children: Principles & practice* (2nd ed., p. 607). Philadelphia: W. B. Saunders.

6. **3**
Rationale: Primary nocturnal enuresis occurs in a child who has never been dry at night for extended periods. The condition is common in children, and most children eventually will outgrow bed-wetting without therapeutic intervention. The child is not able to sense a full bladder and does not awaken to void. The child may have delayed maturation of the central nervous system. The condition is not caused by a psychiatric problem.
Test-Taking Strategy: Use the process of elimination, noting the relationship between the words "enuresis" in the question and "bed-wetting" in the correct option. If you had difficulty with this question, review the characteristics associated with enuresis.
Level of Cognitive Ability: Comprehension
Client Needs: Physiological Integrity
Integrated Process: Nursing Process—planning
Content Area: Child health
Reference: James, S., Ashwill, J., & Droske, S. (2002). *Nursing care of children: Principles & practice* (2nd ed., p. 595). Philadelphia: W. B. Saunders.

7. **4**
Rationale: The most common complications associated with orchiopexy are bleeding and infection. The parents are instructed in postoperative home care measures, including preventing infection, pain control, and activity restrictions. Anticholinergics are prescribed for the relief of bladder spasms and are not necessary following orchiopexy. Measurement of intake and output is not required. Cold wet compresses are not prescribed. In addition, the moisture from a wet compress presents a potential for infection.
Test-Taking Strategy: Note the key word "priority" in the stem of the question. Use Maslow's hierarchy of needs theory to answer the question. Of the options presented, the potential for infection is the physiological priority. Review home care instructions following orchiopexy if you had difficulty with this question.
Level of Cognitive Ability: Application
Client Needs: Health Promotion and Maintenance
Integrated Process: Teaching/Learning
Content Area: Child health
Reference: Wong, D., Hockenberry-Eaton, M. (2000). *Wong's essentials of pediatric nursing* (6th ed., p. 1043). St. Louis: Mosby.

8. **2**
Rationale: All vigorous activities should be restricted for 2 weeks following surgery to promote healing and prevent injury. This will prevent dislodging of the suture, which is internal.

Normally, 2-year-olds will want to be active; therefore allowing the child to decide when to return to his play activities may prevent healing and cause injury. The parent should be taught to monitor the temperature, provide analgesics as needed, and monitor the urine output.

Test-Taking Strategy: Use the process of elimination. Note the key words "further teaching is necessary." Option 1 is an important action to recognize signs of infection. Option 3 is appropriate to keep pain to a minimum. Option 4 monitors voiding pattern, which is also important following this type of surgery. If you had difficulty with this question, review the discharge instructions following surgical correction of cryptorchidism.

Level of Cognitive Ability: Analysis
Client Needs: Health Promotion and Maintenance
Integrated Process: Teaching/Learning
Content Area: Child health
Reference: Wong, D., Hockenberry-Eaton, M. (2000). *Wong's essentials of pediatric nursing* (6th ed., p. 1043). St. Louis: Mosby.

9. 3
Rationale: Epispadias is a congenital defect involving abnormal placement of the urethral orifice of the penis. The urethral opening is located anywhere on the dorsum of the penis. This anatomical characteristic leads to the easy entry of bacteria into the urine. Options 1, 2, and 4 are not characteristically noted in this condition.

Test-Taking Strategy: Use knowledge regarding the anatomical characteristic of epispadias and the process of elimination to answer the question. Options 1, 2, and 4 do not relate to the potential for infection, which can be present in the condition of epispadias. If you had difficulty with this question, review the diagnostic findings associated with epispadias.

Level of Cognitive Ability: Analysis
Client Needs: Physiological Integrity
Integrated Process: Nursing Process—assessment
Content Area: Child health
Reference: James, S., Ashwill, J., & Droske, S. (2002). *Nursing care of children: Principles & practice* (2nd ed., p. 603). Philadelphia: W. B. Saunders.

10. 1
Rationale: At the age of 1 year, a child's fears of separation are great because the child is facing the developmental task of trusting others. Options 3 and 4 may be issues if the child was older. No data in the question allow one to determine that siblings exist.

Test-Taking Strategy: Use the process of elimination and knowledge regarding the stages of growth and development to answer the question. Options 3 and 4 can be eliminated easily. Next, eliminate option 2 because no data in the question allow one to determine that siblings exist. If you had difficulty with this question, review the stages of growth and development.

Level of Cognitive Ability: Analysis
Client Needs: Health Promotion and Maintenance
Integrated Process: Nursing Process—planning
Content Area: Child health
Reference: Wong, D., Hockenberry-Eaton, M. (2000). *Wong's essentials of pediatric nursing* (6th ed., pp. 680, 1043). St. Louis: Mosby.

11. 3
Rationale: After hypospadias repair, the parents are instructed to avoid giving the child a tub bath until the stent has been removed to prevent infection. Diapers are placed on the child to prevent contamination of the surgical site. Fluids should be encouraged to maintain hydration. Toilet training should not be an issue during this stressful period.

Test-Taking Strategy: Use the process of elimination. Option 1 is eliminated first because toilet training should not be initiated during times of stress, such as following surgery. Option 2 is inappropriate because fluids should be encouraged rather than restricted. Eliminate option 4 because this action can cause contamination of the surgical site. If you had difficulty with this question, review the postoperative care following surgical repair of hypospadias.

Level of Cognitive Ability: Application
Client Needs: Health Promotion and Maintenance
Integrated Process: Teaching/Learning
Content Area: Child health
References: Wong, D., Hockenberry-Eaton, M. (2000). *Wong's essentials of pediatric nursing* (6th ed., p. 1043). St. Louis: Mosby. Wong, D., Perry, S., & Hockenberry, M. (2002). *Maternal child nursing care* (2nd ed., p. 936). St. Louis: Mosby.

12. 1
Rationale: Hypospadias is a congenital defect involving abnormal placement of the urethral orifice of the penis. In hypospadias the urethral orifice is located below the glans penis along the ventral surface. The infant should not be circumcised because the dorsal foreskin tissue will be used for surgical repair of the hypospadias. Options 2, 3, and 4 are unrelated to this disorder.

Test-Taking Strategy: Use the process of elimination. Note the key words "indicates their understanding." Recalling that hypospadias is a congenital defect involving abnormal placement of the urethral orifice of the penis will direct you to option 1. Review the treatment plan related to the repair of the hypospadias, if you had difficulty with this question.

Level of Cognitive Ability: Analysis
Client Needs: Health Promotion and Maintenance
Integrated Process: Teaching/Learning
Content Area: Child health
Reference: James, S., Ashwill, J., & Droske, S. (2002). *Nursing care of children: Principles & practice* (2nd ed., p. 603). Philadelphia: W. B. Saunders.

13. 4
Rationale: Bladder exstrophy is a congenital anomaly characterized by the extrusion of the urinary bladder to the outside of the body through a defect in the lower abdominal wall. The cause in not known, and a higher incidence occurs in the male. Options 1, 2, and 3 are not characteristics of this disorder.

Test Taking Strategy: Use the process of elimination. If you are unfamiliar with this condition, note the relationship of *exstrophy* in the name of the disorder to the word *extrusion* in the correct option. This should remind you that this condition is located external to the body. If you had difficulty with this question, review the characteristics of bladder exstrophy.

Level of Cognitive Ability: Comprehension
Client Needs: Physiological Integrity

Integrated Process: Nursing Process—planning
Content Area: Child health
Reference: Wong, D., Hockenberry-Eaton, M. (2000). *Wong's essentials of pediatric nursing* (6th ed., p. 1042). St. Louis: Mosby.

14. 2
Rationale: In bladder exstrophy the bladder is exposed and external to the body. The highest priority is impaired tissue integrity related to the exposed bladder mucosa. Although the infant needs to be monitored for elimination patterns and kidney function, option 1 is not a concern for this condition. Parental knowledge deficit related to the diagnosis and treatment of the condition will need to be addressed but again is not the priority. Although infection related to the anatomical location of the defect is an appropriate nursing diagnosis, it is a potential problem and not an actual one.
Test-Taking Strategy: Use the process of elimination. Eliminate option 4 first because this addresses a potential problem rather than an actual one. Eliminate option 3 next because physiological needs take precedence over psychosocial needs. From the remaining options, knowledge that the bladder mucosa is exposed in this condition should direct you to the correct option. Review this disorder if you had difficulty with this question.
Level of Cognitive Ability: Analysis
Client Needs: Physiological Integrity
Integrated Process: Nursing Process—analysis
Content Area: Child health
Reference: Wong, D., Hockenberry-Eaton, M. (2000). *Wong's essentials of pediatric nursing* (6th ed., p. 1044). St. Louis: Mosby.

15. 3
Rationale: In this disorder, one must take care to protect the exposed bladder tissue from drying while allowing the drainage of urine. This is accomplished best by covering the bladder with a nonadhering plastic wrap. The use of petroleum jelly gauze should be avoided because this type of dressing can dry out, adhere to the mucosa, and damage the delicate tissue when removed. Dry sterile dressings and dressings soaked in solutions (that can dry out) also damage the mucosa when removed.
Test-Taking Strategy: Use the process of elimination. Also note the key word "nonadhering" in the correct option. If you had difficulty with this question, review care of the infant with bladder exstrophy.
Level of Cognitive Ability: Application
Client Needs: Physiological Integrity
Integrated Process: Nursing Process—planning
Content Area: Child health
Reference: James, S., Ashwill, J., & Droske, S. (2002). *Nursing care of children: Principles & practice* (2nd ed., p. 605). Philadelphia: W. B. Saunders.

CRITICAL THINKING: FILL IN THE BLANK
Answer: Dark, frothy urine
Rationale: Nephrotic syndrome is a kidney disorder characterized by massive proteinuria, hypoalbuminemia, and edema. The urine volume is decreased, and the urine is dark and frothy in appearance.
Test-Taking Strategy: Focus on the probable diagnosis of the child and think about the definition of nephrotic syndrome and its associated characteristics to answer the question. Review the clinical manifestations associated with nephrotic syndrome if you had difficulty with this question.
Level of Cognitive Ability: Analysis
Client Needs: Physiological Integrity
Integrated Process: Nursing Process—assessment
Content Area: Child health
Reference: James, S., Ashwill, J., & Droske, S. (2002). *Nursing care of children: Principles & practice* (2nd ed., p. 608). Philadelphia: W. B. Saunders.

REFERENCES

James, S., Ashwill, J., & Droske, S. (2002). *Nursing care of children: Principles & practice* (2nd ed.). Philadelphia: W. B. Saunders.
McKinney, E., Ashwill, J., Murray, S., James, S., Gorrie, T., & Droske, S. (2000). *Maternal-child nursing.* Philadelphia: W. B. Saunders.
Wong, D., Hockenberry-Eaton, M. (2000). *Wong's essentials of pediatric nursing* (6th ed.). St. Louis: Mosby.
Wong, D., Perry, S., & Hockenberry, M. (2002). *Maternal child nursing care* (2nd ed.). St. Louis: Mosby.

Integumentary Disorders

I. ECZEMA (ATOPIC DERMATITIS)

A. Description

1. Eczema is a superficial inflammatory process involving primarily the epidermis.
2. The major goals of management are to relieve pruritus, hydrate the skin, reduce inflammation, and prevent or control secondary infections.

B. Forms of eczema (Box 42-1)

C. Assessment

1. Redness
2. Itching
3. Minute papules and vesicles
4. Weeping, oozing, and crusting of lesions

D. Interventions

1. Avoid exposure to skin irritants such as soaps, detergents, fabric softeners, diaper wipes, and powder.
2. Improve skin hydration.
3. Apply cool, wet compresses to soothe the skin.
4. Administer antihistamines and topical corticosteroids as prescribed; corticosteroids are applied in a thin layer and are rubbed into the area thoroughly.
5. Prevent or minimize scratching; keep the nails short and clean, and place gloves or cotton socks over the hands.
6. Eliminate conditions that increase itching, such as heat, woolen clothes or blankets, rough fabrics, or furry stuffed animals.
7. Instruct the parents to wash clothing in a mild detergent and rinse thoroughly; putting the clothes through a second complete wash cycle without detergent will minimize the amount of residue remaining on the fabric.
8. Instruct the parents in the measures to prevent skin infections.
9. Instruct the parents to monitor the lesions for signs of infection (honey-colored crusts with surrounding erythema).

II. IMPETIGO

A. Description

1. Impetigo is a highly contagious bacterial infection of the skin caused by β-hemolytic streptococci or *Staphylococcus aureus* or both.
2. The most common sites of infection are the face, around the mouth, the hands, the neck, and the extremities.
3. The lesions begin as vesicles or pustules surrounded by edema and redness, usually at a site that has been injured; this progresses to an exudative and crusting stage.
4. After the crusting of the lesions, the initially serous vesicular fluid becomes cloudy, and the vesicle ruptures, leaving a honey-colored crust covering an ulcerated base.

B. Assessment

1. Lesions

BOX 42-1

Forms of Eczema

INFANTILE
Usually begins at 2 to 6 months of age and generally undergoes spontaneous remission by 3 years of age.

CHILDHOOD
May follow the infantile form and occurs at 2 to 3 years of age.

PREADOLESCENT AND ADOLESCENT
Begins at about 12 years of age and may continue into the early adult years or indefinitely.

2. Pruritus
3. Burning
4. Secondary lymph node involvement

C. Interventions

1. Contact isolation; use standard precautions and implement agency-specific isolation procedures for the hospitalized child.
2. Allow lesions to dry by air exposure.
3. Assist the child with daily bathing with antibacterial soap, such as pHisoHex, as prescribed.
4. Apply warm compresses to lesions 2 or 3 times per day, as prescribed, to remove crusts and to allow for healing.
5. Apply and instruct the parents in the use of antibiotic ointments; the infection is communicable for 48 hours after antibiotic ointment treatment is begun.
6. Administer oral antibiotics, which may be prescribed if there is no response to topical antibiotic treatment.
7. Apply and instruct the parents in the use of emollients, as prescribed, to prevent skin cracking.
8. Instruct the parents in the methods to prevent the spread of the infection, especially careful hand washing.
9. Inform the parents that the child needs to use separate towels, linens, and dishes.
10. Inform the parents that all linens and clothing should be washed separately with detergent in hot water.

III. PEDICULOSIS CAPITIS (LICE)

A. Description

1. Pediculosis capitis is an infestation of the hair and scalp with lice.
2. The most common sites of involvement are the occipital area, behind the ears at the nape of the neck, and occasionally the eyebrows and eyelashes.
3. The female louse lays her eggs (nits) on the hair shaft, close to the scalp; the incubation period is 8 to 10 days.
4. Head lice live and reproduce only on human beings and are transmitted by direct and indirect contact, such as sharing of brushes, hats, towels, and bedding.
5. All contacts of the infested child should be examined.

B. Assessment (Box 42-2)

C. Interventions

1. Use a pediculicide shampoo; towel dry the hair, remove the nits with a fine-toothed comb, and repeat the treatment in 7 days.
2. Use permethrin (Nix) rinse.
   a. Apply to washed and towel-dried hair, leave in place for 10 minutes, and then rinse.
   b. After rinsing, towel dry the hair, and remove the nits with a fine-toothed comb.

BOX 42-2

Assessment Findings: Pediculosis Capitis

Person has intense pruritis.
Adult lice are difficult to see and appear as small gray specks, which may crawl fast.
Nits are visible and firmly attached to the hair shaft near the scalp; they are tiny silver or gray specks resembling dandruff.

3. Instruct the parents in the use of shampoo and rinse as prescribed.
4. Instruct the parents that bedding and clothing used by the child should be changed daily, laundered in hot water with detergent, and dried in a hot dryer for 20 minutes.
5. Instruct the parents that nonessential bedding and clothing can be stored in a tightly sealed bag for 10 days to 2 weeks and then washed.
6. Instruct the parents to seal toys that cannot be washed or dry cleaned in a plastic bag for 2 weeks.
7. Instruct the parents that hairbrushes or combs should be discarded or soaked in hot water (54.4° C [130° F]).
8. Instruct the parents that furniture and carpets need to be vacuumed frequently.
9. Teach the child not to share clothing, headwear, or brushes and combs.

IV. SCABIES (REFER TO CHAPTER 49 FOR ADDITIONAL INFORMATION RELATED TO SCABIES.)

A. Description

1. A parasitic skin disorder caused by an infestation of *Sarcoptes scabiei* (itch mite)
2. Endemic among schoolchildren and institutionalized populations as a result of close personal contact
3. Incubation period
   a. Female mite burrows into epidermis, lays eggs, and dies in the burrow after 4 to 5 weeks.
   b. The eggs hatch in 3 to 5 days, and larvae mature and complete their life cycle.
4. Infectious period: During the course of the infestation
5. Transmission: By close personal contact with infected person

B. Assessment (Box 42-3)

BOX 42-3

Assessment Findings: Scabies

Intense pruritis, especially at night
Burrows (fine grayish red lines that may be difficult to see) on the skin

C. Interventions
   1. Topical application of a scabicide such as lindane cream (Kwell, Scabene), crotamiton (Eurax), or permethrin 5% (Elimite) kills the mites.
   2. Lindane cream (Kwell, Scabene) should not be used in children younger than age 2 because of the risk of neurotoxicity and seizures.
   3. Instruct the parents in the application of the scabicide.
      a. Application should be preceded by a warm soap-and-water bath.
      b. Skin must be cool and dry before the application of the lotion.
      c. Lotion is left in place for 8 to 14 hours before it is washed off.
   4. When permethrin 5% (Elimite, Nix) is used, the cream is massaged thoroughly and gently into all skin surfaces (not just the areas that have the rash) from the head to the soles of the feet; care should be taken to avoid contact with the eyes.
   5. Household members and contacts of the infected child need to be treated at the same time.
   6. Instruct the parents about the importance of frequent hand washing.
   7. Instruct the parents that all clothing, bedding, and pillowcases used by the child need to be changed daily, washed in hot water with detergent, dried in a hot dryer, and ironed before reuse.
   8. Instruct the parents that nonwashable toys and other items should be sealed in plastic bags for 4 days.

V. THE BURNED CHILD (REFER TO CHAPTER 49 FOR ADDITIONAL INFORMATION RELATED TO BURNS.)

A. Pediatric differences
   1. Very young children who have been burned severely have a higher mortality rate than older children and adults with comparable burns.
   2. Lower burn temperatures and shorter exposure to heat can cause a more severe burn in a child than in an adult because a child's skin is thinner
   3. Severely burned children are at increased risk for fluid and heat loss, dehydration, and metabolic acidosis than an adult.
   4. The higher proportion of body fluid to mass in children increases the risk of cardiovascular problems.
   5. Burns involving more than 10% of total body surface area require some form of fluid resuscitation.
   6. Infants and children are at increased risk for protein and calorie deficiency because they have smaller muscle mass and less body fat than adults.
   7. Scarring is more severe in a child.
   8. An immature immune system presents an increased risk of infection for infants and young children.
   9. A delay in **growth** may occur following a burn.

B. Extent of burn injury
   1. The rule of nines, used for an adult with a burn injury, gives an inaccurate estimate because of the differences in body proportion between children and adults.
   2. A modified rule of nines may be used for the pediatric population (Fig. 42-1).

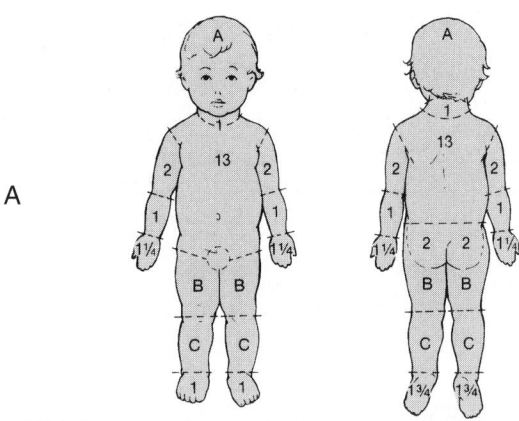

A

RELATIVE PERCENTAGES OF AREAS AFFECTED BY GROWTH

AREA	BIRTH	AGE 1 YR	AGE 5 YR
A = 1/2 of head	9 1/2	8 1/2	6 1/2
B = 1/2 of one thigh	2 3/4	3 1/4	4
C = 1/2 of one leg	2 1/2	2 1/2	2 3/4

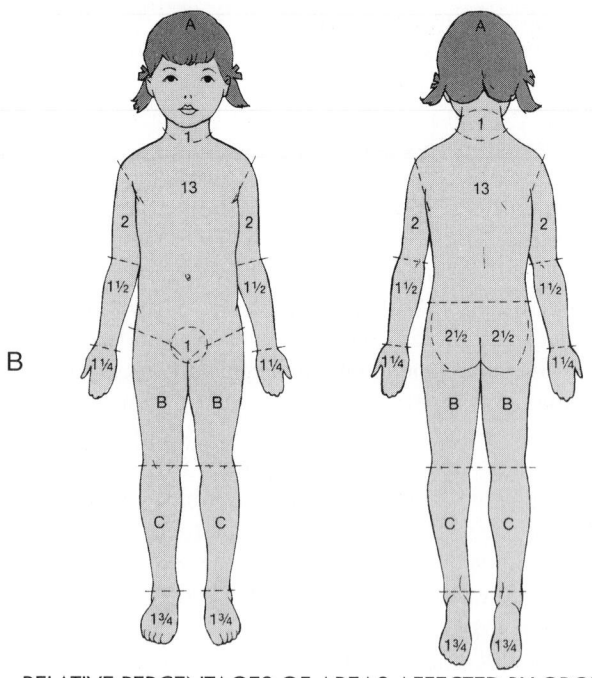

B

RELATIVE PERCENTAGES OF AREAS AFFECTED BY GROWTH

AREA	AGE 10 YR	AGE 15 YR	ADULT
A = 1/2 of head	5 1/2	4 1/2	3 1/2
B = 1/2 of one thigh	4 1/2	4 1/2	4 3/4
C = 1/2 of one leg	3	3 1/4	3 1/2

FIG. 42-1 Estimation of distribution of burns in children. **A,** Children from birth to age 5 years. **B,** Older children. (From Wong, D., Perry, S., & Hockenberry, M. [2002]. *Maternal child nursing care* [2nd ed.]. St. Louis: Mosby.)

BOX 42-4

Parkland Formula for Fluid Resuscitation

4 mL Ringer's lactate solution × kilograms of body mass × percent total body surface area burned

One half of the total is administered in the first 8 hours after the burn.

One fourth of the total is administered in the second 8 hours after the burn.

One fourth of the total is administered in the third 8 hours after the burn.

Time is calculated from the time of injury, not the time of admission to the hospital.

The criterion for successful burn, shock, and fluid resuscitation is a urine output of 1 mL/kg per hour in children.

C. Formulas of fluid resuscitation

1. Several formulas are available that can be used to calculate the rate of fluid administration.

2. The Parkland formula for fluid resuscitation is one method to calculate fluid replacement (Box 42-4).

PRACTICE QUESTIONS

1. Corticream is prescribed by a physician for a child with atopic dermatitis (eczema). A nurse instructs the mother in how to apply the cream appropriately and tells the mother to
   1. Avoid cleansing the area before application of the cream.
   2. Apply the cream over the entire body.
   3. Apply a thin layer of cream and rub into the area thoroughly.
   4. Apply a thick layer of cream in affected areas only.

2. A school nurse has provided an instructional session about impetigo to parents of the children attending the school. Which statement if made by a parent indicates a need for further instructions?
   1. "It is most common in humid weather."
   2. "It begins in an area of broken skin, such as an insect bite."
   3. "It is extremely contagious."
   4. "Lesions most often are located on the arms and chest."

3. A clinic nurse provides instructions to the mother of a child with impetigo regarding the application of antibiotic ointment. The mother asks the nurse when the child can return to school. The most appropriate response to the mother is
   1. 24 hours after using antibiotic ointment.
   2. 48 hours after using antibiotic ointment.
   3. 1 week after using antibiotic ointment.
   4. 10 days after using antibiotic ointment.

4. A school nurse has provided instructions regarding the use of permethrin 1% (Nix) to the parents of children diagnosed with pediculosis capitis (head lice). Which statement if made by a parent indicates a need for further instructions?
   1. "The Nix can be obtained over the counter in a local pharmacy."
   2. "It is applied to the hair after shampooing and left on for 24 hours."
   3. "It is applied to the hair after shampooing, left on for 10 minutes, and then rinsed out."
   4. "The hair should not be shampooed for 24 hours following treatment."

5. A school nurse prepares a list of home care instructions for the parents of schoolchildren diagnosed with pediculosis capitis. Which of the following will the nurse include in the list?
   1. Use antilice sprays on all bedding and furniture.
   2. Bring all bedding and linens to the cleaners to be dry cleaned.
   3. Soak combs and brushes in warm water.
   4. Vacuum floors, play areas, and furniture to remove any hairs that might carry live nits.

6. A mother of a 3-year-old child arrives at a clinic and tells a nurse that the child has been scratching the skin continuously and has developed a rash. The nurse assesses the child and suspects the presence of scabies. The nurse bases this suspicion on which finding noted on assessment of the child's skin?
   1. Clusters of fluid-filled vesicles
   2. Fine threadlike lines
   3. Purple-colored lesions
   4. Thick, honey-colored crusts

7. Permethrin 5% (Elimite) is prescribed for a 4-year-old child with a diagnosis of scabies. A clinic nurse instructs the mother regarding the use of this treatment and tells the mother
   1. That the lotion should be applied to areas of the rash only.
   2. To apply the lotion and leave it on for 6 hours.
   3. To apply the lotion to cool, dry skin at least one half hour after bathing.
   4. To avoid clothing the child while the lotion is in place.

8. A 2-year-old child is admitted to a burn unit with partial- and full-thickness burns over 35% of the body. After admission assessment and review of the physician's orders, the priority nursing intervention focuses on
   1. Sedating with morphine sulfate.
   2. Restricting intravenously administered fluids.
   3. Inserting a nasogastric tube.
   4. Inserting a Foley catheter.

9. A clinic nurse is reviewing the physician's orders for a child who has been diagnosed with scabies. Lindane

(Kwell, Scabene) has been prescribed for the child. The nurse questions the order if which of the following is noted in the child's record?
1. The child is 18 months old.
2. The child has a history of frequent respiratory infections.
3. A sibling is using lindane for the treatment of scabies.
4. The child is being bottle-fed.

10. A nurse is monitoring a child with burns during the treatment for burn shock. The nurse understands that which of the following assessments provides the most accurate guide to determining the adequacy of fluid resuscitation?
1. Skin turgor
2. Level of edema at burn site
3. Adequacy of peripheral pulses
4. Neurological assessment

CRITICAL THINKING: FILL IN THE BLANK

A 10-kg child sustains a burn from a house fire, and the total body surface area of the burn is determined to be 50%. The Parkland formula for fluid resuscitation is used to determine the amount of fluid that this child requires. A nurse determines that the child will receive how many milliliters of fluid in the first 8 hours from the time of the injury?

Answer: _____

ANSWERS

1. 3

Rationale: Corticream is a topical corticosteroid. Corticream should be applied sparingly (thin layer) and rubbed into the area thoroughly. The affected area should be cleansed gently before application. Corticream should not be applied over extensive areas. Systemic absorption is more likely to occur with extensive application.
Test-Taking Strategy: Use the process of elimination. Eliminate option 1 first because it does not make sense not to cleanse an affected area. Eliminate option 2 because cream should be applied only to areas that are affected. Eliminate option 4 because of the word "thick." Review the procedure for the application of a topical corticosteroid if you had difficulty with this question.
Level of Cognitive Ability: Application
Client Needs: Physiological Integrity
Integrated Process: Teaching/Learning
Content Area: Child health
Reference: Wong, D., Hockenberry-Eaton, M. (2000). *Wong's essentials of pediatric nursing* (6th ed., p. 1156). St. Louis: Mosby.

2. 4

Rationale: Impetigo is most common during hot, humid summer months. Impetigo begins in an area of broken skin, such as an insect bite or atopic dermatitis. Infection may be caused by *Staphylococcus aureus*, group A β-hemolytic streptococci, or a combination of these bacteria. Impetigo is extremely contagious. Lesions usually are located around the mouth and nose but may be present on the extremities.
Test-Taking Strategy: Use the process of elimination, noting the key words "need for further instructions." Knowledge regarding the cause and manifestations of impetigo will direct you easily to option 4. If you are unfamiliar with this disorder, review this content.
Level of Cognitive Ability: Analysis
Client Needs: Safe, Effective Care Environment
Integrated Process: Teaching/Learning
Content Area: Child health
Reference: James, S., Ashwill, J., & Droske, S. (2002). *Nursing care of children: Principles & practice* (2nd ed., p. 811). Philadelphia: W. B. Saunders.

3. 2

Rationale: The child should not attend school for 24 to 48 hours after the initiation of systemic antibiotics or 48 hours after the use of antibiotic ointment. The school should be notified of the diagnosis. Options 1, 3, and 4 are incorrect time frames.
Test-Taking Strategy: Use general principles related to the administration of antibiotics to answer the question. Eliminate options 3 and 4 first because these time frames are closely related and rather lengthy. From the remaining options, noting the key word "ointment" in the question should assist in directing you to option 2. Review home care measures related to the administration of antibiotics if you had difficulty with this question.
Level of Cognitive Ability: Application
Client Needs: Safe, Effective Care Environment
Integrated Process: Teaching/Learning
Content Area: Child health
Reference: James, S., Ashwill, J., & Droske, S. (2002). *Nursing care of children: Principles & practice* (2nd ed., p. 810). Philadelphia: W. B. Saunders.

4. 2

Rationale: Nix is an over-the-counter scabicide that kills lice and eggs with one application and has residual activity for 10 days. Nix is applied to the hair after shampooing and left for 10 minutes before rinsing out. The hair should not be shampooed for 24 hours after the treatment.
Test-Taking Strategy: Use the process of elimination, noting the key words "need for further instructions." Recalling the instructions for the use of this scabicide product will direct you to option 2. Review the procedure for using this product if you had difficulty with this question.
Level of Cognitive Ability: Analysis
Client Needs: Safe, Effective Care Environment
Integrated Process: Teaching/Learning
Content Area: Child health
Reference: James, S., Ashwill, J., & Droske, S. (2002). *Nursing care of children: Principles & practice* (2nd ed., p. 821). Philadelphia: W. B. Saunders.

5. 4

Rationale: Thorough home cleaning is necessary to remove any remaining lice or nits. Antilice sprays are unnecessary.

In addition, they should never be used on a child. Bedding and linens should be washed with hot water and dried on a hot setting. Items that cannot be washed should be dry cleaned or sealed in plastic bags in a warm place for 2 weeks. Combs and brushes should be soaked in the scabicide shampoo or hot water.
Test-Taking Strategy: Use the process of elimination. Eliminate option 1 first, knowing that antilice sprays should not be used. Eliminate option 2 next, knowing that bedding and linens can be washed. Also note the absolute term "all" in this option and in option 1. From the remaining options, eliminate option 3 because of the words "warm water." If you had difficulty with this question, review these important home care instructions.
Level of Cognitive Ability: Application
Client Needs: Safe, Effective Care Environment
Integrated Process: Teaching/Learning
Content Area: Child health
Reference: James, S., Ashwill, J., & Droske, S. (2002). *Nursing care of children: Principles & practice* (2nd ed., p. 821). Philadelphia: W. B. Saunders.

6. **2**
Rationale: Scabies appears as burrows or fine, grayish, thread-like lines. They may be difficult to see if they are obscured by excoriation and inflammation. Clusters of fluid-filled vesicles are seen in herpesvirus. Thick, honey-colored crusts are characteristic of impetigo. Purple-colored lesions may indicate various disorders, including systemic conditions.
Test-Taking Strategy: Use the process of elimination. Recalling that scabies infestation produces burrows will assist in directing you to option 2. If you are unfamiliar with the clinical manifestations associated with scabies, review this content.
Level of Cognitive Ability: Analysis
Client Needs: Physiological Integrity
Integrated Process: Nursing Process—assessment
Content Area: Child health
Reference: James, S., Ashwill, J., & Droske, S. (2002). *Nursing care of children: Principles & practice* (2nd ed., p. 822). Philadelphia: W. B. Saunders.

7. **3**
Rationale: Permethrin is massaged thoroughly and gently into all skin surfaces (not just the areas that have the rash) from the head to the soles of the feet. One should take care to avoid contact with the eyes. The lotion should be kept on for 8 to 14 hours, and then the child should be given a bath. The lotion should not be applied until at least one half hour after bathing and should be applied only to cool, dry skin. The child should be clothed during treatment.
Test-Taking Strategy: Use the process of elimination. Options 1 and 4 can be eliminated easily. Also, note the absolute word "only" in option 1. Knowledge regarding the procedure for the application of this lotion will direct you to option 3. Review this treatment if you had difficulty with this question.
Level of Cognitive Ability: Application
Client Needs: Physiological Integrity
Integrated Process: Teaching/Learning
Content Area: Child health

Reference: James, S., Ashwill, J., & Droske, S. (2002). *Nursing care of children: Principles & practice* (2nd ed., p. 823). Philadelphia: W. B. Saunders.

8. **4**
Rationale: A Foley catheter is inserted into the child's bladder so that urine output can be measured accurately each hour. Although pain medication may be required, the child should not be sedated. Intravenously administered fluids are not restricted and are administered at a rate sufficient to keep the child's urine output at 1 mL/kg of body mass per hour, thus reflecting adequate tissue perfusion. A nasogastric tube may or may not be required, but this is not the priority intervention.
Test-Taking Strategy: Use the process of elimination. Option 1 can be eliminated first because the child should not be sedated. Eliminate option 2 next, knowing that fluid resuscitation is an important component of therapy to prevent burn shock. From the remaining options, knowledge that urine output reflects adequate tissue perfusion will direct you to option 4. Review the treatment of burns if you had difficulty with this question.
Level of Cognitive Ability: Analysis
Client Needs: Physiological Integrity
Integrated Process: Nursing Process—implementation
Content Area: Child health
Reference: Wong, D., Hockenberry-Eaton, M. (2000). *Wong's essentials of pediatric nursing* (6th ed., p. 777). St. Louis: Mosby.

9. **1**
Rationale: Lindane is contraindicated for children younger than 2 years of age. These children have more permeable skin, and high systemic absorption may occur, placing the child at risk for central nervous system toxicity and seizures. Lindane also is used with caution in children between the ages of 2 and 10. Siblings and other household members also should be treated at the same time. Options 2 and 4 are unrelated to the use of lindane. Lindane is not recommended for use by a woman who is breast-feeding because the medication is secreted into breast milk.
Test-Taking Strategy: Use the process of elimination. Recall the concepts related to the body surface area of children and medication administration. These concepts will direct you easily to option 1. If you are unfamiliar with this medication, review the contraindications associated with its use.
Level of Cognitive Ability: Analysis
Client Needs: Physiological Integrity
Integrated Process: Analysis
Content Area: Child health
Reference: James, S., Ashwill, J., & Droske, S. (2002). *Nursing care of children: Principles & practice* (2nd ed., p. 823). Philadelphia: W. B. Saunders.

10. **4**
Rationale: Sensorium is an accurate guide to determine the adequacy of fluid resuscitation. The burn injury itself does not affect the sensorium, so the child should be alert and oriented. Any alteration in sensorium should be evaluated further. A neurological assessment would determine the level of sensorium in the child. Options 1, 2, and 3 would not provide an accurate assessment of the adequacy of fluid resuscitation.

Test-Taking Strategy: Note the key words "most accurate" in the stem of the question. Although options 1, 2, and 3 may provide some information related to fluid volume, in a burn injury, from the options provided, neurological assessment is most accurate. Review assessments during fluid resuscitation and treatment for burn shock if you had difficulty with this question.
Level of Cognitive Ability: Analysis
Client Needs: Physiological Integrity
Integrated Process: Nursing Process—evaluation
Content Area: Child health
Reference: Wong, D., Hockenberry-Eaton, M. (2000). *Wong's essentials of pediatric nursing* (6th ed., p. 1194). St. Louis: Mosby.

CRITICAL THINKING: FILL IN THE BLANK

Answer: 1000 mL
Rationale: The Parkland formula is calculated as 4 mL Ringer's lactate solution multiplied by kilograms of body mass multiplied by percent total body surface area (TBSA) of the burn.

One half of the total is administered in the first 8 hours after the burn. One fourth of the total is administered in the second 8 hours after the burn. One fourth of the total is administered in the third 8 hours after the burn: 4 mL × 10 kg × 50% TBSA burn = 2000 mL Ringer's lacate solution in 24 hours. The child would receive 1000 mL in the first 8 hours at 125 mL/hr, 500 mL in the second 8 hours at 62 mL/hr, and 500 mL in the third 8 hours at 62 mL/hr.
Test-Taking Strategy: Knowledge regarding the calculation of the amount of fluid required by the Parkland formula is required to answer this question. If you are unfamiliar with this method of calculation, review the formula.
Level of Cognitive Ability: Analysis
Client Needs: Physiological Integrity
Integrated Process: Nursing Process—analysis
Content Area: Child health
Reference: James, S., Ashwill, J., & Droske, S. (2002). *Nursing care of children: Principles & practice* (2nd ed., p. 845). Philadelphia: W. B. Saunders.

REFERENCES

Hodgson, B., & Kizior, R. (2003). *Saunders nursing drug handbook 2003.* Philadelphia: W. B. Saunders.

James, S., Ashwill, J., & Droske, S. (2002). *Nursing care of children: Principles & practice* (2nd ed.). Philadelphia: W. B. Saunders.

McKinney, E., Ashwill, J., Murray, S., James, S., Gorrie, T., & Droske, S. (2000). *Maternal-child nursing.* Philadelphia: W. B. Saunders.

Wong, D., Hockenberry-Eaton, M. (2000). *Wong's essentials of pediatric nursing* (6th ed.). St. Louis: Mosby.

Wong, D., Perry, S., & Hockenberry, M. (2002). *Maternal child nursing care* (2nd ed.). St. Louis: Mosby.

Musculoskeletal Disorders

I. DYSPLASIA OF THE HIP

A. Description
1. Dysplasia of the hip is a condition in which the head of the femur is seated improperly in the acetabulum, or hip socket, of the pelvis.
2. Dysplasia can range from mild to severely dislocated.
3. Dysplasia can be congenital or can develop after birth.

B. Assessment (Fig. 43-1)
1. Neonates: laxity of the ligaments around the hip, which allows the femoral head to be displaced from the acetabulum on manipulation
2. Infants beyond the newborn period
   a. Asymmetry of the gluteal and thigh skinfolds when the child is placed prone and the legs are extended against the examining table
   b. Limited range of motion in the affected hip
   c. Asymmetric abduction of the affected hip when the child is placed supine with the knees and hips flexed
   d. Apparent short femur on the affected side
3. Positive Barlow or Ortolani maneuver
4. The walking child: minimal to pronounced variations in gait with lurching toward the affected side; positive Trendelenburg's sign

C. Interventions
1. In the neonatal period, splinting of the hips with Pavlik harness to maintain flexion and abduction and external rotation
2. Following the neonatal period, traction and/or surgery to release muscles and tendons
3. Following surgery, positioning and immobilization in a spica cast until healing is achieved, then use of an abduction splint
4. Operative reduction possibly required in the older child
5. Instruction to parents regarding proper care of a Pavlik harness or spica cast (Fig. 43-2)

II. CONGENITAL CLUBFOOT

A. Description
1. Clubfoot is a congenital malformation of the lower extremities.
2. The defect may be unilateral or bilateral.
3. Defects are rigid and cannot be manipulated into a neutral position.
4. Long-term interval follow-up is required until the child reaches skeletal maturity.

B. Assessment: The foot is plantar flexed with an inverted heel and adducted forefoot.

C. Interventions
1. Treatment begins as soon after birth as possible.
2. Serial manipulation and casting are performed weekly, and if correction is not achieved in 3 to 6 months, surgery is indicated.
3. Monitor for pain.
4. Monitor neurovascular status of the toes.
5. Instruct parents in cast care and the signs of neurovascular impairment that requires physician notification.

III. SCOLIOSIS

A. Description
1. Scoliosis is a lateral curvature of the spine.
2. Surgical and nonsurgical interventions are used, and the type of treatment depends on the degree of curvature, the age of the child, and the amount of **growth** that is anticipated.
3. Long-term monitoring is essential to detect any progression of the curve.

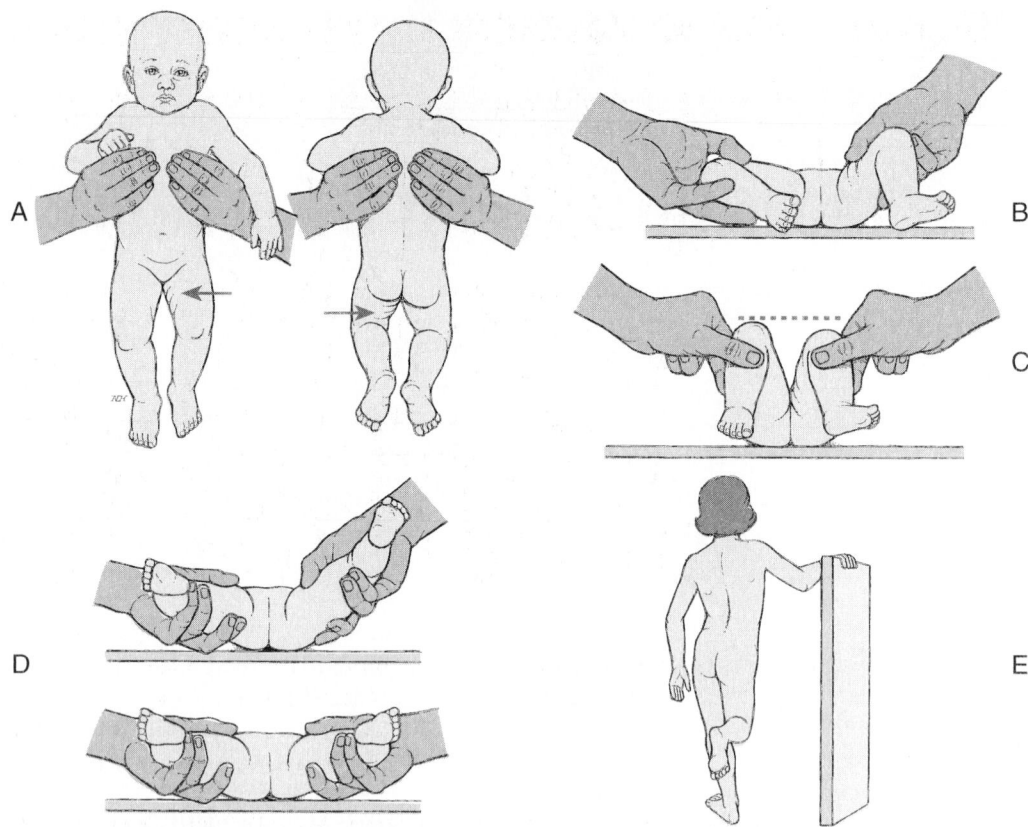

FIG. 43-1   Signs of developmental dysplasia of the hip. **A,** Asymmetry of gluteal and thigh folds. **B,** Limited hip abduction, as seen in flexion. **C,** Apparent shortening of the femur, as indicated by the level of the knees in flexion. **D,** Ortolani click (if infant is under 4 weeks of age). **E,** Positive Trendelenburg's sign or gait (if child is weight bearing). (From Hockenberry MJ. [2005]. *Wong's essentials of pediatric nursing* [7th ed.]. St. Louis: Mosby.)

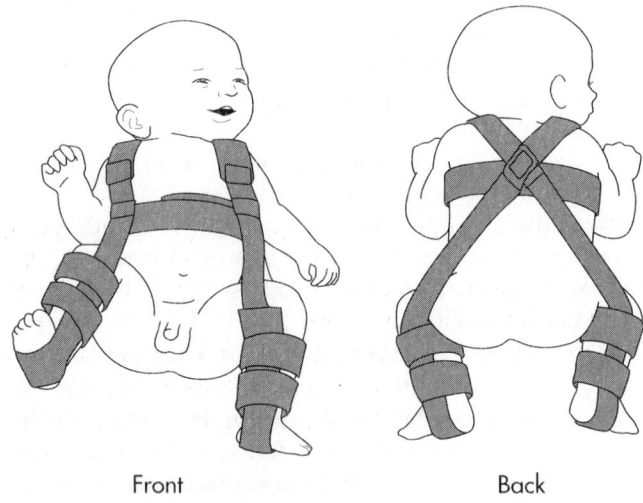

Front   Back

FIG. 43-2   Child in Pavlik harness. (From Ball JW. [1998]. *Mosby's pediatric patient teaching guides.* St Louis: Mosby.)

B. Assessment
   1. Visible curve fails to straighten when the child bends forward and hangs arms down toward feet.
   2. Hips, ribs, and shoulders are asymmetrical.
   3. Leg length discrepancy is apparent.

C. Interventions
   1. Monitor progression of the curvature.
   2. Prepare the child and parents for the use of a brace if prescribed.
   3. Prepare the child and parents for surgery (spinal fusion; placement of internal instrumentation rods) if prescribed.

D. Braces
   1. Braces usually are worn from 16 to 23 hours a day.
   2. Inspect the skin for signs of redness or breakdown.
   3. Keep the skin clean and dry, avoiding lotions and powders.
   4. Advise the child to wear soft nonirritating clothing under the brace.
   5. Instruct in prescribed exercises.
   6. Encourage verbalization about body image.

E. Postoperative interventions (spinal fusion)
   1. Maintain proper alignment; avoid twisting movements.
   2. Logroll the child when turning to maintain alignment.
   3. Assess extremities for neurovascular status.
   4. Encourage coughing and deep breathing and use of incentive spirometry.

5. Assess pain and administer prescribed analgesics.
6. Monitor for incontinence.
7. Monitor for superior mesenteric artery syndrome disorder, caused by mechanical changes in the position of the child's abdominal contents during surgery, and notify the physician if it occurs; symptoms include emesis and abdominal distention similar to that which occurs with intestinal obstruction or paralytic ileus.
8. Instruct in activity restrictions.
9. Instruct the child to roll from a side-lying position to a sitting position, and assist with ambulation.
10. Prepare the child for the use of a molded plastic jacket to provide external stability of the spine when resuming activities.

IV. JUVENILE RHEUMATOID ARTHRITIS
A. Description
   1. Juvenile rheumatoid arthritis is an inflammatory disease affecting the joints; it occurs most often in girls.
   2. The cause is unknown.
   3. Iridocyclitis (inflammation of the iris and ciliary body) can occur.
   4. Treatment of juvenile rheumatoid arthritis is supportive and directed toward preserving joint function, controlling inflammation, minimizing deformity, and reducing the impact that the disease may have on the development of the child.
   5. Therapy includes medications, physical and occupational therapies, and child and family education.
   6. Surgical intervention may be implemented when the child has problems with joint contractures and unequal **growth** of extremities.
B. Assessment (Box 43-1)
C. Interventions
   1. Facilitate social and emotional development.
   2. Instruct the parents and child in the administration of medications (Box 43-2).
   3. Instruct the parent regarding the signs of aspirin toxicity; instruct to stop aspirin if signs of toxicity occur and to notify the physician.
   4. Assist the child with range-of-motion exercises and instruct in prescribed exercises.
   5. Encourage normal performance of activities of daily living.

6. Instruct the parents and child in the use of hot or cold packs, splinting, and positioning the affected joint in a neutral position during painful episodes.
7. Encourage and support prescribed physical and occupational therapy.
8. Instruct in the importance of preventive eye care and reporting visual disturbances.
9. Assess the child's perception regarding the chronic illness.

V. FRACTURES
A. Description
   1. A fracture is a break in the continuity of the bone as a result of trauma, twisting, or bone decalcification.
   2. Fractures in children usually occur as a result of increased mobility and inadequate or immature motor and cognitive skills.
   3. Fractures in children may result from trauma or bone diseases.
   4. Fractures in infancy are generally rare and warrant further investigation to rule out the possibility of child **abuse.**
B. Assessment
   1. Pain or tenderness over the involved area
   2. Loss of function
   3. Obvious deformity
   4. Crepitation
   5. Ecchymosis
   6. Edema
   7. Muscle spasm
C. Initial care of a fracture (Box 43-3)
D. Interventions
   1. Reduction
      a. Restoring the bone to proper alignment
      b. Closed reduction: accomplished by manual alignment of the fragments, followed by immobilization

---

BOX 43-1

Assessment Findings: Juvenile Rheumatoid Arthritis

Stiffness, swelling, and limited motion occur in the affected joints.
Affected joints are warm to touch.
Morning stiffness is present on arising in the morning and after inactivity.
Affected joints may be painful and tender.

BOX 43-2

Medications Used in Juvenile Rheumatoid Arthritis

Acetylsalicylic acid (aspirin)
Corticosteroids
Cytotoxic medications
Immunologic modulators
Nonsteroidal antiinflammatory drugs
Slower-acting antirheumatic drugs

BOX 43-3

Initial Care of a Fracture

Assess the extent of injury and immobilize affected extremity.
If a compound fracture exists, splint the extremity and cover the wound with a sterile dressing.

c. Open reduction: the surgical insertion of internal fixation devices, such as rods, wires, or pins, that help maintain alignment while healing occurs

2. Retention: the application of traction or a cast to maintain alignment until healing occurs

E. Traction

1. Russell skin traction
   a. Used to stabilize a fractured femur before surgery
   b. Similar to Buck's traction but provides a double pull with the use of a knee sling
   c. Traction that pulls at the knee and the foot

2. Balanced suspension
   a. Balanced suspension is used with skin or skeletal traction.
   b. Balanced suspension is used to approximate fractures of the femur, tibia, or fibula.
   c. Balanced suspension is produced by a counterforce other than the child.
   d. Types include Thomas ring splint with Pearson attachment, Steinmann pin, Kirschner wires.
   e. Protect the skin from breakdown.
   f. Provide pin care if pins are used with the skeletal traction.

3. 90-degree-90-degree
   a. The lower leg is supported by a boot cast or a calf sling.
   b. A skeletal Steinmann pin or Kirschner wire is placed in the distal fragment of the femur, allowing a 90 degree flexion at both the hip and the knee.

4. Interventions
   a. Maintain correct amount of weight as ordered.
   b. Ensure that weights hang freely.
   c. Check ropes for fraying and be sure that they are appropriately on the pulleys.
   d. Monitor neurovascular status of involved extremity.
   e. Monitor for signs and symptoms of immobilization; constipation, skin breakdown, disuse syndrome of unaffected extremities.
   f. Provide therapeutic and diversional play.

F. Casts

1. Description
   a. Casts are made of plaster or fiberglass to provide immobilization of bone and joints after a fracture or injury.
   b. Fractures of the hip or the knee may require a spica cast.

2. Interventions
   a. Examine the cast for pressure areas.
   b. Monitor the extremity for circulatory impairment, such as pain, swelling, discoloration, tingling, numbness or coolness, or diminished pulse.
   c. Notify the physician if circulatory impairment occurs.

d. Prepare for bivalving or cutting the cast if circulatory impairment occurs.
e. Instruct the child not to stick objects down the cast.
f. Teach the child to keep the cast clean and dry.
g. Instruct the child in isometric exercises to prevent muscle atrophy.

PRACTICE QUESTIONS

1. A 1-month-old infant is seen in a clinic and is diagnosed with unilateral hip dysplasia. A nurse assesses the infant, knowing that which of the following findings would be noted in this condition?
   1. An apparent lengthened femur on the affected side
   2. Limited range of motion in the affected hip
   3. Asymmetric adduction of the affected hip when the infant is placed supine with the knees and hips flexed
   4. Symmetry of the gluteal skinfolds when the infant is placed prone and the legs are extended against the examining table

2. A nurse is assisting a physician during the examination of an infant with hip dysplasia. The physician performs an Ortolani maneuver. The nurse is aware that this maneuver is performed to
   1. Push the unstable femoral head out of the acetabulum.
   2. Reduce the dislocated femoral head back into the acetabulum.
   3. Determine the extent of range of motion.
   4. Assess for asymmetry on the affected side.

3. A clinic nurse provides instructions to the parents of an infant with hip dysplasia regarding care of the Pavlik harness. Which of the following does the nurse include in the instructions?
   1. The harness should be worn 12 hours a day.
   2. The harness needs be removed for diaper changes and for feeding.
   3. The harness should be removed only to check the skin and for bathing.
   4. The infant should not be moved when out of the harness.

4. A mother brings her 2-week-old infant to a clinic for treatment following a diagnosis of clubfoot made at the time of birth. Which of the following statements, if made by the mother, indicates a need for further teaching regarding this disorder?
   1. "I need to bring my infant back to the clinic in 1 month for a new cast."
   2. "Treatment needs to be started as soon as possible."
   3. "I need to come to the clinic every week with my infant for the casting."
   4. "I realize my infant will require follow-up care until full grown."

5. A nurse is caring for a child after spinal fusion for the treatment of scoliosis. The child complains of

abdominal discomfort and begins to have episodes of vomiting. On further assessment, the nurse notes abdominal distention. Which of the following nursing actions would be most appropriate?

1. Administer an antiemetic.
2. Place the child in a Sims' position.
3. Notify the physician.
4. Increase the intravenous fluids.

6. A nurse is providing instructions to the parents of a child with scoliosis regarding the use of a brace. Which statement by parents indicates a need for further instructions?

1. "I should apply lotion under the brace to prevent skin breakdown."
2. "I should avoid the use of powder because it will cake under the brace."
3. "I will have my child wear soft-fabric clothing under the brace."
4. "I will encourage my child to perform prescribed exercises."

7. A pediatric nurse educator provides a teaching session to the nursing staff regarding juvenile rheumatoid arthritis (JRA). Which statement by a nursing staff member indicates a need for further education?

1. "JRA most often occurs before the age of 16."
2. "JRA is twice as likely to occur in boys than in girls."
3. "A complication of JRA is iridocyclitis."
4. "Clinical manifestations of JRA include morning stiffness and painful, stiff, swollen joints."

8. The mother of a child with juvenile rheumatoid arthritis calls the clinic nurse because the child is experiencing a painful exacerbation of the disease. The mother asks the nurse if the child should perform range-of-motion exercises at this time. The most appropriate nursing response is

1. "The range-of-motion exercises must be performed every day."
2. "Avoid all exercise during painful periods."
3. "Administer additional pain medication before performing range-of-motion exercises."
4. "Have the child perform simple isometric exercises during this time."

9. A child is placed in skeletal traction for treatment of a fractured femur. The nurse develops a plan of care for the child and includes which intervention in the plan?

1. Ensure that the weights are resting lightly on the floor.
2. Check the physician's orders for the amount of weight to be applied.
3. Ensure that all ropes are outside of the pulleys.
4. Restrict diversional and play activities until the child is out of traction.

10. A 4-year-old child sustains a fall at home and is brought to the emergency room by the mother. After an x-ray examination, the child is determined to have a fractured arm and a plaster cast is applied. The nurse provides instructions to the mother regarding cast care for the child. Which statement by the mother indicates a need for further instructions?

1. "The cast may feel warm as the cast dries."
2. "If the cast becomes wet, a blow drier set on the cool setting may be used to dry the cast."
3. "A small amount of white shoe polish can touch up a soiled white cast."
4. "I can use lotion or powder around the cast edges to relieve itching."

CRITICAL THINKING: MULTIPLE RESPONSE

A nurse prepares a list of home care instructions for the parents of a child who has a plaster cast applied to the left forearm. Select all instructions that would be included on the list.

____ Keep small toys and sharp objects away from the cast.

____ Use fingertips to lift the cast while it is drying.

____ Use a padded ruler or another padded object to scratch the skin under the cast if it itches.

____ Contact the physician if the child complains of numbness or tingling in the extremity.

____ Elevate the extremity on pillows for the first 24 to 48 hours after casting to prevent swelling.

ANSWERS

1. 2

Rationale: Asymmetric abduction of the affected hip, when the child is placed supine with the knees and hips flexed, would be an assessment finding in hip dysplasia in infants beyond the newborn period. Other findings include an apparent short femur on the affected side, asymmetry of the gluteal skinfolds, and limited range of motion in the affected extremity.

Test-Taking Strategy: Note the age of the infant and focus on the infant's diagnosis. Visualizing each of the assessment findings described in the options will direct you to option 2. If you had difficulty with this question, review the assessment findings in hip dysplasia.

Level of Cognitive Ability: Analysis
Client Needs: Physiological Integrity
Integrated Process: Nursing Process—assessment
Content Area: Child health
Reference: James, S., Ashwill, J., & Droske, S. (2002). *Nursing care of children: Principles & practice* (2nd ed., p. 864). Philadelphia: W. B. Saunders.

2. 2

Rationale: In the Barlow maneuver the examiner pushes the unstable femoral head out of the acetabulum. In the Ortolani maneuver, the examiner reduces the dislocated femoral head back into the acetabulum. A positive finding is a palpable click on entry or exit of the femoral head over the acetabular ring. Options 3 and 4 are done to assess for hip dysplasia.

Test-Taking Strategy: Use the process of elimination. Options 3 and 4 can be eliminated first because they are specific assessments performed to determine the presence of hip dysplasia. From the remaining options, you must know the purpose of the Ortolani maneuver. Review this maneuver if you had difficulty with this question.

Level of Cognitive Ability: Comprehension
Client Needs: Physiological Integrity
Integrated Process: Nursing Process—implementation
Content Area: Child health
Reference: James, S., Ashwill, J., & Droske, S. (2002). *Nursing care of children: Principles & practice* (2nd ed., p. 864). Philadelphia: W. B. Saunders.

3. 3

Rationale: The harness should be worn 16 to 23 hours a day and should be removed only to check the skin and for bathing. The infant can be moved when out of the harness, but the hips and buttocks should be supported carefully. The harness does not need to be removed for diaper changes or feedings.

Test-Taking Strategy: Use the process of elimination. Attempt to visualize this harness to assist in eliminating options 2 and 4. Select option 3 over option 1 because the time frame in option 1 is short. Review home care instruction regarding this harness if you had difficulty with this question.

Level of Cognitive Ability: Application
Client Needs: Health Promotion and Maintenance
Integrated Process: Teaching/Learning
Content Area: Child health
References: James, S., Ashwill, J., & Droske, S. (2002). *Nursing care of children: Principles & practice* (2nd ed., p. 867). Philadelphia: W. B. Saunders.
Wong, D., Hockenberry-Eaton, M. (2000). *Wong's essentials of pediatric nursing* (6th ed., p. 1224). St. Louis: Mosby.

4. 1

Rationale: Treatment for clubfoot is started as soon as possible after birth. Serial manipulation and casting are performed at least weekly. If sufficient correction is not achieved in 3 to 6 months, surgery usually is indicated. Because clubfoot can recur, all children with clubfoot require long-term interval follow-up until they reach skeletal maturity to ensure an optimal outcome.

Test-Taking Strategy: Use the process of elimination. Note the key words "indicates a need for further teaching." This will assist you in eliminating options 2 and 4. Recalling that serial manipulations and casting are required weekly will assist in directing you to option 1. Review these treatment procedures if you had difficulty with this question.

Level of Cognitive Ability: Analysis
Client Needs: Health Promotion and Maintenance
Integrated Process: Teaching/Learning

Content Area: Child health
References: James, S., Ashwill, J., & Droske, S. (2002). *Nursing care of children: Principles & practice* (2nd ed., p. 863). Philadelphia: W. B. Saunders.
Wong, D., Hockenberry-Eaton, M. (2000). *Wong's essentials of pediatric nursing* (6th ed., p. 1225). St. Louis: Mosby.

5. 3

Rationale: A complication after surgical treatment of scoliosis is superior mesenteric artery syndrome. This disorder is caused by mechanical changes in the position of the child's abdominal contents, resulting from lengthening of the child's body. The disorder results in a syndrome of emesis and abdominal distention similar to that which occurs with intestinal obstruction or paralytic ileus. Postoperative vomiting in children with body casts or those who have undergone spinal fusion warrants attention because of the possibility of superior mesenteric artery syndrome.

Test-Taking Strategy: Use the process of elimination. Eliminate option 4 first because it should not be implemented without a prescribed order. Eliminate option 2 next because this child requires logrolling, and Sims' position may cause injury following surgery. From the remaining options, note the assessment signs and symptoms in the question. These should alert you that physician notification is necessary. Review superior mesenteric artery syndrome if you had difficulty with this question.

Level of Cognitive Ability: Analysis
Client Needs: Physiological Integrity
Integrated Process: Nursing Process—implementation
Content Area: Child health
References: James, S., Ashwill, J., & Droske, S. (2002). *Nursing care of children: Principles & practice* (2nd ed., p. 892). Philadelphia: W. B. Saunders.
McKinney, E., Ashwill, J., Murray, S., James, S., Gorrie, T., & Droske, S. (2000). *Maternal-child nursing* (p. 1424). Philadelphia: W. B. Saunders.

6. 1

Rationale: The use of lotions or powders should be avoided because they can become sticky and cake under the brace, causing irritation. Options 2, 3, and 4 are appropriate interventions in the care of a child with a brace.

Test-Taking Strategy: Use the process of elimination. Note the key words "need for further instructions" in the stem of the question. Careful reading of the options will assist in directing you to option 1. Review home care instructions regarding the care of a child in a brace if you had difficulty with this question.

Level of Cognitive Ability: Analysis
Client Needs: Health Promotion and Maintenance
Integrated Process: Teaching/Learning
Content Area: Child health
Reference: James, S., Ashwill, J., & Droske, S. (2002). *Nursing care of children: Principles & practice* (2nd ed., p. 839). Philadelphia: W. B. Saunders.

7. 2

Rationale: Juvenile rheumatoid arthritis is twice as likely to occur in girls than in boys. Options 1, 3, and 4 are accurate regarding this disorder.

Test-Taking Strategy: Use the process of elimination. Note the key words "need for further education" in the stem of the question. Simply recalling that juvenile rheumatoid arthritis is twice as likely to occur in girls than in boys will direct you to option 2. Review this disorder if you are unfamiliar with it.
Level of Cognitive Ability: Analysis
Client Needs: Physiological Integrity
Integrated Process: Teaching/Learning
Content Area: Child health
Reference: Wong, D., Hockenberry-Eaton, M. (2000). *Wong's essentials of pediatric nursing* (6th ed., p. 1238). St. Louis: Mosby.

8. **4**
Rationale: During painful episodes, hot or cold packs and splinting and positioning the affected joint in a neutral position help reduce the pain. Although resting the extremity is appropriate, beginning simple isometric or tensing exercises as soon as the child is able is important. These exercises do not involve joint movement.
Test-Taking Strategy: Use the process of elimination. Eliminate options 1, 2, and 3 because of the words "must," "all," and "additional" in these options. Review pain management and care during exacerbations if you had difficulty with this question.
Level of Cognitive Ability: Application
Client Needs: Health Promotion and Maintenance
Integrated Process: Teaching/Learning
Content Area: Child health
Reference: James, S., Ashwill, J., & Droske, S. (2002). *Nursing care of children: Principles & practice* (2nd ed., p. 886). Philadelphia: W. B. Saunders.

9. **2**
Rationale: When a child is in traction, the nurse would check the physician's orders to verify the prescribed amount of traction weight. The nurse would maintain the correct amount of weight as ordered, ensure that the weights hang freely, check the ropes for fraying and be sure that they are appropriately on the pulleys, monitor the neurovascular status of involved extremity, and monitor for signs and symptoms of immobilization such as constipation, skin breakdown, or disuse syndrome of unaffected extremities. The nurse would provide therapeutic and diversional play activities for the child.
Test-Taking Strategy: Use the process of elimination. Recalling the general principles related to traction will direct you to option 2. Review care to the child in traction if you had difficulty with this question.
Level of Cognitive Ability: Application
Client Needs: Physiological Integrity
Integrated Process: Nursing Process—planning
Content Area: Child health

Reference: James, S., Ashwill, J., & Droske, S. (2002). *Nursing care of children: Principles & practice* (2nd ed., p. 861). Philadelphia: W .B. Saunders.

10. **4**
Rationale: The mother needs to be instructed not to use lotion or powders on the skin around the cast edges or inside the cast. Lotions or powders can become sticky or caked and cause skin irritation. Options 1, 2, and 3 are appropriate instructions.
Test-Taking Strategy: Use the process of elimination. Note the key words "indicates a need for further instructions." Remember that lotions or powders can become sticky or caked and cause skin irritation. Review home care instructions regarding cast care if you had difficulty with this question.
Level of Cognitive Ability: Analysis
Client Needs: Health Promotion and Maintenance
Integrated Process: Teaching/Learning
Content Area: Child health
Reference: McKinney, E., Ashwill, J., Murray, S., James, S., Gorrie, T., & Droske, S. (2000). *Maternal-child nursing* (p. 1934). Philadelphia: W. B. Saunders.

CRITICAL THINKING: MULTIPLE RESPONSE
Answer:
Keep small toys and sharp objects away from the cast.
Contact the physician if the child complains of numbness or tingling in the extremity.
Elevate the extremity on pillows for the first 24 to 48 hours after casting to prevent swelling.
Rationale: While the cast is drying, the palms of the hands are used to lift the cast. If the fingertips are used, indentations in the cast could occur and cause pressure on the underlying skin. Small toys and sharp objects are kept away from the cast and no objects (including padded objects) are placed inside of the cast because of the risk of altered skin integrity. The extremity is elevated to prevent swelling and the physician is notified immediately if any signs of neurovascular impairment develop.
Test-Taking Strategy: Use of the ABCs—airway, breathing, and circulation—and safety principles, related to care of a child with a cast will assist in answering the question. Review these general principles if you had difficulty with this question.
Level of Cognitive Ability: Application
Client Needs: Health Promotion and Maintenance
Integrated Process: Teaching/Learning
Content Area: Child health
Reference: James, S., Ashwill, J., & Droske, S. (2002). *Nursing care of children: Principles & practice* (2nd ed., p. 861). Philadelphia: W. B. Saunders.

REFERENCES

James, S., Ashwill, J., & Droske, S. (2002). *Nursing care of children: Principles & practice* (2nd ed.). Philadelphia: W. B. Saunders.
McKinney, E., Ashwill, J., Murray, S., James, S., Gorrie, T., & Droske, S. (2000). *Maternal-child nursing.* Philadelphia: W. B. Saunders.

Wong, D., Hockenberry-Eaton, M. (2000). *Wong's essentials of pediatric nursing* (6th ed.). St. Louis: Mosby.
Wong, D., Perry, S., & Hockenberry, M. (2002). *Maternal child nursing care* (2nd ed.). St. Louis: Mosby.

Hematological Disorders

I. SICKLE CELL DISEASE

A. Description
1. Sickle cell disease is a group of diseases collectively termed *hemoglobinopathies*, in which hemoglobin (hemoglobin A) is partly or completely replaced by abnormal sickle hemoglobin S.
2. Sickle cell disease is caused by the inheritance of a gene for a structurally abnormal portion of the hemoglobin chain.
3. Hemoglobin S is sensitive to changes in the oxygen content of the red blood cell.
4. Insufficient oxygen causes the cells to assume a sickle shape; and the cells become rigid and clumped together, obstructing capillary blood flow.
5. Situations that precipitate sickling include fever and emotional or physical stress; any condition that increases the need for oxygen or alters the transport of oxygen can result in sickle cell crisis.
6. Risk factors include having parents heterozygous for hemoglobin S or being black.
7. The sickling response is reversible under conditions of adequate oxygenation and hydration; after repeated sickling, the cell becomes permanently sickled.
8. The clinical manifestations are primarily the result of obstruction caused by sickled red blood cells and increased red blood cell destruction.
9. Sickle cell crises are acute exacerbations of the disease, which vary considerably in severity and frequency; these include vasoocclusive crisis, splenic sequestration, and aplastic crisis.
10. Care focuses on the prevention (preventing exposure to infection and maintaining normal hydration) and treatment (oxygen, hydration, pain management, and bed rest) of the crisis.

B. Assessment of the crisis (Box 44-1)
C. Interventions
1. Maintain adequate hydration and blood flow with intravenously administered normal saline as prescribed and with oral fluids.
2. Administer oxygen and blood transfusions as prescribed to increase tissue perfusion.
3. Administer analgesics as prescribed (around the clock); administration of meperidine (Demerol) is avoided because of the risk of normeperidine-induced seizures.
4. Assist the child to assume a comfortable position so that the child keeps the extremities extended to promote venous return; elevate the head of the bed no more than 30 degrees, avoid putting strain on painful joints, and do not raise the knee gatch of the bed.

BOX 44-1

Sickle Cell Crisis

VASOOCCLUSIVE CRISIS
Vasoocclusive crisis is the most common type of crisis.
The crisis is caused by stasis of blood with clumping of the cells in the microcirculation, ischemia, and infarction.
Signs include fever, pain, and tissue engorgement.

SPLENIC SEQUESTRATION
Life-threatening crisis is caused by the pooling of blood in the spleen.
Signs include profound anemia, hypovolemia, and shock.

APLASTIC CRISIS
Aplastic crisis is caused by the diminished production and increased destruction of red blood cells, triggered by viral infection or the depletion of folic acid.
Signs include profound anemia and pallor.

5. Encourage consumption of a high-calorie, high-protein diet with folic acid supplementation.
6. Administer antibiotics as prescribed to prevent infection.
7. Monitor for signs of increasing anemia and shock (mental status changes, pallor, vital sign changes).
8. Instruct the child and parents about the early signs and symptoms of crisis and the measures to prevent crisis.
9. Inform the parents of the **hereditary** aspects of the disorder.

II. IRON DEFICIENCY ANEMIA
A. Description
   1. Iron stores are depleted, resulting in a decreased supply of iron for the manufacture of hemoglobin in red blood cells.
   2. Iron deficiency anemia commonly results from blood loss, increased metabolic demands, syndromes of gastrointestinal malabsorption, and dietary inadequacy.
B. Assessment
   1. Pallor
   2. Weakness and fatigue
   3. Irritability
C. Interventions
   1. Increase the oral intake of iron.
   2. Instruct the child and parents in food choices that are high in iron (Box 44-2).
   3. Administer iron supplements as prescribed.
   4. Teach parents how to administer the iron supplements.
      a. Give iron supplements between meals for maximum absorption.
      b. Give iron supplements with a multivitamin or fruit juice because vitamin C increases absorption.
      c. Do not give iron supplements with milk or antacids because these items decrease absorption.
   5. Teach the child and parents that liquid iron preparation stains the teeth and should be taken through a straw.
   6. Instruct the child and parents about the side effects of iron supplements (black stools, constipation, and foul aftertaste).

BOX 44-2

Iron-rich Foods

Breads and cereals
Dark green, leafy vegetables
Egg yolks
Kidney beans
Liver
Meats
Raisins

III. APLASTIC ANEMIA
A. Description
   1. Aplastic anemia is a deficiency of circulating erythrocytes resulting from the arrested development of red blood cells within the bone marrow.
   2. Several possible causes exist, including chronic exposure to myelotoxic agents, viruses, infection, autoimmune disorders, and allergic states.
   3. The definitive diagnosis is determined by bone marrow aspiration (demonstrates conversion of red bone marrow to fatty red bone marrow).
   4. Therapeutic management focuses on restoring function to the bone marrow and involves immunosuppressive therapy and bone marrow transplant (treatment of choice if a suitable donor exists).
B. Assessment
   1. Pancytopenia (a deficiency of erythrocytes, leukocytes, and thrombocytes).
   2. Petechiae, purpura, bleeding, pallor, weakness, tachycardia, and fatigue.
C. Interventions
   1. Prepare the child for bone marrow transplant if planned.
   2. Administer immunosuppressive medications as prescribed; antilymphocyte globulin or antithymocyte globulin may be prescribed to suppress the autoimmune response.
   3. Colony-stimulating factors may be prescribed to enhance bone marrow production.
   4. Corticosteroids and cyclosporine (Sandimmune) may be prescribed.
   5. Administer blood transfusions if prescribed and monitor for transfusion reactions.
   6. Advise the parents to obtain a Medic-Alert bracelet for the child.

IV. HEMOPHILIA
A. Description (Box 44-3)
   1. Hemophilia is an X-linked recessive trait.
   2. Males inherit hemophilia from their mothers, and females inherit the carrier status from their fathers.
   3. Some females who are carriers have an increased tendency to bleed, and although rare, females can have hemophilia if their fathers have the disorder and their mothers are carriers of the genetic disorder.

BOX 44-3

Hemophilia

HEMOPHILIA A (CLASSIC HEMOPHILIA)
Results from a deficiency of factor VIII

HEMOPHILIA B (CHRISTMAS DISEASE)
Results from a deficiency of factor IX

4. The primary treatment is replacement of the missing clotting factor; products used are factor VIII concentrate and desmopressin (DDAVP).

▲ B. Assessment
   1. Abnormal bleeding in response to trauma or surgery
   2. Joint bleeding causing pain, tenderness, swelling, and limited range of motion
   3. Tendency to bruise easily
   4. Prolonged partial thromboplastin time
   5. Normal bleeding time, prothrombin time, and platelet count

▲ C. Interventions
   1. Monitor for bleeding and maintain bleeding precautions.
   2. Prepare to administer factor VIII concentrate or desmopressin (DDAVP).
   3. Monitor for joint pain; immobilize the affected extremity if joint pain occurs.
   4. Assess neurological status (child is at risk for intracranial hemorrhage).
   5. Monitor urine for hematuria.
   6. Control bleeding by immobilization, elevation, and the application of ice; in addition, apply pressure (15 minutes) for superficial bleeding.
   7. Instruct the child and parents about the signs of internal bleeding.
   8. Instruct the parents in how to control the bleeding.
   9. Instruct the parents regarding activities for the child, emphasizing the avoidance of contact sports.
   10. Instruct the child to wear protective devices such as helmets, knee, and elbow pads when participating in sports such as bicycling and skating.
   11. Instruct the parents to obtain a Medic-Alert bracelet for the child.

V. β-THALASSEMIA MAJOR

A. Description
   1. Thalassemia major is an autosomal recessive disorder.
   2. The disorder also is called *Cooley's anemia* and includes a group of disorders characterized by the reduced production of one of the globin chains in the synthesis of hemoglobin.
   3. The incidence is highest in individuals of Mediterranean descent.
   4. Treatment is supportive, and the goal of therapy is to maintain normal hemoglobin levels by the administration of blood transfusions.
   5. Bone marrow transplantation may be offered as an alternative therapy.
   6. A splenectomy may be performed in a child with severe splenomegaly who requires repeated transfusions (assists in relieving abdominal pressure and may increase the life span of supplemental red blood cells).

B. Assessment
   1. Frontal bossing
   2. Maxillary prominence
   3. Wide-set eyes with a flattened nose
   4. Greenish yellow skin tone
   5. Hepatosplenomegaly
   6. Severe anemia
   7. Microcytic, hypochromic red blood cells

C. Interventions
   1. Administer blood transfusions as prescribed; monitor for transfusion reactions.
   2. Monitor for iron overload and administer chelation therapy with deferoxamine (Desferal) as prescribed to treat iron overload and to prevent organ damage from the elevated levels of iron caused by the multiple transfusion therapy.
   3. If the child had a splenectomy, instruct the parents to report any signs of infection because of the risk of sepsis.
   4. Provide genetic counseling.

PRACTICE QUESTIONS

1. A child suspected of having sickle cell disease is seen in a clinic, and laboratory studies are performed. A nurse checks the laboratory results, knowing that which of the following would be increased in this disease?
   1. Platelet count
   2. Hematocrit level
   3. Reticulocyte count
   4. Hemoglobin level

2. A pediatric nursing instructor asks a nursing student to describe the cause of the clinical manifestations that occur in sickle cell disease. The student responds correctly by telling the instructor that
   1. Sickled cells increase the blood flow through the body and cause a great deal of pain.
   2. Sickled cells mix with the unsickled cells and cause the immune system to become depressed.
   3. Bone marrow depression occurs because of the development of sickled cells.
   4. Sickled cells are unable to flow easily through the microvasculature and their clumping obstructs blood flow.

3. A clinic nurse instructs the mother of a child with sickle cell disease about the precipitating factors related to pain crisis. Which of the following, if identified by the mother as a precipitating factor, indicates the need for further instructions?
   1. Infection
   2. Trauma
   3. Fluid overload
   4. Stress

4. Laboratory studies are performed for a child suspected of having iron deficiency anemia. The nurse reviews the laboratory results, knowing that which of the following results would indicate this type of anemia?
   1. An elevated hemoglobin level
   2. A decreased reticulocyte count
   3. An elevated red blood cell count
   4. Red blood cells that are microcytic and hypochromic

5. A home care nurse is instructing the parents of a child with iron deficiency anemia regarding the administration of a liquid oral iron supplement. The nurse tells the mother to
   1. Administer the iron through a straw.
   2. Administer the iron at mealtimes.
   3. Add the iron to the formula for easy administration.
   4. Mix the iron with cereal to administer.

6. A pediatric nurse educator provides a teaching session to the nursing staff regarding hemophilia. Which of the following information regarding this disorder would the nurse plan to include in the discussion?
   1. Hemophilia is a Y-linked hereditary disorder.
   2. Males inherit hemophilia from their fathers.
   3. Females inherit hemophilia from their mothers.
   4. Hemophilia A results from deficiency of factor VIII.

7. A nurse analyzes the laboratory results of a child with hemophilia. The nurse understands that which of the following would most likely be abnormal in this child?
   1. Bleeding time
   2. Platelet count
   3. Prothrombin time
   4. Partial thromboplastin time

8. A nurse is providing home care instructions to the mother of a 10-year-old child with hemophilia. In which of the following activities would the nurse suggest that the child could participate safely with peers?
   1. Basketball
   2. Swimming
   3. Soccer
   4. Field hockey

9. A nursing student is presenting a clinical conference and discusses the etiology of β-thalassemia. The nursing student informs the group that the child at greatest risk of developing this disorder is
   1. A child whose intake of iron is extremely poor.
   2. A breast-fed child of a mother with chronic anemia.
   3. A child of Mediterranean descent.
   4. A child of Mexican descent.

10. A child with β-thalassemia is receiving long-term blood transfusion therapy for the treatment of this disorder. Chelation therapy is prescribed to prevent organ damage from the presence of too much iron in the body as a result of the transfusions. Which of the following medications would the nurse anticipate to be prescribed in chelation therapy?
    1. Dalteparin sodium (Fragmin)
    2. Meropenem (Merrem)
    3. Molindone (Moban)
    4. Deferoxamine (Desferal)

CRITICAL THINKING: FILL IN THE BLANK

A nurse is reviewing a physician's orders for a child with sickle cell anemia who was admitted to the hospital for the treatment of vasoocclusive crisis. The nurse notes that the physician has prescribed an increased fluid intake, intravenous fluids, oxygen, heat to the affected areas, and meperidine (Demerol) for pain. Which order documented by the physician will the nurse question?

Answer: _____

ANSWERS

1. **3**

Rationale: A diagnosis is established based on a complete blood count, examination for sickled red blood cells in the peripheral smear, and hemoglobin electrophoresis. Laboratory studies will show decreased hemoglobin and hematocrit levels and a decreased platelet count, an increased reticulocyte count, and the presence of nucleated red blood cells. Increased reticulocyte counts occur in children with sickle cell disease because the life span of their sickled red blood cells is shortened.

Test-Taking Strategy: Use the process of elimination. Recalling that the life span of the sickled red blood cells is shortened in sickle cell disease and recalling the relationship between this concept and the reticulocytes will direct you to the correct option. Review the laboratory tests that are diagnostic for this disorder if you had difficulty with this question.

Level of Cognitive Ability: Analysis
Client Needs: Physiological Integrity
Integrated Process: Nursing Process—assessment
Content Area: Child health
References: James, S., Ashwill, J., & Droske, S. (2002). *Nursing care of children: Principles & practice* (2nd ed., p. 747). Philadelphia: W. B. Saunders.
Wong, D., Hockenberry-Eaton, M. (2000). *Wong's essentials of pediatric nursing* (6th ed., p. 989). St. Louis: Mosby.

2. **4**

Rationale: All of the clinical manifestations of sickle cell disease result from the sickled cells being unable to flow easily through the microvasculature, and their clumping obstructs blood flow. With reoxygenation, most of the sickled red blood cells resume their normal shape. Options 1, 2, and 3 are incorrect statements.

Test-Taking Strategy: Use the process of elimination. Recalling that sickled cells clump will direct you to the correct option. Review the pathophysiology associated with sickle cell disease if you had difficulty with this question.
Level of Cognitive Ability: Comprehension
Client Needs: Physiological Integrity
Integrated Process: Teaching/Learning
Content Area: Child health
Reference: Wong, D., Hockenberry-Eaton, M. (2000). *Wong's essentials of pediatric nursing* (6th ed., p. 990). St. Louis: Mosby.

3. **3**
Rationale: Pain crisis may be precipitated by infection, dehydration, hypoxia, trauma, or physical or emotional stress. The mother of a child with sickle cell disease should encourage fluid intake of 1½ to 2 times the daily requirement to prevent dehydration.
Test-Taking Strategy: Use the process of elimination. Note the key words "the need for further instructions." Recalling that fluids are a main component of treatment in sickle cell disease to prevent pain crisis will direct you to option 3. Remember that fluids are required to prevent dehydration. Review the precipitating factors of pain crisis if you had difficulty with this question.
Level of Cognitive Ability: Analysis
Client Needs: Health Promotion and Maintenance
Integrated Process: Teaching/Learning
Content Area: Child health
Reference: James, S., Ashwill, J., & Droske, S. (2002). *Nursing care of children: Principles & practice* (2nd ed., p. 749). Philadelphia: W. B. Saunders.

4. **4**
Rationale: The results of a complete blood count in children with iron deficiency anemia will show decreased hemoglobin levels and microcytic and hypochromic red blood cells. The red blood cell count is decreased. The reticulocyte count is usually normal or slightly elevated.
Test-Taking Strategy: Use the process of elimination. Eliminate options 1 and 3 first, knowing that the hemoglobin and red blood cell counts would be decreased. From the remaining options, select option 4 over option 2 because of the relationship between anemia and red blood cells. Review the laboratory findings in iron deficiency anemia if you had difficulty with this question.
Level of Cognitive Ability: Analysis
Client Needs: Physiological Integrity
Integrated Process: Nursing Process—assessment
Content Area: Child health
Reference: James, S., Ashwill, J., & Droske, S. (2002). *Nursing care of children: Principles & practice* (2nd ed., p. 745). Philadelphia: W. B. Saunders.

5. **1**
Rationale: An oral iron supplement should be administered through a straw or medicine dropper placed at the back of the mouth because the iron will stain the teeth. The parents should be instructed to brush or wipe the teeth after administration. Iron is administered between meals because absorption is decreased if there is food in the stomach. Iron requires an acid environment to facilitate its absorption in the duodenum. Iron is not added to formula or mixed with cereal or other food items.
Test-Taking Strategy: Use the process of elimination. Eliminate options 3 and 4 first because they are similar and because medication should not be added to formula and food. Note the key word "liquid" in the question. This should assist you in recalling that iron in liquid form stains teeth. Review the teaching points related to this medication if you had difficulty with this question.
Level of Cognitive Ability: Application
Client Needs: Physiological Integrity
Integrated Process: Teaching/Learning
Content Area: Child health
Reference: Wong, D., Hockenberry-Eaton, M. (2000). *Wong's essentials of pediatric nursing* (6th ed., p. 989). St. Louis: Mosby.

6. **4**
Rationale: Males inherit hemophilia from their mothers, and females inherit the carrier status from their fathers. Hemophilia is inherited in a recessive manner via a genetic defect on the X chromosome. Hemophilia A results from a deficiency of factor VIII. Hemophilia B (Christmas disease) is a deficiency of factor IX.
Test-Taking Strategy: Use the process of elimination. Read each option carefully, and use knowledge regarding hemophilia and its related etiology to answer the question. Review this important disorder if you had difficulty with this question.
Level of Cognitive Ability: Application
Client Needs: Physiological Integrity
Integrated Process: Teaching/Learning
Content Area: Child health
References: James, S., Ashwill, J., & Droske, S. (2002). *Nursing care of children: Principles & practice* (2nd ed., p. 755). Philadelphia: W. B. Saunders.
Wong, D., Hockenberry-Eaton, M. (2000). *Wong's essentials of pediatric nursing* (6th ed., p. 989). St. Louis: Mosby.

7. **4**
Rationale: Abnormal laboratory results in hemophilia indicate a prolonged partial thromboplastin time. The bleeding time, prothrombin time, and platelet count are normal in hemophilia.
Test-Taking Strategy: Use the process of elimination and knowledge regarding the laboratory tests used to monitor hemophilia. Recalling the pathophysiology associated with this disorder will direct you to option 4. Review these laboratory tests if you had difficulty with this question.
Level of Cognitive Ability: Analysis
Client Needs: Physiological Integrity
Integrated Process: Nursing Process—analysis
Content Area: Child health
Reference: James, S., Ashwill, J., & Droske, S. (2002). *Nursing care of children: Principles & practice* (2nd ed., p. 756). Philadelphia: W. B. Saunders.

8. **2**
Rationale: Children with hemophilia need to avoid contact sports and to take precautions such as wearing elbow and knee pads and helmets with other sports. The safest activity for them is swimming.

Test-Taking Strategy: Use the process of elimination. Note the key word "safely" in the stem of the question. Recalling that bleeding is a major concern in this condition will assist in directing you to option 2. Eliminate options 1, 3, and 4 because these activities present the potential for injury. Review home care instructions for the child with hemophilia if you had difficulty with this question.
Level of Cognitive Ability: Application
Client Needs: Safe, Effective Care Environment
Integrated Process: Teaching/Learning
Content Area: Child health
Reference: Wong, D., Hockenberry-Eaton, M. (2000). *Wong's essentials of pediatric nursing* (6th ed., p. 998). St. Louis: Mosby.

9. **3**
Rationale: β-Thalassemia is inherited as an autosomal recessive pattern. This disorder is found primarily in individuals of Mediterranean descent. The disease has been reported in the Asian and African populations as well. Options 1, 2, and 4 are incorrect.
Test-Taking Strategy: Use the process of elimination. Recalling that this disorder occurs primarily in individuals of Mediterranean descent will direct you to the correct option. If you are unfamiliar with this disorder, review the information associated with its incidence and cause.
Level of Cognitive Ability: Application
Client Needs: Physiological Integrity
Integrated Process: Teaching/Learning
Content Area: Child health
References: James, S., Ashwill, J., & Droske, S. (2002). *Nursing care of children: Principles & practice* (2nd ed., p. 753). Philadelphia: W. B. Saunders.
Wong, D., Hockenberry-Eaton, M. (2000). *Wong's essentials of pediatric nursing* (6th ed., p. 994). St. Louis: Mosby.

10. **4**
Rationale: The major complication of chronic transfusion therapy is hemosiderosis. To prevent organ damage from too much iron in the blood, chelation therapy with a medication called deferoxamine (Desferal) is used. Desferoxamine is classified as an antidote for acute iron toxicity. Dalteparin is an anticoagulant used as prophylaxis for postoperative deep vein thrombosis. Meropenem is an antibiotic. Molindone is an antipsychotic.
Test-Taking Strategy: Use the process of elimination and knowledge regarding the antidote for iron toxicity. If you had difficulty with this question, review these medications.
Level of Cognitive Ability: Analysis
Client Needs: Physiological Integrity
Integrated Process: Nursing Process—analysis
Content Area: Child health
References: Hodgson, B., & Kizior, R. (2003). *Saunders nursing drug handbook 2003.* (pp. 304, 315, 707, 762). Philadelphia: W. B. Saunders.
Wong, D., Hockenberry-Eaton, M. (2000). *Wong's essentials of pediatric nursing* (6th ed., p. 995). St. Louis: Mosby.

CRITICAL THINKING: FILL IN THE BLANK

Answer: Meperidine (Demerol) for pain
Rationale: Meperidine (Demerol) is not recommended for the child with sickle cell disease because of the risk for normeperidine-induced seizures. Normeperidine, a metabolite of meperidine, is a central nervous system stimulant that produces anxiety, tremors, myoclonus, and generalized seizures when it accumulates with repetitive dosing. The nurse would question the order for this pain control medication. Fluids, oxygen, and heat to affected areas are used to treat vasoocclusive crisis.
Test-Taking Strategy: Focus on the pathophysiology that occurs in sickle cell disease to assist in identifying the order that needs to be questioned. Recalling the effects of meperidine will assist in identifying the answer. Review care of the child with sickle cell disease experiencing a crisis if you had difficulty with this question.
Level of Cognitive Ability: Analysis
Client Needs: Physiological Integrity
Integrated Process: Nursing Process—analysis
Content Area: Child health
Reference: Wong, D., Hockenberry-Eaton, M. (2000). *Wong's essentials of pediatric nursing* (6th ed., p. 992). St. Louis: Mosby.

REFERENCES

Agency for Healthcare Research and Quality. http://www.ahcpr.gov.
Cooley's Anemia Foundation. http://www.thalassemia.org.
Hodgson, B., & Kizior, R. (2003). *Saunders nursing drug handbook 2003.* Philadelphia: W. B. Saunders.
James, S., Ashwill, J., & Droske, S. (2002). *Nursing care of children: Principles & practice* (2nd ed.). Philadelphia: W. B. Saunders.

McKinney, E., Ashwill, J., Murray, S., James, S., Gorrie, T., & Droske, S. (2000). *Maternal-child nursing.* Philadelphia: W. B. Saunders.
Wong, D., Hockenberry-Eaton, M. (2000). *Wong's essentials of pediatric nursing* (6th ed.). St. Louis: Mosby.
Wong, D., Perry, S., & Hockenberry, M. (2002). *Maternal child nursing care* (2nd ed.). St. Louis: Mosby.

Oncological Disorders

I. LEUKEMIA (BOX 45-1)

A. Description
1. Leukemia is a malignant exacerbation in the number of leukocytes, usually at an immature stage, in the bone marrow.
2. Leukemia affects the bone marrow, causing anemia from decreased erythrocytes, infection from neutropenia, and bleeding from decreased platelet production.
3. The cause is unknown and appears to involve gene damage of cells, leading to the transformation of cells from a normal state to a malignant state.
4. Risk factors include genetic, viral, immunological, and environmental factors and exposure to radiation, chemicals, and medications.
5. Acute lymphocytic leukemia is the most frequent type of cancer in children; peak onset is age 2 to 6 years.
6. Leukemia is more common in boys than girls after 1 year of age.
7. Treatment involves the use of chemotherapeutic agents with or without cranial radiation.
8. The phases of treatment include induction, which achieves a complete remission or disappearance of leukemic cells; intensification or consolidation therapy, which further decreases the tumor burden; central nervous system prophylactic therapy, which prevents leukemic cells from invading the central nervous system; and maintenance, which serves to maintain the remission phase.
9. Bone marrow transplantation also may be performed to treat some children with leukemia.

B. Assessment
1. Infiltration of the bone marrow causes fever, pallor, fatigue, anorexia, hemorrhage (usually petechiae), and bone and joint pain; pathological fractures can occur as a result of bone marrow invasion with leukemic cells.
2. Signs of infection occur as a result of neutropenia.
3. Child experiences hepatosplenomegaly and lymphadenopathy.
4. Child has normal, elevated, or low white blood cell count.
5. Child has decreased hemoglobin and hematocrit levels.
6. Child has decreased platelet count.
7. Positive bone marrow biopsy identifies leukemic blast (immature) phase cells.
8. Signs of increased intracranial pressure, such as severe headache, vomiting, papilledema, irritability, lethargy, and eventually coma occur as a result of central nervous system involvement.
9. Child shows signs of cranial nerve (cranial nerve VII, or the facial nerve, is most commonly affected) or spinal nerve involvement; clinical manifestations relate to the area involved.
10. Clinical manifestations indicate the invasion of leukemic cells to the kidneys, testes, prostate, ovaries, gastrointestinal tract, and lungs.

C. Infection (Box 45-2)
1. Infection is a major cause of death in the immunosuppressed child.

BOX 45-1

Classification of Leukemia

ACUTE LYMPHOCYTIC LEUKEMIA
Mostly lymphoblasts present in bone marrow
Age of onset less than 15 years

ACUTE MYELOGENOUS LEUKEMIA
Mostly myeloblasts present in bone marrow
Age of onset between 15 and 39 years

BOX 45-2

Protecting the Child from Infection

Initiate protective isolation procedures.

Maintain frequent and thorough hand washing.

Maintain the child in a private room and a room with high-efficiency particulate air filtration or laminar air flow system if possible.

Be sure that the child's room is cleaned daily.

Use strict aseptic technique for all nursing procedures.

Limit the number of caregivers entering the child's room, and ensure that anyone entering the child's room is wearing a mask.

Keep supplies for the child separate from supplies for other children.

Reduce exposure to environmental organisms by eliminating raw fruits and vegetables and fresh flowers and by not leaving standing water in the child's room.

Assist the child with daily bathing using antimicrobial soap.

Assist the child to perform oral hygiene frequently.

Assess for signs and symptoms of infection.

Monitor temperature, pulse, and blood pressure.

Change wound dressings daily and inspect wounds for redness, swelling, or drainage.

Assess urine for color and cloudiness.

Assess the skin and oral mucous membranes for signs of infection.

Auscultate lung sounds.

Encourage the child to cough and deep breathe.

Monitor the white blood cell and the neutrophil counts.

Notify the physician if signs of infection are present, and prepare to obtain specimens for culture of open lesions, urine, and sputum.

Initiate a bowel program to prevent constipation and rectal trauma.

Avoid invasive procedures such as injections, rectal temperatures, and urinary catheterization.

Administer antibiotic, antifungal, and antiviral medication as prescribed.

Administer granulocyte colony-stimulating factor as prescribed.

Instruct the parents to keep the child away from crowds and those with infections.

Instruct the parents that the child should not receive immunization with a live virus.

Keep any child with chickenpox or any child who has been exposed to the virus away from the child with leukemia.

Instruct the parents to inform the teacher that they should be notified immediately if a case of chickenpox occurs in another child at school.

2. Infection can occur through autocontamination or cross-contamination.

3. Most common sites of infection are the skin (any break in the skin is a potential site of infection), respiratory tract, and gastrointestinal tract.

▲ D. Bleeding (Box 45-3)

1. Children with platelet counts less than 20,000 cells/µl may need a platelet transfusion.

2. For children with severe blood loss, packed red blood cells may be prescribed.

▲ E. Fatigue and nutrition

1. Assist the child in selecting a well-balanced diet.

2. Provide small meals that require little chewing.

3. Assist the child in self-care and mobility activities.

4. Allow adequate rest periods during care.

5. Do not perform activities unless they are essential.

F. Chemotherapy

▲ 1. Monitor for severe bone marrow suppression; during the period of greatest bone marrow suppression (the nadir), blood counts will be extremely low.

▲ 2. Monitor for infection and bleeding.

▲ 3. Protect the child from life-threatening infections.

4. Monitor for nausea, vomiting, and diarrhea.

5. Administer antiemetics as prescribed.

6. Monitor for signs of dehydration.

7. Monitor for signs of hemorrhagic cystitis.

8. Monitor for signs of peripheral neuropathy.

9. Assess oral mucous membranes for mucositis; administer frequent mouth rinses (normal saline

BOX 45-3

Protecting the Child from Bleeding

Examine the child for signs and symptoms of bleeding.

Handle the child gently.

Measure abdominal girth, which can indicate internal hemorrhage.

Instruct the child to use a soft toothbrush and to avoid dental floss.

Provide soft foods that are cool to warm in temperature.

Avoid injections, if possible, to prevent trauma to the skin and bleeding.

Apply firm and gentle pressure to a needlestick site for at least 10 minutes.

Pad side rails and sharp corners of the bed and furniture.

Discourage the child from engaging in activities involving the use of sharp objects.

Instruct the child to avoid constrictive or tight clothing.

Use caution when taking the blood pressure to prevent skin injury.

Instruct the child to avoid blowing the nose.

Avoid rectal suppositories, enemas, and rectal thermometers.

Examine all body fluids and excrement for the presence of blood.

Count the number of pads or tampons used if the female adolescent is menstruating.

Instruct the child in the signs and symptoms of bleeding.

Instruct the parents to avoid administering nonsteroidal antiinflammatory drugs and products that contain aspirin to the child.

with or without sodium bicarbonate solution) to promote healing as prescribed.

10. Instruct the parents in signs and symptoms to watch for after chemotherapy and when to notify the physician.

11. Inform the parents that hair loss may occur from chemotherapy (hair will regrow in 3 to 6 months and may be a slightly different color or texture).

12. Instruct the parents about the care of a central venous access device as necessary.

13. Listen to the child and family, and encourage them to verbalize their feelings and express their concerns.

14. Introduce the family to other families of children with cancer.

15. Consult social services and chaplains as necessary.

II. HODGKIN'S DISEASE (BOX 45-4)

A. Description
1. Hodgkin's disease (a type of lymphoma) is a malignancy of the lymph nodes that originates in a single lymph node or a single chain of nodes.
2. The disease predictably metastasizes to nonnodal or extralymphatic sites, especially the spleen, liver, bone marrow, lungs, and mediastinum.
3. Hodgkin's disease is characterized by the presence of the Reed-Sternberg cell in the lymph nodes.
4. Possible causes include viral infections and previous exposure to alkalating chemical agents.
5. The prognosis depends on the stage of the disease; the prognosis is excellent in children with localized disease.
6. The primary treatment modalities are radiation and chemotherapy; each may be used alone or in combination, depending on the clinical staging of the disease.
7. Bone marrow transplantation may be a consideration in treating Hodgkin's disease.

B. Assessment
1. Painless enlargement of lymph nodes
2. Enlarged, firm, nontender, movable nodes in the supraclavicular area; in children, the "sentinel" node located near the left clavicle may be the first enlarged node
3. Nonproductive cough as a result of mediastinal lymphadenopathy
4. Abdominal pain as a result of enlarged retroperitoneal nodes
5. Advanced lymph node and extralymphatic involvement that may cause systemic symptoms such as low-grade or intermittent fever, anorexia, nausea, weight loss, night sweats, and pruritus
6. Positive biopsy of lymph node (presence of Reed-Sternberg cell) and positive bone marrow biopsy
7. Computed tomography scan of the liver, spleen, and bone marrow to detect metastasis

C. Interventions
1. For stages I and II without mediastinal node involvement, the treatment of choice is extensive external radiation of the involved lymph node regions.
2. With more extensive disease, radiation along with multiagent chemotherapy is used.
3. Monitor for drug-induced pancytopenia, which increases the risk for infection, bleeding, and anemia.
4. Monitor for signs of infection and bleeding.
5. Protect the child from infection.
6. Provide a safe, hazard-free environment.
7. Monitor for side effects related to chemotherapy or radiation; the most common complication of radiation to the neck area is hypothyroidism.
8. Monitor for nausea and vomiting, and administer antiemetics as prescribed.
9. Monitor for skin irritation and breakdown as a result of radiation therapy.

III. NEPHROBLASTOMA (WILMS' TUMOR)

A. Description
1. Wilms' tumor is a tumor of the kidney that may present unilaterally and localized or bilaterally, sometimes with metastasis to other organs.
2. The peak incidence is at 3 years of age.
3. The occurrence is associated with a genetic inheritance and with several congenital anomalies.
4. Therapeutic management includes a combined treatment of surgery (partial to total nephrectomy) and chemotherapy with or without radiation, depending on the clinical stage and histologic pattern.

BOX 45-4

Staging of Hodgkin's Disease

STAGE I
Involvement of a single lymph node region or only one extralymphatic organ or site such as the liver, kidneys, lungs, or intestines

STAGE II
Involvement of two or more lymph node regions on the same side of the diaphragm or one additional extralymphatic organ or site on the same side of the diaphragm

STAGE III
Involvement of lymph node regions on both sides of the diaphragm or one extralymphatic organ or site or spleen or both

STAGE IV
Diffuse or disseminated involvement of one or more extralymphatic organs with or without associated lymph node involvement

B. Assessment
   1. Swelling or mass within the abdomen (mass is characteristically firm, nontender, confined to one side, and deep within the flank)
   2. Abdominal pain
   3. Urinary retention and/or hematuria
   4. Anemia (caused by hemorrhage within the tumor)
   5. Pallor, anorexia, lethargy (resulting from anemia)
   6. Hypertension (caused by secretion of excess amounts of renin by the tumor)
   7. Weight loss and fever
   8. Symptoms of lung involvement such as dyspnea, shortness of breath, and pain in the chest, if metastasis has occurred
C. Interventions preoperatively
   1. Monitor vital signs, particularly blood pressure.
   2. Place a sign at the bedside: "Do Not Palpate Abdomen."
   3. Avoid palpation of the abdomen.
   4. Measure abdominal girth.
D. Interventions postoperatively
   1. Monitor temperature and blood pressure closely.
   2. Monitor for signs of hemorrhage and infection.
   3. Monitor intake and output and urine output closely.
   4. Monitor for abdominal distention; monitor bowel sounds and for other signs of gastrointestinal activity because of the risk for intestinal obstruction.

IV. NEUROBLASTOMA
A. Description
   1. Neuroblastoma is an embryonal tumor found in children that arises from the neural crest.
   2. The primary site is in the abdomen because the tumor arises from the adrenal gland or from the retroperitoneal sympathetic chain; other sites may be within the head, neck, chest, or pelvis.
   3. Most presenting signs are caused by the tumor compressing adjacent normal tissue and organs.
   4. Diagnostic evaluation is aimed at locating the primary site of the tumor.
   5. The prognosis is poor because of the frequency of invasiveness of the tumor and because in most cases a diagnosis is not made until after metastasis has occurred.
   6. Therapeutic management
      a. Surgery is performed to remove as much of the tumor as possible and to obtain biopsies; in stages I and II, complete surgical removal of the tumor is the treatment of choice.
      b. Surgery usually is limited to biopsy in stages III and IV because of the extensive metastasis.
      c. Radiation is used commonly with stage III disease and provides palliation for metastatic lesions in bones, lungs, liver, or brain.
      d. Chemotherapy is the mainstay of treatment for extensive local or disseminated disease.

B. Assessment
   1. Firm, nontender, irregular mass in the abdomen that crosses the midline
   2. Urinary frequency or retention from compression of the kidney, ureter, or bladder
   3. Lymphadenopathy, especially in the cervical and supraclavicular area
   4. Bone pain if skeletal involvement occurs
   5. Supraorbital ecchymosis, periorbital edema, and exophthalmos as a result of invasion of retrobulbar soft tissue
   6. Pallor, weakness, irritability, anorexia, weight loss
   7. Signs of respiratory impairment (thoracic lesion)
   8. Signs of neurological impairment (intracranial lesion)
   9. Paralysis from compression of the spinal cord
C. Interventions preoperatively
   1. Monitor for signs and symptoms related to the location of the tumor.
   2. Provide emotional support to the child and parents.
D. Interventions postoperatively
   1. Monitor for postoperative complications related to the location (organ) of the surgery.
   2. Monitor for complications related to chemotherapy or radiation if prescribed.
   3. Provide support to the parents and encourage them to express their feelings; many parents suffer from guilt for not having recognized signs in the child earlier.
   4. Refer the parents to appropriate community services.

V. OSTEOGENIC SARCOMA
A. Description
   1. Osteogenic sarcoma is the most common bone cancer in children.
   2. Cancer usually is found in the metaphysis of long bones, especially in the lower extremities, with most tumors occurring in the femur.
   3. Peak age of incidence is between 10 and 25 years.
   4. Symptoms in the earliest stage are almost always attributed to extremity injury or normal growing pains.
   5. Treatment may include surgical resection by limb salvage to remove affected tissue or amputation.
   6. Chemotherapy plays a vital role in treatment and may be used before and after surgery.
B. Assessment
   1. Localized pain at the affected site (may be severe or dull) that may be attributed to trauma or the vague complaint of "growing pains"; pain often is relieved by a flexed position
   2. Palpable mass
   3. Limping if weight-bearing limb is affected
   4. Progressive limited range of motion and the child's curtailing of physical activity
   5. Child may be unable to hold heavy objects
   6. Pathological fractures at the tumor site

C. Interventions
1. Prepare the child and family for prescribed treatment modalities, which may include surgical resection by limb salvage to remove affected tissue, amputation, and chemotherapy.
2. Provide honesty and support for the child and family.
3. Prepare for prosthetic fitting as necessary.
4. Assist the child in dealing with problems of self-image

VI. BRAIN TUMORS
A. Description
1. An infratentorial (below the tentorium cerebelli) tumor is located in the posterior third of the brain (primarily in the cerebellum or brainstem) and accounts for the frequency of symptoms resulting from increased intracranial pressure (ICP).
2. A supratentorial tumor is located within the anterior two thirds of the brain, mainly the cerebrum.
3. The signs and symptoms of a brain tumor depend on its anatomical location and size and to some extent on the age of the child.
4. Therapeutic management includes surgery, radiation, and chemotherapy; the treatment of choice is total removal of the tumor without residual neurological damage.
B. Assessment
1. Headache that is worse on awakening and improves during the day
2. Vomiting that is unrelated to feeding or eating
3. Ataxia
4. Seizures
5. Behavioral changes
6. Clumsiness; awkward gait or difficulty walking
7. Diplopia
8. Facial weakness
C. Interventions preoperatively
1. Perform a neurological assessment.
2. Institute safety measures.
3. Assess weight loss and nutritional status.
4. Initiate seizure precautions.
5. The child's head will be shaved (provide a favorite cap or hat for the child).
6. Prepare the child as much as possible; tell the child that he or she will wake up with a large head dressing.
D. Interventions postoperatively
1. Assess neurological and motor function and level of consciousness.
2. Monitor temperature closely, which may be elevated because of hypothalamus or brainstem involvement during surgery; maintain a cooling blanket by the bedside.
3. Monitor for signs of respiratory infection.
4. Monitor for signs of meningitis (opisthotonos, Kernig's and Brudzinski's signs).

BOX 45-5

Positioning Following Craniotomy

Assess the physician's order for positioning, including the degree of neck flexion.

If a large tumor was removed, the child is not placed on the operative side because the brain may shift suddenly to that cavity.

In an infratentorial procedure the child usually is positioned flat and on either side.

In a supratentorial procedure the head usually is elevated above the heart level to facilitate cerebrospinal fluid drainage and to decrease excessive blood flow to the brain to prevent hemorrhage.

Never place the child in the Trendelenburg's position because it increases intracranial pressure and the risk of hemorrhage.

---

5. Monitor for signs of increased intracranial pressure (ICP) or hemorrhage (check the back of the head dressing for posterior pooling of blood).
6. Assess pupillary response; sluggish, dilated, or unequal pupils are reported immediately because they may indicate increased intracranial pressure (ICP) and potential brainstem herniation.
7. Monitor for colorless drainage on the dressing or from the ears or nose, which indicates cerebrospinal fluid and should be reported immediately.
8. Assess the physician's order for positioning, including the degree of neck flexion (Box 45-5).
9. Monitor intravenous fluids carefully.
10. Promote measures that prevent vomiting (vomiting increases intracranial pressure and the risk for incisional rupture).
11. Provide a quiet environment.
12. Administer analgesics as prescribed.
13. Provide emotional support to the child and parents, and promote maximum functioning in the child.

PRACTICE QUESTIONS

1. A pediatric nurse clinician is discussing the pathophysiology related to childhood leukemia with a class of nursing students. Which statement made by a nursing student indicates a lack of understanding of the pathophysiology of this disease?
   1. Normal bone marrow is replaced by blast cells.
   2. Red blood cell production is affected.
   3. The platelet count is decreased.
   4. The presence of a Reed-Sternberg cell is found on biopsy.
2. A 4-year-old child is admitted to the hospital for abdominal pain. The mother reports that the child has been pale and excessively tired and is bruising easily. On physical examination, lymphadenopathy and hepatosplenomegaly are noted. Diagnostic studies

are being performed on the child because acute lymphocytic leukemia is suspected. The nurse understands that which diagnostic study will confirm this diagnosis?

1. White blood cell count
2. A lumbar puncture
3. Bone marrow biopsy
4. A platelet count

3. A nurse instructs the parents of a child with leukemia regarding measures related to monitoring for infection. Which statement if made by a parent indicates a need for further instructions?

1. "I will perform proper hand-washing techniques."
2. "I will take a rectal temperature daily."
3. "I will inspect the skin daily for redness."
4. "I will inspect the mouth daily for lesions."

4. A 6-year-old child with leukemia is hospitalized and is receiving combination chemotherapy. Laboratory results indicate that the child is neutropenic, and protective isolation procedures are initiated. The grandmother of the child visits and brings a fresh bouquet of flowers picked from her garden and asks the nurse for a vase for the flowers. The nurse responds to the grandmother by telling her

1. "I have a vase in the utility room, and I will get it for you."
2. "The flowers from your garden are beautiful but should not be placed in the child's room at this time."
3. "I will get the vase and wash it well before you put the flowers in it."
4. "When you bring the flowers into the room, place them on the bedside stand as far away from the child as possible."

5. A 9-year-old child with leukemia is in remission and has returned to school. The school nurse calls the mother of the child and tells the mother that a classmate has just been diagnosed with chickenpox. The mother immediately calls the clinic nurse because the leukemic child has never had chickenpox. The most appropriate response by the clinic nurse to the mother is

1. "Monitor the child for an elevated temperature, and call the clinic if a temperature occurs."
2. "Keep the child out of school for a 2-week period."
3. "There is no need to be concerned."
4. "Bring the child into the clinic for a vaccine."

6. The nurse analyzes the laboratory values of a child with leukemia who is receiving chemotherapy. The nurse notes that the platelet count is 20,000 cells/μl. Based on this laboratory result, which intervention will the nurse document in the plan of care?

1. Initiate protective isolation precautions.
2. Monitor the temperature every 4 hours.
3. Monitor closely for signs of infection.
4. Use a soft small toothbrush for mouth care.

7. A child with leukemia is complaining of nausea. A nurse suspects that the nausea is related to the chemotherapy. The nurse, concerned about the child's nutritional status, most appropriately would offer which of the following during this episode of nausea?

1. The child's favorite foods
2. Cool, clear liquids
3. Low-protein foods
4. Low-calorie foods

8. A 12-year-old child is seen in a clinic, and a diagnosis of Hodgkin's disease is suspected. Several diagnostic studies are performed to determine the presence of this disease. When evaluating the diagnostic results, a nurse would expect to note which of the following, if this child had Hodgkin's disease?

1. The presence of blast cells in the bone marrow
2. The presence of Reed-Sternberg cells in the lymph nodes
3. The presence of Epstein-Barr virus in the blood
4. Elevated vanillylmandelic acid urinary levels

9. A nurse is performing an assessment on a 10-year-old child suspected of having Hodgkin's disease. The nurse understands that which data are most characteristic of this disease?

1. Painful, enlarged inguinal lymph nodes
2. Fever and malaise
3. Painless, firm, and movable adenopathy in the cervical area
4. Anorexia and weight loss

10. A pediatric nurse is assigned to care for a child with a diagnosis of Wilms' tumor. In planning care for the child, the nurse understands that this tumor is

1. An abdominal tumor.
2. A renal tumor.
3. A brain tumor.
4. A bone tumor.

11. The mother of a 4-year-old child brings the child to a clinic and tells a pediatric nurse specialist that the child's abdomen seems to be swollen. During further assessment of subjective data, the mother tells the nurse that the child is eating well and that the activity level of the child is unchanged. The nurse, suspecting the possibility of Wilms' tumor, would avoid which of the following during the physical assessment?

1. Palpating the abdomen for a mass
2. Assessing the urine for the presence of hematuria
3. Monitoring the temperature for the presence of fever
4. Monitoring the blood pressure for the presence of hypertension

12. A pediatric nurse specialist provides a teaching session to the nursing staff regarding osteogenic sarcoma. Which statement by a member of the nursing staff indicates a need for clarifying the information presented?

1. "The symptoms of the disease in the early stage are almost always attributed to normal growing pains."
2. "The femur is the most common site of this sarcoma."
3. "Limping, if a weight-bearing limb is affected, is a clinical manifestation."
4. "The child does not experience pain at the primary tumor site."

13. A nurse is caring for a child after surgical removal of a brain tumor. The nurse assesses the child for which of the following signs that would indicate that brainstem involvement occurred during the surgical procedure?
    1. Elevated temperature
    2. Orthostatic hypotension
    3. Inability to swallow
    4. Altered hearing ability

14. A nurse is monitoring a child for bleeding following surgery for removal of a brain tumor. The nurse checks the head dressing for the presence of blood and notes a colorless drainage on the back of the dressing. Which of the following would be the most appropriate nursing intervention?
    1. Circle the area of drainage and continue to monitor.
    2. Reinforce the dressing.
    3. Notify the physician.
    4. Document the findings and continue to monitor.

15. After surgical removal of a brain tumor, the physician writes an order to maintain the child in a flat position. In the postoperative period a nurse is monitoring the child and notes that the child is restless, the pulse rate is elevated, and the blood pressure has dropped significantly from the baseline value. The nurse suspects that the child is in shock. Which of the following would be the most appropriate nursing action?
    1. Place the child in the Trendelenburg's position.
    2. Elevate the head of the bed.
    3. Increase the intravenous fluids.
    4. Notify the physician.

CRITICAL THINKING: FILL IN THE BLANK

A pediatric nurse assists a physician in performing a lumbar puncture on a 3-year-old child with leukemia who is suspected of having central nervous system metastasis. The nurse places the child in which position for this procedure?

Answer: _____

ANSWERS

1. **4**

Rationale: In leukemia, normal bone marrow is replaced by malignant blast cells. As the blast cells take over the bone marrow, eventually red blood cell and platelet production is affected and the child becomes anemic and thrombocytopenic. The Reed-Sternberg cell is found in Hodgkin's disease.

Test-Taking Strategy: Use the process of elimination. Note the key words "lack of understanding" in the stem of the question. Recalling that the Reed-Sternberg cell is found in Hodgkin's disease will direct you easily to option 4. Review the pathophysiology related to leukemia if you had difficulty with this question.

Level of Cognitive Ability: Comprehension
Client Needs: Physiological Integrity
Integrated Process: Teaching/Learning
Content Area: Child health
Reference: Wong, D., Hockenberry-Eaton, M. (2000). *Wong's essentials of pediatric nursing* (6th ed., p. 1002). St. Louis: Mosby.

2. **3**

Rationale: The confirmatory test for leukemia is microscopic examination of bone marrow obtained by bone marrow aspirate and biopsy. A lumbar puncture may be done to look for blast cells in the spinal fluid that indicate central nervous system disease. The white blood cell count may be normal, high, or low in leukemia. An altered platelet count occurs as a result of the disease but also may occur as a result of chemotherapy and does not confirm the diagnosis.

Test-Taking Strategy: Use the process of elimination. Note the key word "confirm" in the stem of the question. This key word and knowledge that the bone marrow is affected in leukemia will direct you to option 3. If you had difficulty with this question, review the significance of the bone marrow biopsy.

Level of Cognitive Ability: Comprehension
Client Needs: Physiological Integrity
Integrated Process: Nursing Process—assessment
Content Area: Child health
Reference: James, S., Ashwill, J., & Droske, S. (2002). *Nursing care of children: Principles & practice* (2nd ed., p. 781). Philadelphia: W. B. Saunders.

3. **2**

Rationale: The risk of injury to fragile mucous membranes is so great in the child with leukemia that only oral or axillary temperatures should be taken. Rectal abscesses can occur easily to damaged rectal tissue. No rectal temperatures should be taken. In addition, oral temperatures should be avoided if the child has oral ulcers. Options 1, 3, and 4 are appropriate measures to prevent infection.

Test-Taking Strategy: Use the process of elimination. Note the key words "a need for further instructions." Options 1 and 3 can be eliminated easily first. From the remaining options, note the word "rectal" in option 2. Recalling that rectal temperatures should be avoided will direct you to this option. Review home care instructions related to infection in the child with leukemia if you had difficulty with this question.

Level of Cognitive Ability: Analysis
Client Needs: Safe, Effective Care Environment

Integrated Process: Teaching/Learning
Content Area: Child health
Reference: James, S., Ashwill, J., & Droske, S. (2002). *Nursing care of children: Principles & practice* (2nd ed., p. 783). Philadelphia: W. B. Saunders.

4. 2
Rationale: For the hospitalized neutropenic child, flowers or plants should not be kept in the room because standing water and damp soil harbor *Aspergillus* and *Pseudomonas,* to which these children are susceptible. In addition, fresh fruits and vegetables harbor molds and should be avoided until the white blood cell count rises.
Test-Taking Strategy: Use the process of elimination. Note that options 1 and 3 are similar and should be eliminated first. From the remaining options, select option 2 over option 4 because this nursing response maintains the protective isolation procedures required. Review protective isolation procedures for the neutropenic child if you had difficulty with this question.
Level of Cognitive Ability: Application
Client Needs: Safe, Effective Care Environment
Integrated Process: Caring
Content Area: Child health
Reference: James, S., Ashwill, J., & Droske, S. (2002). *Nursing care of children: Principles & practice* (2nd ed., p. 784). Philadelphia: W. B. Saunders.

5. 4
Rationale: Immunocompromised children are unable to fight varicella adequately. Chickenpox can be deadly to the immunocompromised child. If an immunocompromised child who has not had chickenpox is exposed to someone with varicella, the child should receive varicella zoster immune globulin within 96 hours of exposure. Options 1, 2, and 3 are incorrect.
Test-Taking Strategy: Use the process of elimination. Note the key words "never had chickenpox" in the question. Recall that a child with leukemia is immunocompromised and is unable to fight infection. This should assist you in eliminating options 1, 2, and 3. Review protective procedures for the immunocompromised child if you had difficulty with this question.
Level of Cognitive Ability: Application
Client Needs: Health Promotion and Maintenance
Integrated Process: Nursing Process—implementation
Content Area: Child health
Reference: James, S., Ashwill, J., & Droske, S. (2002). *Nursing care of children: Principles & practice* (2nd ed., p. 784). Philadelphia: W. B. Saunders.

6. 4
Rationale: If a child is severely thrombocytopenic and has a platelet count less than 20,000 cells/μl, precautions need to be taken because of the increased risk of bleeding. The precautions include limiting activity that could result in head injury, using soft toothbrushes or Toothettes, checking urine and stools for blood, and administering stool softeners to prevent straining with constipation. In addition, suppositories and rectal temperatures are avoided. Options 1, 2, and 3 are related to the prevention of infection rather than bleeding.

Test-Taking Strategy: Use the process of elimination. Noting that the platelet count is low and that a low platelet count places the child at risk for bleeding will assist in directing you to option 4. In addition, note that options 1, 2, and 3 are similar because they relate to prevention of and monitoring for infection.
Level of Cognitive Ability: Analysis
Client Needs: Physiological Integrity
Integrated Process: Communication and Documentation
Content Area: Child health
Reference: James, S., Ashwill, J., & Droske, S. (2002). *Nursing care of children: Principles & practice* (2nd ed., p. 785). Philadelphia: W. B. Saunders.

7. 2
Rationale: When the child is nauseated, offering cool, clear liquids is best because they are soothing and better tolerated. One should not offer favorite foods when the child is nauseated because foods eaten during times of nausea will be associated with being sick. Supportive nutritional measures also should include oral supplements with high-protein and high-calorie foods.
Test-Taking Strategy: The issue of the question relates to the nutritional status in a child with nausea. Focusing on this issue will assist in eliminating options 3 and 4. From the remaining options, you may be tempted to select option 1. Remember that it is best not to offer favorite foods when the child is nauseated because foods eaten during times of nausea will be associated with being sick. Review these interventions related to nutrition if you had difficulty with this question.
Level of Cognitive Ability: Application
Client Needs: Physiological Integrity
Integrated Process: Nursing Process—implementation
Content Area: Child health
Reference: James, S., Ashwill, J., & Droske, S. (2002). *Nursing care of children: Principles & practice* (2nd ed., p. 786). Philadelphia: W. B. Saunders.

8. 2
Rationale: Hodgkin's disease is a neoplasm of lymphatic tissue. The presence of giant, multinucleated cells (Reed-Sternberg cells) is the hallmark of this disease. The presence of blast cells in the bone marrow indicates leukemia. The Epstein-Barr virus is associated with infectious mononucleosis. Elevated levels of vanillylmandelic acid in the urine may be found in children with neuroblastoma.
Test-Taking Strategy: Use the process of elimination. Recalling that the Reed-Sternberg cell is characteristic of Hodgkin's disease will direct you easily to option 2. Review the clinical manifestations associated with Hodgkin's disease if you had difficulty with this question.
Level of Cognitive Ability: Analysis
Client Needs: Physiological Integrity
Integrated Process: Nursing Process—assessment
Content Area: Child health
References: James, S., Ashwill, J., & Droske, S. (2002). *Nursing care of children: Principles & practice* (2nd ed., p. 796). Philadelphia: W. B. Saunders.
Wong, D., Hockenberry-Eaton, M. (2000). *Wong's essentials of pediatric nursing* (6th ed., p. 1017). St. Louis: Mosby.

9. 3

Rationale: Clinical manifestations specifically associated with Hodgkin's disease include painless, firm, and movable adenopathy in the cervical and supraclavicular area. Hepatosplenomegaly also is noted. Although fever, malaise, anorexia, and weight loss are associated with Hodgkin's disease, these manifestations are seen in many disorders.

Test-Taking Strategy: Use the process of elimination. Note the key words "most characteristic" in the stem of the question. Eliminate options 2 and 4 first because these symptoms are general and vague. Recalling that painless adenopathy is associated with Hodgkin's disease will direct you to option 3. Review the clinical manifestations related to Hodgkin's disease if you had difficulty with this question.

Level of Cognitive Ability: Analysis
Client Needs: Physiological Integrity
Integrated Process: Nursing Process—assessment
Content Area: Child health
Reference: Wong, D., Hockenberry-Eaton, M. (2000). *Wong's essentials of pediatric nursing* (6th ed., p. 1018). St. Louis: Mosby.

10. 2

Rationale: Wilms' tumor, or nephroblastoma, is the most common renal tumor in children. Arising from the renal parenchyma of the kidney, this tumor grows rapidly. The tumor may be present unilaterally and localized or bilaterally, sometimes with metastasis to other organs. Options 1, 3, and 4 are incorrect.

Test-Taking Strategy: Knowledge regarding the location of Wilms' tumor is required to answer this question. If you are unfamiliar with this type of tumor, review this content.

Level of Cognitive Ability: Application
Client Needs: Physiological Integrity
Integrated Process: Nursing Process—planning
Content Area: Child health
Reference: Wong, D., Hockenberry-Eaton, M. (2000). *Wong's essentials of pediatric nursing* (6th ed., p. 1049). St. Louis: Mosby.

11. 1

Rationale: If Wilms' tumor is suspected, the tumor mass should not be palpated by the nurse. Excessive manipulation can cause seeding of the tumor and spread of the cancerous cells. Fever, hematuria, and hypertension are clinical manifestations associated with Wilms' tumor.

Test-Taking Strategy: Use the process of elimination. Note the key word "avoid." Knowledge that this tumor is located in the kidney will assist in eliminating options 2, 3, and 4 because of the relationship of these options to renal function. Review the significant assessment procedures in the child with Wilms' tumor if you had difficulty with this question.

Level of Cognitive Ability: Application
Client Needs: Physiological Integrity
Integrated Process: Nursing Process—assessment
Content Area: Child health
Reference: Wong, D., Hockenberry-Eaton, M. (2000). *Wong's essentials of pediatric nursing* (6th ed., p. 1049). St. Louis: Mosby.

12. 4

Rationale: A clinical manifestation of osteogenic sarcoma is progressive, insidious, and intermittent pain at the tumor site.

By the time these children receive medical attention, they may be in considerable pain from the tumor. Options 1, 2, and 3 are accurate regarding osteogenic sarcoma.

Test-Taking Strategy: Use the process of elimination. Note the key words "need for clarifying the information presented" in the stem of the question. Knowledge that osteogenic sarcoma is a malignant tumor of the bone will direct you easily to option 4. Review the clinical manifestations associated with osteogenic sarcoma if you had difficulty with this question.

Level of Cognitive Ability: Analysis
Client Needs: Physiological Integrity
Integrated Process: Teaching/Learning
Content Area: Child health
Reference: James, S., Ashwill, J., & Droske, S. (2002). *Nursing care of children: Principles & practice* (2nd ed., p. 798). Philadelphia: W. B. Saunders.

13. 1

Rationale: Vital signs and neurological status are assessed frequently. Special attention is paid to the child's temperature, which may be elevated because of hypothalamus or brainstem involvement during surgery. A cooling blanket should be in place on the bed or readily available if the child becomes hyperthermic. Options 3 and 4 are related to functional deficits following surgery. An elevated blood pressure and a widened pulse pressure may be associated with increased intracranial pressure.

Test-Taking Strategy: Use the process of elimination. Recalling the functions of the hypothalamus and the brainstem will direct you easily to option 1. If you had difficulty with this question, review the complications that can occur following surgical removal of a brain tumor.

Level of Cognitive Ability: Analysis
Client Needs: Physiological Integrity
Integrated Process: Nursing Process—assessment
Content Area: Child health
Reference: Wong, D., Hockenberry-Eaton, M. (2000). *Wong's essentials of pediatric nursing* (6th ed., p. 1089). St. Louis: Mosby.

14. 3

Rationale: Colorless drainage on the dressing would indicate the presence of cerebrospinal fluid and should be reported to the physician immediately. Options 1, 2, and 4 are inaccurate nursing interventions.

Test-Taking Strategy: Use the process of elimination. Eliminate options 1 and 4 first because they are similar. Note the key words "colorless drainage." This should alert you quickly to the possibility of the presence of cerebrospinal fluid and direct you to option 3. If you had difficulty with this question, review the significance of the presence of colorless drainage following cranial surgery.

Level of Cognitive Ability: Application
Client Needs: Physiological Integrity
Integrated Process: Nursing Process—implementation
Content Area: Child health
Reference: Wong, D., Hockenberry-Eaton, M. (2000). *Wong's essentials of pediatric nursing* (6th ed., p. 1089). St. Louis: Mosby.

15. **4**

Rationale: The child is never placed in the Trendelenburg's position because it increases intracranial pressure (ICP) and the risk of bleeding. In the event of shock, the physician is notified immediately before changing the child's position or increasing intravenous fluids. Increasing intravenous fluids can cause an increase in ICP.

Test-Taking Strategy: Recall the complications associated with cranial surgery to answer this question. Eliminate option 1 because this position increases ICP. Eliminate option 2 because this intervention will not assist in alleviating shock. In fact, this action could cause harm to the child. Eliminate option 3 because this action could increase ICP. In addition, the nurse should not increase intravenous fluids without a physician's order. Review care to the client after surgical removal of a brain tumor if you had difficulty with this question.

Level of Cognitive Ability: Application
Client Needs: Physiological Integrity
Integrated Process: Nursing Process—implementation
Content Area: Child health
Reference: Wong, D., Hockenberry-Eaton, M. (2000). *Wong's essentials of pediatric nursing* (6th ed., p. 1090). St. Louis: Mosby.

CRITICAL THINKING: FILL IN THE BLANK

Answer: Lateral recumbent with the knees flexed to the abdomen and the head bent with the chin resting on the chest

Rationale: This position separates the spinal processes and facilitates needle insertion into the subarachnoid space.

Test-Taking Strategy: Note the key word "lumbar" in the question. Visualize the position needed to access the subarachnoid space to obtain cerebrospinal fluid. Review this procedure if you are unfamiliar with it.

Level of Cognitive Ability: Application
Client Needs: Physiological Integrity
Integrated Process: Nursing Process—implementation
Content Area: Child health
Reference: Wong, D., Hockenberry-Eaton, M. (2000). *Wong's essentials of pediatric nursing* (6th ed., p. 774). St. Louis: Mosby.

REFERENCES

American Cancer Society. http://www.cancer.org.

James, S., Ashwill, J., & Droske, S. (2002). *Nursing care of children: Principles & practice* (2nd ed.). Philadelphia: W. B. Saunders.

National Brain Tumor Foundation. http://www.braintumor.org.

Perry, A., & Potter, P. (2002), *Clinical nursing skills and techniques* (5th ed.). St. Louis: Mosby.

Wong, D., Hockenberry-Eaton, M. (2000). *Wong's essentials of pediatric nursing* (6th ed.). St. Louis: Mosby.

Wong, D., Perry, S., & Hockenberry, M. (2002). *Maternal child nursing care* (2nd ed.). St. Louis: Mosby.

Acquired Immunodeficiency Syndrome

I. ACQUIRED IMMUNODEFICIENCY SYNDROME (AIDS)

A. Description
1. Acquired immunodeficiency syndrome is a disorder caused by the human immunodeficiency virus (HIV) and characterized by generalized dysfunction of the immune system.
2. Cellular and humoral immunity are compromised.
3. Horizontal transmission of HIV occurs through intimate sexual contact or parenteral exposure to blood or body fluids containing visible blood.
4. Vertical (perinatal) transmission occurs when an HIV-infected pregnant woman passes the infection to her fetus.
5. The most common opportunistic infection of children infected with HIV is *Pneumocystis carinii* pneumonia (PCP), which occurs most frequently between the ages of 3 and 6 months, when HIV status maybe indeterminate.
6. The goals of therapy include slowing the growth of the virus, preventing and treating opportunistic infections, and providing nutritional support and symptomatic treatment.

B. Assessment
1. During neonatal period
    a. Lymphadenopathy
    b. Hepatosplenomegaly
    c. PCP
    d. Progressive encephalopathy
    e. Microcephaly
2. Infants
    a. Failure to thrive
    b. Diarrhea
    c. Developmental delays
    d. Oral candidiasis
    e. Hepatosplenomegaly
    f. Chronic cough and lymphoid interstitial pneumonia
    g. Chronic otitis media
3. Children/adolescents
    a. Malaise and fatigue
    b. Night sweats
    c. Weight loss
    d. Diarrhea
    e. Fever
    f. **Regression** of developmental milestones
    g. Generalized lymphadenopathy
    h. Nephropathy
    i. PCP and lymphoid interstitial pneumonia
    j. Encephalopathy

C. Diagnostic tests (Box 46-1)
1. Enzyme-linked immunosorbent assay (ELISA)
    a. The ELISA determines the response of antibodies to the HIV virus.
    b. The assay is useful in children older than 18 months.
2. Western blot
    a. Western blot confirms the presence of HIV antibodies.
    b. The test is useful in children older than 18 months.
    c. A positive HIV antibody test in children younger than 18 months indicates only that the mother is infected; other diagnostic tests will be used,

---

BOX 46-1

Diagnostic and Evaluative Tests

CD4+
Enzyme-linked immunosorbent assay
p24 antigen detection
Polymerase chain reaction
Virus culture
Western blot

---

including the virus culture, polymerase chain reaction for detection of proviral DNA, and p24 antigen detection, which is HIV specific.

3. p24 antigen
   a. The test is used to detect HIV antigen in children younger than 18 months.
   b. Test can be useful at any age.
   c. Only a positive result is significant.
   d. Two or more positive results are diagnostic for HIV infection.

4. CD4+: Used to assess a child's immune status, risk for disease progression, and the need for PCP prophylaxis after 1 year of age

II. CARE OF THE CHILD WITH HIV OR AIDS

A. Prophylaxis
1. Provide prophylaxis as prescribed against PCP during the first year of life to the infant born to an HIV-infected woman; after 1 year of age, the need for prophylaxis is determined by the presence of severe immunosuppression or a history of PCP.
2. Provide continued prophylaxis through 12 months of age for children diagnosed with HIV.
3. For HIV-infected children older than 12 months, continued prophylaxis is based on CD4+ counts and whether PCP has previously occurred.

B. Antiretroviral therapy: The goal is to suppress viral replication to preserve immune function and to delay disease progression.

C. Highly active antiretroviral therapy
1. Combination therapy usually includes two nucleoside analogs, which target viral replication during the reverse transcription phase, and a protease inhibitor, which targets viral replication at a different phase.
2. The therapy usually is prescribed for an HIV-infected infant or child who exhibits clinical signs of infection or whose immune status in depressed or for an HIV-infected infant younger than 1 year of age when the diagnosis is confirmed.

D. Parent instructions
1. Wash hands frequently.
2. Assess for fever, malaise, fatigue, weight loss, vomiting and diarrhea, altered activity level, and oral lesions; notify the physician if any these occurs.
3. Assess for the signs and symptoms of opportunistic infections.
4. Administer antiretroviral medications as prescribed.
5. The child should avoid exposure to other illnesses.
6. Keep immunizations up to date.
7. Keep the child home when sick.
8. Avoid kissing the child on the mouth.
9. Monitor the child's weight.
10. Provide a high-calorie and high-protein diet.
11. Do not share eating utensils.
12. Wash eating utensils in the dishwasher.
13. Cover unused food and formula and refrigerate.
14. Discard unused refrigerated formula and food after 24 hours.
15. Wear gloves for care, especially when in contact with body fluids and changing diapers.
16. Change diapers frequently, away from food areas.
17. Fold soiled disposable diapers inward and tab, and dispose in a tightly covered plastic-lined container.
18. Dispose of trash daily.
19. Cover sandboxes when not in use to create a barrier to germs.
20. Clean up spills with bleach solution (10:1 ratio of water to bleach).

E. Immunizations
1. Immunizations against common childhood illnesses are recommended for all children exposed to or infected with HIV.
2. Avoid the varicella (chickenpox) vaccine.
3. Ensure administration of pneumococcal and influenza vaccines.
4. Measles, mumps, rubella (MMR) vaccine is administered if the child is not severely immunocompromised (the child receiving intravenous gamma globulin prophylaxis may not respond to the MMR vaccine).
5. Refer to Chapter 47 for additional information regarding immunizations.

PRACTICE QUESTIONS

1. A pediatric nurse educator provides a teaching session to the nursing staff regarding human immunodeficiency virus (HIV) and acquired immunodeficiency syndrome (AIDS). The nurse educator includes which information in the teaching session?
   1. Most newborn infants of HIV-positive women test positive for the HIV virus.
   2. HIV primarily attacks the hematological system.
   3. In AIDS, the B cells are depleted and cannot signal the T4 cells to form protective antibodies.
   4. The virus attacks the immune system by destroying T lymphocytes.

2. A newborn infant of a mother who has human immunodeficiency virus (HIV) is tested for the presence of HIV antibodies. An enzyme-linked immunosorbent assay (ELISA) is performed, and the results are positive. A nurse interprets these results as
   1. Positive for HIV virus.
   2. Indicating the presence of maternal infection.
   3. Indicating the absence of maternal infection.
   4. Negative for HIV virus.

3. A physician prescribes laboratory studies for an infant of a woman who has human immunodeficiency virus (HIV) to determine the presence of HIV antigen. The nurse anticipates that which laboratory study will be prescribed?
   1. Western blot
   2. Chest x-ray

3. CD4+ count

4. p24 antigen assay

4. A mother with human immunodeficiency virus (HIV) infection brings her 10-month-old infant to the clinic for a routine checkup. The physician has documented that the infant is asymptomatic for HIV infection. After the checkup the mother tells the nurse that she is so pleased that the infant will not get HIV. The most appropriate nursing response to the mother is

1. "I am so pleased also that everything has turned out fine."

2. "Everything looks great, but be sure that you return with your infant next month for the scheduled visit."

3. "Most children infected with HIV develop symptoms within the first 9 months of life, and some become symptomatic sometime before age 3."

4. "Since symptoms have not developed, it is unlikely that your infant will develop HIV infection."

5. An infant of a mother infected with human immunodeficiency virus (HIV) is seen in the clinic each month and is being monitored for symptoms indicative of HIV. The nurse assesses the infant, knowing that the most common opportunistic infection of children infected with HIV is

1. Gastroenteritis

2. Meningitis

3. *Pneumocystis carinii* pneumonia

4. Lymphoid interstitial pneumonia

6. A clinic nurse is instructing the mother of a child with human immunodeficiency virus (HIV) infection regarding immunizations. The nurse tells the mother that

1. Household members need to avoid receiving the varicella vaccine.

2. Pneumococcal and influenza vaccines are recommended.

3. The hepatitis B vaccine will not be given to the child.

4. A Western blot needs to be performed and the results evaluated before immunizations.

7. A child with acquired immunodeficiency syndrome (AIDS) is hospitalized for the treatment of *Pneumocystis carinii* pneumonia. The child will be receiving nebulizer treatments at home when discharged. The nurse instructs the mother regarding the maintenance of the nebulizer equipment and tells the mother to

1. Clean the nebulizer pieces after each treatment with one-fourth strength bleach and water.

2. Clean the nebulizer pieces with warm water after each treatment and allow to air dry.

3. Boil the nebulizer pieces for 15 minutes after each treatment.

4. Clean the mouthpiece with alcohol after each use and soak in alcohol for 30 minutes at the end of each day.

8. A child with human immunodeficiency virus (HIV) infection is receiving zidovudine (AZT, Retrovir). The nurse monitors which laboratory study to determine whether the child is experiencing an adverse reaction from the medication?

1. Sedimentation rate

2. Complete blood count

3. Calcium level

4. Potassium level

9. A nurse is caring for a 4-year-old child with a diagnosis of human immunodeficiency virus (HIV) infection. In planning care to address the psychosocial issues, the nurse would expect that this child

1. Is unable to grasp the concept of illness and death.

2. Begins to understand that something is wrong.

3. Begins to conceptualize the death process as involving physical harm.

4. Will express fear, withdrawal, and denial.

10. A home care nurse provides instructions regarding basic infection control to the mother of a child with human immunodeficiency virus (HIV) infection. Which statement if made by the mother indicates the need for further instructions?

1. "I will carefully wash all fresh fruits and vegetables."

2. "I will wash baby bottles, nipples, and pacifiers in the dishwasher."

3. "I will clean up any spills from the diaper with full-strength alcohol."

4. "I will rub the inside of the nipple with salt and rinse well if it becomes slimy."

CRITICAL THINKING: FILL IN THE BLANK

A young child with acquired immunodeficiency syndrome is scheduled for a CD4+ blood test. The child's mother asks the nurse about the purpose of the test. The nurse tells the mother that the blood test assesses the status of which specific body system?

Answer: _____

ANSWERS

1. **4**

Rationale: The human immunodeficiency virus (HIV) virus attacks the immune system by destroying T lymphocytes. Infants born to HIV-positive women test positive for HIV antibody, not HIV virus. This is actually a measure of maternal antibody and not indicative of true infection in the infant.

The virus attacks the immune system. T4 cells are depleted in number and cannot signal B cells to form protective antibodies to fight off the invading virus.

Test-Taking Strategy: Use the process of elimination. Eliminate option 2 first, knowing that HIV attacks the immune system. Eliminate option 1 next with the knowledge that newborn infants test positive for HIV antibody, but not the virus.

Recalling that T4 cells are depleted will assist in eliminating option 3. Review the physiological occurrences in HIV and acquired immunodeficiency syndrome (AIDS) if you had difficulty with this question.
Level of Cognitive Ability: Application
Client Needs: Physiological Integrity
Integrated Process: Teaching/Learning
Content Area: Child health
Reference: Wong, D., Hockenberry-Eaton, M. (2000). *Wong's essentials of pediatric nursing* (6th ed., p. 1019). St. Louis: Mosby.

2. 2
Rationale: A positive antibody test in a child younger than 18 months indicates only that the mother is infected because maternal immunoglobulin G antibodies persist in infants for 6 to 9 months and, in some cases, as long as 18 months. A positive enzyme-linked immunosorbent assay (ELISA) does not indicate true infection.
Test-Taking Strategy: Use the process of elimination. Noting the key words "newborn infant" in the question, and recalling that a positive antibody test in a child younger than 18 months indicates only that the mother is infected will assist in directing you to the correct option. Review tests associated with HIV infection if you had difficulty with this question.
Level of Cognitive Ability: Analysis
Client Needs: Physiological Integrity
Integrated Process: Nursing Process—analysis
Content Area: Child health
References: Chernecky, C., & Berger, B. (2001). *Laboratory tests and diagnostic procedures* (3rd ed., p. 60). Philadelphia: W. B. Saunders.
Wong, D., Hockenberry-Eaton, M. (2000). *Wong's essentials of pediatric nursing* (6th ed., p. 1020). St. Louis: Mosby.

3. 4
Rationale: True infections in infants are confirmed by the detection of HIV by a p24 antigen assay, virus culture of HIV, or polymerase chain reaction. A Western blot confirms the presence of HIV antibodies. The CD4+ count indicates how well the immune system is working. A chest x-ray evaluates the presence of other manifestations associated HIV infection such as pneumonia.
Test-Taking Strategy: Knowledge regarding the laboratory tests used to determine the presence of HIV infection is required to answer this question. If you are unfamiliar with these laboratory tests, review them. Specific laboratory tests to review include ELISA, Western blot, CD4+ counts, and p24 antigen assay.
Level of Cognitive Ability: Analysis
Client Needs: Physiological Integrity
Integrated Process: Nursing Process—analysis
Content Area: Child health
Reference: Wong, D., Hockenberry-Eaton, M. (2000). *Wong's essentials of pediatric nursing* (6th ed., p. 1020). St. Louis: Mosby.

4. 3
Rationale: Most children infected with HIV develop symptoms within the first 9 months of life. The remainder of these infected children become symptomatic sometime before age 3. Children, with their immature immune systems, have a much shorter incubation period than adults. Options 1, 2, and 4 are incorrect.
Test-Taking Strategy: Use the process of elimination. Eliminate options 1, 2, and 4 because they are similar in content. Option 3 is the only option that provides specific and accurate data regarding HIV infection in the infant. Review assessment findings associated with HIV infection if you had difficulty with this question.
Level of Cognitive Ability: Application
Client Needs: Psychosocial Integrity
Integrated Process: Nursing Process—implementation
Content Area: Child health
Reference: James, S., Ashwill, J., & Droske, S. (2002). *Nursing care of children: Principles & practice* (2nd ed., p. 488). Philadelphia: W. B. Saunders.

5. 3
Rationale: The most common opportunistic infection of children infected with HIV is *Pneumocystis carinii* pneumonia, which occurs most frequently between the ages of 3 and 6 months, when HIV status may be indeterminate. Lymphoid interstitial pneumonia is a form of chronic pneumonitis and is also characteristic of HIV infection; however, it is not the most common opportunistic infection. Although gastrointestinal disturbances and neurological abnormalities may occur in the child with HIV infection, options 1 and 2 are not specific opportunistic infections noted in the HIV-infected child.
Test-Taking Strategy: Use the process of elimination and note the key words "most common opportunistic infection." This focus will direct you to option 3. Review the common manifestations associated with HIV, if you had difficulty with this question.
Level of Cognitive Ability: Analysis
Client Needs: Physiological Integrity
Integrated Process: Nursing Process—assessment
Content Area: Child health
Reference: Wong, D., Hockenberry-Eaton, M. (2000). *Wong's essentials of pediatric nursing* (6th ed., p. 1020). St. Louis: Mosby.

6. 2
Rationale: Immunizations against common childhood illnesses are recommended for all children exposed to or infected with HIV. Pneumococcal and influenza vaccines also are recommended. The varicella (chickenpox) vaccine is avoided in the child who is HIV infected. The hepatitis B vaccine is administered according to the recommended immunization schedule. Option 4 is not necessary and is inaccurate.
Test-Taking Strategy: Use the process of elimination. Option 4 can be eliminated easily first. From the remaining options, recalling that *Pneumocystis carinii* is the most common opportunistic infection in the child infected with HIV will assist in directing you to option 2. Review immunizations in the immunodeficient child if you had difficulty with this question.
Level of Cognitive Ability: Application
Client Needs: Health Promotion and Maintenance
Integrated Process: Teaching/Learning
Content Area: Child health
Reference: Wong, D., Hockenberry-Eaton, M. (2000). *Wong's essentials of pediatric nursing* (6th ed., p. 1020). St. Louis: Mosby.

7. 2

Rationale: Nebulizer pieces are cleaned with warm water after each treatment and allowed to air dry. They are soaked in white vinegar and water for 30 minutes at the end of each day. Options 1, 3, and 4 are inaccurate and would damage the nebulizer equipment.

Test-Taking Strategy: Use the process of elimination. Options 1, 3, and 4 are similar in that they will damage the equipment. Options 1 and 4 should be eliminated first because these cleaning agents are strong and will damage the equipment. Next eliminate option 3 because boiling also may cause damage. Review home care instructions regarding respiratory treatments if you had difficulty with this question.

Level of Cognitive Ability: Application
Client Needs: Safe, Effective Care Environment
Integrated Process: Teaching/Learning
Content Area: Child health
Reference: James, S., Ashwill, J., & Droske, S. (2002). *Nursing care of children: Principles & practice* (2nd ed., p. 492). Philadelphia: W. B. Saunders.

8. 2

Rationale: Zidovudine effectively interferes with HIV replication but can cause bone marrow suppression. Anemia occurs most commonly after 4 to 6 weeks of therapy. Hematology studies need to be monitored for anemia and granulocytopenia. Renal and liver function tests also should be monitored. Options 1, 3, and 4 are not associated with the use of zidovudine.

Test-Taking Strategy: Use the process of elimination. Recalling that anemia is a concern with the administration of this medication will direct you easily to option 2. Review the adverse effects related to this medication if you had difficulty with this question.

Level of Cognitive Ability: Analysis
Client Needs: Physiological Integrity
Integrated Process: Nursing Process—analysis
Content Area: Pharmacology
Reference: Hodgson, B., & Kizior, R. (2003). *Saunders nursing drug handbook 2003* (p. 1177). Philadelphia: W. B. Saunders.

9. 3

Rationale: The preschool child will begin to conceptualize the death process as involving physical harm. A child from birth to 2 years of age will be unable to grasp the concept of illness and death. A school-aged child will begin to understand that something is wrong. An adolescent will express fear, withdrawal, and denial.

Test-Taking Strategy: Use concepts of growth and development and the related psychosocial issues to answer the question.

Noting the age of the child will assist in directing you to the correct option. Review these concepts if you had difficulty with this question.

Level of Cognitive Ability: Analysis
Client Needs: Psychosocial Integrity
Integrated Process: Nursing Process—analysis
Content Area: Child health
References: James, S., Ashwill, J., & Droske, S. (2002). *Nursing care of children: Principles & practice* (2nd ed., p. 489). Philadelphia: W. B. Saunders.
Wong, D., Hockenberry-Eaton, M. (2000). *Wong's essentials of pediatric nursing* (6th ed., 1022). St. Louis: Mosby.

10. 3

Rationale: The mother should be instructed to use a bleach solution for disinfecting contaminated objects or cleaning up spills from the child's diaper. Options 1, 2, and 4 are accurate instructions related to basic infection control.

Test-Taking Strategy: Use the process of elimination and note the key words "need for further instructions." Knowledge regarding basic infection control measures will direct you easily to option 3. Review these measures if you had difficulty with this question.

Level of Cognitive Ability: Analysis
Client Needs: Health Promotion and Maintenance
Integrated Process: Teaching/Learning
Content Area: Child health
Reference: James, S., Ashwill, J., & Droske, S. (2002). *Nursing care of children: Principles & practice* (2nd ed., p. 489). Philadelphia: W. B. Saunders.

CRITICAL THINKING: FILL IN THE BLANK

Answer: Immune system

Rationale: A CD4+ count is a useful tool specifically to assess an infected young child's immune status. The test also determines a child's response to therapy, risk for disease progression, and need for *Pneumocystis carinii* pneumonia prophylaxis after 1 year of age.

Test-Taking Strategy: Specific knowledge regarding the purpose of the CD4+ blood test is needed to answer this question. Review this blood test if you had difficulty with this question.

Level of Cognitive Ability: Application
Client Needs: Physiological Integrity
Integrated Process: Nursing Process—implementation
Content Area: Child health
Reference: James, S., Ashwill, J., & Droske, S. (2002). *Nursing care of children: Principles & practice* (2nd ed., p. 486). Philadelphia: W. B. Saunders.

REFERENCES

Chernecky, C., & Berger, B. (2001). *Laboratory tests and diagnostic procedures* (3rd ed.). Philadelphia: W. B. Saunders.

Hodgson, B., & Kizior, R. (2003). *Saunders nursing drug handbook 2003*. Philadelphia: W. B. Saunders.

James, S., Ashwill, J., & Droske, S. (2002). *Nursing care of children: Principles & practice* (2nd ed.). Philadelphia: W. B. Saunders.

McKinney, E., Ashwill, J., Murray, S., James, S., Gorrie, T., & Droske, S. (2000). *Maternal-child nursing*. Philadelphia: W. B. Saunders.

Wong, D., Hockenberry-Eaton, M. (2000). *Wong's essentials of pediatric nursing* (6th ed.). St. Louis: Mosby.

Wong, D., Perry, S., & Hockenberry, M. (2002). *Maternal child nursing care* (2nd ed.). St. Louis: Mosby.

Infectious and Communicable Diseases

I. RUBEOLA (MEASLES)

A. Description
1. Agent: virus
2. Incubation period: 10 to 20 days
3. Communicable period: from 4 days before to 5 days after the rash appears; mainly during prodromal (catarrhal) stage
4. Source: respiratory tract secretions, blood, or urine of infected person
5. Transmission: airborne or direct contact with infectious droplets

B. Assessment
1. Fever
2. Malaise
3. Coryza and cough
4. Rash appears as red, discrete maculopapules that blanch easily with pressure and gradually turn a brownish color (lasts 6 to 7 days); rash begins behind the ears and spreads downward to the feet.
5. Koplik's spots: small, red spots with a bluish white center and a red base; located on the mucosa and last 3 days

C. Interventions
1. Use respiratory precautions if the child is hospitalized.
2. Restrict child to quiet activities and bed rest.
3. Use a cool mist vaporizer for cough and coryza.
4. Dim lights if photophobia is present.
5. Administer antipyretics for fever.

II. ROSEOLA (EXANTHEMA SUBITUM)

A. Description
1. Agent: human herpesvirus type 6
2. Incubation period: 5 to 15 days
3. Communicable period: unknown but thought to extend from the febrile stage to the time the rash first appears
4. Source: unknown
5. Transmission: unknown

B. Assessment
1. Fever lasts for 3 to 5 days, followed by a rash (rose-pink maculas that blanch with pressure).
2. The rash appears 2 to 3 days after the onset of fever and lasts 1 to 2 days.

C. Interventions: supportive

III. RUBELLA (GERMAN MEASLES)

A. Description
1. Agent: rubella virus
2. Incubation period: 14 to 21 days
3. Communicable period: 7 days before to about 5 days after the rash appears
4. Source: nasopharyngeal secretions; virus is also present in blood, stool, and urine
5. Transmission
   a. Airborne or direct contact with infectious droplets
   b. Indirectly via articles freshly contaminated with nasopharyngeal secretions, feces, or urine
   c. Transplacental

B. Assessment
1. Low-grade fever
2. Malaise
3. Pinkish red maculopapular rash that begins on the face and spreads to the entire body
4. Petechial spots may occur on the soft palate

C. Interventions
1. Provide supportive treatment.
2. Isolate the infected child from pregnant women.

IV. MUMPS
A. Description
   1. Agent: paramyxovirus
   2. Incubation period: 14 to 21 days
   3. Communicable period: immediately before and after the swelling begins
   4. Source: saliva of infected person and possibly urine
   5. Transmission
      a. Direct contact with infected person
      b. Droplet spread from infected person
B. Assessment
   1. Fever
   2. Headache and malaise
   3. Anorexia
   4. Earache aggravated by chewing, followed by parotid glandular swelling
C. Interventions
   1. Use respiratory precautions.
   2. Provide bed rest until the parotid glandular swelling subsides.
   3. Avoid foods that require chewing.
   4. Apply hot or cold compresses as prescribed to the neck.
   5. To relieve orchitis, apply warmth and local support with tight-fitting underpants.

V. CHICKENPOX (VARICELLA)
A. Description
   1. Agent: varicella-zoster virus
   2. Incubation period: 13 to 17 days
   3. Communicable period: 1 to 2 days before the onset of the rash to 6 days after the first crop of vesicles, when crusts have formed
   4. Source: respiratory tract secretions of infected person; skin lesions
   5. Transmission: direct contact, droplet (airborne) spread, and contaminated objects
B. Assessment
   1. Slight fever, malaise, and anorexia are followed by a macular rash that first appears on the trunk and scalp and moves to the extremities.
   2. Lesions become pustules, begin to dry, and develop a crust.
   3. Lesions may appear on the mucous membranes of the mouth, the genital area, and the rectal area.
C. Interventions
   1. In the hospital setting, ensure strict isolation (contact and airborne precautions).
   2. In the home setting, isolate the infected child until the vesicles have dried; isolate high-risk children from the infected child.

VI. PERTUSSIS (WHOOPING COUGH)
A. Description
   1. Agent: *Bordetella pertussis*
   2. Incubation period: 5 to 21 days (usually 10 days)

   3. Communicable period: greatest during the catarrhal stage
   4. Source: discharge from the respiratory tract of the infected person
   5. Transmission: direct contact or droplet spread from infected person; indirect contact with freshly contaminated articles
B. Assessment: symptoms of respiratory infection followed by increased severity of cough
C. Interventions
   1. Isolate child during the catarrhal stage; if the child is hospitalized, institute respiratory precautions.
   2. Administer antimicrobial therapy as prescribed.
   3. Administer pertussis immune globulin as prescribed.
   4. Reduce environmental factors that promote paroxysms of coughing, such as dust, smoke, and sudden changes in temperature.
   5. Encourage fluid intake.
   6. Provide high humidity with the use of a humidifier or tent.

VII. DIPHTHERIA
A. Description
   1. Agent: *Corynebacterium diphtheriae*
   2. Incubation period: 2 to 5 days
   3. Communicable period: variable; until virulent bacilli are no longer present (three negative cultures), usually 2 weeks but as long as 4 weeks
   4. Source: discharge from the mucous membrane of the nose and nasopharynx, skin, and other lesions of the infected person
   5. Transmission: direct contact with infected person, carrier, or contaminated articles
B. Assessment
   1. Low-grade fever, malaise, sore throat
   2. Foul-smelling, mucopurulent nasal discharge
   3. Gray membrane on the tonsils and pharynx
   4. Lymphadenitis (neck edema)
C. Interventions
   1. Ensure strict isolation of the hospitalized child.
   2. Administer antitoxin as prescribed (preceded by a skin or conjunctival test to rule out sensitivity to horse serum).
   3. Provide bed rest.
   4. Administer antibiotics as prescribed.

VIII. POLIOMYELITIS
A. Description
   1. Agent: enteroviruses
   2. Incubation period: 7 to 14 days
   3. Communicable period: not exactly known; the virus is present in the throat and feces shortly after infection and persists for about 1 week in the throat and 4 to 6 weeks in the feces
   4. Source: oropharyngeal secretions and feces of the infected person

5. Transmission: direct contact with infected person; fecal-oral and oropharyngeal routes

B. Assessment
   1. Fever, malaise, anorexia, nausea, headache, sore throat
   2. Abdominal pain followed by soreness and stiffness of the trunk, neck, and limbs that progresses to flaccid paralysis

C. Interventions
   1. Enteric precautions
   2. Supportive treatment
   3. Bed rest
   4. Monitoring for respiratory paralysis
   5. Physical therapy

IX. SCARLET FEVER

A. Description
   1. Agent: group A β-hemolytic streptococci
   2. Incubation period: 1 to 7 days
   3. Communicable period: during the incubation period and clinical illness, about 10 days; during the first 2 weeks of the carrier stage, although may persist for months
   4. Source: nasopharyngeal secretions of infected person and carriers
   5. Transmission: direct contact with infected person or droplet spread; indirectly by contact with contaminated articles, ingestion of contaminated milk, or other foods

B. Assessment
   1. Child has abrupt high fever, vomiting, headache, malaise, and abdominal pain.
   2. A red, fine papular rash develops in the axilla, groin, and neck that spreads to cover the entire body.
   3. The rash blanches with pressure except in areas of deep creases and folds of the joints (Pastia's sign).
   4. The tongue is coated and papillae become red and swollen (white strawberry tongue); by the fourth to fifth day the white coat sloughs off, leaving prominent papillae (red strawberry tongue).
   5. Tonsils are edematous and covered with a gray-white exudate.
   6. Pharynx is edematous and beefy red.

C. Interventions
   1. Use respiratory precautions until 24 hours after the initiation of treatment.
   2. Provide supportive therapy.
   3. Provide bed rest.
   4. Encourage fluid intake.
   5. Administer antibiotics as prescribed.

X. ERYTHEMA INFECTIOSUM (FIFTH DISEASE)

A. Description
   1. Agent: human parvovirus B19

2. Incubation period: 4 to 14 days; may be as long as 20 days
3. Communicable period: uncertain but before the onset of symptoms in most children
4. Source: infected person
5. Transmission: unknown; possibly respiratory secretions and blood

B. Assessment
   1. Fever, myalgia, lethargy, nausea, vomiting, abdominal pain
   2. Stages of the rash
      a. Erythema of the face (slapped-face appearance) develops, chiefly on the cheeks, and disappears by 1 to 4 days.
      b. About 1 day after the rash appears on the face, maculopapular red spots appear, symmetrically distributed in the extremities; rash progresses from proximal to distal surfaces and may last a week or more.
      c. Rash subsides but may reappear if the skin becomes irritated or traumatized by factors such as the sun, heat, cold, or friction.

C. Interventions
   1. Ensure respiratory isolation of the hospitalized child.
   2. Pregnant women should not be in contact with or care for the infected person.
   3. Provide supportive care.
   4. Administer antipyretics, analgesics, and antiinflammatory medications as prescribed.

XI. INFECTIOUS MONONUCLEOSIS

A. Description
   1. Agent: Epstein-Barr virus
   2. Incubation period: 4 to 6 weeks
   3. Communicable period: unknown; the virus is shed before the onset of the disease until 6 months or longer after recovery
   4. Source: oral secretions
   5. Transmission: direct intimate contact, infected blood

B. Assessment
   1. Fever, sore throat, malaise, headache, fatigue, nausea, abdominal pain
   2. Lymphadenopathy and hepatosplenomegaly

C. Interventions
   1. Provide supportive care.
   2. Monitor for signs of splenic rupture, which include abdominal pain, left upper quadrant pain, or left shoulder pain.

XII. ROCKY MOUNTAIN SPOTTED FEVER

A. Description
   1. Agent: *Rickettsia rickettsii*
   2. Incubation period: 2 to 14 days
   3. Source: tick; mammal source: wild rodents, dogs
   4. Transmission: bite of infected tick

B. Assessment
  1. Fever, malaise, anorexia, vomiting, headache, myalgia
  2. Maculopapular or petechial rash primarily on the extremities (ankles and wrists) but may spread to other areas, characteristically on the palms and soles
C. Interventions
  1. Provide vigorous supportive care.
  2. Administer antibiotics as prescribed.
  3. Teach child and parents about protection from tick bites.

XIII. ENTEROBIASIS (PINWORM)
A. Description
  1. Agent: *Enterobius vermicularis*
  2. Source
    a. The nematode is universally present in temperate climatic zones.
    b. Eggs are ingested or inhaled (eggs float in the air), hatch in the upper intestine, mature in 2 to 8 weeks, and migrate to the cecal area; females then mate, migrate out the anus, and lay eggs.
  3. Transmission
    a. Favored in crowded conditions
    b. Ingestion or inhalation of eggs
    c. Hands to mouth or fecal-oral route
    d. Contaminated items (pinworm eggs persist in the environment for 2 to 3 weeks)
B. Assessment: intense perianal itching, irritability, restlessness, poor sleep, bed-wetting, distractibility, short attention span; in females, the worm may migrate to the vagina and urethra and cause infection
C. Interventions
  1. Identify the worms.
    a. Use a flashlight to inspect the anal area 2 to 3 hours after the child is asleep.
    b. Tape test: Use transparent, sticky tape to obtain a specimen from the child's perianal area; collect the specimen in the morning as soon as the child awakens and before a bowel movement or a bath.
  2. Use enteric precautions.
  3. Administer anthelmintic medications (all household members are treated) as prescribed; course of medication is repeated in 2 weeks following the first course to prevent reinfection.
  4. Teach home care measures to prevent reinfection.

XIV. IMMUNIZATIONS
A. Guidelines
  1. In the United States, the recommended age for beginning primary immunizations of infants is at birth.
  2. Children born prematurely should receive the full dose of each vaccine at the appropriate chronological age.

  3. Children who began primary immunizations at the recommended age but failed to receive all of the doses, do not need to begin the series again but instead receive only the missed doses.
  4. If one suspects that the parent will not bring the child to the pediatrician or health care clinic for follow-up immunizations according to the optimal immunization schedule, any of the recommended vaccines can be administered simultaneously.
B. General contraindications (Box 47-1)
C. Guidelines for administration (Box 47-2)

XV. RECOMMENDED IMMUNIZATIONS: CHILD AND ADOLESCENT (BOX 47-3)
A. Hepatitis B vaccine
  1. The vaccine protects against hepatitis B.
  2. The first dose of hepatitis B should be administered soon after birth and before hospital

---

BOX 47-1

General Contraindications to Immunizations

Moderate or severe illnesses with or without a fever
Anaphylactic reaction to a previously administered vaccine or a substance in the vaccine
Live virus vaccines generally are not administered to anyone with an altered immune system

---

BOX 47-2

Guidelines for Administration

Follow manufactures recommendations for route of administration, storage, and reconstitution of the vaccine.
If refrigeration is necessary, store on a center shelf and not on the door; frequent temperature increases from opening the refrigerator door can alter the potency of the vaccine.
For protection against light, wrap the vial in aluminum foil.
A vaccine information statement needs to be given to the parents or individual, and informed consent for administration needs to be obtained.
Check expiration date on vaccine bottle.
Parenteral vaccines are given in separate syringes in different injection sites.
Vaccines administered intramuscularly are given in the vastus lateralis muscle (best site) in newborns and in the deltoid for older infants and children (dorsogluteal site is avoided).
Maintain immunization record; document day, month, year of administration; manufacturer and lot number of vaccine; name, address, title of person administering vaccine; and site and route of administration.
A Vaccine Adverse Event Report (VAERS form) needs to be filed and the health department needs to be notified if an adverse reaction to an immunization occurs.

BOX 47-3

Recommended Childhood and Adolescent Immunizations

Birth	Hepatitis B
1 month	Hepatitis B
2 months	Inactivated poliovirus vaccine (IPV), diphtheria, tetanus, acellular pertussis (DTaP), *Haemophilus influenzae* type b conjugate vaccine (Hib), pneumococcal vaccine (PCV)
4 months	DTaP, Hib, IPV, (PCV)
6 months	DTaP, Hib, hepatitis B, IPV, (PCV)
12-15 months	Hib; mumps, measles, rubella vaccine (MMR), (PCV)
12-18 months	varicella-zoster
15-18 months	DTaP
4-6 years	DTaP, IPV, MMR
11-12 years	MMR (if not administered at 4-6 years), tetanus and diphtheria toxoids (Td)

discharge; the first dose also may be given by age 2 if the infant's mother tests negative for hepatitis B surface antigen (HBsAg).

3. Only monovalent hepatitis B vaccine can be used for the birth dose, and monovalent or combination vaccine containing hepatitis B may be used to complete the series.

4. The second dose is administered at least 4 weeks after the first dose (except for combination vaccines which cannot be administered before age 6 weeks).

5. The last dose in the vaccination series should not be administered before age 6 months.

6. All children from birth through 18 years of age need three doses of hepatitis B vaccine if they have not already received them.

7. Vaccine is administered intramuscularly in the vastus lateralis muscle in newborns and in the deltoid for older infants and children (dorsogluteal site is avoided).

8. Anaphylactic reaction to common baker's yeast is a contraindication.

9. HBsAg-positive mothers
   a. Infant should receive hepatitis B vaccine and hepatitis B immune globulin within 12 hours of birth at two different injection sites.
   b. The second dose is recommended at age 1 to 2 months.
   c. The last dose should not be administered before age 6 months.
   d. Infant should be tested for HBsAg and antibody to hepatitis B surface antigen at 9 to 15 months of age.

10. Mother whose HBsAg status is unknown
   a. Infant should receive the first dose of hepatitis vaccine series within 12 hours of birth.

   b. Maternal blood should be drawn as soon as possible to determine the mother's HBsAg status.
   c. If the HBsAg test is positive, the infant should receive hepatitis B immune globulin as soon as possible (no later than age 1 week).
   d. The second dose of hepatitis B vaccine is recommended at age 1 to 2 months.
   e. The last dose of hepatitis B vaccine should not be administered before age 6 months.

B. Diphtheria, tetanus, acellular pertussis (DTaP) and tetanus and diphtheria toxoids (Td)
   1. The vaccines protect against diphtheria, tetanus, and pertussis.
   2. The DTaP is administered at 2 months, 4 months, 6 months, between 15 and 18 months of age, and between 4 and 6 years of age.
   3. The fourth dose of DTaP can be given at 12 months of age if 6 months have elapsed since the previous dose and if the child might not return for follow-up by 18 months of age.
   4. The Td is given at 11 to 12 years of age if at least 5 years have passed since the last dose of tetanus and diphtheria toxoid-containing vaccine.
   5. Subsequent routine Td boosters are recommended every 10 years.
   6. Encephalopathy within 7 days of administration of previous dose of DTaP is a contraindication.

C. *Haemophilus influenzae* type b (Hib) conjugate vaccine
   1. The vaccine protects against a number of serious infections caused by *H. influenzae* type b, such as bacterial meningitis, epiglottitis, bacterial pneumonia, septic arthritis, and sepsis.
   2. The Hib is administered at 2 months, 4 months, 6 months, and between 12 and 15 months of age.
   3. Depending on the brand of Hib vaccine used for the first and second doses, a dose at 6 months of age may not be needed.
   4. The DTaP/Hib combination products should not be used for primary immunization in infants ages 2, 4, or 6 months but can be used as boosters following any Hib vaccine.
   5. The Hib vaccines are administered by intramuscular injection and are given at a separate site from any concurrent vaccinations.
   6. No contraindications have been identified.

D. Inactivated poliovirus vaccine (IPV)
   1. The IPV protects against polio.
   2. The IPV is administered at 2 months, 4 months, 6 months, and between 4 and 6 years of age.
   3. The third dose of IPV may be administered between 6 and 18 months of age.
   4. Anaphylactic reaction to neomycin or streptomycin is a contraindication.

E. Measles, mumps, rubella vaccine (MMR)
   1. The MMR protects against measles, mumps, and rubella (German measles).

2. The first dose of MMR is administered between 12 and 15 months of age; the second dose is administered at 4 to 6 years of age (the second dose may be administered during any visit as long as at least 4 weeks have elapsed since the first dose and both doses are administered beginning at or after age 12 months).

3. If the second dose was not given by 4 to 6 years of age, it should be given at the next scheduled pediatrician or health care clinic visit.

4. Those who have not received the second dose previously should complete the schedule at the 11- to 12-year-old pediatric or health care clinic visit.

5. The MMR contains minute amounts of neomycin; measles and mumps vaccines, which are grown on chick embryo tissue cultures, are not believed to contain significant amounts of egg cross-reacting proteins.

6. Contraindications
   a. Pregnancy
   b. Known altered immunodeficiency
   c. Allergy to contents of immunization (before the administration of MMR vaccine, assess for a known history of allergy to neomycin or related antibiotics)
   d. Presence of recently acquired **passive immunity** through blood transfusions, immunoglobulin, or maternal antibodies (MMR should be postponed for a minimum of 3 months after passive immunization with immunoglobulins or blood transfusions, except washed blood cells, which do not interfere with the immune response)

F. Varicella-zoster vaccine
   1. Vaccine protects against chickenpox.
   2. Varicella-zoster vaccine is administered between 12 and 18 months of age.
   3. Susceptible children 13 years of age and older (who have not had chickenpox or have not been previously vaccinated) need two doses given at least 4 weeks apart.
   4. Vaccine is administered by subcutaneous injection.
   5. The vaccine should be kept frozen and used within 30 minutes of reconstitution to ensure viral potency.
   6. Contraindications
      a. Pregnancy
      b. Immunocompromised individuals
      c. Children receiving corticosteroids

G. Pneumococcal vaccine
   1. A heptavalent pneumococcal conjugate vaccine is recommended for all children ages 2 to 23 months.
   2. The vaccine can be given concurrently with other childhood vaccines at 2, 4, 6, and 12 to 15 months of age.
   3. It is also recommended for certain children age 24 to 59 months.

4. Pneumococcal polysaccharide vaccine is recommended in addition to pneumococcal conjugate vaccine for certain high-risk groups.

XVI. REACTIONS TO A VACCINE
A. Local reactions
   1. Tenderness, erythema, and swelling at the injection site
   2. Low grade fever
   3. Behavioral changes such as drowsiness, unusual crying, eating less
B. Minimizing local reactions
   1. Select a needle of adequate length (1 inch in infants) to deposit the antigen deep into the muscle mass.
   2. Inject into the vastus lateralis muscle or ventrogluteal muscle; one may use the deltoid in children 18 months of age or older.
   3. Use an air bubble when administering the vaccine.
C. Anaphylactic reactions
   1. The goals of treatment are to provide ventilation, restore adequate circulation, and prevent further exposure to the antigen.
   2. For a mild reaction with no evidence of respiratory distress or cardiovascular compromise, subcutaneous injection of an antihistamine such as diphenhydramine (Benadryl) and epinephrine (Adrenalin) may be administered.
   3. For moderate or severe distress, establish an airway; provide cardiopulmonary resuscitation if the child is not breathing; elevate the head; administer epinephrine, fluids, and vasopressors as prescribed; monitor vital signs; and monitor urine output.

XVII. VACCINES FOR SELECTED POPULATIONS
A. Hepatitis A vaccine
   1. Vaccine is recommended for children and adolescents in selected states and regions (communities with high-infection rates) and for certain high-risk groups.
   2. Vaccine is given intramuscularly in the deltoid muscle.
B. Influenza vaccine
   1. Vaccine is recommended annually for children from age 6 months with certain risk factors such as asthma, sickle cell disease, human immunodeficiency virus infection, diabetes mellitus, and household members of persons in groups at high risk.
   2. Annual vaccinations are recommended for adult groups at high risk.
      a. Anyone 50 years of age or older
      b. Adults of any age with a chronic cardiac or pulmonary disease
      c. Residents of long-term care facilities
      d. Immunocompromised adults
      e. Women who will be in the second or third trimester of pregnancy during influenza season

3. Administer vaccine by intramuscular injection.
4. Vaccination is contraindicated in persons with anaphylactic hypersensitivity to eggs.

C. Pneumococcal vaccine
1. Vaccine is recommended for persons 65 years of age or older and those with chronic cardiovascular disease, chronic pulmonary disease, or diabetes mellitus.
2. Revaccination is advised if the individual was less than 65 years of age at the time of vaccination.
3. In immunocompromised persons, an initial vaccination is recommended, followed by revaccination every 5 years.

D. Meningococcal vaccine
1. Vaccine is recommended for persons with medical indications, such as adults with terminal complement component deficiencies, persons with anatomic or functional asplenia, or persons traveling to countries where the disease is hyperendemic or epidemic (revaccination at 3 to 5 years may be indicated for persons at high risk for infection).
2. College freshman should be counseled about meningococcal disease so that they can make an informed decision about receiving the vaccine.
3. Administer vaccine by subcutaneous injection.

E. Smallpox vaccine
1. Vaccine protects persons who work with smallpox or related viruses in laboratories.
2. The vaccinia virus is the "live virus" used in the smallpox vaccine that is a pox-type virus related to smallpox.
3. The vaccine does not contain the smallpox virus and cannot cause smallpox.
4. Recommendations for use (Box 47-4)
5. Getting the vaccine before exposure most likely will prevent smallpox.

6. Getting the vaccine within 3 days after exposure will help to prevent the disease or make it less severe.
7. Getting the vaccine within a week after exposure also can make the disease less severe.
8. Protection from infection lasts 3 to 5 years, and protection from severe illness and death can last 10 years or more.
9. Vaccinated persons may need to be revaccinated after 3 to 10 years, depending on risk.
10. Site should be checked at around 7 days after vaccination to make sure that the vaccine is working (a successful vaccination is characterized by a pustular lesion or an area of definite induration or congestion surrounding a central lesion, which might be a scab or ulcer).
11. Expected reactions
   a. Formation of a blister and then a scar
   b. Swelling and tenderness of the lymph nodes lasting 2 to 4 weeks after the blister has healed, itching at the site, fatigue, mild fever, headache, or muscle aches
12. Adverse reactions
   a. Mild to moderate reactions: mild rash, lasting 2 to 4 days, temperature of more than 100° F, blisters on the body
   b. Moderate to severe reactions: eye infection (spread of the vaccine to the eye), rash on entire body
   c. Potentially life threatening reactions: severe rash that can lead to scarring, encephalitis that can lead to permanent brain damage and death,

---

BOX 47-4

Recommendations for Smallpox Vaccine

ROUTINE NONEMERGENCY USE
Laboratory workers who handle cultures or animals contaminated with vaccinia or other related viruses such as monkeypox, cowpox, and variola should be vaccinated.
Public health, hospital, and other personnel, generally 18 to 65 years of age, who may have to respond to a smallpox case or outbreak should be vaccinated.

EMERGENCY USE (SMALLPOX OUTBREAK)
Anyone directly exposed to smallpox virus should get one dose of the vaccine as soon as possible after exposure.
Anyone at risk of exposure to smallpox virus may need to get one dose of the vaccine when the risk occurs or becomes known.

BOX 47-5

Contraindications to Smallpox Vaccine

Anyone who has eczema or atopic dermatitis or has a history of either condition
Anyone with a skin condition that causes breaks in the skin should wait until the condition clears up
Anyone whose immune system is weakened
Pregnancy (women should avoid getting pregnant for 4 weeks after getting smallpox vaccine)
Breast-feeding mothers
Individuals who live with or who have close physical contact with someone with a skin condition or with a compromised immune system, someone who is pregnant, or someone less than 1 year of age should not get the smallpox vaccine because it poses a risk to that person
Not recommended for anyone under 18 years of age
History of anaphylaxis reaction to polymyxin B, streptomycin, chlortetracycline, neomycin, or a previous dose of smallpox vaccine
Persons using steroid drops in their eyes
Persons who are moderately or severely ill at the time of vaccination usually should wait until they recover before getting the vaccine

BOX 47-6

Care of the Vaccination Site

A scab will form in the spot where the vaccination was administered; this scab should be left alone so that the vaccinia virus in the vaccine does not spread to other parts of the body.

Hands need to be washed frequently and whenever the site is touched or the bandage is changed (the eyes or any other part of the body should not be touched after changing the bandage or touching the vaccination site).

The site should be covered loosely with a gauze bandage; and health care workers may need additional measures, such as placing a semipermeable dressing over the gauze bandage.

Gauze bandage should be covered with a waterproof bandage while bathing.

Clothing should be worn over the vaccination site as an extra precaution.

Used bandages should be discarded in a plastic zip bag (the scab is discarded in the same manner).

Avoid sharing towels and launder items that have touched the vaccination site.

Avoid scratching or putting ointment on the vaccination site.

   severe progressive infection that can lead to death
   d. Possibly can cause heart inflammation (myocarditis, pericarditis, myopericarditis)
13. Contraindications (Box 47-5)
14. Care of the vaccination site (Box 47-6)

PRACTICE QUESTIONS

1. A child with rubeola (measles) is being admitted to the hospital. In preparing for the admission of the child, a nurse plans to place the child on which precautions?
   1. Contact
   2. Enteric
   3. Respiratory
   4. Protective

2. Several children have contracted rubeola (measles) in a local school. The school nurse conducts a teaching session for the mothers of the schoolchildren. Which statement made by a mother indicates a need for further teaching regarding this communicable disease?
   1. "Respiratory symptoms such as a profuse runny nose, cough, and fever occur before the development of a rash."
   2. "Small blue-white spots with a red base may appear in the mouth."
   3. "The rash usually begins behind the ears and spreads downward toward the feet."
   4. "The communicable period ranges from 10 days before the onset of symptoms to 15 days after the rash appears."

3. The mother of a 15-month-old child brings the child to a clinic and reports that the child has a fever and has developed a rash on the neck and trunk. Roseola is diagnosed. The mother is concerned that her other children will contract the disease. A nurse provides which of the following instructions to the mother regarding the prevention of transmission of the disease?
   1. The disease is transmitted through the urine and feces, so the other children should use a separate bathroom.
   2. Disease transmission is unknown.
   3. The disease is transmitted through the respiratory tract, so the child should be isolated from the other children as much as possible.
   4. The disease is transmitted by contact with body fluids, so any items contaminated with body fluids need to discarded in a separate receptacle.

4. A nurse provides instructions to the mother of a child with mumps regarding respiratory precautions. The mother asks the nurse about the length of time required for the respiratory precautions. The nurse most appropriately responds
   1. "Respiratory precautions are not necessary once the swelling appears."
   2. "Respiratory precautions are not neccessary before the swelling begins."
   3. "Respiratory precautions are indicated during the period of communicability."
   4. "Respiratory precautions are indicated for 18 days following the onset of parotid swelling."

5. A mother brings her 6-year-old child to the clinic because the child has developed a rash on the trunk and on the scalp. The mother reports that the child has had a low-grade fever, has not felt like eating, and generally has been tired. The child is diagnosed with chickenpox. The mother inquires about the communicable period associated with chickenpox. A nurse plans to base the response on which of the following?
   1. The communicable period is unknown.
   2. The communicable period is 1 to 2 days before the onset of the rash to 6 days after the first crop of vesicles, when crusts have formed.
   3. The communicable period is 10 days before the onset of symptoms to 15 days after the rash appears.
   4. The communicable period ranges from 2 weeks or less to several months.

6. A nurse provides home care instructions to the parents of a child hospitalized with pertussis. The child is in the convalescent stage and is being prepared for discharge. Which statement by a parent indicates a need for further instructions?
   1. "We need to maintain respiratory precautions and a quiet environment for at least 2 weeks."
   2. "Coughing spells may be triggered by dust or smoke."
   3. "We need to encourage our child to drink fluids."
   4. "Good hand-washing techniques must be instituted to prevent spreading the disease to others."

7. A 6-month-old infant receives a diphtheria, tetanus, and acellular pertussis immunization at a well-baby clinic. The mother returns home and calls the clinic to report that the infant has developed swelling and redness at the site of injection. The nurse tells the mother to
   1. Apply a warm pack to the injection site.
   2. Bring the infant back to the clinic.
   3. Apply an ice pack to the injection site.
   4. Monitor the infant for a fever.

8. A child diagnosed with scarlet fever is being cared for at home. A home health nurse performs an assessment on the child, knowing that which of the following is not a clinical manifestation associated with this disease?
   1. Pastia's sign
   2. White strawberry tongue
   3. Edematous and beefy-red pharynx
   4. Koplik's spots

9. A home health nurse visits a child with infectious mononucleosis and provides home care instructions to the parents about the care of the child. The nurse tells the parents to
   1. Maintain the child on bed rest for 2 weeks.
   2. Maintain respiratory precautions for 1 week.
   3. Notify the physician if the child develops a fever.
   4. Notify the physician if the child develops abdominal pain or left shoulder pain.

10. The mother of a preschooler who attends day care calls a clinic nurse and tells the nurse that the child is constantly scratching the perianal area and that the area is irritated. The nurse suspects the possibility of pinworm infection (enterobiasis). The nurse instructs the mother to obtain a tape test rectal specimen and tells the mother to obtain the specimen
    1. When the child is put to bed.
    2. After toileting.
    3. After bathing.
    4. In the morning when the child awakens.

11. A nursing student is assigned to administer immunizations to children in a clinic. The nursing instructor asks the student about the contraindications to receiving an immunization. The student responds correctly by telling the instructor that a contraindication to receiving an immunization is if a child has
    1. A cold.
    2. Otitis media.
    3. Mild diarrhea.
    4. A severe febrile illness.

12. A mother brings her 4-month-old infant to a well-baby clinic for immunizations. A nurse would prepare to administer which of the following immunizations to this infant?
    1. DTaP (diphtheria, tetanus, acellular pertussis), MMR (measles, mumps, rubella), IPV (inactivated poliovirus vaccine)
    2. MMR, Hib (*Haemophilus influenzae* type b), DTaP
    3. DTaP, Hib, IPV
    4. Varicella and hepatitis B vaccines

13. A clinic nurse prepares to administer a measles, mumps, rubella (MMR) vaccine to a 5-year-old child. The nurse administers this vaccine
    1. Intramuscularly in the anterolateral aspect of the thigh.
    2. Intramuscularly in the deltoid muscle.
    3. Subcutaneously in the outer aspect of the upper arm.
    4. Subcutaneously in the gluteal muscle.

14. A child is scheduled to receive a measles, mumps, rubella (MMR) vaccine. The nurse preparing to administer the vaccine reviews the child's record and questions the order if which of the following is documented in the child's record?
    1. A local reaction at the site of injection of a previous MMR vaccine
    2. A history of an anaphylactic reaction to neomycin
    3. A history of frequent respiratory infections
    4. Recent recovery from a cold

15. A 15-year-old child is scheduled to receive a series of the hepatitis B vaccine. The child arrives at a clinic for the first dose. Before administering the vaccine, a nurse performs an assessment on the child and asks the child about a history of an allergy to
    1. Baker's yeast.
    2. Eggs.
    3. Penicillin.
    4. Sulfonamides.

CRITICAL THINKING: FILL IN THE BLANK

A nurse is preparing to care for a child with rubella (German measles) and anticipates contact with infectious material during care. The nurse enters the supply closet where the masks, gloves, gowns, and goggles are kept. Which item(s) does the nurse obtain to care for this child?

Answer: _____

ANSWERS

1. 3
Rationale: Rubeola is transmitted via airborne particles or direct contact with infectious droplets. Respiratory precautions are required, and those in contact with the child should wear masks. Gowns and gloves are not indicated. Articles that are contaminated should be bagged and labeled. Options 1, 2, and 4 are not indicated in rubeola.
Test-Taking Strategy: Use the process of elimination. Recalling that rubeola is transmitted via the airborne route will direct you easily to option 3. Review the route of transmission and therapeutic management of rubeola if you had difficulty with this question.
Level of Cognitive Ability: Application
Client Needs: Safe, Effective Care Environment
Integrated Process: Nursing Process—planning
Content Area: Child health
Reference: Wong, D., Hockenberry-Eaton, M. (2000). *Wong's essentials of pediatric nursing* (6th ed., p. 461). St. Louis: Mosby.

2. 4
Rationale: The communicable period for rubeola ranges from 4 days before to 5 days after the rash appears, mainly during the prodromal (catarrhal) stage. Options 1, 2, and 3 are accurate descriptions of rubeola. The small blue-white spots found in this communicable disease are called Koplik's spots. Option 4, the incorrect option, describes the incubation period for rubella, not rubeola.
Test-Taking Strategy: Note the key words "need for further teaching" in the stem of the question. Recalling that the communicable period for rubeola ranges from 4 days before to 5 days after the rash appears will direct you to option 4. Review the clinical manifestations associated with rubeola if you had difficulty with this question.
Level of Cognitive Ability: Analysis
Client Needs: Safe, Effective Care Environment
Integrated Process: Teaching/Learning
Content Area: Child health
References: James, S., Ashwill, J., & Droske, S. (2002). *Nursing care of children: Principles & practice* (2nd ed., p. 450). Philadelphia: W. B. Saunders.
Wong, D., Hockenberry-Eaton, M. (2000). *Wong's essentials of pediatric nursing* (6th ed., p. 461). St. Louis: Mosby.

3. 2
Rationale: The method of transmission of roseola is unknown. Options 1, 3, and 4 are not accurate transmission routes of roseola.
Test-Taking Strategy: Use the process of elimination. Eliminate options 1 and 4 first because they are similar. From the remaining options, recall that the method of transmission of roseola is unknown. Review the characteristics of roseola if you had difficulty with this question.
Level of Cognitive Ability: Application
Client Needs: Safe, Effective Care Environment
Integrated Process: Teaching/Learning
Content Area: Child health
Reference: Wong, D., Hockenberry-Eaton, M. (2000). *Wong's essentials of pediatric nursing* (6th ed., p. 458). St. Louis: Mosby.

4. 3
Rationale: Mumps is transmitted via direct contact with or droplet spread from an infected person and possibly by contact with the urine. Respiratory precautions are indicated during the period of communicability (immediately before and after swelling begins).
Test-Taking Strategy: Use the process of elimination. Options 1 and 2 can be eliminated first because they are similar. From the remaining options, select option 3 because it is the global option and addresses communicability. Also, the time frame indicated in option 4 seems rather lengthy. Review the infectious period related to mumps if you had difficulty with this question.
Level of Cognitive Ability: Application
Client Needs: Safe, Effective Care Environment
Integrated Process: Teaching/Learning
Content Area: Child health
Reference: Wong, D., Hockenberry-Eaton, M. (2000). *Wong's essentials of pediatric nursing* (6th ed., pp. 460-461). St. Louis: Mosby.

5. 2
Rationale: The communicable period for chickenpox is 1 to 2 days before the onset of the rash to 6 days after the first crop of vesicles, when crusts have formed. In roseola the communicable period is unknown. Option 3 describes rubella. Option 4 describes diphtheria.
Test-Taking Strategy: Use the process of elimination. Option 1 can be eliminated easily. Eliminate options 3 and 4 next because the time frames in these two options seem rather lengthy and are similar. If you had difficulty with this question, review the communicable period for chickenpox.
Level of Cognitive Ability: Application
Client Needs: Safe, Effective Care Environment
Integrated Process: Teaching/Learning
Content Area: Child health
Reference: James, S., Ashwill, J., & Droske, S. (2002). *Nursing care of children: Principles & practice* (2nd ed., p. 456). Philadelphia: W. B. Saunders.

6. 1
Rationale: Pertussis is transmitted by direct contact or respiratory droplets from coughing. The communicable period occurs primarily during the catarrhal stage. Respiratory precautions are not required during the convalescent phase. Options 2, 3, and 4 are components of home care instructions.
Test-Taking Strategy: Use the process of elimination. Note the key words "convalescent" in the question and "need for further instructions" in the stem of the question. Options 3 and 4 can be eliminated easily because they are general interventions associated with convalescence. Knowing that coughing spells are associated with pertussis will assist in directing you to option 1. In addition, 2 weeks of respiratory precautions is not required. If you had difficulty with this question, review home care instructions for the child with pertussis.
Level of Cognitive Ability: Analysis
Client Needs: Health Promotion and Maintenance
Integrated Process: Teaching/Learning
Content Area: Child health
Reference: James, S., Ashwill, J., & Droske, S. (2002). *Nursing care of children: Principles & practice* (2nd ed., p. 465). Philadelphia: W. B. Saunders.

7. 3

Rationale: Occasionally, tenderness, redness, or swelling may occur at the site of the injection. This can be relieved with ice packs for the first 24 hours, followed by warm compresses if the inflammation persists. Bringing the infant back to the clinic is not necessary. Option 4 may be an appropriate intervention but is not specific to the issue of the question.

Test-Taking Strategy: Use the process of elimination. Option 4 can be eliminated first because it does not relate specifically to the issue of the question. Eliminate option 2 next as an unnecessary intervention. From the remaining options, general principles related to the effects of heat and cold will direct you easily to option 3. Review interventions following immunizations and injections if you had difficulty with this question.

Level of Cognitive Ability: Application
Client Needs: Health Promotion and Maintenance
Integrated Process: Nursing Process—implementation
Content Area: Child health
Reference: McKinney, E., Ashwill, J., Murray, S., James, S., Gorrie, T., & Droske, S. (2000). *Maternal-child nursing* (p. 73). Philadelphia: W. B. Saunders.

8. 4

Rationale: Pastia's sign describes a rash seen in scarlet fever that will blanch with pressure except in areas of deep creases and the folds of joints. The tongue initially is coated with a white furry covering with red projecting papillae (white strawberry tongue). By the fourth to fifth day, the white strawberry tongue sloughs off, leaving a red swollen tongue (strawberry tongue). The pharynx is edematous and beefy red. Koplik's spots are associated with rubeola.

Test-Taking Strategy: Use the process of elimination, noting the key word "not" in the stem of the question. Recalling that Koplik's spots are associated with rubeola will assist you in answering this question. Review the clinical manifestations associated with scarlet fever if you had difficulty with this question.

Level of Cognitive Ability: Analysis
Client Needs: Physiological Integrity
Integrated Process: Nursing Process—assessment
Content Area: Child health
Reference: Wong, D., Hockenberry-Eaton, M. (2000). *Wong's essentials of pediatric nursing* (6th ed., p. 465). St. Louis: Mosby.

9. 4

Rationale: The parents need to be instructed to notify the physician if abdominal pain, especially in the left upper quadrant, or left shoulder pain occurs because this may indicate splenic rupture. Children with enlarged spleens also are instructed to avoid contact sports until splenomegaly resolves. Bed rest is not necessary, and children usually self-limit their activity. Respiratory precautions are not required, although transmission can occur via direct intimate contact or contact with infected blood. Fever is treated with acetaminophen (Tylenol).

Test-Taking Strategy: Use the process of elimination and knowledge regarding the organs affected in mononucleosis. Options 1 and 2 can be eliminated first because they are unnecessary interventions in this disease. From the remaining options, knowledge that splenic rupture is a concern will

direct you to option 4. Review the complications associated with mononucleosis if you had difficulty with this question.

Level of Cognitive Ability: Application
Client Needs: Physiological Integrity
Integrated Process: Teaching/Learning
Content Area: Child health
Reference: Wong, D., Perry, S., & Hockenberry, M. (2002). *Maternal child nursing care* (2nd ed., p. 1197). St. Louis: Mosby.

10. 4

Rationale: Diagnosis is confirmed by direct visualization of the worms. Parents can view the sleeping child's anus with a flashlight. The worm is white, thin, about ½ inch long, and moves. A simple technique, the tape test, is used to capture worms and eggs. Transparent tape is lightly touched to the anus and then applied to a slide for examination. The best specimens are obtained as the child awakens, before toileting or bathing.

Test-Taking Strategy: Use the process of elimination. Thinking about the test and the purpose of the test (to obtain a specimen that contains worms and eggs) will direct you easily to option 4. Review the procedure for this test if you are unfamiliar with it.

Level of Cognitive Ability: Application
Client Needs: Physiological Integrity
Integrated Process: Nursing Process—implementation
Content Area: Child health
References: Wong, D., Hockenberry-Eaton, M. (2000). *Wong's essentials of pediatric nursing* (6th ed., p. 472). St. Louis: Mosby. Wong, D., Perry, S., & Hockenberry, M. (2002). *Maternal child nursing care* (2nd ed., p. 1267). St. Louis: Mosby.

11. 4

Rationale: A severe febrile illness is a reason to delay immunization but only until the child has recovered from the acute stage of the illness. Minor illnesses such as a cold, otitis media, or mild diarrhea are not contraindications to immunization.

Test-Taking Strategy: Use the process of elimination, focusing on the issue of the question, a contraindication to receiving an immunization. Reviewing each option carefully will direct you easily to option 4. If you had difficulty with this question, review the contraindications associated with immunizations.

Level of Cognitive Ability: Comprehension
Client Needs: Physiological Integrity
Integrated Process: Teaching/Learning
Content Area: Child health
Reference: Wong, D., Perry, S., & Hockenberry, M. (2002). *Maternal child nursing care* (2nd ed., p. 858). St. Louis: Mosby.

12. 3

Rationale: Diphtheria, tetanus, acellular pertussis vaccine (DTaP), *Haemophilus influenzae* type b conjugate vaccine (Hib), and inactivated poliovirus vaccine (IPV) are administered at 4 months of age. The DTaP is administered at 2 months, 4 months, 6 months, between 15 and 18 months of age, and between 4 and 6 years of age. The Hib is administered at 2 months, 4 months, 6 months, and between 12 and 15 months of age. The IPV is administered at 2 months, 4 months, 6 months, and between 4 and 6 years of age. The first dose of measles, mumps, rubella vaccine (MMR) is administered between 12 and 15 months of age; the second dose is administered at 4 to 6 years of age (if the second dose was not given by 4 to 6 years of age, it should be given at the next visit). The first dose of hepatitis B vaccine is administered between the ages of birth and 2 months, the second dose is administered between the ages of 1 and 4 months, and the third dose is administered between the ages of 6 and 18 months. Varicella-zoster vaccine is administered between 12 and 18 months of age.

Test-Taking Strategy: Knowledge regarding the immunization schedule for infants and children is required to answer this question. Noting the age of the infant in the question will assist in directing you to option 3. Learn the immunization schedule if you are unfamiliar with it.

Level of Cognitive Ability: Application
Client Needs: Health Promotion and Maintenance
Integrated Process: Nursing Process—implementation
Content Area: Child health
References: Centers for Disease Control and Prevention. (2004). *Recommended childhood and adolescent immunization schedule.* Atlanta: CDC. Retrieved January 16, 2004, from http://www.cdc.gov/nip.

13. 3

Rationale: The MMR is administered subcutaneously in the outer aspect of the upper arm. The gluteal muscle most often is used for intramuscular injections. The MMR is not administered by the intramuscular route.

Test-Taking Strategy: Use the process of elimination. Knowledge that MMR is administered subcutaneously will assist you in eliminating options 1 and 2. From the remaining options, recalling that the gluteal muscle most often is used for intramuscular injections will assist in directing you to option 3. Review the procedures related to the administration of MMR if you had difficulty with this question.

Level of Cognitive Ability: Application
Client Needs: Physiological Integrity
Integrated Process: Nursing Process—implementation
Content Area: Child health
Reference: Wong, D., Hockenberry-Eaton, M. (2000). *Wong's essentials of pediatric nursing* (6th ed., p. 366). St. Louis: Mosby.

14. 2

Rationale: The MMR contains minute amounts of neomycin. A history of an anaphylactic reaction to neomycin is considered a contraindication to the MMR vaccine. The general contraindication to all immunizations is a severe febrile illness. The presence of minor illnesses such as a common cold is not a contraindication. In addition, a history of frequent respiratory infections is not a contraindication to receiving a vaccine. A local reaction to an immunization is treated with ice packs for the first 24 hours after injection, followed by warm compresses if the inflammation persists.

Test-Taking Strategy: Use the process of elimination. Recalling that a general contraindication to all immunizations is a

severe febrile illness will assist you in eliminating options 3 and 4. From the remaining options, note that option 1 identifies a local reaction. This will direct you to option 2, the systemic reaction, and a potential life-threatening condition. Review the contraindications to receiving immunizations if you had difficulty with this question.

Level of Cognitive Ability: Analysis
Client Needs: Physiological Integrity
Integrated Process: Nursing Process—analysis
Content Area: Child health
Reference: Wong, D., Hockenberry-Eaton, M. (2000). *Wong's essentials of pediatric nursing* (6th ed., p. 367). St. Louis: Mosby.

15. 1

Rationale: A contraindication to receiving the hepatitis B vaccine is a previous anaphylactic reaction to common baker's yeast. An allergy to eggs, penicillin, and sulfonamides is unrelated to the contraindication to receiving this vaccine.

Test-Taking Strategy: Use the process of elimination and knowledge regarding the contraindications associated with the administration of vaccines. You must know that a contraindication to receiving the hepatitis B vaccine is an anaphylactic reaction to common baker's yeast. Review the contraindication to receiving the hepatitis B vaccine if you had difficulty with this question.

Level of Cognitive Ability: Analysis
Client Needs: Physiological Integrity
Integrated Process: Nursing Process—assessment
Content Area: Child health
Reference: Wong, D., Hockenberry-Eaton, M. (2000). *Wong's essentials of pediatric nursing* (6th ed., p. 368). St. Louis: Mosby.

CRITICAL THINKING: FILL IN THE BLANK

Answer: Mask, gown, and gloves

Rationale: The rubella virus is primarily present in nasopharyngeal secretions. The virus is also present in blood, stool, and urine. The virus is transmitted via the airborne route, by direct contact with infectious droplets, or indirectly via articles freshly contaminated with nasopharyngeal secretions, feces, or urine. Care for the child with rubella involves contact isolation. Contact isolation requires masks, gowns, and gloves if contact with infectious material is anticipated.

Test-Taking Strategy: Think about the source and route of transmission of the rubella virus. Recalling that contact precautions are required will assist in identifying the protective items needed in caring for this child. Review the modes of transmission of rubella if you had difficulty with this question.

Level of Cognitive Ability: Application
Client Needs: Safe, Effective Care Environment
Integrated Process: Nursing Process—implementation
Content Area: Child health
Reference: McKinney, E., Ashwill, J., Murray, S., James, S., Gorrie, T., & Droske, S. (2000). *Maternal-child nursing* (p. 1033). Philadelphia: W. B. Saunders.

REFERENCES

American Academy of Family Physicians. http://www.aafp.org.

American Academy of Pediatrics. http://www.aap.org.

Centers for Disease Control and Prevention. (2004). *Recommended childhood and adolescent immunization schedule.* Atlanta: CDC. Retrieved January 16, 2004, from http://www.cdc.gov/nip.

Centers for Disease Control and Prevention. (2004). *Smallpox pre-vaccination information packet.* Atlanta: CDC. Retrieved August 12, 2003 from http://www.bt.cdc.gov/agent/smallpox/basics/index.asp.

Centers for Disease Control and Prevention. Retrieved January 16, 2004, from http://www2.cdc.gov/mmwr/.

Immunization Action Coalition. http://www.immunize.org.

James, S., Ashwill, J., & Droske, S. (2002). *Nursing care of children: Principles & practice* (2nd ed.). Philadelphia: W. B. Saunders.

Lewis, S., Heitkemper, M., & Dirksen, S. (2004). *Medical-surgical nursing: Assessment and management of clinical problems* (6th ed.). St. Louis: Mosby.

McKinney, E., Ashwill, J., Murray, S., James, S., Gorrie, T., & Droske, S. (2000). *Maternal-child nursing.* Philadelphia: W. B. Saunders.

U.S. Department of Health & Human Services. (2003). *Smallpox vaccine: What you need to know* (pp. 1-2). Atlanta: Centers for Disease Control and Prevention, National Immunization Program.

Wong, D., Hockenberry-Eaton, M. (2000). *Wong's essentials of pediatric nursing* (6th ed.). St. Louis: Mosby.

Wong, D., Perry, S., & Hockenberry, M. (2002). *Maternal child nursing care* (2nd ed.). St. Louis: Mosby.

Pediatric Medication Administration and Calculations

I. ORAL MEDICATIONS

A. Most oral pediatric medications are in liquid or suspension form because children usually are not able to swallow a tablet.

B. Solutions may be measured by using an oral syringe; if an oral syringe is not available, hypodermic syringes without the needle can be used for dosage measurement.

C. When volumes are minute, orally administered liquids are measured by using a calibrated medication dropper.

D. Medications in suspension settle to the bottom of the bottle between uses, and thorough mixing is required before pouring of the medication.

E. Suspensions must be administered immediately after measurement to prevent settling and administration of an incomplete dose.

F. Administer oral medications with the child sitting in an upright position and with the head elevated to prevent aspiration if the child cries or resists.

G. Never pinch the infant or child's nostrils when administering medication.

H. Do not place medication in a baby's bottle.

I. Draw the required dose of an unpleasant medication into a small syringe, and place the syringe into the side and toward the back of the infant's mouth; administer the medication slowly, allowing the infant to swallow.

J. Place the small child sideways on the lap; the child's closest arm should be placed under the adult's arm and behind the adult's back; cradle the child's head and hold the child's hand, and administer the medication slowly with a plastic spoon or small plastic cup.

K. Mix liquid medications with less than an ounce of fluid to disguise the taste if necessary.

L. If a tablet or capsule has been administered, check the child's mouth to ensure that it has been swallowed; if swallowing is a problem, some tablets can be crushed and given in small amounts of pureed food or flavored syrup (enteric-coated tablets, timed-release tablets, and capsules should not be crushed).

II. PARENTERAL MEDICATIONS

A. Subcutaneously and intramuscularly administered medications

1. Medications most often given via the subcutaneous route are insulin and most immunizations.

2. Any site with sufficient subcutaneous tissue may be used for subcutaneous injections; common sites include the central third of the lateral aspect of the upper arm, the abdomen, and the center third of the anterior thigh.

3. The safe use of all injection sites is based on normal muscle development and the size of the child; the preferred site for intramuscular injections in infants is the vastus lateralis.

4. Usually not more than 0.5 mL (infant) to 2 mL (child) is injected per intramuscular or subcutaneous site, and the site of injection is rotated if frequent injections are necessary.

5. The usual needle length and gauge for pediatric clients are $\frac{1}{2}$ to 1 inch and 22 to 25 gauge.

6. Needle length also can be estimated by grasping the muscle for injection between the thumb and forefinger; half the resulting distance between thumb and forefinger would be the needle length.

7. Pediatric dosages for subcutaneous and intramuscular administration are calculated to the nearest hundredth and measured by using a tuberculin syringe.

8. For the toddler or preschooler, place an adhesive bandage or decorated Band-Aid over the puncture site.

B. Intravenously administered medications
1. Intravenous (IV) medications are diluted for administration.
2. When an infant or child is receiving an IV medication, the IV site needs to be assessed for signs of infiltration and inflammation immediately before, during, and after completion of each medication (Box 48-1).
3. Intravenous medication may be administered continuously by adding the medication to an IV solution bag and infusing it through a primary infusion line.
4. Intravenous medications may be administered intermittently, involving several doses within a 24-hour period.
5. Medications for IV administration are diluted according to the directions accompanying the medication and according to the physician's orders and agency procedures.
6. Infusion time for IV medications is determined based on the directions accompanying the medication, the physician's orders, and agency procedures.
7. Determine agency procedures related to the volume of flush for peripheral IV lines and for central lines.
8. The flush volume (3 to 20 mL) must be included in the child's intake; the flush is started after the IV medication is completed and is infused at the same rate as the medication.

C. Intermittent IV medication administration
1. Children receiving IV medications intermittently may or may not have a primary IV solution infusing.
2. If a primary IV solution is infusing, the medication may be administered by IV piggyback via a secondary line.
3. If a primary IV solution does not exist, an indwelling infusion catheter is used for medication administration.
4. All intermittent medication administrations are preceded and followed by a flush to ensure that the medication has cleared the IV tubing and that the total dose has been administered.

5. Electronic controllers and pumps are used to regulate and administer IV fluids and intermittent IV medications.

D. Special IV administration sets
1. Special IV administration sets, referred to by their trade names (Burretrol, Soluset, Volutrol), may be used for medication preparation and administration.
2. These special sets are all microdrip sets calibrated to deliver 60 gtt/mL.
3. The total capacity of these special IV administration sets is between 100 and 150 mL, calibrated in 1-mL increments so that exact measurements of small volumes are possible.
4. The medication is mixed with the appropriate amount of diluent and added to the special IV administration set, and the medication is allowed to infuse at the prescribed rate.
5. Label the special IV administration set to identify the medication and fluid dosage added.
6. Attach a label that states "medication infusing" during the medication infusion time.
7. Attach a label that states "flush infusing" during the flush infusion time.

E. Retrograde IV injection
1. The medication is mixed with the appropriate amount of diluent in a syringe.
2. The IV tubing is clamped close to the child, the medication is injected through the port in the direction of the burette, the tubing is unclamped, the prescribed rate is set, and the medication is allowed to infuse over the prescribed time.

F. Syringe pump for IV medication administration
1. A syringe containing the medication is fitted into a pump that is connected to the IV tubing through a Y-connector.
2. The medication is administered over the prescribed time.

III. CALCULATION OF MEDICATION DOSAGE BY BODY WEIGHT
A. Conversion of body weight (Box 48-2)
B. Calculation of daily dosages
1. Abbreviations (Box 48-3)

BOX 48-1

Intravenous Site: Signs of Inflammation and Infiltration

INFLAMMATION
Redness, heat, swelling, and tenderness

INFILTRATION
Swelling, coolness, pain, and lack of blood return
Note: If inflammation or infiltration occurs, the intravenous line is discontinued and restarted at a new site.

BOX 48-2

Conversion of Body Weight

POUNDS TO KILOGRAMS
1 kg = 2.2 lb
To convert from pounds to kilograms, divide by 2.2.
Kilograms are expressed to the nearest tenth.

KILOGRAMS TO POUNDS
1 kg = 2.2 lb
To convert from kilograms to pounds, multiply by 2.2.
Pounds are expressed to the nearest tenth.

BOX 48-3

Abbreviations

gr, grain(s)
mcg, microgram(s)
mg, milligram(s)
g, gram(s)
kg, kilogram(s)
lb, pound(s)
mL, milliliter(s)
BSA, body surface area
SA, surface area
m^2, square meters

2. Dosages are expressed in terms of milligrams per kilogram per day, milligrams per pound per day, or milligrams per kilogram per dose.
3. The total daily dosage usually is administered in divided (more than one) doses per day.
4. Express the child's body weight in kilograms or pounds to correlate with the dosage specifications.
5. Calculate the total daily dosage.
6. Divide the total daily dosage by the number of doses to be administered in 1 day.

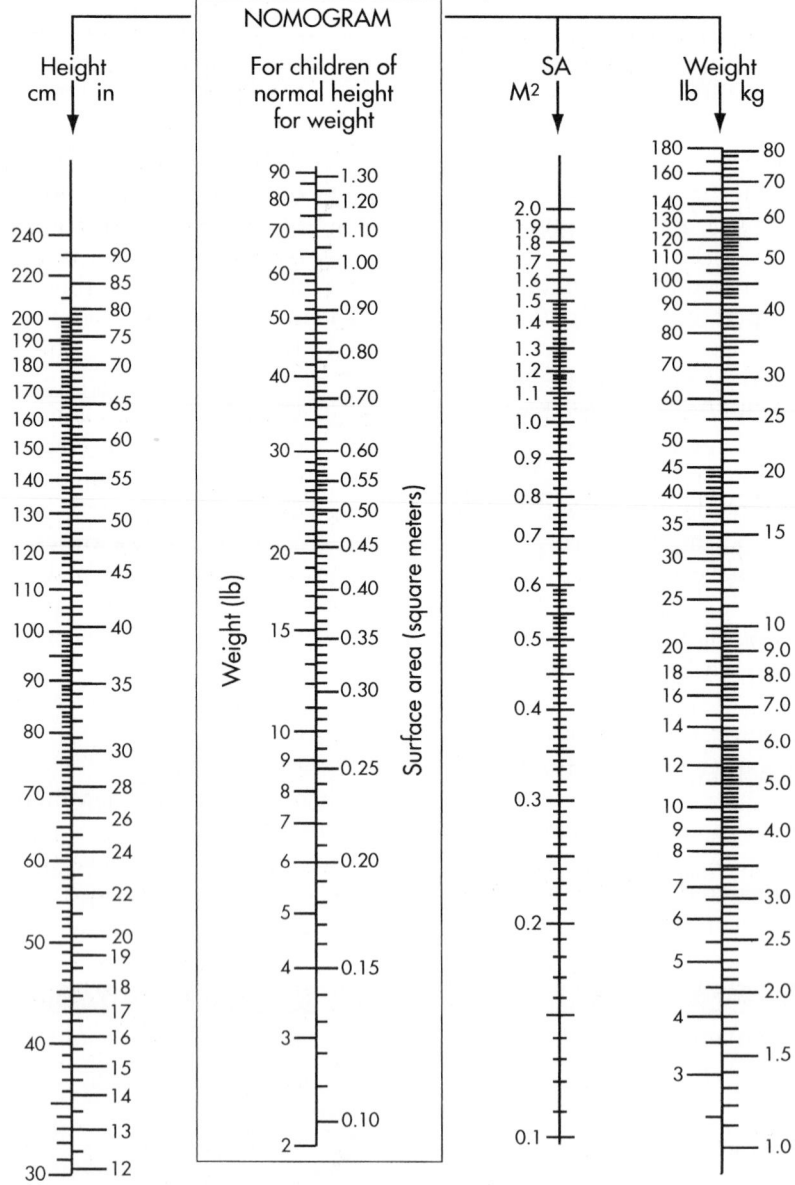

FIG. 48-1   West nomogram for infants and children. Directions: (1) Find height; (2) find weight; (3) draw a straight line connecting the height and weight. Where the line intersects on the SA column is the body surface area (square meters). (Modified from data of Boyd, E., & West, C. D. [1996]. In R. E. Behrman, R. M. Lkiegman, & A. M. Alvin [Eds.], *Nelson textbook of pediatrics* (15th ed). Philadelphia: W. B. Saunders.)

IV. CALCULATION OF BODY SURFACE AREA (BSA)

A. The BSA is determined by comparing body weight and height with averages or norms on a graph called a nomogram.

B. Not all children are the same size at the same age; therefore the nomogram is used to determine the BSA of a child.

C. Look at the nomogram (Fig. 48-1), and note that the height is on the left-hand side of the chart and the weight is on the right-hand side.

D. Place a ruler on the chart.

E. Line up the left side of the ruler on the height and the right side of the ruler on the weight; read the BSA at the point where the straight edge of the ruler intersects the surface area (SA) column.

F. The estimated surface area is given in square meters.

G. See Box 48-4 for an example.

V. CALCULATION BASED ON BSA

A. When dosage recommendations for children specify milligrams, micrograms, or units per square meter, calculating the dosage is simple multiplication (Box 48-5).

B. When dosages are specified only for adults, a formula is used to calculate a child's dosage from the adult dosage (Box 48-6).

BOX 48-4

How to Use the Nomogram

Example: Use the nomogram and calculate the body surface area for a child whose height is 58 inches and weight is 12 kg.

Look at the nomogram chart and note that the height is on the left-hand side of the chart and the weight is on the right-hand side.

Place a ruler on the chart and line up the left side of the ruler on the height and the right side of the ruler on the weight; read the body surface area at the point where the straight edge of the ruler intersects the surface area (SA) column.

The estimated surface area is given in square meters.

Answer: 0.66 m^2

BOX 48-5

Calculating Medication Dosage

When dosage recommendations for children specify milligrams, micrograms, or units per square meter, calculating the dosage is simple multiplication.

Example: The dosage recommendation is 4 mg/m^2. The child has a body surface area of 1.1 m^2. What is the dosage to be administered?

Answer: 1.1 × 4 mg = 4.4 mg

BOX 48-6

Calculating a Child's Dosage from the Adult Dosage

When dosages are specified only for adults, a formula is used to calculate a child's dosage from the adult dosage.

Example: A physician has prescribed an antibiotic for a child. The average adult dose is 250 mg. The child has a body surface area (BSA) of 0.41 m^2. What is the dose for the child?

Answer: 59.24 mg

Formula:

$$\frac{\text{BSA of child (m}^2)}{1.73 \text{ m}^2} \times \text{Adult dose} = \text{Child's dose}$$

$$\frac{0.41}{1.73} \times 250 \text{ mg} = 59.24 \text{ mg}$$

PRACTICE QUESTIONS

1. Penicillin V (Veetids), 250 mg PO every 8 hours, is prescribed for a child with a respiratory infection. The child's weight is 45 lb. The safe pediatric dosage is 25 to 50 mg/kg per day. The nurse determines that
   1. The dose prescribed is too low.
   2. The dose prescribed is too high.
   3. The dose prescribed is within the safe dosage range.
   4. There is not enough information to determine the safe dose.

2. A physician has prescribed phenobarbital sodium (Luminal), 25 mg PO bid, for a child with febrile seizures. The medication label reads "phenobarbital sodium, 20 mg per 5 mL." A nurse has determined that the dosage prescribed is safe for the child. The nurse prepares to administer how many milliliters per dose to the child?
   1. 2 mL
   2. 4.5 mL
   3. 6.25 mL
   4. 7 mL

3. Cloxacillin (Tegopen), 100 mg PO every 8 hours, is prescribed for a child with an elevated temperature who is suspected of having a respiratory tract infection. The child weighs 17 lb. The safe pediatric dosage is 50 mg/kg per day. The nurse determines that
   1. The dose prescribed is too low.
   2. The dose prescribed is too high.
   3. The dose prescribed is safe.
   4. There is not enough information to determine the safe dose.

4. Sulfisoxazole (Gantrisin), 1 g PO qid, is prescribed for an adolescent with a urinary tract infection. The medication label reads "500-mg tablets." A nurse has determined that the dosage prescribed is safe. The nurse administers how many tablets per dose to the adolescent?
   1. ½ tablet
   2. 1 tablet

3. 2 tablets
4. 3 tablets

5. Diphenhydramine hydrochloride (Benadryl), 25 mg PO every 6 hours, is prescribed for a child with an allergic reaction. The child weighs 25 kg. The safe pediatric dosage is 5 mg/kg per day. The nurse determines that
   1. The dose prescribed is too low.
   2. The dose prescribed is too high.
   3. The dose prescribed is safe.
   4. There is not enough information to determine the safe dose.

6. Penicillin G procaine (Wycillin), 1,000,000 units IM (intramuscularly), is prescribed for a child with an infection. The medication label reads "1,200,000 units per 2 mL." A nurse has determined that the dose prescribed is safe. The nurse prepares to administer how many milliliters per dose to the child?
   1. 0.8 mL
   2. 1.2 mL
   3. 1.44 mL
   4. 1.66 mL

7. Morphine sulfate, 2.5 mg, IV piggyback, is prescribed for a child with cancer. The safe pediatric dose is 0.05 to 0.1 mg/kg per dose. The child weighs 50 kg. The nurse determines that
   1. The dose prescribed is too low.
   2. The dose prescribed is too high.
   3. The dose prescribed is within the safe dosage range.
   4. There is not enough information to determine the safe dosage range.

8. Morphine sulfate, 2.5 mg, IV piggyback, in 10 mL of normal saline, is prescribed for a child postoperatively. The medication label reads "$\frac{1}{15}$ gr per mL." The nurse has determined that the dosage is safe. The nurse prepares to add how many milliliters of morphine sulfate to the 10 mL of normal saline solution?
   1. 0.62 mL
   2. 0.82 mL
   3. 1.35 mL
   4. 1.62 mL

9. A physician's order reads "ampicillin (Omnipen), 125 mg IV every 6 hours." The medication label reads "1 g and reconstitute with 7.4 mL of bacteriostatic water." A nurse prepares to draw up how many milliliters to administer one dose?
   1. 0.54 mL
   2. 0.92 mL
   3. 1.1 mL
   4. 7.4 mL

10. A pediatric client with ventricular septal defect repair is placed on a maintenance dosage of digoxin (Lanoxin) elixir. The dosage is 0.07 mg/kg per day, and the client's weight is 7.2 kg. The physician orders the digoxin to be given twice daily. A nurse prepares how much digoxin to administer to the client at each dose?
   1. 0.25 mg
   2. 0.37 mg
   3. 0.5 mg
   4. 2.5 mg

CRITICAL THINKING: FILL IN THE BLANK

Atropine sulfate, 0.2 mg IM (intramuscularly), is prescribed for a child preoperatively. The medication label reads: 0.4 mg per mL. A nurse has determined that the dose prescribed is safe. The nurse prepares to administer how many milliliters to the child?

Answer: _____

ANSWERS

1. **3**
   Rationale: Convert pounds to kilograms by dividing by 2.2.
   Pounds to kilograms:
   45 lb ÷ 2.2 lb/kg = 20.45 kg
   Dosage parameters:
   25 mg/kg per day × 20.45 kg = 511.25 mg/day
   50 mg/kg per day × 20.45 kg = 1022.5 mg/day
   Dosage frequency:
   250 mg × 3 doses (every 8 hours) = 750 mg/day
   Dose is within the safe dosage range.
   Test-Taking Strategy: Identify the key components of the question and what the question is asking. In this case, the question asks for the safe dosage range for medication. Change pounds to kilograms. Calculate the dosage parameters by using the safe dosage range identified in the question and the child's weight in kilograms. Remember to determine the total daily dosage before selecting an option. Review this formula if you had difficulty with this question.

Level of Cognitive Ability: Analysis
Client Needs: Physiological Integrity
Integrated Process: Nursing Process—analysis
Content Area: Child health
Reference: Kee, J., & Marshall, S. (2004). *Clinical calculations: With applications to general and specialty areas* (5th ed., p. 235). Philadelphia: W. B. Saunders.

2. **3**
   Rationale:
   Formula:
   $$\frac{Desired}{Available} \times Volume = \frac{25 \text{ mg}}{20 \text{ mg}} \times 5 \text{ mL} = 6.25 \text{ mL per dose}$$
   Test-Taking Strategy: Identify the key components of the question and what the question is asking. In this case, the question asks for the milliliters per dose. Use the formula to determine the correct dosage. Review this formula if you had difficulty with this question.
   Level of Cognitive Ability: Application

Client Needs: Physiological Integrity
Integrated Process: Nursing Process—planning
Content Area: Child health
Reference: Kee, J., & Marshall, S. (2004). *Clinical calculations: With applications to general and specialty areas* (5th ed., p. 80). Philadelphia: W. B. Saunders.

3. 3
Rationale:
Convert pounds to kilograms by dividing by 2.2.
Pounds to kilograms:
17 lb ÷ 2.2 lb/kg = 7.72 kg
Dosage parameters:
50 mg/kg per day × 7.72 kg = 386 mg/day
Dosage frequency:
100 mg × 3 doses (every 8 hours) = 300 mg/day
The dose is safe.
Test-Taking Strategy: Identify the key components of the question and what the question is asking. In this case, the question asks for the safe dose of the medication. Convert pounds to kilograms. Calculate the dose by using the safe dosage identified in the question and the child's weight in kilograms. Remember to determine the total daily dosage before selecting an option. Review this formula if you had difficulty with this question.
Level of Cognitive Ability: Analysis
Client Needs: Physiological Integrity
Integrated Process: Nursing Process—analysis
Content Area: Child health
Reference: Kee, J., & Marshall, S. (2004). *Clinical calculations: With applications to general and specialty areas* (5th ed., p. 235). Philadelphia: W. B. Saunders.

4. 3
Rationale: Change 1 g to milligrams, knowing that 1000 mg = 1 g. Also, when converting from grams to milligrams (larger to smaller), move the decimal point three places to the right. Therefore, 1 g = 1000 mg.
Formula:
$$\frac{Desired}{Available} \times Tablet = \frac{1000\ mg}{500\ mg} \times Tablet = 2\ tablets$$
Test-Taking Strategy: Identify the key components of the question and what the question is asking. In this case, the question asks for tablets per dose. Convert grams to milligrams first. Then use the formula to determine the correct dose. Review this formula if you had difficulty with this question.
Level of Cognitive Ability: Application
Client Needs: Physiological Integrity
Integrated Process: Nursing Process—implementation
Content Area: Child health
Reference: Kee, J., & Marshall, S. (2004). *Clinical calculations: With applications to general and specialty areas* (5th ed., p. 80). Philadelphia: W. B. Saunders.

5. 3
Rationale:
Dosage parameters:
5 mg/kg per day × 25 kg = 125 mg/day
Dosage frequency:
25 mg × 4 doses (every 6 hours) = 100 mg/day
Dose is within the safe dosage range.

Test-Taking Strategy: Identify the key components of the question and what the question is asking. In this case, the question asks for the safe dose of the medication. Calculate the dosage parameters by using the safe dosage identified in the question and the child's weight in kilograms. Remember to determine the total daily dosage before selecting an option. Review this formula if you had difficulty with this question.
Level of Cognitive Ability: Analysis
Client Needs: Physiological Integrity
Integrated Process: Nursing Process—analysis
Content Area: Child health
Reference: Kee, J., & Marshall, S. (2004). *Clinical calculations: With applications to general and specialty areas* (5th ed., p. 235). Philadelphia: W. B. Saunders.

6. 4
Rationale:
Formula:
$$\frac{Desired}{Available} \times Volume = \frac{1,000,000}{1,200,000} \times 2\ mL = 1.66\ mL\ per\ dose$$
Test-Taking Strategy: Identify the key components of the question and what the question is asking. In this case, the question asks for the milliliters per dose. Use the formula to determine the correct dose. Review this formula if you had difficulty with this question.
Level of Cognitive Ability: Application
Client Needs: Physiological Integrity
Integrated Process: Nursing Process—planning
Content Area: Child health
Reference: Kee, J., & Marshall, S. (2004). *Clinical calculations: With applications to general and specialty areas* (5th ed., p. 80). Philadelphia: W. B. Saunders.

7. 3
Rationale:
Dosage parameters:
0.05 mg/kg per dose × 50 kg = 2.5 mg/dose
0.1 mg/kg per dose × 50 kg = 5 mg/dose
Dosage is within the safe dosage range.
Test-Taking Strategy: Identify the key components of the question and what the question is asking. In this case, the question asks for the safe dose of the medication. Calculate the dosage parameters, using the safe dosage range identified in the question and the child's weight in kilograms. Review this formula if you had difficulty with this question.
Level of Cognitive Ability: Analysis
Client Needs: Physiological Integrity
Integrated Process: Nursing Process—analysis
Content Area: Child health
Reference: Kee, J., & Marshall, S. (2004). *Clinical calculations: With applications to general and specialty areas* (5th ed., p. 235). Philadelphia: W. B. Saunders.

8. 1
Rationale:
Convert grains to milligrams:
60 mg = 1 gr
$\frac{1}{15}$ gr × 60 mg = 4 mg
Formula:
$$\frac{Desired}{Available} \times Volume = \frac{2.5\ mg}{4\ mg} \times 1\ mL = 0.62\ mL$$

Test-Taking Strategy: Identify the key components of the question and what the question is asking. In this case, the question asks for the milliliters per dose. Begin by converting grains to milligrams. Then use the formula to determine the correct dose. Review this formula if you had difficulty with this question.
Level of Cognitive Ability: Application
Client Needs: Physiological Integrity
Integrated Process: Nursing Process—planning
Content Area: Child health
Reference: Kee, J., & Marshall, S. (2004). *Clinical calculations: With applications to general and specialty areas* (5th ed., p. 80). Philadelphia: W. B. Saunders.

9. **2**
Rationale: Convert 1 g to milligrams. In the metric system, to convert larger to smaller, multiply by 1000 or move the decimal point three places to the right.
1 g = 1000 mg
Formula:

$$\frac{\text{Desired}}{\text{Available}} \times \text{Volume} = \frac{125 \text{ mg}}{1000 \text{ mg}} \times 7.4 \text{ mL} = 0.925 \text{ mL}$$
$$= 0.92 \text{ mL per dose}$$

Test-Taking Strategy: Identify the key components of the question and what the question is asking. In this case, the question asks for the milliliters per dose. Convert grams to milligrams first. Next, use the formula to determine the correct dose, knowing that 1000 mg = 7.4 mL. Review this formula if you had difficulty with this question.
Level of Cognitive Ability: Application
Client Needs: Physiological Integrity
Integrated Process: Nursing Process—planning
Content Area: Fundamental skills
Reference: Kee, J., & Marshall, S. (2004). *Clinical calculations: With applications to general and specialty areas* (5th ed., p. 80). Philadelphia: W. B. Saunders.

10. **1**
Rationale:
Calculate the dosage by weight first:
0.07 mg/day × 7.2 kg = 0.5 mg/day
The physician orders digoxin twice daily; therefore two doses in 24 hours will be administered.
0.50 mg/day ÷ 2 doses = 0.25 mg for each dose

Test-Taking Strategy: Identify the key components of the question and what the question is asking. Read the question carefully, noting that the question states "twice daily" and "each dose." Calculate the dosage by weight first, and then determine the milligrams per each dose.
Level of Cognitive Ability: Application
Client Needs: Physiological Integrity
Integrated Process: Nursing Process—planning
Content Area: Child health
Reference: Kee, J., & Marshall, S. (2004). *Clinical calculations: With applications to general and specialty areas* (5th ed., p. 80). Philadelphia: W. B. Saunders.

CRITICAL THINKING: FILL IN THE BLANK
Answer: 0.5 mL
Rationale:
Formula:

$$\frac{\text{Desired}}{\text{Available}} \times \text{Volume} = \frac{0.2 \text{ mg}}{0.4 \text{ mg}} \times 1 \text{ mL} = 0.5 \text{ mL}$$

Test-Taking Strategy: Identify the key components of the question and what the question is asking. In this case, the question asks for the milliliters to be administered. Use the formula to determine the correct dose. Review this formula if you had difficulty with this question.
Level of Cognitive Ability: Application
Client Needs: Physiological Integrity
Integrated Process: Nursing Process—planning
Content Area: Child health
Reference: Kee, J., & Marshall, S. (2004). *Clinical calculations: With applications to general and specialty areas* (5th ed., p. 80). Philadelphia: W. B. Saunders.

REFERENCES

Hodgson, B., & Kizior, R. (2004). *Saunders nursing drug handbook 2004*. Philadelphia: W. B. Saunders.
James, S., Ashwill, J., & Droske, S. (2002). *Nursing care of children: Principles & practice* (2nd ed.). Philadelphia: W. B. Saunders.
Joint Commission on Accreditation of Healthcare Organizations. (2004). *2004 national patient safety goals*. Oakbrook Terrace, IL: JCAHO.

Retrieved March 1, 2004, from http://www.jcaho.org/accredited+ organizations/patient+safety/04+npsg/04_faqs.htm
Kee, J., & Marshall, S. (2004). *Clinical calculations: With applications to general and specialty areas* (5th ed.). Philadelphia: W. B. Saunders.
Wong, D., Perry, S., & Hockenberry, M. (2002). *Maternal child nursing care* (2nd ed.). St. Louis: Mosby.

The Adult Client with an Integumentary Disorder

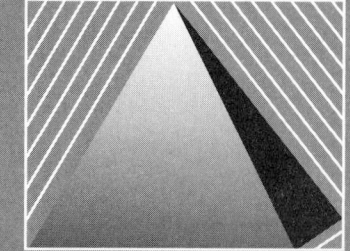

PYRAMID TERMS

burns Cell destruction of the layers of the skin and the resultant depletion of fluid and electrolytes.

carbon monoxide poisoning Carbon monoxide is a colorless, odorless, and tasteless gas that has an affinity for hemoglobin 200 times greater than that of oxygen. Oxygen molecules are displaced, and carbon monoxide reversibly binds to hemoglobin to form carboxyhemoglobin. Tissue hypoxia occurs.

chemical burns Tissue injury caused by tissue contact with strong acids, alkalis, or organic compounds. Systemic toxicity from cutaneous absorption can occur.

decubitus Localized areas of skin breakdown that occurs as a result of poor circulation to the area; also called a pressure ulcer.

deep full-thickness burn Similar to a fourth-degree burn and involving injury to the muscle and bone. Injured area appears black. Edema is absent.

electrical burns Tissue injury caused by heat generated from electrical energy as it passes through the body; results in internal tissue damage.

full-thickness burn Similar to a third-degree burn. The injured area appears deep red, black, white, yellow, or brown. Injured surface appears dry. Tissue disruption is noted with fat exposed. Skin is edematous.

herpes zoster (shingles) An acute viral infection of the nerve structure caused by varicella-zoster. Herpes zoster is contagious to individuals who have not had chickenpox.

Kaposi's sarcoma Skin lesions that occur in individuals with a compromised immune system.

Lyme disease An infection acquired from a tick bite. Ticks live in wooded areas and survive by attaching to a host.

partial-thickness superficial burn Similar to a second-degree burn. A mottled red base and broken epidermis with a wet shiny and weeping surface is present. Large blisters cover an extensive area. Skin is edematous and painful.

skin cancer A malignant lesion of the skin that may or may not metastasize. Causes include chronic friction and irritation to a skin area and exposure to ultraviolet rays. Diagnosis is confirmed by a skin biopsy that is positive for cancer cells.

smoke inhalation injury Respiratory injury resulting when the victim is trapped in an enclosed, smoke-filled space.

superficial-thickness burn Similar to a first-degree burn. Mild to severe erythema is noted, and the skin blanches with pressure.

thermal burns Tissue injury caused by exposure to flames, hot liquids, steam, or hot objects.

▲ PYRAMID TO SUCCESS

The Pyramid to Success focuses on the concept that the integumentary system provides the first line of defense against infections. Focus on the protective measures necessary to prevent infection. Pyramid Points address the risk factors related to the development of integumentary disorders, the preventive measures related to skin cancer, and the content related to Kaposi's sarcoma and Lyme disease. Focus on the emergency measures related to a client with a burn, fluid resuscitation, monitoring for complications, and skin grafting. Psychosocial issues relate to the body image disturbances that can occur as a result of the integumentary disorder. The Integrated Processes addressed in this unit include Nursing Process, Caring, Communication and Documentation, and Teaching/Learning.

▲ CLIENT NEEDS

Safe, Effective Care Environment

Confidentiality related to the disorder
Consultation with members of the health care team
Establishing priorities
Handling of infectious materials
Informed consent for treatments and procedures
Medical and surgical asepsis; preventing infection
Referrals
Standard and other precautions

Health Promotion and Maintenance

Disease prevention measures
Health promotion programs
Health screening
Instructions to the client regarding care to integumentary disorder
Physical assessment of the integumentary system

Psychosocial Integrity

Coping mechanisms
End-of-life issues
Situational role changes
Unexpected body image changes
Use of support systems

Physiological Integrity

Adequate nutrition for healing
Alteration in body systems
Basic care and comfort
Expected effects of treatments
Fluid and electrolyte imbalances
Monitoring for complications
Monitoring laboratory values
Providing emergency care

REFERENCES

Chernecky, C., & Berger, B. (2004). *Laboratory tests & diagnostic procedures* (4th ed.). Philadelphia: W. B. Saunders.

Harkreader, H., & Hogan, M. A. (2004). *Fundamentals of nursing: caring and clinical judgment* (2nd ed.). Philadelphia: W. B. Saunders.

Ignatavicius, D., & Workman, M. (2002). *Medical-surgical nursing: Critical thinking for collaborative care* (4th ed.). Philadelphia: W. B. Saunders.

Lewis, S., Heitkemper, M., & Dirksen, S. (2004). *Medical-surgical nursing: Assessment and management of clinical problems* (6th ed.). St. Louis: Mosby.

National Council of State Boards of Nursing (Eds.). (2003). *Test Plan for the National Council Licensure Examination for Registered Nurses* (effective date: April 2004). Chicago: Author.

Perry, A., & Potter, P. (2002). *Clinical nursing skills and techniques* (5th ed.). St. Louis: Mosby.

Phipps, W., Monahan, F., Sands, J., Marek, J., & Neighbors, M. (2003). *Medical-surgical nursing: Health and illness perspectives* (7th ed.). St. Louis: Mosby.

Potter, P., & Perry, A. (2001). *Fundamentals of nursing* (5th ed.). St. Louis: Mosby.

Varcarolis, E. M. (2002). *Foundations of psychiatric mental health nursing.* (4th ed.). Philadelphia: W. B. Saunders.

Integumentary System

I. ANATOMY AND PHYSIOLOGY

A. The skin is the largest sensory organ of the body, with a surface area of 15 to 20 square feet and a weight of about 9 lb.

B. Functions
  1. The skin is the first line of defense against infections.
  2. The skin protects underlying tissues and organs from injury.
  3. The skin receives stimuli from the external environment; detects touch, pressure, pain, and temperature stimuli; and relays that information to the nervous system.
  4. The skin maintains normal body temperature.
  5. The skin excretes salts, water, and organic wastes.
  6. The skin protects the body from excessive water loss.
  7. The skin synthesizes vitamin D_3, which converts to calcitriol, for normal calcium metabolism.
  8. The skin stores nutrients.

C. Layers
  1. Epidermis
  2. Dermis
  3. Hypodermis (subcutaneous fat)

D. Epidermal appendages
  1. Nails
  2. Hair
  3. Glands
    a. Sebaceous
    b. Sweat

E. Normal bacterial flora
  1. Types of normal bacterial flora include the following:
    a. Gram-positive and gram-negative staphylococci
    b. *Pseudomonas*
    c. Streptococcus

2. Organisms are shed with normal exfoliation.
3. A pH of 4.2 to 5.6 halts the growth of bacteria.

II. RISK FACTORS FOR INTEGUMENTARY DISORDERS

A. Exposure to chemical and environmental pollutants
B. Exposure to radiation
C. Exposure to the sun
D. Lack of personal hygiene habits
E. Use of cosmetics and harsh soaps
F. Medications, such as long-term corticosteroid and anticoagulant therapy
G. Nutritional deficiencies
H. Moderate to severe emotional stress
I. Infection, with injured areas as the potential entry points for infection
J. Changes associated with developmental stages and aging

III. PSYCHOSOCIAL IMPACT

A. Change in body image and decreased self-esteem
B. Social isolation and fear of rejection (from embarrassment about changes in skin appearance)
C. Restrictions in physical activity
D. Pain
E. Disruption or loss of employment
F. Cost of medications, hospitalizations, and follow-up care including dressing supplies

IV. DIAGNOSTIC TESTS

A. Skin biopsy
  1. Description
    a. Skin biopsy is collection of a small piece of skin tissue for histopathologic study.
    b. Methods include punch, excisional, incisional, and shave.

2. Interventions preprocedure
   a. Obtain informed consent.
   b. Cleanse site as prescribed.
3. Interventions postprocedure
   a. Place specimen when obtained by physician in the appropriate container and send to pathology laboratory for analysis.
   b. Use surgically aseptic technique for biopsy site dressings.
   c. Assess the biopsy site for bleeding and infection.
   d. Instruct the client to keep dressing in place for at least 8 hours, and then clean daily as prescribed and use antibiotic ointment as prescribed.

B. Skin cultures
   1. Description
      a. Noninvasive procedure
      b. A small skin culture sample is obtained using a sterile applicator and appropriate type of culture tube (bacterial versus viral).
      c. Viral culture is placed immediately on ice.
      d. Sample is sent to laboratory to identify an existing organism.
   2. Intervention preprocedure: Obtain skin culture samples before instituting antibiotic therapy.
   3. Intervention postprocedure: Send skin culture sample to the laboratory.

C. Wood's light examination
   1. Description: Skin is viewed under ultraviolet light through a special glass (Wood's glass) to identify superficial infections of the skin.
   2. Intervention preprocedure: Darken room before the examination.
   3. Intervention postprocedure: Assist the client during adjustment from the darkened room.

D. Skin testing
   1. Description
      a. The administration of an allergen to the surface of the skin or into the dermis
      b. Administered by patch, scratch, or intradermal techniques
   2. Interventions preprocedure
      a. Discontinue systemic corticosteroids or antihistamine therapy 5 days before the test as prescribed.
      b. Obtain informed consent.
      c. Have resuscitation equipment available if a scratch test is performed, for it may induce an anaphylactic reaction.
   3. Interventions postprocedure
      a. Instruct the client to keep skin-testing area dry.
      b. Instruct the client to avoid activities that may produce sweating if a patch test was performed (if the patch loosens or falls off, it should not be reapplied).
      c. Record the site, date, and time of the test.
      d. Record the date and the time for follow-up site reading.

   e. Inspect the site for erythema, papules, vesicles, edema, and induration.
   f. Provide the client with a list of potential allergens, if identified.

V. SKIN DISORDERS

A. Skin cancer
   1. Description
      a. **Skin cancer** is a malignant lesion of the skin, which may or may not metastasize.
      b. **Skin cancer** causes include chronic friction and irritation to a skin area and exposure to ultraviolet rays.
      c. Diagnosis is confirmed by a skin biopsy that is positive for cancer cells.
   2. Types
      a. Basal cell: The most common type, basal cell cancer arises from the basal cells contained in the epidermis.
      b. Squamous cell: The second most common type of **skin cancer** in whites, squamous cell cancer is a tumor of the epidermal keratinocytes and can infiltrate surrounding structures, metastasize to lymph nodes, and be subsequently fatal.
      c. Malignant melanoma: Cancer of the melanocytes can metastasize to the brain, lungs, bone, liver, and skin and is ultimately fatal.
   3. Assessment (Box 49-1)
      a. Change in color, size, or shape of preexisting lesion
      b. Pruritus
      c. Local soreness
   4. Interventions
      a. Instruct the client regarding preventative measures.
      b. Instruct the client to monitor for lesions that do not heal or that change characteristics.
      c. Instruct the client to have moles or lesions removed that are subject to chronic irritation.
      d. Instruct the client to avoid contact with chemical irritants.
      e. Instruct the client to wear layered clothing and use sunscreening lotions with an appropriate skin protection factor when outdoors.
      f. Instruct the client to avoid sun exposure between 11 AM and 3 PM.

BOX 49-1

Appearance of Skin Cancer Lesions

A waxy nodule
An irregular, circular, bordered lesion with hues of tan, black, or blue
A small, red, nodular lesion
An oozing, bleeding, crusting lesion

g. Assist with surgical excision of the lesion as prescribed.

B. Contact dermatitis
1. Description: An inflammatory response of the skin that produces skin changes after contact with a specific antigen
2. Assessment
   a. Pruritus and burning
   b. Edema
   c. Erythema at the point of contact
   d. Signs of infection
   e. Vesicles with drainage
3. Interventions
   a. Elevate the extremity to reduce edema.
   b. Apply cool, wet dressings and tepid baths as prescribed.
   c. Maintain a cool environment.
   d. Protect the affected area from trauma.
   e. Prevent scratching and rubbing of the affected area.
   f. Assist with skin testing as prescribed to determine allergen(s).
   g. Instruct the client to avoid contact with the allergen when determined.
   h. Instruct the client to avoid harsh soaps.
   i. Instruct the client to avoid using heating pads or blankets.
   j. Administer antibiotic for infection, antipruritic or antihistamine for itching, and corticosteroids for inflammation as prescribed.

C. Poison ivy, poison oak, and poison sumac
1. Description: A dermatitis that develops from contact with urushiol from poison ivy, oak, or sumac plants
2. Assessment
   a. Papulovesicular lesions
   b. Severe itching
3. Interventions
   a. Cleanse the skin of the plant oils.
   b. Apply cool, wet dressings with Burow's solution, as prescribed to relieve the itching.
   c. Apply lotion or topical corticosteroids as prescribed.
   d. Administer oral corticosteroids as prescribed for severe reaction.

D. **Lyme disease**
1. Description
   a. **Lyme disease** is an infection caused by the spirochete *Borrelia burgdorferi*, acquired from a tick bite.
   b. Ticks live in wooded areas and survive by attaching to a host.
2. Assessment (Box 49-2)
3. Interventions
   a. Gently remove the tick with tweezers, wash skin with antiseptic, and dispose of the tick by flushing it down the toilet.

BOX 49-2

Assessment and Stages of Lyme Disease

FIRST STAGE
Symptoms can occur several days to months following the bite.
A small red pimple develops that spreads into a ring-shaped rash.
Rash may be large or small or may not occur at all.
Flulike symptoms occur, such as headaches, stiff neck, muscle aches, and fatigue.

SECOND STAGE
This stage occurs several weeks following the bite.
Joint pain occurs.
Neurological complications occur.
Cardiac complications occur.

THIRD STAGE
Large joints become involved.
Arthritis progresses.

---

   b. Obtain a blood test 4 to 6 weeks after a bite to detect the presence of the disease (testing before this time is not reliable).
   c. Instruct the client in the administration of antibiotics as prescribed if the disease is confirmed.
   d. Instruct the client to avoid areas that contain ticks, such as wooded grassy areas, especially in the summer months.
   e. Instruct the client to wear long-sleeved tops, long pants, closed shoes, and hats while outside.
   f. Instruct the client to spray the body with tick repellent before going outside.
   g. Instruct the client to examine the body when returning inside.

E. Erysipelas and cellulitis
1. Description
   a. Erysipelas is an acute, superficial, rapidly spreading inflammation of the dermis and lymphatics caused by β-hemolytic streptococcus group A that enters the tissue via an abrasion, bite, trauma, or wound.
   b. Cellulitis is a skin infection into the deeper dermis and subcutaneous fat, and the causative organism is usually *Streptococcus pyogenes*.
2. Assessment
   a. Pain
   b. Itching
   c. Swelling
   d. Redness and warmth
3. Interventions
   a. Promote rest.
   b. Apply warm compresses as prescribed (usually twice a day) to promote circulation and to decrease discomfort, erythema, and edema.
   c. Administer antibiotics as prescribed for infection following a culture of the area.

d. Clean skin daily with an antibacterial type of soap as prescribed.

F. Psoriasis

1. Description
   a. Psoriasis is a chronic, noninfectious skin inflammation involving keratin synthesis that results in psoriatic patches.
   b. Various forms exist, with psoriasis vulgaris being the most common.
   c. Possible causes of the disorder include stress, trauma, infection, and changes in climate.
   d. The disorder also may be exacerbated by the use of certain medications.
   e. Koebner's phenomenon is the development of psoriatic lesions at a site of injury, such as a scratched or sunburned area.

2. Assessment
   a. Pruritus
   b. Shedding, silvery, white scales on a raised, reddened, round plaque that usually affects the scalp, knees, elbows, extensor surfaces of arms and legs, and sacral regions
   c. A yellow discoloration, pitting, and a thickening of nails if they are affected
   d. Joint inflammation with psoriatic arthritis

3. Interventions
   a. Administer daily soaks and tepid, wet compresses to the affected areas to remove scales; oils or coal tar preparations may be added to the bath water.
   b. Assist the client to remove the scales during the soak, using a soft washcloth and gentle, circular motions; emollient creams or salicylic acid may be applied to affected areas after the bath to continue to soften thick scales.

4. Topical pharmacological therapy
   a. Pharmacological therapy includes tar preparations, anthralin, salicylic acid, and corticosteroids; vitamin D preparation, calcipotriene (Dovonex), and a retinoid compound, tazarotene (Tazorac), suppress epidermopoiesis and cause sloughing of the rapidly growing epidermal cells
   b. Occlusive dressings may be applied following application of the corticosteroid to increase its effectiveness.
   c. Use plastic wrap or bags as the occlusive dressing, and use rubber gloves on the client's hands, plastic bags on the feet, and a shower cap on the head if affected; a plastic vinyl jogging suit may be used for the client being treated at home.

5. Intralesional therapy involves injections of triamcinolone acetonide (Aristocort, Kenalog-10, Trymex) into highly visible or isolated patches of psoriasis that are resistant to other forms of therapy.

6. Systemic therapy
   a. Systemic medications may be prescribed to treat extensive psoriasis that does not respond to other forms of therapy.
   b. Prescribed medications may include methotrexate, (Folex), hydroxyurea (Hydrea), and cyclosporine A (CyA).

7. Photochemotherapy
   a. A combination of psoralens and ultraviolet A light therapy decreases cellular proliferation.
   b. The client takes a photosensitizing medication (8-methoxypsoralen) and subsequently is exposed to long-wave ultraviolet light.

8. Client education
   a. Instruct the client not to scratch the affected areas and to keep the skin lubricated to minimize itching.
   b. Monitor for and instruct the client to recognize the signs and symptoms of infection.
   c. Instruct the client to wear light cotton clothing over affected areas.
   d. Instruct the client regarding prescribed treatments and medications and to avoid over-the-counter medications.
   e. Assist the client to identify ways to reduce stress.

G. **Kaposi's sarcoma**
   1. Description: Skin lesions that occur primarily in individuals with a compromised immune system
   2. Assessment
      a. **Kaposi's sarcoma** is a slow-growing tumor that appears as raised, oblong, purplish, reddish-brown lesion and may be tender or nontender.
      b. Organ involvement includes the lymph nodes, airways or lungs, or any part of the gastrointestinal tract from the mouth to anus.
   3. Interventions
      a. Maintain standard precautions.
      b. Provide protective isolation if the immune system is depressed.
      c. Prepare the client for radiation therapy or chemotherapy as prescribed.
      d. Administer immunotherapy, as prescribed, to stabilize the immune system.

H. **Herpes zoster (shingles)**
   1. Description
      a. **Shingles** is an acute viral infection of the dorsal nerve root ganglion caused by the varicella-zoster virus.
      b. **Shingles** can be caused by the reactivation of the varicella-zoster virus or exposure to varicella-zoster or can occur during any immunocompromised state.
      c. Diagnosis is determined by visual examination, skin cultures, and skin stains that identify the organism and by an antinuclear antibody blood test that will produce a positive result.

d. A culture provides the definitive diagnosis.

e. **Herpes zoster** is contagious to individuals who have not had chickenpox.

2. Assessment

a. Unilaterally clustered skin vesicles along peripheral sensory nerves on the trunk, thorax, or face

b. Fever

c. Burning and neuralgia

d. Pruritus

e. Paresthesia

3. Interventions

a. Isolate the client because exudate from the lesions contains the virus (maintain standard and other precautions, such as contact precaurions).

b. Assess neurovascular status and seventh cranial nerve function.

c. Assess for signs and symptoms of infection.

d. Keep blisters intact if formed.

e. Assist the client with acetic acid compresses; cool, wet compresses; and tepid baths as prescribed.

f. Prepare to assist physician with a nerve block using lidocaine (Xylocaine) if prescribed.

g. Administer antiviral agents, analgesics, antianxiety agents, antipruritics, and corticosteroids as prescribed.

h. Use an air mattress and a bed cradle on the client's bed and keep environment cool; warmth and touch aggravate pain.

i. Prevent the client from scratching and rubbing the affected area.

j. Instruct the client to wear lightweight, loose cotton clothing and to avoid wool and synthetic clothing

I. Paronychia

1. Description: An infection of the tissue around the nail plate that most commonly occurs in middle-aged women and in the client with diabetes mellitus

2. Assessment

a. Redness and swelling around the nailbed

b. Soreness at the nailbed

3. Interventions

a. Monitor temperature.

b. Monitor for infection around the nails.

c. Monitor for cellulitis in the affected area.

d. Assist the client with warm soaks as prescribed.

e. Prepare to assist with incision and drainage of infected area if prescribed.

f. Administer antibiotic or fungicidal ointments as prescribed.

J. Impetigo: Refer to Chapter 42 for information on this disorder.

K. Boils

1. Description

a. Boils are a deep bacterial inflammation of hair follicles caused by staphylococcus.

b. Boils commonly occur on the face, neck, arms, legs, and groin.

2. Assessment

a. Redness on skin

b. Tender and painful furuncle

c. Skin swelling at the site

d. A yellow or white center at the furuncle

3. Interventions

a. Instruct the client in good hand-washing technique to prevent the spread of infection.

b. Apply hot moist compresses until drainage occurs.

c. Assist the physician in incision and drainage, which relieves pain and allows the escape of purulent drainage.

d. Instruct the client in daily cleanliness, the use of separate bath linens, and in the administration of antibiotics if prescribed.

L. Frostbite

1. Description

a. Frostbite is damage to tissues and blood vessels as a result of prolonged exposure to cold.

b. Fingers, toes, nose, and ears often are affected.

2. Assessment

a. Numbness

b. Paresthesia

c. Pallor

d. Severe pain, swelling, erythema, and blistering that occur once the client is in a warm environment

e. Necrosis and gangrene may develop in severe cases

3. Interventions

a. Handle the tissues gently.

b. Rewarm the affected part rapidly and continuously with a warm water bath (90° to 107° F) for 15 to 20 minutes or until skin flushing occurs.

c. Avoid slow thawing, interrupted periods of warmth, or massage (may result in further tissue damage).

d. Do not débride blisters.

e. Leave area exposed initially for continued assessment, and then apply bulky dressings as prescribed to provide protection.

M. Scabies

1. Description

a. Scabies is a parasitic skin disorder caused by an infestation of the *Sarcoptes scabiei* (itch mite).

b. Scabies is endemic among schoolchildren and institutionalized populations because of close personal contact.

c. Risk factors include close personal contact with an infected person or contaminated article.

d. Usually a 1-month delay occurs between the initial infestation and onset of pruritus in the host.

2. Assessment
   a. Erythematous papules and pustules
   b. Threadlike, brownish, linear burrows up to 1 cm long
   c. Secondary lesions consist of vesicles, crusts, reddish-brown nodules, and excoriations
   d. Intense pruritus that worsens at night
3. Interventions
   a. Administer antihistamines or topical steroids to relieve itching as prescribed.
   b. Apply topical antiscabies creams or lotions such as lindane (Kwell, Scabene), crotamiton (Eurax), or permethrin 5% (Elimite) as prescribed.
   c. Lindane should not be used in children younger than age 2 because of the risk of neurotoxicity and seizures.
   d. Instruct the client to apply the antiscabies preparation thinly to the entire skin from the neck down (face and scalp are not affected in scabies) and to leave on for 12 to 24 hours, as prescribed.
   e. Instruct the client to apply antiscabies preparations to dry skin because moist skin increases absorption and the potential for central nervous system side effects such as seizures.
   f. Following treatment with antiscabies preparations, instruct the client to remove the medication by thoroughly washing with soap and water.
   g. All family members and close contacts should be treated simultaneously.
   h. Instruct the client that all bedding and clothing should be washed in hot water and dried on the hot dryer cycle or dry-cleaned (mites can survive up to 36 hours on linen).

N. Acne vulgaris
1. Description
   a. Acne is a common, self-limiting, multifactorial disorder.
   b. Acne requires active treatment for control until it spontaneously resolves.
   c. The types of lesions include comedones (open and closed), pustules, papules, and nodules.
   d. The exact cause is unknown but may include androgenic influence on sebaceous glands, increased sebum production, and proliferation of *Propionibacterium acnes* (the enzymes of which reduce lipids to irritating fatty acids).
   e. Exacerbations coincide with the menstrual cycle from hormonal activity.
   f. Heat, humidity, and excessive perspiration have a role in increased acne.
2. Assessment
   a. Closed comedones are whiteheads and noninflamed lesions that develop as a follicle and enlarge with the retention of horny cells
   b. Open comedones are blackheads that result from continuing accumulation of horny cells and sebum, which dilates the follicles.
   c. Pustules and papules result as the inflammatory process progresses.
   d. Nodules result from total disintegration of a comedone and subsequent collapse of the follicle.
   e. Deep scarring can result from nodules.
3. Interventions
   a. Instruct the client in the administration (provide written instructions) of topical or oral antibiotics as prescribed.
   b. Instruct the client in the use of isotretinoin (Accutane) or other medications, if prescribed to inhibit sebum production and reduce sebaceous gland size.
   c. Instruct the client about the adverse effects of isotretinoin, which include cheilitis (lip inflammation), skin dryness, elevated triglycerides, and eye discomfort.
   d. Instruct the client to stop taking vitamin A supplements during treatment with isotretinoin.
   e. Inform the client that improvement may not be apparent for 4 to 6 weeks.
   f. Instruct the client in appropriate skin-cleansing methods, with emphasis on not scrubbing the face and using only the agreed-on topical agents.
   g. Instruct the client not to squeeze, prick, or pick at lesions.
   h. Instruct the client to use products labeled noncomedogenic and cosmetics that are water-based and to avoid contact with excessively oil-based products.
   i. Instruct the client on the importance of follow-up treatment.

O. **Decubitus**
1. Description
   a. **Decubitus** is an impairment of skin integrity.
   b. Localized areas of necrosis of the skin and subcutaneous tissue are caused by pressure.
   c. Prevention of skin breakdown is a major role of the nurse, particularly in caring for the bedridden or immobile client.
2. Risk factors
   a. Malnutrition
   b. Incontinence
   c. Immobility
   d. Skin-shearing
   e. Decreased sensory perception
3. Assessment (Box 49-3)
4. Interventions
   a. Institute measures to prevent **decubitus.**
   b. Assess the nutritional status of the client.
   c. Provide adequate nutritional intake to promote tissue integrity.
   d. Monitor for an alteration in skin integrity.
   e. Relieve or remove pressure on the skin.
   f. Turn and reposition the immobile client every 2 hours or more frequently if necessary.

BOX 49-3

Stages of Decubitus Ulcers

STAGE 1

Ulcer is a reddened area that returns to normal skin color after 15 to 20 minutes of pressure relief, such as turning the client to another position.

The skin is intact.

Area is red and does does not blanche with external pressure.

STAGE 2

Ulcer is an area in which the top layer of skin is missing.

The ulcer usually is shallow with a pink to red base, and a white or yellow eschar may be present.

STAGE 3

A deep ulcer that extends into the dermis and subcutaneous tissues.

White, gray, or yellow eschar usually is present at the bottom of the ulcer, and the ulcer may have a lip or edge.

Purulent drainage is common.

STAGE 4

A deep ulcer that extends into muscle and bone.

Ulcer is foul-smelling.

Brown or black eschar is present.

Purulent drainage is common.

BOX 49-4

Methods to Estimate Extent of Burn Injury

RULE OF NINES (ADULT)

Head and neck: 9%
Anterior trunk: 18%
Posterior trunk: 18%
Arms (9% each): 18%
Legs (18% each): 36%
Perineum: 1%

LUND-BROWDER CLASSIFICATION

Modifies percentages for body segments according to age.

Provides a more accurate estimate of the burn size.

Uses a diagram of the body divided into sections, with the representative percentage of the total body surface area for ages greater than 1 year.

Should be reevaluated after initial wound débridement.

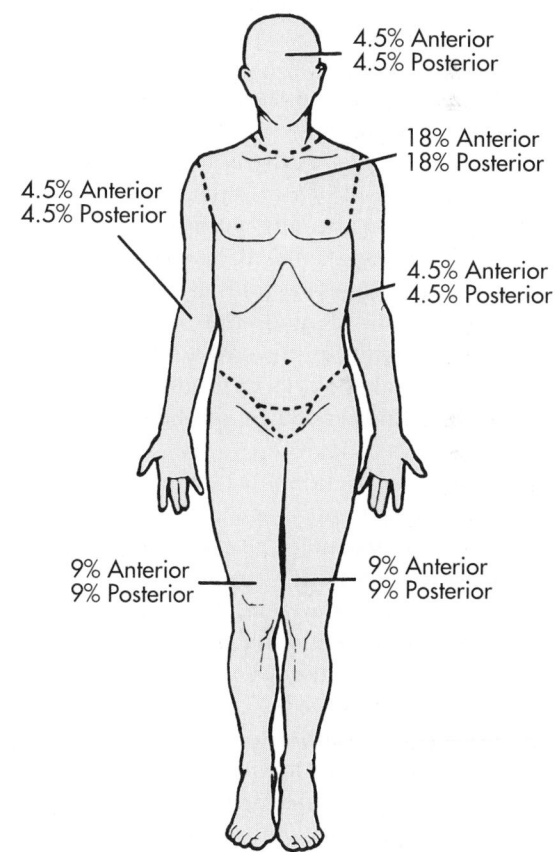

FIG. 49-1 The rule of nines for estimating burn percentage. (From Ignatavicius, D., & Workman, M. [2002]. *Medical-surgical nursing: Critical thinking for collaborative care* [4th ed.]. Philadelphia: W .B. Saunders.)

g. Help the client ambulate.

h. Provide active and passive exercises every 8 hours.

i. Keep the skin clean and dry and the sheets wrinkle free.

j. Apply moisture barrier as prescribed to protect the skin.

k. Use assistive devices to prevent pressure such as an alternating air pressure mattress or sheepskin padding.

l. Apply medications or dressings to the wound as prescribed.

VI. BURN INJURIES

A. Description: Cell destruction of the layers of the skin and the resultant depletion of fluid and electrolytes

B. Burn size

1. Small **burns**: The response of the body to injury is localized to the injured area.

2. Large or extensive **burns**

a. Large **burns** consist of 25% or more of the total body surface area

b. The response of the body to the injury is systemic.

c. The burn affects all of the major systems of the body.

C. Estimating the extent of injury (Box 49-4 and Fig. 49-1)

D. Burn depth

1. **Superficial-thickness burn** (similar to first-degree burn)

a. Mild to severe erythema (pink to red) is present, but no blisters.

b. Skin blanches with pressure.

c. Burn is painful, with tingling sensation.

d. Pain is eased by cooling.

e. Discomfort lasts about 48 hours; healing occurs in about 3 to 7 days.

f. Skin grafts are not required.

2. **Partial-thickness superficial burn** (similar to second-degree burn)

a. Large blisters cover an extensive area.

b. Edema is present.

c. Mottled red base and broken epidermis, with a wet, shiny, and weeping surface are characteristic.

d. Burn is painful.

e. Injured area is sensitive to cold air.

f. Superficial partial thickness burn heals in 2 to 3 weeks.

g. Deep partial thickness burn heals in 3 to 6 weeks.

h. Grafts may be used if the healing process is prolonged.

3. **Full-thickness burn** (similar to third-degree burn)

a. Burn leaves a deep red, black, white, yellow, or brown area.

b. Injured surface appears dry.

c. Edema is present.

d. Burn causes tissue disruption with fat exposed.

e. Burn causes little or no pain.

f. Spontaneous healing will not occur.

g. Burn requires removal of eschar and split- or full-thickness skin grafting.

h. Scarring and wound contractures are likely to develop without preventive measures.

i. Healing takes weeks to months.

4. **Deep full-thickness burn** (similar to fourth-degree burn)

a. Burn involves injury to the muscle and bone.

b. Injured area appears black.

c. Edema is absent.

d. Pain is absent.

e. No blisters are present.

f. Eschar is hard and inelastic.

g. Healing time takes weeks to months.

h. Grafts are required.

E. Age and general health

1. Mortality rates are higher for children less than 4 years of age, particularly in the birth to 1-year age group, and for clients over the age of 65 years.

2. Debilitating disorders, such as cardiac, respiratory, endocrine, and renal disorders, negatively influence the client's response to injury and treatment.

3. Mortality rate is higher when the client has a pre-existing disorder at the time of the burn injury.

F. Burn location

1. **Burns** of the head, neck, and chest are associated with pulmonary complications.

2. **Burns** of the face are associated with corneal abrasion.

3. **Burns** of the ear are associated with auricular chondritis.

4. Hands and joints require intensive therapy to prevent disability.

5. The perineal area is prone to autocontamination by urine and feces.

6. Circumferential **burns** of the extremities can produce a tourniquet-like effect and lead to vascular compromise (compartment syndrome).

7. Circumferential thorax **burns** lead to inadequate chest wall expansion and pulmonary insufficiency.

VII. TYPES OF BURNS

A. **Thermal burns** are caused by exposure to flames, hot liquids, steam, or hot objects.

B. **Chemical burns**

1. **Burns** are caused by tissue contact with strong acids, alkalis, or organic compounds.

2. Systemic toxicity from cutaneous absorption can occur.

C. **Electrical burns**

1. **Burns** are caused by heat generated by an electrical energy as it passes through the body.

2. **Electrical burns** result in internal tissue damage.

3. Cutaneous **burns** cause muscle and soft tissue damage that may be extensive, particularly in high-voltage electrical injuries.

4. The voltage, type of current, contact site, and duration of contact are important to identify.

5. Alternating current is more dangerous than direct current because it is associated with cardiopulmonary arrest, ventricular fibrillation, tetanic muscle contractions, and long bone or vertebral fractures.

D. Radiation **burns** are caused by exposure to ultraviolet light, x-rays, or a radioactive source.

VIII. INHALATION INJURIES

A. **Smoke inhalation injury**

1. Description: Injury results when the victim is trapped in an enclosed, hot, smoke-filled space.

2. Assessment

a. Facial burns

b. Erythema

c. Swelling of oropharynx and nasopharynx

d. Singed nasal hairs

e. Flaring nostrils

f. Stridor, wheezing, and dyspnea

g. Hoarse voice

h. Sooty (carbonaceous) sputum and cough

i. Agitation and anxiety

j. Tachycardia

B. **Carbon monoxide poisoning**

1. Description

a. Carbon monoxide is a colorless, odorless, and tasteless gas that has an affinity for hemoglobin 200 times greater than that of oxygen.

b. Oxygen molecules are displaced and carbon monoxide reversibly binds to hemoglobin to form carboxyhemoglobin.

TABLE 49-1

Carbon Monoxide Poisoning

Blood Level (%)	Clinical Manifestation
1-10	Impaired visual acuity
11-20	Flushing; headache
21-30	Nausea
	Impaired dexterity
31-40	Vomiting
	Dizziness
	Syncope
41-50	Tachypnea
	Tachycardia
Greater than 50	Coma and death

    c. Tissue hypoxia occurs.

  2. Assessment (Table 49-1)

C. Smoke poisoning

  1. Description

    a. Smoke poisoning is caused by the inhalation of the by-products of combustion.

    b. A localized inflammatory reaction occurs, causing a decrease in bronchial ciliary action and a decrease in surfactant.

  2. Assessment

    a. Mucosal edema occurs in the airways.

    b. Wheezing is evident on auscultation.

    c. After several hours, sloughing of the tracheobronchial epithelium may occur, and hemorrhagic bronchitis may develop.

    d. Adult respiratory distress syndrome can result.

D. Direct thermal heat injury

  1. Description

    a. Thermal heat injury can occur to the lower airways by the inhalation of steam or explosive gases or the aspiration of scalding liquids.

    b. Injury can occur to the upper airways, which appear erythematous and edematous, with mucosal blisters and ulcerations.

    c. Mucosal edema can lead to upper airway obstruction, especially during the first 24 to 48 hours.

    d. All clients with head or neck **burns** should be monitored closely for the development of airway obstruction and are considered immediately for endotracheal intubation if obstruction occurs.

  2. Assessment

    a. Erythema and edema of the upper airways

    b. Mucosal blisters and ulcerations

IX. PATHOPHYSIOLOGY OF BURNS

A. Following the burn, vasoactive substances are released from the injured tissue; and these substances cause an increase in the capillary permeability, allowing the plasma to seep to the surrounding tissues.

B. The direct injury to the vessels increases capillary permeability (capillary permeability decreases 18 to 26 hours after the burn but does not normalize until 2 to 3 weeks following the injury).

C. Extensive **burns** result in generalized body edema and a decrease in circulating intravascular blood volume.

D. The fluid losses result in a decrease in organ perfusion.

E. The heart rate increases, cardiac output decreases, and the blood pressure drops.

F. Initially hyponatremia and hyperkalemia occur.

G. The hematocrit level increases as a result of plasma loss; this initial increase falls to below normal at the third to fourth day after the burn as a result of the red blood cell damage and loss at the time of injury.

H. Initially, the body shunts blood from the kidneys, causing oliguria; then the body begins to reabsorb fluid, and diuresis of the excess fluid occurs over the next days to weeks.

I. Blood flow to the gastrointestinal tract is diminished, leading to intestinal ileus and gastrointestinal dysfunction.

J. Immune system function is depressed, resulting in immunosuppression and thus increasing the risk of infection and sepsis.

K. Pulmonary hypertension can develop, resulting in a decrease in the arterial oxygen tension level and a decrease in lung compliance.

L. Evaporative fluid losses through the burn wound are greater than normal, and the losses continue until complete wound closure occurs.

M. If the intravascular space is not replenished with intravenously administered fluids, hypovolemic shock and ultimately death will occur.

X. MANAGEMENT OF THE BURN INJURY (BOX 49-5)

A. Emergent phase

  1. Description

    a. The emergent phase begins at the time of injury and ends with the restoration of capillary permeability (fluid resuscitation), usually at 48 to 72 hours following the injury; the phase includes prehospital and emergency room care.

    b. The primary goal is to prevent hypovolemic shock and preserve vital organ functioning.

  2. Prehospital care

    a. Prehospital care begins at the scene of the accident and ends when emergency care is obtained.

    b. Remove the victim from the source of the burn.

    c. Remove the source of heat.

    d. Assess airway, breathing, and circulation.

    e. Assess for associated trauma.

    f. Conserve body heat.

    g. Cover **burns** with sterile or clean cloths.

    h. Remove constricting jewelry and clothing.

    i. Assess the need for intravenous fluids.

    j. Transport.

BOX 49-5

Phases of Management of the Burn Injury

EMERGENT PHASE

The emergent phase begins at the time of injury and ends with the restoration of capillary permeability, usually at 48 to 72 hours following the injury.

The primary goal is to prevent hypovolemic shock and preserve vital organ functioning.

This phase includes prehospital care and emergency room care.

RESUSCITATIVE PHASE

The resuscitative phase begins with the initiation of fluids and ends when capillary integrity returns to near-normal levels and the large fluid shifts have decreased.

The amount of fluid administered is based on the client's weight and extent of injury.

Most fluid replacement formulas are calculated from the time of injury and not from the time of arrival at the hospital.

The goal is to prevent shock by maintaining adequate circulating blood volume and maintaining vital organ perfusion.

ACUTE PHASE

The acute phase begins when the client is hemodynamically stable, capillary permeability is restored, and diuresis has begun.

This phase usually begins 48 to 72 hours after the time of injury.

Emphasis during this phase is placed on restorative therapy, and the phase continues until wound closure is achieved.

The focus is on infection control, wound care, wound closure, nutritional support, pain management, and physical therapy.

REHABILITATIVE PHASE

Rehabilitation is the final phase of burn care.

The phase overlaps the acute care phase and goes well beyond hospitalization.

Goals of this phase are designed so that the client can gain independence and achieve maximal function.

3. Emergency room care is a continuation of care administered at the scene of the injury.
4. Major **burns**
   a. Evaluate the degree and extent of the burn and treat life-threatening conditions.
   b. Ensure a patent airway and administer 100% oxygen as prescribed if the burn occurred in an enclosed area.
   c. Monitor for respiratory distress and assess the need for intubation.
   d. Assess oropharynx for blisters and erythema.
   e. Monitor arterial blood gases and carboxyhemoglobin levels.
   f. For an inhalation injury, administer 100% oxygen via a tight-fitting non-rebreather face mask as prescribed until carboxyhemoglobin levels fall below 15%.
   g. Initiate peripheral intravenous (IV) access to nonburned skin proximal to any extremity burn, or prepare for the insertion of a central venous pressure line as prescribed.
   h. Assess for hypovolemia and prepare to administer fluids intravenously to maintain fluid balance.
   i. Monitor vital signs closely.
   j. Insert a Foley catheter as prescribed, and maintain urine output at 30 to 50 mL per hour.
   k. Maintain NPO status.
   l. Insert a nasogastric tube as prescribed to remove gastric secretions and prevent aspiration.

   m. Administer tetanus prophylaxis as prescribed.
   n. Administer pain medication, as prescribed, by the IV route.
   o. Prepare the client for an escharotomy or fasciotomy as prescribed.
5. Minor **burns**
   a. Administer pain medication with small doses of morphine sulfate or meperidine (Demerol) as prescribed.
   b. Instruct the client in the use of oral analgesics as prescribed.
   c. Administer tetanus prophylaxis as prescribed.
   d. Administer wound care as prescribed, which may include cleansing, débriding loose tissue, and removing any damaging agents, followed by the application of topical antimicrobial cream and a sterile dressing.
   e. Instruct the client in follow-up care, including active range of motion exercises and wound care treatments.
B. Resuscitative phase
   1. Description
      a. The resuscitative phase begins with the initiation of fluids and ends when capillary integrity returns to near-normal levels and the large fluid shifts have decreased.
      b. The amount of fluid administered is based on client's weight and extent of injury.
      c. Most fluid replacement formulas are calculated from the time of injury and not from the time of arrival at the hospital.

TABLE 49-2

Common Fluid Resuscitation Formulas for First 24 Hours after a Burn Injury

Formula	Solution	Infusion Rate
MODIFIED BROOKE		
2.0 mL/kg per percent TBSA* burned	Lactated Ringer's	Half in first 8 hours Half in next 16 hours
PARKLAND (BAXTER)		
4 mL/kg per percent TBSA burned	Lactated Ringer's	Half in first 8 hours One-quarter each next 8 hours

*Total body surface area.

d. The goal is to prevent shock by maintaining adequate circulating blood volume and maintaining vital organ perfusion.

2. Fluid resuscitation (Table 49-2)

a. The amount of fluid administered depends on how much intravenous fluid per hour is required to maintain a urinary output of 30 to 50 mL per hour.

b. Successful fluid resuscitation is evaluated by stable vital signs, an adequate urine output, palpable peripheral pulses, and a clear sensorium.

c. Urinary output is the most common and most sensitive noninvasive assessment parameter for cardiac output and tissue perfusion.

d. Intravenous fluid replacement may be titrated (adjusted) based on urinary output plus serum electrolyte levels to meet the perfusion needs of the client with **burns**.

e. If the hemoglobin and hematocrit levels decrease or if the urinary output exceeds 50 mL/hr, the rate of IV fluid administration may be decreased.

3. Interventions

a. Monitor for tracheal or laryngeal edema and administer respiratory treatments as prescribed.

b. Monitor pulse oximetry and prepare for arterial blood gases and carboxyhemoglobin levels if inhalation injury is suspected.

c. Elevate the head of the bed to 30 degrees or more for **burns** of the face and head.

d. Initiate electrocardiogram monitoring.

e. Monitor temperature and assess for infection.

f. Initiate protective isolation techniques; maintain strict hand washing; use sterile sheets and linens when caring for the client; and use gloves, cap, masks, shoe covers, scrub clothes, and plastic aprons.

g. Shave or cut body hair around wound margins.

h. Monitor daily weights, expecting a weight gain of 15 to 20 lb in the first 72 hours.

i. Monitor gastric output and pH levels and for gastric discomfort and bleeding, indicating a stress ulcer.

j. Administer antacids, H_2-receptor antagonists, and the antiulcer medications such as sucralfate (Carafate) as prescribed.

k. Auscultate bowel sounds for ileus and monitor for abdominal distention and gastrointestinal dysfunction.

l. Monitor stools for occult blood.

m. Obtain urine specimen for myoglobin and hemoglobin levels.

n. Monitor IV fluids and hourly intake and output to determine the adequacy of fluid replacement therapy; notify the physician if urine output is less than 30 or greater than 50 mL per hour.

o. Elevate circumferential **burns** of the extremities on pillows above the level of the heart to reduce dependent edema if no obvious fractures are present.

p. Monitor pulses and capillary refill of the affected extremities and assess perfusion of the distal extremity with a circumferential burn.

q. Prepare for chest and other radiographs to rule out fractures or associated trauma.

r. Keep the room temperature warm.

s. Place the client on an air-fluidized bed and use a bed cradle to keep sheets off the client's skin.

4. Pain management

a. Administer morphine sulfate or meperidine (Demerol) as prescribed by the IV route.

b. Avoid intramuscular or subcutaneous routes because absorption through the soft tissue is unreliable when hypovolemia and large fluid shifts are occurring.

c. Avoid administering medication by the oral route because of the possibility of gastrointestinal dysfunction.

d. Medicate the client before painful procedures.

5. Nutrition

a. Proper nutrition is essential to promote wound healing and prevent infection.

b. The basal metabolic rate is 40 to 100 times higher than normal.

c. Maintain NPO status until the bowel sounds are heard, and then advance to clear liquids as prescribed.

d. Nutrition may be provided via enteral tube feeding, peripheral parenteral nutrition, or total parenteral nutrition.

e. Provide a diet high in protein, carbohydrates, fats, and vitamins.

f. Monitor calorie intake.

6. Escharotomy

a. A lengthwise incision is made through the burn eschar to relieve constriction and pressure and to improve circulation.

b. Escharotomy is performed for circulatory compromise caused by circumferential **burns.**

c. Escharotomy is performed at the bedside without anesthesia because nerve endings have been destroyed by the burn injury.

d. Escharotomy can be performed on the thorax to improve ventilation.

e. Following the escharotomy, assess pulses, color, movement, and sensation of affected extremity and control any bleeding with pressure.

f. Pack incision gently with fine mesh gauze for 24 hours after escharotomy as prescribed.

g. Apply topical antimicrobial agents to the area as prescribed following the procedure.

7. Fasciotomy

a. An incision is made extending through the subcutaneous tissue and fascia.

b. The procedure is performed if adequate tissue perfusion does not return following an escharotomy.

c. Fasciotomy is performed in the operating room with the client under general anesthesia.

d. Following the procedure, assess pulses, color, movement, and sensation of affected extremity and control any bleeding with pressure.

e. Apply topical antimicrobial agents and dressings to the area, as prescribed, following the procedure.

C. Acute phase

1. Description

a. The acute phase begins when the client is hemodynamically stable, capillary permeability is restored, and diuresis has begun.

b. The acute phase usually begins 48 to 72 hours after the time of injury.

c. Emphasis during this phase is placed on restorative therapy, and the phase continues until wound closure is achieved.

d. The focus is on infection control, wound care, wound closure, nutritional support, pain management, and physical therapy.

2. Interventions

a. Continue with protective isolation techniques.

b. Provide wound care as prescribed and prepare for wound closure.

c. Provide pain management.

d. Provide adequate nutrition as prescribed.

e. Prepare client for rehabilitation.

D. Wound care (Table 49-3)

1. Description: The cleansing, débridement, and dressing of the burn wounds

2. Hydrotherapy

a. Wounds are cleansed by immersion, showering, or spraying.

b. Hydrotherapy occurs for 30 minutes or less to prevent increased sodium loss through the burn wound, heat loss, pain, and stress.

c. Client should be premedicated before procedure.

d. Hydrotherapy generally is not used for clients who are hemodynamically unstable or those with new skin grafts.

e. Care is taken to minimize bleeding and maintain body temperature during the procedure.

TABLE 49-3

Open Method versus Closed Method of Wound Care

Method	Advantages	Disadvantages
OPEN		
Antimicrobial cream is applied, and wound is left open to the air without a dressing. Antimicrobial cream is applied every 12 hours.	Visualization of the wound Easier mobility and joint range of motion Simplicity in wound care	Increased chance of hypothermia from exposure
CLOSED		
Gauze dressings are wrapped carefully from the distal to the proximal area of the extremity to ensure circulation is not compromised. No two burn surfaces should be allowed to touch; touching can promote webbing of digits, contractures, and poor cosmetic outcome. Dressings are changed every 8-12 hours.	Decreases evaporative fluid and heat loss Aids in débridement	Mobility limitations Prevents effective range of motion exercises Wound assessment is limited

---

BOX 49-6

Débridement

MECHANICAL

Use of scissors and forceps to lift and trim away loose
  eschar
Wet-to-dry or wet-to-wet dressing changes
A painful procedure
Requires a moist environment to be effective; dressings
  applied directly to the burn wound
Major problems: pain and bleeding

ENZYMATIC

Application of prepared proteolytic and fibrinolytic
  topical enzymes that digest necrotic tissue, which
  facilitates eschar removal

SURGICAL

Excision of eschar and coverage of wound
Tangential
Shaving of thin layers of eschar until viable tissue is
  reached
Fascial
Used for deep burns and removal of burn tissue and
  underlying fat down to the fascia

BOX 49-7

Temporary Wound Coverings

BIOLOGICAL

Amnion
Amniotic membranes from human placenta are used.
Dressing is changed every 48 hours with amnion.
Allograft Homograft
Donated human cadaver skin is provided through
  a skin bank
Monitor for wound exudate and signs of infection.
Rejection can occur within 24 hours.
Xenograft Heterograft
Porcine skin is harvested after slaughter and preserved
  for storage.
Rejection can occur within 24 to 72 hours.
Xenograft over granulation tissue is replaced every 2 to
  5 days until the wound heals naturally or until closure
  with autograft is complete.

BIOSYNTHETIC AND SYNTHETIC

Visual inspection of wound is possible because dressings
  are transparent or translucent.
Monitor for wound exudate and signs of infection.

BOX 49-8

Types of Skin Grafts

SPLIT THICKNESS
Graft of half of the epidermis; applied in sheets or
postage stamp–like pieces

FULL THICKNESS
Graft consisting of epidermis and dermis; commonly
used for reconstructive surgery months or years after the
initial injury

PEDICLE FLAP
Commonly used for reconstructive surgery months or
years after the initial injury

CULTURED EPITHELIUM
Use of the client's unburned skin
Isolation of keratinocytes and culturing of epithelial cells
in a laboratory; these cells then are attached to the burn
wound

---

f. If hydrotherapy is not used, wounds are
   washed and rinsed in bed before the application of antimicrobial agents.
3. Débridement (Box 49-6)
   a. Débridement is removal of eschar to prevent
      bacterial proliferation under the eschar and to
      promote wound healing.
   b. Débridement may be mechanical, enzymatic,
      or surgical.
   c. **Deep partial- or full-thickness burns:** Wound is
      cleansed and débrided, and topical antimicro-
      bial agents are applied once or twice daily.
E. Wound closure
   1. Description
      a. Wound closure prevents infection and loss of
         fluid.
      b. Closure promotes healing.
      c. Closure prevents contractures.
      d. Wound closure is performed on the fifth to
         twenty-first day, depending on the extent of the
         burn.
   2. Temporary wound coverings (Box 49-7)
   3. Autografting (Box 49-8)
      a. Autografting provides permanent wound
         coverage.
      b. Autografting is surgical removal of a thin layer
         of the client's own unburned skin, which then
         is applied to the excised burn wound.
      c. Autografting is performed in the operating room
         under anesthesia.

d. Monitor for bleeding following the graft
   because bleeding beneath an autograft can prevent adherence.
e. If prescribed, small amounts of blood or serum
   can be removed by gently rolling the fluid from
   the center of the graft to the periphery with a
   sterile gauze pad, where it can be absorbed.
f. For large accumulations of blood, the physician will aspirate the blood using a small-gauge
   needle and syringe.

g. Autografts are immobilized following surgery for 3 to 7 days to allow time to adhere and attach to the wound bed.

h. Position for immobilization and elevation of the graft site to prevent movement and shearing of the graft.

4. Care to the graft site
   a. Elevate and immobilize graft site.
   b. Keep site free from pressure.
   c. Avoid weight bearing.
   d. When graft takes, roll a cotton-tipped applicator over the graft to remove exudate because exudate can lead to infection and prevent graft adherence.
   e. Monitor for foul-smelling drainage, increased temperature, increased white blood cell count, hematoma, or fluid accumulation.
   f. Instruct the client to avoid using fabric softeners and harsh detergents in the laundry.
   g. Instruct the client to lubricate healing skin with cocoa butter as prescribed.
   h. Instruct the client to protect the affected area from sunlight.
   i. Instruct the client to use splints and support garments as prescribed.

5. Care to the donor site
   a. Method of care varies depending on physician's preference.
   b. A moist gauze dressing is applied at the time of the surgery to maintain pressure and stop any oozing.
   c. The physician may prescribe site treatment with single-layer gauze impregnated with petrolatum or with a biosynthetic dressing such as Biobrane.
   d. Keep the donor site clean, dry, and free from pressure.
   e. Prevent the client from scratching the donor site.
   f. Apply lubricating lotions to soften the area and reduce the itching after the donor site is healed.
   g. Donor site can be reused once healing has occurred (heals spontaneously within 7 to 14 days with proper care).

F. Physical therapy
   1. An individualized program of splinting, positioning, exercises, ambulation, and activities of daily living is implemented early in the acute phase of recovery to maximize functional and cosmetic outcomes.
   2. Perform range of motion exercises as prescribed to reduce edema and maintain strength and joint function.
   3. Ambulate the client as prescribed to maintain the strength of the lower extremities.
   4. Apply splints as prescribed to maintain proper joint position and prevent contractures.
      a. Static splints immobilize the joint and are applied for periods of immobilization, during

---

BOX 49-9

Surgical Options for Contractures and Scarring

Skin flaps
Split-thickness and full-thickness skin grafts
Tissue expansion
Z-plasties

---

sleeping, and for clients who cannot maintain proper positioning.
      b. Dynamic splints exercise the affected joint.
      c. Avoid pressure to skin areas when applying splints, which could lead to further tissue and nerve damage.
   5. Scarring is controlled by elastic wraps and bandages that apply continuous pressure to the healing skin during the period of time when the skin is vulnerable to shearing.
   6. Antiburn scar support garments are worn 23 hours a day until the burn scar tissue has matured, which takes 18 months to 2 years.

G. Rehabilitative phase (Box 49-9)
   1. Description
      a. Rehabilitation is the final phase of burn care.
      b. Rehabilitation overlaps the acute care phase and goes well beyond hospitalization.
      c. Goals of this phase are designed so that the client can gain independence and achieve maximal function.
   2. Goals
      a. Promote wound healing.
      b. Minimize deformities.
      c. Increase strength and function.
      d. Provide emotional support.

PRACTICE QUESTIONS

1. The nurse is reviewing the health care record of the clients scheduled to be seen at the health care clinic. The nurse determines that which of the following individuals is at the greatest risk for development of an integumentary disorder?
   1. An older female
   2. An adolescent
   3. An outdoor construction worker
   4. A physical education teacher

2. The client scheduled for a skin biopsy is concerned and asks the nurse how painful the procedure is. The most appropriate response by the nurse is
   1. "There is no pain associated with this procedure."
   2. "There is some pain, but the physician will prescribe an analgesic following the procedure."
   3. "The local anesthetic may cause a burning or stinging sensation."
   4. "A preoperative medication will be given so you will be sleeping and will not feel any pain."

3. The nurse is reviewing the discharge instructions for the client who had a skin biopsy. Which of the following statements, if made by the client, would indicate a need for further instruction?
   1. "I will call the physician if I see any drainage from the wound."
   2. "I will return in 7 days to have the sutures removed."
   3. "I will use the antibiotic ointment as prescribed."
   4. "I will remove the dressing as soon as I get home and wash it with tap water."

4. The nurse prepares to assist the physician to examine the client's skin with a Wood's light. The nurse includes which of the following in the plan for this procedure?
   1. Obtain an informed consent.
   2. Darken the room for the examination.
   3. Shave the skin and scrub with povidone-iodine solution.
   4. Prepare a local anesthetic.

5. The clinic nurse provides instructions to a client who is to return to the clinic in 1 week for a scratch skin test. The test will be done to identify the allergen causing the dermatitis. The nurse provides which instruction to the client?
   1. Do not ingest anything before the test.
   2. Shower using an antibacterial soap on the morning of the test.
   3. Discontinue the prescribed antihistamine 5 days before the test.
   4. Consume only fluids on the day of the test.

6. The nurse provides discharge instructions to a client following patch testing. Which statement if made by the client would indicate the need for further instruction?
   1. "I will return to the clinic in 2 days for the initial reading."
   2. "If the patch comes off, I need to reapply it."
   3. "I need to avoid activities that will cause me to sweat."
   4. "I need to keep the test sites dry at all times."

7. The clinic nurse implements a teaching plan for the client who has complained of chronic dry skin and episodes of pruritus. Which of the following if stated by the client would indicate a need for further teaching?
   1. "I should drink 8 to 10 glasses of water a day."
   2. "I need to avoid using astringents on my skin."
   3. "I should limit myself to one shower a day and apply emollient to my skin after the shower."
   4. "I should use a dehumidifier especially during the winter months."

8. The camp nurse prepares to instruct a group of children about Lyme disease. Which of the following information would the nurse include in the instructions?
   1. Lyme disease can be contagious by skin contact with an infected individual.
   2. Lyme disease can be caused by the inhalation of spores from bird droppings.

   3. Lyme disease is caused by contamination from cat feces.
   4. Lyme disease is caused by a tick carried by deer.

9. The client is diagnosed with stage I of Lyme disease. The nurse assesses the client for which characteristic of this stage?
   1. Signs of neurological disorders
   2. Enlarged and inflamed joints
   3. Arthralgias
   4. Flulike symptoms

10. A female client arrives at the health care clinic and tells the nurse that she was just bitten by a tick and would like to be tested for Lyme disease. The client tells the nurse that she removed the tick and flushed it down the toilet. Which of the following nursing actions is most appropriate?
   1. Refer the client for a blood test immediately.
   2. Inform the client that there is not a test available for Lyme disease.
   3. Instruct the client to return in 4 to 6 weeks to be tested because testing before this time is not reliable.
   4. Tell the client that testing is not necessary unless arthralgia develops.

11. Following diagnosis of stage I Lyme disease, the nurse would anticipate that which of the following will be part of the treatment plan for the client?
   1. No treatment unless symptoms develop.
   2. A 3-week course of oral antibiotic therapy.
   3. Treatment with intravenously administered antibiotics.
   4. Daily oatmeal baths for a period of 2 weeks.

12. A Cub Scout leader who is a nurse is preparing a group of Cub Scouts for an overnight camping trip instructs the scouts about the methods to prevent Lyme disease. Which statement by one of the Cub Scouts indicates a need for further instructions?
   1. "I should not use insect repellents because it will attract the ticks."
   2. "I should wear long-sleeved tops and long pants."
   3. "I need to bring a hat to wear during the trip."
   4. "I need to wear closed shoes and socks that can be pulled up over my pants."

13. A male client calls the emergency room and tells the nurse that he has been cleaning a wooded area in the backyard and has discovered that he came directly in contact with poison ivy shrubs. The client tells the nurse that he cannot see anything on the skin and asks the nurse what to do. Which of the following is the most appropriate nursing response?
   1. "Come to the emergency room."
   2. "It is not necessary to do anything if you cannot see anything on your skin."
   3. "Take a shower immediately, lathering and rinsing several times."
   4. "Apply calamine lotion immediately to the exposed skin areas."

14. The client with acquired immunodeficiency syndrome is diagnosed with cutaneous Kaposi's sarcoma. Based on this diagnosis, the nurse understands that this has been confirmed by which of the following?
    1. Appearance of reddish blue lesions noted on the skin
    2. Swelling in the lower extremities
    3. Punch biopsy of the cutaneous lesions
    4. Swelling in the genital area

15. Which of the following individuals is least likely at risk for the development of Kaposi's sarcoma?
    1. A male with a history of same-sex partners
    2. A kidney transplant client
    3. A client receiving antineoplastic medications
    4. An individual working in an environment where exposure to asbestos exists

16. The nurse prepares to give a bath and change the bed linens on a client with cutaneous Kaposi's sarcoma lesions. The lesions are open and draining a scant amount of serous fluid. Which of the following would the nurse most appropriately incorporate in the plan during the bathing of this client?
    1. Wearing a gown, gloves, and a mask
    2. Wearing a gown and gloves
    3. Wearing gloves
    4. Wear a gown and gloves to change the bed linens and gloves only for the bath

17. The client is being admitted to the hospital for treatment of acute cellulitis of the lower left leg. The client asks the admitting nurse to explain what cellulitis means. The nurse bases the response on the understanding that the characteristics of cellulitis include
    1. A skin infection into the dermis and subcutaneous tissue.
    2. An acute superficial infection.
    3. An inflammation of the epidermis.
    4. An epidermal infection caused by staphylococcus.

18. The nurse prepares to care for a client with acute cellulitis of the lower leg. The nurse anticipates that which of the following will be prescribed for the client?
    1. Warm compresses to the affected area
    2. Cold compresses to the affected area
    3. Intermittent heat lamp treatments 4 times daily
    4. Alternating hot to cold compresses continuously

19. The clinic nurse assesses the skin of a white client with a diagnosis of psoriasis. The nurse understands that which characteristic is associated with this skin disorder?
    1. Clear, thin nail beds
    2. Silvery white, scaly patches on the scalp, elbows, knees, and sacral regions
    3. Oily skin and no episodes of pruritus
    4. Red-purplish scaly lesions

20. Ultraviolet light therapy is prescribed as a component of the treatment plan for a client with psoriasis. The nurse provides instructions to the client regarding the treatment. Which statement if made by the client indicates a need for further instructions?
    1. "Eye goggles need to be worn to prevent exposure to ultraviolet light."
    2. "Treatments are limited to 2 to 3 times a week."
    3. "The ultraviolet light treatments are given on consecutive days."
    4. "Just the area requiring treatment should be exposed to the ultraviolet light."

21. The clinic nurse notes that the physician has documented a diagnosis of herpes zoster (shingles) in the client's chart. Based on an understanding of the cause of this disorder, the nurse would determine that this definitive diagnosis was made following which diagnostic test?
    1. Skin biopsy
    2. Wood's light examination
    3. Culture of the lesion
    4. Patch test

22. The nurse is assigned to care for a client with herpes zoster (shingles). Which of the following characteristics would the nurse expect to note when assessing the lesions of this infection?
    1. A generalized body rash
    2. Small, blue-white spots with a red base
    3. A fiery red, edematous rash on the cheeks
    4. Clustered skin vesicles

23. The nurse manager is planning the clinical assignments for the day. The nurse manager avoids assigning which of the following staff members to the client with herpes zoster?
    1. The nurse who never had mumps.
    2. An experienced registered nurse who never had chickenpox.
    3. The nurse who never had roseola.
    4. The nurse who never had German measles.

24. A client returns to the clinic for follow-up treatment following a skin biopsy of a suspicious lesion performed 1 week ago. The biopsy report indicates that the lesion is a melanoma. The nurse understands that which of the following describes the characteristic of this type of a lesion?
    1. Melanoma is highly metastatic.
    2. Metastasis is rare.
    3. Melanoma is characterized by local invasion.
    4. Melanoma is encapsulated.

25. When assessing a lesion diagnosed as malignant melanoma, the nurse most likely would expect to note which of the following?
    1. A small papule with a dry, rough scale
    2. A firm, nodular lesion topped with crust
    3. A pearly papule with a central crater and a waxy border
    4. An irregularly shaped lesion

26. The nurse prepares discharge instructions for a client following cryosurgery for the treatment of a

malignant skin lesion. Which of the following would the nurse include in the plan of care?
1. To clean the site with hydrogen peroxide to prevent infection
2. To apply ice to the site to prevent discomfort
3. To apply alcohol-soaked dressings twice a day
4. To avoid showering for 7 to 10 days

27. The health education nurse provides instructions to a group of clients regarding measures that will assist in preventing skin cancer. Which statement if made by a client indicates a need for further education?
1. "I will use sunscreen when participating in outdoor activities."
2. "I will examine my body monthly for any lesions that may be suspicious."
3. "I will wear a hat, opaque clothing, and sunglasses when in the sun."
4. "I will avoid sun exposure after 3 PM."

28. The clinic nurse reviews the client's chart and notes that the physician has documented a diagnosis of paronychia. Based on this diagnosis, which of the following would the nurse expect to note during the assessment?
1. Swelling of the skin near the parotid gland
2. Red, shiny skin around the nailbed
3. White, silvery patches on the elbows
4. White, taut skin in the popliteal area

29. The nurse provides home care instructions to a client diagnosed with impetigo. Which statement by the client indicates the need for further instructions?
1. "I need to continue with the antibiotics as prescribed."
2. "I should wash my dishes separately from those of other household members."
3. "It is not necessary to separate my linen and towels from other household members."
4. "I need to wash my hands thoroughly and frequently throughout the day."

30. The client arrives at the emergency room and has experienced frostbite to the right hand. Which of the following would the nurse note on assessment of the client's hand?
1. A fiery red skin with edema in the nailbeds
2. A pink, edematous hand
3. Black fingertips surrounded by an erythematous rash
4. A white color to the skin, which is insensitive to touch

31. The nurse prepares to treat a client with frostbite of the toes. Which of the following does the nurse anticipate to be prescribed for this condition?
1. Rapid and continuous rewarming of the toes in a warm water bath until flushing of the skin occurs
2. Rapid and continuous rewarming of the toes in hot water for 15 to 20 minutes
3. Rapid and continuous rewarming of the toes after flushing returns

4. Rapid and continuous rewarming of the toes in cold water for 45 minutes

32. The evening nurse reviews the nursing documentation in the client's chart and notes that the day nurse has documented that the client has a stage 2 pressure ulcer (decubitus) in the sacral area. Which of the following would the nurse expect to note on assessment of the client's sacral area?
1. Intact skin
2. Partial-thickness skin loss of the epidermis
3. A deep, craterlike appearance
4. The presence of sinus tracts

33. The nurse is assessing for the presence of cyanosis in a dark-skinned client. The nurse understands that which body area would provide the best assessment?
1. Back of the hands
2. Earlobes
3. Palms of the hands
4. Sacrum

34. Which of the following individuals is least likely to be at risk of developing psoriasis?
1. A 32-year-old African American
2. A client with a family history of the disorder
3. An individual who has experienced a significant amount of emotional distress
4. A woman experiencing menopause

35. Which of the following clients would least likely be at risk of developing skin breakdown?
1. A client who is unable to move about and is confined to bed
2. A client incontinent of urine and feces
3. A client with chronic nutritional deficiencies
4. A client with a lowered mental awareness status

36. The nurse is implementing a teaching plan to a group of adolescents regarding the causes of acne. Which of the following is the most appropriate nursing statement regarding the cause of this disorder?
1. "Acne is caused by eating chocolate."
2. "Acne is caused by oily skin."
3. "The actual cause is not known."
4. "Acne is caused as a result of exposure to heat and humidity."

37. Isotretinoin (Accutane) is prescribed for a client with severe cystic acne. The nurse provides instructions to the client regarding administration of the medication. Which of the following if stated by the client would indicate a need for further teaching regarding this medication?
1. "I need to continue to take my vitamin A supplements."
2. "I need to use emollients and lip balms for my dry skin and lips."
3. "The medication may cause dryness and burning in my eyes."
4. "I will need to return for a blood test to check my triglyceride level."

38. The clinic nurse inspects the skin of a client suspected of having scabies. Which of the following assessment findings would the nurse note if this disorder was present?
    1. The appearance of vesicles or pustules with a thick honey-colored crust
    2. The presence of white patches scattered about the trunk
    3. Multiple straight or wavy, threadlike lines beneath the skin
    4. Patchy hair loss and round red macules with scales
39. The home health nurse visits a client suspected of having scabies. Which of the following precautions will the nurse institute during the assessment of the client?
    1. Wear a mask and gloves.
    2. Wear gloves only.
    3. Wear a gown and gloves.
    4. Avoid touching client's home furnishings.
40. The nurse inspects the oral cavity of a client with candidiasis (thrush). Which of the following would the nurse expect to note?
    1. The presence of numerous small red pinpoint lesions
    2. The presence of blisters
    3. The presence of white patches
    4. The presence of purple-colored patches
41. The client was burned at 7 AM. The client states that before the burn, the body weight was 198 lb (90 kg). The physician has estimated that the total body surface area burned is 83%. Using the Parkland (Baxter) formula, the nurse determines that the total amount of intravenous lactated Ringer's solution that the client will receive by 3 PM of the same day that the burn occurred is which of the following?
    1. 3735 mL
    2. 7470 mL
    3. 14,940 mL
    4. 29,880 mL
42. The nurse is preparing to care for a burn client scheduled for an escharotomy procedure being performed for a third-degree circumferential arm burn. The nurse understands that the anticipated therapeutic outcome of the escharotomy is
    1. Brisk bleeding from the site.
    2. Formation of granulation tissue.
    3. Decreasing edema formation.
    4. Return of distal pulses.
43. The client sustained a burn from cutaneous exposure to lye. At the site of injury, copious irrigation to the site was performed for 1 hour. On admission to the emergency department, the nurse assesses the burn site and determines that the presence of which of the following indicates that the chemical burn process is continuing?
    1. Eschar
    2. Liquefaction necrosis

    3. Cherry red, firm tissue
    4. Intact blisters
44. The client is undergoing radiation therapy to treat lung cancer. Following the treatment, the nurse notes erythema on the client's chest and neck, and the client is complaining of pain at the radiation site. The nurse interprets this assessment data as
    1. A superficial injury to tissue from the radiation
    2. An allergic reaction to the radiation
    3. A cutaneous reaction to products formed by the of lysis of the neoplastic cells
    4. An ischemic injury, much like decubitus formation, caused by pressure from the linear accelerator
45. The nurse is caring for a client who sustained second- and third-degree burns on the anterior lower legs and anterior thorax. Which of the following does the nurse expect to note during the emergent phase of the burn injury?
    1. Decreased heart rate
    2. Increased blood pressure
    3. Elevated hematocrit levels
    4. Increased urinary output
46. The nurse is caring for a client who suffered an inhalation injury from a wood stove. The carbon monoxide blood report reveals a level of 12%. Based on this level, the nurse would anticipate which of the following signs in the client?
    1. Flushing
    2. Dizziness
    3. Tachycardia
    4. Coma
47. The client arrives at the emergency room following a burn injury that occurred in the basement at home. An inhalation injury is suspected. Which of the following would the nurse anticipate to prescribed for the client?
    1. 100% oxygen via an aerosol mask
    2. Oxygen via nasal cannula at 15 L/min
    3. 100% oxygen via a tight-fitting, non-rebreather face mask
    4. Oxygen via nasal cannula at 10 L/min
48. The nurse is administering fluids intravenously as prescribed to a client who sustained second- and third-degree burn injuries of the back and legs. In evaluating the adequacy of fluid resuscitation, the nurse understands that which of the following would provide the most reliable indicator for determining the adequacy?
    1. Vital signs
    2. Urine output
    3. Peripheral pulses
    4. Mental status
49. The nurse manager is observing a new nursing graduate caring for a burn client in protective isolation. The nurse manager intervenes if the new nursing graduate planned to implement which incorrect component of protective isolation technique?

1. Using sterile sheets and linens
2. Performing strict hand-washing technique
3. Wearing gloves and a gown only when giving direct care to the client
4. Wearing protective garb, including a mask, gloves, cap, shoe covers, scrub clothes, and plastic aprons

50. The nurse is caring for a client following an autograft and grafting to a burn wound on the right knee. Which of the following would the nurse anticipate to be prescribed for the client?
   1. Immobilization of the affected leg
   2. Out of bed
   3. Placing the affected leg in a dependent position
   4. Bathroom privileges

CRITICAL THINKING: FILL IN THE BLANK

The adult client was burned as a result of an explosion. The burn initially affected the client's entire face (anterior half of the head), and the upper half of the anterior torso, and there were circumferential burns to the lower half of both of the arms. The client's clothes caught on fire, and the client ran, causing subsequent burn injuries to the posterior surface of the head and the upper half of the posterior torso. Using the rule of nines, what would be the extent of the burn injury?

Answer: _____

ANSWERS

1. 3
Rationale: Prolonged exposure to the sun, unusual cold, or other conditions can damage the skin. The outdoor construction worker would fit into a high-risk category for the development of an integumentary disorder. Immobility and lack of nutrition would increase the older person's risk but the older client is not at as high a risk as the outdoor construction worker. An adolescent may be prone to the development of acne, but this does not occur in all adolescents. The physical education teacher is at low or no risk of developing an integumentary problem.
Test-Taking Strategy: Use the process of elimination. Note the key words "greatest risk." Eliminate option 4 first. Eliminate options 1 and 2 next because not all older clients or adolescents are at risk for the development of integumentary disorders. Noting the key word "outdoor" in option 3 should direct you easily to this option. If you had difficulty with this question, review the risk factors associated with integumentary disorders.
Level of Cognitive Ability: Analysis
Client Needs: Health Promotion and Maintenance
Integrated Process: Nursing Process—assessment
Content Area: Adult health—integumentary
Reference: Lewis, S., Heitkemper, M., & Dirksen, S. (2004). *Medical-surgical nursing: Assessment and management of clinical problems* (6th ed., p. 487). St. Louis: Mosby.

2. 3
Rationale: Depending on the size and location of the lesion, a biopsy is usually a quick and almost painless procedure. The most common source of pain is the initial local anesthetic, which can produce a burning or stinging sensation. Preoperative medication is not necessary with this procedure.
Test-Taking Strategy: Use the process of elimination. Eliminate option 1 first because of the words "no pain." Eliminate option 2 because this option addresses postprocedure, which is not the issue of the client's question to the nurse. Eliminate option 4 because a preoperative medication that puts the client to sleep is not a part of the procedure for a skin biopsy. If you had difficulty with this question, review the procedure related to a skin biopsy.
Level of Cognitive Ability: Application
Client Needs: Psychosocial Integrity

Integrated Process: Caring
Content Area: Adult health—integumentary
Reference: Ignatavicius, D., & Workman, M. (2002). *Medical-surgical nursing: Critical thinking for collaborative care* (4th ed., p. 1512). Philadelphia: W. B. Saunders.

3. 4
Rationale: Following a skin biopsy, the nurse instructs the client to keep the dressing dry and in place for a minimum of 8 hours. After the dressing is removed, the site is cleaned once a day with tap water or saline to remove any dry blood or crusts. The physician may prescribe an antibiotic ointment to minimize local bacterial colonization. The nurse instructs the client to report any redness or excessive drainage at the site. Sutures usually are removed 7 to 10 days after biopsy.
Test-Taking Strategy: Use the process of elimination. Note the key words "indicate a need for further instruction." Eliminate option 3 first because of the words "as prescribed." Eliminate options 1 and 2 next. A client needs to report signs of drainage and needs to return to the physician for follow-up and suture removal. Consider the alteration in skin integrity that occurs with a skin biopsy. This should assist in directing you to option 4. Review care to the client following this procedure if you had difficulty with this question.
Level of Cognitive Ability: Analysis
Client Needs: Health Promotion and Maintenance
Integrated Process: Teaching/Learning
Content Area: Adult health—integumentary
Reference: Ignatavicius, D., & Workman, M. (2002). *Medical-surgical nursing: Critical thinking for collaborative care* (4th ed., p. 1512). Philadelphia: W. B. Saunders.

4. 2
Rationale: Examination of the skin under a Wood's light is always carried out in a darkened room. This is a noninvasive examination; therefore an informed consent is not required. A handheld long wavelength ultraviolet light or Wood's light is used. The skin does not need to be shaved, and a local anesthetic is not necessary. Areas of blue-green or red fluorescence are associated with certain skin infections. The procedure is painless.
Test-Taking Strategy: Use the process of elimination. Knowing that this is a noninvasive procedure will assist in eliminating

options 1, 3, and 4. Review this procedure if you had difficulty answering this question.
Level of Cognitive Ability: Application
Client Needs: Physiological Integrity
Integrated Process: Nursing Process—planning
Content Area: Adult health—integumentary
Reference: Ignatavicius, D., & Workman, M. (2002). *Medical-surgical nursing: Critical thinking for collaborative care* (4th ed., p. 1513). Philadelphia: W. B. Saunders.

5. **3**
Rationale: Client preparation for a scratch skin test includes informing the client to discontinue the administration of systemic corticosteroids or antihistamines for at least 5 days before the test. These medications must be discontinued to prevent suppression of the inflammatory response to the allergen. Topical steroid therapy may be continued as long as the agent is not applied on the area to be tested. There is no need to restrict fluids or to avoid ingesting anything before the procedure. This test does not require a body shower with an antibacterial soap.
Test-Taking Strategy: Use the process of elimination. Eliminate options 1 and 4 first because these options are similar. From the remaining options, note the relationship between "allergen" in the question and "antihistamine" in the correct option. Review client preparation for a scratch test if you had difficulty with this question.
Level of Cognitive Ability: Application
Client Needs: Physiological Integrity
Integrated Process: Teaching/Learning
Content Area: Adult health—integumentary
Reference: Ignatavicius, D., & Workman, M. (2002). *Medical-surgical nursing: Critical thinking for collaborative care* (4th ed., p. 394). Philadelphia: W. B. Saunders.

6. **2**
Rationale: If the client reapplies patches that come loose, this can interfere with an accurate interpretation of the allergic reactions. The nurse reinforces the necessity of removing loose or nonadherent test patches for reapplication at a later date. The initial reading is performed 2 days after application, and the final reading is performed 2 to 5 days later. The nurse instructs the client to keep the test sites dry at all times. The nurse also discourages excessive physical activity that will result in sweating.
Test-Taking Strategy: Use the process of elimination. Note the key words "the need for further instruction." Eliminate options 3 and 4 first because keeping the test site dry and avoiding sweating are similar. Knowledge that follow-up is important after any procedure should assist in directing you to option 2. If you had difficulty with this question, review the client teaching points following a patch test.
Level of Cognitive Ability: Analysis
Client Needs: Health Promotion and Maintenance
Integrated Process: Teaching/Learning
Content Area: Adult health—integumentary
Reference: Black, J., Hawks, J., & Keene, A. (2001). *Medical-surgical nursing: Clinical management for positive outcomes* (6th ed., p. 1277). Philadelphia: W. B. Saunders.

7. **4**
Rationale: The client should avoid using a dehumidifier because this will dry room air further. Instead, the client should use a room humidifier during the winter months or whenever the furnace is in use. The client should be taught to maintain a daily fluid intake of 3000 mL, unless contraindicated and should avoid alcohol and caffeine ingestion. The client should avoid applying rubbing alcohol, astringents, or other drying agents to the skin. One bath or one shower per day for 15 to 20 minutes with warm water and a mild soap should be followed immediately by the application of an emollient to prevent evaporation of water from the hydrated epidermis.
Test-Taking Strategy: Use the process of elimination. Note the key words "a need for further teaching." Recalling that a dehumidifier is going to dry the air in the environment will assist in directing you to option 4. If you had difficulty with this question, review the client-teaching points related to dry skin and pruritus.
Level of Cognitive Ability: Analysis
Client Needs: Health Promotion and Maintenance
Integrated Process: Teaching/Learning
Content Area: Adult health—integumentary
Reference: Ignatavicius, D., & Workman, M. (2002). *Medical-surgical nursing: Critical thinking for collaborative care* (4th ed., p. 1515). Philadelphia: W. B. Saunders.

8. **4**
Rationale: Lyme disease is a multisystem infection that results from a bite by a tick carried by several species of deer. Persons bitten by the *Ixodes* ticks are infected with the spirochete *Borrelia burgdorferi*. Lyme disease cannot be transmitted from one person to another. Histoplasmosis is caused by the inhalation of spores from bat or bird droppings. Toxoplasmosis is caused from the ingestion of cysts from contaminated cat feces.
Test-Taking Strategy: Use the process of elimination. Recalling that this disease is caused by a bite will assist in eliminating the incorrect options. If you had difficulty with this question, review the cause of Lyme disease.
Level of Cognitive Ability: Application
Client Needs: Health Promotion and Maintenance
Integrated Process: Teaching/Learning
Content Area: Adult health—integumentary
Reference: Lewis, S., Heitkemper, M., & Dirksen, S. (2004). *Medical-surgical nursing: Assessment and management of clinical problems* (6th ed., p. 1736). St. Louis: Mosby.

9. **4**
Rationale: The hallmark of stage I is the development of a skin rash within 2 to 30 days of infection, generally at the site of the tick bite. The rash develops into a concentric ring, giving it a bull's-eye appearance. The lesion enlarges up to 50 to 60 cm, and smaller lesions develop farther away from the original tick bite. In stage I, most infected persons develop flulike symptoms that last 7 to 10 days; these symptoms may reoccur later. Neurological deficits occur in stage II. Arthralgias and joint enlargements are most likely to occur in stage III.
Test-Taking Strategy: Use the process of elimination and eliminate options 2 and 3 first because they are similar. Next, note

that the question asks for the characteristic of stage I. From the remaining two options, select the least serious one because the issue of the question relates to stage I. Expect neurological disorders to occur with progression of the disease. If you had difficulty with this question, review the stages of Lyme disease.
Level of Cognitive Ability: Analysis
Client Needs: Physiological Integrity
Integrated Process: Nursing Process—assessment
Content Area: Adult health—integumentary
Reference: Ignatavicius, D., & Workman, M. (2002). *Medical-surgical nursing: Critical thinking for collaborative care* (4th ed., p. 361). Philadelphia: W. B. Saunders.

10. **3**
Rationale: A blood test is available to detect Lyme disease; however, the test is not reliable if performed before 4 to 6 weeks following the tick bite. Antibody formation takes place in the following manner: immunoglobulin M is detected 3 to 4 weeks after Lyme disease onset, peaks at 6 to 8 weeks, and then gradually disappears; immunoglobulin G is detected 2 to 3 months after infection and may remain elevated for years. Options 1, 2, and 4 are incorrect.
Test-Taking Strategy: Use the process of elimination. Eliminate option 1 first. The word "immediately" should indicate that this is potentially an incorrect option. A blood test is available; therefore eliminate option 2. Eliminate option 4 because treatment should begin before the arthralgia develops. If you had difficulty with this question, review the method of diagnosing Lyme disease.
Level of Cognitive Ability: Application
Client Needs: Physiological Integrity
Integrated Process: Nursing Process—implementation
Content Area: Adult health—integumentary
Reference: Ignatavicius, D., & Workman, M. (2002). *Medical-surgical nursing: Critical thinking for collaborative care* (4th ed., p. 361). Philadelphia: W. B. Saunders.

11. **2**
Rationale: Prevention, public education, and early diagnosis are vital to the control and treatment of Lyme disease. A 3-week course of oral antibiotic therapy is recommended during stage I. Later stages of Lyme disease may require therapy with intravenously administered antibiotics, such as penicillin G. Options 1 and 4 are incorrect.
Test-Taking Strategy: Use the process of elimination. Note that the question addresses stage I. Eliminate option 3 because intravenous antibiotics will not be administered in this stage. Eliminate option 4, because although oatmeal baths **may** be helpful for pruritus, they would not be helpful for a systemic disorder. Waiting for symptoms to develop is an incorrect option. Review the treatment associated with Lyme disease if you had difficulty with this question.
Level of Cognitive Ability: Analysis
Client Needs: Physiological Integrity
Integrated Process: Nursing Process—planning
Content Area: Adult health—integumentary
Reference: Ignatavicius, D., & Workman, M. (2002). *Medical-surgical nursing: Critical thinking for collaborative care* (4th ed., p. 361). Philadelphia: W. B. Saunders.

12. **1**
Rationale: In the prevention of Lyme disease, individuals need to be instructed to use an insect repellent on the skin and clothes when in an area where ticks are likely to be found. Long-sleeve tops and long pants, closed shoes, and a hat or cap should be worn. If possible, one should avoid heavily wooded areas or areas with thick underbrush. Socks can be pulled up and over the pant legs to the prevent ticks from entering under clothing.
Test-Taking Strategy: Use the process of elimination. Note the key words "need for further instructions." Note that option 1 uses the words "should not." Reading carefully will assist in directing you to this option. If you had difficulty with this question, review the measures to prevent contact with ticks.
Level of Cognitive Ability: Analysis
Client Needs: Safe, Effective Care Environment
Integrated Process: Teaching/Learning
Content Area: Adult health—integumentary
Reference: Ignatavicius, D., & Workman, M. (2002). *Medical-surgical nursing: Critical thinking for collaborative care* (4th ed., p. 361). Philadelphia: W. B. Saunders.

13. **3**
Rationale: When an individual comes in contact with a poison ivy plant, the sap from the plant forms an invisible film on the human skin. The client should be instructed to shower immediately and to lather the skin several times and rinse each time in running water. Calamine lotion is a treatment used if dermatitis develops. The client does not need to be seen in the emergency room at this time.
Test-Taking Strategy: Use the process of elimination. Recalling that dermatitis can develop from contact with an allergen and that contact with poison ivy results in an invisible film will assist in directing you to option 3. Review the immediate treatment for contact with poison ivy, if you had difficulty with this question.
Level of Cognitive Ability: Application
Client Needs: Physiological Integrity
Integrated Process: Nursing Process—implementation
Content Area: Adult health—integumentary
Reference: Phipps, W., Monahan, F., Sands, J., Marek, J., & Neighbors, M. (2003). *Medical-surgical nursing: Health and illness perspectives* (7th ed., p.1957). St. Louis: Mosby.

14. **3**
Rationale: Kaposi's sarcoma lesions begin as red, dark blue, or purple macules on the lower legs that change into plaques. These large plaques ulcerate or open and drain. The lesions spread by metastasis through the upper body and then to the face and oral mucosa. They can move to the lymphatic system, lungs, and gastrointestinal tract. Late disease results in swelling and pain in the lower extremities, penis, scrotum, or face. Diagnosis is made by punch biopsy of cutaneous lesions and biopsy of pulmonary and gastrointestinal lesions.
Test-Taking Strategy: Use the process of elimination. Eliminate options 2 and 4 first because these symptoms occur late in the development of Kaposi's sarcoma. From the remaining options, note the key word "confirmed." This key word will assist in directing you to the option that will confirm the diagnosis,

the biopsy of the lesions. Review diagnostic measures for Kaposi's sarcoma if you had difficulty with this question.
Level of Cognitive Ability: Analysis
Client Needs: Physiological Integrity
Integrated Process: Nursing Process—assessment
Content Area: Adult health—integumentary
Reference: Phipps, W., Monahan, F., Sands, J., Marek, J., & Neighbors, M. (2003). *Medical-surgical nursing: Health and illness perspectives* (7th ed., p. 1684). St. Louis: Mosby.

15. **4**
Rationale: Kaposi's sarcoma is a vascular malignancy that presents as a skin disorder and is a common acquired immunodeficiency syndrome indicator. Malignancy is seen most frequently in men with a history of same-sex partners. Although the cause of Kaposi's sarcoma is not known, it is considered to be due to an alteration or failure in the immune system. The renal transplant client and the client receiving antineoplastic medications are at risk for immunosuppression. Exposure to asbestos is not related to the development of Kaposi's sarcoma.
Test-Taking Strategy: Use the process of elimination. Note the key words "least likely at risk." Option 1 can be eliminated easily. Note the similarity between options 2 and 3. These clients are at risk for immunosuppression. With this in mind, these options can be eliminated. If you had difficulty with this question, review the risk factors associated with Kaposi's sarcoma.
Level of Cognitive Ability: Analysis
Client Needs: Physiological Integrity
Integrated Process: Nursing Process—assessment
Content Area: Adult health—integumentary
Reference: Phipps, W., Monahan, F., Sands, J., Marek, J., & Neighbors, M. (2003). *Medical-surgical nursing: Health and illness perspectives* (7th ed., p. 1684). St. Louis: Mosby.

16. **2**
Rationale: Gowns and gloves are required if the nurse anticipates contact with soiled items such as wound drainage or in caring for a client who is incontinent with diarrhea or a client who has an ileostomy or colostomy. Masks are not required unless droplet or airborne precautions are necessary. Regardless of the amount of wound drainage, a gown and gloves must be worn.
Test-Taking Strategy: Use the process of elimination and think about the method of transmission of infection when answering a question of this type. Read the question, noting the task that is presented; in this case, it is bathing and changing linens. Eliminate option 1 because the method of transmission is not respiratory. Eliminate options 3 and 4 because neither provide adequate protection based on the method of transmission. If you had difficulty with this question, review standard and transmission-based precautions.
Level of Cognitive Ability: Application
Client Needs: Safe, Effective Care Environment
Integrated Process: Nursing Process—planning
Content Area: Adult health—integumentary
Reference: Potter, P., & Perry, A. (2001). *Fundamentals of nursing* (5th ed., pp. 858-859). St. Louis: Mosby.

17. **1**
Rationale: Cellulitis is a skin infection into deeper dermis and subcutaneous tissue that results in a deep red erythema

without sharp borders and spreads widely through tissue spaces. The skin is erythematous, edematous, tender, and sometimes nodular. Erysipelas is an acute, superficial, rapidly spreading inflammation of the dermis and lymphatics.
Test-Taking Strategy: Use the process of elimination. Eliminate options 2, 3, and 4 because they are similar. If you had difficulty with this question, review the characteristics of cellulitis and erysipelas.
Level of Cognitive Ability: Comprehension
Client Needs: Physiological Integrity
Integrated Process: Nursing Process—planning
Content Area: Adult health—integumentary
Reference: Lewis, S., Heitkemper, M., & Dirksen, S. (2004). *Medical-surgical nursing: Assessment and management of clinical problems* (6th ed., p. 494). St. Louis: Mosby.

18. **1**
Rationale: Warm compresses may be used to decrease the discomfort, erythema, and edema. After tissue and blood cultures are obtained, antibiotics will be initiated. The nurse should provide supportive care as prescribed to manage symptoms such as fatigue, fever, chills, headache, and myalgia. Heat lamps can cause more disruption to already inflamed tissue. Cold compresses and alternating cold and hot compresses are not the best measures.
Test-Taking Strategy: Use the process of elimination noting that option 1 is different from the other options. The words *cold, heat,* and *hot* identify extremes in temperature. If you had difficulty with this question, review the treatment associated with cellulitis.
Level of Cognitive Ability: Analysis
Client Needs: Physiological Integrity
Integrated Process: Nursing Process—planning
Content Area: Adult health—integumentary
Reference: Lewis, S., Heitkemper, M., & Dirksen, S. (2004). *Medical-surgical nursing: Assessment and management of clinical problems* (6th ed., p. 494). St. Louis: Mosby.

19. **2**
Rationale: Psoriatic patches are covered with silvery white scales. Affected areas include the scalp, elbows, knees, shins, sacral area, and trunk. Thickening, pitting, and discoloration of the nails occurs. Pruritus may occur. The lesions in psoriasis are not red, purplish scaly lesions.
Test-Taking Strategy: Use the process of elimination. Recalling that psoriasis is associated with the presence of silvery white, scaly patches will direct you easily to option 2. If you had difficulty with this question, review the manifestations associated with psoriasis.
Level of Cognitive Ability: Comprehension
Client Needs: Physiological Integrity
Integrated Process: Nursing Process—assessment
Content Area: Adult health—integumentary
Reference: Lewis, S., Heitkemper, M., & Dirksen, S. (2004). *Medical-surgical nursing: Assessment and management of clinical problems* (6th ed., p. 506). St. Louis: Mosby.

20. **3**
Rationale: Ultraviolet light (UVL) treatments are limited to 2 to 3 times a week and are not given on consecutive days.

Safety precautions are required during UVL therapy. Exposure of only those areas requiring treatment to the UVL is best. Protective wraparound goggles prevent exposure of the eyes to UVL. The face should be shielded with a loosely applied pillow case if it is unaffected. Direct contact with the light bulbs of the treatment unit should be avoided to prevent burning of the skin.
Test-Taking Strategy: Use the process of elimination. Note the key words "indicates a need for further instructions." Recalling that safety precautions are necessary for this treatment and noting the words "given on consecutive days" will direct you to this option. If you had difficulty with this question, review client education for UVL treatments.
Level of Cognitive Ability: Analysis
Client Needs: Health Promotion and Maintenance
Integrated Process: Teaching/Learning
Content Area: Adult health—integumentary
Reference: Ignatavicius, D., & Workman, M. (2002). *Medical-surgical nursing: Critical thinking for collaborative care* (4th ed., p. 1543). Philadelphia: W. B. Saunders.

21. 3
Rationale: With classic presentation of herpes zoster, the clinical examination is diagnostic. A viral culture of the lesion provides the definitive diagnosis. Herpes zoster (shingles) is caused by a reactivation of the varicella-zoster virus, the cause of the virus for chickenpox. A biopsy would provide a cytological examination of tissue. In a Wood's light examination, the skin is viewed under ultraviolet light to identify superficial infections of the skin. A patch test is a skin test that involves the administration of an allergen to the surface of the skin to identify specific allergies.
Test-Taking Strategy: Use the process of elimination. Recalling that herpes zoster is caused by a virus will assist in directing you to the correct option. Remember that a biopsy will determine tissue type, whereas a culture will identify an organism. Review the diagnostic measures for herpes zoster (shingles) if you had difficulty with this question.
Level of Cognitive Ability: Comprehension
Client Needs: Physiological Integrity
Integrated Process: Nursing Process—assessment
Content Area: Adult health—integumentary
Reference: Black, J., Hawks, J., & Keene, A. (2001). *Medical-surgical nursing: Clinical management for positive outcomes* (6th ed., p. 1312). Philadelphia: W. B. Saunders.

22. 4
Rationale: The primary lesion of herpes zoster is a vesicle. The classic presentation is grouped vesicles on an erythematous base along a dermatome. Because the lesions follow nerve pathways, they do not cross the midline of the body. Options 1, 2, and 3 are incorrect descriptions of herpes zoster.
Test-Taking Strategy: Use the process of elimination. Remembering that these lesions occur as grouped vesicles along a nerve pathway will assist in answering the question. If you had difficulty with this question, review the characteristics of herpes zoster lesions.
Level of Cognitive Ability: Comprehension
Client Needs: Physiological Integrity
Integrated Process: Nursing Process—assessment

Content Area: Adult health—integumentary
Reference: Lewis, S., Heitkemper, M., & Dirksen, S. (2004). *Medical-surgical nursing: Assessment and management of clinical problems* (6th ed., p. 496). St. Louis: Mosby.

23. 2
Rationale: Herpes zoster (shingles) is caused by a reactivation of the varicella-zoster virus, the causative virus for chickenpox. Individuals who have not been exposed to the varicella-zoster virus are susceptible to chickenpox. Health care workers who are unsure of their immune status should have varicella titers done before exposure to a person with herpes zoster. Options 1, 3, and 4 are unrelated to the herpes zoster virus.
Test-Taking Strategy: Use the process of elimination. Recalling that herpes zoster is caused by a reactivation of the varicella-zoster virus, the causative virus for chickenpox, will direct you to the correct option. Review the relationship between herpes zoster virus and chickenpox if you had difficulty with this question.
Level of Cognitive Ability: Application
Client Needs: Safe, Effective Care Environment
Integrated Process: Nursing Process—planning
Content Area: Adult health—integumentary
Reference: Lewis, S., Heitkemper, M., & Dirksen, S. (2004). *Medical-surgical nursing: Assessment and management of clinical problems* (6th ed., p. 496). St. Louis: Mosby.

24. 1
Rationale: Melanomas are pigmented, malignant lesions originating in the melanin-producing cells of the epidermis. This skin cancer is highly metastatic, and a person's survival depends on early diagnosis and treatment. Options 2, 3, and 4 are not characteristics of a melanoma.
Test-Taking Strategy: Use the process of elimination. Note the similarity between options 2, 3, and 4. Also, recalling that melanomas are highly metastatic will assist in directing you to the correct option. If you had difficulty with this question, review the characteristics of skin cancers.
Level of Cognitive Ability: Comprehension
Client Needs: Physiological Integrity
Integrated Process: Nursing Process—assessment
Content Area: Adult health—integumentary
Reference: Ignatavicius, D., & Workman, M. (2002). *Medical-surgical nursing: Critical thinking for collaborative care* (4th ed., p. 1546). Philadelphia: W. B. Saunders.

25. 4
Rationale: A melanoma is a irregularly shaped, pigmented papule or plaque with a red-, white-, or blue-toned color. Basal cell carcinoma appears as a pearly papule with a central crater and rolled waxy border. Squamous cell carcinoma is a firm, nodular lesion topped with a crust or a central area of ulceration. Actinic keratosis, a premalignant lesion, appears as a small macule or papule with a dry, rough, adherent yellow, or brown scale.
Test-Taking Strategy: Use the process of elimination. Remembering that irregularly shaped lesions are a cause for concern will assist in directing you to option 4. If you had difficulty with this question, review the characteristics of malignant skin lesions.

Level of Cognitive Ability: Comprehension
Client Needs: Physiological Integrity
Integrated Process: Nursing Process—assessment
Content Area: Adult health—integumentary
Reference: Lewis, S., Heitkemper, M., & Dirksen, S. (2004). *Medical-surgical nursing: Assessment and management of clinical problems* (6th ed., p. 492). St. Louis: Mosby.

26. **1**

Rationale: Cryosurgery involves the local application of liquid nitrogen to isolated lesions and causes cell death and tissue destruction. The nurse prepares the client for swelling and increased tenderness of the treated area when the skin thaws. Tissue freezing is followed by hemorrhagic blister formation in 1 to 2 days. The nurse instructs the client to clean the treatment site with hydrogen peroxide to prevent secondary infection. A topical antibiotic also may be prescribed. Application of a warm, damp wash cloth intermittently to the site will provide relief from any discomfort. Alcohol-soaked dressings will cause irritation. The client does not need to avoid showering.

Test-Taking Strategy: Use the process of elimination. Eliminate option 4 first because there is no reason for the client to avoid showers. Eliminate option 3 next because alcohol-soaked dressings will cause irritation. From the remaining options, note that option 1 addresses the prevention of infection. Therefore this is the best option to select. If you had difficulty with this question, review client education following cryosurgery.

Level of Cognitive Ability: Application
Client Needs: Health Promotion and Maintenance
Integrated Process: Teaching/Learning
Content Area: Adult health—integumentary
Reference: Ignatavicius, D., & Workman, M. (2002). *Medical-surgical nursing: Critical thinking for collaborative care* (4th ed., p. 1547). Philadelphia: W. B. Saunders.

27. **4**

Rationale: The client should be instructed to avoid sun exposure between the hours of 11 AM and 3 PM. Sunscreen, a hat, opaque clothing, and sunglasses should be worn for outdoor activities. The client should be instructed to examine the body monthly for the appearance of any possible cancerous or any precancerous lesions.

Test-Taking Strategy: Use the process of elimination. Note the key words "a need for further education." Note the key word "avoid" in option 4 to assist in directing you to this option. Review client education in the prevention of skin cancer if you had difficulty with this question.

Level of Cognitive Ability: Analysis
Client Needs: Health Promotion and Maintenance
Integrated Process: Teaching/Learning
Content Area: Adult health—integumentary
References: Ignatavicius, D., & Workman, M. (2002). *Medical-surgical nursing: Critical thinking for collaborative care* (4th ed., p. 1548). Philadelphia: W. B. Saunders.
Lewis, S., Heitkemper, M., & Dirksen, S. (2004). *Medical-surgical nursing: Assessment and management of clinical problems* (6th ed., p. 490). St. Louis: Mosby.

28. **2**

Rationale: Paronychia, or infection around the nail, is characterized by red, shiny skin, often associated with painful swelling. These infections frequently result from trauma, picking at the nail, or disorders such as dermatitis. Often these become secondarily infected with bacteria or fungus, which later involves the nail. Warm soaks 3 to 4 times a day may reduce pain and pressure; however, incision and drainage of the inflamed site frequently is required. Options 1, 3, and 4 are incorrect.

Test-Taking Strategy: Use the process of elimination. Recalling that this disorder relates to an infection of the nail will direct you easily to the correct option. If you had difficulty with this question, review the definition of this disorder.

Level of Cognitive Ability: Comprehension
Client Needs: Physiological Integrity
Integrated Process: Nursing Process—assessment
Content Area: Adult health—integumentary
Reference: Phipps, W., Monahan, F., Sands, J., Marek, J., & Neighbors, M. (2003). *Medical-surgical nursing: Health and illness perspectives* (7th ed., p. 1940). St. Louis: Mosby.

29. **3**

Rationale: The client needs to separate his or her linen and towels from other household members. Thorough hand washing, separating linens and towels, and separating washing of the client's dishes is required because the infection is contagious as long as skin lesions are present. Antibiotics are administered and should be continued as prescribed.

Test-Taking Strategy: Use the process of elimination. Note the key words "need for further instructions." Recalling that the infection is contagious as long as skin lesions are present will direct you to the correct option. If you had difficulty with this question, review client teaching related to home care and the prevention of transmission.

Level of Cognitive Ability: Analysis
Client Needs: Safe, Effective Care Environment
Integrated Process: Teaching/Learning
Content Area: Adult health—integumentary
Reference: Phipps, W., Monahan, F., Sands, J., Marek, J., & Neighbors, M. (2003). *Medical-surgical nursing: Health and illness perspectives* (7th ed., p. 1951). St. Louis: Mosby.

30. **4**

Rationale: Assessment findings in frostbite include a white or blue color; the skin will be hard, cold, and insensitive to touch. As thawing occurs, flushing of the skin, the development of blisters or blebs, or tissue edema appears. Options 1, 2, and 3 are incorrect.

Test-Taking Strategy: Use the process of elimination. Noting the key words "insensitive to touch" in option 4 should direct you to this option. If you had difficulty with this question, review the characteristics associated with frostbite.

Level of Cognitive Ability: Comprehension
Client Needs: Physiological Integrity
Integrated Process: Nursing Process—assessment
Content Area: Adult health—integumentary
Reference: Lewis, S., Heitkemper, M., & Dirksen, S. (2004). *Medical-surgical nursing: Assessment and management of clinical problems* (6th ed., p. 1854). St. Louis: Mosby.

31. **1**

Rationale: Acute frostbite is treated ideally with rapid and continuous rewarming of the tissue in a warm water bath for 15 to 20 minutes or until flushing of the skin occurs. Slow thawing or interrupted periods of warmth are avoided because this can contribute to increased cellular damage. Cold or hot water is not used. Thawing can cause considerable pain, and the nurse administers analgesics as prescribed.

Test-Taking Strategy: Use the process of elimination. Eliminate options 2 and 4 because of the words "hot" and "cold." Eliminate option 3 because intervention would begin immediately. If you had difficulty with this question, review the interventions associated with frostbite.

Level of Cognitive Ability: Comprehension
Client Needs: Physiological Integrity
Integrated Process: Nursing Process—planning
Content Area: Adult health—integumentary
Reference: Lewis, S., Heitkemper, M., & Dirksen, S. (2004). *Medical-surgical nursing: Assessment and management of clinical problems* (6th ed., p. 1854). St. Louis: Mosby.

32. **2**

Rationale: In a stage 2 pressure ulcer the skin is not intact. Partial-thickness skin loss of the epidermis or dermis has occurred. The ulcer is superficial and may be characterized as an abrasion, blister, or shallow crater. The skin is intact in stage 1. A deep craterlike appearance occurs in stage 3, and sinus tracts develop in stage 4.

Test-Taking Strategy: Use the process of elimination. Focus on the key words "stage 2." If you had difficulty with this question, review the characteristics associated with each stage of pressure ulcers.

Level of Cognitive Ability: Comprehension
Client Needs: Physiological Integrity
Integrated Process: Nursing Process—assessment
Content Area: Adult health—integumentary
References: Lewis, S., Heitkemper, M., & Dirksen, S. (2004). *Medical-surgical nursing: Assessment and management of clinical problems* (6th ed., p. 226). St. Louis: Mosby.
Phipps, W., Monahan, F., Sands, J., Marek, J., & Neighbors, M. (2003). *Medical-surgical nursing: Health and illness perspectives* (7th ed., p. 1974). St. Louis: Mosby.

33. **3**

Rationale: In a dark-skinned client, the nurse examines the lips, tongue, nailbeds, conjunctiva, and palms of the hands and soles of the feet at regular intervals for subtle color changes. In a client with cyanosis, the lips and tongue are gray; the palms, soles, conjunctiva, and nailbeds have a bluish tinge.

Test-Taking Strategy: Use the process of elimination focusing on the issue, cyanosis in a dark-skinned client. Attempt to visualize assessment of the areas identified in each option to assist in directing you to option 3. Review this important assessment technique if you had difficulty with this question.

Level of Cognitive Ability: Comprehension
Client Needs: Physiological Integrity
Integrated Process: Nursing Process—assessment
Content Area: Adult health—integumentary

Reference: Phipps, W., Monahan, F., Sands, J., Marek, J., & Neighbors, M. (2003). *Medical-surgical nursing: Health and illness perspectives* (7th ed., p. 1938). St. Louis: Mosby.

34. **1**

Rationale: Psoriasis occurs equally among women and men, although the incidence is lower in darker-skinned races. A genetic predisposition has been recognized in some cases. Emotional distress, trauma, systemic illness, seasonal changes, and hormonal changes are linked to exacerbations.

Test-Taking Strategy: Note the key words "least likely." Use the process of elimination and knowledge regarding what psoriasis is and the risk factors associated with the disorder to answer the question. If you had difficulty with the question, review the risk factors of the disorder and the factors that affect exacerbations.

Level of Cognitive Ability: Analysis
Client Needs: Health Promotion and Maintenance
Integrated Process: Nursing Process—assessment
Content Area: Adult health—integumentary
Reference: Phipps, W., Monahan, F., Sands, J., Marek, J., & Neighbors, M. (2003). *Medical-surgical nursing: Health and illness perspectives* (7th ed., p. 1962). St. Louis: Mosby.

35. **4**

Rationale: Bed or chair confinement, inability to move, loss of bowel or bladder control, poor nutrition, absent or inconsistent caregiving, and a lowered mental awareness can contribute to the development of skin breakdown. The least likely risk, as presented in the options, is the lowered mental awareness status. Options 1, 2, and 3 identify physiological conditions, which are the risk priorities.

Test-Taking Strategy: Note the key words "least likely." Use Maslow's hierarchy of needs theory to answer the question. Remember that physiological needs are the priority. This will assist you in eliminating options 1, 2, and 3. Review the risk factors associated with skin breakdown if you had difficulty with this question.

Level of Cognitive Ability: Analysis
Client Needs: Physiological Integrity
Integrated Process: Nursing Process—assessment
Content Area: Delegating/Prioritizing
Reference: Potter, P., & Perry, A. (2001). *Fundamentals of nursing* (5th ed., p. 1547). St. Louis: Mosby.

36. **3**

Rationale: The actual cause of acne is unknown. Oily skin or the consumption of foods such as chocolate, nuts, or fatty foods are not causes of acne. Exacerbations that coincide with the menstrual cycle result from hormonal activity. Heat, humidity, and excessive perspiration may play a role in exacerbating acne but does not cause it.

Test-Taking Strategy: Use the process of elimination. Note that the question asks for the "cause" of acne. Options 1, 2, and 4 relate specifically to factors that exacerbate acne. Review the cause of and factors that exacerbate acne, if you had difficulty with this question.

Level of Cognitive Ability: Comprehension
Client Needs: Health Promotion and Maintenance

Integrated Process: Teaching/Learning
Content Area: Adult health—integumentary
Reference: Phipps, W., Monahan, F., Sands, J., Marek, J., & Neighbors, M. (2003). *Medical-surgical nursing: Health and illness perspectives* (7th ed., p. 1954). St. Louis: Mosby.

37. 1
Rationale: In severe cystic acne, isotretinoin (Accutane) is used to inhibit inflammation. Adverse effects include elevated triglycerides, skin dryness, eye discomfort such as dryness and burning, and cheilitis (lip inflammation). Close medical follow-up is required, and dry skin and cheilitis can be decreased by the use of emollients and lip balms. Vitamin A supplements are stopped during this treatment.
Test-Taking Strategy: Use the process of elimination. Note the key words "a need for further teaching." Recalling that vitamin A supplements need to be discontinued during this treatment will direct you to the correct option. If you had difficulty with this question review the action, side effects, and adverse effects related to this medication.
Level of Cognitive Ability: Analysis
Client Needs: Health Promotion and Maintenance
Integrated Process: Teaching/Learning
Content Area: Pharmacology
Reference: Hodgson, B., & Kizior, R. (2004). *Saunders nursing drug handbook 2004* (p. 564). Philadelphia: W. B. Saunders.

38. 3
Rationale: Scabies can be identified by the multiple straight or wavy, threadlike lines noted beneath the skin. The skin lesions are caused by the female mite, which burrows beneath the skin and lays her eggs. The eggs hatch in a few days, and the baby mites find their way to the skin surface, where they mate and complete the life cycle. Options 1, 2, and 4 are not characteristics of scabies.
Test-Taking Strategy: Use the process of elimination. Recalling that scabies burrows beneath the skin surface will provide direction toward selection of the correct option. If you had difficulty with this question, review the characteristics associated with scabies.
Level of Cognitive Ability: Comprehension
Client Needs: Physiological Integrity
Integrated Process: Nursing Process—assessment
Content Area: Adult health—integumentary
Reference: Phipps, W., Monahan, F., Sands, J., Marek, J., & Neighbors, M. (2003). *Medical-surgical nursing: Health and illness perspectives* (7th ed., p. 1947). St. Louis: Mosby.

39. 3
Rationale: The Centers for Disease Control and Prevention recommends the wearing of gowns and gloves for close contact with a person infested with scabies. Masks are not necessary. Transmission via clothing and other inanimate objects is uncommon. Scabies usually is transmitted from person to person by direct skin contact. All contacts that the client has had should be treated at the same time.
Test-Taking Strategy: Consider the mode of transmission of scabies and use the process of elimination. Because scabies is transmitted by direct skin contact, eliminate options 1, 2,

and 4. If you had difficulty with question, review standard precautions and the transmission mode of scabies.
Level of Cognitive Ability: Application
Client Needs: Safe, Effective Care Environment
Integrated Process: Nursing Process—implementation
Content Area: Adult health—integumentary
Reference: Black, J., Hawks, J., & Keene, A. (2001). *Medical-surgical nursing: Clinical management for positive outcomes* (6th ed., p. 1056). Philadelphia: W. B. Saunders.

40. 3
Rationale: Assessment of candidiasis (thrush) reveals white patches on the tongue, palate, and buccal mucosa. The lesions adhere firmly to the tissues and are difficult to remove. The lesions often are referred to as *milk curds* because of their appearance. Clients often describe the lesions as dry and hot. Options 1, 2, and 4 are not characteristics of thrush.
Test-Taking Strategy: Use the process of elimination. Recalling that candidiasis (thrush) presents as white patches will assist you in answering the question. If you had difficulty with this question, review the characteristics associated with candidiasis (thrush).
Level of Cognitive Ability: Comprehension
Client Needs: Physiological Integrity
Integrated Process: Nursing Process—assessment
Content Area: Adult health—integumentary
Reference: Lewis, S., Heitkemper, M., & Dirksen, S. (2004). *Medical-surgical nursing: Assessment and management of clinical problems* (6th ed., p. 1008). St. Louis: Mosby.

41. 3
Rationale: The Parkland (Baxter) formula for estimating fluid requirements is 4 mL × kilograms body mass × percent total body surface area. Half of this total is administered in the first 8 hours following the burn. Therefore, 4 × 90 × 83 = 29,880 mL, divided by 2 = 14,940 mL.
Test-Taking Strategy: Knowledge of the Parkland (Baxter) formula is required to answer the question. Read the question carefully and remember that half of the total is administered in the first 8 hours following the burn. Review this formula if you had difficulty with this question.
Level of Cognitive Ability: Analysis
Client Needs: Physiological Integrity
Integrated Process: Nursing Process—analysis
Content Area: Adult health—integumentary
Reference: Lewis, S., Heitkemper, M., & Dirksen, S. (2004). *Medical-surgical nursing: Assessment and management of clinical problems* (6th ed., pp. 519, 527). St. Louis: Mosby.

42. 4
Rationale: Escharotomies are performed to alleviate the compartment syndrome that can occur when edema forms under nondistensible eschar in a circumferential third-degree burn. Escharotomies are performed through avascular eschar to subcutaneous fat. Although bleeding may occur from the site, it is considered a complication rather that an anticipated therapeutic outcome. Usually direct pressure with a bulky dressing and elevation will control the bleeding, but occasionally an artery is damaged and may require ligation. Formation of

granulation tissue is not the intent of an escharotomy. Escharotomy will not affect the formation of edema.
Test-Taking Strategy: Use the ABCs—airway, breathing, and circulation—to answer the question. The only option that addresses circulation is option 4. If you had difficulty with this question, review the purpose of an escharotomy.
Level of Cognitive Ability: Analysis
Client Needs: Physiological Integrity
Integrated Process: Nursing Process—evaluation
Content Area: Adult health—integumentary
Reference: Lewis, S., Heitkemper, M., & Dirksen, S. (2004). *Medical-surgical nursing: Assessment and management of clinical problems* (6th ed., p. 523). St. Louis: Mosby.

43. 2
Rationale: Alkalis, such as lye, cause a liquefaction necrosis, and exposure to fat forms a soapy coagulum. Thick, leathery eschar forms with exposure to acids or heat. Cherry red, firm tissue can occur as a result of thermal injury. Intact blisters indicate a partial-thickness thermal injury.
Test-Taking Strategy: Use the process of elimination and focus on the issue of the question. Remembering that alkali burns cause a liquefaction necrosis and form a soapy coagulum will assist you in answering the question. If you had difficulty with this question, review assessment findings in chemical burns.
Level of Cognitive Ability: Analysis
Client Needs: Physiological Integrity
Integrated Process: Nursing Process—assessment
Content Area: Adult health—integumentary
Reference: Lewis, S., Heitkemper, M., & Dirksen, S. (2004). *Medical-surgical nursing: Assessment and management of clinical problems* (6th ed., pp. 515-516). St. Louis: Mosby.

44. 1
Rationale: Superficial injury from radiation can manifest with erythema (probably caused by capillary damage), hyperpigmentation (from stimulation of melanocytes), dry desquamation (caused by basal cell destruction), or moist desquamation (also caused by basal cell destruction). Moist desquamation is comparable to a second-degree burn in histology, appearance, and sensation.
Test-Taking Strategy: Use the process of elimination and note the relationship between "erythema" in the question and "superficial" in the correct option. If you had difficulty with this question, review the effects of radiation burns.
Level of Cognitive Ability: Analysis
Client Needs: Physiological Integrity
Integrated Process: Nursing Process—assessment
Content Area: Adult health—integumentary
Reference: Black, J., Hawks, J., & Keene, A. (2001). *Medical-surgical nursing: Clinical management for positive outcomes* (6th ed., p. 1332). Philadelphia: W. B. Saunders.

45. 3
Rationale: The emergent phase begins at the time of injury and ends with the restoration of capillary permeability, usually at 48 to 72 hours following the injury. During the emergent phase, the hematocrit increases to above normal because of hemoconcentration from the large fluid shifts. Hematocrit levels

of 50% to 55% are expected during the first 24 hours after injury, with return to normal by 36 hours after injury. Initially, blood is shunted away from the kidneys, and renal perfusion and glomerular filtration are decreased, resulting in low urine output. Pulse rates are typically higher than normal, and the blood pressure is decreased as a result of the large fluid shifts.
Test-Taking Strategy: Use the process of elimination and think about how the body would react in such a traumatizing event. Eliminate options 1 and 4 first. Knowledge that the blood pressure would decrease as a result of the decrease in circulating blood volume will direct you to option 3. Review pathophysiology related to burn injuries if you had difficulty with this question.
Level of Cognitive Ability: Analysis
Client Needs: Physiological Integrity
Integrated Process: Nursing Process—analysis
Content Area: Adult health—integumentary
Reference: Lewis, S., Heitkemper, M., & Dirksen, S. (2004). *Medical-surgical nursing: Assessment and management of clinical problems* (6th ed., p. 522). St. Louis: Mosby.

46. 1
Rationale: Carbon monoxide levels between 1% and 10 % result in impaired visual acuity; levels of 11% to 20% result in flushing and headache; levels of 21% to 30% result in nausea and impaired dexterity. Levels of 31% to 40% result in vomiting, dizziness, and syncope; levels of 41% to 50% result in tachypnea and tachycardia; and levels greater than 50% result in coma and death.
Test-Taking Strategy: Use the process of elimination and focus on the carbon monoxide level presented in the question. If you had difficulty with this question, review these clinical manifestations.
Level of Cognitive Ability: Analysis
Client Needs: Physiological Integrity
Integrated Process: Nursing Process—assessment
Content Area: Adult health—integumentary
Reference: Ignatavicius, D., & Workman, M. (2002). *Medical-surgical nursing: Critical thinking for collaborative care* (4th ed., p. 1566). Philadelphia: W. B. Saunders.

47. 3
Rationale: If an inhalation injury is suspected, administration of 100% oxygen via a tight-fitting non-rebreather face mask is prescribed until carboxyhemoglobin levels fall below 15%. In inhalation injuries the oropharynx is inspected for evidence of erythema, blisters, or ulcerations. The need for endotracheal intubation also is assessed. Options 1, 2, and 4 are incorrect.
Test-Taking Strategy: Use the process of elimination. Recalling that 100% oxygen is required following an inhalation injury will assist you in eliminating options 2 and 4. From the remaining options, recall that with a tight-fitting mask, a non-rebreather is preferred so that the client will not rebreath exhaled air. If you had difficulty with this question, review care to the client following an inhalation injury.
Level of Cognitive Ability: Analysis
Client Needs: Physiological Integrity
Integrated Process: Nursing Process—analysis

Content Area: Adult health—integumentary
Reference: Lewis, S., Heitkemper, M., & Dirksen, S. (2004). *Medical-surgical nursing: Assessment and management of clinical problems* (6th ed., p. 516). St. Louis: Mosby.

48. **2**
Rationale: Successful or adequate fluid resuscitation in the adult is signaled by stable vital signs, adequate urine output, palpable peripheral pulses, and clear sensorium. The most reliable indicator for determining adequacy of fluid resuscitation is the urine output. For an adult, the hourly urine volume should be 30 to 50 mL.
Test-Taking Strategy: Use the process of elimination. Note the key words "most reliable." Note the issue of the question, fluid resuscitation. Urine output is most similar to the issue of administering fluids. Review care to the burn client during fluid resuscitation if you had difficulty with this question.
Level of Cognitive Ability: Analysis
Client Needs: Physiological Integrity
Integrated Process: Nursing Process—evaluation
Content Area: Adult health—integumentary
Reference: Phipps, W., Monahan, F., Sands, J., Marek, J., & Neighbors, M. (2003). *Medical-surgical nursing: Health and illness perspectives* (7th ed., p. 1995). St. Louis: Mosby.

49. **3**
Rationale: Thorough hand washing should be done before and after each contact with the burn-injured client. Sterile sheets and linens are used. Protective garb, including gloves, cap, masks, shoe covers, scrub clothes, and plastic aprons need to be worn when in the client's room and when directly caring for the client.
Test-Taking Strategy: Use the process of elimination noting the key word "incorrect" in the stem of the question. Option 2 can be eliminated easily. Note the absolute word "only" in option 3. Also, option 3 identifies the least thorough technique to prevent infection. If you had difficulty with this question, review protective isolation techniques when caring for a burn client.
Level of Cognitive Ability: Analysis
Client Needs: Safe, Effective Care Environment
Integrated Process: Nursing Process—implementation
Content Area: Leadership/Management
References: Lewis, S., Heitkemper, M., & Dirksen, S. (2004). *Medical-surgical nursing: Assessment and management of clinical problems* (6th ed., p. 857). St. Louis: Mosby.

Phipps, W., Monahan, F., Sands, J., Marek, J., & Neighbors, M. (2003). *Medical-surgical nursing: Health and illness perspectives* (7th ed., p. 202). St. Louis: Mosby.

50. **1**
Rationale: Autografts placed over joints or on the lower extremities often are elevated and immobilized following surgery for 3 to 7 days. This period of immobilization allows the autograft time to adhere and attach to the wound bed. Options 2, 3, and 4 are incorrect.
Test-Taking Strategy: Use the process of elimination. Eliminate options 2 and 4 first because they are similar. From the remaining options, note that the autograft was placed over a joint. This should direct you to option 1. If you had difficulty with this question, review care to an autograft placed over a joint.
Level of Cognitive Ability: Analysis
Client Needs: Physiological Integrity
Integrated Process: Nursing Process—analysis
Content Area: Adult health—integumentary
Reference: Ignatavicius, D., & Workman, M. (2002). *Medical-surgical nursing: Critical thinking for collaborative care* (4th ed., p. 1530). Philadelphia: W. B. Saunders.

CRITICAL THINKING: FILL IN THE BLANK
Answer: 36%
Rationale: According to the rule of nines, with the initial burn, the anterior half of the head equals 4.5%, the upper half of the anterior torso equals 9%, and the lower half of both arms equals 9%. The subsequent burn included the posterior half of head, equaling 4.5%, and the upper half of posterior torso, equaling 9%. This totals 36%.
Test-Taking Strategy: Knowledge regarding the rule of nines is required to answer this question. The entire head equals 9%, each entire arm equals 9% (both arms equal 18%), anterior or posterior torso each equals 18% (36% for entire torso), each entire leg equals 18% (both legs equal 36%), and the perineum equals 1%. Remember, 9 (head), 18 (arms), 36 (torso), 36 (legs), and 1 (perineum) equals 100. If you had difficulty with this question, learn the rule of nines.
Level of Cognitive Ability: Analysis
Client needs: Physiological Integrity
Integrated Process: Nursing Process—assessment
Content Area: Adult health—integumentary
Reference: Lewis, S., Heitkemper, M., & Dirksen, S. (2004). *Medical-surgical nursing: Assessment and management of clinical problems* (6th ed., p. 519). St. Louis: Mosby.

REFERENCES

Black, J., Hawks, J., & Keene, A. (2001). *Medical-surgical nursing: Clinical management for positive outcomes.* (6th ed.). Philadelphia: W. B. Saunders.

Hodgson, B., & Kizior, R. (2004). *Saunders nursing drug handbook 2004.* Philadelphia: W. B. Saunders.

Ignatavicius, D., & Workman, M. (2002). *Medical-surgical nursing: Critical thinking for collaborative care* (4th ed.). Philadelphia: W. B. Saunders.

Lewis, S., Heitkemper, M., & Dirksen, S. (2004). *Medical-surgical nursing: Assessment and management of clinical problems* (6th ed.). St. Louis: Mosby.

Phipps, W., Monahan, F., Sands, J., Marek, J., & Neighbors, M. (2003). *Medical-surgical nursing: Health and illness perspectives* (7th ed.). St. Louis: Mosby.

Potter, P., & Perry, A. (2001). *Fundamentals of nursing* (5th ed.). St. Louis: Mosby.

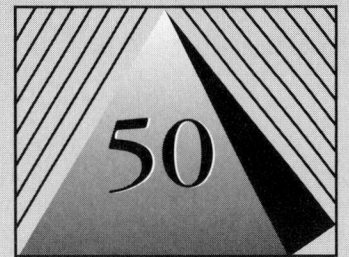

Integumentary Medications

I. EMOLLIENTS AND LOTIONS

A. Emollients (Box 50-1)
   1. Oily or fatty substances that soften and soothe irritated skin by allowing the skin to retain water
   2. Available as creams or ointments
   3. Used for dry, scaly, itchy inflammatory conditions

B. Solutions and lotions (Box 50-2)
   1. Solutions and lotions are liquid suspensions or dispersions.
   2. Solutions and lotions require shaking before application.
   3. Although lotions are predominantly water, they have a drying effect on the skin when the water evaporates.
   4. Solutions and lotions are used as a wash for the skin, as soaks, or as wet dressings on ulcers or **burns.**
   5. Solutions and lotions are used for subacute inflammatory lesions after the severe exudate phase has ceased.
   6. Medicated lotions are often used as antiinflammatory agents because they provide a drying, protective, and cooling effect.

II. RUBS AND LINIMENTS (BOX 50-3)

A. Rubs and liniments are used for the temporary relief of muscular aches, rheumatism, arthritis, sprains, and neuralgia.

B. Over-the-counter products contain combinations of antiseptics, local anesthetics, analgesics, and counterirritants.

C. Some products contain salicylates and, if used over a large area of the skin, may cause salicylate side effects such as tinnitus, nausea, or vomiting.

D. A heating pad is not used with these products because irritation or burning of the skin may occur.

III. ANTIINFECTIVE AGENTS

A. Description
   1. Antiinfective agents include antiseptics and antibacterial, antifungal, antiviral, and antiparasitic medications.
   2. Topical antibiotics are safe and effective in certain conditions; extensive use may encourage the emergence of resistant bacteria.

BOX 50-1

Emollients

Cold cream
Glycerin
Lanolin
Lubriderm
Petrolatum
Vitamin A and D ointment
Zinc ointment

BOX 50-2

Solutions and Lotions

Aluminum acetate solution (Burow's solution)
Calamine lotion (Caladryl lotion)

BOX 50-3

Rubs and Liniments

Aspercreme
Ben-Gay
Icy Hot
Myoflex

566 UNIT VIII The Adult Client with an Integumentary Disorder

B. Antiseptics
1. Sodium hypochlorite (Dakin's solution)
   a. Dakin's solution is a chloride solution that loosens, dissolves, and deodorizes necrotic tissue and blood clots.
   b. The solution kills most common bacteria, including spores, amebas, fungi, protozoa viruses, and yeast.
   c. The solution is used for irrigating and cleaning necrotic or purulent wounds.
   d. The solution loses its potency during storage, so fresh solution is prepared frequently.
   e. The solution should not be in contact with healing or normal tissue.
2. Chlorhexidine gluconate (Hibiclens)
   a. Chlorhexidine is effective for cleaning wounds caused by staphylococci and other gram-positive bacteria.
   b. Chlorhexidine is used for irrigating and cleansing wounds but not for packing wounds because it may cause contact dermatitis.
3. Acetic acid
   a. Acetic acid is effective for irrigating, cleansing, and packing wounds infected by *Pseudomonas aeruginosa*.
   b. Healthy skin surrounding the wound must be protected with a petroleum barrier because acetic acid excoriates the skin.
4. Hydrogen peroxide
   a. As a 3% solution, hydrogen peroxide has effervescent action that releases gas and breaks up necrotic tissue.
   b. Hydrogen peroxide is used to irrigate and clean necrotic tissue and pus from open wounds.
   c. Hydrogen peroxide is not used to pack wounds because it decomposes too rapidly.

d. When epithelial tissue begins to form, use of hydrogen peroxide is discontinued because it inhibits tissue formation.
5. Hexachlorophene (pHisoHex, Septisol)
   a. Hexachlorophene solution is a combination of hexachlorophene and alcohol.
   b. Hexachlorophene is a bacteriostatic agent with activity against staphylococci and other gram-positive bacteria.
   c. Hexachlorophene absorbs through broken skin and can cause neurotoxicity; it should not be used on wounds.
   d. The alcohol component dries and irritates tissue, is not an effective germicide, and forms a film that actually can promote infection.
   e. All hexachlorophene products should be rinsed well from the skin after their use to prevent systemic absorption.
C. Antibacterials (Box 50-4)
1. Description: used for superficial skin infections
2. Mupirocin (Bactroban)
   a. Topical antibacterial active against *Staphylococcus aureus*, β-hemolytic streptococci, or *Streptococcus pyogenes*
   b. Usually applied 3 times daily; if improvement is not observed within 3 to 5 days, mupirocin is discontinued
D. Antifungals
1. Antifungal agents may cause erythema, stinging, blistering, peeling, pruritis, urticaria, and general skin irritation.
2. Client is reevaluated if no results are obtained after 4 weeks of treatment.
E. Antiviral: Acyclovir (Zovirax)
1. Acyclovir inhibits DNA replication in the virus.

BOX 50-4

Antibacterials, Antifungals, and Antiparasitics

ANTIBACTERIALS
Bacitracin (Baciguent ointment)
Chloramphenicol
Chlortetracycline
Erythromycin
Gentamicin
Mupirocin (Bactroban)
Mycitracin Triple Antibiotic (neomycin, bacitracin, polymixin B)
Neomycin

ANTIFUNGALS
Amphotericin B (Fungizone)
Betamethasone and clotrimazole (Lotrisone)
Ciclopirox olamine (Loprox)
Clioquinol (Vioform)
Clotrimazole (Lotrimin, Mycelex)

Econazole nitrate (Spectazole)
Haloprogin (Halotex)
Ketoconazole (Nizoral)
Miconazole (Micatin)
Nystatin (Mycostatin)
Tolnaftate (Tinactin)
Triacetin (Fungoid)
Undecylenic acid (Desenex)

ANTIVIRAL
Acyclovir (Zovirax)

ANTIPARASITICS
Crotamiton (Eurax)
Lindane (Kwell)
Malathion (Ovide)
Permethrin (Elimite, Nix)

2. Acyclovir is used for herpes simplex types 1 and 2, varicella-zoster, Epstein-Barr virus, and cytomegalovirus.
3. Acyclovir can cause mild pain and transient burning and stinging.
4. Acyclovir is applied completely over the lesion usually every 3 hours 6 times daily for 1 week.
5. Rubber gloves are used to apply the ointment to prevent the spread of infection.

F. Antiparasitics
1. Antiparasitic agents are used to treat scabies (mites) and pediculosis (lice).
2. Antiparasitic agents may be harmful during pregnancy and in young children.
3. Antiparasitic agents may irritate the skin, eyes, and mucous membranes.
4. Antiparasitic agents may cause allergic reactions.

IV. ANTIPRURITICS (BOX 50-5)
A. Antipuritic agents are used to allay itching.
B. Antipuritic agents are applied as wet dressings, pastes, lotions, creams, or ointments.
C. Persons with dry skin should be instructed to bathe less frequently.

V. KERATOLYTICS (BOX 50-6)
A. Description
1. Preparations that dissolve keratin
2. Soften scales and loosen the horny layer of the skin, resulting in minimal peeling or extensive desquamation
3. For treatment of superficial fungal infections, dermatitis, psoriasis, and localized dermatitis
B. Salicylic acid
1. Salicylic acid is used to treat seborrheic dermatitis, acne, and psoriasis and to thin and remove calluses.

BOX 50-5

Antipruritics

Calamine lotion
Corn starch or oatmeal baths
Solutions of bismuth salts, aluminum acetate, or
  boric acid

BOX 50-6

Keratolytics

Cantharidin (Cantharone)
Imiquimod (Aldara)
Masoprocol (Actinex)
Podophyllum resin
Podofilox (Condylox)
Resorcinol
Salicylic acid

---

2. Salicylic acid can be absorbed systematically and can cause salicylism, which is characterized by dizziness and tinnitus; salicylic acid is not applied to large surface areas or open wounds.
C. Podophyllum resin
1. Podophyllum resin is used for various types of **skin cancer.**
2. Podophyllum resin causes lesions to slough off, leaving a superficial ulcer and moderate dermatitis.
3. After the therapy is discontinued, the lesions are treated with a mild antiseptic ointment; healing usually occurs within a few days.
D. Cantharidin (Cantharone)
1. Cantharidin is used to treat warts.
2. Cantharidin has an exfoliation effect only on the epidermal cells.
3. Cantharidin may cause tingling, itching, and burning.
4. Site may be tender for 2 to 6 days.
E. Masoprocol (Actinex)
1. Masoprocol has antiproliferative activity against keratinocytes and is used to treat keratosis.
2. Occlusive dressings are not to be used with masoprocol.
3. Client may experience transient burning after administration.

VI. STIMULANTS AND IRRITANTS (BOX 50-7)
A. Description: Stimulants and irritants produce a mild irritation to the surface of the skin, causing hyperemia and inflammation that promote the healing process.
B. Coal tar
1. Coal tar is used to treat psoriasis, seborrheic dermatitis, and atopic dermatitis.
2. Coal tar has an unpleasant odor and frequently stains the skin and hair.
3. Coal tar can cause phototoxicity.
C. Compound benzoin tincture
1. The tincture protects the skin when the client has bed sores, ulcers, cracked nipples, and fissures of any orifice.
2. The tincture causes a mild irritation that produces increased blood flow and healing.

VII. PROTECTIVES (BOX 50-8)
A. Description
1. Protectives are preparations that provide a film on the skin to protect it from irritations such as light, moisture, air, and dust.

BOX 50-7

Stimulants and Irritants

Coal tar
Compound benzoin tincture

BOX 50-8

Protectives

Benzoin
DuoDerm
Ensure-It (Deseret)
Mediskin and Silver
Op-Site
Polyskin
Tegaderm
Tegasorb
Uniflex
Vigilon
Zinc oxide paste (Unna's boot)

2. Protectives promote natural healing without the usual formation of dry crust over the wound.
3. Protectives allow exudate to collect beneath the dressing, forming an artificial blister.
4. Protectives are designed to be left in place for up to 7 days or until leakage occurs around the dressing.
5. Uniflex, PolySkin, and Ensure-It may be used to cover central and peripheral intravenous sites.
6. Op-Site, Tegasorb, Mediskin and Silver, and Vigilon may be used for skin burns.
B. Sunscreens
1. Sunscreens act by absorbing ultraviolet rays.
2. Sunscreens are most effective when applied about 30 minutes to 1 hour before exposure to the sun and should be reapplied every 2 to 3 hours after swimming or sweating.
3. Sunscreens can cause contact dermatitis and photosensitivity reactions.
C. Nonadherent dressings
1. Woven or nonwoven dressings may be impregnated with saline, petrolatum, or antimicrobials.
2. Nonadherent dressings include Adaptic, Exu-Dry, Sofsorb, Telfa, vaseline gauze, and Xeroform.

VIII. GROWTH FACTORS

A. Description
1. Growth factors are used to promote wound healing.
2. Growth factors stimulate cells to divide and migrate, which results in wound healing, formation of granulation tissue, and new epidermis.
B. Procuren solution
1. Procuren solution promotes healing by actively stimulating growth and granulation tissue, capillaries, and epithelium.
2. Procuren solution is applied to the wound and covered with petrolatum-impregnated gauze.
3. The material is left in place for 12 hours and then washed off; during the remaining 12 hours of the day, the wound is covered with sulfadiazine (Silvadene).

IX. ENZYMES

A. Description
1. Enzymes are used to promote healing of wounds and to débride skin ulcers.
2. Enzymes reduce inflammation resulting from trauma and infection.
3. Enzymes dissolve fibrin clots, which helps reduce the size of surface hematomas.
4. To be effective, enzymes must be in contact with affected tissue in adequate concentrations for a sufficient length of time.
5. Wound may need to be débrided surgically before application; if enzymes are not administered to a clean, débrided wound, healing may be delayed.
B. Enzymes that promote wound healing (Box 50-9)
1. Papain (Panafil, Panafil White)
a. Papain does not injure or affect healthy tissue or cells.
b. Enzyme must be in immediate contact with the purulent wound material.
c. Wounds are cleansed with prescribed irrigating solution between applications.
d. Hydrogen peroxide cannot be used to irrigate the wound because it inactivates the papain.
e. Light dressings and cellophane wrap may be used over the wound to prevent soiling of clothing.
f. Dressings are changed frequently to prevent contamination and to remove necrotic debris.
2. Hyaluronidase (Wydase)
a. Hyaluronidase facilitates the absorption of fluid administered by subcutaneous hypodermoclysis.
b. Hyaluronidase can be injected subcutaneously into an infiltrated intravenous site when a potent vasoconstrictor such as norepinephrine (Levophed) or metaraminol (Aramine) has infiltrated.
c. Hyaluronidase reduces the sloughing of tissue likely to occur following infiltration.
C. Enzymes to débride and remove exudates (Box 50-10)
1. Description

BOX 50-9

Enzymes That Promote Wound Healing

Hyaluronidase (Wydase)
Papain (Panafil, Panafil White)

BOX 50-10

Enzymes to Débride and Remove Exudates

Collagenase (Santyl)
Dextranomer (Debrisan)
Fibrinolysin and desoxyribonuclease (Elase)
Sutilains (Travase)

a. Enzymes alter the thick, purulent drainage to a thin, liquid material that can be wiped or irrigated easily off the wound.

b. Enzyme contact with the wound is necessary to promote wound healing.

c. Wound needs to be cleansed, and crosshatching of eschar on burns is performed before application.

2. Sutilains (Travase)

a. Sutilains is used to remove nonviable or necrotic tissue and purulent enzymes from burns, ulcers, traumatic injury, and peripheral vascular disease wounds.

b. Sutilains is inactive on viable tissue.

3. Collagenase (Santyl)

a. Collagenase is used at a topical débriding agent.

b. Collagenase provides effective débridement of the collagen tissue at the wound edges where necrotic tissue is anchored.

c. Collagenase encourages the formation of granulation tissue at the wound edges and quicker epithelization of wounds.

d. Apply collagenase with a tongue depressor directly into deep wounds.

e. Before application, cleanse wound of debris by gently rubbing with a gauze pad with sterile water or Dakin's solution, followed by sterile normal saline.

f. Remove all excess ointment each time dressing is changed.

g. Apply only to injured area; collagenase causes erythema in healthy tissues.

h. Protect healthy tissue by applying zinc oxide paste.

i. Discontinue use of collagenase when necrotic tissue is gone.

4. Fibrinolysin and desoxyribonuclease (Elase)

a. Elase is used to débride wounds, including **burns, decubitus** ulcers, and inflamed or infected lesions.

b. Clean wound with sterile water, pat dry; flush away necrotic debris with normal saline and then apply a thin layer of Elase and cover with petrolatum gauze.

D. Dextranomer (Debrisan)

1. Dextranomer is not a débriding agent but is a cleansing agent that actually absorbs peptides and proteins.

2. Dextranomer is effective in wet wounds only.

3. Dextranomer is not packed tightly into the wound because maceration of surrounding tissue may occur from contact with the agent.

X. CORTICOSTEROIDS

A. Corticosteroids have antiinflammatory, antipruritic, and vasoconstrictive actions.

B. Contraindications

1. Clients demonstrating previous sensitivity to corticosteroids

2. Clients with current systemic fungal, viral, or bacterial infections

3. Clients with current complications related to corticosteroid therapy

C. Local adverse effects

1. Hypopigmentation

2. Acneform eruptions

3. Contact dermatitis

4. Burning, dryness, irritation, itching

5. Overgrowth of bacteria, fungi, and viruses

6. Skin atrophy

D. Systemic adverse effects

1. Rare occurence

2. Adrenal suppression

3. Cushing's syndrome

4. Striae, skin atrophy

5. Ocular effects (glaucoma and cataracts)

E. Topical steroids

1. Monitor plasma cortisol levels if prolonged therapy is necessary.

2. Wash area just before application to increase medication penetration.

3. Apply sparingly in a light film, rubbing gently.

4. May apply to skin alone or with a dry occlusive dressing if prescribed by the physician.

5. Instruct the client to report burning, irritation, or signs of infection to the physician.

XI. ACNE PRODUCTS (BOX 50-11)

A. Description

1. Mild acne can be treated with bar soaps, soap-free cakes, liquid cleansers, lotions, gels, and creams.

2. For moderate acne, topical antiinflammatory medication such as benzoyl peroxide, tretinoin (Retin-A), isotretinoin (Accutane), azelaic acid (Azelex), and adapalene (Differin) may be prescribed; antibiotics also may be prescribed.

3. Side effects can include excessive redness, extreme dryness of the skin leading to blistering and crusting, temporary pigmentation changes, and peeling of the skin.

4. All products are kept away from the eyes, inside the nose, mucous membranes, and hair.

B. Benzoyl peroxide is a keratolytic agent that is bacteriostatic and may decrease the production of irritant free fatty acids in the follicle.

C. Tretinoin and adapalene are acids of vitamin A that are used to treat acne vulgaris and also may be used to treat skin cancer and aging of the skin.

D. Tretinoin (Retin-A)

1. Tretinoin decreases cohesiveness of the epithelial cells, increasing cell mitosis and turnover; tretinoin is potentially irritating, and mild redness and skin peeling is expected with topical use.

BOX 50-11

Acne Products

CLEANSERS
Acnomel
Brasivol
Clearasil Medicated Astringent
Fostex
pHisoDerm
Stri-Dex

DRYING AGENTS
Acnomel
Dry and Clear
Ionax
Listerex

MISCELLANEOUS
Adapalene (Differin)
Alpha-hydroxyl acids
Antibiotics
Azelaic acid (Azelex)
Bensulfoid cream (benzoyl peroxide and sulfur)
Benzamycin gel (benzoyl peroxide and sulfur)
Benzoyl peroxide wash, gel
Isotretinoin (Accutane)
Resorcinol (as an ingredient in other preparations)
Salicylic acid (as an ingredient in other preparations)
Tazarotene (Tazorac)
Trentinoin (Retin-A)

---

2. Within 48 hours of use, the skin generally becomes red and begins to peel.
3. Temporary hyperpigmentation and hypopigmentation can occur.
4. Client should avoid sun exposure because photosensitivity may occur.
5. Tretinoin is applied liberally to the skin; the hands should be washed thoroughly immediately after applying tretinoin.
6. Therapeutic results should be seen after 2 to 3 weeks but may not be optimal until after 6 weeks.
7. Client may use cosmetics, but the skin needs to be cleaned thoroughly before applying the cosmetics.

E. Isotretinoin (Accutane)
1. Isotretinoin is a metabolite of vitamin A.
2. Isotretinoin is used to treat severe cystic acne, and its use is reserved for persons who have not responded to other therapies, including systemic antibiotics.
3. Isotretinoin can cause xerosis and facial desquamation, palmoplantar desquamation, pruritus, brittle nails, and hair loss.
4. Isotretinoin is administered with meals 2 times daily for a 15- to 20-week course; if another course of therapy is needed, an 8-week lapse of time should occur.
6. Photosensitivity may occur, so the client needs to be instructed to decrease sun exposure.
7. Alcohol consumption should be eliminated during therapy because alcohol may potentiate serum triglyceride elevation.

F. Local antibiotics
1. Antibiotics are used to treat acne; include clindamycin (Cleocin T), erythromycin, tetracycline (Topicycline), and meclocycline (Meclan).
2. Therapeutic response generally requires 6 to 12 weeks of therapy.
3. Side effects include acute contact dermatitis, transient stinging or burning, staining of the skin, erythema, and skin tenderness.

XII. POISON IVY TREATMENT (SEE BOX 50-12.)

XIII. BURN PRODUCTS (BOX 50-13)
A. Nitrofurazone (Furacin)
1. Nitrofurazone is applied topically to the burn as a solution, ointment, or cream.
2. Nitrofurazone has a broad spectrum of antibacterial activity.
3. Nitrofurazone is used in **burns** when bacterial resistance to other agents is a problem.
4. Topical: Apply $\frac{1}{16}$-inch film directly to burn.
5. Side effects: Contact dermatitis, rash
6. Less common side effects: Pruritus, local edema
B. Mafenide (Sulfamylon)
1. Mafenide is a water-soluble cream that is bacteriostatic for gram-negative and gram-positive organisms.
2. Mafenide is used to treat **burns** to reduce the bacteria present in avascular tissues.
3. Mafenide diffuses through the devascularized areas of the skin and may precipitate metabolic acidosis (usually compensated for by hyperventilation).

BOX 50-12

Poison Ivy Treatment Products

Calamine lotion
Calomox
IV-Chex
Ivy-Rid
Rhuli cream, spray, or gel

BOX 50-13

Burn Products

Mafenide (Sulfamylon)
Nitrofurazone (Furacin)
Silver nitrate
Silver sulfadiazine (Silvadene)

4. Apply $\frac{1}{16}$-inch film directly to the burn.
5. Side effects can include local pain and rash.
6. Systemic effects include bone marrow depression, hemolytic anemia, and metabolic acidosis.
7. Keep burn covered with mafenide at all times.
8. Notify physician if hyperventilation occurs; if acidosis develops, mafenide is washed off the skin.

C. Silver sulfadiazine (Silvadene)
1. Sulfadiazine has a broad spectrum of activity against gram-negative bacteria, gram-positive bacteria, and yeast.
2. Sulfadiazine is released slowly from the cream, which is selectively toxic to bacteria.
3. Sulfadiazine is used primarily to prevent sepsis in clients with **burns.**
4. Sulfadiazine is not a carbonic anhydrase inhibitor and therefore does not cause acidosis.
5. Apply $\frac{1}{16}$-inch film (keep burn covered at all times with silver sulfadiazine).
6. Side effects include rash and itching.
7. Systemic effects include leukopenia and interstitial nephritis.
8. Monitor complete blood cell count, particularly the white blood cells, frequently; if leukopenia develops, the medication is discontinued.

D. Silver nitrate
1. Silver nitrate is an antiseptic solution active against gram-negative bacteria.
2. Dressings are applied to the **burn** and then are kept moist with silver nitrate, which stains anything with which it comes in contact; this discoloration is not usually permanent.
3. Silver nitrate is used on extensive **burns** that may precipitate fluid and electrolyte imbalances.
4. Apply silver nitrate to the dressing; do not apply directly to wounds, cuts, or broken skin.

PRACTICE QUESTIONS

1. The physician has prescribed Myoflex topical cream for a client with a diagnosis of rheumatism who is complaining of muscular aches. Which of the following information does the nurse provide to the client regarding this medication?
   1. Apply a heating pad to the area after applying the medication.
   2. The medication acts by decreasing muscle spasms.
   3. The medication is prescribed to cause the skin to peel.
   4. The medication will act as a local anesthetic.

2. An outbreak of pediculosis capitus has occurred at the local school. The school nurse is providing instructions to the mothers of the children attending the school regarding the application of permethrin (Elimite, Nix). The nurse tells the mothers to
   1. Apply at bedtime and rinse off in the morning.
   2. Apply before washing the hair.
   3. Avoid saturating the hair and scalp when applying.
   4. Allow to remain on the hair 10 minutes and then rinse with water.

3. A client is seen in the clinic for complaints of skin itchiness that has been persistent over the past several weeks. Following an assessment, the client has been determined to have scabies. Lindane (Kwell) is prescribed, and the nurse provides instructions to the client regarding the use of the medication. The nurse tells the client to
   1. Leave the cream on for 8 to12 hours and then remove by washing.
   2. Apply a thick layer of cream to the entire body.
   3. Apply the cream for 2 days in a row.
   4. Apply to the entire body and scalp, excluding the face.

4. A topical corticosteroid is prescribed for the client with dermatitis. The nurse provides instructions to the client regarding the use of the medication. Which of the following, if stated by the client, would indicate a need for further instruction?
   1. "I need to apply the medication in a thin film."
   2. "I should gently rub the medication into the skin."
   3. "I should place a bandage over the site after applying the medication."
   4. "The medication will help to relieve the inflammation and itching."

5. The nurse is applying a topical corticosteroid to a client with eczema. The nurse would be concerned about the potential for systemic absorption of the medication if the medication were being applied to which of the following body areas?
   1. Back
   2. Axilla
   3. Palms of the hands
   4. Soles of the feet

6. Salicylic acid is prescribed for a client with a diagnosis of psoriasis. The nurse monitors the client knowing that which of the following would indicate the presence of systemic toxicity from this medication?
   1. Decreased respirations
   2. Diarrhea
   3. Constipation
   4. Tinnitus

7. The client is diagnosed with herpes simplex type 1. The physician prescribes a topical medication for treatment. The nurse anticipates that which of the following medications will be prescribed?
   1. Triple antibiotic
   2. Acyclovir (Zovirax)
   3. Mupirocin (Bactroban)
   4. Masoprocol (Actinex)

8. The physician has prescribed coal tar treatments for the client with psoriasis, and the nurse provides information to the client about the treatments.

Which statement made by the client indicates a lack of understanding about the treatments?
1. "The medication has an unpleasant odor."
2. "The medication can stain the skin and hair."
3. "The medication can cause systemic toxicity."
4. "The medication can cause phototoxicity."

9. The camp nurse asks the children preparing to swim in the lake if they have applied sunscreen. The nurse reminds the children that chemical sunscreens are most effective when applied
   1. 30 minutes to 1 hour before exposure to the sun.
   2. Immediately before exposure to the sun.
   3. 15 minutes before exposure to the sun.
   4. Immediately before swimming.

10. Mafenide (Sulfamylon) is prescribed for the client with a burn injury. When applying the medication, the client complains of local discomfort and burning. Which of the following is the most appropriate nursing action?
    1. Discontinue the medication.
    2. Notify the physician.
    3. Apply a thinner film than prescribed to the burn site.
    4. Inform the client that this is normal.

11. The burn client is receiving treatments of topical mafenide (Sulfamylon) to the site of injury. The nurse monitors the client knowing, that which of the following indicates that a systemic effect has occurred?
    1. Local pain at the burn site
    2. Local rash at the burn site
    3. Hyperventilation
    4. Elevated blood pressure

12. Sodium hypochlorite (Dakin's solution) is prescribed for a client with a leg wound that is draining purulent material. The home health nurse teaches a family member how to perform these treatments. Which statement if made by the family member indicates a need for further teaching?
    1. "The solution should not come in contact with normal skin tissue."
    2. "I should rinse the solution off immediately following the irrigation."
    3. "I will soak a sterile dressing with solution and pack it into the wound."
    4. "I will prepare the solution before use."

13. The nurse has provided instructions to a client regarding the use of tretinoin (Retin-A). Which statement if made by the client indicates the need for further instructions?
    1. "I will wash my hands thoroughly after applying the medication."
    2. "Optimal results will be seen after 6 weeks."
    3. "I must apply a thin layer to the skin."
    4. "I will cleanse the skin thoroughly before applying the medication."

14. Isotretinoin (Accutane) is prescribed for a client with severe acne. Before the administration of this medication, the nurse would anticipate that which laboratory test will be prescribed?
    1. Complete blood count
    2. White blood cell count
    3. Triglyceride level
    4. Platelet count

15. A client with severe acne is seen in the clinic. The physician prescribes isotretinoin (Accutane). The nurse reviews the client's medication record and would contact the physician if the client is taking which medication?
    1. Digoxin (Lanoxin)
    2. Phenytoin (Dilantin)
    3. Vitamin A
    4. Furosemide (Lasix)

16. The registered nurse is observing a newly hired nurse perform a dressing change on a client with a leg ulcer. Sutilains (Travase) is being used to treat the ulcer. Which observation by the registered nurse would indicate an inaccurate action by the newly hired nurse when performing the dressing change?
    1. The nurse cleans the wound with a sterile solution.
    2. The nurse dries the wound and covers the sutilains application with a dry sterile dressing.
    3. The nurse moistens the wound with sterile normal saline and then applies the sutilains.
    4. The nurse places the sutilains in the refrigerator following use.

17. Dextranomer (Debrisan) is prescribed for a client with a decubitus ulcer. The nursing instructor asks the nursing student preparing to perform the treatment about the medication and the procedure. Which statement if made by the student indicates a need for further research?
    1. "It is effective in wet wounds only."
    2. "It should be packed lightly into the wound."
    3. "Maceration of tissue surrounding the wound can occur from the medication."
    4. "The wound bed must be dried thoroughly before applying the medication."

18. Fibrinolysin and desoxyribonuclease (Elase) dry powder is prescribed to treat a skin ulcer, and the nurse is observing a nursing student perform the treatment. The nurse intervenes if the nursing student is observed doing which of the following?
    1. Cleans the wound with a sterile solution before applying Elase.
    2. Prepares the solution just before use.
    3. Applies a thick layer of medication and covers with a dry sterile dressing.
    4. Applies a thin layer of medication and covers with a petrolatum gauze.

19. The clinic nurse is performing an admission assessment on a client. The nurse notes that the client is taking azelaic acid (Azelex). Because of the medication prescription, the nurse would suspect that the client is being treated for

1. Herpes simplex.
2. Acne.
3. Eczema.
4. Hair loss.

20. Minoxidil (Rogaine) is prescribed for the client to treat hair loss. The client asks the nurse if the hair will continue to grow when the medication is stopped. The most appropriate nursing response is
   1. "The hair will continue to grow."
   2. "Newly gained hair is lost in 3 to 4 months."
   3. "It depends on how long you have been taking the Rogaine."
   4. "I'm not sure, you need to ask your physician."

CRITICAL THINKING: FILL IN THE BLANK

The home health care nurse makes a home visit to a client who has an ulcer on the medial aspect of the left ankle. The wound is being treated with Duoderm. The nurse removes the Duoderm, cleanses the wound as prescribed, and reapplies the Duoderm. The nurse schedules the next visit for wound care and for changing the Duoderm in how many days?

Answer: _____

ANSWERS

1. **4**
Rationale: Myoflex is one of the many products used for the temporary relief of muscular aches, rheumatism, arthritis, sprains, and neuralgia. These products contain combinations of antiseptics, local anesthetics, analgesics, and counterirritants. A heating pad should not be applied because irritation or burning of the skin may occur. The medication does not act in a systemic manner (option 2). They are not prescribed to cause the skin to peel and if this sort of reaction occurs, the physician should be notified.
Test-Taking Strategy: Use the process of elimination. Noting the key words "topical cream" may assist in eliminating option 2. Eliminate option 3, knowing that this is not an expected therapeutic effect. Recalling the principles related to the application of heat will assist in eliminating option 1. Review this medication if you had difficulty with this question.
Level of Cognitive Ability: Application
Client Needs: Physiological Integrity
Integrated Process: Teaching/Learning
Content Area: Pharmacology
Reference: Kee, J., & Hayes, E. (2003). *Pharmacology: A nursing process approach* (4th ed., pp. 254-255). Philadelphia: W. B. Saunders.

2. **4**
Rationale: The instructions for the use of permethrin include wash, rinse, and towel dry hair; apply sufficient volume to saturate hair and scalp; allow to remain on hair 10 minutes; and then rinse with water.
Test-Taking Strategy: Use the process of elimination. Note that options 1 and 4 address a time frame for allowing the medication to remain on the hair. Recognizing this may provide you with the clue that one of these options is correct. Review this treatment if you are unfamiliar with it.
Level of Cognitive Ability: Application
Client Needs: Physiological Integrity
Integrated Process: Teaching/Learning
Content Area: Pharmacology
Reference: Kee, J., & Hayes, E. (2003). *Pharmacology: A nursing process approach* (4th ed., p. 852). Philadelphia: W. B. Saunders.

3. **1**
Rationale: Kwell is applied in a thin layer to the entire body below the head. No more than 30 g (1 oz) should be used. The medication is removed by washing 8 to 12 hours later. In most cases, only one application is required.
Test-Taking Strategy: Use the process of elimination. Eliminate option 2 because of the word "thick." Eliminate option 4 because of the word "entire." From the remaining options, eliminate option 3 knowing that only one application is required. Review this medication, if you are unfamiliar with it.
Level of Cognitive Ability: Application
Client Needs: Physiological Integrity
Integrated Process: Teaching/Learning
Content Area: Pharmacology
Reference: Gutierrez, K., & Queener, S. (2003). *Pharmacology for nursing practice* (p. 1119). St. Louis: Mosby.

4. **3**
Rationale: Clients should be advised not to use occlusive dressings (bandages or plastic wraps) to cover the affected site following the application of the topical corticosteroid, unless the physician specifically prescribes wound coverage. Options 1, 2, and 4 are accurate statements related to the use of this medication.
Test-Taking Strategy: Use the process of elimination. Note the key words "need for further instruction." Eliminate option 4 knowing that this is the action of a corticosteroid. The words "thin" in option 1 and "gently" in option 2 should assist you in eliminating these options. If you had difficulty with this question, review this medication.
Level of Cognitive Ability: Analysis
Client Needs: Physiological Integrity
Integrated Process: Teaching/Learning
Content Area: Pharmacology
Reference: Lehne, R. (2001). *Pharmacology for nursing care* (4th ed., p. 789). Philadelphia: W. B. Saunders.

5. **2**
Rationale: Topical corticosteroids can be absorbed into the systemic circulation. Absorption is higher from regions where the skin is especially permeable (scalp, axilla, face, eyelids, neck,

perineum, genitalia),and lower from regions where penetrability is poor (back, palms, soles).

Test-Taking Strategy: Use the process of elimination. Focus on the issue of the question "permeability and the potential for systemic absorption." Eliminate options 3 and 4 because these body areas are similar in terms of skin substance. From the remaining options, think about permeability of the skin area. This should direct you to option 2. Review the principles related to the administration of topical corticosteroids if you had difficulty with this question.
Level of Cognitive Ability: Analysis
Client Needs: Physiological Integrity
Integrated Process: Nursing Process—analysis
Content Area: Pharmacology
Reference: Hodgson, B., & Kizior, R. (2004). *Saunders nursing drug handbook 2004* (p. 8C). Philadelphia: W. B. Saunders.

6. 4
Rationale: Salicylic acid is absorbed readily through the skin, and systemic toxicity (salicylism) can result. Symptoms include tinnitus, dizziness, hyperpnea, and psychological disturbances. Constipation and diarrhea are not associated with salicylism.
Test-Taking Strategy: Use the process of elimination. Noting the name of the medication will assist in directing you to the correct option if you can recall the toxic effects that occur with acetyl*salicylic* acid (Aspirin). Review the toxic effects of salicylic acid if you are unfamiliar with them.
Level of Cognitive Ability: Analysis
Client Needs: Physiological Integrity
Integrated Process: Nursing Process—assessment
Content Area: Pharmacology
Reference: Lehne, R. (2001). *Pharmacology for nursing care* (4th ed., p. 1153). Philadelphia: W. B. Saunders.

7. 2
Rationale: Acyclovir is a topical antiviral agent that inhibits DNA replication in the virus. Acyclovir has activity against herpes simplex types 1 and 2, varicella-zoster, Epstein-Barr virus and cytomegalovirus. Triple antibiotic would not be effective in treating herpes virus. Bactroban is a topical antibacterial active against *Staphylococcus aureus*, β-hemolytic streptococci, or *Streptococcus pyogenes*. Actinex is a keratolytic.
Test-Taking Strategy: Use the process of elimination. Knowledge that herpes simplex is a virus will direct you to the option that identifies an antiviral medication. Review these medications if you are unfamiliar with them.
Level of Cognitive Ability: Analysis
Client Needs: Physiological Integrity
Integrated Process: Nursing Process—analysis
Content Area: Pharmacology
Reference: Hodgson, B., & Kizior, R. (2004). *Saunders nursing drug handbook 2004* (p. 12). Philadelphia: W. B. Saunders.

8. 3
Rationale: Coal tar is used to treat psoriasis and other chronic disorders of the skin. Coal tar suppresses DNA synthesis, mitotic activity, and cell proliferation. Coal tar has an unpleasant odor, frequently stains the skin and hair, and can cause phototoxicity. Systemic toxicity does not occur.

Test-Taking Strategy: Use the process of elimination. Note the key words "lack of understanding" in the stem of the question. The name of the medication will assist in eliminating options 1 and 2. From the remaining options, you must know that the medication does not cause systemic toxicity. If you had difficulty with this question, review this treatment.
Level of Cognitive Ability: Analysis
Client Needs: Physiological Integrity
Integrated Process: Teaching/Learning
Content Area: Pharmacology
Reference: Lehne, R. (2001). *Pharmacology for nursing care* (4th ed., p. 1157). Philadelphia: W. B. Saunders.

9. 1
Rationale: Sunscreens are most effective when applied about 30 minutes to 1 hour before exposure to the sun so that they can penetrate the skin. All sunscreens should be reapplied after swimming or sweating.
Test-Taking Strategy: Use the process of elimination. Knowledge that sunscreens need to penetrate the skin will assist in eliminating options 2 and 3. Noting the key words "most effective" will assist in directing you to option 1. Review protective skin measures if you had difficulty with this question.
Level of Cognitive Ability: Application
Client Needs: Physiological Integrity
Integrated Process: Teaching/Learning
Content Area: Pharmacology
Reference: Lehne, R. (2001). *Pharmacology for nursing care* (4th ed., p. 1160). Philadelphia: W. B. Saunders.

10. 4
Rationale: Mafenide is bacteriostatic for gram-negative and gram-positive organisms and is used to treat burns to reduce bacteria present in avascular tissues. The client should be informed that the medication will cause local discomfort and burning.
Test-Taking Strategy: Use the process of elimination. Eliminate options 1 and 3 because it is not within the scope of nursing practice to alter or discontinue a medication therapy. Recalling that this is a normal expected occurrence will direct you easily to option 4. If you had difficulty with this question, review the effects of this medication.
Level of Cognitive Ability: Application
Client Needs: Physiological Integrity
Integrated Process: Nursing Process—implementation
Content Area: Pharmacology
References: Kee, J., & Hayes, E. (2003). *Pharmacology: A nursing process approach* (4th ed., p. 706). Philadelphia: W. B. Saunders.
Lehne, R. (2001). *Pharmacology for nursing care* (4th ed., p. 966). Philadelphia: W. B. Saunders.

11. 3
Rationale: Mafenide is a carbonic anhydrase inhibitor and can suppress renal excretion of acid, thereby causing acidosis. Clients receiving this treatment should be monitored for acid-base imbalance. If acidosis becomes severe, the medication should be discontinued for 1 to 2 days. Options 1 and 2 describe local rather than systemic effects. An elevated blood pressure may be expected in the client with pain.

Test-Taking Strategy: Use the process of elimination. Note the key words "systemic effect." Options 1 and 2 can be eliminated because these are local rather than systemic effects. From the remaining options, recall that the client in pain would likely have an elevated blood pressure. This should direct you to option 3. Review the systemic effects of this medication if you had difficulty with this question.
Level of Cognitive Ability: Analysis
Client Needs: Physiological Integrity
Integrated Process: Nursing Process—assessment
Content Area: Pharmacology
References: Kee, J., & Hayes, E. (2003). *Pharmacology: A nursing process approach* (4th ed., p. 706). Philadelphia: W B. Saunders. Lehne, R. (2001). *Pharmacology for nursing care* (4th ed. p. 966). Philadelphia: W. B. Saunders.

12. **3**
Rationale: Sodium hypochlorite is a chloride solution that is used for irrigating and cleaning necrotic or purulent wounds. Although sodium hypochlorite can be used for packing necrotic wounds, it cannot be used to pack purulent wounds because the solution is inactivated by copious pus. The solution should not come in contact with healing or normal tissue and should be rinsed off immediately if used for irrigation. Solutions are unstable and must be prepared fresh for each use.
Test-Taking Strategy: Use the process of elimination. Note the key words "need for further teaching." Eliminate options 1 and 2 first because they are similar and indicate avoiding healthy tissue. Preparing the solution before use makes sense; therefore eliminate option 4. If you are unfamiliar with the use of this solution, review these concepts.
Level of Cognitive Ability: Analysis
Client Needs: Physiological Integrity
Integrated Process: Teaching/Learning
Content Area: Pharmacology
Reference: Lehne, R. (2001). *Pharmacology for nursing care* (4th ed., p. 1074). Philadelphia: W. B. Saunders.

13. **3**
Rationale: Tretinoin is applied liberally to the skin. The hands are washed thoroughly immediately after applying. Therapeutic results should be seen after 2 to 3 weeks but may not be optimal until after 6 weeks. The skin needs to be cleansed thoroughly before applying the medication.
Test-Taking Strategy: Use the process of elimination. Note the key words "need for further instructions." Eliminate options 1 and 4 first using the principles of asepsis. Recalling that the medication is applied liberally to the skin and noting the absolute word "must" in option 3 will direct you to this option. Review this medication if you had difficulty with this question.
Level of Cognitive Ability: Analysis
Client Needs: Physiological Integrity
Integrated Process: Teaching/Learning
Content Area: Pharmacology
Reference: Hodgson, B., & Kizior, R. (2004). *Saunders nursing drug handbook 2004* (p. 1016). Philadelphia: W. B. Saunders.

14. **3**
Rationale: Isotretinoin can elevate triglyceride levels. Blood triglyceride content should be measured before treatment and

periodically thereafter until the effect on the triglycerides have been evaluated. Options 1, 2, and 4 do not need to be monitored specifically during this treatment.
Test-Taking Strategy: Use the process of elimination. Eliminate options 1 and 2 first because a complete blood count also will measure the white blood cell count. From the remaining options, recall that the medication can affect the triglyceride level in the client. Review this medication if you had difficulty with this question
Level of Cognitive Ability: Analysis
Client Needs: Physiological Integrity
Integrated Process: Nursing Process—analysis
Content Area: Pharmacology
Reference: Hodgson, B., & Kizior, R. (2004). *Saunders nursing drug handbook 2004* (p. 563). Philadelphia: W. B. Saunders.

15. **3**
Rationale: Vitamin A, being a relative of isotretinoin, can produce generalized intensification of isotretinoin toxicity. Because of the potential for increased toxicity, vitamin A supplements should be discontinued before isotretinoin therapy. Options 1, 2, and 4 are not contraindicated with the use of isotretinoin.
Test-Taking Strategy: Use the process of elimination. Recalling that isotretinoin is a derivative of vitamin A will direct you easily to the correct option. If you are unfamiliar with this medication, review the contraindications associated with its use.
Level of Cognitive Ability: Analysis
Client Needs: Physiological Integrity
Integrated Process: Nursing Process—analysis
Content Area: Pharmacology
Reference: Hodgson, B., & Kizior, R. (2003). *Saunders nursing drug handbook 2003* (p. 622). Philadelphia: W. B. Saunders.

16. **2**
Rationale: The wound should be cleansed with a sterile solution before treatment. The nurse then thoroughly moistens the wound with normal saline or sterile water, applies a thin film of sutilains extending ¼ to ½ inch beyond the area to be débrided, and then applies a loose thin dressing. The ointment should be refrigerated.
Test-Taking Strategy: Use the process of elimination. Note the key word "inaccurate" in the stem of the question. Recalling that the wound is moistened before applying the sutilains will direct you to the correct option. Review the method of application of sutilains if you had difficulty with this question.
Level of Cognitive Ability: Analysis
Client Needs: Physiological Integrity
Integrated Process: Teaching/Learning
Content Area: Leadership/Management
Reference: McKenry, L., & Salerno, E. (2001). *Mosby's pharmacology in nursing* (21st ed., p. 1146). St. Louis: Mosby.

17. **4**
Rationale: Dextranomer is a cleansing rather than a débriding agent that is effective in wet wounds only. Dextranomer is not packed tightly into the wound because maceration of surrounding tissue may result.
Test-Taking Strategy: Use the process of elimination. Note the key words "indicates a need for further research." Noting that

option 1 indicates that the wound should be wet and option 4 indicates that the wound should be dry provides the clue that one of these options is correct. If you are unfamiliar with the use of dextranomer, review the procedure associated with its use.
Level of Cognitive Ability: Analysis
Client Needs: Physiological Integrity
Integrated Process: Teaching/Learning
Content Area: Pharmacology
Reference: McKenry, L., & Salerno, E. (2001). *Mosby's pharmacology in nursing* (21st ed., p. 1147). St. Louis: Mosby.

18. **3**
Rationale: The wound should be cleansed with a sterile solution and gently patted dry. A thin layer of Elase is applied and covered with a petrolatum gauze. If a dry powder is used, for best effects, the solution should be prepared just before use.
Test-Taking Strategy: Use the process of elimination. Note the word "intervenes" in the stem of the question. Also, noting the key word "thick" in option 3 will direct you to this option. Review the method of application of Elase if you had difficulty with this question.
Level of Cognitive Ability: Application
Client Needs: Physiological Integrity
Integrated Process: Teaching/Learning
Content Area: Leadership/Management
Reference: McKenry, L., & Salerno, E. (2001). *Mosby's pharmacology in nursing* (21st ed., p. 1146). St. Louis: Mosby.

19. **2**
Rationale: Azelaic acid is a topical medication used to treat mild to moderate acne. The acid appears to work by suppressing growth of *Propionibacterium acnes* and by decreasing proliferation of keratinocytes. Options 1, 3, and 4 are incorrect.
Test-Taking Strategy: Use the process of elimination. You must know that azelaic acid is used to treat acne to answer this question correctly. Review this medication if you are unfamiliar with it.
Level of Cognitive Ability: Analysis
Client Needs: Physiological Integrity
Integrated Process: Nursing Process—analysis
Content Area: Pharmacology

Reference: Kee, J., & Hayes, E. (2003). *Pharmacology: A nursing process approach* (4th ed., p.702). Philadelphia: W. B. Saunders.

20. **2**
Rationale: Hair regrowth with the use of Rogaine is most likely to occur when baldness has developed recently and has been limited to a small area. On discontinuation of the medication, newly gained hair is lost in 3 to 4 months, and the natural progression of hair loss resumes. Options 1 and 3 are incorrect. Option 4 places the client's question on hold and is inappropriate.
Test-Taking Strategy: Use the process of elimination. Option 4 can be eliminated easily because it places the client's question on hold. Knowledge regarding the clinical response and effects of this medication is required to select the correct answer from the remaining options. If you are unfamiliar with this medication, review its effects.
Level of Cognitive Ability: Application
Client Needs: Psychosocial Integrity
Integrated Process: Nursing Process—implementation
Content Area: Pharmacology
Reference: Hodgson, B., & Kizior, R. (2004). *Saunders nursing drug handbook 2004* (p. 679). Philadelphia: W. B. Saunders.

CRITICAL THINKING: FILL IN THE BLANK
Answer: 7 days
Rationale: The nurse would schedule the next home care visit in 7 days. Protective dressings such as Duoderm are designed to be left in place for 7 days unless leakage occurs around the dressing.
Test-Taking Strategy: Note the key word "Duoderm." Recalling that protective dressings are designed to be left in place for 7 days will assist you easily in answering this question. Review the purpose and procedure for using protective dressings if you had difficulty with this question.
Level of Cognitive Ability: Application
Client Needs: Physiological Integrity
Integrated Process: Nursing Process—planning
Content Area: Pharmacology
Reference: McKenry, L., & Salerno, E. (2001). *Mosby's pharmacology in nursing* (21st ed.). St. Louis: Mosby, 1147.

REFERENCES

Gutierrez, K., & Queener, S. (2003). *Pharmacology for nursing practice.* St. Louis: Mosby.

Hodgson, B., & Kizior, R. (2003). *Saunders nursing drug handbook 2003.* Philadelphia: W. B. Saunders.

Hodgson, B., & Kizior, R. (2004). *Saunders nursing drug handbook 2004.* Philadelphia: W. B. Saunders.

Kee, J., & Hayes, E. (2003). *Pharmacology: A nursing process approach.* (4th ed.). Philadelphia: W. B. Saunders.

Lehne, R. (2001). *Pharmacology for nursing care* (4th ed.). Philadelphia: W. B. Saunders.

McKenry, L., & Salerno, E. (2001). *Mosby's pharmacology in nursing* (21st ed.). St. Louis: Mosby.

The Adult Client with an Oncological Disorder

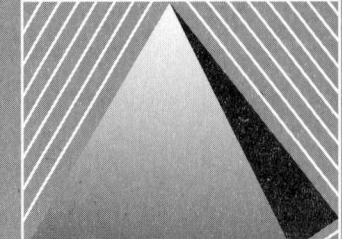

PYRAMID TERMS

benign   Usually a reference to growths that are encapsulated, remain localized, and are slow growing.

cancer   A neoplastic disorder that can involve all body organs. Cells lose their normal growth-controlling mechanism, and the growth of cells is uncontrolled.

carcinogen   A physical, chemical, or biological stressor that causes neoplastic changes in normal cells.

carcinoma   A new growth or malignant tumor that originates from epithelial cells, the skin, gastrointestinal tract, lungs, uterus, breast, and other organs.

carcinoma in situ   A lesion with all the histological characteristics of malignancies, except invasion.

hospice   A concept of care for terminally ill clients that includes the idea of intensive caring rather than intensive care. The family and the client are the focus of nursing care, and the goal is to relieve pain and facilitate the optimal quality of life.

lymphomas   Neoplasms that originate from lymphoid tissue.

leukemias or myelomas   Neoplasms that originate from blood-forming organs.

malignant   Term for growths that are not encapsulated but metastasize and grow. These growths are cancerous lesions having the characteristics of disorderly, uncontrolled, and chaotic proliferation of cells.

metastasis   The transfer of disease from one organ or part to another not directly connected with it. Secondary malignant lesions, originating from the primary tumor, are located in anatomically distant places.

nadir   The period of time during which an antineoplastic medication has its most profound effects on the bone marrow.

neoplasm   A new growth, which may be benign or malignant.

sarcomas   Neoplasms that originate from muscle, bone, fat, the lymph system, or connective tissues.

staging   A method of classifying malignancies based on the presence and extent of the tumor within the body.

tumor markers   Specific bodily substances that seem to indicate tumor progression or regression.

undifferentiated cells   Cells that have lost the capacity for specialized functions.

⯈ PYRAMID TO SUCCESS

Pyramid Points focus on treatment modalities related to an oncological disorder, such as pain management, internal and external radiation, and chemotherapy and on oncological disorders such as skin cancer, leukemia, breast cancer, and lung cancer. Specific focus relates to the nursing care related to these treatment modalities and disorders and to client adaptation and the impact of the treatment or the disorder. Specifically, focus on the complications related to chemotherapy and the nursing measures required in monitoring for these complications and in preventing life-threatening conditions such as infection and bleeding. Specific laboratory values include the white blood cell count and the platelet count. The Integrated Processes addressed in this unit include Nursing Process, Caring, Communication and Documentation, and Teaching/Learning.

CLIENT NEEDS

Safe, Effective Care Environment

Advance directives
Advocacy related to client's decisions
Client rights
Confidentiality regarding diagnosis
Establishing priorities
Ethical practice
Handling of hazardous and infectious materials related to radiation and chemotherapy
Informed consent for treatments and procedures
Medical and surgical asepsis
Oncology-related consultations and referrals
Protective precautions
Standard and other precautions

Health Promotion and Maintenance

Client and family instructions regarding home care
Client lifestyle choices
Expected body image changes related to chemotherapy and treatments
Health screening measures for cancer
Health promotion programs regarding risks for cancer
Instructions regarding monthly breast or testicular self-examinations
Prevention of disease related to infection

Psychosocial Integrity

Ability to cope, adapt, and/or problem solve during illness or stressful events
Assisting the client and family to cope with the alteration in body image
End-of-life issues
Grief and loss related to death and the dying process
Mobilizing appropriate support and resource systems
Promoting a positive environment to maintain optimal quality of life
Religious and cultural preferences

Physiological Integrity

Administration of blood and blood products
Central venous access devices
Chemotherapy
Diagnostic tests and laboratory values such as white blood cell and platelet counts
Management of pain
Monitoring for expected and unexpected responses to radiation and chemotherapy
Promotion of nutrition
Protecting the client from the life-threatening side effects of treatments
Provision of basic care and comfort
Radiation therapy

REFERENCES

Chernecky, C., & Berger, B. (2004). *Laboratory tests & diagnostic procedures* (4th ed.). Philadelphia: W. B. Saunders.

Harkreader, H., & Hogan, M.A. (2004). *Fundamentals of nursing: caring and clinical judgment* (2nd ed.). Philadelphia: W. B. Saunders.

Ignatavicius, D., & Workman, M. (2002). *Medical-surgical nursing: Critical thinking for collaborative care* (4th ed.). Philadelphia: W. B. Saunders.

Lewis, S., Heitkemper, M., & Dirksen, S. (2004). *Medical-surgical nursing: Assessment and management of clinical problems* (6th ed.). St. Louis: Mosby.

National Council of State Boards of Nursing (Eds.). (2003). *Test Plan for the National Council Licensure Examination for Registered Nurses* (effective date: April 2004). Chicago: Author.

Perry, A., & Potter, P. (2002). *Clinical nursing skills and techniques* (5th ed.). St. Louis: Mosby.

Phipps, W., Monahan, F., Sands, J., Marek, J., & Neighbors, M. (2003). *Medical-surgical nursing: Health and illness perspectives* (7th ed.). St. Louis: Mosby.

Potter, P., & Perry, A. (2001). *Fundamentals of nursing* (5th ed.). St. Louis: Mosby.

Varcarolis, Elizabeth M. (2002). *Foundations of psychiatric mental health nursing* (4th ed.). Philadelphia: W. B. Saunders.

Oncological Disorders

I. CANCER
A. Description
   1. **Cancer** is a neoplastic disorder that can involve all body organs.
   2. Cells lose their normal growth-controlling mechanism, and the growth of cells is uncontrolled.
   3. **Cancer** produces serious health problems such as impaired immune and hematopoietic (blood-producing) function, altered gastrointestinal tract structure and function, motor and sensory deficits, and decreased respiratory function.
B. **Metastasis** (Box 51-1)
   1. **Cancer** cells move from their original location to other sites.
   2. Routes of **metastasis**
      a. Local seeding: Distribution of shed **cancer** cells occurs in the local area of the primary tumor.
      b. Blood-borne **metastasis**: Tumor cells enter the blood, which is the most common cause of **cancer** spread.
      c. Lymphatic spread: Primary sites rich in lymphatics are more susceptible to early metastatic spread.
C. **Cancer** classification
   1. Solid tumors: Associated with the organs from which they develop, such as breast **cancer** or lung **cancer**
   2. Hematological cancers: Originate from blood cell-forming tissues, such as the **leukemias** and the **lymphomas**
D. Grading and **staging** (Box 51-2)
   1. Grading and **staging** are methods used to describe the tumor.

BOX 51-1

Common Sites of Metastasis

BREAST CANCER
Bone
Lung

LUNG CANCER
Brain

COLORECTAL CANCER
Liver

PROSTATE CANCER
Bone
Spine and legs

BRAIN TUMORS
Central nervous system

BOX 51-2

Grading and Staging

GRADING
Grade I: Cells differ slightly from normal cells and are well differentiated (mild dysplasia).
Grade II: Cells are more abnormal and are moderately differentiated (moderate dysplasia).
Grade III: Cells are very abnormal and are poorly differentiated (severe dysplasia).
Grade IV: Cells are immature (anaplasia) and undifferentiated; cell of origin is difficult to determine.

STAGING
Stage 0: Carcinoma in situ
Stage I: Tumor limited to the tissue of origin; localized tumor growth
Stage II: Limited local spread
Stage III: Extensive local and regional spread
Stage IV: Metastasis

2. These methods describe the extent of the tumor, the extent to which malignancy has increased in size, the involvement of regional nodes, and metastatic development.

3. Grading a tumor classifies the cellular aspects of the **cancer**.

4. **Staging** classifies the clinical aspects of the **cancer**.

E. Factors that influence **cancer** development

1. Environmental factors

a. Chemical **carcinogen**: Factors include industrial chemicals, drugs, and tobacco.

b. Physical **carcinogen**: Factors include ionizing radiation (diagnostic and therapeutic x-rays) and ultraviolet radiation (sun, tanning beds, and germicidal lights), chronic irritation, and tissue trauma.

c. Viral **carcinogen**: Viruses capable of causing **cancer** are known as oncoviruses (Epstein-Barr virus, hepatitis B virus, human papillomavirus).

2. Dietary factors: Factors include high-fat and low-fiber diets; high animal fat intake; preservatives, contaminants, and additives; and nitrates.

3. Genetic predisposition: Factors include an inherited predisposition to specific cancers, inherited conditions associated with **cancer,** familial clustering, and chromosomal abberations.

4. Age: Advancing age is a significant risk factor for the development of **cancer**.

5. Immune function: Incidences of **cancer** are higher in immunosuppressed individuals, organ transplant recipients who are taking immunosuppressive medication, and individuals with acquired immunodeficiency syndrome.

F. Prevention: Avoidance of known or potential carcinogens and avoidance or modification of the factors associated with the development of **cancer** cells

G. Early detection (Box 51-3)

1. Mammography
2. Papanicolaou's ("Pap") test
3. Stools for occult blood
4. Sigmoidoscopy; colonoscopy
5. Breast self-examination
6. Testicular self-examination
7. Skin inspection

BOX 51-3

Seven Warning Signs of Cancer

Change in bowel or bladder habits
Any sore that does not heal
Unusual bleeding or discharge
Thickening or lump in breast or elsewhere
Indigestion
Obvious change in wart or mole
Nagging cough or hoarseness

II. BREAST SELF-EXAMINATION (BSE)

A. Performing BSE

1. Perform 7 to 10 days after menses.

2. Postmenopausal clients or clients who have had a hysterectomy should select a specific day of the month and perform BSE monthly on that day.

B. Procedure: See Figure 51-1.

III. TESTICULAR SELF-EXAMINATION

A. Performing testicular self-examination: Select a day of the month and perform the examination on the same day each month.

B. Procedure: See Figure 51-2.

IV. DIAGNOSTIC TESTS

A. Diagnostic tests to be performed depend on the suspected primary or metastatic site(s) of the **cancer** (Box 51-4).

B. Biopsy

1. Description

a. Biopsy is the definitive means of diagnosing **cancer** and provides histological proof of malignancy.

b. Biopsy involves the surgical incision of a small piece of tissue for microscopic examination.

2. Types

a. Needle: Aspiration of cells

b. Incisional: Removal of a wedge of suspected tissue from a larger mass

c. Excisional: Complete removal of the entire lesion

d. **Staging**: Multiple needle or incisional biopsies in tissues where **metastasis** is suspected or likely (Refer to Box 51-2.)

3. Tissue examination

a. Following excision, a frozen section or a permanent paraffin section is prepared to examine the specimen.

b. The advantage of the frozen section is the speed with which the section can be prepared and the diagnosis made because only minutes are required for this test.

c. Permanent paraffin section takes about 24 hours; however, it provides clearer details than does the frozen section.

4. Interventions

a. The procedure usually is performed in an outpatient surgical setting.

b. Prepare the client for the diagnostic procedure, following the physician's instructions.

c. Obtain an informed consent.

V. PAIN CONTROL

A. Causes of pain

1. Bone destruction
2. Obstruction of an organ
3. Compression of peripheral nerves

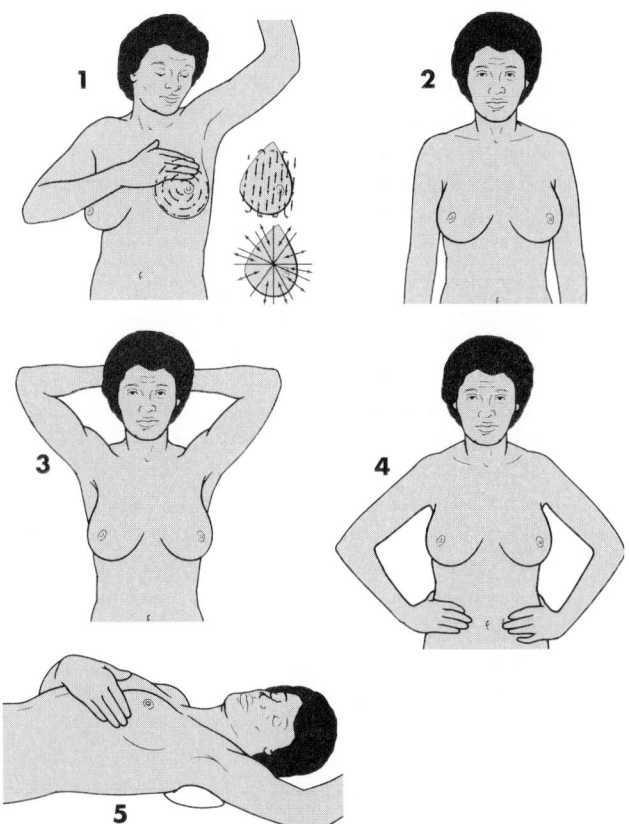

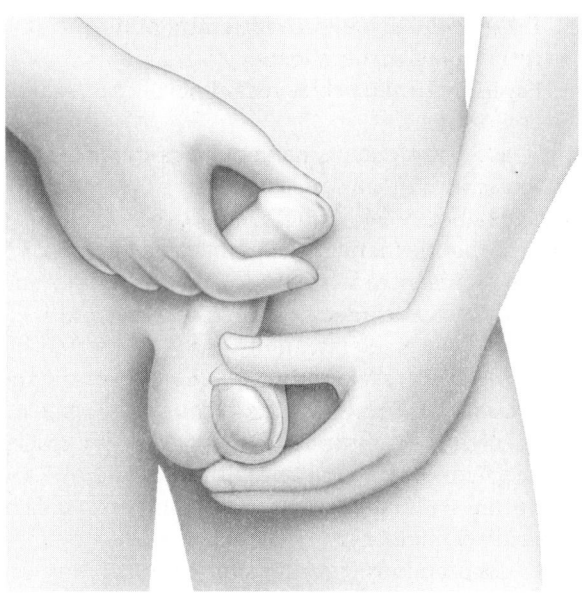

FIG. 51-2   Testicular self-examination. (1) The best time to perform this examination is right after a shower when your scrotal skin is moist and relaxed, making the testicles easy to feel. (2) Gently lift each testicle. Each one should feel like an egg, firm but not hard, and smooth with no lumps. (3) Using both hands, place your middle fingers on the underside of each testicle and your thumbs on top. (4) Gently roll the testicle between the thumb and fingers to feel for any lumps, swelling, or mass. (5) If you notice any changes from one month to the next, notify your physician or nurse practitioner. (From Harkreader, H., & Hogan, M. A. [2004]. *Fundamentals of nursing: Caring and clinical judgment* [2nd ed.]. Philadelphia: W. B. Saunders.)

FIG. 51-1   Breast self-examination and patient instruction. *1,* While in the shower or bath, when the skin is slippery with soap and water, examine your breasts. Use the pads of your second, third, and fourth fingers to press firmly every part of the breast. Use your right hand to examine your left breast, and use your left hand to examine your right breast. Using the pads of the fingers on your left hand, examine the entire breast using small circular motions in a spiral or in an up-and-down motion so that the entire breast area is examined. Repeat the procedure using your right hand to examine your left breast. Repeat pattern of palpation under the arm. Check for any lump, hard knot, or thickening of the tissue. *2,* Look at your breasts in a mirror. Stand with your arms at your side. *3,* Raise your arms overhead and check for any changes in the shape of your breasts, dimpling of the skin, or any changes in the nipple. *4,* Next, place your hands on your hips and press down firmly, tightening the pectoral muscles. Observe for asymmetry or changes, keeping in mind that your breasts probably do not match exactly. *5,* While lying down, feel your breasts as described in step 1. When examining your right breast, place a folded towel under your right shoulder and put your right hand behind your head. Repeat the procedure while examining your left breast. Mark your calendar that you have completed your breast-self-examination; note any changes or unique characteristics you want to check with your health care provider. (From Lewis, S., Heitkemper, M., & Dirksen, S. [2004]. *Medical-surgical nursing: Assessment and management of clinical problems* [6th ed.]. St. Louis: Mosby.)

BOX 51-4

Diagnostic Tests

Biopsy
Bone marrow examination (if a hematolymphoid malignancy is suspected)
Chest radiograph
Complete blood count
Computed tomography scan
Cytological studies (Papanicolaou's smear)
Liver function studies
Magnetic resonance imaging
Presence of oncofetal antigens such as carcinoembryonic antigen and alpha fetoprotein
Proctoscopic examination (including guaiac for occult blood)
Radiographic studies (mammogram)
Radioisotope scans (liver, brain, bone, lung)

4. Infiltration/distention of tissue
5. Inflammation/necrosis
6. Psychological, such as fear or anxiety
B. Interventions
1. Assess the client's pain; pain is what the client describes or says that it is.
2. Collaborate with other members of the health care team to develop a pain management program.
3. Administer oral preparations if possible and if they provide adequate relief of pain.
4. Mild or moderate pain may be treated with salicylates, acetaminophen (Tylenol), and nonsteroidal antiinflammatory drugs.
5. Severe pain is treated with narcotics, such as codeine sulfate, meperidine (Demerol), morphine sulfate, and hydromorphone hydrochloride (Dilaudid).
6. Subcutaneous injections and continuous intravenous (IV) infusions of narcotics provide better pain control than via the oral route.
7. Monitor vital signs and for side effects of medications.
8. Monitor for effectiveness of medications.
9. Provide nonpharmacological techniques of pain control, such as relaxation, guided imagery, biofeedback, and diversion.
10. Do not undermedicate the **cancer** client who is in pain.

VI. SURGERY

A. Description: Surgery is used to diagnose, stage, and treat **cancer.**
B. Prophylactic surgery
1. Prophylactic surgery is performed in clients with an existing premalignant condition or a known family history that strongly predisposes the person to the development of **cancer.**
2. An attempt is made to remove the tissue or organ at risk and thus prevent the development of **cancer.**
C. Curative surgery: All gross and microscopic tumor is removed or destroyed.
D. Control (cytoreductive) surgery
1. Control surgery is a "debulking" procedure that consists of removing part of the tumor.
2. Surgery decreases the number of **cancer** cells and increases the chance that other therapies will be successful.
E. Palliative surgery
1. Palliative surgery is performed to improve quality of life during the survival time.
2. Palliative surgery is performed to reduce pain, relieve airway obstruction, relieve obstructions in the gastrointestinal or urinary tract, relieve pressure on the brain or spinal cord, prevent hemorrhage, remove infected or ulcerated tumors, or drain abscesses.

F. Reconstructive or rehabilitative surgery is performed to improve quality of life by restoring maximal function and appearance, such as breast reconstruction after mastectomy.
G. Side effects of surgery
1. Loss or loss of function of a specific body part
2. Reduced function as a result of organ loss
3. Scarring or disfigurement
4. Grieving about altered body image or imposed change in lifestyle

VII. CHEMOTHERAPY

A. Description
1. Chemotherapy kills or inhibits the reproduction of neoplastic cells and also attacks and kills normal cells.
2. The effects are systemic; chemotherapy affects healthy cells and cancerous cells.
3. Normal cells most profoundly affected include those of the skin, hair, and lining of the gastrointestinal tract, spermatocytes, and hematopoietic cells.
4. Cell cycle phase-specific medications affect cells only during a certain phase of the reproductive cycle, and cell cycle phase-nonspecific medications affect cells in any phase of the reproductive cycle.
5. Usually several medications are used in combination (combination therapy) to increase the therapeutic response.
6. Combination chemotherapy is planned to avoid prescribing medications with nadirs (the time during which bone marrow activity and white blood cell counts are at their lowest) at or near the same time to minimize immunosuppression.
7. Antineoplastic therapy may be combined with other treatments, such as surgery and radiation.
8. The preferred route of administration is intravenously.
9. Side effects include alopecia, nausea and vomiting, mucositis, skin changes, immunosuppression, anemia, and thrombocytopenia.
10. Refer to Chapter 52 for information regarding the care of the client receiving chemotherapy.

VIII. RADIATION THERAPY

A. Description
1. Radiation therapy destroys **cancer** cells with minimal exposure of normal cells to the damaging effects of radiation; the cells damaged die or become unable to divide.
2. Radiation therapy is effective on tissues directly within the path of the radiation beam.
3. Side effects include skin changes and irritation, alopecia, fatigue, and altered taste sensation; also, the effects vary according to the site of treatment.
4. Teletherapy and brachytherapy are the types of radiation therapy most commonly used to treat **cancer.**

BOX 51-5

Teletherapy: Client Education

Wash area with water or mild soap and water, using the hand rather than a washcloth; rinse the soap thoroughly, and pat dry with a soft towel or cloth.

Do not remove the radiation markings from the skin.

Use no powders, ointments, lotions, or creams on the area unless prescribed.

Wear soft clothing over the area, avoiding belts, buckles, straps, or any clothing that binds or rubs the skin.

Avoid sun and heat exposure.

Monitor for moist desquamation (weeping of the skin).

If moist desquamation occurs, cleanse the area with warm water and pat dry, apply antibiotic ointment or steroid cream as prescribed, and expose the site to air.

BOX 51-6

Care of the Client with a Sealed Radiation Source

Place the client in a private room with a private bath.

Place a caution sign on the client's door.

Organize nursing tasks to minimize exposure to the radiation source.

Nursing assignments to a client with a radiation implant should be rotated.

Limit time to 30 minutes per care provider per shift.

Wear a dosimeter film badge to measure radiation exposure.

Wear a lead shield to reduce the transmission of radiation.

A nurse should never care for more than one client with a radiation implant at one time.

Do not allow a pregnant nurse to care for the client.

Do not allow children under the age of 16 or a pregnant woman to visit the client.

Limit visitors to 30 minutes per day; visitors should be at least 6 feet from the source.

Save bed linens and dressings until the source is removed; then dispose of in the usual manner.

Other equipment can be removed from the room at any time.

BOX 51-7

A Dislodged Radiation Source

Do not touch a dislodged radiation source with bare hands.

If the radiation source dislodges, use long-handled forceps to place the source in the lead container kept in the client's room, and call the physician.

If unable to locate the radiation source, bar visitors and notify the physician.

B. Teletherapy (Box 51-5)
  1. Teletherapy also is called beam radiation; the actual radiation source is external to client.
  2. The client does not emit radiation and does not pose a hazard to anyone else.
C. Brachytherapy
  1. The radiation source comes into direct, continuous contact with tumor tissues for a specific time.
  2. The radiation source is within the client; for a period of time, the client emits radiation and can pose a hazard to others.
  3. Brachytherapy includes an unsealed source or a sealed source of radiation.
  4. Unsealed radiation source
    a. Administration is via the oral or IV route or by instillation into body cavities.
    b. The source is not confined completely to one body area, and it enters body fluids and eventually is eliminated via various excreta, which are radioactive and harmful to others; most of the source is eliminated from the body within 48 hours; then neither the client nor the excreta are radioactive or harmful.
  5. Sealed radiation source (Boxes 51-6 and 51-7)
    a. A sealed, temporary or permanent radiation source (solid implant) is implanted within the tumor target tissues.
    b. The client emits radiation while the implant is in place, but the excreta are not radioactive.
  6. Removal of sealed radiation sources
    a. The client is no longer radioactive.
    b. Inform the client that sexual partners cannot "catch" **cancer.**
    c. Inform the female client that she may resume sexual intercourse after 7 to 10 days, if the implant was cervical or vaginal.
    d. Provide a povidone-iodine douche if prescribed, if the implant was placed in the cervix.
    e. Administer a Fleet enema if prescribed.
    f. Advise the client who had a cervical or vaginal implant to notify the physician if nausea, vomiting, diarrhea, frequent urination, vaginal or rectal bleeding, hematuria, foul-smelling vaginal discharge, abdominal pain or distention, or a fever occurs.

IX. BONE MARROW TRANSPLANTATION
A. Description
  1. Bone marrow transplantation is used to treat **leukemia** in clients who have closely matched donors and who are experiencing temporary remission with chemotherapy.
  2. The goal of treatment is to rid the client of all leukemic or other **malignant** cells through treatment with high doses of chemotherapy and whole-body irradiation.
  3. Because these treatments are lethal to bone marrow, without the replacement of bone marrow function through transplantation, the client would die of infection or hemorrhage.

B. Types of donor marrow
1. Allogeneic: Marrow donor is usually a sibling or parent with a similar tissue type.
2. Syngeneic: Bone marrow is from an identical twin.
3. Autologous
   a. Autologous donation is the most common type.
   b. The marrow donor is also the recipient.
   c. Marrow is harvested during disease remission and is stored frozen to be reinfused later.
C. Procedure
1. Harvest
   a. Marrow is harvested through multiple aspirations from the iliac crest to retrieve sufficient bone marrow for the transplant.
   b. Five hundred to 1000 mL of marrow is aspirated.
   c. Marrow is filtered for any residual **cancer** cells and to deplete cells that may cause graft-versus-host disease.
   d. Allogeneic marrow is transfused immediately; autologous marrow is frozen for later use.
   e. Harvest is obtained before the initiation of the conditioning regimen.
2. Conditioning refers to an immunosuppression therapy regimen used to eradicate all **malignant** cells, provide a state of immunosuppression, and create space in the bone marrow for the engraftment of the new marrow.
3. Transplantation
   a. Bone marrow is administered through the client's central line in a manner similar to a blood transfusion.
   b. Marrow is infused over a 30-minute period or may be administered by IV push directly into the central line.
4. Engraftment
   a. The transfused bone marrow cells move to the marrow-forming sites of the recipient's bones.
   b. Engraftment occurs when the white blood cell, erythrocyte, and platelet counts begin to rise.
   c. When successful, the engraftment process takes 2 to 5 weeks.
D. Posttransplantation period
1. The client remains without any natural immunity until the donor marrow begins to proliferate and engraftment occurs.
2. Infection and severe thrombocytopenia are major concerns until engraftment occurs.
E. Complications
1. Failure to engraft: If the transplanted bone marrow fails to engraft, the client will die unless another transplantation is attempted and is successful.
2. Graft-versus-host disease
   a. Although the recipient cannot recognize the donated bone marrow cells as foreign or non-self because of the total immunosuppression, the immune competent cells of the donated

marrow recognize the client's cells as foreign and mount an immune offense against them.
   b. The graft actually is trying to attack the host.
   c. Graft-versus-host disease is managed with immunosuppressive agents with caution to avoid suppressing the new immune system to the extent that the client becomes more susceptible to infection or the transplanted cells stop engrafting.
3. Venoocclusive disease
   a. The disease involves occlusion of the hepatic venules by thrombosis or phlebitis.
   b. Signs include right upper quadrant abdominal pain, jaundice, ascites, weight gain, and hepatomegaly.
   c. Early detection is critical because there is no known way to open the hepatic vessels.
   d. The client will be treated with fluids and supportive therapy.

X. SKIN CANCER (REFER TO CHAPTER 49.)

XI. LEUKEMIA (BOX 51-8)
A. Description
1. **Leukemia** is **malignant** exacerbation in the number of leukocytes, usually at an immature stage, in the bone marrow.
2. **Leukemia** may be acute, with a sudden onset and short duration, or chronic, with a slow onset and persistent symptoms over a period of years.
3. **Leukemia** affects the bone marrow, causing anemia, leukopenia, the production of immature cells, thrombocytopenia, and a decline in immunity.
4. The cause is unknown and appears to involve gene damage of cells, leading to the transformation of cells from a normal state to a **malignant** state.
5. Risk factors include genetic, viral, immunological, and environmental factors and exposure to radiation, chemicals, and medications.

BOX 51-8

Classification of Leukemia

ACUTE LYMPHOCYTIC LEUKEMIA
Mostly lymphoblasts present in bone marrow
Age of onset is less than 15 years

ACUTE MYELOGENOUS LEUKEMIA
Mostly myeloblasts present in bone marrow
Age of onset is between 15 and 39 years

CHRONIC MYELOGENOUS LEUKEMIA
Mostly granulocytes present in bone marrow
Age of onset is after 50 years

CHRONIC LYMPHOCYTIC LEUKEMIA
Mostly lymphocytes present in bone marrow
Age of onset is after 50 years

B. Assessment
   1. Anorexia, fatigue, weakness, weight loss
   2. Anemia
   3. Bleeding (nosebleeds, gum bleeding, rectal bleeding, hematuria, increased menstrual flow)
   4. Petechiae
   5. Prolonged bleeding after minor abrasions or lacerations
   6. Elevated temperature
   7. Lymphadenopathy and splenomegaly
   8. Palpitations, tachycardia, orthostatic hypotension
   9. Pallor and dyspnea on exertion
   10. Headache
   11. Bone pain and joint swelling
   12. Normal, elevated, or reduced white blood cell count
   13. Decreased hemoglobin and hematocrit levels
   14. Decreased platelet count
   15. Positive bone marrow biopsy identifying leukemic blast phase cells
C. Infection
   1. Infection is a major cause of death in the immunosuppressed client.
   2. Infection can occur through autocontamination or cross-contamination.
   3. Common sites of infection are the skin, respiratory tract, and gastrointestinal tract.
   4. Initiate protective isolation procedures.
   5. Ensure frequent and thorough hand washing.
   6. Ensure that anyone entering the client's room is wearing a mask.
   7. Use strict aseptic technique for all procedures.
   8. Keep supplies for the client separate from supplies for other clients; keep frequently used equipment in the room for the client's use only.
   9. Limit the number of caregivers entering the client's room.
   10. Maintain the client in a private room.
   11. Place the client in a room with high-efficiency particulate air filtration or laminar air flow system if possible.
   12. Reduce exposure to environmental organisms by eliminating fresh or raw fruits and vegetables (low-bacteria diet) from the diet and fresh flowers from the client's room and by not leaving standing water in the client's room.
   13. Be sure that the client's room is cleaned daily.
   14. Assist the client with daily bathing, using an antimicrobial soap.
   15. Assist the client to perform oral hygiene frequently.
   16. Initiate a bowel program to prevent constipation and prevent rectal trauma.
   17. Avoid invasive procedures such as injections, rectal temperatures, and urinary catheterization.
   18. Change wound dressings daily, and inspect the wounds for redness, swelling, or drainage.
   19. Assess the urine for color and cloudiness.

BOX 51-9

Mouth Care for the Client with Mucositis

Inspect mouth daily.
Offer complete mouth care before and after every meal and at bedtime.
Brush teeth and tongue with a soft-bristled toothbrush or sponges.
Provide mouth rinses every 12 hours (saline or sodium bicarbonate and water, as prescribed).
Administer topical anesthetic agents to the mouth sores as prescribed.
Avoid the use of alcohol- or glycerin-based mouthwashes or swabs.
Avoid foods that are hard or spicy.

---

   20. Assess skin and oral mucous membranes for signs of infection (Box 51-9).
   21. Auscultate lung sounds, and encourage the client to cough and deep breathe.
   22. Monitor temperature, pulse, and blood pressure.
   23. Monitor white blood cell and neutrophil counts.
   24. Notify the physician if signs of infection are present, and prepare to obtain specimens for culture of open lesions, urine, and sputum.
   25. Administer prescribed antibiotic, antifungal, and antiviral medication.
   26. Instruct the client to avoid crowds and those with infections.
   27. Instruct the client about a low-bacteria diet and to avoid drinking water that has been standing for longer than 15 minutes.
   28. Instruct the client to avoid activities that expose the client to infection, such as changing a pet's litter box or working with houseplants or in the garden.
   29. Instruct clients that neither they nor their household contacts should receive immunization with a live virus.
D. Bleeding
   1. During the period of greatest bone marrow suppression (the **nadir**), the platelet count may be low, fewer than 10,000 cells/mm^3.
   2. The client is at risk for bleeding when the platelet count falls below 50,000 cells/mm^3, and spontaneous bleeding frequently occurs when the platelet count is fewer than 20,000 cells/mm^3.
   3. Clients with platelet counts fewer than 20,000 cells/mm^3 may need a platelet transfusion.
   4. For clients with anemia and fatigue, packed red blood cells may be prescribed.
   5. Monitor laboratory values.
   6. Examine the client for signs and symptoms of bleeding; examine all body fluids and excrement for the presence of blood.
   7. Handle the client gently; use caution when taking blood pressures to prevent skin injury.

8. Measure abdominal girth, which can provide an indication of internal hemorrhage.
9. Provide soft foods that are cool to warm.
10. Avoid injections, if possible, to prevent trauma to the skin and bleeding; apply firm and gentle pressure to a needle stick site for at least 10 minutes.
11. Pad side rails and sharp corners of the bed and furniture.
12. Avoid rectal suppositories, enemas, and thermometers.
13. If the female client is menstruating, count the number of pads or tampons used.
14. Administer blood products as prescribed.
15. Instruct the client to use a soft toothbrush and avoid dental floss.
16. Instruct the client to use only an electric razor for shaving.
17. Instruct the client to avoid blowing the nose.
18. Instruct the client to avoid constrictive or tight clothing or shoes
19. Discourage the client from engaging in activities involving the use of sharp objects.
20. Instruct the client to avoid using nonsteroidal antiinflammatory drugs and products that contain aspirin.

E. Fatigue and nutrition
1. Assist the client in selecting a well-balanced diet.
2. Provide small, frequent meals (high calorie, high protein, high carbohydrate) that require little chewing.
3. Assist the client in self-care and mobility activities.
4. Allow adequate rest periods during care.
5. Do not perform activities unless they are essential.
6. Administer blood products for anemia as prescribed.

F. Additional interventions
1. Chemotherapy
   a. Induction therapy is aimed at achieving a rapid, complete remission of all manifestations of the disease.
   b. Consolidation therapy is administered early in remission with the aim of cure.
   c. Maintenance therapy may be prescribed for months or years following successful induction and consolidation therapy; the aim is to maintain remission.
2. Administer antibiotic, antibacterial, antiviral, and antifungal medications as prescribed.
3. Administer blood replacements as prescribed.
4. Prepare the client for transplantation as prescribed.
5. Administer colony-stimulating factors as prescribed.
6. Maintain infection and bleeding precautions.
7. Provide an adequate diet.
8. Provide an activity schedule that will conserve energy.
9. Instruct the client in appropriate home care measures.
10. Provide psychosocial support and support services for home care.

XII. HODGKIN'S DISEASE

A. Description
1. Hodgkin's disease (**lymphoma**) is a malignancy of the lymph nodes that originates in a single lymph node or a single chain of nodes.
2. **Metastasis** occurs to other, adjacent lymph structures and eventually invades nonlymphoid tissue.
3. The disease usually involves lymph nodes, tonsils, spleen, and bone marrow and is characterized by the presence of the Reed-Sternberg cell in the nodes.
4. Possible causes include viral infections and previous exposure to alkylating chemical agents.
5. Prognosis depends on the stage of the disease (Box 51-10).

B. Assessment
1. Fever
2. Malaise, fatigue, and weakness
3. Night sweats
4. Loss of appetite and significant weight loss
5. Anemia and thrombocytopenia
6. Enlarged lymph nodes, spleen, and liver
7. Positive biopsy of lymph nodes, with cervical nodes most often affected first
8. Presence of Reed-Sternberg cell in nodes
9. Positive computed tomography scan of the liver and spleen

C. Interventions
1. For stages I and II without mediastinal node involvement, the treatment of choice is extensive external radiation of the involved lymph node regions.
2. With more extensive disease, radiation along with multiagent chemotherapy is used.

BOX 51-10

Staging in Hodgkin's Disease

STAGE I
Involvement of a single lymph node region or an extralymphatic organ or site

STAGE II
Involvement of two or more lymph node regions on the same side of the diaphragm or localized involvement of an extralymphatic organ or site

STAGE III
Involvement of lymph node regions on both sides of the diaphragm

STAGE IV
Diffuse or disseminated involvement of one or more extralymphatic organs with or without associated lymph node involvement

3. Monitor for side effects related to chemotherapy or radiation therapy.
4. Monitor for signs of infection and bleeding.
5. Maintain infection and bleeding precautions.
6. Discuss the possibility of sterility with the male client receiving radiation, and inform the client of options related to sperm banks.

XIII. MULTIPLE MYELOMA

A. Description
1. A **malignant** proliferation of plasma cells and tumors within the bone.
2. An excessive number of abnormal plasma cells invade the bone marrow, develop into tumors, and ultimately destroy bone; invasion of the lymph nodes, spleen, and liver occurs.
3. The abnormal plasma cells produce an abnormal antibody (**myeloma** protein or the Bence Jones protein) that is found in the blood and urine.
4. Multiple myeloma causes decreased production of immunoglobulin and antibodies and increased levels of uric acid and calcium, which can lead to renal failure.
5. The cause of the disease is unknown.

B. Assessment
1. Bone (skeletal) pain, especially in the pelvis, spine, and ribs
2. Weakness and fatigue
3. Recurrent infections
4. Anemia
5. Bence Jones proteinuria and elevated total serum protein level
6. Osteoporosis (bone loss and the development of pathological fractures)
7. Thrombocytopenia and granulocytopenia
8. Elevated calcium and uric acid levels
9. Renal failure
10. Spinal cord compression and paraplegia

C. Interventions
1. Administer chemotherapy as prescribed.
2. Provide supportive care to control symptoms and prevent complications, especially bone fractures, renal failure, and infections.
3. Maintain neutropenic and bleeding precautions as necessary.
4. Monitor for signs of bleeding, infection, and skeletal fractures.
5. Encourage fluids up to 3 to 4 L a day to offset potential problems associated with hypercalcemia, hyperuricemia, and proteinuria.
6. Monitor for signs of renal failure.
7. Encourage ambulation to prevent renal problems and to slow down bone resorption.
8. Provide skeletal support during moving, turning, and ambulating to prevent pathological fractures; provide a hazard-free environment.

9. Administer IV fluids and diuretics as prescribed to increase renal excretion of calcium.
10. Administer blood transfusions as prescribed for anemia.
11. Administer analgesics as prescribed to control pain.
12. Administer antibiotics as prescribed for infection.
13. Prepare the client for local radiation therapy if prescribed.
14. Instruct the client in home care measures and the signs and symptoms of infection.

XIV. TESTICULAR CANCER

A. Description
1. Testicular **cancer** arises from germinal epithelium from the sperm-producing germ cells or from nongerminal epithelium from other structures in the testicles (Box 51-11).
2. Testicular **cancer** most often occurs between the ages of 15 and 40.
3. **Metastasis** occurs to the lung, liver, bone, and adrenal glands.

B. Prevention: Routine testicular self-examination

C. Assessment
1. Painless testicular swelling occurs.
2. Dragging sensation is evident in the scrotum.
3. Palpable lymphadenopathy, abdominal masses, and gynecomastia may indicate **metastasis**.
4. Late signs include back or bone pain and respiratory symptoms.

D. Interventions
1. Administer chemotherapy as prescribed.
2. Prepare the client for radiation therapy as prescribed.
3. Prepare the client for unilateral orchiectomy, if prescribed, for diagnosis and primary surgical management.
4. Prepare the client for radical retroperitoneal lymph node dissection, if prescribed, to stage the disease and reduce tumor volume so that chemotherapy and radiation therapy are more effective.
5. Discuss reproduction, sexuality, and fertility information and options with the client.
6. Identify reproductive options such as sperm storage, donor insemination, and adoption.

BOX 51-11

Types of Testicular Cancer

GERMINAL TUMORS
Seminomas
Nonseminomas

NONGERMINAL TUMORS
Interstitial cell tumors
Androblastoma

E. Postoperative interventions
 1. Monitor for signs of bleeding and wound infection.
 2. Monitor intake and output.
 3. Notify the physician if chills, fever, increasing pain or tenderness at the incision site, or drainage of the incision occurs.
 4. Instruct the client that he may resume normal activities within 1 week, except for lifting objects heavier than 20 lb or stair climbing.
 5. Instruct the client to perform a monthly testicular self-examination on the remaining testicle.
 6. Inform the client that sutures will be removed 7 to 10 days after surgery.

XV. CERVICAL CANCER

A. Description
 1. Preinvasive **cancer** is limited to the cervix (Box 51-12).
 2. Invasive **cancer** is in the cervix and other pelvic structures.
 3. **Metastasis** usually is confined to the pelvis, but distant **metastasis** occurs through lymphatic spread.
 4. Premalignant changes are described on a continuum from dysplasia, which is the earliest premalignancy change, to **carcinoma in situ**, the most advanced premalignant change.
B. Precipitating factors
 1. Low socioeconomic groups
 2. Early first marriage
 3. Early and frequent intercourse
 4. Multiple sex partners
 5. High parity
 6. Poor hygiene
C. Assessment
 1. Painless vaginal bleeding postmenstrually and postcoitally
 2. Foul-smelling or serosanguineous vaginal discharge
 3. Pelvic, lower back, leg, or groin pain
 4. Anorexia and weight loss
 5. Leakage of urine and feces from the vagina
 6. Dysuria
 7. Hematuria
 8. Cytological changes on Papanicolaou's test
D. Interventions (Box 51-13)
E. Laser therapy
 1. Laser therapy is used when all boundaries of the lesion are visible during colposcopic examination.
 2. Energy from the beam is absorbed by fluid in the tissues, causing them to vaporize.

BOX 51-12

Preinvasive Cancers: Cervical Intraepithelial Neoplasia

I: Mild dysplasia
II: Moderate dysplasia
III: Severe dysplasia to carcinoma in situ

BOX 51-13

Treatment for Cervical Cancer

NONSURGICAL
Chemotherapy
Cryosurgery
External radiation
Internal radiation implants (intracavitary)
Laser therapy

SURGICAL
Conization
Hysterectomy
Pelvic exenteration

---

 3. Minimal bleeding is associated with the procedure.
 4. Slight vaginal discharge is expected following the procedure, and healing occurs in 6 to 12 weeks.
F. Cryosurgery
 1. Cryosurgery involves freezing of the tissues by a probe with subsequent necrosis.
 2. No anesthesia is required, although cramping may occur during the procedure.
 3. A heavy, watery discharge will occur for several weeks following the procedure.
 4. Instruct the client to avoid intercourse and the use of tampons while the discharge is present.
G. Conization
 1. A cone-shaped area of the cervix is removed.
 2. Conization is performed in women who desire further childbearing.
 3. Long-term follow-up care is needed because new lesions can develop.
 4. The risks of the procedure include hemorrhage, uterine perforation, incompetent cervix, cervical stenosis, and preterm labor in future pregnancies.
H. Hysterectomy
 1. Description
  a. Hysterectomy is performed for microinvasive **cancer** if childbearing is not desired.
  b. A vaginal approach is most commonly performed.
  c. A radical hysterectomy and bilateral lymph node dissection may be performed for **cancer** that has spread beyond the cervix but not to the pelvic wall.
 2. Postoperative interventions
  a. Monitor vital signs
  b. Assist with coughing and deep-breathing exercises.
  c. Assist with range-of-motion exercises and provide early ambulation.
  d. Apply antiembolism stockings as prescribed.
  e. Monitor intake and output, Foley catheter drainage, and hydration status.

f. Monitor bowel sounds.

g. Monitor vaginal bleeding; more than one saturated pad per hour may indicate excessive bleeding.

h. Assess incision site for signs of infection.

i. Administer pain medication as prescribed.

j. Instruct the client to avoid stair climbing for 1 month and to avoid tub baths and sitting for long periods.

k. Avoid strenuous activity or lifting anything weighing more than 20 lb.

l. Instruct the client to consume foods that aid in the healing.

m.Instruct the client to avoid sexual intercourse for 3 to 6 weeks as prescribed.

n. Instruct the client in the signs associated with complications.

I. Pelvic exenteration (Box 51-14)

1. Description

a. Exenteration is a radical surgical procedure performed for recurrent **cancer** if no evidence of tumor outside the pelvis and no lymph node involvement exists.

b. When the bladder is removed, an ileal conduit is created and located on the right side of the abdomen to divert urine.

c. A colostomy may need to be created and is located on the left side of the abdomen for the passage of feces.

2. Postoperative interventions

a. Monitor for atelectasis and pneumonia.

b. Assist with coughing and deep-breathing exercises.

c. Monitor for hemorrhage, shock, and deep vein thrombosis.

d. Apply antiembolism stockings as prescribed.

e. Administer prophylactic heparin infusion as prescribed.

f. Monitor bowel sounds.

g. Monitor intake and output and for signs of dehydration.

h. Monitor incision site for infection.

BOX 51-14

Types of Pelvic Exenteration

ANTERIOR
Removal of the uterus, ovaries, fallopian tubes, vagina, bladder, urethra, and pelvic lymph nodes

POSTERIOR
Removal of the uterus, ovaries, fallopian tubes, descending colon, rectum, and anal canal

TOTAL
Combination of anterior and posterior

---

i. Administer perineal irrigations with half-strength normal saline (NS) and hydrogen peroxide as prescribed.

j. Provide sitz baths as prescribed.

k. Administer analgesics as prescribed for pain.

l. Instruct the client to avoid strenuous activity for 6 months.

m.Instruct the client that the perineal opening, if present, may drain for several months.

n. Instruct the client in the care of the ileal conduit and colostomy, if created.

o. Provide sexual counseling because vaginal intercourse is not possible after anterior and total pelvic exenteration.

XVI. OVARIAN CANCER

A. Description

1. Ovarian cancer grows rapidly, spreads fast, and is often bilateral.

2. **Metastasis** occurs by direct spread to the organs in the pelvis, by distal spread through lymphatic drainage, or by peritoneal seeding.

3. Prognosis is usually poor because the tumor usually is detected late.

4. An exploratory laparotomy is performed to diagnose and stage the tumor.

B. Assessment

1. Abdominal discomfort or swelling

2. Gastrointestinal disturbances

3. Dysfunctional vaginal bleeding

4. Abdominal mass

C. Interventions

1. External radiation is used if the tumor has invaded other organs.

2. Chemotherapy is used postoperatively for all stages of ovarian **cancer.**

3. Intraperitoneal chemotherapy involves the instillation of chemotherapy into the abdominal cavity.

4. Immunotherapy alters the immunological response of the ovary and promotes tumor resistance.

5. Total abdominal hysterectomy and bilateral salpingo-oophorectomy may be necessary.

XVII. ENDOMETRIAL CANCER

A. Description

1. Endometrial cancer is a slow-growing tumor associated with the menopausal years.

2. **Metastasis** occurs through the lymphatic system to the ovaries and pelvis; via the blood to the lungs, liver, and bone; or intraabdominally to the peritoneal cavity.

B. Precipitating factors

1. History of uterine polyps

2. Nulliparity

3. Polycystic ovary disease

4. Estrogen stimulation

5. Late menopause
6. Family history
C. Assessment
1. Postmenopausal bleeding
2. Watery, serosanguineous discharge
3. Low back, pelvic, or abdominal pain
4. Enlarged uterus in advanced stages
D. Nonsurgical interventions
1. External radiation or internal radiation is used alone or in combination with surgery, depending on the stage of **cancer.**
2. Chemotherapy is used to treat advanced or recurrent disease.
3. Progestational therapy with medication such as medroxyprogesterone (Depo-Provera) or megestrol acetate (Megace) is used for estrogen-dependent tumors.
4. Tamoxifen (Nolvadex), an antiestrogen, also may be prescribed.
E. Surgical interventions: Total abdominal hysterectomy and bilateral salpingo-oophorectomy

XVIII. BREAST CANCER
A. Description
1. Breast **cancer** is classified as invasive when it penetrates the tissue surrounding the mammary duct and grows in an irregular pattern.
2. **Metastasis** occurs via lymph nodes.
3. Common sites of **metastasis** are the bone lungs; **metastasis** also occurs to the brain and liver.
4. Diagnosis is made by breast biopsy through a needle aspiration or by surgical removal of the tumor with microscopic examination for **malignant** cells.
B. Precipitating factors
1. Family history
2. Early menarche and late menopause
3. Previous **cancer** of the breast, uterus, or ovaries
4. Nulliparity
5. Obesity
6. High-dose radiation exposure to chest
C. Assessment
1. Mass felt during BSE
2. Mass usually felt in the upper outer quadrant or beneath the nipple
3. A fixed, irregular nonencapsulated mass
4. A painless mass except in the late stages
5. Nipple retraction or elevation
6. Asymmetry, with the affected breast being higher
7. Bloody or clear nipple discharge
8. Skin dimpling, retraction, or ulceration
9. Skin edema or peau d'orange skin
10. Axillary lymphadenopathy
11. Lymphedema of affected arm
12. Symptoms of bone or lung **metastasis**
13. Presence of the lesion on mammography
D. Prevention: Monthly BSE

E. Nonsurgical interventions
1. Chemotherapy
2. Radiation therapy
3. Hormonal manipulation via the use of medication in postmenopausal women or other medications such as tamoxifen (Nolvadex) for estrogen receptor-positive tumors
F. Surgical interventions
1. Surgical breast procedures with possible breast reconstruction (Box 51-15)
2. Oophorectomy for estrogen receptor-positive tumors
3. Ablative therapy with adrenalectomy or chemical ablation, which blocks the production of cortisol, androstenedione, and aldosterone
G. Postoperative interventions
1. Monitor vital signs.
2. Position in semi-Fowler position; turn from back to unaffected side, with the affected arm elevated above the level of the heart to promote drainage and prevent lymphedema.
3. Encourage coughing and deep breathing.
4. If a drain (usually Jackson-Pratt) is in place, maintain suction and record the amount of drainage and drainage characteristics.
5. Assess operative site for infection, swelling, or the presence of fluid collection under the skin flaps.
6. Monitor incision site for restriction of dressing, impaired sensation, or color changes of the skin.
7. If breast reconstruction was performed, the client will return from surgery with a surgical brassiere and the temporary prosthesis in place.
8. Place a sign above the bed stating "No IVs, No Injections, No BPs, No Venipunctures in Affected Arm"; the affected arm is protected for life, and any intervention that could traumatize the affected arm is avoided.

BOX 51-15

Surgical Breast Procedures

LUMPECTOMY
Tumor is excised and removed.
Lymph node dissection may also be performed.

SIMPLE MASTECTOMY
Breast tissue and the nipple are removed.
Lymph nodes are left intact.

MODIFIED RADICAL MASTECTOMY
Breast tissue, nipple, and lymph nodes are removed.
Muscles are left intact.

HALSTED RADICAL MASTECTOMY
Breast tissue, nipple, underlying muscles, and lymph nodes are removed.

9. Provide the use of a pressure sleeve as prescribed if edema is severe.
10. Administer diuretics and provide a low-salt diet as prescribed for severe lymphedema.
11. Consult with the physician and the physical therapist regarding the appropriate exercise program.
12. Assist with exercise as prescribed to decrease lymphedema and muscle weakness.
13. Instruct the client about home care measures (Box 51-16).

XIX. GASTRIC CANCER

A. Description
1. Gastric cancer is a **malignant** growth in the stomach.
2. Risk factors include a diet high in complex carbohydrates, grains, and salt, and low in fresh, green, leafy vegetables and fresh fruit; smoking; alcohol ingestion; the use of nitrates; and a history of gastric ulcers.
3. Complications include hemorrhage, obstruction, **metastasis**, and dumping syndrome.
4. The goal of treatment is to remove the tumor and provide a nutritional program.
B. Assessment
1. Fatigue
2. Anorexia and weight loss
3. Nausea and vomiting
4. Indigestion and epigastric discomfort
5. A sensation of pressure in the stomach
6. Dysphagia
7. Anemia
8. Ascites
9. Palpable mass
C. Interventions
1. Monitor vital signs.
2. Monitor hemoglobin and hematocrit and administer blood transfusions as prescribed.
3. Monitor weight.
4. Assess nutritional status; encourage small, bland, easily digestible meals with vitamin and mineral supplements.
5. Administer pain medication as prescribed.
6. Prepare the client for chemotherapy or radiation therapy as prescribed.
7. Prepare the client for surgical resection of the tumor as prescribed (Box 51-17).
D. Postoperative interventions
1. Monitor vital signs.
2. Place in Fowler's position for comfort.
3. Monitor intake and output; administer fluids and electrolyte replacement by IV as prescribed.
4. Maintain NPO status as prescribed for 1 to 3 days until peristalsis returns.
5. Monitor nasogastric suction.
6. Do not irrigate or remove the nasogastric tube; assist the physician with irrigation or removal.
7. Assess for bowel sounds.
8. Advance the diet from NPO to sips of clear water to six small bland meals a day, as prescribed.
9. Monitor for complications of hemorrhage, dumping syndrome, diarrhea, hypoglycemia, and vitamin B_{12} deficiency.

XX. PANCREATIC CANCER

A. Description
1. Pancreatic **cancer** is the most common **neoplasm** affecting the pancreas.
2. Pancreatic **cancer** is more common in blacks than in whites, in smokers, and in men.

BOX 51-16

Client Instructions Following Mastectomy

Avoid overuse of the arm during the first few months.
To prevent lymphedema, keep the affected arm elevated.
Provide incision care with lanolin to soften and prevent wound contracture.
Encourage use of Reach for Recovery volunteers.
Encourage the client to perform breast self-examination on the remaining breast.
Protect the affected hand and arm.
Avoid strong sunlight to the affected arm.
Do not let the affected arm hang dependent.
Do not carry a pocketbook or anything heavy over the affected arm.
Avoid trauma, cuts, bruises, or burns to the affected side.
Avoid wearing constricted clothing or jewelry on the affected side.
Wear gloves when gardening.
Use thick oven mitts when cooking.
Use a thimble when sewing.
Apply lanolin hand cream several times daily.
Use cream cuticle remover.
Call the physician if signs of inflammation occur in the affected arm.
Wear a Medic-Alert bracelet stating lymphedema arm.

BOX 51-17

Surgical Interventions for Gastric Cancer

SUBTOTAL GASTRECTOMY
Billroth I
Also called gastroduodenostomy
Partial gastrectomy, with remaining segment anastomosed to the duodenum
Billroth II
Also called gastrojejunostomy
Partial gastrectomy, with remaining segment anastomosed to the jejunum

TOTAL GASTRECTOMY
Also called esophagojejunostomy
Removal of the stomach with attachment of the esophagus to the jejunum or duodenum

3. The occurrence of pancreatic **cancer** has been linked to diabetes mellitus, alcohol use, history of previous pancreatitis, smoking, ingestion of a high-fat diet, and exposure to environmental chemicals.

4. Symptoms usually do not occur until the tumor is large; therefore the prognosis is poor.

B. Assessment
   1. Nausea and vomiting
   2. Jaundice
   3. Unexplained weight loss
   4. Clay-colored stools
   5. Glucose intolerance
   6. Abdominal pain

C. Interventions
   1. Radiation
   2. Chemotherapy
   3. Whipple's procedure, which involves a pancreaticoduodenectomy with removal of the distal third of the stomach, pancreaticojejunostomy, gastrojejunostomy, and choledochojejunostomy
   4. Postoperative care measures are similar to care of a client with pancreatitis and the client following gastric surgery

XXI. INTESTINAL TUMORS

A. Description
   1. Intestinal tumors are **malignant** lesions that develop in the cells lining the bowel wall or develop as polyps in the colon or rectum.
   2. Complications include bowel perforation with peritonitis, abscess and fistula formation, hemorrhage, and complete intestinal obstruction.
   3. **Metastasis** occurs via the circulatory or lymphatic system or by direct extension to other areas in the colon or other organs.

B. Assessment
   1. Blood in stools
   2. Anorexia, vomiting, and weight loss
   3. Malaise
   4. Anemia
   5. Abnormal stools
      a. Ascending colon tumor: Diarrhea
      b. Descending colon tumor: Constipation or some diarrhea, or flat, ribbonlike stool resulting from a partial obstruction
      c. Rectal tumor: Alternating constipation and diarrhea
   6. Guarding or abdominal distention
   7. Abdominal mass (a late sign)
   8. Cachexia (a late sign)

C. Interventions
   1. Monitor for signs of complications, which include bowel perforation with peritonitis, abscess or fistula formation, hemorrhage, and complete intestinal obstruction.
   2. Monitor for signs of bowel perforation, which include low blood pressure, rapid and weak pulse, distended abdomen, and elevated temperature.
   3. Monitor for signs of intestinal obstruction, which include vomiting (may be fecal contents), pain, constipation, and abdominal distention.
   4. Note that an early sign of intestinal obstruction is increased peristaltic activity, which produces an increase in bowel sounds; as the obstruction progresses, hypoactive sounds are heard.
   5. Prepare for radiation preoperatively to facilitate surgical resection, and postoperatively to decrease the risk of recurrence or to reduce pain, hemorrhage, bowel obstruction, or **metastasis.**
   6. Chemotherapy is used postoperatively to assist in the control of symptoms and the spread of the disease.

D. Surgical interventions: Bowel resection and creation of colostomy or ileostomy

E. Colostomy/ileostomy
   1. Preoperative interventions
      a. Consult with the enterostomal therapist to assist in identifying optimal placement of ostomy.
      b. Instruct the client to eat a low-residue diet for 1 to 2 days before surgery as prescribed.
      c. Administer intestinal antiseptics and antibiotics, as prescribed, to decrease the bacterial content of the colon and to reduce the risk of infection from the surgical procedure.
      d. Administer laxatives and enemas as prescribed.
   2. Postoperative: colostomy
      a. Place a petroleum jelly gauze over the stoma to keep it moist, followed by a dry sterile dressing if a pouch system is not in place.
      b. Place a pouch system on the stoma as soon as possible.
      c. Monitor the stoma for size, unusual bleeding, or necrotic tissue.
      d. Monitor for color changes in the stoma.
      e. Note that the normal stoma color is red or pink, indicating high vascularity.
      f. Note that a pale pink stoma indicates low hemoglobin and hematocrit levels, and a purple-black stoma indicates compromised circulation, requiring physician notification.
      g. Monitor the pouch system for proper fit and signs of leakage.
      h. Assess the functioning of the colostomy.
      i. Expect that stool will be liquid postoperatively but will become more solid, depending on the area of the colostomy.
      j. Ascending colon colostomy: Expect liquid stool.
      k. Transverse colon colostomy: Expect loose to semiformed stool.
      l. Descending colon colostomy: Expect close to normal stool.
      m. Fecal matter should not be allowed to remain on the skin.

n. Empty pouch when one third full.

o. Administer analgesics and antibiotics as prescribed.

p. Irrigate perineal wound if present and if prescribed, and monitor for signs of infection.

q. Instruct the client to avoid foods that cause excessive gas formation and odor.

r. Instruct the client in stoma care and irrigations as prescribed.

s. Instruct the client that normal activities may be resumed when approved by the physician.

3. Postoperative: ileostomy

a. Healthy stoma is red; a color change to dark blue or black should be reported to the physician.

b. Postoperative drainage will be dark green and progress to yellow as the client begins to eat.

c. Stool is liquid.

d. Risk for dehydration and electrolyte imbalance exists.

e. Do not give suppositories through ileostomy.

XXII. LUNG CANCER

A. Description

1. Lung cancer is a **malignant** tumor of the lung that may be primary or metastatic.

2. The lungs are a common target for **metastasis** from other organs.

3. Bronchiogenic **carcinoma** spreads through direct extension and lymphatic dissemination.

4. The four major types of lung **cancer** include small cell (oat cell), epidermal (squamous cell), adeno**carcinoma,** and large cell anaplastic **carcinoma.**

5. Diagnosis is made by a chest x-ray, which will show a lesion or mass, and bronchoscopy and sputum studies, which will demonstrate a positive cytological study for **cancer** cells.

B. Causes

1. Cigarette smoking

2. Exposure to environmental pollutants

3. Exposure to occupational pollutants

C. Assessment

1. Cough

2. Dyspnea

3. Hoarseness

4. Hemoptysis

5. Chest pain

6. Anorexia and weight loss

7. Weakness

D. Interventions

1. Monitor vital signs.

2. Monitor breathing patterns and breath sounds and for signs of respiratory impairment.

3. Assess for tracheal deviation.

4. Administer analgesics as prescribed for pain management.

5. Place in Fowler's position for ease in breathing.

6. Administer oxygen as prescribed and humidification to moisten and loosen secretions.

7. Monitor pulse oximetry.

8. Provide respiratory treatments as prescribed.

9. Administer bronchodilators and corticosteroids as prescribed to decrease bronchospasm, inflammation, and edema.

10. Provide a high-calorie, high-protein, high-vitamin diet.

11. Provide activity as tolerated, rest periods, and active and passive range-of-motion exercises.

12. Monitor for bleeding, infection, and electrolyte imbalances.

E. Nonsurgical interventions

1. Radiation therapy for localized intrathoracic lung cancers and for palliation of hemoptysis, obstructions, dysphagia, and pain

2. Chemotherapy

3. Immunotherapy directed at enhancing an effective immune response, which favorably affects the course of the disease

F. Surgical interventions

1. Laser therapy: To relieve endobronchial obstruction

2. Thoracentesis and pleurodesis: To remove pleural fluid and relieve hypoxia

3. Thoracotomy with pneumonectomy: Surgical removal of a lung

4. Thoracotomy with lobectomy: Surgical removal of one lobe of the lung for tumors confined to a single lobe

5. Thoracotomy with segmental resection: Surgical removal of a lobe segment for clients unable to tolerate lobectomy or pneumonectomy

G. Preoperative interventions

1. Explain the potential postoperative need for chest tubes.

2. Note that closed chest drainage usually is not used for a pneumonectomy, and the serum fluid that accumulates in the empty thoracic cavity eventually consolidates, preventing shifts of the mediastinum, heart, and remaining lung.

H. Postoperative interventions

1. Monitor vital signs.

2. Assess cardiac and respiratory status; monitor for the absence and presence of lung sounds.

3. Maintain chest tube drainage system, which will drain air and blood that accumulates in the pleural space.

4. Assess chest tube insertion site for crepitus (subcutaneous emphysema) and drainage.

5. Administer oxygen as prescribed.

6. Check physician's orders regarding client positioning; avoid complete lateral turning.

7. Monitor pulse oximetry.

8. Provide activity as tolerated.

9. Encourage active range-of-motion exercises of the operative shoulder as prescribed.

10. Refer to Chapter 21 for care of the client with a chest tube.

XXIII. LARYNGEAL CANCER

A. Description
   1. Laryngeal cancer is a **malignant** tumor of the larynx.
   2. Laryngeal **cancer** presents as **malignant** ulcerations with underlying infiltration.
   3. **Metastasis** to the lung is common.
   4. Diagnosis is made by laryngoscopy and biopsy showing a positive cytological study for **cancer** cells.

B. Causes
   1. Cigarette smoking
   2. Exposure to environmental pollutants
   3. Exposure to radiation
   4. Voice strain

C. Assessment
   1. Persistent hoarseness and sore throat
   2. Painless neck mass
   3. A feeling of a lump in the throat
   4. Burning sensation in the throat
   5. Dysphagia
   6. Change in voice quality
   7. Dyspnea
   8. Weakness and weight loss
   9. Hemoptysis
   10. Foul breath odor

D. Interventions
   ▲ 1. Place in Fowler's position to promote optimal air exchange.
   2. Monitor respiratory status.
   ▲ 3. Monitor for signs of aspiration of food and fluid.
   4. Administer oxygen as prescribed.
   5. Provide respiratory treatments as prescribed.
   6. Provide activity as tolerated.
   7. Provide a high-calorie, high-protein, high-vitamin diet.
   8. Provide nutritional support via total parenteral nutrition, nasogastric tube feedings, or gastrostomy or jejunostomy tube, as prescribed.
   9. Administer analgesics as prescribed for pain.

E. Nonsurgical interventions
   1. Radiation therapy if the **cancer** is limited to a small area in one vocal cord
   2. Chemotherapy, which may be done in combination with radiation and surgery

F. Surgical interventions
   1. Surgical intervention depends on the tumor size and the amount of tissue to be resected.
   2. Types of resection include cordal stripping, cordectomy, partial laryngectomy, and total laryngectomy.
   3. A tracheostomy is performed with a total laryngectomy; this airway opening is always permanent and is referred to as a laryngectomy stoma.

G. Preoperative interventions
   1. Establish methods of communication for the client. ▲
   2. Encourage the client to express feelings about changes in body image and loss of voice.
   3. Describe the rehabilitation program and information about the tracheostomy and suctioning.

H. Postoperative interventions
   1. Monitor vital signs.
   2. Monitor respiratory status; monitor airway ▲ patency and provide frequent suctioning to remove bloody secretions.
   3. Place the client in high Fowler's position. ▲
   4. Maintain mechanical ventilator support or a tracheostomy collar with humidification, as prescribed.
   5. Monitor pulse oximetry.
   6. Maintain surgical drains in the neck area if present.
   7. Observe for hemorrhage and edema in the neck ▲
   8. Monitor IV fluids or total parenteral nutrition until nutrition is administered via nasogastric, gastrostomy, or jejunostomy tube.
   9. Provide oral hygiene.
   10. Assess gag and cough reflexes and ability to ▲ swallow.
   11. Increase activity as tolerated.
   12. Assess the color, amount, and consistency of sputum.
   13. Provide stoma and laryngectomy care (Box 51-18).
   14. Provide consultation with speech and language pathologist as prescribed.
   15. Reinforce method of communication established preoperatively.
   16. Prepare the client for rehabilitation and speech therapy (Box 51-19).

BOX 51-18

Stoma Care Following Laryngectomy

Teach the client the clean suctioning technique.
Instruct the client how to clean the incision and provide stoma care.
Protect the neck from injury.
Instruct the client to wear a stoma guard to shield the stoma.
Avoid swimming, showering, and using aerosol sprays.
Demonstrate ways to prevent debris from entering the stoma.
Advise the client to wear loose-fitting, high-collar clothing to cover the stoma.
Advise the client to increase humidity in the home.
Instruct the client in range-of-motion exercises for arms, shoulders, and neck as prescribed.
Avoid exposure to persons with infections.
Alternate rest periods with activity.
Increase fluid intake to 3000 mL/day as prescribed.
Advise the client to wear a Medic-Alert bracelet.

Speech Rehabilitation Following Laryngectomy

ESOPHAGEAL SPEECH
Client produces esophageal speech by "burping" the air swallowed.
Voice produced is monotone, cannot be raised or lowered, and carries no pitch.
Client must have adequate hearing because the client uses the mouth to shape the words as they are heard.

MECHANICAL DEVICES
The devices are known as electrolarynges.
The devices are placed against the side of the neck; the air inside the neck and pharynx is vibrated, and the client articulates.
A Cooper-Rand device consists of a plastic tube that is placed inside the client's mouth and vibrates on articulation.

TRACHEOESOPHAGEAL FISTULA
Surgical creation of a fistula between the trachea and the esophagus, with eventual placement of a prosthesis used to produce speech.
The prosthesis provides the client with a means to divert the air from the lungs through the trachea, into the esophagus, and out of the mouth.
Lip and tongue movement produces the speech.

XXIV. PROSTATE CANCER

A. Description
1. This slow-growing **cancer** of the prostate gland is usually a androgen-dependent type of **adenocarcinoma**.
2. The risk increases in men with each decade after age 50.
3. Prostate **cancer** can spread via direct invasion of surrounding tissues or by **metastasis**, through the bloodstream and lymphatics, to the bony pelvis and spine.
4. Bone **metastasis** is a concern.

B. Assessment
1. Asymptomatic in early stages
2. Hard, pea-sized nodule palpated on rectal examination
3. Hematuria
4. Late symptoms such as weight loss, urinary obstruction, and pain radiating from the lumbosacral area down the leg
5. Prostate-specific antigen test is not necessarily an indicator of malignancy and use is routine to monitor the client's response to therapy
6. Spread and **metastasis** is indicated by elevated serum acid phosphatase

C. Nonsurgical interventions
1. Prepare the client for hormone manipulation therapy as prescribed.

2. Administer luteinizing hormone, such as leuprolide acetate (Lupron), flutamide (Eulexin), or diethylstilbestrol (DES), as prescribed to slow the rate of growth of the tumor.
3. Goserelin acetate (Zoladex) may be prescribed for palliation in advanced prostatic **cancer** when orchiectomy or estrogen administration is not acceptable or indicated for the client.
4. Prepare the client for radiation (internal or external), which may be prescribed alone or along with surgery and may be prescribed preoperatively or postoperatively to reduce the lesion and limit **metastasis**.
5. Prepare the client for the administration of chemotherapy in cases of hormone-resistant tumors.

D. Surgical interventions
1. Prepare the client for orchiectomy (palliative) if prescribed, which will limit the production of testosterone.
2. Prepare the client for transurethral resection of the prostate (TURP) or prostatectomy if prescribed.
3. Cyrosurgical ablation is a minimally invasive procedure that may be an alternative to radical prostatectomy; liquid nitrogen freezes the gland, and the dead cells are absorbed by the body.

E. TURP
1. The procedure involves insertion of a scope into the urethra to excise prostatic tissue.
2. Bleeding is common following TURP, and monitoring for hemorrhage is an important nursing intervention.
3. Continuous bladder irrigation (CBI) is prescribed postoperatively to maintain the urine at a pink color.
4. Bladder spasms are common following surgery, and antispasmodics may be prescribed.
5. Dribbling or incontinence may occur postoperatively, and it is important for the nurse to instruct the client to monitor for these occurrences.
6. Sterility may or may not occur following the surgical procedure.

F. Suprapubic prostatectomy
1. Suprapubic prostatectomy is removal of the prostate gland by an abdominal incision with a bladder incision.
2. The client will have an abdominal dressing that may drain copious amounts of urine, and the abdominal dressing will need to be changed frequently.
3. Severe hemorrhage is possible, and monitoring for blood loss is an important nursing intervention.
4. Bladder spasms are common, and antispasmodics may be prescribed.
5. Continous bladder irrigation is prescribed and administered to keep the urine pink.
6. A longer healing process is involved as compared with the TURP.
7. Sterility occurs with this procedure.

G. Retropubic prostatectomy
1. Retropubic prostatectomy is removal of the prostate gland by a low abdominal incision without opening the bladder.
2. Less bleeding occurs with this procedure compared with the suprapubic procedure, and the client experiences fewer bladder spasms.
3. Abdominal drainage is minimal.
4. Continuous bladder irrigation may be used.
5. Sterility occurs with this procedure.

H. Perineal prostatectomy
1. The prostate gland is removed through an incision made between the scrotum and anus.
2. Minimal bleeding occurs with this procedure.
3. The client needs to be monitored closely for infection, because the risk of infection is increased with this type of prostatectomy.
4. Urinary incontinence is common.
5. The procedure causes sterility.
6. Teach the client how to perform perineal exercises.
7. Avoid inserting rectal tubes, taking the temperature rectally, or administering enemas.

I. Postoperative interventions
1. Monitor vital signs.
2. Monitor urinary output.
3. Monitor urine for hemorrhage and clots.
4. Increase fluids to 2400 to 3000 mL a day unless contraindicated.
5. Monitor for arterial bleeding as evidenced by bright red urine with numerous clots, and if it occurs, increase CBI and notify the physician immediately.
6. Monitor for venous bleeding as evidenced by burgundy-colored urine output; if it occurs, inform the physician, who may apply traction on the catheter.
7. Monitor hemoglobin and hematocrit levels.
8. Expect red to light pink urine for 24 hours, turning to amber in 3 days.
9. Ambulate the client as early as possible and as soon as urine begins to clear in color.
10. Inform the client that a continuous feeling of an urge to void is normal.
11. Instruct the client to avoid attempts to void around the catheter because this will cause bladder spasms.
12. Administer antibiotics, analgesics, stool softeners, and antispasmodics as prescribed.
13. Monitor three-way Foley catheter, which will have a 30- to 45-mL retention balloon.
14. Maintain CBI with sterile bladder irrigation solution as prescribed to keep the catheter free of obstruction and maintain the urine pink in color (Box 51-20).

J. Postoperative interventions: suprapubic prostatectomy
1. Monitor suprapubic and Foley catheter drainage.
2. Monitor CBI if prescribed.
3. Note that the Foley catheter will be removed 2 to 4 days postoperatively if the client has a suprapubic catheter.
4. If prescribed, clamp the suprapubic catheter after the Foley catheter is removed, and instruct client to attempt to void; after the client has voided, assess the residual urine in the bladder by unclamping the suprapubic catheter and measuring the output.
5. Prepare for removal of suprapubic catheter when client consistently empties bladder and residual urine is 75 mL or less.
6. Monitor suprapubic incision dressing, which may become saturated with urine, until the incision heals.

K. Postoperative interventions: retropubic prostatectomy
1. Note that because the bladder is not entered, there is no urinary drainage on the abdominal dressing.
2. Assess for urinary or purulent drainage on the dressing; if this occurs, notify the physician.
3. Monitor for fever and increased pain, which may indicate an infection.

L. Postoperative interventions: perineal prostatectomy
1. Note that the client will have an incision, which may or may not have a drain.
2. Avoid use of rectal thermometers, rectal tubes, and enemas because they may cause trauma and bleeding.

XXV. BLADDER CANCER

A. Description
1. Bladder **cancer** is papillomatous growths in the bladder urothelium that undergo **malignant** changes and that may infiltrate the bladder wall.
2. Predisposing factors include cigarette smoking, exposure to industrial chemicals, and exposure to radiation.
3. Common sites of **metastasis** include the liver, bones, and lungs.
4. As the tumor progresses, it can extend into the rectum, vagina, other pelvic soft tissues, and retroperitoneal structures.

B. Assessment
1. Gross, painless hematuria
2. Frequency, urgency, dysuria
3. Clot-induced obstruction
4. Bladder biopsy confirms diagnosis

C. Radiation
1. Most bladder cancers are poorly radiosensitive and require high doses of radiation.
2. Radiation therapy is more acceptable for advanced disease that cannot be eradicated by surgery.
3. Palliative radiation may be used to relieve pain and bowel obstruction and control potential hemorrhage and leg edema caused by venous or lymphatic obstruction.
4. Intracavitary radiation may be prescribed, which protects adjacent tissue.

BOX 51-20

Postoperative Care Following Transurethral Resection of the Prostate

CONTINUOUS BLADDER IRRIGATION (CBI)
A three-way (lumen) irrigation is used to decrease bleeding and to keep the bladder free from clots:
One lumen for inflating the balloon (30 mL)
One lumen for instillation (inflow)
One lumen for outflow

INTERVENTIONS
Maintain traction on the catheter if applied to prevent bleeding by pulling the catheter taut and taping it to the abdomen or thigh.
Instruct the client to keep the leg straight if traction is applied to the catheter and it is taped to the thigh.
Catheter traction is not released without a physician's order and usually is released after any bright red drainage has diminished.
Use normal saline or prescribed solution only to prevent water intoxication.
Run the solution at a rate, as prescribed, to keep the urine pink.
Run the solution rapidly if bright red drainage or clots are present.
Run the solution at about 40 gtt/min when the bright red drainage clears.
If the urinary catheter becomes obstructed, turn off the CBI and irrigate the catheter with 30 to 50 mL of normal saline if prescribed; notify physician if obstruction does not resolve.

Monitor for transurethral resection syndrome or severe hyponatremia (water intoxication) caused by the excessive absorption of bladder irrigation during surgery (altered mental status, bradycardia, increased blood pressure, and confusion).
Discontinue CBI and Foley catheter as prescribed, usually 24 to 48 hours after surgery.
Monitor for continence and urinary retention when the catheter is removed.
Inform the client that some burning, frequency, and dribbling may occur following catheter removal.
Inform the client that he should be voiding 150 to 200 mL of clear yellow urine every 3 to 4 hours by 3 days after surgery.
Inform the client that he may pass small clots and tissue debris for several days.
Teach the client to avoid heavy lifting, stressful exercise, driving, Valsalva's maneuver, and sexual intercourse for 2 to 6 weeks to prevent strain, and to call the physician if bleeding occurs or there is a decrease in urinary stream.
Instruct the client to drink 2400 to 3000 mL of fluid each day, preferably before 8 PM.
Instruct the client to avoid alcohol, caffeinated beverages, and spicy foods and to avoid overstimulation of the bladder.
Instruct the client that if the urine becomes bloody, to rest and increase fluid intake, and that if the bleeding does not subside, to notify the physician.

5. External radiation combined with chemotherapy or surgery may be prescribed because the external radiation alone may be ineffective.
6. Complications of radiation
   a. Abacterial cystitis
   b. Proctitis
   c. Fistula formation
   d. Ileitis or colitis
   e. Bladder ulceration and hemorrhage
D. Chemotherapy
1. Intravesical instillation
   a. An alkylating chemotherapeutic agent is instilled into the bladder.
   b. This method provides a concentrated topical treatment with little systemic absorption.
   c. Chemotherapeutic agents used may include thiotepa, mitomycin (Mutamycin), doxorubicin (Adriamycin), cyclophosphamide (Cytoxan), and bacille Calmette-Guérin.
   d. The medication is injected into a urethral catheter and retained for 2 hours.
   e. Following instillation, the client's position is rotated every 15 to 30 minutes, starting in the supine position to avoid lying on a full bladder.
   f. After 2 hours, the client voids in a sitting position and is instructed to increase fluids to flush the bladder.

   g. Treat the urine as biohazard and send to the radioisotope laboratory for monitoring.
   h. For 6 hours following intravesical chemotherapy, disinfect the toilet with household bleach after the client has voided.
2. Systemic chemotherapy
   a. Systemic chemotherapy is used to treat inoperable or late tumors.
   b. Agents used may include cisplatin (Platinol), doxorubicin (Adriamycin), cyclophosphamide (Cytoxan), methotrexate (Folex), and pyridoxine.
3. Complications of chemotherapy
   a. Bladder irritation
   b. Hemorrhagic cystitis
E. Surgical interventions
1. Transurethral resection of bladder tumor
   a. Local resection and fulguration (destruction of tissue by electrical current through electrodes placed in direct contact with the tissue)
   b. Performed for early tumors for cure or for inoperable tumors for palliation
2. Partial cystectomy
   a. Partial cystectomy is the removal of up to half of the bladder.
   b. The procedure is done for early tumors and for clients who cannot tolerate a radical cystectomy.

c. During the initial postoperative period, bladder capacity is reduced greatly to about 60 mL; however, as the bladder tissue expands, the capacity increases to 200 to 400 mL.

d. Maintenance of a continuous output of urine following surgery is critical to prevent bladder distention and stress on the suture line.

e. A urethral catheter and a suprapubic catheter may be in place, and the suprapubic catheter may be left in place for 2 weeks until healing occurs.

3. Cystectomy and urinary diversion
   a. The procedure involves removal of the bladder and the urethra in women, and the bladder, the urethra, and usually the prostate and seminal vesicles in men.
   b. When the bladder and urethra are removed, permanent urinary diversion is required.
   c. The surgery may be performed in two stages if the tumor is extensive, with the creation of the urinary diversion first and the cystectomy several weeks later.
   d. If a radical cystectomy is performed, lower extremity lymphedema may occur as a result of lymph node dissection, and impotence may occur in the male client.

4. Ileal conduit
   a. The ileal conduit also is called ureteroileostomy or Bricker's procedure.
   b. Ureters are implanted into a segment of the ileum, with the formation of an abdominal stoma.
   c. The urine flows into the conduit and is propelled continually out through the stoma by peristalsis.
   d. The client is required to wear an appliance over the stoma to collect the urine.
   e. Complications include obstruction, pyelonephritis, leakage at the anastomosis site, stenosis, hydronephrosis, calculuses, skin irritation and ulceration, and stomal defects.

5. Kock pouch
   a. The Kock pouch is a continent internal ileal reservoir created from a segment of the ileum and ascending colon.
   b. The ureters are implanted into the side of the reservoir, and a special nipple valve is constructed to attach the reservoir to the skin.
   c. Postoperatively, the client will have a 24 to 26 Foley catheter in place to drain urine continuously until the pouch has healed.
   d. The catheter is irrigated gently with NS to prevent obstruction from mucus or clots.
   e. Following removal of the catheter, the client is instructed in how to self-catheterize and to drain the reservoir at 4- to 6-hour intervals.

6. Indiana pouch
   a. A continent reservoir is created from the ascending colon and terminal ileum, making a pouch larger than the Kock pouch.
   b. Postoperatively, the client will have a 24 to 26 Foley catheter in place to drain urine continuously until the pouch has healed.
   c. The Foley catheter is irrigated gently with NS to prevent obstruction from mucus or clots.
   d. Following removal of the Foley catheter, the client is instructed in how to self-catheterize and to drain the reservoir at 4- to 6-hour intervals.

7. Creation of a neobladder
   a. Creation of a neobladder is similar to the creation of an internal reservoir, with the difference being that instead of emptying through an abdominal stoma, the bladder empties through a pelvic outlet into the urethra.
   b. The client empties the neobladder by relaxing the external sphincter and creating abdominal pressure or by intermittent self-catheterization.

8. Percutaneous nephrostomy or pyelostomy
   a. These procedures are used when the **cancer** is inoperable to prevent obstruction.
   b. The procedures involve a percutaneous or surgical insertion of a nephrostomy tube into the kidney for drainage.
   c. Nursing interventions involves stabilizing the tube to prevent dislodgment and monitoring output.

9. Ureterostomy
   a. Ureterstomy may be performed as a palliative procedure if the ureters are obstructed by the tumor.
   b. The ureters are attached to the surface of the abdomen, where the urine flows directly into a drainage appliance without a conduit.
   c. Potential problems include infection, skin irritation, and obstruction to urinary flow as a result of strictures at the opening.

10. Vesicostomy
    a. The bladder is sutured to the abdomen, and a stoma is created in the bladder wall.
    b. The bladder empties through the stoma.

F. Preoperative interventions
   1. Administer bowel preparation as prescribed, which may include a clear liquid diet, laxatives and enemas, and antibiotics to lower the bacterial count in the bowel.
   2. Assist the surgeon and the enterostomal nurse in selecting an appropriate skin site for creation of the abdominal stoma.
   3. Encourage the client to talk about his or her feelings related to the stoma creation.

G. Postoperative interventions
   1. Monitor vital signs.

BOX 51-21

Urinary Stoma Care

Instruct the client to change the appliance in the morning, when urinary production is slowest.

Collect equipment, remove collection bag, use water or commercial solvent to loosen adhesive.

Hold a rolled gauze pad against the stoma to collect and absorb urine during the procedure.

Cleanse the skin around stoma and under the drainage bag with mild nonresidue soap and water.

Inspect the skin for excoriation, and instruct the client to prevent urine from coming into contact with the skin.

After the skin is dry, apply skin adhesive around the appliance.

Instruct the client to cut the stoma opening of the skin barrier just large enough to fit over the stoma (no more that 3 mm larger than the stoma).

Instruct the client that the stoma will begin to shrink, requiring a smaller stoma opening on the skin barrier.

Apply skin barrier before attaching the pouch or face plate.

Place the appliance over the stoma and secure in place.

Encourage self-care; teach the client to use mirror.

Instruct the client that the pouch may be drained by a bedside bag or leg bag, especially at night.

Instruct the client to empty the urinary collection bag when it is one third to one half full to prevent pulling of the appliance and leakage.

Instruct the client to check the appliance seal if perspiring occurs.

Instruct the client to leave the urinary pouch in place as long as it is not leaking and to change it every 5 to 7 days.

During appliance changes, leave the skin open to air as long as possible.

Use a nonkaraya gum product because urine erodes karaya gum.

To control odor, instruct the client to drink adequate fluids, to wash the appliance thoroughly with soap and lukewarm water, and to soak the collection pouch in dilute white vinegar for 20 to 30 minutes or place a special deodorant tablet into the pouch while it is being worn.

Instruct the client who takes baths to keep the level of the water below the stoma and to avoid oily soaps.

If the client plans to shower, instruct the client to direct the flow of water away from the stoma.

---

2. Assess incision site.
3. Assess stoma (should be red and moist) every hour for the first 24 hours (Box 51-21).
4. Monitor for edema in the stoma, which may be present in the immediate postoperative period.
5. If the stoma appears dark and dusky, notify the physician immediately because this indicates necrosis.
6. Monitor for prolapse or retraction of the stoma.
7. Assess for return of bowel function; monitor for peristalsis, which will return in 3 to 4 days.
8. Maintain NPO status as prescribed until bowel sounds return.
9. Monitor urine flow, which is continuous (30 to 60 mL per hour) following surgery.
10. Notify the physician if the urine output is less than 30 mL an hour or if no urine output occurs for more than 15 minutes.
11. Ureteral stents or catheters may be in place for 2 to 3 weeks or until healing occurs; maintain stability with catheters to prevent dislodgment.
12. Monitor urinary output closely and irrigate catheter (if present) gently to prevent obstruction, as prescribed, with 60 mL of NS (Box 51-22).
13. Monitor for hematuria.
14. Monitor for signs of peritonitis.
15. Monitor for bladder distention following a partial cystectomy.
16. Monitor for shock, hemorrhage, thrombophlebitis, and lower extremity lymphedema following a radical cystectomy.
17. Monitor the urinary drainage pouch for leaks, and check skin integrity.
18. Monitor the pH of the urine (do not place the dipstick in the stoma) because strong alkali urine can cause skin irritation and facilitate crystal formation.
19. Instruct the client regarding the potential for urinary tract infection or the development of calculuses.
20. Instruct the client to assess the skin for irritation and to monitor the urinary drainage pouch for any leakage.
21. Encourage the client to express feelings about changes in body image, embarrassment, and sexual dysfunction.

XXVI. ONCOLOGICAL EMERGENCIES

A. Sepsis and disseminated intravascular coagulation (DIC)
   1. Description: The client with an oncological disorder is at increased risk for infection; DIC is caused by sepsis.
   2. Interventions
      a. Maintain strict aseptic technique with the immunocompromised client and monitor closely for infection.

BOX 51-22

Self-Irrigation and Catheterization of Stoma

IRRIGATION

Instruct the client to wash hands and use clean technique.

Instruct the client to use a catheter and syringe and to instill 60 mL of normal saline or water into the reservoir and to aspirate gently or allow to drain.

Instruct the client to irrigate until the drainage remains free of mucus but to be cautious not to overirrigate.

CATHETERIZATION

Instruct the client to wash hands and use clean technique.

Initially, the client is taught to insert a catheter every 2 to 3 hours to drain the reservoir; during each week thereafter, the interval is increased by 1 hour until the catheterization is done every 4 to 6 hours.

Lubricate the catheter well with water-soluble lubricant, and instruct the client never to force the catheter into the reservoir.

If resistance is met, instruct the client to pause, rotate the catheter, and apply gentle pressure to insert.

Instruct the client to notify the physician if the client is unable to insert the catheter.

When urine has stopped, instruct the client to take several deep breaths and move the catheter in and out 2 to 3 inches to ensure that the pouch is empty.

Instruct the client to withdraw the catheter slowly, and to pinch the catheter when withdrawn so that it does not leak urine.

Instruct the client to carry catheterization supplies with him or her.

---

　　b. Administer antibiotics intravenously as prescribed.

　　c. Administer anticoagulants as prescribed during the early phase of DIC.

　　d. Administer cryoprecipitated clotting factors, as prescribed, when DIC progresses and hemorrhage is the primary problem.

B. Syndrome of inappropriate antidiuretic hormone

　1. Description

　　a. Tumors can produce, secrete, or stimulate the brain to synthesize antidiuretic hormone.

　　b. Mild symptoms include weakness, muscle cramps, loss of appetite, and fatigue; serum sodium levels range from 115 to 120 mEq/L.

　　c. More serious signs and symptoms relate to water intoxication and include weight gain, personality changes, confusion, and extreme muscle weakness.

　　d. As the serum sodium level approaches 110 mEq/L, seizures, coma, and eventually death will occur, unless the condition is treated rapidly.

　2. Interventions

　　a. Initiate fluid restriction and increased sodium intake as prescribed.

　　b. Administer demeclocycline (Declomycin) as prescribed, an antagonist to antidiuretic hormone.

　　c. Monitor serum sodium levels.

C. Spinal cord compression

　1. Description

　　a. Spinal cord compression occurs when a tumor directly enters the spinal cord or when the vertebral column collapses from tumor entry.

　　b. Spinal cord compression causes back pain, usually before neurological deficits occur.

　　c. Neurological deficits relate to the spinal level of compression and include numbness; tingling; loss of urethral, vaginal, and rectal sensation; and muscle weakness.

　2. Interventions

　　a. Assess for back pain and neurological deficits.

　　b. Prepare the client for radiation and/or chemotherapy to reduce the size of the tumor and relieve compression.

　　c. Surgery may need to be performed to remove the tumor and relieve the pressure on the spinal cord.

　　d. Instruct the client in the use of neck or back braces if they are prescribed.

D. Hypercalcemia

　1. Description

　　a. Hypercalcemia is a late manifestation of extensive malignancy that occurs most often in clients with bone **metastasis.**

　　b. Decreased physical mobility contributes to or worsens hypercalcemia.

　　c. Early signs include fatigue, anorexia, nausea, vomiting, constipation, and polyuria.

　　d. More serious signs and symptoms include severe muscle weakness, diminished deep tendon reflexes, paralytic ileus, dehydration, and electrocardiogram changes.

　2. Interventions

　　a. Monitor serum calcium level.

　　b. Administer oral or parenteral (NS) fluids as prescribed.

　　c. Administer medications to lower the calcium level as prescribed.

　　d. Prepare the client for dialysis if the condition becomes life threatening or is accompanied by renal impairment.

E. Superior vena cava syndrome

　1. Description

a. Superior vena cava syndrome cccurs when the vein is compressed or obstructed by tumor growth.

b. Signs and symptoms result from blockage of blood flow in the venous system of the head, neck, and upper trunk.

c. Early signs and symptoms generally occur in the morning and include edema of the face, especially around the eyes, and tightness of the shirt or blouse collar (Stokes' sign).

d. As the condition worsens, edema in the arms and hands, dyspnea, erythema of the upper body, and epistaxis occur.

e. Life-threatening signs and symptoms include hemorrhage, cyanosis, mental status changes, decreased cardiac output, and hypotension.

2. Interventions

a. Assess for signs and symptoms of superior vena cava syndrome.

b. Prepare the client for radiation therapy to the mediastinal area.

F. Tumor lysis syndrome

1. Description

a. Tumor lysis syndrome occurs when large quantities of tumor cells are destroyed rapidly and are released into the bloodstream faster than the homeostatic mechanisms of the body can handle them.

b. Tumor lysis syndrome is a positive sign that **cancer** treatment is effective; however, if left untreated, it can cause severe tissue damage and death.

c. Hyperkalemia and hyperuricemia occur; hyperuricemia can lead to acute renal failure.

2. Interventions

a. Encourage oral hydration; IV hydration may be prescribed for the client experiencing nausea.

b. Instruct the client regarding the importance of fluid intake during chemotherapy.

c. Administer diuretics to increase the urine flow through the kidneys as prescribed.

d. Administer medications that increase the excretion of purines, such as allopurinol (Zyloprim), as prescribed.

e. Prepare to administer IV infusion of glucose and insulin to treat hyperkalemia.

f. Prepare the client for dialysis if hyperkalemia and hyperuricemia persist despite treatment.

PRACTICE QUESTIONS

1. The nurse is instructing the client to perform a testicular self-examination. The nurse tells the client
   1. To examine the testicles while lying down.
   2. That the best time for the examination is after a shower.
   3. To gently feel the testicle with one finger to feel for a growth.
   4. That testicular examinations should be done at least every 6 months.

2. The community nurse is conducting a health promotion program at a local school and is discussing the risk factors associated with cancer. Which of the following, if identified by the client as a risk factor, indicates a need for further instructions?
   1. Viral factors
   2. Stress
   3. Low-fat and high-fiber diets
   4. Exposure to radiation

3. The client with cancer is receiving chemotherapy and develops thrombocytopenia. The nurse identifies which intervention as the highest priority in the nursing plan of care?
   1. Ambulation 3 times daily
   2. Monitoring temperature
   3. Monitoring the platelet count
   4. Monitoring for pathological fractures

4. The nurse is monitoring the laboratory results of a client preparing to receive chemotherapy. The nurse would determine that the white blood cell count is normal if which of the following results were present?
   1. 3000 to 8000 cells/mm^3
   2. 5000 to 10,000 cells/mm^3
   3. 7000 to 15,000 cells/mm^3
   4. 2000 to 5000 cells/mm^3

5. The community health nurse is instructing a group of female clients about breast self-examination. The nurse would instruct the clients to perform the examination
   1. At the onset on menstruation.
   2. 1 week after menstruation begins.
   3. Every month during ovulation.
   4. Weekly at the same time of day.

6. The nurse is caring for a client who has undergone a vaginal hysterectomy. The nurse avoids which of the following in the care of this client?
   1. Removal of antiembolism stockings twice daily
   2. Assisting with range-of-motion leg exercises
   3. Elevating the knee gatch on the bed
   4. Checking placement of pneumatic compression boots

7. The client suspected of an ovarian tumor is scheduled for a pelvic ultrasound. The nurse provides which preprocedure instructions to the client?
   1. Maintain an NPO status before the procedure.
   2. Eat a light breakfast only.
   3. Drink six to eight glasses of water without voiding before the test.
   4. Wear comfortable clothing and shoes for the procedure.

8. The client is diagnosed as having a bowel tumor. Several diagnostic tests are prescribed. The nurse

understands that which of the following tests will confirm the diagnosis of malignancy?

1. Magnetic resonance imaging
2. Computerized tomography scan
3. Abdominal ultrasound
4. Biopsy of the tumor

9. A client is diagnosed with multiple myeloma. The client asks the nurse about the diagnosis. The nurse bases the response on which of the following descriptions of this disorder?

1. Malignant exacerbation in the number of leukocytes
2. Altered red blood cell production
3. Altered production of lymph nodes
4. Malignant proliferation of plasma cells and tumors within the bone

10. The nurse is reviewing the laboratory results of a client diagnosed with multiple myeloma. Which of the following would the nurse expect to note specifically in this disorder?

1. Decreased number of plasma cells in the bone marrow
2. Increased white blood cells
3. Increased calcium level
4. Decreased blood urea nitrogen

11. The nurse is developing a plan of care for the client with multiple myeloma. The nurse includes which priority intervention in the plan of care?

1. Coughing and deep breathing
2. Encouraging fluids
3. Monitoring the red blood cell count
4. Providing frequent oral care

12. The oncology nurse specialist provides an educational session to nursing staff regarding the characteristics of Hodgkin's disease. The nurse determines that further education is needed if a nursing staff member states that which of the following is a characteristic of the disease?

1. Presence of Reed-Sternberg cells
2. Involvement of lymph nodes, spleen, and liver
3. Occurs most often in the older client
4. Prognosis depends on the stage of the disease

13. The community health nurse conducts a health promotion program regarding testicular cancer to community members. The nurse determines that further information needs to be provided if a community member states that which of the following is a sign of testicular cancer?

1. Painless testicular swelling
2. Heavy sensation in the scrotum
3. Alopecia
4. Back pain

14. The client is receiving external radiation to the neck for cancer of the larynx. The most likely side effect to be expected is

1. Constipation.
2. Dyspnea.
3. Sore throat.
4. Diarrhea.

15. The nurse is caring for a client with an internal radiation implant. When caring for the client, the nurse should observe which of the following principles?

1. Limit the time with the client to 1 hour per shift.
2. Do not allow pregnant women into the client's room.
3. Individuals less than 16 years old may be allowed to go in the room as long as they are 6 feet away from the client.
4. Remove dosimeter badge when entering the client's room.

16. A cervical radiation implant is placed in the client for treatment of cervical cancer. The nurse initiates what most appropriate activity order for this client?

1. Out of bed in a chair only
2. Ambulate to the bathroom only
3. Bedrest
4. Out of bed ad lib

17. The client is hospitalized for insertion of a internal cervical radiation implant. While giving care, the nurse finds the radiation implant in the bed. The initial action by the nurse is to

1. Call the physician.
2. Pick up the implant with gloved hands and flush it down the toilet.
3. Reinsert the implant into the vagina immediately.
4. Pick up the implant with long handled forceps and place it in a lead container.

18. The nurse is caring for a client experiencing hematologic toxicity as a result of chemotherapy. The nurse develops a plan of care for the client. The nurse plans to

1. Restrict all visitors.
2. Restrict fluid intake.
3. Insert an indwelling urinary catheter to prevent skin breakdown.
4. Restrict fresh fruits and vegetables in the diet.

19. The nurse is reviewing the laboratory results of a client receiving chemotherapy. The platelet count is 10,000 cells/mm³. Based on this laboratory value, the priority nursing assessment is which of the following?

1. Assess level of consciousness.
2. Assess temperature.
3. Assess bowel sounds.
4. Assess skin turgor.

20. The home health care nurse is caring for a client with cancer. The client is complaining of acute pain. The most appropriate nursing assessment of the client's pain would include which of the following?

1. The client's pain rating
2. The nurse's impression of the client's pain
3. Nonverbal cues from the client
4. Pain relief after appropriate nursing intervention

21. The nurse is caring for a client who is 4 days post-operative following a pelvic exenteration. The physician has changed the client's diet from NPO to clear liquids. The nurse makes which priority assessment before administering the diet?
    1. Ability to ambulate
    2. Urine specific gravity
    3. Incision appearance
    4. Bowel sounds

22. The client is admitted to the hospital with a suspected diagnosis of Hodgkin's disease. Which of the following assessment signs would the nurse expect to note specifically in the client?
    1. Weakness
    2. Fatigue
    3. Weight gain
    4. Enlarged lymph nodes

23. During the admission assessment of a client with advanced ovarian cancer, the nurse recognizes which symptom as typical of the disease?
    1. Hypermenorrhea
    2. Abdominal distention
    3. Diarrhea
    4. Abnormal bleeding

24. The nurse is reviewing the complications of conization with a client who has microinvasive cervical cancer. Which complication if identified by the client indicates a need for further teaching?
    1. Infection
    2. Infertility
    3. Ovarian perforation
    4. Hemorrhage

25. When assessing the laboratory results of the client with bladder cancer and bone metastasis, the nurse notes a calcium level of 12 mg/dL. The nurse recognizes that this is consistent with which oncological emergency?
    1. Hyperkalemia
    2. Spinal cord compression
    3. Superior vena cava syndrome
    4. Hypercalcemia

26. The client reports to the nurse that when performing testicular self-examination, he found a lump the size and shape of a pea. The most appropriate response to the client is which of the following?
    1. "That's important to report even though it might not be serious."
    2. "That could be cancer. I'll ask the doctor to examine you."
    3. "Let me know if it gets bigger next month."
    4. "Lumps like that are normal; don't worry."

27. The hospice nurse visits a client dying of ovarian cancer. During the visit, the client expresses that "If I can just live long enough to attend my daughter's graduation, I'll be ready to die." Which phase of coping is this client experiencing?
    1. Denial

2. Bargaining
3. Depression
4. Anger

28. The nurse is caring for a client following a modified radical mastectomy. Which assessment finding would indicate that the client is experiencing a complication related to the surgery?
    1. Sanguineous drainage in the Jackson-Pratt drain
    2. Pain at the incisional site
    3. Complaints of decreased sensation near the operative site
    4. Arm edema on the operative side

29. The nurse is admitting a client with laryngeal cancer to the nursing unit. The nurse assesses for which most common risk factor for this type of cancer?
    1. Use of chewing tobacco
    2. Cigarette smoking
    3. Urban living
    4. Alcohol abuse

30. The female client who has been receiving radiation therapy for bladder cancer tells the nurse that it feels as if she is voiding through the vagina. The nurse interprets that the client may be experiencing
    1. Extreme stress caused by the diagnosis of cancer.
    2. Altered perineal sensation as a side effect of radiation therapy.
    3. The development of a vesicovaginal fistula.
    4. Rupture of the bladder.

31. The client with leukemia is receiving busulfan (Myleran). Allopurinol (Zyloprim) is prescribed for the client. The nurse tells the client that the purpose of the allopurinol (Zyloprim) is to
    1. Prevent alopecia.
    2. Prevent hyperuricemia.
    3. Prevent vomiting.
    4. Prevent nausea.

32. The client receiving chemotherapy is experiencing stomatitis. The nurse advises the client to use which of the following as the best substance to rinse the mouth?
    1. Hydrogen peroxide mixture
    2. Weak salt and bicarbonate mouth rinse
    3. Lemon-flavored mouthwash
    4. Alcohol-based mouthwash

33. The community nurse is conducting a health promotion program and the topic of the discussion relates to the risk factors of gastric cancer. Which risk factor if identified by a client indicates a need for further discussion?
    1. History of gastric polyps
    2. History of pernicious anemia
    3. A diet of smoked, highly salted, and spiced food
    4. High meat and carbohydrate consumption

34. A gastrectomy is performed on a client with gastric cancer. In the immediate postoperative period the nurse notes bloody drainage from the nasogastric

tube. Which of the following is the most appropriate nursing intervention?
1. Notify the physician.
2. Continue to monitor the drainage.
3. Measure abdominal girth.
4. Irrigate the nasogastric tube.

35. The nurse is teaching a client about the risk factors associated with colorectal cancer. The nurse determines that further teaching is necessary if the client identifies which of the following as an associated risk factor?
1. A history of inflammatory bowel disease
2. Family history of colon cancer
3. A high-fiber diet
4. A diet high in fats and carbohydrates

36. The nurse is performing an admission assessment on a client diagnosed with a right colon tumor. The nurse asks the client about which characteristic symptom of this type of a tumor?
1. Alternating constipation and diarrhea
2. Flat, ribbonlike stools
3. Crampy, colicky abdominal pain
4. Rectal bleeding

37. The nurse is reviewing the preoperative orders of a client with a colon tumor who is scheduled for abdominal perineal resection. The nurse notes that the physician has prescribed neomycin (Mycifradin) for the client. The nurse determines that this medication has been prescribed primarily
1. Because the client has an infection.
2. To prevent an infection.
3. To decrease the bacteria in the bowel.
4. Because the client is allergic to penicillin.

38. The nurse is assessing the perineal wound in a client who has returned from the operating room following an abdominal perineal resection. The nurse notes serosanguineous drainage from the wound. Which of the following nursing interventions is most appropriate?
1. Notify the physician.
2. Change the dressing as prescribed.
3. Clamp the Penrose drain.
4. Remove and replace the perineal packing.

39. The nurse is assessing the colostomy of a client who had an abdominal perineal resection for a bowel tumor. Which of the following assessment findings indicate that the colostomy is beginning to function?
1. Blood drainage from the colostomy
2. The client's ability to tolerate food
3. Absent bowel sounds
4. The passage of flatus

40. The nurse is caring for a client following a radical neck dissection and creation of a tracheostomy performed for laryngeal cancer. The nurse is providing discharge instructions to the client. Which statement if made by the client indicates a need for further instructions?

1. "I need to apply a thin layer of petrolatum to the skin around the stoma to prevent cracking."
2. "I will protect the stoma from water."
3. "I need to use an air conditioner to provide cool air to assist in breathing."
4. "I need to keep powders and sprays away from the stoma site."

41. The nurse is caring for a client with a suspected diagnosis of cancer of the prostate. The nurse analyzes the laboratory values and notes that the serum acid phosphatase level is elevated. The nurse determines that this laboratory test is most often useful in determining
1. The diagnosis of prostate cancer.
2. Complications associated with cancer.
3. The progression or regression of the cancer.
4. The likelihood of associated bone cancer.

42. Hormone therapy is prescribed as the mode of treatment for a client with prostatic cancer. The nurse understands that the goal of this form of treatment is to
1. Limit the amount of circulating androgens.
2. Increase the amount of circulating androgens.
3. Increase testosterone levels.
4. Increase prostaglandin levels.

43. The nurse is caring for a client with cancer of the prostate following a prostatectomy. The nurse provides discharge instructions to the client and tells the client to
1. Notify the physician if small blood clots are noticed during urination.
2. Avoid driving the car for 1 week.
3. Restrict fluid intake to prevent incontinence.
4. Avoid lifting objects heavier than 20 lb for at least 6 weeks.

44. The oncology nurse is providing a teaching session to a group of nursing students regarding the risks and causes of bladder cancer. Which statement if made by a student indicates a need for further teaching?
1. "Bladder cancer most often occurs in women."
2. "Bladder cancer generally is seen in clients older than age 40."
3. "Environmental health hazards have been attributed as a cause."
4. "Using cigarettes, artificial sweeteners, and coffee drinking can increase the risk."

45. The nurse is reviewing the history of a client with bladder cancer. The nurse expects to note documentation of which most common symptom of this type of cancer?
1. Frequency of urination
2. Urgency on urination
3. Hematuria
4. Dysuria

46. The nurse is caring for a client following intravesical instillation of an alkalating chemotherapeutic agent into the bladder for the treatment of bladder

cancer. Following the instillation, the nurse most appropriately would instruct the client to
1. Urinate immediately.
2. Maintain strict bed rest.
3. Retain the instillation fluid for 30 minutes.
4. Change position every 15 minutes.

47. The nurse is assessing the stoma of a client following a ureterostomy. Which of the following would the nurse expect to note?
1. A pale stoma
2. A red and moist stoma
3. A dry stoma
4. A dark-colored stoma

48. The nurse is caring for a client following a radical mastectomy. Which of the following nursing interventions would assist in preventing lymphedema of the affected arm?
1. Placing cool compresses on the affected arm
2. Elevating the affected arm on a pillow above heart level
3. Maintaining an intravenous site below the antecubital area on the affected side
4. Avoiding arm exercises in the immediate postoperative period

49. The nurse is preparing a client for a mammography. The nurse tells the client
1. That mammography takes about 1 hour.
2. To avoid the use of deodorants, powders, or creams on the day of the test.

3. That there is no discomfort associated with the procedure.
4. To maintain a nothing-by-mouth status on the day of the test.

50. A nurse is monitoring a client for signs and symptoms related to superior vena cava syndrome. Which of the following is an early sign of this oncological emergency?
1. Periorbital edema
2. Arm edema
3. Mental status changes
4. Cyanosis

CRITICAL THINKING: MULTIPLE RESPONSE

A client with carcinoma of the lung develops syndrome of inappropriate antidiuretic hormone as a complication of the cancer. The nurse anticipates that which of the following may be prescribed?

____ Increased fluid intake

____ Decreased oral sodium intake

____ Serum sodium blood levels

____ Medication that is antagonistic to antidiuretic hormone

____ Radiation or chemotherapy

ANSWERS

1. 2

Rationale: The testicular-self examination is recommended monthly after a warm bath or shower when the scrotal skin is relaxed. The client should stand to examine the testicles. Using both hands, with fingers under the scrotum and thumbs on top, the client should gently roll the testicles, feeling for any lumps.

Test-Taking Strategy: Use the process of elimination. Eliminate option 4 first because of the words "6 months." Next eliminate option 3 because of the word "one." From the remaining options, eliminate option 1 by trying to visualize the process of the self-examination. If you had difficulty with this question, review the procedure for this self-examination.

Level of Cognitive Ability: Application
Client Needs: Health Promotion and Maintenance
Integrated Process: Teaching/Learning
Content Area: Adult health—oncology
Reference: Potter, P., & Perry, A. (2001). *Fundamentals of nursing* (5th ed., pp. 811-813). St. Louis: Mosby.

2. 3

Rationale: Viruses may be one of multiple agents acting to initiate carcinogenesis and have been associated with several types of cancer. Increased stress has been associated with

causing the growth and proliferation of cancer cells. Two forms of radiation, ultraviolet and ionizing, can lead to cancer. A diet high in fat may be a factor in the development of breast, colon, and prostate cancers. High-fiber diets may reduce the risk of colon cancer.

Test-Taking Strategy: Use the process of elimination. Note the key words "indicates a need for further instructions" in the stem of the question. Read each option carefully, using the process of elimination. Familiarity with the risk factors related to cancer will direct you easily to option 3. Review these risk factors if you had difficulty with this question.

Level of Cognitive Ability: Analysis
Client Needs: Health Promotion and Maintenance
Integrated Process: Teaching/Learning
Content Area: Adult health—oncology
Reference: Ignatavicius, D., & Workman, M. (2002). *Medical-surgical nursing: Critical thinking for collaborative care* (4th ed., p. 421). Philadelphia: W. B. Saunders.

3. 3

Rationale: Thrombocytopenia indicates a decrease in the number of platelets in the circulating blood. A major concern is monitoring for and preventing bleeding. Option 2 relates to monitoring for infection particularly if leukopenia is present. Options 1 and 4, although important in the plan of care are not related directly to thrombocytopenia.

Test-Taking Strategy: Use the process of elimination. Note the key word "thrombocytopenia" in the question. Recalling that this condition places the client at risk of bleeding will assist in eliminating options 1, 2, and 4. Review the nursing interventions related to this disorder if you had difficulty with this question.
Level of Cognitive Ability: Application
Client Needs: Physiological Integrity
Integrated Process: Nursing Process—planning
Content Area: Adult health—oncology
Reference: Lewis, S., Heitkemper, M., & Dirksen, S. (2004). *Medical-surgical nursing: Assessment and management of clinical problems* (6th ed., p. 306). St. Louis: Mosby.

4. 2
Rationale: The normal white blood cell count ranges from 5000 to 10,000 cells/mm³. Option 1 indicates a low value. Option 3 and 4 indicate elevated values.
Test-Taking Strategy: Use the process of elimination. Knowledge regarding the normal white blood cell count is required to answer this question. Learn this value if you are unfamiliar with it.
Level of Cognitive Ability: Comprehension
Client Needs: Physiological Integrity
Integrated Process: Nursing Process—assessment
Content Area: Adult health—oncology
Reference: Phipps, W., Monahan, F., Sands, J., Marek, J., & Neighbors, M. (2003). *Medical-surgical nursing: Health and illness perspectives* (7th ed., p. 807). St. Louis: Mosby.

5. 2
Rationale: The breast self-examination should be performed monthly seven days after the menstrual period. Performing the examination weekly is not recommended. At the onset of menstruation and during ovulation, hormonal changes occur that may alter breast tissue.
Test-Taking Strategy: Use the process of elimination. Option 4 can be eliminated easily because of the word "weekly." Eliminate options 1 and 3 next because of the similarity that exists regarding the hormonal changes that occur during these times. Review the procedure for performing breast self-examination, if you had difficulty with this question.
Level of Cognitive Ability: Application
Client Needs: Health Promotion and Maintenance
Integrated Process: Teaching/Learning
Content Area: Adult health—oncology
Reference: Lewis, S., Heitkemper, M., & Dirksen, S. (2004). *Medical-surgical nursing: Assessment and management of clinical problems* (6th ed., p. 1361). St. Louis: Mosby.

6. 3
Rationale: The client is at risk of deep vein thrombosis or thrombophlebitis after this surgery, as for any other major surgery. For this reason, the nurse implements measures that will prevent this complication. Range of motion exercises, antiembolism stockings, and pneumatic compression boots are helpful. The nurse should avoid using the knee gatch in the bed, which inhibits venous return, thus placing the client more at risk for deep vein thrombosis or thrombophlebitis.

Test-Taking Strategy: Use the process of elimination. Note the key word "avoids." This tells you that the correct option is an incorrect nursing action. Review postoperative nursing interventions following vaginal hysterectomy if you had difficulty with this question.
Level of Cognitive Ability: Application
Client Needs: Physiological Integrity
Integrated Process: Nursing Process—implementation
Content Area: Adult health—oncology
Reference: Phipps, W., Monahan, F., Sands, J., Marek, J., & Neighbors, M. (2003). *Medical-surgical nursing: Health and illness perspectives* (7th ed., p. 1774). St. Louis: Mosby.

7. 3
Rationale: A pelvic ultrasound requires the ingestion of large volumes of water just before the procedure. A full bladder is necessary so that this organ will be visualized as such and not mistaken as a possible pelvic growth. An abdominal ultrasound may require that the client abstain from food or fluid for several hours before the procedure. Option 4 is unrelated to this specific procedure.
Test-Taking Strategy: Use the process of elimination. Noting the key word "pelvic" will assist in eliminating options 1, 2, and 4. From the remaining options, focusing on the key word will assist in directing you to option 3. Review preparation for a pelvic ultrasound if you had difficulty with this question.
Level of Cognitive Ability: Application
Client Needs: Physiological Integrity
Integrated Process: Nursing Process—implementation
Content Area: Adult health—oncology
Reference: Chernecky, C., & Berger, B. (2001). *Laboratory tests and diagnostic procedures* (3rd ed., p. 578). Philadelphia: W. B. Saunders.

8. 4
Rationale: A biopsy is done to determine whether a tumor is malignant or benign. Magnetic resonance imaging, computed tomography scan, and ultrasound will visualize the presence of a mass but will not confirm a diagnosis of malignancy.
Test-Taking Strategy: Use the process of elimination. Note the key word "confirm." This key word should direct you easily to option 4. Review the purpose of the tests identified in the options if you had difficulty with this question.
Level of Cognitive Ability: Analysis
Client Needs: Physiological Integrity
Integrated Process: Nursing Process—analysis
Content Area: Adult health—oncology
Reference: Ignatavicius, D., & Workman, M. (2002). *Medical-surgical nursing: Critical thinking for collaborative care* (4th ed., p. 425). Philadelphia: W. B. Saunders.

9. 4
Rationale: Multiple myeloma is a B cell neoplastic condition characterized by abnormal malignant proliferation of plasma cells and the accumulation of mature plasma cells in the bone marrow. Option 1 describes the leukemic process. Option 2 and 3 are not characteristics of multiple myeloma.
Test-Taking Strategy: Use the process of elimination. Focus on the name of the disorder, multiple myeloma, to direct you to

option 4. Review this information if you are unfamiliar with this oncological disorder.
Level of Cognitive Ability: Analysis
Client Needs: Physiological Integrity
Integrated Process: Teaching/Learning
Content Area: Adult health—oncology
Reference: Lewis, S., Heitkemper, M., & Dirksen, S. (2004). *Medical-surgical nursing: Assessment and management of clinical problems* (6th ed., p. 744). St. Louis: Mosby.

10. 3
Rationale: Findings indicative of multiple myeloma are an increased number of plasma cells in the bone marrow, anemia, hypercalcemia caused by the release of calcium from the deteriorating bone tissue, and an elevated blood urea nitrogen level. An increased white blood cell count may or may not be present and is not related specifically to multiple myeloma.
Test-Taking Strategy: Use the process of elimination. Noting the name of the disorder will direct you to option 3. Review this information if you are unfamiliar with this oncological disorder.
Level of Cognitive Ability: Analysis
Client Needs: Physiological Integrity
Integrated Process: Nursing Process—assessment
Content Area: Adult health—oncology
Reference: Phipps, W., Monahan, F., Sands, J., Marek, J., & Neighbors, M. (2003). *Medical-surgical nursing: Health and illness perspectives* (7th ed., p. 1629). St. Louis: Mosby.

11. 2
Rationale: Hypercalcemia caused by bone destruction is a priority concern in the client with multiple myeloma. The nurse should administer fluids in adequate amounts to maintain an output of 1.5 to 2 L/day. Clients require about 3 L of fluid per day. The fluid is needed not only to dilute the calcium overload but also to prevent protein from precipitating in the renal tubules. Options 1, 3, and 4 may be components of the plan of care but are not the priority in this client.
Test-Taking Strategy: Use the process of elimination. Recalling the pathophysiology of this disorder and that encouraging fluids is specific to the care of a client with this disorder will direct you to option 2. Review the specific manifestations of this disorder if you had difficulty with this question.
Level of Cognitive Ability: Application
Client Needs: Physiological Integrity
Integrated Process: Nursing Process—planning
Content Area: Delegating/Prioritizing
Reference: Lewis, S., Heitkemper, M., & Dirksen, S. (2004). *Medical-surgical nursing: Assessment and management of clinical problems* (6th ed., p. 746). St. Louis: Mosby.

12. 3
Rationale: Hodgkin's disease is a disorder of young adults. Options 1, 2, and 4 are characteristics of this disease.
Test-Taking Strategy: Use the process of elimination. Note the key words "further education is needed" in the stem of the question. Recalling that Hodgkin's occurs in the young adult will direct you easily to option 3. Review the characteristics of this disorder if you had difficulty with this question.

Level of Cognitive Ability: Analysis
Client Needs: Physiological Integrity
Integrated Process: Teaching/Learning
Content Area: Adult health—oncology
Reference: Lewis, S., Heitkemper, M., & Dirksen, S. (2004). *Medical-surgical nursing: Assessment and management of clinical problems* (6th ed., p. 741). St. Louis: Mosby.

13. 3
Rationale: Alopecia is not an assessment finding in testicular cancer. Alopecia may occur, however, as a result of radiation or chemotherapy. Options 1, 2, and 4 are assessment findings in testicular cancer. Back pain may indicate metastasis to the retroperitoneal lymph nodes.
Test-Taking Strategy: Note the key words "further information needs to be provided" in the stem of the question. Use the process of elimination remembering that alopecia occurs as a result of chemotherapy rather than from the disease. Review the manifestations associated with testicular cancer if you had difficulty with this question.
Level of Cognitive Ability: Analysis
Client Needs: Health Promotion and Maintenance
Integrated Process: Teaching/Learning
Content Area: Adult health—oncology
Reference: Lewis, S., Heitkemper, M., & Dirksen, S. (2004). *Medical-surgical nursing: Assessment and management of clinical problems* (6th ed., p.1454). St. Louis: Mosby.

14. 3
Rationale: In general, only the area in the treatment field is affected by the radiation. Skin reactions, fatigue, nausea, and anorexia may occur with radiation to any site, whereas other side effects occur only when specific areas are involved in treatment. A client receiving radiation to the larynx is most likely to experience a sore throat. Options 1 and 4 may occur with radiation to the gastrointestinal tract. Dyspnea may occur with lung involvement.
Test-Taking Strategy: Use the process of elimination. Eliminate options 1 and 4 first because they are similar and gastrointestinal related. Consider the anatomical location of the radiation therapy to assist you in selecting option 3. Review the effects of radiation therapy if you had difficulty with this question.
Level of Cognitive Ability: Analysis
Client Needs: Physiological Integrity
Integrated Process: Nursing Process—assessment
Content Area: Adult health—oncology
Reference: Ignatavicius, D., & Workman, M. (2002). *Medical-surgical nursing: Critical thinking for collaborative care* (4th ed., p. 429). Philadelphia: W. B. Saunders.

15. 2
Rationale: The time that the nurse spends in a room of a client with an internal radiation implant is 30 minutes per 8-hour shift. The dosimeter badge must be worn when in the client's room. Children younger than 16 years of age and pregnant women are not allowed in the client's room.
Test-Taking Strategy: Use the process of elimination. Option 4 can be eliminated first. Knowledge of the time frame related

to exposure to the client will assist in eliminating option 1. From the remaining options, select option 2 because of the possible risks associated with exposure to the mother and fetus. Review these principles if you had difficulty with this question.
Level of Cognitive Ability: Application
Client Needs: Safe, Effective Care Environment
Integrated Process: Nursing Process—implementation
Content Area: Adult health—oncology
Reference: Ignatavicius, D., & Workman, M. (2002). *Medical-surgical nursing: Critical thinking for collaborative care* (4th ed., p. 1771). Philadelphia: W. B. Saunders.

16. **3**
Rationale: The client with a cervical radiation implant should be maintained on bed rest in the dorsal position to prevent movement of the radiation source. The head of the bed is elevated to a maximum of 10 to 15 degrees for comfort. The nurse avoids turning the client on the side. If turning is absolutely necessary, a pillow is placed between the knees and, with the body in straight alignment, the client is logrolled.
Test-Taking Strategy: Use the process of elimination. Consider the anatomical location of the implant and the risk of dislodgment to answer the question. Additionally, note that options 1, 2, and 4 are similar. If you had difficulty with this question, review care to the client with a radiation implant.
Level of Cognitive Ability: Application
Client Needs: Physiological Integrity
Integrated Process: Nursing Process—implementation
Content Area: Adult health—oncology
Reference: Ignatavicius, D., & Workman, M. (2002). *Medical-surgical nursing: Critical thinking for collaborative care* (4th ed., p. 1771). Philadelphia: W. B. Saunders.

17. **4**
Rationale: A lead container and long-handled forceps should be kept in the client's room at all times during internal radiation therapy. If the implant becomes dislodged, the nurse should pick up the implant with long-handled forceps and place it in the lead container. Options 1, 2, and 3 are inaccurate interventions.
Test-Taking Strategy: Use the process of elimination. Note the key word "initial" in the stem of the question. Option 3 is not an appropriate action. Eliminate option 2 next because the implant would not be discarded. Although the physician would be notified, the initial action is option 4. Review the initial measures related to a dislodged implant if you had difficulty with this question.
Level of Cognitive Ability: Application
Client Needs: Safe, Effective Care Environment
Integrated Process: Nursing Process—implementation
Content Area: Adult health—oncology
Reference: Ignatavicius, D., & Workman, M. (2002). *Medical-surgical nursing: Critical thinking for collaborative care* (4th ed., p. 429). Philadelphia: W. B. Saunders.

18. **4**
Rationale: In the immunocompromised client, a low-bacteria diet is implemented. This includes avoiding fresh fruits and vegetables and thorough cooking of all foods. Not all visitors are restricted, but the client is protected from persons with known infections. Fluids should be encouraged. Invasive measures such as an indwelling urinary catheter should be avoided to prevent infections.
Test-Taking Strategy: Use the process of elimination. Eliminate option 1 because of the word "all." Next, eliminate option 2 because it is not reasonable to eliminate fluids in a client receiving chemotherapy who is at risk for fluid and electrolyte imbalances. Eliminate option 3 because of the risk of infection that exists with this measure. Review interventions for the client with hematologic toxicity if you had difficulty with this question.
Level of Cognitive Ability: Application
Client Needs: Physiological Integrity
Integrated Process: Nursing Process—planning
Content Area: Adult health—oncology
Reference: Ignatavicius, D., & Workman, M. (2002). *Medical-surgical nursing: Critical thinking for collaborative care* (4th ed., p. 437). Philadelphia: W. B. Saunders.

19. **1**
Rationale: A high risk of hemorrhage exists when the platelet count is fewer than 20,000 cells/mm³. Fatal central nervous system hemorrhage or massive gastrointestinal hemorrhage can occur when the platelet count is fewer than 10,000 cells/mm³. The client should be assessed for changes in level of consciousness, which may be an early indication of an intracranial hemorrhage. Option 2 is a priority nursing assessment when the white blood cell count is low and the client is at risk for an infection. Although options 3 and 4 are important to assess, they are not the priority in this situation.
Test-Taking Strategy: Use the process of elimination. Note the key word "priority" in the stem of the question. Recalling the normal platelet count and determining that a low count places the client at risk for bleeding will assist in eliminating options 2, 3, and 4 as assessment measures for bleeding. Review the normal platelet count and the nursing interventions for a client with a low count if you had difficulty with this question.
Level of Cognitive Ability: Analysis
Client Needs: Physiological Integrity
Integrated Process: Nursing Process—assessment
Content Area: Adult health—oncology
Reference: Ignatavicius, D., & Workman, M. (2002). *Medical-surgical nursing: Critical thinking for collaborative care* (4th ed., p. 436). Philadelphia: W. B. Saunders.

20. **1**
Rationale: The client's self report is a critical component of pain assessment. The nurse should ask the client about the description of the pain and listen carefully to the client's words used to describe the pain. The nurse's impression of the client's pain is not appropriate in determining the client's level of pain. Nonverbal cues from the client are important but are not the most appropriate pain assessment measure. Assessing pain relief is an important measure, but this option is not related to the issue of the question.
Test-Taking Strategy: Use the process of elimination. Noting the issue of the question will assist in eliminating option 4. Eliminate option 2 because the nurse is not the client of the question. From the remaining two options, the subjective data from

the client will provide the most accurate description of the pain. Review pain assessment techniques if the question was difficult.
Level of Cognitive Ability: Analysis
Client Needs: Physiological Integrity
Integrated Process: Caring
Content Area: Adult health—oncology
Reference: Ignatavicius, D., & Workman, M. (2002). *Medical-surgical nursing: Critical thinking for collaborative care* (4th ed., pp. 63-65). Philadelphia: W. B. Saunders.

21. **4**
Rationale: The client is kept NPO until peristalsis returns, usually in 4 to 6 days. When signs of bowel function return, clear fluids are given to the client. If no distention occurs, the diet is advanced as tolerated. The most important assessment is to assess bowel sounds before feeding the client. Options 1, 2, and 3 are unrelated to the issue of the question.
Test-Taking Strategy: Use the process of elimination. Note the key word "priority" and the key words "NPO to clear liquids" in the stem of the question. Knowledge regarding general postoperative care measures will assist in selecting the correct option. Option 4 is the only option that relates to gastrointestinal function, which is the issue of the question.
Level of Cognitive Ability: Analysis
Client Needs: Physiological Integrity
Integrated Process: Nursing Process—assessment
Content Area: Adult health—oncology
Reference: Potter, P., & Perry, A. (2001). *Fundamentals of nursing* (5th ed., p. 1711). St. Louis: Mosby.

22. **4**
Rationale: Hodgkin's disease is a chronic progressive neoplastic disorder of lymphoid tissue characterized by the painless enlargement of lymph nodes with progression to extralymphatic sites such as the spleen and liver. Weight loss is most likely to be noted. Fatigue and weakness may occur but are not related significantly to the disease.
Test-Taking Strategy: Use the process of elimination. Knowledge that Hodgkin's affects the lymph nodes will direct you easily to option 4. Option 3 easily can be eliminated first because in such a disorder, weight loss is most likely to occur. Options 1 and 2 are similar and rather vague symptoms that can occur in many disorders. Review the manifestations associated with Hodgkin's disease if you had difficulty with this question.
Level of Cognitive Ability: Analysis
Client Needs: Physiological Integrity
Integrated Process: Nursing Process—assessment
Content Area: Adult health—oncology
Reference: Black, J., Hawks, J., & Keene, A. (2001). *Medical-surgical nursing: Clinical management for positive outcomes* (6th ed., p. 2173). Philadelphia: W. B. Saunders.

23. **2**
Rationale: Clinical manifestations of ovarian cancer include abdominal distention, urinary frequency and urgency, pleural effusion, malnutrition, pain from pressure caused by the growing tumor and the effects of urinary or bowel obstruction, constipation, ascites with dyspnea and ultimately general severe pain. Abnormal bleeding, often resulting in hypermenorrhea, is associated with uterine cancer.

Test-Taking Strategy: Use the process of elimination. Eliminate options 1 and 4 first because they are similar. From the remaining options, consider the anatomical location of the cancer. This will assist in directing you to option 2. Review the manifestations associated with ovarian cancer if you had difficulty with this question.
Level of Cognitive Ability: Analysis
Client Needs: Physiological Integrity
Integrated Process: Nursing Process—assessment
Content Area: Adult health—oncology
Reference: Ignatavicius, D., & Workman, M. (2002). *Medical-surgical nursing: Critical thinking for collaborative care* (4th ed., p. 1776). Philadelphia: W. B. Saunders.

24. **3**
Rationale: Conization generally is not performed on women who desire to bear children because it can lead to incompetence of the cervix or infertility. Complications of the procedure include hemorrhage, infection, and less frequently cervical stenosis.
Test-Taking Strategy: Use the process of elimination. Note the key words "need for further teaching" and the words "cervical cancer" in the question. Select option 3 because this option addresses an "ovarian" condition not a cervical one. Review the complications associated with this procedure if you had difficulty with this question.
Level of Cognitive Ability: Analysis
Client Needs: Physiological Integrity
Integrated Process: Teaching/Learning
Content Area: Adult health—oncology
Reference: Ignatavicius, D., & Workman, M. (2002). *Medical-surgical nursing: Critical thinking for collaborative care* (4th ed., p. 1774). Philadelphia: W. B. Saunders.

25. **4**
Rationale: Hypercalcemia is a serum calcium level greater than 10 mg/dL, most often occurs in clients who have bone metastasis, and is a late manifestation of extensive malignancy. The presence of cancer in the bone causes the bone to release calcium into the bloodstream.
Test-Taking Strategy: Use the process of elimination. Knowledge regarding the normal calcium level will direct you easily to option 4. Note the relationship of "calcium level" in the question and "hypercalcemia" in the correct option. Review oncological emergencies if you had difficulty with this question.
Level of Cognitive Ability: Analysis
Client Needs: Physiological Integrity
Integrated Process: Nursing Process—assessment
Content Area: Adult health—oncology
Reference: Ignatavicius, D., & Workman, M. (2002). *Medical-surgical nursing: Critical thinking for collaborative care* (4th ed., p. 441). Philadelphia: W. B. Saunders.

26. **1**
Rationale: Testicular cancer almost always occurs in only one testicle and is usually a pea-sized painless lump. The cancer is highly curable when found early. The finding should be reported to the physician.
Test-Taking Strategy: Use the process of elimination. Eliminate option 4 because it does not address the client's concern and

is a block to communication. Option 3 places the client's concern on hold and is an inappropriate and inaccurate response. Option 2 is nontherapeutic and may cause concern in the client. Review testicular self-examination and therapeutic communication techniques if you had difficulty with this question.
Level of Cognitive Ability: Application
Client Needs: Psychosocial Integrity
Integrated Process: Caring
Content Area: Adult health—oncology
Reference: Ignatavicius, D., & Workman, M. (2002). *Medical-surgical nursing: Critical thinking for collaborative care* (4th ed., p. 1795). Philadelphia: W. B. Saunders.

27. **2**
Rationale: Denial, bargaining, anger, depression, and acceptance are recognized stages that a person facing a life-threatening illness experiences. Bargaining identifies a behavior in which the individual is willing to do anything to avoid loss or change prognosis or fate. Denial is expressed as shock and disbelief and may be the first response to hearing bad news. Depression may be manifested by hopelessness, weeping openly or remaining quiet or withdrawn. Anger also may be a first response to upsetting news and the predominant theme is "why me?" or the blaming of others.
Test-Taking Strategy: Use the process of elimination. Focus on the client's statement as identified in the question to assist in selecting the correct option. From this point, you should be able easily to eliminate options 1, 3, and 4. Review these stages if you had difficulty with this question.
Level of Cognitive Ability: Analysis
Client Needs: Psychosocial Integrity
Integrated Process: Nursing Process—assessment
Content Area: Adult health—oncology
Reference: Perry, A., & Potter, P. (2002). *Clinical nursing skills & techniques* (5th ed., p. 633). St. Louis: Mosby.

28. **4**
Rationale: Arm edema on the operative side (lymphedema) is a complication following mastectomy and can occur immediately postoperatively or may occur months or even years after surgery. Options 1, 2, and 3 are expected occurrences following mastectomy and do not indicate a complication.
Test-Taking Strategy: Use the process of elimination considering the normal expected occurrences following a mastectomy. You should be able to eliminate options 1, 2, and 3 easily. If you had difficulty with this question, review the complications following mastectomy.
Level of Cognitive Ability: Analysis
Client Needs: Physiological Integrity
Integrated Process: Nursing Process—assessment
Content Area: Adult health—oncology
Reference: Lewis, S., Heitkemper, M., & Dirksen, S. (2004). *Medical-surgical nursing: Assessment and management of clinical problems* (6th ed., p. 1376). St. Louis: Mosby.

29. **2**
Rationale: The most common risk factor associated with laryngeal cancer is cigarette smoking. Approximately ¾ of those

diagnosed with this form of cancer smoke currently or have done so in the past. Alcohol abuse seems to have a synergistic effect with cigarette smoking. Air pollution is also a contributing cause, as is chronic laryngitis and voice abuse.
Test-Taking Strategy: Note the key words "most common" in the question. Begin to answer this question by eliminating options 3 and 4. Because cancer of the upper and lower airway most often is related to tobacco, these are the options that are most likely correct. To discriminate between the last two options, knowing that cigarettes are the most harmful guides you to choose this option over the chewing tobacco. Review the causes of lung cancer if this question was difficult.
Level of Cognitive Ability: Analysis
Client Needs: Physiological Integrity
Integrated Process: Nursing Process—analysis
Content Area: Adult health—oncology
Reference: Lewis, S., Heitkemper, M., & Dirksen, S. (2004). *Medical-surgical nursing: Assessment and management of clinical problems* (6th ed., pp. 586-587). St. Louis: Mosby.

30. **3**
Rationale: A vesicovaginal fistula is a genital fistula that occurs between the bladder and the vagina. The fistula is an abnormal opening between these two body parts and if this occurs, the client may experience drainage of urine through the vagina. The client's complaint is not associated with options 1, 2, and 4.
Test-Taking Strategy: Use the process of elimination. Noting the key words "voiding through the vagina" should direct you easily to option 3. Review the symptoms associated with vesicovaginal fistula if you had difficulty with this question.
Level of Cognitive Ability: Analysis
Client Needs: Physiological Integrity
Integrated Process: Nursing Process—analysis
Content Area: Adult health—oncology
Reference: Phipps, W., Monahan, F., Sands, J., Marek, J., & Neighbors, M. (2003). *Medical-surgical nursing: Health and illness perspectives* (7th ed., p. 1758). St. Louis: Mosby.

31. **2**
Rationale: Allopurinol decreases uric acid production and reduces uric acid concentrations in serum and urine. In the client receiving chemotherapy, uric acid levels increase as a result of the massive cell destruction that occurs from the chemotherapy. This medication prevents or treats hyperuricemia caused by chemotherapy. Allopurinol is not used to prevent alopecia, nausea, or vomiting.
Test-Taking Strategy: Use the process of elimination. Recalling that hyperuricemia occurs as a result of chemotherapy will assist in directing you to option 2. If you had difficulty with this question or are unfamiliar with this medication, review its action in the client receiving chemotherapy.
Level of Cognitive Ability: Application
Client Needs: Physiological Integrity
Integrated Process: Nursing Process—implementation
Content Area: Adult health—oncology
Reference: Hodgson, B., & Kizior, R. (2004). *Saunders nursing drug handbook 2004* (p. 23). Philadelphia: W. B. Saunders.

32. 2

Rationale: An acidic environment in the mouth is favorable for bacterial growth, particularly in an area already compromised from chemotherapy. Therefore the client is advised to rinse the mouth before every meal and at bedtime with a weak salt and sodium bicarbonate mouth rinse. This lessens the growth of bacteria and limits plaque formation. The other substances are irritating to oral tissue. If hydrogen peroxide must be used because of severe plaque, it should be a weak solution because it dries the mucous membranes.

Test-Taking Strategy: Use the process of elimination. Options 3 and 4 can be eliminated first because of the irritating effects of these solutions. From the remaining options, note the word "weak" in the correct option. Review the treatment measures for stomatitis if you had difficulty with this question.

Level of Cognitive Ability: Application
Client Needs: Physiological Integrity
Integrated Process: Nursing Process—implementation
Content Area: Adult health—oncology
References: Ignatavicius, D., & Workman, M. (2002). *Medical-surgical nursing: Critical thinking for collaborative care* (4th ed., p. 506). Philadelphia: W. B. Saunders.
Lewis, S., Heitkemper, M., & Dirksen, S. (2004). *Medical-surgical nursing: Assessment and management of clinical problems* (6th ed., p. 1181). St. Louis: Mosby.

33. 4

Rationale: High meat and carbohydrate consumption plays a role in the development of cancer of the pancreas. Options 1, 2, and 3 are risk factors related to gastric cancer. Additionally, an increased risk exists in the male population in clients 50 years of age and older and in clients with a history of precancerous lesions and chronic gastritis.

Test-Taking Strategy: Use the process of elimination. Note that the question asks about the risk factors associated with gastric cancer. Note the key words "indicates a need for further discussion." Eliminate options 1 and 2 because they are related directly to gastric disorders. Eliminate option 3 knowing that spicy foods cause gastric irritation. Review the risk factors associated with gastric cancer if you had difficulty with this question.

Level of Cognitive Ability: Analysis
Client Needs: Health Promotion and Maintenance
Integrated Process: Teaching/Learning
Content Area: Adult health—oncology
Reference: Ignatavicius, D., & Workman, M. (2002). *Medical-surgical nursing: Critical thinking for collaborative care* (4th ed., p. 1235). Philadelphia: W. B. Saunders.

34. 2

Rationale: Following gastrectomy, drainage from the nasogastric tube is normally bloody for 24 hours postoperatively and then changes to brown-tinged and then to yellow or clear. Because bloody drainage is expected in the immediate postoperative period, the nurse should continue to monitor the drainage. The nurse does not need to notify the physician at this time. Measuring abdominal girth is performed to detect the development of distention. Following gastrectomy,

a nasogastric tube should not be irrigated unless there are specific physician orders to do so.

Test-Taking Strategy: Use the process of elimination. Note the key word "immediate" and the words "most appropriate" in the question. These key items should direct you easily to option 2. If you had difficulty with this question, review the postoperative expected findings following gastrectomy.

Level of Cognitive Ability: Application
Client Needs: Physiological Integrity
Integrated Process: Nursing Process—implementation
Content Area: Adult health—oncology
Reference: Phipps, W., Monahan, F., Sands, J., Marek, J., & Neighbors, M. (2003). *Medical-surgical nursing: Health and illness perspectives* (7th ed., p. 1048). St. Louis: Mosby.

35. 3

Rationale: Colorectal cancer most often occurs in populations with diets low in fiber and high in refined carbohydrates, fats, and meats. Other risk factors include a family history of the disease, rectal polyps, and active inflammatory disease of at least 10 years' duration.

Test-Taking Strategy: Use the process of elimination. Note the key words "further teaching is necessary" in the stem of the question. Eliminate options 1 and 2 because they are similar and directly related to the issue of colorectal cancer. Knowledge that a high-fiber diet is recommended as a preventative measure will assist you in selecting the correct option. Review the risk factors associated with colorectal cancer if you had difficulty with this question.

Level of Cognitive Ability: Analysis
Client Needs: Health Promotion and Maintenance
Integrated Process: Teaching/Learning
Content Area: Adult health—oncology
Reference: Lewis, S., Heitkemper, M., & Dirksen, S. (2004). *Medical-surgical nursing: Assessment and management of clinical problems* (6th ed., p. 1082). St. Louis: Mosby.

36. 3

Rationale: Vague abdominal discomfort or crampy, colicky abdominal pain is a characteristic symptom of a right colon tumor. Options 1, 2, and 4 are symptoms associated with left colon tumors.

Test-Taking Strategy: Use the process of elimination. Note the key words "right colon tumor." Knowledge regarding the signs of right and left colon tumors is required to answer this question. If you are not familiar with the differences, review these types of tumors.

Level of Cognitive Ability: Analysis
Client Needs: Physiological Integrity
Integrated Process: Nursing Process—assessment
Content Area: Adult health—oncology
Reference: Lewis, S., Heitkemper, M., & Dirksen, S. (2004). *Medical-surgical nursing: Assessment and management of clinical problems* (6th ed., p. 1083). St. Louis: Mosby.

37. 3

Rationale: To reduce the risk of contamination at the time of surgery, the bowel is emptied and cleansed. Laxatives and enemas are given to empty the bowel. Intestinal antiinfectives such as neomycin or kanamycin (kantrex) are administered to decrease the bacteria in the bowel.

Test-Taking Strategy: Use the process of elimination. Eliminate options 1 and 4 first because no reference is made to this information in the question. Recalling the concepts related to the flora of the intestinal tract will assist in directing you to option 3 as the primary purpose of this medication. Review this important preoperative intervention if you had difficulty with this question.

Level of Cognitive Ability: Analysis
Client Needs: Physiological Integrity
Integrated Process: Nursing Process—analysis
Content Area: Adult health—oncology
Reference: Black, J., Hawks, J., & Keene, A. (2001). *Medical-surgical nursing: Clinical management for positive outcomes* (6th ed., p. 784). Philadelphia: W. B. Saunders.

38. 2
Rationale: Immediately after surgery, profuse serosanguineous drainage from the perineal wound is expected. The nurse does not need to notify the physician at this time. A Penrose drain should not be clamped because this action will cause the accumulation of drainage within the tissue. Penrose drains and packing are removed gradually over a period of 5 to 7 days as prescribed. The nurse should not remove the perineal packing.

Test-Taking Strategy: Use the process of elimination. Note the key words "most appropriate." Eliminate options 3 and 4 knowing that these are inappropriate interventions. Knowledge of the normal expectations following this type of surgery will assist in directing you to option 2 as the most appropriate action. Review postoperative expectations following abdominal perineal resection if you had difficulty with this question.

Level of Cognitive Ability: Application
Client Needs: Physiological Integrity
Integrated Process: Nursing Process—implementation
Content Area: Adult health—oncology
Reference: Lewis, S., Heitkemper, M., & Dirksen, S. (2004). *Medical-surgical nursing: Assessment and management of clinical problems* (6th ed., p. 1087). St. Louis: Mosby.

39. 4
Rationale: Following abdominal perineal resection, the nurse would expect the colostomy to begin to function within 72 hours after surgery, although it may take up to 5 days. The nurse should assess for a return of peristalsis and listen for bowel sounds and check for the passage of flatus. Absent bowel sounds would not indicate the return of peristalsis. The client would remain NPO until bowel sounds return and the colostomy is functioning. Bloody drainage is not expected from a colostomy.

Test-Taking Strategy: Use the process of elimination. Note the key words "beginning to function." These key words should assist in eliminating option 3. Knowledge of general postoperative measures will assist in eliminating option 2. Focus on the issue of the question to assist in eliminating option 1 as a correct option. Review postoperative care of a client following abdominal perineal resection if you had difficulty with this question.

Level of Cognitive Ability: Analysis
Client Needs: Physiological Integrity

Integrated Process: Nursing Process—assessment
Content Area: Adult health—oncology
Reference: Black, J., Hawks, J., & Keene, A. (2001). *Medical-surgical nursing: Clinical management for positive outcomes* (6th ed., 784). Philadelphia: W. B. Saunders.

40. 3
Rationale: Air conditioners need to be avoided to protect from excessive coldness. A humidifier in the home should be used if excessive dryness is a problem. Options 1, 2, and 4 are appropriate interventions regarding stoma care following radical neck dissection and creation of a tracheotomy.

Test-Taking Strategy: Use the process of elimination. Note the key words "need for further instructions." You should be able easily to eliminate options 2 and 4. From the remaining options, recalling that a humidifier rather than an air conditioner is recommended will assist you in selecting the correct option. If you had difficulty with this question, review discharge instructions following radical neck dissection.

Level of Cognitive Ability: Analysis
Client Needs: Health Promotion and Maintenance
Integrated Process: Teaching/Learning
Content Area: Adult health—oncology
Reference: Black, J., Hawks, J., & Keene, A. (2001). *Medical-surgical nursing: Clinical management for positive outcomes* (6th ed., p. 1669). Philadelphia: W. B. Saunders.

41. 3
Rationale: Serum acid phosphatase levels are elevated in clients with prostatic cancer because acid phosphatase, which is produced by the acinar cells, is absorbed into the circulation rather than secreted into the seminal fluid and kept in the prostate. This makes measurement of serum acid phosphatase a useful biochemical test for monitoring the progression or regression of prostatic cancer.

Test-Taking Strategy: Use the process of elimination. Option 1 can be eliminated first, knowing that biopsy is necessary to confirm the diagnosis of cancer. From the remaining options, select option 3 because it is the most global response. Review this serum test if you had difficulty with this question.

Level of Cognitive Ability: Analysis
Client Needs: Physiological Integrity
Integrated Process: Nursing Process—analysis
Content Area: Adult health—oncology
Reference: Lewis, S., Heitkemper, M., & Dirksen, S. (2004). *Medical-surgical nursing: Assessment and management of clinical problems* (6th ed., p. 1445). St. Louis: Mosby.

42. 1
Rationale: Hormone therapy (androgen deprivation) is a mode of treatment for prostatic cancer. The goal is to limit the amount of circulating androgens because prostate cells depend on androgen for cellular maintenance. Deprivation of androgen often can lead to regression of disease and improvement of symptoms.

Test-Taking Strategy: Use the process of elimination. Note that options 2, 3, and 4 indicate an "increase." Review the goal of this form of therapy if you had difficulty with this question.

Level of Cognitive Ability: Analysis
Client Needs: Physiological Integrity

Integrated Process: Nursing Process—analysis
Content Area: Adult health—oncology
Reference: Ignatavicius, D., & Workman, M. (2002). *Medical-surgical nursing: Critical thinking for collaborative care* (4th ed., p. 1793). Philadelphia: W. B. Saunders.

43. 4
Rationale: Small pieces of tissue or blood clots can be passed during urination for up to 2 weeks after surgery. Driving a car and sitting for long periods of time are restricted for at least 3 weeks. A high daily fluid intake should be maintained to limit clot formation and prevent infection. Option 4 is an accurate discharge instruction following prostatectomy.
Test-Taking Strategy: Use the process of elimination. Option 3 easily can be eliminated first. Eliminate option 2 next, because 1 week is a rather short time. Recalling that blood clots are expected following this type of surgery will assist in directing you to option 4. Review client teaching points following prostatectomy if you had difficulty with this question.
Level of Cognitive Ability: Application
Client Needs: Health Promotion and Maintenance
Integrated Process: Teaching/Learning
Content Area: Adult health—oncology
Reference: Phipps, W., Monahan, F., Sands, J., Marek, J., & Neighbors, M. (2003). *Medical-surgical nursing: Health and illness perspectives* (7th ed., p. 1846). St. Louis: Mosby.

44. 1
Rationale: The incidence of bladder cancer is 3 times greater in men than in women and affects the white population twice as often as blacks. Options 2, 3, and 4 are associated with the incidence of bladder cancer.
Test-Taking Strategy: Use the process of elimination. Note the key words "need for further teaching." Basic information regarding the risks associated with cancer will assist in eliminating options 2, 3, and 4. If you had difficulty with this question, review these risks.
Level of Cognitive Ability: Analysis
Client Needs: Physiological Integrity
Integrated Process: Teaching/Learning
Content Area: Adult health—oncology
Reference: Lewis, S., Heitkemper, M., & Dirksen, S. (2004). *Medical-surgical nursing: Assessment and management of clinical problems* (6th ed., p. 1194). St. Louis: Mosby.

45. 3
Rationale: The most common symptom in clients with cancer of the bladder is hematuria. The client also may experience irritative voiding symptoms such as frequency, urgency, and dysuria, and these symptoms often are associated with carcinoma in situ.
Test-Taking Strategy: Use the process of elimination. Note the key words "most common" in the stem of the question. Options 1, 2, and 4 are symptoms that are associated most often with bladder infection. Review the clinical manifestations associated with bladder cancer if you had difficulty with this question.
Level of Cognitive Ability: Analysis
Client Needs: Physiological Integrity

Integrated Process: Nursing Process—assessment
Content Area: Adult health—oncology
Reference: Phipps, W., Monahan, F., Sands, J., Marek, J., & Neighbors, M. (2003). *Medical-surgical nursing: Health and illness perspectives* (7th ed., p. 1226). St. Louis: Mosby.

46. 4
Rationale: Normally the medication is injected into the bladder through a urethral catheter, the catheter is clamped or removed, and the client is asked to retain the fluid for 2 hours. The client changes position every 15 to 30 minutes from side to side and from supine to prone or resumes all activity immediately. The client then voids and is instructed to drink water to flush the bladder.
Test-Taking Strategy: Use the process of elimination. Note the key words "intravesical instillation" and think about the purpose of this treatment to direct you to option 4. If you are unfamiliar with this treatment measure, review the nursing interventions.
Level of Cognitive Ability: Application
Client Needs: Physiological Integrity
Integrated Process: Nursing Process—implementation
Content Area: Adult health—oncology
Reference: Lewis, S., Heitkemper, M., & Dirksen, S. (2004). *Medical-surgical nursing: Assessment and management of clinical problems* (6th ed., p. 1195). St. Louis: Mosby.

47. 2
Rationale: Following ureterostomy, the stoma should be red and moist. A pale stoma may indicate an inadequate amount of vascular supply. A dry stoma may indicate a body fluid deficit. Any sign of darkness or duskiness in the stoma may indicate a loss of vascular supply and must be reported immediately or necrosis can occur.
Test-Taking Strategy: Use the process of elimination. You should be able to eliminate options 1 and 4 easily. From the remaining options, note the key word "moist" in option 2. This should indicate that this is an expected and positive assessment. If you had difficulty with this question, review expected and unexpected findings following ureterostomy.
Level of Cognitive Ability: Analysis
Client Needs: Physiological Integrity
Integrated Process: Nursing Process—assessment
Content Area: Adult health—oncology
Reference: Black, J., Hawks, J., & Keene, A. (2001). *Medical-surgical nursing: Clinical management for positive outcomes* (6th ed., p. 816). Philadelphia: W. B. Saunders.

48. 2
Rationale: Following mastectomy, the arm should be elevated above the level of the heart. Simple arm exercises should be encouraged. No blood pressure readings, injections, intravenous lines, or blood draws should be performed on the affected arm. Cool compresses are not a suggested measure to prevent lymphedema from occurring.
Test-Taking Strategy: Note the key words "assist in preventing." Use the process of elimination and note the relationship between the words lymph"edema" in the question and "elevating" in the correct option. Review these important measures if you had difficulty with this question.

Level of Cognitive Ability: Application
Client Needs: Physiological Integrity
Integrated Process: Nursing Process—implementation
Content Area: Adult health—oncology
Reference: Ignatavicius, D., & Workman, M. (2002). *Medical-surgical nursing: Critical thinking for collaborative care* (4th ed., p. 1744). Philadelphia: W. B. Saunders.

49. **2**
Rationale: Mammography takes about 15 to 30 minutes to complete. Some discomfort may be experienced because of the breast compression required to obtain a clear image. There is no reason to maintain an NPO status before the procedure. Option 2 is an accurate instruction.
Test-Taking Strategy: Use the process of elimination. Eliminate options 3 and 4 first. Attempt to visualize the procedure to assist in selecting the correct option. If you are unfamiliar with this screening test, review this information.
Level of Cognitive Ability: Application
Client Needs: Physiological Integrity
Integrated Process: Nursing Process—implementation
Content Area: Adult health—oncology
Reference: Ignatavicius, D., & Workman, M. (2002). *Medical-surgical nursing: Critical thinking for collaborative care* (4th ed., p. 1725). Philadelphia: W. B. Saunders.

50. **1**
Rationale: Superior vena cava syndrome occurs when the superior vena cava is compressed or obstructed by tumor growth. Early signs and symptoms generally occur in the morning and include edema of the face, especially around the eyes, and client complaints of tightness of a shirt or blouse collar. As the compression worsens, the client experiences edema of the hands and arms. Mental status changes and cyanosis are late signs.
Test-Taking Strategy: Use the process of elimination. Note the key word "early" in the stem of the question. This key word should assist in eliminating options 2, 3, and 4. If you are unfamiliar with vena cava syndrome, review this oncological emergency.

Level of Cognitive Ability: Analysis
Client Needs: Physiological Integrity
Integrated Process: Nursing Process—assessment
Content Area: Adult health—oncology
Reference: Ignatavicius, D., & Workman, M. (2002). *Medical-surgical nursing: Critical thinking for collaborative care* (4th ed., p. 442). Philadelphia: W. B. Saunders.

CRITICAL THINKING: MULTIPLE RESPONSE
Answer:
___ Serum sodium blood levels
___ Medication that is antagonistic to antidiuretic hormone
___ Radiation or chemotherapy
Rationale: Cancer is a common cause of syndrome of inappropriate antidiuretic hormone (SIADH). In SIADH, excessive amounts of water are reabsorbed by the kidney and put into the systemic circulation. The increased water causes hyponatremia (decreased serum sodium levels) and some degree of fluid retention. The syndrome is managed by treating the condition and cause and usually includes fluid restriction, increased sodium intake, and medication with a mechanism of action that is antagonistic to antidiuretic hormone. Sodium levels are monitored closely because hypernatremia can develop suddenly as a result of treatment. The immediate institution of appropriate cancer therapy, usually radiation or chemotherapy, can cause such tumor regression that antidiuretic hormone synthesis and release processes return to normal.
Test-Taking Strategy: Focusing on the client's diagnosis and recalling that in SIADH, excessive amounts of water are reabsorbed by the kidney and put into the systemic circulation will assist in answering this question. Review the treatment for SIADH if you had difficulty with this question.
Level of Cognitive Ability: Analysis
Client Needs: Physiological Integrity
Integrated Process: Nursing Process—analysis
Content Area: Adult health—oncology
Reference: Ignatavicius, D., & Workman, M. (2002). *Medical-surgical nursing: Critical thinking for collaborative care* (4th ed., p. 441). Philadelphia: W. B. Saunders.

REFERENCES

Black, J., Hawks, J., & Keene, A. (2001). *Medical-surgical nursing: Clinical management for positive outcomes* (6th ed.). Philadelphia: W. B. Saunders.

Chernecky, C., & Berger, B. (2001). *Laboratory tests and diagnostic procedures* (3rd ed.). Philadelphia: W. B. Saunders.

Hodgson, B., & Kizior, R. (2004). *Saunders nursing drug handbook 2004.* Philadelphia: W. B. Saunders.

Ignatavicius, D., & Workman, M. (2002). *Medical-surgical nursing: Critical thinking for collaborative care* (4th ed.). Philadelphia: W. B. Saunders.

Lewis, S., Heitkemper, M., & Dirksen, S. (2004). *Medical-surgical nursing: Assessment and management of clinical problems* (6th ed.). St. Louis: Mosby.

Phipps, W., Monahan, F., Sands, J., Marek, J., & Neighbors, M. (2003). *Medical-surgical nursing: Health and illness perspectives* (7th ed.). St. Louis: Mosby.

Potter, P., & Perry, A. (2001). *Fundamentals of nursing* (5th ed.). St. Louis: Mosby.

Antineoplastic Medications

I. ANTINEOPLASTIC MEDICATIONS

A. Description
1. Antineoplastic medications kill or inhibit the reproduction of neoplastic cells.
2. The effect of antineoplastic medications may not be limited to neoplastic cells; normal cells also are affected by the medication.
3. Cell cycle phase-specific medications affect cells only during a certain phase of the reproductive cycle.
4. Cell cycle phase-nonspecific medications affect cells in any phase of the reproductive cycle.
5. Usually several medications are used in combination to increase the therapeutic response.
6. Antineoplastic medications may be combined with other treatments, such as surgery and radiation.
7. The routes of antineoplastic medication administration can vary; the intravenous (IV) route is preferred.
8. Side effects result from the effects of the antineoplastic medication on normal cells.

B. Side effects
1. Mucositis
2. Alopecia
3. Anorexia, nausea, and vomiting
4. Diarrhea
5. Anemia
6. Low white blood cell count (neutropenia)
7. Thrombocytopenia
8. Infertility

C. Interventions
1. Physiological Integrity
a. Monitor complete blood count (CBC), white blood cell count, platelet count, and electrolytes.
b. Initiate bleeding precautions if thrombocytopenia occurs.
c. When the platelet count is fewer than 50,000 cells/µL, any small trauma can lead to episodes of prolonged bleeding; when fewer than 20,000 cells/µL, spontaneous and uncontrollable bleeding can occur.
d. Monitor for petechiae, ecchymosis, bleeding of the gums, and nosebleeds because the decreased platelet count can precipitate bleeding tendencies.
e. Avoid intramuscular injections and venipunctures as much as possible to prevent bleeding.
f. Initiate neutropenic precautions if the white blood cell count decreases.
g. Monitor for fever, sore throat, unusual bleeding, or signs and symptoms of infection.
h. Inform the client that loss of appetite also may be due to a bitter taste in the mouth from the medications.
i. Monitor for nausea and vomiting, and provide a high-calorie diet with protein supplements.
j. Administer antiemetics several hours before chemotherapy and for 12 to 48 hours after as prescribed because antineoplastic medications stimulate the vomiting center in the brain.
k. Encourage hydration; IV fluids will be administered before and during therapy.
l. Promote a fluid intake of at least 2000 mL a day to maintain adequate renal function.
m. Administer allopurinol (Zyloprim) as prescribed to lower the serum uric acid that occurs from the rapid destruction of cells by the antineoplastic medication.

2. Safe, Effective Care Environment
a. Prepare IV chemotherapy in an air-vented space (biohazard cabinet area).
b. Wear gloves, a gown, eye protectors, and a mask when handling IV medications.

c. Nurses who are pregnant should not prepare or administer IV chemotherapy.

d. Discard IV equipment in designated (biohazard) containers.

e. Prepare to administer the antineoplastic medication in short, high-dose, intermittent courses as prescribed to maximize antineoplastic effects while allowing normal cells to recover.

f. Monitor for phlebitis with IV administration because these medications irritate the veins.

g. Monitor for extravasation (leakage of medication into surrounding skin and subcutaneous tissue), which causes tissue necrosis, and notify the physician if this occurs; heat or ice is applied depending on the medication and an antidote may be injected into the site.

3. Psychosocial Integrity

a. Instruct the client in the potential for hair loss and that varying degrees of hair loss may occur after the first or second treatment.

b. Discuss the purchase of a wig before treatment starts.

c. Inform the client that new hair growth will occur several months after the final treatment.

d. Instruct the client about the need for contraception because these medications have teratogenic effects.

e. Discuss the potential effect of infertility, which may be irreversible.

f. Encourage pretreatment counseling.

4. Health Promotion and Maintenance

a. Instruct the client that if diarrhea is a problem, avoid hot foods and high-fiber foods, which increase peristalsis

b. Instruct the client to inspect the oral mucosa for erythema and ulcers, to rinse mouth after meals, and to provide good oral hygiene.

c. Instruct the client to use saline or sodium bicarbonate mouth rinses for mouth sores.

d. Instruct the client in the use of antifungal medications for mouth sores, if prescribed for the development of a superinfection.

e. Instruct the client to avoid crowds and persons with infections and to report signs of infection such as fever, chills, or sore throat.

f. Instruct individuals with colds or infections to wear a mask when visiting or to avoid visiting the client.

g. Instruct the client to use a soft toothbrush and an electric razor to minimize the risk of bleeding.

h. Instruct the client to avoid aspirin-containing products to minimize the risk of bleeding.

i. Instruct the client to avoid alcohol to minimize the risk of toxicity.

j. Instruct the client to consult the physician before receiving vaccinations.

D. Anaphylactic reactions

1. Precautions

a. Obtain an allergy history.

b. Administer a test dose when prescribed by the physician.

c. Stay with the client during the administration of medication.

d. Monitor vital signs.

e. Have emergency equipment and medications readily available.

f. Provide an IV line for the administration of emergency medications if needed.

2. Signs of anaphylactic reaction

a. Dyspnea

b. Chest tightness or pain

c. Pruritis/urticaria

d. Tachycardia

e. Dizziness

f. Anxiety/agitation

g. Flushed appearance

h. Hypotension

i. Decreased sensorium

j. Cyanosis

3. Interventions for anaphylactic reaction

a. Stop medication.

b. Maintain airway.

c. Notify physician.

d. Maintain IV access with 0.9 % normal saline.

e. Place client in supine position with legs elevated if not contraindicated.

f. Monitor vital signs.

g. Administer prescribed emergency medications.

II. ALKYLATING MEDICATIONS (BOX 52-1)

A. Description

1. Affects the synthesis of DNA by causing cross-linking of DNA to inhibit cell reproduction

2. Cell cycle phase-nonspecific medications

B. Side effects

1. Anorexia, nausea, and vomiting may occur.

2. Stomatitis may occur.

3. Skin rash may occur.

4. Client may feel IV site pain during IV administration.

5. Busulfan (Myleran) may cause hyperuricemia.

6. Chlorambucil (Leukeran) and mechlorethamine (Mustargen) may cause gonadal suppression and hyperuricemia.

7. Cisplatin (Platinol) may cause ototoxicity, tinnitus, hypokalemia, hypocalcemia, hypomagnesemia, and nephrotoxicity (amifostine [Ethyol] may be administered before cisplatin to reduce the potential for renal toxicity).

8. Cyclophosphamide (Cytoxan) may cause alopecia, gonadal suppression, hemorrhagic cystitis, and hematuria.

BOX 52-1

Alkylating Medications

NITROGEN MUSTARDS
Chlorambucil (Leukeran)
Cyclophosphamide (Cytoxan)
Ifosfamide (Ifex)
Mechlorethamine (Mustargen)
Melphalan (Alkeran)
Uracil mustard (Uracil Mustard)

NITROSOUREAS
Carmustine (BiCNU)
Lomustine (CeeNU)
Streptozocin (Zanosar)

ALKYLATING-LIKE MEDICATIONS
Altretamine (Hexalen)
Busulfan (Myleran)
Carboplatin (Paraplatin)
Cisplatin (Platinol)
Dacarbazine (DTIC-Dome)
Thiotepa (Thioplex)

C. Interventions
   1. Assess vital signs and the temperature for signs of infection.
   2. Monitor CBC; white blood cell and platelet counts; and uric acid and electrolyte levels.
   3. Withhold medication if the platelet count is fewer than 75,000 cells/μL or the white blood cell count is fewer than 4000 cells/μL, and notify the physician.
   4. Assess results of pulmonary function tests.
   5. Assess results of chest radiographs and renal and liver function studies.
   6. Hydrate the client with IV and/or oral fluids before administering the antineoplastic medication as prescribed.
   7. Administer antiemetic 30 to 60 minutes before the antineoplastic medication as prescribed.
   8. As prescribed, reduce IV site pain by altering IV rates, diluting the medication, or warming the injection site to distend vein and increase blood flow.
   9. Monitor IV site for irritation and phlebitis.
   10. When administering cisplatin (Platinol), assess the client for dizziness, tinnitus, hearing loss, incoordination, and numbness or tingling of extremities.
   11. Monitor for signs of hemorrhagic cystitis, such as hematuria or dysuria, during cyclophosphamide (Cytoxan) or ifosfamide (Ifex) therapy, and encourage the client to drink increased fluids (2 to 3 L per day).
   12. Mesna (Mesnex) may be administered with ifosfamide (Ifex) to reduce the potential of ifosfamide-induced cystitis.
   13. Instruct the client that cyclophosphamide (Cytoxan), when prescribed orally, is administered without food.
   14. Instruct the client to follow a diet low in purines to alkalize urine and lower uric acid blood levels.
   15. Instruct the client how to avoid infection.
   16. Instruct the client to report signs of infection or bleeding.
   17. Instruct the client about good oral hygiene and use of a soft toothbrush.

III. ANTITUMOR ANTIBIOTIC MEDICATIONS (BOX 52-2)

A. Description
   1. Interfere with DNA and RNA synthesis
   2. Cell cycle phase-nonspecific medications
B. Side effects
   1. Nausea and vomiting
   2. Fever
   3. Bone marrow depression
   4. Skin rash
   5. Alopecia
   6. Stomatitis
   7. Gonadal suppression
   8. Hyperuricemia
   9. Vesication (blistering of tissue at IV site)
   10. Plicamycin (Mithracin) affects bleeding time.
   11. Daunorubicin (Cerubidine) may cause congestive heart failure and dysrhythmias.
   12. Doxorubicin (Adriamycin) and idarubicin (Idamycin) may cause cardiotoxicity, cardiomyopathy, and electrocardiographic changes (Dexrazoxane [Zinecard] may be administered with doxorubicin to reduce cardiomyopathy).
   13. Pulmonary toxicity can occur with bleomycin sulfate (Blenoxane).
C. Interventions
   1. Assess vital signs and temperature for signs of infection.
   2. Monitor CBC; white blood cell and platelet counts; and uric acid, bleeding time, and electrolytes.
   3. Withhold medication if the platelets are fewer than 75,000 cells/μL or the white blood cell

BOX 52-2

Antitumor Antibiotic Medications

Bleomycin sulfate (Blenoxane)
Dactinomycin (Actinomycin D, Cosmegan)
Daunorubicin (Cerubidine, DaunoXome)
Doxorubicin (Adriamycin)
Idarubicin (Idamycin)
Mitomycin (Mutamycin)
Mitoxantrone (Novantrone)
Pentostatin (Nipent)
Plicamycin (Mithracin)
Valrubicin (Valstar)

count is fewer than 4000 cells/μL, and notify physician.

4. Assess results of pulmonary function tests.
5. Monitor for electrocardiographic changes.
6. Assess lung sounds for crackles.
7. Assess for signs of congestive heart failure, including dyspnea, crackles, peripheral edema, and weight gain.
8. Assess results of chest radiographs and renal and liver function studies.
9. Hydrate the client with IV and/or oral fluids before the antineoplastic medication.
10. Administer antiemetic 30 to 60 minutes before the antineoplastic medication.
11. As prescribed, reduce IV site pain by altering IV rates, diluting the medication, or warming injection site to distend vein and increase blood flow.
12. Monitor IV site for irritation, phlebitis, and vesication.
13. Assess for myocardial toxicity, dyspnea, dysrhythmias, hypotension, and weight gain when administering doxorubicin (Adriamycin) or idarubicin (Idamycin).
14. Monitor pulmonary status when administering bleomycin (Blenoxane).
15. Avoid the use of aspirin, anticoagulants, and thrombolytic agents with plicamycin (Mithracin).

IV. ANTIMETABOLITE MEDICATIONS (BOX 52-3)

A. Description
1. Antimetabolite medications halt the synthesis of cell protein.
2. Antimetabolite medications replace normal proteins required for DNA synthesis.
3. Antimetabolite medications are cell cycle phase-specific and affect the S phase.
B. Side effects
1. Anorexia, nausea, and vomiting
2. Diarrhea
3. Alopecia
4. Stomatitis

BOX 52-3

Antimetabolite Medications

Capecitabine (Xeloda)
Cladribine (Leustatin)
Cytarabine (ara-C; Cytosar-U)
Floxuridine (FUDR)
Fludarabine (Fludara)
5-Fluorouracil (Adrucil)
Hydroxyurea (Hydrea)
6-Mercaptopurine (Purinethol)
Methotrexate (Folex)
Procarbazine (Matulane)
Thioguanine

---

5. Depression of bone marrow
6. Cytarabine (ara-C, Cytosar-U) may cause alopecia, stomatitis, hyperuricemia, and hepatotoxicity.
7. 5-Fluorouracil (Adrucil) may cause alopecia, stomatitis, diarrhea, phototoxicity reactions, and cerebellar dysfunction.
8. 6-Mercaptopurine (Purinethol) may cause hyperuricemia and hepatotoxicity.
9. Methotrexate (Folex) may cause alopecia, stomatitis, hyperuricemia, photosensitivity, hepatotoxicity, and hematological, gastrointestinal, and skin toxicity.
C. Interventions
1. Monitor vital signs and temperature for signs of infection.
2. Assess CBC, white blood cell count, uric acid, and platelet count.
3. Hold medication if the white blood cell count is fewer than 4000 cells/μL or the platelet count is fewer than 75,000 cells/μL, and notify the physician.
4. Monitor renal function studies.
5. Monitor for cerebellar dysfunction.
6. Assess for photosensitivity.
7. Administer antiemetics 30 to 60 minutes before the antineoplastic medication as prescribed.
8. Monitor IV site for extravasation.
9. Encourage fluid intake of 2 to 3 L a day.
10. Encourage good oral hygiene.
11. Instruct the client how to avoid infections and bleeding.
12. When administering 5-fluorouracil (Adrucil), assess for signs of cerebellar dysfunction, such as dizziness, weakness, and ataxia, and assess for stomatitis and diarrhea, which may necessitate medication discontinuation.
13. When administering methotrexate (Folex) in large doses, prepare to administer leucovorin (folinic acid or citrovorum factor) as prescribed to prevent toxicity (known as leucovorin rescue).
14. When administering 5-fluorouracil (Adrucil) or methotrexate (Folex), instruct the client to use sunscreen and wear protective clothing to prevent photosensitivity reactions.

V. MITOTIC INHIBITORS (VINCA ALKALOIDS) (BOX 52-4)

A. Description
1. Mitotic inhibitors prevent mitosis, causing cell death.
2. Mitotic inhibitors prevent cell division.
3. Mitotic inhibitors are cell cycle phase-specific and act on the M phase.
B. Side effects
1. Leukopenia

BOX 52-4

Miotic Inhibitors (Vinca Alkaloids)

Docetaxel (Taxotere)
Etoposide (VePesid)
Teniposide (Vumon)
Vinblastine sulfate (Velban)
Vincristine sulfate (Oncovin)
Vinorelbine (Navelbine)

---

2. Neurotoxicity with vincristine sulfate (Oncovin), manifested as numbness and tingling in the fingers and toes.
3. Ptosis
4. Hoarseness
5. Motor instability
6. Anorexia, nausea, and vomiting
7. Constipation
8. Peripheral neuropathy
9. Alopecia
10. Stomatitis
11. Hyperuricemia
12. Phlebitis at IV site

C. Interventions
   1. Monitor vital signs.
   2. Monitor white blood cell count, CBC, uric acid, and platelet count.
   3. Monitor for hoarseness.
   4. Assess eyes for ptosis.
   5. Assess motor stability and initiate safety precautions as necessary.
   6. Monitor for neurotoxicity with vincristine sulfate (Oncovin), manifested as numbness and tingling in the fingers and toes.

VI. HORMONAL MEDICATIONS AND ENZYMES (BOX 52-5)

A. Description
   1. Hormonal medications suppress the immune system and block normal hormones in hormone-sensitive tumors.
   2. Hormonal medications change the hormonal balance and slow the growth rates of certain tumors.
B. Side effects
   1. Anorexia, nausea, and vomiting
   2. Leukopenia
   3. Impaired pancreatic function with asparaginase (Elspar)
   4. Gynecomastia
   5. Breast swelling
   6. Hot flashes
   7. Weight gain
   8. Hemorrhagic cystitis, hypouricemia, and hypercholesterolemia, with mitotane (Lysodren)
   9. Hypertension
   10. Thromboembolitic disorders
   11. Edema
   12. Sex characteristic alterations
   13. Electrolyte imbalances
   14. Tamoxifen citrate (Nolvadex) may cause edema, hypercalcemia, and elevated cholesterol and triglyceride levels.
   15. Tamoxifen citrate decreases the effects of estrogen.
   16. Diethylstilbestrol (Stilphostrol) may cause impotence and gynecomastia in men.
   17. Diethylstilbestrol may alter effects of insulin, orally administered anticoagulants, and orally administered hypoglycemic agents.

BOX 52-5

Hormonal Medications and Enzymes

ESTROGENS
Diethylstilbestrol (Stilphostrol)
Estramustine (Emcyt)
Ethinyl estradiol (Estinyl)
Polyestradiol (Estradurin)

ANTIESTROGENS
Anastrozole (Arimidex)
Exemestane (Aromasin)
Letrozole (Femara)
Raloxifene (Evista)
Tamoxifen citrate (Nolvadex)
Testolactone (Teslac)
Toremifene (Fareston)

ANDROGENS
Fluoxymesterone (Halotestin)
Testosterone

ANTIANDROGENS
Bicalutamide (Casodex)
Flutamide (Eulexin)
Goserelin acetate (Zoladex)
Nilutamide (Nilandron)
Triptorelin (Trelstar)

PROGESTINS
Medroxyprogesterone (Depo-Provera)
Megestrol acetate (Megace)

OTHER HORMONAL ANTAGONISTS AND ENZYMES
Aminoglutethimide (Cytadren)
Asparaginase (Elspar)
Leuprolide acetate (Lupron)
Mitotane (Lysodren)

▶ C. Interventions
   1. Monitor vital signs.
   2. Assess medications that the client is taking currently.
   3. Monitor serum calcium levels with androgens.
   4. Monitor for signs of alterations in sexual characteristics.
   5. Monitor pancreatic function with asparaginase (Elspar).
   6. Encourage an oral intake of 2 to 3 L of fluids per day.
   7. Monitor uric acid and cholesterol levels.
   8. Monitor for signs of hemorrhagic cystitis.

VII. IMMUNOMODULATOR AGENTS: BIOLOGICAL RESPONSE MODIFIERS (BOX 52-6)

A. Description
   1. Immunomodulators stimulate the immune system to recognize **cancer** cells and take action to eliminate or destroy them.
   2. Interleukins help different immune system cells to recognize and destroy abnormal body cells.
   3. Interferons slow down tumor cell division, stimulate proliferation, cause **cancer** cells to differentiate into nonproliferative forms.
B. Colony-stimulating factors induce more rapid bone marrow recovery after suppression by chemotherapy (Box 52-7).

BOX 52-6

Immunomodulator Agents

Aldesleukin (Proleukin, interleukin-2)
Interferon alfa-2a
Interferon alfa-2b
Interferon alfa-n3 (Alferon N)
Levamisole (Ergamisole)
Recombinant interferon-α (Intron A)
Recombinant interferon-α (Roferon-A)
Rituximab (Rituxan)

BOX 52-7

Colony-Stimulating Factors

GRANULOCYTE-MACROPHAGE COLONY-STIMULATING FACTOR
Sargramostim (Leukine, Prokine)

GRANULOCYTE COLONY-STIMULATING FACTOR
Filgrastim (Neupogen)

ERYTHROPOIETIN
Epoetin alfa (Epogen)

BOX 52-8

Other Antineoplastic Medications

Alemtuzumab (Campath)
Arsenic trioxide (Trisenox)
Gemtuzumab ozogamicin (Mylotarg)
Imatinib (Gleevec)
Porfimer (Photofrin)
Temozolomide (Temodar)

VIII. OTHER ANTINEOPLASTIC MEDICATIONS (BOX 52-8)

A. Altretamine (Hexalen): cytotoxic agent used to treat ovarian **cancer**
B. Denileukin difitox (Ontak): recombinant DNA-derived medication used to treat cutaneous T-cell lymphoma
C. Gemcitabine (Gemzar): Used to treat non–small cell lung **cancer** and adenocarcinoma of the pancreas
D. Irinotecan (Camptosar): Used to treat colorectal or rectal **cancer**
E. Paclitaxel (Taxol): Used to treat ovarian or metastatic breast **cancer**
F. Pegaspargase (Oncaspar): Used in combination chemotherapies for acute lymphoblastic leukemia in clients unable to take L-asparaginase
G. Topotecan (Hycamtin): Indicated for the treatment of relapsed or refractory metastatic ovarian **cancer** after other therapies have failed
H. Trastuzumab (Herceptin): Used in combination chemotherapy to treat breast **cancer**
I. Tretinoin (Vesanoid): Used to treat acute promyelocytic leukemia
J. Bexarotene (Targretin): Use to treat advanced stage cutaneous T-cell lymphoma

PRACTICE QUESTIONS

1. The client with breast cancer is being treated with cyclophosphamide (Cytoxan). The nurse administering this medications understands that this medication is
   1. Cell cycle phase-specific, affecting cells only during a certain phase of the cell reproductive cycle.
   2. Cell cycle phase-nonspecific, affecting cells in any phase of the reproductive cell cycle.
   3. Cell cycle phase-specific, affecting the S phase of the reproductive cell cycle.
   4. Cell cycle phase-specific, affecting the M phase of the reproductive cell cycle.
2. The client with bladder cancer is receiving cisplatin (Platinol) and vincristine (Oncovin). The nurse preparing to give the medication understands that the purpose of administering both of these medications is to
   1. Prevent gastrointestinal side effects.

2. Prevent alopecia.

3. Decrease the destruction of cells.

4. Increase the therapeutic response.

3. The nurse is monitoring the laboratory results on a client receiving an antineoplastic medication by the intravenous route. The nurse plans to initiate bleeding precautions if which laboratory result is noted?

1. A white blood cell count of 5000 cells/μL

2. A platelet count of 50,000 cells/μL

3. A clotting time of 10 minutes

4. An ammonia level of 20 mcg/dL

4. The nurse is analyzing the laboratory results of a client with leukemia who received a regimen of chemotherapy. Which of the following laboratory values would the nurse specifically note as a result of the massive cell destruction that occurred from the chemotherapy?

1. Anemia

2. Decreased platelets

3. Decreased leukocyte count

4. Increased uric acid level

5. The client with leukemia is receiving busulfan (Myleran). The physician prescribes allopurinol (Zyloprim) for the client. The nurse prepares to administer the medication and understands that the purpose of the allopurinol is to prevent

1. Arthritis.

2. Hyperuricemia.

3. Alopecia.

4. Diarrhea.

6. The nurse is providing medication instructions to a client with breast cancer who is receiving cyclophosphamide (Cytoxan). The nurse tells the client to

1. Take the medication with food.

2. Increase fluid intake to 2000 to 3000 mL daily.

3. Decrease sodium intake while taking the medication.

4. Increase potassium intake while taking the medication.

7. The client with non–Hodgkin's lymphoma is receiving daunorubicin (Cerubidine). Which of the following would indicate to the nurse that the client is experiencing a toxic effect related to the medication?

1. Complaints of nausea and vomiting

2. Fever

3. Crackles on auscultation of the lungs

4. Diarrhea

8. The nurse is assigned to care for a client with testicular cancer who is receiving plicamycin (Mithracin). The nurse reviews the client's record and would question which prescribed medication if noted written in the physician's orders?

1. Warfarin (Coumadin)

2. Allopurinol (Zyloprim)

3. Acetaminophen (Tylenol)

4. Ondansetron (Zofran)

9. The client with squamous cell carcinoma of the larynx is receiving bleomycin sulfate (Blenoxane)

intravenously. The nurse caring for the client anticipates that which diagnostic study will be prescribed?

1. Pulmonary function studies

2. Electrocardiogram

3. Cervical radiographs

4. Echocardiogram

10. Cytarabine (Cytosar) is prescribed for the client with acute lymphocytic leukemia. The nurse administering this medication understands that this medication is classified as an antimetabolite and is a

1. Cell cycle phase-nonspecific medication.

2. Cell cycle phase-specific medication affecting the M phase.

3. Cell cycle phase-specific medication affecting the S phase.

4. Medication that affects cells in any phase of the reproductive cell cycle.

11. The clinic nurse prepares a teaching plan for the client receiving an antineoplastic medication. When implementing the plan, the nurse tells the client to

1. Take aspirin (acetylsalicylic acid) as needed for headache.

2. Drink beverages containing alcohol in moderate amounts.

3. Consult with the physician before receiving immunizations.

4. Be sure to receive the flu and pneumonia vaccine.

12. The client with lung cancer is receiving a high dose of methotrexate (Folex). Leucovorin (citrovorum factor, folic acid) also is prescribed. The nurse caring for the client understands that the purpose of administering the leucovorin is to

1. Preserve normal cells.

2. Promote DNA synthesis.

3. Promote medication excretion.

4. Promote the synthesis of nucleic acids.

13. The client with ovarian cancer is being treated with vincristine (Oncovin). The nurse monitors the client knowing that which of the following indicates a side effect specific to this medication?

1. Diarrhea

2. Numbness and tingling in the fingers and toes

3. Chest pain

4. Hair loss

14. The nurse is reviewing the history and physical of a client who will be receiving asparaginase (Elspar), an antineoplastic agent. The nurse contacts the physician before administering the medication if which of the following is documented in the client's history?

1. Myocardial infarction

2. Chronic obstructive pulmonary disease

3. Diabetes mellitus

4. Pancreatitis

15. Tamoxifen (Nolvadex) is prescribed for the client with metastatic breast carcinoma. The nurse administering the medication understands that the primary action of this medication is to

1. Increase DNA and RNA synthesis.
2. Compete with estradiol for binding to estrogen in tissues containing high concentrations of receptors.
3. Increase estrogen concentration and estrogen response.
4. Promote the biosynthesis of nucleic acids.

16. The client with metastatic breast cancer is receiving Tamoxifen (Nolvadex). The nurse specifically monitors which of the following laboratory values while the client is taking this medication?
    1. Potassium level
    2. Glucose level
    3. Calcium level
    4. Prothrombin time

17. Megestrol acetate (Megace), an antineoplastic medication, is prescribed for the client with metastatic endometrial carcinoma. The nurse reviews the client's history and contacts the physician if which of the following is documented in the client's history?
    1. Asthma
    2. Myocardial infarction
    3. Thrombophlebitis
    4. Gout

18. A female client with carcinoma of the breast is admitted to the hospital for treatment with intravenously administered vincristine (Oncovin). The client tells the nurse that she has been told by her friends that she is going to lose all of her hair. The most appropriate nursing response is which of the following?
    1. "You will not lose your hair."
    2. "Your friends are correct."
    3. "Hair loss may occur, but it will grow back just as it is now."

4. "Hair loss may occur, and it will grow back, but it may have a different color or texture."

19. The clinic nurse prepares instructions for a client who developed stomatitis following the administration of a course of antineoplastic medications. The nurse tells the client to
    1. Rinse the mouth with baking soda or saline.
    2. Avoid foods and fluids for the next 24 hours.
    3. Swab the mouth daily with lemon and glycerin pads.
    4. Brush the teeth and use waxed dental floss 3 times a day.

20. The client with acute myelocytic leukemia is being treated with busulfan (Myleran). Which of the following laboratory values would the nurse specifically monitor during treatment with this medication?
    1. Blood glucose
    2. Uric acid level
    3. Potassium level
    4. Clotting time

CRITICAL THINKING: FILL IN THE BLANK

The nurse is monitoring the intravenous infusion of an antineoplastic medication. During the infusion, the client complains of pain at the insertion site. On inspection of the site the nurse notes redness and swelling and that the infusion of the medication has slowed in rate. Based on this assessment data, what is the nurse's initial action?

Answer: _____

ANSWERS

1. **2**

Rationale: Cyclophosphamide (Cytoxan) is an antineoplastic medication of the alkylating classification. Medications in this classification affect all phases of the reproductive cell cycle. Cell cycle phase-specific medications affect cells only during a certain phase of the reproductive cycle. Antimetabolite medications are cell cycle phase-specific and affect the S phase. Vinca alkaloids are cell cycle phase-specific and act on the M phase.

Test-Taking Strategy: Use the process of elimination. Note that option 2 is the option that is different. Option 2 addresses the action as cell cycle phase-nonspecific, whereas options 1, 3, and 4 address a cell cycle phase-specific action. If you had difficulty with this question, review the action of alkylating medications.

Level of Cognitive Ability: Comprehension
Client Needs: Physiological Integrity
Integrated Process: Nursing Process—implementation
Content Area: Pharmacology
Reference: Lehne, R. (2001). *Pharmacology for nursing care* (4th ed., p. 752). Philadelphia: W. B. Saunders.

2. **4**

Rationale: Cisplatin (Platinol) is an alkylating-like medication, and vincristine (Oncovin) is a vinca (plant) alkaloid. Alkylating medications are cell cycle phase-nonspecific. Vinca alkaloids are cell cycle phase-specific and act on the M phase. Combinations of medications are used to enhance tumoricidal effects and increase the therapeutic response.

Test-Taking Strategy: Use the process of elimination. Option 3 easily can be eliminated first. Eliminate options 1 and 2 next. It may be possible, with some specific interventions, to reduce gastrointestinal effects and alopecia, but these occurrences are unlikely be prevented. Review the purpose of combination medication therapy if you had difficulty with this question.

Level of Cognitive Ability: Analysis
Client Needs: Physiological Integrity
Integrated Process: Nursing Process—planning
Content Area: Pharmacology
Reference: Hodgson, B., & Kizior, R. (2004). *Saunders nursing drug handbook 2004* (p. 216). Philadelphia: W. B. Saunders.

3. 2

Rationale: Bleeding precautions need to be initiated when the platelet count decreases. The normal platelet count is 150,000 to 450,000 cells/μL. When the platelets are fewer than 50,000 cells/μL, any small trauma can lead to episodes of prolonged bleeding. The normal white blood cell count is 5000 to 10,000 cells/μL. When the white blood cell count drops, neutropenic precautions need to be implemented. The normal clotting time is 8 to 15 minutes. The normal ammonia value is 15 to 45 mcg/dL.

Test-Taking Strategy: Use the process of elimination and knowledge regarding normal laboratory values. Options 1, 3, and 4 identify normal laboratory values. Remember, correlate a low platelet count with the need for bleeding precautions and a low white blood cell count with the need for neutropenic precaution. Review the indications to implement bleeding precautions in a client receiving chemotherapy if you had difficulty with this question.

Level of Cognitive Ability: Analysis
Client Needs: Physiological Integrity
Integrated Process: Nursing Process—planning
Content Area: Pharmacology
References: Kee, J., & Hayes, E. (2003). *Pharmacology: A nursing process approach* (4th ed., p. 504). Philadelphia: W. B. Saunders. Lehne, R. (2001). *Pharmacology for nursing care* (4th ed., p. 1006). Philadelphia: W. B. Saunders.

4. 4

Rationale: Hyperuricemia is especially common following treatment for leukemias and lymphomas because chemotherapy results in massive cell kill. Although options 1, 2, and 3 also may be noted, an increased uric acid level is related specifically to cell destruction.

Test-Taking Strategy: Note the key words "massive cell destruction" in the question. Recalling the cell response to destruction will assist in directing you to option 4. Review this concept, if you had difficulty with this question.

Level of Cognitive Ability: Analysis
Client Needs: Physiological Integrity
Integrated Process: Nursing Process—assessment
Content Area: Pharmacology
Reference: Lehne, R. (2001). *Pharmacology for nursing care* (4th ed., pp. 74, 577). Philadelphia: W. B. Saunders.

5. 2

Rationale: Busulfan (Myleran) is an alkylating medication used to treat acute myelocytic leukemia and in the palliative treatment of chronic myelogenous leukemia. Hyperuricemia can result from the use of this medication. Allopurinol (Zyloprim), an antigout medication, is used with chemotherapy to prevent or treat hyperuricemia that occurs from the rapid destruction of cells by the antineoplastic medication. Allopurinol is not used to prevent alopecia and diarrhea.

Test-Taking Strategy: Use the process of elimination, recalling that hyperuricemia occurs from the rapid destruction of cells by the antineoplastic medication. This knowledge will direct you easily to option 2. Review the purpose of administering allopurinol to a client receiving chemotherapy if you had difficulty with this question.

Level of Cognitive Ability: Analysis

Client Needs: Physiological Integrity
Integrated Process: Nursing Process—planning
Content Area: Pharmacology
Reference: Hodgson, B., & Kizior, R. (2004). *Saunders nursing drug handbook 2004* (p. 23). Philadelphia: W. B. Saunders.

6. 2

Rationale: Hemorrhagic cystitis is a toxic effect that can occur with the use of cyclophosphamide (Cytoxan). The client needs to be instructed to drink copious amounts of fluid during the administration of this medication. Clients also should monitor urine output for hematuria. The medication should be taken on an empty stomach, unless gastrointestinal upset occurs. Hyperkalemia can result from the use of the medication; therefore the client would not be told to increase potassium intake. The client would not be instructed to alter sodium intake.

Test-Taking Strategy: Use the process of elimination. Recalling that cyclophosphamide can cause hemorrhagic cystitis will direct you easily to option 2. If you had difficulty with this question, review the toxic effects associated with this medication.

Level of Cognitive Ability: Application
Client Needs: Health Promotion and Maintenance
Integrated Process: Teaching/Learning
Content Area: Pharmacology
Reference: Hodgson, B., & Kizior, R. (2004). *Saunders nursing drug handbook 2004* (p. 258). Philadelphia: W. B. Saunders.

7. 3

Rationale: Cardiotoxicity noted by abnormal electrocardiographic findings or cardiomyopathy manifested as congestive heart failure is a toxic effect of daunorubicin. Bone marrow depression is also a toxic effect. Nausea and vomiting is a frequent side effect associated with the medication that begins a few hours after administration and lasts 24 to 48 hours. Fever is a frequent side effect and diarrhea can occur occasionally. Options 1, 2, and 4, however, are not toxic effects.

Test-Taking Strategy: Use the process of elimination keeping in mind that the question is asking about a toxic effect. Use of the ABCs—airway, breathing, and circulation—will direct you easily to option 3. If you had difficulty with this question, review the toxic effects associated with daunorubicin.

Level of Cognitive Ability: Analysis
Client Needs: Physiological Integrity
Integrated Process: Nursing Process—analysis
Content Area: Pharmacology
References: Gutierrez, K., & Queener, S. (2003). *Pharmacology for nursing practice* (p. 584). St. Louis: Mosby. Hodgson, B., & Kizior, R. (2004). *Saunders nursing drug handbook 2004* (p. 278). Philadelphia: W. B. Saunders.

8. 1

Rationale: Plicamycin (Mithracin) is an antitumor antibiotic chemotherapeutic agent. Because plicamycin affects bleeding time, the use of aspirin, anticoagulants, and thrombolytic agents should be avoided. Warfarin (Coumadin) is an anticoagulant and the risk of hemorrhage is increased if administered during plicamycin (Mithracin) therapy. Allopurinol (Zyloprim), an antigout medication, may be used with chemotherapy to prevent or treat hyperuricemia from cell destruction caused by cancer chemotherapy. Acetaminophen (Tylenol) may be

used to treat mild discomfort. Ondansetron (Zofran) is an antiemetic used to prevent or treat nausea and vomiting during chemotherapy.
Test-Taking Strategy: Use the process of elimination, recalling the classifications of the medications identified in the options. Recalling that plicamycin affects bleeding time will direct you to option 1. If you are unfamiliar with these medications, review their classifications and purposes for use. Additionally, review the medication interactions associated with plicamycin.
Level of Cognitive Ability: Analysis
Client Needs: Physiological Integrity
Integrated Process: Nursing Process—implementation
Content Area: Pharmacology
Reference: Hodgson, B., & Kizior, R. (2004). *Saunders nursing drug handbook 2004* (p. 1063). Philadelphia: W. B. Saunders.

9. 1
Rationale: Bleomycin sulfate (Blenoxane) is an antineoplastic medication that can cause interstitial pneumonitis that can progress to pulmonary fibrosis. Pulmonary function studies along with hematological, hepatic, and renal function tests need to be monitored. The nurse needs to monitor lung sounds for dyspnea and crackles that indicate pulmonary toxicity. The medication needs to be discontinued immediately if pulmonary toxicity occurs. Options 2, 3, and 4 are unrelated to the specific use of this medication.
Test-Taking Strategy: Use the process of elimination. Eliminate options 2 and 4 first because they are cardiac related and are therefore similar. From the remaining options, use the ABCs—airway, breathing, and circulation—to direct you to option 1. If you had difficulty with this question, review the toxic effects of this medication.
Level of Cognitive Ability: Analysis
Client Needs: Physiological Integrity
Integrated Process: Nursing Process—analysis
Content Area: Pharmacology
Reference: Hodgson, B., & Kizior, R. (2004). *Saunders nursing drug handbook 2004* (p. 118). Philadelphia: W. B. Saunders.

10. 3
Rationale: Cytarabine (Cytosar) is an antimetabolite. Antimetabolites are classified as cell cycle phase-specific and affect the S phase (DNA synthesis and metabolism) of the reproductive cell cycle. Alkylating medications affect all phases of the cell reproductive cycle. Vinca alkaloids are cell cycle phase-specific and act on the M phase of the cell reproductive cycle.
Test-Taking Strategy: Use the process of elimination. Eliminate options 1 and 4 first because they are similar. From this point, knowledge regarding the action of an antimetabolite is required to answer the question. Review the specific action of an antimetabolite if you had difficulty with this question.
Level of Cognitive Ability: Comprehension
Client Needs: Physiological Integrity
Integrated Process: Nursing Process—implementation
Content Area: Pharmacology
Reference: Clark, J., Queener, S., & Karb, V. (2000). *Pharmacologic basis of nursing practice* (6th ed., p. 580). St. Louis: Mosby.

11. 3
Rationale: Because antineoplastic medications lower the resistance of the body, clients must be informed not to receive immunizations without a physician's approval. Clients also need to avoid contact with individuals who recently have received a live virus vaccine. Clients need to avoid aspirin and aspirin-containing products to minimize the risk of bleeding, and they need to avoid alcohol to minimize the risk of toxicity.
Test-Taking Strategy: Use the process of elimination. Remember that antineoplastic medications lower the resistance of the body. Review the client teaching points regarding these medications, if you had difficulty with this question.
Level of Cognitive Ability: Application
Client Needs: Health Promotion and Maintenance
Integrated Process: Teaching/Learning
Content Area: Pharmacology
Reference: Kee, J., & Hayes, E. (2003). *Pharmacology: A nursing process approach* (4th ed., p. 504). Philadelphia: W. B. Saunders.

12. 1
Rationale: High concentrations of methotrexate (Folex) causes harm and damage to normal cells. To save normal cells, leucovorin is given, which is known as leucovorin rescue. Leucovorin bypasses the metabolic block caused by methotrexate, thereby permitting normal cells to synthesize. One should note that leucovorin rescue is potentially hazardous. Failure to administer leucovorin in the right dose at the right time can be fatal.
Test-Taking Strategy: Use the process of elimination. Eliminate options 2 and 4 first because they are similar. Nucleic acids include RNA and DNA. Eliminate option 3 because increased fluids and diuretics normally are administered to promote medication excretion. This leaves option 1 as the correct answer. If you had difficulty with this question, review the purpose of leucovorin rescue.
Level of Cognitive Ability: Analysis
Client Needs: Physiological Integrity
Integrated Process: Nursing Process—analysis
Content Area: Pharmacology
Reference: Lehne, R. (2001). *Pharmacology for nursing care* (4th ed., p. 1121). Philadelphia: W. B. Saunders.

13. 2
Rationale: A side effect specific to vincristine (Oncovin) is peripheral neuropathy, which occurs in nearly every client. Peripheral neuropathy can be manifested as numbness and tingling in the fingers and toes. Depression of Achilles' tendon reflex may be the first clinical sign indicating peripheral neuropathy. Constipation rather than diarrhea is most likely to occur with this medication, although diarrhea may occur occasionally. Hair loss occurs with nearly all of the antineoplastic medications. Chest pain is unrelated to this medication.
Test-Taking Strategy: Use the process of elimination. Eliminate options 1 and 4 first because these side effects are associated with many of the antineoplastic agents. Note that the question asks for the side effect "specific" to this medication. Correlate peripheral neuropathy with vincristine (Oncovin).
Level of Cognitive Ability: Analysis
Client Needs: Physiological Integrity
Integrated Process: Nursing Process—assessment

Content Area: Pharmacology
References: Hodgson, B., & Kizior, R. (2004). *Saunders nursing drug handbook 2004* (p. 1053). Philadelphia: W. B. Saunders. Kee, J., & Hayes, E. (2003). *Pharmacology: A nursing process approach* (4th ed., p. 508). Philadelphia: W. B. Saunders.

14. **4**
Rationale: Asparaginase (Elspar) is contraindicated if hypersensitivity exists, in pancreatitis, or if the client has a history of pancreatitis. The medication impairs pancreatic function, and pancreatic function tests should be performed before therapy begins, and when a week or more has elapsed between the administration of the doses. The client needs to be monitored for signs of pancreatitis, which include nausea, vomiting, and abdominal pain.
Test-Taking Strategy: Use the process of elimination. Recalling that this medication affects pancreatic function will direct you to option 4. Review this medication if you had difficulty answering this question.
Level of Cognitive Ability: Analysis
Client Needs: Physiological Integrity
Integrated Process: Nursing Process—assessment
Content Area: Pharmacology
Reference: Lehne, R. (2001). *Pharmacology for nursing care* (4th ed., p. 1128). Philadelphia: W. B. Saunders.

15. **2**
Rationale: Tamoxifen (Nolvadex) is an antineoplastic medication that competes with estradiol for binding to estrogen in tissues containing high concentrations of receptors. Tamoxifen is used to treat metastatic breast carcinoma in women and men. Tamoxifen is also effective in delaying the recurrence of cancer following mastectomy. Tamoxifen reduces DNA synthesis and estrogen response.
Test-Taking Strategy: Use the process of elimination. Eliminate options 1 and 4 first because they are similar. Nucleic acids include DNA and RNA. From this point, select option 2, because it is unlikely that treatment of metastatic breast carcinoma would focus toward increasing estrogen concentration and estrogen response. If you had difficulty with this question, review the action of this medication.
Level of Cognitive Ability: Analysis
Client Needs: Physiological Integrity
Integrated Process: Nursing Process—implementation
Content Area: Pharmacology
Reference: Hodgson, B., & Kizior, R. (2004). *Saunders nursing drug handbook 2004* (p. 951). Philadelphia: W. B. Saunders.

16. **3**
Rationale: Tamoxifen (Nolvadex) may increase calcium, cholesterol, and triglyceride levels. Before the initiation of therapy, a complete blood count, platelet count, and serum calcium levels should be assessed. These blood levels along with the cholesterol and triglyceride levels should be monitored periodically during therapy. The nurse should assess for hypercalcemia while the client is taking this medication. Signs of hypercalcemia include increased urine volume, excessive thirst, nausea, vomiting, constipation, hypotonicity of muscles, deep bone, or flank pain.

Test-Taking Strategy: Use the process of elimination. Recalling that this medication causes hypercalcemia will direct you to option 3. Review this medication if you had difficulty answering this question.
Level of Cognitive Ability: Analysis
Client Needs: Physiological Integrity
Integrated Process: Nursing Process—assessment
Content Area: Pharmacology
Reference: Hodgson, B., & Kizior, R. (2004). *Saunders nursing drug handbook 2004* (p. 952). Philadelphia: W. B. Saunders.

17. **3**
Rationale: Megestrol acetate (Megace) suppresses the release of luteinizing hormone from the anterior pituitary by inhibiting pituitary function and regressing tumor size. Megestrol is used with caution if the client has a history of thrombophlebitis.
Test-Taking Strategy: Use the process of elimination. Recalling that megestrol acetate (Megace) is a hormonal antagonist enzyme and that a side effect is thrombolytic disorders will direct you to option 3. Review this medication if you had difficulty answering this question.
Level of Cognitive Ability: Analysis
Client Needs: Physiological Integrity
Integrated Process: Nursing Process—implementation
Content Area: Pharmacology
Reference: Hodgson, B., & Kizior, R. (2004). *Saunders nursing drug handbook 2004* (p. 630). Philadelphia: W. B. Saunders.

18. **4**
Rationale: Alopecia (hair loss) can occur following the administration of many antineoplastic medications. Alopecia is reversible, but new hair growth may have a different color and texture.
Test-Taking Strategy: Use the process of elimination. Eliminate option 2 because it is a nontherapeutic response. Next, eliminate options 1 and 3 because they are incorrect. Review content related to hair loss and antineoplastic medications, if you had difficulty with this question.
Level of Cognitive Ability: Application
Client Needs: Psychosocial Integrity
Integrated Process: Caring
Content Area: Pharmacology
Reference: Hodgson, B., & Kizior, R. (2004). *Saunders nursing drug handbook 2004* (p. 1053). Philadelphia: W. B. Saunders.

19. **1**
Rationale: Stomatitis (ulceration in the mouth) can result from the administration of antineoplastic medications. The client should be instructed to examine the mouth daily and to report any signs of ulceration. If stomatitis occurs, the client should be instructed to rinse the mouth with baking soda or saline. Food and fluid is important and should not be restricted. If chewing and swallowing are painful, the client may switch to a liquid diet that includes milk shakes and ice cream. Instruct the client to avoid spicy foods and foods with hard crusts or edges. The client should avoid toothbrushing and flossing when stomatitis is severe. Lemon and glycerin swabs may cause pain and further irritation.
Test-Taking Strategy: Knowing that stomatitis involves ulcerations in the mucous membrane of the mouth will assist you

in the process of eliminating the incorrect options. Eliminate option 2 first because foods and fluids would not be restricted in a client that received antineoplastic medication. Eliminate option 3 because lemon can be irritating to ulcerated lesions. Eliminate option 4 because a toothbrush and floss also will irritate ulcerations and may cause bleeding. If you had difficulty with this question, review the client teaching points related to stomatitis.
Level of Cognitive Ability: Application
Client Needs: Physiological Integrity
Integrated Process: Teaching/Learning
Content Area: Pharmacology
Reference: Kee, J., & Hayes, E. (2003). *Pharmacology: A nursing process approach* (4th ed., p. 500). Philadelphia: W. B. Saunders.

20. **2**
Rationale: Busulfan (Myleran) can cause an increase in the uric acid level. Hyperuricemia can produce uric acid nephropathy, renal stones, and acute renal failure. Options 1, 3, and 4 are not specifically related to this medication.
Test-Taking Strategy: Use the process of elimination. Recall that busulfan (Myleran) increases uric acid levels. If you had difficulty with this question, review the effects of busulfan (Myleran).

Level of Cognitive Ability: Analysis
Client Needs: Physiological Integrity
Integrated Process: Nursing Process—assessment
Content Area: Pharmacology
Reference: Hodgson, B., & Kizior, R. (2004). *Saunders nursing drug handbook 2004* (p. 132). Philadelphia: W. B. Saunders.

CRITICAL THINKING: FILL-IN-THE BLANK
Answer: Stop the infusion and notify the physician.
Rationale: Redness and swelling and a slowed infusion indicate signs of extravasation. If extravasation occurs during the intravenous administration of an antineoplastic medication, the infusion is stopped and the physician is notified.
Test-Taking Strategy: Focus on the assessment signs in the question. Attempt to visualize the situation to identify the initial nursing action. Review nursing actions if extravasation occurs if you had difficulty with this question.
Level of Cognitive Ability: Application
Client Needs: Physiological Integrity
Integrated Process: Nursing Process—implementation
Content Area: Pharmacology
Reference: Kee, J., & Hayes, E. (2003). *Pharmacology: A nursing process approach* (4th ed., pp. 500, 507). Philadelphia: W. B. Saunders.

REFERENCES

Clark, J., Queener, S., & Karb, V. (2000). *Pharmacologic basis of nursing practice* (6th ed.). St. Louis: Mosby.

Gutierrez, K., & Queener, S. (2003). *Pharmacology for nursing practice.* St. Louis: Mosby.

Hodgson, B., & Kizior, R. (2004). *Saunders nursing drug handbook 2004.* Philadelphia: W. B. Saunders.

Kee, J., & Hayes, E. (2003). *Pharmacology: A nursing process approach* (4th ed.). Philadelphia: W. B. Saunders.

Lehne, R. (2001). *Pharmacology for nursing care* (4th ed.). Philadelphia: W. B. Saunders.

McKenry, L., & Salerno, E. (2003). *Mosby's pharmacology in nursing* (21st ed.). St. Louis: Mosby.

The Adult Client with an Endocrine Disorder

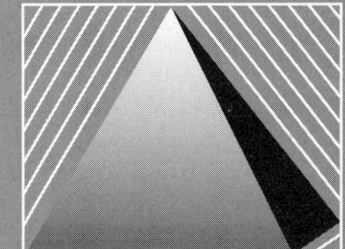

PYRAMID TERMS

addisonian crisis A life-threatening disorder caused by adrenal hormone insufficiency. Crisis is precipitated by infection, trauma, stress, or surgery. Death can occur from shock, vascular collapse, or hyperkalemia.

Addison's disease Hyposecretion of adrenal cortex hormones (glucocorticoids and mineralocorticoids) from the adrenal gland, resulting in deficiency of the steroid hormones. The condition is fatal if left untreated.

adrenalectomy The surgical removal of an adrenal gland. Lifelong replacement of glucocorticoids and mineralocorticoids is necessary with a bilateral adrenalectomy. Temporary replacement may be necessary for up to 2 years for a unilateral adrenalectomy.

Chvostek's sign A spasm of the facial muscles elicited by tapping the facial nerve just anterior to the ear. The sign is noted in hypocalcemia.

Cushing's syndrome A condition resulting from the hypersecretion of glucocorticoids from the adrenal cortex.

dawn phenomenon A nocturnal release of growth hormone, which may cause blood glucose elevations before breakfast. Treatment includes administering an evening dose of intermediate-acting insulin at 10 PM.

diabetes insipidus The hyposecretion of antidiuretic hormone from the posterior pituitary gland, which results in failure of tubular reabsorption of water in the kidneys.

diabetic ketoacidosis A life-threatening complication of diabetes mellitus that develops when a severe insulin deficiency occurs. Hyperglycemia progresses to ketoacidosis over a period of several hours to several days. Acidosis occurs in clients with type 1 diabetes mellitus, persons with undiagnosed diabetes, and persons who stop prescribed treatment for diabetes.

diabetes mellitus A chronic disorder of glucose intolerance and impaired carbohydrate, protein, and lipid metabolism caused by a deficiency of insulin or resistance to the action of insulin. A deficiency of effective insulin results in hyperglycemia.

hyperglycemia Elevated blood glucose level.

hyperglycemic hyperosmolar nonketotic syndrome Extreme hyperglycemia without acidosis. A complication of type 2 diabetes mellitus, which may result in dehydration or vascular collapse but does not include the acidosis component of diabetic ketoacidosis. Onset is usually slow, taking from hours to days.

hyperthyroidism A condition that occurs as a result of excessive thyroid hormone secretion.

hypoglycemia Low blood glucose level (less than 60 mg/dL) that results from too much insulin, not enough food, or excess activity.

hypophysectomy The removal of the pituitary gland.

insulin waning A progressive rise in the blood glucose level from bedtime to morning. Treatment includes increasing the evening (predinner or bedtime) dose of intermediate- or long-acting insulin, or instituting a dose of insulin before the evening meal if one is not prescribed already.

myxedema (hypothyroidism) A hypothyroid state resulting from a hyposecretion of thyroid hormone. The condition occurs in adulthood.

myxedema coma A rare but serious disorder that results from persistently low thyroid production. Coma can be precipitated by acute illness, rapid withdrawal of thyroid medication, anesthesia and surgery, hypothermia, and the use of sedatives and narcotics.

Somogyi phenomenon A rebound phenomenon that occurs in clients with type 1 diabetes mellitus. Normal or elevated blood glucose levels are present at bedtime; hypoglycemia occurs at about 2 to 3 AM. Counterregulatory hormones, produced to prevent further hypoglycemia, result in hyperglycemia (evident in the prebreakfast blood glucose level). Treatment includes decreasing the evening (predinner or bedtime) dose of intermediate-acting insulin or increasing the bedtime snack.

thyroidectomy Surgical removal of the thyroid gland to treat persistent hyperthyroidism or thyroid tumors.

thyroid storm An acute, potentially fatal exacerbation of hyperthyroidism that may result from manipulation of the thyroid gland during surgery, severe infection, or stress.

Trousseau's sign A sign of hypocalcemia. Carpal spasm can be elicited by compressing the brachial artery with a blood pressure cuff for 3 minutes.

▲ PYRAMID TO SUCCESS

The endocrine system is made up of organs or glands that secrete hormones and release them directly into the circulation. The endocrine system can be understood easily if you remember that basically one of two situations can occur: hypersecretion or hyposecretion of hormones from the organ or gland. When an excess of the hormone occurs, treatment is aimed at blocking the hormone release through medication or surgery. When a deficit of the hormone exists, treatment is aimed at replacement therapy. Pyramid Points focus on diabetes mellitus, including the prevention and treatment of complications, insulin therapy, hypoglycemic and hyperglycemic reactions, and diabetic ketoacidosis; Addison's disease and addisonian crisis; Cushing's syndrome; thyroid disorders and thyroid storm; and care of the client after thyroidectomy or adrenalectomy. The Integrated Processes addressed in this unit include Nursing Process, Caring, Communication and Documentation, and Teaching/Learning.

▲ CLIENT NEEDS

Safe, Effective Care Environment

Accident prevention
Advocacy
Confidentiality
Consultation
Establishing priorities
Handling of hazardous and infectious materials
Informed consent
Medical and surgical asepsis

Health Promotion and Maintenance

Disease prevention
Expected body image changes
Health screening
Human sexuality
Lifestyle choices
Principles of teaching/learning
Self-care
Techniques of physical assessment

Psychosocial Integrity

Coping mechanisms
Grief and loss
Sensory/perceptual alterations
Situational role changes
Support systems
Unexpected body image changes

Physiological Integrity

Alterations in body systems
Diagnostic tests
Elimination
Expected outcomes/effects of medication administration
Fluid and electrolyte imbalances
Identification of potential complications
Laboratory values
Nonpharmacological comfort interventions
Nutrition and oral hydration
Potential for complications of diagnostic tests/treatments/
  procedures
Unexpected response to therapies

REFERENCES

Chernecky, C., & Berger, B. (2004). *Laboratory tests & diagnostic procedures* (4th ed.). Philadelphia: W. B. Saunders.

Ignatavicius, D., & Workman, M. (2002). *Medical surgical nursing: Critical thinking for collaborative care* (4th ed.). Philadelphia: W. B. Saunders.

Lewis, S., Heitkemper, M., & Dirksen, S. (2004). *Medical-surgical nursing: Assessment and management of clinical problems* (6th ed.). St. Louis: Mosby.

National Council of State Boards of Nursing (Eds.) (2003). *Test Plan for the National Council Licensure Examination for Registered Nurses* (effective date: April 2004). Chicago: Author.

Perry, A., & Potter, P. (2002). *Clinical nursing skills and techniques* (5th ed.). St. Louis: Mosby.

Phipps, W., Monahan, F., Sands, J., Marek, J., & Neighbors, M. (2003). *Medical-surgical nursing: Health and illness perspectives* (7th ed.). St. Louis: Mosby.

Potter, P., & Perry, A. (2001). *Fundamentals of nursing* (5th ed.). St. Louis: Mosby.

Varcarolis, E. M. (2002). *Foundations of psychiatric mental health nursing* (4th ed.). Philadelphia: W. B. Saunders.

53

Endocrine System

I. ANATOMY AND PHYSIOLOGY OF ENDOCRINE GLANDS (BOX 53-1)

A. Functions (Box 53-2)
1. Maintenance and regulation of vital functions
2. Response to stress and injury
3. Growth and development
4. Energy metabolism
5. Reproduction
6. Fluid, electrolyte, and acid-base balance

B. Pituitary gland (Box 53-3)
1. The pituitary gland is the master gland.
2. The pituitary gland is located at the base of the brain.
3. The pituitary gland is influenced by the hypothalamus.
4. The pituitary gland directly affects the function of the other endocrine glands.
5. The pituitary gland promotes growth of body tissue.
6. The pituitary gland influences water absorption by the kidney.
7. The pituitary gland controls sexual development and function.

C. Adrenal gland
1. One adrenal gland is on top of each kidney.
2. The adrenal gland regulates sodium and electrolyte balance.
3. The adrenal gland affects carbohydrate, fat, and protein metabolism.
4. The adrenal gland influences the development of sexual characteristics.
5. The adrenal gland sustains the "flight or fight" response.
6. Adrenal cortex
   a. The cortex is the outer shell of the adrenal gland.

BOX 53-1

Endocrine Glands

Adrenal
Ovaries
Pancreas
Parathyroid
Pituitary
Testes
Thyroid

BOX 53-2

Risk Factors for Endocrine Disorders

Heredity
Congenital
Trauma
Environmental
Consequence of other disorders

BOX 53-3

Pituitary Gland

ANTERIOR LOBE PRODUCTION
Adrenocorticotropic hormone
Follicle-stimulating hormone
Growth hormone
Luteinizing hormone
Melanocyte-stimulating hormone
Prolactin
Somatotropic growth-stimulating hormone
Thyroid-stimulating hormone

POSTERIOR LOBE PRODUCTION
Oxytocin
Vasopressin, antidiuretic hormone

BOX 53-4

Adrenal Cortex

GLUCOCORTICOIDS: CORTISOL, CORTISONE, CORTICOSTERONE
Responsible for glucose metabolism, protein metabolism, fluid and electrolyte balance, suppression of the inflammatory response to injury, the protective immune response to invasion by infectious agents, and resistance to stress

MINERALOCORTICOIDS: ALDOSTERONE
Regulation of electrolyte balance by promoting sodium retention and potassium excretion

---

  b. The cortex synthesizes glucocorticoids and mineralocorticoids and secretes small amounts of sex hormones (androgens, estrogens) (Box 53-4).
 7. Adrenal medulla
  a. The medulla is the inner core of the adrenal gland.
  b. The medulla works as part of the sympathetic nervous system.
  c. The medulla produces epinephrine and norepinephrine.
D. Thyroid gland
 1. The thyroid gland is located in the anterior part of the neck.
 2. The thyroid gland controls the rate of body metabolism and growth.
 3. The thyroid gland produces thyroxine (T_4), triiodothyronine (T_3), and thyrocalcitonin.
E. Parathyroid glands
 1. The parathyroid glands are located on the thyroid gland.
 2. The parathyroid glands control calcium and phosphorus metabolism.
 3. The parathyroid glands produce parathyroid hormone.
F. Pancreas
 1. The pancreas is located posterior to the stomach.
 2. The pancreas influences carbohydrate metabolism.
 3. The pancreas indirectly influences fat and protein metabolism.
 4. The pancreas produces insulin and glucagon.
G. Ovaries and testes
 1. Ovaries
  a. The ovaries are located in the pelvic cavity.
  b. The ovaries produce estrogen and progesterone.
 2. Testes
  a. The testes are located in the scrotum.
  b. The testes control the development of the secondary sex characteristics.
  c. The testes produce testosterone.

II. DIAGNOSTIC TESTS
A. Stimulation/suppression tests
 1. Stimulation testing
  a. In the client with suspected underactivity of an endocrine gland, a stimulus may be provided to determine whether the gland is capable of normal hormone production.
  b. Measured amounts of selected hormones or substances are administered to stimulate the target gland to produce its hormone.
  c. Hormone levels produced by the target gland are measured.
  d. Failure of the hormone level to increase with stimulation indicates hypofunction.
 2. Suppression tests
  a. Suppression tests are used when hormone levels are high or in the upper range of normal.
  b. Failure of hormone production to be suppressed during standardized testing indicates hyperfunction.
B. Radioactive iodine uptake
 1. This thyroid function test measures the absorption of the iodine isotope to determine how the thyroid gland is functioning.
 2. A small dose of radioactive iodine is given by mouth or intravenously; the amount of radioactivity is measured in 2 to 4 hours and again at 24 hours.
 3. Normal values are 3% to 10% at 2 to 4 hours, and 5% to 30% in 24 hours.
 4. Elevated values indicate **hyperthyroidism**, decreased iodine intake, or increased iodine excretion.
 5. Decreased values indicate a low T_4, the use of antithyroid medications, thyroiditis, **myxedema**, or **hypothyroidism**.
 6. The test is contraindicated in pregnancy.
C. T_3 and T_4 resin uptake test
 1. Blood tests are used to diagnose thyroid disorders.
 2. T_3 and T_4 regulate thyroid-stimulating hormone.
 3. Normal values (normal findings vary between laboratory settings)
  a. T_3: 80 to 230 ng/dL
  b. T_4: 5 to 12 mcg/dL
  c. Thyroxine, free (FT_4): 0.8 to 2.4 ng/dL
 4. The T_3 is elevated in **hyperthyroidism**, decreases with the aging process, and may be decreased in **hypothyroidism**.
 5. The T_4 is elevated in **hyperthyroidism** and decreased in **hypothyroidism**.
D. Thyroid-stimulating hormone
 1. Blood test is used to differentiate the diagnosis of primary **hypothyroidism**.
 2. Normal value is 0.2 to 5.4 microunits/mL (normal findings vary between laboratory settings).
 3. Elevated values indicate primary **hypothyroidism**.
 4. Decreased values indicate **hyperthyroidism** or secondary **hypothyroidism**.
E. Thyroid scan
 1. A thyroid scan is performed to identify nodules or growths in the thyroid gland.

2. A radioisotope of iodine or technetium is administered before the scanning of the thyroid gland.

3. Reassure the client that the level of radioactive medication is not dangerous to self or others.

4. Determine whether the client has received radiographic contrast agents within the past 3 months because these may invalidate the scan.

5. Check with the physician regarding discontinuing medications containing iodine for 14 days before the test and the need to discontinue thyroid medication before the test.

6. Instruct the client to maintain an NPO status after midnight on the day before the test; if iodine is used, the client will fast for an additional 45 minutes after ingestion of the oral isotope and the scan will be performed in 24 hours.

7. If technetium is used, it is administered by the intravenous (IV) route 30 minutes before the scan.

F. Needle aspiration of thyroid tissue

1. Aspiration of thyroid tissue is done for cytological examination.

2. No client preparation is necessary.

3. Light pressure is applied to the aspiration site after the procedure.

G. Glucose tolerance test

1. The glucose tolerance test aids in the diagnosis of **diabetes mellitus.**

2. If the glucose levels peak at higher than normal at 1 and 2 hours after injection or ingestion of glucose and are slower than normal to return to fasting levels, then **diabetes mellitus** is confirmed.

3. Client preparation (Box 53-5)

H. Glycosylated hemoglobin

1. Description

a. Glycosylated hemoglobin is blood glucose bound to hemoglobin.

b. Glycosylated hemoglobin A (HbA_{1c}) is a reflection of how well blood glucose levels have been controlled for up to the prior 3 to 4 months.

c. **Hyperglycemia** in a client with **diabetes mellitus** is usually a cause of an increase in HbA_{1c}.

BOX 53-5

Client Preparation: Glucose Tolerance Test

Eat a diet with adequate carbohydrates for 3 days before the test.

Avoid alcohol, coffee, and smoking for 36 hours before testing.

Fast for 10 to 16 hours before the test.

Avoid strenuous exercise for 8 hours before and after the test.

Withhold morning insulin or oral hypoglycemic medication (client with diabetes mellitus).

The test will take 3 to 5 hours, requires intravenous or oral administration of glucose, and multiple blood samples.

---

2. Values

a. Values are expressed as a percentage of total hemoglobin.

b. Goal for client with diabetes mellitus is 7.5% or less.

c. For clients without diabetes, normal range is 4% to 6%.

3. Nursing consideration: Fasting is not required.

III. DISORDERS OF PITUITARY GLAND (BOX 53-6)

A. Hypopituitarism

1. Description: Hypopituitarism is the hyposecretion of one or more of the pituitary hormones caused by tumors, trauma, encephalitis, autoimmunity, or stroke.

2. Hormones most often affected are growth hormone and the gonadotropins (luteinizing hormone and follicle-stimulating hormone), but thyroid-stimulating hormone, adrenocorticotropic hormone (ACTH), or antidiuretic hormone (ADH) may be involved.

3. Assessment

a. Mild to moderate obesity (growth hormone, thyroid-stimulating hormone)

b. Reduced cardiac output (growth hormone, ADH)

c. Infertility, sexual dysfunction (gonadotropins, ACTH)

d. Fatigue, low blood pressure

e. Tumors of the pituitary also may cause headaches and visual defects (pituitary is located near the optic nerve).

4. Interventions

a. Provide emotional support to client and family.

b. Encourage client and family to express feelings related to altered body image or sexual dysfunction.

c. Client may need hormone replacement for specific deficient hormones.

B. Acromegaly

1. Description: Acromegaly is the hypersecretion of growth hormone by the anterior pituitary gland in an adult and is caused primarily by pituitary tumors.

2. Assessment

a. Large hands and feet

BOX 53-6

Disorders of the Pituitary Gland

ANTERIOR PITUITARY
Hyperpituitarism
Hypopituitarism

POSTERIOR PITUITARY
Diabetes insipidus
Syndrome of inappropriate antidiuretic hormone

b. Thickening and protrusion of the jaw

c. Arthritic changes

d. Visual disturbances

e. Diaphoresis

f. Oily, rough skin

g. Organomegaly

h. Hypertension

i. Dysphagia

j. Deepening of the voice

3. Interventions

a. Provide emotional support to client and family, and encourage client and family to express feelings related to altered body image.

b. Provide frequent skin care.

c. Provide pharmacological and nonpharmacological interventions for joint pain.

d. Prepare the client for radiation of the pituitary gland if prescribed.

e. Prepare the client for **hypophysectomy** if planned.

C. **Hypophysectomy** (pituitary adenectomy, transsphenoidal pituitary surgery)

1. Description

a. **Hypophysectomy** is the removal of the pituitary tumor via craniotomy or via transsphenoidal (endoscopic transnasal) approach (the latter approach is preferred because it is associated with few complications).

b. Complications for craniotomy include increased intracranial pressure, bleeding, meningitis, and hypopituitarism.

c. Complications for the transsphenoidal surgery include cerebrospinal fluid leak, infection, and hypopituitarism.

2. Postoperative interventions

a. Initiate postoperative care similar to craniotomy care.

b. Monitor vital signs, neurological status, and level of consciousness.

c. Elevate the head of the bed.

d. Monitor for increased intracranial pressure.

e. Monitor for bleeding.

f. Monitor for any postnasal drip or nasal drainage, which might indicate leakage of cerebrospinal fluid in transsphenoidal approach (check the nasal drainage for glucose).

g. Instruct the client to avoid sneezing, coughing, and blowing the nose.

h. Monitor electrolyte values for temporary **diabetes insipidus** resulting from ADH disturbances.

i. Monitor intake and output, and avoid water intoxication.

j. Administer glucocorticoids and other hormone replacements as prescribed.

k. Administer antibiotics, analgesics, and antipyretics as prescribed.

l. Instruct the client in the administration of prescribed medications, which may include vasopressin (synthetic ADH), levothyroxine, gonadotropic hormones, growth hormone (somatotropin), and glucocorticoids if the entire gland was removed.

D. **Diabetes insipidus**

1. Description

a. **Diabetes insipidus** is hyposecretion of ADH caused by strokes, trauma, or idiopathic causes.

b. Kidney tubules fail to reabsorb water.

2. Assessment

a. Polyuria of 4 to 24 L per day

b. Polydipsia

c. Dehydration

d. Decreased skin turgor, dry mucous membranes

e. Inability to concentrate urine

f. A low urinary specific gravity: 1.006 or less

g. Fatigue

h. Muscle pain and weakness

i. Headache

j. Postural hypotension that may progress to vascular collapse without rehydration

k. Tachycardia

3. Interventions

a. Monitor vital signs and neurological and cardiovascular status.

b. Provide a safe environment, particularly for the client with a change in level of consciousness or mental status.

c. Monitor electrolyte values and for signs of dehydration.

d. Monitor intake and output, weight, and specific gravity of urine.

e. Maintain the intake of adequate fluids, and monitor for signs of dehydration.

f. Instruct the client to avoid foods or liquids that produce diuresis.

g. Administer chlorpropamide (Diabinese) if prescribed for mild diabetes insipidus.

h. Administer vasopressin tannate (Pitressin) or desmopressin acetate (DDAVP, Stimate) as prescribed; these are used when the ADH deficiency is severe or chronic.

i. Instruct the client in the administration of medications as prescribed (DDAVP may be administered by injection, intranasally, or orally).

j. Instruct the client to wear a Medic-Alert bracelet.

E. Syndrome of inappropriate antidiuretic hormone

1. Description

a. Excess ADH is released, but not in response to a bodily need for it.

b. Causes include trauma, stroke, malignancies (often in the lungs or pancreas), medications, and stress.

c. The syndrome results in hyponatremia.

2. Assessment
   a. Signs of fluid volume overload
   b. Changes in level of consciousness and mental status changes
   c. Weight gain
   d. Hypertension
   e. Tachycardia
   f. Anorexia, nausea, and vomiting
   g. Hyponatremia
3. Interventions
   a. Monitor vital signs and cardiac and neurological status.
   b. Provide a safe environment, particularly for the client with changes in level of consciousness or mental status.
   c. Monitor intake and output and obtain weight daily.
   d. Monitor fluid and electrolyte balance.
   e. Restrict fluid intake as prescribed.
   f. Administer diuretics and IV fluids as prescribed; monitor IV fluids carefully because of the risk for water intoxication.
   g. Administer demeclocycline (Declomycin) as prescribed (inhibits ADH-induced water reabsorption and produces water diuresis).

IV. DISORDERS OF ADRENAL GLANDS (BOX 53-7)

A. **Addison's disease**
   1. Description
      a. **Addison's disease** is hyposecretion of adrenal cortex hormones (glucocorticoids and mineralocorticoids).
      b. The condition is fatal if left untreated.
   2. Assessment
      a. Lethargy, fatigue, and muscle weakness
      b. Gastrointestinal disturbances
      c. Weight loss
      d. Menstrual changes in women; impotence in men
      e. **Hypoglycemia**
      f. Hyperkalemia
      g. Postural hypotension
      h. Dehydration
      i. Emotional disturbances

3. Interventions
   a. Monitor vital signs, particularly blood pressure, weight, and intake and output.
   b. Monitor blood glucose and potassium levels.
   c. Administer glucocorticoid or mineralocorticoid medications as prescribed.
   d. Observe for **addisonian crisis** caused by stress, infection, trauma, or surgery.
4. Client education
   a. Avoid individuals with an infection.
   b. Diet: high protein and carbohydrate; normal sodium intake.
   c. Avoid strenuous exercise and stressful situations.
   d. Need for lifelong glucocorticoid therapy.
   e. Avoid over-the-counter medications.
   f. Wear a Medic-Alert bracelet.

B. **Addisonian crisis**
   1. Description (Box 53-8)
   2. Assessment
      a. Severe headache
      b. Severe abdominal, leg, and lower back pain
      c. Generalized weakness
      d. Irritability and confusion
      e. Severe hypotension
      f. Shock
   3. Interventions
      a. Prepare to administer glucocorticoids intravenously as prescribed; hydrocortisone sodium succinate (Solu-Cortef) usually is prescribed initially.
      b. Following resolution of the crisis, administer glucocorticoid and mineralocorticoid orally as prescribed.
      c. Monitor vital signs, particularly blood pressure.
      d. Monitor neurological status, noting irritability and confusion.
      e. Monitor intake and output.
      f. Monitor laboratory values, particularly the sodium, potassium, and blood glucose.
      g. Administer IV fluids as prescribed to restore electrolyte balance.
      h. Protect the client from infection.
      i. Maintain bed rest and provide a quiet environment.

C. **Cushing's syndrome**
   1. Description

BOX 53-7

Disorders of the Adrenal Glands

ADRENAL CORTEX
Addison's disease
Aldosteronism (Conn's syndrome)
Cushing's syndrome

ADRENAL MEDULLA
Pheochromocytoma

BOX 53-8

Addisonian Crisis

Addisonian crisis is a life-threatening disorder caused by acute adrenal insufficiency.
Crisis is precipitated by stress, infection, trauma, or surgery.
Addisonian crisis can cause hyponatremia, hyperkalemia, hypoglycemia, and shock.

a. **Cushing's syndrome** is a condition resulting from the hypersecretion of glucocorticoids from the adrenal cortex.
b. **Cushing's syndrome** can be caused by an increased pituitary secretion of ACTH, a pituitary adenoma, or an adrenal adenoma.

2. Assessment
a. Truncal obesity with thin extremities
b. Moonface
c. Buffalo hump
d. Supraclavicular fat pads
e. Generalized muscle wasting and weakness
f. Fragile skin that easily bruises
g. Reddish-purple striae on the abdomen and upper thighs
h. Hirsutism (masculine characteristics in female)
i. Hypertension
j. Elevated blood glucose, sodium, and white blood cell counts
k. Decreased calcium and potassium levels

3. Interventions
a. Monitor vital signs, particularly blood pressure.
b. Monitor intake and output and weight
c. Monitory laboratory values, particularly the blood glucose, white blood cell count, and sodium, potassium, and calcium levels.
d. Provide good skin care.
e. Allow the client to discuss feelings related to body appearance.
f. Administer chemotherapeutic agents as prescribed for inoperable adrenal tumors.
g. Prepare the client for radiation as prescribed if the condition results from a pituitary adenoma.
h. Prepare the client for removal of pituitary tumor (**hypophysectomy**, transsphenoidal adenectomy) if the condition results from increased pituitary secretion of ACTH.
i. Prepare the client for **adrenalectomy** if the condition results from an adrenal adenoma; glucocorticoid replacement may be required following **adrenalectomy**.

D. Hyperaldosteronism (Conn's syndrome)
1. Description
a. A hypersecretion of aldosterone from the adrenal cortex of the adrenal gland
b. Most commonly caused by an adenoma
2. Assessment
a. Symptoms related to hypokalemia and hypertension
b. Headache, fatigue, muscle weakness, nocturia
c. Polydipsia and polyuria
d. Paresthesias
e. Visual changes
f. Hypernatremia
g. Low urine specific gravity and increased urinary aldosterone

3. Interventions
a. Monitor vital signs, particularly blood pressure.
b. Monitor for signs of hypokalemia.
c. Monitor intake and output and urine for specific gravity.
d. Administer spironolactone (Aldactone) as prescribed to promote fluid balance; medication is a potassium-sparing diuretic and aldosterone antagonist.
e. Administer potassium supplements as prescribed.
f. Administer antihypertensives as prescribed.
g. Prepare the client for **adrenalectomy**.
h. Maintain sodium restriction, if prescribed, preoperatively.
i. Administer glucocorticoids preoperatively, as prescribed, to prevent adrenal hypofunction.
j. Instruct the client regarding the need for glucocorticoid therapy following **adrenalectomy**.
k. Instruct the client about the need to wear a Medic-Alert bracelet.

E. Pheochromocytoma
1. Description
a. Pheochromocytoma is a catecholamine-producing tumor usually found in the adrenal medulla, but extraadrenal locations include the chest, bladder, abdomen, and brain.
b. Excessive amounts of epinephrine and norepinephrine are secreted.
c. Pheochromocytoma is typically a benign tumor but can be malignant.
d. Surgical excision of adrenal gland is the primary treatment.
e. Symptomatic treatment is initiated if surgical excision is not possible.
f. The complications associated with pheochromocytoma include hypertensive retinopathy and nephropathy, cardiac enlargement, congestive heart failure, increased platelet aggregation, and cerebrovascular accident.
g. Death can occur from shock, cerebrovascular accident, renal failure, dysrhythmias, or dissecting aortic aneurysm.

2. Assessment
a. Paroxysmal or sustained hypertension
b. Severe headaches
c. Palpitations
d. Profuse diaphoresis
e. Flushing
f. Pain in the chest or abdomen with nausea and vomiting
g. Heat intolerance
h. Weight loss
i. Tremors
j. **Hyperglycemia** and glycosuria

3. Interventions
a. Monitor vital signs, particularly the blood pressure and heart rate.

b. Monitor for hypertensive crisis; monitor for complications that can occur with hypertensive crisis such as cerebrovascular accident, cardiac dysrhythmias, myocardial infarction.

c. Be alert to stimuli that can precipitate a hypertensive crisis, such as increased abdominal pressure, urination, and vigorous abdominal palpation (avoid these stimuli).

d. Instruct the client not to smoke, drink caffeine-containing beverages, or change position suddenly.

e. Prepare to administer an α-adrenergic blocking agent, phenoxybenzamine (Dibenzyline) as prescribed to control blood pressure.

f. Monitor blood glucose and urine for ketones.

g. Promote rest and a nonstressful environment.

h. Provide a diet high in calories, vitamins, and minerals.

i. Prepare the client for **adrenalectomy.**

F. **Adrenalectomy**

1. Description (Box 53-9)

2. Preoperative interventions

   a. Monitor electrolytes and correct electrolyte imbalances.

   b. Assess for dysrhythmias.

   c. Monitor for **hyperglycemia.**

   d. Protect the client from infections.

   e. Administer glucocorticoids as prescribed.

3. Postoperative interventions

   a. Monitor vital signs.

   b. Monitor intake and output, and if the urinary output is less that 30 mL per hour, notify the physician, because this may indicate renal failure and impending shock.

   c. Monitor weight daily.

   d. Monitor electrolytes.

   e. Monitor for signs of shock and hemorrhage, particularly during first 24 to 48 hours.

   f. Assess the dressing for drainage.

   g. Monitor for paralytic ileus, as manifested by abdominal distention and pain, nausea, vomiting, and diminished or absent bowel sounds (paralytic ileus can develop from internal bleeding).

   h. Administer IV fluids as prescribed to maintain blood volume.

   i. Administer glucocorticoids as prescribed.

   j. Administer pain medication as prescribed.

   k. Instruct the client in the importance of glucocorticoid therapy following surgery.

   l. Instruct the client regarding the need to wear a Medic-Alert bracelet.

V. DISORDERS OF THE THYROID GLAND (BOX 53-10)

A. **Hypothyroidism** (myxedema)

1. Description

   a. **Hypothyroidism** is a hypothyroid state resulting from a hyposecretion of the thyroid hormones T_4 and T_3.

   b. **Hypothyroidism** is characterized by a decreased rate of body metabolism.

2. Assessment

   a. Lethargy and fatigue

   b. Weakness, muscle aches, paresthesias

   c. Intolerance to cold

   d. Weight gain

   e. Dry skin and hair

   f. Loss of body hair

   g. Bradycardia

   h. Constipation

   i. Generalized puffiness and edema around the eyes and face

   j. Forgetfulness and loss of memory

   k. Menstrual disturbances

   l. Cardiac enlargement, tendency to develop congestive heart failure

3. Interventions

   a. Monitor vital signs, including heart rate and rhythm.

   b. Administer thyroid replacement; levothyroxine sodium (Synthroid) is most commonly prescribed.

   c. Instruct the client about thyroid replacement therapy.

   d. Instruct the client in low-calorie, low-cholesterol, low-saturated-fat diet.

   e. Assess the client for constipation; provide roughage and fluids to prevent constipation.

   f. Provide a warm environment for the client.

   g. Avoid sedatives and narcotics because of increased sensitivity to these medications.

BOX 53-9

Adrenalectomy

Adrenalectomy is the surgical removal of an adrenal gland.

Lifelong glucocorticoid replacement is necessary with a bilateral adrenalectomy.

Temporary glucocorticoid replacement, up to 2 years, is necessary for a unilateral adrenalectomy.

Catecholamine levels drop as a result of surgery, which can result in cardiovascular collapse, hypotension, and shock, and the client needs to be monitored closely.

Hemorrhage also can occur because of the high vascularity of the adrenal glands.

BOX 53-10

Disorders of the Thyroid Gland

Hyperthyroidism
Hypothyroidism

h. Monitor for overdose of thyroid medications, characterized by tachycardia, restlessness, nervousness, and insomnia.

i. Instruct the client to report episodes of chest pain immediately.

▲ B. **Myxedema coma**
1. Description (Box 53-11)
2. Assessment
   a. Hypotension
   b. Bradycardia
   c. Hypothermia
   d. Hyponatremia
   e. **Hypoglycemia**
   f. Respiratory failure
   g. Coma
3. Interventions
   a. Maintain a patent airway.
   b. Administer IV fluids as prescribed.
   c. Administer levothyroxine sodium (Synthroid) intravenously as prescribed.
   d. Administer glucose intravenously as prescribed.
   e. Assess client's temperature frequently.
   f. Monitor blood pressure.
   g. Keep client warm.
   h. Monitor for changes in mental status.
   i. Monitor electrolytes and glucose level.

▲ C. **Hyperthyroidism**
1. Description
   a. **Hyperthyroidism** is a hyperthyroid state resulting from hypersecretion of thyroid hormones (T_3 and T_4).
   b. **Hyperthyroidism** is characterized by an increased rate of body metabolism.
   c. A common cause is Graves' disease, also known as toxic diffuse goiter.
   d. Clinical manifestations are referred to as thyrotoxicosis.
2. Assessment for **hyperthyroidism** caused by Graves' disease
   a. Enlarged thyroid gland (goiter)
   b. Palpitations, cardiac dysrhythmias, such as tachycardia or atrial fibrillation
   c. Protruding eyeballs (exophthalmos) possibly present
   d. Hypertension
   e. Heat intolerance
   f. Diaphoresis

g. Weight loss
h. Diarrhea
i. Smooth, soft skin and hair
j. Nervousness and fine tremors of hands
k. Personality changes
l. Irritability and agitation
m. Mood swings
3. Interventions
   a. Provide adequate rest.
   b. Administer sedatives as prescribed.
   c. Provide a cool and quiet environment.
   d. Obtain weight daily.
   e. Provide a high-calorie diet.
   f. Avoid the administration of stimulants.
   g. Administer antithyroid medications (propylthiouracil [PTU]) that block thyroid synthesis, as prescribed.
   h. Administer iodine preparations that inhibit the release of thyroid hormone as prescribed.
   i. Administer propranolol (Inderal) for tachycardia as prescribed.
   j. Prepare the client for radioactive iodine therapy, as prescribed, to destroy thyroid cells.
   k. Prepare the client for **thyroidectomy** if prescribed.

D. **Thyroid storm**
1. Description (Box 53-12)
2. Assessment
   a. Elevated temperature (fever)
   b. Tachycardia
   c. Systolic hypertension
   d. Nausea, vomiting, and diarrhea
   e. Agitation, tremors, anxiety
   f. Irritability, agitation, restlessness, confusion, and seizures as the condition progresses
   g. Delirium and coma
3. Interventions
   a. Maintain a patent airway and adequate ventilation.
   b. Administer antithyroid medications, sodium iodide solution, propranolol (Inderal), and glucocorticoids as prescribed.
   c. Monitor vital signs.

BOX 53-11

Myxedema Coma

Myxedema coma is a rare but serious disorder that results from persistently low thyroid production.
Coma can be precipitated by acute illness, rapid withdrawal of thyroid medication, anesthesia and surgery, hypothermia, or the use of sedatives and narcotics.

BOX 53-12

Thyroid Storm

Thyroid storm is an acute and life-threatening condition that occurs in a client with uncontrollable hyperthyroidism.
Thyroid storm can occur from manipulation of the thyroid gland during surgery and the release of thyroid hormone into the bloodstream; it also can occur from severe infection and stress.
Antithyroid medications, β-blockers, glucocorticoids, and iodides are administered to the client before thyroid surgery to prevent its occurrence.

d. Monitor continually for cardiac dysrhythmias.

e. Administer nonsalicylate antipyretics as prescribed (salicylates increase free thyroid hormone levels).

f. Use a cooling blanket to decrease temperature as prescribed.

E. **Thyroidectomy**

1. Description

   a. Removal of the thyroid gland

   b. Performed when persistent hyperthryoidism exists

2. Preoperative interventions

   a. Obtain vital signs and weight.

   b. Assess electrolyte levels.

   c. Assess for **hyperglycemia** and glycosuria.

   d. Instruct the client in how to perform coughing and deep-breathing exercises and how to support the neck in the postoperative period when coughing and moving.

   e. Administer antithyroid medications, sodium iodide solution, propranolol (Inderal), and glucocorticoids as prescribed to prevent the occurrence of **thyroid storm.**

3. Postoperative interventions

   a. Monitor for respiratory distress.

   b. Have a tracheotomy set, oxygen, and suction at the bedside.

   c. Maintain client in semi-Fowler position.

   d. Monitor surgical site for edema and for signs of bleeding; check dressing anteriorly and at the back of the neck.

   e. Limit client talking, and assess level of hoarseness.

   f. Monitor for laryngeal nerve damage, as evidenced by respiratory obstruction, dysphonia, high-pitched voice, stridor, dysphagia, and restlessness.

   g. Monitor for signs of hypocalcemia and tetany, which can be due to trauma to the parathyroid gland (Box 53-13).

   h. Prepare to administer calcium gluconate as prescribed for tetany.

   i. Monitor for **thyroid storm.**

BOX 53-13

Signs of Tetany

Cardiac dysrhythmias
Carpopedal spasm
Dysphagia
Muscle and abdominal cramps
Numbness and tingling of the face and extremities
Positive Chvostek's sign
Positive Trousseau's sign
Seizures
Visual disturbances (photophobia)
Wheezing and dyspnea (bronchospasm, laryngospasm)

BOX 53-14

Disorders of the Parathyroid Gland

Hyperparathyroidism
Hypoparathyroidism

VI. DISORDERS OF THE PARATHYROID GLAND (BOX 53-14)

A. Hypoparathyroidism

1. Description

   a. Hypoparathyroidism is a condition caused by hyposecretion of parathyroid hormone by the parathyroid gland.

   b. Hypoparathyroidism can occur following **thyroidectomy** because of removal of parathyroid tissue.

2. Assessment

   a. Hypocalcemia and hyperphosphatemia

   b. Numbness and tingling in the face

   c. Muscle cramps and cramps in the abdomen or in the extremities

   d. Positive **Trousseau's sign** or **Chvostek's sign**

   e. Signs of overt tetany, such as bronchospasm, laryngospasm, carpopedal spasm, dysphagia, photophobia, cardiac dysrhythmias, seizures

   f. Hypotension

   g. Anxiety, irritability, depression

3. Interventions

   a. Monitor vital signs.

   b. Monitor for signs of hypocalcemia and tetany.

   c. Initiate seizure precautions.

   d. Place a tracheotomy set, oxygen, and suctioning at the bedside.

   e. Prepare to administer calcium gluconate intravenously for hypocalcemia.

   f. Provide a high-calcium, low-phosphorus diet.

   g. Instruct the client in the administration of calcium supplements as prescribed.

   h. Instruct the client in the administration of vitamin D supplements as prescribed; vitamin D enhances the absorption of calcium from the gastrointestinal tract.

   i. Instruct the client in the administration of phosphate binders as prescribed to promote the excretion of phosphate through the gastrointestinal tract.

   j. Instruct the client to wear a Medic-Alert bracelet.

B. Hyperparathyroidism

1. Description: A condition caused by hypersecretion of parathyroid hormone by the parathyroid gland

2. Assessment

   a. Hypercalcemia and hypophosphatemia

   b. Fatigue and muscle weakness

   c. Skeletal pain and tenderness

   d. Bone deformities that result in pathological fractures

e. Anorexia, nausea, vomiting, epigastric pain
f. Weight loss
g. Constipation
h. Hypertension
i. Cardiac dysrhythmias
j. Renal stones

3. Interventions
   a. Monitor vital signs, particularly the blood pressure.
   b. Monitor for cardiac dysrhythmias.
   c. Monitor intake and output and for signs of renal stones.
   d. Monitor for skeletal pain; move client slowly and carefully.
   e. Encourage fluid intake.
   f. Administer furosemide (Lasix) as prescribed to lower calcium levels.
   g. Administer normal saline intravenously as prescribed to maintain hydration.
   h. Administer phosphates as prescribed, which interfere with calcium resorption.
   i. Administer calcitonin (Calcimar) as prescribed to decrease skeletal calcium release and increase renal clearance of calcium.
   j. Monitor calcium and phosphorus levels.
   k. Notify the physician immediately if a precipitous drop in the calcium level occurs; assess for tingling and numbness in the face and extremities and signs of hypocalcemia.
   l. Prepare the client for parathyroidectomy as prescribed.

C. Parathyroidectomy
   1. Description: Removal of one or more of the parathyroid glands
   2. Preoperative interventions
      a. Monitor electrolytes, calcium, phosphate, and magnesium levels.
      b. Ensure that calcium levels are decreased to near normal.
      c. Inform the client that talking may be painful for the first day or two after surgery.
   3. Postoperative interventions
      a. Monitor for respiratory distress.
      b. Place a tracheotomy set, oxygen, and suctioning at the bedside.
      c. Monitor vital signs.
      d. Position the client in the semi-Fowler position.
      e. Assess neck dressing for bleeding.
      f. Monitor for hypocalcemic crisis, as evidenced by tingling and twitching in the extremities and face.
      g. Assess for positive **Trousseau's** or **Chvostek's sign,** which signals the potential for tetany.
      h. Monitor for changes in voice pattern and hoarseness.
      i. Monitor for laryngeal nerve damage.
      j. Instruct the client in the administration of calcium and vitamin D supplements as prescribed.

BOX 53-15

Major Types of Diabetes Mellitus

Type 1: insulin-dependent diabetes mellitus
Type 2: non–insulin-dependent diabetes mellitus

VII. DISORDERS OF THE PANCREAS
A. **Diabetes mellitus** (Box 53-15)
   1. Description
      a. **Diabetes mellitus** is a chronic disorder of impaired carbohydrate, protein, and lipid metabolism that is caused by a deficiency of insulin.
      b. A deficiency of insulin results in **hyperglycemia.**
      c. Type 1 **diabetes mellitus** is a nearly absolute deficiency of insulin; if insulin is not given, fats are metabolized, resulting in ketonemia (acidosis).
      d. Type 2 **diabetes mellitus** is a relative lack of insulin or resistance to the action of insulin; usually insulin is sufficient to stabilize fat and protein metabolism but not to deal with carbohydrate metabolism.
      e. Macrovascular complications include coronary artery disease, cardiomyopathy, hypertension, cerebrovascular disease, peripheral vascular disease, and infection.
      f. Microvascular complications include retinopathy, nephropathy, and neuropathy.
   2. Assessment
      a. Polyuria, polydipsia, polyphagia (more common in type 1 **diabetes mellitus**)
      b. **Hyperglycemia**
      c. Weight loss (common in type 1 **diabetes mellitus,** rare in type 2 **diabetes mellitus**)
      d. Blurred vision
      e. Slow wound healing
      f. Vaginal infections
      g. Weakness and paresthesias
      h. Signs of inadequate circulation to the feet
      i. Signs of accelerated atherosclerosis (renal, cerebral, cardiac, peripheral)
   3. Diet
      a. The total number of calories is individualized based on the client's current or desired weight and the presence of other existing health problems.
      b. As prescribed by the physician, the client may be advised to follow the food exchange from the American Diabetic Association diet or the dietary guidelines for Americans (Food Guide Pyramid) issued by the U.S. Departments of Agriculture and Health and Human Services.
      c. Incorporate diet into individual client needs, lifestyle, and cultural and socioeconomic patterns.

4. Exercise
   a. Exercise lowers blood glucose level.
   b. Exercise reduces cardiovascular risks.
   c. Exercise improves circulation and muscle tone.
   d. Exercise decreases total cholesterol and triglyceride levels.
   e. Exercise encourages weight loss.
   f. Instruct the client in dietary adjustments when exercising; dietary adjustments are individualized.
   g. Instruct the client to monitor blood glucose before exercising; if the client plans to participate in extended periods of exercise, blood glucose levels should be checked before, during, and after the exercise period.
   h. Initially, the client who requires insulin should be instructed to eat a 15-g carbohydrate snack (a fruit exchange) or a snack of complex carbohydrate with a protein before engaging in moderate exercise so as to prevent **hypoglycemia.**
   i. If the client requires extra food during exercise to prevent **hypoglycemia,** it need not be deducted from the regular meal plan.
   j. If the blood glucose level is greater than 250 mg/dL and urinary ketones (type 1 **diabetes mellitus**) are present, the client is instructed not to exercise until the blood glucose is closer to normal and urinary ketones are absent.
5. Oral hypoglycemic medications
   a. Oral medications are prescribed for clients with **diabetes mellitus** type 2.
   b. Assess the client's knowledge of **diabetes mellitus** and the use of oral hypoglycemic agents.
   c. Assess vital signs and blood glucose levels.
   d. Assess the medications that the client is currently taking.
   e. Aspirin, alcohol, sulfonamides, oral contraceptives, and monoamine oxidase inhibitors increase the hypoglycemic effect, causing a decrease in blood glucose levels.
   f. Glucocorticoids, thiazide diuretics, and estrogen increase blood glucose levels.
   g. Teach the client to recognize symptoms of **hypoglycemia** and **hyperglycemia.**
   h. Teach the client to avoid over-the-counter medications unless prescribed by the physician.
   i. Teach the client to avoid alcohol if taking sulfonylureas.
   j. Inform the client with type 2 **diabetes mellitus** that insulin may be needed during stress, surgery, or infection.
   k. Teach the client about the importance of compliance with the prescribed medication.
   l. Advise the client to wear a Medic-Alert bracelet.
6. Insulin
   a. Insulin is used to treat type 1 **diabetes mellitus** and type 2 **diabetes mellitus** when diet and

weight control therapy have failed to maintain satisfactory blood glucose levels.
   b. Regular insulin is the only insulin that can be administered intravenously in the emergency treatment of **diabetic ketoacidosis.**
   c. Aspirin, alcohol, oral anticoagulants, oral hypoglycemic drugs, β-blockers, tricyclic antidepressants, tetracycline, and monoamine oxidase inhibitors increase the hypoglycemic effect of insulin, causing further decrease in blood glucose levels.
   d. Glucocorticoids, thiazide diuretics, thyroid agents, oral contraceptives, and estrogen increase blood glucose levels.
   e. Illness, infection, and stress increase blood glucose levels and the need for insulin; insulin should not be withheld during illness, infection, or stress because **hyperglycemia** and ketoacidosis can result.
   f. Instruct the client to recognize symptoms of **hypoglycemia** and **hyperglycemia.**
   g. The peak action time of insulin is important because of the possibility of hypoglycemic reactions occurring during that time.
B. Complications of insulin therapy
   1. Local allergic reactions
      a. Redness, swelling, tenderness, and induration or a wheal at the site of injection may occur 1 to 2 hours after administration.
      b. Reactions usually occur during the early stages of insulin therapy.
      c. Instruct the client to avoid the use of alcohol to cleanse the skin before injection.
      d. The physician may prescribe an antihistamine to be taken 1 hour before injection.
   2. Insulin lipodystrophy
      a. Lipoatrophy is loss of subcutaneous fat and appears as slight dimpling or more serious pitting of subcutaneous fat; the use of human insulin helps to prevent this complication.
      b. Lipohypertrophy is the development of fibrous fatty masses at the injection site and is caused by repeated use of an injection site.
      c. Instruct the client to avoid injecting insulin into affected sites.
      d. Instruct the client about the importance of rotating insulin injection sites.
   3. Insulin resistance
      a. The client receiving insulin develops immune antibodies that bind the insulin, thereby decreasing the insulin available for use in the body.
      b. Treatment consists of administering a purer insulin preparation.
      c. Insulin resistance is also the term used for lack of tissue sensitivity to the insulin from the body, which results in hyperglycemia.

4. **Dawn phenomenon**
    a. **Dawn phenomenon** results from reduced tissue sensitivity to insulin that develops between 5 and 8 AM (prebreakfast hyperglycemia occurs) and may be caused by nocturnal release of growth hormone.
    b. Treatment includes administering an evening dose of intermediate-acting insulin at 10 PM.
5. **Somogyi phenomenon**
    a. Normal or elevated blood glucose levels are present at bedtime; **hypoglycemia** occurs at 2 to 3 AM, which causes an increase in the production of counterregulatory hormones.
    b. By 7 AM, in response to the counterregulatory hormones, the blood glucose rebounds significantly to the hyperglycemic range.
    c. Treatment includes decreasing the evening (predinner or bedtime) dose of intermediate-acting insulin, or increasing the bedtime snack.
6. **Insulin waning**
    a. **Insulin waning** is a progressive rise in the blood glucose level from bedtime to morning.
    b. Treatment includes increasing the evening (predinner or bedtime) dose of intermediate- or long-acting insulin or instituting a dose of insulin before the evening meal if one is not already prescribed.
C. Insulin administration
1. Subcutaneous injections and mixing insulin: Refer to Chapter 54.
2. Insulin pens
    a. An insulin pen is a device that uses a small, prefilled insulin cartridge that is loaded into a penlike holder; a disposable needle is attached to the device for injection.
    b. The client inserts the needle for injection, and the insulin is delivered by dialing in a dose or pushing a button for every 1- to 2-unit increment administered.
3. Jet injectors
    a. A jet injector is a device that delivers insulin through the skin under pressure in an extremely fine stream.
    b. Insulin administered by this device usually absorbs faster.
    c. The injector can cause bruising at the site of insulin delivery.
4. Insulin pumps
    a. Continuous subcutaneous insulin infusion is administered by an externally worn device that contains a syringe attached to a long, thin, narrow-lumen tube with a needle or Teflon catheter attached to the end.
    b. The client inserts the needle or Teflon catheter into the subcutaneous tissue (usually on the abdomen) and secures it with tape or a transparent dressing; the pump is worn on a belt or

in a pocket; the needle or Teflon catheter is changed at least every 3 days.
    c. A continuous basal rate of insulin infuses; in addition, based on the blood glucose level, the anticipated food intake, and the activity level, the client delivers a bolus of insulin before each meal.
    d. The pump uses regular insulin (buffered to prevent the precipitation of insulin crystals within the catheter); some physicians may prescribe the use of lispro insulin.
5. Implantable insulin delivery
    a. An insulin pump is implanted in the peritoneal cavity, where insulin can be absorbed in a more physiological manner.
    b. Implants are not widely used because of mechanical problems associated with the pump, the catheter, and the insulin delivery.
6. Pancreas transplants
    a. The goal of pancreatic transplantation is to halt or reverse the complications of **diabetes mellitus.**
    b. Transplants are performed on a limited number of clients (mostly clients receiving kidney transplantations simultaneously).
    c. Immunosuppressive therapy is prescribed to prevent and treat rejection.
D. Self-monitoring of blood glucose
1. Self-monitoring provides the client with the current blood glucose level and information to maintain good glycemic control.
2. Monitoring requires a finger prick to obtain a drop of blood for testing.
3. Tests must be used with caution in clients with diabetic retinopathy and neuropathy.
4. Client instructions (Box 53-16)
E. Urine testing
1. Urine testing is a less reliable indicator compared with blood glucose monitoring.

BOX 53-16

Client Instructions: Monitoring of Blood Glucose

Use the proper procedure for obtaining the blood glucose level.
Perform the procedure precisely to obtain accurate results.
Follow the manufacturer's instructions for the glucometer.
Wash hands before and after performing the procedure to prevent infection.
Calibrate the monitor as instructed by the manufacturer.
Check the expiration date on the test strips.
If the blood glucose results do not seem reasonable, reread the instructions, reassess technique, check the expiration date of the test strips, and perform the procedure again to verify results.

2. Instruct the client in the procedure for testing urine for glucose and ketones.
3. Inform the client that the second voided urine specimen is most accurate.
4. The presence of ketones may indicate impending **ketoacidosis.**
5. Urine ketone testing should be performed during illness and whenever the client with type 1 **diabetes mellitus** has glycosuria or persistently elevated blood glucose levels (greater than 240 mg/dL for two consecutive testing periods).

VIII. ACUTE COMPLICATIONS OF DIABETES MELLITUS

A. Hypoglycemia
1. Description
   a. **Hypoglycemia** occurs when the blood glucose level falls below 60 mg/dL.
   b. **Hypoglycemia** is caused by too much insulin or oral hypoglycemic agents, too little food, or excessive activity.
   c. The client needs to be instructed always to carry some form of fast-acting simple carbohydrate with them.
   d. If the client has a hypoglycemic reaction and does not have any of the recommended emergency foods available, any available food should be eaten; high-fat foods slow the absorption of glucose and the hypoglycemic symptoms may not resolve quickly.
2. Assessment (Box 53-17)
   a. Mild **hypoglycemia:** A blood glucose level less than 60 mg/dL
   b. Moderate **hypoglycemia:** A blood glucose level less than 40 mg/dL
   c. Severe **hypoglycemia:** A blood glucose level less than 20 mg/dL (the client is unable to swallow, is unconscious, or is experiencing seizures)

BOX 53-18

Simple Carbohydrates to Treat Hypoglycemia

Commercially prepared glucose tablets
6 to 10 Life Savers or hard candy
4 tsp of sugar
4 sugar cubes
1 Tbs of honey or syrup
½ cup of fruit juice or regular (nondiet) soft drink
8 oz low-fat milk
6 saltine crackers
3 graham crackers

---

3. Interventions: mild **hypoglycemia**
   a. Give 10 to 15 g of a fast-acting simple carbohydrate (Box 53-18).
   b. Retest the blood glucose level in 15 minutes and repeat the treatment if symptoms do not resolve.
   c. Once symptoms resolve, a snack containing protein and carbohydrates, such as milk or cheese and crackers, is recommended unless the client plans to eat a regular meal within 60 minutes.
4. Interventions: moderate **hypoglycemia**
   a. Administer 15 to 30 g of a fast-acting simple carbohydrate.
   b. Administer additional food such as low-fat milk or cheese after 10 to 15 minutes.
5. Interventions for severe **hypoglycemia**
   a. If the client is unconscious and cannot swallow, an injection of glucagon is administered subcutaneously or intramuscularly.
   b. Administer a second dose in 10 minutes if the client remains unconscious.
   c. A small meal is given to the client when the client awakens as long as the client is not nauseated.
   d. The physician is notified if a severe hypoglycemic reaction occurs.

BOX 53-17

Assessment of Hypoglycemia

MILD	
Hunger	Impaired coordination
Nervousness	Inability to concentrate
Palpitations	Irrational or combative behavior
Sweating	Light-headedness
Tachycardia	Memory lapses
Tremor	Numbness of the lips and tongue
	Slurred speech
MODERATE	**SEVERE**
Confusion	Difficulty arousing from sleep
Double vision	Disoriented behavior
Drowsiness	Loss of consciousness
Emotional changes	Seizures
Headache	

e. In the hospital or emergency department, the client may be treated with an IV injection of 25 to 50 mL of 50% dextrose in water.

f. Family members need to be instructed on the administration of glucagon.

B. **Diabetic ketoacidosis (DKA)**

1. Description
   a. **Diabetic ketoacidosis** is a life-threatening complication of type 1 **diabetes mellitus** that develops when a severe insulin deficiency occurs.
   b. The main clinical manifestations include **hyperglycemia**, dehydration and electrolyte loss, and acidosis.
   c. The major causes include a decreased or missed dose of insulin, illness or infection, and undiagnosed and untreated type 1 **diabetes mellitus.**
   d. Ketoacidosis develops over a period several hours to days.

2. Assessment (Box 53-19)
   a. Blood glucose levels may vary from 300 to 800 mg/dL.
   b. Low serum bicarbonate and a low pH are present.
   c. Sodium and potassium levels may be low, normal, or high, depending on the amount of water loss and dehydration status.

3. Interventions
   a. Restore circulating volume and protect against cerebral, coronary, or renal hypoperfusion.
   b. Treat dehydration with rapid IV infusions of 0.9% or 0.45% saline as prescribed; dextrose is added to IV fluids (D_5NS, or 5% dextrose in 0.45% saline) when the blood glucose level reaches 250 to 300 mg/dL.
   c. Treat **hyperglycemia** with regular insulin administered intravenously as prescribed.
   d. Correct electrolyte imbalances (potassium level may be elevated as a result of dehydration and acidosis).
   e. Monitor potassium level closely because when the client receives treatment for the dehydration and acidosis, the serum potassium will decrease and potassium replacement may be required.

4. Insulin IV administration
   a. Use regular insulin only.
   b. A dose of 5 to 10 units of regular insulin by IV bolus may be prescribed before a continuous infusion is begun.
   c. Mix the prescribed IV dose of regular insulin for continuous infusion in 0.9% or 0.45% saline as prescribed.
   d. Flush the insulin solution through the entire intravenous infusion set and discard the first 50 mL of solution before connecting and administering to the client; insulin molecules adhere to the plastic of IV infusion sets.
   e. Always place the insulin infusion on an IV infusion controller.
   f. Insulin is infused continuously until subcutaneous administration resumes.
   g. Monitor vital signs and for signs of fluid overload.
   h. Monitor potassium levels, glucose levels, and urinary output and for signs of increased intracranial pressure.
   i. If the blood glucose level falls too far, too fast before the brain has time to equilibrate, water is pulled from the blood to the cerebrospinal fluid and the brain, causing cerebral edema and increased intracranial pressure.
   j. The potassium level will fall rapidly within the first hour of treatment as the dehydration and the acidosis are treated.
   k. Potassium is administered intravenously in a diluted solution as prescribed when the potassium reaches normal level to prevent hypokalemia; ensure adequate renal function before administering potassium.

5. Client education (Box 53-20)

C. **Hyperglycemic hyperosmolar nonketotic syndrome (HHNS)**

1. Description

BOX 53-19

Assessment of Diabetic Ketoacidosis

Acetone breath (a fruity odor)
Anorexia, nausea, vomiting, and abdominal pain
Blurred vision
Headache
Hypotension
Kussmaul's respirations
Mental status changes
Polydipsia
Polyuria
Weak, rapid pulse
Weakness

BOX 53-20

Client Education: Guidelines during Illness

Take insulin or oral antidiabetic medications as prescribed.
Test blood glucose and test the urine for ketones every 3 to 4 hours.
If the usual meal plan cannot be followed, substitute soft foods 6 to 8 times a day.
If vomiting, diarrhea, or fever occurs, consume liquids every ½ to 1 hour to prevent dehydration and to provide calories.
Notify the physician if vomiting, diarrhea, or fever persists; if blood glucose levels are greater than 250 to 300 mg/dL; when ketonuria is present for more than 24 hours; when unable to take food or fluids for a period of 4 hours; or when illness persists for more than 2 days.

a. Extreme **hyperglycemia** occurs without ketosis and acidosis.

b. The syndrome occurs most often in individuals with type 2 **diabetes mellitus.**

c. The major difference between HHNS and DKA is that ketosis and acidosis do not occur with HHNS.

d. Onset is usually slow and takes hours to days to develop.

2. Assessment

a. Blood glucose level from 600 to 1200 mg/dL

b. Hypotension

c. Dehydration

d. Tachycardia

e. Mental status changes

f. Neurological deficits

g. Seizures

3. Interventions

a. Treatment is similar to that for DKA.

b. Treatment includes fluid replacement, correction of electrolyte imbalances, and insulin administration.

c. Insulin plays a less critical role in the treatment of HHNS than it does for the treatment of DKA because insulin is not needed for reversal of acidosis in HHNS.

IX. CHRONIC COMPLICATIONS OF DIABETES MELLITUS

A. Diabetic retinopathy

1. Description

a. Diabetic retinopathy is a chronic and progressive impairment of the retinal circulation that eventually causes hemorrhage.

b. Permanent vision changes and blindness can occur.

c. The client has difficulty with carrying out the daily tasks of blood glucose testing and insulin injections.

2. Assessment

a. A change in vision is caused by the rupture of small microaneurysms in retinal blood vessels.

b. Blurred vision results from macular edema.

c. Sudden loss of vision results from retinal detachment.

d. Cataracts results from lens opacity.

3. Interventions

a. Maintain safety.

b. Early prevention is by the control of hypertension and blood glucose levels.

c. Photocoagulation (laser therapy) removes hemorrhagic tissue to decrease scarring.

d. Vitrectomy removes vitreous hemorrhages and thus decreases tension on the retina, preventing detachment.

e. Cataract removal with lens implant improves vision.

B. Diabetic nephropathy

1. Description: a progressive decrease in kidney function

2. Assessment

a. Microalbuminuria

b. Thirst

c. Fatigue

d. Anemia

e. Weight loss

f. Signs of malnutrition

g. Frequent urinary tract infections

h. Signs of a neurogenic bladder

3. Interventions

a. Early prevention measures include the control of hypertension and blood glucose levels.

b. Assess vital signs.

c. Monitor intake and output.

d. Monitor serum blood urea nitrogen and creatinine levels and urine albumin levels.

e. Restrict dietary protein, sodium, and potassium intake as prescribed.

f. Avoid nephrotoxic medications.

g. Prepare the client for dialysis procedures as prescribed.

h. Prepare the client for kidney transplant as prescribed.

i. Prepare the client for pancreas transplant as prescribed.

C. Diabetic neuropathy

1. Description

a. Diabetic neuropathy is general deterioration of the nervous system throughout the body.

b. Complications include the development of nonhealing ulcers of the feet, gastric paresis, erectile dysfunction.

2. Assessment

a. Paresthesias

b. Decreased or absent reflexes

c. Decreased sensation to vibration or light touch

d. Pain, aching, and burning in the lower extremities

e. Poor peripheral pulses

f. Skin breakdown and signs of infection

g. Weakness or loss of sensation in cranial nerves III, IV, V, or VI

h. Dizziness and postural hypotension

i. Nausea and vomiting

j. Diarrhea or constipation

k. Incontinence

l. Dyspareunia

m. Impotence

n. Hypoglycemic unawareness

3. Interventions

a. Early prevention measures include the control of hypertension and blood glucose levels.

b. Careful foot care is required to prevent trauma (Box 53-21).

Preventive Foot Care Instructions

Provide meticulous skin care and proper foot care.

Inspect feet daily and monitor feet for redness, swelling, or break in skin integrity.

Notify the physician if redness or a break in the skin occurs.

Avoid thermal injuries from hot water, heating pads, and baths.

Wash feet with warm (not hot) water and dry thoroughly (avoid foot soaks).

Do not soak feet.

Do not treat corns, blisters, or ingrown toenails.

Do not cross legs or wear tight garments that may constrict blood flow.

Apply moisturizing lotion to the feet but not between the toes.

Prevent moisture from accumulating between the toes.

Wear loose socks and well-fitting (not tight) shoes, and instruct the client not to go barefoot.

Change into clean cotton socks daily.

Wear socks to keep feet warm.

Do not wear the same pair of shoes 2 days in a row.

Do not wear open-toed shoes or shoes with a strap that goes between the toes.

Check shoes for cracks or tears in the lining and for foreign objects before putting them on.

Break in new shoes gradually.

Cut toenails straight across and smooth nails with an emery board.

Do not smoke.

c. Administer medications as prescribed for pain relief.
d. Initiate bladder-training programs.
e. Instruct in the use of estrogen-containing lubricants for women with dyspareunia.
f. Prepare the male client with impotence for penile injections or implantable devices as prescribed.
g. Prepare for surgical decompression for compression lesions related to the cranial nerves as prescribed.

X. OPERATIVE CARE FOR THE DIABETIC CLIENT

A. Preoperative care
1. Check with physician regarding withholding oral hypoglycemic medications or insulin.
2. Some long-acting oral antidiabetic medications are discontinued 24 to 48 hours before surgery.
3. Insulin dose may be adjusted or may be withheld if IV insulin administration during surgery is planned.
4. Monitor blood glucose level.
5. Administer IV fluids as prescribed.

B. Postoperative care
1. Administer IV glucose and regular insulin infusions as prescribed until the client can tolerate oral feedings.

2. Administer supplemental short-acting insulin as prescribed based on blood glucose results.
3. Monitor blood glucose levels frequently if the client is receiving total parenteral nutrition.
4. When the client is tolerating food, ensure that the client receives an adequate amount of carbohydrates daily to prevent **hypoglycemia** and ketosis.

PRACTICE QUESTIONS

1. After hypophysectomy, a client complains of being thirsty and having to urinate frequently. The initial nursing action is to
   1. Document the complaints.
   2. Increase fluid intake.
   3. Assess urine specific gravity.
   4. Assess for urinary glucose.

2. A nurse is caring for a client after hypophysectomy. The nurse notices clear nasal drainage from the client's nostril. The initial nursing action would be to
   1. Continue to observe the drainage.
   2. Test the drainage for glucose.
   3. Lower the head of the bed.
   4. Obtain a culture of the drainage.

3. After several diagnostic tests, a client is diagnosed with diabetes insipidus. A nurse performs an assessment on the client, knowing that which symptom is indicative of this disorder?
   1. Diarrhea
   2. Polydipsia
   3. Weight gain
   4. Fatigue

4. A nurse develops a plan of care for a client with hyperthyroidism and includes which of the following in the plan?
   1. Provide small meals.
   2. Provide extra blankets.
   3. Provide a high-fiber diet.
   4. Provide a restful environment.

5. A nurse is performing an assessment on a client following a thyroidectomy. The nurse notes that the client has developed hoarseness and a weak voice. Which nursing action is most appropriate?
   1. Notify the physician immediately.
   2. Reassure the client that this is usually a temporary condition.
   3. Check for signs of bleeding.
   4. Administer calcium gluconate.

6. A client is admitted to an emergency room, and a diagnosis of myxedema coma is made. Which action would the nurse prepare to carry out initially?
   1. Warm the client.
   2. Administer fluid replacement.
   3. Maintain an airway.
   4. Administer thyroid hormone.

7. A client is taking NPH insulin daily every morning. The nurse instructs the client that the most likely time for a hypoglycemic reaction to occur is
   1. 2 to 4 hours after administration.
   2. 6 to 14 hours after administration.
   3. 16 to 18 hours after administration.
   4. 18 to 24 hours after administration.

8. A nurse is preparing a teaching plan for a client with diabetes mellitus regarding proper foot care. Which instruction is included in the plan?
   1. Soak feet in hot water.
   2. Apply a moisturizing lotion to dry feet but not between the toes.
   3. Always have a podiatrist cut your toenails; never cut them yourself.
   4. Avoid using a mild soap on the feet.

9. A client is brought to the emergency room in an unresponsive state, and a diagnosis of hyperglycemic hyperosmolar nonketotic syndrome is made. The nurse would prepare immediately to initiate which of the following anticipated physician's orders?
   1. 100 units of NPH insulin
   2. Endotracheal intubation
   3. Intravenous replacement of sodium bicarbonate
   4. Intravenous infusion of normal saline

10. An external insulin pump is prescribed for a client with diabetes mellitus. The client asks the nurse about the functioning of the pump. The nurse bases the response on the information that the pump
    1. Gives a small continuous dose of regular insulin subcutaneously, and the client can self-administer a bolus with an additional dosage from the pump before each meal.
    2. Is timed to release programmed doses of regular or NPH insulin into the bloodstream at specific intervals.
    3. Is surgically attached to the pancreas and infuses regular insulin into the pancreas, which in turn releases the insulin into the bloodstream.
    4. Continuously infuses small amounts of NPH insulin into the bloodstream while regularly monitoring blood glucose levels.

11. A client newly diagnosed with diabetes mellitus has been stabilized with insulin injections daily. A nurse prepares a discharge teaching plan regarding the insulin. The teaching plan should reinforce which of the following concepts?
    1. Increase the amount of insulin before unusual exercise.
    2. Ketones in the urine signify a need for less insulin.
    3. Always keep insulin vials refrigerated.
    4. Systematically rotate insulin injection sites.

12. A client with a diagnosis of diabetic ketoacidosis (DKA) is being treated in an emergency room. Which finding would a nurse expect to note as confirming this diagnosis?

1. Elevated blood glucose level and a low plasma bicarbonate
2. Decreased urine output
3. Increased respirations and an increase in pH
4. Comatose state

13. A nurse teaches a client with diabetes mellitus about differentiating between hypoglycemia and ketoacidosis. The client demonstrates an understanding of the teaching by stating that glucose will be taken if which of the following symptoms develops?
   1. Fruity breath odor
   2. Shakiness
   3. Blurred vision
   4. Polyuria

14. A client with diabetes mellitus demonstrates acute anxiety when first admitted for the treatment of hyperglycemia. The most appropriate intervention to decrease the client's anxiety would be to
   1. Administer a sedative.
   2. Make sure the client knows all the correct medical terms to understand what is happening.
   3. Ignore the signs and symptoms of anxiety so that they will soon disappear.
   4. Convey empathy, trust, and respect toward the client.

15. A nurse provides instructions to a client newly diagnosed with type 1 diabetes mellitus. The nurse recognizes accurate understanding of measures to prevent diabetic ketoacidosis when the client states,
   1. "I will stop taking my insulin if I'm too sick to eat."
   2. "I will decrease my insulin dose during times of illness."
   3. "I will notify my physician if my blood glucose level is greater than 250 mg/dL."
   4. "I will adjust my insulin dose according to the level of glucose in my urine."

16. A client is admitted to a hospital with a diagnosis of diabetic ketoacidosis (DKA). The initial blood glucose level was 950 mg/dL. A continuous intravenous infusion of regular insulin is initiated along with intravenous rehydration with normal saline. The serum glucose level is now 240 mg/dL. The nurse would next prepare to administer which of the following?
   1. Intravenous fluids containing 5% dextrose
   2. NPH insulin subcutaneously
   3. An ampule of 50% dextrose
   4. Phenytoin (Dilantin) for the prevention of seizures

17. A physician has prescribed propylthiouracil (PTU) for a client with hyperthyroidism. A nurse develops a plan of care for the client. A priority nursing assessment to be included in the plan regarding this medication is to assess for
   1. Signs and symptoms of hypothyroidism.
   2. Signs and symptoms of hyperglycemia.

3. Relief of pain.

4. Signs of renal toxicity.

18. A nurse develops a plan of care for a client with hyperparathyroidism who is receiving calcitonin salmon (Calcimar). Which of the following outcome criteria has the highest priority regarding this medication?

    1. Absence of side effects

    2. Achievement of normal serum calcium levels

    3. Relief of pain

    4. Verbalization of appropriate medication knowledge

19. A physician prescribes levothyroxine sodium (Synthroid), 0.15 mg PO daily, for a client with hypothyroidism. A nurse will prepare to administer this medication

    1. 3 times a day in equal doses of 0.5 mg each to ensure consistent serum drug levels.

    2. In the morning to prevent sleeplessness.

    3. Only when the client complains of fatigue and cold intolerance.

    4. At various times during the day to prevent tolerance from occurring.

20. A nurse is monitoring a client receiving chlorpropamide (Diabinese). The nurse knows that which of the following is not a therapeutic outcome for this client?

    1. A decrease in polyuria

    2. A fasting blood glucose of 110 mg/dL

    3. A decrease in polyphagia

    4. A glycosylated hemoglobin of 10%

21. A nurse is monitoring a client with diabetes insipidus. Desmopressin (DDAVP, Stimate) has been prescribed for the client. Which of the following outcomes reflects a therapeutic effect of this medication?

    1. Serum osmolality greater than 320 mOsm/kg

    2. Increased blood pressure

    3. Decreased urine output

    4. Urine osmolality less than 100 mOsm/kg

22. A nurse is monitoring a client newly diagnosed with diabetes mellitus for signs of complications. Which of the following, if exhibited in the client, would indicate hyperglycemia and warrant physician notification?

    1. Hypertension

    2. Diaphoresis

    3. Polyuria

    4. Increased pulse rate

23. A nurse is preparing a plan of care for a client with diabetes mellitus who has hyperglycemia. The priority nursing diagnosis would be

    1. High risk for deficient fluid volume.

    2. Deficient Knowledge: Disease Process and Treatment.

    3. Imbalanced Nutrition: Less Than Body Requirements.

    4. Disabled Family Coping: Compromised.

24. A home health nurse visits a client with a diagnosis of type 1 diabetes mellitus. The client relates a history of vomiting and diarrhea and tells the nurse that no food or medication has been consumed for 36 hours. Which additional statement by the client indicates a need for further teaching?

    1. "I need to stop my insulin."

    2. "I need to increase my fluid intake."

    3. "I need to call the physician because of these symptoms."

    4. "I need to monitor my blood glucose every 3 to 4 hours."

25. A nurse is assisting a client with diabetes mellitus who is recovering from diabetic ketoacidosis (DKA) to develop a plan to prevent a recurrence. Which of the following is most important to include in the plan of care?

    1. Eat six small meals per day.

    2. Receive appropriate follow-up health care.

    3. Monitor blood glucose levels frequently.

    4. Test urine for ketone levels.

26. A nurse is caring for a client admitted to the emergency room with diabetic ketoacidosis (DKA). In the acute phase the priority nursing action is to prepare to

    1. Administer regular insulin intravenously.

    2. Administer 5% dextrose intravenously.

    3. Correct the acidosis.

    4. Apply an electrocardiogram monitor.

27. A client with type 2 diabetes mellitus has a blood glucose greater than 600 mg/dL and is complaining of polydipsia, polyuria, weight loss, and weakness. A nurse reviews the physician's documentation and would expect to note which of the following diagnoses?

    1. Diabetic ketoacidosis (DKA)

    2. Hypoglycemia

    3. Hyperglycemic hyperosmolar nonketotic syndrome (HHNS)

    4. Pheochromocytoma

28. The family of a bedridden client with type 2 diabetes mellitus calls a nurse to report the following symptoms: blood glucose of 400 mg/dL (by fingerstick), polydipsia, and increased lethargy. To determine a possible diagnosis, the nurse asks the family which most important question?

    1. "Has there been any change in the dietary intake?"

    2. "Have there been any ketones in the urine?"

    3. "Has there been any fever?"

    4. "Have you increased the amount of fluids provided?"

29. A nurse performs a physical assessment on a client with type 2 diabetes mellitus. Findings include a fasting blood glucose of 120 mg/dL, temperature of 101° F, pulse of 88, respirations of 22, and blood pressure of 140/84 mm Hg. Which finding would be of most concern to the nurse?

1. Pulse
2. Blood pressure
3. Respiration
4. Temperature

30. A nurse is interviewing a client with type 2 diabetes mellitus. Which statement by the client indicates an understanding of the treatment for this disorder?
    1. "I am taking oral insulin instead of shots."
    2. "The medications I'm taking help release the insulin I already make."
    3. "By taking these medications, I am able to eat more."
    4. "When I become ill, I need to increase the number of pills I take."

31. A nurse is providing discharge instructions to a client who has Cushing's syndrome. Which statement by the client indicates that instructions related to dietary management were understood?
    1. "I am fortunate that I do not need to follow any special diet."
    2. "I will need to limit the amount of protein in my diet."
    3. "I am fortunate that I can eat all the salty foods I enjoy."
    4. "I can eat foods that have a lot of potassium in them."

32. A client with type 1 diabetes mellitus calls the nurse to report recurrent episodes of hypoglycemia with exercising. Which statement by the client indicates an inadequate understanding of the peak action of NPH insulin and exercise?
    1. "The best time for me to exercise is every afternoon."
    2. "The best time for me to exercise is after I eat."
    3. "The best time for me to exercise is after breakfast."
    4. "The best time for me to exercise is after my morning snack."

33. A nurse is completing an assessment on an older client who is being admitted for a diagnostic workup for primary hyperparathyroidism. Which client complaint would be characteristic of this disorder?
    1. Diarrhea
    2. Polyuria
    3. Polyphagia
    4. Weight gain

34. A nurse is caring for a postoperative parathyroidectomy client. Which client complaint would indicate that a serious, life-threatening complication may be developing, requiring immediate notification of the physician?
    1. Difficulty in voiding
    2. Abdominal cramps
    3. Laryngeal stridor
    4. Mild to moderate incisional pain

35. A nurse notes that a client with type 1 diabetes mellitus has lipodystrophy on both upper thighs. The nurse would appropriately inquire if the client
    1. Cleanses the skin with alcohol before each injection.
    2. Rotates sites for injection.
    3. Aspirates for blood before injection into the subcutaneous tissue.
    4. Administers the insulin at a 45-degree angle.

36. A nurse is caring for a client with type 1 diabetes mellitus. Which client complaint would alert the nurse to the presence of a possible hypoglycemic reaction?
    1. Hot, dry skin
    2. Muscle cramps
    3. Anorexia
    4. Tremors

37. A nurse needs to maintain food and fluid intake to minimize the risk of dehydration in a frail, older, client with diabetes mellitus who has gastroenteritis. The most appropriate nursing intervention is to
    1. Offer water only, until the client is able to tolerate solid foods.
    2. Withhold all fluids until vomiting has ceased for at least 4 hours.
    3. Encourage the client to take 8 to 12 oz of fluid every hour while awake.
    4. Maintain a clear liquid diet for at least 5 days before advancing to solids to allow inflammation of the bowel to dissipate.

38. A client who currently is taking levothyroxine sodium (Synthroid) complains of cold intolerance, constipation, dry skin, weight gain, and puffy eyes. Based on these findings, the nurse would anticipate which of the following prescriptions?
    1. Increase levothyroxine sodium dosage after checking the T_4 level
    2. Decrease levothyroxine sodium dosage after checking the T_4 level
    3. Discontinue levothyroxine sodium because the client is having an adverse reaction
    4. No change in medication because these are common side effects that will diminish with time

39. A client with diabetes mellitus visits a health care clinic. The client's diabetes mellitus previously had been well controlled with glyburide (DiaBeta), 5 mg PO daily, but recently the fasting blood glucose has been running 180 to 200 mg/dL. Which medication, if added to the client's regimen, may have contributed to the hyperglycemia?
    1. Prednisone (Deltasone)
    2. Atenolol (Tenormin)
    3. Phenelzine (Nardil)
    4. Allopurinol (Zyloprim)

40. A nurse is caring for a client with diabetes insipidus who is receiving vasopressin (Pitressin). The nurse monitors the client, knowing that which of the following is a therapeutic effect of this medication?

1. Decreased gastrointestinal tract smooth muscle tone and contractions
2. Increased urine output
3. Increased rebasorption of water by the renal tubules
4. Vasodilation of vascular vessels

41. A client is diagnosed with pheochromocytoma. A nurse prepares a plan of care for the client, and in the planning the nurse understands that pheochromocytoma is a condition that
    1. Causes profound hypotension.
    2. Causes the release of excessive amounts of catecholamines.
    3. Is not curable and is treated symptomatically.
    4. Is manifested by severe hypoglycemia.

42. A nurse is performing an admission assessment on a client admitted with a diagnosis of pheochromocytoma. The nurse assesses for the major symptom associated with pheochromocytoma when the nurse
    1. Tests the client's urine for glucose.
    2. Obtains the client's weight.
    3. Palpates the skin for its temperature.
    4. Takes the client's blood pressure.

43. A nurse collects urine specimens for catecholamine testing from a client with suspected pheochromocytoma. The results of the catecholamine test are reported as 20 mcg/100 mL urine. The nurse analyzes these results as
    1. Normal.
    2. Lower than normal, ruling out pheochromocytoma.
    3. Higher than normal, indicating pheochromocytoma.
    4. Insignificant and unrelated to pheochromocytoma.

44. A nurse is caring for a client with pheochromocytoma. The client is scheduled for adrenalectomy. In the preoperative period the priority nursing action would be to monitor
    1. Vital signs.
    2. Urine for glucose and acetone.
    3. Intake and output.
    4. Blood urea nitrogen results.

45. A nurse is caring for a client with pheochromocytoma. As part of the nursing care plan, the nurse monitors for hypertensive crisis. In the event that hypertensive crisis occurs, the nurse would anticipate that the most likely medication to be prescribed would be
    1. Propranolol (Inderal).
    2. Phentolamine mesylate (Regitine).
    3. Phenoxybenzamine hydrochloride (Dibenzyline).
    4. Prazosin hydrochloride (Minipress).

46. A nurse is caring for a client with pheochromocytoma. The client asks for a snack and something warm to drink. The most appropriate choice for this client to meet nutritional needs would be which of the following?
    1. Graham crackers and warm milk
    2. Toast with peanut butter and cocoa
    3. Crackers with cheese and tea
    4. Vanilla wafers and coffee with cream and sugar

47. A nurse is performing an assessment on a client with pheochromocytoma. Which of the following assessment data would indicate a potential complication associated with this disorder?
    1. A urinary output of 50 mL per hour
    2. An irregular heart rate
    3. A blood urea nitrogen of 20 mg/dL
    4. A coagulation time of 5 minutes

48. A community health nurse visits a client at home. Prednisone (Deltasone), 10 mg PO daily, has been prescribed for the client. The nurse teaches the client about the medication. Which statement, if made by the client, indicates that further teaching is necessary?
    1. "I need to take the medication every day at the same time."
    2. "I can take aspirin or my antihistamine if I need it."
    3. " If I gain more than 5 pounds a week, I will call my doctor."
    4. "I need to avoid coffee, tea, cola, and chocolate in my diet."

49. A nurse is preparing to provide instructions to a client with Addison's disease regarding diet therapy. The nurse knows that which of the following diets most likely would be prescribed for this client?
    1. High fat intake
    2. Normal sodium intake
    3. Low protein intake
    4. Low carbohydrate intake

50. A nursing instructor asks a student to describe the pathophysiology that occurs in Cushing's disease. Which statement by the student indicates an accurate understanding of this disorder?
    1. "Cushing's disease is characterized by an oversecretion of glucocorticoid hormones."
    2. "Cushing's disease is characterized by an undersecretion of glucocorticoid hormones."
    3. "Cushing's disease is characterized by an oversecretion of insulin."
    4. "Cushing's disease is characterized by an undersecretion of corticotropic hormones."

CRITICAL THINKING: PRIORITIZING (ORDERED RESPONSE)

A hospitalized client with type 1 diabetes mellitus received NPH and regular insulin 2 hours ago (at 7:30 AM). The client calls the nurse and reports that he is feeling hungry, shaky, and weak. The client ate breakfast at 8 AM and is due to eat lunch at noon. List in order of priority the actions that the nurse would take. (Number 1 is the first action.)

___ Give the client ½ cup of fruit juice to drink.

___ Check the client's blood glucose level.

___ Take the client's vital signs.

___ Give the client a small snack of carbohydrate and protein.

___ Document the client's complaints, actions taken, and outcome.

ANSWERS

1. 3

Rationale: After hypophysectomy, diabetes insipidus can occur temporarily because of antidiuretic hormone deficiency. This deficiency is related to surgical manipulation. The nurse should assess specific gravity of the urine and notify the physician if the results are less than 1.006.

Test-Taking Strategy: Use the process of elimination. Recalling that diabetes insipidus is a complication of this type of surgery will assist in eliminating option 4. Note the key word "initial." Knowledge of the nursing assessment measures in diabetes insipidus will easily direct you to option 3. Review the complications of hypophysectomy if you had difficulty with this question.

Level of Cognitive Ability: Application
Client Needs: Physiological Integrity
Integrated Process: Nursing Process—implementation
Content Area: Adult health—endocrine
Reference: Ignatavicius, D., & Workman, M. (2002). *Medical-surgical nursing: Critical thinking for collaborative care* (4th ed., p. 1407). Philadelphia: W. B. Saunders.

2. 2

Rationale: After hypophysectomy the client should be monitored for rhinorrhea, which could indicate a cerebrospinal fluid leak. If this occurs, the drainage should be collected and tested for the presence of cerebrospinal fluid. The head of the bed should not be lowered so as to prevent increased intracranial pressure. Clear nasal drainage would not indicate the need for a culture. Continuing to observe the drainage without taking action could result in a serious complication.

Test-Taking Strategy: Use the process of elimination. Note the key word "initial." This indicates that an action is required. Option 3 can be eliminated easily. Option 4 can be eliminated easily because the drainage is clear. Because an action is required, eliminate option 1. Review the complications following hypophysectomy if you had difficulty with this question.

Level of Cognitive Ability: Application
Client Needs: Physiological Integrity
Integrated Process: Nursing Process—implementation
Content Area: Adult health—endocrine
Reference: Ignatavicius, D., & Workman, M. (2002). *Medical-surgical nursing: Critical thinking for collaborative care* (4th ed., p. 1407). Philadelphia: W. B. Saunders.

3. 2

Rationale: Polydipsia and polyuria are classic symptoms of diabetes insipidus. The urine is pale, and the specific gravity is low. Anorexia and weight loss occur. Options 1 and 4 are not specific to this disorder.

Test-Taking Strategy: Use the process of elimination. Eliminate option 4 first because this symptom is rather vague and occurs in many conditions. Knowledge of the manifestations of diabetes insipidus will assist you in eliminating options 1 and 3. If you had difficulty with this question, review the clinical manifestations associated with diabetes insipidus.

Level of Cognitive Ability: Analysis
Client Needs: Physiological Integrity
Integrated Process: Nursing Process—assessment
Content Area: Adult health—endocrine
Reference: Black, J., Hawks, J., & Keene, A. (2001). *Medical-surgical nursing: Clinical management for positive outcomes* (6th ed., p. 887). Philadelphia: W. B. Saunders.

4. 4

Rationale: Because of the hypermetabolic state, the client with hyperthyroidism needs to be provided with an environment that is restful physically and mentally. Six full meals a day that are well balanced and high in calories are required because of the accelerated metabolic rate. Foods that increase peristalsis, such as high-fiber foods, need to be avoided. These clients suffer from heat intolerance and require a cool environment.

Test-Taking Strategy: Use the process of elimination. The key concept to bear in mind when answering this question is that clients with hyperthyroidism experience an accelerated metabolic rate. This concept should assist you in eliminating options 1, 2, and 3. Review the plan of care for the client with hyperthyroidism if you had difficulty with this question.

Level of Cognitive Ability: Application
Client Needs: Physiological Integrity
Integrated Process: Nursing Process—planning
Content Area: Adult health—endocrine
Reference: Phipps, W., Monahan, F., Sands, J., Marek, J., & Neighbors, M. (2003). *Medical-surgical nursing: Health and illness perspectives* (7th ed., p. 893). St. Louis: Mosby.

5. 2

Rationale: Weakness and hoarseness of the voice can occur as a result of trauma from the surgery. If this develops, the client should be reassured that the problem will subside in a few days. Unnecessary talking should be discouraged. The nurse does not need to notify the physician immediately. These signs do not indicate bleeding or the need to administer calcium gluconate.

Test-Taking Strategy: Use the process of elimination. Options 3 and 4 can be eliminated easily because they are unrelated to the signs presented in the question. No data are presented requiring immediate physician notification. Review care of the client following thyroidectomy if you had difficulty with this question.

Level of Cognitive Ability: Application
Client Needs: Physiological Integrity
Integrated Process: Nursing Process—implementation
Content Area: Adult health—endocrine
Reference: Ignatavicius, D., & Workman, M. (2002). *Medical-surgical nursing: Critical thinking for collaborative care* (4th ed., p. 1429). Philadelphia: W. B. Saunders.

6. **3**
Rationale: The initial nursing action would be to maintain a patent airway. Oxygen would be administered, followed by fluid replacement, keeping the client warm, monitoring vital signs, and administering thyroid hormones by the intravenous (IV) route.
Test-Taking Strategy: Use the process of elimination. Note the key word "initially." All of the options are appropriate interventions, but use the ABCs—airway, breathing, and circulation—in selecting the correct option. Review the initial interventions for myxedema coma if you had difficulty with this question.
Level of Cognitive Ability: Application
Client Needs: Physiological Integrity
Integrated Process: Nursing Process—implementation
Content Area: Delegating/Prioritizing
Reference: Black, J., Hawks, J., & Keene, A. (2001). *Medical-surgical nursing: Clinical management for positive outcomes* (6th ed., p. 1093). Philadelphia: W. B. Saunders.

7. **2**
Rationale: NPH is an intermediate-acting insulin. The onset of action is 1 to 2 hours, it peaks in 6 to 14 hours, and its duration of action is 24 hours. Hypoglycemic reactions most likely occur during peak time.
Test-Taking Strategy: Use the process of elimination and knowledge regarding the onset, peak, and duration of action for NPH insulin. If you had difficulty with this question, review the characteristics of NPH insulin.
Level of Cognitive Ability: Application
Client Needs: Physiological Integrity
Integrated Process: Teaching/Learning
Content Area: Adult health—endocrine
Reference: Lehne, R. (2001). *Pharmacology for nursing care* (4th ed., p. 617). Philadelphia: W. B. Saunders.

8. **2**
Rationale: The client is instructed to use a moisturizing lotion on the feet and to avoid applying the lotion between the toes. The client should be instructed not to soak the feet and should avoid hot water to prevent burns. The client may cut the toenails straight across and even with the toe itself and would consult a podiatrist if the toenails were thick or hard to cut or if vision was poor. The client should be instructed to wash the feet daily with a mild soap.
Test-Taking Strategy: Use the process of elimination. Eliminate option 3 because of the word "always" and option 1 because of the word "hot." Eliminate option 4 next because of the words "avoid" and "mild." Review diabetic foot care instructions if you had difficulty with this question.
Level of Cognitive Ability: Application
Client Needs: Health Promotion and Maintenance

Integrated Process: Nursing Process—planning
Content Area: Adult health—endocrine
Reference: Ignatavicius, D., & Workman, M. (2002). *Medical-surgical nursing: Critical thinking for collaborative care* (4th ed., p. 1474). Philadelphia: W. B. Saunders.

9. **4**
Rationale: The primary goal of treatment in hyperglycemic hyperosmolar nonketotic syndrome (HHNS) is to rehydrate the client to restore fluid volume and to correct electrolyte deficiency. Intravenous fluid replacement is similar to that administered in diabetic ketoacidosis (DKA) and begins with IV infusion of normal saline. Regular, not NPH, insulin would be administered. The use of sodium bicarbonate to correct acidosis is avoided because it can precipitate a further drop in serum potassium levels. Intubation and mechanical ventilation are not required to treat HHNS.
Test-Taking Strategy: Use the process of elimination. If you can recall the treatment for DKA, you will be able to answer this question easily. Treatment for HHNS is similar to the treatment for DKA. Review the treatment for HHNS if you had difficulty with this question.
Level of Cognitive Ability: Application
Client Needs: Physiological Integrity
Integrated Process: Nursing Process—planning
Content Area: Adult health—endocrine
Reference: Black, J., Hawks, J., & Keene, A. (2001). *Medical-surgical nursing: Clinical management for positive outcomes* (6th ed., p. 1177). Philadelphia: W. B. Saunders.

10. **1**
Rationale: An insulin pump provides a small continuous dose of regular insulin subcutaneously throughout the day and night, and the client can self-administer a bolus with additional dosage from the pump before each meal as needed. Regular insulin is used in an insulin pump. An external pump is not attached surgically to the pancreas.
Test-Taking Strategy: Use the process of elimination. Knowledge that regular insulin is used in an insulin pump will assist in eliminating options 2 and 4. Noting the word "external" in the question will assist in eliminating option 3. Review the use of the insulin pump if you are unfamiliar with it.
Level of Cognitive Ability: Application
Client Needs: Physiological Integrity
Integrated Process: Teaching/Learning
Content Area: Adult health—endocrine
Reference: Lewis, S., Heitkemper, M., & Dirksen, S. (2004). *Medical-surgical nursing: Assessment and management of clinical problems* (6th ed., pp. 1276-1277). St. Louis: Mosby.

11. **4**
Rationale: Insulin dosages should not be adjusted and should not be increased before unusual exercise. If acetone is found in the urine, it possibly may indicate the need for additional insulin. To minimize the discomfort associated with insulin injections, insulin should be administered at room temperature. Injection sites should be rotated systematically from one area to another.
Test-Taking Strategy: Use the process of elimination. Eliminate option 3 first because of the word "always."

Knowledge regarding insulin administration and the significance of acetone in the urine will assist in eliminating options 1 and 2. If you had difficulty with this question, review the components of insulin management.
Level of Cognitive Ability: Application
Client Needs: Health Promotion and Maintenance
Integrated Process: Teaching/Learning
Content Area: Adult health—endocrine
Reference: Lewis, S., Heitkemper, M., & Dirksen, S. (2004). *Medical-surgical nursing: Assessment and management of clinical problems* (6th ed., p. 1274). St. Louis: Mosby.

12. 1
Rationale: In DKA the arterial pH is less than 7.35, plasma bicarbonate is less than 15 mEq/L, the blood glucose level is higher than 250 mg/dL, and ketones are present in the blood and urine. The client would be experiencing polyuria, and Kussmaul's respirations would be present. A comatose state may occur if DKA is not treated, but coma would not confirm the diagnosis.
Test-Taking Strategy: Use the process of elimination. Note the key word "confirming" in the stem of the question. Eliminate option 4 because a comatose state can exist is many conditions. Eliminate option 3 because in acidosis the pH would be low. Remember that polyuria exists in DKA. Review the clinical manifestations of DKA if you had difficulty with this question.
Level of Cognitive Ability: Analysis
Client Needs: Physiological Integrity
Integrated Process: Nursing Process—assessment
Content Area: Adult health—endocrine
Reference: Lewis, S., Heitkemper, M., & Dirksen, S. (2004). *Medical-surgical nursing: Assessment and management of clinical problems* (6th ed., p. 1291). St. Louis: Mosby.

13. 2
Rationale: Shakiness is a sign of hypoglycemia and would indicate the need for food or glucose. A fruity breath odor, blurred vision, and polyuria are signs of hyperglycemia.
Test-Taking Strategy: Focus on the issue of the question, the treatment of hypoglycemia. Recalling the signs of hypoglycemia will direct you to option 2. Review these signs if you had difficulty with this question.
Level of Cognitive Ability: Analysis
Client Needs: Health Promotion and Maintenance
Integrated Process: Teaching/Learning
Content Area: Adult health—endocrine
Reference: Black, J., Hawks, J., & Keene, A. (2001). *Medical-surgical nursing: Clinical management for positive outcomes* (6th ed., p. 1178). Philadelphia: W. B. Saunders.

14. 4
Rationale: The most appropriate intervention is to address the client's feelings related to the anxiety. Administering a sedative is not the most appropriate intervention. The nurse should not ignore the client's anxious feelings. A client will not relate to medical terms, particularly when anxiety exists.
Test-Taking Strategy: Use therapeutic communication techniques to answer the question. Remember that the client's feelings come first. Keeping this in mind will direct you easily

to option 4. Review therapeutic communication techniques if you had difficulty with this question.
Level of Cognitive Ability: Application
Client Needs: Psychosocial Integrity
Integrated Process: Caring
Content Area: Adult health—endocrine
Reference: Ignatavicius, D., & Workman, M. (2002). *Medical-surgical nursing: Critical thinking for collaborative care* (4th ed., p. 1487). Philadelphia: W. B. Saunders.

15. 3
Rationale: During illness, the client should monitor blood glucose levels and should notify the physician if the level is greater than 250 mg/dL. Insulin should never be stopped. In fact, insulin may need to be increased during times of illness. Doses should not be adjusted without the physician's advice to do so.
Test-Taking Strategy: Use the process of elimination. Note that options 1, 2, and 4 are similar and all relate to adjustment of insulin doses. Review diabetic management during illness if you had difficulty with this question.
Level of Cognitive Ability: Analysis
Client Needs: Health Promotion and Maintenance
Integrated Process: Teaching/Learning
Content Area: Adult health—endocrine
Reference: Ignatavicius, D., & Workman, M. (2002). *Medical-surgical nursing: Critical thinking for collaborative care* (4th ed., p. 1483). Philadelphia: W. B. Saunders.

16. 1
Rationale: During management of DKA, when the blood glucose level falls to 250 to 300 mg/dL, the infusion rate is reduced and 5% dextrose is added to maintain a blood glucose level of about 250 mg/dL or until the client recovers from ketosis. NPH insulin is not used to treat DKA. Fifty percent dextrose is used to treat hypoglycemia. Phenytoin (Dilantin) is not a usual treatment measure for DKA.
Test-Taking Strategy: Use the process of elimination. Eliminate option 2 first, knowing that regular insulin is used in the management of DKA. Eliminate option 3 next, knowing that this is the treatment for hypoglycemia. Note the key words "the serum glucose level is now 240 mg/dL." This should indicate that the IV solution of 5% dextrose is the next step in management of care. Review care of the client with DKA if you had difficulty with this question.
Level of Cognitive Ability: Application
Client Needs: Physiological Integrity
Integrated Process: Nursing Process—planning
Content Area: Adult health—endocrine
Reference: Lewis, S., Heitkemper, M., & Dirksen, S. (2004). *Medical-surgical nursing: Assessment and management of clinical problems* (6th ed., p. 1293). St. Louis: Mosby.

17. 1
Rationale: Excessive dosing with propylthiouracil (PTU) may convert the client from a hyperthyroid state to a hypothyroid state. If this occurs, the dosage should be reduced. Temporary administration of thyroid hormone may be required. Propylthiouracil is not used for pain and does not cause hyperglycemia or renal toxicity.

Test-Taking Strategy: Read the question carefully, noting the client's diagnosis. Noting that propylthiouracil is used to treat hyperthyroidism should direct you easily to option 1. If you had difficulty with this question, review the side effects and adverse effects of this medication.
Level of Cognitive Ability: Application
Client Needs: Physiological Integrity
Integrated Process: Nursing Process—assessment
Content Area: Adult health—endocrine
Reference: Hodgson, B., & Kizior, R. (2004). *Saunders nursing drug handbook 2004* (p. 852). Philadelphia: W. B. Saunders.

18. **2**
Rationale: Calcitonin can lower plasma calcium levels in clients with hypercalcemia caused by hyperparathyroidism. The therapeutic effect in this client situation would be a reduction in serum calcium levels. Options 1, 3, and 4 are incorrect outcome criteria.
Test-Taking Strategy: Use the process of elimination. Reading the question carefully, noting the client's diagnosis, will assist in directing you to option 2. In addition, note the relationship between the name of the medication and the word "calcium" in option 2. Review the action of this medication if you are unfamiliar with it.
Level of Cognitive Ability: Analysis
Client Needs: Physiological Integrity
Integrated Process: Nursing Process—evaluation
Content Area: Adult health—endocrine
Reference: Hodgson, B., & Kizior, R. (2004). *Saunders nursing drug handbook 2004* (p. 137). Philadelphia: W. B. Saunders.

19. **2**
Rationale: Levothyroxine (Synthroid) is a synthetic thyroid hormone that increases cellular metabolism. Levothyroxine should be given in the morning in a single dose to prevent sleeplessness and should be given at the same time each day to maintain an adequate drug level.
Test-Taking Strategy: Use the process of elimination. Focus on the key word "daily" in the question to direct you to option 2. Review the administration of this medication if you had difficulty with this question.
Level of Cognitive Ability: Application
Client Needs: Physiological Integrity
Integrated Process: Nursing Process—planning
Content Area: Adult health—endocrine
Reference: Hodgson, B., & Kizior, R. (2004). *Saunders nursing drug handbook 2004* (p. 598). Philadelphia: W. B. Saunders.

20. **4**
Rationale: Chlorpropamide (Diabinese) is an oral hypoglycemic agent given to reduce the serum glucose level and the signs and symptoms of hyperglycemia. Therefore a decrease in polyuria and polyphagia and symptoms of hyperglycemia would denote a beneficial response to chlorpropamide. Laboratory values also are used to assess the client's response to treatment. A fasting blood glucose level of 110 mg/dL is within normal limits. However, a glycosylated hemoglobin of 10% denotes poor glycemic control.
Test-Taking Strategy: Use the process of elimination. Note the key word "not" in the stem of the question. Knowledge that

chlorpropamide is an oral hypoglycemic agent tells you to look for an option that would denote hyperglycemia (lack of response to medication). Options 1 and 3 are similar and can be eliminated first. Knowledge of the normal blood glucose level will assist in eliminating option 2. Review the action and expected therapeutic outcome of chlorpropamide if you had difficulty with this question.
Level of Cognitive Ability: Analysis
Client Needs: Physiological Integrity
Integrated Process: Nursing Process—evaluation
Content Area: Adult health—endocrine
References: Chernecky, C., & Berger, B. (2004). *Laboratory tests & diagnostic procedures* (4th ed., p. 615). Philadelphia: W. B. Saunders.
Hodgson, B., & Kizior, R. (2003). *Saunders nursing drug handbook 2003* (p. 39C). Philadelphia: W. B. Saunders.

21. **3**
Rationale: Desmopressin (DDAVP, Stimate) is a synthetic form of antidiuretic hormone that causes increased reabsorption of water with a resultant decrease in urine output. The therapeutic response to DDAVP or Stimate would demonstrate a decrease in serum osmolality, because more fluid is retained, and an increase in urine osmolality, because less fluid is excreted. Increased blood pressure is a side effect rather than a therapeutic effect of DDAVP or Stimate.
Test-Taking Strategy: Use the process of elimination and note the client's diagnosis. Focus on the issue, therapeutic effect. Knowledge of the therapeutic effects of the medication will direct you to the correct option. Review these therapeutic effects if you had difficulty with this question.
Level of Cognitive Ability: Analysis
Client Needs: Physiological Integrity
Integrated Process: Nursing Process—evaluation
Content Area: Adult health—endocrine
Reference: Hodgson, B., & Kizior, R. (2004). *Saunders nursing drug handbook 2004* (p. 286). Philadelphia: W. B. Saunders.

22. **3**
Rationale: Classic symptoms of hyperglycemia include polydipsia, polyuria, and polyphagia. Options 1, 2, and 4 are not signs of hyperglycemia.
Test-Taking Strategy: Use the process of elimination. Remember the three P's: polyuria, polydipsia, polyphagia. Learn the signs of hyperglycemia if you had difficulty with this question.
Level of Cognitive Ability: Analysis
Client Needs: Physiological Integrity
Integrated Process: Nursing Process—assessment
Content Area: Adult health—endocrine
Reference: Lewis, S., Heitkemper, M., & Dirksen, S. (2004). *Medical-surgical nursing: Assessment and management of clinical problems* (6th ed., p. 1272). St. Louis: Mosby.

23. **1**
Rationale: Increased blood glucose will cause the kidneys to excrete the glucose in the urine. This glucose is accompanied by fluids and electrolytes, causing an osmotic diuresis leading to dehydration. This fluid loss must be replaced when it becomes severe. Options 2, 3, and 4 are not related specifically to the issue of the question.

Test-Taking Strategy: Use Maslow's hierarchy of needs to answer this question. Option 1 indicates a physiological need and is the priority. Options 2, 3, and 4 are nursing diagnoses that may need to be addressed after providing for the high-priority physiological needs.
Level of Cognitive Ability: Analysis
Client Needs: Physiological Integrity
Integrated Process: Nursing Process—analysis
Content Area: Delegating/Prioritizing
Reference: Lewis, S., Heitkemper, M., & Dirksen, S. (2004). *Medical-surgical nursing: Assessment and management of clinical problems* (6th ed., p. 1291). St. Louis: Mosby.

24. 1
Rationale: When a client with diabetes mellitus is unable to eat normally because of illness, the client still should take the prescribed insulin or oral medication. The client should consume additional fluids and should notify the physician. The client should monitor the blood glucose level every 3 to 4 hours.
Test-Taking Strategy: Use the process of elimination and knowledge regarding the guidelines related to illness in the diabetic client to answer this question. Remembering that the client needs to take insulin will direct you easily to option 1. Review these guidelines if you had difficulty with this question.
Level of Cognitive Ability: Analysis
Client Needs: Health Promotion and Maintenance
Integrated Process: Teaching/Learning
Content Area: Adult health—endocrine
Reference: Lewis, S., Heitkemper, M., & Dirksen, S. (2004). *Medical-surgical nursing: Assessment and management of clinical problems* (6th ed., p. 1285). St. Louis: Mosby.

25. 3
Rationale: Client education following DKA should emphasize the need for home glucose monitoring 2 to 4 times per day. Instructing the client to notify the health care provider when illness occurs also is important. The presence of urine ketones indicates that DKA has occurred already. The client should eat well-balanced meals with snacks as prescribed.
Test-Taking Strategy: Use the process of elimination and focus on the issue "prevent a recurrence." Option 1 is not an accurate component of the dietary measures for a client with diabetes mellitus. Option 2 will not prevent DKA, and option 4 does not prevent DKA but actually confirms the diagnosis. Review the measures to prevent DKA if you had difficulty with this question.
Level of Cognitive Ability: Application
Client Needs: Health Promotion and Maintenance
Integrated Process: Nursing Process—planning
Content Area: Adult health—endocrine
Reference: Phipps, W., Monahan, F., Sands, J., Marek, J., & Neighbors, M. (2003). *Medical-surgical nursing: Health and illness perspectives* (7th ed., p. 975). St. Louis: Mosby.

26. 1
Rationale: Lack (absolute or relative) of insulin is the primary cause of DKA. Treatment consists of insulin administration (regular insulin), IV fluid administration (normal saline initially), and potassium replacement, followed by

correcting acidosis. Applying an electrocardiogram monitor is not a priority action.
Test-Taking Strategy: Use the process of elimination and focus on the client's diagnosis. Note the key word "priority." Remember that in DKA, the initial treatment is regular insulin. Normal saline is administered initially; therefore option 2 is incorrect. Options 3 and 4 may be components of the treatment plan but are not the priority. Review the initial treatment for DKA if you had difficulty with this question.
Level of Cognitive Ability: Application
Client Needs: Physiological Integrity
Integrated Process: Nursing Process—implementation
Content Area: Adult health—endocrine
Reference: Phipps, W., Monahan, F., Sands, J., Marek, J., & Neighbors, M. (2003). *Medical-surgical nursing: Health and illness perspectives* (7th ed., p. 975). St. Louis: Mosby.

27. 3
Rationale: Hyperglycemic hyperosmolar nonketotic syndrome occurs in clients with type 2 diabetes mellitus. The onset of symptoms may be gradual. The symptoms may include polyuria, polydipsia, dehydration, mental status alterations, weight loss, and weakness. Options 1, 2, and 4 are incorrect interpretations of the client's symptoms.
Test-Taking Strategy: Use the process of elimination and note the key words "with a blood glucose greater than 600 mg/dL." This will assist you in eliminating options 2 and 4. Recalling that HHNS most commonly occurs in type 2 diabetes mellitus will direct you easily to option 3. Review the clinical manifestations of HHNS if you had difficulty with this question.
Level of Cognitive Ability: Analysis
Client Needs: Physiological Integrity
Integrated Process: Nursing Process—analysis
Content Area: Adult health—endocrine
Reference: Phipps, W., Monahan, F., Sands, J., Marek, J., & Neighbors, M. (2003). *Medical-surgical nursing: Health and illness perspectives* (7th ed., p. 974). St. Louis: Mosby.

28. 2
Rationale: Hyperglycemic hyperosmolar nonketotic syndrome (HHNS) is differentiated from diabetic ketoacidosis (DKA) by the absence of ketones in the urine. Options 1, 3, and 4 will not assist in determining a potential diagnosis.
Test-Taking Strategy: Use the process of elimination and note the signs and symptoms presented in the question. Eliminate options 1 and 4 first because they are similar. From the remaining options, option 2 is related most specifically to a client with diabetes mellitus. Review the differences between DKA and HHNS if you had difficulty with this question.
Level of Cognitive Ability: Analysis
Client Needs: Health Promotion and Maintenance
Integrated Process: Nursing Process—assessment
Content Area: Adult health—endocrine
Reference: Phipps, W., Monahan, F., Sands, J., Marek, J., & Neighbors, M. (2003). *Medical-surgical nursing: Health and illness perspectives* (7th ed., p. 974). St. Louis: Mosby.

29. 4
Rationale: An elevated temperature may indicate infection. Infection is a leading cause of hyperglycemic hyperosmolar

nonketotic syndrome or diabetic ketoacidosis. The other findings noted in the question are within normal limits.

Test-Taking Strategy: Use the process of elimination and knowledge of the normal values of vital signs to direct you to option 4. The client's temperature is the only abnormal value. Remember that an elevated temperature can indicate an infectious process that can lead to complications in the client with diabetes mellitus. Review normal and abnormal findings in the client with diabetes mellitus if you had difficulty with this question.

Level of Cognitive Ability: Analysis
Client Needs: Physiological Integrity
Integrated Process: Nursing Process—analysis
Content Area: Adult health—endocrine
Reference: Lewis, S., Heitkemper, M., & Dirksen, S. (2004). *Medical-surgical nursing: Assessment and management of clinical problems* (6th ed., p. 1290). St. Louis: Mosby.

30. 2
Rationale: Clients with type 2 diabetes mellitus have decreased or impaired insulin secretion. Oral hypoglycemic agents are given to these clients to facilitate glucose utilization. Insulin injections may be given during times of stress-induced hyperglycemia. Oral insulin is not available because of the breakdown of the insulin by digestion. Options 1, 3, and 4 are incorrect.

Test-Taking Strategy: Use the process of elimination, focusing on the issue, type 2 diabetes mellitus. Eliminate option 1 because "oral insulin" is not available. Treatment with medication does not mean that the client can eat more; therefore eliminate option 3. Recalling that during times of illness insulin may be required will eliminate option 4. Review treatment measures for type 2 diabetes mellitus if you had difficulty with this question.

Level of Cognitive Ability: Analysis
Client Needs: Physiological Integrity
Integrated Process: Nursing Process—evaluation
Content Area: Adult health—endocrine
Reference: Lewis, S., Heitkemper, M., & Dirksen, S. (2004). *Medical-surgical nursing: Assessment and management of clinical problems* (6th ed., p. 1271). St. Louis: Mosby.

31. 4
Rationale: A diet low in carbohydrates and sodium but ample in protein and potassium is encouraged for a client with Cushing's syndrome. Such a diet promotes weight loss, reduction of edema and hypertension, control of hypokalemia, and rebuilding of wasted tissue.

Test-Taking Strategy: Use the process of elimination. Eliminate option 1 because it reflects that no dietary change is necessary. Eliminate option 2 next because protein most likely is limited in liver or renal disorders. From the remaining options, eliminate option 3 because excess sodium is not normally healthy. Review dietary management in Cushing's syndrome if you had difficulty with this question.

Level of Cognitive Ability: Analysis
Client Needs: Health Promotion and Maintenance
Integrated Process: Teaching/Learning
Content Area: Adult health—endocrine
References: Black, J., Hawks, J., & Keene, A. (2001). *Medical-surgical nursing: Clinical management for positive outcomes* (6th ed., p. 1131). Philadelphia: W. B. Saunders.

Ignatavicius, D., & Workman, M. (2002). *Medical-surgical nursing: Critical thinking for collaborative care* (4th ed., p. 1419). Philadelphia: W. B. Saunders.

32. 1
Rationale: A hypoglycemic reaction may occur in response to increased exercise. Clients should avoid exercise during the peak time of insulin. NPH insulin peaks at 6 to 14 hours; therefore afternoon exercise will occur during the peak of the medication. Options 2, 3, and 4 do not address peak action times.

Test-Taking Strategy: Use the process of elimination and note the key words "inadequate understanding." Focus on the issue, "peak action of the NPH." Recalling that NPH peaks at 6 to 14 hours will direct you to option 1. Review the peak action time of NPH if you had difficulty with this question.

Level of Cognitive Ability: Analysis
Client Needs: Physiological Integrity
Integrated Process: Nursing Process—evaluation
Content Area: Adult health—endocrine
Reference: Lewis, S., Heitkemper, M., & Dirksen, S. (2004). *Medical-surgical nursing: Assessment and management of clinical problems* (6th ed., p. 1282). St. Louis: Mosby.

33. 2
Rationale: Hypercalcemia is the hallmark of hyperparathyroidism. Elevated serum calcium levels produce osmotic diuresis and thus polyuria. This diuresis leads to dehydration (weight loss rather than weight gain). Options 1 and 3 are gastrointestinal symptoms and are not associated with the common gastrointestinal symptoms typical of hyperparathyroidism (nausea, vomiting, anorexia, constipation).

Test-Taking Strategy: Use the process of elimination. Note that options 1, 3, and 4 are gastrointestinal symptoms and are similar. Review the clinical manifestations of hyperparathyroidism if you had difficulty with this question.

Level of Cognitive Ability: Analysis
Client Needs: Physiological Integrity
Integrated Process: Nursing Process—assessment
Content Area: Adult health—endocrine
Reference: Black, J., Hawks, J., & Keene, A. (2001). *Medical-surgical nursing: Clinical management for positive outcomes* (6th ed., p. 1109). Philadelphia: W. B. Saunders.

34. 3
Rationale: During the postoperative period, the nurse carefully observes the client for signs of hemorrhage, which causes swelling and compression of adjacent tissue. Laryngeal stridor is a harsh, high-pitched sound heard on inspiration and expiration; stridor is caused by compression of the trachea, leading to respiratory distress. Stridor is an acute emergency situation that requires immediate attention to avoid complete obstruction of the airway. Options 1, 2, and 4 do not identify signs of a life-threatening complication.

Test-Taking Strategy: Consider the anatomical location of the surgical procedure and use the ABCs—airway, breathing, and circulation—to select the correct option. Options 1, 2, and 4 are usual postoperative findings that are not life threatening. Option 3 addresses airway. Review postoperative care of the parathyroidectomy client if you had difficulty with this question.

Level of Cognitive Ability: Analysis
Client Needs: Physiological Integrity
Integrated Process: Nursing Process—assessment
Content Area: Adult health—endocrine
References: Black, J., Hawks, J., & Keene, A. (2001). *Medical-surgical nursing: Clinical management for positive outcomes* (6th ed., p. 1113). Philadelphia: W. B. Saunders.
Ignatavicius, D., & Workman, M. (2002). *Medical surgical nursing: Critical thinking for collaborative care* (4th ed., p. 1438). Philadelphia: W. B. Saunders.

35. **2**
Rationale: Lipodystrophy (hypertrophy of subcutaneous tissue at the injection site) occurs in some clients with diabetes mellitus when injection sites are used for a prolonged period of time. Thus clients are instructed to adhere to a plan of rotating injection sites to avoid tissue changes. Cleansing with alcohol, aspiration, and angle of insulin administration do not produce this complication.
Test-Taking Strategy: Use the process of elimination and knowledge of the definition of lipodystrophy to answer this question. This will direct you easily to option 2. Review this complication of insulin therapy if you had difficulty with this question.
Level of Cognitive Ability: Analysis
Client Needs: Physiological Integrity
Integrated Process: Nursing Process—assessment
Content Area: Adult health—endocrine
Reference: Ignatavicius, D., & Workman, M. (2002). *Medical-surgical nursing: Critical thinking for collaborative care* (4th ed., p. 1460). Philadelphia: W. B. Saunders.

36. **4**
Rationale: Decreased blood glucose levels produce autonomic nervous system symptoms, which are manifested classically as nervousness, irritability, and tremors. Option 1 is more likely to occur with hyperglycemia. Options 2 and 3 are unrelated to the signs of hypoglycemia.
Test-Taking Strategy: Use the process of elimination and focus on the issue, hypoglycemic reaction. Recalling the signs of this type of reaction will direct you easily to option 4. Review the signs of hypoglycemia if you had difficulty with this question.
Level of Cognitive Ability: Analysis
Client Needs: Physiological Integrity
Integrated Process: Nursing Process—assessment
Content Area: Adult health—endocrine
References: Black, J., Hawks, J., & Keene, A. (2001). *Medical-surgical nursing: Clinical management for positive outcomes* (6th ed., p. 1178). Philadelphia: W. B. Saunders.
Ignatavicius, D., & Workman, M. (2002). *Medical-surgical nursing: Critical thinking for collaborative care* (4th ed., p. 1479). Philadelphia: W. B. Saunders.

37. **3**
Rationale: Small amounts of fluid may be tolerated even when vomiting is present. The nurse should encourage liquids containing glucose and electrolytes every hour. Options 1, 2, and 4 will not provide the adequate intake needed by the client with diabetes mellitus.
Test-Taking Strategy: Use the process of elimination. Eliminate options 1 and 2 because of the words "only" and "all." The time

frame in option 4 (5 days) is unreasonable; therefore select option 3. Review care of the client with diabetes mellitus during times of illness if you had difficulty with this question.
Level of Cognitive Ability: Application
Client Needs: Physiological Integrity
Integrated Process: Nursing Process—implementation
Content Area: Adult health—endocrine
Reference: Phipps, W., Monahan, F., Sands, J., Marek, J., & Neighbors, M. (2003). *Medical-surgical nursing: Health and illness perspectives* (7th ed., p. 245). St. Louis: Mosby.

38. **1**
Rationale: Manifestations of hypothyroidism include cold intolerance, constipation, loss of initiative, thick dry skin, weight gain, a notably puffy appearance of the skin around the eyes, slowed intellectual function, including retarded speech and apathy, and low metabolic rate. Levothyroxine (Synthroid) is used to correct hypothyroidism. The dosage needs to be increased.
Test-Taking Strategy: Use the process of elimination. Note the key words "currently is taking." Knowledge that the signs presented in the question relate to the manifestations associated with hypothyroidism will direct you easily to option 1. The dosage needs to be increased. Review the expected therapeutic effect of levothyroxine if you had difficulty with this question.
Level of Cognitive Ability: Analysis
Client Needs: Physiological Integrity
Integrated Process: Nursing Process—analysis
Content Area: Adult health—endocrine
Reference: Lewis, S., Heitkemper, M., & Dirksen, S. (2004). *Medical-surgical nursing: Assessment and management of clinical problems* (6th ed., 1320). St. Louis: Mosby.

39. **1**
Rationale: Prednisone may decrease the effect of oral hypoglycemics, insulin, diuretics, and potassium supplements. Options 2, a β-blocker, and 3, a monoamine oxidase inhibitor, have their own intrinsic hypoglycemic activity. Option 4 decreases urinary excretion of sulfonylurea agents, causing increased levels of the oral agents, which can lead to hypoglycemia.
Test-Taking Strategy: Use the process of elimination and recall that prednisone decreases the effects of oral hypoglycemics. Review medication interactions with hypoglycemics if you had difficulty with this question.
Level of Cognitive Ability: Analysis
Client Needs: Physiological Integrity
Integrated Process: Nursing Process—analysis
Content Area: Adult health—endocrine
Reference: Hodgson, B., & Kizior, R. (2004). *Saunders nursing drug handbook 2004* (p. 831). Philadelphia: W. B. Saunders.

40. **3**
Rationale: Vasopressin, an antidiuretic hormone, increases reabsorption of water by the renal tubules; causes vasoconstriction with reduced blood flow in coronary, peripheral, cerebral, and pulmonary vessels; increases gastrointestinal smooth muscle tone and contractions; and decreases urine output.

Test-Taking Strategy: Use the process of elimination. Recalling the pathophysiology associated with diabetes insipidus will direct you to the correct option. If you had difficulty with this question, review this disorder and the effects of this medication.
Level of Cognitive Ability: Analysis
Client Needs: Physiological Integrity
Integrated Process: Nursing Process—evaluation
Content Area: Adult health—endocrine
Reference: Hodgson, B., & Kizior, R. (2004). *Saunders nursing drug handbook 2004* (p. 1043). Philadelphia: W. B. Saunders.

41. **2**
Rationale: Pheochromocytoma is a catecholamine-producing tumor and causes secretion of excessive amounts of epinephrine and norepinephrine. Hypertension is the principal manifestation, and the client has episodes of a high blood pressure accompanied by pounding headaches. The excessive release of catecholamine also results in excessive conversion of glycogen into glucose in the liver. Consequently, hyperglycemia and glucosuria occur during attacks. Pheochromocytoma is curable. The primary treatment is surgical removal of one or both of the adrenal glands, depending on whether the tumor is unilateral or bilateral.
Test-Taking Strategy: Use the process of elimination and knowledge of the manifestations of pheochromocytoma to answer this question. If you are unfamiliar with this disorder, review this content.
Level of Cognitive Ability: Comprehension
Client Needs: Physiological Integrity
Integrated Process: Nursing Process—planning
Content Area: Adult health—endocrine
Reference: Black, J., Hawks, J., & Keene, A. (2001). *Medical-surgical nursing: Clinical management for positive outcomes* (6th ed., p. 1135). Philadelphia: W. B. Saunders.

42. **4**
Rationale: Hypertension is the major symptom associated with pheochromocytoma. Taking the client's blood pressure would assess the blood pressure status. Glycosuria, weight loss, and diaphoresis are also clinical manifestations of pheochromocytoma, yet hypertension is the major symptom.
Test-Taking Strategy: Use the process of elimination, noting the key words "major symptom." Use the ABCs—airway, breathing, and circulation. A method of assessing circulation is to take the blood pressure. Review the clinical manifestations of pheochromocytoma if you had difficulty with this question.
Level of Cognitive Ability: Analysis
Client Needs: Physiological Integrity
Integrated Process: Nursing Process—assessment
Content Area: Delegating/Prioritizing
Reference: Black, J., Hawks, J., & Keene, A. (2001). *Medical-surgical nursing: Clinical management for positive outcomes* (6th ed., p. 1137). Philadelphia: W. B. Saunders.

43. **3**
Rationale: Assays of catecholamines are performed on single-voided urine specimens, 2- to 4-hour specimens, and 24-hour urine specimens. The normal range of urinary catecholamines

is up to 14 mcg/100 mL of urine, with higher levels occurring in pheochromocytoma.
Test-Taking Strategy: Recall that pheochromocytoma is a catecholamine-producing tumor. Because the question addresses urine specimens for catecholamine testing, expect the results to indicate higher than normal amounts of catecholamine. In addition, the question addresses that the client is suspected of having pheochromocytoma, so if you need to select an answer and you are not sure, select the option that has similarity to a thought in the question. In this case, suspected pheochromocytoma is similar to "indicating pheochromocytoma" in option 3. Review diagnostic tests for pheochromocytoma if you had difficulty with this question.
Level of Cognitive Ability: Analysis
Client Needs: Physiological Integrity
Integrated Process: Nursing Process—analysis
Content Area: Adult health—endocrine
Reference: Black, J., Hawks, J., & Keene, A. (2001). *Medical-surgical nursing: Clinical management for positive outcomes* (6th ed., p. 1136). Philadelphia: W. B. Saunders.

44. **1**
Rationale: Hypertension is the hallmark of pheochromocytoma. Severe hypertension can precipitate a cerebrovascular accident or sudden blindness. Although all of the options are accurate nursing interventions for the client with pheochromocytoma, the priority nursing action is to monitor the vital signs, particularly the blood pressure.
Test-Taking Strategy: Use the process of elimination. Note the key words "priority nursing action." Use the ABCs—airway, breathing, and circulation. Monitoring vital signs is the nursing action that would assess airway, breathing, and circulation. Also, options 2, 3, and 4 refer to the assessment of the renal system, whereas option 1 does not. Review preoperative care of the client with pheochromocytoma if you had difficulty with this question.
Level of Cognitive Ability: Application
Client Needs: Physiological Integrity
Integrated Process: Nursing Process—implementation
Content Area: Delegating/Prioritizing
Reference: Black, J., Hawks, J., & Keene, A. (2001). *Medical-surgical nursing: Clinical management for positive outcomes* (6th ed., p. 1137). Philadelphia: W. B. Saunders.

45. **2**
Rationale: The most likely medication to be prescribed in hypertensive crisis is phentolamine mesylate (Regitine). This medication is a short-acting α-adrenergic blocker and would be given by IV bolus or drip for hypertensive crisis. Phenoxybenzamine hydrochloride (Dibenzyline) is an oral medication and produces long-acting α-adrenergic blockade. Phenoxybenzamine is used to manage pheochromocytoma and is most suitable for preoperative management of hypertension and prevention of hypertensive crisis. Prazosin hydrochloride (Minipress), an α-blocker, is used less frequently for the preoperative pheochromocytoma client because of its shorter duration of action. The physician would not prescribe β-receptor blocking agents in clients with suspected or confirmed pheochromocytoma until after α-adrenergic blockade has been initiated because these medications may cause the

blood pressure to rise. After α-adrenergic blockade, low doses of propranolol (Inderal) may be used to treat tachycardia and dysrhythmias.

Test-Taking Strategy: Use the process of elimination. Note that the question asks about hypertensive crisis, and such a situation requires immediate intervention. Recalling that phentolamine mesylate (Regitine) is a short-acting medication will direct you to this option. Review medications to treat hypertensive crisis if you had difficulty with this question.

Level of Cognitive Ability: Analysis
Client Needs: Physiological Integrity
Integrated Process: Nursing Process—analysis
Content Area: Adult health—endocrine
Reference: Ignatavicius, D., & Workman, M. (2002). *Medical-surgical nursing: Critical thinking for collaborative care* (4th ed., p. 1420). Philadelphia: W. B. Saunders.

46. 1
Rationale: The client with pheochromocytoma needs to be provided with a diet high in vitamins, minerals, and calories. Of particular importance are the foods or beverages that contain caffeine, such as cocoa, coffee, tea, or colas. These foods are prohibited because they can precipitate a hypertensive crisis.

Test-Taking Strategy: Use the process of elimination. Note that options 2, 3, and 4 are similar in that they include a drink that contains caffeine; therefore, eliminate these options. Review dietary measures for the client with pheochromocytoma if you had difficulty with this question.

Level of Cognitive Ability: Application
Client Needs: Physiological Integrity
Integrated Process: Nursing Process—implementation
Content Area: Adult health—endocrine
Reference: Ignatavicius, D., & Workman, M. (2002). *Medical-surgical nursing: Critical thinking for collaborative care* (4th ed., p. 1421). Philadelphia: W.B. Saunders.

47. 2
Rationale: The complications associated with pheochromocytoma include hypertensive retinopathy and nephropathy, myocarditis, increased platelet aggregation, and cerebrovascular accident. Death can occur from shock, cerebrovascular accident, renal failure, dysrhythmias, or dissecting aortic aneurysm. An irregular heart rate indicates the presence of a dysrhythmia. A urinary output of 50 mL per hour is an adequate output. A blood urea nitrogen level of 20 mg/dL is a normal finding. A coagulation time of 5 minutes is normal.

Test-Taking Strategy: Use the process of elimination and the ABCs—airway, breathing, and circulation. An irregular heart rate is associated with circulation. In addition, if you knew the normal hourly expectations associated with urinary output and the normal laboratory values for coagulation time and blood urea nitrogen, you would be directed easily to option 2. Review the complications associated with pheochromocytoma if you had difficulty with this question.

Level of Cognitive Ability: Analysis
Client Needs: Physiological Integrity
Integrated Process: Nursing Process—analysis
Content Area: Adult health—endocrine

Reference: Black, J., Hawks, J., & Keene, A. (2001). *Medical-surgical nursing: Clinical management for positive outcomes* (6th ed., p. 1136). Philadelphia: W. B. Saunders.

48. 2
Rationale: Aspirin and other over-the-counter medications should not be taken unless the client consults with the physician. The client needs to take the medication at the same time every day and should be instructed not to stop the medication. A slight weight gain as a result of an improved appetite is expected, but after the dosage is stabilized, a weight gain of 5 lb or more weekly should be reported to the physician. Caffeine-containing foods and fluids need to be avoided because they may contribute to steroid-ulcer development.

Test-Taking Strategy: Use the process of elimination, noting the key words "further teaching is necessary." Remember that a client should not take other medications, especially over-the-counter medications, without first consulting with his or her physician. Review teaching points for the client taking prednisone if you had difficulty with this question.

Level of Cognitive Ability: Analysis
Client Needs: Health Promotion and Maintenance
Integrated Process: Teaching/Learning
Content Area: Adult health—endocrine
Reference: Kee, J., & Hayes, E. (2003). *Pharmacology: A nursing process approach* (4th ed., p. 728). Philadelphia: W. B. Saunders.

49. 2
Rationale: A high-complex-carbohydrate and high-protein diet will be prescribed for the client with Addison's disease. To prevent excess fluid and sodium loss, the client is instructed to maintain a normal salt intake daily (3 g) and to increase salt intake during hot weather, before strenuous exercise, and in response to fever, vomiting, or diarrhea.

Test-Taking Strategy: Use the process of elimination and knowledge regarding the pathophysiology associated with Addison's disease to answer this question. If you are unfamiliar with this disorder, review the pathophysiology and dietary measures associated with Addison's disease.

Level of Cognitive Ability: Analysis
Client Needs: Physiological Integrity
Integrated Process: Nursing Process—planning
Content Area: Adult health—endocrine
References: Lewis, S., Heitkemper, M., & Dirksen, S. (2004). *Medical-surgical nursing: Assessment and management of clinical problems* (6th ed., p. 1334). St. Louis: Mosby.
Phipps, W., Monahan, F., Sands, J., Marek, J., & Neighbors, M. (2003). *Medical-surgical nursing: Health and illness perspectives* (7th ed., p. 922). St. Louis: Mosby.

50. 1
Rationale: Cushing's syndrome is characterized by an oversecretion of glucocorticoid hormones. Addison's disease is characterized by the failure of the adrenal cortex to produce and secrete adrenocorticol hormones. Options 3 and 4 are inaccurate regarding Cushing's syndrome.

Test-Taking Strategy: Use the process of elimination. Options 2 and 4 can be eliminated easily if you remember that in Cushing's (up) syndrome there is an oversecretion and in Addison's disease there is an undersecretion. Next eliminate

option 3 because this disease is unrelated to insulin. Review the pathophysiology associated with Cushing's syndrome if you had difficulty with this question.
Level of Cognitive Ability: Comprehension
Client Needs: Physiological Integrity
Integrated Process: Teaching/Learning
Content Area: Adult health—endocrine
Reference: Black, J., Hawks, J., & Keene, A. (2001). *Medical-surgical nursing: Clinical management for positive outcomes* (6th ed., p. 1126). Philadelphia: W. B. Saunders.

CRITICAL THINKING: PRIORITIZING (ORDERED RESPONSE)

Answer: 21345
Rationale: The client is experiencing symptoms of mild hypoglycemia. If symptoms such as hunger, irritability, shakiness, or weakness occur, the nurse first would check the client's blood glucose level to verify that the client is experiencing hypoglycemia. Once this is verified, the nurse would give the client 10 to 15 g of carbohydrates. The nurse would retest the blood glucose in 15 minutes. In the meantime, the nurse would check the client's vital signs. The nurse would give the client another 10- to 15-g carbohydrate food item if the client's symptoms do not resolve. Otherwise, the nurse would provide a small snack of carbohydrates and protein if the client's next scheduled meal is more than an hour away from the time of the occurrence. Following treatment and resolution of the hypoglycemic event, the nurse would document the occurrence, actions taken, and outcome.
Test-Taking Strategy: Focus on the client's symptoms. Noting that the client is hospitalized will assist you in determining that the first action would be to check the client's blood glucose. Once this has been done, treating the hypoglycemia is necessary. Recalling that an outcome cannot be determined until treatment has been instituted will assist you in selecting the documentation action as the last action. From the remaining two actions, select taking the vital signs as the third action. The nurse would not give the client a carbohydrate and protein item immediately after giving the client a 10- to 15-g carbohydrate item. Review management of hypoglycemia if you had difficulty with this question.
Level of Cognitive Ability: Application
Client Needs: Physiological Integrity
Integrated Process: Nursing Process—implementation
Content Area: Delegating/Prioritizing
Reference: Ignatavicius, D., & Workman, M. (2002). *Medical-surgical nursing: Critical thinking for collaborative care* (4th ed., p. 1479). Philadelphia: W. B. Saunders.

REFERENCES

Black, J., Hawks, J., & Keene, A. (2001). *Medical-surgical nursing: Clinical management for positive outcomes* (6th ed.). Philadelphia: W. B. Saunders.

Chernecky, C., & Berger, B. (2004). *Laboratory tests and diagnostic procedures* (4th ed.). Philadelphia: W. B. Saunders.

Hodgson, B., & Kizior, R. (2003). *Saunders nursing drug handbook 2003.* Philadelphia: W. B. Saunders.

Hodgson, B., & Kizior, R. (2004). *Saunders nursing drug handbook 2004.* Philadelphia: W. B. Saunders.

Ignatavicius, D., & Workman, M. (2002). *Medical-surgical nursing: Critical thinking for collaborative care* (4th ed.). Philadelphia: W. B. Saunders.

Kee, J., & Hayes, E. (2003). *Pharmacology: A nursing process approach* (4th ed.). Philadelphia: W. B. Saunders.

Lehne, R. (2001). *Pharmacology for nursing care* (4th ed.). Philadelphia: W. B. Saunders.

Lewis, S., Heitkemper, M., & Dirksen, S. (2004). *Medical-surgical nursing: Assessment and management of clinical problems* (6th ed.). St. Louis: Mosby.

Phipps, W., Monahan, F., Sands, J., Marek, J., & Neighbors, M. (2003). *Medical-surgical nursing: Health and illness perspectives* (7th ed.). St. Louis: Mosby.

54

Endocrine Medications

I. PITUITARY MEDICATIONS

A. Description
1. The anterior pituitary gland secretes growth hormone, thyroid-stimulating hormone, adreno-corticotropic hormone, and gonadotropins (follicle-stimulating hormone and luteinizing hormone).
2. The posterior pituitary gland secretes antidiuretic hormones (vasopressin) and oxytocin.

B. Growth hormones and related medications
1. Uses and side effects (Table 54-1)
2. Interventions
   a. Assess child's physical growth and compare growth with standards.
   b. Recommend annual bone age determinations for children receiving growth hormones.
   c. Monitor blood and urine glucose levels.
   d. Teach the client and family about the importance of follow-up regarding blood and urine glucose testing.

II. ANTIDIURETIC HORMONES (BOX 54-1)

A. Description
1. Antidiuretic hormones enhance reabsorption of water in the kidneys, promoting an antidiuretic effect and regulating fluid balance.
2. Antidiuretic hormones are used in **diabetes insipidus.**

B. Side effects
1. Flushing
2. Headache
3. Nausea and abdominal cramps
4. Water intoxication
5. Hypertension with water intoxication
6. Nasal congestion with nasal administration

BOX 54-1

Antidiuretic Hormones

Desmopressin acetate (DDAVP, Stimate)
Vasopressin (Pitressin)

TABLE 54-1

Growth Hormones and Related Medications

Medication(s)	Use	Side Effects
Somatrem (Protropin)	Growth failure (adults)	Development of antibodies to growth hormone
Somatropin (Humatrope)	Growth failure (children)	Headache, muscle pain, weakness, mild hyperglycemia, hypertension, allergic reaction (rash, swelling), pain at injection site
Bromocriptine (Parlodel)	Acromegaly	Nausea, headache, dizziness
Octreotide (Sandostatin)	Acromegaly	Diarrhea, nausea, abdominal discomfort, increased or decreased glucose

C. Interventions
1. Monitor weight.
2. Monitor intake and output and urine osmolality.
3. Monitor electrolytes.
4. Restrict fluid intake as prescribed to prevent water intoxication.
5. Monitor for signs of water intoxication, such as drowsiness, listlessness, and headache.
6. Monitor blood pressure.
7. Instruct the client in how to use the intranasal medication.
8. Instruct the client to report signs of water intoxication or symptoms of headache or shortness of breath.

III. THYROID HORMONES (BOX 54-2)
A. Description
1. Thyroid hormones control the metabolic rate of tissues and accelerate heat production and oxygen consumption.
2. Thyroid hormones are used to replace the thyroid hormone deficit in the treatment of **hypothyroidism, myxedema,** or cretinism.
3. Thyroid hormones enhance the action of oral anticoagulants, sympathomimetics, and antidepressants and decreases the action of insulin, oral hypoglycemics, and digitalis preparations; the action of thyroid hormones is decreased by phenytoin (Dilantin) and carbamazine (Tegretol).
4. Thyroid hormones should be given at least 4 hours apart from multivitamins, aluminum hydroxide and magnesium hydroxide, simethicone, calcium carbonate, bile acid sequestrants, iron, and sucralfate (Carafate) because these medications decrease the absorption of thyroid replacements.
B. Side effects
1. Nausea and decreased appetite
2. Cramps and diarrhea
3. Weight loss
4. Nervousness and tremors
5. Headache
6. Hypertension
7. Tachycardia and dysrhythmias
8. Sweating and heat intolerance
9. Insomnia
10. Toxicity: **hyperthyroidism**
C. Interventions
1. Assess client for history of medications currently being taken.

2. Monitor vital signs.
3. Monitor weight.
4. Monitor triiodothyronine, thyroxine, and thyroid-stimulating hormone levels.
5. Instruct the client to take the medication at the same time each day, preferably in the morning without food.
6. Instruct the client in how to monitor pulse rate.
7. Advise the client to report symptoms of **hyperthyroidism,** such as tachycardia, chest pain, palpitations, and excessive sweating.
8. Instruct the client to avoid foods that can inhibit thyroid secretion, such as strawberries, peaches, pears, cabbage, turnips, spinach, kale, Brussels sprouts, cauliflower, radishes, and peas.
9. Advise the client to avoid over-the-counter medications.
10. Instruct the client to wear a Medic-Alert bracelet.

IV. ANTITHYROID MEDICATIONS (BOX 54-3)
A. Description
1. Antithyroid medications inhibit the synthesis of thyroid hormone.
2. Antithyroid medications are used for **hyperthyroidism,** or Graves' disease.
B. Side effects
1. Nausea and vomiting
2. Diarrhea
3. Hypersensitivity with skin rash
4. Agranulocytosis with leukopenia
5. Toxicity: **hypothyroidism**
6. Iodism: characterized by vomiting, abdominal pain, metallic or brassy taste in the mouth, rash, and sore gums and salivary glands
C. Interventions
1. Monitor vital signs.
2. Monitor triiodothyronine, thyroxine, and thyroid-stimulating hormone levels.
3. Monitor weight.
4. Instruct the client to take medication with meals to avoid gastrointestinal upset.
5. Instruct the client in how to monitor the pulse rate.
6. Inform the client of side effects and when to notify the physician.
7. Advise the client to contact the physician if a fever or sore throat develops.
8. Instruct the client in the signs of **hypothyroidism.**
9. Instruct the client regarding the importance of medication compliance and that abruptly

---

BOX 54-2

Thyroid Hormones

Levothyroxine (Synthroid, Levothroid, Levoxyl)
Liothyronine (Cytomel)
Liotrix (Thyrolar)
Thyroid (Thyrar)

BOX 54-3

Antithyroid Medications

Methimazole (Tapazole)
Propylthiouracil (PTU)
Strong iodine solution (Lugol's solution)

stopping the medication could cause **thyroid storm.**

10. Instruct the client to monitor for signs and symptoms of **thyroid storm** (fever, flushed skin, confusion and behavioral changes, tachycardia, dysrhythmias, and signs of heart failure).

11. Instruct the client to monitor for signs of iodism.

12. Advise the client to consult physician before eating iodized salt and iodine-rich foods.

13. Instruct the client to avoid acetylsalicylic acid (aspirin) and medications containing iodine.

V. PARATHYROID MEDICATIONS (BOX 54-4)

A. Description

1. Parathyroid hormone regulates serum calcium levels.

2. Low serum levels of calcium stimulate parathyroid hormone release.

3. Hyperparathyroidism results in a high serum calcium level and bone demineralization, and medication is used to lower the serum calcium level.

4. Hypoparathyroidism results in a low serum calcium level, which increases neuromuscular excitability, and the treatment includes calcium and vitamin D supplements.

5. Parathyroid and antihypercalcemic agents may cause hypermagnesemia.

BOX 54-4

Medications to Treat Calcium Disorders

CALCIUM SUPPLEMENTS
Calcium carbonate (BioCal, Caltrate 600, Rolaids, Tums)
Calcium carbonate, oyster-shell derived (OsCal 500, Oysco, Oyst-Cal)
Calcium citrate (Citracal)
Calcium glubionate (Calcionate, Neo-Calglucon)
Calcium gluconate
Calcium lactate
Dibasic calcium phosphate
Tribasic calcium phosphate (Posture)

VITAMIN D SUPPLEMENTS
Calcifediol (Calderol)
Calcitriol (Calcijex, Rocaltrol)
Dihydrotachysterol (DHT, Hytakerol)
Ergocalciferol (Calciferol, Drisdol)

CALCIUM REGULATORS
Alendronate (Fosamax)
Calcitonin human (Cibacalcin)
Calcitonin salmon (Calcimar, Miacalcin)
Etidronate (Didronel)
Pamidronate (Aredia)
Risedronate (Actonel)
Tiludronate (Skelid)

ANTIHYPERCALCEMICS
Gallium nitrate (Ganite)

---

6. Calcium salts administered with digoxin (Lanoxin) increases the risk of digoxin toxicity.

7. Oral calcium salts reduce the absorption of tetracycline hydrochloride.

B. Interventions

1. Monitor electrolyte and calcium levels.

2. Assess for signs and symptoms of hypocalcemia and hypercalcemia.

3. Assess for symptoms of tetany in the client with hypocalcemia.

4. Instruct the client in the signs and symptoms of hypercalcemia and hypocalcemia.

5. Instruct the client to check over-the-counter medication labels for the possibility of calcium content.

6. Instruct the client receiving oral calcium supplements to maintain an adequate intake of vitamin D because vitamin D enhances absorption of calcium.

7. Instruct clients receiving calcium regulators such as alendronate sodium (Fosamax) to swallow the tablet whole with water at least 30 minutes before breakfast and not to lie down for at least 30 minutes.

VI. ADRENOCORTICOTROPIC HORMONES (BOX 54-5)

A. Description

1. Adrenocorticotropic hormones stimulate the adrenal cortex to secrete cortisol.

2. Adrenocorticotropic hormones produce an antiinflammatory effect.

3. Adrenocorticotropic hormones are used to diagnose adrenocortical disorders (Box 54-6).

4. Adrenocorticotropic hormones are used to treat acute multiple sclerosis.

B. Side effects

1. Nausea and vomiting

BOX 54-5

Medications for Adrenal Replacement Therapy

Betamethasone (Celestone)
Cortisone (Cortone, Cortistan)
Dexamethasone (Decadron)
Fludrocortisone (Florinef)
Hydrocortisone (Cortef)
Methylprednisolone (Medrol dose pack, Depo-Medrol, Solu-Medrol)
Prednisolone (Delta-Cortef, Prelone, Orapred, Pediapred)
Prednisone (Orasone, Deltasone, Meticorten)
Triamcinolone (Aristocort, Kenacort)

BOX 54-6

Medications Used in Diagnosing Adrenal Gland Dysfunction

Corticotropin (Acthàr, ACTH)
Corticotropin repository (Acthar gel, ACTH gel)
Cosyntropin (Cortrosyn)

2. Gastric irritation with tendency to develop peptic ulcer disease
3. Mood swings
4. Petechiae
5. Water and sodium retention, hypertension
6. Hypokalemia
7. Hypocalcemia, osteoporosis
8. Increased susceptibility to infection
9. Cataracts
10. Hirsuitism, acne, fragile skin, bruising

C. Interventions
1. Monitor vital signs.
2. Monitor intake and output and weight and for edema.
3. Monitor for signs of infection.
4. Monitor electrolyte and calcium levels.
5. Avoid administering adrenocorticotropic hormones to the client with adrenocortical hyperfunction.
6. Instruct the client to decrease salt intake.
7. Instruct the client to report side effects such as muscle weakness, edema, petechiae, ecchymosis, decrease in growth, decreased wound healing, and menstrual irregularities.
8. Monitor for adverse effects when the medication is discontinued; dose should be tapered and not stopped abruptly because adrenal hypofunction may result.
9. Advise the client to wear Medic-Alert bracelet.

VII. CORTICOSTEROIDS (GLUCOCORTICOIDS) (BOX 54-5)

A. Description
1. Corticosteroids produce metabolic effects.
2. Corticosteroids alter the normal immune response and suppress inflammation.
3. Corticosteroids promote sodium and water retention and potassium excretion.
4. Corticosteroids produce antiinflammatory, antiallergic, and antistress effects.
5. Corticosteroids may be used as a replacement for adrenocortical insufficiency.

B. Side effects
1. **Hyperglycemia**
2. Hypokalemia
3. Sodium and water retention
4. Edema
5. Possible effects: muscle wasting, osteoporosis, growth retardation in children, peptic ulcer, increased serum glucose levels, hypertension, convulsions, mood swings, cataracts, glaucoma, fragile skin, hirsutism, and altered fat distribution
6. Masking of the signs and symptoms of infection

C. Contraindications and cautions
1. Corticosteroids are contraindicated in clients with hypersensitivity, psychosis, and fungal infections.
2. Corticosteroids should be used with caution in clients with **diabetes mellitus.**

3. Dexamethasone (Decadron) decreases the effects of orally administered anticoagulants and antidiabetic agents.
4. Corticosteroids increase the potency of medications taken concurrently, such as aspirin, and nonsteroidal antiinflammatory drugs, thus increasing the risk of gastrointestinal bleeding and ulceration.
5. Use of potassium-wasting diuretics increases potassium loss, resulting in hypokalemia.
6. Barbiturates, phenytoin (Dilantin), and rifampin (Rifadin) decrease the effect of prednisone.
7. Use of phenytoin (Dilantin), theophylline, rifampin (Rifadin), barbiturates, and antacids decreases the action of dexamethasone (Decadron).
8. Nonsteroidal antiinflammatory drugs, aspirin, and estrogen increase the effect of dexamethasone (Decadron).
9. Corticosteroids should be used with extreme caution in clients with infections because they mask the signs and symptoms of an infection.
10. Advise the client to wear Medic-Alert bracelet.

D. Interventions
1. Monitor vital signs.
2. Monitor serum electrolytes and blood glucose level.
3. Monitor for hypokalemia and **hyperglycemia.**
4. Monitor intake and output and weight and for edema.
5. Monitor for hypertension.
6. Assess medical history for glaucoma, cataracts, peptic ulcer, mental health disorders, or **diabetes mellitus.**
7. Monitor the older client for signs and symptoms of increased osteoporosis.
8. Assess for changes in muscle strength.
9. Prepare a schedule for the client on short-term, tapered doses.
10. Instruct the client to take at mealtime or with food.
11. Advise the client to eat foods high in potassium.
12. Instruct the client to avoid individuals with respiratory infections.
13. Advise the client to inform all health care providers of the medication regimen.
14. Instruct the client to report signs and symptoms of a medication overdose or **Cushing's syndrome,** including a moon face, puffy eyelids, edema in the feet, increased bruising, dizziness, bleeding, and menstrual irregularities.
15. Note that the client may need additional doses during periods of stress, such as surgery.
16. Instruct the client not to stop medication abruptly because abrupt withdrawal can result in severe adrenal insufficiency.

17. Advise the client to consult with the physician before receiving vaccinations.
18. Advise the client to wear a Medic-Alert bracelet.

E. Mineralocorticoids
1. Description
   a. Mineralocorticoids are steroid hormones that enhance the reabsorption of sodium and chloride and promote the excretion of potassium and hydrogen from the renal tubules, thereby helping to maintain fluid and electrolyte balance.
   b. Mineralocorticoids are used for replacement therapy in primary and secondary adrenal insufficiency in **Addison's disease.**
2. Medication: fludrocortisone (Florinef)
3. Side effects
   a. Sodium and water retention, hypertension
   b. Hypokalemia
   c. Hypocalcemia
   d. Increased susceptibility to infection
   e. Delayed wound healing
   f. Gastrointestinal distress, tendency to develop peptic ulcer
   g. Osteoporosis, compression fractures
   h. Increased appetite
   i. Weight gain
   j. Insomnia
   k. Mood swings
   l. Abdominal distention
4. Interventions
   a. Monitor vital signs.
   b. Monitor weight.
   c. Monitor electrolytes and calcium level.
   d. Instruct the client to take medication with food or milk.
   e. Instruct the client to consume a high-potassium diet.
   f. Instruct the client not to stop the medication abruptly.
   g. Instruct the client to notify the physician if signs of infection, muscle aches, sudden weight gain, or headaches occur.
   h. Instruct the client to avoid exposure to disease or trauma.
   i. Instruct the client not to take aspirin or any other medication without consulting the physician.
   j. Instruct the client to wear a Medic-Alert bracelet.

VIII. ANDROGENS (BOX 54-7)

A. Description
1. Androgens are used to replace deficient hormones or to treat hormone-sensitive disorders.
2. Androgens can cause bleeding if the client is taking oral anticoagulants (increase the effect of anticoagulants).
3. Androgens cause decreased serum glucose concentration, thereby reducing insulin requirements in the client with **diabetes mellitus.**

BOX 54-7

Androgens

Fluoxymesterone (Ora Testryl, Halotestin)
Methyltestosterone (Android, Testred, Virilon)
Testosterone (Andro, Histerone, Testaqua)
Testosterone, pellets (Testopel)
Testosterone, transdermal (Androderm, Testoderm)
Testosterone cypionate (Andronate, Depo-Testosterone)
Testosterone enanthate (Delatest, Delatestryl)

---

4. Hepatotoxic medications are avoided with the use of androgens because of the risk of additive damage to the liver.
5. Androgens usually are avoided in men with known prostatic or breast carcinoma because androgens often stimulate growth of these tumors.

B. Side effects
1. Masculine secondary sexual characteristics (body hair growth, lowered voice, muscle growth)
2. Bladder irritation and urinary tract infections
3. Breast tenderness
4. Gynecomastia
5. Priapism
6. Menstrual irregularities
7. Virilism
8. Sodium and water retention with edema
9. Nausea, vomiting, or diarrhea
10. Acne
11. Changes in libido
12. Hepatotoxicity, jaundice
13. Hypercalcemia

C. Interventions
1. Monitor vital signs.
2. Monitor for edema, weight gain, and skin changes.
3. Assess mental status and neurological function.
4. Assess for signs of liver dysfunction, including right upper quadrant abdominal pain, malaise, fever, jaundice, and pruritus.
5. Assess for the development of secondary sexual characteristics.
6. Instruct the client to take with meals or a snack.
7. Instruct the client to notify the physician if priapism develops.
8. Instruct the client to notify the physician if fluid retention occurs
9. Instruct women to use a nonhormonal contraceptive while on therapy.
10. For women, monitor for menstrual irregularities and decreased breast size.

IX. ESTROGENS AND PROGESTINS

A. Description
1. Estrogens are steroids that stimulate female reproductive tissue.
2. Progestins are steroids that specifically stimulate the uterine lining.

3. Estrogen and progestin preparations may be used to stimulate the endogenous hormones to restore hormonal balance or to treat hormone-sensitive tumors (suppress tumor growth) or for contraception (Boxes 54-8 and 54-9).

B. Contraindications and cautions
1. Estrogens
   a. Estrogens are contraindicated in clients with breast cancer, endometrial hyperplasia, endometrial cancer, history of thromboembolism, known or suspected pregnancy, or lactation.
   b. Use estrogens with caution in clients with hypertension, gall bladder disease, or liver or kidney dysfunction.
   c. Estrogens increase the risk of toxicity when used with hepatotoxic medications.
   d. Barbiturates, phenytoin (Dilantin), and rifampin (Rifadin) decrease the effectiveness of estrogen.
2. Progestins are contraindicated in clients with thromboembolitic disorders and should be avoided in clients with breast tumors or hepatic disease.

C. Side effects
1. Breast tenderness, menstrual changes
2. Nausea, vomiting, and diarrhea
3. Malaise, depression, excessive irritability
4. Weight gain
5. Edema and fluid retention
6. Atherosclerosis

BOX 54-8

Estrogens

Diethylstibesterol
Estradiol (Estrace, Climara, Estraderm, FemPatch, Vivelle)
Estradiol cypionate (Depo-Estradiol, Depogen)
Estradiol valerate (Delestrogen)
Estrogens, congugated (Premarin)
Estrogens, esterified (Estratab)
Estrone (Kestrone 5)
Estropipate (Ogen Ortho-Est)
Ethinyl estradiol (Estinyl)

BOX 54-9

Progestins

Hydroxyprogesterone (Hylutin)
Levonorgestrel (Norplant)
Medroxyprogesterone (Cycrin, Depo-Provera, Provera)
Medroxyprogesterone and conjugated estrogens (Premphase, Prempro)
Megestrol (Megace)
Norethindrone acetate (Aygestin)
Progesterone (Gesterol, Crinone, Progestasert, Prometrium)

---

7. Hypertension, stroke, myocardial infarction
8. Thromboembolism (estrogen)
9. Migraine headaches and vomiting (estrogen)

D. Interventions
1. Monitor vital signs.
2. Monitor for hypertension.
3. Assess for edema and weight gain.
4. Advise the client not to smoke.
5. Advise the client to undergo routine breast and pelvic examinations.

X. ORAL CONTRACEPTIVES
A. Description
1. These medications contain a combination of estrogen and a progestin or a progestin alone.
2. Estrogen-progestin combinations suppress ovulation and change the cervical mucus, making it difficult for sperm to enter.
3. Medications that contain only progestins are less effective than the combined medications.
4. Oral contraceptives usually are taken for 21 consecutive days and stopped for 7 days; then the administration cycle is repeated.
5. Oral contraceptives provide reversible prevention of pregnancy.
6. Oral contraceptives are useful in controlling irregular or excessive menstrual cycles.
7. Risk factors associated with the development of complications related to the use of oral contraceptives include smoking, obesity, and hypertension.
8. Oral contraceptives are contraindicated in women with hypertension, thromboembolitic disease, cerebrovascular or coronary disease, estrogen dependent cancers, and pregnancy.
9. Oral contraceptives should be avoided with the use of hepatotoxic medications.
10. Oral contraceptives interfere with the activity of bromocriptine (Parlodel) and anticoagulants and increase the toxicity of tricyclic antidepressants.
11. Oral contraceptives may alter blood glucose levels.

B. Side effects
1. Breakthrough bleeding
2. Excessive cervical mucus formation
3. Breast tenderness
4. Hypertension
5. Nausea, vomiting

C. Interventions
1. Monitor vital signs and weight.
2. Instruct the client in the administration of the medication (it may take up to 1 week for full contraceptive effect to occur when the medication is begun).
3. Instruct the client with **diabetes mellitus** to monitor blood glucose levels carefully.
4. Instruct the client to report signs of thromboembolitic complications.

5. Instruct the client to notify the physician if vaginal bleeding or menstrual irregularities occur or if pregnancy is suspected.
6. Inform the client that many medications interfere with the effectiveness of birth control pills.
7. Instruct the client to perform breast self-examination monthly and about the importance of yearly physical examinations.
8. If the client decides to discontinue the oral contraceptive to become pregnant, recommend that the client use an alternative form of birth control for 2 months after discontinuation to ensure more complete excretion of hormonal agents before conception.

XI. FERTILITY MEDICATIONS (BOX 54-10)
A. Description
1. Fertility medications act to stimulate follicle development and ovulation in functioning ovaries and are combined with human chorionic gonadotropin to maintain the follicles once ovulation has occurred.
2. Fertility medications are contraindicated in the presence of primary ovarian dysfunction, thyroid or adrenal dysfunction, ovarian cysts, pregnancy, or idiopathic uterine bleeding.
3. Fertility medications should be used with caution in clients with thromboembolitic or respiratory diseases.
B. Side effects
1. Risk of multiple births and birth defects
2. Ovarian overstimulation (abdominal pain, distention, ascites, pleural effusion)
3. Headache, irritability
4. Fluid retention and bloating
5. Nausea, vomiting
6. Uterine bleeding
7. Ovarian enlargement
8. Gynecomastia
9. Rash
10. Orthostatic hypotension
11. Febrile reactions
C. Interventions
1. Instruct the client regarding administration of the medication.

BOX 54-10

Fertility Medications

Bromocriptine (Parlodel)
Chorionic gonadotropin (A.P.L., Profasi HP)
Clomiphene (Clomid)
Follitropin alfa (Gonal-F)
Follitropin beta (Follistim)
Menotropins (Humegon, Pergonal)

---

2. Provide a calendar of treatment days and instructions on when intercourse should occur to increase therapeutic effectiveness of the medication.
3. Provide information about the risks and hazards of multiple births.
4. Instruct the client to notify the physician if signs of ovarian stimulation occur.
5. Inform the client about the need for regular follow-up for evaluation.

XII. MEDICATIONS FOR PENILE ERECTION DYSFUNCTION
A. Description
1. Alprostadil (Caverject, Muse) is a prostaglandin that relaxes smooth muscle and promotes blood flow into the corpus cavernosum.
2. Sildenafil (Viagra), tadalafil (Cialis), vardenafil (Levitra) cause smooth muscle relaxation and allow blood flow into the corpus cavernosum.
3. Erectile dysfunction medications are contraindicated in the presence of any anatomical obstruction or condition that might predispose to priapism and in clients with penile implants.
4. Caution should be used in clients with bleeding disorders.
5. Sildenafil, tadalafil, and vardenafil are used cautiously in clients with coronary artery disease, active peptic ulcer, bleeding disorders, or retinitis pigmentosa.
6. Sildenafil, tadalafil, and vardenafil cannot be administered to clients taking nitrates, nitroprusside, or α-blockers.
B. Side effects
1. Alprostadil: Pain at the injection site, infection, priapism, fibrosis, rash, hypertension
2. Sildenafil, tadalafil, and vardenafil: Headache, flushing, dyspepsia, urinary tract infection, diarrhea, dizziness, rash, neuralgia, insomnia
C. Interventions
1. Perform a thorough assessment of health and medication history.
2. Instruct the client regarding administration of the medication; alprostadil is injected, and sildenafil, tadalafil, and vardenafil are taken orally.
3. Inform the client of the side effects necessitating the need to notify the physician.

XIII. MEDICATIONS FOR DIABETES MELLITUS
A. Insulin and oral hypoglycemic medications
1. Description
   a. Insulin increases glucose transport into cells and promotes conversion of glucose to glycogen, decreasing serum glucose levels.
   b. Oral hypoglycemic agents stimulate the pancreas to produce more insulin, increase the sensitivity of peripheral receptors to insulin, decrease hepatic glucose output or delay intestinal

absorption of glucose, thus decreasing serum glucose levels.

2. Contraindications and concerns
   a. Insulin is contraindicated in clients with hypersensitivity.
   b. Oral hypoglycemic agents are contraindicated in type 1 **diabetes mellitus.**
   c. Sulfonylureas can affect cardiac function and oxygen consumption and lead to cardiac dysrhythmias.
   d. Use of hypoglycemic medications with β-adrenergic blocking agents masks signs and symptoms of **hypoglycemia.**
   e. Anticoagulants, chloramphenicol (Chloromycetin), salicylates, propranolol (Inderal), monoamine oxidase inhibitors, pentamidine (Pentam 300), and sulfonamides may cause hypoglycemia.
   f. Corticosteroids, sympathomimetics, thiazide diuretics, phenytoin (Dilantin), thyroid preparations, oral contraceptives, and estrogen compounds may cause **hyperglycemia.**
   g. Side effects of the sulfonylureas include gastrointestinal symptoms and dermatological reactions; **hypoglycemia** can occur when an excessive dose is administered or when meals are omitted or delayed, food intake is decreased, or activity is increased.
   h. Sulfonylureas, such as chlorpropamide (Diabinese), can cause a disulfiram (Antabuse) type of reaction when alcohol is ingested.

B. Oral hypoglycemic medications
   1. Prescribed for clients with type 2 **diabetes mellitus**
   2. Sulfonylureas (Box 54-11)
      a. Sulfonylureas may be classified as first- or second-generation sulfonylureas.
      b. Sulfonylureas stimulate the beta cells to produce more insulin.
   3. Nonsulfonylureas (Box 54-11)
      a. Nonsulfonylureas affect the hepatic and gastrointestinal production of glucose.
      b. Nonsulfonylureas may be used alone or in combination with a sulfonylurea.
   4. Interventions
      a. Assess the client's knowledge of **diabetes mellitus** and the use of oral antidiabetic agents.
      b. Obtain a medication history regarding the medications that the client is taking currently.
      c. Assess vital signs and blood glucose levels.
      d. Instruct the client to recognize symptoms of **hypoglycemia** and **hyperglycemia.**
      e. Instruct the client to avoid over-the-counter medications unless prescribed by the health care provider.
      f. Instruct the client not to ingest alcohol with sulfonylureas.

BOX 54-11

Sulfonylureas and Nonsulfonylureas

SULFONYLUREAS
Acetohexamide (Dymelor)
Chlorpropamide (Diabinese)
Glimepiride (Amaryl)
Glipizide (Glucotrol)
Glyburide (DiaBeta, Micronase)
Tolazamide (Tolinase)
Tolbutamide (Orinase)

NONSULFONYLUREAS
Alpha Glucosidase Inhibitor
Acarbose (Precose)
Miglitol (Glyset)
Biguanide
Metformin (Glucophage)
Meglitinide
Nateglinide (Starlix)
Repaglinide (Prandin)
Thiozolidinediones
Pioglitazone (Actos)
Rosiglitazone (Avandia)

---

   g. Inform the client that insulin may be needed during stress, surgery, or infection.
   h. Instruct the client in the necessity of compliance with prescribed medication.
   i. Advise the client to wear a Medic-Alert bracelet.

C. Insulin (Table 54-2)
   1. Insulin primarily acts in the liver, muscle, and adipose tissue by attaching to receptors on cellular membranes and facilitating the passage of glucose, potassium, and magnesium.
   2. Insulin is prescribed for clients with type 1 **diabetes mellitus.**
   3. Storing of insulin (Box 54-12)
   4. Insulin injection sites
      a. The main areas for injections are the abdomen, arms (posterior surface), thighs (anterior surface), and hips.
      b. Insulin injected into the abdomen may absorb more evenly and rapidly than at other sites.
      c. Systematic rotation within one anatomical area is recommended to prevent lipodystrophy; client should be instructed not to use the same site more than once in a 2- to 3-week period.
      d. Injections should be 1½ inches apart within the anatomical area.
      e. Heat, massage, and exercise of the injected area can increase absorption rates and may result in **hypoglycemia.**
      f. Injection into scar tissue may delay absorption of insulin.

TABLE 54-2

Common Types of Insulin

Type	Onset	Peak (Hours)	Duration (Hours)
RAPID-ACTING INSULIN			
Lispro (Humalog)	15 minutes	½-1½	4-5
Insulin aspart (NovoLog)	5 to 10 minutes	1-3	3-5
SHORT-ACTING INSULIN			
Regular (Humulin R, Novolin R)	½-1 hour	2-4	5-7
INTERMEDIATE-ACTING INSULIN			
NPH (Humulin N, Novolin N)	1-2 hours	6-14	24
Lente (Humulin L, Novolin L)	1-3 hours	6-14	24
LONG-ACTING INSULIN			
Ultralente (Humulin U)	6 hours	18-24	36
Insulin glargine (Lantus)	—	—	24
PREMIXED INSULIN			
70% NPH/30% regular (Humulin 70/30)	½-1 hour	2-12	18-24
50% NPH/50% regular (Humulin 50/50)	½ hour	3-5	24
75% lispro protamine/25% lispro	10-15 minutes	1-6	24

BOX 54-12

Storing Insulin

Avoid exposing insulin to extremes in temperature.
Insulin should not be frozen or kept in direct sunlight or a hot car.
Before injection, insulin should be at room temperature.
If a vial of insulin will be used up in a month, it may be kept at room temperature; otherwise, the vial should be refrigerated.

---

5. Administering insulin
   a. To prevent dosage errors, be certain that there is a match between the insulin concentration noted on the vial and the calibration of units on the insulin syringe; the usual concentration of insulin is U 100 (100 units/mL).
   b. Most insulin syringes have a 27- to 29-gauge needle that is about ½ inch long.
   c. Before use, roll the insulin bottle to ensure that the insulin and ingredients are mixed well; otherwise, an inaccurate dose will be drawn; shaking the bottle will cause bubbles to form.
   d. Premixed insulins (NPH to regular insulin) are available as 70/30 (most commonly used) and 50/50; (premixed insulin lispro protamine and insulin lispro 75/25 are also available).
   e. Mixtures of insulin in prefilled syringes should be kept in the refrigerator, where they will be stable for at least 1 week; prefilled syringes should be kept flat or with the needle in an upright position to avoid clogging of the needle.
   f. Inject air into the insulin bottle (a vacuum makes it difficult to draw up the insulin).
   g. When mixing insulins, draw up the regular (shorter-acting) insulin first.
   h. Regular insulin may be mixed with any other type of insulin.
   i. Insulin zinc suspensions may be mixed only with each other and regular insulin, not with other types of insulin.
   j. Administer a mixed dose of insulin within 5 to 15 minutes of preparation; after this time the regular insulin binds with the NPH insulin and its action is reduced.
   k. Aspiration generally is not recommended with self-injection of insulin.
   l. Administer insulin at a 45- to 90-degree angle and at a 45- to 60-degree angle in thin persons.
   m. *Remember:* Regular insulin is the only type of insulin that can be administered intravenously.

D. Glucagon
   1. Glucagon is a hormone secreted by the alpha cells of the islets of Langerhans in the pancreas.
   2. Glucagon increases blood glucose by stimulating glycogenolysis in the liver.
   3. Glucagon can be administered subcutaneously, intramuscularly, or intravenously.
   4. Glucagon is used to treat insulin-induced **hypoglycemia** when the client is semiconscious or unconscious and is unable to ingest liquids.
   5. The blood glucose level begins to increase within 5 to 20 minutes after administration.
   6. Instruct the family in the procedure for administration.

7. Refer to Chapter 53 for additional information regarding interventions for severe **hypoglycemia.**

E. Diazoxide (Proglycem)

1. Diazoxide increases blood glucose by inhibiting insulin release from the beta cells and stimulating the release of epinephrine from the adrenal medulla.

2. Diazoxide is used to treat chronic **hypoglycemia** caused by hyperinsulinism resulting from islet cell cancer or hyperplasia.

3. Diazoxide is not used for hypoglycemic reactions from insulin

PRACTICE QUESTIONS

1. Somatren (Protropin) is administered to a client with pituitary dwarfism. A nurse monitors the client, knowing that the expected therapeutic effect of this medication is to
   1. Promote weight gain.
   2. Stimulate linear growth.
   3. Increase bone density.
   4. Decrease the mobilization of fats.

2. Desmopressin acetate (DDAVP, Stimate) is prescribed for the treatment of diabetes insipidus. The nurse administering the medication monitors the client, knowing that the primary action of the medication is to
   1. Decrease permeability in the kidneys to water.
   2. Decrease water reabsorption.
   3. Increase renal excretion of water.
   4. Promote renal conservation of water.

3. A nurse is monitoring a client receiving desmopressin acetate (DDAVP, Stimate) for adverse reactions to the medication. Which of the following indicates the presence of an adverse reaction?
   1. Increased urination
   2. Weight loss
   3. Drowsiness
   4. Insomnia

4. Vasopressin (Pitressin) is prescribed for a client with diabetes insipidus. A nurse is particularly cautious in monitoring the client receiving this medication if the client has which of the following preexisting conditions?
   1. Depression
   2. Endometriosis
   3. Coronary artery disease
   4. Pheochromocytoma

5. A nurse provides instructions to a client who is taking levothyroxine (Synthroid). The nurse tells the client to take the medication
   1. With food.
   2. On an empty stomach.
   3. At bedtime with a snack.
   4. At lunchtime.

6. A nurse provides medication instructions to a client who is taking levothyroxine (Synthroid). The nurse instructs the client to notify the physician if which of the following occurs?
   1. Cold intolerance
   2. Tremors
   3. Excessively dry skin
   4. Fatigue

7. A nurse performs an admission assessment on a client who visits a health care clinic for the first time. The client tells the nurse that propylthiouracil (PTU) is taken daily. The nurse continues to collect data from the client, suspecting that the client has a history of
   1. Cushing's syndrome
   2. Addison's disease
   3. Myxedema
   4. Graves' disease

8. A nurse is instructing a client regarding intranasal desmopressin (DDVAP). The nurse tells the client that which of the following is a side effect of the medication?
   1. Flushed skin
   2. Headache
   3. Runny nose
   4. Vulval pain

9. A client is receiving somatropin (Humatrope). The nurse monitors which most significant laboratory study during therapy with this medication?
   1. Amylase
   2. Lipase
   3. Blood urea nitrogen
   4. Thyroid-stimulating hormone

10. A client is scheduled for a subtotal thyroidectomy. Strong iodine solution (Lugol's solution) is prescribed. A nurse prepares to administer the medication, knowing that the therapeutic effect of this medication is to
    1. Increase thyroid hormone production.
    2. Suppress thyroid hormone production.
    3. Replace thyroid hormone.
    4. Prevent the oxidation of iodide.

11. Strong iodine solution (Lugol's solution) is prescribed for a client with thyrotoxic crisis. The client calls a clinic nurse and complains of a brassy taste and burning sensations in the mouth. The most appropriate instruction to the client is which of the following?
    1. Continue with the medication.
    2. Take half of the prescribed dose for the next 24 hours.
    3. Stop the medication for the next 24 hours and then continue as prescribed.
    4. Stop the medication and notify the physician.

12. A nurse provides instructions to a client taking fludrocortisone (Florinef). The nurse instructs the client to notify the physician if which of the following occurs?
    1. Weight loss

2. Nausea

3. Swelling of the feet

4. Fatigue

13. Calcium carbonate (OsCal) is prescribed for a client with hypocalcemia. A nurse instructs the client to take the medication
1. With meals.
2. 1 hour after meals.
3. Just before meals.
4. Every 4 hours.

14. Calcitriol (Rocaltrol) is prescribed for a client with hypocalcemia. A nurse provides dietary instructions to the client. Which of the following food items would the nurse instruct the client to avoid while taking this medication?
1. Dark green, leafy vegetables
2. Milk
3. Whole-grain cereals
4. Sardines

15. A daily dose of prednisone (Deltasone) is prescribed for a client. A nurse provides instructions to the client regarding administration of the medication. The nurse instructs the client that the best time to take this medication is
1. At bedtime.
2. At noon.
3. Early morning.
4. Anytime, at the same time, each day.

16. Prednisone (Deltasone) is prescribed for a client with diabetes mellitus who is taking NPH insulin daily. Which of the following prescriptions does the nurse anticipate during therapy with the prednisone?
1. A decreased amount of daily NPH insulin.
2. An increased amount of daily NPH insulin.
3. An additional dose of prednisone daily.
4. The addition of an oral hypoglycemic medication daily.

17. A nurse is teaching a client how to mix regular insulin and NPH insulin in the same syringe. Which of the following actions, if performed by the client, indicates the need for further teaching?
1. Injects air into NPH insulin vial first.

2. Injects an amount of air equal to the desired dose of insulin into the vial.

3. Withdraws the NPH insulin first.

4. Withdraws the regular insulin first.

18. A home care nurse visits a client recently diagnosed with diabetes mellitus. The client is taking NPH insulin daily. The client asks the nurse how to store the unopened vials of insulin. The nurse tells the client to
1. Freeze the insulin.
2. Refrigerate the insulin.
3. Keep the insulin at room temperature.
4. Store the insulin in a dark, dry place.

19. Tolbutamide (Orinase) is prescribed for a client with diabetes mellitus. A nurse instructs the client to avoid which of the following while taking this medication?
1. Carbonated beverages
2. Organ meats
3. Alcohol
4. Whole-grain cereals

20. Sildenafil citrate (Viagra) is prescribed to treat a client with erectile dysfunction. A nurse reviews the client's medical record and would question the prescription if which of the following is noted in the client's history?
1. Neuralgia
2. Use of nitroglycerin
3. Use of multivitamins
4. Insomnia

CRITICAL THINKING: FILL IN THE BLANK

A home care nurse prefills syringes containing NPH and regular insulin for a client with diabetes mellitus who has difficulty with seeing and accurately preparing dosages. The client can administer the injection. Considering the stability of insulin, how many prefilled syringes should the nurse prepare for the client for self-administration?

Answer: _____

ANSWERS

1. **2**

Rationale: Somatrem (Protropin) is a growth stimulator used in the long-term treatment of growth failure resulting from endogenous growth hormone deficiency. Somatrem stimulates linear growth and increases the number and size of muscle cells and red cell mass. Somatrem affects carbohydrate metabolism by antagonizing the action of insulin, increases mobilization of fats, and increases cellular protein synthesis. Options 1, 3, and 4 are not actions of this medication.

Test-Taking Strategy: Focus on the client's diagnosis to assist in the process of elimination. Note the relationship between "dwarfism" in the question and "growth" in the correct option. Review the action of this medication if you had difficulty with this question.
Level of Cognitive Ability: Analysis
Client Needs: Physiological Integrity
Integrated Process: Nursing Process—evaluation
Content Area: Pharmacology
Reference: Hodgson, B., & Kizior, R. (2004). *Saunders nursing drug handbook 2004* (p. 928). Philadelphia: W. B. Saunders.

2. 4

Rationale: Desmopressin promotes renal conservation of water. The hormone accomplishes this by acting on the collecting ducts of the kidney to increase their permeability to water, which results in increased water reabsorption.

Test-Taking Strategy: Use the process of elimination. Focus on the diagnosis in the question to assist you in answering the question. Recalling the manifestations related to the loss of large volumes of urine in this disorder will assist in directing you to option 4. Review diabetes insipidus and the action of desmopressin if you had difficulty with this question.

Level of Cognitive Ability: Analysis
Client Needs: Physiological Integrity
Integrated Process: Nursing Process—analysis
Content Area: Pharmacology
Reference: Hodgson, B., & Kizior, R. (2004). *Saunders nursing drug handbook 2004* (p. 286). Philadelphia: W. B. Saunders.

3. 3

Rationale: Water intoxication (overhydration) or hyponatremia is an adverse reaction to desmopressin. Early signs include drowsiness, listlessness, and headache. Decreased urination, rapid weight gain, confusion, seizures, and coma also may occur in overhydration.

Test-Taking Strategy: Use the process of elimination. Knowledge that this medication is used to treat diabetes insipidus will assist you in eliminating options 1 and 2. Recalling the action of the medication will assist you in determining that water intoxication is an adverse reaction. This thought process will direct you to option 3. Review the adverse reactions related to this medication if you had difficulty with this question.

Level of Cognitive Ability: Analysis
Client Needs: Physiological Integrity
Integrated Process: Nursing Process—assessment
Content Area: Pharmacology
Reference: Hodgson, B., & Kizior, R. (2004). *Saunders nursing drug handbook 2004* (p. 287). Philadelphia: W. B. Saunders.

4. 3

Rationale: Because of its powerful vasoconstrictor actions, vasopressin can cause adverse cardiovascular effects. By constricting arteries of the heart, vasopressin can cause angina pectoris and even myocardial infarction, especially if administered to clients with coronary artery disease. In addition, vasopressin may cause gangrene by decreasing blood flow in the periphery. Options 1, 2, and 4 are incorrect.

Test-Taking Strategy: Use the process of elimination. Attempt to make a relationship between the name of the medication, *vaso*pressin, and coronary artery disease, the correct option. Review the cautions associated with the administration of this medication if you had difficulty with this question.

Level of Cognitive Ability: Analysis
Client Needs: Physiological Integrity
Integrated Process: Nursing Process—analysis
Content Area: Pharmacology
Reference: Lehne, R. (2001). *Pharmacology for nursing care* (4th ed., p. 655). Philadelphia: W. B. Saunders.

5. 2

Rationale: Oral doses of levothyroxine (Synthroid) should be taken on an empty stomach to enhance absorption. Dosing is usually done in the morning before breakfast.

Test-Taking Strategy: Use the process of elimination. Note the similarity between options 1, 3, and 4 in that these options address administering the medication with food. Review client teaching points regarding the administration of levothyroxine if you had difficulty with this question.

Level of Cognitive Ability: Application
Client Needs: Health Promotion and Maintenance
Integrated Process: Teaching/Learning
Content Area: Pharmacology
Reference: Lehne, R. (2001). *Pharmacology for nursing care* (4th ed., p. 641). Philadelphia: W. B. Saunders.

6. 2

Rationale: Excessive doses of levothyroxine (Synthroid) can produce signs and symptoms of hyperthyroidism. These include tachycardia, angina, tremors, nervousness, insomnia, hyperthermia, heat intolerance, and sweating. The client should be instructed to notify the physician if these occur. Options 1, 3, and 4 are signs of hypothyroidism.

Test-Taking Strategy: Use the process of elimination, recalling the symptoms associated with hypothyroidism, the purpose of administering levothyroxine, and the effects of the medication. Options 1, 3, and 4 are symptoms related to hypothyroidism. Review the adverse effects of this medication if you are unfamiliar with them.

Level of Cognitive Ability: Application
Client Needs: Physiological Integrity
Integrated Process: Teaching/Learning
Content Area: Pharmacology
Reference: Lehne, R. (2001). *Pharmacology for nursing care* (4th ed., p. 641). Philadelphia: W. B. Saunders.

7. 4

Rationale: Propylthiouracil (PTU) inhibits thyroid hormone synthesis and is used to treat hyperthyroidism, or Graves' disease. Myxedema indicates hypothyroidism. Cushing's syndrome and Addison's disease are disorders related to adrenal function.

Test-Taking Strategy: Use the process of elimination and knowledge regarding the action of the medication and the treatment measures for Graves' disease to answer the question. Review this medication and Graves' disease if you had difficulty with this question.

Level of Cognitive Ability: Analysis
Client Needs: Physiological Integrity
Integrated Process: Nursing Process—assessment
Content Area: Pharmacology
References: Hodgson, B., & Kizior, R. (2004). *Saunders nursing drug handbook 2004* (p. 852). Philadelphia: W. B. Saunders. Lehne, R. (2001). *Pharmacology for nursing care* (4th ed., p. 642). Philadelphia: W. B. Saunders.

8. 3

Rationale: Desmopressin administered by the intranasal route can cause a runny or stuffy nose. Options 1, 2, and 4 are side effects of IV administration.

Test-Taking Strategy: Note the relationship between the words "intranasal" in the question and "runny nose" in option 3. Review this medication if you are unfamiliar with it.
Level of Cognitive Ability: Application
Client Needs: Physiological Integrity
Integrated Process: Teaching/Learning
Content Area: Pharmacology
Reference: Lehne, R. (2001). *Pharmacology for nursing care* (4th ed., p. 655). Philadelphia: W. B. Saunders.

9. 4
Rationale: An adverse reaction to somatropin (Humatrope) is hypothyroidism. Thyroid function is monitored throughout therapy. Options 1 and 2 would evaluate pancreatic function, and option 3 evaluates renal function.
Test-Taking Strategy: Use the process of elimination. Eliminate options 1 and 2 first because both evaluate pancreatic function and therefore are similar. Next, eliminate option 3 because it evaluates renal function. Recalling that somatropin is a growth hormone will assist in directing you to option 4. If you had difficulty with this question, review interventions associated with the administration of somatropin.
Level of Cognitive Ability: Analysis
Client Needs: Physiological Integrity
Integrated Process: Nursing Process—assessment
Content Area: Pharmacology
Reference: Hodgson, B., & Kizior, R. (2004). *Saunders nursing drug handbook 2004* (p. 928). Philadelphia: W. B. Saunders.

10. 2
Rationale: Lugol's solution is administered to hyperthyroid individuals in preparation for thyroidectomy to suppress thyroid function. Initial effects develop within 24 hours; peak effects develop in 10 to 15 days. In most cases, plasma levels of thyroid hormone are reduced with propylthiouracil(PTU) before Lugol's solution therapy is initiated. Then Lugol's solution along with propylthiouracil is administered for the last 10 days before surgery.
Test-Taking Strategy: Use the process of elimination. Eliminate options 1 and 3 first because they are similar. From the remaining options, select option 2 because of its relationship to the issue of the question. If you had difficulty with this question, review the purpose of this medication for the client scheduled for subtotal thyroidectomy.
Level of Cognitive Ability: Analysis
Client Needs: Physiological Integrity
Integrated Process: Nursing Process—planning
Content Area: Pharmacology
Reference: Lehne, R. (2001). *Pharmacology for nursing care* (4th ed., p. 644). Philadelphia: W. B. Saunders.

11. 4
Rationale: Chronic ingestion of iodine can produce iodism. The client needs to be instructed about the symptoms of iodism, which includes a brassy taste, burning sensations in the mouth, soreness of gums and teeth, frontal headache, vomiting, and abdominal pain. The client needs to be instructed to notify the physician if these symptoms occur.
Test-Taking Strategy: Use the process of elimination. Eliminate options 2 and 3 first because the nurse cannot

legally alter medication prescriptions without a physician's order. Consider the client symptoms presented in the question, and eliminate option 1. Review the adverse effects of iodine solution if you had difficulty with this question.
Level of Cognitive Ability: Application
Client Needs: Physiological Integrity
Integrated Process: Nursing Process—implementation
Content Area: Pharmacology
Reference: Lehne, R. (2001). *Pharmacology for nursing care* (4th ed., p. 644). Philadelphia: W. B. Saunders.

12. 3
Rationale: Excessive doses of fludrocortisone (Florinef) cause retention of sodium and water and excessive excretion of potassium, resulting in expansion of blood volume, hypertension, cardiac enlargement, edema, and hypokalemia. The client needs to be informed about the signs of sodium and water retention, such as unusual weight gain or swelling of the feet or lower legs. If these signs occur, the physician needs to be notified.
Test-Taking Strategy: Use the process of elimination. Recalling that fludrocortisone can cause water retention will direct you easily to option 3. Review client teaching points related to this medication if you had difficulty with this question.
Level of Cognitive Ability: Application
Client Needs: Health Promotion and Maintenance
Integrated Process: Teaching/Learning
Content Area: Pharmacology
References: Hodgson, B., & Kizior, R. (2004). *Saunders nursing drug handbook 2004* (p. 418). Philadelphia: W.B. Saunders. Lehne, R. (2001). *Pharmacology for nursing care* (4th ed., p. 664). Philadelphia: W. B. Saunders.

13. 2
Rationale: The client should be instructed to take the medication exactly as prescribed. When used as a calcium supplement, calcitriol should be taken 1 to 1½ hours after meals. The client should take the tablets with a full glass of water; however, calcitriol can be taken with milk.
Test-Taking Strategy: Use the process of elimination. Option 4 easily can be eliminated first. From the remaining options, eliminate options 1 and 3 because they are similar. If you are unfamiliar with the administration of calcium supplements, review this information.
Level of Cognitive Ability: Application
Client Needs: Health Promotion and Maintenance
Integrated Process: Teaching/Learning
Content Area: Pharmacology
Reference: Hodgson, B., & Kizior, R. (2004). *Saunders nursing drug handbook 2004* (p. 140). Philadelphia: W. B. Saunders.

14. 3
Rationale: The client who is taking an antihypocalcemic medication should be instructed to avoid eating too much spinach, rhubarb, bran, or whole-grain cereals because they decrease calcium absorption. Good dietary sources of calcium are milk products; dark green, leafy vegetables (although spinach needs to be avoided); clams; oysters; sardines; and orange juice fortified with calcium.

Test-Taking Strategy: Note that the client diagnosis is "hypocalcemia." Note the key word "avoid" in the stem of the question. Use the process of elimination and knowledge regarding food items high in calcium to assist in selecting the correct option. This should assist in eliminating options 1, 2, and 4. Review this medication and food sources high in calcium if you had difficulty with this question.
Level of Cognitive Ability: Application
Client Needs: Health Promotion and Maintenance
Integrated Process: Teaching/Learning
Content Area: Pharmacology
Reference: Gutierrez, K., & Queener, S. (2003). *Pharmacology for nursing practice* (p. 1031). St. Louis: Mosby.

15. **3**
Rationale: Glucocorticoids should be administered before 9 AM. Administration at this time helps minimize adrenal insufficiency and mimics the burst of glucocorticoids released naturally by the adrenal glands each morning. Options 1, 2, and 4 are incorrect.
Test-Taking Strategy: Use the process of elimination. Recalling that this medication is a glucocorticoid will direct you to option 3. If you had difficulty with this question, review the administration of glucocorticoids.
Level of Cognitive Ability: Application
Client Needs: Physiological Integrity
Integrated Process: Teaching/Learning
Content Area: Pharmacology
Reference: Hodgson, B., & Kizior, R. (2004). *Saunders nursing drug handbook 2004* (p. 831). Philadelphia: W. B. Saunders.

16. **2**
Rationale: Glucocorticoids can elevate blood glucose levels. Clients with diabetes mellitus may need their dosages of insulin or oral hypoglycemic medications increased during glucocorticoid therapy.
Test-Taking Strategy: Use the process of elimination. Recalling that glucocorticoids can increase blood glucose levels will direct you easily to option 2. Review the effects of glucocorticoids if you had difficulty with this question.
Level of Cognitive Ability: Analysis
Client Needs: Physiological Integrity
Integrated Process: Nursing Process—analysis
Content Area: Pharmacology
Reference: Kee, J., & Hayes, E. (2003). *Pharmacology: A nursing process approach* (4th ed., pp. 724, 730). Philadelphia: W. B. Saunders.

17. **3**
Rationale: When preparing a mixture of regular insulin with another insulin preparation, draw the regular insulin into the syringe first. This sequence will avoid contaminating the vial of regular insulin with insulin of another type. Options 1, 2, and 4 identify the correct actions for preparing NPH and regular insulin.
Test-Taking Strategy: Use the process of elimination, noting the key words "need for further teaching." Remember "RN"; draw up the *R*egular insulin before the *N*PH insulin. Review the procedure for preparing NPH and regular insulin if you had difficulty with this question.

Level of Cognitive Ability: Analysis
Client Needs: Health Promotion and Maintenance
Integrated Process: Teaching/Learning
Content Area: Pharmacology
References: Kee, J. & Hayes, E. (2003). *Pharmacology: A nursing process approach* (4th ed., p. 737). Philadelphia: W. B. Saunders. Lehne, R. (2001). *Pharmacology for nursing care* (4th ed., p. 619). Philadelphia: W. B. Saunders.

18. **2**
Rationale: Insulin in unopened vials should be stored under refrigeration until needed. Vials should not be frozen. When stored unopened under refrigeration, insulin can be used up to the expiration date on the vial.
Test-Taking Strategy: Use the process of elimination. Note the key words "store the unopened vials" in the question. Remembering that insulin should not be frozen will assist in eliminating option 1. Options 3 and 4 are similar and should be eliminated. Review client teaching points related to insulin if you had difficulty with this question.
Level of Cognitive Ability: Application
Client Needs: Health Promotion and Maintenance
Integrated Process: Teaching/Learning
Content Area: Pharmacology
Reference: Hodgson, B., & Kizior, R. (2004). *Saunders nursing drug handbook 2004* (p. 538). Philadelphia: W. B. Saunders.

19. **3**
Rationale: When alcohol is combined with tolbutamide, a disulfiram-like reaction may occur. This syndrome includes flushing, palpitations, and nausea. Alcohol can potentiate the hypoglycemic effects of tolbutamide. Clients need to be instructed to avoid alcohol consumption while taking this medication.
Test-Taking Strategy: Use the process of elimination. Eliminate options 1, 2, and 4 because these food items are allowed in a diabetic diet. Remembering that alcohol can affect the action of many medications will assist in directing you to option 3. Review this medication if you had difficulty with this question.
Level of Cognitive Ability: Application
Client Needs: Physiological Integrity
Integrated Process: Teaching/Learning
Content Area: Pharmacology
Reference: Lehne, R. (2001). *Pharmacology for nursing care* (4th ed., p. 625). Philadelphia: W. B. Saunders.

20. **2**
Rationale: Sildenafil citrate (Viagra) enhances the vasodilation effect of nitric oxide in the corpus cavernosum of the penis, thus sustaining an erection. Because of the effect of the medication, it is contraindicated with concurrent use of organic nitrates and nitroglycerin. Sildenafil is not contraindicated with the use of vitamins. Neuralgia and insomnia are side effects of the medication.
Test-Taking Strategy: Use the process of elimination, noting the key words "would question the prescription." Recalling the action of the medication will direct you easily to option 2. If you had difficulty with this question, review the contraindications associated with the use of this medication.

Level of Cognitive Ability: Analysis
Client Needs: Physiological Integrity
Integrated Process: Nursing Process—analysis
Content Area: Pharmacology
Reference: Hodgson, B., & Kizior, R. (2004). *Saunders nursing drug handbook 2004* (p. 915). Philadelphia: W. B. Saunders.

CRITICAL THINKING: FILL IN THE BLANK

Answer: Seven prefilled syringes or a 1 week supply.
Rationale: Mixtures of insulin in prefilled syringes should be stored in a refrigerator, where they will be stable for 1 week. The syringe should be stored vertically with the needle pointing up to avoid clogging the needle. Before administration,

the syringe should be agitated gently to resuspend the insulin.
Test-Taking Strategy: You must know the concepts related to insulin stability and storage to answer this question. Review these concepts if you are unfamiliar with the principles related to prefilling insulin syringes.
Level of Cognitive Ability: Application
Client Needs: Health Promotion and Maintenance
Integrated Process: Nursing Process—implementation
Content Area: Pharmacology
References: Hodgson, B., & Kizior, R. (2003). *Saunders nursing drug handbook 2003* (p. 591). Philadelphia: W. B. Saunders. Lehne, R. (2001). *Pharmacology for nursing care* (4th ed., p. 620). Philadelphia: W. B. Saunders.

REFERENCES

Gutierrez, K., & Queener, S. (2003). *Pharmacology for nursing practice.* St. Louis: Mosby.

Hodgson, B., & Kizior, R. (2003). *Saunders nursing drug handbook 2003.* Philadelphia: W. B. Saunders.

Hodgson, B., & Kizior, R. (2004). *Saunders nursing drug handbook 2004.* Philadelphia: W. B. Saunders.

Ignatavicius, D., & Workman, M. (2002). *Medical-surgical nursing: Critical thinking for collaborative care* (4th ed.). Philadelphia: W. B. Saunders.

Kee, J., & Hayes, E. (2003). *Pharmacology: A nursing process approach* (4th ed.). Philadelphia: W. B. Saunders.

Lehne, R. (2001). *Pharmacology for nursing care* (4th ed.). Philadelphia: W.B. Saunders.

Lewis, S., Heitkemper, M., & Dirksen, S. (2004). *Medical-surgical nursing: Assessment and management of clinical problems* (6th ed.). St. Louis: Mosby.

Phipps, W., Monahan, F., Sands, J., Marek, J., & Neighbors, M. (2003). *Medical-surgical nursing: Health and illness perspectives* (7th ed.). St. Louis: Mosby.

The Adult Client with a Gastrointestinal Disorder

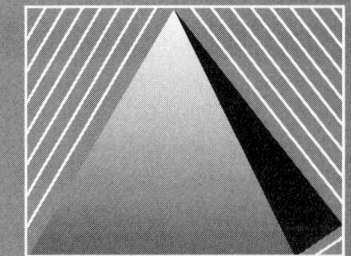

PYRAMID TERMS

ascites The accumulation of fluid within the peritoneal cavity that results in venous congestion of the hepatic capillaries, which leads to plasma leaking directly from the liver surface and portal vein.

asterixis A coarse tremor characterized by rapid, nonrhythmic extensions and flexions in the wrist and fingers. Also termed liver flap.

Billroth I Partial gastrectomy with the remaining segment being anastomosed to duodenum. Also called gastroduodenostomy.

Billroth II Partial gastrectomy with the remaining segment being anastomosed to the jejunum. Also called gastrojejunostomy.

cholecystectomy Removal of the gallbladder.

cholecystitis An inflammation of the gallbladder that may occur as an acute or chronic process. Acute inflammation is associated with gallstones (cholelithiasis). Chronic cholecystitis results when inefficient bile emptying and gallbladder muscle wall disease causes a fibrotic and contracted gallbladder.

choledochotomy Incision into the common bile duct to remove the stone.

cirrhosis A chronic, progressive disease of the liver characterized by diffuse damage to cells with fibrosis and nodular regeneration. Repeated destruction of hepatic cells causes the formation of scar tissue.

Crohn's disease An inflammatory disease that can occur anywhere in the gastrointestinal tract but most often affects the terminal ileum and leads to thickening and scarring, a narrowed lumen, fistulas, ulcerations, and abscesses. The disease is characterized by remissions and exacerbations.

Cullen's sign Bluish discoloration of the abdomen and periumbilical area seen in acute hemorrhagic pancreatitis.

diverticulitis Inflammation of one or more diverticula that results when the diverticulum perforates, with local abscess formation. A perforated diverticulum can progress to intraabdominal perforation with generalized peritonitis.

diverticulosis Outpouching or herniations of the intestinal mucosa that can occur in any part of the intestine but are most common in the sigmoid colon.

dumping syndrome Rapid emptying of the gastric contents into the small intestine, which occurs following gastric resection.

esophageal varices Dilated and tortuous veins in the submucosa of the esophagus that are caused by portal hypertension, often are associated with liver cirrhosis, and are at high risk for rupture if portal circulation pressure rises.

fetor hepaticus The fruity, musty breath odor associated with chronic liver disease.

gastrectomy Removal of the stomach with attachment of the esophagus to the jejunum or duodenum. Also called esophagojejunostomy.

gastric resection Removal of the lower half of the stomach, usually including a vagotomy. Also called antrectomy.

hiatal hernia A portion of the stomach that herniates through the diaphragm and into the thorax. Herniation results from weakening of the muscles of the diaphragm and is aggravated by factors that increase abdominal pressure, such as pregnancy, ascites, obesity, tumors, and heavy lifting. Also known as esophageal or diaphragmatic hernia.

Kock ileostomy (continent ileostomy) An intraabdominal pouch that is constructed from the terminal ileum. The pouch is connected to the stoma with a nipplelike valve constructed from a portion of the ileum. The stoma is flush with the skin.

Murphy's sign A sign of gallbladder disease consisting of pain on taking a deep breath when the examiner's fingers are on the approximate location of the gallbladder.

pancreatitis An acute or chronic inflammation of the pancreas, with associated escape of pancreatic enzymes into surrounding tissue. Acute pancreatitis occurs suddenly as one attack or can be recurrent with resolution. Chronic pancreatitis is a continual inflammation and destruction of the pancreas, with scar tissue replacing pancreatic tissue.

peristalsis Wavelike rhythmic contractions that propels material through the gastrointestinal tract.

portal hypertension A persistent increase in pressure within the portal vein that develops as a result of obstruction to flow.

pyloroplasty Enlarging the pylorus to prevent or decrease pyloric obstruction, thereby enhancing gastric emptying.

Turner's sign A gray-blue discoloration of the flanks seen in acute hemorrhagic pancreatitis.

ulcerative colitis Ulcerative and inflammatory disease of the bowel that results in poor absorption of nutrients. Acute ulcerative colitis results in vascular congestion, hemorrhage, edema, and ulceration of the bowel mucosa. Chronic ulcerative colitis causes muscular hypertrophy, fat deposits, and fibrous tissue with bowel thickening, shortening, and narrowing.

vagotomy Surgical division of the vagus nerve to eliminate the vagal impulses that stimulate hydrochloric acid secretion in the stomach.

▲ PYRAMID TO SUCCESS

Pyramid Points focus on diagnostic tests and nursing care related to the various gastric or intestinal tubes, gastric surgery, cirrhosis, hepatitis, pancreatitis, and colostomy care. Focus on preprocedure and postprocedure care of the client undergoing a gastrointestinal diagnostic test. Remember that an informed consent is required for any invasive procedure. Focus on diet restrictions before and after the diagnostic test and remember that the gag reflex or bowel sounds must return before allowing a client to consume food or fluids. Pyramid Points include instructions to the client and family regarding the prevention of gastrointestinal disorders and the complications associated with the disorder. Focus on teaching the client and family about diet and nutrition specific to the disorder, tube and wound care, preventing the transmission of infection, and care to a colostomy or ileostomy. Remember that body image disturbances can occur in clients with a gastrointestinal disorder. Specific focus relates to the client with a diversion, such as an ileostomy or colostomy, and to the social isolation issues that can occur, and coping strategies. The Integrated Processes addressed in this unit include Nursing Process, Caring, Communication and Documentation, and Teaching/Learning.

▲ CLIENT NEEDS

Safe, Effective Care Environment

Confidentiality issues related to the gastrointestinal disorder
Consultation related to nutritional status
Establishing priorities
Handling of infectious drainage and secretions
Informed consent for treatments and surgical procedures
Prevention of disease transmission
Referrals to home care and community services
Standard precautions

Health Promotion and Maintenance

Health screening related to gastrointestinal disorders
Health promotion programs related to gastrointestinal disorders
Physical assessment techniques of the gastrointestinal system
Teaching related to prescribed dietary and other treatment measures
Teaching related to colostomy or ileostomy care
Teaching related to preventing the transmission of disease

Psychosocial Integrity

Coping mechanisms
End of life issues
Grief and loss
Support systems
Unexpected body image changes related to colostomy or ileostomy

Physiological Integrity

Care of gastrointestinal tubes
Diagnostic tests related to the gastrointestinal system
Elimination
Fluid and electrolyte imbalances
Infectious diseases of the gastrointestinal tract
Medication therapy specific to the gastrointestinal disorder
Monitoring for complications related to tests, procedures, and surgical interventions
Nonpharmacological and pharmacological comfort measures
Nutrition and oral hydration
Parenterally administered fluids
Personal hygiene
Total parenteral nutrition

REFERENCES

Chernecky, C., & Berger, B. (2004). *Laboratory tests & diagnostic procedures* (4th ed.). Philadelphia: W. B. Saunders.

Harkreader, H., & Hogan, M. A. (2004). *Fundamentals of nursing: Caring and clinical judgment* (2nd ed.). Philadelphia: W. B. Saunders.

Ignatavicius, D., & Workman, M. (2002). *Medical-surgical nursing: Critical thinking for collaborative care* (4th ed.). Philadelphia: W. B. Saunders.

Lewis, S., Heitkemper, M., & Dirksen, S. (2004). *Medical-surgical nursing: Assessment and management of clinical problems* (6th ed.). St. Louis: Mosby.

McKenry, L., & Salerno, E. (2003). *Mosby's pharmacology in nursing* (21st ed.) St. Louis: Mosby.

National Council of State Boards of Nursing (Eds.). (2003). *Test Plan for the National Council Licensure Examination for Registered Nurses* (effective date: April 2004). Chicago: Author.

Perry, A., & Potter, P. (2002). *Clinical nursing skills and techniques* (5th ed.). St. Louis: Mosby.

Phipps, W., Monahan, F., Sands, J., Marek, J., & Neighbors, M. (2003). *Medical-surgical nursing: Health and illness perspectives* (7th ed.). St. Louis: Mosby.

Potter, P., & Perry, A. (2001). *Fundamentals of nursing* (5th ed.). St. Louis: Mosby.

Varcarolis, E. M. (2002). *Foundations of psychiatric mental health nursing* (4th ed.). Philadelphia: W. B. Saunders.

Gastrointestinal System

I. ANATOMY AND PHYSIOLOGY

A. Functions of the gastrointestinal system
 1. Process food substances.
 2. Absorb the products of digestion into the blood.
 3. Excrete unabsorbed materials.
 4. Provide an environment for microorganisms to synthesize nutrients, such as vitamin K.
 5. For risk factors associated with the gastrointestinal system, see Box 55-1.

B. Mouth
 1. The mouth contains the lips, cheeks, palate, tongue, teeth, salivary glands, muscles, and maxillary bones.
 2. Saliva contains the amylase enzyme (ptyalin) that aids in digestion.

BOX 55-1

Risk Factors Associated with the Gastrointestinal System

Family history of gastrointestinal disorders
Chronic laxative use
Tobacco use
Chronic alcohol use
Chronic high stress levels
Allergic reactions to food or medications
Chronic use of aspirin or nonsteroidal antiinflammatory drugs
Long-term gastrointestinal conditions such as ulcerative colitis that may predispose to colorectal cancer
Previous abdominal surgery or trauma, which may lead to adhesions
Neurological disorders that can impair movement, particularly with chewing and swallowing
Cardiac, respiratory, and endocrine disorders that may lead to constipation
Diabetes mellitus, which may predispose to oral candidal infections

---

C. Esophagus
 1. The esophagus is a collapsible muscular tube about 10 inches long.
 2. The esophagus carries food from the pharynx to the stomach.

D. The stomach contains the cardia, fundus, the body, and the pylorus.
 1. Mucous glands
  a. Mucous glands are located in the mucosa.
  b. Mucous glands prevent autodigestion by providing an alkaline protective covering.
 2. The lower esophageal (cardiac) sphincter prevents reflux of gastric contents into the esophagus.
 3. The pyloric sphincter regulates the rate of stomach emptying into the small intestine.
 4. Hydrochloric acid kills microorganisms, breaks food into small particles, and provides a chemical environment that is required by the gastric enzymes.
 5. Pepsin is the chief coenzyme of gastric juice, which converts proteins into proteases and peptones.
 6. Intrinsic factor is necessary for the absorption of vitamin B_{12}.
 7. Gastrin controls gastric acidity.

E. Small intestine
 1. The duodenum contains the openings of the bile and pancreatic ducts.
 2. The jejunum is about 8 feet long.
 3. The ileum is about 12 feet long.
 4. The small intestine terminates into the cecum.

F. Pancreatic intestinal juice enzymes
 1. Amylase digests starch to maltose.
 2. Maltase reduces maltose to monosaccharide glucose
 3. Lactase splits lactose into galactose and glucose.
 4. Sucrase reduces sucrose to fructose and glucose.
 5. Nucleoses split nucleic acids to nucleotides.
 6. Enterokinase activates trypsinogen to trypsin.

G. Large intestine
   1. The large intestine is about 5 feet long.
   2. The large intestine absorbs water and eliminates wastes.
   3. Intestinal bacteria play a vital role in the synthesis of some B vitamins and vitamin K.
   4. Colon
      a. Ascending
      b. Transverse
      c. Descending
      d. Sigmoid
      e. Rectum
   5. The ileocecal valve prevents contents of large intestine from entering ileum.
   6. The anal sphincters guard the anal canal.
H. Peritoneum
   1. The peritoneum lines the abdominal cavity.
   2. The peritoneum forms the mesentery that supports the intestines and blood supply.
I. Liver
   1. The liver is the largest gland in the body, weighing 3 to 4 lb.
   2. The liver contains Kupffer's cells, which remove bacteria in the portal venous blood.
   3. The liver removes excess glucose and amino acids from the portal blood.
   4. The liver synthesizes glucose, amino acids, and fats.
   5. The liver aids in the digestion of fats, carbohydrates, and proteins.
   6. The liver stores and filters blood (200 to 400 mL of blood stored).
   7. The liver stores vitamins A, D, and B and iron.
   8. The liver secretes bile to emulsify fats (500 to 1000 mL of bile a day).
   9. Hepatic ducts
      a. The hepatic ducts deliver bile to the gallbladder via the cystic duct.
      b. The hepatic ducts deliver bile to the duodenum via the common bile duct.
      c. The common bile duct opens into the duodenum, with the pancreatic duct at the ampulla of Vater.
      d. The sphincter prevents the reflux of intestinal contents into the common bile duct and pancreatic duct.
J. Gallbladder
   1. The gallbladder stores and concentrates bile.
   2. The gallbladder contracts to force bile into the duodenum during the digestion of fats.
   3. The cystic duct joins the hepatic duct to form the common bile duct.
   4. The sphincter of Oddi guards the entrance into the duodenum.
   5. The presence of fatty materials in the duodenum stimulates the liberation of cholecystokinin, which causes contraction of the gallbladder and relaxation of the sphincter of Oddi.

K. Pancreas
   1. Exocrine gland
      a. The pancreas secretes sodium bicarbonate to neutralize the acidity of the stomach contents that enter the duodenum.
      b. Pancreatic juices contain enzymes for digesting carbohydrates, fats, and proteins.
   2. Endocrine gland
      a. The islets of Langerhans secrete insulin.
      b. Insulin is secreted into the bloodstream and is important for carbohydrate metabolism.
      c. The pancreas secretes glucagon to raise blood glucose levels.
      d. The pancreas secretes somatostatin to exert a hypoglycemic effect.

II. DIAGNOSTIC PROCEDURES (BOX 55-2)
A. Upper gastrointestinal tract study (barium swallow)
   1. Description: An examination of the upper gastrointestinal tract under fluoroscopy after the client drinks barium sulfate
   2. Preprocedure: NPO after midnight before the day of the test
   3. Postprocedure
      a. A laxative may be prescribed.
      b. Instruct the client to increase oral fluid intake to help pass the barium.
      c. Monitor stools for the passage of barium (stools will appear chalky white) because barium can cause a bowel obstruction.
B. Lower gastrointestinal tract study (barium enema)
   1. Description
      a. A fluoroscopic and radiographic examination of the large intestine is performed after rectal instillation of barium sulfate.
      b. The study may be done with or without air.

BOX 55-2

Gastrointestinal System Diagnostic Studies

Anoscopy, proctoscopy, and sigmoidoscopy
Cholecystography
Defecography
Endoscopic retrograde cholangiopancreatography
Fiberoptic colonoscopy
Gastric analysis
Gastrointestinal motility studies
Hydrogen and urea breath test
Laparoscopy (peritoneoscopy)
Liver and pancreas laboratory studies
Liver biopsy
Lower gastrointestinal tract study (barium enema)
Paracentesis
Percutaneous transhepatic cholangiography
Stool specimens
Upper gastrointestinal fiberoscopy
Upper gastrointestinal tract study (barium swallow)

2. Preprocedure
   a. A low-residue diet for 1 to 2 days before the test
   b. A clear liquid diet and a laxative the evening before the test
   c. NPO after midnight before the day of the test
   d. Cleansing enemas on the morning of the test
3. Postprocedure
   a. Instruct the client to increase oral fluid intake to help pass the barium.
   b. Administer a mild laxative as prescribed to facilitate emptying of the barium.
   c. Monitor stools for the passage of barium.
   d. Notify the physician if a bowel movement does not occur within 2 days.

C. Gastric analysis
1. Description
   a. Gastric analysis requires the passage of a nasogastric tube into the stomach to aspirate gastric contents for the analysis of acidity (pH), appearance, and volume; the entire gastric contents are aspirated, and then specimens are collected every 15 minutes for 1 hour.
   b. Histamine or pentagastrin may be administered subcutaneously to stimulate gastric secretions and may produce a flushed feeling.
   c. Esophageal reflux of gastric acid may be performed by ambulatory pH monitoring; a probe is placed just above the lower esophageal sphincter, is connected to an external recording device, and provides a computer analysis and graphic display of results.
2. Preprocedure
   a. Fasting for 8 to 12 hours is required before the test.
   b. Avoid tobacco and chewing gum for 6 hours before the test.
   c. Medications that stimulate gastric secretions are withheld for 24 to 48 hours.
3. Postprocedure
   a. Client may resume normal activities.
   b. Refrigerate gastric samples if not tested within 4 hours.

D. Upper gastrointestinal fiberoscopy
1. Description
   a. Upper gastrointestinal fiberoscopy also is known as esophagogastroduodenoscopy.
   b. Following sedation, an endoscope is passed down the esophagus to view the gastric wall, sphincters, and duodenum; tissue specimens can be obtained.
2. Preprocedure
   a. The client must be NPO for 6 to 12 hours before the test.
   b. A local anesthetic (spray or gargle) is administered along with midazolam (Versed) intravenously (provides conscious sedation and relieves anxiety) just before the scope is inserted.

c. Atropine may be administered to reduce secretions, and glucagon may be administered to relax smooth muscle.
   d. Client is positioned on the left side to facilitate saliva drainage and to provide easy access of the endoscope.
   e. Airway patency is monitored during the test and pulse oximetry is used to monitor oxygen saturation; emergency equipment should be readily available.
3. Postprocedure
   a. Client must be NPO until the gag reflex returns (1 to 2 hours).
   b. Monitor for signs of perforation (pain, bleeding, unusual difficulty swallowing, elevated temperature).
   c. Maintain bedrest for the sedated client until alert.
   d. Lozenges, saline gargles, or oral analgesics can relieve minor sore throat, after the gag reflex returns.

E. Anoscopy, proctoscopy, and sigmoidoscopy
1. Description
   a. Anoscopy requires use of a rigid scope to examine the anal canal; client is placed in the knee-chest position with the back inclined at a 45-degree angle.
   b. Proctoscopy and sigmoidoscopy require use of a flexible scope to examine the rectum and sigmoid colon; client is placed on the left side with the right leg bent and placed anteriorly.
   c. Biopsies and polypectomies can be performed.
2. Preprocedure: Enemas are given until the returns are clear.
3. Postprocedure: Monitor for rectal bleeding and signs of perforation.

F. Fiberoptic colonoscopy
1. Description
   a. Colonoscopy is a fiberoptic endoscopy study in which the lining of the large intestine is visually examined; biopsies and polypectomies can be performed.
   b. Cardiac and respiratory function is monitored continuously during the test.
   c. Colonoscopy is performed with the client lying on the left side with the knees drawn up to the chest; position may be changed during the test to facilitate passing of the scope.
2. Preprocedure
   a. Adequate cleansing of the colon is necessary, as prescribed by the physician.
   b. A clear liquid diet is started at noon on the day before the test.
   c. Consult with the physician regarding medications that must be withheld before the test.
   d. Client is NPO after midnight on the day before the test.

e. Midazolam (Versed) is administered intravenously to provide sedation.

f. Glucagon may be administered to relax smooth muscle.

3. Postprocedure

a. Provide bedrest until alert.

b. Monitor for signs of perforation.

c. Instruct the client to report any bleeding to the physician.

G. Laparoscopy (peritoneoscopy) is performed with a fiberoscopic laparoscope that allows direct visualization of organs and structures within the abdomen; biopsies may be obtained.

H. Cholecystography

1. Description: Performed to detect gallstones and to assess the ability of the gallbladder to fill, concentrate its contents, contract, and empty.

2. Preprocedure

a. Assess allergies to iodine or seafood.

b. Contrast agents such as iopanoic acid (Telepaque), iodipamide meglumine (Cholografin), or sodium ipodate (Oragrafin) may be administered 10 to 12 hours (evening before) before the test.

c. Client is NPO after the contrast agent is administered.

d. Instruct the client that if a rash, itching, hives, or difficulty in breathing occurs after taking the contrast agent, to report to the emergency room.

3. Postprocedure

a. Inform the client that dysuria is common because the contrast agent is excreted in the urine.

b. A normal diet may be resumed (a fatty meal may enhance excretion of the contrast agent).

I. Endoscopic retrograde cholangiopancreatography (ERCP)

1. Description

a. Examination of the hepatobiliary system is performed via a flexible endoscope inserted into the esophagus to the descending duodenum; multiple positions are required during the procedure to pass the endoscope.

b. If medication is administered before the procedure, the client is monitored closely for signs of respiratory and central nervous system depression, hypotension, oversedation, and vomiting.

2. Preprocedure

a. Client is NPO for several hours before the procedure.

b. Sedation is administered before the procedure.

3. Postprocedure

a. Monitor vital signs.

b. Monitor for the return of the gag reflex.

c. Monitor for signs of perforation or infection.

J. Percutaneous transhepatic cholangiography

1. Description

a. The examination involves the injection of dye directly into the biliary tree.

b. The hepatic ducts within the liver, the entire length of the common bile duct, the cystic duct, and the gallbladder are outlined clearly.

2. Preprocedure

a. Client is NPO.

b. Sedating medication is administered.

3. Postprocedure

a. Monitor vital signs.

b. Monitor for signs of bleeding, peritonitis, and septicemia; report the presence of pain immediately.

c. Administer antibiotics as prescribed to reduce the risk of sepsis.

K. Paracentesis

1. Description: Transabdominal removal of fluid from the peritoneal cavity for analysis

2. Preprocedure

a. Obtain informed consent.

b. Have client void before the start of procedure to empty bladder and to move bladder out of the way of the paracentesis needle.

c. Measure abdominal girth, weight, and baseline vital signs.

d. Note that the client is positioned upright on the edge of the bed with the back supported and the feet resting on a stool (Fowler's position is used for the client confined to bed).

3. Postprocedure

a. Monitor vital signs.

b. Measure fluid collected, describe, and record.

c. Label fluid samples and send to the laboratory for analysis.

d. Apply a dry sterile dressing to the insertion site; monitor site for bleeding.

e. Measure abdominal girth and weight.

f. Monitor for hypovolemia, electrolyte loss, mental status changes, or encephalopathy.

g. Monitor for hematuria caused by bladder trauma.

h. Instruct the client to notify the physician if the urine becomes bloody, pink, or red.

L. Liver biopsy

1. Description: A needle is inserted through the abdominal wall to the liver to obtain a tissue sample for biopsy and microscopic examination.

2. Preprocedure

a. Obtained informed consent.

b. Assess results of coagulation tests (prothrombin time, partial thromboplastin time, platelet count).

c. Administer a sedative as prescribed.

d. Note that the client is placed in the supine or left lateral position during the procedure to expose the right side of the upper abdomen.

3. Postprocedure
   a. Assess vital signs.
   b. Assess biopsy site for bleeding.
   c. Monitor for peritonitis.
   d. Maintain bed rest for several hours.
   e. Place client on the right side with a pillow under the costal margin to decrease the risk of hemorrhage, and instruct the client to avoid coughing and straining.
   f. Instruct the client to avoid heavy lifting and strenuous exercise for 1 week.

M. Gastrointestinal motility studies
   1. Radionuclide testing assesses gastric emptying and colonic emptying time; a capsule containing radioactive material is administered to the client and the time it takes for the radioactive material to move through the colon indicates colonic motility.
   2. Esophageal manometry detects motility disorders of the esophagus and lower esophageal sphincter; client is NPO for 8 to 12 hours before the test and medications that affect gastrointestinal motility are withheld.
   3. Gastrointestinal, small intestinal, and colonic manometry evaluates delayed gastric emptying and gastric and intestinal motility disorders; often this is an ambulatory outpatient procedure that lasts 24 to 72 hours.
   4. Anorectal manometry measures the resting tone and contractibility of the anal sphincters to evaluate the client with chronic constipation or fecal incontinence; phosphosoda or a cleansing enema is administered 1 hour before the test.
   5. Electrogastrography is used to detect motor or neurological dysfunction in the stomach and records gastric electrical activity.
   6. Rectal sensory function test evaluates rectal sensory function and neuropathy to evaluate the client with chronic constipation, diarrhea, or incontinence.

N. Defecography
   1. Defecography measures anorectal function.
   2. Thick barium is instilled into the rectum, fluoroscopy is performed, and the function of the rectum and anal sphincter is visualized while the client attempts to pass the barium.
   3. Digital subtraction methods may be used for more rapid imaging and mapping of rectal evacuation.
   4. No preparation is required.

O. Stool specimens
   1. Testing of stool specimens includes inspecting the specimen for consistency and color and testing for occult blood.
   2. Tests for fecal urobilinogen, fat, nitrogen, parasites, pathogens, food substances, and other substances may be performed; these tests require that the specimen be sent to the laboratory.
   3. Random specimens are sent promptly to the laboratory.

4. Quantitative 24- to 72-hour collections must be kept refrigerated until they are taken to the laboratory.
   5. Some specimens require that a certain diet be followed or that certain medications be withheld; check agency guidelines regarding specific procedures.

P. Hydrogen breath test
   1. The hydrogen breath test evaluates carbohydrate absorption by determining the amount of hydrogen expelled in the breath after it is produced in the colon and absorbed in the blood.
   2. The hydrogen breath test is used to aid in the diagnosis of bacterial overgrowth in the intestine.

Q. Urea breath test
   1. The urea breath test detects the presence of *Helicobacter pylori*, the bacteria that causes peptic ulcer disease.
   2. The client consumes a capsule of carbon-labeled urea and provides a breath sample 10 to 20 minutes later.
   3. Client is instructed to avoid antibiotics or bismuth subsalicylate (Pepto-Bismol) for 1 month before the test; sucralfate (Carafate) and omeprazole (Prilosec) for 1 week before the test; and cimetidine (Tagamet), famotidine (Pepcid), ranitidine (Zantac), or nizatidine (Axid) for 24 hours before breath testing.
   4. *Helicobacter pylori* also can be detected by assessing serum antibody levels.

R. Liver and pancreas laboratory studies (Refer to Chapter 11.)
   1. Alkaline phosphatase is released during liver damage or biliary obstruction.
   2. Prothrombin time is prolonged with liver damage.
   3. Serum ammonia assesses the ability of the liver to deaminate protein by-products.
   4. Liver enzymes (transaminase studies) are elevated with liver damage.
   5. An increase in cholesterol indicates **pancreatitis** or biliary obstruction.
   6. An increase in bilirubin indicates liver damage or biliary obstruction.
   7. Increased values for amylase and lipase indicate **pancreatitis.**

III. ASSESSMENT

A. Abdominal assessment (Box 55-3)
   1. Inspect skin for color, abnormalities, contour, and tautness, and the abdomen for distention.

BOX 55-3

Order for Performing the Abdominal Assessment

1. Inspect
2. Auscultate
3. Percuss
4. Palpate

2. Auscultate for bowel sounds
3. Percuss for air or solids.
4. Palpate for tenderness.

B. Bowel sounds
1. Auscultate bowel sounds before percussion and palpation.
2. Normal bowel sounds occur 5 to 30 times a minute or every 5 to 15 seconds.
3. Auscultate in all abdominal quadrants.
4. Listen at least 5 minutes in each quadrant before assuming sounds are absent.

IV. GASTROINTESTINAL TUBES (REFER TO CHAPTER 21.)

V. GASTROESOPHAGEAL REFLUX DISEASE

A. Description
1. Gastroesophageal reflux is the backflow of gastric and duodenal contents into the esophagus.
2. The reflux is caused by an incompetent lower esophageal sphincter, pyloric stenosis, or a motility disorder.
3. Symptoms may mimic those of a heart attack.

B. Assessment
1. Pyrosis
2. Dyspepsia
3. Regurgitation
4. Pain and difficulty with swallowing
5. Hypersalivation

C. Interventions
1. Instruct the client to avoid factors that decrease lower esophageal sphincter pressure or cause esophageal irritation.
2. Instruct the client to eat a low-fat, high-fiber diet; avoid caffeine, tobacco, and carbonated beverages; avoid eating and drinking 2 hours before bedtime; avoid wearing tight clothes; and elevate the head of the bed on 6- to 8- inch blocks.
3. Avoid the use of anticholinergics, which delay stomach emptying.
4. Instruct the client regarding prescribed medications, such as antacids, histamine H_2 receptor antagonists, or gastric acid pump inhibitors.
5. Instruct the client regarding the administration of prokinetic medications, if prescribed, which accelerate gastric emptying.
6. If medical management is unsuccessful, surgery may be required and involves a fundoplication (wrapping a portion of the gastric fundus around the sphincter area of the esophagus); surgery may be performed by laparoscopy.

VI. HIATAL HERNIA

A. Description
1. A **hiatal hernia** also is known as esophageal or diaphragmatic hernia.
2. A portion of the stomach herniates through the diaphragm and into the thorax.
3. Hernation results from weakening of the muscles of the diaphragm and is aggravated by factors that increase abdominal pressure such as pregnancy, **ascites,** obesity, tumors, and heavy lifting.
4. Complications include ulceration, hemorrhage, regurgitation and aspiration of stomach contents, strangulation, and incarceration of the stomach in the chest with possible necrosis, peritonitis, and mediastinitis.

B. Assessment
1. Heartburn
2. Regurgitation or vomiting
3. Dysphagia
4. Feeling of fullness

C. Interventions
1. Medical and surgical management is similar to that for gastroesophageal reflux disease.
2. Provide small frequent meals and minimize the amount of liquids.
3. Advise the client not to recline for 1 hour after eating.
4. Avoid anticholinergics, which delay stomach emptying.

VII. GASTRITIS

A. Description
1. Inflammation of the stomach or gastric mucosa
2. Acute gastritis is caused by the ingestion of food contaminated with disease-causing microorganisms or food that is irritating or too highly seasoned, the overuse of aspirin or other nonsteroidal antiinflammatory drugs (NSAIDs), excessive alcohol intake, bile reflux, or radiation therapy.
3. Chronic gastritis is caused by benign or malignant ulcers or by the bacteria *H. pylori* and also may be caused by autoimmune diseases, dietary factors, medications, alcohol, smoking, or reflux.

B. Assessment (Box 55-4)

C. Interventions
1. Acute gastritis: Food and fluids may be withheld until symptoms subside; afterward, ice chips,

---

BOX 55-4

Assessment Findings in Acute and Chronic Gastritis

ACUTE
Abdominal discomfort
Anorexia, nausea, and vomiting
Headache
Hiccuping

CHRONIC
Anorexia, nausea, and vomiting
Belching
Heartburn after eating
Sour taste in the mouth
Vitamin B_{12} deficiency

followed by clear liquids, and then solid food is introduced.

2. Monitor for signs of hemorrhagic gastritis such as hematemesis, tachycardia, and hypotension, and notify the physician if these signs occur.

3. Instruct the client to avoid irritating foods, fluids, and other substances such as spicy and highly seasoned foods, caffeine, alcohol, and nicotine.

4. Instruct the client in the use of prescribed medications, such as antibiotics and bismuth salts (Pepto-Bismol).

5. Provide the client with information about the importance of vitamin B_{12} injections, if a deficiency is present.

VIII. PEPTIC ULCER DISEASE

A. Description
1. A peptic ulcer is an ulceration in the mucosal wall of the stomach, pylorus, duodenum, or esophagus in portions that are accessible to gastric secretions; erosion may extend through the muscle.
2. The ulcer may be referred to as gastric, duodenal, or esophageal depending on its location.
3. The most common peptic ulcers are gastric ulcers and duodenal ulcers.

B. Gastric ulcers
1. Description
   a. A gastric ulcer involves ulceration of the mucosal lining that extends to the submucosal layer of the stomach.
   b. Predisposing factors include stress, smoking, the use of corticosteroids, NSAIDs, alcohol, a history of gastritis, a family history of gastric ulcers, or infection with *H. pylori*.
   c. Complications include hemorrhage, perforation, and pyloric obstruction.
2. Assessment (Box 55-5)
3. Interventions
   a. Monitor vital signs and for signs of bleeding.
   b. Administer small, frequent bland feedings during the active phase.

BOX 55-5

Assessment: Gastric and Duodenal Ulcers

GASTRIC
Gnawing, sharp pain in or left of the midepigastric region 1 to 2 hours after eating
Hematemesis
Nausea and vomiting

DUODENAL
Burning pain in the midepigastric area 2 to 4 hours after eating and during the night
Melena
Pain that often is relieved by eating

---

c. Administer histamine H_2 receptor antagonists as prescribed to decrease the secretion of gastric acid.
d. Administer antacids as prescribed to neutralize gastric secretions.
e. Administer anticholinergics as prescribed to reduce gastric motility.
f. Administer mucosal barrier protectants as prescribed 1 hour before each meal.
g. Administer prostaglandins as prescribed for their protective and antisecretory actions.

4. Client education
   a. Avoid consuming alcohol and substances that contain caffeine or chocolate.
   b. Avoid smoking.
   c. Avoid aspirin or NSAIDs.
   d. Obtain adequate rest and reduce stress.

5. Interventions during active bleeding
   a. Monitor vital signs closely.
   b. Assess for signs of dehydration, hypovolemic shock, sepsis, and respiratory insufficiency.
   c. Maintain NPO status and administer intravenous (IV) fluid replacement as prescribed; monitor intake and output.
   d. Monitor hemoglobin and hematocrit.
   e. Administer blood transfusions as prescribed.
   f. Assist with the insertion of a nasogastric tube for decompression and for lavage access.
   g. Assist with normal saline or tap water lavage at room temperature to reduce active bleeding.
   h. Prepare to assist with administering vasopressin (Pitressin) intravenously as prescribed to induce vasoconstriction and reduce bleeding.

6. Surgical interventions
   a. Total **gastrectomy**: removal of the stomach with attachment of the esophagus to the jejunum or duodenum; also called esophagojejunostomy
   b. **Vagotomy**: surgical division of the vagus nerve to eliminate the vagal impulses that stimulate hydrochloric acid secretion in the stomach
   c. **Gastric resection**: removal of the lower half of the stomach and usually including a **vagotomy**; also called antrectomy.
   d. **Billroth I**: partial **gastrectomy**, with the remaining segment anastomosed to the duodenum; also called gastroduodenostomy.
   e. **Billroth II**: partial **gastrectomy**, with the remaining segment anastomosed to the jejunum; also called gastrojejunostomy.
   f. **Pyloroplasty**: enlargement of the pylorus to prevent or decrease pyloric obstruction, thereby enhancing gastric emptying.

7. Postoperative interventions
   a. Monitor vital signs.
   b. Position in Fowler's for comfort and to promote drainage.

c. Administer fluids and electrolyte replacements intravenously as prescribed; monitor intake and output.

d. Assess bowel sounds.

e. Monitor nasogastric suction as prescribed.

f. Do not irrigate or remove the nasogastric tube.

g. Assist the physician with nasogastric irrigation or removal of the nasogastric tube.

h. Maintain NPO status as prescribed for 1 to 3 days until **peristalsis** returns.

i. Progress the diet from NPO to sips of clear water to 6 small, bland meals a day as prescribed when bowel sounds return.

j. Monitor for postoperative complications of hemorrhage, **dumping syndrome**, diarrhea, hypoglycemia, and vitamin B_{12} deficiency.

C. Duodenal ulcers

1. Description

a. A duodenal ulcer is a break in the mucosa of the duodenum.

b. Risk factors and causes include alcohol intake; smoking; stress; caffeine; the use of aspirin, corticosteroids, and NSAIDs; and infection with *H. pylori*.

c. Complications include bleeding, perforation, gastric outlet obstruction, and intractable disease.

2. Assessment (Box 55-5)

3. Interventions

a. Monitor vital signs.

b. Perform abdominal assessment.

c. Instruct the client in a bland diet with small frequent meals.

d. Provide for adequate rest.

e. Encourage the cessation of smoking.

f. Instruct the client to avoid alcohol intake, caffeine, the use of aspirin, corticosteroids, and NSAIDs.

g. Administer antacids as prescribed to neutralize acid secretions.

h. Administer histamine H_2 receptor antagonists as prescribed to block the secretion of acid.

4. Surgical interventions: Surgery is performed only if the ulcer is unresponsive to medications or if hemorrhage, obstruction, or perforation occurs.

D. **Dumping syndrome**

1. Description

a. **Dumping syndrome** is rapid emptying of the gastric contents into the small intestine.

b. **Dumping syndrome** occurs following **gastric resection**.

2. Assessment

a. Symptoms occurring 30 minutes after eating

b. Nausea and vomiting

c. Feelings of abdominal fullness and abdominal cramping

d. Diarrhea

e. Palpitations and tachycardia

f. Perspiration

g. Weakness and dizziness

h. Borborygmi

3. Client education (Box 55-6)

IX. VITAMIN B_{12} DEFICIENCY

A. Description

1. Vitamin B_{12} deficiency results from an inadequate intake of vitamin B_{12} or a lack of absorption of ingested vitamin B_{12} from the intestinal tract.

2. Pernicious anemia results from a deficiency of intrinsic factor, which is necessary for intestinal absorption of vitamin B_{12}.

B. Assessment

1. Severe pallor

2. Fatigue

3. Weight loss

4. Smooth, beefy red tongue

5. Slight jaundice

6. Paresthesias of the hands and feet

7. Disturbances with gait and balance

C. Interventions

1. Increase dietary intake of foods rich in vitamin B_{12} if the anemia is the result of a dietary deficiency (Box 55-7).

2. Administer vitamin B_{12} injections as prescribed weekly initially and then monthly for maintenance (lifelong) if the anemia is the result of a deficiency of the intrinsic factor.

X. GASTRIC CANCER (REFER TO CHAPTER 51.)

XI. ESOPHAGEAL VARICES

A. Description

BOX 55-6

Client Education: Preventing Dumping Syndrome

Eat a high-protein, high-fat, low-carbohydrate diet.
Eat small meals and avoid consuming fluids with meals.
Avoid sugar and salt.
Lie down after meals.
Take antispasmodic medications as prescribed to delay gastric emptying.

BOX 55-7

Foods Rich in Vitamin B_{12}

Brewer's yeast
Citrus fruits
Dried beans
Green, leafy vegetables
Liver
Nuts
Organ meats

1. **Esophageal varices** are dilated and tortuous veins in the submucosa of the esophagus.
2. Varices are caused by **portal hypertension**, often are associated with liver **cirrhosis**, and are at high risk for rupture if portal circulation pressure rises.
3. Bleeding varices are an emergency.
4. The goal of treatment is to control bleeding, prevent complications, and prevent the reoccurrence of bleeding.

B. Assessment
1. Hematemesis
2. Melena
3. Tarry stools
4. **Ascites**
5. Jaundice
6. Hepatomegaly and splenomegaly
7. Dilated abdominal veins
8. Hemorrhoids
9. Signs of shock

C. Interventions
1. Monitor vital signs.
2. Elevate the head of the bed.
3. Monitor for orthostatic hypotension.
4. Monitor lung sounds and for the presence of respiratory distress.
5. Administer oxygen as prescribed to prevent tissue hypoxia.
6. Monitor level of consciousness.
7. Maintain NPO status.
8. Administer fluids intravenously as prescribed to restore fluid volume and electrolyte imbalances; monitor intake and output.
9. Monitor hemoglobin, hematocrit, and coagulation factors.
10. Administer blood transfusions or clotting factors as prescribed.
11. Assist in inserting a nasogastric tube or a balloon tamponade as prescribed.
12. Assist with the administration of iced saline irrigations to achieve vasoconstriction of the varices.
13. Prepare to assist with administering vasopressin (Pitressin) by IV or intraarterial infusion as prescribed to induce vasoconstriction and reduce bleeding.
14. Prepare to assist with administering nitroglycerin (Tridil) with the vasopressin (Pitressin) if prescribed to prevent vasoconstriction of the coronary arteries.
15. Instruct the client to avoid activities that will initiate vasovagal responses.
16. Prepare the client for endoscopic procedures or surgical procedures as prescribed.

D. Endoscopic injection (sclerotherapy)
1. Sclerotherapy is injection of a sclerosing agent into and around bleeding varices.

2. Complications include chest pain, pleural effusion, aspiration pneumonia, esophageal stricture, and perforation of the esophagus.

E. Endoscopic variceal ligation
1. The procedure involves ligation of the varices with an elastic rubber band.
2. Sloughing, followed by superficial ulceration, occurs in the area of ligation within 3 to 7 days.

F. Surgical shunt procedures
1. Splenorenal involves splenectomy, with anastomosis of the splenic vein to the left renal vein.
2. Portacaval shunting is shunting of the blood from the portal vein to the inferior vena cava.
3. Mesocaval shunting involves a side anastomosis of the superior mesenteric vein to the proximal end of the inferior vena cava.
4. Transjugular intrahepatic portal/systemic
   a. The procedure uses the normal vascular anatomy of the liver to create a shunt with the use of a metallic stent.
   b. The shunt is between the portal and systemic venous system within the liver and is aimed at relieving **portal hypertension**.

XII. ULCERATIVE COLITIS
A. Description
1. Colitis is an ulcerative and inflammatory disease of the bowel that results in poor absorption of nutrients.
2. Colitis commonly begins in the rectum and spreads upward toward the cecum.
3. The colon becomes edematous and may develop bleeding lesions and ulcers; the ulcers may lead to perforation.
4. Scar tissue develops and causes loss of elasticity and loss of ability to absorb nutrients.
5. Colitis is characterized by various periods of remissions and exacerbations.
6. Acute **ulcerative colitis** results in vascular congestion, hemorrhage, edema, and ulceration of the bowel mucosa.
7. Chronic **ulcerative colitis** causes muscular hypertrophy, fat deposits, and fibrous tissue with bowel thickening, shortening, and narrowing.
8. Surgical intervention involves creation of an ostomy; the ostomy can be created within the ileum or at various sites within the large bowel.
9. An ileostomy is the surgical creation of an opening into the ileum or small intestine that allows for drainage of fecal matter from the ileum to the outside of the body.
10. A colostomy is the surgical creation of an opening into the colon that allows for drainage of fecal matter from the colon to the outside of the body.

B. Assessment
1. Anorexia

2. Weight loss
3. Malaise
4. Abdominal tenderness and cramping
5. Severe diarrhea that may contain blood and mucus
6. Dehydration and electrolyte imbalances
7. Anemia
8. Vitamin K deficiency

C. Interventions

1. Acute phase: Maintain NPO status and administer fluids and electrolytes intravenously or total parenteral nutrition as prescribed.
2. Restrict the client's activity to reduce intestinal activity.
3. Monitor bowel sounds and for abdominal tenderness and cramping.
4. Monitor stools, noting color, consistency, and the presence or absence of blood.
5. Monitor for perforation, peritonitis, and hemorrhage.
6. Following the acute phase, the diet progresses from clear liquids to low-residue as tolerated.
7. Instruct the client to consume a low-residue, high-protein diet; vitamins and iron supplements may be prescribed.
8. Instruct the client to avoid gas-forming foods and milk products, and foods such as whole wheat grains, nuts, raw fruits and vegetables, pepper, alcohol, and caffeine-containing products.
9. Instruct the client to avoid smoking.
10. Administer bulk-forming agents such as bran, psyllium, or methylcellulose to decrease diarrhea and relieve symptoms.
11. Administer antimicrobial agents, corticosteroids, and immunosuppressants as prescribed to prevent infection and reduce inflammation.

D. Surgical interventions

1. Total proctocolectomy with permanent ileostomy
   a. The procedure is curative and involves the removal of the entire colon (colon, rectum, and anus with anal closure).
   b. The end of the terminal ileum forms the stoma, which is located in the right lower quadrant.
2. **Kock ileostomy** (continent ileostomy)
   a. The **Kock ileostomy** is an intraabdominal pouch that stores the feces and is constructed from the terminal ileum.
   b. The pouch is connected to the stoma with a nipplelike valve constructed from a portion of the ileum; the stoma is flush with the skin.
   c. A catheter is used to empty the pouch, and a small dressing or adhesive bandage is worn over the stoma between emptyings.
3. Ileoanal reservoir
   a. Creation of an ileoanal reservoir is a two-stage procedure that involves the excision of the rectal mucosa, an abdominal colectomy, construction

of a reservoir to the anal canal, and a temporary loop ileostomy.
   b. The ileostomy is closed in 3 to 4 months after the capacity of the reservoir is increased.
4. Ileoanal anastomosis (ileorectostomy)
   a. Ileorectostomy does not require an ileostomy.
   b. A 12- to 15-cm rectal stump is left after the colon is removed, and the small intestine is inserted into this rectal sleeve and anastomosed.
   c. Ileorectostomy requires a large, compliant rectum.
5. Preoperative colostomy/ileostomy interventions
   a. Consult with enterostomal therapist to assist in identifying optimal placement of the ostomy.
   b. Instruct the client to eat a low-residue diet for 1 to 2 days before surgery as prescribed.
   c. Administer intestinal antiseptics and antibiotics as prescribed to cleanse the bowel and to decrease the bacterial content of the colon.
   d. Administer laxatives and enemas as prescribed.
6. Postoperative colostomy interventions
   a. Place a petrolatum gauze over the stoma as prescribed to keep it moist, followed by a dry sterile dressing if a pouch (external) system is not in place.
   b. Place a pouch system on the stoma as soon as possible.
   c. Monitor the stoma for size, unusual bleeding, or necrotic tissue.
   d. Monitor for color changes in the stoma.
   e. Note that the normal stoma color is pink to bright red and shiny, indicating high vascularity.
   f. Note that a pale pink stoma indicates low hemoglobin and hematocrit levels and a purple-black stoma indicates compromised circulation, requiring physician notification.
   g. Assess the functioning of the colostomy.
   h. Expect that stool is liquid in the immediate postoperative period but becomes more solid depending on the area of the colostomy: ascending colon—liquid; transverse colon—loose to semiformed; and descending colon—close to normal.
   i. Monitor the pouch system for proper fit and signs of leakage.
   j. Empty the pouch when it is one-third full.
   k. Fecal matter should not be allowed to remain on the skin.
   l. Administer analgesics and antibiotics as prescribed.
   m. Irrigate the perineal wound (if present) as prescribed and monitor for signs of infection.
   n. Instruct the client to avoid foods that cause excess gas formation and odor.
   o. Instruct the client about stoma care and irrigations as prescribed (Box 55-8).

BOX 55-8
Colostomy Irrigation

PURPOSE
An enema is given through the stoma to stimulate bowel emptying.

DESCRIPTION
Irrigation is performed by instilling 500 to 1000 mL of lukewarm tap water through the stoma and allowing the water and stool to drain into a collection bag.

PROCEDURE
If ambulatory, position the client sitting on toilet.
If on bedrest, position the client on the side.
Hang the irrigation bag so that the bottom of the bag is at the level of the client's shoulder or slightly higher.
Insert the irrigation tube carefully without force.
Begin the flow of irrigation.
Clamp tubing if cramping occurs; release tubing as cramping subsides.
Avoid frequent irrigations with water, which can lead to loss of fluids and electrolytes.
Perform irrigation around the same time each day.
Perform irrigation preferably 1 hour after a meal.

p. Instruct the client that normal activities may be resumed when approved by the physician.
  7. Postoperative ileostomy interventions
    a. Note that normal stool is liquid.
    b. Monitor for dehydration and electrolyte imbalance.
    c. Do not give suppositories through an ileostomy.

XIII. CROHN'S DISEASE (REGIONAL ENTERITIS)
A. Description
  1. **Crohn's disease** is an inflammatory disease that can occur anywhere in the gastrointestinal tract but most often affects the terminal ileum and leads to thickening and scarring, a narrowed lumen, fistulas, ulcerations, and abscesses.
  2. **Crohn's disease** is characterized by remissions and exacerbations.
B. Assessment
  1. Fever
  2. Cramplike and colicky pain after meals
  3. Diarrhea (semisolid), which may contain mucus and pus
  4. Abdominal distention
  5. Anorexia, nausea, and vomiting
  6. Weight loss
  7. Anemia
  8. Dehydration
  9. Electrolyte imbalances
C. Interventions: Care is similar to the client with ulcerative colitis; however, surgery is avoided as much as

possible because recurrence of the disease process in the same region is likely to occur.

XIV. PANCREATIC TUMORS, INTESTINAL TUMORS, AND BOWEL OBSTRUCTIONS (REFER TO CHAPTER 51.)

XV. DIVERTICULOSIS AND DIVERTICULITIS
A. Description
  1. **Diverticulosis**
    a. **Diverticulosis** is an outpouching or herniation of the intestinal mucosa.
    b. The disorder can occur in any part of the intestine but is most common in the sigmoid colon.
  2. **Diverticulitis**
    a. **Diverticulitis** is inflammation of one or more diverticula that results when a diverticulum perforates.
    b. A perforated diverticulum can progress to intraabdominal perforation with generalized peritonitis.
B. Assessment
  1. Left lower quadrant abdominal pain that increases with coughing, straining, or lifting
  2. Elevated temperature
  3. Nausea and vomiting
  4. Flatulence
  5. Cramplike pain
  6. Abdominal distention and tenderness
  7. Palpable, tender rectal mass
  8. Blood in the stools
C. Interventions
  1. Provide bed rest during the acute phase.
  2. Maintain NPO status or provide clear liquids during the acute phase as prescribed.
  3. Introduce a fiber-containing diet gradually, when the inflammation has resolved.
  4. Administer antibiotics, analgesics, and anticholinergics to reduce bowel spasms as prescribed.
  5. Instruct the client to refrain from lifting, straining, coughing, or bending to avoid increased intraabdominal pressure.
  6. Monitor for perforation, hemorrhage, fistulas, and abscesses.
  7. Instruct the client to increase fluid intake to 2500 to 3000 mL daily, unless contraindicated.
  8. Instruct the client to eat soft high-fiber foods such as whole grains.
  9. Instruct the client to avoid gas-forming foods or foods containing indigestible roughage, seeds, or nuts because these food substances become trapped in diverticula and cause inflammation.
  10. Instruct the client to consume a small amount of bran daily and to take bulk-forming laxatives as prescribed to increase stool mass.
  11. Instruct the client to avoid high-fiber foods when inflammation occurs because these foods will irritate the mucosa further.

D. Surgical interventions
   1. Colon resection with primary anastomosis is one option.
   2. Temporary or permanent colostomy may be required for increased bowel inflammation.

XVI. HEMORRHOIDS

A. Description
   1. Hemorrhoids are dilated varicose veins of the anal canal.
   2. Hemorrhoids may be internal, external, or prolapsed.
   3. Internal hemorrhoids lie above the anal sphincter and cannot be seen on inspection of the perianal area.
   4. External hemorrhoids lie below the anal sphincter and can be seen on inspection.
   5. Prolapsed hemorrhoids can become thrombosed or inflamed.
   6. Hemorrhoids are caused from **portal hypertension,** straining, irritation, increased venous or abdominal pressure.

B. Assessment
   1. Bright red bleeding with defecation
   2. Rectal pain
   3. Rectal itching

C. Interventions
   1. Apply cold packs to the anal/rectal area followed by sitz baths as prescribed.
   2. Apply witch hazel soaks and topical anesthetics as prescribed.
   3. Encourage a high-fiber diet and fluids to promote bowel movements without straining.
   4. Administer stool softeners as prescribed.

D. Endoscopic procedures
   1. Sclerotherapy
   2. Endoscopic ligation

E. Surgical procedures
   1. Cryosurgery
   2. Hemorrhoidectomy

F. Postoperative interventions
   1. Assist the client to a prone or side-lying position to prevent bleeding.
   2. Maintain ice packs over the dressing as prescribed until the packing is removed by the physician.
   3. Monitor for urinary retention.
   4. Administer stool softeners as prescribed.
   5. Instruct the client to increase fluids and high-fiber foods.
   6. Instruct the client to limit sitting to short periods of time.
   7. Instruct the client in the use of sitz baths 3 to 4 times a day as prescribed.

XVII. APPENDICITIS

A. Description
   1. Appendicitis is inflammation of the appendix.

   2. When the appendix becomes inflamed or infected, rupture may occur within a matter of hours, leading to peritonitis and sepsis.

B. Assessment
   1. Pain in the periumbilical area that descends to the right lower quadrant
   2. Abdominal pain that is most intense at McBurney's point
   3. Rebound tenderness and abdominal rigidity
   4. Low-grade fever
   5. Elevated white blood cell count
   6. Anorexia, nausea, and vomiting
   7. Client in side-lying position, with abdominal guarding and legs flexed
   8. Constipation or diarrhea

C. Peritonitis: inflammation of the peritoneum (Box 55-9)

D. Appendectomy: surgical removal of the appendix
   1. Preoperative interventions
     a. Maintain NPO status.
     b. Administer fluids intravenously to prevent dehydration.
     c. Monitor for changes in level of pain.
     d. Monitor for signs of ruptured appendix and peritonitis.
     e. Position right side-lying or low to semi-Fowler position to promote comfort.
     f. Monitor bowel sounds.
     g. Apply ice packs to the abdomen for 20 to 30 minutes every hour as prescribed.
     h. Administer antibiotics as prescribed.
     i. Avoid the application of heat to the abdomen.
     j. Avoid laxatives or enemas.
   2. Postoperative interventions
     a. Monitor temperature for signs of infection.
     b. Assess incision for signs of infection such as redness, swelling, and pain.
     c. Maintain NPO status until bowel function has returned.
     d. Advance diet gradually as tolerated and as prescribed, when bowel sounds return.
     e. If rupture of the appendix occurred, expect a Penrose drain to be inserted, or the incision may be left open to heal from the inside out.
     f. Expect that drainage from the Penrose drain may be profuse for the first 12 hours.

BOX 55-9

Signs of Peritonitis

Increased fever and chills
Pallor
Progressive abdominal distention and abdominal pain
Restlessness
Right guarding of the abdomen
Tachycardia and tachypnea

g. Position the client in right side-lying or low to semi-Fowler position, with legs flexed, to facilitate drainage.

h. Change the dressing as prescribed and record the type and amount of drainage.

i. Perform wound irrigations if prescribed.

j. Maintain nasogastric suction and patency of nasogastric tube if present.

k. Administer antibiotics and analgesics as prescribed.

XVIII. CIRRHOSIS (BOX 55-10)

A. Description

1. **Cirrhosis** is a chronic, progressive disease of the liver characterized by diffuse damage to cells with fibrosis and nodular regeneration.

2. Repeated destruction of hepatic cells causes the formation of scar tissue.

B. Complications

1. **Portal hypertension**: A persistent increase in pressure within the portal vein that develops as a result of obstruction to flow

2. **Ascites**

   a. **Ascites** is the accumulation of fluid within the peritoneal cavity that results in venous congestion of the hepatic capillaries.

   b. Capillary congestion leads to plasma leaking directly from the liver surface and portal vein.

3. Bleeding **esophageal varices**: fragile, thin-walled, distended esophageal veins that become irritated and rupture

---

BOX 55-10

Types of Cirrhosis

LAËNNEC'S CIRRHOSIS
Cirrhosis is alcohol-induced, nutritional, or portal.
Cellular necrosis causes eventual widespread scar tissue, with fibrotic infiltration of the liver.

POSTNECROTIC CIRRHOSIS
Cirrhosis occurs after massive liver necrosis.
Cirrhosis results as a complication of acute viral hepatitis or exposure to hepatotoxins.
Scar tissue causes destruction of liver lobules and entire lobes.

BILIARY CIRRHOSIS
Cirrhosis develops from chronic biliary obstruction, bile stasis, and inflammation resulting in severe obstructive jaundice.

CARDIAC CIRRHOSIS
Cirrhosis is associated with severe, right-sided congestive heart failure and results in an enlarged, edematous, congested liver.
The liver becomes anoxic, resulting in liver cell necrosis and fibrosis.

---

4. Coagulation defects

   a. Decreased synthesis of bile fats in the liver prevents the absorption of fat-soluble vitamins.

   b. Without vitamin K and clotting factors II, VII, IX, and X, the client is prone to bleeding.

5. Jaundice: Occurs because the liver is unable to metabolize bilirubin and because the edema, fibrosis, and scarring of the hepatic bile ducts interfere with normal bile and bilirubin secretion.

6. Portal systemic encephalopathy: End-stage hepatic failure and **cirrhosis** characterized by altered level of consciousness, neurological symptoms, impaired thinking, and neuromuscular disturbances.

7. Hepatorenal syndrome

   a. Progressive renal failure associated with hepatic failure

   b. Characterized by a sudden decrease in urinary output, elevated blood urea nitrogen and creatinine, decreased urine sodium excretion, and increased urine osmolarity

C. Assessment

1. Anorexia and weight loss

2. Early morning nausea and vomiting (presence of blood in vomitus)

3. Dyspepsia

4. Flatulence and changes in bowel habits

5. Emaciation

6. Fatigue

7. Jaundice

8. Abdominal pain or tenderness

9. **Ascites**

10. Peripheral edema

11. Dry skin and rashes

12. Petechiae or ecchymosis

13. Spider angiomas on the nose, cheeks, upper thorax, and shoulders

14. Hepatomegaly

15. Protruding umbilicus

16. Dilated abdominal veins

17. **Fetor hepaticus**, the fruity, musty breath odor of chronic liver disease

18. **Asterixis** (liver flap): A course tremor characterized by rapid, nonrhythmic extension and flexions in the wrist and fingers

19. Delirium

D. Interventions

1. Elevate the head of the bed to minimize shortness of breath.

2. If **ascites** and edema is absent and the client does not exhibit signs of impending coma, a high-protein diet supplemented with vitamins is prescribed.

3. Provide supplemental vitamins (B complex; vitamins A, C, and K; folic acid; and thiamine) as prescribed.

4. Restrict sodium intake and fluid intake as prescribed.

5. Initiate enteral feedings or total parenteral nutrition as prescribed.
6. Administer diuretics as prescribed.
7. Monitor intake and output and electrolyte balance.
8. Weigh client and measure abdominal girth daily.
9. Monitor level of consciousness; assess for precoma state (tremors, delirium).
10. Monitor for **asterixis.**
11. Maintain gastric intubation to assess bleeding or esophagogastric balloon tamponade to control bleeding varices if prescribed.
12. Administer blood products as prescribed.
13. Monitor coagulation laboratory results; administer vitamin K if prescribed.
14. Administer low sodium antacids as prescribed.
15. Administer lactulose (Chronulac) as prescribed, which decreases the pH of the bowel, decreases production of ammonia by bacteria in the bowel, and facilitates the excretion of ammonia.
16. Administer neomycin (Mycifradin) as prescribed to inhibit protein synthesis in bacteria and decrease the production of ammonia.
17. Avoid medications such as narcotics, sedatives, and barbiturates and any hepatotoxic medications or substances.
18. Instruct the client about the restriction of alcohol intake.
19. Prepare the client for paracentesis to remove abdominal fluid.
20. Prepare the client for surgical shunting procedures if prescribed.

XIX. CHOLECYSTITIS

A. Description
1. **Cholecystitis** is an inflammation of the gallbladder that may occur as an acute or chronic process.
2. Acute inflammation is associated with gallstones (cholelithiasis).
3. Chronic **cholecystitis** results when inefficient bile emptying and gallbladder muscle wall disease cause a fibrotic and contracted gallbladder.
4. Acalculus **cholecystitis** occurs in the absence of gallstones and is due to bacterial invasion via the lymphatic or vascular systems.

B. Assessment
1. Nausea and vomiting
2. Indigestion
3. Belching
4. Flatulence
5. Epigastric pain that radiates to the scapula 2 to 4 hours after eating fatty foods and may persist for 4 to 6 hours.
6. Pain localized in right upper quadrant
7. Guarding, rigidity, and rebound tenderness
8. Mass palpated in the right upper quadrant

9. **Murphy's sign** (cannot take a deep breath when the examiner's fingers are passed below the hepatic margin)
10. Elevated temperature
11. Tachycardia
12. Signs of dehydration

C. Biliary obstruction
1. Jaundice
2. Dark orange and foamy urine
3. Steatorrhea and clay-colored feces
4. Pruritus

D. Interventions
1. Maintain NPO status during nausea and vomiting episodes.
2. Maintain nasogastric decompression as prescribed for severe vomiting.
3. Administer antiemetics as prescribed for nausea and vomiting.
4. Administer analgesics as prescribed to relieve pain and reduce spasm (note: although morphine sulfate or codeine sulfate may be prescribed, they generally are avoided because they can cause spasm of the sphincter of Oddi and increase pain).
5. Administer antispasmodic (anticholinergics) as prescribed to relax smooth muscle.
6. Instruct the client with chronic **cholecystitis** to eat low-fat meals more frequently in small amounts.
7. Instruct the client to avoid gas-forming foods.
8. Prepare the client for nonsurgical and surgical procedures as prescribed.

E. Nonsurgical interventions
1. Dissolution therapy
   a. Dissolution therapy is done to remove cholesterol stones.
   b. Medications such as chenodeoxycholic acid (Chenodiol) or ursodiol (Actigall) may be administered orally to decrease the size of the stones or to dissolve small stones.
   c. Direct contact with repeated injections and aspirations of a dissolution agent via percutaneous catheter may be performed.
2. Extracorporeal shock wave lithotripsy
   a. Shock waves are administered that disintegrate stones in the biliary system.
   b. Oral dissolution follows.

F. Surgical interventions
1. **Cholecystectomy** is removal of the gallbladder.
2. **Choledochotomy** requires incision into the common bile duct to remove the stone.
3. Surgical procedures may be performed by laparoscopy.

G. Postoperative interventions
1. Monitor for respiratory complications caused by pain at the incisional site.
2. Encourage coughing and deep breathing.
3. Encourage early ambulation.

4. Instruct the client about splinting the abdomen to prevent discomfort during coughing.
5. Administer antiemetics as prescribed for nausea and vomiting.
6. Administer analgesics as prescribed for pain relief.
7. Maintain NPO status and nasogastric tube suction as prescribed.
8. Advance diet from clear liquids to solids when prescribed and as tolerated by the client.
9. Maintain and monitor drainage from the T-tube, if present (Box 55-11).

XX. PANCREATITIS

A. Description
1. **Pancreatitis** is an acute or chronic inflammation of the pancreas with associated escape of pancreatic enzymes into surrounding tissue.
2. Acute **pancreatitis** occurs suddenly as one attack or can be recurrent with resolutions.
3. Chronic **pancreatitis** is a continual inflammation and destruction of the pancreas, with scar tissue replacing pancreatic tissue.
4. Precipitating factors include trauma, the use of alcohol, biliary tract disease, viral or bacterial disease, hyperlipedemia, hypercalcemia, cholelithiasis, hyperparathyroidism, ischemic vascular disease, and peptic ulcer disease.

BOX 55-11

Care of a T-Tube

PURPOSE AND DESCRIPTION
A T-tube is placed after surgical exploration of the common bile duct. The tube preserves the patency of the duct and ensures drainage of bile until edema resolves and bile is effectively draining into the duodenum. A gravity drainage bag is attached to the T-tube to collect the drainage.

INTERVENTIONS
Position client in semi-Fowler position to facilitate drainage.
Monitor the amount, color, consistency, and odor of drainage.
Report sudden increases in bile output to the physician.
Monitor for inflammation and protect the skin from irritation.
Keep the drainage system below the level of the gallbladder.
Monitor for foul odor and purulent drainage and report to the physician.
Avoid irrigation, aspiration, or clamping of the T-tube without a physician's order.
As prescribed, clamp the tube before a meal, and observe for abdominal discomfort and distention, nausea, chills, or fever; unclamp the tube if nausea or vomiting occurs.

B. Acute **pancreatitis**
1. Assessment
   a. Abdominal pain, including a sudden onset at the midepigastric or left upper quadrant location with radiation to the back
   b. Pain that is aggravated by a fatty meal, alcohol, or lying in a recumbent position
   c. Abdominal tenderness and guarding
   d. Nausea and vomiting
   e. Weight loss
   f. **Cullen's sign** (discoloration of the abdomen and periumbilical area)
   g. **Turner's sign** (bluish discoloration of the flanks)
   h. Absent or decreased bowel sounds
   i. Elevated white blood cell count, glucose, bilirubin, alkaline phosphatase, urinary amylase
   j. Elevated lipase and amylase
2. Interventions
   a. Maintain NPO status and maintain hydration with IV fluids as prescribed.
   b. Administer total parenteral nutrition for severe nutritional depletion.
   c. Administer supplemental preparations and vitamins and minerals to increase caloric intake if prescribed.
   d. Maintain nasogastric tube to decrease gastric distention and suppress pancreatic secretion.
   e. Administer meperidine hydrochloride (Demerol) as prescribed for pain because it causes less incidence of smooth muscle spasm of the pancreatic ducts and sphincter of Oddi (note: although morphine sulfate or codeine sulfate may be prescribed, they generally are avoided because they can cause spasm of the sphincter of Oddi and increase pain).
   f. Administer antacids as prescribed to neutralize gastric secretions.
   g. Administer histamine H_2 receptor antagonists as prescribed to decrease hydrochloric acid production and prevent activation of pancreatic enzymes.
   h. Administer anticholinergics as prescribed to decrease vagal stimulation, decrease gastrointestinal motility, and inhibit pancreatic enzyme secretion.
   i. Instruct the client in the importance of avoiding alcohol.
   j. Instruct the client in the importance of follow-up visits with the physician.
   k. Instruct the client to notify the physician if acute abdominal pain, jaundice, clay-colored stools, or dark urine develops.
C. Chronic **pancreatitis**
1. Assessment
   a. Abdominal pain and tenderness
   b. Left upper quadrant mass

c. Steatorrhea and foul-smelling stools that may increase in volume as pancreatic insufficiency increases
d. Weight loss
e. Muscle wasting
f. Jaundice
g. Signs and symptoms of diabetes mellitus
2. Interventions
a. Instruct the client in the prescribed dietary measures (fat and protein intake may be limited).
b. Instruct the client to avoid heavy meals.
c. Instruct the client about the importance of avoiding alcohol.
d. Provide supplemental preparations and vitamins and minerals to increase caloric intake.
e. Administer pancreatic enzymes as prescribed to aid in the digestion and absorption of fat and protein.
f. Administer insulin or oral hypoglycemic medications as prescribed to control diabetes mellitus, if present.
g. Instruct the client in the use of pancreatic enzyme medications.
h. Instruct the client in the treatment plan for glucose management.
i. Instruct the client to notify the physician if increased steatorrhea occurs or if abdominal distention or cramping and skin breakdown develops.
j. Instruct the client in the importance of follow-up visits.

XXI. HEPATITIS

A. Description
1. An inflammation of the liver caused by a virus, bacteria, or exposure to medications or hepatotoxins.
2. The goals of treatment include resting the inflamed liver to reduce metabolic demands and increasing the blood supply, thus promoting cellular regeneration and preventing complications.
B. Types of viral hepatitis
1. Hepatitis A virus (HAV), infectious hepatitis
2. Hepatitis B virus (HBV), serum hepatitis
3. Hepatitis C virus (HCV), non-A, non-B hepatitis or posttransfusion hepatitis
4. Hepatitis D virus (HDV), delta agent hepatitis
5. Hepatitis E virus (HEV), enterically transmitted or epidemic non-A, non-B hepatitis
6. Hepatitis G virus, non-A, non-B, non-C hepatitis
C. Stages of viral hepatitis (Box 55-12)
D. Assessment
1. Preicteric stage
a. Flulike symptoms: malaise, fatigue
b. Anorexia, nausea, vomiting, diarrhea
c. Pain: headache, muscle aches, polyarthritis
d. Serum bilirubin and enzyme levels are elevated

BOX 55-12

Stages of Viral Hepatitis

PREICTERIC STAGE
The first stage of hepatitis preceding the appearance of jaundice

ICTERIC STAGE
The second stage of hepatitis, which includes the appearance of jaundice and associated symptoms such as elevated bilirubin levels, dark or tea-colored urine, and clay-colored stools

POSTICTERIC STAGE
The convalescent stage in which the jaundice decreases and the color of the urine and stool return to normal

---

2. Icteric stage
a. Jaundice
b. Pruritus
c. Brown-colored urine
d. Lighter-colored stools
e. Decrease in preicteric phase symptoms
3. Posticteric stage
a. Increased energy levels
b. Subsiding of pain
c. Minimal to absent gastrointestinal symptoms
d. Serum bilirubin and enzyme levels returned to normal
E. Laboratory assessment
1. Alanine aminotransferase: elevated to more than 1000 milliunits/mL and may rise to as high as 4000 milliunits/mL
2. Aspartate aminotransferase: may rise to 1000 to 2000 milliunits/mL
3. Alkaline phosphatase levels: may be normal or mildly elevated
4. Total bilirubin levels: elevated in serum and urine

XXII. HEPATITIS A

A. Description
1. Formerly known as infectious hepatitis
2. Commonly seen during the fall and early winter
B. Individuals at increased risk
1. Commonly seen in young children
2. Individuals in institutionalized settings
3. Health care personnel
C. Transmission
1. Fecal-oral route
2. Person-to-person contact
3. Parenteral
4. Contaminated fruits, vegetables, or uncooked shellfish
5. Contaminated water or milk
6. Poorly washed utensils
D. Incubation period
1. Incubation period is 2 to 6 weeks.

2. Infectious period is 2 to 3 weeks before and 1 week after development of jaundice

E. Testing
1. Infection is established by the presence of HAV antibodies (anti-HAV) in the blood.
2. Immunoglobulin M (IgM) and IgG are normally present in the blood, and increased levels indicate infection and inflammation.
3. Ongoing inflammation of the liver is evidenced by the presence of elevated IgM antibodies, which persist in the blood for 4 to 6 weeks.
4. Previous infection is indicated by the presence of elevated IgG antibodies.

F. Complication: fulminant hepatitis

G. Prevention
1. Strict hand washing
2. Stool and needle precautions
3. Treatment of municipal water supplies
4. Serological screening of food handlers
5. Hepatitis A vaccine (Havrix)
6. Immune globulin: For individuals exposed to HAV who have never received the hepatitis A vaccine; administer immunoglobulin during the period of incubation and within 2 weeks of exposure.
7. Immunoglobulin is recommended for household members and sexual contacts of individuals with hepatitis A.
8. Preexposure prophylaxis with immunoglobulin is recommended to individuals traveling to countries with poor or uncertain sanitation conditions.

XXIII. HEPATITIS B

A. Description
1. Hepatitis B is nonseasonal.
2. All age groups are affected.

B. Individuals at increased risk
1. Drug addicts
2. Clients undergoing long-term hemodialysis
3. Health care personnel

C. Transmission
1. Blood or body fluid contact
2. Infected blood products
3. Infected saliva or semen
4. Contaminated needles
5. Sexual contact
6. Parenteral
7. Perinatal period
8. Blood or body fluids contact at birth

D. Incubation period: 6 to 24 weeks

E. Testing
1. Infection is established by the presence of hepatitis B antigen-antibody systems in the blood.
2. Presence of hepatitis B surface antigens (HBsAg) is the serological marker to establish the diagnosis of hepatitis B.
3. The client is considered infectious if these antigens are present in the blood.

4. If the serological marker (HBsAg) is present after 6 months, it indicates a carrier state or chronic hepatitis.
5. Normally the serological marker (HBsAg) level declines and disappears after the acute hepatitis B episode.
6. The presence of antibodies to HBsAg (anti-HBs) indicates recovery and immunity to hepatitis B.
7. Hepatitis B early antigen (HBeAG) is detected in the blood about 1 week after the appearance of HBsAg and its presence determines the infective state of the client.

F. Complications
1. Fulminant hepatitis
2. Chronic liver disease
3. **Cirrhosis**
4. Primary hepatocellular carcinoma

G. Prevention
1. Strict hand washing
2. Screening blood donors
3. Testing of all pregnant women
4. Needle precautions
5. Avoiding intimate sexual contact if test for hepatitis B surface antigen (HBsAg) is positive in a person
6. Hepatitis B vaccine: Engerix-B, Recombivax HB
7. Hepatitis B immune globulin is for individuals exposed to HBV through sexual contact or through the percutaneous or transmucosal routes, who have never had hepatitis B and have never received hepatitis B vaccine.

XXIV. HEPATITIS C

A. Description
1. Hepatitis C virus infection occurs year-round.
2. Infection can occur in any age group.
3. Infection with HCV is common among drug abusers and is the major cause of posttransfusion hepatitis.
4. Risk factors are similar to those for HBV because hepatitis C also is transmitted parenterally.

B. Individuals at increased risk
1. Parenteral drug users
2. Clients receiving frequent transfusions
3. Health care personnel

C. Transmission: Same as for HBV; primarily through blood

D. Incubation period: 5 to 10 weeks

E. Testing: Anti-HCV is the antibody to HCV and is most accurate in detecting chronic states of hepatitis C.

F. Complications
1. Chronic liver disease
2. **Cirrhosis**
3. Primary hepatocellular carcinoma

G. Prevention
1. Strict hand washing
2. Needle precautions
3. Screening of blood donors

XXV. HEPATITIS D

A. Description
 1. Hepatitis D is common in the Mediterranean and Middle Eastern areas.
 2. Hepatitis D occurs with hepatitis B and may cause infection only in the presence of active HBV infection.
 3. Coinfection with the delta-agent intensifies the acute symptoms of hepatitis B.
 4. Transmission and risk of infection are the same as for HBV, via contact with blood and blood products.
 5. Prevention of HBV infection with vaccine also prevents HDV infection because HDV depends on HBV for replication.
B. High-risk individuals
 1. Drug users
 2. Clients receiving hemodialysis
 3. Clients receiving frequent blood transfusions
C. Transmission: Same as for HBV
D. Incubation period: 7 to 8 weeks
E. Testing: Serological HDV determination is made by detection of the hepatitis D (HDAg) antigen early in the course of the infection and by detection of anti-HDV antibody in the later disease stages.
F. Complications
 1. Chronic liver disease
 2. Fulminant hepatitis
G. Prevention: Because hepatitis D must coexist with hepatitis B, the precautions that help prevent hepatitis B are also useful in preventing delta hepatitis.

XXVI. HEPATITIS E

A. Description
 1. Hepatitis E is a waterborne virus.
 2. Hepatitis E is prevalent in areas where sewage disposal is inadequate or where communal bathing in contaminated rivers is practiced.
 3. Risk of infection is the same as for HAV.
 4. Infection with HEV presents as a mild disease except in infected women in the third trimester of pregnancy, with whom the mortality rate is high.
B. Individuals with increased risk
 1. Travelers to countries that have a high incidence of Hepatitis E such as India, Burma (Myanmar), Afghanistan, Algeria, and Mexico
 2. Eating or drinking of food or water contaminated with the virus
C. Transmission: Same as for HAV
D. Incubation period: 2 to 9 weeks
E. Testing: Specific serological tests for HEV include detection of IgM and IgG antibodies to hepatitis E (anti-HEV).
F. Complications
 1. High mortality rate in pregnant women
 2. Fetal demise
G. Prevention
 1. Strict hand washing

BOX 55-13

Client and Family Education for Hepatitis

Hand washing must be strict and frequent.
Do not share bathrooms unless the client strictly adheres to personal hygiene measures.
Individual washcloths, towels, drinking and eating utensils, and toothbrushes and razors must be labeled and identified.
The client must not prepare food for other family members.
The client should avoid alcohol and over-the-counter medications, particularly acetaminophen (Tylenol) and sedatives because these medications are hepatotoxic.
The client should increase activity gradually to prevent fatigue.
The client should consume small, frequent, high-carbohydrate, low-fat foods.
The client is not to donate blood.
The client may maintain normal contact with persons as long as proper personal hygiene is maintained.
Close personal contact such as kissing should be discouraged until hepatitis B surface antigen test results are negative.
The client is to avoid sexual activity until hepatitis B surface antigen results are negative.
The client needs to carry a Medic-Alert card noting the date of hepatitis onset.
The client needs to inform other health professionals, such as medical or dental personnel, of the onset of hepatitis.
The client needs to keep follow-up appointments with the health care provider.

---

 2. Treatment of water supplies and sanitation measures

XXVII. HEPATITIS G

A. Hepatitis G is non-A, non-B, non-C hepatitis.
B. Autoantibodies are absent.
C. Risk factors are similar to those for hepatitis C.
D. Hepatitis G virus has been found in some blood donors, IV drug users, hemodialysis clients, and clients with hemophilia; however, hepatitis G virus does not appear to cause significant liver disease.

XXVIII. INSTRUCTION FOR HOME CARE FOR THE CLIENT AND FAMILY (BOX 55-13)

PRACTICE QUESTIONS

1. The nurse is participating in a health screening clinic and is preparing teaching materials about colorectal cancer. The nurse plans to include which of the following in a list of risk factors for colorectal cancer?
 1. Age over 30 years
 2. High-fiber, low-fat diet
 3. Distant relative with colorectal cancer

4. Personal history of ulcerative colitis or gastrointestinal polyps

2. The hospitalized client with gastroesophageal reflux disease is complaining of chest discomfort that feels like heartburn following a meal. After administering an ordered antacid, the nurse encourages the client to lie in which of the following positions?
   1. Supine with the head of bed flat
   2. On the stomach with the head flat
   3. On the left side with the head of bed elevated 30 degrees
   4. On the right side with the head of bed elevated 30 degrees

3. The nurse is planning to teach the client with gastroesophageal reflux disease about substances that will increase the lower esophageal sphincter pressure. Which of the following items would the nurse include on this list?
   1. Fatty foods
   2. Nonfat milk
   3. Chocolate
   4. Coffee

4. The client has undergone esophagogastroduodenoscopy. The nurse places highest priority on which of the following items as part of the client's care plan?
   1. Assessing for the return of the gag reflex
   2. Giving warm gargles for a sore throat
   3. Monitoring the temperature
   4. Monitoring complaints of heartburn

5. The nurse has taught the client about an upcoming endoscopic retrograde cholangiopancreatography procedure. The nurse determines that the client needs further information if the client makes which of the following statements?
   1. "I know I must sign the consent form."
   2. "I'm glad I don't have to lie still for this procedure."
   3. "I'm glad some IV medication will be given to relax me."
   4. "I hope the throat spray keeps me from gagging."

6. The client being seen in a physician's office has just been scheduled for a barium swallow the next day. The nurse writes down which of the following instructions for the client to follow before the test?
   1. Fast for 8 hours before the test.
   2. Eat a regular supper and breakfast.
   3. Continue to take all oral medications as scheduled.
   4. Monitor own bowel movement pattern for constipation.

7. The nurse has given postprocedure instructions to a client who underwent colonoscopy. The nurse determines that the client needs further instructions if the client stated that
   1. Intake should be light at first and then progress to regular intake.
   2. It is normal to feel gassy or bloated after the procedure.

3. The abdominal muscles may be tender from the procedure.
   4. It is all right to drive once the client has been home for an hour or so.

8. The nurse is performing an abdominal assessment. The nurse performs which assessment technique first?
   1. Auscultation
   2. Inspection
   3. Palpation
   4. Percussion

9. Polyethylene glycol–electrolyte solution (GoLYTELY) is prescribed for the client scheduled for a colonoscopy. The client begins to experience diarrhea following administration of the solution. What action by the nurse is most appropriate?
   1. Cancel the diagnostic test.
   2. Start an IV infusion.
   3. Administer an enema.
   4. Explain that diarrhea is expected.

10. The nurse is caring for a client with a diagnosis of chronic gastritis. The nurse monitors the client, knowing that this client is at risk for which of the following vitamin deficiencies?
    1. Vitamin A
    2. Vitamin B_{12}
    3. Vitamin C
    4. Vitamin E

11. The nurse is reviewing the medication record of a client with acute gastritis. Which medication if noted on the client's record, would the nurse question?
    1. Digoxin (Lanoxin)
    2. Indomethacin (Indocin)
    3. Furosemide (Lasix)
    4. Propranolol hydrochloride (Inderal)

12. The nurse is assessing a client 24 hours following a cholecystectomy. The nurse notes that the T-tube has drained 750 mL of green-brown drainage. Which nursing intervention is most appropriate?
    1. Notify the physician.
    2. Document the findings.
    3. Irrigate the T-tube.
    4. Clamp the T-tube.

13. The nurse is monitoring a client with a diagnosis of peptic ulcer. Which assessment finding would most likely indicate perforation of the ulcer?
    1. Bradycardia
    2. Numbness in the legs
    3. Nausea and vomiting
    4. A rigid, boardlike abdomen

14. The nurse provides medication instructions to a client with peptic ulcer disease. Which statement, if made by the client, indicates the best understanding of the medication therapy?
    1. "The cimetidine (Tagamet) will cause me to produce less stomach acid."
    2. "Sucralfate (Carafate) will change the fluid in my stomach."

3. "Antacids will coat my stomach."

4. "Omeprazole (Prilosec) will coat the ulcer and help it heal."

15. The client with peptic ulcer disease is scheduled for a pyloroplasty. The client asks the nurse about the procedure. The nurse plans to respond knowing that a pyloroplasty involves

1. Cutting the vagus nerve.

2. Removing the distal portion of the stomach.

3. Removal of the ulcer and a large portion of the cells that produce hydrochloric acid.

4. An incision and resuturing of the pylorus to relax the muscle and enlarge the opening from the stomach to the duodenum.

16. A client with a peptic ulcer is scheduled for a vagotomy. The client asks the nurse about the purpose of this procedure. The nurse tells the client that the procedure

1. Decreases food absorption in the stomach.

2. Heals the gastric mucosa.

3. Halts stress reactions.

4. Reduces the stimulus to acid secretions.

17. The nurse is caring for a client following a Billroth II procedure. On review of the postoperative orders, which of the following, if prescribed, would the nurse question and verify?

1. Irrigating the nasogastric tube

2. Coughing and deep breathing exercises

3. Leg exercises

4. Early ambulation

18. The nurse is providing discharge instructions to a client following gastrectomy. Which measure will the nurse instruct the client to follow to assist in preventing dumping syndrome?

1. Eat high carbohydrate foods.

2. Limit the fluids taken with meals.

3. Ambulate following a meal.

4. Sit in a high Fowler's position during meals.

19. The nurse is monitoring a client for the early signs and symptoms of dumping syndrome. Which symptom indicates this occurrence?

1. Abdominal cramping and pain

2. Bradycardia and indigestion

3. Sweating and pallor

4. Double vision and chest pain

20. The nurse is preparing a discharge teaching plan for the client who had an umbilical hernia repair. Which of the following would the nurse include in the plan?

1. Restricting pain medication

2. Maintaining bedrest

3. Avoiding coughing

4. Irrigating the drain

21. The nurse is instructing the client who had an inguinal hernia repair how to reduce postoperative swelling following the procedure. The nurse tells the client to

1. Apply heat to the abdomen.

2. Elevate the scrotum.

3. Limit oral fluids.

4. Remain on a low-fiber diet.

22. The nurse is caring for a hospitalized client with a diagnosis of ulcerative colitis. Which finding, if noted on assessment of the client, would the nurse report to the physician?

1. Bloody diarrhea

2. Hypotension

3. A hemoglobin level of 12 mg/dL

4. Rebound tenderness

23. The nurse is caring for a client postoperatively following creation of a colostomy. Which of the following nursing diagnoses would the nurse include in the plan of care?

1. Imbalanced Nutrition: More Than Body Requirements

2. Disturbed Body Image

3. Fear Related to Poor Prognosis

4. Sexual Dysfunction

24. The nurse is reviewing the record of a client with Crohn's disease. Which of the following stool characteristics would the nurse expect to note documented in the client's record?

1. Chronic constipation

2. Diarrhea

3. Constipation alternating with diarrhea

4. Stool constantly oozing from the rectum

25. The nurse is performing a colostomy irrigation on a client. During the irrigation, the client begins to complain of abdominal cramps. Which of the following is the most appropriate nursing action?

1. Notify the physician.

2. Increase the height of the irrigation.

3. Stop the irrigation temporarily.

4. Medicate for pain and resume the irrigation.

26. The nurse is teaching a client how to perform a colostomy irrigation. To enhance the effectiveness of the irrigation and fecal returns, what measure should the nurse instruct the client to do?

1. Increase fluid intake.

2. Reduce the amount of irrigation solution.

3. Perform the irrigation in the evening.

4. Place heat on the abdomen.

27. The nurse is reviewing the record of a client with a diagnosis of cirrhosis and notes that there is documentation of the presence of asterixis. To assess for the presence of this sign, the nurse would do which of the following?

1. Ask the client to extend the arms.

2. Assess for the presence of Homans' sign.

3. Instruct the client to lean forward.

4. Measure the abdominal girth.

28. The client with ascites is scheduled for a paracentesis. The nurse is assisting the physician in performing the procedure. Which of the following positions

will the nurse assist the client to assume for this procedure?

1. Supine
2. Left side-lying
3. Right side-lying
4. Upright position

29. The nurse is reviewing the laboratory results in a client with cirrhosis and notes that the ammonia level is elevated. Which of the following diets would the nurse anticipate would most likely be prescribed for this client?

1. High-carbohydrate
2. Moderate-fat
3. High-protein
4. Low-protein

30. The client is admitted to the hospital for treatment of acute hepatitis B. Which activity order would the nurse expect to be prescribed?

1. Bedrest
2. Encourage ambulation
3. Out of bed in a chair
4. No activity restrictions

31. The physician has determined that the client with hepatitis has contracted the infection from contaminated food. The nurse understands that this client is most likely experiencing what type of hepatitis?

1. Hepatitis A
2. Hepatitis B
3. Hepatitis C
4. Hepatitis D

32. A client is suspected of having hepatitis. Which diagnostic test results will assist in confirming this diagnosis?

1. Decreased erythrocyte sedimentation rate
2. Elevated serum bilirubin
3. Elevated hemoglobin
4. Elevated blood urea nitrogen

33. The nurse is reviewing the physician's orders written for a client admitted with acute pancreatitis. Which physician order would the nurse question if noted on the client's chart?

1. NPO status
2. Insert a nasogastric tube
3. An anticholinergic medication
4. Morphine sulfate for pain

34. The nurse is doing an admission assessment on a client with a history of duodenal ulcer. To determine whether the problem is currently active, the nurse would assess the client for which of the following most frequent symptom(s) of duodenal ulcer?

1. Pain that is relieved by food intake
2. Pain that radiates down the right arm
3. Nausea and vomiting
4. Weight loss

35. The client with peptic ulcer disease needs dietary modification to reduce episodes of epigastric pain. The nurse tells the client that which of the following

items does not need to be limited or eliminated with this disease?

1. Wine
2. Baked chicken
3. Coffee
4. Fresh fruit

36. The medication history of a client with peptic ulcer disease reveals intermittent use of several medications. The nurse would teach the client to avoid which of these medications due to the irritating effects on the lining of the gastrointestinal tract?

1. Omeprazole (Prilosec)
2. Ibuprofen (Motrin)
3. Sucralfate (Carafate)
4. Nizatidine (Axid)

37. The nurse instructs the ileostomy client to do which of the following as part of essential care of the stoma?

1. Cleanse the peristomal skin meticulously.
2. Take in high-fiber foods such as nuts.
3. Massage the area below the stoma.
4. Limit fluid intake to prevent diarrhea.

38. The client with hiatal hernia chronically experiences heartburn following meals. The nurse would plan to teach the client to avoid which of the following, which is contraindicated with a hiatal hernia?

1. Taking in small, frequent, bland meals
2. Lying recumbent following meals
3. Raising the head of bed on 6-inch blocks
4. Taking histamine H_2 receptor antagonist medication

39. The client who has undergone creation of a colostomy has a nursing diagnosis of Disturbed Body Image. The nurse would evaluate that the client is making the most significant progress toward identified goals if the client:

1. Watches the nurse empty the ostomy bag.
2. Looks at the ostomy site.
3. Reads the ostomy product literature.
4. Practices cutting the ostomy appliance.

40. The nurse is assessing for stoma prolapse in a client with a colostomy. The nurse would observe which of the following if stoma prolapse occurred?

1. Sunken and hidden stoma
2. Dark- and bluish-colored stoma
3. Narrowed and flattened stoma
4. Protruding stoma

41. The client has had a new colostomy created 2 days earlier. The client is beginning to pass malodorous flatus from the stoma. The nurse interprets that

1. This indicates inadequate preoperative bowel preparation.
2. This is a normal, expected event.
3. The client is experiencing early signs of ischemic bowel.
4. The client should not have the nasogastric tube removed.

42. The client with a new colostomy is concerned about the odor from stool in the ostomy drainage bag. The nurse teaches the client to include which of the following foods in the diet to reduce odor?
    1. Yogurt
    2. Broccoli
    3. Cucumbers
    4. Eggs

43. The nurse has given instructions to the client with an ileostomy about foods to eat to thicken the stool. The nurse determines that the client needs further instructions if the client stated to eat which of the following foods to make the stool less watery?
    1. Pasta
    2. Boiled rice
    3. Bran
    4. Low-fat cheese

44. The client has just had surgery to create an ileostomy. The nurse assesses the client in the immediate post-operative period for which of the following most frequent complications of this type of surgery?
    1. Intestinal obstruction
    2. Fluid and electrolyte imbalance
    3. Malabsorption of fat
    4. Folate deficiency

45. The nurse is doing preoperative teaching with the client who is about to undergo creation of a Kock pouch. The nurse interprets that the client has the best understanding of the nature of the surgery if the client makes which of the following statements?
    1. "I will need to drain the pouch regularly with a catheter."
    2. "I will need to wear a drainage bag for the rest of my life."
    3. "The drainage from this type of ostomy will be formed."
    4. "I will be able to pass stool by the rectum eventually."

46. The client with a colostomy has an order for irrigation of the colostomy. The nurse uses which solution for the irrigation?
    1. Distilled water
    2. Tap water
    3. Sterile water
    4. Lactated Ringer's

47. The nurse is monitoring a client admitted to the hospital with a diagnosis of appendicitis. The client is scheduled for surgery in 2 hours. The client begins to complain of increased abdominal pain and begins to vomit. On assessment the nurse notes that the abdomen is distended and bowel sounds are diminished. Which of the following is the most appropriate nursing intervention?
    1. Administer the prescribed pain medication.
    2. Notify the physician.
    3. Call and ask the operating room team to perform the surgery as soon as possible.

    4. Reposition the client and apply a heating pad on warm setting to the client's abdomen.

48. The client has been admitted with a diagnosis of acute pancreatitis. The nurse would assess this client for pain that is
    1. Severe and unrelenting, located in the epigastric area and radiating to the back.
    2. Severe and unrelenting, located in the left lower quadrant and radiating to the groin.
    3. Burning and aching, located in the epigastric area and radiating to the umbilicus.
    4. Burning and aching, located in the left lower quadrant and radiating to the hip.

49. The client with chronic pancreatitis needs information on dietary modification to manage the health problem. The nurse teaches the client to limit which of the following items in the diet?
    1. Carbohydrate
    2. Protein
    3. Fat
    4. Water soluble vitamins

50. The nurse had taught the client with chronic pancreatitis about risk factor modification to reduce the incidence of recurrences. The nurse determines that the client has understood the information if the client states it will be necessary to control which of the following?
    1. Diabetes mellitus
    2. Alcohol intake
    3. Duodenal ulcer
    4. Crohn's disease

51. The nurse is evaluating the effect of dietary counseling on the client with cholecystitis. The nurse would evaluate that the client understands the instructions given if the client stated that which of the following food items is acceptable in the diet?
    1. Baked scrod
    2. Sauces and gravies
    3. Fried chicken
    4. Fresh whipped cream

52. The nurse would assess the client experiencing an acute episode of cholecystitis for pain that is located in the right
    1. Upper quadrant and radiates to the left scapula and shoulder.
    2. Upper quadrant and radiates to the right scapula and shoulder.
    3. Lower quadrant and radiates to the umbilicus.
    4. Lower quadrant and radiates to the back.

53. The client with cirrhosis is beginning to show signs of hepatic encephalopathy. The nurse would plan a dietary consult to limit the amount of which of the following ingredients in the client's diet?
    1. Fat
    2. Carbohydrate
    3. Protein
    4. Minerals

54. The client with cirrhosis complicated by ascites is admitted to the hospital. The client has stated a 10-lb weight gain over the last week and a half. The client has edema of the feet and ankles. The abdomen is distended, taut, and shiny with striae. The nurse would select which of the following as the most appropriate nursing diagnosis for this client?
    1. Imbalanced Nutrition: More Than Body Requirements
    2. Impaired Gas Exchange
    3. Risk for Impaired Skin Integrity
    4. Excess Fluid Volume

55. The client with Crohn's disease has a nursing diagnosis of Acute Pain. The nurse would teach the client to avoid which of the following in managing this problem?
    1. Lying supine with the legs straight
    2. Massaging the abdomen
    3. Using antispasmodic medication
    4. Using relaxation techniques

56. The client with ulcerative colitis has an order to begin a salicylate medication to reduce inflammation. The nurse instructs the client to take the medication:
    1. 30 minutes before meals
    2. On an empty stomach
    3. After meals
    4. On arising

57. The client with hepatitis is scheduled for a liver biopsy. The nurse implements which of the following to assess for the most common symptom of bile peritonitis following the liver biopsy?
    1. Monitoring for bloody diarrhea
    2. Assessing for rebound tenderness
    3. Assessing for increased flatulence
    4. Monitoring for abdominal pain

58. The client is admitted to the hospital with viral hepatitis, complaining of "no appetite" and "losing my taste for food." To provide adequate nutrition, the nurse would instruct the client to
    1. Eat a good supper when anorexia is not as severe.
    2. Eat less often, preferably only three large meals daily.
    3. Increase intake of fluids including juices.
    4. Select foods high in fat.

59. A client has developed hepatitis A after eating contaminated oysters. The nurse assesses the client for which of the following?
    1. Dark stools
    2. Left upper quadrant discomfort
    3. Malaise
    4. Weight gain

60. The nurse is caring for a black client who has a diagnosis of acute viral hepatitis. The nurse assesses for jaundice by checking which specific area?
    1. Flexor surfaces of the extremities
    2. Hard palate of the mouth
    3. Nailbeds
    4. Skin

CRITICAL THINKING: MULTIPLE RESPONSE

A nurse is reviewing the orders of a client admitted to the hospital with a diagnosis of acute pancreatitis. Select the interventions that the nurse would expect to be prescribed for the client.

____ Small, frequent high calorie feedings

____ Meperidine (Demerol) as prescribed for pain

____ Maintain the client in a supine and flat position.

____ Encourage coughing and deep breathing.

____ Administer antacids as prescribed.

____ Administer anticholinergics as prescribed.

ANSWERS

1. **4.**
Rationale: Common risk factors for colorectal cancer include age over 40 years; first-degree relative with colorectal cancer; high-fat, low-fiber diet; and history of bowel problems, such as ulcerative colitis or familial polyposis.
Test-Taking Strategy: Use the process of elimination, reading each option carefully. Eliminate option 1 because of the age. Eliminate option 2 because this diet is healthful. Eliminate option 3 because of the word "distant." Review risk factors for colorectal cancer if you had difficulty with this question.
Level of Cognitive Ability: Application
Client Needs: Health Promotion and Maintenance
Integrated Process: Teaching/Learning
Content Area: Adult health—gastrointestinal

Reference: Ignatavicius, D., & Workman, M. (2002). *Medical-surgical nursing: Critical thinking for collaborative care* (4th ed., pp. 1245-1246). Philadelphia: W. B. Saunders.

2. **3**
Rationale: The discomfort of reflux is aggravated by positions that compress the abdomen and the stomach. These include lying flat on the back or on the stomach after a meal or lying on the right side. The left side-lying position with the head of bed elevated is most likely to give relief to the client.
Test-Taking Strategy: Use the process of elimination. To answer this question correctly, evaluate each of the positions described in terms of their ability to put pressure on the stomach and cause reflux. Using knowledge of anatomy and these basic nursing positions, you should be able to eliminate each

of the incorrect options. Review care to the client with gastroesophageal reflux disease if you had difficulty with this question.

Level of Cognitive Ability: Application
Client Needs: Physiological Integrity
Integrated Process: Nursing Process—implementation
Content Area: Adult health—gastrointestinal
Reference: Ignatavicius, D., & Workman, M. (2002). *Medical-surgical nursing: Critical thinking for collaborative care* (4th ed., p. 1195). Philadelphia: W. B. Saunders.

3. 2

Rationale: Foods that increase the lower esophageal sphincter (LES) pressure will decrease reflux, and lessen the symptoms of gastroesophageal reflux disease (GERD). The food substance that will increase the LES pressure is nonfat milk. The other substances listed decrease the LES pressure, thus increasing reflux symptoms. Aggravating substances include chocolate, coffee, fatty foods and alcohol.

Test-Taking Strategy: Use the process of elimination. You must understand the effect of various food substances on LES pressure and GERD. However, if you were unsure, select the option that identifies the most healthful food item. Review the dietary regimen for a client with GERD if you had difficulty with this question.

Level of Cognitive Ability: Application
Client Needs: Physiological Integrity
Integrated Process: Teaching/Learning
Content Area: Adult health—gastrointestinal
Reference: Ignatavicius, D., & Workman, M. (2002). *Medical-surgical nursing: Critical thinking for collaborative care* (4th ed., p.1196). Philadelphia: W. B. Saunders.

4. 1

Rationale: The nurse places highest priority on assessing for return of the gag reflex. This assessment addresses the client's airway. The nurse also monitors the client's vital signs, and a sudden sharp increase in temperature could indicate perforation of the gastrointestinal tract. This complication would be accompanied by other signs as well, such as pain. Monitoring for sore throat and heartburn are also important; however, the client's airway is the priority.

Test-Taking Strategy: Use the ABCs: airway, breathing, and circulation. Note the key words "highest priority." Option 1 addresses airway. Review care to the client following esophagogastroduodenoscopy if you had difficulty with this question.

Level of Cognitive Ability: Application
Client Needs: Physiological Integrity
Integrated Process: Nursing Process—planning
Content Area: Delegating/Prioritizing
Reference: Lewis, S., Heitkemper, M., & Dirksen, S. (2004). *Medical-surgical nursing: Assessment and management of clinical problems* (6th ed., p. 963). St. Louis: Mosby.

5. 2

Rationale: The client does have to lie still for endoscopic retrograde cholangiopancreatography (ERCP), which takes about an hour to perform. The client also has to sign a consent form. Intravenous sedation is given to relax the client, and an anesthetic spray is used to help keep the client from gagging as the endoscope is passed.

Test-Taking Strategy: Use the process of elimination. Note the key words "needs further information." Invasive procedures require consent, so option 1 can be eliminated. Noting the name of the procedure and considering the anatomical location will assist you in eliminating options 3 and 4. Review this procedure, if you had difficulty with this question.

Level of Cognitive Ability: Analysis
Client Needs: Physiological Integrity
Integrated Process: Teaching/Learning
Content Area: Adult health—gastrointestinal
Reference: Ignatavicius, D., & Workman, M. (2002). *Medical-surgical nursing: Critical thinking for collaborative care* (4th ed., p. 1174). Philadelphia: W. B. Saunders.

6. 1

Rationale: A barium swallow is an x-ray study that uses a substance called barium for contrast to highlight abnormalities in the gastrointestinal tract. The client should fast for 8 to 12 hours before the test, depending on physician instructions. Most oral medications also are withheld before the test. After the procedure the nurse must monitor for constipation, which can occur as a result of the presence of barium in the gastrointestinal tract.

Test-Taking Strategy: Note the key words "barium swallow" and "before." This tells you that the correct option is an item that the client needs to comply with before the test is done. Eliminate option 4 first because it is a part of aftercare. Knowing that the procedure is a type of x-ray study that involves barium for contrast allows you to eliminate options 2 and 3. Review preprocedure client instructions for this test if you had difficulty with this question.

Level of Cognitive Ability: Application
Client Needs: Physiological Integrity
Integrated Process: Nursing Process—implementation
Content Area: Adult health—gastrointestinal
Reference: Chernecky, C., & Berger, B. (2001). *Laboratory tests and diagnostic procedures* (3rd ed., p. 202). Philadelphia: W. B. Saunders.

7. 4

Rationale: The client should not drive for several hours after discharge because the client would have received sedative medications during the procedure. Important decisions also should be delayed for at least 24 hours for the same reason. The client should resume intake slowly and progress as tolerated. The client may experience gas or abdominal tenderness for a short while after the procedure, and this is normal.

Test-Taking Strategy: Use the process of elimination. Note the key words "needs further instructions." Recalling that sedating medications are administered will direct you to option 4. Review postprocedure instructions following colonoscopy if you had difficulty with this question.

Level of Cognitive Ability: Analysis
Client Needs: Physiological Integrity
Integrated Process: Teaching/Learning
Content Area: Adult health—gastrointestinal
Reference: Phipps, W., Monahan, F., Sands, J., Marek, J., & Neighbors, M. (2003). *Medical-surgical nursing: Health and illness perspectives* (7th ed., p. 1001). St. Louis: Mosby.

8. 2
Rationale: The appropriate sequence for abdominal examination is inspection, auscultation, percussion, and palpation. Auscultation is performed after inspection to ensure that the motility of the bowel and bowel sounds are not altered by percussion or palpation.
Test-Taking Strategy: Use the process of elimination and visualize this procedure. Remember that the sequence for abdominal assessment is different than the usual systematic assessment approach. Review this technique, if you had difficulty with this question.
Level of Cognitive Ability: Application
Client Needs: Health Promotion and Maintenance
Integrated Process: Nursing Process—assessment
Content Area: Adult health—gastrointestinal
Reference: Potter, P., & Perry, A. (2001). *Fundamentals of nursing* (5th ed., p. 800). St. Louis: Mosby.

9. 4
Rationale: The solution GoLYTELY is a bowel evacuant used to prepare a client for a colonoscopy by cleansing the bowel. The solution is expected to cause a mild diarrhea and will clear the bowel in 4 to 5 hours. Options 1, 2, and 3 are inappropriate actions.
Test-Taking Strategy: Use the process of elimination. Knowledge regarding the purpose of this medication will assist you in eliminating option 3 and easily direct you to option 4. Options 1 and 2 are not within the scope of nursing practice and should be eliminated. Review the action and purpose of this medication if you had difficulty with this question.
Level of Cognitive Ability: Application
Client Needs: Physiological Integrity
Integrated Process: Nursing Process—implementation
Content Area: Adult health—gastrointestinal
Reference: Hodgson, B., & Kizior, R. (2004). *Saunders nursing drug handbook 2004* (p. 819). Philadelphia: W. B. Saunders.

10. 2
Rationale: Chronic gastritis causes deterioration and atrophy of the lining of the stomach, leading to the loss of the function of the parietal cells. The source of the intrinsic factor is lost, which results in the inability to absorb vitamin B_{12}. This leads to the development of pernicious anemia.
Test-Taking Strategy: Recalling the pathophysiology related to pernicious anemia and vitamin B_{12} deficiency will direct you to option 2. If you are unfamiliar with vitamin B_{12} deficiency and its relationship to gastric disorders, review this content.
Level of Cognitive Ability: Analysis
Client Needs: Physiological Integrity
Integrated Process: Nursing Process—assessment
Content Area: Adult health—gastrointestinal
Reference: Ignatavicius, D., & Workman, M. (2002). *Medical-surgical nursing: Critical thinking for collaborative care* (4th ed., pp. 1215, 1217). Philadelphia: W. B. Saunders.

11. 2
Rationale: Indomethacin (Indocin) is a nonsteroidal antiinflammatory drug and can cause ulceration of the esophagus, stomach, duodenum, or small intestine. Indomethacin is contraindicated in a client with gastrointestinal disorders.

Furosemide (Lasix) is a loop diuretic. Digoxin is an antidysrhythmic. Propranolol (Inderal) is a β-adrenergic blocker. Furosemide, digoxin, and propranolol are not contraindicated in clients with gastric disorders.
Test-Taking Strategy: Identify the classification of each of the medications listed. Use the process of elimination selecting option 2 because this medication is the one that would affect the gastrointestinal tract. Review these medications if you are unfamiliar with them.
Level of Cognitive Ability: Analysis
Client Needs: Physiological Integrity
Integrated Process: Nursing Process—analysis
Content Area: Adult health—gastrointestinal
Reference: Ignatavicius, D., & Workman, M. (2002). *Medical-surgical nursing: Critical thinking for collaborative care* (4th ed., p. 1217). Philadelphia: W. B. Saunders.

12. 2
Rationale: Following cholecystectomy, drainage from the T-tube is initially bloody and then turns to green-brown. The drainage is measured as output. The amount of expected drainage will range from 500 to 1000 mL per day. The nurse would document the output.
Test-Taking Strategy: Use the process of elimination. Options 3 and 4 can be eliminated because a T-tube is not irrigated and would not be clamped with this amount of drainage. From the remaining options, you must know normal expected findings following this surgical procedure. Review postoperative assessment findings following cholecystectomy if you had difficulty with this question.
Level of Cognitive Ability: Application
Client Needs: Physiological Integrity
Integrated Process: Nursing Process—implementation
Content Area: Adult health—gastrointestinal
Reference: Ignatavicius, D., & Workman, M. (2002). *Medical-surgical nursing: Critical thinking for collaborative care* (4th ed., p. 1332). Philadelphia: W. B. Saunders.

13. 4
Rationale: Perforation is a surgical emergency and is characterized by sudden, sharp, intolerable severe pain beginning in the midepigastric area and spreading over the abdomen, which becomes rigid and boardlike. Nausea and vomiting may occur. Tachycardia may occur as hypovolemic shock develops. Numbness in the legs is not an associated finding.
Test-Taking Strategy: Use the process of elimination. Note the key words "most likely." Option 2 can be eliminated easily. Eliminate option 1 next because tachycardia rather than bradycardia would develop if the client is bleeding. From the remaining two options, focusing on the key words will assist in directing you to option 4. Review the signs of a perforated ulcer if you had difficulty with this question.
Level of Cognitive Ability: Analysis
Client Needs: Physiological Integrity
Integrated Process: Nursing Process—assessment
Content Area: Adult health—gastrointestinal
Reference: Ignatavicius, D., & Workman, M. (2002). *Medical-surgical nursing: Critical thinking for collaborative care* (4th ed., p. 1222). Philadelphia: W. B. Saunders.

14. 1
Rationale: Cimetidine (Tagamet), a histamine H$_2$ receptor antagonist, will decrease the secretion of gastric acid. Sucralfate (Carafate) promotes healing by coating the ulcer. Antacids neutralize acid in the stomach. Omeprazole (Prilosec) inhibits gastric acid secretion.
Test-Taking Strategy: Use the process of elimination and knowledge regarding the actions of the medications identified in the options. If you are unfamiliar with these medications or their actions, review this content.
Level of Cognitive Ability: Analysis
Client Needs: Physiological Integrity
Integrated Process: Teaching/Learning
Content Area: Adult health—gastrointestinal
Reference: Hodgson, B., & Kizior, R. (2004). *Saunders nursing drug handbook 2004* (pp. 211-212). Philadelphia: W. B. Saunders.

15. 4
Rationale: Option 4 describes the procedure for a pyloroplasty. A vagotomy involves cutting the vagus nerve. A subtotal gastrectomy involves removing the distal portion of the stomach. A Billroth II procedure involves removal of the ulcer and a large portion of the tissue that produces hydrochloric acid.
Test-Taking Strategy: Use the process of elimination. Note the relationship between the words "pyloroplasty" and "pylorus" in the correct option. Review this procedure if you had difficulty with this question.
Level of Cognitive Ability: Comprehension
Client Needs: Physiological Integrity
Integrated Process: Nursing Process—planning
Content Area: Adult health—gastrointestinal
Reference: Lewis, S., Heitkemper, M., & Dirksen, S. (2004). *Medical-surgical nursing: Assessment and management of clinical problems* (6th ed., p. 1040). St. Louis: Mosby.

16. 4
Rationale: A vagotomy, or cutting of the vagus nerve, is done to eliminate parasympathetic stimulation of gastric secretion. Options 1, 2, and 3 are incorrect descriptions of a vagotomy.
Test-Taking Strategy: Knowledge regarding the purpose of a vagotomy is required to answer this question. If you are unfamiliar with this procedure, review this content.
Level of Cognitive Ability: Comprehension
Client Needs: Physiological Integrity
Integrated Process: Teaching/Learning
Content Area: Adult health—gastrointestinal
Reference: Ignatavicius, D., & Workman, M. (2002). *Medical-surgical nursing: Critical thinking for collaborative care* (4th ed., p. 1229). Philadelphia: W. B. Saunders.

17. 1
Rationale: In a Billroth II procedure the proximal remnant of the stomach is anastamosed to the proximal jejunum. Patency of the nasogastric tube is critical for preventing the retention of gastric secretions. The nurse should never irrigate or reposition the gastric tube after gastric surgery, unless specifically ordered by the physician. In this situation the nurse should clarify the order. Options 2, 3, and 4 are appropriate postoperative interventions.
Test-Taking Strategy: Use the process of elimination. Eliminate options 2, 3, and 4 because they are general postoperative measures. Consider the anatomical location of the surgical procedure to assist in directing you to option 1. Review postoperative measures following a Billroth II if you had difficulty with this question.
Level of Cognitive Ability: Analysis
Client Needs: Physiological Integrity
Integrated Process: Nursing Process—implementation
Content Area: Adult health—gastrointestinal
Reference: Ignatavicius, D., & Workman, M. (2002). *Medical-surgical nursing: Critical thinking for collaborative care* (4th ed., p. 1230). Philadelphia: W. B. Saunders.

18. 2
Rationale: The nurse should instruct the client to decrease the amount of fluid taken at meals and to avoid high-carbohydrate foods including fluids such as fruit nectars; to assume a low Fowler's position during meals; to lie down for 30 minutes after eating to delay gastric emptying; and to take antispasmotics as prescribed.
Test-Taking Strategy: Use the process of elimination. Eliminate options 3 and 4 first because these measures will promote gastric emptying. From the remaining options, select option 2 because this measure will delay gastric emptying. If you are unfamiliar with this syndrome, review the important client teaching points.
Level of Cognitive Ability: Application
Client Needs: Physiological Integrity
Integrated Process: Teaching/Learning
Content Area: Adult health—gastrointestinal
Reference: Ignatavicius, D., & Workman, M. (2002). *Medical-surgical nursing: Critical thinking for collaborative care* (4th ed., p. 1230). Philadelphia: W. B. Saunders.

19. 3
Rationale: Early manifestations of dumping syndrome occur 5 to 30 minutes after eating. Symptoms include vertigo, tachycardia, syncope, sweating, pallor, palpitations, and the desire to lie down.
Test-Taking Strategy: Use the process of elimination. Focus on the key word "early" to direct you to option 3. Review the early manifestations of this syndrome if you had difficulty with this question.
Level of Cognitive Ability: Analysis
Client Needs: Physiological Integrity
Integrated Process: Nursing Process—assessment
Content Area: Adult health—gastrointestinal
Reference: Ignatavicius, D., & Workman, M. (2002). *Medical-surgical nursing: Critical thinking for collaborative care* (4th ed., p. 1230). Philadelphia: W. B. Saunders.

20. 3
Rationale: Bedrest is not required following this surgical procedure. The client should take analgesics as needed and as prescribed to control pain. A drain is not used in this surgical procedure, although the client may be instructed in simple dressing changes. Coughing is avoided to prevent disruption of the tissue integrity, which can occur because of the location of this surgical procedure.

Test-Taking Strategy: Use the process of elimination. General postoperative measures will assist you in eliminating options 1 and 2. From the remaining options, consider the anatomical location of the surgery and the surgical procedure to assist you in selecting option 3. Review postoperative measures following this surgical procedure if you had difficulty with this question.
Level of Cognitive Ability: Application
Client Needs: Physiological Integrity
Integrated Process: Nursing Process—planning
Content Area: Adult health—gastrointestinal
Reference: Ignatavicius, D., & Workman, M. (2002). *Medical-surgical nursing: Critical thinking for collaborative care* (4th ed., p. 1244). Philadelphia: W. B. Saunders.

21. **2**
Rationale: Following herniorrhaphy, the client should be instructed to elevate the scrotum and apply ice packs while in bed to decrease pain and swelling. The nurse also should instruct the client to apply a scrotal support when out of bed. Heat will increase swelling.
Test-Taking Strategy: Focus on the issue, to reduce swelling. Basic knowledge regarding the effects of heat and cold will assist you in eliminating option 1. Options 3 and 4 can be eliminated next because they are similar and these actions will cause constipation. Limiting oral fluids and consuming a low-fiber diet also can cause constipation. Straining with a bowel movement needs to be avoided. Review postoperative care following herniorrhaphy, if you had difficulty with this question.
Level of Cognitive Ability: Application
Client Needs: Physiological Integrity
Integrated Process: Teaching/Learning
Content Area: Adult health—gastrointestinal
Reference: Ignatavicius, D., & Workman, M. (2002). *Medical-surgical nursing: Critical thinking for collaborative care* (4th ed., p. 1244). Philadelphia: W. B. Saunders.

22. **4**
Rationale: Rebound tenderness may indicate peritonitis. Bloody diarrhea is expected to occur in ulcerative colitis. Because of the blood loss, the client may be hypotensive and the hemoglobin level may be lower than normal. Signs of peritonitis must be reported to the physician.
Test-Taking Strategy: Use the process of elimination. Consider the expected manifestations that would occur in ulcerative colitis. This will assist in eliminating option 1. Recalling that bleeding would cause a lowered hemoglobin and hypotension will assist you in eliminating options 2 and 3. Review the normal assessment findings in ulcerative colitis, if you had difficulty with this question.
Level of Cognitive Ability: Analysis
Client Needs: Physiological Integrity
Integrated Process: Nursing Process—analysis
Content Area: Adult health—gastrointestinal
Reference: Ignatavicius, D., & Workman, M. (2002). *Medical-surgical nursing: Critical thinking for collaborative care* (4th ed., p. 1274). Philadelphia: W. B. Saunders.

23. **2**
Rationale: Disturbed Body Image relates to loss of bowel control, the presence of a stoma, the release of fecal material

onto the abdomen, the passage of flatus, odor, and the need for an appliance (external pouch). No data in the question support options 3 and 4. A risk for imbalanced nutrition less than body requirements is the more likely nursing diagnosis.
Test-Taking Strategy: Use the process of elimination. Use the data presented in the question to assist you in selecting the correct option. No data in the question support options 3 and 4. Reading option 1 carefully will assist you in eliminating this option. Review care to the client following a colostomy if you had difficulty with this question.
Level of Cognitive Ability: Analysis
Client Needs: Psychosocial Integrity
Integrated Process: Nursing Process—analysis
Content Area: Adult health—gastrointestinal
Reference: Lewis, S., Heitkemper, M., & Dirksen, S. (2004). *Medical-surgical nursing: Assessment and management of clinical problems* (6th ed., p. 1093). St. Louis: Mosby.

24. **2**
Rationale: Crohn's disease is characterized by nonbloody diarrhea of usually not more than four to five stools daily. Over time, the diarrhea episodes increase in frequency, duration, and severity. Options 1, 3, and 4 are not characteristics of Crohn's disease.
Test-Taking Strategy: Use the process of elimination. Eliminate option 4 first as the most unlikely occurrence. From the remaining options, you must be familiar with the characteristics of Crohn's disease. If you are unfamiliar with this disorder, review this content.
Level of Cognitive Ability: Analysis
Client Needs: Physiological Integrity
Integrated Process: Nursing Process—assessment
Content Area: Adult health—gastrointestinal
Reference: Lewis, S., Heitkemper, M., & Dirksen, S. (2004). *Medical-surgical nursing: Assessment and management of clinical problems* (6th ed., p. 1067). St. Louis: Mosby.

25. **3**
Rationale: If cramping occurs during a colostomy irrigation, the irrigation flow is stopped temporarily and the client is allowed to rest. Cramping may occur from an infusion that is too rapid or is causing too much pressure. Increasing the height of the irrigation will cause further discomfort. The physician does not need to be notified. Medicating the client for pain is not the most appropriate action.
Test-Taking Strategy: Focus on the issue, abdominal cramping during irrigation. This will assist in eliminating options 1, 2, and 4. If you had difficulty answering this question, review the procedure for colostomy irrigation.
Level of Cognitive Ability: Application
Client Needs: Physiological Integrity
Integrated Process: Nursing Process—implementation
Content Area: Adult health—gastrointestinal
Reference: Lewis, S., Heitkemper, M., & Dirksen, S. (2004). *Medical-surgical nursing: Assessment and management of clinical problems* (6th ed., p. 1092). St. Louis: Mosby.

26. **1**
Rationale: To enhance effectiveness of the irrigation and fecal returns, the client is instructed to increase fluid intake

and prevent constipation. Options 2, 3, and 4 will not enhance the effectiveness of this procedure.

Test-Taking Strategy: Focus on the issue of the question, which is the measure that will enhance the effectiveness of the irrigation. This focus will assist in eliminating options 2, 3, and 4. If you are unfamiliar with this procedure, review this content.

Level of Cognitive Ability: Application
Client Needs: Health Promotion and Maintenance
Integrated Process: Teaching/Learning
Content Area: Adult health—gastrointestinal
Reference: Elkin, M., Perry, A., & Potter, P. (2004). *Nursing interventions & clinical skills* (3rd ed., p. 836). St. Louis: Mosby.

27. **1**
Rationale: Asterixis is irregular flapping movements of the fingers and wrists when the hands and arms are outstretched, with the palms down, wrists bent up, and fingers spread. Asterixis is the most common and reliable sign that hepatic encephalopathy is developing. Options 2, 3, and 4 are incorrect.
Test-Taking Strategy: Use the process of elimination and knowledge regarding the procedure for this assessment to answer this question. Review this assessment procedure if you had difficulty with this question.
Level of Cognitive Ability: Application
Client Needs: Health Promotion and Maintenance
Integrated Process: Nursing Process—assessment
Content Area: Adult health—gastrointestinal
Reference: Lewis, S., Heitkemper, M., & Dirksen, S. (2004). *Medical-surgical nursing: Assessment and management of clinical problems* (6th ed., p. 1120). St. Louis: Mosby.

28. **4**
Rationale: An upright position allows the intestine to float posteriorly and helps prevent intestinal laceration during catheter insertion. Options 1, 2, and 3 are incorrect positions.
Test-Taking Strategy: Attempt to visualize this procedure in selecting the correct option. Knowing that fluid will be aspirated from the abdominal cavity will assist in directing you to option 4. If you had difficulty with this question, review this procedure.
Level of Cognitive Ability: Application
Client Needs: Physiological Integrity
Integrated Process: Nursing Process—implementation
Content Area: Adult health—gastrointestinal
Reference: Linton, A., & Maebius, N. (2003). *Introduction to medical-surgical nursing* (3rd ed., p. 725). Philadelphia: W. B. Saunders.

29. **4**
Rationale: Most of the ammonia in the body is found in the gastrointestinal tract. Protein provided by the diet is transported to the liver by the portal vein. The liver breaks down protein, and this results in the formation of ammonia. If the client has hepatic encephalopathy, a low-protein diet would be prescribed.
Test-Taking Strategy: Recall the physiology of the liver in answering this question. Note the key words "most likely." You should be directed easily to option 4. Also note that options 3 and 4 are opposite, which should provide you with

the clue that one of these options is correct. Review dietary measures for the client with a high ammonia level if you had difficulty with this question.
Level of Cognitive Ability: Analysis
Client Needs: Physiological Integrity
Integrated Process: Nursing Process—analysis
Content Area: Adult health—gastrointestinal
Reference: Lewis, S., Heitkemper, M., & Dirksen, S. (2004). *Medical-surgical nursing: Assessment and management of clinical problems* (6th ed., p. 1125). St. Louis: Mosby.

30. **1**
Rationale: Fatigue is a normal response to hepatic cellular damage. During the acute stage, rest is an essential intervention to reduce the metabolic demands on the liver and increase its blood supply. Options 2, 3, and 4 are incorrect.
Test-Taking Strategy: Use the process of elimination. Note the key word "acute" in the question. Knowing that the liver will need to rest to heal will direct you easily to option 1. If you are unfamiliar with the care of a client with hepatitis, review this content.
Level of Cognitive Ability: Analysis
Client Needs: Physiological Integrity
Integrated Process: Nursing Process—analysis
Content Area: Adult health—gastrointestinal
Reference: Ignatavicius, D., & Workman, M. (2002). *Medical-surgical nursing: Critical thinking for collaborative care* (4th ed., p. 1319). Philadelphia: W. B. Saunders.

31. **1**
Rationale: Hepatitis A is transmitted by the fecal-oral route via contaminated food or infected food handlers. Hepatitis B, C, and D are transmitted most commonly via infected blood or body fluids.
Test-Taking Strategy: Knowledge regarding the modes of transmission of the various types of hepatitis is required to answer this question. Review this content if you are unfamiliar with it.
Level of Cognitive Ability: Comprehension
Client Needs: Safe, Effective Care Environment
Integrated Process: Nursing Process—assessment
Content Area: Adult health—gastrointestinal
Reference: Ignatavicius, D., & Workman, M. (2002). *Medical-surgical nursing: Critical thinking for collaborative care* (4th ed., p. 1314). Philadelphia: W. B. Saunders.

32. **2**
Rationale: Laboratory indicators of hepatitis include elevated liver enzyme levels, elevated serum bilirubin levels, elevated erythrocyte sedimentation rates, and leukopenia. An elevated blood urea nitrogen may indicate renal dysfunction. A hemoglobin level is unrelated to this diagnosis.
Test-Taking Strategy: Use the process of elimination. Eliminate option 4 because blood urea nitrogen identifies renal rather than hepatic dysfunction. Thinking about the organ that is involved in hepatitis should assist in directing you to option 2, the liver function test. Review diagnostic tests for hepatitis if you had difficulty with this question.
Level of Cognitive Ability: Analysis
Client Needs: Physiological Integrity

Integrated Process: Nursing Process—assessment
Content Area: Adult health—gastrointestinal
Reference: Lewis, S., Heitkemper, M., & Dirksen, S. (2004). *Medical-surgical nursing: Assessment and management of clinical problems* (6th ed., p. 1110). St. Louis: Mosby.

33. **4**

Rationale: Meperidine (Demerol) rather than morphine sulfate is the medication of choice because morphine sulfate can cause spasms in the sphincter of Oddi. Options 1, 2, and 3 are appropriate interventions for the client with acute pancreatitis.
Test-Taking Strategy: Note the key word "acute" in the question. Recalling the pathophysiology associated with this disorder will direct you to option 4. Review the treatment for acute pancreatitis if you had difficulty with this question.
Level of Cognitive Ability: Analysis
Client Needs: Physiological Integrity
Integrated Process: Nursing Process—analysis
Content Area: Adult health—gastrointestinal
Reference: Lewis, S., Heitkemper, M., & Dirksen, S. (2004). *Medical-surgical nursing: Assessment and management of clinical problems* (6th ed., p. 1135). St. Louis: Mosby.

34. **1**

Rationale: The most frequent symptom of duodenal ulcer is pain that is relieved by food intake. These clients generally describe the pain as a burning, heavy, sharp, or "hungry" pain that often localizes in the midepigastric area. The client with duodenal ulcer usually does not experience weight loss or nausea and vomiting. These symptoms are more typical in the client with a gastric ulcer.
Test-Taking Strategy: Use the process of elimination. To answer this question accurately, you must be able to discriminate between symptoms of duodenal and gastric ulcer. This will allow you to eliminate options 3 and 4 first. Choose option 1 over option 2, knowing that the pain does not radiate down the right arm and by knowing that a pattern of pain-food-relief occurs with duodenal ulcer. Review the clinical manifestations of a duodenal ulcer if you had difficulty with this question.
Level of Cognitive Ability: Application
Client Needs: Physiological Integrity
Integrated Process: Nursing Process—assessment
Content Area: Adult health—gastrointestinal
Reference: Potter, P., & Perry, A. (2001). *Fundamentals of nursing* (5th ed., p. 1440). St. Louis: Mosby.

35. **2**

Rationale: Dietary modification for the client with peptic ulcer disease includes eliminating foods that are irritating to the client. Items that generally are eliminated or avoided are highly spiced foods, alcohol, caffeine, chocolate, and fresh fruits. Other foods may be taken according to the client's tolerance of that specific food.
Test-Taking Strategy: Use the process of elimination noting the key words "does not need to be limited." Recalling which types of foods and beverages are irritating to the gastrointestinal mucosa will direct you to option 2. If this question was difficult, review this content.
Level of Cognitive Ability: Application

Client Needs: Physiological Integrity
Integrated Process: Teaching/Learning
Content Area: Adult health—gastrointestinal
References: Lewis, S., Heitkemper, M., & Dirksen, S. (2004). *Medical-surgical nursing: Assessment and management of clinical problems* (6th ed., p. 1038). St. Louis: Mosby.
Potter, P., & Perry, A. (2001). *Fundamentals of nursing* (5th ed., p. 1374). St. Louis: Mosby.

36. **2**

Rationale: Ibuprofen is a nonsteroidal antiinflammatory drug that typically is irritating to the lining of the gastrointestinal tract and should be avoided by clients with a history of peptic ulcer disease. The other medications listed frequently are used to treat peptic ulcer disease. Omeprazole is a proton-pump inhibitor, which blocks transport of hydrogen ions into the lumen of the gastrointestinal tract. Sucralfate coats the surface of an ulcer to promote healing. Nizatidine is a histamine H_2 receptor antagonist that reduces the secretion of gastric acid.
Test-Taking Strategy: Use the process of elimination. Recalling the types of medications that are irritating to the gastrointestinal tract or knowing which medications are used to treatment peptic ulcer disease will direct you to option 2. Review the pharmacological treatment measures for peptic ulcer disease if you had difficulty with this question.
Level of Cognitive Ability: Application
Client Needs: Physiological Integrity
Integrated Process: Teaching/Learning
Content Area: Adult health—gastrointestinal
Reference: Hodgson, B., & Kizior, R. (2004). *Saunders nursing drug handbook 2004* (, pp. 516-517). Philadelphia: W. B. Saunders.

37. **1**

Rationale: The peristomal skin must receive meticulous cleansing because the ileostomy drainage has more enzymes and is more caustic to the skin than colostomy drainage. Foods such as nuts and those with seeds will pass through the ileostomy. The client should be taught that these foods will remain undigested. The area below the ileostomy may be massaged if needed if the ileostomy becomes blocked by high-fiber foods. Fluid intake should be maintained to at least six to eight glasses of water per day to prevent dehydration.
Test-Taking Strategy: Use the process of elimination and focus on the issue. Note the key words "essential care" and "stoma." This tells you that the correct answer will be the option that deals with the stoma directly. Review client instructions regarding ileostomy care if you had difficulty with this question.
Level of Cognitive Ability: Application
Client Needs: Physiological Integrity
Integrated Process: Teaching/Learning
Content Area: Adult health—gastrointestinal
Reference: Ignatavicius, D., & Workman, M. (2002). *Medical-surgical nursing: Critical thinking for collaborative care* (4th ed., p. 1252). Philadelphia: W. B. Saunders.

38. **2**

Rationale: Hiatal hernia is due to a protrusion of a portion of the stomach above the diaphragm where the esophagus usually is positioned. The client usually experiences pain caused

by reflux with ingestion of irritating foods, lying flat following meals or at night, and with large or fatty meals. Relief is obtained with intake of small, frequent, and bland meals; with use of histamine H_2 antagonists and antacids; and with elevation of the thorax following meals and during sleep.
Test-Taking Strategy: Use the process of elimination noting the key word "contraindicated." Thinking about the pathophysiology that occurs in hiatal hernia will direct you to option 2. Review this pathophysiology if you had difficulty with this question.
Level of Cognitive Ability: Application
Client Needs: Physiological Integrity
Integrated Process: Teaching/Learning
Content Area: Adult health—gastrointestinal
Reference: Ignatavicius, D., & Workman, M. (2002). *Medical-surgical nursing: Critical thinking for collaborative care* (4th ed., p. 1201). Philadelphia: W. B. Saunders.

39. **4**
Rationale: The client is expected to have a body image disturbance after colostomy. The client progresses through normal grieving stages to adjust to this change. The client demonstrates the greatest deal of acceptance when the client participates in the actual colostomy care. Each of the incorrect options represents an interest in colostomy care but is a passive activity. The correct option shows the client participating in self-care.
Test-Taking Strategy: Use the process of elimination. Note the key words "colostomy" and "most significant progress." Eliminate options 1, 2, and 3 because they are similar and indicate passive activities. Review psychosocial adjustment in a client with colostomy if you had difficulty with this question.
Level of Cognitive Ability: Analysis
Client Needs: Psychosocial Integrity
Integrated Process: Nursing Process—evaluation
Content Area: Adult health—gastrointestinal
Reference: Ignatavicius, D., & Workman, M. (2002). *Medical-surgical nursing: Critical thinking for collaborative care* (4th ed., p. 1253). Philadelphia: W. B. Saunders.

40. **4**
Rationale: A prolapsed stoma is one in which the bowel protrudes through the stoma. A stoma retraction is characterized by sinking of the stoma. Ischemia of the stoma would be associated with dusky or bluish color. A stoma with a narrowed opening at the level of the skin or fascia is said to be stenosed.
Test-Taking Strategy: Use the process of elimination. Focus on the key word "prolapse" to direct you to option 4. If this question was difficult, review the complications associated with a colostomy stoma.
Level of Cognitive Ability: Analysis
Client Needs: Physiological Integrity
Integrated Process: Nursing Process—assessment
Content Area: Adult health—gastrointestinal
Reference: Linton, A., & Maebius, N. (2003). *Introduction to medical-surgical nursing* (3rd ed., p. 335). Philadelphia: W. B. Saunders.

41. **2**
Rationale: As peristalsis returns following creation of a colostomy, the client begins to pass malodorous flatus.

This indicates returning bowel function and is an expected event. Within 72 hours of surgery, the client should begin passing stool via the colostomy. Options 1, 3, and 4 are incorrect.
Test-Taking Strategy: Use the process of elimination. Recalling the normal progression of bowel activity following ostomy formation will direct you to option 2. Review the expected findings following a creation of a colostomy if you had difficulty with this question.
Level of Cognitive Ability: Analysis
Client Needs: Physiological Integrity
Integrated Process: Nursing Process—analysis
Content Area: Adult health—gastrointestinal
Reference: Ignatavicius, D., & Workman, M. (2002). *Medical-surgical nursing: Critical thinking for collaborative care* (4th ed., p. 1251). Philadelphia: W. B. Saunders.

42. **1**
Rationale: The client should be taught to include deodorizing foods in the diet, such as beet greens, parsley, buttermilk, and yogurt. Spinach also reduces odor but is a gas-forming food as well. Broccoli, cucumbers, and eggs are gas-forming foods.
Test-Taking Strategy: Use the process of elimination. Recalling the effect of various foods on the gastrointestinal tract of the client with an ostomy will direct you to option 1. If this question was difficult, review which foods cause odor or gas and those that have a deodorizing effect.
Level of Cognitive Ability: Application
Client Needs: Physiological Integrity
Integrated Process: Teaching/Learning
Content Area: Adult health—gastrointestinal
Reference: Ignatavicius, D., & Workman, M. (2002). *Medical-surgical nursing: Critical thinking for collaborative care* (4th ed., p. 1253). Philadelphia: W. B. Saunders.

43. **3**
Rationale: Foods that help to thicken the stool of the client with an ileostomy include pasta, boiled rice, and low-fat cheese. Bran is high in dietary fiber and thus will increase output of watery stool by increasing propulsion through the bowel. Ileostomy output is liquid. Addition or elimination of various foods can help to thicken or loosen this liquid drainage.
Test-Taking Strategy: Use the process of elimination noting the key words "needs further instructions." Recalling that high-fiber foods such as bran can cause watery stools in the client with an ileostomy will direct you to the correct option. Review dietary measures for the client with an ileostomy if you had difficulty with this question.
Level of Cognitive Ability: Analysis
Client Needs: Physiological Integrity
Integrated Process: Teaching/Learning
Content Area: Adult health—gastrointestinal
Reference: Ignatavicius, D., & Workman, M. (2002). *Medical-surgical nursing: Critical thinking for collaborative care* (4th ed., p. 1282). Philadelphia: W. B. Saunders.

44. **2**
Rationale: A major complication that occurs most frequently following ileostomy is fluid and electrolyte imbalance. The client requires constant monitoring of intake and output to

prevent this from occurring. Losses require replacement by intravenous infusion until the client can tolerate a diet orally. Intestinal obstruction is a less frequent complication. Fat malabsorption and folate deficiency are complications that could occur later in the postoperative period.

Test-Taking Strategy: Use the process of elimination. Note the key words "ileostomy," "complications," and "immediate postoperative period." This tells you that the correct option is one that occurs early in the postoperative course, and which occurs with relative frequency. If you had difficulty with this question, review the postoperative complications following this surgical procedure.

Level of Cognitive Ability: Analysis
Client Needs: Physiological Integrity
Integrated Process: Nursing Process—assessment
Content Area: Adult health—gastrointestinal
Reference: Ignatavicius, D., & Workman, M. (2002). *Medical-surgical nursing: Critical thinking for collaborative care* (4th ed., p. 1282). Philadelphia: W. B. Saunders.

45. 1
Rationale: A Kock pouch is a continent ileostomy. As the ileostomy begins to function, the client drains it every 3 to 4 hours and then decreases the draining to about 3 times a day or as needed when full. The client does not need to wear a drainage bag but should wear an absorbent dressing to absorb mucous drainage from the stoma. Ileostomy drainage is liquid. The client would be able to pass stool only from the rectum if an ileal-anal pouch or anastamosis were created. This type of operation is a two-stage procedure.

Test-Taking Strategy: Use the process of elimination. Focusing on the key word "pouch" will assist in directing you to option 1. If this question was difficult, review this content.

Level of Cognitive Ability: Analysis
Client Needs: Physiological Integrity
Integrated Process: Teaching/Learning
Content Area: Adult health—gastrointestinal
Reference: Elkin, M., Perry, A., & Potter, P. (2004). *Nursing interventions & clinical skills* (3rd ed., p. 833). St. Louis: Mosby.

46. 2
Rationale: Warm tap water or saline solution is used to irrigate a colostomy. If the tap water is not suitable for drinking, then bottled water should be used. Options 1, 3, and 4 are incorrect solutions.

Test-Taking Strategy: Use the process of elimination. Recalling that the irrigation involves the gastrointestinal tract and that the gastrointestinal tract is not a sterile organ will direct you to option 2. Review the procedure for performing colostomy irrigation if you had difficulty with this question.

Level of Cognitive Ability: Application
Client Needs: Physiological Integrity
Integrated Process: Nursing Process—implementation
Content Area: Adult health—gastrointestinal
Reference: Ignatavicius, D., & Workman, M. (2002). *Medical-surgical nursing: Critical thinking for collaborative care* (4th ed., p. 1279). Philadelphia: W. B. Saunders.

47. 2
Rationale: Based on the signs and symptoms presented in the question, the nurse should suspect peritonitis and should

notify the physician. Administering pain medication is not an appropriate intervention. Heat should never be applied to the abdomen of a client with suspected appendicitis. Scheduling surgical time is not within the scope of nursing practice, although the physician probably would perform the surgery earlier than the prescheduled time.

Test-Taking Strategy: Use the process of elimination. Focus on the signs and symptoms in the question and consider the complications that can occur with appendicitis. Options 3 and 4 can be eliminated easily. Noting that the signs presented in the question indicate a complication will assist in directing you to option 2. Review care to the client with appendicitis if you had difficulty with this question.

Level of Cognitive Ability: Application
Client Needs: Physiological Integrity
Integrated Process: Nursing Process—implementation
Content Area: Adult health—gastrointestinal
Reference: Ignatavicius, D., & Workman, M. (2002). *Medical-surgical nursing: Critical thinking for collaborative care* (4th ed., pp. 1269-1270). Philadelphia: W. B. Saunders.

48. 1
Rationale: The pain associated with acute pancreatitis is often severe and unrelenting, is located in the epigastric region, and radiates to the back. The other options are incorrect.

Test-Taking Strategy: Use the process of elimination. Noting the key word "acute" will assist in eliminating options 3 and 4. From the remaining options, recalling the anatomical location of the pancreas will direct you to option 1. Review the manifestations in acute pancreatitis if you had difficulty with this question.

Level of Cognitive Ability: Analysis
Client Needs: Physiological Integrity
Integrated Process: Nursing Process—assessment
Content Area: Adult health—gastrointestinal
Reference: Ignatavicius, D., & Workman, M. (2002). *Medical-surgical nursing: Critical thinking for collaborative care* (4th ed., p. 1341). Philadelphia: W. B. Saunders.

49. 3
Rationale: The client should limit fat in the diet. The client also should take in small meals, which also will reduce the amount of carbohydrates and protein that the client must digest at any one time. The client does not need to limit water-soluble vitamins in the diet.

Test-Taking Strategy: Use the process of elimination. Note the key word "limit". Recalling the function of the pancreas will direct you easily to option 3. Review dietary measures for the client with pancreatitis if you had difficulty with this question.

Level of Cognitive Ability: Application
Client Needs: Physiological Integrity
Integrated Process: Teaching/Learning
Content Area: Adult health—gastrointestinal
Reference: Ignatavicius, D., & Workman, M. (2002). *Medical-surgical nursing: Critical thinking for collaborative care* (4th ed., p. 1347). Philadelphia: W. B. Saunders.

50. 2
Rationale: Chronic pancreatitis is aggravated by continued alcohol intake. Each of the other options is not associated with pancreatitis.

Test-Taking Strategy: Use the process of elimination. Remember that options that are similar are not likely to be correct. In this instance, two of the incorrect options (3 and 4) represent other disorders of the digestive system. Choose option 2 over option 1 by recalling that diabetes mellitus is an endocrine disorder of the pancreas, whereas pancreatitis is an exocrine disorder. Review the factors that contribute to a recurrence of pancreatitis if you had difficulty with this question.
Level of Cognitive Ability: Analysis
Client Needs: Physiological Integrity
Integrated Process: Teaching/Learning
Content Area: Adult health—gastrointestinal
Reference: Phipps, W., Monahan, F., Sands, J., Marek, J., & Neighbors, M. (2003). *Medical-surgical nursing: Health and illness perspectives* (7th ed., p. 1129). St. Louis: Mosby.

51. **1**
Rationale: The client with cholecystitis should decrease overall intake of dietary fat. Foods that should be avoided to achieve this end include sauces and gravies, fatty meats, fried foods, products made with cream, and heavy desserts. The correct option is baked scrod, which is low in fat.
Test-Taking Strategy: Use the process of elimination. Recalling the function of the gallbladder and knowledge of the foods that are low in fat will direct you to option 1. Review dietary measures for the client with cholecystitis if you had difficulty with this question.
Level of Cognitive Ability: Analysis
Client Needs: Physiological Integrity
Integrated Process: Teaching/Learning
Content Area: Adult health—gastrointestinal
Reference: Ignatavicius, D., & Workman, M. (2002). *Medical-surgical nursing: Critical thinking for collaborative care* (4th ed., pp. 1330, 1382). Philadelphia: W. B. Saunders.

52. **2**
Rationale: During an acute "gallbladder attack," the client may complain of severe right upper quadrant pain that radiates to the right scapula and shoulder. This is governed by the pattern on dermatomes in the body. The other options are incorrect.
Test-Taking Strategy: Use the process of elimination. Knowledge of the anatomical location of the gallbladder will direct you to option 2. Review the characteristics of the pain associated with cholecystitis if you had difficulty with this question.
Level of Cognitive Ability: Application
Client Needs: Physiological Integrity
Integrated Process: Nursing Process—assessment
Content Area: Adult health—gastrointestinal
Reference: Phipps, W., Monahan, F., Sands, J., Marek, J., & Neighbors, M. (2003). *Medical-surgical nursing: Health and illness perspectives* (7th ed., p. 1117). St. Louis: Mosby.

53. **3**
Rationale: Ammonia is yielded as a product of protein metabolism. Clients with hepatic encephalopathy have high serum ammonia levels, which is responsible for the symptoms of encephalopathy. Limiting protein intake will curb the elevation in serum ammonia and prevent further deterioration of the client's mental status.

Test-Taking Strategy: Recalling the function of the liver and the pathophysiology associated with cirrhosis will direct you to option 3. Review this content if you had difficulty with this question.
Level of Cognitive Ability: Application
Client Needs: Health Promotion and Maintenance
Integrated Process: Nursing Process—planning
Content Area: Adult health—gastrointestinal
Reference: Phipps, W., Monahan, F., Sands, J., Marek, J., & Neighbors, M. (2003). *Medical-surgical nursing: Health and illness perspectives* (7th ed., p. 1183). St. Louis: Mosby.

54. **4**
Rationale: The client with weight gain who also has cirrhosis complicated by ascites most often is retaining fluid. This is especially true when the client has not demonstrated an appreciable increase in food intake or when the weight gain is massive in relation to the time frame given. Therefore Excess Fluid Volume is the most appropriate nursing diagnosis. The client does not have an Imbalanced Nutrition: More Than Body Requirements; in fact, this client is most likely malnourished as part of the overall clinical picture. No data are given to support Impaired Gas Exchange, although in some clients, upward pressure on the diaphragm from ascites does impair respiration. Risk for Impaired Skin Integrity assumes a lower priority than diagnoses that are actual.
Test-Taking Strategy: Focus on the data provided in the question. Note the key words "most appropriate." Begin to answer this question by eliminating option 3 because it is not an actual nursing diagnosis. Eliminate option 2 next because there are no supportive data. Choose correctly between the remaining options, knowing that the weight gain is due to fluid retention. Review the complications associated with cirrhosis if you had difficulty with this question.
Level of Cognitive Ability: Analysis
Client Needs: Physiological Integrity
Integrated Process: Nursing Process—analysis
Content Area: Adult health—gastrointestinal
References: Ignatavicius, D., & Workman, M. (2002). *Medical-surgical nursing: Critical thinking for collaborative care* (4th ed., p. 1299). Philadelphia: W. B. Saunders.
Phipps, W., Monahan, F., Sands, J., Marek, J., & Neighbors, M. (2003). *Medical-surgical nursing: Health and illness perspectives* (7th ed., p. 1140). St. Louis: Mosby.

55. **1**
Rationale: Pain associated with Crohn's disease is alleviated by the use of analgesics and antispasmodics and also is reduced by having the client practice relaxation techniques, applying local cold or heat to the abdomen, massaging the abdomen, and lying with the legs flexed. Lying with the legs extended is not useful because it increases the muscle tension in the abdomen, which could aggravate inflamed intestinal tissues as the abdominal muscles are stretched.
Test-Taking Strategy: Note the key word "avoid." Use the process of elimination and use general knowledge of pain management strategies, application of cold or heat, and client positioning to answer this question. If this question was difficult, review pain management techniques for the client with Crohn's disease.

Level of Cognitive Ability: Application
Client Needs: Physiological Integrity
Integrated Process: Teaching/Learning
Content Area: Adult health—gastrointestinal
Reference: Ignatavicius, D., & Workman, M. (2002). *Medical surgical nursing: Critical thinking for collaborative care* (4th ed., p. 1277). Philadelphia: W. B. Saunders.

56. 3

Rationale: Salicylate compounds such as sulfasalazine (Azulfidine) act by inhibiting prostaglandin synthesis and reducing inflammation. The nurse teaches the client to take the medication with a full glass of water and to increase fluid intake throughout the day. The medication needs to be taken after meals to reduce gastrointestinal irritation. The other options are incorrect.
Test-Taking Strategy: Use the process of elimination. Eliminate options 1, 2, and 4 because they are similar and indicate taking the medication on an empty stomach. Review the administration of salicylate medications if you had difficulty with this question.
Level of Cognitive Ability: Application
Client Needs: Physiological Integrity
Integrated Process: Teaching/Learning
Content Area: Adult health—gastrointestinal
Reference: Ignatavicius, D., & Workman, M. (2002). *Medical surgical nursing: Critical thinking for collaborative care* (4th ed., p. 1277). Philadelphia: W. B. Saunders.

57. 4

Rationale: Abdominal pain is the most common symptom of peritonitis. Although tenderness over the involved area is a universal sign, rebound tenderness is most often associated with appendicitis. Bloody diarrhea is a major symptom of ulcerative colitis. Increased flatulence commonly occurs with irritable bowel syndrome.
Test-Taking Strategy: Use the process of elimination and focus on the issue, on assessment finding that indicates peritonitis. Recalling the signs associated with peritonitis will direct you to option 4. Review the assessment findings associated with peritonitis, if you had difficulty with this question.
Level of Cognitive Ability: Application
Client Needs: Physiological Integrity
Integrated Process: Nursing Process—assessment
Content Area: Adult health—gastrointestinal
Reference: Lewis, S., Heitkemper, M., & Dirksen, S. (2004). *Medical-surgical nursing: Assessment and management of clinical problems* (6th ed., p. 1129). St. Louis: Mosby.

58. 3

Rationale: Although no special diet is required to treat viral hepatitis, it is generally recommended that clients consume a diet with low-fat content because fat may be tolerated poorly because of decreased bile production. Small, frequent meals are preferable and may even prevent nausea. Frequently, appetite is better in the morning, so it is easier to eat a good breakfast. An adequate fluid intake of 2500 to 3000 mL per day that includes nutritional juices is also important.
Test-Taking Strategy: Use the process of elimination. Knowledge regarding the nutritional problems associated with hepatitis will assist in directing you to the correct option.

Review measures to provide adequate nutrition in the client with hepatitis if you had difficulty with this question.
Level of Cognitive Ability: Application
Client Needs: Physiological Integrity
Integrated Process: Teaching/Learning
Content Area: Adult health—gastrointestinal
References: Lewis, S., Heitkemper, M., & Dirksen, S. (2004). *Medical-surgical nursing: Assessment and management of clinical problems* (6th ed., p. 1113). St. Louis: Mosby.
Phipps, W., Monahan, F., Sands, J., Marek, J., & Neighbors, M. (2003). *Medical-surgical nursing: Health and illness perspectives* (7th ed., p. 1163). St. Louis: Mosby.

59. 3

Rationale: Hepatitis causes gastrointestinal symptoms such as anorexia, nausea, right upper quadrant discomfort, and weight loss. Fatigue and malaise are common. Stools will be light- or clay-colored if conjugated bilirubin is unable to flow out of the liver because of inflammation or obstruction of the bile ducts.
Test-Taking Strategy: Use the process of elimination. Recalling the function of the liver will easily direct you to option 3. If you had difficulty with this question, review the signs and symptoms of hepatitis.
Level of Cognitive Ability: Analysis
Client Needs: Physiological Integrity
Integrated Process: Nursing Process—assessment
Content Area: Adult health—gastrointestinal
References: Ignatavicius, D., & Workman, M. (2002). *Medical-surgical nursing: Critical thinking for collaborative care* (4th ed., p. 1318). Philadelphia: W. B. Saunders.
Lewis, S., Heitkemper, M., & Dirksen, S. (2004). *Medical-surgical nursing: Assessment and management of clinical problems* (6th ed., p. 1113). St. Louis: Mosby.

60. 2

Rationale: Jaundice occurs in the skin and mucous membranes. In light-skinned persons, jaundice first is seen in the sclera of the eyes and later in the skin. In dark-skinned persons, jaundice is observed in the inner canthus of the eyes and hard palate of the mouth. Pallor is detected in the nailbeds, and flushing associated with increased body temperature is best noted in the flexor surfaces of the extremities.
Test-Taking Strategy: Use the process of elimination. Recalling that jaundice is not observed in the skin of a dark-skinned client will assist you in eliminating options 1 and 4. Knowing that pallor is assessed in the nailbeds will direct you to option 2. Review assessment techniques if you had difficulty with this question.
Level of Cognitive Ability: Analysis
Client Needs: Physiological Integrity
Integrated Process: Nursing Process—assessment
Content Area: Adult health—gastrointestinal
Reference: Lewis, S., Heitkemper, M., & Dirksen, S. (2004). *Medical-surgical nursing: Assessment and management of clinical problems* (6th ed., p. 483). St. Louis: Mosby.

CRITICAL THINKING: MULTIPLE RESPONSE

Answer:
____ Meperidine (Demerol) as prescribed for pain
____ Encourage coughing and deep breathing.

___ Administer antacids as prescribed.

___ Administer anticholinergics as prescribed.

Rationale: The client with acute pancreatitis normally is placed on an NPO status to rest the pancreas and suppress gastrointestinal secretions. Because abdominal pain is a prominent symptom of pancreatitis, pain medication such as meperidine will be prescribed. Some clients experience lessened pain by assuming positions that flex the trunk and draw the knees up to the chest. A side-lying position with the head elevated 45 degrees decreases tension on the abdomen and also may help to ease the pain. The client is susceptible to respiratory infections because the retroperitoneal fluid raises the diaphragm, which causes the client to take shallow, guarded abdominal breaths. Therefore measures such as turning, coughing, and deep breathing are instituted. Antacids and anticholinergics may be prescribed to suppress gastrointestinal secretions.

Test-Taking Strategy: Focus on the pathophysiology associated with pancreatitis. This will assist in answering the question. Review treatment measures for acute pancreatitis if you had difficulty with this question.

Level of Cognitive Ability: Analysis

Client Needs: Physiological Integrity

Integrated Process: Nursing Process—analysis

Content Area: Adult health—gastrointestinal

Reference: Lewis, S., Heitkemper, M., & Dirksen, S. (2004). Medical-surgical nursing: Assessment and management of clinical problems (6th ed., p. 1138). St. Louis: Mosby.

REFERENCES

Chernecky, C., & Berger, B. (2001). *Laboratory tests and diagnostic procedures* (3rd ed.). Philadelphia: W. B. Saunders.

Elkin, M., Perry, A., & Potter, P. (2004). *Nursing interventions & clinical skills* (3rd ed.). St. Louis: Mosby.

Harkreader, H., & Hogan, M. A. (2004). *Fundamentals of nursing: Caring and clinical judgment* (2nd ed.). Philadelphia: W. B. Saunders.

Hodgson, B., & Kizior, R. (2004). *Saunders nursing drug handbook 2004*. Philadelphia: W. B. Saunders.

Ignatavicius, D., & Workman, M. (2002). *Medical-surgical nursing: Critical thinking for collaborative care* (4th ed.). Philadelphia: W. B. Saunders.

Lewis, S., Heitkemper, M., & Dirksen, S. (2004). *Medical-surgical nursing: Assessment and management of clinical problems* (6th ed.). St. Louis: Mosby.

Linton, A., & Maebius, N. (2003). *Introduction to medical-surgical nursing* (3rd ed.). Philadelphia: W. B. Saunders.

Perry, A., & Potter, P. (2002). *Clinical nursing skills and techniques* (5th ed.). St. Louis: Mosby.

Phipps, W., Monahan, F., Sands, J., Marek, J., & Neighbors, M. (2003). *Medical-surgical nursing: Health and illness perspectives* (7th ed.). St. Louis: Mosby.

Potter, P., & Perry, A. (2001). *Fundamentals of nursing* (5th ed.). St. Louis: Mosby.

Gastrointestinal Medications

I. ANTACIDS AND MUCOSAL PROTECTIVE MEDICATIONS (BOX 56-1)

A. Description
  1. React with gastric acid to produce neutral salts or salts of low acidity.
  2. Inactivate pepsin and enhance mucosal protection but do not coat the ulcer crater to protect it from the acid and pepsin.
  3. These medications are used for peptic ulcer disease and gastroesophageal reflux disease.
  4. These medications should be taken on a regular schedule.
  5. These medications usually are administered 7 times a day, 1 and 3 hours after each meal and at bedtime.
  6. To provide maximum benefit, treatment should elevate the gastric pH above 5.
  7. Antacid tablets should be chewed thoroughly and followed with a glass of water or milk.
  8. Liquid preparations should be shaken before dispensing.
  9. Interactions with other medications can be minimized by allowing 1 hour between antacid administration and the administration of other medications.

BOX 56-1

Antacids and Mucosal Protective Medications

Aluminum hydroxide gel (Amphojel, AlternaGEL)
Aluminum carbonate gel (Basaljel)
Bismuth subsalicylate (Pepto-Bismol)
Calcium carbonate (Tums)
Magnesium hydroxide (Milk of Magnesia, MOM)
Misoprostol (Cytotec)
Sucralfate (Carafate)

  10. These medications can interfere with the action of sucralfate (Carafate), and to minimize this interaction, the medications should be administered 1 hour apart from each other.

B. Sucralfate (Carafate)
  1. Sucralfate creates a protective barrier against acid and pepsin.
  2. Sucralfate is administered orally and should be taken on an empty stomach.
  3. Administer sucralfate at least 60 minutes apart from an antacid.
  4. Sucralfate may cause constipation.
  5. Sucralfate may impede absorption of warfarin sodium (Coumadin), phenytoin (Dilantin), theophylline, digoxin (Lanoxin), and some antibiotics and should be administered at least 2 hours apart from these medications.

C. Misoprostol (Cytotec)
  1. Misoprostol is used to prevent gastric ulcers caused by long-term therapy with nonsteroidal antiinflammatory drugs.
  2. Misoprostol suppresses secretion of gastric acid.
  3. Misoprostol promotes secretion of bicarbonate and cytoprotective mucus.
  4. Misoprostol maintains submucosal blood flow by promoting vasodilation.
  5. Misoprostol is administered with meals.
  6. Misoprostol causes diarrhea and abdominal pain.
  7. Misoprostol is contraindicated for use in pregnancy.

D. Magnesium hydroxide
  1. Magnesium hydroxide is rapid-acting.
  2. Magnesium hydroxide is also referred to as *Milk of Magnesia*.
  3. The most prominent side effect is diarrhea.
  4. Magnesium hydroxide usually is administered in combination with aluminum hydroxide, an antacid that assists in preventing diarrhea.

5. Magnesium hydroxide is contraindicated in clients with intestinal obstruction, appendicitis, or undiagnosed abdominal pain.
6. In clients with renal impairment, magnesium can accumulate to high levels, causing signs of toxicity.

E. Aluminum hydroxide (Amphojel, Alu-Cap, Dialume)
1. Aluminum hydroxide is slow-acting.
2. Aluminum hydroxide contains significant amounts of sodium.
3. Aluminum hydroxide should be used with caution in clients with hypertension and heart failure.
4. The most common side effect is constipation.
5. Aluminum hydroxide can reduce the effects of tetracyclines, warfarin sodium (Coumadin), and digoxin (Lanoxin).
6. Aluminum hydroxide can reduce phosphate absorption and thereby cause hypophosphatemia.

F. Calcium carbonate (Tums)
1. Calcium carbonate is rapid-acting.
2. A common side effect is constipation.
3. Calcium carbonate releases carbon dioxide in the stomach causing belching and flatulence; milk-alkali syndrome (headache, urinary frequency, anorexia, nausea/vomiting, fatigue) can occur.

G. Sodium bicarbonate
1. Sodium bicarbonate has a rapid onset.
2. Sodium bicarbonate liberates carbon dioxide, increases intradominal pressure, and promotes flatulence.
3. Sodium bicarbonate should be used with caution in clients with hypertension and heart failure.
4. Sodium bicarbonate can cause systemic alkalosis in clients with renal impairment.
5. Sodium bicarbonate is useful for treating acidosis and elevating urinary pH to promote excretion of acidic medications following overdose.

II. HISTAMINE H₂ RECEPTOR ANTAGONISTS (BOX 56-2)

A. Description
1. Histamine H_2 receptor antagonists suppress secretion of gastric acid.
2. These medications alleviate symptoms of heartburn and assist in preventing complications of peptic ulcer disease.
3. These medications prevent stress ulcers and reduce the recurrence of all ulcers.

BOX 56-2

Histamine H₂ Receptor Antagonists

Cimetidine (Tagamet)
Famotidine (Pepcid)
Nizatidine (Axid)
Ranitidine (Zantac)

---

4. These medications promote healing in gastroesophageal reflux disease.
5. These medications are contraindicated in hypersensitive clients.
6. These medications should be used with caution in clients with impaired renal or hepatic function.

B. Cimetidine (Tagamet)
1. Cimetidine can be administered orally, intramuscularly, or intravenously.
2. Food reduces the rate of absorption; if taken with meals, absorption will be slowed.
3. By the intravenous route, a 300-mg dose can be diluted in a total volume of 20 mL and injected slowly over not less than 2 minutes, or it may be diluted in 100 mL and infused over 15 to 20 minutes.
4. Antacids can decrease the absorption of oral cimetidine.
5. Cimetidine and antacids should be administered at least 1 hour apart from each other.
6. Cimetidine passes the blood-brain barrier, and central nervous system side effects can occur.
7. Cimetidine may cause mental confusion, agitation, psychosis, depression, anxiety, and disorientation.
8. Dosage should be reduced in clients with renal impairment.
9. Intravenous administration can cause hypotension and dysrhythmias.
10. If cimetidine is administered with warfarin sodium (Coumadin), phenytoin (Dilantin), theophylline, or lidocaine, the dosages of these medications should be reduced.

C. Ranitidine (Zantac)
1. Ranitidine can be administered orally, intramuscularly, or intravenously.
2. Side effects are uncommon.
3. Ranitidine does not penetrate the blood brain-barrier as cimetidine does.
4. Ranitidine is not affected by food.
5. For intravenous injection, ranitidine should be diluted with 20 mL and administered slowly over 5 minutes or more, or diluted in 100 mL and administered over 15 to 20 minutes.

D. Famotidine (Pepcid) and nizatidine (Axid)
1. Famotidine and nizatidine are similar to Ranitidine and cimetidine.
2. These medications do not need to be administered with food.

E. Ranitidine bismuth citrate (Tritec)
1. Used to treat active duodenal ulcers associated with *Helicobacter pylori*.
2. Administered with an antibiotic such as clarithromycin (Biaxin) (Box 56-3).

III. PROTON PUMP INHIBITORS (BOX 56-4)

A. Proton pump inhibitors suppress gastric acid secretion.

BOX 56-3

Antimicrobials Effective against *Helicobacter pylori*

Amoxicillin (Amoxil)
Clarithromycin (Biaxin)
Metronidazole (Flagyl)
Tetracycline (Achromycin)

BOX 56-4

Proton Pump Inhibitors

Esomeprazole (Nexium)
Lansoprazole (Prevacid)
Omeprazole (Prilosec)
Pantoprazole (Protonix)
Rabeprazole (Aciphex)

BOX 56-5

Gastrointestinal Stimulants

Bethanechol chloride (Urecholine, Duvoid)
Dexpanthenol (Ilopan, Ilopan-Choline)
Metoclopramide (Reglan)
Neostigmine methylsulfate (Prostigmin)

B. Proton pump inhibitors are used with active ulcer disease, erosive esophagitis, and pathological hypersecretory conditions.
C. Proton pump inhibitors are contraindicated in hypersensitivity.
D. Common side effects include headache, diarrhea, abdominal pain, and nausea.

IV. GASTROINTESTINAL STIMULANTS (BOX 56-5)

A. These medications stimulate motility of the upper gastrointestinal tract and increase the rate of gastric emptying without stimulating gastric, biliary, or pancreatic secretions.
B. Gastrointestinal stimulants are used for gastroesophageal reflux.
C. Gastrointestinal stimulants may cause restlessness, drowsiness, extrapyramidal reactions, dizziness, insomnia, and headache.
D. Gastrointestinal stimulants usually are administered 30 minutes before meals and at bedtime.
E. Gastrointestinal stimulants are contraindicated in clients with sensitivity.
F. Gastrointestinal stimulants are contraindicated in clients with mechanical obstruction, perforation, or gastrointestinal hemorrhage.
G. Gastrointestinal stimulants can precipitate hypertensive crisis in clients with pheochromocytoma.
H. Safety in pregnancy is not established.

I. Metoclopramide (Reglan) can cause Parkinson-like reactions, and if this occurs, the medication is discontinued.
J. Anticholinergics and narcotic analgesics antagonize the effects of metoclopramide.
K. Alcohol, sedatives, cyclosporine (Sandimmune), and tranquilizers produce an additive effect.

V. BILE ACID SEQUESTRANTS (BOX 56-6)

A. Description
   1. Bile acid sequestrants are used to treat pruritis associated with biliary disease.
   2. Bile acid sequestrants act by absorbing and combining with intestinal bile salts, which then are secreted in the feces, preventing intestinal reabsorption.
   3. Bile acid sequestrants may be used to treat hypercholesterolemia in adults.
   4. Bile acid sequestrants should be used cautiously in clients with bowel obstruction or severe constipation because of the adverse gastrointestinal effects.
   5. Taste and palatability are often reasons for noncompliance and can be improved by the use of flavored products or mixing the medication with various juices.
   6. Stool softeners and other sources of fiber can be used to abate the gastrointestinal side effects.
B. Side effects
   1. Constipation
   2. Bloating
   3. Flatulence
   4. Nausea
   5. Fecal impaction and intestinal obstruction
   6. Exacerbation of hemorrhoids
   7. Hypoprothrombinemia
   8. Decreased vitamin absorption

VI. MEDICATIONS FOR CHOLELITHIASIS (BOX 56-7)

A. Chenodiol (Chenix)

BOX 56-6

Bile Acid Sequestrants

Cholestyramine (Questran, Prevalite)
Colestipol (Colestid)

BOX 56-7

Medications for Cholelithiasis

Chenodiol (Chenix)
Monoctanoin (Moctanin)
Ursodiol (Actigall)

1. Chenodiol decreases cholesterol production, lowering content of bile, and thus facilitates dissolution of gallstones.
2. Chenodiol can cause diarrhea and possibly hepatotoxicity.
3. Baseline liver function studies should be performed.
4. Client should be instructed to contact the physician if abdominal pain, sudden right upper quadrant pain, nausea, or vomiting occurs.
5. Administer chenodiol with food or milk.
6. Avoid aluminum-containing antacids.
B. Ursodiol (Actigall)
1. Ursodiol is a naturally occurring bile salt.
2. Ursodiol suppresses hepatic synthesis and secretion of cholesterol and inhibits intestinal absorption of cholesterol.
3. Ursodiol requires months of therapy for dissolution of gallstone to occur.
4. Ultrasound images are obtained within 6 month to determine effectiveness of therapy.
5. Clients should be instructed to report nausea, vomiting, diarrhea, or rash to the physician.
6. Administer ursodiol with food or milk.
7. Avoid aluminum-containing antacids.
C. Monoctanoin (Moctanin)
1. Monoctanoin is used when stones made of calcium are resistant to dissolution by orally administered chenodiol.
2. Monoctanoin is administered through a T-tube, nasal biliary catheter, or percutaneous transhepatic catheter.
3. Monoctanoin is effective only when in contact with the stone.
4. Major side effects include diarrhea, nausea, and abdominal pain.

VII. MEDICATIONS TO TREAT HEPATIC ENCEPHALOPATHY (BOX 56-8)

A. Lactulose (Cephulac)
1. Lactulose reduces ammonia levels.
2. Lactulose improves protein tolerance in clients with advanced hepatic **cirrhosis.**
3. Lactulose lowers the colonic pH from 7 to 5; this acidification pulls ammonia into the bowel to be excreted in the feces, thus lowering the ammonia level.
4. Lactulose is administered orally in the form of a syrup.

BOX 56-8

Medications to Treat Hepatic Encephalopathy

Lactulose (Chronulac, Duphalac)
Neomycin (Mycifradin)

B. Neomycin (Mycifradin)
1. Neomycin reduces the number of colonic bacteria that normally convert urea and amino acids into ammonia.
2. Neomycin is administered orally or via nasogastric tube.
3. Neomycin is used with caution in clients with kidney impairment.

VIII. PANCREATIC ENZYME REPLACEMENTS (BOX 56-9)

A. These medications are used to supplement or replace pancreatic enzymes.
B. These medications should be taken with meals or a snack (food helps to buffer the stomach acid).
C. A high-fiber diet may increase the efficacy of the medication.
D. Side effects include abdominal cramps or pain, nausea, and diarrhea.
E. Products that contain calcium carbonate or magnesium hydroxide interfere with the action of the medication.

IX. ANTIEMETICS (BOX 56-10)

A. Antiemetics are medications used to control vomiting.
B. The choice of the antiemetic is determined by the cause of the nausea and vomiting.
C. Monitor for drowsiness and protect the client from injury.
D. Monitor vital signs and intake and output.
E. Limit odors in the client's room when the client is nauseated or vomiting.

BOX 56-9

Pancreatic Enzyme Replacements

Pancreatin (Entozyme, Donnazyne)
Pancrelipase (Pancrease, Viokase)

BOX 56-10

Commonly Administered Antiemetics

Diphenidol hydrochloride (Vontrol)
Dolasetron (Anzemet)
Dronabinol (Marinol)
Granisetron (Kytril)
Hydroxyzine hydrochloride (Atarax)
Hydroxyzine pamoate (Vistaril)
Meclizine hydrochloride (Antivert)
Metoclopramide (Reglan)
Ondansetron (Zofran)
Prochlorperazine (Compazine)
Promethazine hydrochloride (Phenergan)
Scopolamine transdermal (Transderm-Scop)
Thiethylperazine malate (Torecan)
Trimethobenzamide hydrochloride (Tigan)

F. Limit oral intake to clear liquids when the client is nauseated or vomiting.

X. LAXATIVES (BOX 56-11)
A. Bulk-forming laxatives
   1. Description
      a. Absorb water into the feces and increase bulk to produce large and soft stools
      b. For short-term use
      c. Contraindicated in bowel obstruction
   2. Side effects
      a. Gastrointestinal disturbances
      b. Dehydration
      c. Electrolyte imbalance
      d. Dependency with chronic use
B. Stimulant cathartics
   1. Description: Stimulate motility of large intestine
   2. Bisacodyl (Dulcolax): Do not administer within 60 minutes of an antacid or milk.
   3. Castor oil: Administer with juice; produces results in 6 to 12 hours.
C. Saline cathartics
   1. Saline cathartics attract water into the large intestine to produce bulk.

2. Saline cathartics stimulate **peristalsis.**
3. Saline cathartics achieve results in 2 to 6 hours.
D. Stool softeners
   1. Stool softeners inhibit absorption of water so fecal mass remains large and soft.
   2. Stool softeners are used to avoid straining.
E. Lubricants
   1. Lubricants act to soften the feces.
   2. Lubricants ease the strain of passing stool.
   3. Lubricants lessen irritation to hemorrhoids.
   4. Mineral oil
      a. Mineral oil can cause lipid pneumonia if accidentally aspirated.
      b. Mineral oil interferes with absorption of the fat-soluble vitamins A, D, E, and K.

XI. MEDICATIONS TO CONTROL DIARRHEA (BOX 56-12)
A. Opioids
   1. Opioids decrease intestinal motility and **peristalsis.**
   2. When poisons, infections, or bacterial toxins are the cause of the diarrhea, opioids worsen the condition by delaying the elimination of toxins.
   3. Tincture of opium has an unpleasant taste and can be diluted with 15 to 30 mL of water for administration.
B. Other antidiarrheals: Refer to Box 56-12.

XII. ANTISPASMODICS (BOX 56-13)
A. Description: Relax smooth muscle of the gastrointestinal tract
B. Side effects
   1. Constipation or diarrhea
   2. Rash
   3. Euphoria
   4. Dizziness

BOX 56-11

Laxatives

BULK-FORMING LAXATIVES
Calcium polycarbophil (FiberCon)
Methylcellulose (Citrucel)
Psyllium hydrophilic mucilloid (Metamucil, Fiberall, Konsyl, Serutan, Modane Bulk)

STIMULANT CATHARTICS
Bisacodyl (Dulcolax)
Cascara sagrada
Castor oil, emulsified (Neoloid)
Docusate sodium (Ex-Lax)
Senna concentrate (Senexon, Senna-Gen)

OSMOTIC CATHARTICS
Senna (Senokot)
Lactulose (Chronulac)
Magnesium citrate (Citroma)
Magnesium hydroxide (Milk of Magnesia, MOM)
Magnesium sulfate (epsom salts)
Polyethylene glycol and electrolytes (GoLYTELY)
Potassium bitartrate and sodium bicarbonate (Coe-Two)
Sodium phosphates (Fleet Enema, Phospho-Soda)

STOOL SOFTENERS
Docusate calcium (Surfak)
Docusate sodium (Colace)
Docusate with casanthranol (Peri-Colace)

LUBRICANT
Mineral oil

BOX 56-12

Medications to Control Diarrhea

OPIOIDS AND RELATED MEDICATIONS
Codeine phosphate; codeine sulfate
Difenoxin with atropine (Motofen)
Diphenoxylate hydrochloride with atropine (Lomotil)
Loperamide hydrochloride (Imodium)
Tincture of opium

ABSORBENT ANTIDIARRHEALS
Bismuth subsalicylate (Pepto-Bismol)
Kaolin and pectin (Kao-Spen, Kapectolin)
Octreotide (Sandostatin)
Somatostatin analog

BOX 56-13

Antispasmodic

Dicyclomine hydrochloride (Antispas, Bentyl)

5. Drowsiness
6. Headache
7. Nausea
8. Weakness

PRACTICE QUESTIONS

1. The client is receiving propantheline bromide (Pro-Banthine) as adjunctive treatment for peptic ulcer disease. The nurse should administer this medication
   1. With meals.
   2. Just after meals.
   3. 30 minutes before meals.
   4. With antacids.
2. The client is taking docusate sodium (Colace). The nurse monitors for which of the following to determine whether the client is having a therapeutic effect from this medication?
   1. Absence of abdominal pain
   2. Hematest negative stools
   3. Reduction in steatorrhea
   4. Regular bowel movements
3. The client is taking cascara sagrada and develops abdominal cramps. The nurse interprets that the client is most likely experiencing
   1. A common side effect of this medication.
   2. Partial bowel obstruction.
   3. A case of influenza.
   4. Peptic ulcer disease.
4. The client taking bisacodyl (Dulcolax) wants to achieve rapid effect from the medication. The nurse then tells the client to take the medication
   1. With a large meal.
   2. On an empty stomach.
   3. At bedtime.
   4. With two glasses of juice.
5. The client who is advised to take senna (Senokot) to treat constipation asks the nurse how this medication works. The nurse would incorporate which of the following when formulating a response?
   1. Senna coats the bowel wall and makes it slippery.
   2. Senna adds fiber and bulk to the stool.
   3. Senna accumulates water and increases peristalsis.
   4. Senna stimulates the vagus nerve to improve bowel tone.
6. The client has a PRN order for loperamide (Imodium). The nurse should plan to administer this medication if the client has
   1. Hematest positive nasogastric tube drainage.
   2. Abdominal pain.
   3. Constipation.
   4. An episode of diarrhea.
7. The nurse has given instructions to the client who just received a prescription for diphenoxylate with atropine (Lomotil). The nurse determines that the client understands the use of the medication and its properties if the client states to

1. Stay within the prescribed dose because it can be habit-forming.
2. Take the medication with a bulk-forming laxative.
3. Expect increased salivation while taking the medication.
4. Anticipate side effects of nervous system excitability.

8. The client has been started on psyllium (Metamucil). The nurse would teach this client to take this medication with
   1. Gelatin, applesauce, or pudding.
   2. A full glass of liquid, followed by a second.
   3. A multivitamin and mineral supplement.
   4. A dose of an antacid.
9. The nurse teaches the client taking metoclopramide (Reglan) to discontinue the medication immediately and call the physician if which of the following occurs with long-term use?
   1. Anxiety or irritability
   2. Dry mouth not minimized by the use of sugar-free hard candy
   3. Excessive drowsiness or excitability
   4. Uncontrolled rhythmic movements of the face or limbs
10. The client has just taken a dose of trimethobenzamide (Tigan). The nurse monitors this client for relief of
    1. Nausea and vomiting.
    2. Abdominal pain.
    3. Heartburn.
    4. Constipation.
11. The client has a PRN order for ondansetron (Zofran). The nurse would administer this medication to the postoperative client for relief of
    1. Urinary retention.
    2. Incisional pain.
    3. Nausea and vomiting.
    4. Paralytic ileus.
12. The client has an order to take magnesium citrate to prevent constipation following a barium study of the upper gastrointestinal tract. The nurse plans to administer this medication
    1. With a full glass of water.
    2. With fruit juice only.
    3. With ice.
    4. At room temperature.
13. The nurse is administering a dose of prochlorperazine (Compazine) to a client for nausea and vomiting. The nurse would assess the client for which of the following frequent side effects of this medication?
    1. Diarrhea
    2. Drooling
    3. Excessive lacrimation
    4. Blurred vision
14. The client has begun medication therapy with pancrelipase (Pancrease). The nurse would evaluate that the medication is having the optimal intended benefit if which of the following effects is observed?

1. Reduction of steatorrhea
2. Absence of abdominal pain
3. Relief of heartburn
4. Weight loss

15. A calcium carbonate antacid has been prescribed for a client and the nurse provides instructions to the client about the medication. The nurse tells the client that it is best to take the antacid with
    1. Milk.
    2. A vitamin D supplement.
    3. Yogurt.
    4. Water.

16. The nurse is giving the client directions for proper use of aluminum hydroxide tablets (Alu-Caps). The nurse tells the client to
    1. Chew the tablets thoroughly and follow with 4 oz of water.
    2. Swallow the tablets whole with a full glass of water.
    3. Take the tablets at the same time as other medications.
    4. Take each dose with a laxative to prevent constipation.

17. The client with history of duodenal ulcer is taking calcium carbonate chewable tablets. The nurse would evaluate that the client is experiencing optimal effects of the medication if
    1. Muscle twitching stops.
    2. Heartburn is relieved.
    3. Serum calcium levels rise.
    4. Serum phosphorus levels decrease.

18. The hospitalized client asks the nurse for sodium bicarbonate to relieve heartburn following a meal. The nurse reviews the client's medical record, knowing that the medication is contraindicated in which of the following conditions?
    1. Urinary calculuses
    2. Chronic bronchitis
    3. Metabolic alkalosis
    4. Respiratory acidosis

19. The client is complaining of gas pains following surgery and requests medication. The nurse selects which of the following medications from the PRN medication list to give to the client?
    1. Magnesium hydroxide (Milk of Magnesia)
    2. Droperidol (Inapsine)
    3. Acetaminophen (Tylenol)
    4. Simethicone (Mylicon)

20. An older client recently has been taking cimetidine (Tagamet). The nurse monitors the client for which of the following most frequent central nervous system side effects of this medication?
    1. Confusion
    2. Dizziness
    3. Tremors
    4. Hallucinations

21. The client with a gastric ulcer has an order for sucralfate (Carafate) 1 g by mouth 4 times a day. The nurse would schedule the medication for which of the following times?
    1. With meals and at bedtime
    2. One hour before meals and at bedtime
    3. Every 6 hours around the clock
    4. One hour after meals and at bedtime

22. The client who chronically uses nonsteroidal anti-inflammatory drugs has been taking misoprostol (Cytotec). The nurse determines that the medication is having the intended therapeutic effect if the client did not experience which of the following symptoms?
    1. Decreased platelet count
    2. Decreased white blood cell count
    3. Epigastric pain
    4. Diarrhea

23. The physician has written an order for ranitidine (Zantac) 300 mg once daily. The nurse would schedule the medication for which of the following times?
    1. Before breakfast
    2. After lunch
    3. With supper
    4. At bedtime

24. The client is taking lansoprazole (Prevacid) for the chronic management of peptic ulcer disease. The nurse advises the client to take which of the following products if needed for headache?
    1. Acetaminophen (Tylenol)
    2. Ibuprofen (Motrin)
    3. Naproxen (Aleve)
    4. Acetylsalicylic acid (aspirin)

25. The client has been taking omeprazole (Prilosec) for 4 weeks. The ambulatory care nurse would evaluate that the client is receiving optimal intended effect of the medication if the client reports absence of which of the following symptoms?
    1. Constipation
    2. Heartburn
    3. Diarrhea
    4. Flatulence

CRITICAL THINKING: FILL-IN-THE-BLANK

The client with esophageal reflex has been given a prescription for metoclopramide (Reglan) 4 times a day. The nurse tells the client to take the medication at which times during the day?

Answer: _____

ANSWERS

1. 3

Rationale: Propantheline bromide is an antimuscarinic anticholinergic medication that decreases gastrointestinal secretions. Propantheline should be administered 30 minutes before meals. The other options are incorrect.

Test-Taking Strategy: Use the process of elimination. Option 4 could be eliminated first because most medications cannot be administered with antacids because of interactive effects. Next, eliminate options 1 and 2 because they are similar. Review this medication if you had difficulty with this question.

Level of Cognitive Ability: Application
Client Needs: Physiological Integrity
Integrated Process: Nursing Process—implementation
Content Area: Pharmacology
Reference: Kee, J., & Hayes, E. (2003). *Pharmacology: A nursing process approach* (4th ed., p. 669). Philadelphia: W. B. Saunders.

2. 4

Rationale: Docusate sodium is a stool softener that promotes absorption of water into the stool, producing a softer consistency of stool. The intended effect is relief or prevention of constipation. The medication does not relieve abdominal pain, stop gastrointestinal bleeding, or decrease the amount of fat in the stools.

Test-Taking Strategy: Use the process of elimination. Recalling that docusate sodium is used to soften the stool will direct you to option 4. Review the expected effects of this medication if you had difficulty with this question.

Level of Cognitive Ability: Analysis
Client Needs: Physiological Integrity
Integrated Process: Nursing Process—analysis
Content Area: Pharmacology
Reference: Hodgson, B., & Kizior, R. (2004). *Saunders nursing drug handbook 2004* (p. 329). Philadelphia: W. B. Saunders.

3. 1

Rationale: Cascara sagrada is a laxative that causes nausea and abdominal cramps as the most frequent side effects. Other health problems (options 2, 3, and 4) are not determined based on a single symptom.

Test-Taking Strategy: Use the process of elimination. Remember that options that are similar are not likely to be correct. This will allow you to eliminate the two gastrointestinal disorders (options 2 and 4). From the remaining options, choose option 1 over option 3, knowing that laxatives can cause abdominal cramping. Review the effects of this medication if you had difficulty with this question.

Level of Cognitive Ability: Analysis
Client Needs: Physiological Integrity
Integrated Process: Nursing Process—analysis
Content Area: Pharmacology
References: Hodgson, B., & Kizior, R. (2004). *Saunders nursing drug handbook 2004* (p. 158). Philadelphia: W. B. Saunders.
Kee, J., & Hayes, E. (2003). *Pharmacology: A nursing process approach* (4th ed., p. 659). Philadelphia: W. B. Saunders.

4. 2

Rationale: Most rapid results from bisacodyl occur when it is taken on an empty stomach. Bisacodyl will not have a rapid effect if taken with a large meal. If bisacodyl is taken at bedtime, the client will have a bowel movement in the morning. Taking the medication with two glasses of juice will not add to its effect.

Test-Taking Strategy: Use the process of elimination noting the key words "rapid effects." Review the administration of this medication if you had difficulty with this question.

Level of Cognitive Ability: Application
Client Needs: Physiological Integrity
Integrated Process: Nursing Process—implementation
Content Area: Pharmacology
Reference: Hodgson, B., & Kizior, R. (2004). *Saunders nursing drug handbook 2004* (p. 111). Philadelphia: W. B. Saunders.

5. 3

Rationale: Senna works by changing the transport of water and electrolytes in the large intestine, which causes accumulation of water in the mass of stool and increased peristalsis. The other options are incorrect.

Test-Taking Strategy: Knowledge regarding the action of this medication is required to answer this question. If you are unfamiliar with this medication, review its action.

Level of Cognitive Ability: Comprehension
Client Needs: Physiological Integrity
Integrated Process: Teaching/Learning
Content Area: Pharmacology
Reference: Hodgson, B., & Kizior, R. (2004). *Saunders nursing drug handbook 2004* (p. 910). Philadelphia: W. B. Saunders.

6. 4

Rationale: Loperamide is an antidiarrheal agent. Loperamide is used to manage acute diarrhea and also chronic diarrhea in conditions such as inflammatory bowel disease. Loperamide also can be used to reduce the volume of drainage from an ileostomy.

Test-Taking Strategy: Recalling that this medication is an antidiarrheal agent will direct you to option 4. Review the action of this medication if you had difficulty with this question.

Level of Cognitive Ability: Application
Client Needs: Physiological Integrity
Integrated Process: Nursing Process—planning
Content Area: Pharmacology
Reference: Kee, J., & Hayes, E. (2003). *Pharmacology: A nursing process approach* (4th ed., p. 655). Philadelphia: W. B. Saunders.

7. 1

Rationale: The client should not exceed the recommended dose because it may be habit-forming. The medication is an antidiarrheal and therefore should not be taken with a laxative. Side effects of the medication include dry mouth and drowsiness.

Test-Taking Strategy: Use the process of elimination. Noting the key word "atropine" will assist in eliminating options 3 and 4. Recalling that the medication is an antidiarrheal will assist in eliminating option 2. Review the properties of this medication if you had difficulty with this question.

Level of Cognitive Ability: Analysis
Client Needs: Physiological Integrity
Integrated Process: Teaching/Learning
Content Area: Pharmacology

Reference: Kee, J., & Hayes, E. (2003). *Pharmacology: A nursing process approach* (4th ed., p. 653). Philadelphia: W. B. Saunders.

8. **2**
Rationale: Metamucil is a bulk-forming laxative and should be taken with a full glass of water or juice, followed by another glass of liquid. This will help prevent impaction of the medication in the stomach or small intestine. The other options are incorrect.
Test-Taking Strategy: Use the process of elimination. Option 4 should be eliminated first because most medications are not taken with antacids. Eliminate options 1 and 3 next because they have no physiological benefit for medication effect. Review client teaching points related to this medication if you had difficulty with this question.
Level of Cognitive Ability: Application
Client Needs: Physiological Integrity
Integrated Process: Teaching/Learning
Content Area: Pharmacology
Reference: Hodgson, B., & Kizior, R. (2004). *Saunders nursing drug handbook 2004* (p. 856). Philadelphia: W. B. Saunders.

9. **4**
Rationale: If the client experiences tardive dyskinesia (rhythmic movements of the face or limbs), the client should stop the medication and call the physician. These side effects may be irreversible. Excitability is not a side effect of this medication. Anxiety, irritability, and dry mouth are side effects that are not so harmful to the client.
Test-Taking Strategy: Use the process of elimination focusing on the key words "discontinue the medication immediately." Select option 4 because these effects are most harmful to the client. Review the side effects and adverse effects of this medication if you had difficulty with this question.
Level of Cognitive Ability: Application
Client Needs: Physiological Integrity
Integrated Process: Teaching/Learning
Content Area: Pharmacology
Reference: Hodgson, B., & Kizior, R. (2004). *Saunders nursing drug handbook 2004* (, p. 661). Philadelphia: W. B. Saunders.

10. **1**
Rationale: Tigan is an antiemetic agent that is used to treat nausea and vomiting. The other options are incorrect.
Test-Taking Strategy: Use the process of elimination. Recalling that this medication is an antiemetic will direct you to option 1. Review this medication if you had difficulty with this question.
Level of Cognitive Ability: Analysis
Client Needs: Physiological Integrity
Integrated Process: Nursing Process—evaluation
Content Area: Pharmacology
Reference: Hodgson, B., & Kizior, R. (2004). *Saunders nursing drug handbook 2004* (, p. 1025). Philadelphia: W. B. Saunders.

11. **3**
Rationale: Ondansetron is an antiemetic that is used to treat postoperative nausea and vomiting, as well as nausea and vomiting associated with chemotherapy. The other options are incorrect.

Test-Taking Strategy: Use the process of elimination. Recalling that this medication is an antiemetic will direct you to option 3. Review this medication if you had difficulty with this question.
Level of Cognitive Ability: Application
Client Needs: Physiological Integrity
Integrated Process: Nursing Process—implementation
Content Area: Pharmacology
References: Hodgson, B., & Kizior, R. (2004). *Saunders nursing drug handbook 2004* (, p. 755). Philadelphia: W. B. Saunders. Kee, J., & Hayes, E. (2003). *Pharmacology: A nursing process approach* (4th ed., p. 867). Philadelphia: W. B. Saunders.

12. **3**
Rationale: Magnesium citrate is available as an oral solution and is used commonly as a laxative in preparation for or following certain studies of the gastrointestinal tract. Magnesium citrate should be served chilled and should not be allowed to stand for prolonged periods, which would reduce the carbonation and make the solution even less palatable. Options 1, 2, and 4 are incorrect.
Test-Taking Strategy: Use the process of elimination. Eliminate options 1 and 2 first, knowing that magnesium citrate is itself a liquid. From the remaining options, you must know that magnesium citrate should be given cold to enhance palatability. Review this medication if you had difficulty with this question.
Level of Cognitive Ability: Application
Client Needs: Physiological Integrity
Integrated Process: Nursing Process—implementation
Content Area: Pharmacology
Reference: McKenry, L., & Salerno, E. (2003). *Mosby's pharmacology in nursing* (21st ed., p. 218). St. Louis: Mosby.

13. **4**
Rationale: The nurse would assess the client for blurred vision as a frequent side effect of prochlorperazine. Other frequent side effects of this phenothiazine-type antiemetic and antipsychotic are dry eyes, dry mouth, and constipation.
Test-Taking Strategy: Use the process of elimination. Recalling that this medication is a phenothiazine-type antiemetic and knowing the side effects of these medications will direct you to option 4. Review this medication if you had difficulty with this question.
Level of Cognitive Ability: Application
Client Needs: Physiological Integrity
Integrated Process: Nursing Process—assessment
Content Area: Pharmacology
Reference: Hodgson, B., & Kizior, R. (2004). *Saunders nursing drug handbook 2004* (p. 840). Philadelphia: W. B. Saunders.

14. **1**
Rationale: Pancrease is a pancreatic enzyme used in clients with pancreatitis as a digestive aid. The medication should reduce the amount of fatty stools (steatorrhea). Another intended effect could be improved nutritional status. Pancrease is not used to treat abdominal pain or heartburn. Use of pancrease could result in weight gain but should not result in weight loss if it is aiding in digestion.
Test-Taking Strategy: Use the process of elimination and focus on the name of the medication. Use knowledge of physiology

of the pancreas to assist in directing you to the correct option. Review this medication if you had difficulty with this question.
Level of Cognitive Ability: Analysis
Client Needs: Physiological Integrity
Integrated Process: Nursing Process—evaluation
Content Area: Pharmacology
Reference: Hodgson, B., & Kizior, R. (2004). *Saunders nursing drug handbook 2004* (p. 776). Philadelphia: W. B. Saunders.

15. **4**
Rationale: Calcium carbonate antacids should not be taken with milk, milk products, or foods or supplements high in vitamin D because milk-alkali syndrome (headache, urinary frequency, anorexia, nausea/vomiting, fatigue) can occur. The best item to consume when taking calcium carbonate is water.
Test-Taking Strategy: Use the process of elimination. Recalling that antacids should not be taken with food items will direct you to option 4. Review this antacid if you had difficulty with this question.
Level of Cognitive Ability: Application
Client Needs: Physiological Integrity
Integrated Process: Teaching/Learning
Content Area: Pharmacology
Reference: McKenry, L., & Salerno, E. (2003). *Mosby's pharmacology in nursing* (21st ed., p. 757). St. Louis: Mosby.

16. **1**
Rationale: Aluminum hydroxide tablets should be chewed thoroughly before swallowing. This prevents them from entering the small intestine undissolved. They should not be swallowed whole. Antacids should be taken at least 1 hour apart from other medications to prevent interactive effects. Constipation is a side effect of the use of aluminum products, but it is not correct for the client to take a laxative with each dose. This promotes laxative abuse; the client first should try other means to prevent constipation.
Test-Taking Strategy: Use the process of elimination. Eliminate option 4 first because this action does not promote healthy bowel function. Next eliminate option 3, using general knowledge of antacid interactive effects. From the remaining options, use principles of digestion and medication use to direct you to option 1. Review this medication if you had difficulty with this question.
Level of Cognitive Ability: Application
Client Needs: Physiological Integrity
Integrated Process: Teaching/Learning
Content Area: Pharmacology
References: Hodgson, B., & Kizior, R. (2004). *Saunders nursing drug handbook 2004* (, p. 35). Philadelphia: W. B. Saunders. Kee, J., & Hayes, E. (2003). *Pharmacology: A nursing process approach* (4th ed., p. 670). Philadelphia: W. B. Saunders.

17. **2**
Rationale: Calcium carbonate can be used as an antacid for the relief of heartburn and indigestion. Calcium carbonate also can be used as a calcium supplement (option 3) or to bind phosphorus in the gastrointestinal tract with renal failure (option 4). Option 1 is incorrect, although adequate calcium levels are needed for proper neurological function.

Test-Taking Strategy: Note the key word "optimal". Focusing on the client's diagnosis will direct you to option 2. Review this medication if you had difficulty with this question.
Level of Cognitive Ability: Analysis
Client Needs: Physiological Integrity
Integrated Process: Nursing Process—evaluation
Content Area: Pharmacology
Reference: Kee, J., & Hayes, E. (2003). *Pharmacology: A nursing process approach* (4th ed., p. 672). Philadelphia: W. B. Saunders.

18. **3**
Rationale: Sodium bicarbonate is an electrolyte modifier and antacid, and it would aggravate metabolic alkalosis, which is a difficult acid-base imbalance to correct. The other options are incorrect.
Test-Taking Strategy: Use the process of elimination. Focusing on the name of the medication "sodium bicarbonate" will direct you to option 3 "metabolic alkalosis." Review the contraindications associated with the use of sodium bicarbonate if you had difficulty with this question.
Level of Cognitive Ability: Analysis
Client Needs: Physiological Integrity
Integrated Process: Nursing Process—analysis
Content Area: Pharmacology
Reference: Hodgson, B., & Kizior, R. (2004). *Saunders nursing drug handbook 2004* (p. 921). Philadelphia: W. B. Saunders.

19. **4**
Rationale: Simethicone is an antiflatulent used to relieve pain caused by excessive gas in the gastrointestinal tract. Magnesium hydroxide is an antacid and laxative. Droperidol is used to treat postoperative nausea and vomiting. Acetaminophen is a nonnarcotic analgesic.
Test-Taking Strategy: Use the process of elimination and focus on the key words "gas pains." Recalling the classifications of the medications in each of the options will direct you to option 4. Review the actions of simethicone if you had difficulty with this question.
Level of Cognitive Ability: Application
Client Needs: Physiological Integrity
Integrated Process: Nursing Process—implementation
Content Area: Pharmacology
References: Hodgson, B., & Kizior, R. (2004). *Saunders nursing drug handbook 2004* (, p. 916). Philadelphia: W. B. Saunders. Kee, J., & Hayes, E. (2003). *Pharmacology: A nursing process approach* (4th ed., p. 979). Philadelphia: W. B. Saunders.

20. **1**
Rationale: Older clients are especially susceptible to central nervous system side effects of cimetidine. The most frequent of these is confusion. Less common central nervous system side effects include headache, dizziness, drowsiness, and hallucinations.
Test-Taking Strategy: Use the process of elimination and note the key words "most frequent." Use knowledge of the older client and medication effects to direct you to option 1. Review the side effects of cimetidine if you had difficulty with this question.
Level of Cognitive Ability: Application
Client Needs: Physiological Integrity

Integrated Process: Nursing Process—assessment
Content Area: Pharmacology
Reference: Hodgson, B., & Kizior, R. (2004). *Saunders nursing drug handbook 2004* (p. 213). Philadelphia: W. B. Saunders.

21. 2
Rationale: The medication should be scheduled for administration 1 hour before meals and at bedtime. The medication is timed to allow it to form a protective coating over the ulcer before food intake stimulates gastric acid production and mechanical irritation. The other options are incorrect.
Test-Taking Strategy: Use the process of elimination. Focus on the diagnosis of the client to assist in directing you to option 2. Review the administration of this medication if you had difficulty with this question.
Level of Cognitive Ability: Application
Client Needs: Physiological Integrity
Integrated Process: Nursing Process—implementation
Content Area: Pharmacology
Reference: Hodgson, B., & Kizior, R. (2004). *Saunders nursing drug handbook 2004* (p. 940). Philadelphia: W. B. Saunders.

22. 3
Rationale: The client who chronically uses nonsteroidal antiinflammatory drugs (NSAIDs) is prone to gastric mucosal injury. Misoprostol is given specifically to prevent this occurrence. Diarrhea can be a side effect of the medication but is not an intended effect. Options 1 and 2 are incorrect.
Test-Taking Strategy: The key words in this question are "intended therapeutic effect" and "did not experience." This tells you that the medication is being given to prevent the occurrence of specific symptoms. Recalling that NSAIDs can cause gastric mucosal injury will direct you to option 3. Review this medication and the side effects of NSAIDs if you had difficulty with this question.
Level of Cognitive Ability: Analysis
Client Needs: Physiological Integrity
Integrated Process: Nursing Process—evaluation
Content Area: Pharmacology
Reference: Hodgson, B., & Kizior, R. (2004). *Saunders nursing drug handbook 2004* (p. 680). Philadelphia: W. B. Saunders.

23. 4
Rationale: A single daily dose of ranitidine is scheduled to be given at bedtime. This allows for a prolonged effect, and the greatest protection of the gastric mucosa. The other options are incorrect.
Test-Taking Strategy: Use the process of elimination. Recalling the action of the medication and focusing on the key words "once daily" will direct you to option 4. Review this medication if you had difficulty with this question.
Level of Cognitive Ability: Application
Client Needs: Physiological Integrity
Integrated Process: Nursing Process—planning
Content Area: Pharmacology
References: Hodgson, B., & Kizior, R. (2004). *Saunders nursing drug handbook 2004* (p. 874). Philadelphia: W. B. Saunders.

Kee, J., & Hayes, E. (2003). *Pharmacology: A nursing process approach* (4th ed., p. 674). Philadelphia: W. B. Saunders.

24. 1
Rationale: The client with peptic ulcer disease should avoid taking medications that are irritating to the stomach lining. Irritants would include aspirin and nonsteroidal antiinflammatory drugs (NSAIDs). The client should be advised to take acetaminophen for a headache.
Test-Taking Strategy: Use the process of elimination. Remember that options that are similar are not likely to be correct. With this in mind, eliminate options 2 and 3 first because both medications are NSAIDs. Choose acetaminophen over aspirin because is least irritating to the stomach. Review this condition and this medication if you had difficulty with this question.
Level of Cognitive Ability: Application
Client Needs: Physiological Integrity
Integrated Process: Teaching/Learning
Content Area: Pharmacology
Reference: Ignatavicius, D., & Workman, M. (2002). *Medical-surgical nursing: Critical thinking for collaborative care* (4th ed., p. 1234). Philadelphia: W. B. Saunders.

25. 2
Rationale: Omeprazole is a gastric pump inhibitor and is classified as an antiulcer agent. The intended effect of the medication is relief of pain from gastric irritation, often referred to as heartburn by clients. Omeprazole is not used to treat the conditions identified in options 1, 3, and 4.
Test-Taking Strategy: Use the process of elimination. Recalling the classification of this medication will direct you to option 2. Review the action of this medication if you had difficulty with this question.
Level of Cognitive Ability: Analysis
Client Needs: Physiological Integrity
Integrated Process: Nursing Process—evaluation
Content Area: Pharmacology
Reference: Hodgson, B., & Kizior, R. (2004). *Saunders nursing drug handbook 2004* (p. 754). Philadelphia: W. B. Saunders.

CRITICAL THINKING: FILL-IN-THE BLANK

Answer: 30 minutes before meals and at bedtime
Rationale: The client should be taught to take this medication 30 minutes before meals and at bedtime. This allows the medication time to begin working before the client takes in food, which requires digestion and movement.
Test-Taking Strategy: Focusing on the client's diagnosis will assist in answering this question. Review administration of this medication if you had difficulty with this question.
Level of Cognitive Ability: Application
Client Needs: Physiological Integrity
Integrated Process: Teaching/Learning
Content Area: Pharmacology
Reference: Hodgson, B., & Kizior, R. (2004). *Saunders nursing drug handbook 2004* (p. 660). Philadelphia: W. B. Saunders.

REFERENCES

Hodgson, B., & Kizior, R. (2004). *Saunders nursing drug handbook 2004*. Philadelphia: W. B. Saunders.

Kee, J., & Hayes, E. (2003). *Pharmacology: A nursing process approach* (4th ed.). Philadelphia: W. B. Saunders.

Ignatavicius, D., & Workman, M. (2002). *Medical-surgical nursing: Critical thinking for collaborative care* (4th ed.). Philadelphia: W. B. Saunders.

McKenry, L., & Salerno, E. (2003). *Mosby's pharmacology in nursing* (21st ed.). St. Louis: Mosby.

The Adult Client with a Respiratory Disorder

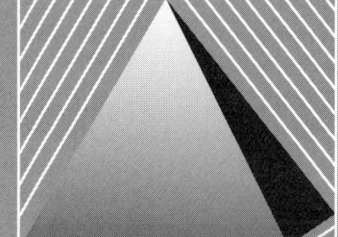

PYRAMID TERMS

bacille Calmette-Guérin vaccine   A vaccine containing attenuated tubercle bacilli that may be given to persons in foreign countries or to those traveling to foreign countries to produce increased resistance to tuberculosis.

chronic airflow limitation, chronic obstructive lung disease, chronic obstructive pulmonary disease   A group of diseases that includes emphysema, asthma, bronchiectasis, and bronchitis and characterized by progressive airflow limitations into and out of the lungs, elevated airway resistance, irreversible lung distention, and arterial blood gas imbalance. These diseases can lead to pulmonary insufficiency, pulmonary hypertension, and cor pulmonale. In emphysema, the stimulus to breathe is a low P_{O_2} instead of an increased P_{CO_2}.

emphysema   A chronic pulmonary disease marked by a narrowing of the small airways and the trapping of air, with destructive changes in their walls. Also known as chronic obstructive pulmonary disease.

Mantoux test   The most reliable determinant of infection with tuberculosis. A small amount (0.1 mL) of intermediate-strength purified protein derivative containing 5 tuberculin units is given intradermally in the forearm. An area of induration measuring 10 mm or more in diameter, 48 to 72 hours after injection, indicates that the individual has been exposed to tuberculosis.

mechanical ventilation   The use of a ventilator if a client is unable to ventilate enough on his or her own to maintain proper levels of oxygen and carbon dioxide in the blood. Types of ventilators include negative-pressure and positive-pressure ventilators. Various ventilator modes are adjusted to the client's individual needs.

multidrug-resistant strain   A multidrug-resistant strain of tuberculosis (MDR-TB) can occur as a result of improper or noncompliant use of treatment programs and the development of mutations in the tubercle bacilli.

Mycobacterium tuberculosis   The causative organism (bacillus) of tuberculosis; an aerobic bacterium that is a nonmotile, nonsporulating, acid-fast rod that secrets niacin.

pneumothorax   The accumulation of atmospheric air in the pleural space, which results in a rise in intrathoracic pressure and reduced vital capacity. The loss of negative intrapleural pressure results in collapse of the lung. Diagnosis of pneumothorax is made by chest radiography.

suctioning   A sterile procedure that involves the removal of respiratory secretions that accumulate in the tracheobronchial airway when the client is unable to expectorate secretions; performed to maintain a patent airway.

tuberculosis   A highly communicable disease caused by Mycobacterium tuberculosis. Tuberculosis is transmitted by the airborne route via droplet infection.

PYRAMID TO SUCCESS

The Pyramid to Success focuses on respiratory acid-base imbalances and reading arterial blood gas results; infectious diseases, particularly tuberculosis; and respiratory care in relation to oxygen delivery systems and mechanical ventilation. Pyramid Points focus on the client with pneumonia, respiratory failure, chronic obstructive pulmonary disease, and pneumothorax. The Pyramid to Success includes the care of the client with tuberculosis, especially regarding the importance of the medication regimen, providing adequate nutrition and adequate rest to promote the healing process, and the prevention of the progression of the disease. Focus on assisting the client to cope with the social isolation issues that exist during the period of illness and on teaching the client and family the critical measures of screening and of preventing respiratory disease and the transmission of disease. The Integrated Processes addressed in this unit include Nursing Process, Caring, Communication and Documentation, and Teaching/Learning.

CLIENT NEEDS
Safe, Effective Care Environment

Asepsis when caring for wounds or tracheostomy sites and during mechanical ventilation or suctioning
Client rights
Confidentiality related to the respiratory disorder
Consultations and referrals related to the respiratory disorder
Establishing priorities
Handling of infectious materials such as sputum or body fluids
Informed consent related to diagnostic and surgical procedures
Respiratory precautions
Standard precautions

Health Promotion and Maintenance

Education related to adequate fluid and nutritional intake
Education related to breathing exercises and respiratory therapy and care
Education related to medication administration
Education related to the need for follow-up care
Education related to the prevention of transmission of infection
Health promotion programs

Health screening related to risks for respiratory disorders
Prevention of respiratory disorders and infectious diseases
Respiratory assessment techniques

Psychosocial Integrity

Body image changes related to tracheostomy if performed
Coping mechanisms
Community resources
End-of-life issues
Grief and loss
Religious, cultural, and spiritual influences
Situational role changes
Support systems

Physiological Integrity

Acid-base imbalances
Alterations in body systems
Comfort interventions
Infectious diseases
Mechanical ventilation
Medical emergencies
Nutrition and oral hygiene
Oxygen delivery systems
Personal hygiene and rest and sleep
Pharmacological therapy
Reading arterial blood gas results
Respiratory care

REFERENCES

Chernecky, C., & Berger, B. (2004). *Laboratory tests & diagnostic procedures* (4th ed.). Philadelphia, W. B. Saunders.

Harkreader, H., & Hogan, M. A. (2004). *Fundamentals of nursing: Caring and clinical judgment* (2nd ed.). Philadelphia, W. B. Saunders.

Ignatavicius, D., & Workman, M. (2002). *Medical-surgical nursing: Critical thinking for collaborative care* (4th ed.). Philadelphia: W. B. Saunders.

Lewis, S., Heitkemper, M., & Dirksen, S. (2004). *Medical-surgical nursing: Assessment and management of clinical problems* (6th ed.). St. Louis: Mosby.

National Council of State Boards of Nursing (Eds.). (2003). *Test Plan for the National Council Licensure Examination for Registered Nurses* (effective date: April 2004). Chicago: Author.

Perry, A., & Potter, P. (2002). *Clinical nursing skills and techniques* (5th ed.). St. Louis: Mosby.

Phipps, W., Monahan, F., Sands, J., Marek, J., & Neighbors, M. (2003). *Medical-surgical nursing: Health and illness perspectives* (7th ed.). St. Louis: Mosby.

Potter, P., & Perry, A. (2001). *Fundamentals of nursing* (5th ed.). St. Louis: Mosby.

Varcarolis, E. M. (2002). *Foundations of psychiatric mental health nursing* (4th ed.). Philadelphia: W. B. Saunders.

Respiratory System

I. ANATOMY AND PHYSIOLOGY

A. Primary functions
   1. The respiratory system provides oxygen for metabolism in the tissues.
   2. The respiratory system removes carbon dioxide, the waste product of metabolism.

B. Secondary functions
   1. The respiratory system facilitates sense of smell.
   2. The respiratory system produces speech.
   3. The respiratory system maintains acid-base balance.
   4. The respiratory system maintains body water levels.
   5. The respiratory system maintains heat balance.

C. Upper respiratory tract
   1. Nose: The nose humidifies, warms, and filters inspired air.
   2. Sinuses
      a. Sinuses are air-filled cavities within the hollow bones that surround the nasal passages.
      b. Sinuses provide resonance during speech.
   3. Pharynx
      a. The pharynx is located behind the oral and nasal cavities.
      b. The pharynx is divided into the nasopharynx, oropharynx, and laryngopharynx.
      c. The pharynx is a passageway for the respiratory and digestive tracts.
   4. Larynx
      a. The larynx is located above the trachea and just below the pharynx at the root of the tongue.
      b. The larynx commonly is called the voice box.
      c. The larynx contains two pairs of vocal cords, the false and true cords.
      d. The opening between the true vocal cords is the glottis.

   e. The glottis plays an important role in coughing, which is the most fundamental defense mechanism of the lungs.
   5. Epiglottis
      a. The epiglottis is a leaf-shaped elastic structure that is attached along one end to the top of the larynx.
      b. The epiglottis prevents food from entering the tracheobronchial tree by closing over the glottis during swallowing.

D. Lower respiratory tract
   1. Trachea
      a. The trachea is located in front of the esophagus.
      b. The trachea branches into the right and left mainstem bronchi at the carina.
   2. Mainstem bronchi
      a. Mainstem bronchi begin at the carina.
      b. The right bronchus is slightly wider, shorter, and more vertical than the left bronchus.
      c. The mainstem bronchi divide into five secondary or lobar bronchi that enter each of the five lobes of the lung.
      d. The bronchi are lined with cilia, which propel mucus up and away from the lower airway to the trachea, where it can be expectorated or swallowed.
   3. Bronchioles
      a. Bronchioles branch from the secondary bronchi and subdivide into the small terminal and respiratory bronchioles.
      b. The bronchioles contain no cartilage and depend on the elastic recoil of the lung for patency.
      c. The terminal bronchioles contain no cilia and do not participate in gas exchange.
   4. Alveolar ducts and alveoli
      a. *Acinus* (plural *acini*) is a term used to indicate all structures distal to the terminal bronchiole.

b. Alveolar ducts branch from the respiratory bronchioles.

c. Alveolar sacs, which arise from the ducts, contain clusters of alveoli, which are the basic units of gas exchange.

d. Cells in the walls of the alveoli secrete surfactant, a phospholipid protein that reduces the surface tension in the alveoli; without surfactant, the alveoli would collapse.

5. Lungs

a. The lungs are located in the pleural cavity in the thorax.

b. The lungs extend from just above the clavicles to the diaphragm, the major muscle of inspiration.

c. The right lung, which is larger than the left, is divided into three lobes, the upper, middle, and lower lobes.

d. The left lung, which is narrower than the right lung to accommodate the heart, is divided into two lobes.

e. Innervation of the respiratory structures is accomplished by the phrenic nerve, the vagus nerve, and the thoracic nerves.

f. The parietal pleura lines the inside of the thoracic cavity, including the upper surface of the diaphragm.

g. The visceral pleura covers the pulmonary surfaces.

h. A thin fluid layer, which is produced by the cells lining the pleura, lubricates the visceral pleura and the parietal pleura, allowing them to glide smoothly and painlessly during respiration.

i. Blood flow through the lungs occurs via the pulmonary system and the bronchial system.

6. Accessory muscles of respiration include the scalene muscles, which elevate the first two ribs; the sternocleidomastoid muscles, which raise the sternum; and the trapezius and pectoralis muscles, which fix the shoulders.

7. The respiratory process

a. The diaphragm descends into the abdominal cavity during inspiration, causing negative pressure in the lungs.

b. The negative pressure draws air from the area of greater pressure, the atmosphere, into the area of lesser pressure, the lungs.

c. In the lungs, air passes through the terminal bronchioles into the alveoli to oxygenate the body tissues.

d. At the end of inspiration, the diaphragm and intercostal muscles relax and the lungs recoil.

e. As the lungs recoil, pressure within the lungs becomes greater than atmospheric pressure, causing the air, which now contains the cellular waste products of carbon dioxide and water, to move from the alveoli in the lungs to the atmosphere.

f. Expiration is a passive process.

II. DIAGNOSTIC TESTS

A. Risk factors for respiratory disorders (Box 57-1)

B. Chest x-ray film (radiograph)

1. Description: provides information regarding the anatomical location and appearance of the lungs

2. Preprocedure

a. Remove all jewelry and other metal objects from the chest area.

b. Assess the client's ability to inhale and hold breath.

c. Question females regarding pregnancy or the possibility of pregnancy.

3. Postprocedure: Assist the client to dress.

C. Sputum specimen

1. Description: a specimen obtained by expectoration or tracheal **suctioning** to assist in the identification of organisms or abnormal cells (Box 57-2)

2. Preprocedure

a. Determine specific purpose of collection and check with institutional policy for appropriate collection of specimen.

b. Obtain an early morning sterile specimen from **suctioning** or expectoration after a respiratory treatment, if a treatment is prescribed.

c. Obtain 15 mL of sputum.

d. Instruct the client to rinse the mouth with water before collection.

BOX 57-1

Risk Factors for Respiratory Disorders

Allergies
Chest injury
Crowded living conditions
Exposure to chemicals and environmental pollutants
Family history of infectious disease
Frequent respiratory illnesses
Geographic residence and travel to foreign countries
Smoking
Surgery
Use of chewing tobacco

BOX 57-2

Suctioning Procedure

Use aseptic technique.
Hyperoxygenate the client by a resuscitation bag, increasing the oxygen flow rate, or by asking the client to take deep breaths.
Lubricate the catheter with sterile water.
Tracheal suctioning: Insert catheter 4 inches.
Nasotracheal suctioning: Insert catheter to induce cough reflex.
Do not apply suction while inserting the catheter.
Apply suction intermittently for 10 seconds; rotate the catheter and withdraw.
Hyperoxygenate the client and encourage deep breaths.

e. Instruct the client to take several deep breaths and then cough deeply to obtain sputum.

f. Always collect the specimen before client begins antibiotic therapy.

3. Postprocedure

a. If a culture of sputum is prescribed, transport specimen to laboratory immediately.

b. Assist the client with mouth care.

D. Bronchoscopy

1. Description: direct visual examination of the larynx, trachea, and bronchi with a fiberoptic bronchoscope

2. Preprocedure

a. Obtain informed consent.

b. Maintain NPO status for client from midnight before the procedure.

c. Obtain vital signs.

d. Assess the results of coagulation studies.

e. Remove dentures or eyeglasses.

f. Prepare suction equipment.

g. Administer medication for sedation as prescribed.

h. Have emergency resuscitation equipment readily available.

3. Postprocedure

a. Monitor vital signs.

b. Maintain client in semi-Fowler position.

c. Assess for the return of the gag reflex.

d. Maintain NPO status until gag reflex returns.

e. Have an emesis basin readily available for client to expectorate sputum.

f. Monitor for bloody sputum.

g. Monitor respiratory status, particularly if sedation was administered.

h. Monitor for complications, such as bronchospasm, bronchial perforation indicated by facial or neck crepitus, dysrhythmias, fever, bacteremia, hemorrhage, hypoxemia, and **pneumothorax.**

i. Notify the physician if fever, difficulty in breathing, or other signs of complications occur following the procedure.

E. Pulmonary angiography

1. Description

a. Pulmonary angiography is an invasive fluoroscopic procedure in which a catheter is inserted through the antecubital or femoral vein into the pulmonary artery or one of its branches.

b. Pulmonary angiography involves an injection of iodine or radiopaque or contrast material.

2. Preprocedure

a. Obtain informed consent.

b. Assess for allergies to iodine, seafood, or other radiopaque dyes.

c. Maintain NPO status of client for 8 hours before the procedure.

d. Monitor vital signs.

e. Assess results of coagulation studies.

f. Establish an intravenous access.

g. Administer sedation as prescribed.

h. Instruct the client to lie still during the procedure.

i. Instruct the client that he or she may feel an urge to cough, flushing, nausea, or a salty taste following injection of the dye.

j. Have emergency resuscitation equipment available.

3. Postprocedure

a. Monitor vital signs.

b. Avoid taking blood pressures for 24 hours in the extremity used for the injection.

c. Monitor peripheral neurovascular status of the affected extremity.

d. Assess insertion site for bleeding.

e. Monitor for delayed reaction to the dye.

F. Thoracentesis

1. Description: removal of fluid or air from the pleural space via a transthoracic aspiration

2. Preprocedure

a. Obtain informed consent.

b. Obtain vital signs.

c. Prepare the client for ultrasound or chest radiograph, if prescribed, before procedure.

d. Assess results of coagulation studies.

e. Note that the client is positioned sitting upright, with the arms and head supported by a table at the bedside during the procedure.

f. If the client cannot sit up, the client is placed lying in bed on the unaffected side with the head of the bed elevated 45 degrees.

g. Instruct the client not to cough, breath deeply, or move during the procedure.

3. Postprocedure

a. Monitor vital signs.

b. Monitor respiratory status.

c. Apply a pressure dressing, and assess the puncture site for bleeding and crepitus.

d. Monitor for signs of **pneumothorax,** air embolism, and pulmonary edema.

G. Pulmonary function test

1. Description: a number of different tests used to evaluate lung mechanics, gas exchange, and acid-base disturbance through spirometric measurements, lung volumes, and arterial blood gases

2. Preprocedure

a. Determine whether an analgesic that may depress the respiratory function is being administered.

b. Consult with the physician regarding holding bronchodilators before testing.

c. Instruct the client to void before the procedure and to wear loose clothing.

d. Remove dentures.

e. Instruct the client to refrain from smoking or eating a heavy meal for 4 to 6 hours before the test.
   3. Postprocedure: Client may resume normal diet and any bronchodilators and respiratory treatments that were held before the procedure.
H. Lung biopsy
   1. Description
      a. A percutaneous lung biopsy is performed to obtain tissue for analysis by culture or cytological examination.
      b. A needle biopsy is done to identify pulmonary lesions, changes in lung tissue, and the cause of pleural effusion.
   2. Preprocedure
      a. Obtain informed consent.
      b. Maintain NPO status of client before the procedure.
      c. Inform the client that a local anesthetic will be used but that a sensation of pressure during needle insertion and aspiration may be felt.
      d. Administer analgesics and sedatives as prescribed.
   3. Postprocedure
      a. Monitor vital signs.
      b. Apply a dressing to the biopsy site and monitor for drainage or bleeding.
      c. Monitor for signs of respiratory distress, and notify the physician if they occur.
      d. Monitor for signs of **pneumothorax** and air emboli, and notify the physician if they occur.
      e. Prepare the client for chest radiography if prescribed.
I. Ventilation perfusion lung scan
   1. Description
      a. The perfusion scan evaluates blood flow to the lungs.
      b. The ventilation scan determines the patency of the pulmonary airways and detects abnormalities in ventilation.
      c. A radionuclide may be injected for the procedure.
   2. Preprocedure
      a. Obtain informed consent.
      b. Assess client for allergies to dye, iodine, or seafood.
      c. Remove jewelry around the chest area.
      d. Review breathing methods that may be required during testing.
      e. Establish an intravenous access.
      f. Administer sedation if prescribed.
      g. Have emergency resuscitation equipment available.
   3. Postprocedure
      a. Monitor client for reaction to the radionuclide.
      b. Instruct client to wash hands carefully with soap and water for 24 hours following the procedure.

J. Skin tests
   1. Description: A skin test is an intradermal injection used to assist in diagnosing various infectious diseases.
   2. Preprocedure: Determine hypersensitivity or previous reactions to skin tests.
   3. Procedure
      a. Use a test site that is free of excessive body hair, dermatitis, and blemishes.
      b. Apply the injection at the upper one third of inner surface of left arm.
      c. Circle and mark the injection test site.
      d. Document the date, time, and test site.
   4. Postprocedure
      a. Advise the client not to scratch the test site so as to prevent infection and abscess formation.
      b. Instruct the client to avoid washing the test site.
      c. Interpret the reaction at the injection site 24 to 72 hours after administration of the test antigen.
      d. Assess the test site for the amount of induration (hard swelling) in millimeters and for the presence of erythema and vesiculation (small blisterlike elevations).
K. Arterial blood gases (ABGs)
   1. Description: measurement of the dissolved oxygen and carbon dioxide in the arterial blood to reveal the acid-base state and how well the oxygen is being carried to the body (Box 57-3)
   2. Preprocedure
      a. Perform Allen's test before drawing radial artery specimens.
      b. Have the client rest for 30 minutes before specimen collection.
      c. Avoid **suctioning** before drawing ABG sample.
      d. Do not turn off oxygen unless the ABG sample is ordered to be drawn with client breathing room air.
   3. Postprocedure
      a. Place the specimen on ice.
      b. Note the client's temperature on laboratory form.
      c. Note the oxygen and type of ventilation that the client is receiving on the laboratory form.
      d. Apply pressure to the puncture site for 5 to 10 minutes and longer if the client is taking anticoagulant therapy or has a bleeding disorder.

BOX 57-3

Normal Arterial Blood Gas Values

pH: 7.35 to 7.45
P_{CO_2}: 35 to 45 mm Hg
HCO_3: 22 to 27 mEq/L
P_{O_2}: 80 to 100 mm Hg
O_2 saturation: 96% to 100%
Oxyhemoglobin dissociation curve: no shift

e. Transport the specimen to the laboratory within 15 minutes.

f. Refer to Chapter 10 for discussion of the analysis of ABG results.

L. Pulse oximetry

1. Description

a. Pulse oximetry is a noninvasive test that registers the oxygen saturation of the client's hemoglobin.

b. This arterial oxygen saturation (SaO_2) is recorded as a percentage.

c. The normal value is 96% to 100%.

d. After a hypoxic client uses up the readily available oxygen (measured as the arterial oxygen pressure, PaO_2, on ABG testing), the reserve oxygen, that oxygen attached to the hemoglobin (SaO_2), is drawn on to provide oxygen to the tissues.

e. A pulse oximeter reading can alert the nurse to hypoxemia before clinical signs occur.

2. Procedure

a. A sensor is placed on the client's finger, toe, nose, ear lobe, or forehead to measure oxygen saturation, which then is displayed on a monitor.

b. Maintain the transducer at heart level.

c. Do not select an extremity with an impediment to blood flow.

d. Results lower than 91% necessitate immediate treatment.

e. If the SaO_2 is less than 85%, the tissues of the body have a difficult time becoming oxygenated; an SaO_2 of less than 70% is life threatening.

III. RESPIRATORY TREATMENTS

A. Chest physiotherapy (CPT)

1. Description: percussion and vibration over the thorax to loosen secretions in the affected area of the lungs

2. Interventions

a. Place a layer of material (gown or pajamas) between the hands and the client's skin.

b. The best time to perform CPT is in the morning on rising, 1 hour before meals, or 2 to 3 hours after meals.

c. If client is receiving a tube feeding, stop the feeding and aspirate the residual before beginning CPT.

d. Stop CPT if pain occurs.

e. Dispose of sputum properly.

f. Provide mouth care after procedure.

3. Contraindications

a. Increase in bronchospasm from CPT

b. History of pathological fractures

c. Rib fractures

d. Chest incisions

B. Postural drainage

1. Description

a. Postural drainage uses gravity to drain secretions from segments of the lungs.

b. Postural drainage may be combined with CPT.

2. Interventions

a. Position the client properly (lung segment to be drained is uppermost).

b. The best time for the procedure is in the morning on arising, 1 hour before meals, or 2 to 3 hours after meals.

c. If client is receiving a tube feeding, stop the feeding and aspirate the residual before beginning postural drainage.

d. Stop postural drainage if cyanosis or exhaustion occurs.

e. Maintain position 5 to 20 minutes after procedure.

f. Dispose of sputum properly.

g. Provide mouth care after the procedure.

3. Contraindications

a. Unstable vital signs

b. Increased intracranial pressure

C. Incentive spirometry (Box 57-4)

IV. OXYGEN

A. Interventions

1. Assess color and vital signs before and during treatment.

2. Place an "OXYGEN IN USE" sign at the client's bedside.

3. Assess for the presence of chronic lung problems.

4. Humidify the oxygen.

B. Nasal cannula (nasal prongs) (Box 57-5)

1. Description

BOX 57-4

Client Instructions for Incentive Spirometry

Instruct the client to assume a sitting or upright position.
Instruct the client to place the mouth tightly around the mouthpiece.
Instruct the client to inhale slowly to raise and maintain the flow rate indicator between the 600 and 900 marks.
Instruct the client to hold the breath for 5 seconds and then to exhale through pursed lips.
Instruct the client to repeat this process 10 times every hour.

BOX 57-5

Fraction of Inspired Oxygen Delivered via Nasal Cannula

24% at 1 L/min
28% at 2 L/min
32% at 3 L/min
36% at 4 L/min
40% at 5 L/min
44% at 6 L/min

a. A nasal cannula is used at flow rates of 1 to 6 L/min, providing approximate oxygen concentrations of 24% (at 1 L/min) to 44% (at 6 L/min).

b. Flow rates higher than 6 L/min do not significantly increase oxygenation because the anatomical reserve or dead space (oral and nasal cavities) is full.

c. A nasal cannula is used for the client with **chronic airflow limitation** and for long-term oxygen use.

d. A client who is hypoxemic and also has chronic hypercarbia requires low levels of oxygen delivery at 1 to 2 L/min; a low arterial oxygen level is the client's primary drive for breathing.

e. Effective oxygen concentration can be delivered to nose breathers and mouth breathers with the use of a nasal cannula.

2. Interventions

a. Place the nasal prongs in the nostrils, with the openings facing the client.

b. Add humidification as prescribed when a flow rate higher than 2 L/min is prescribed.

c. Check the water level and change the humidifier as needed.

d. Assess the client for changes in respiratory rate or depth.

e. Assess the mucosa because high flow rates have a drying effect and increase mucosal irritation.

f. Assess skin integrity because the oxygen tubing can irritate the skin.

g. Provide water-soluble jelly to the nares as needed.

C. Simple face mask (Box 57-6)

1. Description

a. A face mask is used to deliver oxygen concentrations of 40% to 60% for short-term oxygen therapy or to deliver oxygen in an emergency.

b. A minimal flow rate of 5 L/min is needed to prevent the rebreathing of exhaled air.

2. Interventions

a. Be sure the mask fits securely over the nose and mouth because a poorly fitting mask reduces the fraction of inspired oxygen (FIO_2) delivered.

b. Assess skin and provide skin care to the area covered by the mask because pressure and moisture under the mask may cause skin breakdown.

c. Monitor the client closely for risk of aspiration because the mask limits the client's ability to clear the mouth, especially if vomiting occurs.

d. Provide emotional support to decrease anxiety in the client who feels claustrophobic.

e. Consult with the physician regarding switching the client from a mask to a nasal cannula during eating.

D. Partial rebreather mask (Box 57-7)

1. Description

a. A partial rebreather mask consists of a mask with a reservoir bag that provides an oxygen concentration of 70% to 90% with flow rates of 6 to 15 L/min.

b. The client rebreathes one third of the exhaled tidal volume, which is high in oxygen, thus providing a high FIO_2.

2. Interventions

a. Make sure that the reservoir does not twist or kink, which results in a deflated bag.

b. Adjust the flow rate to keep the reservoir bag inflated two-thirds full during inspiration because deflation results in decreased oxygen delivered and rebreathing of exhaled air.

E. Non-rebreather mask

1. Description

a. A non-rebreather mask provides the highest concentration of the low-flow systems and can deliver an FIO_2 greater than 90%, depending on the client's ventilatory pattern.

b. A non-rebreather mask most frequently is used in the client with deteriorating respiratory status who might require intubation.

c. The non-rebreather mask has a one-way valve between the mask and the reservoir and two flaps over the exhalation ports.

d. The valve allows the client to draw the entire quantity of oxygen from the reservoir bag.

e. The flaps prevent room air from entering through the exhalation ports.

f. During exhalation, air leaves through these exhalation ports while the one-way valve prevents exhaled air from reentering the reservoir bag.

2. FIO_2 delivered: 60% to 100% FIO_2 at a liter flow that maintains the bag two-thirds full

---

BOX 57-6

Fraction of Inspired Oxygen Delivered via Simple Face Mask

40% at 5 L/min
45% to 50% at 6 L/min
55% to 60% at 8 L/min
Pyramid Point: Flow rate must be set to at least 5 L/min to flush the mask of carbon dioxide.

BOX 57-7

Fraction of Inspired Oxygen Delivered via Partial Rebreather Mask

70% to 90% FIO_2 delivered at 6 to 15 L/min
Pyramid Point: A flow rate high enough to maintain the bag two-thirds full during inspiration is needed.

3. Interventions
   a. Remove mucus or saliva from the mask.
   b. Assess the client closely.
   c. Ensure that the valve and flaps are intact and functional during each breath.
   d. Valves should open during expiration and close during inhalation.
   e. Suffocation can occur if the reservoir bag kinks or if the oxygen source disconnects.

F. Face tent
   1. A face tent fits over the client's chin, with the top extending halfway across the face.
   2. The oxygen concentration varies, but the face tent is useful instead of a tight-fitting mask for the client who has facial trauma or burns.

G. Aerosol mask: used for the client who requires high humidity after extubation or upper airway surgery or for the client who has thick secretions.

H. Tracheostomy collar and T piece
   1. The tracheostomy collar can be used to deliver high humidity and the desired oxygen to the client with a tracheostomy.
   2. A special adapter, called the T piece, can be used to deliver any desired FIO_2 to the client with a tracheostomy, laryngectomy, or endotracheal tube.
   3. Refer to Chapter 21 for information on endotracheal and tracheostomy tubes.

I. Interventions for face tent, aerosol mask, tracheostomy collar, and T piece
   1. Change delivery system to a nasal cannula during mealtimes.
   2. Assess that the aerosol mist escapes from the vents of the delivery system during inspiration and expiration.
   3. Empty condensation from the tubing to prevent the client from being lavaged with water and to promote an adequate flow rate.
   4. Ensure that sufficient water is in the canister, and change the aerosol water container as needed.
   5. Keep the exhalation port on the T piece open and uncovered (if the port is occluded, the client can suffocate).
   6. Position the T piece so that it does not pull on the tracheostomy or endotracheal tube and cause erosion of skin at the tracheostomy insertion site.
   7. Make sure the humidifier creates enough mist; a mist should be seen during inspiration and expiration.

J. Venturi mask
   1. Description
      a. A Venturi mask provides a high-flow oxygen delivery system.
      b. Operation of the Venturi mask is based on a mechanism that pulls in a specific proportional amount of room air for each liter flow of oxygen.

      c. An adapter is located between the bottom of the mask and the oxygen source; the adapter contains holes of different sizes that allow only specific amounts of air to mix with the oxygen.
      d. The adapter allows selection of the amount of oxygen desired.
   2. FIO_2 delivered: 24% to 55% FIO_2 with flow rates of 4 to 10 L/min
   3. Interventions
      a. Monitor client closely to ensure an accurate flow rate for specific FIO_2.
      b. Keep the orifice for the Venturi adapter open and uncovered to ensure adequate oxygen delivery.
      c. Ensure that the mask fits snugly and that tubing is free of kinks because the FIO_2 is altered if kinking occurs or if the mask fits poorly.
      d. Assess the client for dry mucous membranes; humidity or aerosol can be added to the system.

V. MECHANICAL VENTILATION

A. Types
   1. Pressure-cycled ventilator
      a. The ventilator pushes air into the lungs until an airway pressure is reached.
      b. The ventilator is used for short periods, as in the postanesthesia care unit and for respiratory therapy.
   2. Time-cycled ventilator
      a. The ventilator pushes air into the lungs until a preset time has elapsed.
      b. The ventilator primarily is used in the pediatric or neonatal client.
   3. Volume-cycled ventilator
      a. The ventilator pushes air into the lungs until a preset volume is delivered.
      b. A constant tidal volume is delivered regardless of the changing compliance of the lungs and chest wall or the airway resistance in the client or ventilator.
   4. Microprocessor ventilator
      a. A computer or microprocessor is built into the ventilator to allow continuous monitoring of ventilatory functions, alarms, and client parameters.
      b. The ventilator is more responsive to clients who have severe lung disease or require prolonged weaning.

B. Modes of ventilation (Box 57-8)
   1. Controlled
      a. The client receives a set tidal volume at a set rate.

BOX 57-8

Modes of Ventilation

Controlled
Assist-control
Synchronized intermittent mandatory ventilation

b. Controlled ventilation is used for clients who cannot initiate respiratory effort.

c. Controlled ventilation is the least used mode; if the client attempts to initiate a breath, the ventilator blocks the effort.

2. Assist-control

a. Assist-control ventilation is the most commonly used mode.

b. Tidal volume and ventilatory rate are preset on the ventilator.

c. The ventilator takes over the work of breathing for the client.

d. The ventilator is programmed to respond to the client's inspiratory effort if the client does initiate a breath.

e. The ventilator delivers the preset tidal volume when the client initiates a breath, while allowing the client to control the rate of breathing.

f. If the client's spontaneous ventilatory rate increases, the ventilator continues to deliver a preset tidal volume with each breath, which may cause hyperventilation and respiratory alkalosis.

3. Synchronized intermittent mandatory ventilation (SIMV)

a. The SIMV is similar to assist-control ventilation in that the tidal volume and ventilatory rate are preset on the ventilator.

b. The SIMV allows clients to breath spontaneously at their own rate and tidal volume between the ventilator breaths.

c. The SIMV can be used as a primary ventilatory mode or as a weaning mode.

d. When SIMV is used as a weaning mode, the number of SIMV breaths is decreased gradually, and the client gradually resumes spontaneous breathing.

C. Ventilator controls and settings (Box 57-9)

1. Tidal volume: the volume of air that the client receives with each breath

2. Rate: number of ventilator breaths delivered per minute

3. Fraction of inspired oxygen (FIO_2): the oxygen concentration delivered to the client, which is determined by the client's condition and the ABGs

---

BOX 57-9

Ventilator Controls and Settings

Continuous positive airway pressure
Fraction of inspired oxygen
Peak airway inspiratory pressure
Positive end-expiratory pressure
Pressure support
Rate
Sighs
Tidal volume

---

4. Sighs

a. Sighs are volumes of air that are 1.5 to 2 times the set tidal volume, delivered 6 to 10 times per hour.

b. Sighs may be used to prevent atelectasis.

5. Peak airway inspiratory pressure

a. Peak airway inspiratory pressure is the pressure needed by the ventilator to deliver a set tidal volume at a given compliance.

b. Monitoring peak airway inspiratory pressure reflects changes in compliance of the lungs and resistance in the ventilator or client.

6. Continuous positive airway pressure

a. Continuous positive airway pressure is application of positive airway pressure throughout the entire respiratory cycle for spontaneously breathing clients.

b. Continuous positive airway pressure keeps the alveoli open during inspiration and prevents alveolar collapse.

c. Continuous positive airway pressure is used primarily as a weaning modality.

d. During continuous positive airway pressure, no ventilator breaths are delivered, but the ventilator delivers oxygen and provides monitoring and an alarm system.

e. The respiratory pattern is determined by the client's efforts.

7. Positive end-expiratory pressure (PEEP)

a. Positive pressure is exerted during the expiratory phase of ventilation.

b. Positive end-expiratory pressure improves oxygenation by enhancing gas exchange and preventing atelectasis.

c. The need for PEEP indicates a severe gas exchange disturbance.

d. Higher amounts of PEEP (more than 15) increase the chance of complications such as barotrauma tension pneumothorax.

8. Pressure support

a. Pressure support is application of positive pressure on inspiration.

b. Pressure support eases the workload of breathing.

c. Pressure support may be used in combination with PEEP as a weaning method.

d. As the warning process ensues, the amount of pressure applied to inspiration is gradually decreased.

9. Interventions

a. Assess the client first and the ventilator second.

b. Assess vital signs, lung sounds, respiratory status, and breathing patterns (the client will never breath at a rate less than the rate set on the ventilator).

c. Monitor skin color, particularly in the lips and nailbeds.

d. Monitor chest for bilateral expansion.

e. Obtain pulse oximetry readings.

f. Monitor ABG results.

g. Assess the need for **suctioning** and observe the type, color, and amount of secretions.

h. Assess ventilator settings.

i. Assess level of water in humidifier and temperature of the humidification system because extremes in temperature can cause damage to the mucosa in the airway.

j. Ensure that the alarms are set.

k. If a cause for an alarm cannot be determined, ventilate the client manually with a resuscitation bag until the problem is corrected.

l. Empty the ventilator tubing when moisture collects.

m. Turn the client at least every 2 hours or get the client out of bed, as prescribed, to prevent complications of immobility.

n. Have resuscitation equipment available at the bedside.

D. Causes of alarms (Box 57-10)

E. Complications

1. Hypotension caused by the application of positive pressure, which increases intrathoracic pressure and inhibits blood return to the heart

2. Respiratory complications such as **pneumothorax** or subcutaneous **emphysema** as a result of positive pressure

3. Gastrointestinal alterations such as stress ulcers

4. Malnutrition if nutrition is not maintained

5. Infections

6. Muscular deconditioning

7. Ventilator dependence or inability to wean

F. Weaning: the process of going from ventilator dependence to spontaneous breathing

1. SIMV

a. The client breathes between the preset breaths per minute rate of the ventilator.

BOX 57-10

Causes of Ventilator Alarms

HIGH-PRESSURE ALARM

Increased secretions are in the airway.

Wheezing or bronchospasm causes decreased airway size.

The endotracheal tube is displaced.

The endotracheal tube is obstructed as a result of water or a kink in the tubing.

Client coughs, gags, or bites on the oral endotracheal tube.

Client is anxious or fights the ventilator.

LOW-PRESSURE ALARM

Disconnection or leak in the ventilator or in the client's airway cuff occurs.

The client stops spontaneous breathing.

---

b. The SIMV rate is decreased gradually until the client is breathing on his or her own without the use of the ventilator.

2. T piece

a. The client is taken off the ventilator, and the ventilator is replaced with a T piece or continuous positive airway pressure, which delivers humidified oxygen.

b. The client is taken off the ventilator for short periods initially and allowed to breathe spontaneously.

c. Weaning progresses as the client is able to tolerate progressively longer periods off the ventilator.

3. Pressure support

a. Pressure support is a predetermined pressure on the ventilator to assist the client in respiratory effort.

b. As weaning continues, the amount of pressure is decreased gradually.

c. With pressure support, pressure may be maintained while the preset breaths per minute of the ventilator gradually are decreased.

VI. CHEST INJURIES

A. Rib fracture

1. Description

a. Rib fracture results from direct blunt chest trauma and causes a potential for intrathoracic injury, such as **pneumothorax** or pulmonary contusion.

b. Pain with movement and chest splinting result in impaired ventilation and inadequate clearance of secretions.

2. Assessment

a. Pain at injury site that increases with inspiration

b. Tenderness at site

c. Shallow respirations

d. Client splints chest

e. Fractures noted on chest x-ray film

3. Interventions

a. Note that ribs usually unite spontaneously.

b. Position the client in high Fowler's position.

c. Administer pain medication as prescribed to maintain adequate ventilatory status.

d. Monitor for increased respiratory distress.

e. Instruct the client to self-splint with hands and arms.

f. Prepare the client for an intercostal nerve block as prescribed if the pain is severe.

B. Flail chest

1. Description

a. Flail chest is blunt chest trauma associated with accidents, which may result in hemothorax and rib fractures.

b. The loose segment of the chest wall becomes paradoxical to the expansion and contraction of the rest of the chest wall.
2. Assessment
   a. Paradoxical respirations (inward movement of a segment of the thorax during inspiration with outward movement during expiration)
   b. Severe pain in chest
   c. Dyspnea
   d. Cyanosis
   e. Tachycardia
   f. Hypotension
   g. Tachypnea, shallow respirations
   h. Diminished breath sounds
3. Interventions
   a. Position the client in high Fowler's position.
   b. Administer humidified oxygen as prescribed.
   c. Monitor for increased respiratory distress.
   d. Encourage coughing and deep breathing.
   e. Administer pain medication as prescribed.
   f. Maintain bed rest and limit activity to reduce oxygen demands.
   g. Prepare for intubation with **mechanical ventilation**, with PEEP for severe flail chest associated with respiratory failure and shock.
C. Pulmonary contusion
1. Description
   a. Pulmonary contusion is characterized by interstitial hemorrhage associated with intraalveolar hemorrhage, resulting in decreased pulmonary compliance.
   b. The major complication is acute respiratory distress syndrome.
2. Assessment
   a. Dyspnea
   b. Hypoxemia
   c. Increased bronchial secretions
   d. Hemoptysis
   e. Restlessness
   f. Decreased breath sounds
   g. Crackles and wheezes
3. Interventions
   a. Maintain a patent airway and adequate ventilation.
   b. Position the client in high Fowler's position.
   c. Administer oxygen as prescribed.
   d. Monitor for increased respiratory distress.
   e. Maintain bed rest and limit activity to reduce oxygen demands.
   f. Prepare for **mechanical ventilation** with PEEP if required.
D. **Pneumothorax**
1. Description
   a. **Pneumothorax** is the accumulation of atmospheric air in the pleural space, which results in a rise in intrathoracic pressure and reduced vital capacity.

b. The loss of negative intrapleural pressure results in collapse of the lung.
   c. A spontaneous **pneumothorax** occurs with the rupture of a bleb.
   d. An open **pneumothorax** occurs when an opening through the chest wall allows the entrance of positive atmospheric pressure into the pleural space.
   e. A tension **pneumothorax** occurs from a blunt chest injury or from **mechanical ventilation** with PEEP when a buildup of positive pressure occurs in the pleural space.
   f. Diagnosis of **pneumothorax** is made by chest x-ray film.
2. Assessment (Box 57-11)
3. Interventions
   a. Apply a dressing over an open chest wound.
   b. Administer oxygen as prescribed.
   c. Position the client in high Fowler's position.
   d. Prepare for chest tube placement until the lung has expanded fully.
   e. Monitor chest tube drainage system.
   f. Monitor for subcutaneous **emphysema**.
   g. Refer to Chapter 21 for information on chest tubes.

VII. RESPIRATORY FAILURE

A. Description
1. Respiratory failure occurs when the client cannot eliminate carbon dioxide from the alveoli.
2. The carbon dioxide retention results in hypoxemia.
3. Oxygen reaches the alveoli but cannot be absorbed or used properly.
4. The lungs can move air sufficiently but cannot oxygenate the pulmonary blood properly.
5. Respiratory failure occurs as a result of a mechanical abnormality of the lungs or chest wall, a defect in the respiratory control center in the brain, or an impairment in the function of the respiratory muscles.
6. The $Paco_2$ level is greater than 45 mm Hg.

BOX 57-11

Assessment Findings: Pneumothorax

Absent breath sounds on affected side
Cyanosis
Decreased chest expansion unilaterally
Dyspnea
Hypotension
Sharp chest pain
Subcutaneous emphysema as evidenced by crepitus on palpation
Sucking sound with open chest wound
Tachycardia
Tachypnea
Tracheal deviation to the unaffected side with tension pneumothorax

B. Assessment
1. Dyspnea
2. Headache
3. Restlessness
4. Confusion
5. Tachycardia
6. Cyanosis
7. Dysrhythmias
8. Decreased level of consciousness
9. Alterations in respirations and breath sounds

C. Interventions
1. Identify and treat the cause of respiratory failure
2. Administer oxygen to maintain the PaO_2 level greater than 60 to 70 mm Hg.
3. Position the client in high Fowler's position.
4. Encourage deep breathing.
5. Administer bronchodilators as prescribed.
6. Prepare the client for **mechanical ventilation** if supplemental oxygen cannot maintain acceptable PaO_2 levels.

VIII. ACUTE RESPIRATORY DISTRESS SYNDROME

A. Description
1. Acute respiratory distress syndrome is a form of acute respiratory failure that occurs as a complication of some other condition, is caused by a diffuse lung injury, and leads to extravascular lung fluid.
2. The major site of injury is the alveolar capillary membrane.
3. The interstitial edema causes compression and obliteration of the terminal airways and leads to reduced lung volume and compliance.
4. The ABGs identify respiratory acidosis and hypoxemia that does not respond to an increased percentage of oxygen.
5. The chest x-ray film shows interstitial edema.
6. Some of the causes include sepsis, fluid overload, shock, trauma, neurological injuries, burns, disseminated intravascular coagulation, drug ingestion, and the inhalation of toxic substances.

B. Assessment
1. Tachypnea
2. Dyspnea
3. Decreased breath sounds
4. Deteriorating blood gas levels
5. Hypoxemia despite high concentrations of delivered oxygen
6. Decreased pulmonary compliance
7. Pulmonary infiltrates

C. Interventions
1. Identify and treat cause of the acute respiratory distress syndrome.
2. Administer oxygen as prescribed.
3. Position client in high Fowler's position.
4. Restrict fluid intake as prescribed.
5. Provide respiratory treatments as prescribed.

6. Administer diuretics, anticoagulants, or corticosteroids as prescribed.
7. Prepare the client for intubation and **mechanical ventilation** using PEEP.

IX. CHRONIC OBSTRUCTIVE PULMONARY DISEASE

A. Description
1. **Chronic obstructive pulmonary disease** also is known as **chronic obstructive lung disease** and chronic airflow limitation.
2. **Chronic obstructive pulmonary disease** is a group of diseases that includes **emphysema**, asthma, bronchiectasis, and bronchitis.
3. **Chronic obstructive pulmonary disease** is characterized by progressive airflow limitations into and out of the lungs, elevated airway resistance, irreversible lung distention, and ABG imbalance.
4. **Chronic obstructive pulmonary disease** leads to pulmonary insufficiency, pulmonary hypertension, and cor pulmonale.
5. In **emphysema**, the stimulus to breathe is a low PO_2 instead of an increased PCO_2.

B. Assessment
1. Cough
2. Exertional dyspnea
3. Wheezing and crackles
4. Sputum production
5. Weight loss
6. Barrel chest (**emphysema**)
7. Use of accessory muscles for breathing
8. Cyanosis
9. Clubbing of fingers
10. Orthopnea
11. Cardiac dysrhythmias
12. Congestion and hyperinflation on chest x-ray film
13. ABGs that indicate respiratory acidosis and hypoxemia
14. Pulmonary function tests that demonstrate decreased vital capacity

C. Interventions
1. Monitor vital signs.
2. Administer a low concentration of oxygen (1 to 2 L/min) as prescribed; the stimulus to breathe is a low arterial PO_2 instead of an increased PCO_2.
3. Monitor pulse oximetry.
4. Provide respiratory treatments and CPT.
5. Instruct the client in diaphragmatic or abdominal and pursed lip breathing techniques.
6. Record the color, amount, and consistency of sputum.
7. Suction fluids from the client's lungs, if necessary, to clear the airway and prevent infection.
8. Monitor weight.
9. Encourage small, frequent meals to prevent dyspnea.

10. Provide a high-calorie, high-protein diet with supplements.
11. Encourage fluid intake up to 3000 mL/day to keep secretions thin, unless contraindicated.
12. Position client in high Fowler's position and leaning forward to aid in breathing.
13. Allow activity as tolerated.
14. Administer bronchodilators as prescribed, and instruct the client in the use of oral and inhalant medications.
15. Administer corticosteroids as prescribed to reduce inflammation.
16. Administer mucolytics as prescribed to thin secretions.
17. Administer antibiotics for infection if prescribed.

D. Client education (Box 57-12)

X. SEVERE ACUTE RESPIRATORY SYNDROME (SARS)

A. Severe acute respiratory syndrome is a respiratory illness caused by the coronavirus, called SARS-associated coronavirus.
B. The syndrome begins with a fever, an overall feeling of discomfort, body aches, and mild respiratory symptoms.
C. After 2 to 7 days, the client may develop a dry cough and dyspnea.
D. Infection is spread by close person-to-person contact by direct contact with infectious material (respiratory secretions or by contact with persons or objects infected with infectious droplets)
E. Prevention includes avoiding contact with those suspected of having SARS, avoiding travel to countries where an outbreak of SARS exists, avoiding close contact with crowds in areas where SARS exists, and frequent hand washing if in an area where SARS exists.

XI. PNEUMONIA

A. Description
1. Pneumonia is an infection of the pulmonary tissue, including the interstitial spaces, the alveoli, and the bronchioles.
2. The edema associated with inflammation stiffens the lung, decreases lung compliance and vital capacity, and causes hypoxemia.
3. Pneumonia can be community acquired or hospital acquired.
4. The chest x-ray film shows diffuse patches throughout the lungs or consolidation in a lobe.
5. A sputum culture identifies the organism.
6. The white blood cells and the erythrocyte sedimentation rate are elevated.

B. Assessment
1. Chills
2. Elevated temperature
3. Pleuritic pain
4. Rhonchi and wheezes
5. Use of accessory muscles for breathing
6. Cyanosis
7. Mental status changes
8. Sputum production

C. Interventions
1. Administer oxygen as prescribed.
2. Monitor respiratory status.
3. Monitor for labored respirations, cyanosis, and cold and clammy skin.
4. Encourage coughing and deep breathing and use of incentive spirometer.
5. Position client in semi-Fowler position to facilitate breathing and lung expansion.
6. Change client's position frequently and ambulate as tolerated to mobilize secretions.
7. Provide CPT.
8. Perform nasotracheal **suctioning** if the client is unable to clear secretions.
9. Monitor pulse oximetry.
10. Monitor and record color, consistency, and amount of sputum.
11. Provide a high-calorie, high-protein diet with small frequent meals.
12. Encourage fluids up to 3 L a day to thin secretions unless contraindicated.
13. Provide a balance of rest and activity, increasing activity gradually.
14. Administer antibiotics as prescribed.
15. Administer antipyretics, bronchodilators, cough suppressants, mucolytic agents, and expectorants as prescribed.
16. Prevent the spread of infection by hand washing and the proper disposal of secretions.

BOX 57-12

Client Education: Chronic Obstructive Pulmonary Disease

Stop smoking.
Recognize the signs and symptoms of respiratory infection and hypoxia.
Adhere to activity limitations, alternating rest periods with activity.
Avoid exposure to individuals with infections and avoid crowds.
Use pursed lip and diaphragmatic or abdominal breathing.
Use medications and inhalers.
Use oxygen therapy.
Meet nutritional requirements.
Avoid eating gas-producing foods, spicy foods, and extremely hot or cold foods.
Receive immunizations as recommended.
When dusting, use a wet cloth.
Avoid powerful odors.
Avoid extremes in temperature.
Avoid fireplaces, pets, feather pillows, and other environmental allergens.

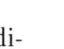

D. Client education
1. Instruct the client about the importance of rest, proper nutrition, and adequate fluid intake.
2. Avoid chilling and exposure to individuals with respiratory infections or viruses.
3. Instruct the client regarding medications and the use of inhalants as prescribed.
4. Instruct the client to notify physician if chills, fever, dyspnea, hemoptysis, or increased fatigue occurs.
5. Instruct the client in the importance of receiving immunizations as recommended.

XII. PLEURAL EFFUSION

A. Description
1. Pleural effusion is the collection of fluid in the pleural space.
2. Any condition that interferes with secretion or drainage of this fluid will lead to pleural effusion.
B. Assessment
1. Pleuritic pain that is sharp and increases with inspiration
2. Dyspnea on exertion
3. Dry, nonproductive cough caused by bronchial irritation or mediastinal shift
4. Tachycardia
5. Elevated temperature
6. Decreased breath sounds
7. Chest x-ray film that shows pleural effusion and a mediastinal shift away from the fluid
C. Interventions
1. Identify and treat underlying cause.
2. Monitor breath sounds.
3. Position the client in high Fowler's position.
4. Encourage coughing and deep breathing.
5. Prepare the client for thoracentesis.
6. If pleural effusion is recurrent, prepare the client for pleurectomy or pleurodesis as prescribed.
D. Pleurectomy
1. Pleurectomy consists of surgically stripping the parietal pleura away from the visceral pleura.
2. This produces an intense inflammatory reaction that promotes adhesion formation between the two layers during healing.
E. Pleurodesis
1. Pleurodesis involves the instillation of a sclerosing substance into the pleural space via a thoracotomy tube.
2. The substance creates an inflammatory response that scleroses tissues together.

XIII. EMPYEMA

A. Description
1. Empyema is the collection of pus within the pleural cavity.
2. The fluid is thick, opaque, and foul smelling.
3. The most common cause is pulmonary infection and lung abscess caused by thoracic surgery or chest trauma, in which bacteria are introduced directly into the pleural space.
4. Treatment focuses on emptying the empyema cavity, reexpanding the lung, and controlling the infection.
B. Assessment
1. Recent febrile illness or trauma
2. Chest pain
3. Cough
4. Dyspnea
5. Anorexia and weight loss
6. Malaise
7. Elevated temperature and chills
8. Night sweats
9. Diminished chest wall movement on the affected side
10. Pleural exudate on chest x-ray film
C. Interventions
1. Monitor breath sounds.
2. Position client in semi-Fowler or high Fowler's position.
3. Encourage coughing and deep breathing.
4. Administer antibiotics as prescribed.
5. Instruct the client to splint the chest as necessary.
6. Assist with chest tube insertion to promote drainage and lung expansion.
7. If marked pleural thickening occurs, prepare the client for decortication, if prescribed; this is a surgical procedure that involves removal of the restrictive mass of fibrin and inflammatory cells.

XIV. PLEURISY

A. Description
1. Pleurisy is inflammation of the visceral and parietal membranes.
2. These membranes rub together during respiration and cause pain.
3. Pleurisy may be caused by pulmonary infarction or pneumonia.
4. Pleurisy usually occurs on one side of the chest, usually in the lower lateral portions in the chest wall.
B. Assessment
1. Knifelike pain that is aggravated on deep breathing and coughing
2. Dyspnea
3. Pleural friction rub heard on auscultation
4. Apprehension
C. Interventions
1. Identify and treat cause.
2. Monitor lung sounds.
3. Administer analgesics as prescribed.
4. Apply hot or cold applications as prescribed.
5. Encourage coughing and deep breathing.
6. Instruct the client to lie on affected side to splint chest.

XV. PULMONARY EMBOLISM

A. Description
   1. Pulmonary embolism occurs when a thrombus that forms in a deep vein detaches and travels to the right side of the heart and then lodges in a branch of the pulmonary artery.
   2. Clients prone to pulmonary embolism are those at risk for deep vein thrombosis, including those with prolonged immobilization, surgery, obesity, pregnancy, congestive heart failure, advanced age, or history of thromboembolism.
   3. Fat emboli can occur as a complication following a fracture of a flat long bone.
   4. Treatment is aimed at preventing venous status and includes range of motion exercises and early ambulation following surgery, the use of antiembolism or pneumatic compression stockings, and preventing pressure under the popliteal space

B. Assessment (Box 57-13)

C. Interventions
   1. Administer oxygen as prescribed.
   2. Position client in high Fowler's position.
   3. Monitor lung sounds.
   4. Maintain bed rest and active and passive range of motion exercises as prescribed.
   5. Encourage use of incentive spirometry as prescribed.
   6. Monitor pulse oximetry.
   7. Prepare for intubation and **mechanical ventilation** for severe hypoxemia.
   8. Administer anticoagulation therapy intravenously with heparin sodium (bolus), followed by continuous infusion during the acute phase.
   9. Administer warfarin (Coumadin) orally, as prescribed, when heparin infusion is discontinued.
   10. Monitor prothrombin time and partial thromboplastin time closely.
   11. Prepare the client for embolectomy, vein ligation, or insertion of an umbrella filter, as prescribed.

XVI. LUNG CANCER AND LARYNGEAL CANCER (REFER TO CHAPTER 51.)

BOX 57-13

Assessment Findings: Pulmonary Embolism

Blood-tinged sputum
Chest pain
Cough
Cyanosis
Distended neck veins
Dyspnea accompanied by anginal and pleuritic pain, exacerbated by inspiration
Hypotension
Wheezes on auscultation
Shallow respirations
Tachypnea and tachycardia

XVII. CARBON MONOXIDE POISONING

A. Description
   1. Carbon monoxide is a colorless, odorless, and tasteless gas that has an affinity for hemoglobin 200 times greater than that of oxygen.
   2. Oxygen molecules are displaced, and carbon monoxide reversibly binds to hemoglobin to form carboxyhemoglobin; tissue hypoxia occurs.

B. Assessment (Table 57-1)

C. Interventions
   1. Remove victim from exposure.
   2. Administer oxygen.
   3. Assess need for basic life support.
   4. Monitor vital signs.
   5. Monitor carbon monoxide levels.

XVIII. HISTOPLASMOSIS

A. Description
   1. Histoplasmosis is a pulmonary fungal infection caused by spores of *Histoplasma capsulatum*.
   2. Transmission occurs by the inhalation of spores, which commonly are located in contaminated soil.
   3. Spores also usually are found in bird droppings.

B. Assessment
   1. Dyspnea
   2. Chills
   3. Elevated temperature
   4. Chest pain
   5. Pulmonary infiltrates on chest x-ray film
   6. Elevated white blood cell count
   7. Positive skin test for histoplasmosis
   8. Positive agglutination test
   9. Splenomegaly, hepatomegaly

C. Interventions
   1. Administer oxygen as prescribed.
   2. Monitor breath sounds.
   3. Administer antiemetics, antihistamines, antipyretics, and corticosteroids as prescribed.
   4. Administer fungicidal medications as prescribed.
   5. Encourage coughing and deep breathing.
   6. Position client in semi-Fowler position.
   7. Monitor vital signs.
   8. Monitor for nephrotoxicity from fungicidal medications.

TABLE 57-1

Assessment: Levels of Carbon Monoxide

Level	Assessment Finding
1% to 10%	Impaired visual acuity
11% to 20%	Flushing; headache
21% to 30%	Nausea and impaired dexterity
31% to 40%	Vomiting, dizziness, and syncope
41% to 50%	Tachypnea and tachycardia
Greater than 50%	Coma and death

9. Instruct the client to spray area with water before sweeping barn and chicken coops.

XIX. SARCOIDOSIS
A. Description
1. Sarcoidosis is the presence of epitheloid cell tubercles in the lung.
2. The cause is unknown.
3. High titer of Epstein-Barr virus may be identified.
4. Virus incidence is highest in blacks and young adults.
B. Assessment
1. Night sweats
2. Fever
3. Weight loss
4. Cough
5. Skin nodules
6. Polyarthritis
7. Kveim test: Sarcoid node antigen is injected intradermally and causes a local nodular lesion in about 1 month.
C. Interventions
1. Administer corticosteroids to control symptoms.
2. Monitor temperature.
3. Increase fluid intake.
4. Provide frequent periods of rest.
5. Encourage small, nutritious meals.

XX. OCCUPATIONAL LUNG DISEASE: SILICOSIS
A. Description
1. Silicosis is known as asbestosis and coal workers' pneumoconiosis.
2. Fibrotic disease of the lungs caused by the inhalation of inorganic dusts over long periods of time.
3. Silicosis is common in miners and sandblasters.
B. Assessment
1. Uncomplicated or simple: asymptomatic with evidence of fibrosis on chest x-ray film
2. Chronic complicated: malaise, anorexia, weight loss, severe dyspnea on exertion, evidence of massive fibrosis on chest x-ray film
C. Interventions
1. Administer antitussive for cough.
2. Administer medication for **tuberculosis** as prescribed (**Tuberculosis** is a complication.)
3. Eliminate the toxic substances.
4. Administer oxygen as prescribed.
5. Encourage coughing and deep breathing.

XXI. TUBERCULOSIS
A. Description
1. Tuberculosis is a highly communicable disease caused by *Mycobacterium tuberculosis.*
2. *Mycobacterium tuberculosis* is a nonmotile, nonsporulating, acid-fast rod that secrets niacin, and when the bacillus reaches a susceptible site, it multiplies freely.
3. Because *M. tuberculosis* is an aerobic bacterium, it primarily affects the pulmonary system, especially the upper lobes where the oxygen content is greatest, but also can affect other areas of the body, such as the brain, intestines, peritoneum, kidney, joints, and liver.
4. An exudative response causes a nonspecific pneumonitis and the development of granulomas in the lung tissue.
5. **Tuberculosis** has an insidious onset, and many clients are not aware of symptoms until the disease is well advanced.
6. A **multidrug-resistant strain** of tuberculosis can exist as a result of improper or noncompliant use of treatment programs and the development of mutations in the tubercle bacilli.
7. The goal of treatment is to prevent transmission, control symptoms, and prevent progression of the disease.
B. Risk factors (Box 57-14)
C. Transmission
1. Transmission of tuberculosis is via the airborne route by droplet infection.
2. When an infected individual coughs, laughs, sneezes, or sings, droplet nuclei containing **tuberculosis** bacteria enter the air and may be inhaled by others.
3. Identification of those individuals in close contact with the infected individual is important so that they can be tested and treated as necessary.
4. When contacts have been identified, these persons are assessed with a tuberculin test and chest x-ray films to determine infection with **tuberculosis.**

BOX 57-14

Risk Factors for Tuberculosis

Alcoholism
Children younger than 5 years of age
Drinking of unpasteurized milk if the cow is infected with bovine tuberculosis
Older client
Homeless
Individuals from a lower socioeconomic group
Individuals in constant, frequent contact with an untreated or undiagnosed individual
Individuals living in crowded areas, such as long-term care facilities, prisons, and mental health facilities
Individuals with immune dysfunction or human immunodeficiency virus infection or individuals who are immunosuppressed as a result of medication therapy
Infection
Intravenous drug use
Malnutrition
Minority groups
Refugees

5. After the infected individual has received **tuberculosis** medication for 2 to 3 weeks, the risk of transmission is reduced greatly.

D. Disease progression
 1. Droplets enter the lungs, and the bacteria form a tubercle lesion.
 2. The defense systems of the body encapsulate the tubercle, leaving a scar.
 3. If encapsulation does not occur, bacteria may enter the lymph system, travel to the lymph nodes, and cause an inflammatory response called granulomatous inflammation.
 4. Primary lesions form; the primary lesions may become dormant but can be reactivated and become a secondary infection when reexposed to the bacterium.
 5. In an active phase, **tuberculosis** can cause necrosis and cavitation in the lesions, leading to rupture and the spread of necrotic tissue, and damage to various parts of the body.

E. Client history
 1. Past exposure to **tuberculosis**
 2. Client's country of origin and travel to foreign countries in which the incidence of **tuberculosis** is high
 3. Recent history of influenza, pneumonia, febrile illness, cough, or foul-smelling sputum production
 4. Previous tests for **tuberculosis** and what the results were
 5. Recent **bacille Calmette-Guérin vaccine** (a vaccine containing attenuated tubercle bacilli that may be given to persons in foreign countries or to persons traveling to foreign countries, to produce increased resistance to **tuberculosis**)
 6. An individual who has received a **bacille Calmette-Guérin vaccine** will have a positive skin test and should be evaluated for **tuberculosis** with a chest x-ray film.

F. Clinical manifestations
 1. May be asymptomatic in primary infection
 2. Fatigue
 3. Lethargy
 4. Anorexia
 5. Weight loss
 6. Low-grade fever
 7. Chills
 8. Night sweats
 9. Persistent cough and the production of mucoid and mucopurulent sputum, which is occasionally streaked with blood
 10. Chest tightness and a dull, aching chest pain may accompany the cough

G. Chest assessment
 1. A physical examination of the chest does not provide conclusive evidence of **tuberculosis**.
 2. Chest x-ray film is not definitive, but the presence of multinodular infiltrates with calcification in the upper lobes suggests **tuberculosis**.

3. If the disease is active, caseation and inflammation may be seen on the chest x-ray film.
 4. Advanced disease
  a. Dullness with percussion over involved parenchymal areas, bronchial breath sounds, rhonchi, and crackles indicate advanced disease.
  b. Partial obstruction of a bronchus caused by endobronchial disease or compression by lymph nodes may produce localized wheezing and dyspnea.

H. Sputum cultures
 1. Sputum specimens are obtained for an acid-fast smear.
 2. A sputum culture identifying *M. tuberculosis* confirms the diagnosis.
 3. After medications are started, sputum samples are obtained again to determine the effectiveness of therapy.
 4. Most clients have negative cultures after 3 months of treatment.

I. **Mantoux test**
 1. The **Mantoux test** is the most reliable determinant of infection with **tuberculosis**.
 2. A positive reaction does not mean that active disease is present but indicates exposure to tuberculosis or the presence of inactive (dormant) disease.
 3. Once the test result is positive, it will be positive in any future tests.
 4. A small amount (0.1 mL) of intermediate-strength purified protein derivative containing 5 tuberculin units is administered intradermally in the forearm.
 5. An area of induration measuring 10 mm or more in diameter, 48 to 72 hours after injection, indicates that the individual has been exposed to **tuberculosis.**
 6. For individuals with human immunodeficiency virus infection or who are immunosuppressed, a reaction of 5 mm or greater is considered positive.
 7. Once an individual's skin test is positive, a chest x-ray film is necessary to rule out active **tuberculosis** or to detect old, healed lesions.

J. The hospitalized client
 1. The client with active **tuberculosis** is placed in respiratory isolation precautions in a negative pressure room; to maintain negative pressure, the door of the room must be tightly closed.
 2. The room should have at least six exchanges of fresh air per hour and should be ventilated to the outside environment if possible.
 3. The nurse wears a particulate respirator (a special individually fitted mask) when caring for the client and a gown when a possibility exists of contamination of clothing.
 4. Always thoroughly wash hands before and after caring for the client.

BOX 57-15

Client Education: Tuberculosis

Provide the client and family with information about tuberculosis and allay concerns about the contagious aspect of the infection.

Instruct the client to follow the medication regimen exactly as prescribed and always to have a supply of the medication on hand.

Advise the client of the side effects of the medication and ways of minimizing them to ensure compliance.

Reassure the client that after 2 to 3 weeks of medication therapy, it is unlikely that the client will infect anyone.

Inform the client to resume activities gradually.

Instruct the client about the need for adequate nutrition and a well-balanced diet to promote healing and to prevent recurrence of infection.

Instruct the client to increase intake of foods rich in iron, protein, and vitamin C.

Inform the client and family that respiratory isolation is not necessary because family members already have been exposed.

Instruct the client to cover the mouth and nose when coughing or sneezing and to confine used tissues to plastic bags.

Instruct the client and family about thorough hand washing.

Inform the client that a sputum culture is needed every 2 to 4 weeks once medication therapy is initiated.

Inform the client that when the results of three sputum cultures are negative, the client is no longer considered infectious and usually can return to former employment.

Advise the client to avoid excessive exposure to silicone or dust because these substances can cause further lung damage.

Instruct the client regarding the importance of compliance with treatment, follow-up care, and sputum cultures, as prescribed.

---

5. If the client needs to leave the room for a test or procedure, the client is required to wear a mask.
6. Isolation is discontinued when the client is no longer considered infectious.
7. After the infected individual has received **tuberculosis** medication for 2 to 3 weeks, the risk of transmission is reduced greatly.

K. Client education (Box 57-15)

L. Medications (Refer to Chapter 58.)

PRACTICE QUESTIONS

1. A nurse is preparing to obtain a sputum specimen from a client. Which of the following nursing actions will facilitate obtaining the specimen?
   1. Limiting fluids
   2. Having the client take three deep breaths
   3. Asking the client to spit into the collection container
   4. Asking the client to obtain the specimen after eating

2. A nurse is caring for a client after a bronchoscopy and biopsy. Which of the following signs if noted in the client should be reported immediately to the physician?
   1. Blood-streaked sputum
   2. Dry cough
   3. Hematuria
   4. Bronchospasm

3. A nurse is suctioning fluids from a client via a tracheostomy tube. When suctioning, the nurse must limit the suctioning to a maximum of
   1. 5 seconds.
   2. 10 seconds.
   3. 30 seconds.
   4. 1 minute.

4. A nurse is suctioning fluids from a client through an endotracheal tube. During the suctioning procedure, the nurse notes on the monitor that the heart rate decreases. Which of the following is the most appropriate nursing intervention?
   1. Continue to suction.
   2. Ensure that the suction is limited to 15 seconds.
   3. Stop the procedure and reoxygenate the client.
   4. Notify the physician immediately.

5. An unconscious client is admitted to an emergency room. Arterial blood gas measurements reveal a pH of 7.30, a low bicarbonate level, a normal carbon dioxide level, and a normal oxygen level. An elevated potassium level is also present. These results indicate the presence of
   1. Metabolic acidosis.
   2. Respiratory acidosis.
   3. Combined respiratory and metabolic acidosis.
   4. Overcompensated respiratory acidosis.

6. An emergency room nurse is assessing a client who sustained a blunt injury to the chest wall. Which of these signs would indicate the presence of a pneumothorax in this client?
   1. A sucking sound at the site of injury
   2. Diminished breath sounds
   3. A low respiratory rate
   4. The presence of a barrel chest

7. A nurse is caring for a client hospitalized with acute exacerbation of chronic obstructive pulmonary disease. Which of the following would the nurse expect to note on assessment of this client?
   1. Increased oxygen saturation with exercise
   2. Hypocapnia
   3. A hyperinflated chest on x-ray film
   4. A widened diaphragm noted on chest x-ray film

8. An oxygen delivery system is prescribed for a client with chronic obstructive pulmonary disease to deliver a precise oxygen concentration. Which of the following types of oxygen delivery systems would the nurse anticipate to be prescribed?

1. Venturi mask
2. Aerosol mask
3. Face tent
4. Tracheostomy collar

9. Theophylline (Theo-Dur) tablets are prescribed for a client with chronic airflow limitation, and the nurse instructs the client about the medication. Which statement by the client indicates a need for further teaching?
   1. "I will take the medication on an empty stomach."
   2. "I will take the medication with food."
   3. "I will continue to take the medication even if I am feeling better."
   4. "Periodic blood levels will need to be obtained."

10. A nurse is instructing a hospitalized client with a diagnosis of emphysema about measures that will enhance the effectiveness of breathing during dyspneic periods. Which of the following positions will the nurse instruct the client to assume?
    1. Side-lying in bed
    2. Sitting in a recliner chair
    3. Sitting up in bed
    4. Sitting on the side of the bed and leaning on an overbed table

11. A community health nurse is conducting an educational session with community members regarding tuberculosis. The nurse tells the group that one of the first symptoms associated with tuberculosis is
    1. A bloody, productive cough.
    2. A cough with the expectoration of mucoid sputum.
    3. Chest pain.
    4. Dyspnea.

12. A nurse performs an admission assessment on a client with a diagnosis of tuberculosis. The nurse reviews the results of which diagnostic test that will confirm this diagnosis?
    1. Bronchoscopy
    2. Chest x-ray film
    3. Sputum culture
    4. Tuberculin skin test

13. A nursing instructor asks a nursing student to describe the route of transmission of tuberculosis. The nursing instructor concludes that the student understands this route of transmission if the student states that tuberculosis is transmitted by
    1. The airborne route.
    2. Blood and body fluids.
    3. The fecal-oral route.
    4. Hand to mouth.

14. A nurse is caring for a client with emphysema. The client is receiving oxygen. The nurse assesses the oxygen flow rate to ensure that it does not exceed
    1. 1 L/min.
    2. 2 L/min.
    3. 6 L/min.
    4. 10 L/min.

15. Which of the following arterial blood gas results indicates metabolic alkalosis?
    1. pH of 7.34, P_{CO_2} of 50 mm Hg, HCO_3 of 32 mEq/L, P_{O_2} of 70 mm Hg
    2. pH of 7.46, P_{CO_2} of 30 mm Hg, HCO_3 of 26 mEq/L, P_{O_2} of 80 mm Hg
    3. pH of 7.38, P_{CO_2} of 45 mm Hg, HCO_3 of 22 mEq/L, P_{O_2} of 50 mm Hg
    4. pH of 7.47, P_{CO_2} of 40 mm Hg, HCO_3 of 36 mEq/L, P_{O_2} of 78 mm Hg

16. A nurse reviews the arterial blood gas values of a client. The results indicate respiratory acidosis. Which of the following values would indicate that this acid-base imbalance exists?
    1. pH of 7.48
    2. P_{CO_2} of 32 mm Hg
    3. pH of 7.30
    4. HCO_3 of 20 mEq/L

17. A nurse instructs a client to use the pursed lip method of breathing. The client asks the nurse about the purpose of this type of breathing. The nurse responds, knowing that the primary purpose of pursed lip breathing is to
    1. Promote oxygen intake.
    2. Strengthen the diaphragm.
    3. Strengthen the intercostal muscles.
    4. Promote carbon dioxide elimination.

18. The low-pressure alarm sounds on a ventilator. A nurse assesses the client and then attempts to determine the cause of the alarm. The nurse is unsuccessful in determining the cause of the alarm and takes what initial action?
    1. Checks the client's vital signs.
    2. Ventilates the client manually.
    3. Administers oxygen.
    4. Starts cardiopulmonary resuscitation.

19. A nurse reviews the arterial blood gas values and notes a pH of 7.50, a P_{CO_2} of 30 mm Hg, and an HCO_3 of 25 mEq/L. The nurse interprets these values as indicating
    1. Respiratory acidosis uncompensated.
    2. Respiratory alkalosis uncompensated.
    3. Metabolic acidosis uncompensated.
    4. Metabolic acidosis partially compensated.

20. Aminophylline (theophylline) is prescribed for a client with acute bronchitis. A nurse administers the medication, knowing that the primary action of this medication is to
    1. Promote expectoration.
    2. Suppress the cough.
    3. Relax smooth muscles of the bronchial airway.
    4. Prevent infection.

21. A nurse evaluates the blood theophylline level of a client receiving aminophylline (theophylline) by intravenous infusion. The nurse would determine that a therapeutic blood level exists if which of the following were noted in the laboratory report?

1. 5 mcg/mL
2. 15 mcg/mL
3. 25 mcg/mL
4. 30 mcg/mL

22. A nurse is caring for a client with acute respiratory distress syndrome. Which of the following would the nurse expect to note in the client?
    1. Decreased respiratory rate
    2. Pallor
    3. Low arterial PaO_2
    4. An elevated arterial PaO_2

23. A client is receiving isoetharine hydrochloride (Bronkosol) via a nebulizer. The nurse monitors the client for which side effect of this medication?
    1. Constipation
    2. Diarrhea
    3. Bradycardia
    4. Tachycardia

24. Isoniazid (INH) and rifampin (Rifadin) have been prescribed for a client with tuberculosis. A nurse reviews the medical record of the client. Which of the following, if noted in the client's history, would require physician notification?
    1. Heart disease
    2. Allergy to penicillin
    3. Hepatitis B
    4. Rheumatic fever

25. A client with tuberculosis is being treated with isoniazid (INH) and rifampin (Rifadin). A nurse is preparing instructions for the client regarding these medications. Which of the following statements would be included in the plan of care?
    1. "You must discontinue the medication if gastrointestinal irritation occurs."
    2. "You must take the medication with meals."
    3. "The entire yearlong course of the medication needs to be completed."
    4. "Fluids must be increased while taking this medication to prevent renal failure."

26. A client exposed to tuberculosis is taking isoniazid (INH) and develops signs and symptoms of the disease. The client is instructed to add rifampin (Rifadin) to the medication regimen. A nurse explains to the client that the purpose of adding this second medication is
    1. That rifampin offsets the side effects of isoniazid.
    2. To be certain that resistant organisms are eliminated.
    3. That these medications potentiate each other.
    4. That isoniazid offsets the side effects of rifampin.

27. A client is suspected of having a pulmonary embolus. A nurse assesses the client, knowing that which of the following is a common clinical manifestation of pulmonary embolism?
    1. Decreased respirations
    2. Bradypnea

3. Dyspnea
4. Bradycardia

28. A nurse teaches a client about the use of a respiratory inhaler. Which action by the client indicates a need for further teaching?
    1. Removes the cap and shakes the inhaler well before use.
    2. Presses the canister down with the finger as he breathes in.
    3. Inhales the mist and quickly exhales.
    4. Waits 1 to 2 minutes between puffs if more than one puff has been prescribed.

29. A female client is scheduled to have a chest radiograph. Which of the following questions is of most importance to the nurse assessing this client?
    1. "Is there any possibility that you could be pregnant?"
    2. "Are you wearing any metal chains or jewelry?"
    3. "Can you hold your breath easily?"
    4. "Are you able to hold your arms above your head?"

30. A client has just returned to a nursing unit following bronchoscopy. A nurse would implement which of the following nursing interventions for this client?
    1. Encouraging additional fluids for the next 24 hours
    2. Ensuring the return of the gag reflex before offering food or fluids
    3. Administering atropine intravenously
    4. Administering small doses of midazolam (Versed)

31. A client has an order to have radial arterial blood gases drawn. Before drawing the sample, a nurse occludes the
    1. Brachial and radial arteries, and then releases them and observes the circulation to the hand.
    2. Radial and ulnar arteries, releases one, evaluates the color of the hand, and repeats the process with the other artery.
    3. Radial artery and observes for color changes in the affected hand.
    4. Ulnar artery and observes for color changes in the affected hand.

32. A nurse is assessing the respiratory status of a client who has suffered a fractured rib. The nurse would expect to note which of the following?
    1. Pain, especially with inspiration
    2. Slow, deep respirations
    3. Rapid, deep respirations
    4. Paradoxical respirations

33. A client with chest injury has suffered flail chest. A nurse assesses the client for which most distinctive sign of flail chest?
    1. Cyanosis
    2. Hypotension
    3. Dyspnea, especially on exhalation
    4. Paradoxical chest movement

34. A client has been admitted with chest trauma after a motor vehicle accident and has undergone

subsequent intubation. A nurse checks the client when the high-pressure alarm on the ventilator sounds, and notes that the client has absence of breath sounds in the right upper lobe of the lung. The nurse immediately assesses for other signs of
1. Displaced endotracheal tube.
2. Acute respiratory distress syndrome.
3. Pulmonary embolism.
4. Right pneumothorax.

35. A client with no history of respiratory disease is admitted with respiratory failure. A nurse assesses the arterial blood gas report for which of the following results that are consistent with this disorder?
1. PaO_2 58 mm Hg, $PaCO_2$ 32 mm Hg
2. PaO_2 60 mm Hg, $PaCO_2$ 45 mm Hg
3. PaO_2 49 mm Hg, $PaCO_2$ 52 mm Hg
4. PaO_2 73 mm Hg, $PaCO_2$ 62 mm Hg

36. A nurse is teaching a client with chronic respiratory failure how to use a metered dose inhaler correctly. The nurse instructs the client to
1. Inhale through the nose.
2. Inhale quickly.
3. Take two inhalations during one breath.
4. Hold the breath after inhalation.

37. A nurse is assessing a client with multiple trauma who is at risk for developing acute respiratory distress syndrome. The nurse assesses for which earliest sign of acute respiratory distress syndrome?
1. Inspiratory crackles
2. Bilateral wheezing
3. Intercostal retractions
4. Increased respiratory rate

38. A nurse is taking pulmonary artery catheter measurements of a client with acute respiratory distress syndrome. The pulmonary capillary wedge pressure reading is 12 mm Hg. The nurse interprets that this reading is
1. High and expected.
2. Low and unexpected.
3. Normal and expected.
4. Uncertain and unexpected.

39. A nurse is assessing a client with chronic airflow limitation and notes that the client has a "barrel chest." The nurse interprets that this client has which of the following forms of chronic airflow limitation?
1. Chronic obstructive bronchitis
2. Emphysema
3. Bronchial asthma
4. Bronchial asthma and bronchitis

40. A client diagnosed with pleurisy is being started on medication therapy with a nonsteroidal antiinflammatory drug. A nurse teaches the client that this medication
1. Will alleviate surface pain.
2. Is a mild narcotic analgesic that will allow the client to deep breathe.

3. Is a glucocorticoid that will decrease the inflammatory response at the site.
4. Will relieve pain and enhance coughing and deep breathing.

41. A client has experienced pulmonary embolism. A nurse assesses for which symptom, which is most commonly reported?
1. Dyspnea when deep breaths are taken
2. Hot, flushed feeling
3. Chest pain that occurs suddenly
4. Sudden chills and fever

42. A client experiencing confusion and tremors is admitted to a nursing unit. An initial arterial blood gas report indicates that the $PaCO_2$ level is 72 mm Hg, whereas the PaO_2 level is 64 mm Hg. A nurse interprets that the client is most likely experiencing
1. Carbon monoxide poisoning.
2. Carbon dioxide narcosis.
3. Respiratory alkalosis.
4. Metabolic acidosis.

43. A client who is human immunodeficiency virus–positive has had a Mantoux skin test. The nurse notes a 7-mm area of induration at the site of the skin test. The nurse interprets the results as:
1. Positive
2. Negative
3. Inconclusive
4. The need for repeat testing

44. A client with uncomplicated or simple silicosis is being monitored yearly at the health care clinic. In this type of silicosis, the nurse would expect that the client would
1. Experience anorexia and weight loss.
2. Experience malaise and fatigue.
3. Complain of severe dyspnea.
4. Be asymptomatic.

45. A nurse is evaluating the respiratory status of a client with carbon dioxide narcosis who is being ventilated mechanically. On evaluation of a set of arterial blood gases, the nurse notes that the client's carbon dioxide level has dropped significantly. The nurse then evaluates the client for which adverse effect of this rapid change?
1. Tachypnea
2. Hyponatremia
3. Seizure activity
4. Confusion

46. A client with acquired immunodeficiency syndrome has histoplasmosis. A nurse assesses the client for which of the following signs and symptoms?
1. Weight gain
2. Dyspnea
3. Hypothermia
4. Headache

47. A client has been admitted to a nursing unit with pulmonary sarcoidosis. A nurse assesses the client

for which of the following signs indicating a complication of the disorder?
1. Bilateral lung crackles
2. Distended neck veins
3. Weak pulse
4. Weight loss

48. A nurse is caring for a client with exacerbation of sarcoidosis who is receiving corticosteroids. A nurse teaches the client about adverse effects of medication therapy, which would include
1. Weight loss
2. Hyperglycemia
3. Hyperkalemia
4. Pruritis

49. A nurse is giving discharge instructions to a client with pulmonary sarcoidosis. The nurse concludes that the client understands the information if the client reports which of the following early signs of exacerbation?
1. Fever
2. Weight loss
3. Fatigue
4. Shortness of breath

50. A nurse is taking the history of a client with silicosis. The nurse assesses whether the client wears which of the following items during periods of exposure to silica particles?
1. Mask
2. Gown
3. Gloves
4. Eye protection

51. A client tells a nurse that a physician has stated a diagnosis of uncomplicated or simple silicosis. The client asks the nurse exactly what this means. In formulating a response, the nurse incorporates the knowledge that
1. There is evidence of silica in the bloodstream but no clinical symptoms.
2. The client has normal pulmonary function studies but has shortness of breath.
3. The client has mild ventilation restriction and has fibrosis on chest x-ray film.
4. Massive pulmonary fibrosis is visible on chest x-ray film, but no extrapulmonary symptoms are apparent.

52. A client has been taking benzonatate (Tessalon Perles) as prescribed. A nurse concludes that the medication is having the intended effect if the client experiences
1. Decreased anxiety level.
2. Increased comfort level.
3. Reduction in nausea and vomiting.
4. Decreased frequency and intensity of cough.

53. A client has been taking pyrazinamide (PMS Pyrazinamide) for 1 month. The client asks a nurse if the therapy is due to be terminated soon. The nurse evaluates that the medication probably will

be continued based on a positive finding in which of the following reports?
1. Blood culture
2. Sputum culture
3. Urine culture
4. Wound culture

54. A nurse working on a medical respiratory nursing unit is caring for several clients with respiratory disorders. The nurse would determine that which of the following clients on the nursing unit is at the least risk for infection with tuberculosis?
1. A newly immigrated woman from Korea
2. An uninsured man who is homeless
3. An older woman admitted from a long-term care facility
4. A man who is an inspector for the U.S. Postal Service

55. A client has an order to receive purified protein derivative, 0.1 mL, intradermally. A nurse administers the medication by using a tuberculin syringe with a
1. 26-gauge, ⅝-inch needle inserted almost parallel to the skin with the bevel side up.
2. 26-gauge, ⅝-inch needle inserted at a 45-degree angle with the bevel side down.
3. 20-gauge, 1-inch needle inserted almost parallel to the skin with the bevel side up.
4. 20-gauge, 1-inch needle inserted at a 30-degree angle with the bevel side down.

56. A nurse is reading a Mantoux skin test for a client with no documented health problems. The site has no induration and a 1 mm area of ecchymosis. The nurse interprets that the result is
1. Positive.
2. Negative.
3. Uncertain.
4. Borderline.

57. A nurse is caring for a client diagnosed with tuberculosis. Which assessment, if made by the nurse, would not be consistent with the usual clinical presentation of tuberculosis and may indicate the development of a concurrent problem?
1. Nonproductive or productive cough
2. Anorexia and weight loss
3. Chills and night sweats
4. High-grade fever

58. A nurse is teaching a client with tuberculosis about dietary elements that should be increased in the diet. The nurse suggests that the client increase intake of
1. Meats and citrus fruits.
2. Grains and broccoli.
3. Eggs and spinach.
4. Potatoes and fish.

59. A nurse has conducted discharge teaching with a client who was diagnosed with tuberculosis. The client has been taking medication for a week and a half. The nurse evaluates that the client has

understood the information if the client makes which of the following statements?

1. "I need to continue drug therapy for 2 months."
2. "I should not be contagious after 2 to 3 weeks of medication therapy."
3. "I can't shop at the mall for the next 6 months."
4. "I can return to work if a sputum culture comes back negative."

60. A nurse is preparing to give a bed bath to an immobilized client with tuberculosis. The nurse should plan to wear which of the following items when performing this care?
    1. Particulate respirator, gown, and gloves.
    2. Particulate respirator and protective eyewear.
    3. Surgical mask and gloves.
    4. Surgical mask, gown, and protective eyewear.

CRITICAL THINKING: MULTIPLE RESPONSE

The nurse is preparing a list of home care instructions for the client who has been hospitalized and treated for tuberculosis. Select the instructions that the nurse will include on the list.

___ Avoid contact with other individuals except family members for at least 6 months.

___ Activities should be resumed gradually.

___ Consume a well-balanced diet and foods rich in iron, protein, and vitamin C.

___ Respiratory isolation is not necessary because family members already have been exposed.

___ Cover the mouth and nose when coughing or sneezing and confine used tissues to plastic bags.

___ A sputum culture is needed every 2 to 4 weeks once medication therapy is initiated.

___ When one sputum cultures is negative, the client is no longer considered infectious and usually can return to former employment.

ANSWERS

1. 2

Rationale: To obtain a sputum specimen, the client should rinse the mouth to reduce contamination, breathe deeply, and then cough into a sputum specimen container. The client should be encouraged to cough and not spit so as to obtain sputum. Sputum can be thinned by fluids or by a respiratory treatment such as inhalation of nebulized saline or water. The optimal time to obtain a specimen is on arising in the morning.

Test-Taking Strategy: Use the process of elimination. Option 1 can be eliminated first because general principles indicate that fluids assist in loosening or thinning secretions. Eliminate option 3 because of the word "spit." Spit is different from sputum. Next eliminate option 4 because of the words "after eating." Review this procedure if you had difficulty with this question.

Level of Cognitive Ability: Application
Client Needs: Physiological Integrity
Integrated Process: Nursing Process—implementation
Content Area: Adult health—respiratory
Reference: Phipps, W., Monahan, F., Sands, J., Marek, J., & Neighbors, M. (2003). *Medical-surgical nursing: Health and illness perspectives* (7th ed., p. 473). St. Louis: Mosby.

2. 4

Rationale: If a biopsy was performed during a bronchoscopy, blood-streaked sputum is expected for several hours. Frank blood indicates hemorrhage. A dry cough may be expected. The client should be assessed for signs of complications, which would include cyanosis, dyspnea, stridor, bronchospasm, hemoptysis, hypotension, tachycardia, and dysrhythmias. Hematuria is unrelated to this procedure.

Test-Taking Strategy: Use the process of elimination. Eliminate option 3 first because it is unrelated to the procedure. Next eliminate option 2 because a dry cough may be expected. Noting that a biopsy has been performed will assist in eliminating option 1 because pink-tinged sputum would be expected. Note that option 4, the correct option, relates to airway. If you had difficulty with this question, review postprocedure care following bronchoscopy with biopsy.

Level of Cognitive Ability: Analysis
Client Needs: Physiological Integrity
Integrated Process: Nursing Process—implementation
Content Area: Adult health—respiratory
Reference: Chernecky, C., & Berger, B. (2001). *Laboratory tests and diagnostic procedures* (3rd ed., p. 276). Philadelphia: W. B. Saunders.

3. 2

Rationale: Hypoxemia can be caused by prolonged suctioning, which stimulates the pacemaker cells within the heart. A vasovagal response may occur, causing bradycardia. The nurse must preoxygenate the client before suctioning and limit the suctioning pass to 10 seconds.

Test-Taking Strategy: Use the process of elimination. Recall that during suctioning, the client's airway is blocked; therefore you should be able to eliminate options 3 and 4 easily. From the remaining options, eliminate option 1 because of the short time frame. Five seconds does not seem reasonable to achieve removal of secretions. Review the procedure for suctioning, if you had difficulty with this question

Level of Cognitive Ability: Application
Client Needs: Physiological Integrity
Integrated Process: Nursing Process—implementation
Content Area: Adult health—respiratory
Reference: Lewis, S., Heitkemper, M., & Dirksen, S. (2004). *Medical-surgical nursing: Assessment and management of clinical problems* (6th ed., p. 579). St. Louis: Mosby.

4. 3

Rationale: During suctioning, the nurse should monitor the client closely for side effects, including hypoxemia, cardiac irregularities such as a decrease in heart rate resulting from vagal stimulation, mucosal trauma, hypotension, and paroxysmal coughing. If side effects develop, especially cardiac irregularities, the procedure is stopped and the client is reoxygenated.

Test-Taking Strategy: Use the process of elimination, recalling that suctioning can cause cardiac irregularities. This principle should direct you easily to option 3. If you had difficulty with this question, review the complications and interventions associated with suctioning procedure.

Level of Cognitive Ability: Application
Client Needs: Physiological Integrity
Integrated Process: Nursing Process—implementation
Content Area: Adult health—respiratory
Reference: Lewis, S., Heitkemper, M., & Dirksen, S. (2004). *Medical-surgical nursing: Assessment and management of clinical problems* (6th ed., p. 579). St. Louis: Mosby.

5. 1

Rationale: In an acidotic condition the pH would be low, indicating the acidosis. In addition, a low bicarbonate level along with the low pH would indicate a metabolic state.

Test-Taking Strategy: Use the Pyramid Steps for evaluating the results of a blood gas. Remember to look at the pH first. This pH of 7.30 would indicate an acidosis. Next look at the CO_2 level, which in this situation is normal; therefore a respiratory condition does not exist. This will assist you in eliminating options 2, 3, and 4. Noting that the bicarbonate level is low, as is the pH, should assist in directing you to option 1, a metabolic condition. Review blood gas analysis if you had difficulty with this question.

Level of Cognitive Ability: Analysis
Client Needs: Physiological Integrity
Integrated Process: Nursing Process—analysis
Content Area: Adult health—respiratory
Reference: Ignatavicius, D., & Workman, M. (2002). *Medical surgical nursing: Critical thinking for collaborative care* (4th ed., p. 227). Philadelphia: W. B. Saunders.

6. 2

Rationale: This client has sustained a blunt or a closed chest injury. Basic symptoms of a closed pneumothorax are shortness of breath and chest pain. A larger pneumothorax may cause tachypnea, cyanosis, diminished breath sounds, and subcutaneous emphysema. Hyperresonance also may occur on the affected side.

Test-Taking Strategy: Use the process of elimination. Note the key word "blunt" in the question. This will assist in eliminating option 1, sucking chest wound injury. Knowing that in a respiratory injury increased respirations will occur will assist you in eliminating option 3. Option 4 can be eliminated because a barrel chest is a characteristic finding in a client with chronic obstructive pulmonary disease. Review the signs of pneumothorax if you had difficulty with this question.

Level of Cognitive Ability: Analysis
Client Needs: Physiological Integrity
Integrated Process: Nursing Process—assessment
Content Area: Adult health—respiratory

Reference: Black, J., Hawks, J., & Keene, A. (2001). *Medical-surgical nursing: Clinical management for positive outcomes* (6th ed., p. 1768). Philadelphia: W. B. Saunders.

7. 3

Rationale: Clinical manifestations of chronic obstructive pulmonary disease (COPD) include hypoxemia, hypercapnia, dyspnea on exertion and at rest, oxygen desaturation with exercise, and the use of accessory muscles of respiration. Chest x-ray films reveal a hyperinflated chest and a flattened diaphragm if the disease is advanced.

Test-Taking Strategy: Use the process of elimination. Eliminate option 1 because oxygen desaturation rather than saturation would occur. Next eliminate option 2 because in the client with COPD, hypercapnia would be noted. From the remaining options, reading carefully will assist in directing you to option 3. If you are unfamiliar with the manifestations associated with COPD, review this content.

Level of Cognitive Ability: Analysis
Client Needs: Physiological Integrity
Integrated Process: Nursing Process—assessment
Content Area: Adult health—respiratory
References: Black, J., Hawks, J., & Keene, A. (2001). *Medical-surgical nursing: Clinical management for positive outcomes* (6th ed., p. 1696). Philadelphia: W. B. Saunders.
Lewis, S., Heitkemper, M., & Dirksen, S. (2004). *Medical-surgical nursing: Assessment and management of clinical problems* (6th ed., p. 662). St. Louis: Mosby.

8. 1

Rationale: The Venturi mask delivers the most accurate oxygen concentration. The Venturi mask is the best oxygen delivery system for the client with chronic airflow limitation because it delivers a precise oxygen concentration. The face tent, the aerosol mask, and the tracheostomy collar are also high-flow oxygen delivery systems but most often are used to administer high humidity.

Test-Taking Strategy: Use the process of elimination. Note the key words "precise oxygen concentration." Eliminate options 2, 3, and 4 because they are similar in that they are used to provide high humidity. Review the various types of oxygen delivery systems if you had difficulty with this question.

Level of Cognitive Ability: Analysis
Client Needs: Physiological Integrity
Integrated Process: Nursing Process—analysis
Content Area: Adult health—respiratory
Reference: Perry, A., & Potter, P. (2002). *Clinical nursing skills and techniques* (5th ed., p. 320). St. Louis: Mosby.

9. 1

Rationale: The medication should be administered with food such as milk and crackers to prevent gastrointestinal irritation. Options 2, 3, and 4 are appropriate instructions regarding the use of this medication.

Test-Taking Strategy: Use the process of elimination, noting the key words "need for further teaching." Noting that options 1 and 2 are opposite in terms of administering the medication should alert you that one of these options is the correct answer. Recalling that the client with chronic airway limitation experiences gastrointestinal upset will direct you easily

to option 1. If you are unfamiliar with this medication, review this content.
Level of Cognitive Ability: Analysis
Client Needs: Physiological Integrity
Integrated Process: Teaching/Learning
Content Area: Pharmacology
Reference: Hodgson, B., & Kizior, R. (2004). *Saunders nursing drug handbook 2004* (p. 44). Philadelphia: W. B. Saunders.

10. **4**
Rationale: Positions that will assist the client with breathing include sitting up and leaning on an overbed table, sitting up and resting the elbows on the knees, and standing and leaning against the wall.
Test-Taking Strategy: Use the process of elimination. Eliminate options 2 and 3 first because they are similar. Next eliminate option 1 because this position will not enhance breathing. If you had difficulty with this question, review the positions that will decrease the work of breathing in a client with emphysema.
Level of Cognitive Ability: Application
Client Needs: Physiological Integrity
Integrated Process: Teaching /Learning
Content Area: Adult health—respiratory
Reference: Lewis, S., Heitkemper, M., & Dirksen, S. (2004). *Medical-surgical nursing: Assessment and management of clinical problems* (6th ed., p. 675). St. Louis: Mosby.

11. **2**
Rationale: One of the first pulmonary symptoms include a slight cough with the expectoration of mucoid sputum. Options 1, 3, and 4 are late symptoms and signify cavitation and extensive lung involvement.
Test-Taking Strategy: Use the process of elimination. Note the key word "first" in the stem of the question. This should direct you easily to option 2. If you are unfamiliar with the signs associated with tuberculosis, review this content.
Level of Cognitive Ability: Application
Client Needs: Health Promotion and Maintenance
Integrated Process: Teaching/Learning
Content Area: Adult health—respiratory
Reference: Lewis, S., Heitkemper, M., & Dirksen, S. (2004). *Medical-surgical nursing: Assessment and management of clinical problems* (6th ed., p. 602). St. Louis: Mosby.

12. **3**
Rationale: Definitive diagnosis of tuberculosis is confirmed through culture and isolation of *Mycobacterium tuberculosis.* A presumptive diagnosis is made based on a tuberculin skin test, a sputum smear that is positive for acid-fast bacteria, a chest x-ray film, and histological evidence of graunulomatous disease on biopsy.
Test-Taking Strategy: Note the key word "confirm" in the stem of the question. Confirmation is made by identifying *M. tuberculosis.* If you had difficulty with this question, review the diagnostic procedures related to tuberculosis.
Level of Cognitive Ability: Analysis
Client Needs: Physiological Integrity
Integrated Process: Nursing Process—assessment

Content Area: Adult health—respiratory
Reference: Lewis, S., Heitkemper, M., & Dirksen, S. (2004). *Medical-surgical nursing: Assessment and management of clinical problems* (6th ed., p. 603). St. Louis: Mosby.

13. **1**
Rationale: Tuberculosis is an infectious disease caused by the bacillus *Mycobacterium tuberculosis* and is spread primarily by the airborne route. Options 2, 3, and 4 are incorrect.
Test-Taking Strategy: Recalling that tuberculosis is a respiratory disease will direct you easily to option 1. If you had difficulty with this question, review the transmission of this disease.
Level of Cognitive Ability: Analysis
Client Needs: Safe, Effective Care Environment
Integrated Process: Teaching/Learning
Content Area: Adult health—respiratory
Reference: Thompson, J., Mcfarland, G., Hirsch, J., & Tucker, S. (2002). *Mosby's clinical nursing* (5th ed., p. 1050). St. Louis: Mosby.

14. **2**
Rationale: One to 3 L/min of oxygen by nasal cannula may be required to raise the PaO_2 to 60 to 80 mm Hg. However, oxygen is used cautiously and should not exceed 2 L/min. Because of the long-standing hypercapnia, the respiratory drive is triggered by low oxygen levels rather than increased carbon dioxide levels, as is the case in a normal respiratory system.
Test-Taking Strategy: Use the process of elimination, focusing on the client's diagnosis. Recalling that in the client with emphysema, respiratory drive is triggered by low oxygen levels will direct you to option 2. If you are unfamiliar with this important concept, review this content.
Level of Cognitive Ability: Analysis
Client Needs: Physiological Integrity
Integrated Process: Nursing Process—assessment
Content Area: Adult health—respiratory
Reference: Black, J., Hawks, J., & Keene, A. (2001). *Medical-surgical nursing: Clinical management for positive outcomes* (6th ed., p. 1702). Philadelphia: W. B. Saunders.

15. **4**
Rationale: In a metabolic alkalosis the pH is elevated along with the bicarbonate level (HCO_3). Option 4 is the only option that reflects these values.
Test-Taking Strategy: Remember that when an alkalotic condition exists, the pH will be elevated. This will assist in eliminating options 1 and 3. Next, recall that in a metabolic condition, the HCO_3 will move in the same direction as the pH. The only option that represents these conditions is option 4. Review the process of blood gas analysis, if you had difficulty with this question.
Level of Cognitive Ability: Analysis
Client Needs: Physiological Integrity
Integrated Process: Nursing Process—analysis
Content Area: Adult health—respiratory
Reference: Ignatavicius, D., & Workman, M. (2002). *Medica-surgical nursing: Critical thinking for collaborative care* (4th ed., p. 231). Philadelphia: W. B. Saunders.

16. 3

Rationale: In respiratory acidosis the pH will be lower than normal and the P_{CO_2} will be elevated. The normal pH is 7.35 to 7.45. The normal P_{CO_2} is 35 to 45 mm Hg. The only option that reflects these conditions is option 3.

Test-Taking Strategy: Remember that when an acidotic condition exists, the pH will be low. Next, recall that in a respiratory acidotic condition, the P_{CO_2} will move in the opposite direction from the pH. The only option that represents these conditions is option 3. Review the process of blood gas analysis, if you had difficulty with this question.

Level of Cognitive Ability: Analysis
Client Needs: Physiological Integrity
Integrated Process: Nursing Process—analysis
Content Area: Adult health—respiratory
Reference: Ignatavicius, D., & Workman, M. (2002). *Medical-surgical nursing: Critical thinking for collaborative care* (4th ed., p. 228). Philadelphia: W. B. Saunders.

17. 4

Rationale: Pursed lip breathing facilitates maximal expiration for clients with obstructive lung disease. This type of breathing allows better expiration by increasing airway pressure that keeps air passages open during exhalation. Options 1, 2, and 3 are not the purposes of this type of breathing.

Test-Taking Strategy: Attempt to visualize the use of this procedure to assist you in answering correctly. Knowledge regarding the respiratory conditions in which this type of breathing is helpful also will assist in directing you to option 4. Review the purpose of this breathing technique, if you had difficulty with this question.

Level of Cognitive Ability: Comprehension
Client Needs: Physiological Integrity
Integrated Process: Teaching/Learning
Content Area: Adult health—respiratory
Reference: Phipps, W., Monahan, F., Sands, J., Marek, J., & Neighbors, M. (2003). *Medical-surgical nursing: Health and illness perspectives* (7th ed., p. 577). St. Louis: Mosby.

18. 2

Rationale: If at any time an alarm is sounding and the nurse cannot quickly ascertain the problem, the client is disconnected from the ventilator and manual resuscitation is used to support respirations until the problem can be corrected. No reason is given to begin cardiopulmonary resuscitation. Checking vital signs is not the initial action. Although oxygen is helpful, it will not provide ventilation to the client.

Test-Taking Strategy: Use the process of elimination. Read the question carefully, and note that the issue relates to adequate ventilation of the client. Focusing on this issue will direct you easily to option 2. If you are unfamiliar with management of ventilators and alarms, review this content.

Level of Cognitive Ability: Application
Client Needs: Physiological Integrity
Integrated Process: Nursing Process—implementation
Content Area: Delegating/Prioritizing
Reference: Phipps, W., Monahan, F., Sands, J., Marek, J., & Neighbors, M. (2003). *Medical-surgical nursing: Health and illness perspectives* (7th ed., p.597). St. Louis: Mosby.

19. 2

Rationale: In respiratory alkalosis the pH will be higher than normal and the P_{CO_2} will be low. The normal pH is 7.35 to 7.45. The normal P_{CO_2} is 35 to 45 mm Hg. The only option that reflects these conditions is option 2.

Test-Taking Strategy: Remember that when an alkalotic condition exists, the pH will be high. Next, recall that in a respiratory alkalotic condition, the P_{CO_2} will move in the opposite direction from the pH. The only option that represents these conditions is option 2. Compensation can be identified if the pH is within normal limits. Review the process of blood gas analysis, if you had difficulty with this question.

Level of Cognitive Ability: Analysis
Client Needs: Physiological Integrity
Integrated Process: Nursing Process—analysis
Content Area: Adult health—respiratory
Reference: Ignatavicius, D., & Workman, M. (2002). *Medical-surgical nursing: Critical thinking for collaborative care* (4th ed., p. 228). Philadelphia: W. B. Saunders.

20. 3

Rationale: Aminophylline is a bronchodilator that directly relaxes the smooth muscles of the bronchial airway. Options 1, 2, and 4 are not direct actions of this medication.

Test-Taking Strategy: Use the process of elimination. Recalling that this medication is a bronchodilator will direct you to option 3. Review this medication if you had difficulty with this question.

Level of Cognitive Ability: Comprehension
Client Needs: Physiological Integrity
Integrated Process: Nursing Process—implementation
Content Area: Pharmacology
Reference: Hodgson, B., & Kizior, R. (2004). *Saunders nursing drug handbook 2004* (p. 44). Philadelphia: W. B. Saunders.

21. 2

Rationale: The therapeutic theophylline blood level range from 10 to 20 mcg/mL. A level of 15 mcg/mL is appropriate. Adverse effects occur at levels above 20 mcg/mL. Options 3 and 4 represent toxic levels. Option 1 indicates that the client may require an increased dose of medication.

Test-Taking Strategy: Note the issue of the question, a therapeutic blood level. Recalling that this level is 10 to 20 mcg/mL will direct you to option 2. Review this therapeutic level if you had difficulty with this question.

Level of Cognitive Ability: Analysis
Client Needs: Physiological Integrity
Integrated Process: Nursing Process—analysis
Content Area: Pharmacology
*Reference:*Kee, J., & Hayes, E. (2003). *Pharmacology: A nursing process approach* (4th ed., p. 556). Philadelphia: W. B. Saunders.

22. 3

Rationale: The earliest clinical sign of acute respiratory distress syndrome is an increased respiratory rate. Breathing becomes labored, and the client may exhibit air hunger, retractions, and cyanosis. Arterial blood gas analysis reveals increasing hypoxemia, with a Pa_{O_2} of less than 60 mm Hg.

Test-Taking Strategy: Use the process of elimination. Note that options 3 and 4 relate to the same issue but present opposite conditions. This may provide you with the clue that one of these options is the correct one. Considering the diagnosis of the client, the best choice is option 3. Review the clinical manifestations associated with acute respiratory distress syndrome if you had difficulty with this question.
Level of Cognitive Ability: Analysis
Client Needs: Physiological Integrity
Integrated Process: Nursing Process—assessment
Content Area: Adult health—respiratory
Reference: Black, J., Hawks, J., & Keene, A. (2001). *Medical-surgical nursing: Clinical management for positive outcomes* (6th ed., p. 1762). Philadelphia: W. B. Saunders.

23. **4**
Rationale: Side effects that can occur from the use of this medication include tremors, nausea, nervousness, palpitations, tachycardia, peripheral vasodilation, and dryness of the mouth or throat.
Test-Taking Strategy: Recalling that this medication causes sympathomimetic stimulation will direct you easily to option 4. If you are unfamiliar with the side effects related to this medication, review this content.
Level of Cognitive Ability: Analysis
Client Needs: Physiological Integrity
Integrated Process: Nursing Process—assessment
Content Area: Pharmacology
Reference: Kee, J., & Hayes, E. (2003). *Pharmacology: A nursing process approach* (4th ed., p. 329). Philadelphia: W. B. Saunders.

24. **3**
Rationale: Isoniazid and rifampin are contraindicated in clients with acute liver disease or a history of hepatic injury. Option 3 is the only option that addresses hepatic dysfunction.
Test-Taking Strategy: Use the process of elimination. Eliminate options 1 and 4 first because they relate to cardiac disorders. From the remaining options, you must know that these medications may cause hepatotoxicity. Review the contraindications associated with the use of these medications if you had difficulty with this question.
Level of Cognitive Ability: Analysis
Client Needs: Physiological Integrity
Integrated Process: Nursing Process—analysis
Content Area: Pharmacology
Reference: Kee, J., & Hayes, E. (2003). *Pharmacology: A nursing process approach* (4th ed., p. 435). Philadelphia: W. B. Saunders.

25. **3**
Rationale: The client needs to be instructed that the entire yearlong course of the medication needs to be completed. The preferable administration is for the client to take the medication 1 hour before or 2 hours after meals. If gastrointestinal irritation occurs, the medication should not be discontinued, and in this situation a small amount of food may be taken to reduce the irritation. Increasing fluid intake during this medication therapy is not necessary.
Test-Taking Strategy: Use the process of elimination. Note that options 1, 2, and 4 contain the absolute word "must."

Review the client teaching points related to these medications, if you had difficulty with this question.
Level of Cognitive Ability: Application
Client Needs: Physiological Integrity
Integrated Process: Teaching/Learning
Content Area: Pharmacology
Reference: Hodgson, B., & Kizior, R. (2004). *Saunders nursing drug handbook 2004* (p. 560). Philadelphia: W. B. Saunders.

26. **2**
Rationale: Clients diagnosed with active tuberculosis usually are started on more than one medication to be certain that the resistant organisms are eliminated. The dosages of some medications initially may be large because the bacilli are difficult to kill. Options 1, 3, and 4 are inaccurate.
Test-Taking Strategy: Use the process of elimination. Recalling the concern related to multidrug-resistant therapy will direct you to option 2. If you are unfamiliar with this therapy, review this content.
Level of Cognitive Ability: Application
Client Needs: Physiological Integrity
Integrated Process: Teaching/Learning
Content Area: Pharmacology
Reference: Phipps, W., Monahan, F., Sands, J., Marek, J., & Neighbors, M. (2003). *Medical-surgical nursing: Health and illness perspectives* (7th ed., p. 536). St. Louis: Mosby.

27. **3**
Rationale: The common clinical manifestations of pulmonary embolism are tachypnea, tachycardia, dyspnea, and chest pain.
Test-Taking Strategy: Use the process of elimination. Eliminate options 1, 2, and 4 because they are similar. Review the clinical manifestations of pulmonary embolism if you had difficulty with this question.
Level of Cognitive Ability: Analysis
Client Needs: Physiological Integrity
Integrated Process: Nursing Process—assessment
Content Area: Adult health—respiratory
References: Black, J., Hawks, J., & Keene, A. (2001). *Medical-surgical nursing: Clinical management for positive outcomes* (6th ed., p. 606). Philadelphia: W. B. Saunders.
Ignatavicius, D., & Workman, M. (2002). *Medical-surgical nursing: Critical thinking for collaborative care* (4th ed., p. 592). Philadelphia: W. B. Saunders.

28. **3**
Rationale: The client should be instructed to hold his or her breath at least 10 to 15 seconds before exhaling the mist. Options 1, 2, and 4 are accurate instructions regarding the use of the inhaler.
Test-Taking Strategy: Use the process of elimination, noting the key words "need for further teaching." Attempt to visualize this procedure to answer the question. If you are unfamiliar with the client teaching points related to the use of an inhaler, review this procedure.
Level of Cognitive Ability: Analysis
Client Needs: Physiological Integrity
Integrated Process: Teaching/Learning
Content Area: Adult health—respiratory

Reference: Lewis, S., Heitkemper, M., & Dirksen, S. (2004). *Medical-surgical nursing: Assessment and management of clinical problems* (6th ed., p. 571). St. Louis: Mosby.

29. **1**

Rationale: The most important item to ask about is the client's pregnancy status because pregnant women should not be exposed to radiation. Clients also are asked to remove any chains or metal objects that could interfere with obtaining an adequate film. A chest radiograph most often is done at full inspiration, which gives optimal lung expansion. If a lateral view of the chest is ordered, the client is asked to raise the arms above the head. Most films are done in posterior-anterior view.

Test-Taking Strategy: Note the key words "most important." Eliminate options 3 and 4 first, because they can be determined by the radiological technologist. Option 1 is a higher priority than option 2 because of potential negative teratogenic consequences to the fetus. Review client preparation for a chest radiograph if you had difficulty with this question.

Level of Cognitive Ability: Application
Client Needs: Physiological Integrity
Integrated Process: Nursing Process—assessment
Content Area: Delegating/Prioritizing
Reference: Potter, P., & Perry, A. (2001). *Fundamentals of nursing* (5th ed., p. 1674). St. Louis: Mosby.

30. **2**

Rationale: After bronchoscopy, the nurse keeps the client on NPO status until the gag reflex returns because the preoperative sedation and the local anesthesia impair swallowing and the protective laryngeal reflexes for a number of hours. Additional fluids is unnecessary because no contrast dye is used that would need flushing from the system. Atropine and midazolam would be administered before the procedure, not after.

Test-Taking Strategy: Use the process of elimination. Recall that the client has lost the protective cough, gag, and swallow reflexes during this procedure. Knowledge of this implication helps you to choose option 2 as the only possible answer. Review nursing care measures following a bronchoscopy, if you had difficulty with this question.

Level of Cognitive Ability: Application
Client Needs: Physiological Integrity
Integrated Process: Nursing Process—implementation
Content Area: Adult health—respiratory
Reference: Chernecky, C., & Berger, B. (2001). *Laboratory tests and diagnostic procedures* (3rd ed., pp. 158, 276). Philadelphia: W. B. Saunders.

31. **2**

Rationale: Before drawing an arterial blood gas, the nurse assesses the collateral circulation to the hand with Allen's test. This involves compressing the radial and ulnar arteries and asking the client to close and open the fist. This should cause the hand to become pale. The nurse then releases pressure on one artery and observes whether circulation is restored quickly. The nurse repeats the process, releasing the other artery. The blood sample may be taken safely if collateral circulation is adequate.

Test-Taking Strategy: Use the process of elimination, recalling that the nurse must ensure collateral circulation to the hand

before drawing a sample for arterial blood gases. Consider the anatomy of the blood vessels that lead to the hand to direct you to option 2. If you are unfamiliar with Allen's test, review this procedure.

Level of Cognitive Ability: Application
Client Needs: Physiological Integrity
Integrated Process: Nursing Process—implementation
Content Area: Adult health—respiratory
Reference: Chernecky, C., & Berger, B. (2001). *Laboratory tests and diagnostic procedures* (3rd ed., p. 229). Philadelphia: W. B. Saunders.

32. **1**

Rationale: Rib fractures are a common injury, especially in the older client, and result from a blunt injury or a fall. Typical signs and symptoms include pain and tenderness that is localized at the fracture site and is exacerbated by inspiration and palpation; shallow respirations; splinting or guarding the chest protectively to minimize chest movement; and possible bruising at the fracture site. Paradoxical respirations are seen with flail chest.

Test-Taking Strategy: Use the process of elimination. Focusing on the anatomical location of the injury will direct you to option 1. Review the assessment findings in rib fractures, if you had difficulty with this question.

Level of Cognitive Ability: Analysis
Client Needs: Physiological Integrity
Integrated Process: Nursing Process—assessment
Content Area: Adult health—respiratory
Reference: Black, J., Hawks, J., & Keene, A. (2001). *Medical-surgical nursing: Clinical management for positive outcomes* (6th ed., p. 1769). Philadelphia: W. B. Saunders.

33. **4**

Rationale: Flail chest results from fracture of two or more ribs in at least two places each. This results in a "floating" section of ribs. Because this section is unattached to the rest of the bony rib cage, this segment results in paradoxical chest movement. This means that the force of inspiration pulls the fractured segment inward, while the rest of the chest expands. Likewise, during exhalation the segment balloons outward, while the rest of the chest moves inward. This is a telltale sign of flail chest.

Test-Taking Strategy: Use the process of elimination, focusing on the key words "most distinctive." Cyanosis and hypotension occur with many different disorders and so eliminate them first. From the remaining options, choose paradoxical chest movement over dyspnea on exhalation by remembering that a flail chest has broken rib segments that move independently of the rest of the rib cage. Review the assessment findings in flail chest if you had difficulty with this question.

Level of Cognitive Ability: Application
Client Needs: Physiological Integrity
Integrated Process: Nursing Process—assessment
Content Area: Adult health—respiratory
Reference: Ignatavicius, D., & Workman, M. (2002). *Medical-surgical nursing: Critical thinking for collaborative care* (4th ed., p. 612). Philadelphia: W. B. Saunders.

34. **4**

Rationale: Pneumothorax is characterized by restlessness, tachycardia, dyspnea, pain with respiration, asymmetrical chest expansion, and diminished or absent breath sounds on the affected side. Pneumothorax can cause increased airway pressure because of resistance to lung inflation. Acute respiratory distress syndrome and pulmonary embolism are not characterized by absent breath sounds. An endotracheal tube that is inserted too far can cause absent breath sounds, but the lack of breath sounds most likely would be on the left side because of the degree of curvature of the right and left mainstem bronchi.

Test-Taking Strategy: Use the process of elimination. Focus on the symptoms presented in the question. Note the relationship between "right" upper lobe and "right" pneumothorax in option 4. Review the manifestations associated with pneumothorax, if you had difficulty with this question.

Level of Cognitive Ability: Analysis
Client Needs: Physiological Integrity
Integrated Process: Nursing Process—assessment
Content Area: Adult health—respiratory
References: Black, J., Hawks, J., & Keene, A. (2001). *Medical-surgical nursing: Clinical management for positive outcomes* (6th ed., p. 1776). Philadelphia: W. B. Saunders.
Lewis, S., Heitkemper, M., & Dirksen, S. (2004). *Medical-surgical nursing: Assessment and management of clinical problems* (6th ed., p. 621). St. Louis: Mosby.

35. 3
Rationale: Respiratory failure is described as a PaO_2 of 50 mm Hg or less and a $PaCO_2$ of 50 mm Hg or greater in a client with no history of respiratory disease. In a client with a history of a respiratory disorder with hypercapnia, increases of 5 mm Hg or more $(PaCO_2)$ from the client's baseline are considered diagnostic.

Test-Taking Strategy: Use the process of elimination. Focusing on the client's diagnosis will direct you to option 3, the option with the lowest PaO_2 level. Review the blood gas findings in a client with respiratory failure if you had difficulty with this question.

Level of Cognitive Ability: Analysis
Client Needs: Physiological Integrity
Integrated Process: Nursing Process—analysis
Content Area: Adult health—respiratory
Reference: Ignatavicius, D., & Workman, M. (2002). *Medical-surgical nursing: Critical thinking for collaborative care* (4th ed., p. 598). Philadelphia: W. B. Saunders.

36. 4
Rationale: Instructions for using a metered dose inhaler include to shake the canister; hold it right side up; inhale slowly and evenly through the mouth; deliver one spray per breath; and hold the breath after inhalation.

Test-Taking Strategy: This question tests a fundamental concept of medication administration using inhalers. Visualize the procedure and use the process of elimination. If you selected the incorrect option, review the key principles of this medication therapy.

Level of Cognitive Ability: Application
Client Needs: Physiological Integrity
Integrated Process: Teaching/Learning
Content Area: Adult health—respiratory
Reference: Ignatavicius, D., & Workman, M. (2002). *Medical-surgical nursing: Critical thinking for collaborative care* (4th ed., p. 537). Philadelphia: W. B. Saunders.

37. 4
Rationale: The earliest detectable sign of acute respiratory distress syndrome is an increased respiratory rate, which can begin anywhere from 1 to 96 hours after the initial insult to the body. This is followed by increasing dyspnea, air hunger, retraction of accessory muscles, and cyanosis. Breath sounds may be clear or may consist of fine inspiratory crackles or diffuse coarse crackles.

Test-Taking Strategy: Use the process of elimination, noting the key word "earliest." Eliminate option 3 first because intercostal retraction is a later sign of respiratory distress. Of the remaining options, recall that adventitious breath sounds (options 1 and 2) would occur later than an increased respiratory rate. Review the early signs of acute respiratory distress syndrome if you had difficulty with this question.

Level of Cognitive Ability: Analysis
Client Needs: Physiological Integrity
Integrated Process: Nursing Process—assessment
Content Area: Adult health—respiratory
Reference: Lewis, S., Heitkemper, M., & Dirksen, S. (2004). *Medical-surgical nursing: Assessment and management of clinical problems* (6th ed., p. 1839). St. Louis: Mosby.

38. 3
Rationale: The normal pulmonary capillary wedge pressure (PCWP) is 8 to 13 mm Hg, and the client is considered to have high readings if they exceed 18 to 20 mm Hg. The client with acute respiratory distress syndrome has a normal PCWP, which is an expected finding because the edema is in the interstitium of the lung and is noncardiac.

Test-Taking Strategy: To answer this question correctly, you must know that the PCWP is normal. This makes sense if you know that in acute respiratory distress syndrome, fluid accumulates in the interstitium of the lung and not in the vascular bed. Learn the normal PCWP reading if you are unfamiliar with it.

Level of Cognitive Ability: Analysis
Client Needs: Physiological Integrity
Integrated Process: Nursing Process—analysis
Content Area: Adult health—respiratory
Reference: Ignatavicius, D., & Workman, M. (2002). *Medical-surgical nursing: Critical thinking for collaborative care* (4th ed., p. 650). Philadelphia: W. B. Saunders.

39. 2
Rationale: The client with emphysema has hyperinflation of the alveoli and flattening of the diaphragm. These lead to increased anteroposterior diameter, which is referred to as "barrel chest." The client also has dyspnea with prolonged expiration and has hyperresonant lungs to percussion.

Test-Taking Strategy: Use the process of elimination. Recall that the "barrel chest" is a result of long-term hyperinflation of the lungs and air trapping. By knowing that emphysema is the only type of chronic airflow limitation in which this occurs, you are able to eliminate each of the other, incorrect options. Review the characteristics of emphysema if you had difficulty with this question.

Level of Cognitive Ability: Analysis
Client Needs: Physiological Integrity
Integrated Process: Nursing Process—assessment

Content Area: Adult health—respiratory
Reference: Lewis, S., Heitkemper, M., & Dirksen, S. (2004). *Medical-surgical nursing: Assessment and management of clinical problems* (6th ed., p. 558). St. Louis: Mosby.

40. 4
Rationale: A nonsteroidal antiinflammatory drug, which has an analgesic effect, will relieve pain and allow the client to cough and deep breathe more effectively. Options 1, 2, and 3 are incorrect.
Test-Taking Strategy: Recalling the action and purpose of a non-steroidal antiinflammatory drug will direct you to option 4. Review this classification of medications if you had difficulty with this question.
Level of Cognitive Ability: Application
Client Needs: Health Promotion and Maintenance
Integrated Process: Teaching/Learning
Content Area: Pharmacology
Reference: Lewis, S., Heitkemper, M., & Dirksen, S. (2004). *Medical-surgical nursing: Assessment and management of clinical problems* (6th ed., p. 630). St. Louis: Mosby.

41. 3
Rationale: The most common initial symptom in pulmonary embolism is chest pain that is sudden in onset. The next most commonly reported symptom is dyspnea, which is accompanied by an increased respiratory rate. Other typical symptoms of pulmonary embolism include tachycardia, fever, diaphoresis, cough, anxiety, and possibly syncope.
Test-Taking Strategy: Use the process of elimination. Because pulmonary embolism does not result from an infectious process or an allergic reaction, eliminate options 2 and 4 first. To discriminate between options 1 and 3, look at them closely. Option 1 states dyspnea when deep breaths are taken. Although dyspnea commonly occurs with pulmonary embolism, dyspnea is not associated only with deep breathing. Therefore eliminate option 1. Review the signs of pulmonary embolism if you had difficulty with this question.
Level of Cognitive Ability: Application
Client Needs: Physiological Integrity
Integrated Process: Nursing Process—assessment
Content Area: Adult health—respiratory
Reference: Ignatavicius, D., & Workman, M. (2002). *Medical-surgical nursing: Critical thinking for collaborative care* (4th ed., p. 592). Philadelphia: W. B. Saunders.

42. 2
Rationale: Carbon dioxide narcosis is a condition that results from extreme hypercapnia, with carbon dioxide levels in excess of 70 mm Hg. The client experiences symptoms such as confusion and tremors, which may progress to convulsions and possibly coma.
Test-Taking Strategy: Use the process of elimination, focusing on the data in the question. Noting that the carbon dioxide (CO_2) level is elevated will direct you easily to the correct option, CO_2 narcosis. Review the clinical manifestations associated with CO_2 narcosis if you had difficulty with this question.
Level of Cognitive Ability: Analysis
Client Needs: Physiological Integrity
Integrated Process: Nursing Process—analysis

Content Area: Adult health—respiratory
Reference: *Mosby's medical, nursing, & allied health dictionary* (6th ed., p. 278). (2002). St. Louis: Mosby.

43. 1
Rationale: The client with human immunodeficiency virus (HIV) infection is considered to have positive results on Mantoux skin testing with an area greater than 5 mm of induration. The client without HIV is positive with induration greater than 10 mm. The client with HIV is immunosuppressed, making a smaller area of induration positive for this type of client. For the client infected with HIV to have false-negative readings is possible because of the immunosuppression factor. Options 2, 3, and 4 are incorrect interpretations.
Test-Taking Strategy: Use the process of elimination. Eliminate options 3 and 4 first because they are similar. From the remaining options, recalling that the client with HIV is immunosuppressed will assist in determining the interpretation of the area of induration. Review results of tuberculosis skin testing in an immunosuppressed client if you had difficulty with this question.
Level of Cognitive Ability: Analysis
Client Needs: Physiological Integrity
Integrated Process: Nursing Process—analysis
Content Area: Adult health—respiratory
Reference: Black, J., Hawks, J., & Keene, A. (2001). *Medical-surgical nursing: Clinical management for positive outcomes* (6th ed., p. 1719). Philadelphia: W. B. Saunders.

44. 4
Rationale: In uncomplicated or simple silicosis, the client would be asymptomatic, although evidence of fibrosis on an x-ray film would be present. Malaise, anorexia, weight loss, and severe dyspnea on exertion would occur in a client with chronic complicated silicosis.
Test-Taking Strategy: Use the process of elimination. Noting the words "uncomplicated or simple" will direct you to option 4. Review the manifestations associated with silicosis if you had difficulty with this question.
Level of Cognitive Ability: Analysis
Client Needs: Physiological Integrity
Integrated Process: Nursing Process—assessment
Content Area: Adult health—respiratory
Reference: Ignatavicius, D., & Workman, M. (2002). *Medical-surgical nursing: Critical thinking for collaborative care* (4th ed., p. 558). Philadelphia: W. B. Saunders.

45. 3
Rationale: With a rapid drop in carbon dioxide levels, the kidneys are unable to excrete bicarbonate ions at the same pace. The client can experience rebound metabolic alkalosis, with resulting seizure activity. The nurse evaluates the client's status carefully during this period.
Test-Taking Strategy: Use the process of elimination and knowledge regarding how the body maintains acid-base balance. Because a rapid decline in carbon dioxide often results in metabolic alkalosis, the client is at risk for seizure activity. Review the basic acid-base abnormalities and their manifestations if you had difficulty with this question.
Level of Cognitive Ability: Analysis

Client Needs: Physiological Integrity
Integrated Process: Nursing Process—evaluation
Content Area: Adult health—respiratory
Reference: Mosby's medical, nursing, & allied health dictionary (6th ed., p. 278). (2002). St. Louis: Mosby.

46. 2
Rationale: Histoplasmosis is an opportunistic fungal infection that can occur in the client with acquired immunodeficiency syndrome. The infection begins as a respiratory infection and can progress to disseminated infection. Typical signs and symptoms include fever, dyspnea, cough, and weight loss. Enlargement of the client's lymph nodes, liver, and spleen may occur as well.
Test-Taking Strategy: Use the process of elimination. Recalling that histoplasmosis is an infectious process will help you to eliminate option 3. Because the client has acquired immunodeficiency syndrome and another infection, weight gain is an unlikely symptom and can be eliminated next. Knowing that histoplasmosis begins as a respiratory infection helps you to choose dyspnea over headache as the correct option. Review the signs of histoplasmosis, if you had difficulty with this question.
Level of Cognitive Ability: Application
Client Needs: Physiological Integrity
Integrated Process: Nursing Process—assessment
Content Area: Adult health—respiratory
Reference: Ignatavicius, D., & Workman, M. (2002). *Medical-surgical nursing: Critical thinking for collaborative care* (4th ed., p. 373). Philadelphia: W. B. Saunders.

47. 2
Rationale: Pulmonary sarcoidosis can lead to cor pulmonale (or failure of the right side of the heart), which is characterized by distended neck veins, elevated central venous pressure, full bounding pulse, weight gain, engorged liver, and peripheral edema. Bilateral lung crackles would indicate failure of the left side of the heart.
Test-Taking Strategy: Recall that sarcoidosis is a restrictive lung disease. A complication of restrictive lung disease is cor pulmonale because the right side of the heart has to work hard continuously to overcome pulmonary resistance. Therefore recalling the signs of failure of the right side of the heart will direct you to option 2. Review the complications of pulmonary sarcoidosis and the signs of failure of the right and left sides of the heart if you had difficulty with this question.
Level of Cognitive Ability: Analysis
Client Needs: Physiological Integrity
Integrated Process: Nursing Process—assessment
Content Area: Adult health—respiratory
References: Ignatavicius, D., & Workman, M. (2002). *Medical-surgical nursing: Critical thinking for collaborative care* (4th ed., p. 556). Philadelphia: W. B. Saunders.
Lewis, S., Heitkemper, M., & Dirksen, S. (2004). *Medical-surgical nursing: Assessment and management of clinical problems* (6th ed., p. 632). St. Louis: Mosby.

48. 2
Rationale: The usual treatment for exacerbations of sarcoidosis includes systemic corticosteroids. Side effects of this

therapy include weight gain, changes in mood, and hyperglycemia. Hyperkalemia and pruritis are unrelated findings.
Test-Taking Strategy: Recall that sarcoidosis is a restrictive lung disease and that exacerbations are treated with corticosteroids. Knowing that corticosteroids cause hyperglycemia will direct you to the correct option. Review the medication therapy used in the treatment of sarcoidosis, if you had difficulty with this question.
Level of Cognitive Ability: Application
Client Needs: Physiological Integrity
Integrated Process: Teaching/Learning
Content Area: Adult health—respiratory
Reference: Lehne, R. (2001). *Pharmacology for nursing care* (4th ed., p. 785). Philadelphia: W. B. Saunders.

49. 4
Rationale: Dry cough and dyspnea are typical signs and symptoms of pulmonary sarcoidosis. Others include chest pain, hemoptysis, and pneumothorax. Systemic signs and symptoms include weakness and fatigue, malaise, fever, and weight loss.
Test-Taking Strategy: Use the process of elimination. Note the key word "early." Because sarcoidosis is a pulmonary problem, eliminate options 1 and 2 first. Select option 4 over option 3 because the shortness of breath (and impaired ventilation) appears first and would cause the fatigue as a secondary symptom. Review the early signs of exacerbation in sarcoidosis if you had difficulty with this question.
Level of Cognitive Ability: Analysis
Client Needs: Physiological Integrity
Integrated Process: Teaching/Learning
Content Area: Adult health—respiratory
References: Black, J., Hawks, J., & Keene, A. (2001). *Medical-surgical nursing: Clinical management for positive outcomes* (6th ed., p. 1726). Philadelphia: W. B. Saunders.
Ignatavicius, D., & Workman, M. (2002). *Medical-surgical nursing: Critical thinking for collaborative care* (4th ed., p. 557). Philadelphia: W. B. Saunders.

50. 1
Rationale: Silicosis results from chronic, excessive inhalation of particles of free crystalline silica dust. The client should wear a mask to limit inhalation of this substance, which can cause restrictive lung disease after years of exposure. Options 2, 3, and 4 are not necessary.
Test-Taking Strategy: Use the process of elimination. Recalling that exposure to silica dust causes the illness and that the dust is inhaled into the respiratory tract will direct you to option 1. If you had difficulty with this question, review the protective measures associated with silicosis.
Level of Cognitive Ability: Analysis
Client Needs: Safe, Effective Care Environment
Integrated Process: Nursing Process—assessment
Content Area: Adult health—respiratory
Reference: Phipps, W., Monahan, F., Sands, J., Marek, J., & Neighbors, M. (2003). *Medical-surgical nursing: health and illness perspectives* (7th ed., p. 547). St. Louis: Mosby.

51. 3
Rationale: The client with simple silicosis may be asymptomatic or have mild ventilatory restriction and has evidence of

fibrosis on chest x-ray film. Pulmonary function studies reveal some decreases in vital capacity and total lung volume. Massive fibrosis is not evident at this stage. This disease is restricted to the respiratory system only.

Test-Taking Strategy: Use the process of elimination. Option 4 has the least amount of "fit" with a disorder that is described as simple or uncomplicated and therefore is eliminated first. Because silicosis is a pulmonary disease, option 1 is eliminated. Option 2 is incongruent; it would be difficult for one to have shortness of breath and have normal pulmonary function tests. Review the pathophysiology associated with simple silicosis, if you had difficulty with this question.

Level of Cognitive Ability: Analysis
Client Needs: Physiological Integrity
Integrated Process: Nursing Process—analysis
Content Area: Adult health—respiratory
Reference: Ignatavicius, D., & Workman, M. (2002). *Medical-surgical nursing: Critical thinking for collaborative care* (4th ed., p. 558). Philadelphia: W. B. Saunders.

52. 4
Rationale: Benzonatate is a locally acting antitussive the effectiveness of which is measured by the degree to which it decreases the intensity and frequency of cough without eliminating the cough reflex. Options 1, 2, and 3 are not effects of this medication.

Test-Taking Strategy: Recalling that the medication is an antitussive will direct you to option 4. Review this medication if you are unfamiliar with it.

Level of Cognitive Ability: Analysis
Client Needs: Physiological Integrity
Integrated Process: Nursing Process—evaluation
Content Area: Pharmacology
Reference: Hodgson, B., & Kizior, R. (2004). *Saunders nursing drug handbook 2004* (p. 99). Philadelphia: W. B. Saunders.

53. 2
Rationale: Pyrazinamide is an antitubercular medication that is given with other antitubercular medications. Use of pyrazinamide might not be discontinued if sputum cultures continue to be positive. Options 1, 3, and 4 are not related directly to the use of this medication.

Test-Taking Strategy: Recalling that this medication is an antitubercular medication will direct you to option 2. If this question was difficult, review this medication.

Level of Cognitive Ability: Analysis
Client Needs: Physiological Integrity
Integrated Process: Nursing Process—evaluation
Content Area: Pharmacology
Reference: Kee, J., & Hayes, E. (2003). *Pharmacology: A nursing process approach* (4th ed., p. 435). Philadelphia: W. B. Saunders.

54. 4
Rationale: Persons at high risk for acquiring tuberculosis include immigrants from Asia, Africa, Latin America, and Oceania; medically underserved populations (ethnic minorities, homeless); those with human immunodeficiency virus or other immunosuppressive disorders; residents in group settings (long-term care, correctional facilities); and health care workers.

Test-Taking Strategy: Use the process of elimination, noting the key words "least risk." Begin to answer this question by eliminating options 1 and 2 because immigrants and the medically underserved more frequently are affected by the disease. From the remaining options, the postal inspector may or may not come into contact with many persons, depending on the job description. The client from the long-term care facility, however, lives in a group setting where a large number of persons share a common environment 24 hours a day. Review the risk factors associated with tuberculosis if you had difficulty with this question.

Level of Cognitive Ability: Analysis
Client Needs: Physiological Integrity
Integrated Process: Nursing Process—assessment
Content Area: Adult health—respiratory
Reference: Black, J., Hawks, J., & Keene, A. (2001). *Medical-surgical nursing: Clinical management for positive outcomes* (6th ed., p. 1718). Philadelphia: W. B. Saunders.

55. 1
Rationale: A Mantoux skin test is administered by giving 0.1 mL of purified protein derivative (PPD) intradermally. Administration involves drawing the medication into a tuberculin syringe with a 25- to 27-gauge, $\frac{5}{8}$-inch needle. The injection is given by inserting the needle as close as possible to a parallel position with the skin and with the needle bevel facing up. This results in formation of a wheal when the PPD is administered correctly.

Test-Taking Strategy: Remember that a tuberculin syringe is small and measures small amounts of medication dosages. Use the process of elimination, eliminating options 3 and 4 first because these options indicate the use of larger syringes and needles. Remembering that the bevel side is up during administration of PPD will assist in directing you to the correct option from the remaining choices. If this question was difficult, review the basics of this injection technique.

Level of Cognitive Ability: Application
Client Needs: Physiological Integrity
Integrated Process: Nursing Process—implementation
Content Area: Adult health—respiratory
Reference: Phipps, W., Monahan, F., Sands, J., Marek, J., & Neighbors, M. (2003). *Medical-surgical nursing: Health and illness perspectives* (7th ed., p. 535). St. Louis: Mosby.

56. 2
Rationale: A positive reading has an induration measuring 10 mm or more and is considered abnormal. A small area of ecchymosis is insignificant and probably is related to injection technique. Options 1, 3, and 4 are incorrect interpretations.

Test-Taking Strategy: Recall that induration is necessary for a positive response. Because the client in this question has no induration, the result can only be negative. Review Mantoux skin testing results if you had difficulty with this question.

Level of Cognitive Ability: Analysis
Client Needs: Physiological Integrity
Integrated Process: Nursing Process—analysis
Content Area: Adult health—respiratory
Reference: Phipps, W., Monahan, F., Sands, J., Marek, J., & Neighbors, M. (2003). *Medical-surgical nursing: Health and illness perspectives* (7th ed., p. 535). St. Louis: Mosby.

57. **4**

Rationale: The client with tuberculosis usually experiences cough (productive or nonproductive), fatigue, anorexia, weight loss, dyspnea, hemoptysis, chest discomfort or pain, chills and sweats (which may occur at night), and a low-grade fever.

Test-Taking Strategy: Use the process of elimination. Eliminate options 1 and 2 first because they are symptoms that are common in the client with tuberculosis. From the remaining options, you need to know that the client may get night sweats or that the fever is low grade. Review the clinical manifestations associated with tuberculosis if you had difficulty with this question.

Level of Cognitive Ability: Analysis
Client Needs: Physiological Integrity
Integrated Process: Nursing Process—assessment
Content Area: Adult health—respiratory
Reference: Phipps, W., Monahan, F., Sands, J., Marek, J., & Neighbors, M. (2003). *Medical-surgical nursing: Health and illness perspectives* (7th ed., p. 537). St. Louis: Mosby.

58. **1**

Rationale: The nurse teaches the client with tuberculosis to increase intake of protein, iron, and vitamin C. Foods rich in vitamin C include citrus fruits, berries, melons, pineapple, broccoli, cabbage, green peppers, tomatoes, potatoes, chard, kale, asparagus, and turnip greens. Food sources that are rich in iron include liver and other meats. Less than 10% of iron is absorbed from eggs, and less than 5% is absorbed from grains and vegetables.

Test-Taking Strategy: Use the process of elimination. Recall that the diet in tuberculosis should be high in protein, vitamin C, and iron. Knowing which types of foods contain these various nutrients will direct you to option 1. If you had difficulty with this question, review these nutritional concepts.

Level of Cognitive Ability: Application
Client Needs: Health Promotion and Maintenance
Integrated Process: Teaching/Learning
Content Area: Adult health—respiratory
Reference: Phipps, W., Monahan, F., Sands, J., Marek, J., & Neighbors, M. (2003). *Medical-surgical nursing: Health and illness perspectives* (7th ed., p. 537). St. Louis: Mosby.

59. **2**

Rationale: The client is continued on medication therapy for 6 to 12 months, depending on the situation. The client generally is considered to be not contagious after 2 to 3 weeks of medication therapy. The client is instructed to wear a mask if there will be exposure to crowds until the medication is effective in preventing transmission. The client is allowed to return to work when the results of three sputum cultures are negative.

Test-Taking Strategy: Use the process of elimination. Knowing that the medication therapy lasts for at least 6 months helps you to eliminate option 1 first. Knowing that three sputum cultures must be negative helps you to eliminate option 4 next. From the remaining options, recalling that the client is not contagious after 2 to 3 weeks of therapy will direct you to option 2. If you had difficulty with this question, review the infectious period of tuberculosis.

Level of Cognitive Ability: Analysis

Client Needs: Physiological Integrity
Integrated Process: Teaching/Learning
Content Area: Adult health—respiratory
Reference: Ignatavicius, D., & Workman, M. (2002). *Medical-surgical nursing: Critical thinking for collaborative care* (4th ed., p. 588). Philadelphia: W. B. Saunders.

60. **1**

Rationale: The nurse who is in contact with a client with tuberculosis should wear an individually fitted particulate respirator. The nurse also would wear gloves as per standard precautions. The nurse wears a gown when a possibility exists that the clothing could become contaminated, such as when giving a bed bath.

Test-Taking Strategy: Use the process of elimination. Knowing that the nurse should wear a particulate respirator eliminates options 3 and 4. Knowledge of basic standard precautions directs you to option 1. Review precautions related to the care of a client with tuberculosis if you had difficulty with this question.

Level of Cognitive Ability: Application
Client Needs: Safe, Effective Care Environment
Integrated Process: Nursing Process—implementation
Content Area: Adult health—respiratory
Reference: Ignatavicius, D., & Workman, M. (2002). *Medical-surgical nursing: Critical thinking for collaborative care* (4th ed., p. 588). Philadelphia: W. B. Saunders.

CRITICAL THINKING: MULTIPLE RESPONSE

Answer:

Activities should be resumed gradually.

Consume a well-balanced diet and foods rich in iron, protein, and vitamin C.

Respiratory isolation is not necessary because family members already have been exposed.

Cover the mouth and nose when coughing or sneezing and confine used tissues to plastic bags.

A sputum culture is needed every 2 to 4 weeks once medication therapy is initiated.

Rationale: The nurse should provide the client and family with information about tuberculosis and allay concerns about the contagious aspect of the infection. Instruct the client to follow the medication regimen exactly as prescribed and always to have a supply of the medication on hand. Advise the client of the side effects of the medication and ways of minimizing them to ensure compliance. Reassure the client that after 2 to 3 weeks of medication therapy, it is unlikely that the client will infect anyone. Inform the client that activities should be resumed gradually and about the need for adequate nutrition and a well-balanced diet that is rich in iron, protein, and vitamin C to promote healing and to prevent recurrence of infection. Inform the client and family that respiratory isolation is not necessary because family members already have been exposed. Instruct the client about thorough hand washing and to cover the mouth and nose when coughing or sneezing and to confine used tissues to plastic bags. Inform the client that a sputum culture is needed every 2 to 4 weeks once medication therapy is initiated and that when the results of three sputum cultures are negative, the client is no longer considered infectious and can usually return to former employment.

Test-Taking Strategy: Knowledge regarding the pathophysiology, transmission, and treatment of tuberculosis is needed to answer this question. Review home care instructions for the client with tuberculosis if you had difficulty with this question.
Level of Cognitive Ability: Application
Client Needs: Health Promotion and Maintenance

Integrated Process: Teaching/Learning
Content Area: Adult health—respiratory
Reference: Ignatavicius, D., & Workman, M. (2002). *Medical-surgical nursing: Critical thinking for collaborative care* (4th ed., pp. 587-588). Philadelphia: W. B. Saunders.

REFERENCES

Black, J., Hawks, J., & Keene, A. (2001). *Medical-surgical nursing: Clinical management for positive outcomes* (6th ed.). Philadelphia: W. B. Saunders.

Chernecky, C., & Berger, B. (2001). *Laboratory tests and diagnostic procedures* (3rd ed.). Philadelphia: W. B. Saunders.

Harkreader, H., & Hogan, M. A. (2004). *Fundamentals of nursing: Caring and clinical judgment* (2nd ed.). Philadelphia: W. B. Saunders.

Hodgson, B., & Kizior, R. (2004). *Saunders nursing drug handbook 2004.* Philadelphia: W. B. Saunders.

Ignatavicius, D., & Workman, M. (2002). *Medical-surgical nursing: Critical thinking for collaborative care* (4th ed.). Philadelphia: W. B. Saunders.

Kee, J., & Hayes, E. (2003). *Pharmacology: A nursing process approach* (4th ed.). Philadelphia: W. B. Saunders.

Lehne, R. (2001). *Pharmacology for nursing care* (4th ed.). Philadelphia: W. B. Saunders.

Lewis, S., Heitkemper, M., & Dirksen, S. (2004). *Medical-surgical nursing: Assessment and management of clinical problems* (6th ed.). St. Louis: Mosby.

Mosby's medical, nursing, & allied health dictionary (6th ed.). (2002). St. Louis: Mosby.

Phipps, W., Monahan, F., Sands, J., Marek, J., & Neighbors, M. (2003). *Medical-surgical nursing: Health and illness perspectives* (7th ed.). St. Louis: Mosby.

Perry, A., & Potter, P. (2002). *Clinical nursing skills and techniques* (5th ed.). St. Louis: Mosby.

Potter, P., & Perry, A. (2001). *Fundamentals of nursing* (5th ed.). St. Louis: Mosby.

Thompson, J., Mcfarland, G., Hirsch, J., & Tucker, S. (2002). *Mosby's clinical nursing* (5th ed.). St. Louis: Mosby.

Respiratory Medications

I. BRONCHODILATORS

A. Description

1. Sympathomimetic bronchodilators dilate the airways of the respiratory tree, making air exchange and respiration easier for the client, and relax the smooth muscle of the bronchi (Box 58-1).

2. Xanthine bronchodilators stimulate the central nervous system and respiration, dilate coronary and pulmonary vessels, cause diuresis, and relax smooth muscle (Box 58-2).

3. Bronchodilators are used to treat allergic rhinitis and sinusitis, acute bronchospasm, acute and chronic asthma, bronchitis, **chronic obstructive pulmonary disease**, and **emphysema.**

4. Bronchodilators are contraindicated in individuals with hypersensitivity, peptic ulcer disease, severe cardiac disease and cardiac dysrhythmias, hyperthyroidism, or uncontrolled seizure disorders.

5. Bronchodilators should be used with caution in clients with hypertension, diabetes mellitus, or narrow-angle glaucoma.

6. Theophylline increases the risk of digitalis toxicity and decreases the effects of lithium and phenytoin (Dilantin).

7. If theophylline and a β-receptor agonist are administered together, cardiac dysrhythmias may result.

8. β-Blockers, cimetidine (Tagamet), and erythromycin increase the effects of theophylline.

9. Barbiturate and carbamazepine (Tegretol) decrease the effects of theophylline.

10. Xanthine bronchodilators are not used as frequently as they previously were; they may be introduced later in therapy.

B. Side effects

1. Palpitations and tachycardia
2. Dysrhythmias
3. Restlessness, nervousness, tremors
4. Anorexia, nausea, and vomiting
5. Headaches and dizziness
6. Hyperglycemia
7. Decreased clotting time
8. Mouth dryness and throat irritation with inhalers

BOX 58-1

Bronchodilators: Sympathomimetics

β-RECEPTOR AGONISTS
Albuterol (Proventil, Ventolin)
Bitolterol mesylate (Tornalate)
Epinephrine (AsthmaHaler Mist)
Epinephrine bitartrate (Adrenalin, Bronkaid, Primatene)
Formoterol fumarate (Foradil)
Isoetharine hydrochloride (Bronkosol, Bronkometer)
Isoproterenol (Isuprel, Medihaler-Iso)
Levalbuterol (Xopenex)
Metaproterenol sulfate (Alupent, Metaprel)
Pirbuterol acetate (Maxair)
Salmeterol (Serevent)
Terbutaline sulfate (Brethine, Brethaire)

ANTICHOLINERGIC
Ipratropium bromide (Atrovent, Combivent)

BOX 58-2

Bronchodilators: Xanthines

Aminophylline (Truphylline)
Oxtriphylline (Choledyl, Choledyl SA)
Theophylline (Aerolate, Slo-Phyllin, Theolair)
Theophylline (Bronkodyl, Elixophyllin)
Theophylline (Theo-Dur, Slo-bid, Theo-24, Uni-Dur, Uniphyl)

9. Tolerance and paradoxic bronchoconstriction with inhalers

▶ C. Interventions
1. Assess vital signs.
2. Monitor for cardiac dysrhythmias.
3. Assess for cough, wheezing, decreased breath sounds, and sputum production.
4. Monitor for restlessness and confusion.
5. Provide adequate hydration.
6. Administer the medication at regular intervals around the clock to maintain a sustained therapeutic level.
7. Administer oral medications with or after meals to decrease gastrointestinal irritation.
8. Instruct the client not to crush enteric-coated or sustained-release tablets or capsules.
9. Instruct the client to avoid caffeine-containing products such as coffee, tea, cola, and chocolate.
10. Instruct the client in the side effects of bronchodilators.
11. Instruct the client in how to monitor the pulse and to report any abnormalities to the physician.
12. Instruct the client in how to use an inhaler or nebulizer and how to monitor the amount of medication remaining in an inhaler canister.
13. Instruct the client to avoid over-the-counter medications.
14. Instruct the client to stop smoking and provide information regarding support resources.
15. Instruct the client with diabetes mellitus to monitor blood glucose levels.
16. Instruct the client with asthma to wear a Medic-Alert bracelet.
▶ 17. Monitor for a therapeutic serum theophylline level of 10 to 20 mcg/mL.
▶ 18. Note that toxicity is likely to occur when the serum level is greater than 20 mcg/mL.
▶ 19. Intravenously administered aminophylline or theophylline preparations should be administered slowly and always via an infusion pump.

II. GLUCOCORTICOIDS (CORTICOSTEROIDS) (BOX 58-3)

A. Glucocorticoids act as antiinflammatory agents and reduce edema of the airways.
B. Refer to Chapter 54 for information on glucocorticoids.

BOX 58-3

Glucocorticoids (Corticosteroids)

Beclomethasone dipropionate (Vanceril, Beclovent)
Budesonide (Pulmicort)
Flunisolide (AeroBid)
Fluticasone (Flonase, Flovent)
Fluticasone and salmeterol (Advair Diskus)
Mometasone intranasal (Nasonex)
Triamcinolone (Azmacort)

III. INHALED NONSTEROIDAL ANTIALLERGY AGENTS (BOX 58-4)

A. Description
1. Antiasthmatic, antiallergic, and mast cell stabilizers inhibit mast cell release after exposure to antigens.
2. These medications are used to treat allergic rhinitis, bronchial asthma, and exercised-induced bronchospasm.
3. These medications are contraindicated in clients with known hypersensitivity.
4. Orally administered cromolyn sodium is used with caution in clients with impaired hepatic or renal function.
B. Side effects
1. Cough or bronchospasm following inhalation ▶
2. Nasal sting or sneezing following inhalation
3. Unpleasant taste in the mouth
C. Interventions
1. Monitor vital signs.
2. Monitor respirations and assess lung sounds for rhonchi, wheezing, and rales.
3. Instruct the client to drink a few sips of water ▶ before and after inhalation to prevent cough and unpleasant taste in the mouth.
4. Administer oral capsules (cromolyn sodium) at least 30 minutes before meals.
5. Instruct the client not to discontinue the medica- ▶ tion abruptly because a rebound asthmatic attack can occur.

IV. LEUKOTRIENE MODIFIERS (BOX 58-5)

A. Description
1. Leukotriene modifiers are used in the prophylaxis and treatment of chronic bronchial asthma.
2. Leukotriene modifiers are not used for acute asthma episodes.
3. Leukotriene modifiers inhibit bronchoconstriction caused by specific antigens.
4. Leukotriene modifiers reduce airway edema and smooth muscle constriction.
5. Leukotriene modifiers are contraindicated in clients with hypersensitivity and in breast-feeding mothers.

BOX 58-4

Inhaled Nonsteroidal Antiallergy Agents: Mast-cell Stabilizers

Cromolyn sodium (Intal)
Nedocromil (Tilade)

BOX 58-5

Leukotriene Modifiers

Montelukast (Singulair)
Zafirlukast (Accolate)
Zileuton (Zyflo)

6. Leukotriene modifiers should be used with caution in clients with impaired hepatic function.
7. Coadministration of inhaled glucocorticoids increases the risk of upper respiratory infection.

B. Side effects
1. Headache
2. Nausea and vomiting
3. Dyspepsia
4. Diarrhea
5. Generalized pain, myalgia
6. Fever
7. Dizziness

C. Interventions
1. Monitor vital signs.
2. Assess lung sounds for rhonchi wheezing.
3. Assess liver function laboratory values.
4. Monitor for cyanosis.
5. Instruct the client to take medication 1 hour before or 2 hours after meals.
6. Instruct the client to increase fluid intake.
7. Instruct the client not to discontinue medication and to take as prescribed even during symptom-free periods.

V. ANTIHISTAMINES (BOX 58-6)

A. Description
1. Antihistamines are called histamine antagonists or H_1 blockers; these medications compete with histamine for receptor sites, thus preventing a histamine response.
2. When the H_1 receptor is stimulated, the extravascular smooth muscles, including those lining the nasal cavity, are constricted.
3. Antihistamines decrease nasopharyngeal secretions by blocking the H_1 receptor and decrease nasal itching that causes sneezing.

BOX 58-6

Antihistamines

Astemizole (Hismanal)
Azatadine maleate (Optimine)
Azelastine hydrochloride (Astelin)
Brompheniramine maleate (Dimetane, Dimetapp)
Cetirizine hydrochloride (Zyrtec)
Chlorpheniramine maleate (Aller-Chlor, Chlor-Trimeton)
Clemastine fumarate (Tavist)
Cyproheptadine hydrochloride (Periactin)
Dexchlorpheniramine maleate (Polaramine)
Dimenhydrinate (Dramamine)
Diphenhydramine (Benadryl)
Doxylamine succinate (Unisom)
Fexofenadine (Allegra)
Loratadine (Claritin)
Phenindamine tartrate (Nolahist)
Tripelennamine (Pyribenzamine)
Triprolidine hydrochloride (Myidil)

---

4. Antihistamines are used for the common cold, rhinitis, nausea and vomiting, motion sickness, urticaria, and as a sleep aid.
5. Antihistamines can cause central nervous system (CNS) depression if taken with alcohol, narcotics, hypnotics, or barbiturates.
6. Antihistamines should be used with caution in clients with **chronic obstructive pulmonary disease** because of their drying effect.
7. Diphenhydramine (Benadryl) has an anticholinergic effect and should be avoided in clients with narrow-angle glaucoma.

B. Side effects
1. Drowsiness and fatigue
2. Dizziness
3. Urinary retention
4. Blurred vision
5. Wheezing
6. Constipation
7. Dry mouth
8. Gastrointestinal irritation
9. Hypotension
10. Hearing disturbances
11. Photosensitivity
12. Nervousness and irritability
13. Confusion
14. Nightmares

C. Interventions
1. Monitor vital signs.
2. Monitor for signs of urinary dysfunction.
3. Administer with food or milk.
4. Avoid subcutaneous injection, and administer intramuscular injection in a large muscle if the intramuscular route is prescribed.
5. Instruct the client to avoid hazardous activities, alcohol, and other CNS depressants.
6. Instruct the client taking medication for motion sickness to take the medication 30 minutes before the event and then before meals and at bedtime during the event.
7. Instruct the client to suck on hard candy or ice chips for dry mouth.

VI. NASAL DECONGESTANTS (BOX 58-7)

A. Description
1. Nasal decongestants stimulate the α-adrenergic receptors, thus producing vasoconstriction of the capillaries within the nasal mucosa.

BOX 58-7

Nasal Decongestants

Oxymetazoline hydrochloride (Afrin)
Phenylephrine hydrochloride (Neo-Synephrine)
Phenylpropanolamine hydrochloride (Dimetapp)
Pseudoephedrine hydrochloride (Sudafed)
Xylometazoline hydrochloride (Otrivin)

2. Nasal decongestants shrink nasal mucosal membranes and reduce fluid secretion.

3. Nasal decongestants are used for allergic rhinitis, hay fever, and acute coryza (profuse nasal discharge).

4. Nasal decongestants are contraindicated or used with extreme caution in clients with hypertension, cardiac disease, hyperthyroidism, or diabetes mellitus.

5. Nasal decongestants can cause tolerance and rebound nasal congestion (vasodilation) caused by irritation of the nasal mucosa and should not be used for more than 48 hours.

B. Side effects

1. Frequent use of decongestants, especially nasal sprays or drops, can result in tolerance and rebound nasal congestion (vasodilation) caused by irritation of the nasal mucosa.

2. Nervousness

3. Restlessness

4. Hypertension

5. Hyperglycemia

C. Interventions

1. Assess the client for existing medical disorders.

2. Monitor for cardiac dysrhythmias.

3. Monitor blood glucose levels.

4. Instruct the client to avoid caffeine in large amounts because it can increase restlessness and palpitations.

5. Instruct the client in the importance of limiting the use of nasal sprays and drops.

VII. EXPECTORANTS AND MUCOLYTIC AGENTS (BOX 58-8)

A. Description

1. Expectorants loosen bronchial secretions so that they can be eliminated with coughing.

2. Expectorants are used for dry, unproductive cough and to stimulate bronchial secretions.

3. Mucolytic agents with dextromethorphan should not be used by clients with **chronic obstructive pulmonary disease** because they suppress the cough.

4. Acetylcysteine (Mucomyst) can increase airway resistance and should not be used in clients with asthma.

B. Side effects

1. Gastrointestinal irritation

2. Skin rash

3. Oropharyngeal irritation

C. Interventions

1. Instruct the client to take medication with a full glass of water to loosen mucus.

2. Instruct the client to maintain an adequate fluid intake.

3. Encourage the client to cough and deep breathe.

4. Acetylcysteine (Mucomyst), administered by nebulization, should not be mixed with another medication.

5. If acetylcysteine is administered with a bronchodilator, the bronchodilator should be administered 5 minutes before the acetylcysteine.

6. Monitor for side effects of acetylcysteine such as nausea and vomiting, stomatitis, and runny nose.

VIII. ANTITUSSIVES (BOX 58-9)

A. Description

1. Antitussives act on the cough control center in the medulla to suppress the cough reflex.

2. Antitussives are used for a cough that is nonproductive and irritating.

B. Side effects

1. Dizziness, drowsiness, sedation

2. Gastrointestinal irritation, nausea

3. Dry mouth

4. Constipation

5. Respiratory depression

C. Interventions

1. Instruct the client that if the cough lasts longer than 1 week and a fever or rash occurs to notify the physician.

2. Encourage the client to take adequate fluids with the medication.

3. Encourage the client to sleep with the head of the bed elevated.

4. Instruct the client to avoid hazardous activities.

5. Note that drug dependency can occur.

6. Avoid administration to the client with a head injury or postoperative cranial surgery.

BOX 58-8

Expectorants and Mucolytic Agents

EXPECTORANTS
Dornase alfa (Pulmozyme)
Guaifenesin (glycerylguaiacolate) (Anti-Tuss, Glycotuss, Humibid, Robitussin)

MUCOLYTIC
Acetylcysteine (Mucomyst)

BOX 58-9

Antitussives

NARCOTICS
Codeine, codeine phosphate, codeine sulfate
Hydrocodone bitartrate (Hycodan)

NONNARCOTICS
Dextromethorphan hydrochloride (Benylin DM, Robitussin)
Diphenhydramine hydrochloride (Benylin Cough Syrup, Benadryl)

BOX 58-10

Narcotic Antagonist

Naloxone hydrochloride (Narcan)

7. Avoid administration to the client using narcotics, sedative hypnotics, barbiturates, or antidepressants because CNS depression can occur.
8. Instruct the client to avoid the use of alcohol.

IX. NARCOTIC ANTAGONIST (BOX 58-10)
A. Description
   1. A narcotic antagonist reverses respiratory depression in narcotic overdose.
   2. Avoid use in nonnarcotic respiratory depression.
B. Side effects
   1. CNS depression
   2. Nausea, vomiting
   3. Tremors
   4. Sweating
   5. Increased blood pressure
   6. Tachycardia
C. Interventions
   1. Assess vital signs, especially respirations.
   2. Have oxygen and resuscitative equipment available during administration.

X. USE OF AN INHALER
A. Client instructions (Fig. 58-1)

B. If two different inhaled medications are prescribed and one of the medications contains a glucocorticoid (corticosteroid), administer the bronchodilator first and the corticosteroid second.
C. Wait 5 minutes following the bronchodilator before inhaling the corticosteroid.

XI. TUBERCULOSIS MEDICATIONS
A. Description
   1. Tuberculosis medications offer the most effective method for treating the disease and preventing transmission.
   2. Treatment of identified lesions depends on whether the individual has active disease or has been exposed to the disease.
   3. Treatment is difficult because the bacterium has a waxy substance on the capsule that makes penetration and destruction difficult.
   4. The use of a multiple-medication regimen destroys organisms as quickly as possible and minimizes the emergence of medication-resistant organisms.
   5. Active **tuberculosis** is treated with a combination of medications to which the organism is susceptible.
   6. Individuals with active **tuberculosis** are treated for 6 to 9 months; however, clients with human immunodeficiency virus infection are treated for a longer period of time.
   7. After the infected individual has received medication for 2 to 3 weeks, the risk of transmission is reduced greatly.

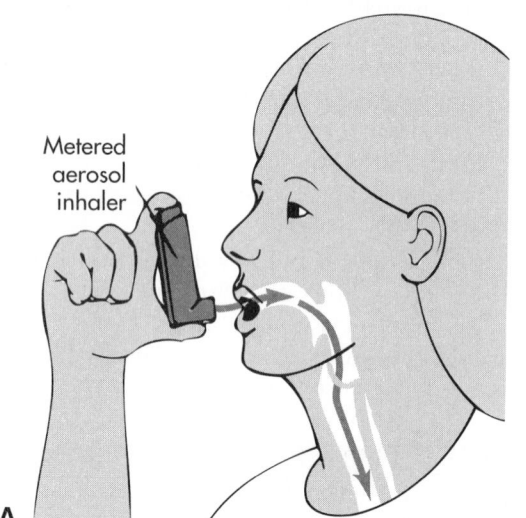
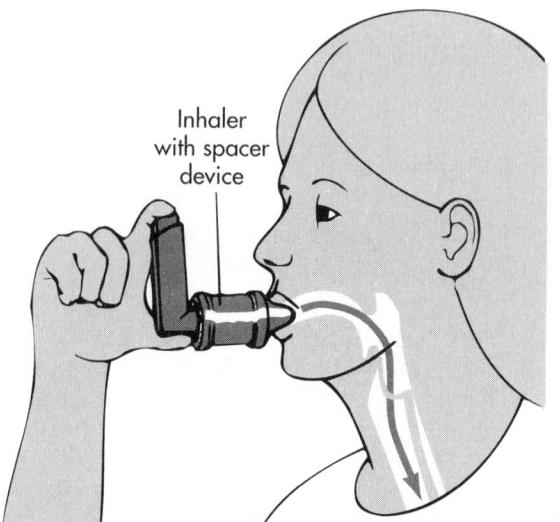

FIG. 58-1   Inhaled drugs commonly used in asthma treatment include β-adrenergic bronchodilators, cromolyn sodium, and aerosol glucocorticoids. Metered dose inhaler (**A**) should not be put in mouth but held about two fingerwidths (1½ inches) in front of mouth. Alternatively, an inhaler with spacer device (**B**) can be used. Patients should breathe deeply once before activating the inhaler and then continue breathing in for about 5 seconds. Patients then should hold the breath for 10 to 15 seconds before breathing out slowly. If second dose is needed, patients should wait 1 to 2 minutes before taking another dose. (From Clark, J. F., Queener, S., Karb, V.B. [2000]. *Pharmacologic basis of nursing practice* [6th ed.]. St Louis: Mosby.)

8. Most clients have negative sputum cultures after 3 months of compliance with medication therapy.
9. Individuals who have been exposed to active **tuberculosis** are treated with preventive isoniazid (INH) for 9 to12 months.
B. First-line or second-line medications
   1. First-line medications provide the most effective antituberculosis activity.
   2. Second-line medications are used in combination with first-line medications but are more toxic.
   3. Current infecting organisms are proving resistant to standard first-line medications, and the resistant organisms develop because individuals with the disease fail to complete the course of treatment; surviving bacteria adapt to the medication and become resistant.
   4. Multidrug therapies are instituted because of the resistant organisms.
C. **Multidrug-resistant strain of tuberculosis (MDR-TB)**
   1. Resistance occurs when a client receiving two medications (first-line and second-line medications) discontinues one of the medications without the physician's knowledge.
   2. The client briefly experiences some response from the single medication but then large numbers of resistant organisms begin to grow.
   3. The client, infectious again, transmits the drug-resistant organism to other individuals.
   4. As this event is repeated, an organism develops that is resistant to many of the first-line **tuberculosis** medications.

XII. FIRST-LINE MEDICATIONS FOR TUBERCULOSIS (BOX 58-11)

A. Isoniazid (INH, Laniazid, Nydrazid)
   1. Description
      a. Isoniazid is bactericidal.
      b. Isoniazid inhibits synthesis of mycolic acids and acts to kill actively growing organisms in the extracellular environment.
      c. Isoniazid inhibits growth of dormant organisms in the macrophages and caseating granulomas.
      d. Isoniazid is active only during cell division.
      e. Isoniazid is used in combination with other antitubercular medications.
   2. Contraindications and cautions
      a. Isoniazid is contraindicated in clients with hypersensitivity or with acute liver disease.
      b. Use isoniazid with caution in clients with chronic liver disease, alcoholism, or renal impairment.
      c. Use isoniazid with caution in clients taking niacin/nicotinic acid (Nicobid).
      d. Use isoniazid with caution in clients taking hepatotoxic medications because the risk for hepatotoxicity increases.
      e. Alcohol increases the risk of hepatotoxicity.

BOX 58-11

First-Line and Second-Line Medications for Tuberculosis

FIRST LINE
Ethambutol (Myambutol)
Isoniazid (INH)
Pyrazinamide
Rifampin (Rifadin)
Streptomycin

SECOND LINE
Capreomycin (Capastat)
Cycloserine (Seromycin)
Ethionamide (Trecator)
Kanamycin (Kantrex)
Para-aminosalicylic acid

OTHER MEDICATIONS
Aminosalicylate sodium (Tubasal) is indicated for the treatment of pulmonary and extrapulmonary tuberculosis in combination with other antituberculosis medications.
Rifabutin (Mycobutin) is an antimycobacterial used for the prophylaxis for disseminated *Mycobacterium avium* complex in persons with advanced human immunodeficiency virus infection.
Rifampin and isoniazid (Rifamate) is used to treat tuberculosis after dosage of separate medications has been established.

---

      f. Isoniazid (INH) may increase the risk of toxicity of carbamazepine (Tegretol) and phenytoin (Dilantin).
      g. Isoniazid (INH) may decrease ketoconazole (Nizoral) concentrations.
   3. Side effects
      a. Hypersensitivity reactions
      b. Peripheral neuritis
      c. Neurotoxicity
      d. Hepatotoxicity; increased liver function levels
      e. Pyridoxine (vitamin B_6) deficiency
      f. Irritation at injection site with intramuscular administration
      g. Nausea and vomiting
      h. Dry mouth
      i. Dizziness
      j. Hyperglycemia
      k. Vision changes
      l. Hepatitis
   4. Interventions
      a. Assess for hypersensitivity.
      b. Assess for hepatic dysfunction.
      c. Assess for sensitivity to niacin/nicotinic acid (Nicobid).
      d. Monitor liver function tests.
      e. Monitor for signs of hepatitis, such as anorexia, nausea, vomiting, weakness, fatigue, dark urine,

or jaundice, and if these symptoms occur, withhold the medication and notify the physician.

▲ f. Monitor for tingling, numbness, or burning of the extremities.

g. Assess mental status.

▲ h. Monitor for visual changes, and notify the physician if they occur.

▲ i. Assess for dizziness and initiate safety precautions.

▲ j. Monitor complete blood count (CBC) and blood glucose levels.

▲ k. Administer isoniazid 1 hour before or 2 hours after a meal because food may delay absorption.

▲ l. Administer isoniazid at least 1 hour before antacids, especially those antacids that contain aluminum.

5. Client education

▲ a. Instruct the client not to skip doses and to take medication for the full length of the prescribed therapy.

b. Instruct the client not to take any other medication without consulting the physician.

c. Advise the client of the importance of follow-up physician visits, vision testing, and laboratory tests.

d. Instruct the client to avoid alcohol.

e. Advise the client to take medication on an empty stomach with 8 oz of water 1 hour before or 2 hours after meals and to avoid taking antacids with the medication.

▲ f. Instruct the client to avoid tyramine-containing foods because they may cause a reaction such as red and itching skin, a pounding heartbeat, light-headedness, a hot or clammy feeling, or a headache, and if this does occur, to notify the physician.

▲ g. Instruct the client in the signs of neurotoxicity, hepatitis, and hepatotoxicity.

▲ h. Instruct the client to notify the physician if signs of neurotoxicity, hepatitis and hepatotoxicity, or visual changes occur.

▲ B. Rifampin (Rifadin)

1. Description

a. Rifampin inhibits bacterial RNA synthesis.

b. Rifampin binds to DNA-dependent RNA polymerase and blocks RNA transcription.

c. Rifampin is used with at least one other antitubercular medication.

2. Contraindications and cautions

a. Rifampin is contraindicated in clients with hypersensitivity.

b. Rifampin should be used with caution in clients with hepatic dysfunction or alcoholism.

c. Use of alcohol or hepatotoxic medications may increase the risk of hepatotoxicity.

d. Rifampin decreases the effects of several medications, including oral anticoagulants,

oral hypoglycemics, chloramphenicol (Chloromycetin), digoxin (Lanoxin), disopyramide phosphate (Norpace), mexiletine (Mexitil), quinidine polygalacturonate (Cardioquin), tocainide hydrochloride (Tonocard), fluconazole (Difulcan), methadone hydrochloride (Dolophine), phenytoin (Dilantin), and verapamil hydrochloride (Calan).

3. Side effects ▲

a. Hypersensitivity reaction including fever, chills, shivering, headache, muscle and bone pain, and dyspnea

b. Heartburn

c. Nausea, vomiting, diarrhea

d. Vision changes ▲

e. Hepatotoxicity and hepatitis ▲

f. Increased uric acid levels ▲

g. Blood dyscrasias ▲

h. Colitis

4. Interventions ▲

a. Assess for hypersensitivity.

b. Evaluate CBC, uric acid, and liver function ▲ tests.

c. Assess for signs of hepatitis, and if they ▲ occur, withhold the medication and notify the physician.

d. Monitor stools for signs of colitis.

e. Monitor mental status.

f. Assess for visual changes. ▲

5. Client education

a. Instruct the client not to skip doses and to take ▲ medication for the full length of the prescribed therapy.

b. Instruct the client not to take any other medication without consulting the physician.

c. Advise the client of the importance of follow- ▲ up physician visits and laboratory tests.

d. Instruct the client to avoid alcohol.

e. Advise the client to take medication on an empty ▲ stomach with 8 oz of water 1 hour before or 2 hours after meals and to avoid taking antacids with the medication.

f. Instruct the client that urine, feces, sweat, and ▲ tears will be red-orange and that soft contact lens can become permanently discolored.

g. Instruct the client to notify the physician if jaun- ▲ dice (yellow eyes or skin) develops or if weakness, fatigue, nausea, vomiting, sore throat, fever, or unusual bleeding occurs.

C. Ethambutol (Myambutol) ▲

1. Description

a. Ethambutol is bacteriostatic.

b. Ethambutol interferes with cell metabolism and multiplication by inhibiting one or more metabolites in susceptible organism.

c. Ethambutol inhibits bacterial RNA synthesis.

d. Ethambutol is active only during cell division.

e. Ethambutol is slow acting and must be used with other bactericidal agents.

2. Contraindications and cautions

a. Ethambutol is contraindicated in clients with hypersensitivity or optic neuritis and in children under 13 years of age.

b. Use with caution in clients with renal dysfunction, gout, ocular defects, diabetic retinopathy, cataracts, or ocular inflammatory conditions.

c. Use with caution in clients taking neurotoxic medications because the risk for neurotoxicity increases.

3. Side effects

a. Hypersensitivity reactions

b. Anorexia, nausea, vomiting

c. Dizziness

d. Malaise

e. Mental confusion

f. Joint pain

g. Dermatitis

h. Optic neuritis

i. Peripheral neuritis

j. Thrombocytopenia

k. Increased uric acid levels

l. Anaphylactoid reaction

4. Interventions

a. Assess client for hypersensitivity.

b. Evaluate results of CBC, uric acid, and renal and liver function tests.

c. Obtain baseline visual acuity and color discrimination, especially to green.

d. Monitor for visual changes such as altered color perception and decreased visual acuity, and if changes occur, withhold the medication and notify the physician.

e. Administer once every 24 hours and administer with food to decrease gastrointestinal upset.

f. Monitor uric acid concentrations and assess for painful or swollen joints or signs of gout.

g. Monitor intake and output and for adequate renal function.

h. Assess mental status.

i. Monitor for dizziness and initiate safety precautions.

j. Assess for peripheral neuritis (numbness, tingling or burning of the extremities), and if it occurs, notify the physician.

5. Client education

a. Inform the client that he or she can prevent nausea related to the medication by taking the daily dose at bedtime or by taking the prescribed antinausea medications.

b. Instruct the client not to skip doses and to take the medication for the full length of the prescribed therapy.

c. Instruct the client not to take any other medication without consulting the physician.

d. Advise the client of the importance of follow-up physician visits, vision testing, and laboratory tests.

e. Instruct the client to notify the physician immediately if any visual problems occur or a rash, swelling and pain in the joints, or numbness, tingling, or burning in the hands or feet occurs.

D. Streptomycin

1. Description

a. Streptomycin is an aminoglycoside antibiotic used with at least one other antitubercular medication.

b. Streptomycin is bactericidal because of receptor-binding action that interferes with protein synthesis in susceptible organisms.

2. Contraindications and cautions

a. Streptomycin is contraindicated in clients with hypersensitivity, myasthenia gravis, parkinsonism, or eighth cranial nerve damage.

b. Use streptomycin with caution in the older client, in neonates because of renal insufficiency and immaturity, and in young infants because the medication may cause CNS depression.

c. The risk of toxicity increases when streptomycin is taken with other aminoglycosides or nephrotoxicity- or ototoxicity-producing medications.

3. Side effects (Box 58-12)

a. Hypersensitivity

b. Visual changes

c. Increased liver and renal function levels

d. Peripheral neuritis such as burning of the face or mouth

BOX 58-12

Side Effects of Streptomycin

NEPHROTOXICITY
Changes in urine output
Decreased appetite
Increased thirst
Nausea, vomiting

NEUROTOXICITY
Muscle numbness
Seizures
Tingling
Twitching

VESTIBULAR OTOTOXICITY
Clumsiness
Dizziness
Unsteadiness

AUDITORY OTOTOXICITY
A full feeling in the ears
Ringing in the ears
Loss of hearing

4. Interventions
   a. Assess for hypersensitivity.
   b. Monitor liver and renal function tests.
   c. Monitor for ototoxic, neurotoxic, and nephrotoxic reactions.
   d. Obtain baseline audiometric test and repeat every 1 to 2 months because the medication impairs the eighth cranial nerve.
   e. Assess hearing acuity.
   f. Monitor for visual changes.
   g. Assess hydration status and maintain adequate hydration during therapy.
   h. Monitor intake and output.
   i. Assess urinalysis results.
   j. Monitor for signs of peripheral neuritis.
5. Client education
   a. Instruct the client not to skip doses and to take medication for the full length of the prescribed therapy.
   b. Instruct the client not to take any other medication without consulting the physician.
   c. Advise the client of the importance of follow-up physician visits and laboratory tests.
   d. Instruct the client to notify the physician if hearing loss, changes in vision, or urinary problems occur.
   E. Pyrazinamide
   1. Description
      a. The exact mechanism of action of pyrazinamide is unknown.
      b. Pyrazinamide may be bacteriostatic or bactericidal, depending on its concentration at the infection site and susceptibility of infecting organism.
      c. Pyrazinamide is used with at least one other antitubercular medication after failure or ineffectiveness of the primary medications occurs.
   2. Contraindications and cautions
      a. Pyrazinamide is contraindicated in clients with hypersensitivity.
      b. Use pyrazinamide with caution in clients with diabetes mellitus, renal impairment, or gout, and in children.
      c. Pyrazinamide may decrease the effects of allopurinol (Zyloprim), colchicine, probenecid (Benemid), and sulfinpyrazone (Anturane).
      d. Cross-sensitivity is possible with isoniazid (INH), ethionamide (Trecator-SC) or niacin/nicotinic acid (Nicobid).
   3. Side effects
      a. Increases liver function and uric acid levels
      b. Arthralgia, myalgia
      c. Photosensitivity
      d. Hepatotoxicity
      e. Thrombocytopenia
   4. Interventions
      a. Assess for hypersensitivity.

b. Evaluate CBC, liver function tests, and uric acid levels.
c. Observe for hepatotoxic effects, and if they occur, withhold the medication and notify the physician.
d. Assess for painful or swollen joints.
e. Evaluate blood glucose levels because diabetes mellitus may be difficult to control while client is taking the medication.
5. Client education
   a. Instruct the client to take the medication with food to reduce gastrointestinal distress.
   b. Instruct the client to avoid sunlight or ultraviolet light until photosensitivity is determined.
   c. Instruct the client to notify the physician if any side effects occur.
   d. Instruct the client not to skip doses and to take the medication for the full length of the prescribed therapy.
   e. Instruct the client not to take any other medication without consulting the physician.
   f. Advise the client of the importance of follow-up physician visits and laboratory tests.

XIII. SECOND-LINE MEDICATIONS FOR TUBERCULOSIS

A. Capreomycin sulfate (Capastat Sulfate)
   1. Description
      a. Mechanism of action for capreomycin is unknown.
      b. Capreomycin is used to treat MDR-TB when significant resistance to other medications is expected.
      c. Capreomycin must be given intramuscularly.
   2. Contraindications and cautions
      a. The risk of nephrotoxicity, ototoxicity, and neuromuscular blockade is increased with the use of aminoglycosides or loop diuretics.
      b. Use capreomycin with caution in clients with renal insufficiency, acoustic nerve impairment, hepatic disorder, myasthenia gravis, or parkinsonism.
      c. Do not administer to clients receiving streptomycin.
   3. Side effects
      a. Nephrotoxicity
      b. Ototoxicity
      c. Neuromuscular blockade
   4. Interventions
      a. Perform baseline audiometric testing.
      b. Assess renal, hepatic, and electrolyte levels before administration.
      c. Monitor intake and output.
      d. Reconstituted medication may be stored for 48 hours at room temperature.
      e. Administer intramuscularly deep in a large muscle mass.

f. Rotate injection sites.

g. Observe injection site for redness, excessive bleeding, and inflammation.

5. Client education

a. Instruct the client not to perform tasks that require mental alertness.

b. Instruct the client to report any hearing loss, balance disturbances, respiratory difficulty, weakness, or signs of hypersensitivity reactions.

B. Kanamycin (Kantrex)

1. Description

a. Kanamycin is an aminoglycoside antibiotic given with at least one other antitubercular medication.

b. Kanamycin is bactericidal because of receptor-binding action, interfering with protein synthesis in susceptible microorganisms.

2. Contraindications and cautions

a. Kanamycin is contraindicated in clients with hypersensitivity, neuromuscular disorders, or eighth cranial nerve damage.

b. Use kanamycin with caution in the older client, in neonates because of renal insufficiency and immaturity, and in young infants because it may cause CNS depression.

c. The risk of toxicity increases when kanamycin is taken with other aminoglycosides or nephrotoxicity- or ototoxicity-producing medications.

3. Side effects

a. Hypersensitivity

b. Pain and irritation at the injection site

c. Nephrotoxicity as evidenced by increased blood urea nitrogen and serum creatinine levels

d. Ototoxicity as evidenced by tinnitus, dizziness, ringing/roaring in the ears, and reduced hearing

e. Neurotoxicity as evidenced by headache, dizziness, lethargy, tremors, and visual disturbances

f. Superinfections

4. Interventions

a. Assess for hypersensitivity.

b. Monitor for ototoxic, neurotoxic, and nephrotoxic reactions.

c. Monitor liver and renal function tests.

d. Obtain baseline audiometric test and repeat every 1 to 2 months because the medication impairs the eighth cranial nerve.

e. Assess acuteness of hearing.

f. Monitor for visual changes.

g. Assess hydration status and maintain adequate hydration during therapy.

h. Monitor intake and output.

i. Assess urinalysis.

j. Monitor for superinfection.

5. Client education

a. Instruct the client not to skip doses and to take medication for the full length of the prescribed therapy.

b. Instruct the client not to take any other medication without consulting the physician.

c. Advise the client of the importance of follow-up physician visits and laboratory tests.

d. Instruct the client to notify the physician if hearing loss, changes in vision, or urinary problems occur.

C. Ethionamide (Trecator-SC)

1. Description

a. Mechanism of action for ethionamide is unknown.

b. Ethionamide is used to treat **MDR-TB** when significant resistance to other medications is expected.

2. Contraindications and cautions

a. Ethionamide is contraindicated in clients with hypersensitivity.

b. Use ethionamide with caution in clients with diabetes mellitus or renal dysfunction.

3. Side effects

a. Anorexia, nausea, vomiting

b. Metallic taste in the mouth

c. Orthostatic hypotension

d. Jaundice

e. Mental changes

f. Peripheral neuritis

g. Rash

4. Interventions

a. Assess liver and renal function tests.

b. Monitor glucose levels in the client with diabetes mellitus.

c. Administer pyridoxine as prescribed to reduce the risk of neurotoxicity.

5. Client education

a. Instruct the client to take medication with food or meals to minimize gastrointestinal irritation.

b. Instruct the client to change positions slowly.

c. Instruct the client to report signs of a rash, which can progress to exfoliative dermatitis if the medication is not discontinued.

d. Instruct the client to avoid alcohol.

e. Instruct the client to report signs of jaundice and other side effects of the medication if they occur.

D. Aminosalicylate sodium (Tubasal)

1. Description

a. Aminosalicylate inhibits folic acid metabolism in mycobacteria.

b. Aminosalicylate is used to treat **MDR-TB** when significant resistance to other medications is expected.

2. Contraindications and cautions

a. Aminosalicylate is contraindicated with hypersensitivity to aminosalicylates, salicylates, or compounds containing para-aminophenyl group.

b. Aminobenzoates block the absorption of aminosalicylate sodium.

3. Side effects
   a. Hypersensitivity
   b. Bitter taste in the mouth
   c. Gastrointestinal tract irritation
   d. Exfoliative dermatitis
   e. Blood dyscrasias
   f. Crystalluria
   g. Changes in thyroid function
4. Interventions
   a. Assess for hypersensitivity.
   b. Offer clear water to rinse the mouth and chewing gum or hard candy to alleviate the bitter taste.
   c. Encourage fluid intake to prevent crystalluria.
   d. Monitor intake and output.
5. Client education
   a. Instruct the client to discard the medication and obtain a new supply if a purplish brown discoloration occurs.
   b. Instruct the client to take the medication with food.
   c. Inform the client that urine may turn red on contact with hypochlorite bleach if bleach was used to clean a toilet.
   d. Instruct the client not to take aspirin or over-the-counter medications without the physician's approval.
   e. Inform the client with diabetes mellitus that a false-positive result can occur in glucose monitoring.
   f. Instruct the client to report signs of a blood dyscrasia, such as sore throat or mouth, malaise, fatigue, bruising, or bleeding.

E. Cycloserine (Seromycin)
1. Description
   a. Cycloserine interferes with cell wall biosynthesis.
   b. Cycloserine is used to treat **MDR-TB** when significant resistance to other medications is expected.
2. Contraindications and cautions
   a. Use of alcohol or ethionamide (Trecator-SC) increases the risk of seizures.
   b. Use cycloserine with caution in clients with epilepsy, depression, severe anxiety, psychosis, or renal insufficiency, or the client who uses alcohol.
3. Side effects
   a. Hypersensitivity
   b. CNS reactions
   c. Neurotoxicity
   d. Seizures
   e. Congestive heart failure
   f. Headache
   g. Vertigo
   h. Altered level of consciousness
   i. Irritability, nervousness, anxiety
   j. Confusion
   k. Mood changes, depression, thoughts of suicide

4. Interventions
   a. Monitor level of consciousness.
   b. Monitor for changes in mental status and thought processes.
   c. Monitor renal and hepatic function tests.
   d. Monitor serum drug level to avoid the risk of neurotoxicity; peak concentrations, measured 2 hours after dosing, should be 25 to 35 mcg/mL.
5. Client education
   a. Instruct the client to take the medication after meals to prevent gastrointestinal upset.
   b. Instruct the client to avoid alcohol.
   c. Instruct the client to report signs of a rash or signs of CNS toxicity.
   d. Instruct the client to avoid driving or performing tasks that require alertness until the reaction to the medication has been determined.
   e. Advise the client of the need for serum drug levels weekly, as prescribed.

PRACTICE QUESTIONS

1. A nurse is preparing to administer albuterol (Proventil) to a client. The nurse assesses which of the following parameters before and during therapy?
   1. Urine output and blood urea nitrogen
   2. Nausea and vomiting
   3. Lung sounds and presence of dyspnea
   4. Headache and level of consciousness
2. A home care nurse has observed a client self-administer a dose of metaproterenol sulfate (Alupent) via metered dose inhaler. Within a short time, the client begins to wheeze loudly. The nurse interprets that this is due to
   1. Insufficient dosage of the medication, which needs to be increased.
   2. Probable interaction of this medication with an over-the-counter cold remedy.
   3. Tolerance to the medication, indicating a need for a stronger type of bronchodilator.
   4. Paradoxical bronchospasm, which must be reported to the physician.
3. A nurse has an order to give a client metaproterenol sulfate (Alupent), two puffs, and beclomethasone (Vanceril), two puffs, by metered dose inhaler. The nurse administers the medication by giving the
   1. Beclomethasone first and then the metaproterenol.
   2. Metaproterenol first and then the beclomethasone.
   3. Alternating a single puff of each, beginning with the beclomethasone.
   4. Alternating a single puff of each, beginning with the metaproterenol.
4. A client receiving theophylline is due to have a theophylline level drawn. A nurse questions the client to ensure that the client has not ingested which of the following substances before the blood sample is drawn?

1. Sedatives
2. Narcotics
3. Glucose
4. Caffeine

5. A client has begun therapy with oxtriphylline (Choledyl). A nurse plans to teach the client to limit the intake of which of the following while taking this medication?
   1. Oysters, lobster, and shrimp
   2. Coffee, cola, and chocolate
   3. Cottage cheese, cream cheese, and dairy creamers
   4. Grapefruit, oranges, and pineapple

6. A nurse has administered a dose of salmeterol (Serevent) to a client. The client develops a generalized rash and urticaria, and the eyelids begin to swell. The nurse should
   1. Call the physician immediately.
   2. Encourage the client to drink fluids quickly.
   3. Apply a lanolin-based cream to the rash.
   4. Assess the client's vision with a Snellen chart.

7. A client is receiving acetylcysteine (Mucomyst) by nebulizer. A nurse should have which of the following items available for possible use after giving this medication?
   1. Suction equipment
   2. Nasogastric tube
   3. Intubation tray
   4. Ambu bag

8. A client has an order to take guaifenesin (Humibid L.A.). A nurse concludes that the client understands the most effective use of this medication if the client states to
   1. Take the tablet with a full glass of water.
   2. Take an extra dose if the cough is accompanied by fever.
   3. Watch for irritability as a side effect.
   4. Crush the sustained-release tablet if immediate relief is needed.

9. A nurse is preparing to administer a dose of naloxone hydrochloride (Narcan) intravenously to a client with an intravenous narcotic overdose. The nurse plans to have which of the following available as supportive equipment in case it is needed?
   1. Nasogastric tube
   2. Paracentesis tray
   3. Central line insertion tray
   4. Resuscitation equipment

10. A nurse teaches a client about the effects of diphenhydramine hydrochloride (Benadryl), which has been ordered as a cough suppressant. The nurse determines that the client needs further instructions if the client states to
    1. Avoid driving or other activities requiring mental alertness while taking this medication.
    2. Use sugarless gum, candy, or oral rinses to decrease dry mouth.
    3. Avoid using alcohol while taking this medication.
    4. Take the medication on an empty stomach.

11. A client has been prescribed a cough formula containing codeine sulfate. A nurse has given the client instructions for its use. The nurse concludes that the client understands the instructions if the client verbalizes to self-assess for
    1. Excitability.
    2. Constipation.
    3. Rapid pulse.
    4. Excessive urination.

12. A cromolyn sodium (Intal) inhaler is prescribed for a client with allergic asthma. A nurse provides instructions regarding the side effects of this medication. Which of the following undesirable side effects is associated with this medication?
    1. Constipation
    2. Hypotension
    3. Insomnia
    4. Bronchospasm

13. Terbutaline sulfate (Brethine) is prescribed for a client with bronchitis. A nurse understands that this medication should be used with caution if which of the following existing medical conditions is present in the client?
    1. Hypothyroidism
    2. Polycystic disease
    3. Osteoarthritis
    4. Diabetes mellitus

14. Zafirlukast (Accolate) is prescribed for a client with bronchial asthma. Which laboratory test does the nurse expect to be prescribed before the administration of this medication?
    1. Platelet count
    2. Complete blood count
    3. Liver function tests
    4. Neutrophil count

15. A client has been taking isoniazid (INH) for a month and a half. The client complains to a nurse about numbness, paresthesias, and tingling in the extremities. The nurse interprets that the client is experiencing
    1. Small blood vessel spasm.
    2. Impaired peripheral circulation.
    3. Hypercalcemia.
    4. Peripheral neuritis.

16. A client is to begin a 6-month course of therapy with isoniazid (INH). A nurse plans to teach the client to
    1. Use alcohol in small amounts only.
    2. Report yellow eyes or skin immediately.
    3. Increase intake of Swiss or aged cheeses.
    4. Avoid vitamin supplements during therapy.

17. A client has been started on long-term therapy with rifampin (Rifadin). A nurse teaches the client that the medication

1. Should be double dosed if one dose is forgotten.
2. May be discontinued independently if symptoms are gone in 3 months.
3. Causes orange discoloration of sweat, tears, urine, and feces.
4. Should always be taken with food or antacids.

18. A nurse has given a client taking ethambutol (Myambutol) information about the medication. The nurse determines that the client understands the instructions if the client states to immediately report
1. Gastrointestinal side effects.
2. Impaired sense of hearing.
3. Orange-red discoloration of body secretions.
4. Difficulty in discriminating the color red from green.

19. Cycloserine (Seromycin) is added to the medication regimen for a client with tuberculosis. Which of the following would the nurse include in the client teaching plan regarding this medication?
1. Take the medication before meals.
2. Return to the clinic weekly for serum drug levels.

3. It is not necessary to call the physician if a skin rash occurs.
4. It is not necessary to restrict alcohol intake with this medication.

20. A client with tuberculosis is being started on anti-tuberculosis therapy with isoniazid (INH). Before giving the client the first dose, a nurse ensures that which of the following baseline studies has been completed?
1. Coagulation times
2. Electrolytes
3. Serum creatinine
4. Liver enzymes

CRITICAL THINKING: FILL IN THE BLANK

A nurse receives a report of the serum theophylline level of a client receiving theophylline by continuous intravenous infusion. The result is 18 mcg/mL. The nurse documents what interpretation regarding this result?

Answer: _____

ANSWERS

1. 3
Rationale: Albuterol is a bronchodilator of the adrenergic type. The nurse assesses respiratory pattern, lung sounds, pulse, and blood pressure before and during therapy. The nurse also notes the color, character, and amount of sputum.
Test-Taking Strategy: Use the process of elimination. Knowing that this medication is a bronchodilator allows you to eliminate each of the incorrect options. Use the ABCs—airway, breathing, and circulation—to answer the question. Option 3 is the only option that addresses airway. Review this medication if you had difficulty with this question.
Level of Cognitive Ability: Application
Client Needs: Physiological Integrity
Integrated Process: Nursing Process—assessment
Content Area: Pharmacology
Reference: Hodgson, B., & Kizior, R. (2004). *Saunders nursing drug handbook 2004* (p. 19). Philadelphia: W. B. Saunders.

2. 4
Rationale: The client taking adrenergic bronchodilators may experience paradoxical bronchospasm, which is evidenced by the client's wheezing. This can occur with excessive use of inhalers. Further medication should be withheld, and the physician should be notified. Options 1, 2, and 3 are incorrect interpretations.
Test-Taking Strategy: Use the process of elimination. Eliminate option 1 first because the client began wheezing after the medication was administered and not before. Option 3 may be eliminated next because tolerance generally does not occur. From the remaining options, knowing that wheezing is associated with bronchospasm will direct you to option 4. Review the side effects associated with the use of inhaled bronchodilators if you had difficulty with this question.

Level of Cognitive Ability: Analysis
Client Needs: Physiological Integrity
Integrated Process: Nursing Process—analysis
Content Area: Pharmacology
Reference: Hodgson, B., & Kizior, R. (2004). *Saunders nursing drug handbook 2004* (p.644). Philadelphia: W. B. Saunders.

3. 2
Rationale: Metaproterenol sulfate is an adrenergic type of bronchodilator. Beclomethasone is a glucocorticoid. Bronchodilators are always administered before glucocorticoids when both are to be given on the same time schedule. This allows for widening of the air passages by the bronchodilator, which then makes the glucocorticoid more effective.
Test-Taking Strategy: Use the process of elimination. To answer this question correctly, you must know two different things. First, you must know that a bronchodilator is always given before a glucocorticoid. This would allow you to eliminate options 3 and 4 because you would not alternate the medications. To discriminate between options 1 and 2, you must know that metaproterenol is a bronchodilator, whereas beclomethasone is a glucocorticoid. Review these medications if you had difficulty with this question.
Level of Cognitive Ability: Application
Client Needs: Physiological Integrity
Integrated Process: Nursing Process—implementation
Content Area: Pharmacology
Reference: Hodgson, B., & Kizior, R. (2004). *Saunders nursing drug handbook 2004* (p. 97). Philadelphia: W. B. Saunders.

4. 4
Rationale: Theophylline is a xanthine bronchodilator. Before drawing of a serum level of the medication, the client should avoid taking in foods or beverages that contain xanthine, such

as colas, coffee, or chocolate. Thus the client is told to avoid caffeine intake before the test.

Test-Taking Strategy: Use the process of elimination. Recalling that this medication is a xanthine bronchodilator will direct you to option 4. Review client teaching points related to this medication if you had difficulty with this question.

Level of Cognitive Ability: Application
Client Needs: Physiological Integrity
Integrated Process: Nursing Process—assessment
Content Area: Pharmacology
Reference: Hodgson, B., & Kizior, R. (2004). *Saunders nursing drug handbook 2004* (p. 44). Philadelphia: W. B. Saunders.

5. 2
Rationale: Oxtriphylline (Choledyl) is a xanthine bronchodilator. The nurse teaches the client to limit the intake of xanthine-containing foods while taking this medication. These foods include coffee, cola, and chocolate.

Test-Taking Strategy: Use the process of elimination. You must understand that oxtriphylline is a xanthine bronchodilator and know that intake of excessive amounts of foods naturally high in xanthines should be curtailed. Review the foods naturally high in xanthines if you had difficulty with this question.

Level of Cognitive Ability: Application
Client Needs: Physiological Integrity
Integrated Process: Teaching/Learning
Content Area: Pharmacology
Reference: McKenry, L., & Salerno, E. (2003). *Mosby's pharmacology in nursing* (21st ed., p. 724) St. Louis: Mosby.

6. 1
Rationale: Hypersensitivity reaction can occur in clients taking ephedrine, epinephrine, isoproterenol, or salmeterol. Signs and symptoms include rash, urticaria, and swelling of the face, lips, or eyelids. The nurse should call the physician immediately if any of these occur. The other options are incorrect.

Test-Taking Strategy: Use the process of elimination. Recognizing that the signs and symptoms listed in the question are typical of a hypersensitivity reaction allows you to eliminate options 3 and 4 first. From the remaining options, recall that the client needs treatment with an antihistamine or epinephrine, not oral fluids. Review this medication if the question was difficult.

Level of Cognitive Ability: Application
Client Needs: Physiological Integrity
Integrated Process: Nursing Process—implementation
Content Area: Pharmacology
Reference: Gutierrez, K., & Queener, S. (2003). *Pharmacology for nursing practice* (p. 850). St. Louis: Mosby.

7. 1
Rationale: Acetylcysteine can be given orally or by a nasogastric tube to treat acetaminophen overdose, or it may be given by inhalation for use as a mucolytic. The nurse administering this medication as a mucolytic should have suction equipment available in case the client cannot manage to clear the increased volume of liquefied secretions.

Test-Taking Strategy: Use the process of elimination. Note the key word "nebulizer." This will assist in directing you to option 1. If you had difficulty with this question, review the purpose of this medication and the related nursing interventions.

Level of Cognitive Ability: Application
Client Needs: Physiological Integrity
Integrated Process: Nursing Process—implementation
Content Area: Pharmacology
Reference: Hodgson, B., & Kizior, R. (2004). *Saunders nursing drug handbook 2004* (p. 11). Philadelphia: W. B. Saunders.

8. 1
Rationale: Guaifenesin (Humibid L.A.) is an expectorant and should be taken with a full glass of water to decrease viscosity of secretions. Sustained-release preparations should not be broken open, crushed, or chewed. The medication occasionally may cause dizziness, headache, or drowsiness as side effects. The client should contact the physician if the cough lasts longer than 1 week or is accompanied by fever, rash, sore throat, or persistent headache.

Test-Taking Strategy: Use the process of elimination. Begin to answer this question by eliminating option 4 first. Sustained-released preparations are not crushed or broken. Option 2 is eliminated next because fever indicates infection, and an "extra dose" of an expectorant is not helpful in treating infection. From the remaining options, knowing that increased fluids helps to liquefy secretions for more effective coughing directs you to option 1 as correct. If you had difficulty with this question, review this medication.

Level of Cognitive Ability: Analysis
Client Needs: Physiological Integrity
Integrated Process: Teaching/Learning
Content Area: Pharmacology
Reference: Gutierrez, K., & Queener, S. (2003). *Pharmacology for nursing practice* (p. 886). St. Louis: Mosby.

9. 4
Rationale: The nurse administering naloxone for suspected narcotic overdose should have resuscitation equipment readily available to support naloxone therapy if it is needed. Other adjuncts that may be needed include oxygen, mechanical ventilator, and vasopressors.

Test-Taking Strategy: Use the process of elimination. Note the key words "intravenous narcotic overdose." Recalling the effects of these medications will direct you to option 4. Option 4 is also the most global response. Review this medication if you had difficulty with this question.

Level of Cognitive Ability: Application
Client Needs: Physiological Integrity
Integrated Process: Nursing Process—planning
Content Area: Pharmacology
Reference: Kee, J., & Hayes, E. (2003). *Pharmacology: A nursing process approach* (4th ed., p. 314). Philadelphia: W. B. Saunders.

10. 4
Rationale: Diphenhydramine (Benadryl) has several uses, including antihistamine, antitussive, antidyskinetic, and sedative/hypnotic. Instructions for use include to take with food or milk to decrease gastrointestinal upset and to use oral rinses or sugarless gum or hard candy to minimize dry mouth. Because the medication causes drowsiness, the client should avoid use of alcohol or central nervous system depressants, operating a car, or engaging in other activities requiring mental awareness during use.

Test-Taking Strategy: Use the process of elimination, noting the key words "needs further instructions." Knowing that the medication has a sedative effect helps you to eliminate options 1 and 3 first. Recalling that the medication causes a dry mouth helps you choose option 4 as the answer to the question, according to the way the question is stated. If you had difficulty with this question, review client education related to this medication.
Level of Cognitive Ability: Analysis
Client Needs: Physiological Integrity
Integrated Process: Teaching/Learning
Content Area: Pharmacology
Reference: Hodgson, B., & Kizior, R. (2004). *Saunders nursing drug handbook 2004* (p. 834). Philadelphia: W. B. Saunders.

11. 2
Rationale: The client is taught about side effects that could occur with the use of codeine sulfate. The most common side effects include drowsiness, confusion, hypotension, nausea and vomiting, and constipation. Others include bradycardia, respiratory depression, and urinary retention.
Test-Taking Strategy: Use the process of elimination. Remember that codeine sulfate causes constipation. Review the side effects of this medication if you had difficulty with this question.
Level of Cognitive Ability: Analysis
Client Needs: Physiological Integrity
Integrated Process: Teaching/Learning
Content Area: Pharmacology
Reference: Hodgson, B., & Kizior, R. (2004). *Saunders nursing drug handbook 2004* (p. 239). Philadelphia: W. B. Saunders.

12. 4
Rationale: The most common undesired side effects associated with inhalation therapy of cromolyn sodium (Intal) are bronchospasm, cough, nasal congestion, throat irritation, and wheezing. Clients receiving this medication orally may experience pruritis, nausea, diarrhea, and myalgia.
Test-Taking Strategy: Use the process of elimination. Note the key words "undesirable side effects." This should assist in directing you to option 4. In addition, use the ABCs—airway, breathing, and circulation—to select the correct option. Option 4 addresses airway. Review the undesirable side effects of this medication if you had difficulty with this question.
Level of Cognitive Ability: Analysis
Client Needs: Physiological Integrity
Integrated Process: Teaching/Learning
Content Area: Pharmacology
Reference: Hodgson, B., & Kizior, R. (2004). *Saunders nursing drug handbook 2004* (p. 253). Philadelphia: W. B. Saunders.

13. 4
Rationale: Terbutaline sulfate (Brethine) is contraindicated in clients with hypersensitivity to sympathomimetics and should be used with caution in clients with impaired cardiac function, diabetes mellitus, hypertension, or hyperthyroidism, and clients with a history of seizures. The medication may increase blood glucose levels.
Test-Taking Strategy: This is a difficult question, and knowledge regarding this medication is required to answer correctly. Review the contraindications associated with this medication

if you are unfamiliar with them.
Level of Cognitive Ability: Analysis
Client Needs: Physiological Integrity
Integrated Process: Nursing Process—analysis
Content Area: Pharmacology
Reference: Kee, J., & Hayes, E. (2003). *Pharmacology: A nursing process approach* (4th ed., p. 329). Philadelphia: W. B. Saunders.

14. 3
Rationale: Zafirlukast (Accolate) is a leukotriene receptor antagonist used in the prophylaxis and long-term treatment of bronchial asthma. Zafirlukast is used with caution in clients with impaired hepatic function. Liver function laboratory tests should be performed to obtain a baseline, and the levels should be monitored during administration of the medication.
Test-Taking Strategy: Use the process of elimination, eliminating options 2 and 4 first because a complete blood count would include a neutrophil count. From the remaining options, you would need to know that this medication would affect hepatic function. If you had difficulty with this question, review this medication.
Level of Cognitive Ability: Analysis
Client Needs: Physiological Integrity
Integrated Process: Nursing Process—analysis
Content Area: Pharmacology
Reference: Hodgson, B., & Kizior, R. (2004). *Saunders nursing drug handbook 2004* (p. 1067). Philadelphia: W. B. Saunders.

15. 4
Rationale: A common side effect of isoniazid (INH) is peripheral neuritis. This is manifested by numbness, tingling, and paresthesias in the extremities. This side effect can be minimized with pyridoxine (vitamin B_6) intake. Options 1, 2, and 3 are incorrect.
Test-Taking Strategy: Use the process of elimination. Options 1 and 2 would not cause the symptoms presented in the question but instead would cause pallor and coolness. From the remaining options, you should know that peripheral neuritis is a side effect of the medication or that these signs and symptoms do not correlate with hypercalcemia. Review the side effects associated with isoniazid if you had difficulty with this question.
Level of Cognitive Ability: Analysis
Client Needs: Physiological Integrity
Integrated Process: Nursing Process—analysis
Content Area: Pharmacology
Reference: Kee, J., & Hayes, E. (2003). Pharmacology: *A nursing process approach* (4th ed., pp. 435-436). Philadelphia: W. B. Saunders.

16. 2
Rationale: Isoniazid (INH) is hepatotoxic, and therefore the client is taught to report signs and symptoms of hepatitis immediately (which include yellow skin and sclera). For the same reason, alcohol should be avoided during therapy. The client should avoid intake of Swiss cheese, fish such as tuna, and foods containing tyramine because they may cause a reaction characterized by redness and itching of the skin, flushing, sweating, tachycardia, headache, or light-headedness. The client can avoid developing peripheral neuritis by increasing

the intake of pyridoxine (vitamin B_6) during the course of isoniazid therapy.

Test-Taking Strategy: Use the process of elimination. Because alcohol intake is prohibited with the use of many medications, eliminate option 1 first. Because the client receiving this medication typically is given supplements of vitamin B_6, option 4 is incorrect and is eliminated next. Recalling that the medication is hepatotoxic will direct you to option 2. If you had difficulty with this question, review this medication.

Level of Cognitive Ability: Application
Client Needs: Physiological Integrity
Integrated Process: Teaching/Learning
Content Area: Pharmacology
Reference: Hodgson, B., & Kizior, R. (2004). *Saunders nursing drug handbook 2004* (p. 560). Philadelphia: W. B. Saunders.

17. 3

Rationale: Rifampin should be taken exactly as directed. Doses should not be doubled or skipped. The client should not stop therapy until directed to do so by a physician. The medication should be administered on an empty stomach unless it causes gastrointestinal upset, and then it may be taken with food. Antacids, if prescribed, should be taken at least 1 hour before the medication. Rifampin causes orange-red discoloration of body secretions and will stain soft contact lenses permanently.

Test-Taking Strategy: Use the process of elimination. Options 1 and 2 are inaccurate in general and are eliminated first. Eliminate option 4 next because of the absolute word "always." If you had difficulty with this question, review the side effects associated with this medication.

Level of Cognitive Ability: Application
Client Needs: Physiological Integrity
Integrated Process: Teaching/Learning
Content Area: Pharmacology
Reference: Kee, J., & Hayes, E. (2003). *Pharmacology: A nursing process approach* (4th ed., p. 436). Philadelphia: W. B. Saunders.

18. 4

Rationale: Ethambutol causes optic neuritis, which decreases visual acuity and the ability to discriminate between the colors red and green. This poses a potential safety hazard when a client is driving a motor vehicle. The client is taught to report this symptom immediately. The client also is taught to take the medication with food if gastrointestinal upset occurs. Impaired hearing results from antitubercular therapy with streptomycin. Orange-red discoloration of secretions occurs with rifampin (Rifadin).

Test-Taking Strategy: Use the process of elimination. Option 1 is the least likely symptom to report; rather it should be managed by taking the medication with food. To discriminate among the other options, you must know that this medication causes optic neuritis, resulting in difficulty with red-green discrimination. If this question was difficult, review antitubercular medications because the incorrect options for this question are typical side effects of other antitubercular medications.

Level of Cognitive Ability: Analysis
Client Needs: Physiological Integrity
Integrated Process: Teaching/Learning
Content Area: Pharmacology

Reference: Hodgson, B., & Kizior, R. (2004). *Saunders nursing drug handbook 2004* (pp. 388, 389). Philadelphia: W. B. Saunders.

19. 2

Rationale: Cycloserine (Seromycin) is an antitubercular medication that requires weekly serum drug level determinations to monitor for the potential of neurotoxicity. Serum drug levels less than 30 mg/mL reduce the incidence of neurotoxicity. The medication needs to be taken after meals to prevent gastrointestinal irritation. The client needs to be instructed to notify the physician if a skin rash or early signs of central nervous system toxicity are noted. Alcohol needs to be avoided because it increases the risk of seizure activity.

Test-Taking Strategy: Use the process of elimination. Eliminate options 3 and 4 first because they are the least likely correct options. From this point, knowing that the medication level needs to be monitored will assist in selecting the correct option. If you had difficulty with this question, review this medication.

Level of Cognitive Ability: Application
Client Needs: Physiological Integrity
Integrated Process: Teaching/Learning
Content Area: Pharmacology
Reference: Kee, J., & Hayes, E. (2003). *Pharmacology: A nursing process approach* (4th ed., p. 435). Philadelphia: W. B. Saunders.

20. 4

Rationale: Isoniazid (INH) therapy can cause an elevation of hepatic enzymes and hepatitis. Therefore liver enzymes are monitored when therapy is initiated and during the first 3 months of therapy. They may be monitored longer in the client who is over age 50 or abuses alcohol.

Test-Taking Strategy: Use the process of elimination. To answer this question correctly, you must know that this medication can be toxic to the liver. Review the adverse effects of the various anti-tuberculosis medications if this is an area that is unfamiliar to you.

Level of Cognitive Ability: Application
Client Needs: Physiological Integrity
Integrated Process: Nursing Process—assessment
Content Area: Pharmacology
Reference: Kee, J., & Hayes, E. (2003). *Pharmacology: A nursing process approach* (4th ed., p. 433). Philadelphia: W. B. Saunders.

CRITICAL THINKING: FILL IN THE BLANK

Answer: The theophylline blood level is within the therapeutic range.

Rationale: The normal therapeutic range for a theophylline level is 10 to 20 mcg/mL. A level greater than 20 mcg/mL is considered toxic. The value of 18 mcg/mL places the client within the therapeutic range.

Test-Taking Strategy: You must know the therapeutic theophylline level to interpret this result. Review this therapeutic range if you had difficulty with this question.

Level of Cognitive Ability: Analysis
Client Needs: Physiological Integrity
Integrated Process: Nursing Process—analysis
Content Area: Pharmacology
Reference: Kee, J., & Hayes, E. (2003). *Pharmacology: A nursing process approach* (4th ed., p. 556). Philadelphia: W. B. Saunders.

REFERENCES

Gutierrez, K., & Queener, S. (2003). *Pharmacology for nursing practice.* St. Louis: Mosby.

Hodgson, B., & Kizior, R. (2004). *Saunders nursing drug handbook 2004.* Philadelphia: W. B. Saunders.

Kee, J., & Hayes, E. (2003). *Pharmacology: A nursing process approach* (4th ed.). Philadelphia: W. B. Saunders.

McKenry, L., & Salerno, E. (2003). *Mosby's pharmacology in nursing* (21st ed.) St. Louis: Mosby.

The Adult Client with a Cardiovascular Disorder

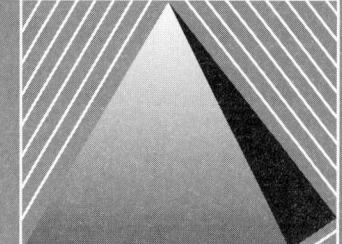

PYRAMID TERMS

afterload The force against which the heart has to pump to eject blood from the ventricle. Factors and conditions that would impede blood flow increase left ventricular afterload.

arterial anastomoses Arterial connections that ensure that when one of the blood-supplying arteries is damaged, flow is maintained from the other arteries. Blood flow to the hands, feet, brain, and other organs is protected by arterial anastomoses.

arterial pressure The pressure of the blood against the arterial walls. Pressure can be measured indirectly by sphygmomanometer or directly by arterial catheter. Readings are expressed as systolic over diastolic. Arterial pressure increases when the cardiac output, peripheral resistance, or blood volume increases.

automaticity The ability of cardiac cells to initiate an impulse spontaneously and repetitively without external neurohormonal control. The pacemaker cells have the highest rate of automaticity of all cardiac cells.

baroreceptors Specialized nerve endings located in the walls of the aortic arch and carotid sinuses that are affected by changes in the arterial blood pressure. Increases in arterial pressure stimulate baroreceptors and the heart rate and arterial pressure decrease. Decreases in arterial pressure lead to a lessened stimulation of the baroreceptors, and vasoconstriction occurs, as does an increase in heart rate. Also called pressoreceptors.

blood pressure The force exerted by the blood against the walls of the blood vessels. If the blood pressure falls too low, blood flow to the tissues, heart, brain, and other organs become inadequate. If the blood pressure becomes too high, the risk of vessel rupture and damage increases.

capillary pressure or hydrostatic pressure The pressure exerted by the blood against the capillary wall. Normal capillary pressure is 25 to 30 mm Hg at the arterial end of the capillaries, and 10 to 15 mm Hg at the venous end.

cardiac output The total volume of blood pumped through the heart in 1 minute. The normal cardiac output is 4 to 8 L per minute. Cardiac output equals stroke volume multiplied by heart rate.

chemoreceptors Nerve endings located in the aortic arch and carotid bodies that are stimulated by hypoxemia and that then transmit impulses to the central nervous system.

conductivity The ability of the heart muscle fibers to propagate electrical impulses along and across cell membranes.

contractility The inherent ability of the myocardium to alter contractile force and velocity. Sympathetic stimulation increases myocardial contractility, thus increases stroke volume. Conditions that decrease myocardial contractility reduce stroke volume.

diastole The phase of the cardiac cycle in which the heart relaxes between contractions. Diastole represents the period of time when the two ventricles are dilated by the blood flowing into them.

diastolic pressure The force of the blood exerted against the artery walls when the heart relaxes or fills.

excitability The ability of cardiac muscle cells to depolarize in response to a stimulus. Excitability is influenced by hormones, electrolytes, nutrition, oxygen supply, medication, infections, and nerve characteristics.

Frank-Starling law The principle that the more the heart fills within reasonable limits during diastole, the greater the force of contraction during systole and the greater the stroke volume. The exception to the law is during heart failure, when increasing blood volume into the ventricle decreases stroke volume. If the left ventricle fills to such an extent that it overdistends the myocardium, cardiac output begins to decrease and the heart begins to fail.

hepatojugular reflux Jugular vein distention induced when pressure is applied over the liver. Position the client with the head of the bed elevated 45 degrees and locate the internal jugular vein. Compress the upper right abdomen for 30 to 40 seconds. Sudden distention of the neck veins after abdominal compression usually indicates failure of the right side of the heart.

mean arterial pressure The equivalent of one third of the pulse pressure plus the diastolic blood pressure. Mean arterial pressure is used in hemodynamic monitoring.

paradoxical blood pressure An exaggerated decrease in systolic pressure by more than 10 mm Hg during the inspiratory phase of the respiratory cycle. Normal value is 3 to 10 mm Hg.

postural (orthostatic) hypotension A blood pressure fall of more than 10 to 15 mm Hg of the systolic pressure or a fall of more than 10 mm Hg of the diastolic pressure and a 10% to 20% increase in heart rate. Postural hypotension occurs when the client's blood pressure is not maintained adequately when moving from a lying to a sitting or standing position.

preload The volume of blood stretching the left ventricle at the end of diastole. Preload is determined by the total circulating blood volume and is increased by an increase in venous return to the heart.

pulse pressure The difference between the systolic and diastolic pressure. Normal pulse pressure is 30 to 40 mm Hg.

refractoriness The inability of the heart to respond to a new stimulus while still in a state of contraction from an earlier stimulus. Refractoriness prevents uncontrolled rapid cardiac contractions and helps to preserve the heart rhythm.

stretch receptors Nerve endings located in the vena cava and the right atrium that respond to pressure changes that affect circulatory blood volume. When the blood pressure decreases because of hypovolemia, a sympathetic response occurs, causing an increased heart rate and blood vessel constriction. When the blood pressure increases because of hypervolemia, an opposite effect occurs.

stroke volume The amount of blood ejected from the left ventricle with each contraction. The normal stroke volume is 70 to 130 mL per heart beat. The stroke volume can be affected by preload, afterload, contractility, and the Frank-Starling law.

systole The phase of contraction of the heart, especially of the ventricles, during which blood is forced into the aorta and pulmonary artery.

systolic pressure The maximum pressure of blood exerted against the artery walls when the heart contracts.

venous pressure The force exerted by the blood against the vein walls. Normal venous pressures are highest in the extremities (5 to 14 cm of H_2O in the arm), and lowest closest to the heart (6 to 8 cm of H_2O in the inferior vena cava).

▶ PYRAMID TO SUCCESS

Pyramid Points focus on assessment data related to cardiovascular risks, health screening and promotion, complications of the various cardiovascular disorders, emergency implementation measures, and client education. Focus on the assessment findings in angina, myocardial infarction, congestive heart failure and pulmonary edema, pericarditis, dysrhythmias, pacemakers, aneurysms, hypertension, and arterial and venous disorders. You must be able to identify the most common dysrhythmias and determine the appropriate interventions for these dysrhythmias. Focus also on the care of the client following diagnostic treatments and surgical procedures. Note appropriate and therapeutic client positions, particularly with arterial and venous disorders of the extremities. Focus on treatments and medications prescribed for the various cardiovascular disorders and client teaching related to prescribed treatment plans. Be familiar with the components related to cardiac rehabilitation. The Integrated Processes addressed in this unit include Nursing Process, Caring, Communication and Documentation, and Teaching/Learning.

CLIENT NEEDS
Safe, Effective Care Environment

Cardiovascular consultations and referrals
Client rights
Consultation with members of the health care team
Establishing priorities
Informed consent related to treatments and procedures
Medical and surgical asepsis
Standard precautions

Health Promotion and Maintenance

Alterations in lifestyle
Cardiac rehabilitation
Cardiovascular assessment techniques
Health screening and health promotion programs
Mobilization of appropriate community resources
Prevention of cardiovascular disease
Teaching related to diet therapy, exercise, and medications

Psychosocial Integrity

Accepting lifestyle changes
Coping mechanisms
End of life
Fear, anxiety, and denial
Grief and loss
Religious, spiritual, and cultural influences on health
Situational role changes
Support systems
Unexpected body image changes

Physiological Integrity

Activity limitations and rest and sleep
Administration of intravenous medications
Assisting with basic care measures
Hemodynamics
Interventions required in emergencies
Medical emergencies
Monitoring for complications related to cardiovascular disorders
Monitoring for therapeutic effects of medications
Monitoring of cardiac enzymes, troponin levels, and laboratory values related to the cardiovascular system
Nonpharmacological and pharmacological comfort interventions

REFERENCES

Chernecky, C., & Berger, B. (2004). *Laboratory tests & diagnostic procedures* (4th ed.). Philadelphia: W. B. Saunders.

Harkreader, H., & Hogan, M. A. (2004). *Fundamentals of nursing: Caring and clinical judgment* (2nd ed.). Philadelphia: W. B. Saunders.

Ignatavicius, D., & Workman, M. (2002). *Medical-surgical nursing: Critical thinking for collaborative care* (4th ed.). Philadelphia: W. B. Saunders.

Jarvis, C. (2000). *Physical examination & health assessment* (3rd ed.). Philadelphia: W. B. Saunders.

Lewis, S., Heitkemper, M., & Dirksen, S. (2004). *Medical-surgical nursing: Assessment and management of clinical problems* (6th ed.). St. Louis: Mosby.

National Council of State Boards of Nursing (Eds.) (2003). *Test Plan for the National Council Licensure Examination for Registered Nurses* (effective date: April 2004). Chicago: Author.

Perry, A., & Potter, P. (2002). *Clinical nursing skills and techniques* (5th ed.). St. Louis: Mosby.

Phipps, W., Monahan, F., Sands, J., Marek, J., & Neighbors, M. (2003). *Medical-surgical nursing: Health and illness perspectives* (7th ed.). St. Louis: Mosby.

Potter, P., & Perry, A. (2001). *Fundamentals of nursing* (5th ed.). St. Louis: Mosby.

Stuart, G., & Laraia, M. (2001). *Principles and practice of psychiatric nursing* (7th ed.). St. Louis: Mosby.

Varcarolis, E. M. (2002). *Foundations of psychiatric mental health nursing* (4th ed.). Philadelphia: W. B. Saunders.

Cardiovascular Disorders

I. ANATOMY AND PHYSIOLOGY

A. Heart and heart layers
1. The heart is located in the left side of the mediastinum.
2. The epicardium covers the outer surface of the heart.
3. The myocardium is the middle layer and is the actual contracting muscle of the heart.
4. The endocardium is the innermost layer and lines the inner chambers and heart valves.

B. Pericardium
1. The pericardium encases and protects the heart from trauma and infection.
2. The parietal pericardium is the tough, fibrous outer membrane that attaches anteriorly to the lower half of the sternum, posteriorly to the thoracic vertebrae, and inferiorly to the diaphragm.
3. The visceral pericardium is the thin, inner layer that closely adheres to the heart.
4. The pericardial space is between the parietal and visceral layers; it holds 5 to 20 mL of pericardial fluid, which lubricates the pericardial surfaces and cushions the heart.

C. Heart chambers
1. The right atrium receives deoxygenated blood from the body via the superior and inferior vena cava.
2. The right ventricle receives blood from the right atrium and pumps it to the lungs via the pulmonary artery.
3. The left atrium receives oxygenated blood from the lungs via four pulmonary veins.
4. The left ventricle is the largest and most muscular chamber; it receives oxygenated blood from the lungs via the left atrium and pumps blood into the systemic circulation via the aorta.

D. Heart valves
1. The atrioventricular valves lie between the atria and the ventricles.
2. The atrioventricular valves close at the beginning of ventricular contraction and prevent blood from flowing back into the atria from the ventricles; these valves open when the ventricle relaxes.
3. The bicuspid or mitral valve is located on the left side of the heart.
4. The tricuspid valve is located on the right side of the heart.
5. The pulmonic semilunar valve lies between the right ventricle and the pulmonary artery.
6. The aortic semilunar valve lies between the left ventricle and the aorta.
7. The semilunar valves prevent blood from flowing back into the ventricles during relaxation; they open during ventricular contraction and close when the ventricles begin to relax.

E. Atrioventricular node
1. The atrioventricular node is located in the lower aspect of the atrial septum.
2. The atrioventricular node receives electrical impulses from the sinoatrial node.

F. The bundle of His (atrioventricular bundle)
1. The bundle of His fuses with the atrioventricular node to form another pacemaker site.
2. The bundle of His branches into the right bundle branch, which extends down the right side of the interventricular septum, and the left bundle branch, which extends into the left ventricle.
3. The right and left bundle branches terminate into Purkinje fibers.
4. If the sinoatrial node fails, the bundle of His can initiate and sustain a heart rate at 40 to 60 beats per minute.

G. Purkinje fibers
   1. Purkinje fibers are a diffuse network of conducting strands located beneath the ventricular endocardium.
   2. These fibers spread the wave of depolarization through the ventricles.

H. Coronary arteries
   1. The coronary arteries supply the capillaries of the myocardium with blood.
   2. The right coronary artery supplies the right atrium and ventricle, the inferior portion of the left ventricle, the posterior septal wall, and the sinoatrial and atrioventricular nodes.
   3. The left coronary artery consists of two major branches, the left anterior descending and the circumflex arteries.
   4. The left anterior descending artery supplies blood to the anterior wall of the left ventricle, the anterior ventricular septum, and the apex of the left ventricle.
   5. The circumflex artery supplies blood to the left atrium and the lateral and posterior surfaces of the left ventricle.

I. Sinoatrial node
   1. The sinoatrial node or pacemaker initiates each heart beat.
   2. The sinoatrial node is located at the junction of the superior vena cava and the right atrium.
   3. The sinoatrial node generates electrical impulses at 60 to 100 times per minute and is controlled by the sympathetic and parasympathetic nervous systems.

J. Heart sounds
   1. The first heart sound is heard as the atrioventricular valves close.
   2. The second heart sound is heard when the semilunar valves close.
   3. A third heart sound may be heard if ventricular wall compliance is decreased and structures in the ventricular wall vibrate; this can occur in conditions such as congestive heart failure or valvular regurgitation; however, a third heart sound may be normal in individuals younger than 30 years of age.
   4. A fourth heart sound may be heard on atrial **systole** if resistance to ventricular filling is present; this is an abnormal finding, and the causes include cardiac hypertrophy, disease, or injury to the ventricular wall.

K. Heart rate
   1. The faster the heart rate, the less time the heart has for filling, and the **cardiac output** decreases.
   2. An increase in heart rate increases oxygen consumption.
   3. The normal heart rate is 60 to 100 beats per minute.
   4. Sinus tachycardia is a rate greater than 100 beats per minute.

5. Sinus bradycardia is a rate less than 60 beats per minute.

L. Autonomic nervous system
   1. Stimulation of sympathetic nerve fibers releases the neurotransmitter norepinephrine, producing an increased heart rate, increased conduction speed through the atrioventricular node, increased atrial and ventricular **contractility**, and peripheral vasoconstriction; stimulation occurs when a decrease in pressure is detected.
   2. Stimulation of the parasympathetic nerve fibers releases the neurotransmitter acetylcholine, which decreases the heart rate and lessens atrial and ventricular contractility and **conductivity**; stimulation occurs when an increase in pressure is detected.

M. **Blood pressure (BP)** control
   1. **Baroreceptors**, also called pressoreceptors, are located in the walls of the aortic arch and carotid sinuses.
   2. **Baroreceptors** are specialized nerve endings that are affected by changes in the arterial **blood pressure.**
   3. Increases in **arterial pressure** stimulate **baroreceptors,** and the heart rate and **arterial pressure** decrease.
   4. Decreases in **arterial pressure** reduce stimulation of the **baroreceptors,** and vasoconstriction occurs, as does an increase in heart rate.
   5. **Stretch receptors,** located in the vena cava and the right atrium, respond to pressure changes that affect circulatory blood volume.
   6. When the **blood pressure** decreases as a result of hypovolemia, a sympathetic response occurs, causing an increased heart rate and blood vessel constriction; when the **blood pressure** increases as a result of hypervolemia, an opposite effect occurs.
   7. The antidiuretic hormone influences **blood pressure** indirectly by regulating vascular volume.
   8. Increases in blood volume result in decreased antidiuretic hormone release, increasing diuresis, and decreasing blood volume and thus **blood pressure.**
   9. Decreases in blood volume result in increased antidiuretic hormone release; this promotes an increase in blood volume and thus **blood pressure.**
   10. Renin, a potent vasoconstrictor, causes the **blood pressure** to increase.
   11. Renin converts angiotensinogen to angiotensin I; angiotensin I then is converted to angiotensin II in the lungs.
   12. Angiotensin II stimulates the release of aldosterone, which promotes water and sodium retention by the kidneys; this action increases blood volume and **blood pressure.**

N. The vascular system
   1. Arteries are vessels through which the blood passes away from the heart to various parts of

the body; they convey highly oxygenated blood from the left side of heart to the tissues.

2. Arterioles control the blood flow into the capillaries.

3. Capillaries allow the exchange of fluid and nutrients between the blood and the interstitial spaces.

4. Venules receive blood from the capillary bed and move blood into the veins.

5. Veins transport deoxygenated blood from the tissues back to the heart and lungs for oxygenation.

6. Valves help return blood to the heart against the force of gravity.

7. The lymphatics drain the tissues and return the tissue fluid to the blood.

II. DIAGNOSTIC TESTS AND PROCEDURES

A. Cardiac enzymes
1. CK-MB (creatine kinase, myocardial muscle)
   a. An elevation in value indicates myocardial damage.
   b. An elevation occurs within 4 to 6 hours and peaks 18 to 24 hours following an acute ischemic attack.
   c. Normal value is 0 to 5% of total; total CK is 26 to 174 units/L.
2. Lactate dehydrogenase (LDH)
   a. Elevations in LDH occur 24 hours following myocardial infarction and peak in 48 to 72 hours.
   b. When the serum concentration of LDH_1 is higher than that for LDH_2, the pattern is indicated as "flipped," signifying myocardial necrosis.
   c. Normal value in conventional units is 140 to 280 international units/L.
3. Troponin
   a. Troponin is composed of three proteins: cardiac troponin, troponin I, and troponin T.
   b. Troponin I especially has a high affinity for myocardial injury; it rises within 3 hours and persists for up to 7 days.
   c. Normal values are low, with troponin T normally ranging from 0 to 0.2 ng/mL, and troponin I being less than 0.6 ng/mL; thus any rise can indicate myocardial cell damage.
4. Myoglobin
   a. Myoglobin is an oxygen-binding protein found in cardiac and skeletal muscle.
   b. Level rises within 1 hour after cell death, peaks in 4 to 6 hours, and returns to normal within 24 to 36 hours (and in some clients even faster).

B. Complete blood count
1. The red blood cell count decreases in rheumatic heart disease and infective endocarditis and increases in conditions characterized by inadequate tissue oxygenation.
2. The white blood cell count increases in infectious and inflammatory diseases of the heart and after

myocardial infarction (MI) because large numbers of white blood cells are needed to dispose of the necrotic tissue resulting from the infarction.
3. An elevated hematocrit can result from vascular volume depletion.
4. Decreases in hematocrit and hemoglobin can indicate anemia.

C. Blood coagulation factors: An increase in coagulation factors can occur during and after MI, which places the client at greater risk of thrombophlebitis and extension of clots in the coronary arteries.

D. Serum lipids
1. The lipid profile measures serum cholesterol, triglycerides, and lipoprotein levels.
2. The lipid profile is used to assess the risk of developing coronary artery disease.
3. The desirable range for serum cholesterol is less than 200 mg/dL, with the low-density lipoprotein cholesterol less than 130 mg/dL and the high-density lipoprotein cholesterol at 30 to 70 mg/dL.

E. Electrolytes
1. Potassium
   a. Hypokalemia causes increased cardiac electrical instability, ventricular dysrhythmias, and increased risk of digitalis toxicity.
   b. In hypokalemia, the electrocardiogram would show flattening and inversion of the T wave, the appearance of a U wave, and ST depression.
   c. Hyperkalemia causes asystole and ventricular dysrhythmias.
2. Sodium
   a. The serum sodium level decreases with the use of diuretics.
   b. The serum sodium level decreases in heart failure, indicating water excess.

F. Calcium
1. Hypocalcemia can cause ventricular dysrhythmias, prolonged ST and QT interval, and cardiac arrest.
2. Hypercalcemia can cause a shortened ST interval, atrioventricular block, tachycardia or bradycardia, digitalis hypersensitivity, and cardiac arrest.

G. Phosphorus level: Phosphorus levels should be interpreted with calcium levels because the kidneys retain or excrete one electrolyte in an inverse relationship to the other.

H. Magnesium
1. A low magnesium level can cause ventricular tachycardia and fibrillation.
2. A high magnesium level can cause muscle weakness, hypotension, bradycardia, and a prolonged PR interval and wide QRS complex.

I. Blood urea nitrogen: The blood urea nitrogen is elevated in heart disorders that adversely affect renal circulation, such as heart failure and cardiogenic shock.

J. Blood glucose: An acute cardiac episode can elevate the blood glucose.

K. Chest x-ray film
1. Description
   a. Radiography of the chest is done to determine the size, silhouette, and position of the heart.
   b. Specific pathological changes are difficult to determine via x-ray film, but anatomical changes can be seen.
2. Interventions
   a. Prepare the client for x-ray film, explaining the purpose and procedure.
   b. Remove jewelry.

▲ L. Electrocardiogram (Box 59-1)
1. Description: a common noninvasive diagnostic test that evaluates the function of the heart by recording electrical activity
2. Interventions
   a. Determine the client's ability to lie still, and advise the client to lie still, breathe normally, and refrain from talking during the test.
   b. Reassure the client that an electrical shock will not occur.
   c. Document any cardiac medications the client is taking.

M. Holter monitoring
1. Description
   a. In this noninvasive test the client wears a Holter monitor and an electrocardiogram tracing is recorded continuously over a period of 24 hours or more.
   b. The Holter monitor identifies dysrhythmias if they occur and evaluates the effectiveness of antidysrhythmics or pacemaker therapy.
▲ 2. Interventions: Instruct the client to resume normal daily activities and to maintain a diary documenting activities and any symptoms that may develop.

N. Echocardiogram
1. Description
   a. An echocardiogram is a noninvasive procedure based on the principles of ultrasound.
   b. An echocardiogram evaluates structural and functional changes in the heart.
2. Interventions: Determine the client's ability to lie still, and advise the client to lie still, breathe normally, and refrain from talking during the test.

O. Exercise testing (stress test)
1. Description
   a. The stress test is a noninvasive test that studies the heart during activity and detects and evaluates coronary artery disease.
   b. Treadmill testing is the most commonly used mode of stress testing.
   c. Stress testing may be used with myocardial radionuclide testing (perfusion imaging), at which point the procedure becomes invasive because a radionuclide must be injected.
   d. If the client is unable to tolerate exercise, an intravenous (IV) infusion of dipyridamole

---

BOX 59-1

Electrocardiogram Basics

An electrocardiogram reflects the electrical activity of cardiac cells and records electrical activity at a speed of 25 mm/sec.

An electrocardiogram strip consists of horizontal squares representing seconds and vertical squares representing voltage.

Each small square represents 0.04 second.

Each large square represents 0.20 second.

The P wave represents atrial depolarization.

The PR interval represents the time it takes an impulse to travel from the atria through the atrioventricular node, bundle of His, and bundle branches to the Purkinje fibers.

Normal PR interval duration ranges from 0.12 to 0.2 second.

The PR interval is measured from the beginning of the P wave to the end of the PR segment.

The QRS complex represents ventricular depolarization.

Normal QRS complex duration ranges from 0.04 to 0.1 second.

The Q wave appears as the first negative deflection in the QRS complex and reflects initial ventricular septal depolarization.

The R wave is the first positive deflection in the QRS complex.

The S wave appears as the second negative deflection in the QRS complex.

The J point marks the end of the QRS complex and the beginning of the ST segment.

The QRS duration is measured from the end of the PR segment to the J point.

The ST segment represents part of ventricular repolarization.

The T wave represents ventricular repolarization and ventricular diastole.

The U wave may follow the T wave.

A prominent U wave may indicate an electrolyte abnormality such as hypokalemia.

The QT interval represents ventricular refractory time, or the total time required for ventricular depolarization and repolarization.

The QT interval is measured from the beginning of the QRS complex to the end of the T wave.

The QT interval normally lasts 0.32 to 0.4 second but varies with the client's heart rate, age, and sex.

(Persantine) is given to dilate the coronary arteries and stimulate the effect of exercise; caffeine and theophylline products are held 12 hours before the test and calcium channel blockers and β-blockers are held for 24 hours.
   e. An informed consent is required if a radionuclide is injected.
2. Preprocedure interventions
   a. Obtain an informed consent if required.
   b. Provide adequate rest the night before the procedure.

c. Instruct the client to eat a light meal 1 to 2 hours before the procedure.

d. Instruct the client to avoid smoking, alcohol, and caffeine before the procedure.

e. Ask the physician about taking prescribed medication on the day of the procedure.

f. Instruct the client to wear nonconstrictive, comfortable clothing and supportive shoes.

3. Postprocedure interventions

a. Instruct the client to notify the physician if any chest pain, dizziness, or shortness of breath occurs.

b. Instruct the client to avoid taking a hot bath or shower for at least 1 to 2 hours.

P. Digital subtraction angiography

1. Description

a. Digital subtraction angiography combines x-ray techniques and a computerized subtraction technique with fluoroscopy for visualization of the cardiovascular system.

b. A contrast medium (dye) is injected.

2. Preprocedure interventions

a. Assess the client for allergy to contrast medium (dye), iodine, or seafood.

b. Obtain informed consent.

3. Postprocedure interventions

a. Monitor vital signs.

b. Assess injection site for bleeding or discomfort.

Q. Nuclear cardiology

1. Description

a. Nuclear cardiology is the use of radionuclide techniques and scanning in cardiovascular assessment.

b. The most common tests include technetium pyrophosphate scanning, thallium imaging, and multigated cardiac blood pool imaging.

2. Preprocedure interventions

a. Obtain informed consent.

b. Inform the client that a small amount of radioisotope will be injected and that the radiation exposure and risks are minimal.

3. Postprocedure interventions

a. Assess vital signs.

b. Assess injection site for bleeding or discomfort.

c. Inform the client that fatigue is possible.

R. Cardiac catheterization

1. Description

a. Cardiac catheterization involves insertion of a catheter into the heart and surrounding vessels.

b. Cardiac catheterization obtains information about the structure and performance of the heart valves and circulatory system.

2. Preprocedure interventions

a. Obtain informed consent.

b. Assess for allergies to seafood, iodine, or radiopaque dyes.

c. Withhold solid food for 6 to 8 hours and liquids for 4 hours to prevent vomiting and aspiration during the procedure.

d. Document the client's height and weight because these data will be needed to determine the amount of dye to be administered.

e. Document baseline vital signs, and note the quality and presence of peripheral pulses for postprocedure comparison.

f. Inform the client that a local anesthetic will be administered before catheter insertion.

g. Inform the client that he or she may feel fatigued because of the need to lie still and quiet on a hard table for up to 2 hours.

h. Inform the client that he or she may feel a fluttery feeling as the catheter passes through the heart, a flushed, warm feeling when the dye is injected, a desire to cough, and palpitations caused by heart irritability.

i. Prepare insertion site by shaving and cleaning with an antiseptic solution if prescribed.

j. Administer preprocedure medications if prescribed.

k. Insert an IV line if prescribed.

3. Postprocedure interventions

a. Monitor vital signs and cardiac rhythm for dysrhythmias at least every 30 minutes for 2 hours initially.

b. Assess for chest pain, and if dysrhythmias or chest pain occurs, notify the physician.

c. Monitor peripheral pulses and the color, warmth, and sensation of the extremity distal to insertion site at least every 30 minutes for 2 hours initially.

d. Notify the physician if the client complains of numbness and tingling, if the extremity becomes cool, pale, or cyanotic, or if loss of the peripheral pulses occurs.

e. Monitor the pressure dressing for bleeding or hematoma formation.

f. Apply a sandbag or compression device to the insertion site to provide additional pressure if required.

g. Monitor for bleeding, and if bleeding occurs, apply pressure immediately and notify the physician.

h. Monitor for hematoma, and if a hematoma develops, notify the physician.

i. Keep extremity extended for 4 to 6 hours, as prescribed, keeping the leg straight to prevent arterial occlusion.

j. Maintain strict bed rest for 6 to 12 hours, as prescribed; however, the client may turn from side to side; do not elevate the head of the bed more than 15 degrees.

k. If the antecubital vessel was used, immobilize the arm with an armboard.

l. Encourage fluid intake, if not contraindicated, to promote renal excretion of the dye.

m. Monitor for nausea, vomiting, rash, or other signs of hypersensitivity to the dye.

S. Central **venous pressure** (CVP)
1. Description
   a. The CVP is the pressure within the superior vena cava and reflects the pressure under which blood is returned to the superior vena cava and right atrium.
   b. The CVP is measured with a central venous line in the superior vena cava or by a balloon flotation catheter in the pulmonary artery.
   c. Normal CVP pressure is about 3 to 8 mm Hg.
   d. An elevated CVP measurement indicates an increase in blood volume as a result of sodium and water retention, excessive IV fluids, alterations in fluid balance, or renal failure.
   e. A decreased CVP measurement indicates a decrease in circulating blood volume and may be due to hemorrhage or severe vasodilation with pooling of blood in the extremities that limits venous return and to fluid imbalances.
2. Measuring CVP
   a. The right atrium is located at the midaxillary line at the fourth intercostal space, and the zero point on the transducer needs to be at the level of the right atrium.
   b. The client needs to be supine, with the head of the bed at 45 degrees.
   c. The client needs to be relaxed; note that activity that increases intrathoracic pressure, such as coughing or straining, will cause false increases in the readings.
   d. If the client is on a ventilator, the reading should be taken at the point of end expiration.
   e. To maintain patency of the line, a constant, small amount of fluid is delivered under pressure.

III. THERAPEUTIC MANAGEMENT

A. Percutaneous transluminal coronary angioplasty (PTCA)
1. Description
   a. One or more arteries are dilated with a balloon catheter to open the vessel lumen and improve arterial blood flow.
   b. The client can experience reocclusion after the procedure, thus the procedure may need to be repeated.
   c. Complications can include arterial dissection or rupture, immobilization of plaque fragments, spasm, and acute MI.
   d. Firm commitment is needed on the client's part to stop smoking, lose weight, alter exercise pattern, and stop any behaviors that lead to progression of artery occlusion.

2. Preprocedure interventions
   a. Maintain NPO status after midnight.
   b. Prepare the groin area with antiseptic soap and shave per institutional procedure and as prescribed.
   c. Assess baseline vital signs and peripheral pulses.
3. Postprocedure interventions
   a. Monitor vital signs closely.
   b. Assess distal pulses in both extremities.
   c. Maintain bed rest as prescribed, keeping the limb straight for 6 to 8 hours.
   d. Administer anticoagulants and antiplatelet agents as prescribed to prevent thrombus formation.
   e. Monitor IV nitroglycerin that may be prescribed to prevent coronary artery spasm.
   f. Instruct the client in the administration of nitrates, calcium channel blockers, antiplatelet agents, and anticoagulants as prescribed.
   g. Instruct the client to take aspirin daily permanently if prescribed.
   h. Assist the client with planning lifestyle modifications.

B. Laser-assisted angioplasty
1. Description
   a. A laser probe is advanced through a cannula similar to that used for PTCA.
   b. Laser-assisted angioplasty is used also for clients with small occlusions in the distal superficial femoral, proximal popliteal, and common iliac arteries.
   c. Heat from the laser vaporizes the plaque to open the occluded artery.
2. Preprocedure and postprocedure care
   a. Care is similar to that for the PTCA.
   b. Monitor for complications of coronary dissection, acute occlusion, perforation, embolism, and MI.

C. Coronary artery stents
1. Description
   a. Coronary artery stents are used instead of PTCA to eliminate the risk of acute coronary vessel closure and to improve long-term patency of the vessel.
   b. A balloon catheter bearing the stent is inserted into the coronary artery and positioned at the site of occlusion.
   c. When placed in the coronary artery, the stent reopens the blocked artery.
2. Postprocedure interventions
   a. Acute thrombosis is a major concern following the procedure, and the client is placed on antiplatelet and anticoagulation therapy for several months following the procedure.
   b. Monitor for complications of the procedure such as stent migration or occlusion, coronary

artery dissection, and bleeding resulting from anticoagulation.

D. Atherectomy
1. Description
   a. Atherectomy removes plaque from an artery by the use of a cutting chamber on the inserted catheter or a rotating blade that pulverizes the plaque.
   b. Atherectomy is used to improve blood flow to ischemic limbs in individuals with peripheral arterial disease.
2. Postprocedure interventions: Monitor for complications of perforation, embolus, and reocclusion.

E. Transmyocardial revascularization
1. Transmyocardial revascularization is used for clients with widespread atherosclerosis involving vessels that are too small and numerous for replacement or balloon catheterization.
2. Transmyocardial revascularization uses a high-powered laser that creates 15 to 30 holes (channels) in the heart.
3. Blood enters these small channels, providing the affected region of the heart with oxygenated blood.
4. Transmyocardial revascularization is performed through a small chest incision.
5. The opening on the surface of the heart heals; however, the main channels remain and perfuse the myocardium.

F. Arterial revascularization
1. Description
   a. Arterial revascularization is performed to increase arterial blood flow to the affected limb.
   b. Inflow procedures involve bypassing the arterial occlusion above the superficial femoral arteries.
   c. Outflow procedures involve bypassing the arterial occlusions at or below the superficial femoral arteries.
   d. Graft material is sutured above and below the occlusion to facilitate blood flow around the occlusion.
2. Preoperative interventions
   a. Assess baseline vital signs and peripheral pulses.
   b. Insert IV line and urinary catheter as prescribed.
   c. Maintain central venous catheter and/or arterial line if inserted.
3. Postoperative interventions
   a. Assess vital signs.
   b. Monitor the **blood pressure** and notify the physician if changes occur.
   c. Monitor for hypotension, which may indicate hypovolemia.
   d. Monitor for hypertension, which may place stress on the graft and facilitate clot formation.
   e. Maintain bed rest for 24 hours as prescribed.
   f. Instruct the client to keep affected extremity straight, limit movement, and avoid bending the knee and hip.
   g. Monitor for warmth, redness, and edema, which often are expected outcomes because of increased blood flow.
   h. Monitor for graft occlusion, which often occurs within the first 24 hours.
   i. Assess peripheral pulses and for adverse changes in color and temperature of the extremity.
   j. Monitor for a sharp increase in pain because pain is frequently the first indicator of postoperative graft occlusion.
   k. If signs of graft occlusion occur, notify the physician immediately.
   l. Encourage coughing and deep breathing and the use of incentive spirometry.
   m. Maintain NPO status, with progression to clear liquids as prescribed.
   n. Use strict aseptic technique when in contact with the incision.
   o. Assess the incision for drainage, warmth, or swelling.
   p. Monitor for excessive bleeding (a small amount of bloody drainage is expected).
   q. Monitor the area over the graft for hardness, tenderness, and warmth, which may indicate infection; if this occurs, notify the physician immediately.
   r. Instruct the client about proper foot care and measures to prevent ulcer formation.
   s. Instruct the client to take medications as prescribed.
   t. Instruct the client in how to care for incision.
   u. Assist the client in modifying lifestyle to prevent further plaque formation.

G. Coronary artery bypass graft
1. Description
   a. The occluded coronary arteries are bypassed with the client's own venous or arterial blood vessels.
   b. The saphenous vein, radial artery, or internal mammary artery is used to bypass lesions in the coronary arteries.
   c. Coronary artery bypass graft is performed when the client does not respond to medical management of coronary artery disease or when disease progression is evident.
2. Preoperative interventions
   a. Familiarize the client and family with the cardiac surgical critical care unit.
   b. Instruct the client in how to splint the chest incision, cough and deep breathe, and perform arm and leg exercises.
   c. Instruct the client to inform the nurse of any postoperative pain because pain medication will be available.

d. Inform the client to expect a sternal incision, possible arm or leg incision(s), one or two chest tubes, a Foley catheter, and several IV fluid catheters.

e. Inform the client that an endotracheal tube will be in place and connected to a ventilator for 6 to 24 hours.

f. Advise the client to breathe with the ventilator and not fight it.

g. Inform the family that the client will not be able to talk while the endotracheal tube is in place.

h. Encourage the client and family to discuss anxieties and fears related to surgery.

i. Note that prescribed medications are to be discontinued preoperatively (usually diuretics 2 to 3 days before surgery, digitalis 12 hours before surgery, and aspirin and anticoagulants 1 week before surgery).

j. Administer medications as prescribed, which may include potassium chloride, antihypertensives, antidysrhythmics, and antibiotics.

3. Cardiac surgical unit postoperative interventions

a. Maintain mechanical ventilation for 6 to 24 hours as prescribed.

b. Monitor heart rate and rhythm, pulmonary artery and arterial pressures, and neurological status.

c. Monitor mediastinal and pericardial tubes and water seal drainage system, and report drainage exceeding 100 to 150 mL per hour.

d. Ground epicardial pacer wires.

e. Assess fluid and electrolyte balance.

f. Restrict fluids, as prescribed, to 1500 to 2000 mL because the client usually has edema.

g. Monitor for hypotension, which can cause collapse of a vein graft.

h. Monitor for hypertension because increased pressure promotes leakage from the suture line and may cause bleeding.

i. Monitor the temperature and initiate rewarming procedures using warm or thermal blankets if the temperature drops below 96.8° F; rewarm the client no faster than 1.8° F per hour to prevent shivering, and discontinue when the temperature approaches 98.6° F.

j. Administer potassium intravenously as prescribed to maintain the potassium level between 4 and 5 mEq/L to prevent dysrhythmias.

k. Monitor for signs of cardiac tamponade, which will include sudden cessation of previously heavy mediastinal drainage, jugular vein distention with clear lung sounds, and pulsus paradoxus.

l. Monitor pain, differentiating sternotomy pain from anginal pain, which would indicate graft failure.

4. Transfer client from the cardiac surgical unit.

a. Monitor vital signs, level of consciousness, and peripheral perfusion.

b. Monitor for dysrhythmias.

c. Auscultate lungs and assess respiratory status.

d. Encourage the client to splint the incision, cough, deep breathe, and use incentive spirometer to raise secretions and prevent atelectasis.

e. Monitor temperature and white blood cell count, which if elevated after 3 to 4 days indicate infection.

f. Provide adequate fluids and hydration as prescribed to liquefy secretions.

g. Assess suture line and chest tube insertion sites for redness, purulent discharge, and signs of infection.

h. Assess sternal suture line for instability, which may indicate an infection.

i. Guide the client to gradually resume activity.

j. Assess the client for tachycardia, **postural (orthostatic) hypotension**, and fatigue before, during, and after activity.

k. Discontinue activities if the **blood pressure** drops more than 10 to 20 mm Hg or if the pulse increases more than 10 beats per minute.

l. Monitor episodes of pain closely.

m. See Box 59-2 for home care instructions.

H. Heart transplant

1. A donor heart from an individual with a comparable body weight and ABO compatibility is transplanted into a recipient within less than 6 hours of procurement.

2. The surgeon removes the diseased heart, leaving the posterior portion of the atria to serve as an anchor for the new heart.

BOX 59-2

Home Care Instructions Following Cardiac Surgery

Progressively return to activities at home.

Limit pushing or pulling activities for 6 weeks following discharge.

Maintain incisional care and record signs of redness, swelling, or drainage.

Sternotomy incision heals in about 6 to 8 weeks.

Avoid crossing legs, wear elastic hose as prescribed until edema subsides, and elevate surgical limb when sitting in a chair.

Use of prescribed medications.

Dietary measures, including the avoidance of saturated fats and cholesterol and the use of salt.

Sexual intercourse can be resumed on the advice of the physician after exercise tolerance is assessed; if the client can walk one block or climb two flights of stairs without symptoms, he or she can resume sexual activity safely.

3. Because a remnant of the client's atria remains, two unrelated P waves are noted on the electrocardiogram.
4. The transplanted heart is denervated and unresponsive to vagal stimulation; because the heart is denervated, clients do not experience angina.
5. Symptoms of heart rejection include hypotension, dysrhythmias, weakness, fatigue, and dizziness.
6. Endomyocardial biopsies are performed at regular scheduled intervals and whenever rejection is suspected.
7. Clients require lifetime immunosuppressive therapy.
8. The heart rate approximates 100 beats per minute and responds slowly to exercise or stress regarding increases in heart rate, **contractility**, and **cardiac output.**

IV. CARDIAC DYSRHYTHMIAS

A. Normal sinus rhythm (Fig. 59-1)
   1. Rhythm originates from the sinoatrial node.
   2. Atrial and ventricular rhythms are regular.
   3. Atrial and ventricular rates are 60 to 100 beats per minute (Fig. 59-2; Box 59-3).
B. Sinus bradycardia
   1. Description
      a. Atrial and ventricular rates are less than 60 beats per minute.

BOX 59-3

Six-Second Strip Method to Determine Heart Rate

The method can be used to determine heart rate for regular and irregular rhythms.
To determine atrial rate, count the number of PP intervals in 6 seconds and multiply by 10 to obtain a full minute rate.
To determine ventricular rate, count the number of RR intervals in 6 seconds and multiply by 10 to obtain a full minute rate.
For accuracy, timing should begin on the P wave or the QRS complex and end exactly at 30 large blocks later.

---

   b. Treatment may be necessary if the client is symptomatic.
   c. Note that a low heart rate may be normal for some individuals.
   2. Interventions
      a. Attempt to determine the cause of sinus bradycardia, and if a medication is suspected of causing the bradycardia, hold the medication and notify the physician.
      b. Administer oxygen as prescribed.
      c. Administer atropine sulfate as prescribed to increase the heart rate to 60 beats per minute.

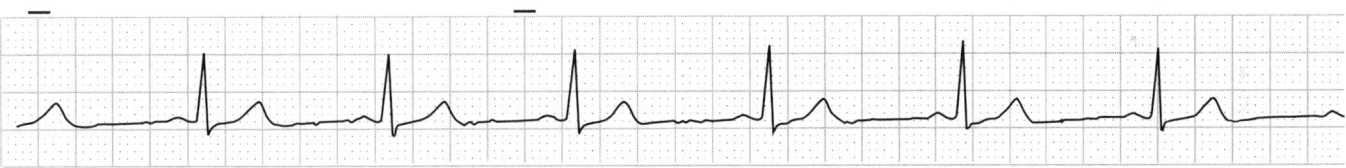

FIG. 59-1 Normal sinus rhythm. (From Paul, S., & Hebra, J. D. [1998]. *The nurse's guide to cardiac rhythm interpretation.* Philadelphia: W. B. Saunders.)

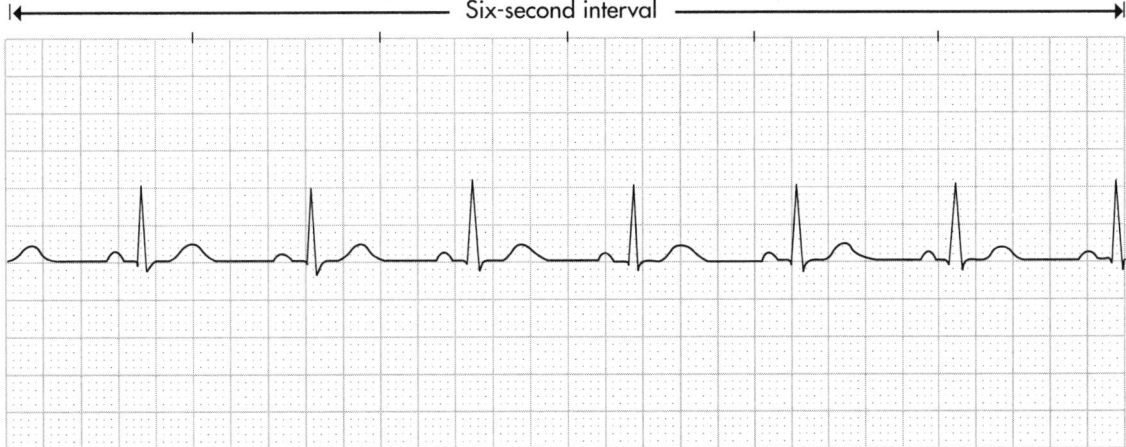

Six-second interval

FIG. 59-2 Six-second method for calculating heart rate: seven QRS complexes in a six-second interval is equal to a heart rate of 70 beats per minute. (From Paul, S., & Hebra, J. D. [1998]. *The nurse's guide to cardiac rhythm interpretation.* Philadelphia: W. B. Saunders.)

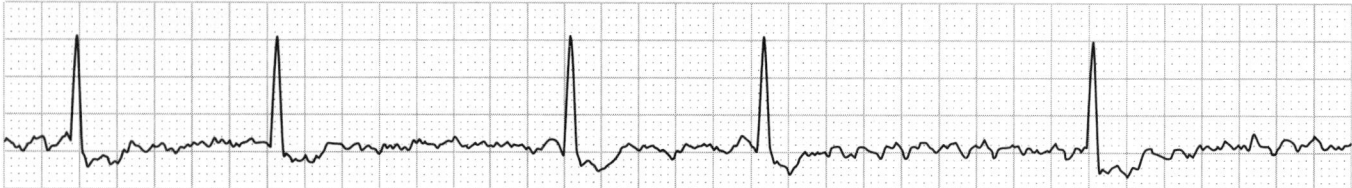

FIG. 59-3 Atrial fibrillation. Note the chaotic undulations of the atria and irregular response of the ventricles. (From Paul, S., & Hebra, J. D. [1998]. *The nurse's guide to cardiac rhythm interpretation.* Philadelphia: W. B. Saunders.)

d. Be prepared to apply a noninvasive pacemaker initially as prescribed if the atropine sulfate does not increase the heart rate sufficiently.

e. Avoid additional doses of atropine sulfate because they will induce tachycardia.

f. Monitor for hypotension and administer fluids intravenously as prescribed.

g. Depending on the cause of the bradycardia, the client may need a permanent pacemaker.

C. Sinus tachycardia

1. Description: atrial and ventricular rates are 100 to180 beats per minute

2. Interventions

a. Identify the cause of the tachycardia.

b. Decrease the heart rate to normal by treating the cause.

D. Atrial fibrillation (Fig. 59-3)

1. Description

a. Multiple rapid impulses from many foci depolarize in the atria in a totally disorganized manner at a rate of 350 to 600 times per minute.

b. The atria quiver, which can lead to the formation of thrombi.

c. P wave shows fibrillatory waves, but no definitive P wave can be observed.

2. Interventions

a. Administer oxygen.

b. Administer anticoagulants as prescribed because of the risk of emboli.

c. Administer cardiac medications as prescribed to control the ventricular rhythm and assist in the maintenance of **cardiac output.**

d. Prepare the client for cardioversion as prescribed.

e. Instruct the client in the use of medications as prescribed to control the dysrhythmia.

E. Premature ventricular contractions (PVCs) (Box 59-4)

1. Description

a. Early ventricular complexes result from increased irritability of the ventricles.

b. Premature ventricular contractions frequently occur in repetitive rhythms such as bigeminy, trigeminy, and quadrigeminy.

c. The QRS complexes may be unifocal or multifocal.

2. Interventions

a. Notify the physician if PVCs occur.

b. Identify the cause and treat based on the cause.

c. Evaluate electrolytes, particularly the potassium level, because hypokalemia can cause PVCs.

d. Administer oxygen as prescribed.

e. Administer lidocaine as prescribed.

f. Notify the physician if the client complains of chest pain or if PVCs increase in frequency, are multifocal, occur on the T wave (R on T), or occur in runs of ventricular tachycardia.

F. Ventricular tachycardia (VT) (Fig. 59-4)

1. Description

a. Ventricular tachycardia occurs because of a repetitive firing of an irritable ventricular ectopic focus at a rate of 140 to 250 beats per minute or more.

b. Ventricular tachycardia may present as a paroxysm of three self-limiting beats or more or may be a sustained rhythm.

c. Ventricular tachycardia can cause cardiac arrest.

2. Stable client with sustained VT

a. Administer oxygen as prescribed.

b. Administer antidysrhythmics as prescribed.

3. Unstable client with VT

a. Administer oxygen and antidysrhythmic therapy as prescribed.

BOX 59-4

Premature Ventricular Contractions

Bigeminy: Premature ventricular contraction (PVC) every other heart beat
Trigeminy: PVC every third heart beat
Quadrigeminy: PVC every fourth heartbeat
Couplet or pair: Two sequential PVCs
Unifocal: Uniform upward or downward deflection, arising from the same ectopic foci
Multifocal: Different shapes, with the impulse generation from different sites
R-on-T phenomenon: PVC falls on preceding beat
T wave, which is considered a vulnerable period, may precipitate ventricular fibrillation.

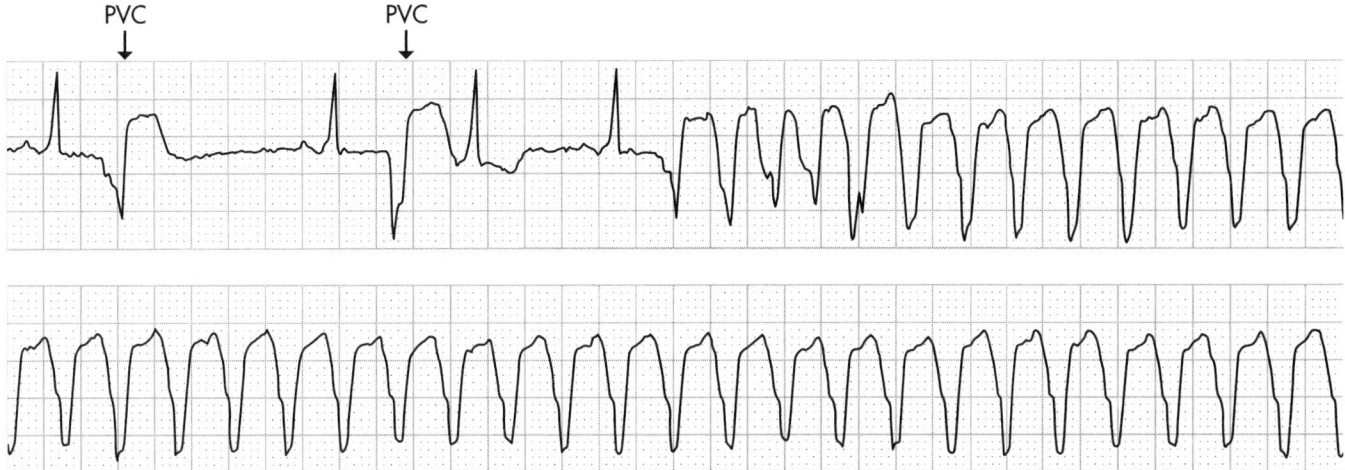

FIG. 59-4   Ventricular tachycardia. Note the premature ventricular contractions (PVCs) before the onset of the tachycardia (second and fourth beats on the strip). The premature ventricular contraction that initiates the tachycardia has the identical morphology (shape) of the first premature ventricular contraction. (From Paul, S., & Hebra, J. D. [1998]. *The nurse's guide to cardiac rhythm interpretation.* Philadelphia: W. B. Saunders.)

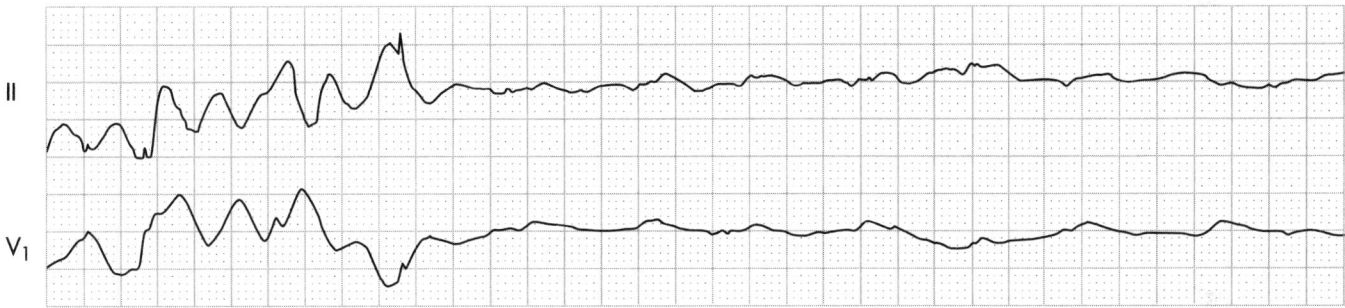

FIG. 59-5   Coarse ventricular fibrillation degenerating into fine ventricular fibrillation. (From Paul, S., & Hebra, J. D. [1998]. *The nurse's guide to cardiac rhythm interpretation.* Philadelphia: W. B. Saunders.)

   b. Prepare for synchronized cardioversion if client is unstable.
   c. Attempt cough cardiopulmonary resuscitation (CPR) by asking the client to cough hard every 1 to 3 seconds.
   4. Pulseless client: defibrillation and CPR
G. Ventricular fibrillation (VF) (Fig. 59-5)
   1. Description
      a. Impulses from many irritable foci fire in a totally disorganized manner.
      b. Ventricular fibrillation is a chaotic rapid rhythm in which the ventricles quiver.
      c. Ventricular fibrillation is rapidly fatal if not successfully terminated within 3 to 5 minutes.
      d. Client lacks a pulse, **BP**, respirations, and heart sounds.
   2. Interventions
      a. Defibrillate the client immediately, up to 3 times consecutively at 200, 300, and 360 Joules (J).
      b. Initiate CPR.

   c. Administer oxygen as prescribed.
   d. Administer epinephrine (Adrenalin) and anti-dysrhythmic therapy with amiodarone (Cordarone) or lidocaine as prescribed; other antidysrhythmics also may be prescribed.

V. MANAGEMENT OF DYSRHYTHMIAS
A. Vagal maneuvers
   1. Description: Vagal maneuvers induce vagal stimulation of the cardiac conduction system and are used to terminate supraventricular tachydysrhythmias.
   2. Carotid sinus massage
      a. The physician instructs the client to turn the head away from the side to be massaged.
      b. The physician massages over the carotid artery for 6 to 8 seconds until a change in cardiac rhythm occurs.
      c. Observe the cardiac monitor for a change in rhythm.

d. Record an electrocardiogram rhythm strip before, during, and after the procedure.

e. Have a defibrillator and resuscitative equipment available.

f. Monitor vital signs, cardiac rhythm, and level of consciousness following the procedure.

3. Valsalva's maneuver

a. The physician instructs the client to bear down or induces a gag reflex in the client, both of which stimulate a vagal reflex.

b. Monitor the heart rate, rhythm, and **BP.**

c. Observe the cardiac monitor for a change in rhythm.

d. Record an electrocardiogram rhythm strip before, during, and after the procedure.

e. Provide an emesis basin if the gag reflex is stimulated, and initiate precautions to prevent aspiration.

f. Have a defibrillator and resuscitative equipment available.

B. Cardioversion

1. Description

a. Cardioversion is synchronized countershock to convert an undesirable rhythm to a stable rhythm.

b. Cardioversion is an elective procedure and is performed by the physician.

c. A lower amount of energy is used than with defibrillation.

d. Defibrillator is synchronized to the client's R wave to avoid discharging the shock during the vulnerable period (T wave).

e. If the defibrillator were not synchronized, it would discharge on the T wave and cause VF.

2. Preprocedure interventions

a. Obtain an informed consent.

b. Administer sedation as prescribed.

c. Hold digoxin (Lanoxin) 48 hours preprocedure as prescribed to prevent postcardioversion ventricular irritability.

3. During the procedure

a. Ensure that the skin is clean and dry in the area where the electrode paddles will be placed.

b. Stop the oxygen during the procedure to avoid the hazard of fire.

c. Be sure that no one is touching the bed or the client when delivering the countershock.

4. Postprocedure interventions

a. Maintain airway patency.

b. Administer oxygen as prescribed.

c. Assess vital signs.

d. Assess level of consciousness.

e. Monitor cardiac rhythm.

f. Monitor for indications of successful response such as conversion to sinus rhythm, strong peripheral pulses, and an adequate **BP.**

C. Defibrillation

1. Description

a. Defibrillation is an asynchronous countershock used to terminate pulseless VT or VF.

b. Three rapid consecutive shocks are delivered, with the first at an energy of 200 J.

c. If unsuccessful, the shock is repeated at 200 to 300 J.

d. The third and subsequent shock will be 360 J.

2. During the procedure

a. Stop the oxygen during the procedure to avoid the hazard of fire.

b. Be sure that no one is touching the bed or the client when delivering the countershock.

D. Use of paddle electrodes

1. Apply conductive pads.

2. One paddle is placed at the third intercostal space to the right of the sternum; the other is placed at the fifth intercostal space on the left midaxillary line.

3. Apply firm pressure with the paddles.

4. Be sure that no one is touching the bed or the client when delivering the countershock.

E. Automatic external defibrillator

1. An automatic external defibrillator is used by laypersons and emergency medical technicians for prehospital cardiac arrest.

2. Place the client on a firm dry surface.

3. Stop CPR.

4. Ensure that no one is touching the client to avoid motion artifact during rhythm analysis.

5. Place the electrode paddles in the correct position on the client's chest.

6. Press the analyzer button to identify the rhythm, which may take 30 seconds; the machine will advise whether a shock is necessary.

7. Shocks are recommended for pulseless VF only.

8. If shock is recommended, the shock initially is delivered at an energy of 200 J.

9. If unsuccessful, the shock is repeated at 200 to 300 J.

10. The third and subsequent shock will be 360 J.

11. If unsuccessful, CPR is continued for 1 minute, and then another series of three shocks is delivered, each at 360 J.

F. Implantable cardioverter defibrillator (ICD)

1. Description

a. An ICD monitors cardiac rhythm and detects and terminates episodes of VT and VF.

b. The ICD senses VT or VF and delivers 25 to 30 J up to 4 times if necessary.

c. An ICD is used in clients with episodes of spontaneous sustained VT or VF unrelated to an MI or in clients whose medication therapy has been unsuccessful in controlling life-threatening dysrhythmias.

d. Electrodes are placed in the right atrium and ventricle and apical pericardium.

e. The generator is implanted in the abdomen.

2. Client education
   a. Instruct the client in the basic functions of the ICD.
   b. Instruct the client in how to perform cough CPR.
   c. Instruct the client in how to take the pulse; the client must take the pulse daily and maintain a diary of pulse rates.
   d. Wear loose-fitting clothing.
   e. Avoid contact sports and strenuous activities.
   f. Report any fever, redness, swelling, or drainage from the insertion site.
   g. Report symptoms of fainting, nausea, weakness, blackouts, and rapid pulse rates to the physician.
   h. During shock discharge, the client may feel faint or short of breath.
   i. Instruct the client to sit or lie down if he or she feels a shock and to notify the physician.
   j. Instruct the client and family in how to access emergency medical system.
   k. Encourage the family to learn CPR.
   l. Advise the client to maintain a diary of any shocks that are delivered, including the date, preceding activity, the number of shocks, and if the shocks were successful.
   m. Instruct the client to avoid electromagnetic fields directly over the ICD because they can inactivate the device.
   n. Instruct the client to move away from the magnetic field immediately if beeping tones are heard, and notify the physician.
   o. Keep a pacemaker ID in the wallet, and obtain and wear a Medic-Alert bracelet.
   p. Inform all health care providers that an ICD has been inserted.

VI. PACEMAKERS

A. Description: a temporary or permanent device that provides electrical stimulation and maintains the heart rate when the client's intrinsic pacemaker fails to provide a perfusing rhythm

B. Settings
   1. A synchronous or demand pacemaker senses the client's rhythm and paces only if the client's intrinsic rate falls below the set pacemaker rate.
   2. Asynchronous or fixed rate paces at a preset rate regardless of the client's intrinsic rhythm.
   3. Overdrive pacing suppresses the underlying rhythm in tachydysrhythmias so that the sinus node will regain control of the heart.

C. Spikes
   1. When a pacing stimulus is delivered to the heart, a spike (straight vertical line) is seen on the monitor or electrocardiogram strip.
   2. The spike should be followed by a P wave indicating atrial depolarization, or a QRS complex indicating ventricular depolarization; this pattern

is referred to as "capture," indicating that the pacemaker successfully depolarized, or captured, the chamber.

3. If the electrode is in the ventricle, the spike is in front of the QRS complex; if the electrode is in the atrium, the spike is before the P wave.
4. If the electrode is in the atrium and the ventricle, the spike is before the P wave and the QRS complex.

D. Temporary pacemakers
   1. Noninvasive temporary pacing
      a. Noninvasive temporary pacing is used as an emergency measure or when a client is being transported and the risk of bradydysrhythmia exists.
      b. A large electrode patch is placed on the chest and back.
      c. Wash the skin with soap and water before applying electrodes.
      d. Do not shave the hair or apply alcohol or tinctures to the skin.
      e. Place the posterior electrode between the spine and left scapula behind the heart, avoiding placement over bone.
      f. Place the anterior electrode between V_2 and V_5 positions over the heart.
      g. Do not place the anterior electrode over female breast tissue; rather, displace breast tissue and place under the breast.
      h. Do not take the pulse or **BP** on the left side; the results will not be accurate because of the muscle twitching and electrical current.
      i. Ensure that electrodes are in good contact with the skin.
      j. If loss of "capture" occurs, assess the skin contact of the electrodes and increase the current until "capture" is regained.
   2. Transvenous invasive temporary pacing
      a. Pacing lead wire is placed through antecubital, femoral, jugular, or subclavian vein into the right atrium for atrial pacing or through the right ventricle and is positioned in contact with the endocardium.
      b. Monitor cardiac rhythm continuously.
      c. Monitor vital signs.
      d. Monitor pacemaker insertion site.
      e. Restrict client movement to prevent lead wire displacement.
   3. Epicardial invasive temporary pacing: applied by using a transthoracic approach; the lead wires are threaded loosely on the epicardial surface of the heart after cardiac surgery
   4. Reducing the risk of microshock
      a. Use only inspected and approved equipment.
      b. Insulate the exposed portion of wires with plastic or rubber material (fingers of rubber gloves) when wires are not attached to the

pulse generator, and cover with nonconductive tape.

   c. Ground all electrical equipment using a three-pronged plug.

   d. Wear gloves when handling exposed wires.

   e. Keep dressings dry.

E. Permanent pacemakers

1. Pulse generator is internal and surgically implanted in a subcutaneous pocket under the clavicle or abdominal wall.

2. The leads are passed transvenously via the cephalic or subclavian vein to the endocardium on the right side of the heart.

3. Permanent pacemakers may be single chambered, in which the lead wire is placed in the chamber to be paced, or may be dual chambered, with lead wires placed in the atrium and right ventricle.

4. A permanent pacemaker is programmed when inserted and can be reprogrammed if necessary by noninvasive transmission from an external programmer to the implanted generator.

5. Pacemakers are powered by a lithium battery that has an average life span of 10 years, are nuclear powered with a life span of 20 years or longer, or are designed to be recharged externally.

6. Pacemaker function can be checked in the physician's office or clinic by a pacemaker interrogater/programmer or from home using telephone transmitter devices.

7. The client may be provided with a device that is placed over the pacemaker battery generator with an attachment to the telephone; the heart rate then can be transmitted to the clinic.

8. Provide client teaching as per Box 59-5.

VII. CORONARY ARTERY DISEASE

A. Description

1. Coronary artery disease is a narrowing or obstruction of one or more coronary arteries as a result of atherosclerosis, an accumulation of lipid-containing plaque in the arteries.

2. Coronary artery disease causes decreased perfusion of myocardial tissue and inadequate myocardial oxygen supply.

3. Coronary artery disease leads to hypertension, angina, dysrhythmias, MI, heart failure, and death.

4. Collateral circulation, more than one artery supplying a muscle with blood, is normally present in the coronary arteries, especially in older persons.

5. The development of collateral circulation takes time and develops when chronic ischemia occurs to meet the metabolic demands; therefore an occlusion of a coronary artery in a younger individual is more likely to be lethal than in an older individual.

6. Symptoms occur when the coronary artery is occluded to the point that inadequate blood supply to the muscle occurs, causing ischemia.

BOX 59-5

Pacemakers: Client Education

Instruct the client about the pacemaker, including the programmed rate.

Instruct the client in the signs of battery failure and when to notify the physician.

Instruct the client to report any fever, redness, swelling, or drainage from the insertion site.

Report signs of dizziness, weakness or fatigue, swelling of the ankles or legs, chest pain, or shortness of breath.

Keep a pacemaker identification card in the wallet and obtain and wear a Medic-Alert bracelet.

Instruct the client in how to take the pulse, to take the pulse daily, and to maintain a diary of pulse rates.

Wear loose-fitting clothing.

Avoid contact sports.

Inform all health care providers that a pacemaker has been inserted.

Instruct the client to inform airport security that he or she has a pacemaker because the pacemaker may set off the security detector.

Instruct the client that most electrical appliances can be used without any interference with the functioning of the pacemaker; however, advise the client not to operate electrical appliances directly over the pacemaker site.

Avoid transmitter towers and antitheft devices in stores.

Instruct the client that if any unusual feelings occur when near any electrical devices to move 5 to 10 feet away and check the pulse.

Instruct the client about the methods of monitoring the function of the device.

Emphasize the importance of follow-up with the physician.

---

7. Coronary artery narrowing is significant if the lumen diameter of the left main artery is reduced at least 50%, or if any major branch is reduced at least 75%.

8. The goal of treatment is to alter the atherosclerotic progression.

B. Assessment

1. Possibly normal findings during asymptomatic periods

2. Chest pain

3. Palpitations

4. Dyspnea

5. Syncope

6. Cough or hemoptysis

7. Excessive fatigue

C. Diagnostic studies

1. Electrocardiogram

   a. When blood flow is reduced and ischemia occurs, ST segment depression or T wave inversion is noted; the ST segment returns to normal when the blood flow returns.

b. With infarction, cell injury results in ST segment elevation, followed by T wave inversion.

2. Cardiac catheterization
   a. Cardiac catheterization provides the most definitive source for diagnosis.
   b. Cardiac catheterization shows the presence of atherosclerotic lesions.

3. Blood lipid levels
   a. Blood lipid levels may be elevated.
   b. Cholesterol-lowering medications may be prescribed to reduce the development of atherosclerotic plaques.

D. Interventions
   1. Instruct the client regarding the purpose of diagnostic medical and surgical procedures and the preprocedure and postprocedure expectations.
   2. Assist the client to identify risk factors that can be modified.
   3. Assist the client to set goals to promote lifestyle changes that will reduce the impact of risk factors.
   4. Assist the client to identify barriers to compliance with the therapeutic plan and to identify methods to overcome barriers.
   5. Instruct the client regarding a low-calorie, low-sodium, low-cholesterol, and low-fat diet, with an increase in dietary fiber.
   6. Stress to the client that dietary changes are not temporary and must be maintained for life; instruct the client regarding prescribed medications.
   7. Provide community resources to the client regarding exercise, smoking reduction, and stress reduction as appropriate.

E. Surgical procedures
   1. PTCA to compress the plaque against the walls of the artery and dilate the vessel
   2. Laser angioplasty to vaporize the plaque
   3. Atherectomy to remove the plaque from the artery
   4. Vascular stent to prevent the artery from closing and to prevent restenosis
   5. Coronary artery bypass graft to improve blood flow to the myocardial tissue that is at risk for ischemia or infarction because of the occluded artery

F. Medications
   1. Nitrates to dilate the coronary arteries and to decrease **preload** and **afterload**
   2. Calcium channel blockers to dilate coronary arteries and reduce vasospasm
   3. Cholesterol-lowering medications to reduce the development of atherosclerotic plaques
   4. β-Blockers to reduce **BP** in individuals who are hypertensive

VIII. ANGINA

A. Description
   1. Angina is chest pain resulting from myocardial ischemia caused by inadequate myocardial blood and oxygen supply.

2. Angina is caused by an imbalance between oxygen supply and demand.
3. Causes include obstruction of coronary blood flow because of atherosclerosis, coronary artery spasm, and conditions increasing myocardial oxygen consumption.
4. The goal of treatment is to provide relief of an acute attack, correct the imbalance between myocardial oxygen supply and demand, and prevent the progression of the disease and further attacks to reduce the risk of MI.

B. Patterns of angina
   1. Stable angina
      a. Stable angina also is called exertional angina.
      b. Stable angina occurs with activities that involve exertion or emotional stress and is relieved with rest or nitroglycerin.
      c. Stable angina usually has a stable pattern of onset, duration, severity, and relieving factors.
   2. Unstable angina
      a. Unstable angina also is called preinfarction angina.
      b. Unstable angina occurs with an unpredictable degree of exertion or emotion and increases in occurrence, duration, and severity over time.
      c. Pain may not be relieved with nitroglycerin.
   3. Variant angina
      a. Variant angina also is called Prinzmetal's or vasospastic angina.
      b. Variant angina results from coronary artery spasm.
      c. Variant angina may occur at rest.
      d. Attacks may be associated with ST segment elevation noted on the electrocardiogram.
   4. Intractable angina is a chronic, incapacitating angina that is unresponsive to interventions.
   5. Preinfarction angina
      a. Preinfarction angina is associated with acute coronary insufficiency.
      b. Preinfarction angina lasts longer than 15 minutes.
      c. Preinfarction angina is a symptom of worsening cardiac ischemia.
   6. Postinfarction angina occurs after an MI, when residual ischemia may cause episodes of angina.

C. Assessment
   1. Pain
      a. Pain can develop slowly or quickly.
      b. Pain usually is described as mild or moderate.
      c. Substernal, crushing, squeezing pain may occur.
      d. Pain may radiate to the shoulders, arms, jaw, neck, and back.
      e. Pain usually lasts less than 5 minutes; however, pain can last up to 15 to 20 minutes.
      f. Pain is relieved by nitroglycerin or rest.

2. Dyspnea
3. Pallor
4. Sweating
5. Palpitations and tachycardia
6. Dizziness and faintness
7. Hypertension
8. Digestive disturbances

D. Diagnostic studies
1. Electrocardiogram: Readings are normal during rest, with ST depression or elevation and/or T wave inversion during an episode of pain.
2. Stress test: Chest pain or changes in the electrocardiogram or vital signs during testing may indicate ischemia.
3. Cardiac enzymes and troponins: Findings are normal in angina.
4. Cardiac catheterization: Catheterization provides a definitive diagnosis by providing information about the patency of the coronary arteries.

E. Interventions
1. Immediate management
   a. Assess pain.
   b. Provide bed rest.
   c. Administer oxygen at 3 L/min by nasal cannula as prescribed.
   d. Administer nitroglycerin as prescribed to dilate the coronary arteries, reduce the oxygen requirements of the myocardium, and relieve the chest pain.
   e. Obtain a 12-lead electrocardiogram.
   f. Provide continuous cardiac monitoring.
2. Following acute episode
   a. Instruct the client regarding the purpose of diagnostic medical and surgical procedures and the preprocedure and postprocedure expectations.
   b. Assist the client to identify angina-precipitating events.
   c. Instruct the client to stop activity and rest if chest pain occurs and to take nitroglycerin as prescribed.
   d. Instruct the client to seek medical attention if pain persists.
   e. Instruct the client regarding prescribed medications.
   f. Provide diet instructions to the client, stressing that dietary changes are not temporary and must be maintained for life.
   g. Assist the client to identify risk factors that can be modified.
   h. Assist the client to set goals that will promote changes in lifestyle to reduce the impact of risk factors.
   i. Assist the client to identify barriers to compliance with therapeutic plan and to identify methods to overcome barriers.
   j. Provide community resources to the client regarding exercise, smoking reduction, and stress reduction.

F. Surgical procedures: Refer to the section Coronary Artery Disease.

G. Medications
1. Refer to the section Coronary Artery Disease.
2. Antiplatelet therapy inhibits platelet aggregation and reduces the risk of developing an acute MI.

IX. MYOCARDIAL INFARCTION

A. Description
1. Myocardial infarction occurs when myocardial tissue is abruptly and severely deprived of oxygen.
2. Ischemia can lead to necrosis of myocardial tissue if blood flow is not restored.
3. Infarction does not occur instantly but evolves over several hours.
4. Obvious physical changes do not occur in the heart until 6 hours after the infarction, when the infarcted area appears blue and swollen.
5. After 48 hours the infarct turns gray with yellow streaks as neutrophils invade the tissue.
6. By 8 to 10 days after infarction, granulation tissue forms.
7. Over 2 to 3 months, the necrotic area develops into a scar; scar tissue permanently changes the size and shape of the entire left ventricle.
8. Not all clients experience the classic symptoms of an MI.
9. Women may experience atypical discomfort, shortness of breath, or fatigue.
10. An older client may experience shortness of breath, pulmonary edema, dizziness, altered mental status, or a dysrhythmia.

B. Location of MI
1. Obstruction of the left anterior descending artery results in anterior or septal MI or both.
2. Obstruction of the circumflex artery results in posterior wall MI or lateral wall MI.
3. Obstruction of the right coronary artery results in inferior wall MI.

C. Risk factors
1. Atherosclerosis
2. Coronary artery disease
3. Elevated cholesterol levels
4. Smoking
5. Hypertension
6. Obesity
7. Physical inactivity
8. Impaired glucose tolerance
9. Stress

D. Diagnostic studies
1. Total creatine kinase level
   a. Level rises within 3 hours after the onset of chest pain.

b. Level peaks within 24 hours after damage and death of cardiac tissue.

2. CK-MB isoenzyme
   a. Peak elevation occurs 18 to 24 hours after the onset of chest pain.
   b. Level returns to normal 48 to 72 hours later.

3. Troponin level
   a. Level rises within 3 hours.
   b. Level remains elevated for up to 7 days.

4. Myoglobin: Level rises within 1 hour after cell death, peaks in 4 to 6 hours, and returns to normal within 24 to 36 hours or less.

5. LDH level
   a. Level rises 24 hours after MI.
   b. Level peaks between 48 and 72 hours and falls to normal in 7 days.
   c. Serum level of LDH_1 isoenzyme rises higher than serum level of LDH_2.

6. White blood cell count: An elevated white blood cell count of 10,000 to 20,000 cells/mm³ appears on the second day following the MI and lasts up to a week.

7. Electrocardiogram
   a. Electrocardiogram shows ST segment elevation, T wave inversion, and an abnormal Q wave.
   b. Hours to days after the MI, ST and T wave changes will return to normal but the Q wave usually remains permanently.

8. Diagnostic tests following the acute stage
   a. Exercise tolerance test or stress test may be prescribed to assess for electrocardiographic changes and ischemia and to evaluate for medical therapy or identify clients who may need invasive therapy.
   b. Thallium scans may be prescribed to assess for ischemia or necrotic muscle tissue.
   c. Multigated cardiac blood pool imaging scans may be used to evaluate left ventricular function.
   d. Cardiac catheterization is performed to determine the extent and location of obstructions of the coronary arteries.

E. Assessment
   1. Pain
      a. Client may experience crushing substernal pain.
      b. Pain may radiate to the jaw, back, and left arm.
      c. Pain may occur without cause, primarily early in the morning.
      d. Pain is unrelieved by rest or nitroglycerin and is relieved only by opioids.
      e. Pain lasts 30 minutes or longer.
   2. Nausea and vomiting
   3. Diaphoresis
   4. Dyspnea
   5. Dysrhythmias
   6. Feelings of fear and anxiety
   7. Pallor, cyanosis, coolness of extremities

F. Complications of MI
   1. Dysrhythmias
   2. Heart failure
   3. Pulmonary edema
   4. Cardiogenic shock
   5. Thrombophlebitis
   6. Pericarditis
   7. Mitral valve insufficiency
   8. Postinfarction angina
   9. Ventricular rupture
   10. Dressler's syndrome (a combination of pericarditis, pericardial effusion, and pleural effusion, which can occur several weeks to months following an MI)

G. Interventions, acute stage
   1. Obtain a description of the chest discomfort.
   2. Assess vital signs.
   3. Assess cardiovascular status and maintain cardiac monitoring.
   4. Place the client in semi-Fowler position to enhance comfort and tissue oxygenation.
   5. Administer oxygen at 2 to 4 L/min by nasal cannula as prescribed.
   6. Establish an IV access route.
   7. Administer nitroglycerin as prescribed.
   8. Administer morphine sulfate as prescribed to relieve chest discomfort that is unresponsive to nitroglycerin.
   9. Obtain a 12-lead electrocardiogram.
   10. Administer IV nitroglycerin and antidysrhythmics as prescribed.
   11. Monitor thrombolytic therapy, which may be prescribed within the first 6 hours of the coronary event.
   12. Monitor for signs of bleeding if the client is receiving thrombolytic therapy.
   13. Monitor laboratory values as prescribed.
   14. Administer β-blockers as prescribed to slow the heart rate and increase myocardial perfusion while reducing the force of myocardial contraction.
   15. Monitor for complications related to the MI.
   16. Monitor for cardiac dysrhythmias because tachycardia and PVCs frequently occur in the first few hours after MI.
   17. Assess distal peripheral pulses and skin temperature because poor **cardiac output** may be identified by cool diaphoretic skin and diminished or absent pulses.
   18. Monitor intake and output.
   19. Assess respiratory rate and breath sounds for signs of heart failure, as indicated by the presence of crackles or wheezes or dependent edema.
   20. Monitor the **BP** closely after the administration of medications; if the **BP** is less than 100 systolic or

25 mm Hg lower than the previous reading, lower the head of the bed and notify the physician.
21. Provide reassurance to the client and family.

H. Interventions following acute episode
1. Maintain bed rest for the first 24 to 36 hours.
2. Allow the client to stand to void or use a bedside commode if prescribed.
3. Provide range of motion exercises to prevent thrombus formation and maintain muscle strength.
4. Progress to dangling legs at the side of the bed or out of bed to the chair for 30 minutes 3 times a day as prescribed.
5. Progress to ambulation in the client's room and to the bathroom and then in the hallway 3 times a day.
6. Monitor for complications.
7. Encourage the client to verbalize feelings regarding the MI.

I. Cardiac rehabilitation: Process of actively assisting the client with cardiac disease to achieve and maintain a vital and productive life within the limitations of the heart disease

X. HEART FAILURE

A. Description
1. Heart failure is the inability of the heart to maintain adequate circulation to meet the metabolic needs of the body because of an impaired pumping capability.
2. **Cardiac output** is diminished, and peripheral tissue is not perfused adequately.
3. Congestion of the lungs and periphery may occur.

B. Classification
1. Acute heart failure occurs suddenly.
2. Chronic heart failure develops over time; however, a client with chronic heart failure can develop an acute episode.

C. Types of heart failure
1. Right ventricular failure/left ventricular failure
   a. Because the two ventricles of the heart represent two separate pumping systems, it is possible for one to fail alone for a short period.
   b. Most heart failure begins with left ventricular failure and progresses to failure of both ventricles.
   c. Acute pulmonary edema, a medical emergency, results from left ventricular failure.
   d. If pulmonary edema is not treated, death will occur from suffocation because the client literally drowns in his or her own fluids.
2. Forward failure/backward failure
   a. In forward failure, an inadequate output of the affected ventricle causes decreased perfusion to vital organs.
   b. In backward failure, blood backs up behind the affected ventricle, causing increased pressure in the atrium behind the affected ventricle.

3. Low output/high output
   a. In low-output failure, not enough **cardiac output** is available to meet the demands of the body.
   b. High-output failure occurs when a condition causes the heart to work harder to meet the demands of the body.
4. Systolic failure/diastolic failure
   a. Systolic failure leads to problems with contraction and the ejection of blood.
   b. Diastolic failure leads to problems with the heart relaxing and filling with blood.

D. Compensatory mechanisms
1. Compensatory mechanisms act to restore **cardiac output** to near-normal levels.
2. Initially these mechanisms increase **cardiac output;** however, they eventually have a damaging effect on pump action.
3. Compensatory mechanisms contribute to an increase in myocardial oxygen consumption, and when this occurs, myocardial reserve is exhausted and clinical manifestations of heart failure develop.
4. Compensatory mechanisms include increased heart rate, improved **stroke volume**, arterial vasoconstriction, sodium and water retention, and myocardial hypertrophy.

E. Assessment
1. Right ventricular failure
   a. Signs of right ventricular failure are evident in the systemic circulation
   b. Pitting, dependent edema in the feet, legs, sacrum, back, and buttocks
   c. Ascites from portal hypertension
   d. Tenderness of right upper quadrant, organomegaly
   e. Distended neck veins
   f. Pulsus alternans (regular alteration of weak and strong beats noted in the pulse)
   g. Abdominal pain, bloating
   h. Anorexia, nausea
   i. Fatigue
   j. Weight gain
   k. Nocturnal diuresis
2. Left ventricular failure
   a. Signs of left ventricular failure are evident in the pulmonary system
   b. Cough, which may become productive with frothy sputum
   c. Dyspnea on exertion
   d. Orthopnea
   e. Paroxysmal nocturnal dyspnea
   f. Presence of crackles on auscultation
   g. Tachycardia
   h. Pulsus alternans
   i. Fatigue
   j. Pallor
   k. Cyanosis

l. Confusion and disorientation

m.Signs of cerebral anoxia

3. Acute pulmonary edema
   a. Severe dyspnea and orthopnea
   b. Pallor
   c. Tachycardia
   d. Expectoration of large amounts of blood-tinged, frothy sputum
   e. Wheezing and crackles on auscultation
   f. Bubbling respirations
   g. Acute anxiety, apprehension, restlessness
   h. Profuse sweating
   i. Cold, clammy skin
   j. Cyanosis
   k. Nasal flaring
   l. Use of accessory breathing muscles
   m.Tachypnea
   n. Hypocapnia, evidenced by muscle cramps, weakness, dizziness, and paresthesias

F. Immediate management
   1. Place the client in high Fowler's position, with the legs in a dependent position, to reduce pulmonary congestion and relieve edema.
   2. Administer oxygen in high concentrations by mask or cannula as prescribed to improve gas exchange and pulmonary function.
   3. Prepare for intubation and ventilator support if required; monitor lung sounds for crackles and decreased breath sounds.
   4. Suction fluids as needed to maintain a patent airway.
   5. Assess level of consciousness.
   6. Provide reassurance to the client.
   7. Monitor vital signs closely, noting tachycardia or pulsus alternans.
   8. Monitor for hypotension resulting from decreased tissue perfusion or hypertension resulting from anxiety or history of hypertension.
   9. Monitor heart rate and for dysrhythmias by using a cardiac monitor.
   10. Assess for edema in dependent areas and in the sacral, lumbar, and posterior thigh region in the client on bed rest.
   11. Insert a Foley catheter as prescribed and monitor urine output closely following administration of a diuretic.
   12. Monitor intake and output.
   13. Avoid the unnecessary IV administration of fluids.
   14. Administer morphine sulfate as prescribed to provide sedation and vasodilation, and monitor for respiratory depression or hypotension after administration.
   15. Administer diuretics as prescribed to reduce **preload,** enhance renal excretion of sodium and water, reduce circulating blood volume, and reduce pulmonary congestion.
   16. Administer digitalis as prescribed to increase ventricular **contractility** and improve **cardiac output.**
   17. Administer bronchodilators as prescribed for severe bronchospasm or bronchoconstriction.
   18. Administer additional inotropic medications, such as dopamine (Intropin) or dobutamine (Dobutrex), as prescribed to facilitate myocardial **contractility** and enhance **stroke** volume.
   19. Administer vasodilators as prescribed to reduce **afterload,** increase the capacity of the systemic venous bed, and decrease venous return to the heart.
   20. Monitor weight to determine a response to treatment.
   21. Assess for hepatomegaly and ascites, and measure and record abdominal girth.
   22. Monitor peripheral pulses.
   23. Analyze arterial blood gas results and electrolyte values for imbalances.
   24. Monitor potassium level closely, which may decrease as a result of diuretic therapy, and administer potassium supplements as prescribed to prevent digitalis toxicity.

G. Following the acute episode
   1. Encourage the client to verbalize feelings about the lifestyle changes required as a result of the heart failure.
   2. Assist the client to identify precipitating risk factors of heart failure and methods of eliminating these risk factors.
   3. Instruct the client in the prescribed medication regimen, which may include digoxin (Lanoxin), a diuretic, and vasodilators.
   4. Advise the client to notify the physician if side effects occur from the medications.
   5. Advise the client to avoid over-the-counter medications.
   6. Instruct the client to contact the physician if he or she is unable to take medications because of illness.
   7. Instruct the client to avoid large amounts of caffeine, found in coffee, tea, cocoa, chocolate, and some carbonated beverages.
   8. Instruct the client about the prescribed low-sodium, low-fat, and low-cholesterol diet.
   9. Provide the client with a list of potassium-rich foods because diuretics can cause hypokalemia (except for potassium-sparing diuretics).
   10. Instruct the client regarding fluid restriction, if prescribed, advising the client to spread the fluid out during the day and to suck on hard candy to reduce thirst.
   11. Instruct the client to balance periods of activity and rest.
   12. Advise the client to avoid isometric activities, which increase pressure in the heart.

13. Instruct the client to monitor daily weight.
14. Instruct the client to report signs of fluid retention such as edema or weight gain.

XI. CARDIOGENIC SHOCK
A. Description
  1. Cardiogenic shock is failure of the heart to pump adequately, thereby reducing **cardiac output** and compromising tissue perfusion.
  2. Necrosis of more than 40% of the left ventricle occurs, usually as a result of occlusion of major coronary vessels.
  3. The goal of treatment is to maintain tissue oxygenation and perfusion and improve the pumping ability of the heart.
B. Assessment
  1. Hypotension: **BP** less than 90 mm Hg systolic or 30 mm Hg less than the client's baseline
  2. Urine output of less than 30 mL/hour
  3. Cold, clammy skin
  4. Poor peripheral pulses
  5. Tachycardia
  6. Pulmonary congestion
  7. Tachypnea
  8. Disorientation, restlessness, and confusion
  9. Continuing chest discomfort
C. Interventions
  1. Administer morphine sulfate intravenously as prescribed to decrease pulmonary congestion and relieve pain.
  2. Administer oxygen as prescribed.
  3. Prepare for intubation and mechanical ventilation.
  4. Administer diuretics and nitrates as prescribed while monitoring **BP** constantly.
  5. Administer vasopressors and positive inotropics as prescribed to maintain organ perfusion.
  6. Prepare the client for insertion of an intraaortic balloon pump, if prescribed, to facilitate emptying of the left ventricle and improve **cardiac output.**
  7. Prepare the client for immediate reperfusion procedures such as PTCA or coronary artery bypass graft.
  8. Monitor arterial blood gas levels and prepare to treat imbalances.
  9. Monitor urinary output.
  10. Assist with the insertion of Swan-Ganz catheter to assess heart failure.
  11. Monitor distal pulses and maintain the transducer at the level of the right atrium if the client has a Swan-Ganz catheter.

XII. INFLAMMATORY DISEASES OF THE HEART
▲ A. Pericarditis
  1. Description
    a. Pericarditis is an acute or chronic inflammation of the pericardium.
    b. Chronic pericarditis, a chronic inflammatory thickening of the pericardium, constricts the heart, causing compression.
    c. The pericardial sac becomes inflamed.
    d. Pericarditis can result in loss of pericardial elasticity or an accumulation of fluid within the sac.
    e. Heart failure or cardiac tamponade may result.
  2. Assessment
    a. Precordial pain in the anterior chest that radiates to the left side of the neck, shoulder, or back
    b. Pain that is aggravated by breathing (particularly inspiration), coughing, and swallowing ▲
    c. Pain that is worse when in the supine position ▲ and may be relieved by leaning forward
    d. Pericardial friction rub (scratchy, high-pitched sound) heard on auscultation and produced by the rubbing of the inflamed pericardial layers
    e. Fever and chills
    f. Fatigue and malaise
    g. Elevated white blood cell count
    h. Electrocardiogram changes
    i. Signs of right ventricular failure in clients with chronic constrictive pericarditis
  3. Interventions
    a. Assess the nature of the pain.
    b. Position the client in high Fowler's, or upright ▲ and leaning forward.
    c. Administer analgesics, nonsteroidal antiinflammatory drugs, or corticosteroids for pain as prescribed.
    d. Avoid the administration of aspirin and anticoagulants because they increase the risk of tamponade.
    e. Auscultate for a pericardial friction rub.
    f. Check results of blood culture to identify causative organism.
    g. Administer antibiotics for bacterial infection as prescribed.
    h. Administer diuretics and digoxin (Lanoxin) as prescribed to the client with chronic constrictive pericarditis.
    i. Monitor for signs of cardiac tamponade, ▲ including pulsus paradoxus, jugular vein distention with clear lung sounds, muffled heart sounds, narrowed **pulse pressure**, tachycardia, and decreased **cardiac output.**
    j. Notify the physician if signs of cardiac tamponade occur.
B. Myocarditis
  1. Description: an acute or chronic inflammation of the myocardium as a result of pericarditis, systemic infection, or allergic response
  2. Assessment
    a. Fever
    b. Pericardial friction rub
    c. A gallop rhythm

d. A murmur that sounds like fluid passing an obstruction
e. Pulsus alternans
f. Signs of heart failure
g. Fatigue
h. Dyspnea
i. Tachycardia
j. Chest pain

3. Interventions
   a. Assist the client to a position of comfort such as sitting up and leaning forward.
   b. Administer analgesics, salicylates, and nonsteroidal antiinflammatory drugs as prescribed to reduce fever and pain.
   c. Administer oxygen as prescribed.
   d. Provide adequate rest periods.
   e. Limit activities to avoid overexertion and to decrease the workload of the heart.
   f. Administer digoxin (Lanoxin) as prescribed, and monitor for signs of digoxin toxicity.
   g. Administer antidysrhythmics as prescribed.
   h. Administer antibiotics as prescribed to treat the causative organism.
   i. Monitor for complications, which can include thrombus, heart failure, or cardiomyopathy.

C. Endocarditis
   1. Description
      a. Endocarditis is an inflammation of the inner lining of the heart and valves.
      b. Endocarditis occurs primarily in clients who are IV drug abusers, have had valve replacements, or have mitral valve prolapse or other structural defects.
      c. Ports of entry for the infecting organism include the oral cavity (especially if the client had a dental procedure in the previous 3 to 6 months), cutaneous invasion, infections, or invasive procedures or surgery.
   2. Assessment
      a. Fever
      b. Anorexia
      c. Weight loss
      d. Fatigue
      e. Cardiac murmurs
      f. Heart failure
      g. Embolic complications from vegetation fragments traveling through the circulation
      h. Petechiae
      i. Splinter hemorrhages in the nailbeds
      j. Osler's nodes (reddish tender lesions) on the pads of the fingers, hands, and toes
      k. Janeway's lesions (nontender hemorrhagic lesions) on the fingers, toes, nose, or ear lobes
      l. Splenomegaly
      m. Clubbing of the fingers
   3. Interventions
      a. Provide adequate rest balanced with activity to prevent thrombus formation.

b. Maintain antiembolism stockings.
c. Monitor cardiovascular status.
d. Monitor for signs of heart failure.
e. Monitor for signs of emboli.
f. Monitor for splenic emboli, as evidenced by sudden abdominal pain radiating to the left shoulder, and the presence of rebound abdominal tenderness on palpation.
g. Monitor for renal emboli, as evidenced by flank pain radiating to the groin, hematuria, and pyuria.
h. Monitor for confusion, aphasia, or dysphagia, which may indicate central nervous system emboli.
i. Monitor for pulmonary emboli as evidenced by pleuritic chest pain, dyspnea, and cough.
j. Assess skin, mucous membranes, and conjunctiva for petechiae.
k. Assess nailbeds for splinter hemorrhages.
l. Assess for Osler's nodes on the pads of the fingers, hands, and toes.
m. Assess for Janeway's lesions on the fingers, toes, nose, or ear lobes.
n. Assess for clubbing of the fingers.
o. Evaluate blood culture results.
p. Administer antibiotics intravenously as prescribed.
q. Plan and arrange for discharge, providing resources required for the continued administration of antibiotics intravenously.

4. Client education
   a. Instruct the client about the signs and symptoms of complications and to notify the physician if they occur.
   b. Inform the client about the importance of good oral hygiene.
   c. Instruct the client to brush teeth twice daily with a soft toothbrush, followed by oral rinses.
   d. Instruct the client to avoid irrigation devices, electric toothbrushes, and flossing because these activities can cause the gums to bleed, allowing bacteria to enter the mucous membranes and bloodstream.
   e. Advise the client of the importance of prophylactic antibiotics before any invasive procedure and the importance of informing all health care professionals of the client's disease history.

XIII. CARDIAC TAMPONADE

A. Description
   1. A pericardial effusion occurs when the space between the parietal and visceral layers of the pericardium fill with fluid.
   2. Pericardial effusion places the client at risk for cardiac tamponade, an accumulation of fluid in the pericardial cavity.
   3. Tamponade restricts ventricular filling, and **cardiac output** drops.

4. Acute tamponade occurs when small volumes (20 to 50 mL) of fluid accumulate in the pericardium.

B. Assessment
1. Pulsus paradoxus
2. Increased CVP
3. Jugular venous distention with clear lungs
4. Distant, muffled heart sounds
5. Decreased **cardiac output**

C. Interventions
1. The client needs to be placed in a critical care unit for hemodynamic monitoring.
2. Administer fluids intravenously as prescribed to manage decreased **cardiac output.**
3. Prepare the client for chest x-ray film or echocardiogram.
4. Prepare the client for pericardiocentesis to withdraw pericardial fluid if prescribed.
5. Monitor for recurrence of tamponade following pericardiocentesis.
6. If the client experiences recurrent tamponade or recurrent effusions or develops adhesions from chronic pericarditis, a portion (pericardial window) or all of the pericardium (pericardiectomy) may be removed to allow adequate ventricular filling and contraction.

XIV. VALVULAR HEART DISEASE

A. Description
1. Valvular heart disease occurs when the heart valves cannot fully open (stenosis) or close completely (insufficiency or regurgitation).
2. Valvular heart disease prevents efficient blood flow through the heart.

B. Types
1. Mitral stenosis: Valvular tissue thickens and narrows the valve opening.
2. Mitral insufficiency/regurgitation: Valve is incompetent, preventing complete valve closure.
3. Mitral valve prolapse: Valve leaflets protrude into the left atrium during **systole.**
4. Aortic stenosis: Valvular tissue thickens and narrows the valve opening.
5. Aortic insufficiency: Valve is incompetent, preventing complete valve closure.

C. Repair procedures
1. Balloon valvuloplasty
   a. Balloon valvuloplasty is an invasive, nonsurgical procedure.
   b. A balloon catheter is passed from the femoral vein through the atrial septum to the mitral valve or through the femoral artery to the aortic valve.
   c. The balloon is inflated to enlarge the orifice.
   d. Institute precautions for arterial puncture if appropriate.
   e. Monitor for bleeding from the catheter insertion site.

f. Monitor for signs of systemic emboli.
g. Monitor for signs of a regurgitant valve by monitoring cardiac rhythm, heart sounds, and **cardiac output.**

2. Mitral annuloplasty: tightening and suturing the malfunctioning valve annulus to eliminate or greatly reduce regurgitation
3. Commissurotomy/valvotomy
   a. The procedure is accomplished with cardiopulmonary bypass during open heart surgery.
   b. The valve is visualized, thrombi are removed from the atria, fused leaflets are incised, and calcium is débrided from the leaflets, thus widening the orifice.

D. Valve replacement procedures
1. Mechanical prosthetic valves
   a. Prosthetic valves are durable.
   b. Thromboembolism is a problem following the valve replacement, and lifetime anticoagulant therapy is required. ▲
2. Bioprosthetic valves
   a. Biological grafts are xenografts (valves from other species): porcine valves (pig), bovine valves (cow), or homografts (human cadavers).
   b. The risk of clot formation is small; therefore long-term anticoagulation is not indicated.
3. Preoperative interventions: Consult with the physician regarding discontinuing anticoagulants 72 hours before surgery.
4. Postoperative interventions
   a. Monitor closely for signs of bleeding.
   b. Monitor **cardiac output** and for signs of heart failure.
   c. Administer digoxin (Lanoxin) as prescribed to maintain **cardiac output** and prevent atrial fibrillation.
   d. Provide client teaching (Box 59-6).

E. Mitral stenosis
1. Assessment
   a. Asymptomatic initially
   b. Symptoms occur when the orifice is reduced by 50%
   c. Dyspnea
   d. Orthopnea
   e. Paroxysmal nocturnal dyspnea
   f. Dry cough
   g. Rumbling apical diastolic murmur
   h. Right ventricular failure
   i. Hepatomegaly
   j. Neck vein distention
   k. Pitting peripheral edema
   l. Hemoptysis and pulmonary edema as pulmonary hypertension and congestion progress
   m. Development of atrial fibrillation, indicating that the client may decompensate (notify physician immediately)

BOX 59-6

Client Instructions Following Valve Replacement

Adequate rest is important, and fatigue is usual.

Anticoagulant therapy is necessary if a mechanical prosthetic valve was inserted.

Instruct the client concerning hazards related to anticoagulant therapy and to notify the physician if bleeding or excessive bruising occurs.

Instruct the client concerning the importance of good oral hygiene to reduce the risk of infective endocarditis.

Brush teeth twice daily with a soft toothbrush, followed by oral rinses.

Avoid irrigation devices, electric toothbrushes, and flossing because these activities can cause the gums to bleed, allowing bacteria to enter the mucous membranes and bloodstream.

Monitor incision and report any drainage or redness.

Avoid any dental procedures for 6 months.

Heavy lifting (greater than 10 lb) is to be avoided, and exercise caution when in an automobile to prevent injury to the sternal incision.

If a prosthetic valve was inserted, a soft audible clicking sound may be heard.

Instruct the client concerning the importance of prophylactic antibiotics before any invasive procedure and the importance of informing all health care professionals of the valvular disease history.

Obtain and wear a Medic-Alert bracelet.

2. Interventions
    a. Administer prescribed treatment for heart failure.
    b. Administer oxygen as prescribed.
    c. Provide a low-sodium diet.
    d. Administer diuretics and digoxin (Lanoxin) as prescribed.
    e. Administer antibiotics as prescribed if infective endocarditis is present.
    f. Administer antidysrhythmics and anticoagulants for atrial fibrillation as prescribed.
    g. Prepare the client for commissurotomy or valve replacement as indicated.
F. Mitral valve prolapse
  1. Assessment
    a. Fatigue
    b. Atypical chest pain
    c. Palpitations
    d. Dizziness and syncope
    e. Tachycardia
    f. Systolic click
  2. Interventions
    a. Administer propranolol (Inderal) for dyspnea and chest pain as prescribed.
    b. Administer prophylactic antibiotics as prescribed.
G. Mitral insufficiency
  1. Assessment
    a. Dyspnea

    b. Orthopnea
    c. Fatigue
    d. Dizziness
    e. Palpitations
    f. Signs of right ventricular failure
    g. Atrial fibrillation
    h. Neck vein distention
    i. Pitting peripheral edema
    j. High-pitched systolic murmur
  2. Interventions
    a. Administer prescribed treatment for heart failure.
    b. Administer oxygen as prescribed.
    c. Provide a low-sodium diet.
    d. Administer diuretics and digoxin (Lanoxin) as prescribed.
    e. Administer antibiotics as prescribed if infective endocarditis is present.
    f. Administer antidysrhythmics and anticoagulants for atrial fibrillation as prescribed.
    g. Prepare the client for commissurotomy or valve replacement as indicated.
H. Aortic stenosis
  1. Assessment
    a. Dyspnea on exertion
    b. Angina
    c. Syncope on exertion
    d. Fatigue
    e. Orthopnea
    f. Paroxysmal nocturnal dyspnea
    g. Harsh systolic crescendo-decrescendo murmur
  2. Interventions
    a. Administer prescribed treatment for heart failure.
    b. Administer oxygen as prescribed.
    c. Provide a low-sodium diet.
    d. Administer diuretics and digoxin (Lanoxin) as prescribed.
    e. Administer antibiotics as prescribed if infective endocarditis is present.
    f. Prepare the client for valve replacement as indicated.
I. Aortic insufficiency
  1. Assessment
    a. Dyspnea
    b. Orthopnea
    c. Paroxysmal nocturnal dyspnea
    d. Fatigue
    e. Angina
    f. Tachycardia
    g. Blowing decresendo diastolic murmur
  2. Interventions
    a. Administer prescribed treatment for heart failure.
    b. Administer oxygen as prescribed.
    c. Provide a low-sodium diet.
    d. Administer diuretics and digoxin (Lanoxin) as prescribed.
    e. Administer antibiotics as prescribed if infective endocarditis is present.

  f. Prepare the client for valve replacement as indicated.

J. Tricuspid stenosis

 1. Assessment

  a. Easily fatigued

  b. Effort intolerance

  c. Complaints of fluttering sensations in the neck (obstructed venous flow)

  d. Cyanosis

  e. Signs of right ventricular failure

  f. Symptoms of decreased **cardiac output**

  g. Ascites

  h. Hepatomegaly

  i. Peripheral edema

  j. Rumbling diastolic murmur

  k. Jugular vein distention with clear lung fields

 2. Interventions

  a. Administer prescribed treatment for heart failure.

  b. Administer oxygen as prescribed.

  c. Provide a low-sodium diet.

  d. Administer diuretics and digoxin (Lanoxin) as prescribed.

  e. Administer antibiotics as prescribed if infective endocarditis is present.

  f. Prepare the client for valve replacement as indicated.

K. Tricuspid insufficiency

 1. Assessment

  a. Asymptomatic in mild situations

  b. Signs of right ventricular failure

  c. Ascites

  d. Hepatomegaly

  e. Pleural effusion

  f. Peripheral edema

  g. Systolic murmur heard at the left sternal border, fourth intercostal space

 2. Interventions

  a. Administer prescribed treatment for heart failure.

  b. Administer oxygen as prescribed.

  c. Provide a low-sodium diet.

  d. Administer diuretics and digoxin (Lanoxin) as prescribed.

  e. Administer antibiotics as prescribed if infective endocarditis is present.

  f. Prepare the client for valve replacement as indicated.

L. Pulmonary stenosis

 1. Assessment

  a. Asymptomatic in a mild condition

  b. Dyspnea

  c. Fatigue

  d. Syncope

  e. Signs of right ventricular failure

  f. Ascites

  g. Hepatomegaly

  h. Peripheral edema

  i. Systolic thrill heard at left sternal border

 2. Interventions

  a. Administer prescribed treatment for heart failure.

  b. Administer oxygen as prescribed.

  c. Provide a low-sodium diet.

  d. Administer diuretics and digoxin (Lanoxin) as prescribed.

  e. Administer antibiotics as prescribed if infective endocarditis is present.

  f. Prepare the client for pulmonary valve commissurotomy as indicated.

M. Pulmonary insufficiency

 1. Assessment

  a. Asymptomatic in mild condition

  b. Dyspnea

  c. Fatigue

  d. Syncope

  e. Signs of right ventricular failure

  f. Ascites

  g. Hepatomegaly

  h. Peripheral edema

  i. Systolic thrill heard at the left sternal border

 2. Interventions

  a. Administer prescribed treatment for heart failure.

  b. Administer oxygen as prescribed.

  c. Provide a low-sodium diet.

  d. Administer diuretics and digoxin (Lanoxin) as prescribed.

  e. Administer antibiotics as prescribed if infective endocarditis is present.

  f. Prepare the client for valve replacement as indicated.

XV. CARDIOMYOPATHY

A. Description

 1. Cardiomyopathy is a subacute or chronic disorder of the heart muscle.

 2. Treatment is palliative, not curative, and the client needs to deal with numerous lifestyle changes and a shortened life span.

B. Dilated cardiomyopathy

 1. Description

  a. Dilated cardiomyopathy is the most common type of cardiomyopathy.

  b. Heart ejects less than 40% of the blood in the left ventricle (normal is 70%), and reduced **cardiac output** leads to heart failure.

 2. Assessment

  a. Symptoms of left ventricular failure

  b. Weakness and fatigue

  c. Activity intolerance

  d. Chest pain

  e. Dysrhythmias

  f. Eventually signs of right ventricular failure

 3. Interventions

  a. Treatment of heart failure is symptomatic.

  b. Diuretics, cardiac glycosides, and vasodilators are administered to increase **cardiac output.**

c. Antidysrhythmics are administered to control dysrhythmias.

d. Instruct the client to report any signs of dizziness or fainting, which may indicate a dysrhythmia.

e. Instruct the client to avoid ingestion of alcohol because of its cardiac depressant effect.

f. Heart transplant may be necessary.

C. Hypertropic cardiomyopathy

1. Description

a. Hypertropic cardiomyopathy is characterized by massive ventricular hypertrophy, leading to hypercontraction of the left ventricle and rigid ventricle walls.

b. Hypertropic cardiomyopathy causes obstruction of the left ventricular outflow.

2. Assessment

a. Exertional dyspnea

b. Syncope

c. Chest pain that occurs at rest, is prolonged, is unrelated to exertion, and is not relieved by nitrates

d. Dysrhythmias

3. Interventions

a. Treatment is symptomatic, similar to the care of a client with MI.

b. Conversion of atrial fibrillation is performed if fibrillation occurs.

c. Instruct the client to report any signs of dizziness or fainting, which may indicate a dysrhythmia.

d. Instruct the client to avoid ingestion of alcohol because of its cardiac depressant effect.

e. β-Blockers and calcium antagonists decrease the outflow obstruction and decrease the heart rate.

f. Vasodilators and cardiac glycosides are contraindicated because vasodilator and positive inotropic effects augment the obstruction.

g. Ventriculomyotomy or muscle resection with mitral valve replacement may be necessary.

D. Restrictive cardiomyopathy

1. Description: Characterized by restriction of filling of the ventricles

2. Assessment

a. Exertional dyspnea

b. Weakness

3. Interventions

a. Treatment of heart failure is symptomatic.

b. Exercise is restricted.

c. Diuretics, cardiac glycosides, and vasodilators are administered to increase cardiac output.

d. Antidysrhythmics are administered to control dysrhythmias.

e. Instruct the client to report any signs of dizziness or fainting, which may indicate a dysrhythmia.

f. Instruct the client to avoid ingestion of alcohol because of its cardiac depressant effect.

XVI. VASCULAR DISORDERS

A. Venous thrombosis

1. Description

a. Thrombus can be associated with an inflammatory process.

b. When a thrombus develops, inflammation occurs, thickening the vein wall and leading to embolization.

2. Types

a. Thrombophlebitis: A thrombus associated with inflammation

b. Phlebothrombus: A thrombus without inflammation

c. Phlebitis: Vein inflammation associated with invasive procedures such as IV lines

d. Deep vein thrombophlebitis: More serious than a superficial thrombophlebitis because of the risk for pulmonary embolism

3. Risks factors for thrombus formation

a. Venous stasis from varicose veins, heart failure, immobility

b. Hypercoagulability disorders

c. Injury to the venous wall from IV injections, fractures, trauma

d. Following surgery, particularly hip surgery and open prostate surgery

e. Pregnancy

f. Ulcerative colitis

g. Use of oral contraceptives

B. Phlebitis

1. Assessment

a. Red, warm area radiating up an extremity

b. Pain and soreness

c. Swelling

2. Interventions

a. Apply warm moist soaks as prescribed to dilate the vein and promote circulation.

b. Assess temperature of soak before applying.

c. Assess for signs of complications such as tissue necrosis, infection, or pulmonary embolus.

C. Deep vein thrombophlebitis

1. Assessment

a. Calf or groin tenderness or pain with or without swelling

b. Positive Homans' sign

c. Warm skin that is tender to touch

2. Interventions

a. Provide bed rest.

b. Elevate the affected extremity above the level of the heart as prescribed.

c. Avoid using the knee gatch or a pillow under the knees.

d. Do not massage the extremity.

e. Provide thigh-high compression or antiembolism stockings as prescribed to reduce venous stasis and to assist in the venous return of blood to the heart.

f. Administer intermittent or continuous warm, moist compresses as prescribed.

g. Palpate the site gently, monitoring for warmth and edema.

h. Measure and record the circumferences of the thighs and calves.

i. Monitor for shortness of breath and chest pain, which can indicate pulmonary emboli.

j. Administer thrombolytic therapy (tissue plasminogen activator) if prescribed, which must be initiated within 5 days after the onset of symptoms.

k. Administer heparin therapy as prescribed to prevent enlargement of the existing clot and prevent the formation of new clots.

l. Monitor activated partial thromboplastin time during heparin therapy.

m. Administer warfarin (Coumadin) as prescribed following heparin therapy when the symptoms of deep vein thrombophlebitis have resolved.

n. Monitor prothrombin time and international normalized ratio during warfarin (Coumadin) therapy.

o. Monitor for the hazards and side effects associated with anticoagulant therapy.

p. Administer analgesics as prescribed to reduce pain.

q. Administer diuretics as prescribed to reduce lower extremity edema.

r. Provide client teaching (Box 59-7).

D. Venous insufficiency
  1. Description
    a. Venous insufficiency results from prolonged venous hypertension, which stretches the veins and damages the valves.

BOX 59-7

Instructions for the Client with Deep Vein Thrombophlebitis

Instruct the client concerning the hazards of anticoagulation therapy.

Recognize the signs and symptoms of bleeding.

Avoid prolonged sitting or standing, constrictive clothing, or crossing legs when seated.

Elevate the legs for 10 to 20 minutes every few hours each day.

Plan a progressive walking program.

Inspect the legs for edema, and measure the circumference of the legs.

Wear antiembolism stockings as prescribed.

Avoid smoking.

Avoid any medications unless prescribed by the physician.

Instruct the client concerning the importance of follow-up physician visits and laboratory studies.

Obtain and wear a Medic-Alert bracelet.

---

b. The resultant edema and venous stasis cause venous stasis ulcers, swelling, and cellulitis.

c. Treatment focuses on decreasing edema and promoting venous return from the affected extremity.

d. Treatment for venous stasis ulcers focuses on healing the ulcer and preventing stasis and ulcer recurrence.

2. Assessment
  a. Stasis dermatitis or brown discoloration along the ankles and extending up to the calf
  b. Edema
  c. Ulcer formation: edges are uneven and ulcer bed is pink

3. Interventions
  a. Instruct the client to wear elastic or compression stockings during the day and evening as prescribed.
  b. Instruct the client to put elastic stockings on upon awakening before getting out of bed.
  c. Advise the client to put a clean pair of elastic stockings on each day and that it will probably be necessary to wear the stockings for the remainder of life.
  d. Instruct the client to avoid prolonged sitting or standing, constrictive clothing, or crossing legs when seated.
  e. Instruct the client to elevate the legs for 10 to 20 minutes every few hours each day.
  f. Instruct the client to elevate legs above the level of the heart when in bed.
  g. Instruct the client in the use of an intermittent sequential pneumatic compression system, if prescribed; instruct the client to apply the compression system twice daily for 1 hour in the morning and evening.
  h. Advise the client with an open ulcer that the compression system is applied over a dressing.

4. Wound care
  a. Provide care to the wound as prescribed by the physician.
  b. Assess the client's ability to care for the wound, and initiate home care resources as necessary.
  c. If an Unna boot (a dressing constructed of gauze moistened with zinc oxide) is prescribed, the physician will change it weekly.
  d. The wound is cleansed with normal saline before application of the Unna boot; providone-iodine (Betadine) and hydrogen peroxide are not used because they destroy granulation tissue.
  e. The Unna boot is covered with an elastic wrap that hardens to promote venous return and prevent stasis.
  f. Monitor for signs of arterial occlusion from an Unna's boot that may be too tight.
  g. Keep tape off of the client's skin.

5. Medications
   a. Apply topical agents to wound as prescribed to débride the ulcer, eliminate necrotic tissue, and promote healing.
   b. When applying topical agents, apply an oil-based agent such as petroleum jelly (Vaseline) on surrounding skin, because débriding agents can injure healthy tissue.
   c. Administer antibiotics as prescribed if infection or cellulitis occurs.

E. Varicose veins
   1. Description
      a. Distended, protruding veins that appear darkened and tortuous are evident.
      b. Vein walls weaken and dilate, and valves become incompetent.
   2. Assessment
      a. Pain in the legs with dull aching after standing
      b. A feeling of fullness in the legs
      c. Ankle edema
   3. Trendelenburg's test
      a. Place the client in a supine position with the legs elevated.
      b. When the client sits up, if varicosities are present, veins fill from the proximal end; veins normally fill from the distal end.
   4. Interventions
      a. Assist with the Trendelenburg's test.
      b. Emphasize the importance of antiembolism stockings as prescribed.
      c. Instruct the client to elevate the legs as much as possible.
      d. Instruct the client to avoid constrictive clothing and pressure on the legs.
      e. Prepare the client for sclerotherapy or vein stripping as prescribed.
   5. Sclerotherapy
      a. A solution is injected into the vein, followed by the application of a pressure dressing.
      b. An incision and drainage of the trapped blood in the sclerosed vein are performed 14 to 21 days after the injection, followed by the application of a pressure dressing for 12 to 18 hours.
   6. Vein stripping
      a. Varicose veins are removed if they are larger than 4 mm in diameter or if they are in clusters.
      b. Preoperatively assist the physician with vein marking.
      c. Evaluate pulses as a baseline for comparison postoperatively.
      d. Maintain elastic (Ace) bandages on the client's legs postoperatively.
      e. Monitor the groin and leg for bleeding through the elastic bandages.
      f. Monitor the extremity for edema, warmth, color, and pulses.

   g. Elevate the legs above the level of the heart postoperatively.
   h. Encourage range of motion exercises of the legs.
   i. Instruct the client to avoid leg dangling or chair sitting.
   j. Instruct the client to elevate the legs when sitting.
   k. Emphasize the importance of wearing elastic stockings after bandage removal.

XVII. ARTERIAL DISORDERS
A. Peripheral arterial disease
   1. Description
      a. Peripheral arterial disease is a chronic disorder in which partial or total arterial occlusion deprives the lower extremities of oxygen and nutrients.
      b. Tissue damage occurs below the level of the arterial occlusion.
      c. Atherosclerosis is the most common cause of peripheral arterial disease.
   2. Assessment
      a. Intermittent claudication (pain in the muscles resulting from an inadequate blood supply)
      b. Rest pain, characterized by numbness, burning, or aching in the distal portion of the lower extremities, which awakens the client at night and is relieved by placing the extremity in a dependent position
      c. Lower back or buttock discomfort
      d. Loss of hair and dry scaly skin on the lower extremities
      e. Thickened toenails
      f. Cold and gray-blue color of skin in the lower extremities
      g. Elevational pallor and dependent rubor in the lower extremities
      h. Decreased or absent peripheral pulses
      i. Signs of arterial ulcer formation occurring on or between the toes or on the upper aspect of the foot that are characterized as painful
      j. **Blood pressure** measurements at the thigh, calf, and ankle are lower than the brachial pressure (normally **BP** readings in the thigh and calf are higher than those in the upper extremities)
   3. Interventions
      a. Assess pain.
      b. Monitor the extremities for color, motion and sensation, and pulses.
      c. Obtain **BP** measurements.
      d. Assess for signs of ulcer formation or signs of gangrene.
      e. Assist in developing an individualized exercise program, which is initiated gradually and slowly increased.
      f. Encourage prescribed exercise, which will improve arterial flow through the development of collateral circulation.

g. Instruct the client to walk to the point of claudication, stop and rest, and then walk a little farther.

h. Because swelling in the extremities prevents arterial blood flow, instruct the client to elevate the feet at rest but to refrain from elevating them above the level of the heart because extreme elevation slows arterial blood flow to the feet.

i. In severe cases of peripheral arterial disease, clients with edema may sleep with the affected limb hanging from the bed or they may sit upright in a chair for comfort.

j. Instruct the client with peripheral arterial disease to avoid crossing the legs, which interferes with blood flow.

k. Instruct the client to avoid exposure to cold (causes vasoconstriction) to the extremities and to wear socks or insulated shoes for warmth at all times.

l. Instruct the client never to apply direct heat to the limb, such as with a heating pad or hot water, because the decreased sensitivity in the limb will cause burning.

m. Instruct the client to inspect the skin on the extremities daily and to report any signs of skin breakdown.

n. Instruct the client to avoid tobacco and caffeine because of their vasoconstrictive effects.

o. Instruct the client in the use of hemorrheologic and antiplatelet medications as prescribed.

p. Inform the client of the importance of taking all medications prescribed by the physician.

4. Procedures to improve arterial blood flow
   a. Percutaneous transluminal coronary angioplasty
   b. Laser-assisted angioplasty
   c. Atherectomy
   d. Bypass surgery (aortofemoral or femoropopliteal)

B. Raynaud's disease
   1. Description
      a. Raynaud's disease is vasospasms of the arterioles and arteries of the upper and lower extremities.
      b. Vasospasm causes constriction of the cutaneous vessels.
      c. Attacks are intermittent and occur with exposure to cold or stress.
      d. Affects primarily fingers, toes, ears, and cheeks.
   2. Assessment
      a. Blanching of the extremity, followed by cyanosis during vasoconstriction
      b. Reddened tissue when the vasospasm is relieved
      c. Numbness, tingling, swelling, and a cold temperature at the affected body part
   3. Interventions
      a. Monitor pulses.
      b. Administer vasodilators as prescribed.

c. Instruct the client regarding medication therapy.
d. Assist the client to identify and avoid precipitating factors such as cold and stress.
e. Instruct the client to avoid smoking.
f. Instruct the client to wear warm clothing, socks, and gloves in cold weather.
g. Advise the client to avoid injuries to fingers and hands.

C. Buerger's disease (thromboangiitis obliterans)
   1. Description
      a. Buerger's disease is an occlusive disease of the median and small arteries and veins.
      b. The distal upper and lower limbs are affected most commonly.
   2. Assessment
      a. Intermittent claudication
      b. Ischemic pain occurring in the digits while at rest
      c. Aching pain that is more severe at night
      d. Cool, numb, or tingling sensation
      e. Diminished pulses in the distal extremities
      f. Extremities that are cool and red in the dependent position
      g. Development of ulcerations in the extremities
   3. Interventions
      a. Instruct the client to stop smoking.
      b. Monitor pulses.
      c. Instruct the client to avoid injury to the upper and lower extremities.
      d. Administer vasodilators as prescribed.
      e. Instruct the client regarding medication therapy.

XVIII. AORTIC ANEURYSMS

A. Description
   1. An aortic aneurysm is an abnormal dilation of the arterial wall caused by localized weakness and stretching in the medial layer or wall of an artery.
   2. The aneurysm can be located anywhere along the abdominal aorta.
   3. The goal of treatment is to limit the progression of the disease by modifying risk factors, controlling the **BP** to prevent strain on the aneurysm, recognizing symptoms early, and preventing rupture.

B. Types of aortic aneurysm
   1. Fusiform: Diffuse dilation that involves the entire circumference of the arterial segment
   2. Saccular: Distinct localized outpouching of the artery wall
   3. Dissecting: Created when blood separates the layers of the artery wall, forming a cavity between them
   4. False (pseudoaneurysm)
      a. Pseudoaneurysm occurs when the clot and connective tissue are outside the arterial wall.
      b. Pseudoaneurysm occurs as a result of vessel injury or trauma to all three layers of the arterial wall.

C. Assessment
   1. Thoracic aneurysm

a. Pain extending to neck, shoulders, lower back, or abdomen

b. Syncope

c. Dyspnea

d. Increased pulse

e. Cyanosis

f. Weakness

2. Abdominal aneurysm

a. Prominent, pulsating mass in abdomen, at or above the umbilicus

b. Systolic bruit over the aorta

c. Tenderness on deep palpation

d. Abdominal or lower back pain

3. Rupturing aneurysm

a. Severe abdominal or back pain

b. Lumbar pain radiating to the flank and groin

c. Hypotension

d. Increased pulse rate

e. Signs of shock

4. Diagnostic tests

a. Diagnostic tests are done to confirm the presence, size, and location of the aneurysm.

b. Tests includes abdominal ultrasound, computed tomography scan, and arteriography.

5. Interventions

a. Monitor vital signs.

b. Assess risk factors for the arterial disease process.

c. Obtain information regarding back or abdominal pain.

d. Question the client regarding the sensation of palpation in the abdomen.

e. Inspect the skin for the presence of vascular disease or breakdown.

f. Check peripheral circulation, including pulses, temperature, and color.

g. Observe for signs of rupture.

h. Note any tenderness over the abdomen.

i. Monitor for abdominal distention.

6. Nonsurgical interventions

a. Modify risk factors.

b. Instruct the client regarding the procedure for monitoring **BP**.

c. Instruct the client on the importance of regular physician visits to follow the size of the aneurysm.

d. Instruct the client that if severe back or abdominal pain or fullness, soreness over the umbilicus, sudden development of discoloration in the extremities, or a persistent elevation of **BP** occurs to notify the physician immediately.

e. Instruct the client with a thoracic aneurysm to report immediately the occurrence of chest or back pain, shortness of breath, difficulty swallowing, or hoarseness.

D. Pharmacological interventions

1. Administer antihypertensives to maintain the **BP** within normal limits and to prevent strain on the aneurysm.

2. Instruct the client in the purpose of the medications.

3. Instruct the client about the side effects and schedule of the medication.

E. Abdominal aneurysm resection

1. Description: Surgical resection or excision of the aneurysm; the excised section is replaced with a graft that is sewn end to end

2. Preoperative interventions

a. Assess all peripheral pulses as a baseline for postoperative comparison.

b. Instruct the client on coughing and deep breathing exercises.

c. Administer bowel preparation as prescribed.

3. Postoperative interventions

a. Monitor vital signs.

b. Monitor peripheral pulses distal to the graft site.

c. Monitor for signs of graft occlusion, including changes in pulses, cool to cold extremities below the graft, white or blue extremities or flanks, severe pain, or abdominal distention.

d. Limit elevation of the head of the bed to 45 degrees to prevent flexion of the graft.

e. Monitor for hypovolemia and renal failure resulting from significant blood loss during surgery.

f. Monitor urine output hourly, and notify the physician if it is less than 50 mL per hour.

g. Monitor serum creatinine and blood urea nitrogen daily.

h. Monitor respiratory status and auscultate breath sounds to identify respiratory complications.

i. Encourage turning, coughing and deep breathing, and splinting the incision.

j. Ambulate as prescribed.

k. Maintain nasogastric tube to low suction until bowel sounds return.

l. Assess for bowel sounds and report their return to the physician

m. Monitor for pain and administer medication as prescribed.

n. Assess incision site for bleeding or signs of infection.

o. Prepare the client for discharge by providing instructions regarding pain management, wound care, and activity restrictions.

p. Instruct the client not to lift objects heavier than 15 to 20 lb for 6 to 12 weeks.

q. Advise the client to avoid activities requiring pushing, pulling, or straining.

r. Instruct the client not to drive a vehicle until approved by the physician.

▲ F. Thoracic aneurysm repair
  1. Description
     a. A thoracotomy or median sternotomy approach is used to enter the thoracic cavity.
     b. The aneurysm is exposed and excised, and a graft or prosthesis is sewn onto the aorta.
     c. Total cardiopulmonary bypass is necessary for excision of aneurysms in the ascending aorta.
     d. Partial cardiopulmonary bypass is used for clients with an aneurysm in the descending aorta.
  2. Postoperative interventions
     a. Monitor vital signs.
     b. Monitor for signs of hemorrhage, such as a drop in **BP** and increased pulse rate and respirations, and report to the physician immediately.
     c. Monitor chest tubes for an increase in chest drainage, which may indicate bleeding or separation at the graft site.
     d. Assess sensation and motion of all extremities and notify the physician if deficits occur, which can be due to a lack of blood supply during surgery.
     e. Monitor respiratory status and auscultate breath sounds to identify respiratory complications.
     f. Encourage turning, coughing, and deep breathing while splinting the incision.
     g. Monitor cardiac status for dysrhythmias.
     h. Monitor for pain and administer medication as prescribed.
     i. Assess the incision site for bleeding or signs of infection.
     j. Prepare the client for discharge by providing instructions regarding pain management, wound care, and activity restrictions.
     k. Instruct the client not to lift objects heavier than 15 to 20 lb for 6 to 12 weeks.
     l. Advise the client to avoid activities requiring pushing, pulling, or straining.
     m. Instruct the client not to drive a vehicle until approved by the physician.

XIX. EMBOLECTOMY
A. Description
  1. Embolectomy is removal of an embolus from an artery using a catheter.
  2. A patch graft may be required to close the artery.
B. Preoperative interventions
  1. Obtain a baseline vascular assessment.
  2. Administer anticoagulants as prescribed.
  3. Administer thrombolytics as prescribed.
  4. Place a bed cradle on the bed.
  5. Avoid bumping or jarring the bed.
  6. Maintain the extremity in slightly dependent position.
C. Postoperative interventions
  1. Assess cardiac, respiratory, and neurological status.

  2. Monitor affected extremity for color, temperature, and pulse.
  3. Assess sensory and motor function of the affected extremity.
  4. Monitor for signs and symptoms of new thrombi or emboli.
  5. Administer oxygen as prescribed.
  6. Monitor pulse oximetry.
  7. Monitor for complications caused by reperfusion of the artery, such as spasms and swelling of the skeletal muscles.
  8. Monitor for signs of swollen skeletal muscles such as edema, pain on passive movement, poor capillary refill, numbness, and muscle tenseness.
  9. Maintain bed rest initially, with the client in semi-Fowler position.
  10. Place a bed cradle on the bed.
  11. Check the incision site for bleeding or hematoma.
  12. Administer anticoagulants as prescribed.
  13. Monitor laboratory values related to anticoagulant therapy.
  14. Instruct the client to recognize the signs and symptoms of infection and edema.
  15. Instruct the client to avoid prolonged sitting or crossing the legs when sitting.
  16. Instruct the client to elevate the legs when sitting.
  17. Instruct the client to wear antiembolism stockings as prescribed and how to remove and reapply the stockings
  18. Instruct the client to ambulate daily.
  19. Instruct the client about anticoagulant therapy ▲ and the hazards associated with anticoagulants.

XX. VENA CAVAL FILTER AND LIGATION OF INFERIOR VENA CAVA
A. Vena caval filter: insertion of an intracaval filter (umbrella) that partially occludes the inferior vena cava and traps emboli to prevent pulmonary emboli
B. Ligation: suturing or placing clips on the inferior vena cava to prevent pulmonary emboli
C. Preoperative interventions: If the client has been taking an anticoagulant, consult with the physician regarding discontinuation of the medication to prevent hemorrhage.
D. Postoperative interventions
  1. Monitor vital signs.
  2. Assess cardiac and respiratory status.
  3. Administer oxygen as prescribed.
  4. Monitor pulse oximetry.
  5. Maintain semi-Fowler position.
  6. Avoid hip flexion.
  7. Provide activity as prescribed.
  8. Check the insertion site for bleeding and hematoma.
  9. Assess for peripheral edema.
  10. Maintain antiembolism stockings as prescribed.

11. Monitor laboratory values related to anticoagulant therapy.
12. Instruct the client to recognize the signs and symptoms of infection and edema.
13. Instruct the client to avoid prolonged sitting or crossing legs when sitting.
14. Instruct the client to elevate the legs when sitting.
15. Instruct the client to wear antiembolism stockings as prescribed and how to remove and reapply the stockings.
16. Instruct the client to ambulate daily.
17. Instruct the client about anticoagulant therapy and the hazards associated with anticoagulants.

XXI. HYPERTENSION

A. Description
1. The classification of prehypertension describes an individual with a systolic **BP** between 120 and 139 mm Hg or a **diastolic pressure** between 80 and 89 mm Hg.
2. In an individual over the age of 50, the **systolic pressure** is a more important value to note than the **diastolic pressure** regarding the need for treatment.
3. Hypertension is a major risk factor for coronary, cerebral, renal, and peripheral vascular disease.
4. The disease is initially asymptomatic.
5. The goals of treatment include to reduce the **BP** and to prevent or lessen the extent of organ damage (Table 59-1).
6. Nonpharmacological approaches, such as lifestyle changes, may be prescribed initially, and if the **BP** cannot be decreased after a reasonable time period (1 to 3 months), then the client may require pharmacological treatment.

B. Primary or essential hypertension
1. No known cause
2. Risk factors
   a. Aging
   b. Family history
   c. Black race, with higher prevalence in males
   d. Obesity
   e. Smoking
   f. Stress

C. Secondary hypertension
1. Treatment depends on the cause and the organs involved.

2. Secondary hypertension occurs as a result of other disorders or conditions.
3. Precipitating disorders or conditions
   a. Cardiovascular disorders
   b. Renal disorders
   c. Endocrine system disorders
   d. Pregnancy
   e. Medications

D. Assessment
1. May be asymptomatic
2. Headache
3. Visual disturbances
4. Dizziness
5. Chest pain
6. Tinnitus
7. Flushed face
8. Epistaxis

E. Interventions
1. Goals
   a. One treatment goal is to reduce the **BP**.
   b. Another treatment goal is to prevent or lessen the extent of organ damage.
2. Question the client regarding the signs and symptoms indicative of hypertension.
3. Obtain the **BP** two or more times on both arms with the client supine and standing.
4. Compare the **BP** with prior documentation.
5. Determine family history of hypertension.
6. Identify current medication therapy.
7. Obtain weight.
8. Evaluate dietary patterns and sodium intake.
9. Assess for visual changes or retinal damage.
10. Assess for cardiovascular changes such as distended neck veins, increased heart rate, dysrhythmias.
11. Evaluate chest x-ray film for heart enlargement.
12. Assess neurological system.
13. Evaluate renal function.
14. Evaluate results of diagnostic and laboratory studies.

F. Nonpharmacological interventions
1. Weight reduction, if necessary, or maintenance of ideal weight.
2. Dietary sodium restriction to 2 g daily as prescribed.
3. Moderate intake of alcohol and caffeine-containing products.
4. Initiation of a regular exercise program.
5. Avoidance of smoking.
6. Relaxation techniques and biofeedback therapy.
7. Elimination of unnecessary medications that may contribute to the hypertension.

G. Stepped-care approach
1. Description
   a. If a pharmacological approach to treating hypertension is required, a single medication is prescribed and monitored for its effectiveness.

TABLE 59-1

Hypertension

Organ Involvement	Complications
Eyes	Visual changes
Brain	Cerebrovascular accident
Cardiovascular system	Heart failure, hypertensive crisis
Kidneys	Renal failure

b. Medications are added to the treatment regimen until the **BP** is controlled.

c. Refer to Chapter 60 for medications to treat hypertension.

2. Step 1: A single medication is prescribed, which may be a diuretic, β-blocker, calcium channel blocker, or angiotensin-converting enzyme inhibitor.

3. Step 2
   a. Step 1 therapy is evaluated after 1 to 3 months.
   b. If the response is not adequate, compliance is evaluated.
   c. The medication may be increased or a new medication may be prescribed or a second medication may be added the treatment plan.

4. Step 3
   a. Compliance is evaluated.
   b. Further evaluation of Step 2.
   c. If a therapeutic response is not adequate, a second medication is substituted or a third medication is added to the treatment plan.

5. Step 4
   a. Compliance is evaluated.
   b. Careful assessment of factors limiting the antihypertensive response is done.
   c. A third or fourth medication may be added to the treatment plan.

H. See Box 59-8 for client education.

XXII. HYPERTENSIVE CRISIS

A. Description
   1. A hypertensive crisis is any clinical condition requiring immediate reduction in **BP**.
   2. A hypertensive crisis is an acute and life-threatening condition.
   3. The accelerated hypertension requires emergency treatment because target organ damage (brain, heart, kidneys, retina of the eye) can occur quickly.
   4. Death can be caused by stroke, renal failure, or cardiac disease.

B. Assessment
   1. A **diastolic pressure** greater than 120 mm Hg
   2. Headache
   3. Drowsiness
   4. Confusion
   5. Changes in neurological status
   6. Tachycardia and tachypnea
   7. Dyspnea
   8. Cyanosis
   9. Seizures

C. Interventions
   1. Maintain a patent airway.
   2. Administer antihypertensive medications intravenously as prescribed, which may include nitroprusside (Nipride), diazoxide (Hyperstat), or trimethaphan camsylate (Arfonad).

BOX 59-8

Client Education for Hypertension

Describe the importance of compliance with the treatment plan.

Describe the disease process, explaining that symptoms usually do not develop until organs have suffered damage.

Initiate and assist the client in planning a regular exercise program, avoiding heavy weight lifting and isometric exercises.

Emphasize the importance of beginning the exercise program gradually.

Encourage the client to express feelings about daily stress.

Assist the client to identify ways to reduce stress.

Teach relaxation techniques.

Instruct the client in how to incorporate relaxation techniques into the daily living pattern.

Instruct the client and family in the technique for monitoring blood pressure.

Instruct the client to maintain a diary of blood pressure readings.

Emphasize the importance of lifelong medication and the need for follow-up treatment.

Instruct the client and family about the dietary restrictions, which may include sodium, fat, calories, and cholesterol.

Instruct the client in how to shop for and prepare low-sodium meals.

Provide a list of products that contain sodium.

Instruct the client to read labels of products to determine sodium content, focusing on substances listed as sodium, NaCl, or MSG (monosodium glutamate).

Instruct the client to bake, roast, or boil foods, avoid salt in preparation of foods, and avoid using salt at the table.

Instruct the client that fresh foods are best to consume and to avoid canned foods.

Instruct the client about the actions, side effects, and scheduling of medications.

Advise the client that if uncomfortable side effects occur to contact the physician and not to stop the medication.

Instruct the client to avoid over-the-counter medications.

Stress the importance of follow-up care.

---

3. Monitor vital signs, assessing **BP** every 5 minutes.

4. Assess for hypotension during the administration of antihypertensives; place the client in a supine position if hypotension occurs.

5. Have emergency medications and resuscitation equipment readily available.

6. Maintain bed rest, with the head of the bed elevated at 45 degrees.

7. Monitor IV therapy, assessing for fluid overload.

8. Monitor intake and output.

9. Insert Foley catheter as prescribed.

10. Monitor urinary output, and if oliguria or anuria occurs, notify the physician.

PRACTICE QUESTIONS

1. A client with angina pectoris has a 12-lead electrocardiogram taken during an episode of chest pain. A nurse examines the tracing for which electrocardiogram change caused by myocardial ischemia?
   1. Prolonged PR interval
   2. Widened QRS complex
   3. ST segment elevation or depression
   4. Tall, peaked T waves

2. A client is scheduled for a cardiac catheterization using a radiopaque dye. Which of the following assessments is most critical before the procedure?
   1. Intake and output
   2. Baseline peripheral pulse rates
   3. Height and weight
   4. Allergy to iodine or shellfish

3. A client is scheduled for a dipyridamole (Persantine) thallium-201 scan. A nurse would assess to make sure that the client avoided which of the following before the procedure?
   1. Milk products
   2. Caffeine
   3. Excess sugar
   4. Fatty meal

4. A client with no history of cardiovascular disease comes the ambulatory clinic with flulike symptoms. The client suddenly complains of chest pain. Which of the following questions would best help a nurse to discriminate pain caused by a noncardiac problem?
   1. "Have you ever had this pain before?"
   2. "Can you describe the pain to me?"
   3. "Does the pain get worse when you breathe in?"
   4. "Can you rate the pain on a scale of 1 to 10, with 10 being the worst?"

5. A client is admitted to an emergency room with chest pain and is being ruled out for myocardial infarction. Vital signs are as follows: at 11 AM, pulse (P) 92, respiratory rate (RR) 24, blood pressure (BP) 140/88 mm Hg; 11:15 AM, P 96, RR 26, BP 128/82 mm Hg; 11:30 AM, P 104, RR 28, BP 104/68 mm Hg; 11:45 AM, P 118, RR 32, BP 88/58 mm Hg. A nurse alerts the physician because these changes are most consistent with
   1. Cardiogenic shock.
   2. Cardiac tamponade.
   3. Pulmonary embolism.
   4. Dissecting thoracic aortic aneurysm.

6. A client with myocardial infarction has been transferred from a coronary care unit to a general medical unit with cardiac monitoring via telemetry. A nurse plans to allow for which of the following client activities?
   1. Strict bed rest for 24 hours after transfer
   2. Bathroom privileges and self-care activities
   3. Unsupervised hallway ambulation with distances under 200 feet
   4. Ad lib activities because the client is monitored

7. A nurse notes bilateral 2+ edema in the lower extremities of a client with myocardial infarction who was admitted 2 days ago. The nurse would plan to do which of the following next?
   1. Review the intake and output records for the last 2 days.
   2. Change the time of diuretic administration from morning to evening.
   3. Request a sodium restriction of 1 g/day from the physician.
   4. Order daily weights starting on the following morning.

8. A nurse is conducting a health history with a client with a primary diagnosis of heart failure. Which of the following disorders reported by the client is unlikely to play a role in exacerbating the heart failure?
   1. Recent upper respiratory infection
   2. Nutritional anemia
   3. Peptic ulcer disease
   4. Atrial fibrillation

9. A nurse is preparing for the admission of a client with heart failure who is being sent directly to the hospital from the physician's office. The nurse would plan on having which of the following medications readily available for use?
   1. Diltiazem (Cardizem)
   2. Digoxin (Lanoxin)
   3. Propranolol (Inderal)
   4. Metoprolol (Lopressor)

10. A client with myocardial infarction suddenly becomes tachycardic, shows signs of air hunger, and begins coughing frothy, pink-tinged sputum. A nurse listens to breath sounds, expecting to hear bilateral
    1. Rhonchi.
    2. Diminished breath sounds.
    3. Crackles.
    4. Wheezes.

11. A nurse caring for a client in one room is told by another nurse that a second client has developed severe pulmonary edema. On entering the second client's room, the nurse would expect the client to be
    1. Slightly anxious.
    2. Mildly anxious.
    3. Moderately anxious.
    4. Extremely anxious.

12. A client with pulmonary edema has been on diuretic therapy. The client has an order for additional furosemide (Lasix) in the amount of 40 mg intravenous push. Knowing that the client also will be started on digoxin (Lanoxin), a nurse checks the client's most recent
    1. Digoxin level.
    2. Sodium level.
    3. Potassium level.
    4. Creatinine level.

13. A client with myocardial infarction is going into cardiogenic shock. Because of myocardial ischemia, a nurse would assess the client carefully for
    1. Ventricular dysrhythmias.
    2. Bradycardia.
    3. Rising diastolic blood pressure.
    4. Falling central venous pressure.

14. A client in cardiogenic shock has a multilumen pulmonary artery catheter placed. The nurse would interpret that the client is most unstable if which of the following cardiac output (CO) and pulmonary capillary wedge pressure (PCWP) readings were obtained?
    1. CO 5 L/min, PCWP low
    2. CO 4 L/min, PCWP high
    3. CO 3 L/min, PCWP high
    4. CO 2 L/min, PCWP low

15. A client in cardiogenic shock had insertion of an intraaortic balloon pump 24 hours ago via the left femoral approach. A nurse notes that the left foot is cool and mottled and the left pedal pulse is weak. The nurse would
    1. Document the data because this is expected because of the catheter size.
    2. Reevaluate the neurovascular status in another hour.
    3. Increase the rate of intravenous nitroglycerin that is infusing.
    4. Call the physician immediately.

16. A nurse assesses the sternotomy incision of a client on the third day after cardiac surgery. The incision shows some slight "puffiness" along the edges and is nonreddened, with no apparent drainage. Temperature is 99° F orally. The white blood cell count is 7500 cells/mm³. The nurse interprets that the incision line
    1. Is slightly edematous but shows no active signs of infection.
    2. Shows no sign of infection, although the white blood cell count is elevated.
    3. Shows early signs of infection, although the temperature is near normal.
    4. Shows early signs of infection, supported by an elevated white blood cell count.

17. A client who had cardiac surgery 24 hours ago has a urine output averaging 20 mL/hour for 2 hours. The client received a single bolus of 500 mL of intravenous fluid. Urine output for the subsequent hour was 25 mL. Daily laboratory results indicate that the blood urea nitrogen is 45 mg/dL and the serum creatinine is 2.2 mg/dL. A nurse interprets that the client is at risk for
    1. Hypovolemia.
    2. Urinary tract infection.
    3. Glomerulonephritis.
    4. Acute renal failure.

18. A nurse is preparing to ambulate a client on the third day after cardiac surgery. The nurse would plan to do which of the following to enable the client to best tolerate the ambulation?
    1. Encourage the client to cough and deep breathe.
    2. Premedicate the client with an analgesic.
    3. Provide the client with a walker.
    4. Remove telemetry equipment.

19. A nurse is assessing an electrocardiogram rhythm strip. The P waves and QRS complexes are regular. The PR interval is 0.16 second, and QRS complexes measure 0.06 second. The overall heart rate is 64 beats per minute. The nurse assesses the cardiac rhythm as
    1. Normal sinus rhythm.
    2. Sinus bradycardia.
    3. Sick sinus syndrome.
    4. First-degree heart block.

20. A client is wearing a continuous cardiac monitor, which begins to sound its alarm. A nurse sees no electrocardiogram complexes on the screen. The first action of the nurse is to
    1. Check the client status and lead placement.
    2. Press the recorder button on the electrocardiogram console.
    3. Call the physician.
    4. Call a code blue.

21. A client's electrocardiogram strip shows atrial and ventricular rates of 80 complexes per minute. The PR interval is 0.14 second, the QRS complex measures 0.08 second, and the PP interval is slightly irregular. The nurse interprets that this rhythm is
    1. Normal sinus rhythm.
    2. Sinus bradycardia.
    3. Sinus tachycardia.
    4. Sinus dysrhythmia.

22. A nurse notices frequent artifact on the electrocardiogram monitor for a client whose leads are connected by cable to a console at the bedside. The nurse examines the client to determine the cause. Which of the following items is unlikely to be responsible for the artifact?
    1. Frequent movement of the client
    2. Tightly secured cable connections
    3. Leads applied over hairy areas
    4. Leads applied to the limbs

23. A nurse is watching the cardiac monitor and notices that the rhythm suddenly changes. There are no P waves, the QRS complexes are wide, and the ventricular rate is regular but over 100. The nurse determines that the client is experiencing
    1. Premature ventricular contractions.
    2. Ventricular tachycardia.
    3. Ventricular fibrillation.
    4. Sinus tachycardia.

24. A client has frequent bursts of ventricular tachycardia on the cardiac monitor. A nurse is most concerned with this dysrhythmia because

1. It is uncomfortable for the client, giving a sense of impending doom.
2. It produces a high cardiac output that quickly leads to cerebral and myocardial ischemia.
3. It is almost impossible to convert to a normal rhythm.
4. It can develop into ventricular fibrillation at any time.

25. A nurse is viewing the cardiac monitor in a client's room and notes that the client has just gone into ventricular tachycardia. The client is awake and alert and has good skin color. The nurse would prepare to do which of the following?
1. Immediately defibrillate.
2. Prepare for pacemaker insertion.
3. Administer amiodarone (Cordarone) intravenously.
4. Administer epinephrine (Adrenalin) intravenously.

26. A nurse is caring for a client with unstable ventricular tachycardia. The nurse instructs the client to do which of the following, if prescribed, during an episode of ventricular tachycardia?
1. Breathe deeply, regularly, and easily.
2. Inhale deeply and cough forcefully every 1 to 3 seconds.
3. Lie down flat in bed.
4. Remove any metal jewelry.

27. A client is having frequent premature ventricular contractions. A nurse would place priority on assessment of which of the following items?
1. Blood pressure and peripheral perfusion
2. Sensation of palpitations
3. Causative factors such as caffeine
4. Precipitating factors such as infection

28. A client has developed atrial fibrillation, with a ventricular rate of 150 beats per minute. A nurse assesses the client for
1. Hypotension and dizziness.
2. Nausea and vomiting.
3. Hypertension and headache.
4. Flat neck veins.

29. A nurse is watching the cardiac monitor, and a client's rhythm suddenly changes. There are no P waves; instead there are wavy lines. The QRS complexes measure 0.08 second, but they are irregular, with a rate of 120 beats per minute. The nurse interprets that this rhythm is
1. Sinus tachycardia.
2. Atrial fibrillation.
3. Ventricular tachycardia.
4. Ventricular fibrillation.

30. A client with rapid-rate atrial fibrillation asks a nurse why the physician is going to perform carotid massage. The nurse responds that this procedure may stimulate the
1. Vagus nerve to slow the heart rate.
2. Vagus nerve to increase the heart rate, overdriving the rhythm.
3. Diaphragmatic nerve to slow the heart rate.
4. Diaphragmatic nerve to overdrive the rhythm.

31. A nurse notes that a client with sinus rhythm has a premature ventricular contraction that falls on the T wave of the preceding beat. The client's rhythm suddenly changes to one with no P waves or definable QRS complexes. Instead there are coarse wavy lines of varying amplitude. The nurse assesses this rhythm to be
1. Ventricular tachycardia.
2. Ventricular fibrillation.
3. Atrial fibrillation.
4. Asystole.

32. A nurse is preparing to defibrillate a client in ventricular fibrillation. The nurse places the paddles on the client's chest and before defibrillating the client assesses that
1. The client has received lidocaine hydrochloride (Xylocaine).
2. The rhythm is actually ventricular fibrillation.
3. The machine has been set to the "synchronize" mode.
4. The client has been intubated.

33. A client in ventricular fibrillation is about to be defibrillated. A nurse knows that to convert this rhythm effectively, the machine should be set at which of the following energy levels for the first delivery?
1. 50 Joules (J)
2. 100 Joules (J)
3. 200 Joules (J)
4. 360 Joules (J)

34. A nurse would evaluate that defibrillation of a client was most successful if which of the following observations was made?
1. Nonarousable, sinus rhythm, blood pressure (BP) 88/60 mm Hg
2. Arousable, sinus rhythm, BP 116/72 mm Hg
3. Nonarousable, supraventricular tachycardia, BP 122/60 mm Hg
4. Arousable, marked bradycardia, BP 86/54 mm Hg

35. A nurse is evaluating a client's response to cardioversion. Which of the following observations would be of highest priority to the nurse?
1. Oxygen flow rate
2. Status of airway
3. Blood pressure
4. Level of consciousness

36. A nurse is performing cardiopulmonary resuscitation on a client who had a cardiac arrest. An automatic external defibrillator is available to treat the client. The nurse uses the defibrillator and assesses the cardiac rhythm by
1. Applying standard electrocardiogram monitoring leads to the client and observing the rhythm.

2. Holding the defibrillator paddles firmly against the chest.

3. Applying the adhesive patch electrodes to the chest and moving away from the client.

4. Connecting standard electrocardiogram electrodes to a transtelephonic monitoring device.

37. A nurse employed in a cardiac unit determines that which of the following clients is the least likely to have implantation of an automatic internal cardioverter-defibrillator?
   1. A client with three episodes of cardiac arrest unrelated to myocardial infarction
   2. A client with ventricular dysrhythmias despite medication therapy
   3. A client with an episode of cardiac arrest related to myocardial infarction
   4. A client with syncopal episodes related to ventricular tachycardia

38. A nurse is caring for a client who has just had implantation of an automatic internal cardioverter-defibrillator. The nurse immediately would assess which of the following items based on priority?
   1. Activation status of the device, heart rate cutoff, and number of shocks it is programmed to deliver
   2. Presence of a Medic-Alert card for the client to carry
   3. Anxiety level of the client and family
   4. Knowledge of restrictions of postdischarge physical activity

39. A nurse is caring for a client immediately after insertion of a permanent demand pacemaker via the right subclavian vein. The nurse takes care to avoid dislodging the pacing catheter by
   1. Limiting movement and abduction of the right arm.
   2. Limiting movement and abduction of the left arm.
   3. Assisting the client to get out of bed and ambulate with a walker.
   4. Having the physical therapist do active range of motion to the right arm.

40. A client diagnosed with thrombophlebitis 1 day ago suddenly complains of chest pain and shortness of breath and is visibly anxious. A nurse immediately assesses the client for other signs and symptoms of
   1. Myocardial infarction.
   2. Pneumonia.
   3. Pulmonary embolism.
   4. Pulmonary edema.

41. A client seeks treatment in a physician's office for unsightly varicose veins, and sclerotherapy is recommended. Before leaving the examining room, the client says to the nurse, "Can you tell me again how this sclerotherapy is done?" In formulating a response, the nurse incorporates the knowledge that sclerotherapy consists of
   1. Injecting an agent into the vein to damage the vein wall and close the vein off.

2. Tying off the vein at the upper end to prevent stasis from occurring.

3. Tying off the vein at the lower end to prevent stasis from occurring

4. Surgical removal of the varicosity

42. A client is having a follow-up physician office visit after vein ligation and stripping. The client describes a sensation of "pins and needles" in the affected leg. Based on evaluation of this comment, the nurse
   1. Reassures the client that this is only temporary.
   2. Advises the client to take acetaminophen (Tylenol) until it is gone.
   3. States that warm packs should help.
   4. Reports the complaint to the physician.

43. A 24-year-old man seeks medical attention for complaints of claudication in the arch of the foot. A nurse also notes superficial thrombophlebitis of the lower leg. The nurse would next assess the client for
   1. Familial tendency toward peripheral vascular disease.
   2. Smoking history.
   3. Recent exposure to allergens.
   4. History of recent insect bites.

44. A nurse has given instructions to the client with Raynaud's disease about self-management of the disease process. The nurse determines that the client needs further reinforcement if the client states that
   1. Smoking cessation is important.
   2. Sources of caffeine should be eliminated from the diet.
   3. Taking nifedipine (Procardia) as prescribed will decrease vessel spasm.
   4. Moving to a warmer climate is needed.

45. A nurse is caring for a client who had a percutaneous insertion of an inferior vena cava filter and was on heparin therapy before surgery. The nurse would inspect the surgical site most closely for signs of
   1. Thrombosis and infection.
   2. Bleeding and infection.
   3. Bleeding and wound dehiscence.
   4. Wound dehiscence and evisceration.

46. A nurse is assessing the blood pressure of a client diagnosed with primary hypertension. The nurse ensures accurate measurement by avoiding which of the following?
   1. Seating the client with arm bared, supported, and at heart level
   2. Measuring the blood pressure after the client has been seated quietly for 5 minutes
   3. Using a cuff with a rubber bladder that encircles at least 80% of the limb
   4. Taking the blood pressure within 15 minutes after nicotine or caffeine ingestion

47. Intravenous heparin therapy is ordered for a client. While implementing this order, a nurse ensures that which of the following medications is available on the nursing unit?

1. Vitamin K (AquaMEPHYTON)
2. Aminocaproic acid (Amicar)
3. Potassium chloride
4. Protamine sulfate

48. A client is at risk for pulmonary embolism and is on anticoagulant therapy with warfarin sodium (Coumadin). The client's prothrombin time is 20 seconds, with a control of 11 seconds. The nurse assesses that this result is
    1. The same as the client's own baseline level.
    2. Lower than the needed therapeutic level.
    3. Within the therapeutic range.
    4. Higher than the therapeutic range.

49. A client who has been receiving heparin therapy also is started on warfarin sodium (Coumadin). The client asks a nurse why both medications are being administered. In formulating a response, the nurse incorporates the understanding that warfarin sodium
    1. Stimulates breakdown of specific clotting factors by the liver, and it takes 2 to 3 days for this to exert an anticoagulant effect.
    2. Inhibits synthesis of specific clotting factors in the liver, and it takes 3 to 4 days for this medication to exert an anticoagulant effect.
    3. Stimulates production of the body's own thrombolytic substances, but it takes 2 to 4 days for this to begin.
    4. Has the same mechanism of action as heparin, and the crossover time is needed for the serum level of warfarin sodium to be therapeutic.

50. A nurse has an order to begin administering warfarin sodium (Coumadin) to a client. While implementing this order, the nurse ensures that which of the following medications is available on the nursing unit as the antidote for Coumadin?
    1. Vitamin K (AquaMEPHYTON)
    2. Aminocaproic acid (Amicar)
    3. Potassium chloride
    4. Protamine sulfate

51. A client is admitted to a hospital with acute myocardial infarction and is started on tissue plasminogen activator (t-PA, Activase) by infusion. Of the following parameters, which one would a nurse determine requires the least frequent assessment to detect complications of therapy with tissue plasminogen activator?
    1. Oxygen saturation
    2. Neurological signs
    3. Blood pressure and pulse
    4. Complaints of abdominal and back pain

52. A client is admitted with pulmonary embolism and is to be treated with streptokinase (Streptase). A nurse would report which of the following assessments to the physician before initiating this therapy?
    1. Adventitious breath sounds
    2. Respiratory rate of 28 breaths per minute

3. Temperature of 99.4° F orally
4. Blood pressure of 198/110 mm Hg

53. A client is receiving thrombolytic therapy with a continuous infusion of streptokinase (Streptase). The client suddenly becomes extremely anxious and complains of itching. A nurse hears stridor and on examination of the client notes generalized urticaria and hypotension. The nurse should
    1. Administer oxygen and protamine sulfate.
    2. Cut the infusion rate in half and sit the client up in bed.
    3. Stop the infusion and call the physician.
    4. Administer diphenhydramine (Benadryl) and continue the infusion.

54. A nurse is assessing the neurovascular status of a client who returned to the surgical nursing unit 4 hours ago after undergoing aortoiliac bypass graft. The affected leg is warm, and the nurse notes redness and edema. The pedal pulse is palpable and unchanged from admission. The nurse interprets that the neurovascular status is
    1. Normal because of increased blood flow through the leg.
    2. Slightly deteriorating and should be monitored for another hour.
    3. Moderately impaired, and the surgeon should be called.
    4. Adequate from an arterial approach, but venous complications are arising.

55. A nurse is evaluating the condition of a client after pericardiocentesis for cardiac tamponade. Which of the following observations would indicate that the procedure was unsuccessful?
    1. Rising central venous pressure
    2. Rising blood pressure
    3. Client expressions of relief
    4. Clearly audible heart sounds

56. A nurse is assessing a client with an abdominal aortic aneurysm. Which of the following assessment findings by the nurse is probably unrelated to the aneurysm?
    1. Pulsatile abdominal mass
    2. Hyperactive bowel sounds in the area
    3. Systolic bruit over the area of the mass
    4. Subjective sensation of "heart beating" in the abdomen

57. A nurse is caring for a client who had a resection of an abdominal aortic aneurysm yesterday. The client has an intravenous infusion with a rate of 150 mL/hour, unchanged for the last 10 hours. The client's urine output for the last 3 hours was 90 mL, 50 mL, and 28 mL (28 mL most recent). The client's blood urea nitrogen is 35 mg/dL, and serum creatinine is 1.8 mg/dL, drawn this morning. Which of the following actions should the nurse take next?
    1. Put the intravenous line on a pump so that the infusion rate is sure to stay stable.

2. Check to see if the client had a serum albumin level drawn.
3. Check the urine specific gravity.
4. Call the physician.

58. A client is admitted with a venous stasis leg ulcer. A nurse assesses the ulcer, expecting to note that the ulcer
   1. Has a pale-colored base.
   2. Is deep, with even edges.
   3. Has little granulation tissue.
   4. Has brown pigmentation surrounding it.

59. A home care nurse is making a routine visit to a client receiving digoxin (Lanoxin) in the treatment of heart failure. The nurse would particularly assess the client for
   1. Thrombocytopenia and weight gain.
   2. Anorexia, nausea, and visual disturbances.
   3. Diarrhea and hypotension.
   4. Fatigue and muscle twitching.

60. A client with angina complains that the anginal pain is prolonged and severe and occurs at the same time each day, most often in the morning. On further assessment a nurse notes that the pain occurs in the absence of precipitating factors. This type of anginal pain is best described as
   1. Stable angina.
   2. Unstable angina.
   3. Variant angina.
   4. Nonanginal pain.

CRITICAL THINKING: MULTIPLE RESPONSE

A nurse in a medical unit is caring for a client with heart failure. The client suddenly develops extreme dyspnea, tachycardia, and lung crackles and the nurse suspects pulmonary edema. The nurse immediately asks another nurse to contact the physician and prepares to implement which priority interventions?

_____ Administering furosemide (Lasix)

_____ Transporting the client to the coronary care unit

_____ Administering oxygen

_____ Placing the client in a low Fowler's side-lying position

_____ Administering morphine sulfate intravenously

ANSWERS

1. **3**

Rationale: An electrocardiogram taken with pain captures ischemic changes, which include ST segment elevation or depression. A prolonged PR interval indicates first-degree heart block. A widened QRS complex indicates delay in intraventricular conduction, such as bundle branch block. Tall, peaked T waves may indicate hyperkalemia.

Test-Taking Strategy: Use the process of elimination. Recalling that myocardial ischemia causes cellular derangements that alter the processes of depolarization will direct you to option 3. Review the electrocardiogram changes that occur with myocardial ischemia if you had difficulty with this question.

Level of Cognitive Ability: Analysis
Client Needs: Physiological Integrity
Integrated Process: Nursing Process—analysis
Content Area: Adult health—cardiovascular
Reference: Ignatavicius, D., & Workman, M. (2002). *Medical-surgical nursing: Critical thinking for collaborative care* (4th ed., pp. 791, 795). Philadelphia: W. B. Saunders.

2. **4**

Rationale: This procedure requires an informed consent because it involves injection of a radiopaque dye into the blood vessel. The risk of allergic reaction and possible anaphylaxis is serious and must be assessed before the procedure. Although options 1, 2, and 3 are accurate, they are not the most critical preprocedure assessments.

Test-Taking Strategy: Use the process of elimination. Note the key words "most critical." Recalling the concern related to allergy to the dye and the risk of anaphylaxis makes option 4 correct. Review preprocedure interventions for a cardiac catheterization if you had difficulty with this question.

Level of Cognitive Ability: Analysis
Client Needs: Physiological Integrity
Integrated Process: Nursing Process—assessment
Content Area: Delegating/Prioritizing
Reference: Ignatavicius, D., & Workman, M. (2002). *Medical-surgical nursing critical thinking for collaborative care* (4th ed., p. 642). Philadelphia: W. B. Saunders.

3. **2**

Rationale: This test is an alternative to the exercise thallium-201 scan. The dipyridamole (Persantine) dilates the coronary arteries as exercise would. Before the procedure, any form of caffeine should be withheld, as should aminophylline or theophylline. Aminophylline may decrease the effects of dipyridamole. The client does not have to avoid the items identified in options 1, 3, and 4.

Test-Taking Strategy: Use the process of elimination, noting the key word "avoided." Factors that put a strain on the heart, such as nicotine and caffeine, can interfere with cardiac diagnostic test results. Look for items such as these in similarly worded questions. Review preprocedure client instructions for this test if you had difficulty with this question.

Level of Cognitive Ability: Analysis
Client Needs: Physiological Integrity
Integrated Process: Nursing Process—assessment
Content Area: Adult health—cardiovascular
References: Chernecky, C., & Berger, B. (2001). *Laboratory tests and diagnostic procedures* (3rd ed., p. 584). Philadelphia: W. B. Saunders.
Ignatavicius, D., & Workman, M. (2002). *Medical-surgical nursing: Critical thinking for collaborative care* (4th ed., p. 649). Philadelphia: W. B. Saunders.

4. **3**

Rationale: Chest pain is assessed by using the standard pain assessment parameters (e.g., characteristics, location, intensity, duration, precipitating and alleviating factors, and associated symptoms). Options 1, 2, and 4 may or may not help discriminate the origin of pain. Pain of pleuropulmonary origin usually worsens on inspiration.

Test-Taking Strategy: Use the process of elimination, focusing on the issue, pain resulting from a noncardiac problem. The three incorrect options, although appropriate to use in practice, are general assessment questions only. Option 3 will discriminate between a cardiac and noncardiac cause of pain. Review pain assessment measures for the client with a cardiovascular problem if you had difficulty with this question.

Level of Cognitive Ability: Analysis
Client Needs: Physiological Integrity
Integrated Process: Nursing Process—assessment
Content Area: Adult health—cardiovascular
Reference: Ignatavicius, D., & Workman, M. (2002). *Medicalsurgical nursing: Critical thinking for collaborative care* (4th ed., pp. 474, 631). Philadelphia: W. B. Saunders.

5. **1**

Rationale: Cardiogenic shock occurs with severe damage (greater than 40%) to the left ventricle. Classic signs include hypotension, rapid pulse that becomes weaker, decreased urine output, and cool, clammy skin. Respiratory rate increases as the body develops metabolic acidosis from shock. Cardiac tamponade is accompanied by distant, muffled heart sounds and prominent neck vessels. Pulmonary embolism presents suddenly with severe dyspnea accompanying the chest pain. Dissecting aortic aneurysms usually are accompanied by back pain.

Test-Taking Strategy: Use the process of elimination. Recalling that the early serious complications of myocardial infarction include dysrhythmias, cardiogenic shock, and sudden death will direct you to option 1. No information in the question would guide you to another option. Review the complications of myocardial infarction if you had difficulty with this question.

Level of Cognitive Ability: Analysis
Client Needs: Physiological Integrity
Integrated Process: Nursing Process—analysis
Content Area: Adult health—cardiovascular
References: Lewis, S., Heitkemper, M., & Dirksen, S. (2004). *Medical-surgical nursing: Assessment and management of clinical problems* (6th ed., p. 1796). St. Louis: Mosby.
Phipps, W., Monahan, F., Sands, J., Marek, J., & Neighbors, M. (2003). *Medical-surgical nursing: Health and illness perspectives* (7th ed., p. 293). St. Louis: Mosby.

6. **2**

Rationale: On transfer from the coronary care unit, the client is allowed self-care activities and bathroom privileges. Supervised ambulation in the hall for brief distances is encouraged, with distances gradually increased (50, 100, 200 feet).

Test-Taking Strategy: Use the process of elimination. Eliminate options 3 and 4 first because they are excessive, given that the client has just transferred from the coronary care unit. Option 1 is not appropriate because the client would be doing less activity than in the coronary care unit before transfer.

Review activity prescriptions for the client with a myocardial infarction, if you had difficulty with this question.

Level of Cognitive Ability: Application
Client Needs: Physiological Integrity
Integrated Process: Nursing Process—planning
Content Area: Adult health—cardiovascular
References: Black, J., Hawks, J., & Keene, A. (2001). *Medicalsurgical nursing: Clinical management for positive outcomes* (6th ed., p. 1597). Philadelphia: W. B. Saunders.
Ignatavicius, D., & Workman, M. (2002). *Medical-surgical nursing: Critical thinking for collaborative care* (4th ed., p. 802). Philadelphia: W. B. Saunders.

7. **1**

Rationale: Edema, the accumulation of excess fluid in the interstitial spaces, can be measured by intake greater than output and by a sudden increase in weight. Diuretics should be given in the morning whenever possible to avoid nocturia. Strict sodium restrictions are reserved for clients with severe symptoms.

Test-Taking Strategy: Use the process of elimination, noting the key word "next." Use the steps of the nursing process to prioritize. Option 1 is the only option that addresses assessment of data. Review care to the client with myocardial infarction if you had difficulty with this question.

Level of Cognitive Ability: Application
Client Needs: Physiological Integrity
Integrated Process: Nursing Process—assessment
Content Area: Adult health—cardiovascular
Reference: Ignatavicius, D., & Workman, M. (2002). *Medicalsurgical nursing: Critical thinking for collaborative care* (4th ed., pp. 631, 702). Philadelphia: W. B. Saunders.

8. **3**

Rationale: Heart failure is precipitated or exacerbated by physical or emotional stress, dysrhythmias, infections, anemia, thyroid disorders, pregnancy, Paget's disease, nutritional deficiencies (thiamine, alcoholism), pulmonary disease, and hypervolemia.

Test-Taking Strategy: Use the process of elimination. Note the key word "unlikely." Remembering that heart failure is exacerbated by factors that increase the workload of the heart will assist you in eliminating options 1, 2, and 4. Review the precipitating factors associated with heart failure if you had difficulty with this question.

Level of Cognitive Ability: Analysis
Client Needs: Physiological Integrity
Integrated Process: Nursing Process—assessment
Content Area: Adult health—cardiovascular
References: Ignatavicius, D., & Workman, M. (2002). *Medicalsurgical nursing: Critical thinking for collaborative care* (4th ed., p. 701). Philadelphia: W. B. Saunders.
Lewis, S., Heitkemper, M., & Dirksen, S. (2004). *Medicalsurgical nursing: Assessment and management of clinical problems* (6th ed., p. 839). St. Louis: Mosby.

9. **2**

Rationale: Digoxin exerts a positive inotropic effect on the heart while slowing the overall rate through a variety of mechanisms. Digoxin is the medication of choice to treat heart failure. Diltiazem (calcium channel blocker) and propranolol

and metoprolol (β-adrenergic blockers) have a negative inotropic effect and would worsen the failing heart.
Test-Taking Strategy: Use the process of elimination. Options 3 and 4 can be eliminated first because they are β-blockers. From the remaining options, use knowledge of the classification and actions of these medications to direct you to option 2. Review these medications if you had difficulty with this question.
Level of Cognitive Ability: Application
Client Needs: Physiological Integrity
Integrated Process: Nursing Process—planning
Content Area: Adult health—cardiovascular
References: Ignatavicius, D., & Workman, M. (2002). *Medical-surgical nursing: Critical thinking for collaborative care* (4th ed., pp. 705-706, 708). Philadelphia: W. B. Saunders.
Lewis, S., Heitkemper, M., & Dirksen, S. (2004). *Medical-surgical nursing: Assessment and management of clinical problems* (6th ed., p. 846). St. Louis: Mosby.

10. 3
Rationale: Pulmonary edema is characterized by extreme breathlessness, dyspnea, air hunger, and production of frothy, pink-tinged sputum. Auscultation of the lungs reveals crackled. Wheezes, rhonchi, and diminished breath sounds are not associated with pulmonary edema.
Test-Taking Strategy: Use the process of elimination. Recall that fluid produces sounds that are called crackles. This will assist you in eliminating options 1, 2, and 4. If you had difficulty with this question, review the manifestations found in pulmonary edema.
Level of Cognitive Ability: Analysis
Client Needs: Physiological Integrity
Integrated Process: Nursing Process—assessment
Content Area: Adult health—cardiovascular
References: Ignatavicius, D., & Workman, M. (2002). *Medical-surgical nursing: Critical thinking for collaborative care* (4th ed., p. 709). Philadelphia: W. B. Saunders.
Lewis, S., Heitkemper, M., & Dirksen, S. (2004). *Medical-surgical nursing: Assessment and management of clinical problems* (6th ed., p. 842). St. Louis: Mosby.

11. 4
Rationale: Pulmonary edema causes the client to be extremely agitated and anxious. The client may complain of a sense of drowning, suffocation, or smothering.
Test-Taking Strategy: Use the process of elimination. Noting the key word "severe" will direct you to option 4. Review the clinical manifestations associated with severe pulmonary edema if you had difficulty with this question.
Level of Cognitive Ability: Analysis
Client Needs: Psychosocial Integrity
Integrated Process: Nursing Process—assessment
Content Area: Adult health—cardiovascular
References: Ignatavicius, D., & Workman, M. (2002). *Medical-surgical nursing: Critical thinking for collaborative care* (4th ed., p. 709). Philadelphia: W. B. Saunders.
Phipps, W., Monahan, F., Sands, J., Marek, J., & Neighbors, M. (2003). *Medical-surgical nursing: Health and illness perspectives* (7th ed., p. 730). St. Louis: Mosby.

12. 3
Rationale: The serum potassium level is measured in the client receiving digoxin and furosemide. Heightened digitalis effect leading to digoxin toxicity can occur in the client with hypokalemia. Hypokalemia also predisposes the client to ventricular dysrhythmias.
Test-Taking Strategy: Use the process of elimination. Eliminate option 1 because the client will just be beginning digoxin therapy. No data indicate the presence of renal insufficiency; therefore eliminate option 4. Furosemide therapy can cause hyponatremia and hypokalemia, but remember that the risk of hypokalemia has more severe consequences in this situation. Review the nursing considerations related to administering furosemide if you had difficulty with this question.
Level of Cognitive Ability: Analysis
Client Needs: Physiological Integrity
Integrated Process: Nursing Process—assessment
Content Area: Adult health—cardiovascular
Reference: Ignatavicius, D., & Workman, M. (2002). *Medical-surgical nursing: Critical thinking for collaborative care* (4th ed., pp. 671, 707). Philadelphia: W. B. Saunders.

13. 1
Rationale: Classic signs of cardiogenic shock as they relate to this question include low blood pressure and tachycardia. The central venous pressure would rise as the backward effects of the left ventricular failure became apparent. Dysrhythmias commonly occur as a result of decreased oxygenation to the myocardium.
Test-Taking Strategy: Use the process of elimination. Focus on the key words "myocardial ischemia." Recall that ischemia makes the myocardium irritable, producing dysrhythmias. Also, knowledge of the classic signs of shock helps you to eliminate the incorrect options. Review the clinical manifestations associated with cardiogenic shock if you had difficulty with this question.
Level of Cognitive Ability: Analysis
Client Needs: Physiological Integrity
Integrated Process: Nursing Process—assessment
Content Area: Adult health—cardiovascular
References: Ignatavicius, D., & Workman, M. (2002). *Medical-surgical nursing: Critical thinking for collaborative care* (4th ed., p. 809). Philadelphia: W. B. Saunders.
Lewis, S., Heitkemper, M., & Dirksen, S. (2004). *Medical-surgical nursing: Assessment and management of clinical problems* (6th ed., p. 814). St. Louis: Mosby.

14. 3
Rationale: The normal cardiac output is 4 to 8 L/min. With cardiogenic shock the cardiac output falls below normal because of failure of the heart as a pump. The pulmonary capillary wedge pressure, however, rises because it is a reflection of the left ventricular end-diastolic pressure which rises with pump failure.
Test-Taking Strategy: Use the process of elimination. Knowing that the normal cardiac output is 4 to 8 L/min helps you eliminate options 1 and 2. From the remaining options, think about what the pressure would do in the lungs behind a failing heart to direct you to option 3. Review these concepts if you had difficulty with this question.

Level of Cognitive Ability: Analysis
Client Needs: Physiological Integrity
Integrated Process: Nursing Process—assessment
Content Area: Adult health—cardiovascular
Reference: Ignatavicius, D., & Workman, M. (2002). *Medical-surgical nursing: Critical thinking for collaborative care* (4th ed., pp. 650-651). Philadelphia: W. B. Saunders.

15. 4
Rationale: The nursing interventions for the client with an intraaortic balloon pump are the same as for any cardiovascular surgery client. The peripheral circulation to the affected limb is monitored for signs of occlusion, such as coolness, mottling, pain, tingling, and decreased or absent distal pulse. Adverse changes are reported immediately.
Test-Taking Strategy: Focus on the data provided in this question. From these data, use the ABCs—airway, breathing, and circulation. Because these data indicate a circulatory problem, select option 4. Review nursing care for a client with an intraaortic balloon pump if you had difficulty with this question.
Level of Cognitive Ability: Application
Client Needs: Physiological Integrity
Integrated Process: Nursing Process—implementation
Content Area: Adult health—cardiovascular
Reference: Lewis, S., Heitkemper, M., & Dirksen, S. (2004). *Medical-surgical nursing: Assessment and management of clinical problems* (6th ed., p. 1774). St. Louis: Mosby.

16. 1
Rationale: Sternotomy incision sites are assessed for signs and symptoms of infection, such as redness, swelling, induration, and drainage. Elevated temperature and white blood cell count after 3 to 4 days postoperatively usually indicate infection.
Test-Taking Strategy: Use the process of elimination. Eliminate options 2 and 4 because the white blood cell count is within normal range. From the remaining options, focus on the data in the question. A nonreddened incision with no apparent drainage indicates no signs of infection. Review the signs of infection if you had difficulty with this question.
Level of Cognitive Ability: Analysis
Client Needs: Physiological Integrity
Integrated Process: Nursing Process—analysis
Content Area: Adult health—cardiovascular
References: Ignatavicius, D., & Workman, M. (2002). *Medical-surgical nursing: Critical thinking for collaborative care* (4th ed., p. 810). Philadelphia: W. B. Saunders.
Lewis, S., Heitkemper, M., & Dirksen, S. (2004). *Medical-surgical nursing: Assessment and management of clinical problems* (6th ed., pp. 402, 825). St. Louis: Mosby.

17. 4
Rationale: The client who undergoes cardiac surgery is at risk for renal injury from poor perfusion, hemolysis, low cardiac output, or vasopressor medication therapy. Renal insult is signaled by decreased urine output, and increased blood urea nitrogen and creatinine. The client may need medications such as dopamine (Intropin) to increase renal perfusion and possibly could need peritoneal dialysis or hemodialysis.

No data in the question indicate the presence of hypovolemia, urinary tract infection, or glomerulonephritis.
Test-Taking Strategy: Use the process of elimination. Eliminate options 2 and 3 first because no data indicate infection or inflammation. Noting that the urine output is inadequate will assist you in eliminating option 1. Review the complications associated with cardiac surgery if you had difficulty with this question.
Level of Cognitive Ability: Analysis
Client Needs: Physiological Integrity
Integrated Process: Nursing Process—analysis
Content Area: Adult health—cardiovascular
References: Black, J., Hawks, J., & Keene, A. (2001). *Medical-surgical nursing: Clinical management for positive outcomes* (6th ed., pp. 1509, 1511). Philadelphia: W. B. Saunders.
Ignatavicius, D., & Workman, M. (2002). *Medical-surgical nursing: Critical thinking for collaborative care* (4th ed., pp. 804, 1668). Philadelphia: W. B. Saunders.

18. 2
Rationale: The nurse should encourage regular use of pain medication for the first 48 to 72 hours after cardiac surgery because analgesia will promote rest, decrease myocardial oxygen consumption resulting from pain, and allow better participation in activities such as coughing, deep breathing, and ambulation. Options 1 and 3 will not help in tolerating ambulation. Removal of telemetry equipment is contraindicated unless prescribed.
Test Taking Strategy: Use the process of elimination. Focus on the issue, how best to tolerate the ambulation. Coughing and deep breathing will not actively help endurance, so eliminate option 1. Removal of telemetry equipment is contraindicated unless ordered. From the remaining options, focusing on the issue will direct you to option 2. Review comfort measures for the client following cardiac surgery if you had difficulty with this question.
Level of Cognitive Ability: Application
Client Needs: Physiological Integrity
Integrated Process: Nursing Process—planning
Content Area: Adult health—cardiovascular
References: Ignatavicius, D., & Workman, M. (2002). *Medical-surgical nursing: Critical thinking for collaborative care* (4th ed., p. 254). Philadelphia: W. B. Saunders.
Lewis, S., Heitkemper, M., & Dirksen, S. (2004). *Medical-surgical nursing: Assessment and management of clinical problems* (6th ed., p. 830). St. Louis: Mosby.

19. 1
Rationale: Normal sinus rhythm is defined as a regular rhythm with an overall rate of 60 to 100 beats per minute. The PR and QRS measurements are normal, measuring 0.12 to 0.20 second and 0.04 to 0.10 second, respectively.
Test-Taking Strategy: A baseline knowledge of normal electrocardiogram measurements is needed to answer this question. Review this content if you are unfamiliar with it.
Level of Cognitive Ability: Analysis
Client Needs: Physiological Integrity
Integrated Process: Nursing Process—assessment
Content Area: Adult health—cardiovascular

Reference: Ignatavicius, D., & Workman, M. (2002). *Medical-surgical nursing: Critical thinking for collaborative care* (4th ed., p. 662). Philadelphia: W. B. Saunders.

20. 1
Rationale: Sudden loss of electrocardiogram complexes indicates ventricular asystole or possibly electrode displacement. Accurate assessment of the client and equipment is necessary to determine the cause and identify the appropriate intervention.
Test-Taking Strategy: Use the steps of the nursing process. Option 1 is the only option that addresses assessment. Review care to the client on a cardiac monitor if you had difficulty with this question. Remember, always assess the client directly before taking any action.
Level of Cognitive Ability: Application
Client Needs: Physiological Integrity
Integrated Process: Nursing Process—implementation
Content Area: Delegating/Prioritizing
Reference: Ignatavicius, D., & Workman, M. (2002). *Medical-surgical nursing: Critical thinking for collaborative care* (4th ed., p. 679). Philadelphia: W. B. Saunders.

21. 4
Rationale: Sinus dysrhythmia has all the characteristics of normal sinus rhythm, except there is an irregular PP interval, which is due to phasic changes in the rate of firing of the sinoatrial node. Sinus dysrhythmia does not affect the cardiac output. Options 1, 2, and 3 identify rhythms that are regular.
Test-Taking Strategy: Use the process of elimination. Eliminate options 1, 2, and 3 because they are similar in that the rhythm of each of these is regular. Review the characteristics of sinus dysrhythmia if you had difficulty with this question.
Level of Cognitive Ability: Analysis
Client Needs: Physiological Integrity
Integrated Process: Nursing Process—analysis
Content Area: Adult health—cardiovascular
Reference: Phipps, W., Monahan, F., Sands, J., Marek, J., & Neighbors, M. (2003). *Medical-surgical nursing: Health and illness perspectives* (7th ed., pp. 680, 682). St. Louis: Mosby.

22. 2
Rationale: Motion artifact, or "noise," can be caused by frequent client movement, electrode placement on limbs, and insufficient adhesion to the skin, such as placing electrodes over hairy areas of the skin. Electrode placement over bony prominences also should be avoided. Signal interference also can occur with electrode removal and cable disconnection.
Test-Taking Strategy: Use the process of elimination, focusing on the issue, artifact. Note the key word "unlikely." Recalling the causes of artifact will direct you to option 2. Review these causes if you had difficulty with this question.
Level of Cognitive Ability: Analysis
Client Needs: Physiological Integrity
Integrated Process: Nursing Process—assessment
Content Area: Adult health—cardiovascular
Reference: Ignatavicius, D., & Workman, M. (2002). *Medical-surgical nursing: Critical thinking for collaborative care* (4th ed., pp. 656, 658). Philadelphia: W. B. Saunders.

23. 2
Rationale: Ventricular tachycardia is characterized by the absence of P waves, wide QRS complexes (usually greater than 0.14 second), and a rate between 100 and 250 impulses per minute. The rhythm is usually regular.
Test-Taking Strategy: Use the process of elimination. Eliminate option 4 first because there are no P waves. Premature ventricular contractions are isolated ectopic beats superimposed on an underlying rhythm, so option 1 is eliminated next. Recalling that there are no true QRS complexes with ventricular fibrillation will direct you to option 2. Review the characteristics of ventricular tachycardia if you are unfamiliar with it.
Level of Cognitive Ability: Analysis
Client Needs: Physiological Integrity
Integrated Process: Nursing Process—assessment
Content Area: Adult health—cardiovascular
References: Ignatavicius, D., & Workman, M. (2002). *Medical-surgical nursing: Critical thinking for collaborative care* (4th ed., p. 677). Philadelphia: W. B. Saunders.
Lewis, S., Heitkemper, M., & Dirksen, S. (2004). *Medical-surgical nursing: Assessment and management of clinical problems* (6th ed., p. 868). St. Louis: Mosby.

24. 4
Rationale: Ventricular tachycardia is a life-threatening dysrhythmia that results from an irritable ectopic focus that takes over as the pacemaker for the heart. The low cardiac output that results can lead quickly to cerebral and myocardial ischemia. Clients frequently experience a feeling of impending death. Ventricular tachycardia is treated with antidysrhythmic medications or magnesium sulfate, cardioversion (client awake), or defibrillation (loss of consciousness). Ventricular tachycardia can deteriorate into ventricular fibrillation at any time.
Test-Taking Strategy: Use the process of elimination. Note the key words "most concerned." Option 3 is incorrect and is eliminated first. From the remaining options, focusing on the key words will direct you to option 4 because this option identifies the life-threatening condition. Review the concerns associated with ventricular tachycardia if you had difficulty with this question.
Level of Cognitive Ability: Analysis
Client Needs: Physiological Integrity
Integrated Process: Nursing Process—analysis
Content Area: Adult health—cardiovascular
References: Ignatavicius, D., & Workman, M. (2002). *Medical-surgical nursing: Critical thinking for collaborative care* (4th ed., pp. 677-678). Philadelphia: W. B. Saunders.
Lewis, S., Heitkemper, M., & Dirksen, S. (2004). *Medical-surgical nursing: Assessment and management of clinical problems* (6th ed., p. 870). St. Louis: Mosby.

25. 3
Rationale: First-line treatment of ventricular tachycardia in a client who is hemodynamically stable is the use of antidysrhythmics such as amiodarone (Cordarone), lidocaine (Xylocaine), and procainamide (Pronestyl). Cardioversion also may be needed to correct the rhythm (cardioversion is recommended for stable ventricular tachycardia). Defibrillation is used with pulseless ventricular tachycardia. Epinephrine would stimulate an already excitable ventricle and is contraindicated.

Test-Taking Strategy: Use the process of elimination. Eliminate option 2, recalling that pacemakers are used most often to treat bradycardias and heart block. Knowing that epinephrine is a sympathomimetic eliminates option 4. From the remaining options, noting that the client is awake and alert will direct you to option 3. Review treatment for ventricular tachycardia if you had difficulty with this question.
Level of Cognitive Ability: Application
Client Needs: Physiological Integrity
Integrated Process: Nursing Process—planning
Content Area: Adult health—cardiovascular
References: Ignatavicius, D., & Workman, M. (2002). *Medical-surgical nursing: Critical thinking for collaborative care* (4th ed., p. 677). Philadelphia: W. B. Saunders.
Lehne, R. (2001). *Pharmacology for nursing care* (4th ed., p. 690). Philadelphia: W. B. Saunders.
Lewis, S., Heitkemper, M., & Dirksen, S. (2004). *Medical-surgical nursing: Assessment and management of clinical problems* (6th ed., p. 869). St. Louis: Mosby.

26. 2
Rationale: Cough cardiopulmonary resuscitation (CPR) sometimes is used in the client with unstable ventricular tachycardia. The nurse tells the client to use cough CPR, if prescribed, by inhaling deeply and coughing forcefully every 1 to 3 seconds. Cough CPR may terminate the dysrhythmia or sustain the cerebral and coronary circulation for a short time until other measures can be implemented. Options 1, 3, and 4 will not assist in terminating the dysrhythmia.
Test-Taking Strategy: To answer this question, you must be familiar with the treatment for unstable ventricular tachycardia. Review the concept of cough CPR if you are not familiar with it.
Level of Cognitive Ability: Application
Client Needs: Physiological Integrity
Integrated Process: Teaching/Learning
Content Area: Adult health—cardiovascular
Reference: Ignatavicius, D., & Workman, M. (2002). *Medical-surgical nursing: Critical thinking for collaborative care* (4th ed., p. 677). Philadelphia: W. B. Saunders.

27. 1
Rationale: Premature ventricular contractions can cause hemodynamic compromise. The shortened ventricular filling time with the ectopic beat leads to decreased stroke volume and, if frequent enough, to decreased cardiac output. The client may be asymptomatic or may feel palpitations. Premature ventricular contractions can be caused by cardiac disorders or by any number of physiological stressors, such as infection, illness, surgery, or trauma, and by intake of caffeine, nicotine, or alcohol.
Test-Taking Strategy: Note the key words "priority on assessment." Use the ABCs—airway, breathing, and circulation—to direct you to option 1. Review the effects of premature ventricular contractions if you had difficulty with this question.
Level of Cognitive Ability: Analysis
Client Needs: Physiological Integrity
Integrated Process: Nursing Process—assessment
Content Area: Delegating/Prioritizing
Reference: Ignatavicius, D., & Workman, M. (2002). *Medical-surgical nursing: Critical thinking for collaborative care* (4th ed., pp. 675, 794). Philadelphia: W. B. Saunders.

28. 1
Rationale: The client with uncontrolled atrial fibrillation with a ventricular rate more than 100 beats per minute is at risk for low cardiac output because of loss of atrial kick. The nurse assesses the client for palpitations, chest pain or discomfort, hypotension, pulse deficit, fatigue, weakness, dizziness, syncope, shortness of breath, and distended neck veins.
Test-Taking Strategy: Use the process of elimination. Flat neck veins are normal or indicate hypovolemia, so eliminate option 4. Nausea and vomiting (option 2) is associated with vagus nerve activity and does not correlate with a tachycardic state. From the remaining options, think of the consequences of falling cardiac output to direct you to option 1. Review the effects of atrial fibrillation if you had difficulty with this question.
Level of Cognitive Ability: Analysis
Client Needs: Physiological Integrity
Integrated Process: Nursing Process—assessment
Content Area: Adult health—cardiovascular
References: Ignatavicius, D., & Workman, M. (2002). *Medical-surgical nursing: Critical thinking for collaborative care* (4th ed., pp. 673-674). Philadelphia: W. B. Saunders.
Phipps, W., Monahan, F., Sands, J., Marek, J., & Neighbors, M. (2003). *Medical-surgical nursing: Health and illness perspectives* (7th ed., p. 685). St. Louis: Mosby.

29. 2
Rationale: Atrial fibrillation is characterized by a loss of P waves; an undulating, wavy baseline; QRS duration that is often within normal limits; and an irregular ventricular rate, which can range from 60 to 100 beats per minute (when controlled with medications) to 100 to 160 beats per minute (when uncontrolled).
Test-Taking Strategy: Use the process of elimination. Noting the key words "there are no P waves" should direct you to option 2. Loss of P waves is characteristic of this dysrhythmia. Review the characteristics of atrial fibrillation if you had difficulty with this question.
Level of Cognitive Ability: Analysis
Client Needs: Physiological Integrity
Integrated Process: Nursing Process—assessment
Content Area: Adult health—cardiovascular
Reference: Phipps, W., Monahan, F., Sands, J., Marek, J., & Neighbors, M. (2003). *Medical-surgical nursing: Health and illness perspectives* (7th ed., pp. 680, 685). St. Louis: Mosby.

30. 1
Rationale: Carotid sinus massage is one of maneuvers used for vagal stimulation to decrease a rapid heart rate and possibly terminate a tachydysrhythmia. The others include inducing the gag reflex and asking the client to strain or bear down. Medication therapy often is needed as an adjunct to keep the rate down or maintain the normal rhythm. Options 2, 3, and 4 are incorrect descriptions of this procedure.
Test-Taking Strategy: Knowledge of anatomy and physiology alone may be sufficient to answer this question. Eliminate options 2 and 4 because a rapid-rate dysrhythmia would need to be slowed. Recalling the functions of the vagus nerve and the diaphragmatic nerve will direct you to option 1. The vagus nerve affects heart rate. The diaphragmatic nerve

affects respiration. If you are unfamiliar with the functions of these nerves, review this content.
Level of Cognitive Ability: Application
Client Needs: Physiological Integrity
Integrated Process: Nursing Process—implementation
Content Area: Adult health—cardiovascular
Reference: Ignatavicius, D., & Workman, M. (2002). *Medical-surgical nursing: Critical thinking for collaborative care* (4th ed., p. 684). Philadelphia: W. B. Saunders.

31. 2
Rationale: Ventricular fibrillation is characterized by irregular, chaotic undulations of varying amplitudes. Ventricular fibrillation has no measurable rate and no visible P waves or QRS complexes and results from electrical chaos in the ventricles.
Test-Taking Strategy: Use the process of elimination and knowledge regarding the characteristics of ventricular fibrillation. The lack of visible QRS complexes eliminates atrial fibrillation and ventricular tachycardia. Recalling that asystole is lack of any electrical activity of the heart will direct you to option 2. Review the characteristics of ventricular fibrillation if you had difficulty with this question.
Level of Cognitive Ability: Analysis
Client Needs: Physiological Integrity
Integrated Process: Nursing Process—assessment
Content Area: Adult health—cardiovascular
Reference: Lewis, S., Heitkemper, M., & Dirksen, S. (2004). *Medical-surgical nursing: Assessment and management of clinical problems* (6th ed., p. 874). St. Louis: Mosby.

32. 2
Rationale: Until the defibrillator is attached and charged, the client is resuscitated by using cardiopulmonary resuscitation. Once the defibrillator has been attached, the electrocardiogram is checked to verify that the rhythm is ventricular fibrillation or pulseless ventricular tachycardia. Leads also are checked for any loose connections. A nitroglycerin patch, if present, is removed. The client does not have to be intubated to be defibrillated. Lidocaine may be given subsequently but is not required before defibrillation. The machine is not set to the synchronous mode because there is no underlying rhythm with which to synchronize.
Test-Taking Strategy: Use the process of elimination, focusing on the issue, ventricular fibrillation. Note that option 2 directly addresses this issue and also addresses assessment of the client. Review the procedure for defibrillation if you had difficulty with this question.
Level of Cognitive Ability: Analysis
Client Needs: Physiological Integrity
Integrated Process: Nursing Process—assessment
Content Area: Adult health—cardiovascular
References: Ignatavicius, D., & Workman, M. (2002). *Medical-surgical nursing: Critical thinking for collaborative care* (4th ed., p. 678). Philadelphia: W. B. Saunders.
Lewis, S., Heitkemper, M., & Dirksen, S. (2004). *Medical-surgical nursing: Assessment and management of clinical problems* (6th ed., p. 874). St. Louis: Mosby.

33. 3
Rationale: The client may be defibrillated up to 3 times in succession. The energy levels used are 200, 300, and 360 J for the first, second, and third attempts, respectively.
Test-Taking Strategy: This is a difficult question to answer unless you are familiar with the defibrillation procedure. As a general rule, though, remember that lower levels of energy are used for cardioversion. Higher levels are used in defibrillation. Review this procedure if you had difficulty with this question.
Level of Cognitive Ability: Application
Client Needs: Physiological Integrity
Integrated Process: Nursing Process—implementation
Content Area: Adult health—cardiovascular
References: Ignatavicius, D., & Workman, M. (2002). *Medical-surgical nursing: Critical thinking for collaborative care* (4th ed., p. 691). Philadelphia: W. B. Saunders.
Lewis, S., Heitkemper, M., & Dirksen, S. (2004). *Medical-surgical nursing: Assessment and management of clinical problems* (6th ed., p. 875). St. Louis: Mosby.

34. 2
Rationale: After defibrillation the client requires continuous monitoring of electrocardiogram rhythm, hemodynamic status, and neurological status. Respiratory and metabolic acidosis develop during ventricular fibrillation because of lack of respiration and cardiac output. These can cause cerebral and cardiopulmonary complications. Arousable status, adequate blood pressure, and a sinus rhythm indicate successful response to defibrillation.
Test-Taking Strategy: Use the process of elimination. Note the key words "most successful." Eliminate options 1 and 3 first because the client is nonarousable. From the remaining options, select option 2 because a sinus rhythm is a more successful response compared with marked bradycardia. Review the expected effects of defibrillation if you had difficulty with this question.
Level of Cognitive Ability: Analysis
Client Needs: Physiological Integrity
Integrated Process: Nursing Process—evaluation
Content Area: Adult health—cardiovascular
Reference: Ignatavicius, D., & Workman, M. (2002). *Medical-surgical nursing: Critical thinking for collaborative care* (4th ed., pp. 678, 691). Philadelphia: W. B. Saunders.

35. 2
Rationale: Nursing responsibilities after cardioversion include maintenance of a patent airway, first, oxygen administration, assessment of vital signs and level of consciousness, and dysrhythmia detection.
Test-Taking Strategy: Use the process of elimination, noting the key words "highest priority." Use the ABCs—airway, breathing, and circulation—to direct you to option 2. Review care of the client following cardioversion if you had difficulty with this question.
Level of Cognitive Ability: Analysis
Client Needs: Physiological Integrity
Integrated Process: Nursing Process—evaluation
Content Area: Delegating/Prioritizing

Reference: Ignatavicius, D., & Workman, M. (2002). *Medical-surgical nursing: Critical thinking for collaborative care* (4th ed., p. 690). Philadelphia: W. B. Saunders.

36. **3**

Rationale: The nurse or rescuer puts two large adhesive patch electrodes on the client's chest in the usual defibrillator positions. The nurse stops cardiopulmonary resuscitation and orders anyone near the client to move away and not touch the client. The defibrillator then analyzes the rhythm, which may take up to 30 seconds. The machine then indicates if defibrillation is necessary.

Test-Taking Strategy: Use the process of elimination. If you are not familiar with this piece of equipment, look first at the word "automatic" in the name. This implies that a person is not as involved in the process as with a conventional defibrillator and will help to eliminate option 2. Because standard electrocardiogram monitoring leads do not play an active role once resuscitation is underway (options 1 and 4), you can eliminate these similar options. Review the procedure related to the use of an automatic external defibrillator if you had difficulty with this question.

Level of Cognitive Ability: Application
Client Needs: Physiological Integrity
Integrated Process: Nursing Process—implementation
Content Area: Adult health—cardiovascular
Reference: Ignatavicius, D., & Workman, M. (2002). *Medical-surgical nursing: Critical thinking for collaborative care* (4th ed., pp. 690-691). Philadelphia: W. B. Saunders.

37. **3**

Rationale: An automatic internal cardioverter-defibrillator (AICD) detects and delivers an electrical shock to terminate life-threatening episodes of ventricular tachycardia and ventricular fibrillation. These devices are implanted in clients who are considered high risk, including those who have survived sudden cardiac death unrelated to myocardial infarction, those who are refractive to medication therapy, and those who have syncopal episodes related to ventricular tachycardia.

Test-Taking Strategy: Use the process of elimination. Note the key words "least likely." Ventricular dysrhythmias that induce syncope or occur while the client is on medication are likely to be true indications for the AICD, so eliminate options 2 and 4 first. From the remaining options, the main difference is whether or not the cardiac arrest was related to myocardial infarction. Of these two, the one most likely to be responsive to AICD would be the client without myocardial infarction because those dysrhythmias are spontaneous. Review the indications for the use of an AICD, if you had difficulty with this question.

Level of Cognitive Ability: Analysis
Client Needs: Physiological Integrity
Integrated Process: Nursing Process—assessment
Content Area: Adult health—cardiovascular
Reference: Ignatavicius, D., & Workman, M. (2002). *Medical-surgical nursing: Critical thinking for collaborative care* (4th ed., p. 693). Philadelphia: W. B. Saunders.

38. **1**

Rationale: The nurse who is caring for the client after insertion of an automatic internal cardioverter-defibrillator needs to assess device settings, similar to after insertion of a permanent pacemaker. Specifically, the nurse needs to know whether the device is activated, the heart rate cutoff above which it will fire, and the number of shocks it is programmed to deliver. Options 2, 3, and 4 are also nursing interventions but are not the priority.

Test-Taking Strategy: Use Maslow's hierarchy of needs theory. Option 1 is the option that identifies the physiological need. Review care to the client following insertion of an automatic internal cardioverter-defibrillator if you had difficulty with this question.

Level of Cognitive Ability: Application
Client Needs: Physiological Integrity
Integrated Process: Nursing Process—assessment
Content Area: Delegating/Prioritizing
Reference: Ignatavicius, D., & Workman, M. (2002). *Medical-surgical nursing: Critical thinking for collaborative care* (4th ed., pp. 693, 696). Philadelphia: W. B. Saunders.

39. **1**

Rationale: In the first several hours after insertion of a permanent or a temporary pacemaker, the most common complication is pacing electrode dislodgment. The nurse helps prevent this complication by limiting the client's activities.

Test-Taking Strategy: Note the key word "avoid". Note that the pacemaker was inserted on the right side. Therefore to prevent pacing electrode dislodgment, motion must be limited on that side. Options 3 and 4 involve movement of the right arm and are eliminated first. Limiting the movement of the left arm (option 2) is of no benefit to the client. Thus option 1 is the correct option. Review care to the client following insertion of a pacemaker if you had difficulty with this question.

Level of Cognitive Ability: Application
Client Needs: Physiological Integrity
Integrated Process: Nursing Process—implementation
Content Area: Adult health—cardiovascular
Reference: Ignatavicius, D., & Workman, M. (2002). *Medical-surgical nursing: Critical thinking for collaborative care* (4th ed., p. 695). Philadelphia: W. B. Saunders.

40. **3**

Rationale: Pulmonary embolism is a life-threatening complication of deep vein thrombosis and thrombophlebitis. Chest pain is the most common symptom, which is sudden in onset, and may be aggravated by breathing. Other signs and symptoms include dyspnea, cough, diaphoresis, and apprehension.

Test-Taking Strategy: Focus on the client's diagnosis to answer the question. Recalling the complications related to thrombophlebitis will direct you to option 3. Review these complications and the associated signs and symptoms if you had difficulty with this question.

Level of Cognitive Ability: Analysis
Client Needs: Physiological Integrity
Integrated Process: Nursing Process—assessment
Content Area: Adult health—cardiovascular
Reference: Ignatavicius, D., & Workman, M. (2002). *Medical-surgical nursing: Critical thinking for collaborative care* (4th ed., p. 763). Philadelphia: W. B. Saunders.

41. 1

Rationale: Sclerotherapy is the injection of a sclerosing agent into a varicosity. The agent damages the vessel and causes aseptic thrombosis, which results in vein closure. With no blood flow through the vessel, there is no distention. The surgical procedure for varicose veins is vein ligation and stripping. This procedure involves tying off the varicose vein and large tributaries and then removal of the vein with the use of hook and wires via multiple small incisions in the leg.

Test-Taking Strategy: Use the process of elimination. Note the name of the procedure, "sclerotherapy." A vessel that is sclerosed is blocked. This will direct you to option 1. Review this procedure, if you had difficulty with this question.

Level of Cognitive Ability: Comprehension
Client Needs: Physiological Integrity
Integrated Process: Teaching/Learning
Content Area: Adult health—cardiovascular
Reference: Ignatavicius, D., & Workman, M. (2002). *Medical-surgical nursing: Critical thinking for collaborative care* (4th ed., p. 768). Philadelphia: W. B. Saunders.

42. 4

Rationale: Hypersensitivity or a sensation of "pins and needles" in the surgical limb may indicate temporary or permanent nerve injury following surgery. The saphenous vein and the saphenous nerve run close together in the distal third of the leg. Because complications from this surgery are relatively rare, this symptom should be reported.

Test-Taking Strategy: Use the process of elimination. Pins and needles sensations usually indicate nerve irritation or damage. If you know this, you can eliminate options 2 and 3. Reassuring the client about something being "only temporary" is not often an appropriate action, unless this is known to be absolutely true. Review the complications associated with vein ligation and stripping if you had difficulty with this question.

Level of Cognitive Ability: Analysis
Client Needs: Physiological Integrity
Integrated Process: Nursing Process—implementation
Content Area: Adult health—cardiovascular
References: Ignatavicius, D., & Workman, M. (2002). *Medical-surgical nursing: Critical thinking for collaborative care* (4th ed., p. 768). Philadelphia: W. B. Saunders.
Lewis, S., Heitkemper, M., & Dirksen, S. (2004). *Medical-surgical nursing: Assessment and management of clinical problems* (6th ed., p. 245). St. Louis: Mosby.

43. 2

Rationale: The mixture of arterial and venous manifestations (claudication and phlebitis, respectively) in the young male client suggests thromboangiitis obliterans (Buerger's disease). This is an uncommon disorder characterized by inflammation and thrombosis of smaller arteries and veins. This disorder typically is found in young adult males who smoke. The cause is not known precisely but is suspected to have an autoimmune component.

Test-Taking Strategy: Use the process of elimination and knowledge of this disorder to answer the question. Eliminate options 3 and 4 because they most likely would cause local skin reactions. From the remaining options, focus on the key words "next assess." To assess a modifiable factor before a

nonmodifiable one often is better. Review this disorder if you had difficulty with this question.

Level of Cognitive Ability: Analysis
Client Needs: Physiological Integrity
Integrated Process: Nursing Process—assessment
Content Area: Adult health—cardiovascular
Reference: Ignatavicius, D., & Workman, M. (2002). *Medical-surgical nursing: Critical thinking for collaborative care* (4th ed., pp. 744, 761). Philadelphia: W. B. Saunders.

44. 4

Rationale: Raynaud's disease responds favorably to eliminating caffeine from the diet and by the cessation of smoking. Medications may inhibit vessel spasm and prevent symptoms. Avoiding exposure to cold through a variety of means is important. However, moving to a warmer climate may not necessarily be beneficial because the symptoms still could occur with the use of air conditioning and during periods of cooler weather.

Test-Taking Strategy: Note the key words "needs further reinforcement." Think about the measures used to treat the disease to direct you to option 4. Also, relocation is the least favorable of all the options from the viewpoints of practicality and encountering new environmental concerns. Review this disorder if this question was difficult.

Level of Cognitive Ability: Analysis
Client Needs: Physiological Integrity
Integrated Process: Teaching/Learning
Content Area: Adult health—cardiovascular
References: Ignatavicius, D., & Workman, M. (2002). *Medical-surgical nursing: Critical thinking for collaborative care* (4th ed., p. 763). Philadelphia: W. B. Saunders.
Phipps, W., Monahan, F., Sands, J., Marek, J., & Neighbors, M. (2003). *Medical-surgical nursing: Health and illness perspectives* (7th ed., p. 778). St. Louis: Mosby.

45. 2

Rationale: After inferior vena cava filter insertion, the nurse inspects the surgical site for bleeding and signs and symptoms of infection. Otherwise, care is the same as for any other postoperative client.

Test-Taking Strategy: Use the process of elimination. Because inferior vena cava filters are inserted percutaneously through a deep vein, options 3 and 4 are eliminated because no abdominal incision is made. From the remaining options, noting that the client has been on anticoagulant therapy before surgery because of the high risk of pulmonary embolism will direct you to option 2. Review care of the client following insertion of an inferior vena cava filter if you had difficulty with this question.

Level of Cognitive Ability: Analysis
Client Needs: Physiological Integrity
Integrated Process: Nursing Process—assessment
Content Area: Adult health—cardiovascular
Reference: Ignatavicius, D., & Workman, M. (2002). *Medical-surgical nursing: Critical thinking for collaborative care* (4th ed., p. 765). Philadelphia: W. B. Saunders.

46. 4

Rationale: Blood pressure should be taken with the client seated with the arm bared, positioned with support and at heart level. The client should sit with the legs on the floor, feet uncrossed, and not speak during the recording. The client should not have smoked tobacco or taken in caffeine in the 30 minutes preceding the measurement. The client should rest quietly for 5 minutes before the reading is taken. The cuff bladder should encircle at least 80% of the limb being measured. Gauges other than a mercury sphygmomanometer should be calibrated every 6 months to ensure accuracy. Finally, two or more readings should be averaged.

Test-Taking Strategy: Use the process of elimination, noting the key word "avoiding." Looking for the option that identifies variables that interfere with accuracy (caffeine and nicotine) will direct you to option 4. Review this skill and procedure if you had difficulty with this question.

Level of Cognitive Ability: Application
Client Needs: Physiological Integrity
Integrated Process: Nursing Process—assessment
Content Area: Adult health—cardiovascular
Reference: Perry, A., & Potter, P. (2002). *Clinical nursing skills and techniques* (5th ed., p. 244). St. Louis: Mosby.

47. **4**

Rationale: The antidote to heparin is protamine sulfate and should be readily available for use if excessive bleeding or hemorrhage should occur. Vitamin K is an antidote for warfarin sodium. Aminocaproic acid is the antidote for thrombolytic therapy. Potassium chloride is administered for a potassium deficit.

Test-Taking Strategy: Knowledge regarding the various antidotes is needed to answer this question. Learn these antidotes if you had difficulty with this question.

Level of Cognitive Ability: Application
Client Needs: Physiological Integrity
Integrated Process: Nursing Process—implementation
Content Area: Adult health—cardiovascular
Reference: Hodgson, B., & Kizior, R. (2003). *Saunders nursing drug handbook 2003* (p. 944). Philadelphia: W. B. Saunders.

48. **3**

Rationale: The therapeutic range for prothrombin time is 1.5 to 2 times the control for clients at high risk for thrombus. Based on the client's control value, the therapeutic range for this individual would be 16.5 to 22 seconds. Therefore the result is within the therapeutic range.

Test Taking Strategy: Use the process of elimination. Look at the control value. Remembering that the purpose of anticoagulant therapy is to prolong clotting times will assist in eliminating options 1 and 2. Because the prothrombin value identified in the question is not even double the control, select option 3 from the remaining options. Review the therapeutic prothrombin level for a client at risk for pulmonary embolism if you had difficulty with this question.

Level of Cognitive Ability: Analysis
Client Needs: Physiological Integrity
Integrated Process: Nursing Process—assessment
Content Area: Adult health—cardiovascular
References: Chernecky, C., & Berger, B. (2001). *Laboratory tests and diagnostic procedures* (3rd ed., p. 865). Philadelphia: W. B. Saunders.

Phipps, W., Monahan, F., Sands, J., Marek, J., & Neighbors, M. (2003). *Medical-surgical nursing: Health and illness perspectives* (7th ed., pp. 630, 808). St. Louis: Mosby.

49. **2**

Rationale: Warfarin sodium works in the liver and inhibits synthesis of four vitamin K-dependent clotting factors (X, IX, VII, and II), but it takes 3 to 4 days before the therapeutic effect of warfarin is exhibited.

Test-Taking Strategy: Use the process of elimination. Heparin and warfarin sodium do not act in the same way, so eliminate option 4 first. Warfarin is an anticoagulant, not a thrombolytic, so eliminate option 3 next. From the remaining options, recalling that the liver synthesizes clotting factors will direct you to option 2. Review the action of warfarin sodium if you had difficulty with this question.

Level of Cognitive Ability: Comprehension
Client Needs: Physiological Integrity
Integrated Process: Teaching/Learning
Content Area: Adult health—cardiovascular
Reference: Ignatavicius, D., & Workman, M. (2002). *Medical-surgical nursing: Critical thinking for collaborative care* (4th ed., p. 826). Philadelphia: W. B. Saunders.

50. **1**

Rationale: The antidote to warfarin (Coumadin) is vitamin K and should be readily available for use if excessive bleeding or hemorrhage should occur. Aminocaproic acid is the antidote for thrombolytic agents. Protamine sulfate is the antidote for heparin. Potassium chloride is administered to treat potassium deficit.

Test-Taking Strategy: Knowledge regarding the various antidotes is needed to answer this question. Review these antidotes if you had difficulty with this question.

Level of Cognitive Ability: Application
Client Needs: Physiological Integrity
Integrated Process: Nursing Process—implementation
Content Area: Adult health—cardiovascular
Reference: Hodgson, B., & Kizior, R. (2003). *Saunders nursing drug handbook 2003* (p. 1168) Philadelphia: W. B. Saunders.

51. **1**

Rationale: Thrombolytic agents dissolve existing clots, and bleeding can occur anywhere in the body. The nurse monitors for any obvious signs of bleeding and also for occult signs of bleeding, which would include hemoglobin and hematocrit, blood pressure and pulse, neurological signs, assessment of abdominal and back pain, and the presence of blood in the urine or stool.

Test-Taking Strategy: Remember that bleeding is the primary complication of thrombolytic therapy. Note the key words "least frequent assessment." Therefore look for the option that is not related to bleeding. A change in neurological signs could indicate cerebral bleeding; abdominal and back pain could indicate abdominal bleeding; change in blood pressure and pulse could be general indicators of hemorrhage. Oxygen saturation is not an indicator of bleeding in the respiratory tract; more likely, hemoptysis would be noted. Review nursing considerations for the client receiving tissue plasminogen activator if you had difficulty with this question.

Level of Cognitive Ability: Analysis
Client Needs: Physiological Integrity
Integrated Process: Nursing Process—assessment
Content Area: Delegating/Prioritizing
Reference: Ignatavicius, D., & Workman, M. (2002). *Medical-surgical nursing: Critical thinking for collaborative care* (4th ed., pp. 799-800). Philadelphia: W. B. Saunders.

52. 4
Rationale: Thrombolytic therapy is contraindicated in a number of preexisting conditions in which there is a risk of uncontrolled bleeding, similar to the case in anticoagulant therapy. Thrombolytic therapy also is contraindicated in severe uncontrolled hypertension because of the risk of cerebral hemorrhage. Therefore the nurse would report the results of the blood pressure to the physician before initiating therapy.
Test-Taking Strategy: Use the process of elimination and focus on the client's diagnosis. Options 1, 2, and 3 may be present in the client with pulmonary embolism and are not necessarily signs that warrant reporting before this therapy is initiated. Review the contraindications associated with the administration of this medication if you had difficulty with this question.
Level of Cognitive Ability: Analysis
Client Needs: Physiological Integrity
Integrated Process: Nursing Process—implementation
Content Area: Adult health—cardiovascular
Reference: Hodgson, B., & Kizior, R. (2003). *Saunders nursing drug handbook 2003* (p. 1035). Philadelphia: W. B. Saunders.

53. 3
Rationale: The client is experiencing an anaphylactic reaction to streptokinase, which is allergenic. The infusion should be stopped, the physician should be notified, and the client should receive treatment with epinephrine, antihistamines, and corticosteroids.
Test-Taking Strategy: Recall that allergic reaction and possible anaphylaxis are risks associated with streptokinase therapy. Also, focusing on the signs and symptoms in the question will assist in answering the question. When a severe allergic reaction occurs, the offending substance should be stopped, and lifesaving treatment should begin. Review the adverse effects of this medication if you had difficulty with this question.
Level of Cognitive Ability: Analysis
Client Needs: Physiological Integrity
Integrated Process: Nursing Process—implementation
Content Area: Adult health—cardiovascular
References: Ignatavicius, D., & Workman, M. (2002). *Medical-surgical nursing: Critical thinking for collaborative care* (4th ed., p. 800). Philadelphia: W. B. Saunders.
Phipps, W., Monahan, F., Sands, J., Marek, J., & Neighbors, M. (2003). *Medical-surgical nursing: Health and illness perspectives* (7th ed., p. 655). St. Louis: Mosby.

54. 1
Rationale: An expected outcome of surgery is warmth, redness, and edema in the surgical extremity because of increased blood flow. Options 2, 3, and 4 are incorrect interpretations.

Test-Taking Strategy: Use the process of elimination. Option 3 can be eliminated because the pedal pulse is unchanged from admission. Venous complications from immobilization resulting from surgery would not be apparent within 4 hours, so eliminate option 4. From the remaining options, think about the effects of sudden reperfusion in an ischemic limb. There would be redness from new blood flow, and edema from the sudden change in pressure in the blood vessels. Review the expected assessment findings following this surgical procedure if you had difficulty with this question.
Level of Cognitive Ability: Analysis
Client Needs: Physiological Integrity
Integrated Process: Nursing Process—assessment
Content Area: Adult health—cardiovascular
References: Ignatavicius, D., & Workman, M. (2002). *Medical-surgical nursing: Critical thinking for collaborative care* (4th ed., pp. 748-749). Philadelphia: W. B. Saunders.
Lewis, S., Heitkemper, M., & Dirksen, S. (2004). *Medical-surgical nursing: Assessment and management of clinical problems* (6th ed., p. 823). St. Louis: Mosby.

55. 1
Rationale: Following pericardiocentesis, a rise in blood pressure and a fall in central venous pressure are expected. The client usually expresses immediate relief. Heart sounds are no longer muffled or distant.
Test-Taking Strategy: Use the process of elimination. Note the key word "unsuccessful." Successful therapy is measured by the disappearance of the original signs and symptoms of cardiac tamponade. Therefore look for the option that identifies a sign consistent with continued tamponade. Review signs of cardiac tamponade and the expected effects of pericardiocentesis if you had difficulty with this question.
Level of Cognitive Ability: Analysis
Client Needs: Physiological Integrity
Integrated Process: Nursing Process—evaluation
Content Area: Adult health—cardiovascular
References: Ignatavicius, D., & Workman, M. (2002. *Medical-surgical nursing: Critical thinking for collaborative care* (4th ed., p. 722). Philadelphia: W. B. Saunders.
Phipps, W., Monahan, F., Sands, J., Marek, J., & Neighbors, M. (2003). *Medical-surgical nursing: Health and illness perspectives* (7th ed., p. 708). St. Louis: Mosby.

56. 2
Rationale: Not all clients with abdominal aortic aneurysm exhibit symptoms. Those who do may describe a feeling of the "heart beating" in the abdomen when supine or being able to feel the mass throbbing. A pulsatile mass may be palpated in the middle and upper abdomen. A systolic bruit may be auscultated over the mass. Hyperactive bowel sounds are not related specifically to an abdominal aortic aneurysm.
Test-Taking Strategy: Use the process of elimination. Note the key word "unrelated." Note that options 1, 3, and 4 are similar in that they identify a circulatory component. Review the signs of abdominal aortic aneurysm if you had difficulty with this question.
Level of Cognitive Ability: Analysis

Client Needs: Physiological Integrity
Integrated Process: Nursing Process—assessment
Content Area: Adult health—cardiovascular
References: Lewis, S., Heitkemper, M., & Dirksen, S. (2004). *Medical-surgical nursing: Assessment and management of clinical problems* (6th ed., p. 914) St. Louis: Mosby.
Phipps, W., Monahan, F., Sands, J., Marek, J., & Neighbors, M. (2003). *Medical-surgical nursing: Health and illness perspectives* (7th ed., p. 708). St. Louis: Mosby.

57. **4**

Rationale: Following abdominal aortic aneurysm resection or repair, the nurse monitors the client for signs of renal failure. Renal failure can occur because often much blood is lost during the surgery, and depending on the aneurysm location, the renal arteries may be hypoperfused for a short period during surgery. The nurse monitors hourly intake and output and notes the results of daily blood urea nitrogen and creatinine levels. Urine output less than 50 mL/hour is reported to the physician.
Test-Taking Strategy: Focus on the information in the question and the abnormal assessment data. This question indicates elevations in blood urea nitrogen and creatinine levels and a significant drop in hourly urine output. These assessment findings should direct you to option 4. Review the complications associated with this surgical procedure if you had difficulty with this question.
Level of Cognitive Ability: Analysis
Client Needs: Physiological Integrity
Integrated Process: Nursing Process—implementation
Content Area: Adult health—cardiovascular
References: Ignatavicius, D., & Workman, M. (2002). *Medical-surgical nursing: Critical thinking for collaborative care* (4th ed., p. 758). Philadelphia: W. B. Saunders.
Lewis, S., Heitkemper, M., & Dirksen, S. (2004). *Medical-surgical nursing: Assessment and management of clinical problems* (6th ed., p. 914) St. Louis: Mosby.

58. **4**

Rationale: Venous leg ulcers, also called stasis ulcers, tend to be more superficial than arterial ulcers, and the ulcer bed is pink. The edges of the ulcer are uneven, and granulation tissue is evident. The skin has a brown pigmentation from accumulation of metabolic waste products resulting from venous stasis. The client also exhibits peripheral edema.
Test-Taking Strategy: Use the process of elimination. You must discriminate between the signs and symptoms of arterial and venous leg ulcers. Knowing that the information in options 1, 2, and 3 is due to tissue malnutrition (and thus an arterial problem) will direct you to option 4. Review the assessment findings in arterial and venous conditions if you had difficulty with this question.
Level of Cognitive Ability: Analysis
Client Needs: Physiological Integrity
Integrated Process: Nursing Process—assessment
Content Area: Adult health—cardiovascular
References: Ignatavicius, D., & Workman, M. (2002). *Medical-surgical nursing: Critical thinking for collaborative care* (4th ed., p. 767). Philadelphia: W. B. Saunders.

Phipps, W., Monahan, F., Sands, J., Marek, J., & Neighbors, M. (2003). *Medical-surgical nursing: Health and illness perspectives* (7th ed., p. 799). St. Louis: Mosby.

59. **2**

Rationale: The first signs and symptoms of digoxin toxicity in adults include abdominal pain, nausea, vomiting, visual disturbances (blurred, yellow, or green vision, halos around lights), bradycardia, and other dysrhythmias. Options 1, 3, and 4 are unrelated to digoxin therapy.
Test Taking Strategy: Use the process of elimination, noting that the client is receiving digoxin. Recalling the signs of digoxin toxicity will direct you to option 2. Review these signs if you had difficulty with this question.
Level of Cognitive Ability: Application
Client Needs: Physiological Integrity
Integrated Process: Nursing Process—assessment
Content Area: Adult health—cardiovascular
References: Hodgson, B., & Kizior, R. (2003). *Saunders nursing drug handbook 2003* (p. 349). Philadelphia: W. B. Saunders.
Ignatavicius, D., & Workman, M. (2002). *Medical-surgical nursing: Critical thinking for collaborative care* (4th ed., p. 708). Philadelphia: W. B. Saunders.

60. **3**

Rationale: Stable angina is induced by exercise and relieved by rest or nitroglycerin tablets. Unstable angina occurs at lower and lower levels of activity or at rest, is less predictable, and is often a precursor of myocardial infarction. Variant angina, or Prinzmetal's angina, is prolonged and severe and occurs at the same time each day, most often in the morning.
Test-Taking Strategy: Use the process of elimination, focusing on the data in the question. Noting the key words "occurs at the same time each day" will direct you to option 3. If you had difficulty with this question, review the characteristics of the various types of angina.
Level of Cognitive Ability: Comprehension
Client Needs: Physiological Integrity
Integrated Process: Nursing Process—assessment
Content Area: Adult health—cardiovascular
Reference: Ignatavicius, D., & Workman, M. (2002). *Medical-surgical nursing: critical thinking for collaborative care* (4th ed., p. 795). Philadelphia: W. B. Saunders.

CRITICAL THINKING: MULTIPLE RESPONSE

Answer:
Administering furosemide (Lasix)
Administering oxygen
Administering morphine sulfate intravenously
Rationale: Pulmonary edema is a life-threatening event that can result from severe heart failure. In pulmonary edema the left ventricle fails to eject sufficient blood, and pressure increases in the lungs because of the accumulated blood. Oxygen is always prescribed, and the client is placed in a high Fowler's position to ease the work of breathing. Furosemide, a rapid-acting diuretic, will eliminate accumulated fluid. Intravenously administered morphine sulfate reduces venous return (preload), decreases anxiety, and also

reduces the work of breathing. Transporting the client to the coronary care unit is not a priority intervention. In fact, this may not be necessary at all if the client's response to treatment is successful.

Test-Taking Strategy: Note the key words "priority interventions" and focus on the client's diagnosis. Recalling the pathophysiology associated with pulmonary edema and using the ABCs—airway, breathing, and circulation—will assist in determining the priority interventions. Review priority interventions for the client with pulmonary edema if you had difficulty with this question.

Level of Cognitive Ability: Application
Client Needs: Physiological Integrity
Integrated Process: Nursing Process—implementation
Content Area: Delegating/Prioritizing
Reference: Ignatavicius, D., & Workman, M. (2002). *Medical-surgical nursing: Critical thinking for collaborative care* (4th ed., p. 709). Philadelphia: W. B. Saunders.

REFERENCES

Black, J., Hawks, J., & Keene, A. (2001). *Medical-surgical nursing: Clinical management for positive outcomes* (6th ed.). Philadelphia: W. B. Saunders.

Chernecky, C., & Berger, B. (2001). *Laboratory tests and diagnostic procedures* (3rd ed.). Philadelphia: W. B. Saunders.

Hodgson, B., & Kizior, R. (2003). *Saunders nursing drug handbook 2003.* Philadelphia: W. B. Saunders.

Ignatavicius, D., & Workman, M. (2002). *Medical-surgical nursing: Critical thinking for collaborative care* (4th ed.). Philadelphia: W. B. Saunders.

Lehne, R. (2001). *Pharmacology for nursing care* (4th ed.). Philadelphia: W. B. Saunders.

Lewis, S., Heitkemper, M., & Dirksen, S. (2004). *Medical-surgical nursing: Assessment and management of clinical problems* (6th ed.). St. Louis: Mosby.

Phipps, W., Monahan, F., Sands, J., Marek, J., & Neighbors, M. (2003). *Medical-surgical nursing: Health and illness perspectives* (7th ed.). St. Louis: Mosby.

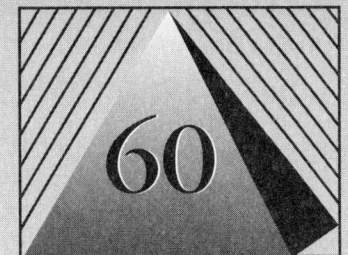

Cardiovascular Medications

I. ANTICOAGULANTS (BOX 60-1)

A. Description
1. Anticoagulants prevent the extension and formation of clots by inhibiting factors in the clotting cascade and decreasing blood coagulability.
2. Anticoagulants are used for thrombosis, pulmonary embolism, and myocardial infarction.
3. Anticoagulants are contraindicated with active bleeding, except for disseminated intravascular coagulation, bleeding disorders or blood dyscrasias, ulcers, liver and kidney disease, and spinal cord or brain injuries.

B. Side effects (Box 60-2)
1. Hemorrhage
2. Hematuria
3. Epistaxis
4. Ecchymosis
5. Bleeding gums
6. Thrombocytopenia
7. Hypotension

C. Heparin sodium (Liquaemin)
1. Description
   a. Heparin prevents thrombin from converting fibrinogen to fibrin.
   b. Heparin prevents thromboembolism.
   c. The therapeutic dose does not dissolve clots but prevents new thrombus formation.
2. Blood levels
   a. The normal activated partial thromboplastin time (aPTT) is 20 to 36 seconds.
   b. Maintain aPTT at 1.5 to 2.5 times normal.
   c. At therapeutic levels, heparin will increase the aPTT by a factor of 1.5 to 2.
   d. Activated partial thromboplastin time therapy should be measured every 4 to 6 hours during initial therapy and then daily.
   e. If the aPTT is too long, greater than 80 seconds, the dosage should be lowered.
   f. If aPTT is too short, less than 60 seconds, the dosage should be increased.
   g. Normal clotting time is 8 to 15 minutes; maintain the clotting time at 15 to 20 minutes.

BOX 60-1

Anticoagulants

ORAL
Anisindione (Miradon)
Warfarin sodium (Coumadin)

PARENTERAL
Ardeparin (Normiflo)
Dalteparin (Fragmin)
Danaparoid (Orgaran)
Enoxaparin (Lovenox)
Heparin sodium (Liquaemin)
Tinzaparin (Innohep)

BOX 60-2

Substances to Avoid with Anticoagulants

Allopurinol (Zyloprim)
Cimetidine (Tagamet)
Corticosteroids
Green leafy vegetables and foods high in vitamin K
Nonsteroidal antiinflammatory drugs
Oral hypoglycemic agents
Phenytoin (Dilantin)
Salicylates
Sulfonamides

3. Interventions
   a. Monitor clotting time and aPTT.
   b. Monitor platelet count.
   c. Observe for bleeding gums, bruises, nosebleeds, hematuria, hematemesis, occult blood in the stool, and petechiae.
   d. When administering heparin subcutaneously, inject into the abdomen with a 5/8 inch needle (25- to 28-gauge) at a 90-degree angle and do not aspirate or rub the injection site.
   e. Instruct the client regarding measures to prevent bleeding.
   f. The antidote to heparin is protamine sulfate.

D. Warfarin sodium (Coumadin)
   1. Description
      a. Warfarin suppresses coagulation by acting as an antagonist of vitamin K.
      b. Warfarin is used for long-term anticoagulation.
      c. Warfarin prolongs clotting time and is monitored by the prothrombin time (PT).
      d. Warfarin is used mainly to prevent thromboembolitic conditions such as thrombophlebitis, pulmonary embolism, and embolism formation caused by atrial fibrillation, thrombosis, myocardial infarction, or heart valve damage.
      e. Warfarin usually is given for 2 to 3 months after a myocardial infarction to decrease the incidence of deep vein thrombosis and thromboembolism.
   2. Blood levels
      a. The normal PT is 9.6 to 11.8 seconds.
      b. Warfarin sodium prolongs the PT.
   3. International normalized ratio (INR)
      a. The normal INR is 1.3 to 2.
      b. The INR is determined by multiplying the observed PT ratio (the ratio of the client's PT to a control PT) by a correction factor specific to a particular thromboplastin preparation used in the testing.
      c. The treatment goal is to raise the INR to an appropriate value.
      d. An INR of 2 to 3 is appropriate for most clients, although for some clients, the target INR is 3 to 4.5.
      e. If the INR is below the recommended range, warfarin sodium should be increased.
      f. If the INR is above the recommended range, warfarin sodium should be reduced.
   4. Interventions
      a. Monitor PT and INR.
      b. Observe for bleeding gums, bruises, nosebleeds, hematuria, hematemesis, occult blood in the stool, and petechiae.
      c. Instruct the client regarding measures to prevent bleeding.
      d. The antidote for warfarin is vitamin K (phytonadione, AquaMEPHYTON).

II. THROMBOLYTIC MEDICATIONS (BOX 60-3)

A. Description
   1. Thrombolytic medications activate plasminogen; plasminogen generates plasmin (the enzyme that dissolves clots).
   2. Thrombolytic medications are used early in the course of myocardial infarct (within 4 to 6 hours of the onset of the infarct) to restore blood flow, limit myocardial damage, preserve left ventricular function, and prevent death.

B. Contraindications
   1. Active internal bleeding
   2. History of cerebrovascular accident
   3. Intracranial problems
   4. Intracranial surgery or trauma within the previous 2 months
   5. History of thoracic, pelvic, or abdominal surgery in the previous 10 days
   6. History of hepatic or renal disease
   7. Uncontrolled hypertension
   8. Recently required, prolonged cardiopulmonary resuscitation

C. Side effects
   1. Bleeding
   2. Dysrhythmias
   3. Fever
   4. Allergic reactions

D. Interventions
   1. Obtain aPTT, PT, fibrinogen level, hematocrit, and platelet count.
   2. Monitor vital signs.
   3. Assess pulses.
   4. Monitor for bleeding.
   5. Monitor all excretions for occult blood.
   6. Monitor for neurological changes such as slurred speech, lethargy, confusion, and hemiparesis.
   7. Monitor for hypotension and tachycardia.
   8. Avoid injections if possible.
   9. Apply direct pressure over a puncture site for 20 to 30 minutes.
   10. Handle the client as little as possible when moving.
   11. Instruct the client to use electric razor for shaving and to brush teeth gently
   12. Discontinue the medication if bleeding develops, and notify the physician.
   13. Antidote
       a. Aminocaproic acid (Amicar)
       b. Used only in acute, life-threatening conditions

BOX 60-3

Thrombolytic Medications

Alteplase (Activase, t-PA)
Anistreplase (APSAC, Eminase)
Reteplase (Retavase)
Streptokinase (Kabikinase, Streptase)
Urokinase (Abbokinase)

III. ANTIPLATELET MEDICATIONS (BOX 60-4)

A. Description
  1. Antiplatelet medications inhibit the aggregation of platelets in the clotting process, thereby prolonging the bleeding time.
  2. Antiplatelet medications may be used with anticoagulants.
  3. Antiplatelet medications are used in the prophylaxis of long-term complications following myocardial infarction, coronary revascularization, stents, and cerebrovascular accidents.
  4. Antiplatelet medications are contraindicated in bleeding disorders and known sensitivity.
B. Side effects
  1. Gastrointestinal bleeding
  2. Bruising
  3. Hematuria
  4. Tarry stools
C. Interventions
  1. Determine sensitivity before administration.
  2. Monitor vital signs.
  3. Instruct the client to take medication with food if gastrointestinal upset occurs.
  4. Monitor bleeding time.
  5. Monitor for side effects related to bleeding.
  6. Instruct the client in the use of the medication.
  7. Instruct the client to monitor for side effects related to bleeding and in the measures to prevent bleeding.

IV. POSITIVE INOTROPIC/CARDIOTONIC MEDICATIONS (BOX 60-5)

A. Description
  1. These medications stimulate myocardial **contractility** and produce a positive inotropic effect.

BOX 60-4

Antiplatelet Medications

Abciximab (ReoPro)
Aspirin (acetylsalicylic acid, A.S.A.)
Clopidolgrel bisulfate (Plavix)
Dipyridamole (Persantine)
Eptifibatide (Integrilin)
Ticlopidine hydrochloride (Ticlid)
Tirofiban (Aggrastat)

BOX 60-5

Positive Inotropic/Cardiotonic Medications

AMRINONE (INOCOR)
Used for short-term management of congestive heart failure in those who have not responded adequately to cardiac glycosides, diuretics, and vasodilators

MILRINONE (PRIMACOR)
Used for short-term management of congestive heart failure or may be given before heart transplantation

---

  2. Used for congestive heart failure; the increase in myocardial **contractility** increases cardiac, peripheral, and kidney function by increasing **cardiac output,** decreasing **preload,** improving blood flow to the periphery and kidneys, decreasing edema, and increasing fluid excretion; as a result, fluid retention in the lungs and extremities is decreased.
B. Side effects
  1. Dysrhythmias
  2. Hypotension
  3. Thrombocytopenia
C. Toxic/adverse reactions
  1. Hepatotoxicity manifested by elevated liver enzyme levels
  2. Hypersensitivity manifested by wheezing, shortness of breath, pruritis, urticaria, clammy skin, and flushing
D. Interventions
  1. Positive inotropic/cardiotonic medications are for intravenous (IV) administration.
    a. Do not dilute with dextrose-containing solutions.
    b. For continuous IV, administer with an infusion pump.
    c. Stop infusion if the client's **blood pressure (BP)** drops or dysrhythmias occur.
  2. Monitor apical pulse and **BP.**
  3. Monitor for hypersensitivity.
  4. Assess lung sounds for wheezing and crackles.
  5. Monitor for edema.
  6. Monitor for relief of congestive heart failure (CHF) as noted by reduction in edema, lessening of dyspnea, orthopnea, and fatigue.
  7. Monitor electrolytes, liver enzymes, platelet count, and renal function studies; the medications may decrease potassium and increase liver enzymes.
E. Milrinone (Primacor)
  1. Side effects
    a. Headache
    b. Hypotension
    c. Angina
  2. Toxic/adverse reactions: dysrhythmias
  3. Interventions
    a. For IV injection of loading dose, administer slowly over 10 minutes.
    b. For continuous IV, administer with an infusion pump.
    c. Monitor apical pulse and **BP.**
    d. Stop infusion if the client's **BP** drops or dysrhythmias occur.
    e. Assess lung sounds for wheezing and crackles.
    f. Monitor for edema.
    g. Monitor for relief of CHF as noted by reduction in edema, lessening of dyspnea, orthopnea, and fatigue.

V. CARDIAC GLYCOSIDES (BOX 60-6)

A. Description

BOX 60-6

Cardiac Glycosides

Digoxin (Lanoxicaps, Lanoxin)
Digitoxin (Crystodigin)

1. Cardiac glycosides inhibit the sodium-potassium pump, thus increasing intracellular calcium, which causes the heart muscle fibers to contract more efficiently.
2. Cardiac glycosides produce a positive inotropic action, which increases the force of myocardial contractions.
3. Cardiac glycosides produce a negative chronotropic action, which depresses the sinoatrial node, reduces conduction of the impulse through the atrioventricular node, and slows the heart rate.
4. Cardiac glycosides produce a negative dromotropic action that slows conduction velocity.
5. The increase in myocardial **contractility** increases cardiac, peripheral, and kidney function by increasing **cardiac output,** decreasing **preload,** improving blood flow to the periphery and kidneys, decreasing edema, and increasing fluid excretion; as a result, fluid retention in the lungs and extremities is decreased.
6. Cardiac glycosides are used for CHF, atrial tachycardia, atrial fibrillation, and atrial flutter.
7. Cardiac glycosides are contraindicated in ventricular dysrhythmias and second- or third-degree heart block.
8. Cardiac glycosides should be used with caution in clients with renal disease, hypothyroidism, and hypokalemia.

B. Side effects and toxic effects
   1. Anorexia, nausea, vomiting
   2. Headache
   3. Visual disturbances: diplopia, blurred vision, yellow-green halos
   4. Photophobia
   5. Drowsiness
   6. Bradycardia
   7. Fatigue, weakness

C. Interventions
   1. Monitor for toxicity as evidenced by anorexia, nausea, vomiting, visual disturbances, confusion, bradycardia, heart block, premature ventricular contractions, and tachydysrhythmias.
   2. Monitor serum digoxin level, electrolyte levels, and renal function tests.
   3. Therapeutic digoxin range is 0.5 to 2 ng/mL, and levels above 2 ng/mL are toxic.
   4. An increased risk of toxicity exists in clients with hypercalcemia, hypokalemia, hypomagnesemia, or hypothyroidism.

5. Monitor potassium level, and if hypokalemia occurs (potassium less than 3.5 mEq/L), notify the physician.
6. Instruct the client to avoid over-the-counter medications.
7. Monitor the client taking a potassium-wasting diuretic or corticosteroids closely for hypokalemia because the hypokalemia can cause digoxin toxicity.
8. Note that older clients are more sensitive to toxicity.
9. Advise the client to eat foods high in potassium, such as fresh and dried fruits, fruit juices, vegetables, and potatoes.
10. Monitor the apical pulse.
11. If the apical pulse rate is less than 60, the medication should be held and the physician notified.
12. Teach the client how to measure pulse.
13. Teach the client to notify physician if the pulse rate is less than 60 or greater than 100.
14. Teach the client the signs and symptoms of toxicity.
15. Antidote: Digoxin immune Fab (Digibind) is used in extreme toxicity.

VI. ANTIHYPERTENSIVE MEDICATIONS (BOX 60-7)
A. Thiazide diuretics (Box 60-8)
   1. Description
      a. Thiazide diuretics increase sodium and water excretion by inhibiting sodium reabsorption in the distal tubule of the kidney.
      b. Thiazide diuretics are used for hypertension and peripheral edema.
      c. Thiazide diuretics are used in clients with normal renal function.
      d. Thiazide diuretics are not effective for immediate diuresis.
      e. Thiazide diuretics are contraindicated in clients with renal failure.

BOX 60-7

Classifications of Diuretics

Carbonic anhydrase inhibitors
Loop diuretics
Osmotic diuretics
Potassium-sparing diuretics
Thiazide diuretics

BOX 60-8

Thiazide and Thiazide-like Diuretics

Chlorothiazide (Diuril)
Chlorthalidone (Hygroton, Thalitone)
Hydrochlorothiazide (Esidrix, Oretic, HydroDIURIL)
Indapamide (Lozol)
Metolazone (Zaroxolyn)

f. Thiazide diuretics should be used with caution in the client taking lithium because lithium toxicity can occur.

g. Thiazide diuretics should be used with caution in the client taking digoxin, corticosteroids, or hypoglycemic medications.

2. Side effects
a. Hypercalcemia, hyperglycemia, hyperuricemia
b. Hypokalemia, hyponatremia
c. Hypovolemia
d. Hypotension
e. Headaches
f. Nausea, vomiting
g. Constipation
h. Rashes
i. Photosensitivity
j. Blood dyscrasias

3. Interventions
a. Monitor vital signs.
b. Monitor weight.
c. Monitor urine output.
d. Monitor electrolytes, glucose, calcium, and uric acid levels.
e. Check peripheral extremities for edema.
f. Instruct the client to take the medication in the morning to avoid nocturia and sleep interruption.
g. Instruct the client in how to record the **BP.**
h. Instruct the client to eat foods rich in potassium.
i. Instruct the client in how to take potassium supplements if prescribed.
j. Instruct the client to take medication with food to avoid gastrointestinal upset.
k. Instruct the client to change positions slowly to prevent **orthostatic hypotension.**
l. Instruct the client to use sunscreen when in direct sunlight.
m. Instruct the client with diabetes mellitus to have the blood glucose checked periodically.

B. Loop diuretics (Box 60-9)
1. Description
a. Loop diuretics inhibit sodium and chloride reabsorption from the loop of Henle and the distal tubule.
b. Loop diuretics have little effect on the blood glucose; however, they cause depletion of water and electrolytes, increased uric acid levels, and the excretion of calcium.

c. Loop diuretics are more potent than the thiazide diuretics, causing rapid diuresis, thus decreasing vascular fluid volume, **cardiac output,** and **blood pressure.**

d. Loop diuretics are used for hypertension, edema associated with CHF, hypercalcemia, and renal disease.

e. Use loop diuretics with caution in the client taking digoxin or lithium.

f. Use loop diuretics with caution in the client on aminoglycosides, anticoagulants, corticosteroids, or amphotericin B.

2. Side effects
a. Hypokalemia, hyponatremia, hypocalcemia, hypomagnesemia
b. Hypochloremia
c. Thrombocytopenia
d. Hyperuricemia
e. **Orthostatic hypotension**
f. Skin disturbances
g. Ototoxicity and deafness
h. Thiamine deficiency
i. Dehydration

3. Interventions
a. Monitor vital signs.
b. Monitor weight.
c. Monitor urine output.
d. Monitor electrolytes, calcium, magnesium, and uric acid levels.
e. Check the peripheral extremities for edema.
f. Monitor for signs of digoxin or lithium toxicity if the client is on these medications.
g. Instruct the client to take the medication in the morning to avoid nocturia and sleep interruption.
h. Instruct the client in how to record the **BP.**
i. Instruct the client to eat foods rich in potassium.
j. Instruct the client in how to take potassium supplements if prescribed.
k. Instruct the client to take medication with food to avoid gastrointestinal upset.
l. Instruct the client to change positions slowly to prevent **orthostatic hypotension.**
m. Administer IV furosemide (Lasix) slowly because hearing loss can occur if injected rapidly.

C. Osmotic diuretics
1. Refer to Chapter 66 for information regarding osmotic diuretics.
2. Refer to Box 60-10 for a list of osmotic diuretics.

BOX 60-9

Loop Diuretics

Bumetanide (Bumex)
Ethacrynic acid (Edecrin)
Furosemide (Lasix)
Torsemide (Demadex)

BOX 60-10

Osmotic Diuretics

Glycerin (Osmoglyn)
Mannitol (Osmitrol)
Urea (Ureaphil)

▶ D. Carbonic anhydrase inhibitors (Box 60-11)
  1. Description
    a. Carbonic anhydrase inhibitors block the action of the enzyme carbonic anhydrase, which is needed to maintain acid-base balance.
    b. Inhibition of this enzyme, carbonic anhydrase, causes increased sodium, potassium, and bicarbonate excretion.
    c. Metabolic acidosis can occur with prolonged use.
    d. Carbonic anhydrase inhibitors are used to decrease intraocular pressure in open-angle (chronic) glaucoma and to produce diuresis, manage epilepsy, and treat high-altitude sickness.
    e. Carbonic anhydrase inhibitors are used to treat metabolic alkalosis.
    f. Carbonic anhydrase inhibitors are contraindicated in narrow-angle or acute glaucoma.
  2. Side effects
    a. Hyperglycemia, hyperuricemia, hypercalcemia
    b. Hypokalemia
    c. Anorexia, nausea, vomiting
    d. **Orthostatic hypotension**
    e. Renal calculi
    f. Hemolytic anemia
  3. Interventions
    a. Monitor vital signs.
    b. Monitor weight.
    c. Monitor urine output.
    d. Monitor electrolytes, glucose, calcium, and uric acid levels.
    e. Monitor mental status.
    f. Instruct the client to monitor for signs of renal calculi.
▶ E. Potassium-sparing diuretics (Box 60-12)
  1. Description
    a. Potassium-sparing diuretics act on the distal tubule to promote sodium and water excretion and potassium retention.

BOX 60-11

Carbonic Anhydrase Inhibitors

Acetazolamide (Diamox)
Dichlorphenamide (Daranide)
Methazolamide (Neptazane)

BOX 60-12

Potassium-Sparing Diuretics

Amiloride (Midamor)
Amiloride hydrochloride and hydrochlorothiazide (Moduretic)
Spironolactone (Aldactone)
Spironolactone and hydrochlorothiazide (Aldactazide)
Triamterene (Dyrenium)

---

    b. Potassium-sparing diuretics are used for edema and hypertension; to increase urine output; to treat fluid retention and overload associated with CHF, hepatic cirrhosis, or nephrotic syndrome; and for diuretic-induced hypokalemia.
    c. Potassium-sparing diuretics are contraindicated in severe kidney or hepatic disease or in severe hyperkalemia.
    d. Potassium-sparing diuretics should be used with caution in the client with diabetes mellitus.
    e. Potassium-sparing diuretics should be used with caution in the client taking antihypertensives or lithium.
    f. Potassium-sparing diuretics should be used with caution in the client taking angiotensin-converting enzyme inhibitors because hyperkalemia can result.
    g. Potassium-sparing diuretics should be used with caution in the client taking potassium supplements.
  2. Side effects
    a. Hyperkalemia
    b. Nausea, vomiting, diarrhea
    c. Rash
    d. Dizziness, weakness
    e. Headache
    f. Dry mouth
    g. Photosensitivity
    h. Anemia
    i. Thrombocytopenia
  3. Interventions
    a. Monitor vital signs.
    b. Monitor urine output.
    c. Monitor for signs and symptoms of hyperkalemia such as nausea, diarrhea, abdominal cramps, tachycardia followed by bradycardia, tall peaked T wave on the electrocardiogram, or oliguria.
    d. Monitor for a potassium level greater than 5.1 mEq/L, which indicates hyperkalemia.
    e. Instruct the client to avoid foods high in potassium.
    f. Instruct the client to avoid exposure to direct sunlight.
    g. Instruct the client to monitor for signs of hyperkalemia.
    h. Instruct the client to avoid salt substitutes because they contain potassium.
    i. Instruct the client to take with or after meals to decrease gastrointestinal irritation.

VII. PERIPHERALLY ACTING α-ADRENERGIC BLOCKERS (BOX 60-13)
A. Description
  1. These medications decrease sympathetic vasoconstriction by reducing the effects of norepinephrine

at peripheral nerve endings, resulting in vasodilation and decreased **BP.**

2. These medications are used to maintain renal blood flow.

3. These medications are used to treat hypertension.

B. Side effects

1. **Orthostatic hypotension**
2. Reflex tachycardia
3. Sodium and water retention
4. Gastrointestinal disturbances
5. Nausea
6. Drowsiness
7. Nasal congestion
8. Edema
9. Weight gain
10. Reserpine (Serpasil) can cause depression, gastrointestinal irritation, and impotence.

C. Interventions

1. Monitor vital signs.
2. Monitor for fluid retention and edema.
3. Instruct the client to change positions slowly to prevent **orthostatic hypotension.**
4. Instruct the client in how to monitor the **BP.**
5. Instruct the client to monitor for edema.
6. Instruct the client to decrease salt intake.
7. Instruct the client to avoid over-the-counter medications.

VIII. CENTRALLY ACTING SYMPATHOLYTICS (ADRENERGIC BLOCKERS) (BOX 60-14)

A. Description

1. Centrally acting sympatholytics stimulate alpha receptors in the central nervous system to inhibit vasoconstriction, thus reducing peripheral resistance.
2. Centrally acting sympatholytics are used to treat hypertension.

BOX 60-13

Peripherally Acting α-Adrenergic Blockers

Doxazosin mesylate (Cardura)
Guanadrel (Hylorel)
Guanethidine (Ismelin)
Phenoxybenzamine (Dibenzyline)
Phentolamine (Regitine)
Prazosin (Minipress)
Reserpine (Serpasil)
Terazosin (Hytrin)
Tolazoline (Priscoline)

BOX 60-14

Centrally Acting Sympatholytics

Clonidine (Catapres)
Guanabenz (Wytensin)
Methyldopa (Aldomet)

---

3. Centrally acting sympatholytics are contraindicated in impaired liver function.

B. Side effects

1. Sodium and water retention
2. Drowsiness, dizziness
3. Dry mouth
4. Bradycardia
5. Edema
6. Impotence
7. Hypotension
8. Depression

C. Interventions

1. Monitor vital signs.
2. Instruct the client not to discontinue medication because abrupt withdrawal can cause severe rebound hypertension.
3. Monitor liver function tests.

IX. ANGIOTENSIN-CONVERTING ENZYME INHIBITORS (BOX 60-15)

A. Description

1. These medications prevent peripheral vasoconstriction by blocking conversion of angiotensin I to angiotensin II.
2. These medications are used to treat hypertension.
3. Avoid use with potassium supplements and potassium-sparing diuretics.

B. Side effects

1. Nausea, vomiting, diarrhea
2. Persistent cough
3. Hypotension
4. Hyperkalemia
5. Tachycardia
6. Headache
7. Dizziness, fatigue
8. Insomnia
9. Hypoglycemic reaction in the client with diabetes mellitus
10. Bruising, petechiae, bleeding
11. Diminished taste

C. Interventions

1. Monitor vital signs.

BOX 60-15

Angiotensin-Converting Enzyme Inhibitors

Benazepril (Lotensin)
Captopril (Capoten)
Enalapril (Vasotec)
Fosinopril (Monopril)
Lisinopril (Prinivil, Zestril)
Moexipril (Univasc)
Perindopril (Aceon)
Quinapril (Accupril)
Ramipril (Altace)
Trandolapril (Mavik)

2. Monitor protein, albumin, blood urea nitrogen, creatinine, white blood cells, and potassium level.
3. Monitor for hypoglycemic reactions in the client with diabetes mellitus.
4. Instruct the client to take captopril (Capoten) 20 minutes to 1 hour before a meal.
5. Monitor for bruising, petechiae, or bleeding with captopril.
6. Instruct the client not to discontinue medications because rebound hypertension can occur.
7. Instruct the client not to take over-the-counter medications.
8. Instruct the client in how to take the BP.
9. Instruct the client that if dizziness occurs and persists to notify the physician.
10. Inform the client that the taste of food may be diminished during the first month of therapy.

▲ **X. ANTIANGINAL MEDICATIONS (BOX 60-16)**
A. Nitrates
1. Description
   a. Nitrates produce vasodilation.
   b. Nitrates decrease **preload** and **afterload** and reduce myocardial oxygen consumption.
   c. Nitrates are contraindicated in the client with significant hypotension, increased intracranial pressure, or severe anemia.
   d. Nitrates should be used with caution with severe renal or hepatic disease.
   e. Avoid abrupt withdrawal of long-acting preparations to prevent the rebound effect of severe pain from myocardial ischemia.
▲ 2. Side effects
   a. Headache
   b. **Orthostatic hypotension**
   c. Dizziness, weakness
   d. Faintness
   e. Nausea, vomiting
   f. Flushing or pallor
   g. Confusion
   h. Rash
   i. Dry mouth
   j. Reflex tachycardia
   k. Paradoxical bradycardia

BOX 60-16

Antianginal Medications

Erythrityl tetranitrate (Cardilate)
Isosorbide dinitrate (Iso-Bid, Isordil, Isotrate, Sorbitrate)
Isosorbide mononitrate (Imdur, Monoket)
Nitroglycerin (Nitrostat, Nitrolingual, Nitrogard, Nitrong, Nitronet)
Nitroglycerin ointment 2% (Nitro-Bid, Nitrol, Nitrong, Nitrodisc, Nitro-Dur, Transderm-Nitro)
Pentaerythritol tetranitrate (Pentylan Duotrate, Peritrate)

---

3. Sublingual medications ▲
   a. Monitor vital signs.
   b. Offer sips of water before giving because dryness may inhibit medication absorption.
   c. Instruct the client to place under the tongue and leave until fully dissolved.
   d. Instruct the client not to swallow the medication.
   e. Instruct the client to take one tablet for pain and repeat every 5 minutes for a total of three doses.
   f. Instruct the client to seek medical help immediately if pain is not relieved in 15 minutes, following the three doses.
   g. Inform the client that a stinging or burning sensation may indicate that the tablet is fresh.
   h. Instruct the client to store medication in a dark, tightly closed bottle.
   i. Instruct the client to check the expiration date on the medication bottle because expiration may occur within 6 months of obtaining medication.
   j. Instruct the client to take acetaminophen (Tylenol) for a headache.
4. Translingual medications (spray) ▲
   a. Instruct the client to direct spray against the oral mucosa.
   b. Instruct the client to avoid inhaling the spray.
5. Sustained-released medications: Instruct the ▲ client to swallow and not to chew or crush the medication.
6. Transmucosal-buccal medications ▲
   a. Instruct the client to place the medication between the upper lip and gum or in the buccal area between the cheek and gum.
   b. Inform the client that the medication will adhere to the oral mucosa and slowly dissolve.
7. Transdermal patch ▲
   a. Instruct the client to apply the patch to a hairless area, using a new patch and a different site each day.
   b. As prescribed, instruct the client to remove the patch after 12 to 14 hours, allowing 10 to 12 "patch-free" hours each day to prevent tolerance.
8. Topical ointments ▲
   a. Instruct the client to remove the ointment on the skin from the previous dose.
   b. Instruct the client to squeeze a ribbon of ointment of the prescribed length onto the applicator paper.
   c. Instruct the client to spread the ointment over a 6 × 6 inch area, using the chest, back, abdomen, upper arm, or anterior thigh (avoiding hairy areas), and cover with a plastic wrap.
   d. Instruct the client to rotate sites and to avoid touching the ointment when applying.

9. Patches and ointments
   a. Wear gloves when applying.
   b. Do not apply on the chest in the area of defibrillator-cardioverter paddle placement because skin burns can result if the paddles needed to be used.

XI. β-ADRENERGIC BLOCKERS (BOX 60-17)

A. Description
   1. β-Adrenergic blockers inhibit response to β-adrenergic stimulation, thus decreasing **cardiac output.**
   2. β-Adrenergic blockers block the release of the catecholamines, epinephrine, and norepinephrine, thus decreasing the heart rate and **blood pressure.**
   3. β-Adrenergic blockers decrease the workload of the heart and decrease oxygen demands.
   4. β-Adrenergic blockers are used for angina, dysrhythmias, hypertension, migraine headaches, prevention of myocardial infarction, and glaucoma.
   5. β-Adrenergic blockers are contraindicated in the client with asthma, bradycardia, CHF, severe renal or hepatic disease, hyperthyroidism, or cerebrovascular accident.
   6. β-Adrenergic blockers should be used with caution in the client with diabetes mellitus because the medication may mask symptoms of hypoglycemia.
   7. β-Adrenergic blockers should be used with caution in the client taking antihypertensive medications.

B. Side effects
   1. Bradycardia
   2. Bronchospasm
   3. Hypotension
   4. Weakness, fatigue
   5. Nausea, vomiting
   6. Dizziness
   7. Hyperglycemia
   8. Agranulocytosis
   9. Behavioral or psychotic response
   10. Depression
   11. Nightmares

BOX 60-17

β-Adrenergic Blockers

Acebutolol (Sectral)
Atenolol (Tenormin)
Betaxolol (Kerlone)
Bisoprolol fumarate (Zebeta)
Carteolol (Cartrol)
Carvedilol (Coreg)
Labetalol (Normodyne, Trandate, Vescal)
Metoprolol (Lopressor, Toprol-XL)
Nadolol (Corgard)
Penbutolol (Levatol)
Pindolol (Visken)
Propranolol (Inderal)
Sotalol (Betapace)
Timolol (Blocadren)

C. Interventions
   1. Monitor vital signs.
   2. Hold the medication if the pulse or **BP** is not within the prescribed parameters.
   3. Monitor for signs of CHF.
   4. Assess for respiratory distress and for signs of wheezing and dyspnea.
   5. Instruct the client to report dizziness, light-headedness, or nasal congestion.
   6. Instruct the client not to stop the medication because rebound hypertension, rebound tachycardia, or an anginal attack can occur.
   7. Advise the client taking insulin that the β-blocker can mask early signs of hypoglycemia such as tachycardia and nervousness.
   8. Instruct the client taking insulin to monitor the blood glucose level.
   9. Instruct the client in how to take pulse and **BP.**
   10. Instruct the client to change positions slowly to prevent **orthostatic hypotension.**
   11. Instruct the client to avoid over-the-counter cold medications and nasal decongestants.

XII. CALCIUM CHANNEL BLOCKERS (BOX 60-18)

A. Description
   1. Calcium channel blockers decrease cardiac **contractility** (negative inotropic effect by relaxing smooth muscle) and the workload of the heart, thus decreasing the need for oxygen.
   2. Calcium channel blockers promote vasodilation of the coronary and peripheral vessels.
   3. Calcium channel blockers are used for angina, dysrhythmias, or hypertension.
   4. Calcium channel blockers should be used with caution in the client with CHF, bradycardia, or atrioventricular block.

B. Side effects
   1. Bradycardia
   2. Hypotension
   3. Reflex tachycardia as a result of hypotension
   4. Headache
   5. Dizziness, light-headedness
   6. Fatigue

BOX 60-18

Calcium Channel Blockers

Amlodipine (Norvasc)
Bepridil (Bepadin, Vascor)
Diltiazem (Cardizem, Cardizem SR)
Felodipine (Plendil)
Isradipine (DynaCirc)
Nicardipine (Cardene)
Nifedipine (Procardia, Procardia XL, Adalat CC)
Nimodipine (Nimotop)
Nisoldipine (Sular)
Verapamil (Calan, Isoptin)

7. Peripheral edema
8. Constipation
9. Flushing of the skin
10. Changes in liver and kidney function

C. Interventions
1. Monitor vital signs.
2. Monitor for signs of CHF.
3. Monitor liver enzyme levels.
4. Monitor kidney function tests.
5. Instruct the client not to discontinue the medication.
6. Instruct the client in how to take a pulse.
7. Instruct the client to notify the physician if dizziness or fainting occurs.
8. Instruct the client not to crush or chew sustained-released tablets.

XIII. PERIPHERAL VASODILATORS (BOX 60-19)

A. Description
1. Peripheral vasodilators decrease peripheral resistance by exerting a direct action on the arteries or on the arteries and the veins.
2. Peripheral vasodilators increase blood flow to the extremities.
3. Peripheral vasodilators are used in peripheral vascular disorders of venous and arterial vessels.
4. Peripheral vasodilators are most effective for disorders resulting from vasospasm (Raynaud's disease).
5. These medications may decrease some of the symptoms of cerebral vascular insufficiency.

B. Side effects
1. Light-headedness, dizziness

BOX 60-19

Peripheral Vasodilators

α-ADRENERGIC BLOCKER
Tolazoline (Priscoline)

β-ADRENERGIC AGONISTS
Isoxsuprine (Vasodilan)
Nylidrin (Arlidin)

α-BLOCKERS
Doxazosin mesylate (Cardura)
Prazosin hydrochloride (Minipress)
Terazosin hydrochloride (Hytrin)

CALCIUM CHANNEL BLOCKERS
Nifedipine (Procardia)
Nimodipine (Nimotop)

DIRECT-ACTING PERIPHERAL VASODILATOR
Ergoloid mesylates (Hydergine)

HEMORRHEOLOGIC
Pentoxifylline (Trental) (increases microcirculation and tissue perfusion)

---

2. **Postural hypotension**
3. Tachycardia
4. Palpitations
5. Flushing
6. Gastrointestinal distress

C. Interventions
1. Monitor vital signs, especially the **BP** and the heart rate.
2. Monitor for **orthostatic hypotension** and tachycardia.
3. Monitor for signs of inadequate blood flow to the extremities such as pallor, coldness of the extremities, and pain.
4. Instruct the client that it may take up to 3 months for a desired therapeutic response.
5. Advise the client not to smoke because smoking increases vasospasm.
6. Instruct the client to avoid aspirin or aspirin-like compounds unless approved by the physician.
7. Instruct the client to take the medication with meals if gastrointestinal disturbances occur.
8. Instruct the client to avoid alcohol because it may cause a hypotensive reaction.
9. Encourage the client to change positions slowly to avoid **orthostatic hypotension.**

XIV. DIRECT-ACTING ARTERIOLAR VASODILATORS (BOX 60-20)

A. Description
1. Direct-acting vasodilators relax the smooth muscles of the blood vessels, mainly the arteries, causing vasodilation.
2. Direct-acting vasodilators promote an increase in blood flow to the brain and kidneys.
3. With vasodilation the **blood pressure** drops and sodium and water are retained, resulting in peripheral edema.
4. Diuretics may be given to decrease the edema.
5. Direct-acting vasodilators are used in the client with moderate to severe hypertension.
6. Direct-acting vasodilators are used during acute hypertensive emergencies.

B. Side effects
1. Hypotension
2. Reflex tachycardia caused by vasodilation and the drop in **BP**

BOX 60-20

Direct-Acting Vasodilators

Diazoxide (Hyperstat)
Fenoldopam (Corlopam)
Hydralazine (Apresoline)
Minoxidil (Loniten)
Nitroglycerin (Nitro-Bid, Nitrol, Nitrostat, Tridil)
Sodium nitroprusside (Nipride, Nitropress)
Trimethaphan camsylate (Arfonad)

3. Palpitations
4. Edema
5. Dizziness
6. Headaches
7. Nasal congestion
8. Gastrointestinal bleeding
9. Neurological symptoms
10. Confusion
11. Excess hair growth with minoxidil (Loniten)
12. With sodium nitroprusside (Nipride), cyanide toxicity, and thiocyanate toxicity can occur.

C. Interventions
1. Monitor vital signs.
2. Sodium nitroprusside
   a. Monitor cyanide and thiocyanate levels.
   b. Protect from light because the medication decomposes.
   c. When administering, solution must be wrapped in aluminum foil and is stable for 24 hours.
   d. Discard if the medication is red or blue.

XV. ANTIDYSRHYTHMIC MEDICATIONS

A. Description: Antidysrhythmic medications suppress dysrhythmias by inhibiting abnormal pathways of electrical conduction through the heart.
B. Group 1A antidysrhythmics
1. Disopyramide phosphate (Norpace)
2. Procainamide hydrochloride (Pronestyl)
3. Quinidine sulfate (Quinora)
C. Group1B antidysrhythmics
1. Lidocaine (Xylocaine)
2. Mexiletine hydrochloride (Mexitil)
3. Tocainide hydrochloride (Tonocard)
D. Group 1C antidysrhythmics
1. Flecainide acetate (Tambocor)
2. Propafenone hydrochloride (Rythmol)
3. Group I (A, B, C): moricizine hydrochloride (Ethmozine)
4. Side effects
   a. Hypotension
   b. Heart failure
   c. Worsened or new dysrhythmias
   d. Nausea, vomiting, or diarrhea
E. Group II antidysrhythmics
1. Acebutolol hydrochloride (Sectral)
2. Esmolol hydrochloride (Brevibloc)
3. Propranolol hydrochloride (Inderal)
4. Side effects
   a. Dizziness
   b. Fatigue
   c. Hypotension
   d. Bradycardia
   e. Heart failure
   f. Dysrhythmias
   g. Heart block
   h. Bronchospasms
   i. Gastrointestinal distress

F. Group III antidysrhythmics
1. Amiodarone hydrochloride (Cordarone)
2. Bretylium tosylate (Bretylol)
3. Dofetilide (Tikosyn)
4. Sotalol hydrochloride (Betapace)
5. Side effects
   a. Hypotension
   b. Bradycardia
   c. Nausea, vomiting
   d. Amiodarone hydrochloride may cause pulmonary fibrosis, photosensitivity, bluish skin discoloration, corneal deposits, peripheral neuropathy, tremor, poor coordination, abnormal gait, and hypothyroidism.
   e. Bretylium tosylate may cause vertigo, syncope, and dizziness.
G. Class IV antidysrhythmics
1. Verapamil hydrochloride (Calan)
2. Diltiazem hydrochloride (Cardizem)
3. Side effects
   a. Dizziness
   b. Hypotension
   c. Bradycardia
   d. Edema
   e. Constipation
H. Other antidysrhythmics
1. Adenosine (Adenocard)
2. Atropine sulfate
3. Digoxin (Lanoxin)
4. Magnesium sulfate
5. Phenytoin (Dilantin)
6. Adenosine can cause dysrhythmias, dyspnea, facial flushing.
7. Atropine sulfate is used to treat sinus bradycardia and is contraindicated in clients with glaucoma, urinary retention, and ileus.
8. Side effects: Atropine sulfate can cause hallucinations, tachycardia, dry mouth, and constipation.
I. Interventions for antidysrhythmics
1. Monitor heart rate, respiratory rate, and **BP.**
2. Monitor electrocardiogram.
3. Provide cardiac monitoring.
4. Maintain therapeutic serum drug levels.
5. Before administering lidocaine, always check the vial label to prevent administering a form that contains epinephrine or preservatives because these solutions are used for local anesthesia only.
6. Do not administer antidysrhythmics with food because food may affect absorption.
7. Mexiletine or tocainide may be administered with food or antacids to reduce gastrointestinal distress.
8. Always administer IV antidysrhythmics via an infusion pump.
9. Monitor for signs of fluid retention such as weight gain, peripheral edema, or shortness of breath.
10. Advise the client to limit fluid and salt intake to minimize fluid retention.

11. Monitor respiratory, thyroid, and neurological function.
12. After administering bretylium, keep the client supine and monitor for hypotension.
13. Instruct the client to change positions slowly to minimize **orthostatic hypotension.**
14. Instruct the client taking amiodarone to use sunscreen and protective clothing to prevent photosensitivity reactions.
15. Encourage the client to increase fiber intake to prevent constipation.
16. When administering atropine sulfate by IV, monitor for paradoxical slowing of the heart.

XVI. ADRENERGIC AGONISTS (BOX 60-21)
A. Dobutamine (Dobutrex)
  1. Dobutamine increases myocardial force and **cardiac output** through stimulation of beta receptors.
  2. Dobutamine is used in clients with CHF and for clients undergoing cardiopulmonary bypass surgery.
B. Dopamine hydrochloride (Intropin)
  1. Dopamine increases **BP** and **cardiac output** through positive inotropic action and increases renal blood flow through its action on alpha and beta receptors.
  2. Dopamine is used to treat mild renal failure caused by low cardiac output.
C. Epinephrine (Adrenalin)
  1. Epinephrine is used for cardiac stimulation in cardiac arrest.
  2. Epinephrine is used for bronchodilation in asthma or allergic reactions.
  3. Epinephrine produces mydriasis.
  4. Epinephrine produces local vasoconstriction when combined with local anesthetics and prolongs anesthetic action by decreasing blood flow to the site.
D. Isoproterenol hydrochloride (Isuprel)
  1. Isoproterenol stimulates beta receptors.
  2. Isoproterenol is used for cardiac stimulation and bronchodilation.
E. Norepinephrine (levarterenol, Levophed)
  1. Norepinephrine stimulates the heart in cardiac arrest.
  2. Norepinephrine vasoconstricts and increases the **BP** in hypotension and shock.

F. Side effects
  1. Dysrhythmias
  2. Tachycardia
  3. Angina
  4. Restlessness
  5. Urgency or urinary incontinence
G. Interventions
  1. Monitor vital signs.
  2. Monitor lung sounds.
  3. Monitor urinary output.
  4. Monitor electrocardiogram.
  5. Administer the medication through a large vein.
  6. If extravasation occurs, infiltrate the site with normal saline and phentolamine (Regitine).

XVII. ANTILIPEMIC MEDICATIONS
A. Description
  1. Antilipemic medications reduce serum levels of cholesterol, triglycerides, or low-density lipoprotein.
  2. When cholesterol, triglycerides, and low-density lipoprotein are elevated, the client is at increased risk for coronary artery disease.
  3. In many cases, diet alone will not lower blood lipid levels; therefore antilipemic medications will be prescribed.
B. Bile sequestrants (Box 60-22)
  1. Description
    a. Bile sequestrants bind with acids in the intestines.
    b. Bile acid sequestrants should not be used as the only therapy in clients with elevated triglycerides because they may raise triglyceride levels.
  2. Side effects
    a. Constipation
    b. Peptic ulcer
  3. Interventions
    a. Cholestyramine (Questran) comes in a gritty powder that must be mixed thoroughly in juice or water before administration.
    b. Monitor the client for early signs of peptic ulcer such as nausea and abdominal discomfort followed by abdominal pain and distention.
    c. Instruct the client that the medication must be taken with and followed by sufficient fluids.
C. HMG-CoA reductase inhibitors (Box 60-23)
  1. Description
    a. Lovastatin (Mevacor) is highly protein bound and should not be administered with anticoagulants.

BOX 60-21

Adrenergic Agonists

Dobutamine (Dobutrex)
Dopamine (Intropin)
Epinephrine (Adrenalin)
Isoproterenol (Isuprel)
Norepinephrine (levarterenol, Levophed)

BOX 60-22

Bile Acid Sequestrants

Cholestyramine (Questran)
Colesevelam (Welchol)
Colestipol (Colestid)

b. Lovastatin should not be administered with gemfibrozil (Lopid).

c. Administer lovastatin with caution to the client taking immunosuppressive medications.

2. Side effects
   a. Nausea
   b. Diarrhea or constipation
   c. Abdominal pain or cramps
   d. Flatulence
   e. Dizziness
   f. Headache
   g. Blurred vision
   h. Rash
   i. Pruritis
   j. Elevated liver enzymes
   k. Gastrointestinal disturbances, headaches, muscle cramps, and fatigue

3. Interventions
   a. Monitor serum liver enzymes.
   b. Instruct the client to receive an annual eye examination because the medication causes cataract formation.
   c. If lovastatin is not effective in lowering the lipid level after 3 months, it should be discontinued.

D. Other antilipemic medications (Box 60-24)

1. Description
   a. Gemfibrozil should not be taken with anticoagulants because they compete for protein sites, and if the client is taking an anticoagulant, the anticoagulant dose should be reduced during antilipemic therapy and the INR should be monitored closely.
   b. Do not administer gemfibrozil with lovastatin.
   c. Clofibrate (Atromid-S) should not be used long term because of its side effects such as

dysrhythmias, angina, thromboembolism, and gallbladder stones.

2. Interventions
   a. Monitor vital signs.
   b. Monitor liver enzyme levels.
   c. Monitor serum cholesterol and triglyceride levels.
   d. Instruct the client to restrict intake of fats, cholesterol, carbohydrates, and alcohol.
   e. Instruct the client to follow an exercise program.
   f. Instruct the client that it will take several weeks before the lipid level declines.
   g. Instruct the client to have an annual eye examination and to report any changes in vision.
   h. Instruct the client with diabetes mellitus who is taking gemfibrozil to monitor blood glucose levels regularly.
   i. Instruct the client to increase fluid intake.
   j. Note that nicotinic acid has numerous side effects, which include gastrointestinal disturbances, flushing of the skin, elevated liver enzymes, hyperglycemia, and hyperuricemia.
   k. Instruct the client that aspirin may assist in reducing the side effects of nicotinic acid.
   l. Instruct the client to take nicotinic acid with meals to reduce gastrointestinal discomfort.

BOX 60-23

HMG-CoA Reductase Inhibitors

Atorvastatin (Lipitor)
Fluvastatin (Lescol)
Lovastatin (Mevacor)
Pravastatin (Pravachol)
Rosuvastatin (Crestor)
Simvastatin (Zocor)

BOX 60-24

Other Antilipemic Medications

Clofibrate (Atromid-S)
Dextrothyroxine (Choloxin)
Exetimibe (Zetia)
Fenofibrate (Tricor)
Gemfibrozil (Lopid)
Nicotinic acid (Niacor)
Probucol (Lorelco)

PRACTICE QUESTIONS

1. A nurse provides discharge instructions to a postoperative client who is taking warfarin sodium (Coumadin). Which statement, if made by the client, reflects the need for further teaching?
   1. "I will take Ecotrin (enteric-coated aspirin) for my headaches because it is coated."
   2. "I will be certain to limit my alcohol consumption."
   3. "I will take my pills every day at the same time."
   4. "I have already called my family to pick up a Medic-Alert bracelet."

2. A client has a serum potassium of 3 mEq/L and is complaining of anorexia. A physician orders a digoxin level to rule out digoxin toxicity. A nurse checks the results, knowing that which of the following is the therapeutic serum level (range) for digoxin?
   1. 0.5 to 2 ng/mL
   2. 1.2 to 2.8 ng/mL
   3. 3 ng/mL
   4. 3.5 ng/mL

3. A client is being treated with procainamide hydrochloride (Pronestyl) for a cardiac dysrhythmia. Following intravenous administration of the medication, the client complains of dizziness. What intervention should the nurse do first?
   1. Administer ordered nitroglycerin tablets.
   2. Auscultate the client's apical pulse and obtain a blood pressure.

3. Measure the heart rate on the rhythm strip.

4. Obtain a 12-lead electrocardiogram immediately.

4. A nurse is monitoring a client who is taking propranolol (Inderal). Which of the following assessment data would indicate a potential serious complication associated with propranolol?

   1. A baseline blood pressure of 150/80 mm Hg followed by a blood pressure of 138/72 mm Hg after two doses of the medication

   2. A baseline resting heart rate of 88 beats per minute followed by a resting heart rate of 72 beats per minute after two doses of the medication

   3. The development of audible expiratory wheezes

   4. The development of complaints of insomnia

5. A home health care nurse is visiting an older client at home. Furosemide (Lasix) is prescribed for the client. The nurse teaches the client about the medication. Which of the following statements, if made by the client, indicates the need for further teaching?

   1. "I will take my medication every morning with breakfast."

   2. "I will call my doctor if my ankles swell or my rings get tight."

   3. "I need to drink lots of coffee and tea to keep myself healthy."

   4. "I will sit up slowly before standing each morning."

6. A nurse is caring for a client receiving a heparin IV infusion. The nurse anticipates that which laboratory study will be prescribed to monitor the therapeutic effect of heparin?

   1. Prothrombin time

   2. Activated partial thromboplastin time

   3. Hematocrit

   4. Hemoglobin

7. A client is diagnosed with an acute myocardial infarction and is receiving tissue plasminogen activator (t-PA). Which of the following is a priority nursing intervention?

   1. Have heparin sodium available.

   2. Monitor for renal failure.

   3. Monitor for signs of bleeding.

   4. Monitor psychosocial status.

8. A home health nurse instructs a client about the use of a nitrate patch. The nurse tells the client which of the following that will prevent client tolerance to nitrates?

   1. Do not remove the patches.

   2. Have a 12-hour "no nitrate" time.

   3. Have a 24-hour "no nitrate" time.

   4. Keep nitrates on 24 hours, then off 24 hours.

9. A client is admitted to a medical unit with nausea and bradycardia. The family hands a nurse a small white envelope labeled "heart pill." The envelope is sent to pharmacy and reveals digoxin (Lanoxin). A family member states, "That doctor doesn't know how to take care of my family." The most therapeutic response by the nurse would be

1. "You are concerned your loved one receives the best care."

2. "You're right! I've never seen a doctor put pills in an envelope."

3. "I think you're wrong. That physician has been in practice over 30 years."

4. "Don't worry about this. I'll take care of everything."

10. A nurse is caring for a client receiving dopamine (Intropin). Which of the following potential nursing diagnoses is appropriate for this client?

    1. Increased cardiac output

    2. Excess fluid volume

    3. Impaired tissue perfusion

    4. Disturbed sensory perception

11. A nurse is planning to administer hydrochlorothiazide (HydroDIURIL) to a client. The nurse understands that which of the following are concerns related to the administration of this medication?

    1. Hyperkalemia, hypoglycemia, penicillin allergy

    2. Hypouricemia, hyperkalemia

    3. Hypokalemia, hyperglycemia, sulfa allergy

    4. Increased risk of osteoporosis

12. A home health care nurse is visiting a client with elevated triglycerides and a serum cholesterol of 398 mg/dL. The client is taking cholestyramine resin (Questran). Which of the following statements, if made by the client, indicates the need for further education?

    1. "Constipation and bloating might be a problem."

    2. "I'll continue to watch my diet and reduce my fats."

    3. "I'll continue my nicotinic acid from the health food store."

    4. "Walking a mile each day will help the whole process."

13. A client with congestive heart failure is on a 1-g sodium diet. A nurse understands that which medication prescribed for the client promotes sodium excretion while conserving potassium?

    1. Spironolactone (Aldactone)

    2. Furosemide (Lasix)

    3. Ethacrynic acid (Edecrin)

    4. Hydrochlorothiazide (HydroDIURIL)

14. A client has developed paroxysmal nocturnal dyspnea. Which of the following medications does a nurse anticipate will be prescribed by the physician?

    1. Lidocaine (Xylocaine)

    2. Propranolol (Inderal)

    3. Bumetanide (Bumex)

    4. Streptokinase (Streptase)

15. A client arrives in the emergency department after complaining of unrelieved chest pain for 2 days. The pain has subsided slightly but never disappeared. When the nurse approaches the client with a 0.4-mg nitroglycerin sublingual tablet, the client states, "I don't need that. My dad takes that for

his heart. There's nothing wrong with my heart." The nurse interprets that the client is exhibiting which type of reaction?

1. Obsessive-compulsive
2. Denial
3. Phobic
4. Angry

16. A nurse has admitted a client who has a diagnosis of syncope to a medical unit. The client is taking enalapril (Vasotec), atenolol (Tenormin), and aspirin (A.S.A.) daily. The client admits that the medications were prescribed by different physicians. The admitting physician wrote in the client's order sheet, "Administer medications as taken at home." Which of the following is the most appropriate action for the nurse to take?

1. Administer the medications as ordered by the physician.
2. Send the client's medication bottles to the pharmacy for identification and then administer the medications as ordered.
3. Call the physician, describe the medications, and request order clarification.
4. Refuse to give any medications, and wait until the physician makes rounds to clarify the orders.

17. A 66-year-old client complaining of not feeling well is seen in a clinic. The client is taking several medications for the control of heart disease and hypertension. These medications include atenolol (Tenormin), digoxin (Lanoxin), and chlorothiazide (Diuril). A tentative diagnosis of digoxin toxicity is made. Which of the following assessment data would support this diagnosis?

1. Chest pain, hypotension, and paresthesia
2. Constipation, dry mouth, and sleep disorder
3. Double vision, loss of appetite, and nausea
4. Dyspnea, edema, and palpitations

18. A client is being treated for acute congestive heart failure with intravenously administered bumetanide (Bumex). The vital signs are as follows: blood pressure, 100/60 mm Hg; pulse, 96 beats per minute; and respirations, 24 breaths per minute. After the initial dose, which of the following is the priority assessment?

1. Monitoring blood pressure.
2. Monitoring potassium level.
3. Monitoring urine output.
4. Monitoring weight loss

19. A client with a diagnosis of congestive heart failure is seen in a clinic. The client is being treated with a variety of medications, including digoxin (Lanoxin) and furosemide (Lasix). Which of the following assessment findings would lead the nurse to suspect that the client is hypokalemic?

1. Diarrhea
2. Intermittent intestinal colic
3. Muscle weakness and leg cramps
4. Tingling of fingers and toes

20. A client is being discharged with a prescription for propranolol hydrochloride (Inderal). In developing a medication teaching plan, a nurse would include which of the following instructions?

1. Exercise will prevent orthostatic hypotension.
2. Hot baths and showers are advised to increase vasodilation.
3. Medication should be taken on an empty stomach to enhance absorption.
4. Medication should be withheld if the pulse rate drops below 60 beats per minute.

CRITICAL THINKING: FILL IN THE BLANK

A client with coronary artery disease complains of substernal chest pain. After assessing the client's heart rate and blood pressure, a nurse administers nitroglycerin, 0.4 mg, sublingually. After 5 minutes, the client states, "My chest still hurts." The nurse checks the client's vital signs, notes that they have remained stable, and does what priority action next?

Answer: _____

ANSWERS

1. **1**

Rationale: Ecotrin is an aspirin-containing product and should be avoided. Excessive alcohol consumption should be avoided by a client taking warfarin sodium. Taking prescribed medication at the same time increases client compliance. The Medic-Alert bracelet provides health care personnel emergency information.

Test-Taking Strategy: Use the process of elimination. Note the key words "need for further teaching." Recalling that warfarin (Coumadin) is an anticoagulant and that Ecotrin is an aspirin-containing product will direct you to option 1. Review client teaching points related to warfarin if you had difficulty with this question.

Level of Cognitive Ability: Analysis
Client Needs: Physiological Integrity
Integrated Process: Teaching/Learning
Content Area: Pharmacology
References: Ignatavicius, D., & Workman, M. (2002). *Medical-surgical nursing: Critical thinking for collaborative care* (4th ed., p. 826). Philadelphia: W. B. Saunders.
Kee, J., & Hayes, E. (2003). *Pharmacology: A nursing process approach* (4th ed., pp. 624, 627). Philadelphia: W. B. Saunders.

2. **1**

Rationale: Therapeutic levels for digoxin range from 0.5 to 2 ng/mL.

Test-Taking Strategy: Knowledge of the therapeutic serum digoxin level will direct you to option 1. If you had difficulty with this question, learn the therapeutic level for digoxin.
Level of Cognitive Ability: Analysis
Client Needs: Physiological Integrity
Integrated Process: Nursing Process—analysis
Content Area: Pharmacology
References: Kee, J., & Hayes, E. (2003). *Pharmacology: A nursing process approach* (4th ed., p. 567). Philadelphia: W. B. Saunders. Lehne, R. (2001). *Pharmacology for nursing care* (4th ed., p. 516). Philadelphia: W. B. Saunders.

3. **2**
Rationale: Signs of toxicity from procainamide include confusion, dizziness, drowsiness, decreased urination, nausea, vomiting, and tachydysrhythmias. If the client complains of dizziness, the nurse should assess the vital signs first.
Test-Taking Strategy: Use the steps of the nursing process to eliminate options 1 and 4. From the remaining options, remember always to assess the client first, not the monitoring devices. Therefore option 2 is correct. Review the signs of toxicity and the nursing interventions if you had difficulty with this question.
Level of Cognitive Ability: Application
Client Needs: Physiological Integrity
Integrated Process: Nursing Process—implementation
Content Area: Pharmacology
Reference: Hodgson, B., & Kizior, R. (2004). *Saunders nursing drug handbook 2004* (pp. 836-837). Philadelphia: W. B. Saunders.

4. **3**
Rationale: Audible expiratory wheezes may indicate a serious adverse reaction, bronchospasm. β-Blockers may induce this reaction, particularly in clients with chronic obstructive pulmonary disease or asthma. Normal decreases in blood pressure and heart rate are expected. Insomnia is a frequent mild side effect and should be monitored.
Test-Taking Strategy: Use the process of elimination, eliminating options 1 and 2 because these are expected effects from the medication. Note the key words "potential serious complication." These key words will direct you to option 3. Review the adverse effects of this medication if you had difficulty with this question.
Level of Cognitive Ability: Analysis
Client Needs: Physiological Integrity
Integrated Process: Nursing Process—assessment
Content Area: Pharmacology
Reference: Lehne, R. (2001). *Pharmacology for nursing care* (4th ed., p. 533). Philadelphia: W. B. Saunders.

5. **3**
Rationale: Tea and coffee are stimulants and mild diuretics. These are a poor choice for hydration. Taking the medication at the same time each day improves compliance. Because furosemide is a diuretic, the morning is the best time to take the medication so as not to interrupt sleep. Notification of the health care provider is appropriate if edema is noticed in the hands, feet, or face or if the client is short of breath. Sitting up slowly prevents postural hypotension.

Test-Taking Strategy: Use the process of elimination, noting the key words "need for further teaching." Recalling that tea and coffee are stimulants and that diuretics potentially can worsen dehydration will direct you to option 3. In addition, coffee and tea are not healthy items to consume. Review client teaching points related to this medication if you had difficulty with this question.
Level of Cognitive Ability: Analysis
Client Needs: Physiological Integrity
Integrated Process: Teaching/Learning
Content Area: Pharmacology
Reference: Kee, J., & Hayes, E. (2003). *Pharmacology: A nursing process approach* (4th ed., pp. 594-595). Philadelphia: W. B. Saunders.

6. **2**
Rationale: The prothrombin time will assess for the therapeutic effect of warfarin sodium (Coumadin), and the activated partial thromboplastin time (aPTT) will assess the therapeutic effect of heparin. Hematocrit and hemoglobin assess red blood cell concentrations. Baseline assessment, including an aPTT value, should be completed, as well as ongoing daily aPTT values while the client is taking heparin. Heparin doses are determined based on the result of the aPTT.
Test-Taking Strategy: Use the process of elimination. Eliminate options 3 and 4 because they are similar and are unrelated to heparin therapy. From the remaining options, recall the relationship between the prothrombin time and warfarin and the aPTT and heparin. Review care of a client on heparin infusion if you had difficulty with this question.
Level of Cognitive Ability: Analysis
Client Needs: Physiological Integrity
Integrated Process: Nursing Process—assessment
Content Area: Pharmacology
Reference: Kee, J., & Hayes, E. (2003). *Pharmacology: A nursing process approach* (4th ed., p. 621). Philadelphia: W. B. Saunders.

7. **3**
Rationale: Tissue plasminogen activator is a thrombolytic. Hemorrhage is a complication of any type of thrombolytic medication. The client is monitored for bleeding. Monitoring for renal failure and monitoring the client's psychosocial status are important but are not the most critical interventions. Heparin is given after thrombolytic therapy, but the question is not asking about follow-up medications.
Test-Taking Strategy: Use the process of elimination. Note the key word "priority." Remember, bleeding is a priority. Review care of the client on tissue plasminogen activator if you had difficulty with this question.
Level of Cognitive Ability: Application
Client Needs: Physiological Integrity
Integrated Process: Nursing Process—implementation
Content Area: Delegating/Prioritizing
Reference: Kee, J., & Hayes, E. (2003). *Pharmacology: A nursing process approach* (4th ed., pp. 630-631). Philadelphia: W. B. Saunders.

8. **2**
Rationale: To help prevent tolerance, clients need a 12-hour "no nitrate" time, sometimes referred to as a pharmacological

vacation away from the medication. Options 1, 3, and 4 are incorrect.

Test-Taking Strategy: Use the process of elimination, focusing on the issue, preventing tolerance to nitrates. This issue and knowledge regarding administering this medication will direct you to option 2. Review the administration of nitrate patches if you had difficulty with this question.

Level of Cognitive Ability: Application
Client Needs: Physiological Integrity
Integrated Process: Teaching/Learning
Content Area: Pharmacology
References: Kee, J., & Hayes, E. (2003). *Pharmacology: A nursing process approach* (4th ed., p. 574). Philadelphia: W. B. Saunders.
Lehne, R. (2001). *Pharmacology for nursing care* (4th ed., p. 497). Philadelphia: W. B. Saunders.

9. 1
Rationale: This is a therapeutic, nonjudgmental response. The statement reflects the family's concern but remains nonjudgmental. Option 2 creates doubt about the physician's practice without actually knowing the circumstances. Option 3 is argumentative and nontherapeutic. Option 4 dismisses the family's concerns and disempowers the family.

Test-Taking Strategy: Use therapeutic communication techniques. Reflection of the client or family's concerns is the most therapeutic. Review therapeutic communication techniques if you had difficulty with this question.

Level of Cognitive Ability: Application
Client Needs: Psychosocial Integrity
Integrated Process: Communication and Documentation
Content Area: Pharmacology
References: Harkreader, H., & Hogan, M. A. (2004). *Fundamentals of nursing: Caring and clinical judgment* (2nd ed., p. 251). Philadelphia: W. B. Saunders.
Kee, J., & Hayes, E. (2003). *Pharmacology: A nursing process approach* (4th ed., pp. 569-570). Philadelphia: W. B. Saunders.

10. 3
Rationale: The client receiving dopamine therapy should be assessed for impaired tissue perfusion related to peripheral vasoconstriction. Options 1, 2, and 4 are not related directly to this medication therapy.

Test-Taking Strategy: Use the process of elimination. Recalling that dopamine causes peripheral vasoconstriction will direct you to option 3. Review the action of this medication if you had difficulty with this question.

Level of Cognitive Ability: Analysis
Client Needs: Physiological Integrity
Integrated Process: Nursing Process—analysis
Content Area: Pharmacology
Reference: Kee, J., & Hayes, E. (2003). *Pharmacology: A nursing process approach* (4th ed., p. 868). Philadelphia: W. B. Saunders.

11. 3
Rationale: Thiazide diuretics like hydrochlorothiazide are sulfa-based medications, and a client with a sulfa allergy is at risk for an allergic reaction. Also, clients are at risk for hypokalemia, hyperglycemia, hypercalcemia, hyperlipidemia, and hyperuricemia.

Test-Taking Strategy: Use the process of elimination. Recalling that thiazide diuretics carry a sulfa ring will direct you to option 3. Review the nursing considerations related to administering this medication if you had difficulty with this question.

Level of Cognitive Ability: Analysis
Client Needs: Physiological Integrity
Integrated Process: Nursing Process—analysis
Content Area: Pharmacology
Reference: Hodgson, B., & Kizior, R. (2004). *Saunders nursing drug handbook 2004* (p. 499). Philadelphia: W. B. Saunders.

12. 3
Rationale: Nicotinic acid, even over-the-counter forms, should be avoided because it may lead to liver abnormalities. All lipid-lowering medications also can cause liver abnormalities, so a combination of nicotinic acid and cholestyramine resin is to be avoided. Constipation and bloating are the two most common side effects. Walking and the reduction of fats in the diet are therapeutic measures to reduce cholesterol and triglyceride levels.

Test-Taking Strategy: Use the process of elimination. Note the key words "need for further education." Remembering that over-the-counter medications should be avoided when a client is taking a prescription medication will direct you to option 3. Review client teaching points related to this medication if you had difficulty with this question.

Level of Cognitive Ability: Analysis
Client Needs: Health Promotion and Maintenance
Integrated Process: Teaching/Learning
Content Area: Pharmacology
Reference: Kee, J., & Hayes, E. (2003). *Pharmacology: A nursing process approach* (4th ed., p. 636). Philadelphia: W. B. Saunders.

13. 1
Rationale: Spironolactone (Aldactone) is a potassium-sparing diuretic that promotes sodium excretion while conserving potassium. Options 2, 3, and 4 identify diuretics that do not conserve potassium.

Test-Taking Strategy: Use the process of elimination. Recalling that spironolactone is a potassium-sparing diuretic will direct you to option 1. Review the potassium-sparing diuretics, if you had difficulty with this question.

Level of Cognitive Ability: Analysis
Client Needs: Physiological Integrity
Integrated Process: Nursing Process—analysis
Content Area: Pharmacology
Reference: Hodgson, B., & Kizior, R. (2004). *Saunders nursing drug handbook 2004* (p. 931). Philadelphia: W. B. Saunders.

14. 3
Rationale: Bumetanide (Bumex) is a diuretic. The paroxysmal nocturnal dyspnea may be due to increased venous return when the client is lying in bed, and the client needs diuresis. Propranolol is a β-blocker, lidocaine is an antidysrhythmic, and streptokinase is a thrombolytic.

Test-Taking Strategy: Use the process of elimination. Knowledge of each medication type and that a diuretic will increase urine output will direct you to option 3. Review the

actions of the medications identified in the options, if you had difficulty with this question.
Level of Cognitive Ability: Analysis
Client Needs: Physiological Integrity
Integrated Process: Nursing Process—analysis
Content Area: Pharmacology
Reference: Hodgson, B., & Kizior, R. (2004). *Saunders nursing drug handbook 2004* (p. 126). Philadelphia: W. B. Saunders.

15. **2**
Rationale: Denial is the most common reaction when a client has a myocardial infarction or anginal pain. Options 1, 3, and 4 are incorrect.
Test-Taking Strategy: Use the process of elimination. Eliminate options 1 and 3 first because both are psychiatric diagnoses. From the remaining options, recalling that denial is the most common reaction when a client has chest pain will direct you to option 2. Review behavioral reactions of a client with chest pain if you had difficulty with this question.
Level of Cognitive Ability: Analysis
Client Needs: Psychosocial Integrity
Integrated Process: Nursing Process—analysis
Content Area: Pharmacology
Reference: Ignatavicius, D., & Workman, M., (2002). *Medical-surgical nursing: Critical thinking for collaborative care* (4th ed., p. 794). Philadelphia: W. B. Saunders.

16. **3**
Rationale: The nurse is responsible for administering the correct medication. When medication orders are vague, the nurse must call the physician to clarify the orders before administering the medication. Waiting for the physician to make rounds delays needed treatment.
Test-Taking Strategy: Use the process of elimination. Options 1 and 2 are similar in that they indicate administering the medication and are eliminated first. Eliminate option 4 next because it is not appropriate to wait to clarify an unclear physician's order. Review the procedures related to clarifying a physician's orders if you had difficulty with this question.
Level of Cognitive Ability: Application
Client Needs: Safe, Effective Care Environment
Integrated Process: Nursing Process—implementation
Content Area: Pharmacology
Reference: Kee, J., & Marshall, S. (2004). *Clinical calculations: With applications to general and specialty areas* (5th ed., p. 52). Philadelphia: W. B. Saunders.

17. **3**
Rationale: Double vision, loss of appetite, and nausea are early signs of digoxin toxicity. Additional signs of digoxin toxicity include bradycardia, difficulty reading, visual alterations such as green and yellow vision or seeing spots or halos, confusion, vomiting, diarrhea, decreased libido, and impotence.
Test-Taking Strategy: Use the process of elimination. Recalling that gastrointestinal and visual disturbances occur with digoxin toxicity will direct you to option 3. If you had difficulty with this question, review the signs of digoxin toxicity.
Level of Cognitive Ability: Analysis

Client Needs: Physiological Integrity
Integrated Process: Nursing Process—assessment
Content Area: Pharmacology
Reference: Kee, J., & Hayes, E. (2003). *Pharmacology: A nursing process approach* (4th ed., p. 569). Philadelphia: W. B. Saunders.

18. **1**
Rationale: Hypotension is a common side effect associated with the use of this medication. Options 2, 3, and 4 also require assessment but are not the priority.
Test-Taking Strategy: Use the process of elimination. Note the key word "priority." Also, note that blood pressure is mentioned in the question and also in option 1. Use of the ABCs—airway, breathing, and circulation—also will direct you to option 1. Review care of the client receiving this medication by the intravenous route if you had difficulty with this question.
Level of Cognitive Ability: Application
Client Needs: Physiological Integrity
Integrated Process: Nursing Process—assessment
Content Area: Delegating/Prioritizing
Reference: Hodgson, B., & Kizior, R. (2004). *Saunders nursing drug handbook 2004* (p. 127). Philadelphia: W. B. Saunders.

19. **3**
Rationale: Clients on potassium-wasting diuretics are at high risk for hypokalemia. Clinical manifestations of hypokalemia include fatigue, anorexia, nausea, vomiting, muscle weakness, leg cramps, decreased bowel motility, paresthesias, and dysrhythmias.
Test-Taking Strategy: Use the process of elimination and knowledge regarding the signs of electrolyte imbalances. Diarrhea and intestinal colic are signs of hyperkalemia. Tingling of the fingers and toes are signs of hypocalcemia. If you had difficulty with this question, review the signs of hypokalemia.
Level of Cognitive Ability: Analysis
Client Needs: Physiological Integrity
Integrated Process: Nursing Process—assessment
Content Area: Pharmacology
References: Ignatavicius, D., & Workman, M., (2002). *Medical-surgical nursing: Critical thinking for collaborative care* (4th ed., p. 174). Philadelphia: W. B. Saunders.
Lehne, R. (2001). *Pharmacology for nursing care* (4th ed., p. 536). Philadelphia: W. B. Saunders.

20. **4**
Rationale: Most β-blockers may be administered with food or on an empty stomach, but propranolol is absorbed best if taken with meals or directly after eating. Exercise will not prevent orthostatic hypotension. Hot showers and baths are not advised. The client needs to be instructed in how to take the pulse rate and to notify the physician if the heart rate falls below 60 beats per minute.
Test-Taking Strategy: Use the process of elimination. Recalling that bradycardia can occur with propranolol will direct you to option 4. If you had difficulty with question, review the client teaching points related to this medication.
Level of Cognitive Ability: Application
Client Needs: Physiological Integrity

Integrated Process: Teaching/Learning
Content Area: Pharmacology
Reference: Hodgson, B., & Kizior, R. (2004). *Saunders nursing drug handbook 2004* (p. 851). Philadelphia: W. B. Saunders.

CRITICAL THINKING: FILL IN THE BLANK

Answer: Administers another nitroglycerin tablet
Rationale: The usual protocol for administering nitroglycerin tablets for chest pain is to administer one tablet every 5 minutes as needed for chest pain for a total dose of three tablets. Because the client still is complaining of chest pain, the nurse would administer a second nitroglycerin tablet.
Test-Taking Strategy: Knowledge regarding the protocol for administering nitroglycerin for chest pain is required to answer this question. Noting that the client's vital signs have remained stable will assist in determining the next priority nursing action. Review care of the client with chest pain and the protocol for the administration of nitroglycerin if you had difficulty with this question.
Level of Cognitive Ability: Application
Client Needs: Physiological Integrity
Integrated Process: Nursing Process—implementation
Content Area: Delegating/Prioritizing
References: Ignatavicius, D., & Workman, M. (2002). *Medical-surgical nursing: Critical thinking for collaborative care* (4th ed., p. 796). Philadelphia: W. B. Saunders.
Kee, J., & Hayes, E. (2003). *Pharmacology: A nursing process approach* (4th ed., p. 576). Philadelphia: W. B. Saunders.

REFERENCES

Harkreader, H., & Hogan, M. A. (2004). *Fundamentals of nursing: Caring and clinical judgment* (2nd ed.). Philadelphia: W. B. Saunders.

Hodgson, B., & Kizior, R. (2004). *Saunders nursing drug handbook 2004*. Philadelphia: W. B. Saunders.

Ignatavicius, D., & Workman, M. (2002). *Medical-surgical nursing: Critical thinking for collaborative care* (4th ed.). Philadelphia: W. B. Saunders.

Kee, J., & Hayes, E. (2003). *Pharmacology: A nursing process approach* (4th ed.). Philadelphia: W. B. Saunders.

Kee, J., & Marshall, S. (2004). *Clinical calculations: With applications to general and specialty areas* (5th ed.). Philadelphia: W. B. Saunders.

Lehne, R. (2001). *Pharmacology for nursing care* (4th ed.). Philadelphia: W. B. Saunders.

The Adult Client with a Renal System Disorder

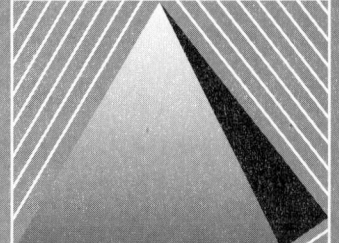

PYRAMID TERMS

acute renal failure The sudden loss of kidney function caused by renal cell damage from ischemia or toxic substances. Acute renal failure occurs abruptly and can be reversible. Acute renal failure leads to hypoperfusion, cell death, and decompensation in renal function. The prognosis depends on the cause and the condition of the client. Near-normal or normal kidney function may resume gradually.

anuria Urine output of less than 100 mL a day.

arterial steal syndrome A syndrome that can develop following the insertion of an arteriovenous fistula when too much blood is diverted to the vein and arterial perfusion to the hand is compromised.

azotemia The retention of nitrogenous waste products in the blood.

chronic renal failure The progressive loss and ongoing deterioration in kidney function that occurs slowly over a period of time. Chronic renal failure is irreversible and results in uremia or end-stage renal disease. Chronic renal failure requires dialysis or kidney transplant to maintain life.

disequilibrium syndrome A rapid change in the composition of the extracellular fluid occurs during hemodialysis. Solutes are removed from the blood faster than from the cerebrospinal fluid and brain. Fluid is pulled into the brain, causing cerebral edema.

hemodialysis The process of cleansing the client's blood; the diffusion of dissolved particles from one fluid compartment into another across a semipermeable membrane. The client's blood flows through one fluid compartment, and the dialysate is in another fluid compartment.

internal arteriovenous fistula Surgical creation by anastomosis of an opening, or fistula, between a large artery and a large vein. The flow of arterial blood into the venous system causes the vein to become engorged (maturity). Maturity is necessary so that the engorged vein can be punctured for the dialysis procedure using a large-bore needle.

nephrolithiasis The formation of kidney stones. Kidney stones are formed in the renal parenchyma.

oliguria Urine output of less than 400 mL a day.

peritoneal dialysis The peritoneum is the dialyzing membrane (semipermeable membrane) and substitutes for kidney function during kidney failure. Dialysis works on the principles of diffusion and osmosis, and the dialysis occurs via the transfer of fluid and solute from the bloodstream through the peritoneum.

renal failure The loss of kidney function. The types of renal failure include acute renal failure and chronic renal failure. The signs and symptoms of renal failure are caused by the retention of wastes, the retention of fluids, and the inability of the kidneys to regulate electrolytes.

urolithiasis The formation of urinary stones or calculuses. Urinary calculuses are formed in the ureter.

▲ PYRAMID TO SUCCESS

Pyramid Points focus on acute renal failure and chronic renal failure, dialysis procedures such as hemodialysis and continuous ambulatory peritoneal dialysis, urinary diversions, and postoperative care following urinary or renal surgery. Focus on the major problems associated with renal failure and the rationale for the prescribed treatment modalities. Be familiar with the complications associated with hemodialysis and peritoneal dialysis, the specific assessment data related to complications, and the expected treatment. Focus on the care of a peritoneal catheter and hemodialysis access devices, the complications associated with these access devices, and the appropriate nursing interventions if a complication is suspected. Review preoperative and postoperative care related to renal transplantation and the assessment data indicating rejection. Be familiar with urinary diversions, care to the client following prostatectomy, and treatment measures for the client with urinary or renal calculuses. The Integrated Processes addressed in this unit include Nursing Process, Caring, Communication and Documentation, and Teaching/Learning.

▲ CLIENT NEEDS
Safe, Effective Care Environment

Accident prevention related to complications associated with disorder
Asepsis related to wound care and dialysis access devices
Client rights
Confidentiality related to the renal disorder
Consultations with members of the health care team
Establishing priorities
Informed consent related to diagnostic and surgical procedures
Renal organ donation
Standard precautions related to care of the client

Health Promotion and Maintenance

Expected body image changes
Instructions regarding care to a urinary diversion, dialysis access device, and dialysis procedures
Instructions regarding postoperative management
Instructions regarding prescribed treatments related to urinary or renal disorder
Instructions regarding the prevention of the recurrence of a urinary and renal disorder
Urinary and renal assessment techniques

Psychosocial Integrity

Body image disturbances
Community resources
Coping mechanisms
End of life
Grief and loss
Loss of function of a body part that occurs in clients with a renal disorder
Religious and spiritual influences
Support systems

Physiological Integrity

Adequate rest and sleep
Assessment data indicating rejection of renal transplant
Care related to dialysis access devices
Care related to hemodialysis and peritoneal dialysis
Care to the client following prostatectomy
Comfort interventions
Diagnostic tests and laboratory results
Elimination measures
Fluid and electrolyte and acid-base disorders
Pharmacological therapy
Preoperative and postoperative care related to renal transplantation
Prescribed nutrition and fluid measures
Prevention of complications arising as a result of dialysis
Treatment measures for the client with urinary or renal calculuses
Urinary diversions

REFERENCES

Harkreader, H. & Hogan, M. A. (2004). *Fundamentals of nursing: Caring and clinical judgment* (2nd ed.). Philadelphia: W.B. Saunders.
Ignatavicius, D., & Workman, M. (2002). *Medical-surgical nursing: Critical thinking for collaborative care.* (4th ed.). Philadelphia: W. B. Saunders.
Lewis, S., Heitkemper, M., & Dirksen, S. (2004). *Medical-surgical nursing: Assessment and management of clinical problems* (6th ed.). St. Louis: Mosby.
National Council of State Boards of Nursing (Eds.). (2003). *Test Plan for the National Council Licensure Examination for Registered Nurses* (effective date: April 2004). Chicago: Author.
Phipps, W., Monahan, F., Sands, J., Marek, J., & Neighbors, M. (2003). *Medical-surgical nursing: Health and illness perspectives* (7th ed.). St. Louis: Mosby
Potter, P., & Perry, A. (2001). *Fundamentals of nursing* (5th ed.). St. Louis: Mosby.
Varcarolis, E. (2002). *Foundations of psychiatric mental health nursing* (4th ed.). Philadelphia: W. B. Saunders.

Renal System

I. ANATOMY AND PHYSIOLOGY

A. Kidneys
1. Each person has two kidneys; each is attached to the abdominal wall at the level of the last thoracic and first three lumbar vertebrae.
2. The kidneys are enclosed in the renal capsule.
3. The cortex is the outer layer of the renal capsule.
4. The medulla is surrounded by the cortex.
5. The nephron makes up the functional unit of the kidneys.
6. Functions of kidneys
   a. The kidneys maintain homeostasis of the blood and acid-base balance.
   b. The kidneys excrete end products of body metabolism.
   c. The kidneys control fluid and electrolyte balance.
   d. The kidneys excrete bacterial toxins, water-soluble drugs, and drug metabolites.
   e. The kidneys secrete renin and erythropoietin, which play a role in the function of the parathyroid hormones and vitamin D.
7. Nephron
   a. The nephron is the functional renal unit.
   b. The nephron is composed of glomerulus and tubules.
8. Glomerulus
   a. The glomerulus is encased in Bowman's capsule.
   b. The glomerulus filters the fluid out of blood.
9. Tubules
   a. The tubules include proximal, distal, and Henle's loop.
   b. Fluid is converted to urine in the tubules, and then the urine moves to the pelvis of the kidney.
   c. The urine flows from the pelvis of the kidney through the ureter and empties into bladder.

B. Bladder
1. The ureterovesical sphincter prevents reflux of urine from the bladder to the ureter.
2. The total capacity of the bladder is 1 L.

C. Prostate gland
1. The prostate gland surrounds the male urethra.
2. The prostate gland contains a duct that opens into the prostatic portion of the urethra and secretes the alkaline portion of seminal fluid.

D. Urine production
1. As fluid flows through the proximal tubules, water and solutes are reabsorbed.
2. Water and solutes that are not reabsorbed become urine.
3. The process of selective reabsorption determines the amount of water and solutes to be secreted.

E. Homeostasis of water
1. The antidiuretic hormone (ADH) is primarily responsible for the reabsorption of water by the kidneys.
2. Antidiuretic hormone is produced by the hypothalamus and secreted from the posterior lobe of the pituitary gland.
3. Secretion of ADH is stimulated by dehydration or high sodium intake and by a fall in blood volume.
4. Antidiuretic hormone increases the permeability to water of the distal convoluted tubules and collecting duct.
5. Water is drawn out of the tubules by osmosis into a high salt concentration of fluid in the medulla and its capillaries; water returns to the blood, and concentrated urine remains in the tubule to be excreted.
6. When the client lacks ADH, the client develops diabetes insipidus.
7. Clients with diabetes insipidus produce large amounts of dilute urine and without treatment are unable to drink sufficient water to survive.

F. Homeostasis of sodium
1. When the amount of sodium increases, extra water is retained to preserve osmotic pressure.
2. An increase in sodium and water produces an increase in the blood volume and blood pressure (BP).
3. When the BP increases, glomerular filtration increases, and extra water and sodium are lost; blood volume is reduced and returns the BP to normal.
4. Reabsorption of sodium in the distal convoluted tubules is controlled by the hormones of the renin-angiotensin system.
5. Renin is secreted when the BP or concentration of fluid in the distal convoluted tubule is low.
6. Renin is an enzyme and splits angiotensin I from angiotensinogen, which converts to angiotensin II as blood flows through the lung.
7. Angiotensin II, a potent vasoconstrictor, stimulates the secretion of aldosterone.
8. Aldosterone stimulates the distal convoluted tubules to reabsorb sodium and secrete potassium.
9. The additional sodium increases water reabsorption and increases blood volume and BP, returning the BP to normal; the stimulus for the secretion of renin then is removed.

G. Homeostasis of potassium
1. Increases in potassium stimulate the secretion of aldosterone.
2. Aldosterone stimulates the distal convoluted tubules to secrete potassium; this acts to return the potassium concentration to normal.

▲ H. Homeostasis of acidity (pH)
1. Blood pH is controlled by maintaining the concentration of buffer systems.
2. Carbonic acid and sodium bicarbonate form the most important buffers for neutralizing acids in the plasma.
3. The concentration of carbonic acid is controlled by the respiratory system.
4. The concentration of sodium bicarbonate is controlled by the kidneys.
5. Normal pH is 7.35 to 7.45, maintained by keeping the ratio of concentrations of sodium bicarbonate to carbon dioxide constant at 20:1.
6. Strong acids are neutralized by sodium bicarbonate to produce carbonic acid and the sodium salts of the strong acid; this process quickly restores the ratio and thus blood pH.
7. The carbonic acid produced dissociates into carbon dioxide and water; because the concentration of carbon dioxide is maintained at a constant level by the respiratory system, the excess carbonic acid is excreted rapidly.
8. Sodium combined with the strong acid is reabsorbed actively in the distal convoluted tubules in exchange for hydrogen or potassium ions; the

strong acid is neutralized by the secretion of ammonia and is excreted as ammonia or potassium salts.
I. Refer to Box 61-1 for risk factors.

II. DIAGNOSTIC TESTS (BOX 61-2)
A. Refer to Chapter 11 for information regarding normal values for renal function studies.
B. Urinalysis
1. Description: a urine test for evaluation of the renal system and for determining renal disease
2. Interventions
   a. Wash perineal area and use a clean container.
   b. Obtain 10 to 15 mL of the first morning sample.
   c. Note that refrigerated samples may alter the specific gravity.
   d. If the client is menstruating, indicate this on the laboratory requisition form.
C. Specific gravity determination
1. Description: a urine test that measures the ability of the kidneys to concentrate urine
2. Interventions
   a. Specific gravity can be measured by multiple-test dipstick (most common method), refractometer (an instrument used in the laboratory setting), or urinometer (least accurate method).
   b. Factors that interfere with an accurate reading include radiopaque contrast agents, glucose, and proteins.
   c. Cold specimens may produce a false high reading.
   d. Normal value is 1.016 to 1.022 (may vary depending on the laboratory).
   e. An increase in specific gravity (more concentrated urine) occurs with insufficient fluid

---

BOX 61-1

Risk Factors Associated with Renal Disorders

Associated medical conditions
Contact sports
Family history of renal disease
Frequent urinary tract infections
High-sodium diet
History of hypertension
Medication use
Trauma and injury

BOX 61-2

Normal Renal Function Tests

Blood urea nitrogen, 8 to 25 mg/dL
Serum creatinine, 0.6 to 1.3 mg/dL
Creatinine clearance, 100 to 120 mL/min
Uric acid, serum, 2.5 to 8.0 mg/dL
Uric acid, urine, 250 to 750 mg per 24 hours

intake, decreased renal perfusion, or the presence of ADH.

    f. A decrease in specific gravity (less concentrated urine) occurs with increased fluid intake, renal failure, and diabetes insipidus.

D. Urine culture and sensitivity

  1. Description: a urine test that identifies the presence of microorganisms and determines the specific antibiotics that will treat the existing microorganism appropriately

  2. Interventions

    a. Clean perineal area and urinary meatus with bacteriostatic solution.

    b. Collect midstream sample in a sterile container.

    c. Send the collected specimen to the laboratory immediately.

    d. Note that urine from the client who forced fluids may be too dilute to provide a positive culture.

    e. Identify any sources of potential contaminants during the collection of the specimen, such as the hands, skin, clothing, hair, or vaginal or rectal secretions.

E. Creatinine clearance test

  1. Description

    a. The creatinine clearance test is a blood and timed urine specimen that evaluates kidney function.

    b. Blood is drawn at the start of the test and the morning of the day that the 24-hour urine specimen collection is complete.

  2. Interventions

    a. Encourage adequate fluids before and during the test.

    b. Instruct the client, as prescribed, to avoid tea, coffee, and medications during testing.

    c. If the client is taking corticosteroids or thyroid medication, check with the physician regarding the administration of these medications during testing.

    d. Maintain the urine specimen on ice or refrigerate, and check with the laboratory regarding the addition of a preservative to the specimen during collection.

F. Vanillylmandelic acid test

  1. Description

    a. The test is a 24-hour urine collection to diagnose pheochromocytoma, a tumor of the adrenal gland.

    b. The test identifies an assay of urinary catecholamines in the urine.

  2. Interventions

    a. Instruct the client to avoid foods such as caffeine, cocoa, vanilla, cheese, gelatin, licorice, and fruits for at least 2 days before beginning the urine collection and during the collection and to avoid taking medications for 2 to 3 days before beginning the test, as prescribed.

    b. Instruct the client to avoid stress and to maintain adequate food and fluid intake during the test.

    c. Save all urine, label the container, add preservative, and place the specimen on ice or refrigerate.

    d. Check with the laboratory regarding medication restrictions.

G. Uric acid test

  1. Description: a 24-hour urine collection to diagnose gout and kidney disease

  2. Interventions

    a. Encourage fluid intake and a regular diet during testing.

    b. Place the specimen on ice or refrigerate, and check with the laboratory regarding the addition of a preservative.

H. KUB (kidneys, ureters, and bladder) radiograph

  1. Description: an x-ray film of the urinary system and adjacent structures that is used to detect urinary calculuses

  2. Interventions: No specific preparation is necessary.

I. Bladder ultrasonography

  1. Bladder ultrasonography is a noninvasive method of measuring the volume of urine in the bladder.

  2. Bladder ultrasonography may be performed for evaluating urinary frequency or inability to urinate.

J. Computed tomography and magnetic resonance imaging

  1. Description: Imaging methods that provide cross-sectional views of the kidney and urinary tract

  2. Interventions: Refer to Chapter 65.

K. Intravenous pyelogram

  1. Description

    a. For an intravenous pyelogram a radiopaque dye is injected that outlines the renal system.

    b. An intravenous pyelogram is performed to identify abnormalities in the system.

  2. Preprocedure interventions

    a. Obtain an informed consent.

    b. Assess the client for allergies to iodine, seafood, and radiopaque dyes.

    c. Withhold food and fluids after midnight on the night before the test.

    d. Administer laxatives as prescribed.

    e. Inform the client about possible throat irritation, flushing of the face, warmth, or a salty taste during the test.

  3. Postprocedure interventions

    a. Monitor vital signs.

    b. Instruct the client to drink at least 1 L of fluid unless contraindicated.

    c. Assess the venipuncture site for bleeding.

    d. Monitor urinary output.

    e. Monitor for signs of a possible allergic reaction to the dye used during the test.

L. Renal angiography
1. Description: the injection of a radiopaque dye through a catheter for examination of the renal arterial supply
2. Preprocedure interventions
   a. Obtain an informed consent.
   b. Assess the client for allergies to iodine, seafood, and radiopaque dyes.
   c. Inform the client about the possible burning feeling or the feeling of heat along the vessel when the dye is injected.
   d. Withhold food and fluids after midnight on the night before the test.
   e. Instruct the client to void immediately before the procedure.
   f. Administer enemas as prescribed.
   g. Shave injection sites as prescribed.
   h. Assess and mark the peripheral pulses.
3. Postprocedure interventions
   a. Assess vital signs and peripheral pulses.
   b. Provide bed rest and use of a sandbag at the insertion site for 4 to 8 hours.
   c. Assess the color and temperature of the involved extremity.
   d. Inspect the catheter insertion site for bleeding or swelling.
   e. Encourage increased fluids unless contraindicated.
   f. Monitor urinary output.

M. Renal scan
1. Description: an intravenous (IV) injection of a radioisotope for visual imaging of renal blood flow
2. Preprocedure interventions
   a. Obtain an informed consent form.
   b. Assess for allergies.
   c. Assist with administering radioisotope as necessary.
   d. Instruct the client that he or she will be required to remain motionless during the test.
   e. Instruct the client that imaging may be repeated at various intervals before the test is complete.
3. Postprocedure interventions
   a. Encourage fluid intake unless contraindicated.
   b. Assess the client for signs of delayed allergic reaction such as itching and hives.
   c. Note that the radioactivity is eliminated in 24 hours.
   d. Follow standard precautions when caring for incontinent clients and double-bag client linens per agency policy.

N. Cystometrogram
1. Description: a graphic recording of the pressures exerted at varying phases of the bladder
2. Preprocedure interventions: Inform the client of the voiding requirements during the procedure.
3. Postprocedure interventions: Monitor the client's voiding after the procedure.

O. Cystoscopy and biopsy
1. Description: The bladder mucosa is examined for inflammation, calculuses, or tumors by means of a cystoscope; a biopsy may be obtained.
2. Preprocedure interventions
   a. Obtain an informed consent.
   b. If a biopsy is planned, withhold food and fluids after midnight on the night before the test.
   c. If a cystoscopy alone is planned, no special preparation is necessary, and the procedure may be performed in the physician's office; postprocedure includes increasing fluid intake.
3. Postprocedure interventions following biopsy
   a. Monitor vital signs.
   b. Increase fluid intake as prescribed.
   c. Monitor intake and output.
   d. Encourage deep-breathing exercises to relieve bladder spasms.
   e. Administer analgesics as prescribed.
   f. Administer sitz baths for back and abdominal pain.
   g. Note that leg cramps are common because of the lithotomy position maintained during the procedure.
   h. Assess the urine for color and consistency.
   i. Note that pink-tinged or tea-colored urine is common.
   j. Monitor for bright red urine or clots, and notify the physician if this occurs.

P. Renal biopsy
1. Description: insertion of a needle into the kidney to obtain a sample of tissue for examination
2. Preprocedure interventions
   a. Assess vital signs.
   b. Assess baseline clotting studies.
   c. Obtain an informed consent.
   d. Withhold food and fluids after midnight on the night before the test.
3. Interventions during the procedure: Position the client prone with a pillow under the abdomen and shoulders.
4. Postprocedure interventions
   a. Monitor vital signs.
   b. Monitor hemoglobin and hematocrit.
   c. Place the client in the supine position and on bed rest for 8 hours as prescribed.
   d. Provide pressure to the biopsy site for 30 minutes.
   e. Check the biopsy site for bleeding.
   f. Encourage fluid intake of 1500 to 2000 mL as prescribed.
   g. Instruct the client to avoid heavy lifting and strenuous activity for 2 weeks.

III. RENAL FAILURE
A. Description
1. **Renal failure** is the loss of kidney function.

2. The types of renal failure include **acute renal failure** and **chronic renal failure.**
3. The signs and symptoms of **renal failure** are caused by the retention of wastes, the retention of fluids, and the inability of the kidneys to regulate electrolytes.
4. Prerenal causes include intravascular volume depletion, decreased cardiac output, and vascular failure caused by vasodilation or obstruction.
5. Intrarenal causes include tubular necrosis, nephrotoxicity, and alterations in renal blood flow.
6. Postrenal causes include obstruction of urine flow between the kidney and urethral meatus and bladder neck obstruction.

B. **Acute renal failure** (Box 61-3)
   1. Description
      a. **Acute renal failure** is the sudden loss of kidney function and is caused by renal cell damage from ischemia or toxic substances.
      b. **Acute renal failure** occurs abruptly and can be reversible.
      c. **Acute renal failure** leads to hypoperfusion, cell death, and decompensation in renal function.
      d. The prognosis depends on the cause and the condition of the client.
      e. Near-normal or normal kidney function may resume gradually.
   2. Causes
      a. Infection
      b. Renal artery occlusion
      c. Obstruction
      d. Acute kidney disease
      e. Dehydration
      f. Diuretic therapy
      g. Ischemia from hypovolemia, heart failure, septic shock, or blood loss
      h. Toxic substances such as medications, particularly antibiotics
   3. Oliguric phase (Box 61-4)
      a. Duration of 8 to 15 days; and the longer the duration, the less chance of recovery
      b. Sudden drop in urine output; urine output less than 400 mL/day
      c. Urine specific gravity of decreased
      d. Anorexia, nausea, and vomiting
      e. Hypertension
      f. Decreased skin turgor
      g. Pruritus
      h. Tingling of the extremities

      i. Drowsiness progressing to disorientation to coma
      j. Edema
      k. Dysrhythmias
      l. Signs of congestive heart failure (CHF) and pulmonary edema
      m. Signs of pericarditis
      n. Signs of acidosis
   4. Diuretic phase (Box 61-4)
      a. Urine output rises slowly, and then diuresis occurs (4 to 5 L/day).
      b. Excessive urine output indicates recovery of damaged nephrons.
      c. Hypotension occurs.
      d. Tachycardia occurs.
      e. Level of consciousness improves.
   5. Recovery phase (convalescent) (Box 61-4)
      a. Recovery is a slow process; complete recovery may take 1 to 2 years.
      b. Urine volume is normal.
      c. Increase in strength occurs.
      d. Level of consciousness occurs.
      e. Blood urea nitrogen is stable and normal.
      f. Client can develop **chronic renal** failure.

C. **Chronic renal failure**
   1. Description
      a. **Chronic renal failure** is the progressive loss and ongoing deterioration in kidney function that occurs slowly over a period of time.
      b. **Chronic renal failure** occurs in stages, is irreversible, and results in uremia or end-stage renal disease (Box 61-5).
      c. **Chronic renal failure** affects all of the major body systems and requires dialysis or kidney transplant to maintain life.
      d. Hypervolemia can occur because of the inability of the kidneys to excrete sodium and water, or

---

BOX 61-3

Phases of Acute Renal Failure

Oliguric
Diuretic
Recovery (convalescent)

BOX 61-4

Acute Renal Failure

OLIGURIC PHASE
Decreased glomerular filtration rate
Hyperkalemia
Sodium level normal or decreased
Fluid overload
Elevated blood urea nitrogen and creatinine

DIURETIC PHASE
Increase in glomerular filtration rate
Hypokalemia
Hyponatremia
Hypovolemia
Gradual decline in blood urea nitrogen and creatinine

RECOVERY PHASE (CONVALESCENT)
Stable and normal blood urea nitrogen
Complete recovery may take 1 to 2 years.

BOX 61-5

Stages of Chronic Renal Failure

STAGE I: DIMINISHED RENAL RESERVE
Renal function is reduced.
No accumulation of metabolic wastes occurs.
The healthier kidney compensates.
Nocturia and polyuria occur as a result of decreased ability to concentrate urine.

STAGE II: RENAL INSUFFICIENCY
Metabolic wastes begin to accumulate.
Oliguria and edema occur as a result of decreased responsiveness to diuretics.

STAGE III: END STAGE
Excessive accumulation of metabolic wastes occurs.
Kidneys are unable to maintain homeostasis.
Dialysis or other renal replacement therapy is required.

hypovolemia can occur because of the inability of the kidneys to conserve sodium and water.

   2. Causes
      a. May follow **acute renal failure**
      b. Renal artery occlusion
      c. Chronic urinary obstruction
      d. Recurrent infections
      e. Hypertension
      f. Metabolic disorders
      g. Diabetes mellitus
      h. Autoimmune disorders
   3. Assessment
      a. Anorexia and nausea
      b. Headache
      c. Weakness and fatigue
      d. Hypertension
      e. Confusion and lethargy, followed by convulsions and coma
      f. Kussmaul's respirations
      g. Diarrhea or constipation
      h. Muscle twitching and numbness of the extremities
      i. Decreased urine output
      j. Decreased or fixed urine specific gravity
      k. Proteinuria
      l. Anemia
      m. **Azotemia**
      n. Fluid overload and signs of heart failure
      o. Uremic frost: a layer of urea crystals from evaporated perspiration that appears on the face, eyebrows, axilla, and groin in clients with advanced uremic syndrome
   D. Interventions
      1. Monitor vital signs.
      2. Monitor urine and intake and output (hourly in **acute renal failure**).
      3. Monitor weight, noting that an increase of ½ to 1 lb daily indicates fluid retention.

   4. Monitor blood urea nitrogen, creatinine, and electrolyte values.
   5. Monitor for acidosis and treat with sodium bicarbonate as prescribed.
   6. Assess urinalysis for protein, hematuria, casts, and specific gravity.
   7. Monitor level of consciousness.
   8. Assess for signs of infection because the client may not demonstrate a temperature or an increased white blood cell count.
   9. Assess for dysrhythmias because a potassium level above 6 mEq/L will cause tall peaked T waves, a prolonged PR interval, and a widened QRS complex.
   10. Monitor for fluid overload; assess lungs for wheezes, and rhonchi.
   11. Monitor for edema.
   12. Administer prescribed diet; usually a moderate protein intake (to decrease the workload on the kidneys) and a high-carbohydrate, low-potassium, and low-phosphorus diet is prescribed.
   13. Restrict sodium intake as prescribed, based on the electrolyte level.
   14. Daily fluid allowances may be 400 mL to 1000 mL plus measured urinary output.
   15. Administer sodium polystyrene sulfonate (Kayexalate) to lower the potassium level as prescribed.
   16. Be alert to the mechanism for metabolism and excretion of all prescribed medication.
   17. Be alert to nephrotoxic medications, such as antibiotics, which may be prescribed.
   18. Prepare the client for dialysis if prescribed.
   E. Special problems in **renal failure** (Box 61-6)
      1. Hypertension
         a. Hypertension is caused by failure of the kidneys to maintain homeostasis of the BP.
         b. Monitor vital signs.

BOX 61-6

Special Problems in Renal Failure

Anemia
Gastrointestinal bleeding
Hypertension
Hypervolemia
Hypovolemia
Infection and injury
Insomnia and fatigue
Low calcium
Metabolic acidosis
Muscle cramps
Neurological changes
Ocular irritation
Phosphorus retention
Potassium retention
Pruritis
Psychosocial problems

c. Maintain fluid and sodium restrictions as prescribed.

d. Administer diuretics and antihypertensives as prescribed.

e. Administer propranolol (Inderal), a β-adrenergic antagonist, as prescribed, which decreases renin release (renin causes vasoconstriction).

2. Hypervolemia

a. Monitor vital signs.

b. Monitor intake and output and weight.

c. Monitor for edema.

d. Monitor electrolytes.

e. Monitor for hypertension.

f. Monitor for CHF and pulmonary edema.

g. Enforce fluid restriction.

h. Avoid the IV administration of fluids.

i. Administer diuretics as prescribed.

j. Instruct the client to avoid foods with sodium.

k. Instruct the client to avoid antacids or cold remedies containing sodium bicarbonate.

3. Hypovolemia

a. Monitor vital signs.

b. Monitor intake and output and weight.

c. Monitor electrolytes.

d. Monitor for hypotension.

e. Monitor for dehydration.

f. Provide replacement therapy based on the electrolyte results.

g. Provide sodium supplements as prescribed, depending on the electrolyte value.

4. Potassium retention

a. Monitor vital signs and apical rate.

b. Monitor potassium level.

c. Monitor for hyperkalemia (tall peaked T waves, a prolonged PR interval, and widened QRS complex) indicating hyperkalemia.

d. Provide a low-potassium diet.

e. Administer medications as prescribed to lower the potassium level.

f. Prepare the client for dialysis.

5. Phosphorus retention

a. Phosphorus level rises and calcium level drops, which leads to stimulation of parathyroid hormone, causing bone demineralization.

b. Treatment is aimed at lowering serum phosphorus levels.

c. Administer aluminum hydroxide preparations or other phosphate binders, as prescribed, that bind phosphorus in the intestine and allow the phosphorus to be eliminated.

d. Administer aluminum hydroxide preparations at meals and not with other medications because they bind medications in the intestinal tract.

e. Administer stools softeners and laxatives as prescribed to prevent constipation because aluminum hydroxide preparations are constipating.

f. Enforce phosphorus restriction in the diet.

6. Low calcium

a. Low calcium level occurs because of the high phosphorus level and because of the inability of the diseased kidney to activate vitamin D.

b. The absence of vitamin D causes a poor absorption of calcium from the intestinal tract.

c. Monitor calcium level.

d. Administer calcium supplements as prescribed.

e. Administer activated vitamin D as prescribed.

7. Metabolic acidosis

a. The kidneys are unable to excrete hydrogen ions or manufacture bicarbonate, resulting in acidosis.

b. Administer alkalyzers such as sodium bicarbonate as prescribed.

c. Note that clients with **chronic renal failure** adjust to low bicarbonate levels and do not become acutely ill.

8. Anemia

a. A decreased rate of production of red blood cells occurs as a result of the diseased kidney and the decreased secretion of erythropoeitin.

b. Monitor hemoglobin and hematocrit.

c. Administer epoetin alfa (Epogen) as prescribed to stimulate the production of red blood cells.

d. Administer folic acid (vitamin B₉) as prescribed instead of orally administered iron because the iron is not well absorbed by the gastrointestinal tract in **chronic renal failure** and causes nausea and vomiting.

e. Administer blood transfusions if prescribed, but blood transfusions are prescribed only when necessary because they decrease the stimulus to produce red blood cells.

f. Monitor bleeding.

g. Instruct the client to use a soft toothbrush.

h. Administer stool softeners as prescribed.

i. Avoid the administration of acetylsalicylic acid (aspirin) because the medication is excreted by the kidneys; and if administered, high toxic levels will occur and prolong bleeding time.

9. Gastrointestinal bleeding

a. Urea is broken down to ammonia by the intestinal bacteria, and ammonia is a mucosal irritant that causes ulceration and bleeding.

b. Monitor hemoglobin and hematocrit levels.

c. Monitor stools for occult blood.

10. Infection and injury

a. Infection and injury need to be monitored and avoided because tissue breakdown causes increased potassium levels.

b. Monitor for signs of infection.

c. Avoid urinary catheters and provide strict asepsis during insertion and catheter care.

d. Instruct the client to avoid fatigue, which decreases body resistance.

e. Instruct the client to avoid persons with infections.

f. Administer antibiotics as prescribed, monitoring for nephrotoxic effects.

11. Pruritis

   a. Urate crystals are excreted through the skin to rid of excess wastes.

   b. This deposit of crystals is called uremic frost and occurs in advanced stages of **renal failure.**

   c. Monitor for skin breakdown, rash, and uremic frost.

   d. Provide good skin care and oral hygiene.

   e. Avoid the use of soaps.

   f. Administer antipruritics as prescribed.

12. Muscle cramps

   a. Muscle cramps occur in the extremities and hands and can be due to electrolyte imbalances.

   b. Monitor electrolytes.

   c. Administer electrolyte replacements as prescribed.

   d. Administer heat and massage as prescribed.

13. Ocular irritation

   a. Calcium deposits in the conjunctiva cause burning and watering of the eyes.

   b. Administer medications to control the calcium and phosphate levels as prescribed.

   c. Administer lubricating eye drops.

14. Insomnia and fatigue

   a. The diseased kidneys cause a buildup of wastes, causing fatigue in the client.

   b. Provide adequate rest periods.

   c. Administer mild central nervous system depressants as prescribed.

15. Neurological changes

   a. The buildup of active particles and fluids causes changes in the brain cells and leads to confusion and impairment in decision-making ability.

   b. Monitor for confusion and monitor level of consciousness.

   c. Protect the client from injury.

   d. Provide a safe and hazard-free environment.

   e. Use side rails as needed.

   f. Provide a calm and restful environment.

   g. Provide comfort measures and backrubs.

16. Psychosocial problems: Monitor the client for psychological problems such as depression, anxiety, suicidal behavior, denial, dependence/independence conflict, and changes in body image.

IV. HEMODIALYSIS

A. Description

1. **Hemodialysis** is the diffusion of dissolved particles from one fluid compartment into another across a **semipermeable membrane.**

2. The client's blood flows through one fluid compartment, and the dialysate is in another fluid compartment.

B. Functions of **hemodialysis**

1. **Hemodialysis** cleanses the blood of accumulated waste products.

2. **Hemodialysis** removes the by-products of protein metabolism such as urea, creatinine, and uric acid.

3. **Hemodialysis** removes excessive fluids.

4. **Hemodialysis** maintains or restores the buffer system of the body.

5. Hemodialysis maintains or restores electrolyte levels.

C. Principles of **hemodialysis**

1. The semipermeable membrane is made of a thin, porous cellophane.

2. The pore size of the membrane allows small particles to pass through, such as urea, creatinine, uric acid, and water molecules.

3. Proteins, bacteria, and some blood cells are too large to pass through the membrane.

4. The client's blood flows into the dialyzer; the movement of substances occurs from the blood to the dialysate.

5. Diffusion is the movement of particles from an area of greater concentration to one of lesser concentration.

6. Osmosis is the movement of fluids across a semipermeable membrane from an area of lesser concentration of particles to an area of greater concentration of particles.

7. Ultrafiltration is the movement of fluid across a semipermeable membrane as a result of an artificially created pressure gradient.

D. Dialysate bath

1. A dialysate bath is composed of water and major electrolytes.

2. The dialysate need not be sterile because bacteria are too large to pass through; however, the dialysate must meet specific standards, and water treatment systems are used to ensure a safe water supply.

E. Interventions

1. Monitor vital signs.

2. Monitor laboratory values before, during, and after dialysis.

3. Assess the client for fluid overload before the procedure.

4. Assess patency of the blood access device.

5. Weigh the client before and after the procedure to determine fluid loss.

6. Hold antihypertensives and other medications that can affect the BP before the procedure as prescribed.

7. Hold medications that could be dialyzed off, such as water-soluble vitamins and certain antibiotics.

8. Monitor for shock and hypovolemia during the procedure.

9. Provide adequate nutrition (client may eat before the procedure).

V. COMPLICATIONS OF HEMODIALYSIS (BOX 61-7)

A. **Disequilibrium syndrome**
   1. Description
      a. A rapid change in the composition of the extracellular fluid occurs during **hemodialysis.**
      b. Solutes are removed from the blood faster than from the cerebrospinal fluid and brain; fluid is pulled into the brain, causing cerebral edema.
   2. Assessment
      a. Nausea
      b. Vomiting
      c. Headache
      d. Hypertension
      e. Restlessness and agitation
      f. Confusion
      g. Seizures
   3. Interventions
      a. Monitor for signs of **disequilibrium syndrome.**
      b. Notify the physician if signs of **disequilibrium syndrome** occur.
      c. Reduce environmental stimuli.
      d. Prepare to dialyze the client for a shorter period at reduced blood flow rates to prevent occurrence.
B. Dialysis encephalopathy
   1. Description: An aluminum toxicity occurs as a result of aluminum in the water sources used in the dialysate and the ingestion of aluminum-containing antacids (phosphate binders).
   2. Assessment
      a. Progressive neurological impairment
      b. Mental cloudiness
      c. Speech disturbances
      d. Dementia
      e. Muscle incoordination
      f. Bone pain
      g. Seizures
   3. Interventions
      a. Monitor for signs of dialysis encephalopathy.
      b. Notify the physician if signs of dialysis encephalopathy occur.

BOX 61-7

Complications of Hemodialysis

Dialysis encephalopathy
Disequilibrium syndrome
Electrolyte changes
Hepatitis
Hypotension and shock
Loss of blood
Muscle cramping
Sepsis

---

c. Administer aluminum-chelating agents as prescribed so that the aluminum is freed up and dialyzed from the body.

VI. ACCESS FOR HEMODIALYSIS

A. Subclavian and femoral catheter (Fig. 61-1)
   1. Description
      a. A subclavian (subclavian vein) or femoral (femoral vein) catheter may be inserted for short term or temporary use in **acute renal failure.**
      b. The catheter may be used until a fistula or graft matures or develops or when the client has fistula or graft access failure because of infection or clotting.
   2. Interventions
      a. Assess insertion site for hematoma, bleeding, dislodging, and infection.
      b. Do not use these catheters for any reason other than dialysis.
      c. Maintain an occlusive dressing.
   3. Subclavian vein catheter
      a. The catheter usually is filled with heparin and capped to maintain patency between dialysis treatments.
      b. The catheter should not be uncapped.
      c. The catheter may be left in place for up to 6 weeks if complications do not occur.
   4. Femoral vein catheter
      a. The client should not sit up more than 45 degrees or lean forward, or the catheter may kink and occlude.
      b. Assess the extremity for circulation, temperature, and pulses.
      c. Prevent pulling or disconnecting of the catheter when giving care.
      d. Use an IV infusion pump with microdrip tubing if a heparin infusion through the catheter is prescribed.
B. External arteriovenous shunt (Fig. 61-1)
   1. Description
      a. Access is formed by the surgical insertion of two Silastic cannulas into an artery and a vein in the forearm or leg to form an external blood path.
      b. The cannulas are connected to form a U shape; blood flows from the client's artery through the shunt into the vein.
      c. A tube leading to the membrane compartment of the dialyzer is connected to the arterial cannula.
      d. Blood fills the membrane compartment and flows back to the client by way of a tube connected to the venous cannula.
      e. When dialysis is complete, the cannulas are clamped and reattached to form their U shape.
   2. Advantages
      a. The external arteriovenous shunt can be used immediately following creation.
      b. No venipuncture is necessary for dialysis.

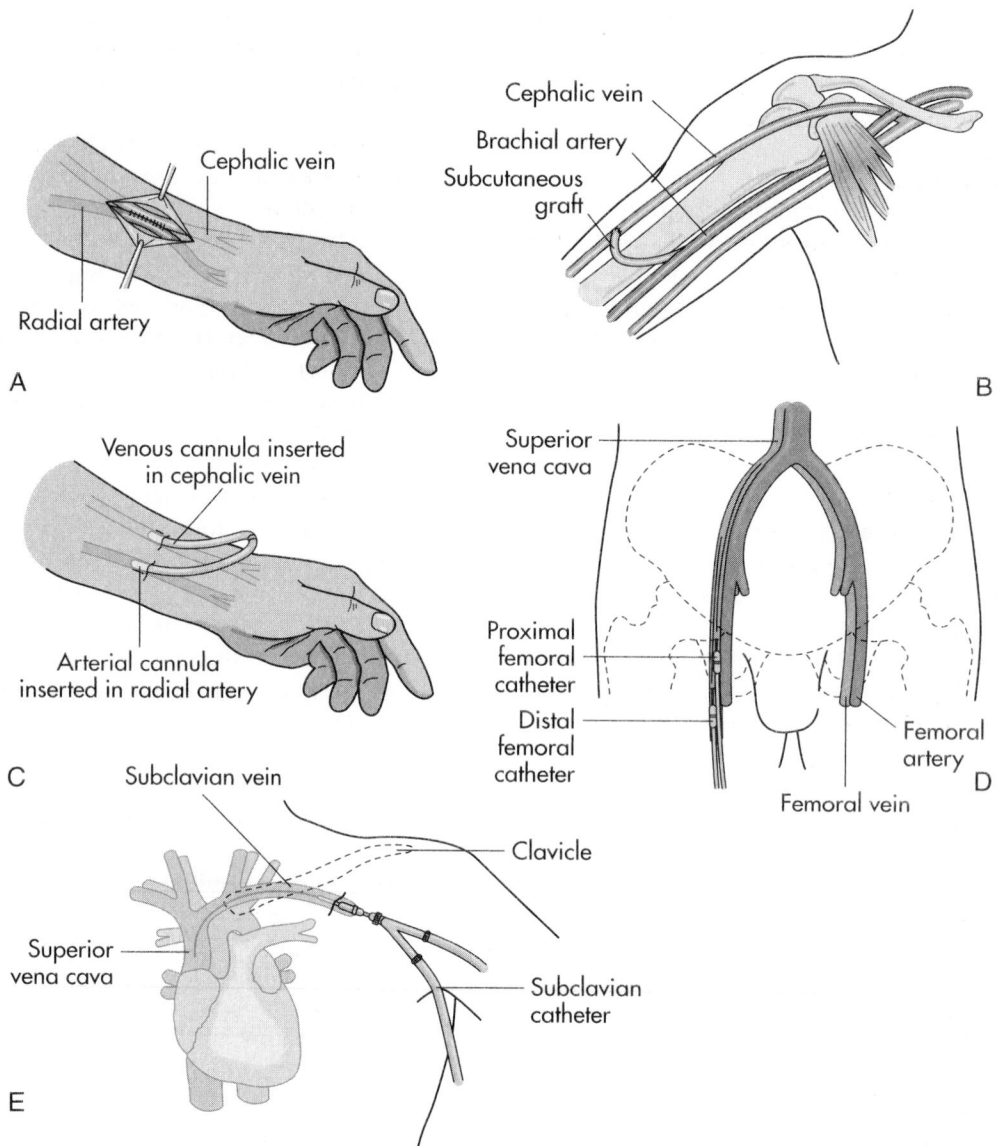

FIG. 61-1   Frequently used means for gaining vascular access for hemodialysis include (**A**) arteriovenous fistula, (**B**) arteriovenous graft, (**C**) external arteriovenous shunt, (**D**) femoral vein catheterization, and (**E**) subclavian vein catheterization. (From Phipps, W., Sands, J., Marek, J. [1999]. *Medical-surgical nursing: Concepts and clinical practice* [6th ed.]. St. Louis: Mosby.)

3. Disadvantages
   a. External danger of disconnecting or dislodging the shunt exists.
   b. Risk of hemorrhage, infection, or clotting exists.
   c. Skin erosion around the catheter site can occur.
4. Interventions
   a. Avoid wetting the shunt.
   b. A dressing is wrapped completely around the shunt and kept dry and intact.
   c. Cannula clamps need to be available at the client's bedside.
   d. Do not take a BP, draw blood, place an IV line, or administer injections in the shunt extremity.

   e. Monitor for hemorrhage, infection, and clotting.
   f. Monitor skin integrity around the insertion site.
   g. Note that the shunt is patent if it is warm to touch.
   h. Auscultate and palpate for a bruit, although a bruit may not be heard and is not always felt with the shunt.
   i. Notify the physician immediately if signs of clotting, hemorrhage, or infection occur.
5. Signs of clotting
   a. Fold back the dressing to expose the shunt tubing and assess for signs of clotting.
   b. Fibrin-white flecks noted in the tubing
   c. The separation of serum and cells

d. The absence of a previously heard bruit

e. Coolness of the tubing or extremity

f. Client complaints of a tingling sensation

C. **Internal arteriovenous fistula** (Fig. 61-1)

1. Description

a. The **internal arteriovenous** fistula provides the access of choice for chronic dialysis clients.

b. The fistula is created surgically by anastomosis of a large artery and a large vein in the arm.

c. The flow of arterial blood into the venous system causes the veins to become engorged (matured or developed).

d. Maturity takes about 1 to 2 weeks and is required before the fistula can be used so that the engorged vein can be punctured with a large-bore needle for the dialysis procedure.

e. Subclavian or femoral catheters, **peritoneal dialysis,** or an external arteriovenous shunt can be used for dialysis while the fistula is maturing or developing.

2. Advantages

a. Because the fistula is internal, the danger of clotting and bleeding is less.

b. The fistula can be used indefinitely.

c. Fistulas have a decreased incidence of infection.

d. No external dressing is required.

e. The fistula allows freedom of movement.

3. Disadvantages

a. The fistula cannot be used immediately after insertion.

b. Needle insertions are required for dialysis.

c. Infiltration of the needles during dialysis can occur and cause hematomas.

d. An aneurysm can form in the fistula.

e. **Arterial steal syndrome** can develop (too much blood is diverted to the vein, and arterial perfusion to the hand is compromised).

f. Congestive heart failure can occur from the increased blood flow in the venous system.

D. Internal arteriovenous graft (Fig. 61-1)

1. Description

a. The internal graft is used primarily for chronic dialysis clients who do not have adequate blood vessels for the creation of a fistula.

b. An artificial graft made of Gore-Tex or a bovine (cow) carotid artery is used to create an artificial vein for blood flow.

c. The procedure involves the anastomosis of the graft to the artery, a tunneling under the skin, and anastomosis to a vein.

d. The graft can be used 2 weeks after insertion

e. Complications of the graft include clotting, aneurysms, and infection.

2. Advantages

a. Because the graft is internal, the danger of clotting and bleeding is less.

b. The graft can be used indefinitely.

c. The graft has a decreased incidence of infection.

d. No external dressing is required.

e. The graft allows freedom of movement.

3. Disadvantages

a. The graft cannot be used immediately after insertion.

b. Needle insertions are required for dialysis.

c. Infiltration of the needles during dialysis can occur and cause hematomas.

d. An aneurysm can form in the graft.

e. Arterial steal syndrome can develop (too much blood is diverted to the vein, and arterial perfusion to the hand is compromised).

f. Congestive heart failure can occur from the increased blood flow in the venous system.

E. Interventions for arteriovenous fistula and arteriovenous graft

1. Do not measure a BP, draw blood, place an IV line, or administer injections in the fistula or graft extremity.

2. Monitor for clotting.

a. Complaints of tingling or discomfort in the extremity

b. Inability to palpate a thrill or auscultate a bruit over the fistula or graft

3. Monitor for **arterial steal syndrome.**

4. Palpate or auscultate for bruit or thrill over the fistula or graft.

5. Palpate pulses below the fistula or graft, and monitor for hand swelling as an indication of ischemia.

6. Note temperature and capillary refill of the extremity.

7. Monitor for infection.

8. Monitor lung and heart sounds for signs of CHF.

9. Notify the physician immediately if signs of clotting, infection, or **arterial steal syndrome** occur.

VII. PERITONEAL DIALYSIS

A. Description

1. The peritoneum is the dialyzing membrane (semipermeable membrane) and substitutes for kidney function during kidney failure.

2. Peritoneal dialysis works on the principles of diffusion and osmosis, and the dialysis occurs via the transfer of fluid and solute from the bloodstream through the peritoneum.

3. The peritoneal membrane is large and porous, allowing solutes and fluid to move via an osmotic gradient from an area of higher concentration in the body to an area of lower concentration in the dialyzing fluid.

4. The peritoneal cavity is rich in capillaries; therefore it provides a ready access to blood supply.

B. Contraindications to **peritoneal** dialysis

1. Peritonitis

2. Recent abdominal surgery

3. Abdominal adhesions
4. Impending renal transplant

C. Dialysate solution
1. Solution is sterile.
2. Solution contains electrolytes and minerals, a specific osmolarity, a specific glucose concentration, and other medication additives as prescribed.
3. The higher the glucose concentration, the greater the amount of fluid removed during an exchange.
4. Increasing the glucose concentration increases the concentration of active particles that cause osmosis and increases the rate of ultrafiltration and the amount of fluid removed.
5. If hyperkalemia is not a problem, potassium may be added to each bag of solution.
6. Heparin is added to the dialysate solution to prevent clotting of the catheter.
7. Prophylactic antibiotics may be added to dialysate to prevent peritonitis.
8. Insulin may be added to the dialysate for the client with diabetes mellitus.

VIII. ACCESS FOR PERITONEAL DIALYSIS (FIG. 61-2)

A. Description
1. A surgical insertion of a siliconized rubber catheter into the abdominal cavity is required to allow infusion of dialysis fluid.
2. The preferred insertion site is 3 to 5 cm below the umbilicus because this area is relatively avascular and has less fascial resistance.
3. The catheters are tunneled under the skin to stabilize the catheter and reduce the risk of infection.
4. Over a period of 1 to 2 weeks following insertion, an ingrowth of fibroblasts and blood vessels occurs into the cuffs of the catheter, which fix the catheter in place and provide an extra barrier against dialysate leakage and bacterial invasion.

B. Types of **peritoneal dialysis**
1. Continuous ambulatory **peritoneal dialysis** (CAPD)
   a. Continuous dialysis closely resembles renal function because it is a continuous process.
   b. Continuous dialysis does not require a machine for the procedure.
   c. Continuous dialysis promotes client independence.
   d. The client performs self-dialysis 24 hours a day, 7 days a week.
   e. Usually four dialysis cycles are administered in 24 hours, including an 8-hour dwell time overnight.
   f. One and a half to 2 L of dialysate are instilled into the abdomen 4 times daily and allowed to dwell as prescribed.

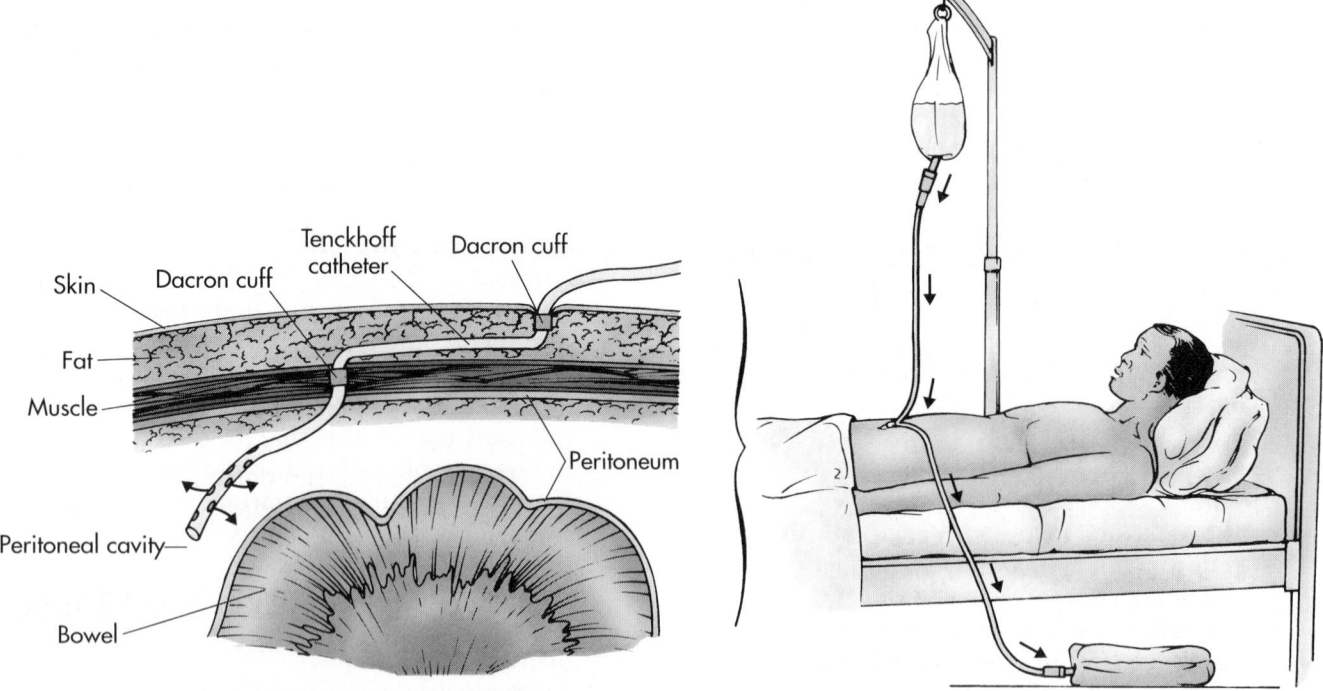

FIG. 61-2   Manual peritoneal dialysis via an implanted abdominal catheter (Tenckhoff catheter). (From Ignatavicius, D., Workman, M., Mishler, M. [1999]. *Medical-surgical nursing across the health care continuum* [3rd ed.]. Philadelphia: W. B. Saunders.)

g. The dialysis bag, attached to the catheter, is folded and carried under the client's clothing until time for outflow.

h. After dwell, the bag is placed lower than the insertion site so that fluid drains by gravity flow

i. When full, the bag is changed, new dialysate is instilled into the abdomen, and the process continues.

2. Automated **peritoneal dialysis** (Box 61-8)

a. Automated **peritoneal dialysis** is similar to continuous ambulatory **peritoneal dialysis** in that it is a continuous dialysis process.

b. Automated dialyis requires a peritoneal cycling machine.

c. Automated dialyis can be done as intermittent **peritoneal dialysis,** continuous cycling **peritoneal dialysis,** or nightly **peritoneal dialysis.**

C. **Peritoneal dialysis** infusion

1. Description

a. One infusion (inflow), dwell, and outflow is considered one exchange.

b. Dialysis infusion uses an open system that presents a risk of infection.

c. Inflow: The infusion of 1 to 2 L of dialysate as prescribed is infused by gravity into the peritoneal space, which usually takes 10 to 20 minutes.

d. Dwell time: The amount of time that the dialysate solution remains in the peritoneal cavity is prescribed by the physician and can last 20 to 30 minutes to 8 or more hours depending on the type of dialysis used.

e. Outflow: Fluid drains out of body by gravity into the drainage bag.

2. Interventions before treatment

a. Monitor vital signs.

b. Obtain weight.

c. Have the client void, if possible.

d. Assess electrolyte and glucose levels.

3. Interventions during treatment

a. Monitor vital signs.

b. Monitor for signs of infection.

c. Monitor for respiratory distress, pain, or discomfort.

d. Monitor for signs of pulmonary edema.

e. Monitor for hypotension and hypertension.

f. Monitor for malaise, nausea, vomiting.

g. Assess the catheter site dressing for wetness or bleeding.

h. Monitor dwell time as prescribed by the physician and initiate outflow.

i. Do not allow dwell time to extend beyond the physician's order because this increases the risk for hyperglycemia.

j. Turn the client from side to side if the outflow is slow to start.

k. Monitor outflow, which should be a continuous stream after the clamp is opened.

l. Monitor outflow for color and clarity.

m. Monitor intake and output accurately.

n. If outflow is less than inflow, the difference is equal to the amount absorbed or retained by the client during dialysis and should be counted as intake.

IX. COMPLICATIONS OF PERITONEAL DIALYSIS (BOX 61-9)

A. Peritonitis

1. Maintain meticulous sterile technique when hooking up or clamping off bags and when caring for the catheter insertion site.

2. Follow institutional procedure for hooking up or clamping off bags, which may include scrubbing the connection sites with an antiseptic solution.

3. Monitor temperature closely.

4. Monitor for fever, cloudy outflow, and rebound abdominal tenderness.

5. If peritonitis is suspected, obtain a culture of the outflow to determine the infective organism.

6. Administer antibiotics as prescribed.

B. Abdominal pain

1. Pain during inflow is common during the first few exchanges, is caused by peritoneal irritation, and

---

BOX 61-8

Types of Automated Peritoneal Dialysis

CONTINUOUS CYCLING PERITONEAL DIALYSIS

Dialysis requires a peritoneal cycling machine.

Dialysis usually consists of three cycles done at night and one cycle with an 8-hour dwell done in the morning.

The sterile catheter system is opened only for the on and off procedures, which reduces the risk of infection.

The client does not need to do exchanges during the day.

INTERMITTENT PERITONEAL DIALYSIS

Dialysis requires a peritoneal cycling machine.

Dialysis is not a continuous procedure.

Dialysis is performed for 10 to 14 hours, 3 to 4 times a week.

NIGHTLY PERITONEAL DIALYSIS

Dialysis is performed 8 to 12 hours each night with no daytime exchanges or dwells.

BOX 61-9

Complications of Peritoneal Dialysis

Abdominal pain

Bladder or bowel perforation

Insufficient outflow

Leakage around the catheter site

Peritonitis

usually disappears after 1 to 2 weeks of dialysis treatments.

2. The cold temperature of the dialysate aggravates the discomfort, and the dialysate should be warmed before use, only with a special dialysate warmer pad.

3. Place a heating pad on the abdomen during the inflow to relieve discomfort; if a heating pad is used, place it on low setting and monitor the client closely.

C. Insufficient outflow

1. Insufficient outflow may be caused by catheter migration out of the peritoneal area; if this occurs, the physician must reposition the catheter.

2. Insufficient outflow also can be caused by a full colon.

3. Maintain the drainage bag below the client's abdomen.

4. Change the client's outflow position by turning the client on his or her side or by ambulating the client.

5. Check for kinks in the tubing.

6. Encourage a high-fiber diet.

7. Administer stool softeners as prescribed.

D. Leakage around the catheter site

1. Over a period of 1 to 2 weeks following insertion of the catheter, an ingrowth of fibroblasts and blood vessels into the cuffs of the catheter occurs that fixes the catheter in place and provides an extra barrier against dialysate leakage and bacterial invasion.

2. It may take up to 2 weeks for the client to tolerate a full 2-L exchange without leaking around the catheter site.

E. Characteristics of outflow

1. During the first or initial exchanges, the outflow may be bloody; outflow should be clear and colorless thereafter.

2. A brown outflow indicates bowel perforation.

3. If the outflow is the same color as urine, this indicates bladder perforation.

4. Cloudy outflow indicates peritonitis.

X. UREMIC SYNDROME

A. Description

1. Uremic syndrome is the accumulation of nitrogenous waste products in the blood because of the inability of the kidneys to filter out these waste products.

2. Uremic syndrome may occur as a result of **acute** or **chronic renal failure.**

B. Assessment

1. **Oliguria**

2. The presence of protein, red blood cells, and casts in the urine

3. A urine specific gravity of 1.010

4. Elevated levels of urea, uric acid, potassium, and magnesium in the urine

5. Hypotension or hypertension

6. Alterations in level of consciousness

7. Electrolyte imbalances

8. Stomatitis

9. Nausea or vomiting

10. Diarrhea or constipation

C. Interventions

1. Monitor vital signs.

2. Monitor electrolyte values.

3. Monitor intake and output.

4. Provide a diet limited in protein as prescribed (protein provided should be high quality).

5. Limit sodium, nitrogen, potassium, and phosphate intake as prescribed.

XI. CYSTITIS/URINARY TRACT INFECTIONS (UTI) (BOX 61-10)

A. Description

1. Cystitis is inflammation of the bladder from infection or obstruction of the urethra.

2. The most common causative organisms are *Escherichia coli, Enterobacter, Pseudomonas,* and *Serratia.*

3. Cystitis is more common in women because women have a shorter urethra than men, and the location of the urethra in the woman is close to the rectum.

4. Sexually active and pregnant women are most vulnerable to cystitis.

B. Assessment

1. Frequency and urgency

2. Burning on urination

3. Voiding in small amounts

4. Inability to void

5. Incomplete emptying of the bladder

6. Lower abdominal discomfort or back discomfort

7. Cloudy, dark, foul-smelling urine

8. Hematuria

BOX 61-10

Causes of Cystitis

Allergens or irritants, such as soaps, sprays, bubble bath, perfumed sanitary napkins

Bladder distention

Calculus

Hormonal changes influencing alterations in vaginal flora

Indwelling urethral catheters

Invasive urinary tract procedures

Loss of bactericidal properties of prostatic secretions in the male

Poor-fitting diaphragms

Sexual intercourse

Synthetic underwear and pantyhose

Urinary stasis

Use of spermicides

Wet bathing suits

9. Bladder spasms
10. Malaise, chills, fever
11. Nausea and vomiting
C. Interventions
1. Obtain a urine specimen for culture and sensitivity, if prescribed, to identify bacterial growth before administering prescribed antibiotics.
2. Instruct the client to increase fluids up to 3000 mL a day, especially if the client is taking a sulfonamide because these medications can form crystals in concentrated urine.
3. Administer medications as prescribed, which may include analgesics, antiseptics, antispasmodics, antibiotics, and antimicrobials.
4. Maintain an acid urine pH (5.5) by an acid-ash diet; instruct the client in foods to consume on an acid-ash diet.
5. Note that if the client is prescribed an aminoglycoside, a sulfonamide, or nitrofurantoin (Macrodantin), the actions of these medications are diminished by acidic urine.
6. Use strict aseptic technique when inserting a urinary catheter into a client.
7. Maintain closed urinary drainage systems for the client with an indwelling catheter.
8. Provide meticulous perineal care for the client with an indwelling catheter.
9. Discourage caffeine products such as coffee, tea, and cola.
10. Instruct the client to avoid alcohol.
11. Provide heat to the abdomen or sitz baths for complaints of discomfort.
12. Instruct the client to take medications as prescribed.
13. Instruct the client to take antibiotics on schedule and to take the entire course of medications as prescribed, which may be a course of 10 to 14 days.
14. Instruct the client in the importance of a follow-up urine culture following treatment.
15. Box 61-11 lists preventive measures.

XII. UROSEPSIS

A. Description
1. Urosepsis is a gram-negative bacteremia originating in the urinary tract.
2. The most common responsible organism is *Escherichia coli.*
3. The most common cause is the presence of an indwelling urinary catheter or an untreated UTI in a client who is medically compromised.
4. The major problem is the ability of this bacterium to develop resistant strains.
5. Urosepsis can lead to septic shock if not treated aggressively.
B. Assessment: Fever is the most common and earliest manifestation.

BOX 61-11

Prevention of Cystitis

Teach the female client good perineal care and to wipe from front to back.
Instruct the female client to avoid bubble baths and tub baths and avoid vaginal deodorants or sprays.
Instruct the client to void every 2 to 3 hours.
Instruct the female client to void and drink a glass of water after intercourse.
Instruct the female client to wear cotton pants and to avoid wearing tight clothes or pantyhose with slacks and to avoid sitting in a wet bathing suit for prolonged periods of time.
Teach pregnant women to void every 2 hours.
Encourage menopausal women to use estrogen vaginal creams to restore pH.
Instruct the female client to use water-soluble lubricants for coitus, especially after menopause.

C. Interventions
1. Obtain a urine specimen for urine culture and sensitivity.
2. Administer antibiotics intravenously as prescribed, usually until the client has been afebrile for 3 to 5 days.
3. Administer oral antibiotics as prescribed after the 3- to 5-day afebrile period.

XIII. URETHRITIS

A. Description
1. Urethritis is an inflammation of the urethra commonly associated with sexually transmitted diseases and may occur with cystitis.
2. In men, urethritis most often is caused by gonorrhea or chlamydial infection.
3. In women, urethritis most often is caused by feminine hygiene sprays, perfumed toilet paper or sanitary napkins, spermicidal jellies, UTIs, or changes in the vaginal mucosal lining.
B. Assessment
1. Males
   a. Burning on urination
   b. Frequency
   c. Urgency
   d. Nocturia
   e. Difficulty voiding
   f. Discharge from the penis
2. Females
   a. Frequency
   b. Urgency
   c. Nocturia
   d. Painful urination
   e. Difficulty voiding
   f. Lower abdominal discomfort
C. Interventions
1. Encourage fluid intake.

2. Prepare the client for testing to determine if a sexually transmitted disease is present.
3. Administer antibiotics as prescribed.
4. Instruct the client in the administration of sitz baths.
5. If stricture occurs, prepare the client for dilation of the urethra and instillation of an antiseptic solution.
6. Instruct the client to avoid intercourse until the symptoms subside or treatment of the sexually transmitted disease is complete.
7. Instruct the female client to avoid the use of perfumed toilet paper or sanitary napkins and feminine hygiene sprays.

XIV. URETERITIS AND PYELONEPHRITIS

A. Ureteritis
1. Ureteritis is an inflammation of the ureter commonly associated with pyelonephritis.
2. Chronic pyelonephritis causes the ureter to become fibrotic and narrowed by strictures.

B. Pyelonephritis
1. Pyelonephritis is an inflammation of the renal pelvis and the parenchyma commonly caused by bacterial invasion.
2. Acute pyelonephritis often occurs after bacterial contamination of the urethra or following an invasive procedure of the urinary tract.
3. Chronic pyelonephritis most commonly occurs following chronic obstruction with reflux or chronic disorders.
4. *Escherichia coli* is the most common bacterial causative organism.

C. Acute pyelonephritis
1. Acute pyelonephritis usually follows a short course that recurs as a relapse of a previous infection or as a new infection.
2. Acute pyelonephritis can progress to bacteremia or chronic pyelonephritis.
3. Assessment
   a. Fever and chills
   b. Nausea
   c. Flank pain on the affected side
   d. Costovertebral angle tenderness
   e. Headache
   f. Muscular pain
   g. Dysuria
   h. Frequency and urgency
   i. Cloudy, bloody, or foul-smelling urine
   j. Increased white blood cells in the urine

D. Chronic pyelonephritis
1. Chronic pyelonephritis is a slow, progressive disease usually associated with recurrent acute attacks.
2. Chronic pyelonephritis causes contraction of the kidney and dysfunctioning of the nephrons, which are replaced by scar tissue.
3. Chronic pyelonephritis can lead to **renal failure.**

4. Assessment
   a. Frequently diagnosed incidentally when a client is being evaluated for hypertension
   b. Poor urine-concentrating ability
   c. Pyuria
   d. **Azotemia**
   e. Proteinuria
   f. Anemia
   g. Acidosis

E. Interventions
1. Monitor vital signs.
2. Monitor intake and output.
3. Monitor weight.
4. Encourage fluid intake up to 3000 mL a day.
5. Encourage adequate rest.
6. Instruct the client in a high-calorie, low-protein diet.
7. Provide warm, moist compresses to the flank area.
8. Encourage the client to take warm baths.
9. Administer analgesics, antipyretics, antibiotics, urinary antiseptics, and antiemetics as prescribed.
10. Monitor for signs of **renal failure.**

XV. GLOMERULONEPHRITIS

A. Description
1. Glomerulonephritis is a term that includes a variety of disorders, most of which are caused by an immunological reaction.
2. Glomerulonephritis results in proliferative and inflammatory changes within the glomerular structure.
3. Destruction, inflammation, and sclerosis of the glomeruli of both kidneys occur.
4. The inflammation of the glomeruli results from an antigen-antibody reaction produced from an infection elsewhere in the body.
5. Loss of kidney function develops.

B. Causes
1. Immunological or autoimmune diseases
2. Streptococcal infection, group A β-hemolytic
3. History of pharyngitis or tonsillitis 2 to 3 weeks before symptoms

C. Types
1. Acute glomerulonephritis occurs 2 to 3 weeks after a streptococcal infection.
2. Chronic glomerulonephritis can occur after the acute phase or slowly over time.

D. Complications
1. Heart failure
2. Hypertensive encephalopathy
3. Pulmonary edema
4. **Renal failure**

E. Assessment
1. Gross hematuria
2. Dark, smoky, cola-colored or red-brown urine
3. Proteinuria that produces a persistent and excessive foam in the urine

4. Urinary debris
5. Moderately elevated to high specific gravity
6. Low urinary pH
7. **Oliguria** or **anuria**
8. Headache
9. Chills and fever
10. Fatigue and weakness
11. Anorexia, nausea, and vomiting
12. Pallor
13. Edema in the face, periorbital area, feet, or generalized
14. Shortness of breath, ascites, pleural effusion, and CHF
15. Abdominal or flank pain
16. Hypertension
17. Reduced visual acuity
18. Increased blood urea nitrogen and creatinine levels
19. Increased antistreptolysin O titer (used to diagnose disorders caused by streptococcal infections)

F. Interventions
1. Monitor vital signs.
2. Monitor intake and output and urine closely.
3. Monitor daily weight.
4. Monitor for edema.
5. Monitor for fluid overload, ascites, pulmonary edema, and CHF.
6. Restrict fluid intake as prescribed.
7. Provide a high-calorie and low-protein diet.
8. Restrict sodium intake as prescribed if edema is present.
9. Provide bed rest and limited activity.
10. Instruct the client to obtain treatment for infections, specifically sore throats and upper respiratory infections.
11. Administer diuretics, antihypertensives, and antibiotics as prescribed.
12. Monitor for signs of **renal failure**, cardiac failure, and hypertensive encephalopathy.
13. Instruct the client to report signs of bloody urine, headache, or edema.

XVI. NEPHROTIC SYNDROME

A. Description: A set of clinical manifestations arising from protein wasting caused by diffuse glomerular damage
B. Assessment
1. Proteinuria
2. Hypoalbuminemia
3. Edema
4. Hyperlipidemia
5. Waxy pallor to the skin
6. Anemia
7. Anorexia
8. Malaise
9. Irritability
10. Amenorrhea or abnormal menses
11. Hematuria may be present

C. Interventions
1. Monitor vital signs.
2. Monitor intake and output.
3. Bed rest is necessary if severe edema is present.
4. Instruct the client in a normal to low-protein diet as prescribed, with adequate carbohydrate and calorie intake.
5. Monitor daily weights.
6. Provide a mild sodium restriction as prescribed.
7. Monitor potassium level; potassium may be restricted from the diet if the potassium rises.
8. Administer diuretics as prescribed.
9. Administer corticosteroids and cytotoxic medications as prescribed.
10. Administer plasma volume expanders, such as albumin, plasma, and dextran, to raise the osmotic pressure.
11. Administer anticoagulants as prescribed for those clients who develop renal vein thrombosis.

XVII. HYDRONEPHROSIS

A. Description
1. Hydronephrosis is distention of the renal pelvis and calices caused by an obstruction of normal urine flow.
2. The urine becomes trapped proximal to the obstruction.
3. The causes include calculus, tumors, scar tissue, and ureter obstructions, and hypertrophy of the prostate.
B. Assessment
1. Hypertension
2. Headache
3. Flank pain
4. Electrolyte imbalances
C. Interventions
1. Monitor vital signs frequently.
2. Monitor for fluid and electrolyte imbalances, including dehydration after the obstruction is relieved.
3. Monitor for diuresis, which can lead to fluid depletion.
4. Monitor weights daily.
5. Monitor urine for specific gravity, albumin, and glucose.
6. Administer fluid replacement as prescribed.

XVIII. POLYCYSTIC KIDNEY DISEASE

A. Description
1. Polycystic kidney disease is a cystic formation and hypertrophy of the kidneys, which lead to cystic rupture, infection, the formation of scar tissue, and damaged nephrons.
2. No way is known to arrest the progress of the destructive cysts.
3. The ultimate result of this disease is **renal failure**.

B. Types
1. Infantile polycystic disease: An inherited autosomal recessive trait that results in the death of the infant within a few months after birth
2. Adult polycystic disease: An autosomal dominant trait that results in end-stage renal disease

C. Assessment
1. Flank, lumbar, or abdominal pain
2. Fever and chills
3. UTIs
4. Hematuria, proteinuria, pyuria
5. Calculuses
6. Hypertension
7. Palpable abdominal masses and enlarged kidneys

▲ D. Interventions
1. Monitor for gross hematuria, which indicates cyst rupture.
2. Increase sodium and water intake because sodium loss rather than retention occurs.
3. Provide bed rest if ruptured cysts and bleeding occur.
4. Prepare the client for percutaneous cyst puncture for relief of obstruction or for draining an abscess.
5. Administer antihypertensives as prescribed.
6. Prepare the client for dialysis or renal transplantation.
7. Encourage the client to seek genetic counseling.

XIX. UROLITHIASIS AND NEPHROLITHIASIS

A. Description
1. Calculuses or stones can form anywhere in the urinary tract; however, the most frequent site is the kidneys.
2. The problems that can occur as a result of calculuses are pain, obstruction, and tissue trauma, with secondary hemorrhage and infection.
3. Kidneys, ureters, and bladder film, intravenous pyelogram, computed tomography scan, and renal ultrasonography will determine the stone location.
4. A stone analysis will be done after passage to determine the type of stone and assist in determining treatment.
5. **Urolithiasis** refers to the formation of urinary stones; urinary calculuses are formed in the ureters.
6. **Nephrolithiasis** refers to the formation of kidney stones; kidney stones are formed in the renal parenchyma.
7. When a calculus occludes the ureter and blocks the flow of urine, the ureter dilates, producing a condition known as hydroureter.
8. If the obstruction is not removed, urinary stasis results in infection, impairment of renal function on the side of the blockage, and resultant hydronephrosis and irreversible kidney damage.

B. Causes
1. Family history of stone formation

2. Diet high in calcium, vitamin D, milk, protein, oxalate, purines, or alkali
3. A high intake of purine-rich food
4. Obstruction and urinary stasis
5. Dehydration
6. Use of diuretics, which can cause volume depletion
7. Urinary tract infections and prolonged urinary catheterization
8. Immobilization ▲
9. Hypercalcemia and hyperparathyroidism
10. Elevated uric acid, such as in gout

C. Assessment
1. Renal colic, which originates in the lumbar ▲ region and radiates around the side and down toward the testicle in men and to the bladder in women
2. Ureteral colic, which radiates toward the geni- ▲ talia and thigh
3. Sharp, severe pain of sudden onset
4. Dull, aching pain in the kidney
5. Nausea and vomiting, pallor, and diaphoresis during acute pain
6. Urinary frequency with alternating retention
7. Signs of a UTI
8. Low-grade fever
9. High numbers of red blood cells, white blood cells, and bacteria in the urinalysis
10. Hematuria

D. Interventions
1. Monitor vital signs.
2. Monitor intake and output.
3. Assess for fever, chills, and infection.
4. Monitor for nausea, vomiting, and diarrhea.
5. Encourage fluid intake up to 3000 mL/day, unless ▲ contraindicated, to facilitate the passage of the stone and prevent infection.
6. Strain all urine for the presence of stones. ▲
7. Send stones to the laboratory for analysis. ▲
8. Provide warm baths and heat to the flank area.
9. Administer analgesics at regularly scheduled intervals as prescribed to relieve pain.
10. Assess the client's response to pain medication.
11. Administer fluids intravenously as prescribed to increase the flow of urine and facilitate the passage of the stone.
12. Assist the client in performing relaxation techniques to assist in relieving pain.
13. Instruct the client in the diet specific to the stone composition.
14. Maintain urinary pH depending on the type of stone.
15. Turn and reposition immobilized clients. ▲
16. Prepare the client for surgical procedures if prescribed.

E. Stone composition (Boxes 61-12 and 61-13)
1. A special diet, such as an alkaline ash or acid ash, may be prescribed depending on the physician's preference.
2. Calcium phosphate stones
   a. Calcium phosphate stones are caused by supersaturation of urine with calcium and phosphate.
   b. Diet includes acid-ash foods because calcium stones have an alkaline chemistry.
   c. Dietary prescription may include to decrease intake of foods high in calcium and phosphate to reduce urinary calcium content and to avoid excess vitamin D intake to prevent stones from forming.
3. Calcium oxalate stones
   a. Calcium oxalate stones are caused by supersaturation of urine with calcium and oxalate.
   b. Diet includes acid-ash foods because calcium stones have an alkaline chemistry.
   c. Dietary prescription may include decreasing intake of foods high in calcium.
   d. Dietary prescription may include avoiding oxalate food sources to reduce urinary oxalate content and the formation of stones.
   e. Oxalate-rich food sources include tea, almonds, cashews, chocolate, cocoa, beans, spinach, and rhubarb.

BOX 61-12

Alkaline-Ash Diet

OUTCOME
Diet increases the pH of the urine.
Diet reduces the acidity of the urine.

FOODS TO INCLUDE
Fruits, except cranberries, plums, and prunes
Milk
Most vegetables
Rhubarb
Small amounts of beef, halibut, veal, trout, and salmon

BOX 61-13

Acid-Ash Diet

OUTCOME
Diet decreases the pH of the urine.
Diet makes the urine more acidic.

FOODS TO INCLUDE
Bread, cereal, whole grains
Cheese, eggs
Corn and legumes
Cranberries, prunes, plums, tomatoes
Meat, fish, oysters, poultry
Pastries

---

4. Struvite stones
   a. Struvite stones also are called triple phosphate stones and are composed of magnesium and ammonium phosphate.
   b. Struvite stones are caused by urea splitting by bacteria.
   c. Struvite stones tend to form in alkaline urine.
   d. Diet includes acid-ash foods.
   e. Dietary prescription includes to limit high-phosphate foods such as dairy products, red and organ meats, and whole grains to reduce urinary phosphate content.
5. Uric acid stones
   a. Uric acid stones are caused by excess dietary purine or from gout.
   b. Uric acid stones tend to form in acidic urine.
   c. Dietary prescription may include alkaline-ash foods and decreased intake of purine sources such as organ meats, gravies, red wines, and sardines to reduce urinary purine content.
   d. Allopurinol (Zyloprim) may be prescribed to lower uric acid levels.
6. Cystine stones
   a. Cystine stone are caused by cystine crystal formation.
   b. Cystine stones tend to form in acidic urine.
   c. Diet includes alkaline-ash foods.
   d. Dietary prescription also may include a low intake of methionine, an essential amino acid that forms cystine, and the client would be instructed to avoid meat, milk, cheese, and eggs.
   e. Dietary measures also focus on encouraging fluid intake up to 3 L a day, unless contraindicated, to help dilute the urine and prevent cystine crystals from forming.

XX. SURGICAL MANAGEMENT OF KIDNEY STONES
A. Cystoscopy
1. Cystoscopy may be done for stones located in the bladder or lower ureter.
2. No incision is made.
3. One or two ureteral catheters are inserted past the stone.
4. The stone may be manipulated and dislodged by the procedure.
5. The catheters may guide the stones mechanically downward as they are removed.
6. Catheters are left in place for 24 hours to drain the urine trapped proximal to the stone and to dilate the ureter.
7. A continuous chemical irrigation may be prescribed to dissolve the stone.
B. Extracorporeal shock wave lithotripsy
1. Extracorporeal shock wave lithotripsy is a noninvasive mechanical procedure for breaking up stones

that are located in the kidney or upper ureter so that they can pass spontaneously or be removed by other methods.
2. Fluoroscopy is used to visualize the stone.
3. No incision is made and no drains are placed.
4. Ultrasonic waves are delivered through a bath of warm water to the areas of the stone to disintegrate it.
5. Stones are passed in the urine within a few days.
6. Preprocedure: Maintain client on NPO status for 8 hours before the procedure.
7. Postprocedure
   a. Monitor vital signs.
   b. Monitor intake and output.
   c. Monitor for bleeding.
   d. Monitor for pain and signs of urinary obstruction.
   e. Instruct the client to increase fluid intake to wash out the stone fragments.
   f. Inform the client that ambulation is important.
C. Percutaneous lithotripsy
   1. Percutaneous lithotripsy is performed for stones in the bladder, ureter, or kidney.
   2. Percutaneous lithotripsy is an invasive procedure in which a guide is inserted under fluoroscopy near the area of the stone.
   3. An ultrasonic wave is aimed at the stone to break it into fragments.
   4. Percutaneous lithotripsy may be performed via cystoscopy or nephroscopy.
   5. No incision is required for cystoscopy; however, a small flank incision is needed for nephroscopy.
   6. The client may possibly have an indwelling catheter.
   7. A nephrostomy tube may be placed to administer chemical irrigations to break up the stone; nephrostomy tube may remain in place for 1 to 5 days.
   8. Encourage the client to drink 3000 to 4000 mL of fluid per day following the procedure.
   9. Monitor for and instruct the client to monitor for complications of infection, hemorrhage, and extravasation of fluid into the retroperitoneal cavity.
D. Ureterolithotomy
   1. Ureterolithotomy is an open surgical procedure performed if lithotripsy is not effective.
   2. Ureterolithotomy is performed if the location of the stone is in the ureter.
   3. Incision into the ureter is made through a lower abdominal or flank incision to remove the stone.
   4. The client may have a Penrose drain, a ureteral stent catheter, and an indwelling bladder catheter.
E. Pyelolithotomy
   1. An incision into the kidney is made to remove stones from the renal pelvis.
   2. A large flank incision is required.
   3. The client may have a Penrose drain and an indwelling bladder catheter.

F. Nephrolithotomy
   1. Incision into the kidney is made to remove the stone.
   2. A large flank incision is required.
   3. The client may have a nephrostomy tube and an indwelling bladder catheter.
G. Partial or total nephrectomy
   1. Partial or total nephrectomy is performed for extensive kidney damage, renal infection, or severe obstruction and to prevent stone recurrence.
   2. Postoperative interventions
      a. The plan of care is focused based on the incision location and the type of drainage tubes present.
      b. Monitor the incision, particularly if a Penrose drain is in place, because it will drain large amounts of urine.
      c. Protect the skin from urinary drainage.
      d. Place an ostomy pouch over the Penrose drain to protect the skin if urinary drainage is excessive.
      e. Monitor the nephrostomy tube, which may be attached to a drainage bag for a free flow of urine.
      f. Do not irrigate catheters unless specifically prescribed.
      g. Monitor indwelling Foley catheter for drainage.
      h. Encourage fluid intake to ensure a urine output of 2500 to 3000 mL or more per day.
      i. Monitor intake and output closely.
      j. Determine the composition of stone from laboratory analysis.
      k. Instruct the client in dietary restrictions if required.
      l. Instruct the client about medications that may be needed for long term to reduce the development of calculuses.
      m. Medications prescribed for calcium stones may include phosphates, thiazide diuretics, and allopurinol (Zyloprim).
      n. Pyridoxine or magnesium oxide may be prescribed for clients with oxalate stones.
      o. Allopurinol (Zyloprim) may be prescribed for clients with oxalate and uric acid stones.
      p. Long-term use of antibiotics may be prescribed for struvite or cystine stones.

XXI. KIDNEY TUMORS
A. Description
   1. Kidney tumors may be benign or malignant, bilateral or unilateral.
   2. Common sites of metastasis include bone, lungs, liver, spleen, or other kidney.
   3. The exact cause of renal carcinoma is unknown.
B. Assessment
   1. Dull flank pain
   2. Palpable renal mass
   3. Painless gross hematuria
C. Radical nephrectomy
   1. Description

a. Radical nephrectomy is removal of the entire kidney, adjacent adrenal gland, and renal artery and vein.

b. Radiation therapy and possibly chemotherapy may follow radical nephrectomy.

2. Postoperative interventions

a. Monitor vital signs

b. Monitor abdomen for distention caused by bleeding.

c. Check bed linens under the client for bleeding.

d. Monitor for hypotension, decreases in urinary output, and alterations in level of consciousness as indicating signs of hemorrhage.

e. Monitor for signs of adrenal insufficiency.

f. In clients with adrenal insufficiency, a large urinary output followed by hypotension and subsequent **oliguria** occurs.

g. Administer fluids and packed red blood cells intravenously as prescribed.

h. Monitor intake and output and daily weight.

i. Monitor for a urinary output of 30 to 50 mL an hour to ensure adequate renal function.

j. Monitor urine for specific gravity.

k. Maintain semi-Fowler position.

l. Monitor for signs of respiratory complications related to surgery.

m. Encourage coughing and deep-breathing exercises.

n. Monitor bowel sounds for paralytic ileus.

o. Apply antiembolism stockings as prescribed.

p. Do not irrigate (unless specifically prescribed) or manipulate the nephrostomy tube if in place.

q. Administer pain medications as prescribed.

XXII. BLADDER TRAUMA

A. Description

1. Bladder trauma occurs following a blunt or penetrating injury to the lower abdomen.

2. Penetrating wounds occur as a result of stabbing, gunshot wound, or other objects piercing the abdominal wall.

3. A fractured pelvis that causes bone fragments to puncture the bladder is the most common cause of bladder trauma.

4. A blunt trauma causes compression of the abdominal wall and the bladder.

B. Assessment

1. **Anuria**

2. Hematuria

3. Pain over the costovertebral area

4. Nausea and vomiting

C. Interventions

1. Monitor vital signs.

2. Monitor for hematuria, hemorrhage, and signs of shock.

3. Promote bed rest.

4. Monitor pain level.

5. Prepare the client for insertion of a suprapubic catheter to aid in urinary drainage if prescribed.

6. Prepare the client for surgical repair of the laceration if prescribed.

XXIII. EPIDIDYMITIS

A. Description

1. Epididymitis is an acute or chronic inflammation of the epididymis that occurs as a result of a UTI, a sexually transmitted disease, prostatitis, or long-term use of a Foley catheter.

2. The infective organism passes upward through the urethra and ejaculatory duct, along the vas deferens to the epididymis.

B. Assessment

1. Scrotal pain

2. Groin pain

3. Swelling in scrotum and groin

4. Pus and bacteria in the urine

5. Fever and chills

6. Abscess development

C. Interventions

1. Encourage fluid intake.

2. Encourage bed rest with the scrotum elevated to prevent traction on the spermatic cord, to facilitate drainage, and to relieve pain.

3. Instruct the client in the intermittent application of cold compresses to scrotum.

4. Instruct the client in the use of sitz baths.

5. Instruct the client in the administration of antibiotics for self and sexual partner if chlamydial or gonorrheal infection is the cause.

6. Instruct the client to avoid lifting, straining, and sexual contact until the infection subsides.

XXIV. PROSTATITIS

A. Description

1. Prostatitis is an inflammation of the prostate gland, which can be caused by an infectious agent (bacterial) or by tissue hyperplasia (abacterial).

2. Bacterial type occurs as a result of the organism reaching the prostate via the urethra or the bloodstream.

3. Abacterial type usually occurs following a viral illness or a decrease in sexual activity.

B. Assessment

1. Bacterial prostatitis

a. Fever and chills

b. Dysuria

c. Urethral discharge

d. Prostate is tender, indurated, and warm to the touch

e. Urethral discharge on palpation of prostate

f. White blood cells found in prostatic secretions

2. Abacterial prostatitis

a. Backache

b. Dysuria

c. Perineal pain

d. Frequency

e. Hematuria

f. Irregularly enlarged, firm, and tender prostate

C. Interventions

1. Encourage adequate fluid intake.

2. Instruct the client in the use of sitz baths to promote comfort.

3. Administer antibiotics, analgesics, antispasmodics, and stool softeners as prescribed.

4. Inform the client of activities to drain the prostate, such as intercourse, masturbation, and prostatic massage.

5. Instruct the client to avoid spicy foods, coffee, alcohol, prolonged automobile rides, and sexual intercourse during an acute inflammation.

XXV. BENIGN PROSTATIC HYPERTROPHY OR HYPERPLASIA

A. Description

1. A slow enlargement of the prostate gland occurs, with hypertrophy and hyperplasia of normal tissue.

2. The enlargement causes narrowing of the urethra and results in partial or complete obstruction.

3. The cause is unknown, and the disorder usually occurs in men older than 50 years.

B. Assessment

1. Urgency, frequency, and hesitancy

2. Changes in size and force of urinary stream

3. Retention

4. Dribbling

5. Nocturia

6. Hematuria

7. Urinary stasis

8. UTIs

C. Interventions

1. Encourage fluid intake of up to 2000 to 3000 mL per day unless contraindicated.

2. Prepare for bladder drainage via urinary catheterization for distention.

3. Avoid administering medications that cause urinary retention, such as anticholinergics, antihistamines, and decongestants.

4. Administer finasteride (Proscar) as prescribed to shrink the prostate gland and improve urine flow.

5. Prepare the client for surgery as prescribed (Box 61-14)

D. Surgical interventions and postoperative care (Refer to Chapter 51.)

BOX 61-14

Surgical Interventions for Benign Prostatic Hyperplasia

Perineal prostatectomy
Retropubic prostatectomy
Suprapubic prostatectomy
Transurethral resection of the prostate

XXVI. KIDNEY TRANSPLANTATION

A. Description

1. A human kidney from a compatible donor is implanted into a recipient.

2. Kidney transplantation is performed for irreversible kidney failure.

3. The recipient must take immunosuppressive medications for life.

B. Living related donors

1. The most desirable source of kidneys for transplant is living related donors who match the client closely.

2. Donors are screened for ABO blood group, tissue-specific antigen, human leukocyte antigen suitability, and mixed lymphocyte culture index (histocompatibility).

3. Donor must be in excellent health with two properly functioning kidneys.

4. The emotional well-being of the donor is determined.

5. Complete understanding of the donation process and outcome is necessary.

C. Cadaver donors

1. Cadaver donors must meet criteria of brain death.

2. Cadaver donors must be under 60 years of age.

3. Cadaver donors must have normal renal function.

4. No malignant disease outside of the central nervous system can be present.

5. No generalized infection can be present.

6. No abdominal or renal trauma can be present.

7. Potential donor must have a negative hepatitis B antigen and negative human immunodeficiency virus antibody.

8. Continuous ventilation and heartbeat are maintained until the kidneys are removed surgically.

9. Normal BP must be present.

10. Once the potential donor has demonstrated cerebral death, restoration of intravascular volume, weaning from vasopressors, and establishing diuresis are crucial.

D. Warm ischemic time

1. Warm ischemic time is the time elapsed between the cessation of perfusion and cooling of the kidney and the time required for anastomosis of the kidney.

2. Maximal allowable warm ischemic time is 30 to 60 minutes.

3. Kidney can be cooled, and then the maximum time for transplantation is increased to 24 to 48 hours.

E. Preoperative interventions

1. Verify histocompatibility tests of identical twin or family member.

2. Administer immunosuppressive medications to recipient as prescribed for 2 days before the transplantation, if this is possible.

3. Maintain protective isolation.

4. Verify that **hemodialysis** of the recipient was completed 24 hours before the transplant.

5. Ensure that the client is free of any infections.
6. Assess renal function studies.
7. Encourage discussion of feelings of the donor and the recipient.

F. Postoperative interventions

1. Kidney begins to function immediately, or it may be delayed a few days.
2. **Hemodialysis** is performed until adequate kidney function is established.
3. Monitor vital signs.
4. Monitor intake and output.
5. Monitor urine output every hour.
6. Monitor daily laboratory studies, urine for blood and specific gravity, daily weight, pulse oximetry, and blood urea nitrogen and creatinine levels.
7. Maintain the client in semi-Fowlers position.
8. Monitor for patency of the Foley catheter.
9. Note that urine is pink and bloody initially but gradually returns to normal within several days to weeks.
10. Monitor for gross hematuria and clots, which are not expected, and notify the physician if they occur.
11. Monitor the three-way bladder irrigation, if prescribed, to prevent blood clot formation.
12. Note that the Foley catheter should be removed as soon as possible to prevent infection.
13. Maintain protective isolation precautions and monitor for infection.
14. Monitor IV fluids closely and for fluid overload.
15. Begin oral fluids as prescribed.
16. Monitor for bowel sounds and initiate diet as prescribed when bowel sounds return.
17. Maintain good oral hygiene, monitoring for stomatitis and bacterial and fungal infections.
18. Encourage coughing and deep-breathing exercises.
19. Maintain strict aseptic technique with wound care.
20. Administer medications as prescribed, which may include antifungal medications, antibiotics, immunosuppressive agents, and corticosteroids.
21. Assess for organ rejection.
22. Promote live donor and recipient relationship.
23. Monitor client and recipient for depression.

G. Graft rejection: Except for identical twin donor and recipient, the major postoperative complication is graft rejection.

1. Assessment
   a. Fever
   b. Malaise
   c. Elevated white blood cell count
   d. Graft tenderness
   e. Signs of deteriorating renal function
   f. Acute hypertension
   g. Anemia
2. Hyperacute rejection
   a. Hyperacute rejection occurs immediately after surgery to 48 hours postoperatively.

BOX 61-15

Client Instructions Following Kidney Transplant

Avoid prolonged periods of sitting.
Recognize the signs and symptoms of infection and rejection.
Avoid contact sports.
Avoid exposure to persons with infections.
Use medications as prescribed, and maintain immunosuppressive therapy for life.
Know the signs and symptoms that require the need to contact the physician.
Ensure follow-up care.

---

   b. Interventions: Removal of rejected kidney.
3. Acute rejection
   a. Acute rejection occurs within 6 weeks postoperative but can occur as late as 2 years.
   b. Acute rejection is potentially reversible with increased immunosuppression.
   c. Interventions: High doses of corticosteroids are administered; if corticosteroids are ineffective, monoclonal antibodies may be administered.
4. Chronic rejection
   a. Chronic rejection occurs slowly months to years after transplant.
   b. Chronic rejection can be irreversible.
   c. Chronic rejection mimics **chronic renal failure.**
   d. Interventions: Immunosuppressive medications
5. Client instructions following kidney transplant (Box 61-15)

PRACTICE QUESTIONS

1. The nurse is caring for the client who has had a renal biopsy. Which of the following interventions would the nurse avoid in the care of the client after this procedure?
   1. Encouraging fluids to at least 3 L in the first 24 hours
   2. Administering narcotics as needed
   3. Testing serial samples with dipsticks for occult blood
   4. Ambulating the client in the room and hall for short distances
2. The client with urolithiasis has a history of chronic urinary tract infections. The nurse concludes that this client most likely has which of the following types of urinary stones?
   1. Calcium oxalate
   2. Uric acid
   3. Struvite
   4. Cystine
3. The client who has a history of gout also is diagnosed with urolithiasis. The stones are determined to be of uric acid type. The nurse gives the client instructions in foods to limit, which include

1. Liver.
2. Apples.
3. Carrots.
4. Milk.

4. The nurse is receiving in transfer from the postanesthesia care unit a client who has had percutaneous ultrasonic lithotripsy for calculuses in the renal pelvis. The nurse anticipates that the client's care will involve monitoring which of the following?
   1. Suprapubic tube
   2. Ureteral stent
   3. Nephrostomy tube
   4. Jackson-Pratt drain

5. The client arrives at the emergency department with complaints of low abdominal pain and hematuria. The client is afebrile. The nurse next assesses the client to determine a history of
   1. Renal cancer in the client's family.
   2. Blow or trauma to the bladder or abdomen.
   3. Glomerulonephritis.
   4. Pyelonephritis.

6. The client is admitted to the emergency department following a motor vehicle accident. The client was wearing a lap seat belt when the accident occurred. The client has hematuria and lower abdominal pain. To determine further whether the pain is due to bladder trauma, the nurse asks the client if the pain is referred to which of the following areas?
   1. Shoulder
   2. Umbilicus
   3. Costovertebral angle
   4. Hip

7. The female client is admitted to the emergency department following a fall from a horse. The physician orders insertion of a Foley catheter. The nurse notes blood at the urinary meatus while preparing for the procedure. The nurse should
   1. Use extra povidone-iodine solution in cleansing the meatus.
   2. Use a smaller size catheter.
   3. Administer pain medication before inserting the catheter.
   4. Notify the physician.

8. A nurse is assessing the patency of an arteriovenous fistula in the left arm of a client who is receiving hemodialysis for the treatment of chronic renal failure. Which finding indicates that the fistula is patent?
   1. Absence of a bruit on auscultation of the fistula
   2. Palpation of a thrill over the fistula
   3. Presence of a radial pulse in the left wrist
   4. Capillary refill less than 3 seconds in the nail beds of the fingers on the left hand

9. The male client has a tentative diagnosis of urethritis. The nurse assesses the client for which of the following manifestations of the disorder?
   1. Hematuria and penile discharge
   2. Hematuria and pyuria
   3. Dysuria and proteinuria
   4. Dysuria and penile discharge

10. The nurse is planning a teaching session with the female client diagnosed with urethritis caused by infection with chlamydia. The nurse would plan to include which of the following points in the teaching session?
    1. The most serious complication of this infection is sterility.
    2. The infection can be prevented by using spermicide to alter the pH in the perineal area.
    3. Medication therapy should be continued for 3 weeks without interruption.
    4. Sexual partners during the last 12 months should be notified and treated.

11. The client with chlamydial infection has received instructions on self-care and prevention of further infection. The nurse determines that the client needs further reinforcement if the client states to
    1. Reduce the chance of reinfection by limiting the number of sexual partners.
    2. Use latex condoms to prevent disease transmission.
    3. Return to the clinic as requested for follow-up culture in 1 week.
    4. Use doxycycline prophylactically to prevent symptoms of chlamydia.

12. The nurse is assessing the client with epididymitis. The nurse anticipates which of the following findings on physical examination?
    1. Fever, diarrhea, groin pain, and ecchymosis
    2. Fever, nausea and vomiting, and painful scrotal edema
    3. Diarrhea, groin pain, and scrotal edema
    4. Nausea and vomiting, and scrotal edema with ecchymosis

13. The client has epididymitis as a complication of urinary tract infection. The nurse is giving the client instructions to prevent a recurrence. The nurse determines that the client needs further instruction if the client states to
    1. Drink increased amounts of fluids.
    2. Continue to take antibiotics until all symptoms are gone.
    3. Limit the force of the stream during voiding.
    4. Use condoms to eliminate contracting chlamydia and gonorrhea.

14. The client complains of fever, perineal pain, and urinary urgency, frequency, and dysuria. To assess whether the client's problem is related to bacterial prostatitis, the nurse would look at the results of the prostate examination, which should reveal that the prostate gland is
    1. Tender, indurated, and warm to the touch.
    2. Soft and swollen.
    3. Tender and edematous with ecchymosis.
    4. Reddened, swollen, and boggy.

15. The nurse is taking the history of a client who has had benign prostatic hyperplasia in the past. To determine whether the client currently is experiencing difficulty, the nurse asks the client about the presence of which of the following early symptoms?
    1. Urge incontinence
    2. Nocturia
    3. Decreased force in the stream of urine
    4. Urinary retention

16. The client who has a cold is seen in the emergency room with inability to void. Because the client has a history of benign prostatic hyperplasia, the nurse determines that the client should be questioned about the use of which of the following medications?
    1. Diuretics
    2. Antibiotics
    3. Antitussives
    4. Decongestants

17. The client with chronic renal failure is at risk of developing dementia related to excessive absorption of aluminum. The nurse teaches the client that this is the reason that the client is being prescribed which of the following phosphate-binding agents?
    1. Alu-Cap (aluminium hydroxide)
    2. Tums (calcium carbonate)
    3. Amphojel (aluminium hydroxide)
    4. Basaljel (aluminium hydroxide)

18. The client newly diagnosed with chronic renal failure recently has begun hemodialysis. Knowing that the client is at risk for disequilibrium syndrome, the nurse assesses the client during dialysis for
    1. Hypertension, tachycardia, and fever
    2. Hypotension, bradycardia, and hypothermia
    3. Restlessness, irritability, and generalized weakness
    4. Headache, deteriorating level of consciousness, and twitching

19. A client with chronic renal failure has completed a hemodialysis treatment. The nurse would use which of the following standard indicators to evaluate the client's status after dialysis?
    1. Potassium level and weight
    2. Blood urea nitrogen and creatinine levels
    3. Vital signs and blood urea nitrogen
    4. Vital signs and weight

20. The hemodialysis client with a left arm fistula is at risk for steal syndrome. The nurse assesses this client for which of the following manifestations?
    1. Warmth, redness, and pain in the left hand
    2. Pallor, diminished pulse, and pain in the left hand
    3. Edema and reddish discoloration of the left arm
    4. Aching pain, pallor, and edema of the left arm

21. The nurse is reviewing the client's record and notes that the physician has documented that the client has a renal disorder. On review of the laboratory results, the nurse most likely would expect to note which of the following?
    1. Elevated blood urea nitrogen

2. Decreased hemoglobin
3. Decreased red blood cell count
4. Decreased white blood cell count

22. The nurse is preparing to care for the client following a renal scan. Which of the following would the nurse include in the plan of care?
    1. Place the client on radiation precautions for 18 hours.
    2. Save all urine in a radiation safe container for 18 hours.
    3. Limit contact with the client to 20 minutes per hour.
    4. No special precautions except to wear gloves if in contact with the client's urine.

23. The client is scheduled for an intravenous pyelogram. Before the test the priority nursing action would be to
    1. Administer an oral preparation of radiopaque dye.
    2. Restrict fluids.
    3. Determine a history of allergies.
    4. Administer a sedative.

24. Following a renal biopsy, the client complains of pain at the biopsy site that radiates to the front of the abdomen. The nurse interprets this complaint and further assesses the client for
    1. Bleeding.
    2. Infection.
    3. Renal colic.
    4. A normal expected pain.

25. A client is admitted to the hospital and has a diagnosis of early stage chronic renal failure. Which of the following would the nurse expect to note on assessment of the client?
    1. Polyuria
    2. Polydypsia
    3. Oliguria
    4. Anuria

26. The client with chronic renal failure returns to the nursing unit following a hemodialysis treatment. On assessment the nurse notes that the client's temperature is 100.2° F. Which of the following is the most appropriate nursing action?
    1. Encourage fluids.
    2. Notify the physician.
    3. Monitor the site of the shunt for infection.
    4. Continue to monitor vital signs.

27. The nurse is performing an assessment on a client who has returned from the dialysis unit following hemodialysis. The client is complaining of a headache and nausea and is extremely restless. Which of the following is the most appropriate nursing action?
    1. Notify the physician.
    2. Monitor the client.
    3. Elevate the head of the bed.
    4. Medicate the client for nausea.

28. The nurse is assisting a client on a low-potassium diet to select food items from the menu. Which of

the following food items, if selected by the client, would indicate an understanding of this dietary restriction?

1. Cantaloupe
2. Spinach
3. Lima beans
4. Strawberries

29. The nurse is reviewing the list of components contained in the peritoneal dialysis solution with the client. The client asks the nurse about the purpose of the glucose contained in the solution. The nurse bases the response knowing that the glucose

1. Prevents excess glucose from being removed from the client.
2. Decreases the risk of peritonitis.
3. Prevents disequilibrium syndrome.
4. Increases osmotic pressure to produce ultra-filtration.

30. The nurse is preparing to care for a client receiving peritoneal dialysis. Which of the following would be included in the nursing plan of care to prevent the major complication associated with peritoneal dialysis?

1. Monitor the client's level of consciousness.
2. Maintain strict aseptic technique.
3. Add heparin to the dialysate solution.
4. Change the catheter site dressing daily.

31. A client newly diagnosed with renal failure is receiving peritoneal dialysis. During the infusion of the dialysate the client complains of abdominal pain. Which action by the nurse is most appropriate?

1. Slow the infusion.
2. Decrease the amount to be infused.
3. Explain that the pain will subside after the first few exchanges.
4. Stop the dialysis.

32. The nurse is instructing a client with diabetes mellitus about peritoneal dialysis. The nurse tells the client that it is important to maintain the dwell time for the dialysis at the prescribed time because of the risk of

1. Infection.
2. Hyperglycemia.
3. Fluid overload.
4. Disequilibrium syndrome.

33. The nurse is monitoring an 88-year-old woman at risk for developing a urinary tract infection. Which of the following, if noted in the client, would alert the nurse to the possibility of the presence of a urinary tract infection?

1. Fever
2. Frequency
3. Confusion
4. Urgency

34. The client passes a urinary stone, and laboratory analysis of the stone indicates that it is composed of calcium oxalate. Based on this analysis, which of

the following would the nurse specifically include in the dietary instructions?

1. Increase intake of meat, fish, plums, and cranberries.
2. Avoid citrus fruits and citrus juices.
3. Avoid green, leafy vegetables such as spinach.
4. Increase intake of dairy products.

35. The client returns to the nursing unit following a pyelolithotomy for removal of a kidney stone. A Penrose drain is in place. Which of the following would the nurse include in the client's postoperative plan of care?

1. Sterile irrigation of the Penrose drain
2. Frequent dressing changes around the Penrose drain
3. Weighing dressings
4. Maintaining the client's position on the affected side

36. The nurse is caring for a client following a kidney transplant. The client develops oliguria. Which of the following would the nurse anticipate to be prescribed as the treatment for the oliguria?

1. Encourage fluid intake
2. Administration of diuretics
3. Irrigation of the Foley catheter
4. Restricting fluids

37. A week after kidney transplantation the client develops a temperature of 101° F, the blood pressure is elevated, and the kidney is tender. The x-ray film results indicate that the transplanted kidney is enlarged. Based on these assessment findings, the nurse would suspect which of the following?

1. Acute rejection
2. Chronic rejection
3. Kidney infection
4. Kidney obstruction

38. The client with benign prostatic hyperplasia undergoes a transurethral resection of the prostate. Postoperatively, the client is receiving continuous bladder irrigations. The nurse assesses the client for signs of transurethral resection syndrome. Which of the following assessment data would indicate the onset of this syndrome?

1. Bradycardia and confusion
2. Tachycardia and diarrhea
3. Decreased urinary output and bladder spasms
4. Increased urinary output and anemia

39. The client is admitted to the hospital with a diagnosis of benign prostatic hyperplasia, and a transurethral resection of the prostate is performed. Four hours after surgery the nurse takes the client's vital signs and empties the urinary drainage bag. Which of the following assessment findings would indicate the need to notify the physician?

1. Red bloody urine
2. Urinary output of 200 mL greater than intake

3. Blood pressure of 100/50 mmHg, pulse 130 beats per minute
4. Pain related to bladder spasms

40. A client is diagnosed with polycystic kidney disease and the nurse provides information to the client about the treatment plan. The nurse determines that the client needs additional information if the client states that which of the following is a component of the treatment plan?
    1. Sodium restriction
    2. Antihypertensive medications
    3. Increased water intake
    4. Genetic counseling

41. The nurse is caring for the client who has undergone renal angiography using the left femoral artery for access. The nurse evaluates that the client is experiencing a complication of the procedure if which of the following observations is made?
    1. Urine output 50 mL/hour
    2. Absence of hematoma in the left groin
    3. Blood pressure 110/74 mmHg
    4. Pallor and coolness of the left leg

42. The nurse has given the client with polycystic disease information about management of the disorder and prevention and recognition of complications. The nurse determines that the client understands the instructions if the client states that there is no reason to be concerned about
    1. A lowered blood pressure.
    2. Onset of shortness of breath.
    3. A fever.
    4. Burning on urination.

43. The client with prostatitis following kidney infection has received instructions on management of the condition at home and prevention of recurrence. The nurse determines that the client understood the instructions if the client verbalized to
    1. Keep fluid intake to a minimum to decrease the need to void.
    2. Exercise as much as possible to stimulate circulation.
    3. Stop antibiotic therapy when pain subsides.
    4. Use warm sitz baths and analgesics to increase comfort.

44. The client with crush injury to the right lower leg develops acute renal failure. The nurse interprets that this type of renal failure is due to
    1. Prerenal causes.
    2. Renal causes.
    3. Postrenal causes.
    4. Extrarenal causes.

45. The client with acute renal failure has a serum potassium level of 5.8 mEq/L. The nurse would plan which of the following as a priority action?
    1. Allow an extra 500 mL fluid intake to dilute the electrolyte concentration.
    2. Encourage increased vegetables in the diet.

3. Place the client on a cardiac monitor.
4. Check the sodium level.

46. The client with chronic renal failure who is scheduled for hemodialysis this morning is due to receive a daily dose of enalapril (Vasotec). The nurse should plan to administer this medication
    1. Just before dialysis.
    2. During dialysis.
    3. On return from dialysis.
    4. The day after dialysis.

47. The client with chronic renal failure has an indwelling catheter for peritoneal dialysis in the abdomen. The client spills water on the catheter dressing while bathing. The nurse should immediately
    1. Reinforce the dressing.
    2. Change the dressing.
    3. Flush the peritoneal dialysis catheter.
    4. Scrub the catheter with povidone-iodine.

48. The client being hemodialyzed suddenly becomes short of breath and complains of chest pain. The client is tachycardic, pale, and anxious. The nurse suspects air embolism. The nurse should
    1. Continue dialysis at a slower rate after checking the lines for air.
    2. Discontinue dialysis and notify the physician.
    3. Monitor vital signs every 15 minutes for the next hour.
    4. Bolus the client with 500 mL normal saline to break up the air embolus.

49. The nurse has completed client teaching with the hemodialysis client about self-monitoring between hemodialysis treatments. The nurse determines that the client best understands the information given if the client states to record daily the
    1. Pulse and respiratory rate.
    2. Intake and output and weight.
    3. Blood urea nitrogen and creatinine levels.
    4. Activity log.

50. The client with an arteriovenous shunt in place for hemodialysis is at risk for bleeding. The nurse would do which of the following as a priority action to prevent this complication from occurring?
    1. Check the results of the prothrombin time as they are ordered.
    2. Observe the site once per shift.
    3. Check the shunt for the presence of bruit and thrill.
    4. Ensure that small clamps are attached to the arteriovenous shunt dressing.

CRITICAL THINKING: FILL IN THE BLANK

The nurse is monitoring a client receiving peritoneal dialysis. The nurse notes that a client's outflow is less than the inflow. Which nursing action is most appropriate initially?

Answer: _____

ANSWERS

1. 4

Rationale: Following renal biopsy, the nurse ensures that the client remains in bed for at least 24 hours. Vital signs and puncture site assessments are done frequently during this time. Encouraging fluids is done to reduce possible clot formation at the biopsy site. Serial urine samples are hematested with urine dipsticks to evaluate bleeding. Narcotic analgesics often are needed to manage the renal colic pain that some clients feel after this procedure.

Test-Taking Strategy: Use the process of elimination. Note the key word "avoid." Eliminate options 2 and 3 by recalling that pain and bleeding are potential concerns after this procedure. From the remaining options, recall that fluids will reduce clotting at the site, whereras ambulation could initiate or enhance bleeding at the biopsy site. Review postprocedure care if you had difficulty with this question.

Level of Cognitive Ability: Application
Client Needs: Physiological Integrity
Integrated Process: Nursing Process—implementation
Content Area: Adult health—renal
Reference: Ignatavicius, D., & Workman, M. (2002). *Medical-surgical nursing: Critical thinking for collaborative care* (4th ed., p. 1610). Philadelphia: W. B. Saunders.

2. 3

Rationale: Struvite stones commonly are referred to as infection stones because they form in urine that is alkaline and rich in ammonia, such as with a urinary tract infection. Calcium oxalate stones result from increased calcium intake or conditions that raise serum calcium concentrations. Uric acid stones occur in clients with gout. Cystine stones are rare and occur in clients with a genetic defect that results in decreased renal absorption of the amino acid cystine.

Test-Taking Strategy: Use the process of elimination. Focus on the data in the question. Noting that the client has a history of chronic urinary tract infections will direct you to option 3. Review the causes of the various types of stones if you had difficulty with this question.

Level of Cognitive Ability: Analysis
Client Needs: Physiological Integrity
Integrated Process: Nursing Process—analysis
Content Area: Adult health—renal
References: Ignatavicius, D., & Workman, M. (2002). *Medical-surgical nursing: Critical thinking for collaborative care* (4th ed., p. 1634). Philadelphia: W. B. Saunders.
Lewis, S., Heitkemper, M., & Dirksen, S. (2004). *Medical-surgical nursing: Assessment and management of clinical problems* (6th ed., p. 1186). St. Louis: Mosby.

3. 1

Rationale: The client with uric acid stones should avoid foods containing high amounts of purines. This includes limiting or avoiding organ meats such as liver, brain, heart, kidney, and sweetbreads. Other foods to avoid include herring, sardines, anchovies, meat extracts, consommés, and gravies. Foods that are low in purines include all fruits, many vegetables, milk, cheese, eggs, refined cereals, sugars and sweets, coffee, tea, chocolate, and carbonated beverages.

Test-Taking Strategy: Use the process of elimination. Begin by examining the options and classifying the types of food sources they represent. Options 2 and 3 represent foods that are grown, whereas options 1 and 4 represent foods that derive from animal sources. Because purines are end products of protein metabolism, you would eliminate options 2 and 3 first. From the remaining options, recall that organ meats such as liver provide a greater quantity of protein than milk. Review foods high in purines if you had difficulty with this question.

Level of Cognitive Ability: Application
Client Needs: Physiological Integrity
Integrated Process: Teaching/Learning
Content Area: Adult health—renal
Reference: Phipps, W., Monahan, F., Sands, J., Marek, J., & Neighbors, M. (2003). *Medical-surgical nursing: Health and illness perspectives* (7th ed., p. 1220). St. Louis: Mosby.

4. 3

Rationale: A nephrostomy tube is put in place after percutaneous ultrasonic lithotripsy to treat calculuses in the renal pelvis. The client also may have a Foley catheter to drain urine produced by the other kidney. The nurse monitors the drainage from each of these tubes and strains the urine to detect elimination of the calculus fragments.

Test-Taking Strategy: Use the process of elimination. Note that the question states that the calculuses are in the renal pelvis. This will direct you to option 3. Review care to the client following this procedure if you had difficulty with this question.

Level of Cognitive Ability: Analysis
Client Needs: Physiological Integrity
Integrated Process: Nursing Process—assessment
Content Area: Adult health—renal
Reference: Ignatavicius, D., & Workman, M. (2002). *Medical-surgical nursing: Critical thinking for collaborative care* (4th ed., p. 1635). Philadelphia: W. B. Saunders.

5. 2

Rationale: Bladder trauma or injury should be considered or suspected in the client with low abdominal pain and hematuria. Renal cancer would not cause pain that is felt in the low abdomen; rather pain would be in the flank area. Glomerulonephritis and pyelonephritis would be accompanied by fever and are thus not applicable to the client in this question.

Test-Taking Strategy: Use the process of elimination. Eliminate options 3 and 4, knowing that any inflammatory disease or infection is accompanied by fever. Because this client is afebrile, these are not possible options. Use knowledge of anatomy and pain assessment to select option 2. Pain from renal cancer is a later finding and is localized in the flank area. Review renal assessment techniques if you had difficulty with this question.

Level of Cognitive Ability: Application
Client Needs: Physiological Integrity
Integrated Process: Nursing Process—assessment
Content Area: Adult health—renal
Reference: Ignatavicius, D., & Workman, M. (2002). *Medical-surgical nursing: Critical thinking for collaborative care* (4th ed., p. 1639). Philadelphia: W. B. Saunders.

6. 1

Rationale: Bladder trauma or injury is characterized by lower abdominal pain that may radiate to one of the shoulders. Bladder injury pain does not radiate to the umbilicus, costovertebral angle, or hip.

Test-Taking Strategy: Use the process of elimination. Recall the concepts related to dermatomes of the body and pain characteristics of bladder trauma. Review the characteristics of bladder trauma if you had difficulty with this question.

Level of Cognitive Ability: Analysis
Client Needs: Physiological Integrity
Integrated Process: Nursing Process—assessment
Content Area: Adult health—renal
Reference: Ignatavicius, D., & Workman, M. (2002). *Medical-surgical nursing: Critical thinking for collaborative care* (4th ed., p. 1639). Philadelphia: W. B. Saunders.

7. 4

Rationale: The presence of blood at the urinary meatus may indicate urethral trauma or disruption. The nurse notifies the physician, knowing that the client should not be catheterized until the cause of the bleeding is determined by diagnostic testing.

Test-Taking Strategy: Use the process of elimination. Noting the key words "blood at the urinary meatus" will direct you to option 4. Review the assessment findings in a client with trauma to the urinary tract if you had difficulty with this question.

Level of Cognitive Ability: Application
Client Needs: Physiological Integrity
Integrated Process: Nursing Process—implementation
Content Area: Adult health—renal
References: Ignatavicius, D., & Workman, M. (2002). *Medical-surgical nursing: Critical thinking for collaborative care* (4th ed., p. 1639). Philadelphia: W. B. Saunders.
Phipps, W., Monahan, F., Sands, J., Marek, J., & Neighbors, M. (2003). *Medical-surgical nursing: Health and illness perspectives* (7th ed., p. 1241). St. Louis: Mosby.

8. 2

Rationale: The nurse assesses the patency of the fistula by palpating for the presence of a thrill or auscultating for a bruit. The presence of a thrill and bruit indicate patency of the fistula. Although the presence of a radial pulse in the left wrist and capillary refill less than 3 seconds in the nail beds of the fingers on the left hand are normal findings, they do not assess fistula patency.

Test-Taking Strategy: Use the process of elimination. Eliminate options 3 and 4 first because they are similar and assess for adequate circulation in the distal portion of the extremity (not the fistula). From the remaining options, focusing on the issue (patency) and noting the word "absence" in option 1 will assist you in eliminating this option. Review the expected findings when assessing an arteriovenous fistula if you had difficulty with this question.

Level of Cognitive Ability: Analysis
Client Needs: Physiological Integrity
Integrated Process: Nursing Process—analysis
Content Area: Adult health—renal

Reference: Ignatavicius, D., & Workman, M. (2002). *Medical-surgical nursing: Critical thinking for collaborative care* (4th ed., p. 1690). Philadelphia: W. B. Saunders.

9. 4

Rationale: Urethritis in the male client often results from chlamydial infection and is characterized by dysuria, which is accompanied by a clear to mucopurulent discharge. Because this disorder often coexists with gonorrhea, diagnostic tests are done for both and include culture and rapid assays.

Test-Taking Strategy: Use the process of elimination. Recalling that urethritis generally is accompanied by dysuria in the male client will assist you in eliminating options 1 and 2. Knowing that the problem originates in the urethra, not the kidney, will assist you in eliminating option 3 because proteinuria indicates a problem with kidney function. Review the clinical manifestations of urethritis if you had difficulty with this question.

Level of Cognitive Ability: Application
Client Needs: Physiological Integrity
Integrated Process: Nursing Process—assessment
Content Area: Adult health—renal
Reference: Ignatavicius, D., & Workman, M. (2002). *Medical-surgical nursing: Critical thinking for collaborative care* (4th ed., p. 1601). Philadelphia: W. B. Saunders.

10. 1

Rationale: The most serious complication of chlamydial infection is sterility. The infection can be prevented by the use of latex condoms. Chlamydial infection is treated with doxycycline for 7 days or with azithromycin (Zithromax) as a single dose. All sexual partners during the 30 days before diagnosis should be notified, examined, and treated as necessary.

Test-Taking Strategy: Use the process of elimination. Eliminate option 2 first using principles of infection control. Knowing that most courses of antibiotic therapy extend from 7 to 10 days in general may help to eliminate option 3. From the remaining options, you must know that sterility is a serious and permanent complication or that partners within the last month should be notified and treated as needed. Review the teaching points for the client with chlamydia if you had difficulty with this question.

Level of Cognitive Ability: Application
Client Needs: Physiological Integrity
Integrated Process: Teaching/Learning
Content Area: Adult health—renal
Reference: Phipps, W., Monahan, F., Sands, J., Marek, J., & Neighbors, M. (2003). *Medical-surgical nursing: Health and illness perspectives* (7th ed., pp. 1857, 1867). St. Louis: Mosby.

11. 4

Rationale: Antibiotics are not taken prophylactically to prevent acquisition of urethritis from chlamydia. The risk of reinfection can be reduced by limiting the number of sexual partners and by the use of condoms. In some instances, follow-up culture is requested in 4 to 7 days to confirm a cure.

Test-Taking Strategy: Use the process of elimination. Note the key words "needs further reinforcement." Knowing the basic principles of antibiotic therapy will direct you to option 4

because antibiotics are not used intermittently at will for prophylaxis of this infection. Review client teaching related to chlamydial infection if you had difficulty with this question.
Level of Cognitive Ability: Analysis
Client Needs: Health Promotion and Maintenance
Integrated Process: Teaching/Learning
Content Area: Adult health—renal
Reference: Phipps, W., Monahan, F., Sands, J., Marek, J., & Neighbors, M. (2003). *Medical-surgical nursing: Health and illness perspectives* (7th ed., p. 1866). St. Louis: Mosby.

12. 2
Rationale: Typical signs and symptoms of epididymitis include scrotal pain and edema, which often are accompanied by fever, nausea and vomiting, and chills. Epididymitis most often is caused by infection, although sometimes it can be caused by trauma. Epididymitis needs to be distinguished correctly from testicular torsion.
Test-Taking Strategy: Use the process of elimination. Any disorder that ends in "itis" results from inflammation or infection. Therefore an expected finding would be elevated temperature. With this in mind, eliminate options 3 and 4 because they do not contain fever as part of the option. Knowing that ecchymosis results from bleeding, which is not part of this clinical picture, directs you to option 2. Review the clinical manifestations of epididymitis if you had difficulty with this question.
Level of Cognitive Ability: Analysis
Client Needs: Physiological Integrity
Integrated Process: Nursing Process—assessment
Content Area: Adult health—renal
Reference: Ignatavicius, D., & Workman, M. (2002). *Medical-surgical nursing: Critical thinking for collaborative care* (4th ed., p. 1803). Philadelphia: W. B. Saunders.

13. 2
Rationale: The client who experiences epididymitis from urinary tract infection should increase intake of fluids to flush the urinary system. Because organisms can be forced into the vas deferens and epididymis from strain or pressure during voiding, the client should limit the force of the stream. Condom use can help to prevent urethritis and epididymitis. Antibiotics are always taken until the full course of therapy is completed.
Test-Taking Strategy: Use the process of elimination. Note the key words "needs further instruction." Careful reading will direct you to option 2. Remember, antibiotics are not stopped when symptoms subside and must be taken until the full course of therapy is completed. Review client instructions regarding epididymitis if you had difficulty with this question.
Level of Cognitive Ability: Analysis
Client Needs: Health Promotion and Maintenance
Integrated Process: Teaching/Learning
Content Area: Adult health—renal
References: Ignatavicius, D., & Workman, M. (2002). *Medical-surgical nursing: Critical thinking for collaborative care* (4th ed., p. 1803). Philadelphia: W. B. Saunders.
Phipps, W., Monahan, F., Sands, J., Marek, J., & Neighbors, M. (2003). *Medical-surgical nursing: Health and illness perspectives* (7th ed., p. 1826). St. Louis: Mosby.

14. 1
Rationale: The client with prostatitis has a prostate gland that is swollen and tender but that is also warm to the touch, firm, and indurated. Systemic symptoms include fever with chills, perineal and low back pain, and signs of urinary tract infection (which often accompany the disorder).
Test-Taking Strategy: Use the process of elimination. Begin to answer this question by reasoning that inflammation of the prostate gland would cause the area to be tender. This would allow you to eliminate options 2 and 4. Recalling that inflammation is accompanied by local warmth will direct you to option 1. Review the signs of prostatitis if you had difficulty with this question.
Level of Cognitive Ability: Analysis
Client Needs: Physiological Integrity
Integrated Process: Nursing process—assessment
Content Area: Adult health—renal
Reference: Ignatavicius, D., & Workman, M. (2002). *Medical-surgical nursing: Critical thinking for collaborative care* (4th ed., p. 1803). Philadelphia: W. B. Saunders.

15. 3
Rationale: Decreased force in the stream of urine is an early sign of benign prostatic hyperplasia. The stream later becomes weak and dribbling. The client then may develop hematuria, frequency, urgency, urge incontinence, and nocturia. If untreated, complete obstruction and urinary retention can occur.
Test-Taking Strategy: Use the process of elimination. Note the key word "early." If you know that benign prostatic hyperplasia can lead to urinary obstruction, look for the option that identifies the least severe symptom. Review early signs of benign prostatic hyperplasia if you had difficulty with this question.
Level of Cognitive Ability: Application
Client Needs: Physiological Integrity
Integrated Process: Nursing Process—assessment
Content Area: Adult health—renal
Reference: Ignatavicius, D., & Workman, M. (2002). *Medical-surgical nursing: Critical thinking for collaborative care* (4th ed., p. 1874). Philadelphia: W. B. Saunders.

16. 4
Rationale: In the client with benign prostatic hyperplasia, episodes of urinary retention can be triggered by certain medications, such as decongestants, anticholinergics, and antidepressants. The client should be questioned about the use of these medications if the client has urinary retention. Retention also can be precipitated by other factors, such as alcoholic beverages, infection, bed rest, and becoming chilled.
Test-Taking Strategy: Use the process of elimination. The question is asking about medications that could exacerbate or contribute to urinary retention in the client with benign prostatic hyperplasia. Diuretics should help voiding, therefore readily eliminate option 1. Antibiotics should have no effect at all, and thus eliminate option 2. From the remaining options, recalling that medications that contain anticholinergics may cause urinary retention will direct you to option 4. Review the factors that can precipitate urinary retention in the

client with benign prostatic hyperplasia if you had difficulty with this question.
Level of Cognitive Ability: Analysis
Client Needs: Physiological Integrity
Integrated Process: Nursing Process—assessment
Content Area: Adult health—renal
Reference: Ignatavicius, D., & Workman, M. (2002). *Medical-surgical nursing: Critical thinking for collaborative care* (4th ed., p. 1785). Philadelphia: W. B. Saunders.

17. 2
Rationale: Phosphate-binding agents that contain aluminum include Alu-Caps, Basaljel, and Amphojel. These products are made from aluminum hydroxide. Tums are made from calcium carbonate and also bind phosphorus. Tums are prescribed to avoid the occurrence of dementia related to high intake of aluminum. Phosphate-binding agents are needed by the client in renal failure because the kidneys cannot eliminate phosphorus.
Test-Taking Strategy: Use the process of elimination. Option 1 may be eliminated because the name of the medication gives a clue as to its ingredients. Otherwise, specific knowledge of the types of antacids is needed to answer this question accurately. Review the various phosphate-binding agents if you had difficulty with this question.
Level of Cognitive Ability: Application
Client Needs: Physiological Integrity
Integrated Process: Teaching/Learning
Content Area: Pharmacology
Reference: McKenry, L., & Salerno, E. (2001). *Mosby's pharmacology in nursing* (21st ed., p. 213). St. Louis: Mosby.

18. 4
Rationale: Disequilibrium syndrome is characterized by headache, mental confusion, decreasing level of consciousness, nausea, vomiting, twitching, and possible seizure activity. Disequilibrium syndrome is caused by rapid removal of solutes from the body during hemodialysis. At the same time, the blood-brain barrier interferes with the efficient removal of wastes from brain tissue. As a result, water goes into cerebral cells because of the osmotic gradient, causing brain swelling and onset of symptoms. The syndrome most often occurs in clients who are new to dialysis and is prevented by dialyzing for shorter times or at reduced blood flow rates.
Test-Taking Strategy: Use the process of elimination. Focus on the name of the syndrome "disequilibrium" to assist in directing you to option 4. Review the manifestations of this syndrome if you had difficulty with this question.
Level of Cognitive Ability: Analysis
Client Needs: Physiological Integrity
Integrated Process: Nursing Process—assessment
Content Area: Adult health—renal
Reference: Ignatavicius, D., & Workman, M. (2002). *Medical-surgical nursing: Critical thinking for collaborative care* (4th ed., p. 1692). Philadelphia: W. B. Saunders.

19. 4
Rationale: Following dialysis, the client's vital signs are monitored to determine whether the client is remaining hemodynamically stable. Weight is measured and compared with the client's predialysis weight to determine effectiveness of fluid extraction. Laboratory studies are done as per protocol but are not necessarily done after the hemodialysis treatment has been ended.
Test-Taking Strategy: Use the process of elimination. Note the issue, measures to determine the client's status after dialysis. Recalling the purpose of the dialysis will direct you to option 4. Review postdialysis nursing assessments if you had difficulty with this question.
Level of Cognitive Ability: Analysis
Client Needs: Physiological Integrity
Integrated Process: Nursing Process—evaluation
Content Area: Adult health—renal
Reference: Ignatavicius, D., & Workman, M. (2002). *Medical-surgical nursing: Critical thinking for collaborative care* (4th ed., p. 1691). Philadelphia: W. B. Saunders.

20. 2
Rationale: Steal syndrome results from vascular insufficiency after creation of a fistula. The client exhibits pallor and a diminished pulse distal to the fistula. The client also complains of pain distal to the fistula, which is due to tissue ischemia. Warmth, redness, and pain more likely would characterize a problem with infection. The manifestations described in options 3 and 4 are incorrect.
Test-Taking Strategy: You must understand steal syndrome and know the signs and symptoms to answer this question. Review this syndrome and associated signs and symptoms if you had difficulty with this question.
Level of Cognitive Ability: Application
Client Needs: Physiological Integrity
Integrated Process: Nursing Process—assessment
Content Area: Adult health—renal
Reference: Lewis, S., Heitkemper, M., & Dirksen, S. (2004). *Medical-surgical nursing: Assessment and management of clinical problems* (6th ed., p. 1233). St. Louis: Mosby.

21. 1
Rationale: The blood urea nitrogen is a frequently used laboratory test to determine renal function. The blood urea nitrogen starts to rise when the glomerular filtration rate falls below 40% to 60%. A decreased hemoglobin and red blood cell count may be noted if bleeding from the urinarytract occurs or if erythropoietic function by the kidney is impaired. An increased white blood cell count is most likely to be noted in renal disease.
Test-Taking Strategy: Use the process of elimination. Recalling the relationship between the blood urea nitrogen and renal function will direct you to option 1. Review significant laboratory tests related to renal function if you had difficulty with this question.
Level of Cognitive Ability: Analysis
Client Needs: Physiological Integrity
Integrated Process: Nursing Process—assessment
Content Area: Adult health—renal
References: Ignatavicius, D., & Workman, M. (2002). *Medical-surgical nursing: Critical thinking for collaborative care* (4th ed., p. 1665). Philadelphia: W. B. Saunders.
Lewis, S., Heitkemper, M., & Dirksen, S. (2004). *Medical-surgical nursing: Assessment and management of clinical problems* (6th ed., p. 1163). St. Louis: Mosby.

22. 4

Rationale: No specific precautions are necessary following a renal scan. Urination into a commode is acceptable without risk from the small amount of radioactive material to be excreted. The nurse wears gloves to maintain body secretion precautions.

Test-Taking Strategy: Use the process of elimination. Recalling that generally no danger exists from the small amount of radioactive material used in this procedure will direct you to option 4. Review this procedure if you had difficulty with this question.

Level of Cognitive Ability: Application
Client Needs: Safe, Effective Care Environment
Integrated Process: Nursing Process—planning
Content Area: Adult health—renal
Reference: Chernecky, C., & Berger, B. (2001). *Laboratory tests and diagnostic procedures* (3rd ed., p. 907). Philadelphia: W. B. Saunders.

23. 3

Rationale: The iodine-based dye used during the intravenous pyelogram can cause allergic reactions such as itching, hives, rash, a tight feeling in the throat, shortness of breath, and bronchospasm. Assessing for allergies is the priority.

Test-Taking Strategy: Use the process of elimination. Note the key word "priority" in the stem of the question. Use the steps of the nursing process as a guide. Options 1, 2, and 4 address implementation. Option 3 is the only option that addresses assessment. Review preprocedure care for an intravenous pyelogram if you had difficulty with this question.

Level of Cognitive Ability: Application
Client Needs: Physiological Integrity
Integrated Process: Nursing Process—assessment
Content Area: Delegating/Prioritizing
Reference: Chernecky, C., & Berger, B. (2001). *Laboratory tests and diagnostic procedures* (3rd ed., p. 653). Philadelphia: W. B. Saunders.

24. 1

Rationale: If pain originates at the biopsy site and begins to radiate to the flank area and around the front of the abdomen, bleeding should be suspected. Hypotension, a decreasing hematocrit level, and gross or microscopic hematuria also would indicate bleeding. Signs of infection would not appear immediately following a biopsy. Pain of this nature is not normal. No data are given to support the presence of renal colic.

Test-Taking Strategy: Use the process of elimination. Focusing on the data in the question will assist in eliminating options 3 and 4. Recalling that signs of infection may not appear immediately following biopsy will assist you in eliminating option 2. Review the complications following renal biopsy if you had difficulty with this question.

Level of Cognitive Ability: Analysis
Client Needs: Physiological Integrity
Integrated Process: Nursing Process—analysis
Content Area: Adult health—renal
Reference: Ignatavicius, D., & Workman, M. (2002). *Medical-surgical nursing: Critical thinking for collaborative care* (4th ed., p. 1610). Philadelphia: W. B. Saunders.

25. 1

Rationale: Polyuria occurs early in chronic renal failure and if untreated can cause severe dehydration. Polyuria progresses to anuria, and the client loses all normal functions of the kidney. Oliguria and anuria are not early signs, and polydipsia is unrelated to chronic renal failure.

Test-Taking Strategy: Use the process of elimination. Note the key word "early" in the question. Eliminate options 3 and 4 because they are similar. From the remaining options, select option 1 because this option relates to renal function. Review the early and the late signs of chronic renal failure if you had difficulty with this question.

Level of Cognitive Ability: Analysis
Client Needs: Physiological Integrity
Integrated Process: Nursing Process—assessment
Content Area: Adult health—renal
Reference: Lewis, S., Heitkemper, M., & Dirksen, S. (2004). *Medical-surgical nursing: Assessment and management of clinical problems* (6th ed., p. 1211). St. Louis: Mosby.

26. 4

Rationale: The client may have an elevated temperature following dialysis because the dialysis machine warms the blood slightly. If the temperature is elevated excessively and remains elevated, sepsis would be suspected and a blood sample would be obtained as prescribed for culture and sensitivity determinations.

Test-Taking Strategy: Use the process of elimination. Note the key words "most appropriate." Recalling that an elevation in temperature is expected following dialysis will direct you to option 4. Review the normal expected findings following dialysis if you had difficulty with this question.

Level of Cognitive Ability: Application
Client Needs: Physiological Integrity
Integrated Process: Nursing Process—implementation
Content Area: Adult health—renal
References: Ignatavicius, D., & Workman, M. (2002). *Medical-surgical nursing: Critical thinking for collaborative care* (4th ed., p. 1691). Philadelphia: W. B. Saunders.
Lewis, S., Heitkemper, M., & Dirksen, S. (2004). *Medical-surgical nursing: Assessment and management of clinical problems* (6th ed., p. 1215). St. Louis: Mosby.

27. 1

Rationale: Disequilibrium syndrome may be due to the rapid decrease in blood urea nitrogen levels during hemodialysis. These changes can cause cerebral edema that leads to increased intracranial pressure. The client is exhibiting early signs of disequilibrium syndrome and appropriate treatments with anticonvulsive medications and barbiturates may be necessary to prevent a life-threatening situation. The physician must be notified.

Test-Taking Strategy: Use the process of elimination and focus on the client's signs and symptoms. Recalling the complications associated with hemodialysis will direct you to option 1. Review the signs and symptoms of disequilibrium syndrome if you had difficulty with this question.

Level of Cognitive Ability: Application
Client Needs: Physiological Integrity
Integrated Process: Nursing Process—implementation

Content Area: Adult health—renal
Reference: Ignatavicius, D., & Workman, M. (2002). *Medical-surgical nursing: Critical thinking for collaborative care* (4th ed., p. 1692). Philadelphia: W. B. Saunders.

28. 3
Rationale: Cantaloupe (¼ small), spinach (½ cup cooked) and strawberries (1¼ cups) are high-potassium foods and average 7 mEq per serving. Lima beans (⅓ cup) averages 3 mEq per serving.
Test-Taking Strategy: Use the process of elimination. Remembering that many fruits and green, leafy vegetables are high in potassium will assist in directing you to option 3. Review foods that are high in potassium if you had difficulty with this question.
Level of Cognitive Ability: Analysis
Client Needs: Physiological Integrity
Integrated Process: Teaching/Learning
Content Area: Adult health—renal
Reference: Peckenpaugh, N. (2003). *Nutrition essentials and diet therapy* (9th ed., p. 295). Philadelphia: W. B. Saunders.

29. 4
Rationale: Increasing the glucose concentration makes the solution increasingly more hypertonic. The more hypertonic the solution, the greater the osmotic pressure for ultrafiltration and thus the greater the amount of fluid removed from the client during an exchange. Options 1, 2, and 3 do not identify the purpose of the glucose.
Test-Taking Strategy: Use the process of elimination. Knowledge regarding the principles related to ultrafiltration will direct you to option 4. If you had difficulty with this question, review dialysate solutions for peritoneal dialysis.
Level of Cognitive Ability: Application
Client Needs: Physiological Integrity
Integrated Process: Teaching/Learning
Content Area: Adult health—renal
Reference: Ignatavicius, D., & Workman, M. (2002). *Medical-surgical nursing: Critical thinking for collaborative care* (4th ed., p. 1695). Philadelphia: W. B. Saunders.

30. 2
Rationale: The major complication of peritoneal dialysis is peritonitis. Strict aseptic technique is required in caring for the client receiving this treatment. Although option 4 may assist in preventing infection, this option relates to an external site. Options 1 and 3 are unrelated to the major complication of peritoneal dialysis.
Test-Taking Strategy: Use the process of elimination. Visualize this procedure and recall the major concern related to peritonitis. This will direct you to option 2. Review the complications associated with peritoneal dialysis if you had difficulty with this question.
Level of Cognitive Ability: Application
Client Needs: Safe, Effective Care Environment
Integrated Process: Nursing Process—planning
Content Area: Adult health—renal
Reference: Phipps, W., Monahan, F., Sands, J., Marek, J., & Neighbors, M. (2003). *Medical-surgical nursing: Health and illness perspectives* (7th ed., p. 1273). St. Louis: Mosby.

31. 3
Rationale: Pain during the inflow of dialysate is common during the first few exchanges because of peritoneal irritation; however, the pain usually disappears after 1 to 2 weeks of treatment. The infusion amount should not be decreased, and the infusion should not be slowed or stopped.
Test-Taking Strategy: Use the process of elimination. Eliminate options 1, 2, and 4 because they are similar actions. Review the complications associated with peritoneal dialysis and the appropriate nursing actions, if you had difficulty with this question.
Level of Cognitive Ability: Application
Client Needs: Physiological Integrity
Integrated Process: Nursing Process—implementation
Content Area: Adult health—renal
Reference: Ignatavicius, D., & Workman, M. (2002). *Medical-surgical nursing: Critical thinking for collaborative care* (4th ed., p. 1696). Philadelphia: W. B. Saunders.

32. 2
Rationale: An extended dwell time increases the risk of hyperglycemia in the client with diabetes mellitus as a result of absorption of glucose from the dialysate and electrolyte changes. Diabetic clients may require extra insulin when receiving peritoneal dialysis.
Test-Taking Strategy: Use the process of elimination. Noting the client's diagnosis and recalling that the dialysate solution contains glucose will direct you to option 2. Review the complications associated with peritoneal dialysis if you had difficulty with this question.
Level of Cognitive Ability: Application
Client Needs: Physiological Integrity
Integrated Process: Teaching/Learning
Content Area: Adult health—renal
References: Ignatavicius, D., & Workman, M. (2002). *Medical-surgical nursing: Critical thinking for collaborative care* (4th ed., p. 1697). Philadelphia: W. B. Saunders.
Lewis, S., Heitkemper, M., & Dirksen, S. (2004). *Medical-surgical nursing: Assessment and management of clinical problems* (6th ed., p. 1232). St. Louis: Mosby.

33. 3
Rationale: In an older client, the only symptom of a urinary tract infection may be something as vague as increasing mental confusion. Frequency and urgency commonly may occur in an older client. Therefore, these symptoms are not specific to urinary tract infection in the older client. Fever can be associated with a variety of conditions.
Test-Taking Strategy: Use the process of elimination. Note the client's age in the question. Eliminate options 2 and 4 because these symptoms commonly may occur in an older client. Eliminate option 1 next because fever can be associated with a variety of conditions. Review the clinical manifestations of urinary tract infection that occur in the older client if you had difficulty with this question.
Level of Cognitive Ability: Analysis
Client Needs: Physiological Integrity
Integrated Process: Nursing Process—assessment
Content Area: Adult health—renal

Reference: Phipps, W., Monahan, F., Sands, J., Marek, J., & Neighbors, M. (2003). *Medical-surgical nursing: Health and illness perspectives* (7th ed., p. 56). St. Louis: Mosby.

34. 3

Rationale: Oxalate is found in dark green foods such as spinach. Other foods that raise urinary oxalate are rhubarb, strawberries, chocolate, wheat bran, nuts, beets, and tea.

Test-Taking Strategy: Use the process of elimination. Remembering the green, leafy foods are high in oxalate will assist in directing you to option 3. Review the foods high in oxalate if you had difficulty with this question.

Level of Cognitive Ability: Application

Client Needs: Physiological Integrity

Integrated Process: Teaching/Learning

Content Area: Adult health—renal

Reference: Peckenpaugh, N. (2003). *Nutrition essentials and diet therapy* (9th ed., p. 301). Philadelphia: W. B. Saunders.

35. 2

Rationale: Frequent dressing changes around the Penrose drain is required to protect the skin against breakdown from the urinary drainage. If urinary drainage is excessive, an ostomy pouch may be placed over the drain to protect the skin. A Penrose drain is not irrigated. Weighting the dressings is not necessary. Placing the client on the affected side will prevent a free flow of urine through the drain.

Test-Taking Strategy: Use the process of elimination. Identify the issue of the question, which relates to the Penrose drain. This should provide you with the clue that drainage is expected. Eliminate option 3 as the least likely answer. Eliminate option 1 because a Penrose drain is not irrigated. Visualize the effect that positioning on the affected side will have on the client. Review postoperative care following a pyelolithotomy if you had difficulty with this question.

Level of Cognitive Ability: Application

Client Needs: Physiological Integrity

Integrated Process: Nursing Process—planning

Content Area: Adult health—renal

References: Ignatavicius, D., & Workman, M. (2002). *Medical-surgical nursing: Critical thinking for collaborative care* (4th ed., p. 290). Philadelphia: W. B. Saunders.

Phipps, W., Monahan, F., Sands, J., Marek, J., & Neighbors, M. (2003). *Medical-surgical nursing: Health and illness perspectives* (7th ed., p. 424). St. Louis: Mosby.

36. 2

Rationale: To increase urinary output, diuretics and osmotic agents are administered. The client should be monitored closely because fluid overload can cause hypertension, congestive heart failure, and pulmonary edema. Fluid intake would not be encouraged or restricted. Irrigation of the Foley catheter will not assist in alleviating this oliguria.

Test-Taking Strategy: Use the process of elimination. Recalling the definition of oliguria will direct you easily to option 2 as the treatment for this occurrence. If you are unfamiliar with the treatment of oliguria following kidney transplant, review this content.

Level of Cognitive Ability: Analysis

Client Needs: Physiological Integrity

Integrated Process: Nursing Process—analysis

Content Area: Adult health—renal

Reference: Ignatavicius, D., & Workman, M. (2002). *Medical-surgical nursing: Critical thinking for collaborative care* (4th ed., p. 1699). Philadelphia: W. B. Saunders.

37. 1

Rationale: Acute rejection most often occurs in the first 2 weeks after transplant. Clinical manifestations include fever, malaise, elevated white blood cell count, acute hypertension, graft tenderness, and manifestations of deteriorating renal function. Chronic rejection occurs gradually during a period of months to years. Although kidney infection or obstruction can occur, the symptoms presented in the question do not relate specifically to these disorders.

Test-Taking Strategy: Use the process of elimination. Note the key words "a week after kidney transplantation." These words should direct you easily to option 1, "acute" rejection. Review the signs of acute rejection if you had difficulty with this question.

Level of Cognitive Ability: Analysis

Client Needs: Physiological Integrity

Integrated Process: Nursing Process—analysis

Content Area: Adult health—renal

Reference: Ignatavicius, D., & Workman, M. (2002). *Medical-surgical nursing: Critical thinking for collaborative care* (4th ed., p. 1700). Philadelphia: W. B. Saunders.

38. 1

Rationale: Transurethral resection syndrome is caused by increased absorption of nonelectrolyte irrigating fluid used during surgery. The client may show signs of cerebral edema and increased intracranial pressure such as increased blood pressure, bradycardia, confusion, disorientation, muscle twitching, visual disturbances, and nausea and vomiting.

Test-Taking Strategy: Use the process of elimination. Recalling that increased intracranial pressure is the concern in this syndrome will direct you to option 1. Review the clinical manifestations of this disorder if you had difficulty with this question.

Level of Cognitive Ability: Analysis

Client Needs: Physiological Integrity

Integrated Process: Nursing Process—assessment

Content Area: Adult health—renal

Reference: Phipps, W., Monahan, F., Sands, J., Marek, J., & Neighbors, M. (2003). *Medical-surgical nursing: Health and illness perspectives* (7th ed., p. 1833). St. Louis: Mosby.

39. 3

Rationale: Frank bleeding (arterial or venous) may occur during the first day after surgery. Some hematuria is usual for several days after surgery. A urinary output of 200 mL greater than intake is adequate. Bladder spasms are expected to occur following surgery. A rapid pulse with a low blood pressure is a potential sign of excessive blood loss. The physician should be notified.

Test-Taking Strategy: Use the process of elimination. Focus on the issue "need to notify the physician." Think about the expected findings following this procedure and note that the vital signs noted in option 3 indicate excessive blood loss.

Review the expected findings following transurethral resection of the prostate if you had difficulty with this question.
Level of Cognitive Ability: Analysis
Client Needs: Physiological Integrity
Integrated Process: Nursing Process—analysis
Content Area: Adult health—renal
Reference: Phipps, W., Monahan, F., Sands, J., Marek, J., & Neighbors, M. (2003). *Medical-surgical nursing: Health and illness perspectives* (7th ed., p. 1838). St. Louis: Mosby.

40. 1
Rationale: Individuals with polycystic kidney disease seem to waste rather than retain sodium. Thus they need an increased sodium and water intake. Aggressive control of hypertension is essential. Genetic counseling is advisable because of the hereditary nature of the disease.
Test-Taking Strategy: Use the process of elimination. Note the key words "needs additional information." Recalling that sodium is wasted in polycystic kidney disease will direct you to option 1. Review the manifestations associated with this disease if you had difficulty with this question.
Level of Cognitive Ability: Analysis
Client Needs: Physiological Integrity
Integrated Process: Teaching/Learning
Content Area: Adult health—renal
Reference: Phipps, W., Monahan, F., Sands, J., Marek, J., & Neighbors, M. (2003). *Medical-surgical nursing: Health and illness perspectives* (7th ed., p. 1204). St. Louis: Mosby.

41. 4
Rationale: Potential complications after renal angiography include allergic reaction to the dye, renal damage from the dye, and a number of vascular complications, which include hemorrhage, thrombosis, or embolism. The nurse detects these complications by noting signs and symptoms of allergic reaction, decreased urine output, hematoma or hemorrhage at the insertion site, or signs of decreased circulation to the affected leg.
Test-Taking Strategy: Use the process of elimination focusing on the issue, a complication. Eliminate options 1 and 3 because they are normal findings. Because a hematoma is abnormal, then "absence of hematoma" is a normal finding, which eliminates option 2 also. Review the signs of a complication following a renal angioplasty if you had difficulty with this question.
Level of Cognitive Ability: Analysis
Client Needs: Physiological Integrity
Integrated Process: Nursing Process—evaluation
Content Area: Adult health—renal
References: Chernecky, C., & Berger, B. (2001). *Laboratory tests and diagnostic procedures* (3rd ed., p. 905). Philadelphia: W. B. Saunders.
Ignatavicius, D., & Workman, M. (2002). *Medical-surgical nursing: Critical thinking for collaborative care* (4th ed., pp. 1609-1610). Philadelphia: W. B. Saunders.
Phipps, W., Monahan, F., Sands, J., Marek, J., & Neighbors, M. (2003). *Medical-surgical nursing: Health and illness perspectives* (7th ed., p. 1198). St. Louis: Mosby.

42. 1
Rationale: The client with polycystic kidney disease should report any signs and symptoms of urinary tract infection so

that treatment may begin promptly. Lowered blood pressure is not a complication of polycystic kidney disease, and it is an expected effect of antihypertensive therapy. The client would be concerned about rises in blood pressure because control of hypertension is essential. The client may experience heart failure as a result of hypertension, and thus any symptoms of heart failure, such as shortness of breath, are also a concern.
Test-Taking Strategy: Use the process of elimination. Note the key words "understands" and "no reason to be concerned." Recalling that the client with polycystic kidney disease is likely to be hypertensive will direct you to option 1. Also note that options 2, 3, and 4 identify signs of complications. Review teaching points for the client with polycystic kidney disease if you had difficulty with this question.
Level of Cognitive Ability: Analysis
Client Needs: Physiological Integrity
Integrated Process: Teaching/Learning
Content Area: Adult health—renal
Reference: Ignatavicius, D., & Workman, M. (2002). *Medical-surgical nursing: Critical thinking for collaborative care* (4th ed., p. 1645). Philadelphia: W. B. Saunders.

43. 4
Rationale: Treatment of prostatitis includes medication with antibiotics, analgesics, and stool softeners. The nurse also teaches the client to rest, increase fluid intake, and use sitz baths for comfort. Antimicrobial therapy is always continued until the prescription is finished.
Test-Taking Strategy: Use the process of elimination. Eliminate option 3 first because stopping medication therapy before the end of the course is contraindicated. Also eliminate option 1 because fluid intake should be increased. From the remaining options, recall that sitz baths provide comfort or that rest is helpful in the healing process. Review home care instructions for the client with prostatitis if you had difficulty with this question.
Level of Cognitive Ability: Analysis
Client Needs: Health Promotion and Maintenance
Integrated Process: Teaching/Learning
Content Area: Adult health—renal
Reference: Phipps, W., Monahan, F., Sands, J., Marek, J., & Neighbors, M. (2003). *Medical-surgical nursing: Health and illness perspectives* (7th ed., p. 1830). St. Louis: Mosby.

44. 2
Rationale: Crush injuries may cause acute tubular necrosis from the accumulation of large amounts of myoglobin and hemoglobin that are released from damaged muscle and blood cells. This type of renal failure is said to be due to renal causes; that is, conditions within the kidney itself. Prerenal causes are conditions that interfere with the perfusion of blood to the kidney. Postrenal causes include conditions that cause urinary obstruction distal to the kidney. The cause and the type of renal failure determines the interventions used in treatment to a certain extent.
Test-Taking Strategy: Use the process of elimination and knowledge of the categories of acute renal failure to answer this question. Eliminate option 4 first because it is not a category of acute renal failure. Next, focus on the nature of the

injury and its effect on the kidney to direct you to option 2. Review the causes of acute renal failure if you had difficulty with this question.
Level of Cognitive Ability: Analysis
Client Needs: Physiological Integrity
Integrated Process: Nursing Process—analysis
Content Area: Adult health—renal
Reference: Phipps, W., Monahan, F., Sands, J., Marek, J., & Neighbors, M. (2003). *Medical-surgical nursing: Health and illness perspectives* (7th ed., p. 1238). St. Louis: Mosby.

45. **3**
Rationale: The client with hyperkalemia is at risk of developing cardiac dysrhythmias and cardiac arrest. Because of this the client should be placed on a cardiac monitor. Fluid intake is not increased because it contributes to fluid overload and would not affect the serum potassium level significantly. Vegetables are a natural source of potassium in the diet, and their use would not be increased. The nurse also may assess the sodium level because sodium is another electrolyte commonly measured with the potassium level. However, this is not a priority action of the nurse.
Test-Taking Strategy: First, note that the potassium level is elevated. Next use the ABCs—airway, breathing, and circulation—to direct you to option 3. Review care to the client with hyperkalemia if you had difficulty with this question.
Level of Cognitive Ability: Application
Client Needs: Physiological Integrity
Integrated Process: Nursing Process—planning
Content Area: Adult health—renal
Reference: Ignatavicius, D., & Workman, M. (2002). *Medical-surgical nursing: Critical thinking for collaborative care* (4th ed., p. 1686). Philadelphia: W. B. Saunders.

46. **3**
Rationale: Antihypertensive medications such as enalapril are given to the client following hemodialysis. This prevents the client from becoming hypotensive during dialysis and also from having the medication removed from the bloodstream by dialysis. No rationale exists for waiting a full day to resume the medication. This would lead to ineffective control of the blood pressure.
Test-Taking Strategy: Use the process of elimination. Begin to answer this question by thinking about the effects of an antihypertensive medication on the blood pressure when fluid is being removed from the body. Because hypotension is much more likely to occur in this circumstance, eliminate options 1 and 2. Eliminate option 4 because this action would lead to ineffective blood pressure control. Review preprocedure hemodialysis measures if you had difficulty with this question.
Level of Cognitive Ability: Application
Client Needs: Physiological Integrity
Integrated Process: Nursing Process—planning
Content Area: Adult health—renal
References: Lewis, S., Heitkemper, M., & Dirksen, S. (2004). *Medical-surgical nursing: Assessment and management of clinical problems* (6th ed., p. 1222). St. Louis: Mosby.
Phipps, W., Monahan, F., Sands, J., Marek, J., & Neighbors, M. (2003). *Medical-surgical nursing: Health and illness perspectives* (7th ed., p. 766). St. Louis: Mosby.

47. **2**
Rationale: Clients with peritoneal dialysis catheters are at high risk for infection. A dressing that is wet is a conduit for bacteria to reach the catheter insertion site. The nurse assures that the dressing is kept dry at all times. Reinforcing the dressing is not a safe practice to prevent infection in this circumstance. Flushing the catheter is not indicated. Scrubbing the catheter with povidone-iodine is done at the time of connection or disconnection of peritoneal dialysis.
Test-Taking Strategy: Use the process of elimination. Note the issue of the question, a wet dressing. Recalling that this client is at risk for infection and knowing that it is better to change a wet dressing than reinforce it will direct you to option 2. Review care to the client receiving peritoneal dialysis if you had difficulty with this question.
Level of Cognitive Ability: Application
Client Needs: Safe, Effective Care Environment
Integrated Process: Nursing Process—implementation
Content Area: Adult health—renal
Reference: Ignatavicius, D., & Workman, M. (2002). *Medical-surgical nursing: Critical thinking for collaborative care* (4th ed., p. 1696). Philadelphia: W. B. Saunders.

48. **2**
Rationale: If the client experiences air embolus during hemodialysis, the nurse should terminate dialysis immediately, notify the physician, and administer oxygen as needed. Options 1, 3, and 4 are incorrect.
Test-Taking Strategy: Use the process of elimination. Recalling that air embolus is an emergency situation that affects the cardiopulmonary system suddenly and profoundly will direct you to option 2. Review the emergency care to a client who develops air embolism if you had difficulty with this question.
Level of Cognitive Ability: Application
Client Needs: Physiological Integrity
Integrated Process: Nursing Process—implementation
Content Area: Adult health—renal
Reference: Ignatavicius, D., & Workman, M. (2002). *Medical-surgical nursing: Critical thinking for collaborative care* (4th ed., p. 207). Philadelphia: W. B. Saunders.

49. **2**
Rationale: The client on hemodialysis should monitor fluid status between hemodialysis treatments by recording intake and output and measuring weight daily. Ideally, the hemodialysis client should not gain more than 0.5 kg of weight per day.
Test-Taking Strategy: Use the process of elimination. Recalling the pathophysiology of renal failure and the impact on the client's bodily functions will assist in answering the question. Also, note that option 2 relates to monitoring of fluid retention. Review teaching points for the client receiving hemodialysis if you had difficulty with this question.
Level of Cognitive Ability: Analysis
Client Needs: Physiological Integrity
Integrated Process: Teaching/Learning
Content Area: Adult health—renal
Reference: Ignatavicius, D.,& Workman, M. (2002). *Medical-surgical nursing: Critical thinking for collaborative care* (4th ed., p. 1701). Philadelphia: W. B. Saunders.

50. **4**

Rationale: An arteriovenous shunt is a less common form of access site but carries a risk for bleeding when it is used because two ends of an external cannula are tunneled subcutaneously into an artery and a vein, and the ends of the cannula are joined. If accidental disconnection occurs, the client could lose blood rapidly. For this reason, small clamps are attached to the dressing that covers the insertion site for use if needed. The shunt site also should be assessed at least every four hours.

Test-Taking Strategy: Use the process of elimination. Focus on the issue, preventing bleeding. Visualize this type of access device. Recalling that the risk of disconnection can occur will direct you to option 4. Review care to the client with an arteriovenous shunt if you had difficulty with this question.

Level of Cognitive Ability: Application
Client Needs: Safe, Effective Care Environment
Integrated Process: Nursing Process—implementation
Content Area: Adult health—renal
Reference: Ignatavicius, D., & Workman, M. (2002). *Medical-surgical nursing: Critical thinking for collaborative care* (4th ed., p. 1691). Philadelphia: W. B. Saunders.

CRITICAL THINKING: FILL IN THE BLANK

Answer: Reposition the client.
Rationale: If outflow drainage is inadequate, the nurse attempts to stimulate outflow by changing the client's position. Turning the client to the other side or making sure that the client is in good body alignment may assist with outflow drainage.

Test-Taking Strategy: Use the process of elimination. Note the key word "initially." Also note that the issue of the question relates to inadequate outflow and the need for a nursing intervention. Review the nursing interventions related to insufficient flow of dialysate, if you had difficulty with this question.

Level of Cognitive Ability: Application
Client Needs: Physiological Integrity
Integrated Process: Nursing Process—implementation
Content Area: Adult health—renal
Reference: Ignatavicius, D., & Workman, M. (2002). *Medical-surgical nursing: Critical thinking for collaborative care* (4th ed., p. 1696). Philadelphia: W. B. Saunders.

REFERENCES

Chernecky, C., & Berger, B. (2001). *Laboratory tests and diagnostic procedures* (3rd ed.). Philadelphia: W. B. Saunders.

Harkreader, H., & Hogan, M. A. (2004). *Fundamentals of nursing: Caring and clinical judgment* (2nd ed.). Philadelphia: W. B. Saunders.

Ignatavicius, D., & Workman, M. (2002). *Medical-surgical nursing: Critical thinking for collaborative care* (4th ed.). Philadelphia: W. B. Saunders.

Lewis, S., Heitkemper, M., & Dirksen, S. (2004). *Medical-surgical nursing: Assessment and management of clinical problems* (6th ed.). St. Louis: Mosby.

McKenry, L., & Salerno, E. (2001). *Mosby's pharmacology in nursing* (21st ed.). St. Louis: Mosby.

Peckenpaugh, N. (2003). *Nutrition essentials and diet therapy* (9th ed.). Philadelphia: W. B. Saunders.

Phipps, W., Monahan, F., Sands, J., Marek, J., & Neighbors, M. (2003). *Medical-surgical nursing: Health and illness perspectives* (7th ed.). St. Louis: Mosby.

Renal Medications

I. URINARY TRACT ANTISEPTICS (BOX 62-1)
A. Description
   1. Antiseptics inhibit the growth of bacteria in the urine.
   2. Antiseptics act as disinfectants within the urinary tract.
   3. Antiseptics are used to treat urinary tract infections.
   4. These medications do not achieve effective antibacterial concentrations in blood or tissues and therefore cannot be used for infections at sites outside the urinary tract.
B. Side effects and nursing considerations
   1. Nitrofurantoin (Furadantin, Macrodantin, Macrobid)
      a. Gastrointestinal effects such as anorexia, nausea, vomiting, and diarrhea can occur; administration with milk or meals minimizes gastrointestinal distress.
      b. Pulmonary reactions such as dyspnea, chest pain, chills, fever, cough, and alveolar infiltrates can occur; these resolve in 2 to 4 days following cessation of treatment.
      c. Hematological effects such as agranulocytosis, leukopenia, thrombocytopenia, and megaloblastic anemia can occur.
      d. Peripheral neuropathy such as muscle weakness, tingling sensations, and numbness can occur.

BOX 62-1

Urinary Tract Antiseptics

Cinoxacin (Cinobac)
Methenamine (Mandelamine)
Methenamine hippurate (Hiprex)
Nalidixic acid (NegGram)
Nitrofurantoin (Furadantin, Macrodantin, Macrobid)

      e. Neurological effects such as headache, vertigo, drowsiness, nystagmus can occur.
      f. Nitrofurantoin imparts a harmless brown color to the urine.
      g. Nitrofurantoin is contraindicated in clients with renal impairment.
      h. Instruct the client in the expected side effects and those warranting notification of the physician.
   2. Methenamine mandelate (Mandelamine) and methenamine hippurate (Hiprex)
      a. Methenamine is relatively safe and well tolerated.
      b. Methenamine may cause gastric distress.
      c. Chronic high-dose therapy can cause bladder irritation.
      d. Methenamine can cause crystalluria and should not be used in clients with renal impairment.
      e. Decomposition of medication generates ammonia; thus it should not be used for clients with liver dysfunction.
      f. Methenamine requires acidic urine with a pH of 5.5 or less.
      g. Ingestion of excessive amounts of fluid will reduce antibacterial effects by diluting the medication and raising the urinary pH.
      h. Methenamine should not be combined with sulfonamides because of the risk of crystalluria and urinary tract injury.
      i. Clients taking this medication should not be given alkalinizing agents.
   3. Nalidixic acid (NegGram)
      a. Nalidixic acid can cause gastrointestinal disturbances such as nausea, vomiting, and abdominal discomfort.
      b. Nalidixic acid can cause rash.
      c. Nalidixic acid can cause visual disturbances.
      d. Nalidixic acid can cause photosensitivity reactions.

e. Nalidixic acid may produce intracranial hypertension in pediatric clients and should not be administered to children under age 3 months.

f. When nalidixic acid is used for more than 2 weeks, complete blood cell counts and liver function tests should be performed.

g. Nalidixic acid can intensify the effects of orally administered anticoagulants.

h. Nalidixic acid is contraindicated in clients with a history of convulsive disorders.

4. Cinoxacin (Cinobac)

a. Side effects are similar to those of nalidixic acid.

b. Dosage should be reduced in clients with renal impairment; failure to do so could result in accumulation of the medication to toxic levels.

II. FLUOROQUINOLONES (BOX 62-2)

A. Significant side effects include dizziness, drowsiness, gastric distress, diarrhea, vaginitis (trovafloxacin), nausea, and vomiting.

B. Adverse effects include psychoses, hallucinations, confusion, tremors, hypersensitivity, and interstitial nephritis.

C. Fluoroquinolones should be used with caution in clients with hepatic, renal, or central nervous system disorders.

D. Monitor client for side effects or signs of adverse reactions.

E. Administer fluoroquinolones with a full glass of water and ensure that the client maintains a urine output of at least 1200 to 1500 mL daily to minimize the occurrence of crystalluria.

F. Enoxacin (Penetrex) and Norfloxacin (Noroxin) are to be taken on an empty stomach.

G. Ciprofloxacin (Cipro), lomefloxacin (Maxaquin), ofloxacin (Floxin), and sparfloxacin (Zagam) may be taken with or without food.

H. Intravenously administered ciprofloxacin (Cipro) and ofloxacin (Floxin) are infused slowly over 60 minutes to minimize discomfort and vein irritation.

I. Advise client to report dizziness, light-headedness, visual disturbances, increased light sensitivity, and feelings of depression because these signs could indicate central nervous system toxicity.

J. Inform client of signs of hepatic and renal toxicity and the importance of reporting these signs to the physician.

III. SULFONAMIDES (BOX 62-3)

A. Description

1. Sulfonamides suppress bacterial growth by inhibiting the synthesis of folic acid.

2. Sulfonamides are active against a broad spectrum of microbes.

B. Side effects and nursing considerations

1. Hypersensitivity reactions include rash, fever, and photosensitivity.

2. Stevens-Johnson syndrome, the most severe hypersensitivity response, produces symptoms that include widespread lesions of the skin and mucous membranes, with fever, malaise, and toxemia.

3. Sulfonamides should be discontinued if a rash is observed.

4. Sulfonamides can cause hemolytic anemia, agranulocytosis, leukopenia, and thrombocytopenia.

5. Instruct the client to take the medication on an empty stomach with a full glass of water.

6. Instruct the client to avoid prolonged exposure to sunlight, wear protective clothing, and apply a sunscreen to exposed skin.

7. Adults should maintain a daily urine output of 1200 mL by consuming 8 to 10 glasses of water each day to minimize the risk of renal damage from the medication.

8. Sulfonamides can intensify the effects of warfarin sodium (Coumadin), phenytoin (Dilantin), and orally administered hypoglycemics.

9. Administer sulfonamides with caution in clients with renal impairment.

10. Sulfonamides are contraindicated if a hypersensitivity exists to sulfonamides, sulfonylureas, or thiazide or loop diuretics.

11. Sulfonamides are contraindicated in infants under age 2 months and in pregnant women or mothers who are breast-feeding.

IV. CHOLINERGIC (BOX 62-4)

A. Description

1. A cholinergic is used to treat nonobstructive urinary retention and neurogenic bladder.

BOX 62-2

Fluoroquinolones

Ciprofloxacin (Cipro)
Enoxacin (Penetrex)
Gatifloxacin (Tequin)
Levofloxacin (Levaquin)
Lomefloxacin (Maxaquin)
Moxifloxacin (Avelox)
Norfloxacin (Noroxin)
Ofloxacin (Floxin)
Sparfloxacin (Zagam)
Trovafloxacin/alatrofloxacin (Trovan)

BOX 62-3

Sulfonamides

Sulfadiazine
Sulfamethizole (Thiosulfil Forte)
Sulfamethoxazole (Gantanol)
Sulfisoxazole (Gantrisin)
Trimethoprim-sulfamethoxazole (Bactrim)

BOX 62-4

Cholinergic

Bethanechol chloride (Urecholine)

2. Cholinergics are used to increase bladder tone and function.
B. Side effects
1. Headache
2. Hypotension
3. Flushing and sweating
4. Increased salivation
5. Abdominal cramps
6. Nausea and vomiting
7. Diarrhea
8. Urinary urgency
9. Bronchoconstriction
C. Nursing considerations
1. Do not administer a cholinergic if the client has a urinary obstruction.
2. Never administer by the intramuscular or intravenous route.
3. Monitor intake and output.
4. Monitor for increased bladder tone and function.
5. Monitor for cholinergic overdose.
6. Have atropine sulfate (antidote) readily available.

V. ANTISPASMODICS
A. Description
1. Oxybutynin chloride (Ditropan) relaxes smooth muscles of the urinary tract.
2. Propantheline bromide (Pro-Banthine) decreases bladder muscle spasms.
B. Oxybutynin chloride (Ditropan)
1. Side effects
a. Constipation
b. Drowsiness
c. Anorexia, nausea, vomiting, dry mouth
d. Decreased sweating
e. Urinary retention
2. Nursing considerations
a. Do not administer oxybutynin to clients with known hypersensitivity, gastrointestinal or genitourinary obstruction, glaucoma, severe colitis, or myasthenia gravis.
b. Instruct the client to avoid hazardous activities.
C. Propantheline bromide (Pro-Banthine)
1. Side effects
a. Palpitations
b. Blurred vision
c. Confusion in older clients
d. Tachycardia
e. Constipation
f. Dry mouth
g. Urinary hesitancy and urgency
h. Decreased sweating

2. Nursing considerations
a. Monitor intake and output.
b. Provide gum or hard candy for dry mouth.
c. Do not administer propantheline bromide to clients with narrow-angle glaucoma, obstructive uropathy, gastrointestinal disease, or ulcerative colitis.

VI. URINARY ANALGESIC (BOX 62-5)
A. Description
1. A urinary tract analgesics is used for pain from urinary tract irritation or infection.
2. A urinary tract analgesic is administered with an antibiotic because it does not treat infection; it only treats pain.
B. Side effects
1. Nausea
2. Headache
3. Vertigo
C. Nursing considerations
1. Instruct the client that the urine will turn red or orange.
2. A urinary tract analgesic is contraindicated in clients with renal or hepatic disease.

VII. HEMATOPOIETIC GROWTH FACTOR (BOX 62-6)
A. Description
1. Hematopoietic growth factor is used to stimulate red blood cell production.
2. Hematopoietic growth factor reverses anemia associated with **chronic renal failure.**
3. Initial effects can be seen within 1 to 2 weeks, and the hematocrit reaches normal levels (30% to 33%) in 2 to 3 months.
B. Side effect: Major side effect is hypertension.
C. Nursing considerations
1. Monitor the complete blood count.
2. Monitor vital signs, especially the blood pressure for hypertension.
3. The extent of hypertension is related directly to the rate of rise in the hematocrit.
4. Hematopoietic growth factor is contraindicated in clients with uncontrolled hypertension or

BOX 62-5

Urinary Tract Analgesic

Phenazopyridine hydrochloride (Pyridium)

BOX 62-6

Hematopoietic Growth Factor

Epoetin alfa (Epogen, Procrit)

hypersensitivity to mammalian cell–derived products or human albumin.

5. Use hematopoietic growth factor with caution in clients with cancers of myeloid origin.

VIII. PREVENTION OF ORGAN REJECTION (BOX 62-7)

A. Description
1. Cyclosporine acts on T lymphocytes to suppress production of interleukin-2, gamma-interferon, and other cytokines.
2. Tracrolimus inhibits calcineurin and thereby prevents T cells from producing interleukin-2, gamma-interferon, and other cytokines.
3. Azathioprine (Imuran) suppresses cell-mediated and humoral immune responses by inhibiting the proliferation of B and T lymphocytes.
4. Mycophenolate mofetil causes selective inhibition of B and T lymphocyte proliferation.
5. Muromonab-CD3 blocks all T cell functions.
6. Daclizumab and basiliximab bind to interleukin-2 receptors on lymphocytes, resulting in diminished cell-mediated immune reactions.

B. Cyclosporine (Sandimmune, Neoral)
1. Cyclosporine is used to prevent rejection of allogenic kidney transplant.
2. Prednisone usually is administered concurrently.
3. Oral administration is preferred; intravenous administration is reserved for clients who cannot take the medication orally.
4. Blood levels of the drug should be measured periodically.
5. The most common adverse effects are nephrotoxicity, infection, hypertension, tremor, and hirsutism.
6. The client should be informed about the possibility of renal damage and liver damage and the need for periodic blood urea nitrogen, creatinine, and liver function tests.
7. The client should be instructed to monitor for early signs of infection and to report these signs immediately.
8. Instruct the client to dispense the oral liquid into a glass container by using a specially calibrated pipette, mix well, and drink immediately; rinse the glass container with diluent and drink it to ensure ingestion of the complete dose; dry the outside of the pipette and return to its cover for storage.
9. Instruct the client to mix the concentrated medication solution with milk, chocolate milk, or orange juice just before administration.
10. Assure the client that hirsutism is reversible.
11. Grapefruit juice can raise cyclosporine levels, thereby increasing the risk of toxicity.
12. Phenytoin (Dilantin), phenobarbital, rifampin (Rifadin), and trimethoprim-sulfamethoxazole can decrease cyclosporine levels.
13. Ketoconazole (Nizoral), erythromycin, and amphotericin B (Fungizone) can elevate cyclosporine levels.
14. Renal damage can be intensified by the concurrent use of other nephrotoxic medications.
15. Cyclosporine is contraindicated in the presence of hypersensitivity, pregnancy and breast-feeding, recent inoculation with live virus vaccines, and recent contact with an active infection such as chickenpox or herpes zoster.
16. Cyclosporine is embryotoxic, and women of childbearing age should use a mechanical form of contraception and avoid oral contraceptives.

C. Tacrolimus (Prograf)
1. Nephrotoxicity is the major concern.
2. Other common reactions include neurotoxicity, gastrointestinal effects, hypertension, hyperkalemia, and hyperglycemia.
3. Tacrolimus increases the risk of infection and lymphomas.
4. Concurrent use of glucocorticoids is recommended.

D. Azathioprine (Imuran)
1. Azathioprine is used as an adjunct to cyclosporine and glucocorticoids to help suppress transplant rejection.
2. Azathioprine can cause neutropenia and thrombocytopenia from bone marrow suppression.
3. Azathioprine is contraindicated in pregnancy and is associated with an increased incidence of neoplasms.

E. Mycophenolate mofetil (CellCept)
1. Mycophenolate mofetil is used along with cyclosporine and glucocorticoids.
2. Major adverse effects include diarrhea, severe neutropenia, vomiting, and sepsis.
3. Mycophenolate mofetil is associated with an increased risk of infection and malignancies.

BOX 62-7

Preventing Organ Rejection

ANTIBODIES
Basiliximab (Simulect)
Daclizumab (Zenapax)
Muromonab-CD3 (Orthoclone OKT3)

CYTOTOXIC MEDICATIONS
Azathioprine (Imuran)
Mycophenolate mofetil (CellCept)

GLUCOCORTICOID
Prednisone (Deltasone)

IMMUNOSUPPRESSANTS
Cyclosporine (Sandimmune, Neoral)
Tacrolimus (Prograf)

4. Absorption is decreased by the use of magnesium and aluminum antacids and by cholestyramine (Questran, Prevalite).
5. Mycophenolate mofetil is contraindicated in pregnancy.

F. Muromonab-CD3 (Orthoclone OKT3)
1. Muromonab-CD3 is used to prevent acute allograft rejection of kidney transplants.
2. Adverse reactions include fever, chills, dyspnea, chest pain, and nausea and vomiting.

G. Daclizumab (Zenapax) and basiliximab (Simulect)
1. These medications are used to prevent acute rejection of transplanted kidneys.
2. These medications are used along with other immunosuppressants such as cyclosporine and glucocorticoids.
3. These medications are administered intravenously.
4. These medications are contraindicated in the client with an allergy to protein.
5. Daclizumab (Zenapax)
   a. Initial dose is administered within 24 hours before transplantation.
   b. Side effects include chest pain, gastrointestinal distress, edema, shortness of breath, pain in the joints, and slow wound healing.
6. Basiliximab (Simulect)
   a. Initial dose is administered within 2 hours before transplantation.
   b. Side effects are similar to those for daclizumab; in addition, headache, insomnia, dizziness, and tremors can occur.

PRACTICE QUESTIONS

1. Trimethoprim-sulfamethoxazole (Bactrim) is prescribed to be administered by intravenous infusion to a client with a recurrent urinary tract infection. A nurse would administer this medication
   1. Over 60 to 90 minutes.
   2. Over 30 minutes.
   3. Piggybacked into the existing infusion of normal saline and potassium chloride.
   4. Piggybacked into the peripheral line containing total parenteral nutrition.

2. Nalidixic acid (NegGram) is prescribed for a client with a urinary tract infection. On review of the client's record, a nurse notes that the client is taking warfarin sodium (Coumadin) daily. Which prescription would the nurse anticipate because the client is taking this anticoagulant orally?
   1. An increase in the anticoagulation dosage
   2. A decrease in the anticoagulation dosage
   3. The need to discontinue the anticoagulant
   4. The need to administer an alternative medication to treat the urinary tract infection.

3. A nurse is providing discharge instructions to a client receiving sulfisoxazole (Gantrisin). Which of the following would be included in the list of instructions?
   1. Restrict fluid intake.
   2. Maintain a high fluid intake.
   3. Decrease the dosage when symptoms are improving to prevent an allergic response.
   4. If the urine turns dark brown, call the physician immediately.

4. Sulfamethoxazole (Gantanol) is prescribed for a client with a urinary tract infection. The client has diabetes mellitus and is receiving tolbutamide (Orinase). Based on the administration of these two medications in combination, which of the following would the nurse anticipate might be prescribed?
   1. A decreased dosage of the tolbutamide
   2. An increased dosage of the tolbutamide
   3. A decreased dosage of the sulfamethoxazole
   4. An increased dosage of the sulfamethoxazole

5. Trimethoprim-sulfamethoxazole (Bactrim) is prescribed for a client. A nurse would instruct the client to report which symptom if it developed during the course of this medication therapy?
   1. Headache
   2. Nausea
   3. Diarrhea
   4. Sore throat

6. Phenazopyridine hydrochloride (Pyridium) is prescribed for a client for symptomatic relief of pain resulting from a lower urinary tract infection. The nurse teaches the client
   1. To take the medication before meals.
   2. That a reddish orange discoloration of the urine may occur.
   3. To discontinue the medication if a headache occurs.
   4. To take the medication at bedtime.

7. Bethanechol chloride (Urecholine) is prescribed for a client with urinary retention. Which disorder would be a contraindication to the administration of this medication?
   1. Neurogenic atony
   2. Urinary strictures
   3. Gastroesophogeal reflux
   4. Gastric atony

8. A nurse who is administering bethanechol chloride (Urecholine) is monitoring for acute toxicity associated with the medication. The nurse checks the client for which sign of toxicity?
   1. Dry mouth
   2. Dry skin
   3. Bradycardia
   4. Signs of dehydration

9. Oxybutynin chloride (Ditropan) is prescribed for a client with neurogenic bladder. Which sign would indicate a possible toxic effect related to this medication?
   1. Bradycardia

2. Pallor

3. Restlessness

4. Drowsiness

10. Propantheline bromide (Pro-Banthine) is prescribed for a client with bladder spasms. Which of the following disorders, if noted in the client's record, would alert a nurse to question the prescription for this medication?

   1. Glaucoma

   2. Hypothyroidism

   3. Myxedema

   4. Coronary artery disease

11. Following kidney transplant, cyclosporine (Sandimmune) is prescribed for a client. Which laboratory result would indicate an adverse effect from the use of this medication?

   1. Decreased white blood cell count

   2. Decreased hemoglobin

   3. Elevated blood urea nitrogen

   4. Decreased creatinine

12. A nurse is providing dietary instructions to a client who has been prescribed cyclosporine (Sandimmune). Which food item would the nurse instruct the client to avoid?

   1. Orange juice

   2. Grapefruit juice

   3. Red meats

   4. Green, leafy vegetables

13. A nurse is caring for a client who will be receiving amphotericin B (Fungizone). The nurse notes that the client is also taking cyclosporine (Sandimmune) to prevent rejection of a kidney transplant performed 2 years ago. Which prescription would the nurse anticipate to be prescribed for this client during the administration of these medications concurrently?

   1. An increased amount of amphotericin B

   2. A decreased amount of amphotericin B

   3. An increased amount of cyclosporine

   4. A decreased amount of cyclosporine

14. A nurse provides instructions to a client who will be taking cyclosporine (Sandimmune) oral solution. The nurse tells the client to

   1. Dilute the concentrate in a Styrofoam cup before administration.

   2. Avoid diluting the concentrate for administration.

   3. Mix the concentrate with chocolate milk.

   4. Mix the concentrate with grapefruit juice.

15. A nurse is monitoring a client receiving cyclosporine (Sandimmune). Which sign or symptom would indicate to the nurse that the client is experiencing an adverse effect from this medication?

   1. Nausea

   2. Alopecia

3. Tremors

4. Hypotension

16. Tacrolimus (Prograf) is prescribed for a client. Which disorder, if noted in the client's record, would indicate that the medication needs to be administered with caution?

   1. Diabetes insipidus

   2. Coronary artery disease

   3. Pancreatitis

   4. Ulcerative colitis

17. A nurse is reviewing the laboratory results for a client receiving tacrolimus (Prograf). Which laboratory result would indicate to the nurse that the client is experiencing an adverse effect of the medication?

   1. White blood cell count of 6000 cells/μL

   2. Blood glucose of 200 mg/dL

   3. Potassium level of 3.8 mEq/L

   4. Platelet count of 300,000 cells/μL

18. Mycophenolate mofetil (CellCept) is prescribed for a client for prophylaxis of organ rejection following allogeneic renal transplant. Which instruction would a nurse provide to the client regarding administration of this medication?

   1. Administer following meals.

   2. Open the capsule and mix with food for administration.

   3. Contact the physician if a sore throat occurs.

   4. Take the medication with a magnesium-type antacid.

19. A client with chronic renal failure is receiving epoetin alfa (Epogen, Procrit). Which laboratory result would indicate a therapeutic effect of the medication?

   1. White blood cell count of 6000 cells/μL

   2. Hematocrit of 32%

   3. Platelet count of 400,000 cells/μL

   4. Blood urea nitrogen of 15 mg/dL

20. A nurse is instructing a client to administer epoetin alfa (Epogen, Procrit) by the subcutaneous route. The nurse tells the client to

   1. Shake the bottle before use.

   2. Freeze the medication before use.

   3. Refrigerate the medication.

   4. Obtain syringes with $1\frac{1}{2}$-inch needles from the pharmacy.

CRITICAL THINKING: FILL IN THE BLANK

A nurse is administering a dose of bethanechol chloride (Urecholine) subcutaneously to a client with urinary retention. The nurse plans to have what medication (antidote) readily available when administering the bethanechol chloride to the client?

Answer: _____

ANSWERS

1. **1**

Rationale: Trimethoprim-sulfamethoxazole (Bactrim) may be administered by intravenous infusion but should not be mixed with any other medications or solutions. Trimethoprim-sulfamethoxazole is infused over 60 to 90 minutes, and bolus infusions or rapid infusions must be avoided.

Test-Taking Strategy: Use the process of elimination. Eliminate options 3 and 4 because they address the issue of mixing the trimethoprim-sulfamethoxazole with other solutions. From the remaining options, option 1 identifies the longer time frame and is the safe and correct choice. Review administration of this medication by intravenous infusion if you had difficulty with this question.

Level of Cognitive Ability: Application
Client Needs: Physiological Integrity
Integrated Process: Nursing Process—implementation
Content Area: Pharmacology
Reference: Hodgson, B., & Kizior, R. (2004). *Saunders nursing drug handbook 2004* (p. 290). Philadelphia: W. B. Saunders.

2. **2**

Rationale: Nalidixic acid can intensify the effects of oral anticoagulants by displacing these agents from binding sites on plasma protein. When an oral anticoagulant is combined with nalidixic acid, a decrease in the anticoagulant dosage may be needed.

Test-Taking Strategy: Knowledge regarding the medication interactions associated with the use of nalidixic acid is needed to answer this question. Review these interactions if you had difficulty with this question.

Level of Cognitive Ability: Analysis
Client Needs: Physiological Integrity
Integrated Process: Nursing Process—analysis
Content Area: Pharmacology
References: Kee, J., & Hayes, E. (2003). *Pharmacology: A nursing process approach* (4th ed., p. 461). Philadelphia: W. B. Saunders. Lehne, R. (2001). *Pharmacology for nursing care* (4th ed., p. 977). Philadelphia: W. B. Saunders.

3. **2**

Rationale: Each dose of sulfisoxazole (Gantrisin) should be administered with a full glass of water, and the client should maintain a high fluid intake. The medication is more soluble in alkaline urine. The client should not be instructed to taper or discontinue the dose. Some forms of Gantrisin, such as Azo-Gantrisin, cause urine to turn dark brown or red. This does not indicate the need to notify the physician.

Test-Taking Strategy: Use the process of elimination. Recalling that this medication is used to treat urinary tract infections will direct you to option 2. Review client instructions regarding this medication if you had difficulty with this question.

Level of Cognitive Ability: Application
Client Needs: Physiological Integrity
Integrated Process: Teaching/Learning
Content Area: Pharmacology
Reference: Hodgson, B., & Kizior, R. (2004). *Saunders nursing drug handbook 2004* (p. 251). Philadelphia: W. B. Saunders.

4. **1**

Rationale: Sulfonamides can intensify the effects of warfarin sodium (Coumadin), phenytoin (Dilantin), and orally administered hypoglycemics such as tolbutamide (Orinase). When combined with sulfonamides, these medications may require a reduction in dosage.

Test-Taking Strategy: Use the process of elimination. Recalling that sulfonamides intensify the action of orally administered hypoglycemics will direct you to option 1. Review the medication interactions associated with sulfonamides if you had difficulty with this question.

Level of Cognitive Ability: Analysis
Client Needs: Physiological Integrity
Integrated Process: Nursing Process—analysis
Content Area: Pharmacology
Reference: Gutierrez, K., & Queener, S. (2003). *Pharmacology for nursing practice* (p. 964). St. Louis: Mosby.

5. **4**

Rationale: Clients taking trimethoprim-sulfamethoxazole should be informed about early signs of blood disorders that can occur from this medication. These signs include sore throat, fever, and pallor, and the client should be instructed to notify the physician if these symptoms occur. The other options do not require physician notification.

Test-Taking Strategy: Use the process of elimination. Knowledge that this medication can cause blood dyscrasias will direct you to option 4. If you are unfamiliar with this medication, review this content.

Level of Cognitive Ability: Application
Client Needs: Physiological Integrity
Integrated Process: Teaching/Learning
Content Area: Pharmacology
Reference: Kee, J., & Hayes, E. (2003). *Pharmacology: A nursing process approach* (4th ed., p. 427). Philadelphia: W. B. Saunders.

6. **2**

Rationale: The nurse should instruct the client that a reddish orange discoloration of urine may occur. The nurse also should instruct the client that this discoloration can stain fabric. The medication should be taken after meals to reduce the possibility of gastrointestinal upset. A headache is an occasional side effect of the medication and does not warrant discontinuation of the medication.

Test-Taking Strategy: Use the process of elimination. Eliminate options 1 and 4 first because they are similar in that they address time schedules for the administration of the medication. From the remaining options, eliminate option 3 because the nurse would not advise the client to discontinue this medication. Review client instructions regarding this medication if you had difficulty with this question.

Level of Cognitive Ability: Application
Client Needs: Physiological Integrity
Integrated Process: Teaching/Learning
Content Area: Pharmacology
Reference: Hodgson, B., & Kizior, R. (2004). *Saunders nursing drug handbook 2004* (p. 797). Philadelphia: W. B. Saunders.

7. 2
Rationale: Bethanechol chloride (Urecholine) can be hazardous to clients with urinary tract obstruction or weakness of the bladder wall. The medication has the ability to contract the bladder and thereby increase pressure within the urinary tract. Elevation of pressure within the urinary tract could rupture the bladder in clients with these conditions.
Test-Taking Strategy: Use the process of elimination. Noting that the medication is used for urinary retention may assist in directing you to option 2. Review the contraindications associated with this medication if you had difficulty with this question.
Level of Cognitive Ability: Analysis
Client Needs: Physiological Integrity
Integrated Process: Nursing Process—analysis
Content Area: Pharmacology
Reference: Kee, J., & Hayes, E. (2003). *Pharmacology: A nursing process approach* (4th ed., p. 339). Philadelphia: W. B. Saunders.

8. 3
Rationale: Toxicity (overdose) produces manifestations of excessive muscarinic stimulation such as salivation, sweating, involuntary urination and defecation, bradycardia, and severe hypotension. Treatment includes supportive measures and the administration of atropine sulfate subcutaneously or intravenously.
Test-Taking Strategy: Use the process of elimination. Noting the similarity in options 1, 2, and 4 will assist in eliminating these options. Review these signs if you had difficulty with this question.
Level of Cognitive Ability: Analysis
Client Needs: Physiological Integrity
Integrated Process: Nursing Process—assessment
Content Area: Pharmacology
Reference: Kee, J., & Hayes, E. (2003). *Pharmacology: A nursing process approach* (4th ed., p. 338). Philadelphia: W. B. Saunders.

9. 3
Rationale: Toxicity (overdosage) of this medication produces central nervous system excitation, such as nervousness, restlessness, hallucinations, and irritability. Other signs of toxicity include hypotension or hypertension, confusion, tachycardia, flushed or red face, and signs of respiratory depression. Drowsiness is a frequent side effect of the medication but does not indicate overdosage.
Test-Taking Strategy: Knowledge regarding the manifestations related to toxicity is required to answer this question. Review the signs that indicate toxicity if you had difficulty with this question.
Level of Cognitive Ability: Analysis
Client Needs: Physiological Integrity
Integrated Process: Nursing Process—assessment
Content Area: Pharmacology
Reference: Hodgson, B., & Kizior, R. (2004). *Saunders nursing drug handbook 2004* (p. 767). Philadelphia: W. B. Saunders.

10. 1
Rationale: Propantheline bromide (Pro-Banthine) is contraindicated in clients with narrow-angle glaucoma, obstructive uropathy, gastrointestinal disease, or ulcerative colitis. The medication decreases bladder muscle spasms.
Test-Taking Strategy: Use the process of elimination. Eliminate options 2 and 3 because they are similar. From the remaining options, you must know the contraindications associated with the medication. Review these contraindications if you had difficulty with this question.
Level of Cognitive Ability: Analysis
Client Needs: Physiological Integrity
Integrated Process: Nursing Process—analysis
Content Area: Pharmacology
Reference: Kee, J., & Hayes, E. (2003). *Pharmacology: A nursing process approach* (4th ed., p. 347). Philadelphia: W. B. Saunders.

11. 3
Rationale: Nephrotoxicity can occur from the use of cyclosporine (Sandimmune). Nephrotoxicity is evaluated by monitoring for elevated blood urea nitrogen and serum creatinine levels. Cyclosporine does not depress the bone marrow.
Test-Taking Strategy: Use the process of elimination. Eliminate options 1 and 2 first because they are unrelated to renal function. Next, eliminate option 4 because the creatinine level would be elevated, not decreased. Option 3 is the only option that indicates an increased level of a renal function test. Review the adverse effects related to this medication if you had difficulty with this question.
Level of Cognitive Ability: Analysis
Client Needs: Physiological Integrity
Integrated Process: Nursing Process—analysis
Content Area: Pharmacology
Reference: Hodgson, B., & Kizior, R. (2004). *Saunders nursing drug handbook 2004* (p. 259). Philadelphia: W. B. Saunders.

12. 2
Rationale: A compound present in grapefruit juice inhibits metabolism of cyclosporine. As a result, consumption of grapefruit juice can raise cyclosporine levels by 50% to 100%, thereby greatly increasing the risk of toxicity.
Test-Taking Strategy: Use the process of elimination, noting the key word "avoid." Use of general pharmacology guidelines will direct you to option 2. If you had difficulty with this question, review this medication and the client instructions regarding its use.
Level of Cognitive Ability: Application
Client Needs: Physiological Integrity
Integrated Process: Teaching/Learning
Content Area: Pharmacology
Reference: Hodgson, B., & Kizior, R. (2004). *Saunders nursing drug handbook 2004* (p. 260). Philadelphia: W. B. Saunders.

13. 4
Rationale: Amphotericin B, erythromycin, and ketoconazole can elevate cyclosporine levels. When either of these medications is combined with cyclosporine, the dosage of cyclosporine must be reduced to prevent accumulation to toxic levels.
Test-Taking Strategy: Knowledge regarding the medications that elevate cyclosporine levels is required to answer this question. If you are unfamiliar with these medications, review these medication interactions.

Level of Cognitive Ability: Analysis
Client Needs: Physiological Integrity
Integrated Process: Nursing Process—analysis
Content Area: Pharmacology
Reference: Kee, J., & Hayes, E. (2003). *Pharmacology: A nursing process approach* (4th ed., p. 439). Philadelphia: W. B. Saunders.

14. 3
Rationale: To improve palatability, the client should be taught to mix the concentrated medication solution with chocolate milk or orange juice just before administration. Grapefruit juice is avoided because it can raise cyclosporine levels. The client is instructed to dilute the concentrate in a glass (not Styrofoam) to ensure ingestion of the complete dose.
Test-Taking Strategy: Knowledge regarding the administration of the oral concentrate of cyclosporine is required to answer this question. Review the client instructions regarding administering this medication if you had difficulty with this question.
Level of Cognitive Ability: Application
Client Needs: Physiological Integrity
Integrated Process: Teaching/Learning
Content Area: Pharmacology
Reference: Hodgson, B., & Kizior, R. (2004). *Saunders nursing drug handbook 2004* (p. 259). Philadelphia: W. B. Saunders.

15. 3
Rationale: The most common adverse effects of cyclosporine are nephrotoxicity, infection, hypertension, tremors, and hirsutism. Of these, nephrotoxicity and infection are the most serious.
Test-Taking Strategy: Knowledge regarding the adverse effects associated with cyclosporine is required to answer this question. If you are unfamiliar with these effects, review this content.
Level of Cognitive Ability: Analysis
Client Needs: Physiological Integrity
Integrated Process: Nursing Process—assessment
Content Area: Pharmacology
Reference: Hodgson, B., & Kizior, R. (2004). *Saunders nursing drug handbook 2004* (p. 260). Philadelphia: W. B. Saunders.

16. 3
Rationale: Tacrolimus (Prograf) is used with caution in immunosuppressed clients and in clients with renal, hepatic, or pancreatic function impairment. Tacrolimus is contraindicated in clients with hypersensitivity to this medication or hypersensitivity to cyclosporine.
Test-Taking Strategy: Use the process of elimination. Many medications affect renal, hepatic, and pancreatic function. If you had to select an option and were unsure, select the option that addresses these body systems. Review the cautions and contraindications associated with the administration of this medication if you had difficulty with this question.
Level of Cognitive Ability: Analysis
Client Needs: Physiological Integrity
Integrated Process: Nursing Process—analysis
Content Area: Pharmacology
Reference: Hodgson, B., & Kizior, R. (2004). *Saunders nursing drug handbook 2004* (p. 949). Philadelphia: W. B. Saunders.

Lehne, R. (2001). *Pharmacology for nursing care* (4th ed., p. 751). Philadelphia: W. B. Saunders.

17. 2
Rationale: Nephrotoxicity is a major concern with this medication. Other common reactions include neurotoxicity evidenced by headache, tremor, and insomnia, gastrointestinal effects such as diarrhea, nausea, and vomiting, hypertension, hyperkalemia, and hyperglycemia.
Test-Taking Strategy: Use the process of elimination, noting that options 1, 3, and 4 represent normal values. Option 2 is the only abnormal value, reflecting an elevation. Review the adverse effects related to this medication if you had difficulty with this question.
Level of Cognitive Ability: Analysis
Client Needs: Physiological Integrity
Integrated Process: Nursing Process—analysis
Content Area: Pharmacology
References: Clark, J., Queener, S., & Karb, V. (2000). *Pharmacologic basis of nursing practice* (6th ed., p. 463). St. Louis: Mosby.
Hodgson, B., & Kizior, R. (2004). *Saunders nursing drug handbook 2004* (p. 950). Philadelphia: W. B. Saunders.

18. 3
Rationale: Mycophenolate mofetil (CellCept) should be administered on an empty stomach. The capsules should not be opened or crushed. The client should contact the physician if unusual bleeding or bruising, sore throat, mouth sores, abdominal pain, or fever occurs. Antacids containing magnesium and aluminum may decrease the absorption of the medication and therefore should not be taken with the medication. The medication is given along with corticosteroids and cyclosporine.
Test-Taking Strategy: Use the process of elimination. Recalling that neutropenia can occur with the use of this medication will direct you to option 3. Review this medication if you had difficulty with this question.
Level of Cognitive Ability: Application
Client Needs: Physiological Integrity
Integrated Process: Teaching/Learning
Content Area: Pharmacology
Reference: Hodgson, B., & Kizior, R. (2004). *Saunders nursing drug handbook 2004* (p. 698). Philadelphia: W. B. Saunders.

19. 2
Rationale: Epoetin alfa is used to reverse anemia associated with chronic renal failure. Therapeutic effect is seen when the hematocrit is between 30% and 33%. Options 1, 3, and 4 are not associated with the action of this medication.
Test-Taking Strategy: Use the process of elimination. Relate the name of the medication, erythropoietin, to the potential action or effect. The only laboratory test that would reflect the effect of this medication is option 2. Review the therapeutic effect of this medication if you had difficulty with this question.
Level of Cognitive Ability: Analysis
Client Needs: Physiological Integrity
Integrated Process: Nursing Process—evaluation
Content Area: Pharmacology

Reference: Hodgson, B., & Kizior, R. (2004). *Saunders nursing drug handbook 2004* (p. 363). Philadelphia: W. B. Saunders.

20. 3
Rationale: The client should be instructed not to shake the bottle. The medication should be refrigerated at all times. The medication should not be frozen. Syringes with a $^5/_8$-inch needle are used for subcutaneous injection. A $1^1/_2$-inch needle may be used for intramuscular injection.
Test-Taking Strategy: Use the process of elimination. Note that options 2 and 3 identify opposite actions. This should provide you with the clue that one of these options may be the correct one. Review the teaching points related to the administration of this medication if you had difficulty with this question.
Level of Cognitive Ability: Application
Client Needs: Physiological Integrity
Integrated Process: Teaching/Learning
Content Area: Pharmacology

Reference: Lehne, R. (2004). *Pharmacology for nursing care* (5th ed., p. 588). Philadelphia: W. B. Saunders.

CRITICAL THINKING: FILL IN THE BLANK
Answer: Atropine sulfate
Rationale: Cholinergic overdose can occur with bethanechol chloride (Urecholine). The antidote is atropine sulfate, administered subcutaneously or intravneously, and it should be readily available for use should overdose occur.
Test-Taking Strategy: Knowledge regarding the antidote for bethanechol chloride is required to answer this question. Review this medication and its antidote if you had difficulty with this question.
Level of Cognitive Ability: Application
Client Needs: Physiological Integrity
Integrated Process: Nursing Process—planning
Content Area: Pharmacology
Reference: Kee, J., & Hayes, E. (2003). *Pharmacology: A nursing process approach* (4th ed., p. 341). Philadelphia: W. B. Saunders.

REFERENCES

Clark, J., Queener, S., & Karb, V. (2000). *Pharmacologic basis of nursing practice* (6th ed.). St. Louis: Mosby.

Gutierrez, K., & Queener, S. (2003). *Pharmacology for nursing practice.* St. Louis: Mosby.

Hodgson, B., & Kizior, R. (2004). *Saunders nursing drug handbook 2004.* Philadelphia: W. B. Saunders.

Kee, J., & Hayes, E. (2003). *Pharmacology: A nursing process approach* (4th ed.). Philadelphia: W. B. Saunders.

Lehne, R. (2001). *Pharmacology for nursing care* (4th ed.). Philadelphia: W. B. Saunders.

Lehne, R. (2004). *Pharmacology for nursing care* (5th ed.). Philadelphia: W. B. Saunders.

UNIT XV

The Adult Client with an Eye or Ear Disorder

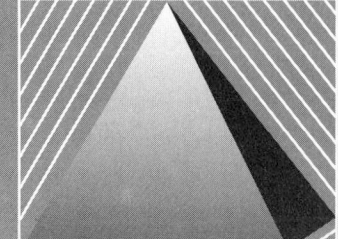

PYRAMID TERMS

accommodation   Process by which a clear visual image is maintained as the gaze is shifted from a distant to a near point.

astigmatism   Corneal curvature; eye may be hyperopic or myopic.

cataract   An opacity of the lens that distorts the image projected onto the retina and that can progress to blindness.

conductive hearing loss   Blockage of sound waves to the inner ear fibers because of external ear or middle ear disorders. Disorders often can be corrected with no damage to hearing or minimal permanent hearing loss.

cycloplegia   The paralysis of the ciliary muscles by medications that block muscarinic receptors. Cycloplegia causes blurred vision because the shape of the lens can no longer be adjusted to near vision.

fenestration   Removal of the stapes with a small hole drilled in the footplate and connection of a prosthesis between the incus and foot plate. Sounds cause the prosthesis to vibrate in the same manner as did the stapes.

glaucoma   Increased intraocular pressure as a result of inadequate drainage of aqueous humor from canal of the Schlemm or overproduction of aqueous humor. The condition damages the optic nerve and can result in blindness.

hyperopia   Farsightedness; objects converge to a point behind the retina. Vision beyond 20 feet is normal, but near vision is poor. Correction is done by a convex lens.

legally blind   The best visual acuity with corrective lenses in the better eye of 20/200 or less or visual acuity of less than 20 degrees of the visual field in the better eye.

Meniere's syndrome   A syndrome also called endolymphatic hydrops that refers to dilation of the endolymphatic system by overproduction or decreased reabsorption of endolymphatic fluid. The syndrome is characterized by tinnitus, unilateral sensorineural hearing loss, and vertigo.

miosis   A constricted pupil achieved primarily by stimulation of the muscarinic receptors of the sphincter muscles.

miotics   Medications that cause contraction of the pupil.

mydriasis   A dilated pupil achieved by blockage of the muscarinic receptors of the sphincter muscles or by stimulation of the alpha receptors of the dilator muscles.

mydriatics   Medications that dilate the pupil.

myopia   Nearsightedness; rays coming from an object are focused in front of the retina. Near vision is normal, but distant vision is defective. A biconcave lens is used for correction.

otosclerosis   Disease of the labyrinthine capsule of the middle ear that results in a bony overgrowth of tissue surrounding the ossicles. Otosclerosis causes the development of irregular areas of new bone formation and causes fixation of the bones. Stapes fixation leads to a conductive hearing loss.

presbycusis   Common cause of sensorineural hearing loss associated with aging.

retinal detachment   Separation of the layers of the retina because of the accumulation of fluid between them or because both retinal layers elevate away from the choroid as a result of a tumor. Partial separation becomes complete if untreated. When detachment becomes complete, blindness occurs.

sensorineural hearing loss   A pathological process of the inner ear or of the sensory fibers that leads to the cerebral cortex. Such hearing loss often is permanent, and measures must be taken to reduce further damage or to attempt to amplify sound as a means of improving hearing to some degree.

▲ PYRAMID TO SUCCESS

Pyramid Points focus on nursing interventions for clients with impairment in sight or hearing and on the nursing care related to disorders such as cataracts, glaucoma, and retinal detachment. Pyramid Points also focus on emergency interventions for eye and ear disorders and injuries. Review nursing care related to organ donation for the donor and the recipient. Pyramid Points also focus on client instructions related to medication administration, sensory perceptual alterations and safety issues, and available support systems. The Integrated Processes addressed in this unit include Nursing Process, Caring, Communication and Documentation, and Teaching/Learning.

▲ CLIENT NEEDS

Safe, Effective Care Environment

Accident prevention related to sensory impairments
Asepsis with procedures and treatments
Client rights
Consultation with members of the health care team
Establishing priorities
Informed consent for invasive procedures
Organ donation
Standard precautions

Health Promotion and Maintenance

Aging process
Expected body image changes
Home care instructions following procedures related to the eye and ear
Instructions regarding the administration of eye and ear medications
Physical assessment of eye and ear disorders
Reinforcement regarding the importance of compliance to the prescribed therapy
The prevention and early detection of health problems and diseases related to the eye and the ear

Psychosocial Integrity

Ability to cope with feelings of isolation and loss of independence

Available community resources
Communication techniques for impaired vision and hearing
Family support systems
Role changes
Sensory perceptual alterations
The threat to vision or hearing loss

Physiological Integrity

Care to assistive devices such as glasses, contact lens, and hearing aids
Complications related to procedures
Expected responses to therapy
Medical emergencies
Pharmacological therapy
Self-care limitations

REFERENCES

Chernecky, C., & Berger, B. (2004). *Laboratory tests & diagnostic procedures* (4th ed.). Philadelphia: W. B. Saunders.

Harkreader, H., & Hogan, M. A. (2004). *Fundamentals of nursing: Caring and clinical judgment* (2nd ed.). Philadelphia: W. B. Saunders.

Ignatavicius, D., & Workman, M. (2002). *Medical-surgical nursing: Critical thinking for collaborative care* (4th ed.). Philadelphia: W. B. Saunders.

Lewis, S., Heitkemper, M., & Dirksen, S. (2004). *Medical-surgical nursing: Assessment and management of clinical problems* (6th ed.). St. Louis: Mosby.

McKenry, L., & Salerno, E. (2003). *Mosby's pharmacology in nursing* (21st ed.) St. Louis: Mosby.

National Council of State Boards of Nursing (Eds.). (2003). *Test Plan for the National Council Licensure Examination for Registered Nurses* (effective date: April 2004). Chicago: Author.

Perry, A., & Potter, P. (2002). *Clinical nursing skills and techniques* (5th ed.). St. Louis: Mosby.

Phipps, W., Monahan, F., Sands, J., Marek, J., & Neighbors, M. (2003). *Medical-surgical nursing: Health and illness perspectives* (7th ed.). St. Louis: Mosby.

Potter, P., & Perry, A. (2001). *Fundamentals of nursing* (5th ed.). St. Louis: Mosby.

Varcarolis, E. M. (2002). *Foundations of psychiatric mental health nursing* (4th ed.). Philadelphia: W. B. Saunders.

The Eye and The Ear

I. ANATOMY AND PHYSIOLOGY OF THE EYE

A. The eye
  1. The eye is 1 inch in diameter.
  2. The eye is located in the anterior portion of the orbit.
  3. The orbit is the bony structure of the skull that surrounds the eye and offers protection to the eye.

B. Layers of the eye
  1. External layer
    a. The external layer is the fibrous coat that supports the eye.
    b. The external layer contains the sclera, which is an opaque white tissue.
    c. The external layer contains the cornea, which is a dense transparent layer.
  2. Middle layer
    a. The middle layer is the second layer of the eyeball.
    b. The middle layer is vascular and heavily pigmented.
    c. The middle layer consists of the choroid, the ciliary body, and the iris.
    d. The choroid is the dark brown membrane located between the sclera and the retina.
    e. The choroid lines most of the sclera and is attached to the retina but can detach easily from the sclera.
    f. The choroid contains many blood vessels and supplies nutrients to the retina.
    g. The ciliary body connects the choroid with the iris and secretes aqueous humor that helps give the eye its shape.
    h. The iris is the colored portion of the eye, is located in front of the lens, and has a central circular opening called the pupil.
  3. Internal layer
    a. The internal layer consists of the retina.
    b. The retina is a thin, delicate structure in which the fibers of the optic nerve are distributed.
    c. The retina is bordered externally by the choroid and sclera and internally by the vitreous.
    d. The retina contains blood vessels and photoreceptors called rods and cones.

C. Vitreous body
  1. The vitreous body contains a gelatinous substance that occupies the vitreous chamber, which is the space between the lens and the retina.
  2. The vitreous body transmits light and gives shape to the posterior eye.

D. Vitreous
  1. Vitreous is a jell-like substance that maintains the shape of the eye.
  2. Vitreous provides additional physical support to the retina.

E. Rods and cones
  1. Rods are responsible for peripheral vision and function at reduced levels of illumination.
  2. Cones function at bright levels of illumination and are responsible for color vision and central vision.

F. Optic disk
  1. The optic disk is a creamy pink to white depressed area in the retina.
  2. The optic nerve enters and exits the eyeball at this area.
  3. This area is called the blind spot because it contains only nerve fibers, lacks photoreceptor cells, and is insensitive to light.

G. Macula lutea
  1. The macula lutea is a small, oval, yellowish pink area located lateral and temporal to the optic disk.
  2. The central depressed part of the macula is the fovea centralis, where most acute vision occurs.

H. Aqueous humor
   1. The aqueous humor is a clear watery fluid that fills the anterior and posterior chambers of the eye.
   2. The aqueous humor is produced by the ciliary processes, and the fluid drains into the canal of Schlemm.
   3. The anterior chamber lies between the cornea and the iris.
   4. The posterior chamber lies between the iris and the lens.
I. Canal of Schlemm
   1. The canal of Schlemm is a passageway that extends completely around the eye.
   2. The canal permits fluid to drain out of the eye into the systemic circulation so a constant intraocular pressure is maintained.
J. Lens
   1. The lens is a transparent circular structure behind the iris and in front of the vitreous body.
   2. The lens bends rays of light so that the light falls on the retina.
K. Pupils
   1. The pupils control the amount of light that enters the eye and reaches the retina.
   2. Darkness produces dilation.
   3. Light produces constriction.
L. Conjunctivae
   1. The conjunctivae are thin transparent mucous membranes.
   2. The conjunctiva lines the posterior surface of each eyelid and is located over the sclera.
M. Lacrimal gland
   1. The larcrimal gland produces tears.
   2. Tears are drained through the punctum into the lacrimal duct and sac.
N. Eye muscles
   1. Muscles do not work independently but work with the muscle that produces the opposite movement.
   2. Rectus muscles exert their pull when the eye turns temporally.
   3. Oblique muscles exert their pull when the eye turns nasally.
O. Nerves
   1. Cranial nerve II: optic nerve (nerve of sight)
   2. Cranial nerve III: oculomotor
   3. Cranial nerve IV: trochlear
   4. Cranial nerve VI: abducens
P. Blood vessels
   1. Ophthalmic artery is the major artery supplying the structures in the eye.
   2. Ophthalmic veins drain the blood from the eye.

▲ II. ASSESSMENT OF VISION (BOX 63-1)
A. Acuity
   1. Visual acuity tests measure the client's distance and near vision.
   2. Snellen's chart

BOX 63-1

Assessment of Vision

Color vision
Confrontational test
Extraocular muscle function
Ophthalmoscopy
Snellen's chart

---

   a. The chart is a simple tool to record visual acuity.
   b. The client stands 20 feet from the chart and covers one eye and uses the other eye to read the line that appears most clearly.
   c. If the client is able to do this accurately, the client reads the next lower line.
   d. This sequence is repeated until the client is unable to identify correctly more than half of the characters on the line.
   e. The procedure is repeated for the other eye.
   f. The findings are recorded as a comparison between what the client can read at 20 feet and the number of feet normally required by an individual to read the same line.
   g. A result of 20/50 means that the client is able to read at 20 feet from the chart what a healthy eye can read at 50 feet.
   h. Clients who wear corrective lenses other than for reading should have their vision tested with the lens in place.
B. Confrontational test
   1. The confrontational test is performed to examine visual fields or peripheral vision.
   2. The examiner and the client sit facing each other.
   3. The client is asked to look directly into the eyes of the examiner throughout the test.
   4. The examiner covers his or her right eye while the client covers his or her left eye.
   5. The examiner moves a finger from a nonvisible area into the client's line of vision.
   6. The examiner and client should see the object at approximately the same time.
   7. When the client sees the object coming into the line of vision, the client informs the examiner.
   8. The procedure is repeated on the opposite eye.
   9. The test assumes that the examiner has normal peripheral vision.
C. Extraocular muscle function
   1. Six cardinal positions of gaze
      a. Client's right (lateral position)
      b. Upward and right (temporal position)
      c. Down and right
      d. Client's left (lateral position)
      e. Upward and left (temporal position)
      f. Down and left
   2. Client holds head still and is asked to move eyes and to follow a small object.

3. The examiner notes for any parallel movements of the eye or for nystagmus, an involuntary rhythmic rapid twitching of the eyeballs.

D. Color vision
1. Tests for color vision involve picking numbers or letters out of a complex and colorful picture.
2. Ishihara chart
   a. The Ishihara chart consists of numbers that are composed of colored dots located within a circle of colored dots.
   b. Client is asked to read the numbers on the chart.
   c. Each eye is tested separately.
   d. The test is sensitive for the diagnosis of red/green blindness but not effective for the detection of the discrimination of blue.

E. Pupils
1. The pupils are round and of equal size.
2. Increasing light causes pupillary constriction.
3. Decreasing light causes pupillary dilation.
4. Constriction of both pupils is a normal response to direct light.
5. The client is asked to look straight ahead while the examiner quickly brings a beam of light (flashlight) in from the side and directs it onto the eye.
6. The constriction of the eye is a direct response to the shining of a light into that eye; constriction of the opposite eye is known as a consensual response.

F. Sclera and cornea
1. Normal sclera color is white.
2. A yellow color to the sclera may indicate jaundice or systemic problems.
3. In a dark skinned person, the sclera may normally appear yellow; pigmented dots may be present.
4. The cornea is transparent, smooth, shiny, and bright.
5. Cloudy areas or specks on the cornea may be the result an accident or eye injury.

G. Ophthalmoscopy
1. The ophthalmoscope is an instrument used to examine the external structures and the interior of the eye.
2. Darken the room so that the pupil will dilate.
3. Hold the instrument with the right hand when examining the right eye and with the left hand when examining the left eye.
4. Ask the client to look straight ahead at an object on the wall.
5. Approach the client's eye from about 12 to 15 inches away and 15 degrees lateral to the client's line of vision.
6. As the instrument is directed at the pupil, a red glare (red reflex) is seen in the pupil.
7. The red reflex is the reflection of light on the vascular retina.
8. Absence of the red reflex may indicate opacity of the lens.
9. The retina, optic disk, optic vessels, fundus, and macula can be examined.

III. DIAGNOSTIC TESTS FOR THE EYE (BOX 63-2)

A. Fluorescein angiography
1. Description: detailed imaging and recording of ocular circulation by a series of photographs after the administration of a dye
2. Preprocedure interventions
   a. Assess the client for allergies and previous reactions to dyes.
   b. Obtain informed consent.
   c. A mydriatic medication, which causes pupil dilation, is instilled in the eye 1 hour before the test.
   d. The dye is injected into a vein of the client's arm.
   e. Inform the client that the dye may cause the skin to appear yellow for several hours after the test and is eliminated gradually through the urine.
   f. The client may experience nausea, vomiting, sneezing, paresthesia of the tongue, or pain at the injection site.
   g. If hives appear, orally or intramuscularly administered antihistamines such as diphenhydramine (Benadryl) are given as prescribed.
3. Postprocedure interventions
   a. Encourage rest.
   b. Encourage fluid intake to assist in eliminating the dye from the client's system.
   c. Remind the client that the yellow skin appearance will disappear.
   d. Instruct the client that the urine will appear bright green until the dye is excreted.
   e. Instruct the client to avoid direct sunlight for a few hours after the test.
   f. Instruct the client that the photophobia will continue until pupil size returns to normal.

B. Computed tomography
1. Description
   a. A beam of x-rays scans the skull and orbits of the eye.
   b. A cross-sectional image is formed by the use of a computer.
   c. Contrast material usually is not administered.
2. Interventions
   a. No special client preparation or follow-up care is required.
   b. Instruct the client that he or she will be positioned in a confined space and will need to keep their heads still during the procedure.

BOX 63-2

Diagnostic Tests for the Eye

Computed tomography
Corneal staining
Fluorescein angiography
Slit lamp
Tonometry

C. Slit lamp
   1. Description
      a. A slit lamp allows examination of the anterior ocular structures under microscopic magnification.
      b. The client leans on a chin rest to stabilize the head while a narrowed beam of light is aimed so that it illuminates only a narrow segment of the eye.
   2. Interventions
      a. Explain the procedure the client.
      b. Advise the client about the brightness of the light and the need to look forward at a point over the examiner's ear.
▲ D. Corneal staining
   1. Description
      a. A topical dye is instilled into the conjuctival sac to outline irregularities of the corneal surface that are not easily visible.
      b. The eye is viewed through a blue filter, and a bright green color indicates areas of a nonintact corneal epithelium.
   2. Interventions
      a. If the client wears contact lenses, the lenses must be removed.
      b. The client is instructed to blink after the dye has been applied to distribute the dye evenly across the cornea.
▲ E. Tonometry
   1. Description
      a. The test is used primarily to assess for an increase of intraocular pressure and potential **glaucoma.**
      b. Normal ocular pressure is 10 to 21 mm Hg.
   2. Interventions
      a. Each eye is anesthetized.
      b. The client is asked to stare forward at a point above the examiner's ear.
      c. A flattened cone is brought in contact with the cornea.
      d. The amount of pressure needed to flatten the cornea is measured.
      e. The client must be instructed to avoid rubbing the eye following the examination if the eye has been anesthetized because the potential for scratching the cornea exists.

▲ **IV. DISORDERS OF THE EYE**
   A. Risk factors related to eye disorders (Box 63-3)
   B. **Legally blind**
      1. Description: the best visual acuity with corrective lenses in the better eye of 20/200 or less or visual acuity of less than 20 degrees of the visual field in the better eye
   ▲ 2. Interventions
      a. When speaking to the client who has limited sight or is blind, the nurse uses a normal tone of voice.
      b. Alert the client when approaching.

BOX 63-3

Risk Factors of Eye Disorders

Aging process
Congenital
Diabetes mellitus
Hereditary
Medications
Trauma

---

      c. Orient the client to the environment.
      d. Use a focal point and provide further orientation to the environment from that focal point.
      e. Allow the client to touch objects in the room.
      f. Use the clock placement of foods on the meal tray to orient the client.
      g. Promote independence as much as is possible.
      h. Provide radios, televisions, and clocks that give the time orally, or provide a braille watch.
      i. When ambulating, allow the client to grasp the nurse's arm at the elbow; the nurse keeps his or her arm close to the body so that the client can detect the direction of movement.
      j. Instruct the client to remain one step behind the nurse when ambulating.
      k. Instruct the client in the use of the cane used for the blind client, which is differentiated from other canes by its straight shape and white color with red tip.
      l. Instruct the client that the cane is held in the dominant hand several inches off the floor.
      m. Instruct the client that the cane sweeps the ground where the client's foot will be placed next to determine the presence of obstacles.
   C. Cataracts   ▲
      1. Description
         a. A **cataract** is an opacity of the lens that distorts the image projected onto the retina and that can progress to blindness.
         b. Causes include the aging process (senile cataracts), inherited (congenital cataracts), and injury (traumatic cataracts); cataracts also can result from another eye disease (secondary cataracts).
         c. Intervention is indicated when visual acuity has been reduced to a level that the client finds to be unacceptable or adversely affects lifestyle.
      2. Assessment
         a. Opaque or cloudy white pupil
         b. Gradual loss of vision
         c. Blurred vision
         d. Decreased color perception
         e. Vision that is better in dim light with pupil dilation
         f. Photophobia
         g. Absence of the red reflex

3. Interventions
   a. Surgical removal of the lens, one eye at a time, is performed.
   b. With extracapsular extraction the lens is lifted out without removing the lens capsule; the procedure may be performed by phacoemulsification in which the lens is broken up by ultrasonic vibrations and is extracted.
   c. With intracapsular extraction the lens is removed within its capsule through a small incision.
   d. A partial iridectomy may be performed with the lens extraction to prevent acute secondary **glaucoma**.
   e. A lens implantation may be performed at the time of the surgical procedure.
4. Preoperative interventions
   a. Instruct the client regarding the postoperative measures to prevent or decrease intraocular pressure.
   b. Administer eye medications preoperatively, including mydriatics and cycloplegics as prescribed.
5. Postoperative interventions

   a. Elevate the head of the bed 30 to 45 degrees.
   b. Turn the client to the back or unoperative side.
   c. Maintain an eye patch; orient the client to the environment.
   d. Position the client's personal belongings to the unoperative side.
   e. Use side rails for safety.
   f. Assist with ambulation.
6. Client education (Box 63-4)

BOX 63-4

Client Education following Cataract Surgery

Avoid eye straining.
Avoid rubbing or placing pressure on the eyes.
Avoid rapid movements, straining, sneezing, coughing, bending, vomiting, or lifting objects of more than 5 lb.
Take measures to prevent constipation.
Follow instructions for dressing changes and prescribed eye drops and medications.
Wipe excess drainage or tearing with a sterile wet cotton ball from the inner to the outward canthus.
Use an eye shield at bedtime.
If a lens implant is not performed, the eye cannot accommodate and glasses must be worn at all times.
Cataract glasses act as magnifying glasses and replace central vision only.
Cataract glasses magnify and objects will appear closer; therefore the client needs to accommodate, judge distance, and climb stairs carefully.
Contact lenses provide sharp visual acuity but dexterity is needed to insert them.
Contact the physician for any decrease in vision, severe eye pain, or increase in eye discharge.

D. Glaucoma
1. Description
   a. Increased intraocular pressure results from inadequate drainage of aqueous humor from the canal of Schlemm or overproduction of aqueous humor.
   b. The condition damages the optic nerve and can result in blindness.
2. Types
   a. Acute closed-angle or narrow-angle **glaucoma** results from obstruction to outflow to aqueous humor.
   b. Chronic closed-angle **glaucoma** follows an untreated attack of acute closed-angle **glaucoma**.
   c. Chronic open-angle **glaucoma** results from overproduction or obstruction to the outflow of aqueous humor.
   d. Acute **glaucoma** is a rapid onset of intraocular pressure greater than 50 to 70 mm Hg.
   e. Chronic **glaucoma** is a slow, progressive, gradual onset of intraocular pressure greater than 30 to 50 mm Hg.
3. Assessment
   a. Progressive loss of peripheral vision followed by loss of central vision
   b. Elevated intraocular pressure (normal pressure is 10 to 21 mm Hg)
   c. Vision worsening in the evening with difficulty adjusting to dark rooms
   d. Blurred vision
   e. Halos around white lights
   f. Frontal headaches
   g. Eye pain
   h. Photophobia
   i. Lacrimation
   j. Progressive loss of central vision
4. Interventions for acute **glaucoma**
   a. Treat acute **glaucoma** as a medical emergency.
   b. Administer medications as prescribed to lower intraocular pressure.
   c. Prepare the client for peripheral iridectomy, which allows aqueous humor to flow from the posterior to anterior chamber.
5. Interventions for chronic **glaucoma**
   a. Instruct the client on the importance of medications (**miotics**) to constrict the pupils, (carbonic anhydrase inhibitors) to decrease the production of aqueous humor, and (β-blockers) to decrease the production of aqueous humor and intraocular pressure.
   b. Instruct the client on the need for lifelong medication use.
   c. Instruct the client to wear a Medic Alert bracelet.
   d. Instruct the client to avoid anticholinergic medications.
   e. Instruct the client to report eye pain, halos around the eyes, and changes in vision to the physician.

f. Instruct the client that when maximal medical therapy has failed to halt the progression of visual field loss and optic nerve damage, surgery will be recommended.

g. Prepare the client for trabeculoplasty as prescribed to facilitate aqueous humor drainage.

h. Prepare the client for trabeculectomy as prescribed, which allows drainage of aqueous humor into the conjunctival spaces by the creation of an opening.

 E. **Retinal detachment**

1. Description

   a. Retinal detachment occurs when the layers of the retina separate because of the accumulation of fluid between them, or when both retinal layers elevate away from the choroid as a result of a tumor.

   b. Partial separation becomes complete if untreated.

   c. When detachment becomes complete, blindness occurs.

2. Assessment

   a. Flashes of light

   b. Floaters

   c. Increase in blurred vision

   d. Sense of a curtain being drawn

   e. Loss of a portion of the visual field

3. Immediate interventions

   a. Provide bed rest.

   b. Cover both eyes with patches to prevent further detachment.

   c. Speak to the client before approaching.

   d. Position the client's head as prescribed.

   e. Protect the client from injury.

   f. Avoid jerky head movements.

   g. Minimize eye stress.

   h. Prepare the client for the surgical procedure as prescribed.

4. Surgical procedures

   a. Draining fluid from the subretinal space so that the retina can return to the normal position

   b. Sealing retinal breaks by cryosurgery, a cold probe applied to the sclera, to stimulate an inflammatory response leading to adhesions

   c. Diathermy, the use of an electrode needle and heat through the sclera, to stimulate an inflammatory response

   d. Laser therapy, to stimulate an inflammatory response, to seal small retinal tears before the detachment occurs

   e. Scleral buckling, to hold the choroid and retina together with a splint until scar tissue forms closing the tear

   f. Insertion of gas or silicone oil to encourage attachment because these agents have a specific gravity less than vitreous or air and can float against the retina

5. Postoperative interventions

   a. Maintain eye patches bilaterally as prescribed.

   b. Monitor for hemorrhage.

   c. Prevent nausea and vomiting and monitor for restlessness, which can cause hemorrhage.

   d. Monitor for sudden, sharp eye pain (notify the physician).

   e. Encourage deep breathing but avoid coughing.

   f. Provide bedrest for 1 to 2 days as prescribed.

   g. Position the client as prescribed.

   h. If gas has been inserted, position client as prescribed on the abdomen and turn the head so unaffected eye is down.

   i. Administer eye medications as prescribed.

   j. Assist the client with activities of daily living.

   k. Avoid sudden head movements or anything that increases intraocular pressure.

   l. Instruct the client to limit reading for 3 to 5 weeks.

   m. Instruct the client to avoid squinting, straining and constipation, lifting heavy objects, and bending from the waist.

   n. Instruct the client to wear dark glasses during the day and an eye patch at night.

   o. Encourage follow-up care because of the danger of recurrence or occurrence in the other eye.

F. Hyphema (Box 63-5)

1. Description

   a. Hyphema is the presence of blood in the anterior chamber.

   b. Hyphema occurs as a result of an injury.

   c. The condition usually resolves in 5 to 7 days.

2. Interventions

   a. Encourage rest with the client in the semi-Fowler position.

   b. Avoid sudden eye movements for 3 to 5 days to decrease the likelihood of bleeding.

   c. Administer cycloplegic eye drops as prescribed to relax the eye muscles and place the eye at rest.

   d. Instruct the client in the use of eye shields or eye patches as prescribed.

   e. Instruct the client to restrict reading and limit watching television.

G. Contusions

1. Description

   a. A contusion is bleeding into the soft tissue as a result of an injury.

BOX 63-5

Types of Eye Injuries

Chemical Burn
Contusion
Foreign Body
Hyphema
Penetrating Object

b. A contusion causes a black eye, and the discoloration disappears in about 10 days.

c. Pain, photophobia, edema, and diplopia may occur.

2. Interventions

a. Place ice on the eye immediately.

b. Instruct the client to receive an eye examination.

H. Foreign bodies

1. Description: an object such as dust that enters the eye

2. Interventions

a. Have the client look upward, expose the lower lid, wet a cotton-tipped applicator with sterile normal saline, and gently twist the swab over the particle and remove it.

b. If the particle cannot be seen, have the client look downward, place a cotton applicator horizontally on the outer surface of the upper eye lid, grasp the lashes, and pull the upper lid outward and over the cotton applicator; if the particle is seen, gently twist swab over it to remove.

I. Penetrating objects

1. Description: an injury that occurs to the eye in which an object penetrates the eye

2. Interventions

a. Never remove the object because it may be holding ocular structures in place; the object must be removed by the physician.

b. Cover the object with a cup.

c. Do not allow the client to bend.

d. Do not place pressure on the eye.

e. Client is to be seen by a physician immediately.

J. Chemical burns

1. Description: an eye injury in which a caustic substance enters the eye

2. Interventions

a. Treatment should begin immediately.

b. Flush the eyes at the site of injury with water for at least 15 to 20 minutes.

c. At the scene of the injury, obtain a sample of the chemical involved.

d. At the emergency room, the eye is irrigated with normal saline solution or an ophthalmic irrigation solution for at least 10 minutes.

e. The solution is directed across the cornea and toward the lateral canthus.

f. Prepare for visual acuity assessment.

g. Apply an antibiotic ointment as prescribed.

h. Cover the eye with a patch as prescribed.

K. Enucleation and exenteration

1. Description

a. Enucleation is removal of the entire eyeball.

b. Exenteration is removal of the eyeball and surrounding tissues and bone.

c. The procedures are performed for the removal of ocular tumors.

d. After the eye is removed, a ball implant is inserted to provide a firm base for socket prosthesis and to facilitate the best cosmetic result.

e. A prosthesis is fitted about 1 month after surgery.

2. Preoperative interventions

a. Provide emotional support to the client.

b. Encourage the client to verbalize feelings related to loss.

3. Postoperative interventions

a. Monitor vital signs.

b. Assess a pressure patch or dressing.

c. Report changes in vital signs or the presence of bright red drainage on the pressure patch or dressing.

L. Organ donation

1. Donor eyes

a. Donor eyes are obtained from cadavers.

b. Donor eyes must be enucleated soon after death because of rapid endothelial cell death.

c. Donor eyes must be stored in a preserving solution.

d. Storage, handling, and coordination of donor tissue with surgeons is provided by a network of state eye bank associations across the country.

2. Care to the deceased client as a potential eye donor

a. Discuss the option of eye donation with the physician and family.

b. Raise the head of the bed 30 degrees.

c. Instill antibiotic eye drops as prescribed.

d. Close the eyes and apply a small ice pack to the closed eyes.

3. Preoperative care to the recipient

a. Recipient may be told of the tissue availability only several hours to 1 day before the surgery.

b. Assist in alleviating client anxiety.

c. Assess eye for signs of infection.

d. Report the presence of any redness, watery or purulent drainage, or edema around the eye to the physician.

e. Instill antibiotic drops into the eye as prescribed to reduce the number of microorganisms present.

f. Administer fluids and medications intravenously as prescribed.

4. Postoperative care to the recipient

a. Eye is covered with a pressure patch and protective shield that is left in place until the next day.

b. Do not remove or change the dressing without a physician's order.

c. Monitor vital signs.

d. Monitor level of consciousness.

e. Assess dressing.

f. Position the client with the head elevated and the nonoperative side to reduce intraocular pressure.

g. Orient the client frequently.

h. Monitor for complications of bleeding, wound leakage, infection, and graft rejection.

i. Instruct the client how to apply a patch and eye shield.

j. Instruct the client to wear the eye shield at night for 1 month and whenever around small children or pets.

k. Advise the client not to rub the eye.

5. Graft rejection (Box 63-6)

a. Rejection can occur at any time.

b. Inform the client of the signs of rejection.

c. Signs include *r*edness, *s*welling, decreased *v*ision, and *p*ain (RSVP).

d. The eye is treated with topical corticosteroids.

V. ANATOMY AND PHYSIOLOGY OF THE EAR

A. Functions
1. Hearing
2. Maintenance of balance

B. External ear
1. The external ear is embedded in the temporal bone bilaterally at the level of the eyes.
2. The external ear extends from the auricle through the external canal to the tympanic membrane or eardrum.
3. The external ear includes the mastoid process, which is the bony ridge located over the temporal bone.

C. Middle ear
1. The middle ear consists of the medial side of the tympanic membrane.
2. The middle ear contains three bony ossicles:
   a. Malleus
   b. Incus
   c. Stapes
3. The tympanic membrane is a thick transparent sheet of tissue that provides a barrier between the external and the middle ear.
4. The middle ear is protected from the inner ear by the round and the oval window membranes.
5. The eustachian tube opens into the middle ear and allows for equalization of pressure on both sides of the tympanic membrane.

D. Inner ear
1. The inner ear contains the semicircular canals, the cochlea, and the distal end of the eighth cranial nerve.
2. The semicircular canals contain fluid and hair cells connected to sensory nerve fibers of the vestibular portion of the eighth cranial nerve.
3. The inner ear maintains sense of balance or equilibrium.
4. The cochlea is the spiral-shaped organ of hearing.
5. The organ of Corti (within the cochlea) is the receptor and organ of hearing.
6. Eighth cranial nerve
   a. The cochlear branch of the nerve transmits neuroimpulses from the cochlea to the brain where they are interpreted as sound.
   b. The vestibular branch maintains balance and equilibrium.

E. Hearing and equilibrium
1. The external ear conducts sound waves to the middle ear.
2. The middle ear, also called the tympanic cavity, conducts sound waves to the inner ear.
3. The middle ear is filled with air, which is kept at atmospheric pressure by the opening of the eustachian tube.
4. The inner ear contains sensory receptors for sound and for equilibrium.
5. The receptors in the inner ear transmit sound waves and changes in body position to the nerve impulses.

VI. ASSESSMENT OF THE EAR (BOX 63-7)

A. Otoscopic examination
1. The speculum is never introduced blindly into the external canal because of the risk of perforating the tympanic membrane.
2. The client's head is tilted slightly away and the otoscope is held upside down as if it were a large pen, for this permits the examiner's hand to lay against the client's head for support.
3. Pull the pinna up and back to straighten the external canal in an adult.
4. Visualize the external canal while slowly inserting the speculum.

BOX 63-6

Signs of Graft Rejection: Corneal Transplant

RSVP:
*R*edness
*S*welling
*V*isual acuity decreased
*P*ain

BOX 63-7

Assessment of Hearing

Otoscopic examination
Tuning fork tests:
   Rinne tuning fork test
   Weber tuning fork test
Vestibular assessment:
   Gaze nystagmus evaluation
   Hallpike's maneuver
   Test for falling
   Test for past pointing
Voice test
Watch test

5. The normal external canal is pink and intact without lesions and with various amounts of cerumen and fine little hairs.
6. Assess the tympanic membrane for intactness; the normal tympanic membrane is intact, without perforations, and should be free from lesions.
7. The tympanic membrane is transparent, opaque, pearly gray, and slightly concave.

B. Auditory assessment
   1. Sound is transmitted by air conduction and bone conduction.
   2. Air conduction takes 2 to 3 times longer than bone conduction.
   3. **Hearing loss** is categorized as **conductive, sensorineural,** and mixed **conductive** and **sensorineural.**
   4. **Conductive hearing loss** is due to any physical obstruction to the transmission of sound waves.
   5. **Sensorineural hearing loss** is due to a defect in the organ of hearing, in the eighth cranial nerve, or in the brain itself.
   6. A mixed **conductive/sensorineural hearing loss** results in profound hearing loss.

C. Voice test
   1. Ask the client to block one external canal.
   2. The examiner stands 1 to 2 feet away and whispers a statement.
   3. Client is asked to repeat the whispered statement.
   4. Each ear is tested separately.

D. Watch test
   1. A ticking watch is used to test for high frequency sounds.
   2. The examiner holds a ticking watch about 5 inches from each ear and asks the client if the ticking is heard.

E. Tuning fork tests
   1. Weber tuning fork test
      a. Place the vibrating tuning fork stem in the middle of the client's head, at the midline of the forehead, or above the upper lip over the teeth.
      b. Hold the fork by the stem only.
      c. The client is asked whether the sound is heard equally in both ears or whether the sound is louder in one ear.
      d. Normal test result is hearing the sound equally in both ears.
      e. If the client hears the sound louder in one ear, the term lateralization is applied to the side hearing the loudest.
      f. Such a finding may indicate that the client has a conductive hearing loss in the ear to which the sound is lateralized or that sensorineural hearing loss has occurred in the opposite ear.
   2. Rinne tuning fork test
      a. The test compares the client's hearing by air conduction and bone conduction.
      b. Air conduction is 2 to 3 times longer than bone conduction.
      c. The vibrating tuning fork stem is placed on the client's mastoid process and the client is asked to indicate when he or she no longer hears the sound.
      d. The examiner quickly brings the tuning fork in front of the pinna without touching the client and asks the client to indicate if he or she still hears the sound.
      e. The client normally continues to hear the sound 2 times longer in front of the pinna; such results are a positive Rinne test.
      f. The examiner records the duration of both phases, bone conduction followed by air conduction and compares the times.
      g. If the client is unable to hear the sound through the ear in front of the pinna, the client may have a **conductive hearing loss** on the side tested; in this situation, the bone conduction is greater than the air conduction (negative Rinne test).
      h. The Rinne test is of no value in determining **sensorineural hearing loss.**

F. Vestibular assessment
   1. Test for falling
      a. The examiner asks the client to stand with the feet together and arms hanging loosely at the side and eyes closed.
      b. The client normally remains erect with only slight swaying.
      c. A significant sway is a positive Romberg's sign.
   2. Test for past pointing
      a. The client sits in front of the examiner.
      b. The client closes the eyes and extends the arms in front, pointing both index fingers at the examiner.
      c. The examiner holds and touches his or her own extended index fingers under the extended index fingers of the client to give the client a point of reference.
      d. The client is instructed to raise both arms and then lower them, attempting to return to the examiner's extended index fingers.
      e. The normal test response is that the client can easily return to the point of reference.
      f. The client with a vestibular function problem lacks a normal sense of position and is unable to return the extended fingers to the point of reference; instead, the fingers deviate to the right or the left of the reference point.
   3. Gaze nystagmus evaluation
      a. The client's eyes are examined as the client looks straight ahead, 30 degrees to each side, upward and downward.
      b. Any spontaneous nystagmus, an involuntary, rhythmic, rapid twitching of the eyeballs,

represents a problem with the vestibular system.
4. Hallpike's maneuver
   a. Assesses for positional vertigo or induced dizziness.
   b. The client assumes a supine position.
   c. The head is rotated to one side for 1 minute.
   d. A positive test results in nystagmus after 5 to 10 seconds.

VII. DIAGNOSTIC TESTS FOR THE EAR (BOX 63-8)

A. Tomography
   1. Description
      a. Tomography may be performed with or without contrast medium.
      b. Tomography assesses the mastoid, middle ear, and inner ear structures.
      c. Multiple radiographs of the head are made.
      d. Tomography is especially helpful in the diagnosis of acoustic tumors.
   2. Interventions
      a. All jewelry is removed.
      b. Lead eye shields are used to cover the cornea to diminish the radiation dose to the eyes.
      c. The client must remain still in a supine position.
      d. No follow-up care is required.
B. Audiometry
   1. Description
      a. Audiometry measures hearing acuity.
      b. Audiometry uses two types, pure tone audiometry and speech audiometry.
      c. Pure tone audiometry is used to identify problems with hearing, speech, music, and other sounds in the environment.
      d. In speech audiometry, the client's ability to hear spoken words is measured.
      e. After testing, audiogram patterns are depicted on a graph to determine the type and level of the hearing loss.
   2. Interventions
      a. Inform the client regarding the procedure.
      b. Instruct the client to identify the sounds as they are heard.
C. Electronystagmography
   1. Description
      a. Electronystagmography is a vestibular test that evaluates spontaneous and induced eye movements known as nystagmus.

   b. Electronystagmography is used to distinguish between normal nystagmus and medication-induced nystagmus or nystagmus caused by a lesion in the central or peripheral vestibular pathway.
   c. Electronystagmography records changing electrical fields with the movement of the eye, as monitored by electrodes placed on the skin around the eye.
   2. Interventions
      a. The client is instructed to remain NPO for 3 hours before testing.
      b. Unnecessary medications are omitted for 24 hours before testing.
      c. Instruct the client that this is a long and tiring procedure.
      d. The client should bring prescription eyeglasses to the examination.
      e. Client sits and is instructed to gaze at lights, focus on a moving pattern, focus on a moving point, and then close the eyes.
      f. While sitting in a chair, the client may be rotated to provide information about vestibular function.
      g. In addition, the client's ears are irrigated with cool and warm water, which may cause nausea and vomiting.
      h. Following the procedure, the client begins taking clear fluids slowly and cautiously because nausea and vomiting may occur.
      i. Assistance with ambulation may also be necessary following the procedure.

VIII. DISORDERS OF THE EAR

A. Risk factors related to ear disorders (Box 63-9)
B. **Conductive hearing loss**
   1. Description
      a. **Conductive hearing loss** occurs when sound waves are blocked to the inner ear fibers because of external ear or middle ear disorders.
      b. Disorders often can be corrected with no damage to hearing or minimal permanent hearing loss.
   2. Causes
      a. Any inflammatory process or obstruction of the external or middle ear
      b. Tumors

BOX 63-8

Diagnostic Tests for the Ear

Audiometry
Electronystagmography
Tomography

BOX 63-9

Risk Factors of Ear Disorders

Aging process
Infection
Medications
Ototoxicity
Trauma
Tumors

c. **Otosclerosis**

d. A buildup of scar tissue on the ossicles from previous middle ear surgery

C. **Sensorineural hearing loss**

1. Description

a. **Sensorineural hearing loss** is a pathological process of the inner ear or of the sensory fibers that lead to the cerebral cortex.

b. **Sensorineural hearing loss** is often permanent, and measures must be taken to reduce further damage or to attempt to amplify sound as a means of improving hearing to some degree.

2. Causes

a. Damage to the inner ear structures

b. Damage to the eighth cranial nerve

c. Prolonged exposure to loud noise

d. Medications

e. Trauma

f. Inherited disorders

g. Metabolic and circulatory disorders

h. Infections

i. Surgery

j. **Meniere's syndrome**

k. Diabetes mellitus

l. Myxedema

D. Mixed hearing loss

1. Mixed hearing loss also is known as **conductive-sensorineural hearing loss.**

2. Client has **sensorineural** and **conductive hearing loss.**

E. Signs of hearing loss and facilitating communication (Boxes 63-10 and 63-11)

F. Cochlear implantation

1. Cochlear implants are used for **sensorineural hearing loss.**

2. A small computer converts sound waves into electrical impulses.

3. Electrodes are placed by the internal ear with a computer device attached to the external ear.

4. Electronic impulses directly stimulate nerve fibers.

G. Hearing aids

1. Hearing aids are used for the client with **conductive hearing loss.**

2. Hearing aids can help the client with **sensorineural hearing loss,** although they are not as effective.

3. A difficulty that exists in the use of hearing aids is the amplification of background noise and of voices.

4. Client education (Box 63-12)

BOX 63-11

Facilitation of Communication

Using written words if the client is able to see, read, and write

Providing plenty of light in the room

Getting the attention of the client before beginning to speak

Facing the client when speaking

Talking in a room without distracting noises

Moving close to the client and speaking slowly and clearly

Keeping hands and other objects away from the mouth when talking to the client

Talking in lower tones because shouting is not helpful

Rephrasing sentences and repeating information

Validating with the client the understanding of statements made by asking the client to repeat what was said

Reading lips

Encouraging the client to wear glasses when talking to someone to improve vision for lip reading

Using sign language, which combines speech with hand movements that signify letters, words, or phrases

Using telephone amplifiers

Flashing lights that are activated by ringing of the telephone or doorbell

Specially trained dogs that help the client to be aware of sound and to alert the client to potential dangers

---

BOX 63-10

Signs of Hearing Loss

Frequently asking others to repeat statements

Straining to hear

Turning head or leaning forward to favor one ear

Shouting in conversation

Ringing in the ears

Failing to respond when not looking in the direction of the sound

Answering questions incorrectly

Raising the volume of the television or radio

Avoiding large groups

Better understanding of speech when in small groups

Withdrawing from social interactions

BOX 63-12

Client Education regarding a Hearing Aid

Encourage client to begin using the hearing aid slowly to adjust to the device.

Adjust the volume to the minimal hearing level to prevent feedback squeaking.

Teach the client to concentrate on the sounds that are to be heard and to filter out background noise.

Instruct the client to clean the ear mold with mild soap and water.

Avoid excessive wetting of the hearing aid and try to keep the hearing aid dry.

Clean the ear cannula of the hearing aid with a toothpick or pipe cleaner.

Turn off the hearing aid and remove the battery when not in use.

Keep extra batteries on hand.

Keep the hearing aid in a safe place.

Prevent hair sprays, oils, or other hair and face products from coming in contact with the receiver of the hearing aid.

▲ H. Presbycusis
  1. Description
     a. **Presbycusis** is associated with aging.
     b. **Presbycusis** leads to degeneration or atrophy of the ganglion cells in the cochlea and a loss of elasticity of the basilar membranes.
     c. **Presbycusis** leads to compromise of the vascular supply to the inner ear with changes in several areas of the ear structure.
  2. Assessment
     a. Hearing loss is gradual and bilateral.
     b. Client states that he or she has no problem with hearing but cannot understand what the words are.
     c. Client thinks that the speaker is mumbling.
 I. External otitis
  1. Description
     a. External otitis is an infective inflammatory or allergic response involving the structure of the external auditory canal or the auricles.
     b. An irritating or infective agent comes in contact with the epithelial layer of the external ear.
     c. Contact leads to an allergic response or signs and symptoms of an infection.
     d. The skin becomes red, swollen, and tender to touch on movement.
     e. The extensive swelling of the canal can lead to **conductive hearing loss** because of obstruction.
     f. External otitis is more common in children, is termed "swimmer's ear," and occurs more often in hot, humid environments.
     g. Prevention includes the elimination of irritating or infecting agents.
  2. Assessment
     a. Pain
     b. Itching
     c. Plugged feeling in the ear
     d. Redness and edema
     e. Exudate
     f. Hearing loss
  3. Interventions
     a. Apply heat locally for 20 minutes 3 times a day.
     b. Encourage rest to assist in reducing pain.
     c. Administer antibiotics or steroids as prescribed.
     d. Administer analgesics such as aspirin or acetaminophen (Tylenol) for the pain as prescribed.
     e. Instruct the client that the ears should be kept clean and dry.
     f. Instruct the client to use earplugs for swimming.
     g. Instruct the client that cotton-tipped applicators should not be used to dry ears because their use can lead to trauma to the canal.
     h. Instruct the client that irritating agents such as hair products or headphones should be discontinued.
 J. Otitis media: Refer to Chapter 36.
  1. Myringotomy

BOX 63-13

Client Education following Myringotomy

Avoid strenuous activities.
Avoid rapid head movements, bouncing, or bending.
Avoid straining on bowel movement.
Avoid drinking through a straw.
Avoid traveling by air.
Avoid forceful coughing.
Avoid contact with persons with colds.
Avoid washing hair, showering, or getting the head wet for 1 week as prescribed.
Instruct the client that if he or she needs to blow the nose, to blow one side at a time with the mouth open.
Instruct the client to keep ears dry by keeping a ball of cotton coated with petroleum jelly in the ear and to change cotton ball daily.
Instruct the client to report excessive ear drainage to the physician.

---

     a. Refer to Chapter 36.
     b. Client education (Box 63-13)
 K. Chronic otitis media
  1. Description
     a. Chronic otitis media is a chronic infective, inflammatory, or allergic response involving the structure of the middle ear.
     b. Surgical treatment is necessary to restore hearing.
     c. The type of surgery can vary and includes a simple reconstruction of the tympanic membrane, a myringoplasty, or replacement of the ossicles within the middle ear.
     d. A tympanoplasty, a reconstruction of the middle ear, may be attempted to improve **conductive hearing loss.**
  2. Preoperative interventions
     a. Administer antibiotic drops as prescribed.
     b. Clean the ear of debris as prescribed; irrigate the ear with a solution of equal parts of vinegar and sterile water as prescribed to restore the normal pH of the ear.
     c. Instruct the client to avoid persons with upper respiratory infections.
     d. Instruct the client to obtain adequate rest, eat a balanced diet, and drink adequate fluids.
     e. Instruct the client in deep breathing and coughing; forceful coughing, which increases pressure in the middle ear, is to be avoided postoperatively.
  3. Postoperative interventions
     a. Inform the client that initial hearing after surgery is diminished because of the packing in the ear canal and that hearing improvement will occur after the ear canal packing is removed.
     b. Keep dressing clean and dry.
     c. Keep the client flat with operative ear up for at least 12 hours.

d. Administer antibiotics as prescribed.

e. Instruct the client that the client may return to work in about 3 weeks postoperatively as prescribed.

L. Mastoiditis

1. Description

a. Mastoiditis may be acute or chronic and results from untreated or inadequately treated chronic or acute otitis media.

b. The pain is not relieved by myringotomy.

2. Assessment

a. Swelling behind the ear and pain with minimal movement of the head

b. Cellulitis on the skin or external scalp over the mastoid process

c. A reddened, dull, thick, immobile tympanic membrane with or without perforation

d. Tender and enlarged postauricular lymph nodes

e. Low-grade fever

f. Malaise

g. Anorexia

3. Interventions

a. Prepare the client for surgical removal of infected material.

b. Monitor for complications.

c. Simple or modified radical mastoidectomy with tympanoplasty is the most common treatment.

d. Once tissue that is infected is removed, the tympanoplasty is performed to reconstruct the ossicles and the tympanic membranes in an attempt to restore normal hearing.

4. Complications

a. Damage to the abducens and facial cranial nerves

b. Damage exhibited by inability to look laterally (cranial nerve VI, abducens) and a drooping of the mouth on the affected side (cranial nerve VII, facial)

c. Meningitis

d. Brain abscess

e. Chronic purulent otitis media

f. Wound infections

g. Vertigo, if the infection spreads into the labyrinth

5. Postoperative interventions

a. Monitor for dizziness.

b. Monitor for signs of meningitis as evidenced by a stiff neck and vomiting.

c. Prepare for a wound dressing change 24 hours postoperatively.

d. Monitor the surgical incision for edema, drainage, and redness.

e. Position the client flat with the operative side up.

f. Restrict the client to bed with bedside commode privileges for 24 hours as prescribed.

g. Assist the client with getting out of bed to prevent falling or injuries from dizziness.

h. With reconstruction of the ossicles via a graft, take precautions to prevent dislodging of the graft.

M. **Otosclerosis**

1. Description

a. **Otosclerosis** is a disease of the labyrinthine capsule of the middle ear that results in a bony overgrowth of the tissue surrounding the ossicles.

b. **Otosclerosis** causes the development of irregular areas of new bone formation and causes the fixation of the bones.

c. Stapes fixation leads to a **conductive hearing loss.**

d. If the disease involves the inner ear, **sensorineural hearing loss** is present.

e. To have bilateral involvement is not uncommon, although hearing loss may be worse in one ear.

f. The cause is unknown, although it is thought to have a familial tendency.

g. Nonsurgical intervention promotes the improvement of hearing through amplification.

h. Surgical intervention involves removal of the bony growth that is causing the hearing loss.

i. A partial stapedectomy or complete stapedectomy with prosthesis (**fenestration**) may be performed surgically.

2. Assessment

a. Slowly progressing **conductive hearing loss**

b. Bilateral hearing loss

c. A ringing or roaring type of constant tinnitus

d. Loud sounds heard in the ear when chewing

e. Pinkish discoloration (Schwartze's sign) of the tympanic membrane, which indicates vascular changes within the ear.

f. Negative Rinne test

g. Weber test that shows lateralization of sound to the ear with the most **conductive hearing loss**

N. Fenestration

1. Description

a. **Fenestration** is removal of the stapes with a small hole drilled in the footplate, and a prosthesis is connected between the incus and footplate.

b. Sounds cause the prosthesis to vibrate in the same manner as did the stapes.

c. Complications include complete hearing loss, prolonged vertigo, infection, or facial nerve damage.

2. Preoperative interventions

a. Instruct the client in measures to prevent middle ear or external ear infections.

b. Instruct the client to avoid excessive nose blowing.

c. Instruct the client not to clean the ear canal with cotton-tipped applicators.

d. Instruct the client to remove the hearing aid 2 weeks before surgery to ensure the integration of local tissue.

3. Postoperative interventions
   a. Inform the client that hearing is initially worse after the surgical procedure because of swelling and that no noticeable improvement in hearing may occur for as long as 6 weeks.
   b. Inform the client that the Gelfoam ear packing interferes with hearing but is used to decrease bleeding.
   c. Assist with ambulating during the first 1 to 2 days after surgery.
   d. Provide side rails when the client is in bed.
   e. Administer antibiotics, antivertiginous, and pain medications as prescribed.
   f. Assess for facial nerve damage, weakness, changes in tactile sensation, changes in taste sensation, vertigo, nausea, and vomiting.
   g. Instruct the client to move the head slowly when changing positions to prevent vertigo.
   h. Instruct the client to avoid persons with upper respiratory tract infections.
   i. Instruct the client to avoid showering and getting the head and wound wet.
   j. Instruct the client to avoid using small objects (cotton-tipped applicators) to clean the external ear canal.
   k. Instruct the client to avoid rapid, extreme changes in pressure caused by quick head movements, sneezing, nose blowing, straining, and changes in altitude.
   l. Instruct the client to avoid changes in middle ear pressure because they could dislodge the graft or prosthesis.

O. Labyrinthitis
   1. Description: infection of the labyrinth that occurs as a complication of acute or chronic otitis media
   2. Assessment
      a. Hearing loss that may be permanent on the affected side
      b. Tinnitus
      c. Spontaneous nystagmus to the affected side
      d. Vertigo
      e. Nausea and vomiting
   3. Interventions
      a. Monitor for signs of meningitis, the most common complication, as evidenced by headache, stiff neck, and lethargy.
      b. Administer systemic antibiotics as prescribed.
      c. Advise the client to rest in bed in a darkened room.
      d. Administer antiemetics and antivertiginous medications as prescribed.
      e. Instruct the client that the vertigo subsides as the inflammation resolves.
      f. Instruct the client that balance problems that persist may require gait training through physical therapy.

P. **Meniere's syndrome**
   1. Description
      a. **Meniere's syndrome** is also called endolymphatic hydrops and refers to dilation of the endolymphatic system by overproduction or decreased reabsorption of endolymphatic fluid.
      b. The syndrome is characterized by tinnitus, unilateral **sensorineural hearing loss,** and vertigo.
      c. Symptoms occur in attacks and last for several days, and the client becomes totally incapacitated during the attacks.
      d. Initial hearing loss is reversible but as the frequency of attacks continues, hearing loss becomes permanent.
      e. Repeated damage to the cochlea caused by increased fluid pressure leads to the permanent hearing loss.
   2. Causes
      a. Any factor that increases endolymphatic secretion in the labyrinth
      b. Viral and bacterial infections
      c. Allergic reactions
      d. Biochemical disturbances
      e. Vascular disturbance producing changes in the microcirculation in the labyrinth
   3. Assessment
      a. Feelings of fullness in the ear
      b. Tinnitus, as a continuous low-pitched roar or humming sound, that is present much of the time but worsens just before and during severe attacks
      c. Hearing loss that is worse during an attack
      d. Vertigo, as periods of whirling, that might cause the client to fall to the ground
      e. Vertigo that is so intense that even while lying down, the client holds the bed or ground in an attempt to prevent the whirling
      f. Nausea and vomiting
      g. Nystagmus
      h. Severe headaches
   4. Nonsurgical interventions
      a. Prevent injury during vertigo attacks.
      b. Provide bedrest in a quiet environment.
      c. Provide assistance with walking.
      d. Instruct the client to move the head slowly to prevent worsening of the vertigo.
      e. Initiate sodium and fluid restrictions as prescribed.
      f. Instruct the client not to stop smoking.
      g. Administer nicotinic acid (niacin) as prescribed for its vasodilatory effect.
      h. Administer antihistamines as prescribed, which will reduce the production of histamine and the inflammation.
      i. Administer antiemetics as prescribed.
      j. Administer tranquilizers and sedatives as prescribed to calm the client and allow the client to rest and to control vertigo, nausea, and vomiting.

5. Surgical interventions
   a. Surgery is performed when medical therapy is ineffective and the functional level of the client has decreased significantly.
   b. Endolymphatic drainage and insertion of a shunt may be performed early in the course of the disease to assist with the drainage of excess fluids.
   c. A resection of the vestibular nerve or total removal of the labyrinth or a labyrinthectomy may be performed.
6. Postoperative interventions
   a. Assess packing and dressing on the ear.
   b. Speak to the client on the side of the unaffected ear.
   c. Perform neurological assessments.
   d. Maintain side rails.
   e. Assist with ambulating.
   f. Encourage the use of a bedside commode.
   g. Administer antivertiginous and antiemetic medications as prescribed.

Q. Acoustic neuroma
1. Description
   a. Acoustic neuroma is a benign tumor of the vestibular or acoustic nerve.
   b. The tumor may cause damage to hearing and to facial movements and sensations.
   c. Treatment includes surgical removal of the tumor via craniotomy.
   d. Care is taken to preserve the function of the facial nerve.
   e. The tumor rarely recurs after surgical removal.
   f. Postoperative nursing care is similar to postoperative craniotomy care.
2. Assessment
   a. Symptoms usually begin with tinnitus and progress to gradual **sensorineural hearing loss.**
   b. As the tumor enlarges, damage to adjacent cranial nerves occurs.

R. Trauma
1. Description
   a. The tympanic membrane has a limited stretching ability and gives way under high pressure.
   b. Foreign objects placed in the external canal may exert pressure on the tympanic membrane and cause perforation.
   c. If the object continues through the canal, the bony structure of the stapes, incus, and malleus may be damaged.
   d. A blunt injury to the basal skull and ear can damage the middle ear structures through fractures extending to the middle ear.
   e. Excessive nose blowing and rapid changes of pressure that occur with nonpressurized air flights can increase pressure in the middle ear.
   f. Depending on the damage to the ossicles, hearing loss may or may not return.

2. Interventions
   a. Tympanic membrane perforations usually heal within 24 hours.
   b. Surgical reconstruction of the ossicles and tympanic membrane through tympanoplasty or myringoplasty may be performed to improve hearing.

S. Cerumen and foreign bodies
1. Description
   a. Cerumen or wax is the most common cause of impacted canals.
   b. Foreign bodies can include vegetables, beads, pencil erasers, or insects.
2. Assessment
   a. Sensation of fullness in the ear with or without hearing loss
   b. Pain, itching, or bleeding
3. Cerumen
   a. Removal of wax by irrigation is a slow process.
   b. Irrigation is contraindicated in clients with a history of tympanic membrane perforation.
   c. To soften cerumen, add three drops of glycerin to the ear at bedtime, and three drops of hydrogen peroxide twice a day as prescribed.
   d. After several days, irrigate the ear.
   e. The maximal amount of solution that should be used for irrigation is 50 to 70 mL.
4. Foreign bodies
   a. With a foreign object of vegetable matter, irrigation is used with care because this material expands with hydration.
   b. Insects are killed before removal, unless they can be coaxed out by flashlight or a humming noise.
   c. Mineral oil or alcohol is instilled to suffocate the insect, which then is removed using ear forceps.
   d. Use a small ear forceps to remove the object and avoid pushing the object farther into the canal and damaging the tympanic membrane.

PRACTICE QUESTIONS

1. The clinic nurse is preparing to test the visual acuity of a client using a Snellen's chart. Which of the following identifies the accurate procedure for this visual acuity test?
   1. Both eyes are assessed together, followed by the assessment of the right and then the left eye.
   2. The right eye is tested followed by the left eye, and then both eyes are tested.
   3. The client is asked to stand at a distance of 40 feet from the chart and is asked to read the largest line on the chart.
   4. The client is asked to stand at a distance of 40 feet from the chart and to read the line that can be read 200 feet away by an individual with unimpaired vision.

2. The client's vision is tested with a Snellen's chart. The results of the tests are documented as 20/60. The nurse interprets this as
   1. The client can read at a distance of 60 feet what a client with normal vision can read at 20 feet.
   2. The client is legally blind.
   3. The client's vision is normal.
   4. The client can read only at a distance of 20 feet what a client with normal vision can read at 60 feet.

3. The clinic nurse notes that following several eye examinations, the physician has documented a diagnosis of legal blindness in the client's chart. The nurse reviews the results of the Snellen's chart test expecting to note which finding?
   1. 20/20 vision
   2. 20/40 vision
   3. 20/60 vision
   4. 20/200 vision

4. Tonometry is performed on the client with a suspected diagnosis of glaucoma. The nurse analyzes the test results as documented in the client's chart and understands that normal intraocular pressure is
   1. 2 to 7 mm Hg
   2. 10 to 21 mm Hg
   3. 22 to 30 mm Hg
   4. 31 to 35 mm Hg

5. The nurse is developing a plan of care for the client scheduled for cataract surgery. The nurse documents which most appropriate nursing diagnosis in the plan of care?
   1. Self-Care Deficit
   2. Imbalanced Nutrition
   3. Disturbed Sensory Perception
   4. Anxiety

6. The nurse is performing an assessment on a client with a suspected diagnosis of cataract. The chief clinical manifestation that the nurse would expect to note in the early stages of cataract formation is
   1. Eye pain.
   2. Floating spots.
   3. Blurred vision.
   4. Diplopia.

7. In preparation for cataract surgery, the nurse is to administer prescribed eye drops. The nurse reviews the physician's orders, expecting which type of eye drops to be prescribed?
   1. An osmotic diuretic
   2. A miotic agent
   3. A mydriatic medication
   4. A thiazide diuretic

8. During the early postoperative period, the client who had a cataract extraction complains of nausea and severe eye pain over the operative site. The initial nursing action is to
   1. Call the physician.
   2. Administer the ordered pain medication and antiemetic.

3. Reassure the client that this is normal.
4. Turn the client on his or her operative side.

9. The client is being discharged from the ambulatory care unit following cataract removal. The nurse provides instructions regarding home care. Which of the following, if stated by the client, indicates an understanding of the instructions?
   1. "I will take aspirin if I have any discomfort."
   2. "I will sleep on the side that I was operated on."
   3. "I will wear my eye shield at night and my glasses during the day."
   4. "I will not lift anything if it weighs more than 10 pounds."

10. The client with glaucoma asks the nurse if complete vision will return. The most appropriate response is
    1. "Although some vision has been lost and cannot be restored, further loss may be prevented by adhering to the treatment plan."
    2. "Your vision will return as soon as the medication begins to work."
    3. "Your vision will never return to normal."
    4. "Your vision loss is temporary and will return in about 3 to 4 weeks."

11. The nurse is developing a teaching plan for the client with glaucoma. Which of the following instructions would the nurse include in the plan of care?
    1. Decrease fluid intake to control the intraocular pressure.
    2. Avoid overuse of the eyes.
    3. Decrease the amount of salt in the diet.
    4. Eye medications will need to be administered lifelong.

12. The nurse is performing an admission assessment on a client with a diagnosis of detached retina. Which of the following is associated with this eye disorder?
    1. Pain in the affected eye
    2. Total loss of vision
    3. A sense of a curtain falling across the field of vision
    4. A yellow discoloration of the sclera

13. The nurse is caring for a client with a diagnosis of detached retina. Which assessment sign would indicate that bleeding has occurred as a result of the retinal detachment?
    1. Complaints of a burst of black spots or floaters
    2. A sudden sharp pain in the eye
    3. Total loss of vision
    4. A reddened conjunctiva

14. The client arrives in the emergency room following an automobile accident. The client's forehead hit the steering wheel and a hyphema is diagnosed. The nurse places the client in which position?
    1. Flat on bed rest
    2. Semi-Fowler on bed rest
    3. Lateral on the affected side
    4. Lateral on the unaffected side

15. The client sustains a contusion of the eyeball following a traumatic injury with a blunt object. Which intervention is initiated immediately?
    1. Notify the physician.
    2. Irrigate the eye with cool water.
    3. Apply ice to the affected eye.
    4. Accompany the client to the emergency room.

16. The client arrives in the emergency room with a penetrating eye injury from wood chips while cutting wood. The nurse assesses the eye and notes a piece of wood protruding from the eye. What is the initial nursing action?
    1. Remove the piece of wood using a sterile eye clamp.
    2. Apply an eye patch.
    3. Perform visual acuity tests.
    4. Irrigate the eye with sterile saline.

17. The client arrives in the emergency room after sustaining a chemical eye injury from a splash of battery acid. The initial nursing action is to
    1. Begin visual acuity testing.
    2. Irrigate the eye with sterile normal saline.
    3. Swab the eye with antibiotic ointment.
    4. Cover the eye with a pressure patch.

18. The nurse is caring for a client following enucleation. The nurse notes the presence of bright red drainage on the dressing. Which nursing action is appropriate?
    1. Notify the physician.
    2. Continue to monitor the drainage.
    3. Document the finding.
    4. Mark the drainage on the dressing and monitor for any increase in bleeding.

19. The nurse is performing a voice test to assess hearing. Which of the following describes the accurate procedure for performing this test?
    1. Stand 4 feet away from the client to ensure that the client can hear at this distance.
    2. Whisper a statement and ask the client to repeat it.
    3. Whisper a statement with the examiner's back facing the client.
    4. Whisper a statement while the client blocks both ears.

20. During a hearing assessment, the nurse notes that the sound lateralizes to the client's left ear with the Weber test. The nurse analyses these results as
    1. A normal finding.
    2. A conductive hearing loss in the right ear.
    3. A sensorineural or conductive loss.
    4. The presence of nystagmus.

21. The nurse is caring for a client that is hearing impaired. Which of the following approaches will facilitate communication?
    1. Speak frequently.
    2. Speak loudly.
    3. Speak directly into the impaired ear.
    4. Speak in a normal tone.

22. A client arrives at the emergency room with a foreign body in the left ear that has been determined to be an insect. Which intervention would the nurse anticipate to be prescribed initially?
    1. Irrigation of the ear.
    2. Instillation of diluted alcohol.
    3. Instillation of antibiotic ear drops.
    4. Instillation of corticosteroid ointment.

23. The nurse notes that the physician has documented a diagnosis of presbycusis on the client's chart. The nurse plans care knowing that the condition is
    1. A sensorineural hearing loss that occurs with aging.
    2. A conductive hearing loss that occurs with aging.
    3. Tinnitus that occurs with aging.
    4. Nystagmus that occurs with aging.

24. The nurse has conducted discharge teaching for a client who had a fenestration procedure for the treatment of otosclerosis. Which of the following, if stated by the client, would indicate that teaching was effective?
    1. "I should drink liquids through a straw for the next 2 to 3 weeks."
    2. "It is okay to take a shower and wash my hair."
    3. "I will take stool softeners as prescribed by my doctor."
    4. "I can resume my tennis lessons starting next week."

25. A client with Meniere's disease is experiencing severe vertigo. Which instruction would the nurse give to the client to assist in controlling the vertigo?
    1. Increase fluid intake to 3000 mL a day.
    2. Avoid sudden head movements.
    3. Lie still and watch the television.
    4. Increase sodium in the diet.

26. The nurse is reviewing the physician's orders for a client with Meniere's disease. Which diet most likely would be prescribed for the client?
    1. Low-cholesterol diet
    2. Low-sodium diet
    3. Low-carbohydrate diet
    4. Low-fat diet

27. The nurse is caring for a client following craniotomy for removal of an acoustic neuroma. Assessment of which of the following cranial nerves would identify a complication specifically associated with this surgery?
    1. Cranial nerve I, olfactory
    2. Cranial nerve III, oculomotor
    3. Cranial nerve IV, trochlear
    4. Cranial nerve VII, facial nerve

28. The nurse assesses the client with a blunt head injury sustained from a motor vehicle accident. Which assessment sign would indicate a basal skull fracture as a result of the injury?
    1. Purulent drainage from the auditory canal
    2. Bloody or clear drainage from the auditory canal
    3. Epistaxis
    4. Periorbital edema

29. The nurse is performing an otoscopic examination on a client with mastoiditis. On examination of the tympanic membrane, which of the following would the nurse expect to observe?
    1. A pink-colored tympanic membrane
    2. A pearly colored tympanic membrane
    3. A red, dull, thick and immobile tympanic membrane
    4. A transparent and clear tympanic membrane
30. The client is diagnosed with a disorder involving the inner ear. Which of the following is the most common client complaint associated with a disorder involving this part of the ear?
    1. Hearing loss
    2. Pruritus
    3. Tinnitus
    4. Burning in the ear

CRITICAL THINKING: MULTIPLE-RESPONSE

The nurse is preparing a teaching plan for a client who is undergoing cataract extraction with intraocular implant. Which home care measures will the nurse include in the plan?

___ To contact the surgeon if eye scratchiness occurs

___ That episodes of sudden severe pain in the eye is expected

___ To place an eye shield on the surgical eye at bedtime

___ To avoid activities that require bending over

___ To contact the surgeon if a decrease in visual acuity occurs

ANSWERS

1. 2
Rationale: Visual acuity is assessed in one eye at a time, and then in both eyes together with the client comfortably standing or sitting. The right eye is tested with the left eye covered; then the left eye is tested with the right eye covered. Both eyes then are tested together. Visual acuity is measured with or without corrective lenses and the client stands at a distance of 20 feet from the chart.
Test-Taking Strategy: Use the process of elimination. Remember that normal visual acuity as measured by a Snellen's chart is 20/20 vision. This should assist in eliminating options 3 and 4. From the remaining options, remember that to test each eye separately first and then test both eyes together is best. This method most accurately assesses visual acuity. Review the procedure for testing visual acuity with a Snellen's chart if you had difficulty with this question.
Level of Cognitive Ability: Application
Client Needs: Health Promotion and Maintenance
Integrated Process: Nursing Process—assessment
Content Area: Adult health—eye
Reference: Jarvis, C. (2000). *Physical examination and health assessment* (3rd ed., p. 307). Philadelphia: W. B. Saunders.

2. 4
Rationale: Vision that is 20/20 is normal, that is, the client is able to read from 20 feet what a person with normal vision can read from 20 feet. A client with a visual acuity of 20/60 only can read at a distance of 20 feet what a person with normal vision can read at 60 feet.
Test-Taking Strategy: Use the process of elimination. Focus on the test result, 20/60, to direct you to option 4. If you had difficulty with this question, review interpretation of visual acuity test results.
Level of Cognitive Ability: Analysis
Client Needs: Physiological Integrity
Integrated Process: Nursing Process—analysis
Content Area: Adult health—eye
Reference: Jarvis, C. (2000). *Physical examination and health assessment* (3rd ed., p. 308). Philadelphia: W. B. Saunders.

3. 4
Rationale: Legal blindness is defined as 20/200 or less with corrected vision (glasses or contact lenses) or visual acuity of less than 20 degrees of the visual field in the better eye.
Test-Taking Strategy: Knowledge of the definition of legal blindness is required to answer this question. Review this definition if you had difficulty with this question.
Level of Cognitive Ability: Comprehension
Client Needs: Physiological Integrity
Integrated Process: Nursing Process—assessment
Content Area: Adult health—eye
Reference: Lewis, S., Heitkemper, M., & Dirksen, S. (2004). *Medical-surgical nursing: Assessment and management of clinical problems* (6th ed., p. 427). St. Louis: Mosby.

4. 2
Rationale: Tonometry is the method of measuring intraocular fluid pressure using a calibrated instrument that indents or flattens the corneal apex. Pressures between 10 and 21 mm Hg are considered within the normal range.
Test-Taking Strategy: Use the process of elimination and knowledge regarding the normal intraocular pressure to answer this question. If you had difficulty with this question, learn this normal value.
Level of Cognitive Ability: Comprehension
Client Needs: Physiological Integrity
Integrated Process: Nursing Process—assessment
Content Area: Adult health—eye
Reference: Ignatavicius, D., & Workman, M. (2002). *Medical-surgical nursing: Critical thinking for collaborative care* (4th ed., p. 1019). Philadelphia: W. B. Saunders.

5. 3
Rationale: The most appropriate nursing diagnosis for the client scheduled for cataract surgery is Disturbed Sensory Perception (visual) related to lens extraction and replacement. Although options 1, 2, and 4 identify nursing diagnoses that may be appropriate, they are not related specifically to cataract surgery.
Test-Taking Strategy: Use the process of elimination. When asked questions regarding nursing diagnosis, use the information

presented in the question to select an option. Remember that disorders of the eye or ear relate to sensory perceptual alterations. Review care to the client scheduled for cataract surgery if you had difficulty with this question.

Level of Cognitive Ability: Analysis
Client Needs: Psychosocial Integrity
Integrated Process: Nursing Process—planning
Content Area: Adult health—eye
Reference: Ignatavicius, D., & Workman, M. (2002). *Medical-surgical nursing: Critical thinking for collaborative care* (4th ed., p. 1032). Philadelphia: W. B. Saunders.

6. 3
Rationale: A gradual, painless blurring of central vision is the chief clinical manifestation of a cataract. Early symptoms include slightly blurred vision and a decrease in color perception. Option 1, 2, and 4 are not signs of a cataract.
Test-Taking Strategy: Use the process of elimination. Remember the pathophysiology related to cataract development. As a cataract develops, the lens of the eye becomes opaque. This description will assist in directing you to the correct option. If you had difficulty with this question, review the assessment signs associated with cataract development.

Level of Cognitive Ability: Analysis
Client Needs: Physiological Integrity
Integrated Process: Nursing Process—assessment
Content Area: Adult health—eye
Reference: Ignatavicius, D., & Workman, M. (2002). *Medical-surgical nursing: Critical thinking for collaborative care* (4th ed., p. 1032). Philadelphia: W. B. Saunders.

7. 3
Rationale: A mydriatic medication produces mydriasis or dilation of the pupil. Mydriatic medications are used preoperatively in the cataract client. These medications act by dilating the pupils. They also constrict blood vessels. An osmotic diuretic may be used to decrease intraocular pressure. A miotic medication constricts the pupil. A thiazide diuretic is not likely to be prescribed for a client with a cataract.
Test-Taking Strategy: Use the process of elimination. Read the question carefully, noting that the client is being prepared for eye surgery. Dilation of the eye is necessary before cataract extraction. Recalling that a mydriatic dilates will direct you to option 3. Review preoperative care for cataract surgery if you had difficulty with this question.

Level of Cognitive Ability: Analysis
Client Needs: Physiological Integrity
Integrated Process: Nursing Process—analysis
Content Area: Adult health—eye
Reference: Ignatavicius, D., & Workman, M. (2002). *Medical-surgical nursing: Critical thinking for collaborative care* (4th ed., p. 1033). Philadelphia: W. B. Saunders.

8. 1
Rationale: Severe pain or pain accompanied by nausea is an indicator of increased intraocular pressure and should be reported to the physician immediately. Option 2, 3, and 4 are inappropriate actions.
Test-Taking Strategy: Use the process of elimination. Note the key word "severe." Eliminate option 3 because this is not a

normal condition. The client should not be turned to the operative side; therefore eliminate option 4. From the remaining options, focusing on the key word will direct you to option 1. If you had difficulty with this question, review the postoperative complications of cataract surgery requiring physician notification.

Level of Cognitive Ability: Application
Client Needs: Physiological Integrity
Integrated Process: Nursing Process—implementation
Content Area: Adult health—eye
Reference: Ignatavicius, D., & Workman, M. (2002). *Medical-surgical nursing: Critical thinking for collaborative care* (4th ed., p. 1034). Philadelphia: W. B. Saunders.

9. 3
Rationale: The client is instructed to wear a metal or plastic shield to protect the eye from accidental injury and is instructed not to rub the eye. Glasses may be worn during the day. Aspirin or medications containing aspirin are not to be administered or taken by the client and the client is instructed to take acetaminophen (Tylenol) as needed for pain. The client is instructed not to sleep on the side of the body on which the operation occurred. The client is not to lift more than 5 lb.
Test-Taking Strategy: Use the process of elimination, noting the key words "understanding of the instructions." Recalling that the operative site needs to be protected will direct you to option 3. If you had difficulty with this question, review the discharge instructions for the client following cataract extraction.

Level of Cognitive Ability: Analysis
Client Needs: Physiological Integrity
Integrated Process: Teaching/Learning
Content Area: Adult health—eye
References: Lewis, S., Heitkemper, M., & Dirksen, S. (2004). *Medical-surgical nursing: Assessment and management of clinical problems* (6th ed., p. 453). St. Louis: Mosby.
Phipps, W., Monahan, F., Sands, J., Marek, J., & Neighbors, M. (2003). *Medical-surgical nursing: Health and illness perspectives* (7th ed., p. 1901). St. Louis: Mosby.

10. 1
Rationale: Vision loss to glaucoma is irreparable. The client should be reassured that although some vision has been lost and cannot be restored, further loss may be prevented by adhering to the treatment plan. Option 3 does not provide reassurance to the client.
Test-Taking Strategy: Use the process of elimination and therapeutic communication techniques. Also note that option 1 is global, addressing the importance of compliance with the treatment plan. Review the effects of glaucoma and therapeutic communication techniques if you had difficulty with this question.

Level of Cognitive Ability: Application
Client Needs: Physiological Integrity
Integrated Process: Communication and Documentation
Content Area: Adult health—eye
Reference: Lewis, S., Heitkemper, M., & Dirksen, S. (2004). *Medical-surgical nursing: Assessment and management of clinical problems* (6th ed., p. 460). St. Louis: Mosby.

11. **4**

Rationale: The administration of eye drops is a critical component of the treatment plan for the client with glaucoma. The client needs to be instructed that medications will need to be taken for the rest of his or her life. Options 1, 2, and 3 are not accurate instructions.

Test-Taking Strategy: Use the process of elimination. Recalling that medications are an integral component of the treatment plan will assist in directing you to the correct option. Review the treatment associated with the care of the client with glaucoma if you had difficulty with this question.

Level of Cognitive Ability: Application
Client Needs: Physiological Integrity
Integrated Process: Nursing Process—planning
Content Area: Adult health—eye
Reference: Phipps, W., Monahan, F., Sands, J., Marek, J., & Neighbors, M. (2003). *Medical-surgical nursing: Health and illness perspectives* (7th ed., p. 1893). St. Louis: Mosby.

12. **3**

Rationale: A characteristic manifestation of retinal detachment described by the client is the feeling that a shadow or curtain is falling across the field of vision. No pain is associated with detachment of the retina. Options 2 and 4 are not characteristics of this disorder. A retinal detachment is an ophthalmic emergency and even more so if visual acuity is still normal.

Test-Taking Strategy: Use the process of elimination focusing on the diagnosis. You must recall the characteristic manifestation associated with this disorder to answer correctly. Review the manifestations associated with this condition if you had difficulty with this question.

Level of Cognitive Ability: Analysis
Client Needs: Physiological Integrity
Integrated Process: Nursing Process—assessment
Content Area: Adult health—eye
References: Lewis, S., Heitkemper, M., & Dirksen, S. (2004). *Medical-surgical nursing: Assessment and management of clinical problems* (6th ed., p. 453). St. Louis: Mosby.
Phipps, W., Monahan, F., Sands, J., Marek, J., & Neighbors, M. (2003). *Medical-surgical nursing: Health and illness perspectives* (7th ed., p. 1902). St. Louis: Mosby.

13. **1**

Rationale: Complaints of a sudden burst of black spots or floaters indicates that bleeding has occurred as a result of the detachment. Options 2, 3, and 4 are not signs of bleeding.

Test-Taking Strategy: Recalling the complications associated with retinal detachment is necessary to answer this question. Review the manifestations associated with the complications of a detached retina if you had difficulty with this question.

Level of Cognitive Ability: Analysis
Client Needs: Physiological Integrity
Integrated Process: Nursing Process—assessment
Content Area: Adult health—eye
Reference: Phipps, W., Monahan, F., Sands, J., Marek, J., & Neighbors, M. (2003). *Medical-surgical nursing: Health and illness perspectives* (7th ed., p. 1902). St. Louis: Mosby.

14. **2**

Rationale: A hyphema is the presence of blood in the anterior chamber. Hyphema is produced when a force is sufficient to break the integrity of the blood vessels in the eye and can be caused by direct injury such as a penetrating injury from a BB or pellet or indirectly such as from striking the forehead on a steering wheel during an accident. The client is treated by bed rest in a semi-Fowler position to assist gravity in keeping the hyphema away from the optical center of the cornea.

Test-Taking Strategy: Use the process of elimination to answer this question. Remember, placing the client flat will produce an increase in pressure at the injured site. Also, note that option 2 is the option that identifies a position different from the other options. Review care to the client with hyphema, if you had difficulty with this question.

Level of Cognitive Ability: Application
Client Needs: Physiological Integrity
Integrated Process: Nursing Process—implementation
Content Area: Adult health—eye
References: Jarvis, C. (2000). *Physical examination and health assessment* (3rd ed., p. 339). Philadelphia: W. B. Saunders.
Lewis, S., Heitkemper, M., & Dirksen, S. (2004). *Medical-surgical nursing: Assessment and management of clinical problems* (6th ed., p. 422). St. Louis: Mosby.

15. **3**

Rationale: Treatment for a contusion begins at the time of injury. Ice is applied immediately. The client then should be seen by a physician and receive a thorough eye examination to rule out the presence of other eye injuries.

Test-Taking Strategy: Use the process of elimination. Focus on the key word "immediately." Recalling the principles related to initial treatment of injuries will direct you to option 3. Review emergency treatment of eye injuries if you had difficulty with this question.

Level of Cognitive Ability: Application
Client Needs: Physiological Integrity
Integrated Process: Nursing Process—implementation
Content Area: Adult health—eye
Reference: Thompson, J., McFarland, G., Hirsch, J., & Tucker, S. (2002). *Mosby's clinical nursing* (5th ed., p. 368). St. Louis: Mosby.

16. **3**

Rationale: If the laceration is the result of a penetrating injury, an object may be noted protruding from the eye. This object must never be removed except by the ophthalmologist because it may be holding ocular structures in place. Application of an eye patch or irrigation of the eye may disrupt the foreign body and cause further tearing of the cornea.

Test-Taking Strategy: Use the process of elimination to answer this question. Note the key word "penetrating." This should indicate that a laceration has occurred and that interventions are directed at preventing further disruption of the integrity of the eye. The only option that will prevent further disruption is to assess visual acuity. Review emergency eye care if you had difficulty with this question.

Level of Cognitive Ability: Application
Client Needs: Physiological Integrity
Integrated Process: Nursing Process—implementation

Content Area: Adult health—eye
Reference: Phipps, W., Monahan, F., Sands, J., Marek, J., & Neighbors, M. (2003). *Medical-surgical nursing: Health and illness perspectives* (7th ed., pp. 1306, 1878). St. Louis: Mosby.

17. 2
Rationale: Emergency care following a chemical burn to the eye includes irrigating the eye immediately with sterile normal saline or ocular irrigating solution. In the emergency department, the irrigation should be maintained for at least 10 minutes. Following this emergency treatment, visual acuity is assessed. Options 3 and 4 are not a component of initial care.
Test-Taking Strategy: Read the question carefully, noting the type of injury to the eye. Noting the key word "splash" will direct you to option 2. Review emergency eye care if you had difficulty with this question.
Level of Cognitive Ability: Application
Client Needs: Physiological Integrity
Integrated Process: Nursing Process—implementation
Content Area: Adult health—eye
Reference: Phipps, W., Monahan, F., Sands, J., Marek, J., & Neighbors, M. (2003). *Medical-surgical nursing: Health and illness perspectives* (7th ed., p. 1891). St. Louis: Mosby.

18. 1
Rationale: If the nurse notes the presence of bright red drainage on the dressing, it must be reported to the physician because this indicates hemorrhage. Options 2, 3, and 4 are inappropriate.
Test-Taking Strategy: Use the process of elimination. Note the key words "bright red." Remember, bright red drainage indicates active bleeding. Review postoperative complications associated with an enucleation if you had difficulty with this question.
Level of Cognitive Ability: Application
Client Needs: Physiological Integrity
Integrated Process: Nursing Process—implementation
Content Area: Adult health—eye
Reference: Lewis, S., Heitkemper, M., & Dirksen, S. (2004). *Medical-surgical nursing: Assessment and management of clinical problems* (6th ed., p. 461). St. Louis: Mosby.

19. 2
Rationale: The examiner stands 1 to 2 feet away from the client and asks the client to block one external ear canal. The nurse whispers a statement and asks the client to repeat it. Each ear is tested separately.
Test-Taking Strategy: Use the process of elimination. Eliminate options 3 and 4 because they are not measures that would assess hearing effectively. Eliminate option 1 because distance hearing is not the issue of the question. Review the procedure for performing a voice test if you had difficulty with this question.
Level of Cognitive Ability: Application
Client Needs: Health Promotion and Maintenance
Integrated Process: Nursing Process—assessment
Content Area: Adult health—ear
Reference: Jarvis, C. (2000). *Physical examination and health assessment* (3rd ed., p. 357). Philadelphia: W. B. Saunders.

20. 3
Rationale: In the Weber tuning fork test the nurse places the vibrating tuning fork in the middle of the client's head, at the midline of the forehead, or above the upper lip over the teeth. Normally, the sound is heard equally in both ears by bone conduction. If the client has a sensorineural hearing loss in one ear, the sound is heard in the other ear. If the client has a conductive hearing loss in one ear, the sound is heard in that ear.
Test-Taking Strategy: Use the process of elimination. This is a difficult question. Knowledge regarding analyzing the results of the Weber tuning fork test is required to answer this question. If you had difficulty with this question, review this hearing test. Also review the Rinne tuning fork test.
Level of Cognitive Ability: Analysis
Client Needs: Physiological Integrity
Integrated Process: Nursing Process—analysis
Content Area: Adult health—ear
Reference: Jarvis, C. (2000). *Physical examination and health assessment* (3rd ed., pp. 375-376). Philadelphia: W. B. Saunders.

21. 4
Rationale: Speaking in a normal tone to the client with impaired hearing and not shouting are important. The nurse should talk directly to the client while facing the client and speak clearly. If the client does not seem to understand what is said, the nurse should express it differently. Moving closer to the client and toward the better ear may facilitate communication, but the nurse should avoid talking directly into the impaired ear.
Test-Taking Strategy: Use the process of elimination and knowledge regarding effective communication techniques for the hearing impaired to answer this question. If you had difficulty with this question, review these techniques.
Level of Cognitive Ability: Application
Client Needs: Psychosocial Integrity
Integrated Process: Communication and Documentation
Content Area: Adult health—ear
Reference: Thompson, J., McFarland, G., Hirsch, J., & Tucker, S. (2002). *Mosby's clinical nursing* (5th ed., p. 584). St. Louis: Mosby.

22. 2
Rationale: Insects are killed before removal unless they can be coaxed out by a flashlight or a humming noise. Mineral oil or diluted alcohol is instilled into the ear to suffocate the insect, which then is removed by using ear forceps. When the foreign object is vegetable matter, irrigation is not used because this material expands with hydration and the impaction becomes worse.
Test-Taking Strategy: Use the process of elimination. Focusing on the key words "foreign body" and "insect" will direct you to option 2. If you had difficulty with this question, review care to the client with a foreign body in the ear.
Level of Cognitive Ability: Analysis
Client Needs: Physiological Integrity
Integrated Process: Nursing Process—planning
Content Area: Adult health—ear
References: Ignatavicius, D., & Workman, M. (2002). *Medical-surgical nursing: Critical thinking for collaborative care* (4th ed., p. 1063). Philadelphia: W. B. Saunders.

Jarvis, C. (2000). *Physical examination and health assessment* (3rd ed., p. 370). Philadelphia: W. B. Saunders.

23. 1
Rationale: Presbycusis is a type of hearing loss that occurs with aging. Presbycusis is a gradual sensorineural loss caused by nerve degeneration in the inner ear or auditory nerve. Options 2, 3, and 4 are incorrect.
Test-Taking Strategy: Knowledge regarding the description of presbycusis is required to answer this question. If you are unfamiliar with this condition, review this age-related disorder.
Level of Cognitive Ability: Comprehension
Client Needs: Physiological Integrity
Integrated Process: Nursing Process—planning
Content Area: Adult health—ear
Reference: Ignatavicius, D., & Workman, M. (2002). *Medical-surgical nursing: Critical thinking for collaborative care* (4th ed., p. 1069). Philadelphia: W. B. Saunders.

24. 3
Rationale: Following ear surgery, the client needs to avoid straining when having a bowel movement. The client needs to be instructed to avoid drinking with a straw for 2 to 3 weeks, air travel, and coughing excessively. The client needs to avoid getting his or her head wet, washing hair, showering for 1 week, and rapidly moving the head, bouncing, and bending over for 3 weeks.
Test-Taking Strategy: Use the process of elimination. Note the key words "teaching was effective." Consider the anatomical area of the client's condition and the surgical procedure in eliminating the incorrect options. If you had difficulty with this question, review client instructions following ear surgery.
Level of Cognitive Ability: Analysis
Client Needs: Physiological Integrity
Integrated Process: Teaching/Learning
Content Area: Adult health—ear
Reference: Phipps, W., Monahan, F., Sands, J., Marek, J., & Neighbors, M. (2003). *Medical-surgical nursing: Health and illness perspectives* (7th ed., p. 1927). St. Louis: Mosby.

25. 2
Rationale: The nurse instructs the client to make slow head movements to prevent worsening of the vertigo. Dietary changes such as salt and fluid restrictions that reduce the amount of endolymphatic fluid sometimes are prescribed. Lying still and watching television will not control vertigo.
Test-Taking Strategy: Use the process of elimination. Identify the issue, vertigo. Note the relationship between vertigo and avoiding sudden head movements in the correct option. If you had difficulty with this question, review the measures that will reduce vertigo in the client with Meniere's disease.
Level of Cognitive Ability: Application
Client Needs: Physiological Integrity
Integrated Process: Nursing Process—implementation
Content Area: Adult health—ear
Reference: Ignatavicius, D, & Workman, M. (2002). *Medical-surgical nursing: Critical thinking for collaborative care* (4th ed., p. 1068). Philadelphia: W. B. Saunders.

26. 2
Rationale: Dietary changes such as salt and fluid restrictions that reduce the amount of endolymphatic fluid sometimes are prescribed. Options 1, 3, and 4 are not specific to the client with Meniere's disease.
Test-Taking Strategy: Use the process of elimination. Recalling the pathophysiology related to Meniere's disease will direct you to option 2. Review the pathophysiology related to this condition and the treatment measures if you had difficulty with this question.
Level of Cognitive Ability: Analysis
Client Needs: Physiological Integrity
Integrated Process: Nursing Process—planning
Content Area: Adult health—ear
Reference: Lewis, S., Heitkemper, M., & Dirksen, S. (2004). *Medical-surgical nursing: Assessment and management of clinical problems* (6th ed., p. 467). St. Louis: Mosby.

27. 4
Rationale: Treatment for acoustic neuroma is surgical removal via a craniotomy. Extreme care is taken to preserve remaining hearing and preserve the function of the facial nerve. Acoustic neuromas rarely recur following surgical removal.
Test-Taking Strategy: Use the process of elimination and knowledge regarding the anatomical location of an acoustic neuroma to direct you to option 4. If you had difficulty with this question, review the complications associated with this surgical procedure.
Level of Cognitive Ability: Analysis
Client Needs: Physiological Integrity
Integrated Process: Nursing Process—assessment
Content Area: Adult health—ear
Reference: Lewis, S., Heitkemper, M., & Dirksen, S. (2004). *Medical-surgical nursing: Assessment and management of clinical problems* (6th ed., p. 1519). St. Louis: Mosby.

28. 2
Rationale: Bloody or clear watery drainage from the auditory canal indicates a cerebrospinal fluid leak following trauma and suggests a basal skull fracture. This warrants immediate attention. Options 1, 3, and 4 are not specific to a basal skull fracture.
Test-Taking Strategy: Use the process of elimination. Recalling the concern related to leakage of cerebrospinal fluid will direct you to option 2. If you had difficulty with this question, review these assessment signs.
Level of Cognitive Ability: Analysis
Client Needs: Physiological Integrity
Integrated Process: Nursing Process—assessment
Content Area: Adult health—ear
Reference: Lewis, S., Heitkemper, M., & Dirksen, S. (2004). *Medical-surgical nursing: Assessment and management of clinical problems* (6th ed., p. 1506). St. Louis: Mosby.

29. 3
Rationale: Otoscopic examination in a client with mastoiditis reveals a red, dull, thick, and immobile tympanic membrane with or without perforation. Postauricular lymph nodes are tender and enlarged. Clients also have a low-grade fever, malaise, anorexia, swelling behind the ear, and pain with minimal movement of the head.

Test-Taking Strategy: Knowledge regarding the pathophysiology associated with mastoiditis is required to answer this question. If you had difficulty with this question, review the assessment findings associated with this disorder.
Level of Cognitive Ability: Analysis
Client Needs: Physiological Integrity
Integrated Process: Nursing Process—assessment
Content Area: Adult health—ear
Reference: Phipps, W., Monahan, F., Sands, J., Marek, J., & Neighbors, M. (2003). *Medical-surgical nursing: Health and illness perspectives* (7th ed., p. 1925). St. Louis: Mosby.

30. **3**
Rationale: Tinnitus is the most common complaint of clients with otological disorders, especially disorders involving the inner ear. Symptoms of tinnitus range from mild ringing in the ear, which can go unnoticed during the day, to a loud roaring in the ear, which can interfere with the client's thinking process and attention span. Options 1, 2, and 4 are not associated specifically with disorders of the inner ear.
Test-Taking Strategy: Use the process of elimination. Recalling the function of the inner ear will direct you to option 3. Review the manifestations associated with an inner ear disorder if you had difficulty with this question.
Level of Cognitive Ability: Analysis
Client Needs: Physiological Integrity
Integrated Process: Nursing Process—assessment
Content Area: Adult health—ear
Reference: Black, J., Hawks, J., & Keene, A. (2001). *Medical-surgical nursing: Clinical management for positive outcomes* (6th ed., pp. 1834-1835). Philadelphia: W. B. Saunders.

CRITICAL THINKING: MULTIPLE RESPONSE
Answer:
___ To place an eye shield on the surgical eye at bedtime
___ To avoid activities that require bending over
___ To contact the surgeon if a decrease in visual acuity occurs
Rationale: Following eye surgery, some scratchiness may occur in the operative eye and usually is relieved by mild analgesics. If the eye pain becomes severe, the client should notify the surgeon because this may indicate hemorrhage, infection, or increased intraocular pressure. The nurse also would instruct the client to notify the surgeon of increased purulent drainage, increased redness, or any decrease in visual acuity. The client is instructed to place an eye shield over the operative eye at bedtime to protect the eye from injury during sleep and to avoid activities that increase intraocular pressure such as bending over.
Test-Taking Strategy: Note that the client has had eye surgery. Recalling that the eye needs to be protected and that a concern is increased intraocular pressure will assist in determining the home care measures to be included in the plan. Review these measures if you had difficulty with this question.
Level of Cognitive Ability: Application
Client Needs: Physiological Integrity
Integrated Process: Teaching/Learning
Content Area: Adult health—eye
Reference: Lewis, S., Heitkemper, M., & Dirksen, S. (2004). *Medical-surgical nursing: Assessment and management of clinical problems* (6th ed., p. 452). St. Louis: Mosby.

REFERENCES

Black, J., Hawks, J., & Keene, A. (2001). *Medical-surgical nursing: Clinical management for positive outcomes* (6th ed.). Philadelphia: W. B. Saunders.

Ignatavicius, D., & Workman, M. (2002). *Medical-surgical nursing: Critical thinking for collaborative care* (4th ed.). Philadelphia: W. B. Saunders.

Jarvis, C. (2000). *Physical examination and health assessment* (3rd ed.). Philadelphia: W. B. Saunders.

Lewis, S., Heitkemper, M., & Dirksen, S. (2004). *Medical-surgical nursing: Assessment and management of clinical problems* (6th ed.). St. Louis: Mosby.

Phipps, W., Monahan, F., Sands, J., Marek, J., & Neighbors, M. (2003). *Medical-surgical nursing: Health and illness perspectives* (7th ed.). St. Louis: Mosby.

Thompson, J., McFarland, G., Hirsch, J., & Tucker, S. (2002). *Mosby's clinical nursing* (5th ed.). St. Louis: Mosby.

Ophthalmic and Otic Medications

I. OPHTHALMIC MEDICATION ADMINISTRATION

A. Guidelines for the use of eye medications
1. Eye medications are usually in the form of drops or ointments.
2. To prevent overflow of medication into the nasal and pharyngeal passages, thus reducing systemic absorption, instruct the client to apply pressure over the inner canthus next to the nose for 30 seconds to 1 minute following administration of the medication.
3. If both an eye drop and an eye ointment are scheduled to be administered at the same time, administer the eye drop first.
4. Wash hands before administering eye medications to avoid contaminating the eye or medication dropper or applicator and after administering eye medications to rinse off any residue.
5. Use a separate bottle or tube of medication for each client to avoid accidental cross-contamination.
6. Place prescribed dose of eye medication in the lower conjunctival sac, never directly onto the cornea.
7. Avoid touching any part of the eye with the dropper or applicator.
8. Administer glucocorticoid preparations before other medications.
9. Monitor the pulse of the client receiving an ophthalmic β-blocker, and instruct the client to do the same; if the pulse is less than 50 to 60 beats per minute (adult), withhold the next dose of eye medication and notify the physician.
10. Instruct the client how to instill medication correctly and supervise instillation until the client can do it safely.
11. Instruct the client to read the medication labels carefully to ensure administration of the correct medication and correct strength.
12. Remind the client to keep these medications out of the reach of children.
13. Instruct the client to avoid driving or operating hazardous equipment if vision is blurred.
14. Inform the client that he or she may be unable to drive home after eye examinations when medications to dilate the pupil **(mydriatics)** or medications to paralyze the ciliary muscle (cycloplegics) are used.
15. If photophobia occurs, instruct the client to wear sunglasses and avoid bright lights.
16. Instruct the client to administer a missed dose of the eye medication as soon as remembered, unless the next dose is scheduled to be administered in 1 to 2 hours.
17. Inform the client with **glaucoma** that the disorder cannot be cured, only controlled.
18. Reinforce the importance of using medications to treat **glaucoma** as prescribed and not to discontinue these medications without consulting the physician.
19. Inform the client that medications used to treat **glaucoma** may cause pain and blurred vision, especially when therapy is begun.
20. Instruct the client to report the development of any eye irritation.
21. Inform the client using eye gel to store the gel at room temperature or in the refrigerator but not to freeze it.
22. Instruct the client to discard unused eye gel kept at room temperature after 8 weeks.
23. Inform the client that soft contact lenses may absorb certain eye medications and that

preservatives in eye medications may discolor the contact lenses.

24. Advise the client wearing contact lenses to question the physician carefully about special precautions to observe.

25. In infants, inform the parents that atropine sulfate eye drops may contribute to abdominal distention.

26. Instruct the parents to keep a record of the infant's bowel movements if atropine sulfate eye drops are being administered.

27. Auscultate bowel sounds of the infant or child receiving atropine sulfate eye drops.

B. Instillation of eye medications

1. Drops

   a. Wash hands.
   b. Put gloves on.
   c. Check the name, strength, and expiration date of the medication.
   d. Instruct the client to tilt the head backward, open the eyes, and look up.
   e. Pull the lower lid down against the cheekbone.
   f. Hold the bottle like a pencil with the tip downward.
   g. Holding the bottle, gently rest the wrist of the hand on the client's cheek.
   h. Squeeze the bottle gently to allow the drop to fall into the conjunctival sac.
   i. Instruct the client to close the eyes gently and not to squeeze the eyes shut.
   j. Wait 3 to 5 minutes before instilling another drop, if more than 1 drop is prescribed, to promote maximal absorption of the medication.
   k. Do not allow the medication bottle, dropper, or applicator to come in contact with the eyeball.

2. Ointments

   a. Hold the ointment tube near, but not touching, the eye or eyelashes.
   b. Squeeze a thin ribbon of ointment along the lining of the lower conjunctival sac from the inner to the outer canthus.
   c. Instruct the client to close the eyes gently.
   d. Instruct the client that vision may be blurred by the ointment.

II. MYDRIATIC/CYCLOPLEGIC AND ANTICHOLINERGIC MEDICATIONS (BOX 64-1)

A. Description

1. **Mydriatics** and **cycloplegics** dilate the pupils (**mydriasis**) and relax the ciliary muscles (**cycloplegia**).

2. Anticholinergics block responses of the sphincter muscle in the ciliary body, producing **mydriasis** and **cycloplegia**.

3. These medications are used preoperatively or for eye examinations to produce **mydriasis**.

4. These medications are contraindicated in clients with **glaucoma** because of the risk of increased intraocular pressure.

BOX 64-1

Mydriatic/Cycloplegic Eye Medications

Atropine sulfate (Isopto Atropine, Ocu-Tropine, Atropair, Atropisol)
Cyclopentolate and phenylephrine (Cyclomydril)
Cyclopentolate hydrochloride (Cyclogyl, AK-Pentolate, Pentolair)
Homatropine hydrobromide (Isopto Homatrine, AK-Homatropine, Spectro-Homatrine)
Scopolamine and phenylephrine (Murocoll 2)
Scopolamine hydrobromide (Isopto-Hyoscine)
Tropicamide (Mydriacyl, I-Piramide, Tropicacyl)
Tropicamide and hydroxyamphetamine (Paremyd)

---

5. **Mydriatics** are contraindicated in cardiac dysrhythmias and cerebral atherosclerosis and should be used with caution in the older client and in clients with prostatic hypertrophy, diabetes mellitus, or parkinsonism.

B. Side effects

1. Tachycardia
2. Photophobia
3. Conjunctivitis
4. Dermatitis

C. Atropine toxicity

1. Dry mouth
2. Blurred vision
3. Photophobia
4. Tachycardia
5. Fever
6. Urinary retention
7. Constipation
8. Headache, brow pain
9. Confusion
10. Hallucinations, delirium
11. Coma
12. Worsening of narrow-angle **glaucoma**

D. Systemic reactions of anticholinergics

1. Dry mouth and skin
2. Fever
3. Thirst
4. Confusion
5. Hyperactivity

E. Interventions

1. Monitor for allergic response.
2. Assess for risk of injury.
3. Assess for constipation and urinary retention.
4. Instruct the client that a burning sensation may occur on instillation.
5. Instruct the client not to drive or perform hazardous activities for 24 hours after instillation of the medication unless otherwise directed by the physician.
6. Instruct the client to wear sunglasses until the effects of the medication wear off.

7. Instruct the client to notify the physician if blurring of vision, loss of sight, difficulty breathing, sweating, or flushing occurs.
8. Instruct the client to report eye pain to the physician.

F. Alpha-Adrenergic blocker
1. Medication: dapiprazole hydrochloride (Rev-Eyes)
2. Use: to counteract **mydriasis**

III. ANTIINFECTIVE EYE MEDICATIONS (BOX 64-2)
A. Description: Antiinfective medications kill or inhibit the growth of bacteria, fungi, and viruses.
B. Side effects
1. Superinfection
2. Global irritation
C. Interventions
1. Assess for risk of injury.
2. Instruct the client how to apply the eye medication.
3. Instruct the client to continue treatment as prescribed.
4. Instruct the client to wash hands thoroughly and frequently.
5. Advise the client that if improvement does not occur to notify the physician.

IV. ANTIINFLAMMATORY EYE MEDICATIONS (BOX 64-3)
A. Description
1. Antiinflammatory medications control inflammation, thereby reducing vision loss and scarring.
2. Antiinflammatory medications are used for uveitis, allergic conditions, and inflammation of the conjunctiva, cornea, and lids.
B. Side effects
1. Cataracts

2. Increased intraocular pressure
3. Impaired healing
4. Masking signs and symptoms of infection
C. Interventions
1. Interventions are the same as for antiinfective medications.
2. Note that dexamethasone (Maxidex) should not be used for eye abrasions and wounds.

V. TOPICAL ANESTHETICS FOR THE EYE (BOX 64-4)
A. Description
1. Topical anesthetics produce corneal anesthesia.
2. Topical anesthetics are used for anesthesia for eye examinations and surgery or to remove foreign bodies from the eye.
B. Side effects
1. Temporary stinging or burning of the eye
2. Temporary loss of corneal reflex
C. Interventions
1. Assess for risk of injury.
2. Note that the medications should not be given to the client for home use and are not to be self-administered by the client.
3. Note that the blink reflex is lost temporarily and that the corneal epithelium needs to be protected.
4. Provide an eye patch to protect the eye from injury until the corneal reflex returns.

VI. EYE LUBRICANTS (BOX 64-5)
A. Description

BOX 64-2
Antiinfective Eye Medications

AMINOGLYCOSIDES
Gentamicin sulfate (Garamycin, Genoptic)
Tobramycin (Nebcin, Tobrex)

ANTIBACTERIAL
Chloramphenicol (Chloromycetin, Chloroptic)
Erythromycin (Ilotycin)

ANTIFUNGAL
Natamycin (Natacyn)

ANTIVIRAL
Idoxuridine (Stoxil, Herplex)
Trifluridine (Viroptic)
Vidarabine (Vira-A)

SULFONAMIDES
Sulfacetamide (Bleph-10, Sulamyd)
Sulfisoxadole (Gantrisin)

BOX 64-3
Antiinflammatory Eye Medications

ANTIALLERGIC AGENTS
Cromolyn sodium (Opticrom)
Ketotifen fumarate (Zaditor)
Levocabastine (Livostin)
Lodoxamide (Alomide)

CORTICOSTEROIDS
Betamethasone (Betnesol)
Dexamethasone (Maxidex)
Fluorometholone (FML-S Ophthalmic Suspension, FML)
Medrysone (HMS Liquifilm)
Prednisolone (Pred-Forte, Predair-A)

NONSTEROIDAL ANTIINFLAMMATORY AGENTS
Diclofenac (Voltaren)
Flurbiprofen sodium (Ocufen)
Ketorolac tromethamine (Acular)

BOX 64-4
Topical Anesthetics for the Eye

Proparacaine hydrochloride (Ophthaine, Ophthetic)
Tetracaine hydrochloride (Pontocaine)

1. Eye lubricants replace tears or add moisture to the eyes.
2. Eye lubricants moisten contact lenses or an artificial eye.
3. Eye lubricants protect the eyes during surgery or diagnostic procedures.
4. Eye lubricants are used for keratitis, during anesthesia, or in a disorder that results in unconsciousness or decreased blinking.

B. Side effects
1. Burning on instillation
2. Discomfort or pain on instillation

C. Interventions
1. Inform the client that burning may occur on instillation.
2. Be alert to allergic responses to the preservatives in the lubricants.

VII. MIOTICS (BOX 64-6)

A. Description
1. **Miotics** reduce intraocular pressure by constricting the pupil and contracting the ciliary muscle, thereby increasing the blood flow to the retina and decreasing retinal damage and loss of vision.
2. **Miotics** open the anterior chamber angle and increase the outflow of aqueous humor.
3. Miotic cholinergic medications reduce intraocular pressure by mimicking the action of acetylcholine.
4. Miotic acetylcholine inhibitors reduce intraocular pressure by inhibiting the action of cholinesterase.
5. **Miotics** are used for chronic open-angle **glaucoma** or acute and chronic closed-angle **glaucoma.**
6. **Miotics** are used to achieve **miosis** during eye surgery.
7. **Miotics** are contraindicated in clients with **retinal detachment,** adhesions between the iris and lens, or inflammatory diseases.
8. Use **miotics** with caution in clients with asthma, hypertension, corneal abrasion, hyperthyroidism, coronary vascular disease, urinary tract obstruction, gastrointestinal obstruction, ulcer disease, parkinsonism, and bradycardia.

B. Side effects
1. **Myopia**
2. Headache
3. Eye pain
4. Decreased vision in poor light
5. Local irritation
6. Systemic effects
   a. Flushing
   b. Diaphoresis
   c. Gastrointestinal upset and diarrhea
   d. Frequent urination
   e. Increased salivation
   f. Muscle weakness
   g. Respiratory difficulty
7. Toxicity
   a. Vertigo and syncope
   b. Bradycardia
   c. Hypotension
   d. Cardiac dysrhythmias
   e. Tremors
   f. Seizures

C. Interventions
1. Assess vital signs.
2. Assess for risk of injury.
3. Assess the client for the degree of diminished vision.
4. Monitor for side effects and toxic effects.
5. Monitor for postural hypotension, and instruct the client to change positions slowly.
6. Assess breath sounds for wheezes and rhonchi because cholinergic medications can cause bronchospasms and increased bronchial secretions.
7. Maintain oral hygiene because of the increase in salivation.
8. Have atropine sulfate available as an antidote for pilocarpine.
9. Instruct the client or family regarding the correct administration of eye medications.
10. Instruct the client not to stop the medication suddenly.
11. Instruct the client to avoid activities such as driving while vision is impaired.
12. Instruct clients with **glaucoma** to read labels on over-the-counter medications and to avoid atropine-like medications because atropine will increase intraocular pressure.

BOX 64-5

Eye Lubricants

Hydroxypropyl methylcellulose (Lacril, Isopto Plain)
Petroleum-based ointment (artificial tears, Liquifilm Tears)

BOX 64-6

Miotics

Carbachol (Carboptic)
Demecarium bromide (Humorsol)
Echothiophate (Phospholine Iodide)
Isoflurophate (Floropryl)
Pilocarpine hydrochloride (Isopto Carpine)

VIII. OCUSERT SYSTEM

A. Description
1. Ocusert is a thin eye wafer (disk) impregnated with a time-release dose of pilocarpine.
2. Ocusert is devised to overcome the frequent application of pilocarpine.
3. Ocusert is placed in the upper or lower cul-de-sac of the eye.

4. The pilocarpine is released over 1 week.
5. The disk is replaced every 7 days.
6. Drawbacks of its use include sudden leakage of pilocarpine, migration of the system over the cornea, and unnoticed loss of the system.

B. Interventions
1. Assess the client's ability to insert the medication disk.
2. Store the medication in the refrigerator.
3. Instruct the client to discard damaged or contaminated disks.
4. Inform the client that temporary stinging is expected but to notify the physician if blurred vision or brow pain occurs.
5. Instruct the client to check for the presence of the disk in the conjunctival sac daily at bedtime and on arising.
6. Because vision may change in the first few hours after the eye system is inserted, instruct the client to replace the disk at bedtime.

◢ IX. β-ADRENERGIC BLOCKING EYE MEDICATIONS (BOX 64-7)

A. Description
1. These medications reduce intraocular pressure by decreasing sympathetic impulses and decreasing aqueous humor production without affecting **accommodation** or pupil size.
2. These medications are used to treat chronic open-angle **glaucoma.**
3. These medications are contraindicated in the client with asthma because systemic absorption can cause increased airway resistance.
4. Use these medications with caution in the client receiving oral β-blockers.

B. Side effects
1. Ocular irritation
2. Visual disturbances
3. Bradycardia
4. Hypotension
5. Bronchospasm

C. Interventions
1. Monitor vital signs, especially blood pressure and pulse, before administering medication.
2. If the pulse is 60 or less or if the systolic blood pressure is less than 90 mm Hg, withhold the medication and contact the physician.
3. Monitor for shortness of breath.

4. Assess for risk of injury.
5. Monitor intake and output.
6. Instruct the client to notify the physician if shortness of breath occurs.
7. Instruct the client not to discontinue the medication abruptly.
8. Instruct the client to change positions slowly because of the potential for orthostatic hypotension.
9. Instruct the client to avoid hazardous activities.
10. Instruct the client to avoid over-the-counter medications without the physician's approval.

D. Adrenergic medications (Box 64-8)
1. Adrenergic medications decrease the production of aqueous humor and lead to a decrease in intraocular pressure.
2. Adrenergic medications may be used to treat **glaucoma.**

X. CARBONIC ANHYDRASE INHIBITORS (BOX 64-9) ◢

A. Description
1. Carbonic anhydrase inhibitors interfere with the production of carbonic acid, which leads to decreased aqueous humor formation and decreased intraocular pressure.
2. These medications are used for long-term treatment of open-angle **glaucoma.**
3. These medications are contraindicated in the client allergic to sulfonamides.

B. Side effects
1. Appetite loss
2. Gastrointestinal upset
3. Paresthesias in the fingers, toes, and face
4. Polyuria
5. Hypokalemia
6. Renal calculuses
7. Photosensitivity
8. Lethargy and drowsiness
9. Depression

BOX 64-7

β-Adrenergic Blocking Eye Medications

Betaxolol hydrochloride (Betoptic)
Carteolol hydrochloride (Ocupress)
Levobunolol hydrochloride (Betagan)
Metipranolol (Optipranolol)
Timolol maleate (Timoptic)

BOX 64-8

Adrenergic Medications

Epinephrine (Epifrin, Glaucon)
Hydroxyamphetamine (Paredrine)
Naphazoline (Allerest, Vasoclear)
Oxymethazoline (OcuClear)
Phenylephrine (AK-Nephrin, Prefin)
Tetrahydrozoline (Murine Plus, Visine)

BOX 64-9

Carbonic Anhydrase Inhibitors: Eye Medications

Acetazolamide (Diamox)
Dichlorphenamide (Daranide)
Dorzolamide hydrochloride (Trusopt)
Methazolamide (Neptazane)

C. Interventions
1. Monitor vital signs.
2. Assess visual acuity.
3. Assess for risk of injury.
4. Monitor intake and output.
5. Monitor weight.
6. Maintain oral hygiene.
7. Monitor for side effects such as lethargy, anorexia, drowsiness, polyuria, nausea, and vomiting.
8. Monitor electrolytes for hypokalemia.
9. Increase fluid intake unless contraindicated.
10. Advise the client to avoid prolonged exposure to sunlight.
11. Encourage the use of artificial tears for dry eyes.
12. Instruct the client not to discontinue the medication abruptly.
13. Instruct the client to avoid hazardous activities while vision is impaired.

XI. OSMOTIC MEDICATIONS (BOX 64-10)
A. Description
1. Osmotic medications lower intraocular pressure.
2. Osmotic medications are used in emergency treatment of acute closed-angle **glaucoma.**
3. Osmotic medications are used preoperatively and postoperatively to decrease vitreous humor volume.
B. Side effects
1. Headache
2. Nausea, vomiting, diarrhea
3. Disorientation
4. Electrolyte imbalances
C. Interventions
1. Assess vital signs.
2. Assess visual acuity.
3. Assess for risk of injury.
4. Monitor intake and output.
5. Monitor weight.
6. Monitor electrolyte imbalances.
7. Increase fluid intake unless contraindicated.
8. Monitor for changes in level of orientation.

XII. OTIC MEDICATION ADMINISTRATION (BOX 64-11)
A. Administration of drops
1. In an adult, pull the pinna up and back to straighten the external canal to instill ear drops.
2. Pull the pinna down and back for infants and children younger than 3 years of age; up and back for older children.

BOX 64-10

Osmotic Medications for the Eye

Glycerin (Osmoglyn)
Mannitol (Osmitrol)

B. Irrigation of the ear
1. Irrigation of the ear needs to be prescribed by the physician.
2. Ensure direct visualization of the tympanic membrane.
3. Warm irrigating solution to 98° F because solutions that are not close to the client's body temperature will cause ear injury, nausea, and vertigo.
4. Irrigation must be done gently to avoid damage to the eardrum.
5. When irrigating, do not direct irrigation solution directly toward the eardrum.
6. If a perforation of the eardrum is suspected, do not perform irrigation.

XIII. ANTIINFECTIVE EAR MEDICATIONS (BOX 64-12)
A. Description
1. Antiinfective medications kill or inhibit the growth of bacteria.
2. Antiinfective medications are used for otitis media or otitis externa.
3. Antiinfective medications are contraindicated if a prior hypersensitivity exists.
B. Side effects: overgrowth of nonsusceptible organisms
C. Interventions
1. Monitor vital signs.
2. Assess for allergies.
3. Asses for pain.
4. Monitor for nephrotoxicity.
5. Instruct the client to report dizziness, fatigue, fever, or sore throat, which may indicate a superimposed infection.

BOX 64-11

Medications that Affect Hearing

ANTIBIOTICS
Amikacin (Amikin)
Chloramphenicol (Chloromycetin, Chloroptic, Ophthoclor)
Erythromycin (E-Mycin, ERYC, Ery-Tab, PCE Dispertabs, Ilotycin)
Gentamicin (Garamycin)
Streptomycin sulfate
Tobramycin sulfate (Nebcin)
Vancomycin (Vancocin)

DIURETICS
Acetazolamide (Diamox)
Ethacrynic acid (Edecrin)
Furosemide (Lasix)

OTHERS
Cisplatin (Platinol, Platinol-AQ)
Nitrogen mustard
Quinine (Quinamm)
Quinidine (Cardioquin, Quinaglute, Quinidex)

BOX 64-12

Antiinfective Ear Medications

Acetic acid and aluminum acetate (Otic Domeboro)
Amoxicillin (Amoxil)
Ampicillin trihydrate (Polycillin)
Cefaclor (Ceclor)
Chloramphenicol (Chloromycetin Otic)
Clarithromycin (Biaxin)
Clindamycin hydrochloride (Cleocin)
Erythromycin (Ilotycin, E-Mycin)
Gentamicin sulfate otic solution (Garamycin)
Loracarbef (Lorabid)
Penicillin V potassium (Pen-V)
Polymyxin B sulfate (Aerosporin)
Tetracycline hydrochloride (Achromycin)
Trimethoprim and sulfamethoxazole (Bactrim, Cotrim, and Septra)

BOX 64-13

Antihistamines and Decongestants

Astemizole (Hismanal)
Brompheniramine (Bromphen, Dimetane)
Cetirizine (Zyrtec)
Chlorpheniramine (Chlor-Trimeton, Teldrin)
Clemastine (Tavist)
Naphazoline hydrochloride (Allerest, Albalon)
Terfenadine (Seldane)
Triprolidine and pseudoephedrine (Actifed)

6. Instruct the client to complete the entire course of the medication.
7. Instruct the client to keep ear canals dry.

XIV. ANTIHISTAMINES AND DECONGESTANTS (BOX 64-13)

A. Description
  1. These medications produce vasoconstriction.
  2. These medications stimulate the receptors of the respiratory mucosa.
  3. These medications reduce respiratory tissue hyperemia and edema to open obstructed eustachian tubes.
  4. These medications are used for acute otitis media.
B. Side effects
  1. Drowsiness
  2. Blurred vision
  3. Dry mucous membranes
C. Interventions
  1. Inform the client that drowsiness, blurred vision, and a dry mouth may occur.
  2. Instruct the client to increase fluid intake unless contraindicated and to suck on hard candy to alleviate the dry mouth.
  3. Instruct the client to avoid hazardous activities if drowsiness occurs.

BOX 64-14

Ceruminolytic Medications

Boric acid (Ear-Dry)
Carbamide peroxide (Debrox)
Trolamine polypeptide oleate—condensate (Cerumenex)

XV. LOCAL ANESTHETICS

A. Description
  1. Local anesthetics block nerve conduction at or near the application site to control pain.
  2. Local anesthetics are used for pain associated with ear infections.
B. Medication: benzocaine (Americaine Otic; Tympagesic)
C. Side effects
  1. Allergic reaction
  2. Irritation
D. Interventions
  1. Monitor for effectiveness if used for pain relief.
  2. Assess for irritation or allergic reaction.

XVI. CERUMINOLYTIC MEDICATIONS (BOX 64-14)

A. Description
  1. Ceruminolytic medications emulsify and loosen cerumen deposits.
  2. Ceruminolytic medications are used to loosen and remove impacted wax from the ear canal.
B. Side effects
  1. Irritation
  2. Redness or swelling of the ear canal
C. Interventions
  1. Instruct the client not to use drops more often than prescribed.
  2. Moisten a cotton plug with medication before insertion.
  3. Keep the container tightly closed and away from moisture.
  4. Avoid touching the ear with the dropper.
  5. Thirty minutes after instillation, gently irrigate the ear as prescribed with warm water using a soft rubber bulb ear syringe.
  6. Irrigation may be done with hydrogen peroxide solution as prescribed to flush cerumen deposits out of the ear canal.
  7. For a chronic cerumen impaction, 1 to 2 drops of mineral oil will soften the wax.
  8. Instruct the client to notify the physician if redness, pain or swelling persists.

PRACTICE QUESTIONS

1. In preparation for cataract surgery the nurse is to administer cyclopentolate (Cyclogyl) eye drops. The nurse administers the eye drops, knowing that the purpose of this medication is to
  1. Provide lubrication to the operative eye.

2. Produce miosis of the operative eye.
3. Dilate the pupil of the operative eye.
4. Constrict the pupil of the operative eye.

2. The home health nurse visits a client at home and instructs the client on the administration of the prescribed eye drops. Which of the following statements by the client indicates a need for further education?
   1. "I can sit and tilt my head back, pull down on the lower lid, and place the drop in the lower lid."
   2. "I can lie down, pull down on the lower lid, and place the drop in the lower lid."
   3. "I can lie down, pull up on the upper lid, and place the drop in the lower lid."
   4. "I can lie on my side opposite to the eye I am going to place the drop. Put the drop in the corner of the lid nearest my nose then slowly turn to my other side while blinking."

3. Ear drops are prescribed for an infant with otitis media. The most appropriate method to administer the ear drops to the infant is to
   1. Pull up and back on the pinna and direct the solution onto the eardrum.
   2. Pull down and back on the pinna and direct the solution onto the eardrum.
   3. Pull down and back on the pinna and direct the solution toward the wall of the canal.
   4. Pull up and back on the ear lobe and direct the solution toward the wall of the canal.

4. The nurse is providing instructions to a client who will be self-administering eye drops. To minimize the systemic effects that eye drops can produce, the nurse instructs the client to
   1. Eat before instilling the drops.
   2. Swallow several times after instilling the drops.
   3. Blink vigorously to encourage tearing after instilling the drops.
   4. Occlude the nasolacrimal duct with a finger for several minutes after instilling the drops.

5. The client is receiving an eye drop and an eye ointment to the right eye. The nurse would most appropriately
   1. Administer the eye drop first, followed by the eye ointment.
   2. Administer the eye ointment first, followed by the eye drop.
   3. Administer the eye drop, wait 10 minutes, and administer the eye ointment.
   4. Administer the eye ointment, wait 10 minutes, and administer the eye drop.

6. The nurse is caring for a client with glaucoma. Which of the following medications, if prescribed for the client, would the nurse question?
   1. Carbachol (Carboptic)

   2. Pilocarpine hydrochloride (Isopto Carpine)
   3. Pilocarpine nitrate (Ocusert Pilo-20, Pilo-40)
   4. Atropine sulfate (Isopto Atropine)

7. A miotic medication has been prescribed for the client with glaucoma. The client asks the nurse about the purpose of the medication. The nurse tells the client that
   1. "The medication causes the pupil to constrict and will lower the pressure in the eye."
   2. "The medication will help to dilate the eye to prevent pressure from occurring."
   3. "The medication will relax the muscles of the eyes and prevent blurred vision."
   4. "The medication will help to block the responses that are sent to the muscles in the eye."

8. Pilocarpine hydrochloride (Isopto Carpine) is prescribed for the client with glaucoma. Which of the following medications does the nurse plan to have available in the event of systemic toxicity?
   1. Naloxone hydrochloride (Narcan)
   2. Pindolol (Visken)
   3. Atropine sulfate
   4. Mesoridazine besylate (Serentil)

9. Betaxolol hydrochloride (Betoptic) eye drops have been prescribed for the client with glaucoma. Which of the following nursing actions is most appropriate related to monitoring for the side effects of this medication?
   1. Monitoring temperature.
   2. Monitoring blood pressure.
   3. Assessing blood glucose level.
   4. Assessing peripheral pulses.

10. The nurse prepares the client for an ear irrigation as prescribed by the physician. In performing the procedure, the nurse
    1. Assists the client to turn his or her head so that the ear to be irrigated is facing upward.
    2. Warms the irrigating solution to 98° F.
    3. Directs a slow steady stream of irrigation solution toward the eardrum.
    4. Positions the client with the affected side up following the irrigation.

CRITICAL THINKING: FILL IN THE BLANK

The nurse is providing instructions to a client with glaucoma regarding the procedure for administering eye drops. The nurse tells the client to perform what specific action following administration of the eye drops to prevent systemic absorption?

Answer: _____

ANSWERS

1. 3

Rationale: Cyclopentolate is a rapidly acting mydriatic and cycloplegic medication. Cyclopentolate is effective in 25 to 75 minutes, and accommodation returns in 6 to 24 hours. Cyclopentolate is used for preoperative mydriasis.

Test-Taking Strategy: Use the process of elimination. Options 2 and 4 are similar and are eliminated first. Miosis refers to a constricted pupil. Note that the question identifies a client being prepared for eye surgery. The pupil would need to be dilated for the surgical procedure. Review the action and purpose of this medication if you had difficulty with this question.

Level of Cognitive Ability: Application
Client Needs: Physiological Integrity
Integrated Process: Nursing Process—implementation
Content Area: Adult health—eye
Reference: Lehne, R. (2001). *Pharmacology for nursing care* (4th ed., p. 1147). Philadelphia: W. B. Saunders.

2. 3

Rationale: The client can lie down or sit with the head tilted back. The lower lid should be pulled downward with the thumb or fingers. The client holds the bottle like a pencil, with the tip downward, and squeezes the bottle gently, allowing 1 drop to fall into the sac. The client gently closes the eye. Options 1, 2, and 4 identify correct methods for administering eye drops.

Test-Taking Strategy: Use the process of elimination. Note the key words "need for further education." Knowing that the client places drops into the eye by pulling down on the lower lid will direct you to the correct option. Review the procedure for the administration of eye medications if you had difficulty with this question.

Level of Cognitive Ability: Analysis
Client Needs: Physiological Integrity
Integrated Process: Teaching/Learning
Content Area: Adult health—eye
Reference: Gutierrez, K., & Queener, S. (2003). *Pharmacology for nursing practice* (p. 1091). St. Louis: Mosby.

3. 3

Rationale: In a child younger than 3 years, the pinna is pulled down and straight back. The infant should be turned on the side with the affected ear uppermost. With the nondominant hand the pinna is pulled down and back. The medication is administered by aiming it at the wall of the canal rather than directly onto the eardrum. The infant should remain with the affected ear uppermost for 10 to 15 minutes to retain the solution. In the adult or a child older than 3 years, the pinna is pulled up and back to straighten the auditory canal.

Test-Taking Strategy: Use the process of elimination. Eliminate options 1 and 2 because you would not direct ear solution directly onto the eardrum. Remembering that in a child younger than 3 years, pulling the pinna down and straight back is the correct procedure for administering ear medications. Review the procedure for the administration of ear medications, if you had difficulty with this question.

Level of Cognitive Ability: Application
Client Needs: Physiological Integrity

Integrated Process: Nursing Process—implementation
Content Area: Adult health—ear
Reference: Gutierrez, K., & Queener, S. (2003). *Pharmacology for nursing practice* (p. 1103). St. Louis: Mosby.

4. 4

Rationale: Applying pressure on the nasolacrimal duct prevents systemic absorption of the medication. Options 1, 2, and 3 will not prevent systemic absorption.

Test-Taking Strategy: Use the process of elimination. Eating and swallowing are similar options and are not related to the systemic absorption of an eye medication. Blinking vigorously to produce tearing may result in the loss of the administered medication. Review the procedure for administering eye drops to prevent systemic absorption if you had difficulty with this question.

Level of Cognitive Ability: Application
Client Needs: Physiological Integrity
Integrated Process: Teaching/Learning
Content Area: Adult health—eye
Reference: Gutierrez, K., & Queener, S. (2003). *Pharmacology for nursing practice* (p. 1091). St. Louis: Mosby.

5. 1

Rationale: When an eye drop and an eye ointment are scheduled to be administered at the same time, the eye drop is administered first. Options 2, 3, and 4 are incorrect.

Test-Taking Strategy: Recalling the guidelines for administering eye medications will direct you to option 1. Review these guidelines if you had difficulty with this question.

Level of Cognitive Ability: Application
Client Needs: Physiological Integrity
Integrated Process: Nursing Process—implementation
Content Area: Adult health—eye
Reference: Harkreader, H., & Hogan, M. A. (2004). *Fundamentals of nursing: Caring and clinical judgment* (2nd ed., p. 438). Philadelphia: W. B. Saunders.

6. 4

Rationale: Options 1, 2, and 3 are miotic agents used to treat glaucoma. Option 4 is a mydriatic and cycloplegic medication, and its use is contraindicated in clients with glaucoma. Mydriatic medications dilate the pupil and can cause an increase in intraocular pressure in the eye.

Test-Taking Strategy: Use the process of elimination. Knowledge regarding the classifications of the medications identified in the options will assist in answering the question. Remember that mydriatics dilate and that these medications are contraindicated in glaucoma. Review the contraindications related to medications in the client with glaucoma if you had difficulty with this question.

Level of Cognitive Ability: Analysis
Client Needs: Physiological Integrity
Integrated Process: Nursing Process—analysis
Content Area: Adult health—eye
Reference: Kee, J., & Hayes, E. (2003). *Pharmacology: A nursing process approach* (4th ed., p. 347). Philadelphia: W. B. Saunders.

7. 1

Rationale: Miotics cause pupillary constriction and are used to treat glaucoma. They lower the intraocular pressure, thereby increasing blood flow to the retina and decreasing retinal damage and loss of vision. Miotics cause a contraction of the ciliary muscle and a widening of trabecular mesh work. Options 2, 3, and 4 are incorrect.

Test-Taking Strategy: Use the process of elimination. Note that the client has glaucoma. Recall that prevention of increased intraocular pressure is the goal in the client with glaucoma. Options 2, 3, and 4 describe actions related to mydriatic medications, which primarily dilate the pupils and relax the ciliary muscles. Review the action of a miotic medication if you had difficulty with this question.

Level of Cognitive Ability: Application
Client Needs: Physiological Integrity
Integrated Process: Nursing Process—implementation
Content Area: Adult health—eye
Reference: McKenry, L., & Salerno, E. (2003). *Mosby's pharmacology in nursing* (21st ed., p. 796). St. Louis: Mosby.

8. 3
Rationale: Systemic absorption of pilocarpine hydrochloride can produce toxicity and includes manifestations of vertigo, bradycardia, tremors, hypotension, syncope, cardiac dysrhythmias, and seizures. Atropine sulfate must be available in the event of systemic toxicity. Mesoridazine besylate is an antipsychotic medication. Pindolol is a β-adrenergic blocker. Naloxone hydrochloride is an opioid antagonist used to reverse narcotic-induced respiratory depression.

Test-Taking Strategy: Use the process of elimination and knowledge regarding antidotes related to various medications to answer this question. Remember atropine sulfate is the antidote for systemic reactions that occur with pilocarpine. Review antidotes if you had difficulty with this question.

Level of Cognitive Ability: Analysis
Client Needs: Physiological Integrity
Integrated Process: Nursing Process—planning
Content Area: Adult health—eye
Reference: Gutierrez, K., & Queener, S. (2003). *Pharmacology for nursing practice* (p. 1082). St. Louis: Mosby.

9. 2
Rationale: Hypotension, dizziness, nausea, diaphoresis, headache, fatigue, constipation, and diarrhea are systemic effects of the medication. Nursing interventions include monitoring the blood pressure for hypotension and assessing the pulse for strength, weakness, irregular rate, and bradycardia. Option 1, 3, and 4 are not specifically associated with this medication.

Test-Taking Strategy: Use the ABCs—airway, breathing, and circulation—to direct you to option 2. Although option 4, peripheral pulses, also is related to circulation monitoring, the blood pressure is the more global option. Review the side effect of this medication if you had difficulty with this question.

Level of Cognitive Ability: Analysis

Client Needs: Physiological Integrity
Integrated Process: Nursing Process—assessment
Content Area: Adult health—eye
Reference: Hodgson, B., & Kizior, R. (2004). *Saunders nursing drug handbook 2004* (p. 106). Philadelphia: W. B. Saunders.

10. 2
Rationale: Irrigation solutions that are not close to the client's body temperature can be uncomfortable and may cause injury, nausea, and vertigo. The client is positioned so that the ear to be irrigated is facing downward because this allows gravity to assist in the removal of the ear wax and solution. Following the irrigation, the client is to lie on the affected side to finish the drainage of the irrigating solution. A slow, steady stream of solution should be directed toward the upper wall of the ear canal and not toward the eardrum. Too much force could cause the tympanic membrane to rupture.

Test-Taking Strategy: Use the process of elimination. Read each option carefully and remember that the nurse's concern is to prevent damage to the tympanic membrane. Additionally, remember that the client should be positioned with the affected side downward to allow drainage of the irrigation solution. Review the procedure for performing an ear irrigation if you had difficulty with this question.

Level of Cognitive Ability: Application
Client Needs: Physiological Integrity
Integrated Process: Nursing process—implementation
Content Area: Adult health—ear
Reference: Harkreader, H., & Hogan, M. A. (2004). *Fundamentals of nursing: Caring and clinical judgment* (2nd ed., p. 992). Philadelphia: W. B. Saunders.

CRITICAL THINKING: FILL IN THE BLANK

Answer: To apply pressure over the inner canthus next to the nose for 30 seconds to 1 minute
Rationale: To prevent overflow of the medication into nasal and pharyngeal passages, thus reducing systemic absorption, the client is taught to apply pressure over the inner canthus next to the nose for 30 seconds to 1 minute following administration of the medication.

Test-Taking Strategy: Focus on the issue, to prevent systemic absorption following administration of the eye drops. Visualize the procedure to determine what specific action will prevent this occurrence. If you are unfamiliar with the procedure for administering eye medications, review these guidelines.

Level of Cognitive Ability: Application
Client Needs: Health Promotion and Maintenance
Integrated Process: Teaching/Learning
Content Area: Adult health—eye
Reference: McKenry, L., & Salerno, E. (2003). *Mosby's pharmacology in nursing* (21st ed., p. 793). St. Louis: Mosby.

REFERENCES

Gutierrez, K., & Queener, S. (2003). *Pharmacology for nursing practice.* St. Louis: Mosby.

Harkreader, H., & Hogan, M. A. (2004). *Fundamentals of nursing: Caring and clinical judgment* (2nd ed.). Philadelphia: W. B. Saunders.

Hodgson, B., & Kizior, R. (2004). *Saunders nursing drug handbook 2004.* Philadelphia: W. B. Saunders.

Kee, J., & Hayes, E. (2003). *Pharmacology: A nursing process approach* (4th ed.). Philadelphia: W. B. Saunders.

Lehne, R. (2001). *Pharmacology for nursing care* (4th ed.). Philadelphia: W. B. Saunders.

McKenry, L., & Salerno, E. (2003). *Mosby's pharmacology in nursing* (21st ed.). St. Louis: Mosby.

The Adult Client with a Neurological Disorder

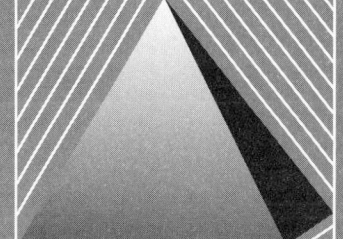

PYRAMID TERMS

agnosia   The inability to use an object correctly.

apraxia   The inability to carry out a purposeful activity.

autonomic dysreflexia   Syndrome characterized by paroxysmal hypertension, bradycardia, excessive sweating, facial flushing, nasal congestion, pilomotor responses, and headache. The syndrome occurs with spinal lesions above T6 after the period of spinal shock is complete. Triggers include visceral distention from a distended bladder or impacted rectum. The syndrome is a neurological emergency and must be treated immediately to prevent a hypertensive stroke. Also known as hyperreflexia.

Babinski's reflex   Dorsiflexion of the ankle and great toe with fanning of the other toes that indicates a disruption of the pyramidal tract.

Brudzinski's sign   Flexion of the head that causes flexion of both thighs at the hips and knee flexion and that indicates meningeal irritation.

decerebrate posturing   Stiff extension of one or both arms and possibly the legs that indicates a brainstem lesion.

decorticate posturing   Flexure of one or both arms on the chest and possibly stiff extension of the legs that indicate a nonfunctioning cortex.

flaccid posturing   No motor response display in any extremity.

Glasgow Coma Scale   A method of assessing a client's neurological condition; a scoring system based on a scale of 1 to 15 points. A score of less than 8 indicates that coma is present. Eye-opening is the most important indicator.

halo traction   Insertion of pins or screws into the client's skull and application of a circular fixation device and halo jacket or cast. Used to immobilize the cervical spine.

hemianopsia   Blindness in half the visual field.

homonymous hemianopsia   Blindness in the same visual field of both eyes.

increased intracranial pressure   An increase in intracranial pressure caused by trauma, hemorrhage, growths or tumors, hydrocephalus, edema, or inflammation. Increased pressure can impede circulation to the brain and absorption of cerebrospinal fluid and can affect the functioning of nerve cells and lead to brainstem compression and death.

Kernig's sign   Flexure of the thigh and knee to right angles and, when they are extended, if spasm of hamstring and pain occurs, it indicates meningeal irritation.

skull tongs   Tongs inserted into the outer aspect of the client's skull, just above the ears, with application of traction.

spinal shock   A sudden depression of reflex activity in the spinal cord below the level of injury (areflexia) that ccurs within the first hour of injury and lasts days to months. The muscles become completely paralyzed and flaccid, and reflexes are absent. Also know as neurogenic shock.

Tensilon test   Test done to diagnose myasthenia gravis and to differentiate between myasthenic crisis and cholinergic crisis.

unconscious client   A state of depressed cerebral functioning with unresponsiveness to sensory and motor function. Causes include head trauma, cerebral toxins, shock, hemorrhage, tumor, and infections.

unilateral neglect   An inability to recognize a physical impairment that occurs most commonly in clients who have had a right cerebral stroke. Also known as neglect syndrome.

▲ PYRAMID TO SUCCESS

Pyramid Points related to neurological disorders focus on monitoring for increased intracranial pressure, assessing level of consciousness, positioning clients, head injuries, spinal cord injuries, spinal shock, autonomic dysreflexia, implementation during a seizure, the client with a cerebrovascular accident, Parkinson's disease, myasthenia gravis, and the Tensilon test. Altered body image and psychosocial issues that occur as a result of the neurological disorder are also a focus of the Pyramid to Success. The Integrated Processes addressed in this unit include Nursing Process, Caring, Communication and Documentation, and Teaching/Learning.

▲ CLIENT NEEDS

Safe, Effective Care Environment

Accident prevention related to neurological deficits
Advance directives
Advocacy
Asepsis with procedures and treatments
Client rights
Confidentiality
Consultation with members of the health care team
Establishing priorities
Informed consent for invasive procedures
Referrals
Standard precautions

Health Promotion and Maintenance

Expected body image changes resulting from neurological deficits
Home care instructions regarding care related to neurological disorder
Neurological assessment
Prevention and early detection of health problems associated with neurological deficits
Reinforcement regarding the importance of prescribed therapy

Psychosocial Integrity

Ability to cope with feelings of isolation and loss of independence
Cultural, religious, and spiritual influences
End-of-life issues
Grief and loss
Mobilization of coping mechanisms
Sensory and perceptual alterations
Support systems and use of community resources
Unexpected body image changes

Physiological Integrity

Alterations in body systems
Complications related to procedures
Emergency care
Fluid and electrolyte imbalances
Measures to promote comfort
Pharmacological therapy
Promotion of normal elimination patterns
Promotion of self-care measures
Use of assistive devices for mobility

REFERENCES

Chernecky, C., & Berger, B. (2004). *Laboratory tests & diagnostic procedures* (4th ed.). Philadelphia: W. B. Saunders.

Harkreader, H., & Hogan, M. A. (2004). *Fundamentals of nursing: Caring and clinical judgment* (2nd ed.). Philadelphia: W. B. Saunders.

Ignatavicius, D., & Workman, M. (2002). *Medical-surgical nursing: Critical thinking for collaborative care* (4th ed.). Philadelphia: W. B. Saunders.

Lewis, S., Heitkemper, M., & Dirksen, S. (2004). *Medical-surgical nursing: Assessment and management of clinical problems* (6th ed.). St. Louis: Mosby.

National Council of State Boards of Nursing (Eds.). (2003). *Test Plan for the National Council Licensure Examination for Registered Nurses* (effective date: April 2004). Chicago: Author.

Perry, A., & Potter, P. (2002). *Clinical nursing skills and techniques* (5th ed.). St. Louis: Mosby.

Phipps, W., Monahan, F., Sands, J., Marek, J., & Neighbors, M. (2003). *Medical-surgical nursing: Health and illness perspectives* (7th ed.). St. Louis: Mosby.

Potter, P., & Perry, A. (2001). *Fundamentals of nursing* (5th ed.). St. Louis: Mosby.

Varcarolis, E. M. (2002). *Foundations of psychiatric mental health nursing* (4th ed.). Philadelphia: W. B. Saunders.

Neurological System

I. ANATOMY AND PHYSIOLOGY OF THE BRAIN AND SPINAL CORD

A. Cerebrum
  1. The cerebrum consists of the right and left hemispheres.
  2. Each hemisphere receives sensory information from the opposite side of the body and controls the skeletal muscles of the opposite side.
  3. The cerebrum governs sensory and motor activity.
  4. The cerebrum governs thought and learning.

B. Cerebral cortex (Box 65-1)
  1. The cerebral cortex is the outer gray layer.
  2. The cortex is divided into four lobes.
  3. The cortex is responsible for the conscious activities of the cerebrum.

C. Basal ganglia
  1. The basal ganglia are cell bodies in white matter.
  2. The basal ganglia assist the cerebral cortex in producing smooth voluntary movements.

BOX 65-1

Cerebral Cortex

FRONTAL LOBE
Broca's area for speech
Prefontal lobe: morals, emotions, and judgments

PARIETAL LOBE
Interpretation of pain, touch, temperature, and pressure

TEMPORAL LOBE
Auditory center
Wenicke's area for sensory and speech

OCCIPITAL LOBE
Visual area

D. Diencephalon
  1. Thalamus
    a. The thalamus relays sensory impulses to the cortex.
    b. The thalamus provides a pain gate.
    c. The thalamus is part of the reticular activating system.
  2. Hypothalamus
    a. The hypothalamus regulates autonomic responses of the sympathetic and parasympathetic nervous systems.
    b. The hypothalamus regulates stress response, sleep, appetite, body temperature, fluid balance, and emotions.
    c. The hypothalamus is responsible for the production of hormones secreted by the pituitary gland and hypothalamus.

E. Brainstem
  1. Midbrain
    a. The midbrain is responsible for motor coordination.
    b. The midbrain contains the visual reflex and auditory relay centers.
  2. Pons
    a. The pons contains the respiratory centers.
    b. The pons regulates breathing.
  3. Medulla oblongata
    a. The medulla oblongata contains all afferent and efferent tracts.
    b. The medulla oblongata contains cardiac, respiratory, vomiting, and vasomotor centers.
    c. The medulla oblongata controls heart rate, respiration, blood vessel diameter, sneezing, swallowing, vomiting, and coughing.

F. Cerebellum
  1. The cerebellum coordinates smooth muscle movement.
  2. The cerebellum coordinates posture, equilibrium, and muscle tone.

G. Spinal cord
   1. The spinal cord provides neuron and synapse networks to produce involuntary responses to sensory stimulation.
   2. The spinal cord allows for control of the number of pain impulses that pass through the spinal cord on their way to the brain.
   3. The spinal cord carries sensory information to and motor information from the brain.
   4. The spinal cord extends from the first cervical to the second lumbar vertebra.
   5. The spinal cord is protected by the meninges, cerebrospinal fluid, and adipose tissue.
   6. Horns
      a. Inner column of gray matter contains two anterior and two posterior horns.
      b. Posterior horns connect with afferent (sensory) nerve fibers.
      c. Anterior horns contain efferent (motor) nerve fibers.
   7. Nerve tracts
      a. White matter contains the nerve tract.
      b. Ascending tracts (sensory pathway)
      c. Descending tract (motor pathway)
H. Meninges
   1. Dura mater is the tough and fibrous membrane.
   2. Arachnoid membrane is the delicate membrane and contains subarachnoid fluid.
   3. Pia mater is the vascular membrane.
   4. Subarachnoid space is formed by the arachnoid membrane and the pia mater.
I. Cerebrospinal fluid
   1. Cerebrospinal fluid is secreted in the ventricles and circulates through the ventricles to the subarachnoid layer of the meninges, where it is reabsorbed.
   2. Cerebrospinal fluid circulates in the subarachnoid space.
   3. Normal pressure is 50 to 175 mm H_2O.
   4. Normal volume is 125 to 150 mL.
   5. Cerebrospinal fluid acts as a protective cushion.
   6. Cerebrospinal fluid aids in the exchange of nutrients and wastes.
J. Ventricles
   1. Four ventricles
   2. The ventricles communicate between the subarachnoid spaces.
   3. The ventricles produce and circulate cerebrospinal fluid.
K. Blood supply
   1. Right and left internal carotids
   2. Right and left vertebral arteries
   3. These arteries supply the brain via an anastamosis at the base of the brain called the circle of Willis.
L. Neurotransmitters
   1. Acetylcholine
   2. Norepinephrine

   3. Dopamine
   4. Serotonin
   5. Amino acids
   6. Polypeptides
M. Neurons
   1. The cell body contains the nucleus.
   2. The neuron contains the axons and dendrites.
   3. Neurons carrying impulses to the central nervous system (CNS) are called sensory neurons.
   4. Neurons carrying impulses away from the CNS are called motor neurons.
   5. Synapse is the chemical transmission of impulses from one neuron to another.
N. Axons and dendrites
   1. The axon conducts impulses from the cell body.
   2. The dendrites receive stimuli from the body and transmit them to the axon.
   3. The neurons are protected and insulated by Schwann cells.
   4. The Schwann cell sheath is called the neurolemma.
   5. Neurons do not reproduce after the neonatal period.
   6. If an axon or dendrite is damaged, it will die and be replaced slowly only if the neurolemma is intact and the cell body has not died.
O. Spinal nerves
   1. The human being has 31 pairs of spinal nerves.
   2. Mixed nerve fibers are formed by the joining of the anterior motor and posterior sensory roots.
   3. Posterior roots contain afferent (sensory) nerve fibers.
   4. Anterior roots contain efferent (motor) nerve fibers.
P. Autonomic nervous system
   1. Sympathetic (adrenergic) fibers dilate pupils, increase heart rate and rhythm, contract blood vessels, and relax smooth muscles of the bronchi.
   2. Parasympathetic (cholinergic) fibers produce the opposite effect.

II. DIAGNOSTIC TESTS
A. Skull and spinal radiography
   1. Description
      a. Radiographs of the skull reveal the size and shape of the skull bones, suture separation in infants, fractures or bony defects, erosion, or calcification.
      b. Spinal radiographs identify fractures, dislocation, compression, curvature, erosion, narrowed spinal cord, and degenerative processes.
   2. Preprocedure interventions
      a. Provide nursing support for the confused, combative, or ventilator-dependent client.
      b. Maintain immobilization of the neck if a spinal fracture is suspected.
      c. Remove metal items from body parts.
      d. If the client has thick and heavy hair, this should be documented because it may affect interpretation of the x-ray film.

3. Postprocedure intervention: Maintain immobilization until results are known.

B. Computed tomography scan

1. Description
   a. Computed tomography is a type of brain scanning that may or may not require an injection of a dye.
   b. Computed tomography is used to detect intracranial bleeding, space-occupying lesions, cerebral edema, infarctions, hydrocephalus, cerebral atrophy, and shifts of brain structures.

2. Preprocedure interventions
   a. Obtain an informed consent if a dye is used.
   b. Assess for allergies to iodine, contrast dyes, or shellfish if a dye is used.
   c. Instruct the client in the need to lie still and flat during the test.
   d. Instruct the client to hold his or her breath when requested.
   e. Initiate an intravenous line if prescribed.
   f. Remove objects from the head, such as wigs, barrettes, earrings, and hairpins.
   g. Assess for claustrophobia.
   h. Inform the client of possible mechanical noises as the scanning occurs.
   i. Inform the client that there may be a hot, flushed sensation and a metallic taste in the mouth when the dye is injected.
   j. Note that some clients may be given the dye even if they report an allergy and are treated with an antihistamine and corticosteroids before the injection to reduce the severity of a reaction.

3. Postprocedure interventions
   a. Provide replacement fluids because diuresis from the dye is expected.
   b. Monitor for an allergic reaction to the dye.
   c. Assess dye injection site for bleeding or hematoma, and monitor extremity for color, warmth, and the presence of distal pulses.

C. Magnetic resonance imaging

1. Description
   a. Magnetic resonance imaging is a noninvasive procedure that identifies types of tissues, tumors, and vascular abnormalities.
   b. Magnetic resonance imaging is similar to the computed tomography scan but provides more detailed pictures.

2. Preprocedure interventions
   a. Remove all metal objects from the client.
   b. Determine whether the client has a pacemaker, implanted defibrillator, or metal implants such as a hip prosthesis or vascular clips because these clients cannot have this test performed.
   c. Remove intravenous fluid pumps during the test.
   d. Provide precautions for the client who is attached to pulse oximeter because it can cause a burn during testing if coiled around the body or a body part.
   e. Provide an assessment of the client with claustrophobia.
   f. Administer medication as prescribed for the client with claustrophobia.
   g. Determine whether a contrast agent is to be used, and follow the prescription related to the administration of food, fluids, and medications.
   h. Instruct the client that he or she will need to remain still during the procedure.

3. Postprocedure interventions
   a. Client may resume normal activities.
   b. Expect diuresis if a contrast agent was used.

D. Lumbar puncture

1. Description
   a. Lumbar puncture is insertion of a spinal needle through the L3-L4 interspace into the lumbar subarachnoid space to obtain cerebrospinal fluid (CSF), measure CSF fluid or pressure, or instill air, dye, or medications.
   b. Lumbar puncture is contraindicated in clients with **increased intracranial pressure** because the procedure will cause a rapid decrease in pressure within the CSF around the spinal cord, leading to brain herniation.

2. Preprocedure interventions
   a. Obtain an informed consent.
   b. Have the client empty the bladder.

3. Interventions during the procedure
   a. Position the client in a lateral recumbent position and have the client draw knees up to the abdomen and chin onto the chest.
   b. Assist with the collection of specimens (label the specimens in sequence).
   c. Maintain strict asepsis.

4. Postprocedure interventions
   a. Monitor vital signs and neurological signs.
   b. Position the client flat as prescribed.
   c. Force fluids.
   d. Monitor intake and output.

E. Myelogram

1. Description: injection of dye or air into the subarachnoid space to detect abnormalities of the spinal cord and vertebrae

2. Preprocedure interventions
   a. Obtain an informed consent.
   b. Provide hydration for at least 12 hours before the test.
   c. Assess for allergies to iodine.
   d. If the client is taking a phenothiazine, hold the medication because this medication lowers the seizure threshold.
   e. Premedicate for sedation as prescribed.

3. Postprocedure interventions
   a. Assess vital signs and neurological condition frequently as prescribed.

b. If a water-based dye is used (most often used), elevate the head 15 to 30 degrees for 6 to 8 hours as prescribed.

c. If an oil-based dye is used, keep the client flat 6 to 8 hours as prescribed.

d. If air is used, keep the head lower than the trunk for up to 48 hours as prescribed.

e. Administer analgesics for headache or backache as prescribed.

f. Encourage fluids.

g. Monitor intake and output.

h. Assess for bladder distention and voiding.

F. Cerebral angiography

1. Description: injection of contrast through the femoral artery into the carotid arteries to visualize the cerebral arteries and assess for lesions

2. Preprocedure interventions

a. Obtain an informed consent.

b. Assess the client for allergies to iodine and shellfish.

c. Encourage hydration for 2 days before the test.

d. Maintain the client on NPO status 4 to 6 hours before the test as prescribed.

e. Obtain a baseline neurological assessment.

f. Mark the peripheral pulses.

g. Remove metal items from the hair.

h. Administer premedication as prescribed.

3. Postprocedure interventions

a. Monitor neurological status and vital signs frequently until stable.

b. Monitor for swelling in the neck and for difficulty swallowing, and notify the physician if these symptoms occur.

c. Maintain bed rest for 12 hours as prescribed.

d. Elevate the head of the bed 15 to 30 degrees only if prescribed.

e. Keep the bed flat if the femoral artery is used, as prescribed.

f. Assess peripheral pulses.

g. Apply sandbags and a pressure dressing to the injection site as prescribed.

h. Place ice on the puncture site as prescribed.

i. Encourage fluids.

G. Electroencephalography

1. Description: a graphic recording of the electrical activity of the superficial layers of the cerebral cortex

2. Preprocedure interventions

a. Wash the client's hair.

b. Inform the client that electrodes are attached to the head and that electricity does not enter the head.

c. Withhold stimulants, antidepressants, tranquilizers, and anticonvulsants for 24 to 48 hours before the test as prescribed.

d. Allow the client to have breakfast if prescribed.

e. Premedicate for sedation as prescribed.

3. Postprocedure interventions

a. Wash the client's hair.

b. Maintain side rails and safety precautions if the client was sedated.

H. Caloric testing (oculovestibular reflex)

1. Description: Caloric testing provides information about the function of the vestibular portion of the eighth cranial nerve and aids in the diagnosis of cerebellum and brainstem lesions.

2. Procedure

a. Patency of the external auditory canal is confirmed.

b. The client is positioned supine with the head of the bed elevated 30 degrees.

c. Cold or warm water is instilled into the auditory canal to stimulate the semicircular canals.

d. A normal response that indicates intact function of cranial nerves III, VI, and VIII is conjugate eye movements toward the side being irrigated, followed by rapid nystagmus to the opposite side.

e. Absent or dysconjugate eye movements indicate brainstem damage.

III. NEUROLOGICAL ASSESSMENT

A. Assessment of risk factors

1. Trauma
2. Hemorrhage
3. Tumors
4. Infection
5. Toxicity
6. Metabolic disorders
7. Hypoxic conditions
8. Aging process
9. Hypertension
10. Cigarette smoking
11. Stress

B. Assessment of the cranial nerves

1. Cranial nerve I (olfactory): sensory, smell

a. Have the client close eyes and occlude one nostril with finger.

b. Ask the client to identify nonirritating odors such as coffee, tea, cloves, soap, chewing gum, and peppermint.

c. Repeat the test on the other nostril.

2. Cranial nerve II (optic): sensory, vision

a. Assess visual acuity with a Snellen's chart or newspaper, or ask the client to count how many fingers the examiner is holding up.

b. Check visual fields by confrontation.

c. Have the client sit directly in front of examiner and stare at examiner's nose.

d. Examiner slowly moves his or her finger from the periphery toward the center until the client says it can be seen.

e. Check color vision by asking the client to name the colors of several nearby objects.

3. Cranial nerve III (oculomotor); cranial nerve IV (trochlear); cranial nerve VI (abducens)
   a. The motor functions of these nerves overlap; therefore they need to be tested together.
   b. First, inspect the eyelids for ptosis (drooping); then assess ocular movements and note any eye deviation.
   c. Test accommodation and direct and consensual light reflexes.
   d. Cranial nerve III (oculomotor; motor): Test assesses pupillary constriction, upper eyelid elevation, and most eye movement.
   e. Cranial nerve IV (trochlear; motor): Test assesses downward and inward eye movement.
   f. Cranial nerve VI (abducens): Test assesses lateral eye movement.

4. Cranial nerve V (trigeminal): sensory and motor
   a. Test assesses sensation to the cornea, nasal and oral mucosa, facial skin, and mastication.
   b. To test motor function, ask the client to close jaws tightly and then try to separate the clenched jaw.
   c. Test the corneal reflex by lightly touching the client's cornea with a cotton wisp.
   d. Check sensory function by asking the client to close the eyes; then lightly touch the forehead, cheeks, and chin, noting whether the client can feel the touch equally on both sides.

5. Cranial nerve VII (facial): sensory and motor
   a. Test taste perception on the anterior two thirds of the tongue.
   b. Have the client show the teeth.
   c. Attempt to close the client's eyes against resistance, and ask the client to puff out the cheeks.
   d. Place sugar, salt, or vinegar on the front of the tongue, and have the client identify these substances by their tastes.

6. Cranial nerve VIII (acoustic): sensory
   a. The ability to hear tests the cochlear portion.
   b. The sense of equilibrium tests the vestibular portion.
   c. Check the client's ability to hear a watch ticking or a whisper.
   d. Observe the client's balance, and observe for swaying when walking or standing.

7. Cranial nerve IX (glossopharyngeal): sensory and motor
   a. Test assesses swallowing ability.
   b. Test assesses sensation to the pharyngeal soft palate and tonsillar mucosa and taste perception on the posterior third of the tongue and salivation.

8. Cranial nerve X (vagus): sensory and motor
   a. Test assesses swallowing and phonation, sensation to the exterior ear's posterior wall, and sensation behind the ear.
   b. Test assesses sensation to the thoracic and abdominal viscera.

9. Cranial nerve IX (glossopharyngeal); cranial nerve X (vagus)
   a. Have the client identify a taste at the back of the tongue.
   b. Inspect the soft palate and observe for symmetrical elevation when the client says "aah."
   c. Touch the posterior pharyngeal wall with a tongue depressor to elicit a gag reflex.

10. Cranial nerve XI (spinal accessory): motor
    a. Test assesses uvula and soft palate movement and sternocleidomastoid and trapezius muscles.
    b. Test assesses upper portion of the trapezius muscle, which governs shoulder movement and neck rotation.
    c. Palpate and inspect the sternocleidomastoid muscle as the client pushes the chin against the examiner's hand.
    d. Palpate and inspect the trapezius muscle as the client shrugs the shoulders against the examiner's resistance.

11. Cranial nerve XII (hypoglossal): motor
    a. Test assesses tongue movements involved in swallowing and speech.
    b. Observe the tongue for asymmetry, atrophy, deviation to one side, and fasciculations.
    c. Ask the client to push the tongue against a tongue depressor and then have the client move the tongue rapidly in and out and from side to side.

C. Assessment of level of consciousness ▲
   1. Test assesses cerebral function.
   2. Test assesses client behavior to determine level of consciousness, such as confusion, delirium, unconsciousness, stupor, and coma.

D. Assessment of vital signs: Monitor for blood pressure or pulse changes, which may indicate **increased intracranial pressure (ICP)**.

E. Assessment of respirations (Box 65-2) ▲

F. Assessment of temperature ▲
   1. An elevated temperature increases the metabolic rate of the brain.
   2. An elevation in temperature may indicate a dysfunction of the hypothalamus or brainstem.
   3. A slow rise in temperature may indicate infection.

G. Assessment of pupils (Fig. 65-1) ▲
   1. Size
   2. Equality
   3. Reactions to light: described as brisk, slow, or fixed
   4. Unusual eye movements
   5. Unilateral pupil dilation indicates compression of the third cranial nerve.

BOX 65-2
Assessment of Respirations

CHEYNE-STOKES
Rhythmical with periods of apnea
Can indicate a metabolic dysfunction or dysfunction in the cerebral hemisphere or basal ganglia

NEUROGENIC HYPERVENTILATION
Regular rapid and deep sustained respirations
Indicates a dysfunction in the low midbrain and middle pons

APNEUSTIC
Irregular respirations with pauses at the end of inspiration and expiration
Indicates a dysfunction in the middle or caudal pons

ATAXIC
Totally irregular in rhythm and depth
Indicates a dysfunction in the medulla

CLUSTER
Clusters of breaths with irregularly spaced pauses
Indicates a dysfunction in the medulla and pons

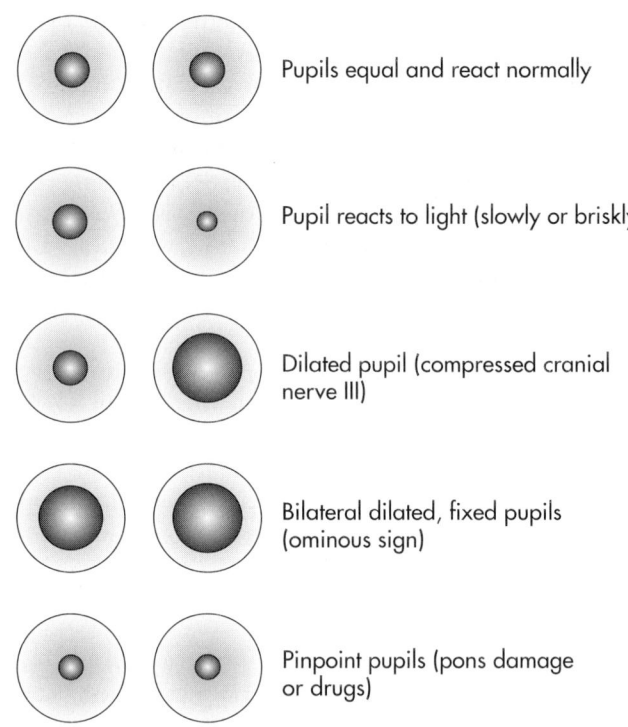

Pupils equal and react normally

Pupil reacts to light (slowly or briskly)

Dilated pupil (compressed cranial nerve III)

Bilateral dilated, fixed pupils (ominous sign)

Pinpoint pupils (pons damage or drugs)

FIG. 65-1 Pupillary check for size and response. (From Lewis, S., Heitkemper, M., & Dirksen, S. [2004]. *Medical-surgical nursing: Assessment and management of clinical problems* [6th ed.]. St. Louis: Mosby.)

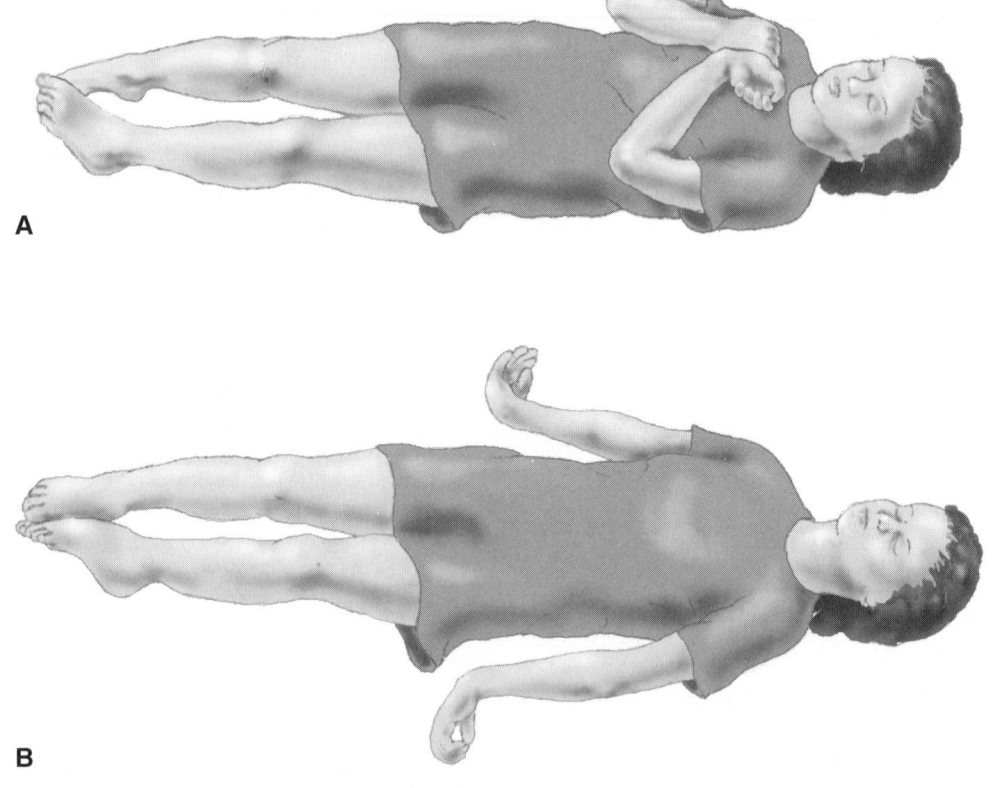

A

B

FIG. 65-2 Posturing. **A,** Decorticate posturing. **B,** Decerebrate posturing. (From Ignatavicius, D., Workman, M., & Mishler, M. [1999]. *Medical-surgical nursing across the health care continuum* [3rd ed.]. Philadelphia: W. B. Saunders.)

6. Midposition fixed pupil indicates midbrain injury.
7. Pinpoint fixed pupil indicates pontine damage.

H. Assessment of motor function
   1. Muscle tone, including strength and equality
   2. Voluntary and involuntary movements
   3. Purposeful and nonpurposeful movements

I. Assessment for posturing (Fig. 65-2)
   1. Posturing indicates a deterioration of the condition.
   2. Flexor (decorticate posturing)
      a. Client flexes one or both arms on the chest and may extend the legs stiffly.
      b. Flexor posturing indicates a nonfunctioning cortex.
   3. Extensor (decerebrate posturing)
      a. Client stiffly extends one or both arms and possibly the legs.
      b. Extensor posturing indicates a brainstem lesion.
   4. Flaccid posturing: Client displays no motor response in any extremity.

J. Assessment of reflexes (Box 65-3)

K. Assessment of meningeal irritation (Box 65-4)
   1. Nuchal rigidity
   2. Irritability
   3. Fever

L. Assessment of the autonomic system
   1. Sympathetic functions/adrenergic responses
      a. Increased pulse and blood pressure
      b. Dilated pupils
      c. Decreased peristalsis
      d. Increased perspiration
   2. Parasympathetic function/cholinergic responses
      a. Decreased pulse and blood pressure
      b. Constricted pupils
      c. Increased salivation
      d. Increased peristalsis
      e. Dilated blood vessels
      f. Bladder contraction

M. Assessment of sensory function
   1. Touch
   2. Pressure
   3. Pain
   4. Bladder control
   5. Bowel control

N. Glasgow Coma Scale (Box 65-5)
   1. The scale is a method of assessing a client's neurological condition.
   2. The scoring system is based on a scale of 1 to 15 points.
   3. A score of less than 8 indicates coma is present.
   4. Eye opening is the most important indicator.

IV. THE UNCONSCIOUS CLIENT

A. Description
   1. The unconscious client is in a state of depressed cerebral functioning with unresponsiveness to sensory and motor function.
   2. Some of the causes include head trauma, cerebral toxins, shock, hemorrhage, tumor, and infection.

B. Assessment
   1. Unarousable
   2. Primitive or no response to painful stimuli

BOX 65-3

Assessment of Reflexes

BABINSKI'S REFLEX
Dorsiflexion of the ankle and great toe with fanning of the other toes
Indicates a disruption of the pyramidal tract

CORNEAL REFLEX
Loss of the blink reflex
Indicates a dysfunction of cranial nerve V

GAG REFLEX
Loss of the gag reflex
Indicates a dysfunction of cranial nerves IX and X

BOX 65-4

Assessment of Meningeal Irritation

BRUDZINSKI'S SIGN
Flexion of the head causes flexion of both thighs at the hips and knee flexion.

KERNIG'S SIGN
Flexion of the thigh and knee to right angles and when the limbs are extended, it causes spasm of the hamstring and pain.

BOX 65-5

Glasgow Coma Scale

MOTOR RESPONSE POINTS
Obeys a simple response = 6
Localizes painful stimuli = 5
Normal flexion (withdrawal) = 4
Abnormal flexion (decorticate posturing) = 3
Extensor response (decerebrate posturing) = 2
No motor response to pain = 1

VERBAL RESPONSE POINTS
Oriented = 5
Confused conversation = 4
Inappropriate words = 3
Responds with incomprehensible sounds = 2
No verbal response = 1

EYE-OPENING POINTS
Spontaneous = 4
In response to sound = 3
In response to pain = 2
No response even to painful stimuli = 1

3. Altered respirations
4. Decreased cranial nerve and reflex activity
C. Interventions (Box 65-6)

V. INCREASED INTRACRANIAL PRESSURE (ICP)

A. Description
  1. An increase in ICP may be caused by trauma, hemorrhage, growths or tumors, hydrocephalus, edema, or inflammation.
  2. **Increased ICP** can impede circulation to the brain, impede the absorption of CSF, affect the functioning of nerve cells, and lead to brainstem compression and death.

B. Assessment
  1. Assess level of consciousness, which is the most sensitive and earliest indication of increasing ICP.
  2. Declining level of consciousness from restlessness to confusion and coma
  3. Headache
  4. Abnormal respirations
  5. Rise in blood pressure with widening pulse pressure
  6. Slowing of pulse
  7. Elevated temperature
  8. Vomiting
  9. Pupil changes
  10. Changes in motor function from weakness to hemiplegia, a positive **Babinski's reflex, decorticate** or **decerebrate posturing,** and seizures
  11. Late signs of **increased ICP** including increased systolic blood pressure, widened pulse pressure, and slowed heart rate

C. Interventions
  1. Elevate the head of the bed 30 to 40 degrees as prescribed.
  2. Avoid Trendelenburg's position.
  3. Prevent flexion of the neck and hips.
  4. Monitor respiratory status and prevent hypoxia.
  5. Avoid the administration of morphine sulfate to prevent the occurrence of hypoxia.
  6. Maintain mechanical ventilation as prescribed; maintaining the $Paco_2$ at 30 to 35 mm Hg will result in vasoconstriction of the cerebral blood vessels, decreased blood flow, and therefore decreased ICP.
  7. Maintain body temperature.
  8. Prevent shivering, which can raise ICP.
  9. Decrease environmental stimuli.
  10. Monitor electrolyte levels and acid-base balance.
  11. Monitor intake and output.
  12. Limit fluid intake to 1200 mL/day.
  13. Instruct the client to avoid straining activities such as coughing and sneezing.
  14. Instruct the client to avoid Valsalva's maneuver.

D. Medications (Box 65-7)

E. Surgical intervention (Box 65-8)

VI. HYPERTHERMIA

A. Description
  1. A temperature of 106° F, which increases the cerebral metabolism and increases the risk of hypoxia.
  2. The causes include infection, heat stroke, exposure to high environmental temperatures, and dysfunction of the thermoregulatory center.

BOX 65-6

Care of the Unconscious Client

Assess patency of airway and keep an airway and emergency equipment at the bedside.
Monitor blood pressure, pulse, and heart sounds.
Assess respiratory and circulatory status.
Maintain a patent airway and ventilation because a high CO_2 level increases intracranial pressure.
Assess lung sounds for the accumulation of secretions.
Suction fluids from airway as needed.
Assess neurological status, including level of consciousness, pupillary reactions, motor and sensory function.
Place the client in semi-Fowler position.
Change position of the client every 2 hours, avoiding injury when turning.
Avoid Trendelenburg's position.
Use side rails at all times.
Assess for edema.
Monitor for dehydration.
Monitor intake and output and daily weight.
Maintain NPO status until consciousness returns.
Maintain nutrition as prescribed, and monitor fluid and electrolyte balance.
Check the gag and swallowing reflex before resuming diet, and begin with ice chips and fluids.

Provide intravenous or enteral feedings as prescribed.
Assess bowel sounds.
Monitor elimination patterns.
Monitor for constipation, impaction, and paralytic ileus.
Maintain urinary output to prevent stasis, infection, and calculus formation.
Monitor the status of skin integrity.
Initiate measures to prevent skin breakdown.
Provide frequent mouth care.
Remove dentures and contact lenses.
Assess the eyes for corneal reflex and irritation, and instill artificial tears or cover the eyes with eye patches.
Monitor drainage from the ears or nose for the presence of cerebrospinal fluid.
Assume that the unconscious client can hear.
Avoid restraints.
Do not leave the client unattended if unstable.
Initiate seizure precautions if necessary.
Provide range of motion exercises to prevent contractures.
Use a footboard or high-top sneakers to prevent foot drop.
Use splints to prevent wrist deformities.
Initiate physical therapy as appropriate.

BOX 65-7

Medications for Intracranial Pressure

ANTICONVULSANTS

Anticonvulsants may be given prophylactically to prevent seizures.

Seizures increase metabolic requirements and cerebral blood flow and volume, thus increasing intracranial pressure.

ANTIPYRETICS AND MUSCLE RELAXANTS

Temperature reduction decreases metabolism, cerebral blood flow, and thus intracranial pressure.

Muscle relaxants prevent shivering.

BLOOD PRESSURE MEDICATION

Blood pressure medication may be required to maintain cerebral perfusion at a normal level.

Notify the physician if the blood pressure range is less than 100 or greater than 150 mm Hg systolic.

CORTICOSTEROIDS

Corticosteriods stabilize the cell membrane and reduce the leakiness in the blood-brain barrier.

Corticosteriods decrease cerebral edema.

A histamine blocker may be administered to counteract the excess gastric secretion that occurs with the corticosteroid.

Clients must be withdrawn slowly from corticosteroid therapy to reduce the risk of adrenal crisis.

INTRAVENOUS FLUIDS

Fluids are administered intravenously via an infusion pump to control the amount administered.

Hypertonic intravenous solutions are avoided because of the risk of promoting additional cerebral edema.

MANNITOL (OSMITROL)

Mannitol is a hyperosmotic agent.

Mannitol increases intravascular pressure by drawing fluid from the interstitial spaces and from the brain cells.

Monitor renal function.

Diuresis is expected.

BOX 65-8

Surgical Intervention for Intracranial Pressure: Ventriculoperitoneal Shunt

DESCRIPTION

Ventriculoperitoneal shunt shunts cerebrospinal fluid from the ventricles into the peritoneum.

POSTPROCEDURE INTERVENTIONS

Position the client supine and turn from back to nonoperative side.

Monitor for signs of increasing intracranial pressure resulting from shunt failure.

Monitor for signs of infection.

BOX 65-9

Medications to Prevent Shivering

CHLORPROMAZINE HYDROCHLORIDE (THORAZINE)

Chlorpromazine depresses thermoregulation in the hypothalamus and reduces peripheral vasoconstriction, muscle tone, and shivering.

MEPERIDINE HYDROCHLORIDE (DEMEROL)

Meperidine relaxes the smooth muscle and reduces shivering.

B. Assessment
1. Temperature of 106° F
2. Shivering
3. Nausea and vomiting
C. Interventions
1. Maintain a patent airway.
2. Initiate seizure precautions.
3. Monitor intake and output and assess skin and mucous membranes for signs of dehydration.
4. Monitor lung sounds.
5. Monitor for dysrhythmias.
6. Assess peripheral pulses for systemic blood flow.
7. Induce normothermia with fluids, cool baths, fans, or hypothermia blanket.
D. Inducement of normothermia
1. Prevent shivering, which will increase intracranial pressure and oxygen consumption.
2. Administer medications as prescribed to prevent shivering.

3. Monitor neurological status.
4. Monitor for infection and respiratory complications because hypothermia may mask signs of infection.
5. Monitor for cardiac dysrhythmias.
6. Monitor intake and output.
7. Prevent trauma to the skin and tissues.
8. Apply lotion to the skin frequently.
9. Inspect for frostbite.
E. Medications to prevent shivering (Box 65-9)

VII. HEAD INJURY

A. Description
1. Head injury is trauma to the skull resulting in mild to extensive damage to the brain.
2. Immediate complications include cerebral bleeding, hematomas, uncontrolled **increased ICP**, infections, and seizures.
3. Changes in personality or behavior, cranial nerve deficits, and any other residual deficits depend on the area of the brain damage and the extent of the damage.

B. Types of head injuries (Box 65-10)
   1. Open
      a. Scalp lacerations
      b. Fractures in the skull
      c. Interruption of the dura mater
   2. Closed
      a. Concussions
      b. Contusions
      c. Fractures
C. Hematoma
   1. Description: Hematoma can occur as a result of a subarachnoid hemorrhage or an intracerebral hemorrhage.
   2. Assessment
      a. Assessment findings depend on the injury.
      b. Clinical manifestations usually result from **increased ICP.**
      c. Changing neurological signs in the client
      d. Changes in level of consciousness
      e. Airway and breathing pattern changes
      f. Vital signs for signs of increasing ICP

BOX 65-10

Types of Head Injuries

CONCUSSION
Concussion is a jarring of the brain within the skull with temporary loss of consciousness.

CONTUSION
Contusion is a bruising type of injury to the brain.
Contusion may occur with subdural or extradural collections of blood.

SKULL FRACTURES
Linear
Depressed
Compound
Comminuted

EPIDURAL HEMATOMA
The most serious type of hematoma, epidural hematoma forms rapidly and results from arterial bleeding.
Epidural hematoma forms between the dura and the skull from a tear in the meningeal artery.
Epidural hematoma is a surgical emergency.

SUBDURAL HEMATOMA
Subdural hematoma forms slowly and results from a venous bleed.
Subdural hematoma occurs under the dura as a result of tears in the veins crossing the subdural space.

INTRACEREBRAL HEMORRHAGE
Multiple hemorrhages occur around a contused area.

SUBARACHNOID HEMORRHAGE
Bleeding occurs directly into the brain, the ventricles, or the subarachnoid space.

---

   g. Headache, nausea, and vomiting
   h. Visual disturbances, pupillary changes, papilledema, and extraocular eye movements
   i. Nuchal rigidity
   j. CSF drainage from the ears or nose
   k. Weakness and paralysis
   l. Posturing
   m. Decreased sensation or absence of feeling
   n. Reflex activity changes
   o. Seizure activity
   3. Interventions
      a. Monitor respiratory status and maintain a patent airway because increased CO_2 levels increase cerebral edema.
      b. Monitor neurological status and vital signs, including temperature.
      c. Monitor for **increased ICP.**
      d. Maintain head elevation to reduce venous pressure.
      e. Prevent neck flexion.
      f. Initiate normothermia measures for increased temperature.
      g. Assess cranial nerve function, reflexes, and motor and sensory function.
      h. Initiate seizure precautions.
      i. Monitor for pain and restlessness.
      j. Avoid the administration of morphine sulfate because it is a respiratory depressant and may increase ICP.
      k. Monitor for drainage from the nose or ears because this fluid may be CSF.
      l. Do not attempt to clean the nose, suction, or allow the client to blow the nose if drainage occurs.
      m. Do not clean the ear if drainage is noted, but apply a loose, dry sterile dressing.
      n. Check drainage for the presence of CSF.
      o. Notify the physician if drainage from ears or nose is noted.
      p. Instruct the client to avoid coughing because this increases ICP.
      q. Monitor for signs of infection.
      r. Prevent complications of immobility.
D. Craniotomy
   1. Description
      a. Craniotomy is a surgical procedure that involves an incision through the cranium to remove accumulated blood or a tumor.
      b. Complications of the procedure include **increased ICP** from cerebral edema, hemorrhage, or obstruction of the normal flow of CSF.
      c. Additional complications include hematomas, hypovolemic shock, hydrocephalus, respiratory and neurogenic complications, pulmonary edema, and wound infections.
      d. Complications related to fluid and electrolyte imbalances include diabetes insipidus

and inappropriate secretion of antidiuretic hormone.

2. Preoperative interventions
   a. Explain the procedure to the client and family.
   b. Ensure that an informed consent has been obtained.
   c. Prepare to shave the client's head as prescribed and cover the head with appropriate covering.
   d. Stabilize the client before surgery.
3. Postoperative interventions (Box 65-11)
4. Postoperative positioning (Box 65-12)

VIII. SPINAL CORD INJURY

A. Description
   1. Trauma to the spinal cord causes partial or complete disruption of the nerve tracts and neurons.
   2. The injury can involve contusion, laceration, or compression of the cord.
   3. Spinal cord edema develops, and necrosis of the spinal cord can develop as a result of compromised capillary circulation and venous return.
   4. Loss of motor function, sensation, reflex activity, and bowel and bladder control may result.

BOX 65-11

Nursing Care following Craniotomy

Monitor vital signs and neurological status every 30 minutes to 1 hour.

Monitor for increased intracranial pressure.

Monitor for decreased level of consciousness, motor weakness or paralysis, aphasia, visual changes, and personality changes.

Maintain mechanical ventilation and slight hyperventilation for the first 24 to 48 hours as prescribed to prevent increased intracranial pressure.

Assess the physician's orders regarding client positioning.

Avoid extreme hip or neck flexion, and maintain the head in a midline neutral position.

Provide a quiet environment.

Monitor the head dressing frequently for signs of drainage.

Mark the area of drainage at least once each nursing shift for baseline comparison.

Monitor the Hemovac or Jackson-Pratt drain, which may be in place for 24 hours.

Maintain suction on the Hemovac or Jackson-Pratt drain.

Measure drainage from the Hemovac or Jackson-Pratt drain every 8 hours, and record the amount and color.

Notify the physician if drainage is greater than the normal of 30 to 50 mL per shift.

Notify the physician immediately of excessive amounts of drainage or a saturated head dressing.

Record strict measurement of hourly intake and output.

Maintain fluid restriction at 1500 mL/day as prescribed.

Monitor electrolyte values.

Monitor for dysrhythmias, which may occur as a result of fluid and electrolyte imbalance.

Apply ice packs or cool compresses as prescribed for periorbital edema and ecchymosis of one or both eyes, which is not an unusual occurrence.

Provide range of motion exercises every 8 hours.

Place antiembolism stockings on the client as prescribed.

Administer anticonvulsants, antacids, corticosteroids, and antibiotics as prescribed.

Administer analgesics such as codeine sulfate and acetaminophen (Tylenol) as prescribed for pain.

BOX 65-12

Client Positioning following Craniotomy

Positions prescribed following craniotomy vary with the type of surgery and the specific postoperative physician's orders.

Always check the physician's orders regarding client positioning.

Incorrect positioning may cause serious and possibly fatal complications.

REMOVAL OF A BONE FLAP FOR DECOMPRESSION

To facilitate brain expansion, the client should be turned from the back to the nonoperative side, but not to the side operated on.

POSTERIOR FOSSA SURGERY

To protect the operative site from pressure and minimize tension on the suture line, position the client on the side, with a pillow under the head for support and not on the back.

INFRATENTORIAL SURGERY

Infratentorial surgery involves surgery below the tentorium of the brain.

The physician may order a flat position without head elevation or may order the head of the bed to be elevated at 30 to 45 degrees.

Do not elevate the head of the bed in the acute phase of care following surgery without a physician's order.

SUPRATENTORIAL SURGERY

Subtentorial surgery involves surgery above the tentorium of the brain.

The physician may order the head of the bed to be elevated at 30 degrees to promote venous outflow through the jugular veins.

Do not lower the head of the bed in the acute phase of care following surgery without a physician's order.

5. The most common causes include motor vehicle accidents, falls, sporting and industrial accidents, and gunshot or stab wounds.
6. Complications related to the injury include respiratory failure, **autonomic dysreflexia, spinal shock,** further cord damage, and death.

B. Most frequently involved vertebrae
   1. Cervical 5, 6, and 7
   2. Thoracic 12
   3. Lumbar 1

C. Transection of the cord
   1. Complete transection of the cord
      a. The spinal cord is severed completely, with total loss of sensation, movement, and reflex activity below the level of injury.
      b. If the cord has not suffered irreparable damage, early treatment is needed to prevent partial damage from developing into total and permanent damage.
   2. Partial transection of the cord
      a. The spinal cord is damaged or severed partially.
      b. The symptoms depend on the extent and location of the damage.

D. Types of injuries
   1. Anterior cord syndrome
      a. Anterior cord syndrome is caused by damage to the anterior portion of the gray and white matter of the spinal cord.
      b. Motor function, pain, and temperature sensation are lost below the level of injury; however, the sensations of touch, position, and vibration remain intact.
   2. Posterior cord injury
      a. Posterior cord injury is caused by damage to the posterior portion of the gray and white matter of the spinal cord.
      b. Motor function remains intact, but the client experiences a loss of vibratory sense, crude touch, and position sensation.
   3. Central cord syndrome
      a. Central cord syndrome cccurs from a lesion in the central portion of the spinal cord.
      b. Loss of motor function is more pronounced in the upper extremities, and varying degrees and patterns of sensation remain intact.
   4. Brown-Séquard's syndrome
      a. Brown-Séquard's syndrome results from penetrating injuries that cause hemisection of the spinal cord or injuries that affect half of the cord.
      b. Motor function, proprioception, vibration, and deep touch sensations are lost on the same side of the body (ipsilateral) as the lesion.
      c. On the opposite side of the body (contralateral) from the injury, the sensations of pain, temperature, and light touch are affected.

5. Conus medullaris syndrome
   a. Conus medullaris syndrome follows damage to the lumbar nerve roots and conus medullaris in the spinal cord.
   b. Client experiences bowel and bladder areflexia and flaccid lower extremities.
   c. If damage is limited to the upper sacral segments of the spinal cord, bulbospongiosus penile (erection) and micturition reflexes will remain.
6. Cauda equina syndrome
   a. Cauda equina syndrome cccurs from injury to the lumbosacral nerve roots below the conus medullaris.
   b. The client experiences areflexia of the bowel, bladder, and lower reflexes.

E. Assessment of spinal cord injuries (Box 65-13)
   1. Dependent on the level of the cord injury
   2. The level of spinal cord injury: the lowest spinal cord segment with intact motor and sensory function
   3. Respiratory status changes
   4. Motor and sensory changes below the level of injury
   5. Total sensory loss and motor paralysis below the level of injury
   6. Loss of reflexes below the level of injury
   7. Loss of bladder and bowel control
   8. Urinary retention and bladder distention
   9. Presence of sweat, which does not occur on paralyzed areas

F. Cervical injuries
   1. Injury at C2 to C3 is usually fatal.
   2. C4 is the major innervation to the diaphragm by the phrenic nerve.
   3. Involvement above C4 causes respiratory difficulty and paralysis of all four extremities.
   4. Client may have movement in the shoulder if the injury is at C5 or below.

G. Thoracic level injuries
   1. Loss of movement of the chest, trunk, bowel, bladder, and legs may occur, depending on the level of injury.
   2. Leg paralysis (paraplegia) may occur.
   3. **Autonomic dysreflexia** with lesions or injuries above T6 and in cervical lesions may occur.

BOX 65-13

Effects of the Spinal Cord Injury

QUADRIPLEGIA
Injury occurring from C1 through C8
Paralysis involving all four extremities

PARAPLEGIA
Injury occurring from T1 through L4
Paralysis involving only the lower extremities

4. Visceral distention from a distended bladder or impacted rectum may cause reactions such as sweating, bradycardia, hypertension, nasal stuffiness, and goose flesh.

H. Lumbar and sacral level injuries

1. Loss of movement and sensation of the lower extremities may occur.
2. S2 and S3 center on micturation; therefore below this level, the bladder will contract but not empty (neurogenic bladder).
3. Injury above S2 in males allows them to have an erection, but they are unable to ejaculate because of sympathetic nerve damage.
4. Injury between S2 and S4 damages the sympathetic and parasympathetic response, preventing erection or ejaculation.

I. Emergency interventions

1. Emergency management is critical because improper handling can cause further damage and loss of neurological function.
2. Maintain a patent airway.
3. Always suspect spinal cord injury until this injury is ruled out.
4. Immobilize the client on a spinal backboard with the head in a neutral position to prevent an incomplete injury from becoming complete.
5. Prevent head flexion, rotation, or extension.
6. During immobilization, maintain traction and alignment on the head by placing hands on either side of the head by the ears.
7. Maintain an extended position.
8. Logroll the client.
9. No part of the body should be twisted or turned, and the client is not allowed to assume a sitting position.
10. In the emergency room, a client who has sustained a severe cervical injury should be placed immediately in skeletal traction via **skull tongs** or **halo traction** to immobilize the cervical spine and reduce the fracture and dislocation.

J. Interventions during hospitalization

1. Respiratory system
   a. Assess respiratory status because paralysis of the intercostal and abdominal muscles occurs with C4 injuries.
   b. Monitor arterial blood gases and maintain mechanical ventilation if prescribed to prevent respiratory arrest, especially with cervical injuries.
   c. Encourage deep breathing and the use of an incentive spirometer.
   d. Monitor for signs of infection, particularly pneumonia.
2. Cardiovascular system
   a. Monitor for cardiac dysrhythmias.
   b. Assess for signs of hemorrhage or bleeding around the fracture site.

c. Assess for signs of shock, such as hypotension, tachycardia, and a weak and thready pulse.
d. Assess the lower extremities for deep vein thrombosis.
e. Measure circumferences of calf and thigh.
f. Apply thigh-high antiembolism stockings as prescribed.
g. Remove antiembolism stockings daily to assess the skin.
h. Monitor for orthostatic hypotension when repositioning the client.

3. Neuromuscular system
   a. Assess neurological status.
   b. Assess motor and sensory status to determine the level of injury.
   c. Assess motor ability by testing the client's ability to squeeze hands, spread the fingers, move the toes, and turn the feet.
   d. Assess sensation by pinching skin or pricking with a pin, starting at the shoulders and working down the extremities.
   e. Monitor for signs of **autonomic dysreflexia** and **spinal shock.**
   f. Immobilize the client to promote healing and prevent further injury.
   g. Assess pain.
   h. Initiate measures to reduce pain.
   i. Administer analgesics as prescribed.
   j. Monitor for complications of immobility.
   k. Prepare the client for decompression laminectomy, spinal fusion, or insertion of steel rods if prescribed.
   l. Collaborate with the physical therapist and occupational therapist to determine appropriate exercise techniques, to assess the need for hand and wrist splints, and to develop an appropriate plan to prevent footdrop.

4. Gastrointestinal system
   a. Assess abdomen for distention and hemorrhage.
   b. Monitor bowel sounds and assess for paralytic ileus.
   c. Prevent bowel retention.
   d. Initiate a bowel control program as appropriate.
   e. Maintain adequate nutrition and a high-fiber diet.

5. Renal system
   a. Prevent urinary retention.
   b. Initiate a bladder control program as appropriate.
   c. Maintain fluid and electrolyte balance.
   d. Maintain adequate fluid intake of 2000 mL daily.
   e. Monitor for urinary tract infection and calculuses.

6. Integumentary system
   a. Assess skin integrity.
   b. Turn the client every 2 hours.

7. Psychosocial integrity
   a. Assess psychosocial status.
   b. Encourage the client to express feelings of anger and depression.
   c. Discuss the sexual concerns of the client.
   d. Promote self-care, setting realistic goals based on the client's potential functional level.
   e. Encourage contact with appropriate community resources.

▶ K. **Spinal shock**
   1. Description
      a. **Spinal shock** also is known as neurogenic shock.
      b. A sudden depression of reflex activity in the spinal cord occurs below the level of injury (areflexia).
      c. **Spinal shock** occurs within the first hour of injury and can last days to months.
      d. The muscles become completely paralyzed and flaccid, and reflexes are absent.
      e. **Spinal shock** ends when the reflexes are regained.
   2. Assessment
      a. Flaccid paralysis
      b. Hypotension
      c. Bradycardia
      d. Loss of reflex activity below the level of injury
      e. Paralytic ileus
   3. Interventions
      a. Monitor for signs of **spinal shock** following a spinal cord injury.
      b. Monitor for hypotension and bradycardia.
      c. Monitor for reflex activity.
      d. Assess bowel sounds.
      e. Monitor for bowel and urinary retention.
      f. Provide supportive measures as prescribed, based on the presence of symptoms.
      g. Monitor for the return of reflexes.

▶ L. **Autonomic dysreflexia**
   1. Description
      a. **Autonomic dysreflexia** also is known as autonomic hyperreflexia.
      b. **Autonomic dysreflexia** commonly is caused by visceral distention from a distended bladder or impacted rectum.
      c. **Autonomic dysreflexia** is a neurological emergency and must be treated immediately to prevent a hypertensive stroke.
      d. **Autonomic dysreflexia** generally occurs after the period of **spinal shock** is resolved.
      e. **Autonomic dysreflexia** occurs with lesions or injuries above T6 and in cervical lesions.
   2. Assessment
      a. Hypertension
      b. Bradycardia
      c. Flushing of the face and neck
      d. Severe, throbbing headache

      e. Nasal stuffiness
      f. Piloerection (goose flesh)
      g. Sweating
      h. Nausea
      i. Restlessness
      j. Dilated pupils and blurred vision
   3. Interventions
      a. Notify the physician if signs of **autonomic dysreflexia** occur.
      b. Assess for the potential cause and remove the stimulus.
      c. Raise the head of the bed to high-Fowler's position.
      d. Loosen tight clothing.
      e. Monitor vital signs, particularly blood pressure, every 15 minutes.
      f. Assess for bladder distention, and prepare for urinary catheterization.
      g. If a urinary catheter is present, check for kinks in the tubing and for drainage.
      h. Assess for a fecal impaction and disimpact immediately.
      i. Administer antihypertensives as prescribed.

M. Cervical traction for cervical injuries (Fig. 65-3)
   1. Description
      a. Skeletal traction is used to stabilize fractures or dislocations of the cervical or upper thoracic spine.
      b. Two types of equipment used for cervical traction are **skull** (cervical) **tongs** and **halo traction** (halo fixation device).
   2. **Skull tongs**
      a. **Skull tongs** are inserted into the outer aspect of the client's skull, and traction is applied.
      b. Weights are attached to the tongs, and the client is used as countertraction.
      c. Monitor neurological status of the client.
      d. Determine the amount of weight prescribed to be added to the traction.
      e. Ensure that weights hang securely and freely at all times.
      f. Ensure that the ropes for the traction remain within the pulley.
      g. Maintain body alignment and maintain care of the client on a special bed (Roto-Rest bed, Stryker, or Foster frame) as prescribed.
      h. Turn the client every 2 hours.
      i. Assess insertion site of the tongs for infection.
      j. Provide sterile pin site care as prescribed.
   3. **Halo traction**
      a. **Halo traction** is a static traction device that consists of a headpiece with four pins, two anterior and two posterior, inserted into the client's skull.
      b. The metal halo ring may be attached to a vest (jacket) or cast when the spine is stable, allowing increased client mobility.

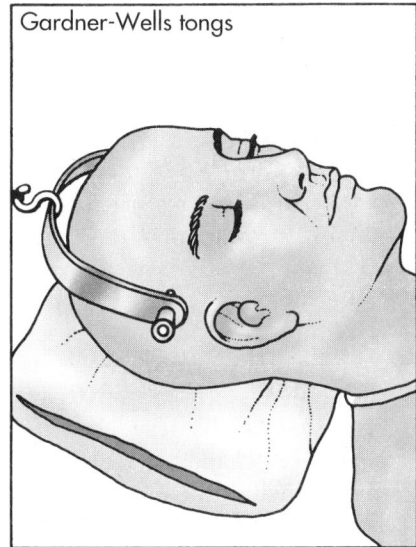

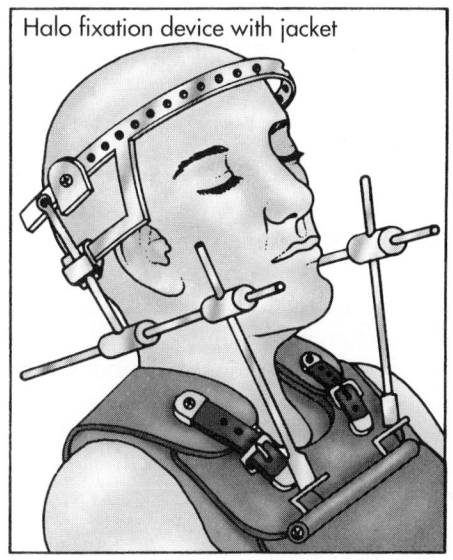

FIG. 65-3 Types of cervical spine traction. (From Ignatavicius, D., Workman, M., & Mishler, M. [1999]. *Medical-surgical nursing across the health care continuum* [3rd ed.]. Philadelphia: W. B. Saunders.)

BOX 65-14

Client Education for a Halo Fixation Device

Notify the physician if the halo vest (jacket) or ring bolts loosen.

Use fleece or foam inserts to relieve pressure points.

Keep the vest lining dry.

Clean the pin site daily.

Notify the physician if redness, swelling, drainage, open areas, pain, tenderness, or a clicking sound occurs from the pin site.

A sponge bath or tub bath is allowed; showers are prohibited.

Assess the skin under the vest daily for breakdown, using a flashlight.

Do not use any products other than shampoo on the hair.

When shampooing the hair, cover the vest with plastic.

When getting out of bed, roll onto the side and push on the mattress with the arms.

Never use the metal frame for turning or lifting.

Use a rolled towel or pillowcase between the back of the neck and the bed or next to the cheek when lying on the side, and raise the head of the bed to increase sleep comfort.

Adapt clothing to fit over the halo device.

Eat foods high in protein and calcium to promote bone healing.

Have the correct-size wrench available at all times for an emergency.

If cardiopulmonary resuscitation is required, the anterior portion of the vest will be loosened and the posterior portion will remain in place to provide stability.

---

   c. Monitor the client's neurological status for changes in movement or decreased strength.
   d. Never move or turn the client by holding or pulling on the **halo traction** device.
   e. Assess for tightness of the jacket by ensuring that one finger can be placed under the jacket.
   f. Assess skin integrity to ensure that the jacket or cast is not causing pressure.
   g. Provide sterile pin site care as prescribed.
   4. Client education for **halo traction** device (Box 65-14)
N. Interventions for thoracic and lumbar/sacral injuries
   1. Bed rest
   2. Immobilization with a body cast
   3. Use of a brace or corset when the client is out of bed

O. Surgical interventions for thoracic and lumbar/sacral injuries
   1. Decompressive laminectomy
      a. Decompressive laminectomy is removal of one or more laminae.
      b. Decompressive laminectomy allows for cord expansion from edema.
      c. Decompressive laminectomy is performed if conventional methods fail to prevent neurological deterioration.
   2. Spinal fusion and rod insertion
      a. Spinal fusion is used for thoracic spinal injuries.
      b. Insertion of a metal or steel rod, such as a Harrington rod, is done to stabilize the thoracic spine.

3. Postoperative interventions
   a. Monitor for respiratory impairment.
   b. Monitor vital signs, motor function, sensation, and circulatory status in the lower extremities.
   c. Encourage breathing exercises.
   d. Assess for signs of fluid and electrolyte imbalance.
   e. Observe for complications of immobility.
   f. Keep the client flat.
   g. Provide cast care if the client is in a full body cast.
   h. Turn and reposition frequently by logrolling side to back to side, using turning sheets and pillows between the legs to maintain alignment.
   i. Administer pain medication as prescribed.
   j. Maintain NPO status until the client is passing flatus.
   k. Monitor bowel sounds.
   l. Provide the use of a fracture bedpan.
   m. Monitor intake and output.
   n. Maintain nutritional status.
P. Medications
   1. Dexamethasone (Decadron)
      a. Dexamethasone is used for its antiinflammatory and edema-reducing effects.
      b. Dexamethasone may interfere with healing.
   2. Dextran
      a. Dextran is a plasma expander.
      b. Dextran is used to increase capillary blood flow within the spinal cord and to prevent or treat hypotension.
   3. Dantrolene (Dantrium)/Baclofen (Lioresal)
      a. These medications are used for clients with upper motor neuron injuries.
      b. These medications control muscle spasticity.

IX. CEREBRAL ANEURYSM
A. Description
   1. Cerebral aneurysm is dilation of the walls of a weakened cerebral artery.
   2. Aneurysm can lead to rupture.
B. Assessment
   1. Headache
   2. Pain
   3. Diplopia
   4. Blurred vision
   5. Tinnitus
   6. Nausea
   7. Hemiparesis
   8. Nuchal rigidity
   9. Irritability
   10. Seizures
C. Interventions
   1. Maintain a patent airway (suction only with a physician's order).
   2. Administer oxygen as prescribed.
   3. Monitor vital signs and for hypertension or dysrhythmias.

4. Avoid taking temperatures via the rectum.
5. Initiate aneurysm precautions.
   a. Maintain bed rest in semi-Fowler or side-lying position.
   b. Maintain a darkened room without stimulation.
   c. Limit visitors.
   d. Maintain fluid restrictions.
   e. Avoid stimulants in the diet.

X. SEIZURES
A. Description
   1. Seizures are an abnormal, sudden, excessive discharge of electrical activity within the brain.
   2. Epilepsy is a disorder characterized by chronic seizure activity and indicates brain or CNS irritation.
   3. Causes include genetic factors, trauma, tumors, circulatory or metabolic disorders, toxicity, and infections.
   4. Status epilepticus involves a rapid succession of epileptic spasms without intervals of consciousness; it is a potential complication that can occur with any type of seizure, and brain damage may result.
B. Types of seizures (Box 65-15)
   1. Generalized seizures
      a. Tonic-clonic (grand mal)
      b. Absence (petit mal)
      c. Myoclonic
      d. Atonic or akinetic (drop attacks)
   2. Partial seizures
      a. Simple partial
      b. Complex partial
C. Assessment
   1. Seizure history
   2. Type of seizure
   3. Occurrences before, during, and after the seizure
   4. Prodromal signs, such as mood changes, irritability, and insomnia
   5. Aura: a sensation that warns the client of the impending seizure
   6. Loss of motor activity or bowel and bladder function or loss of consciousness during the seizure
   7. Occurrences during the postictal state, such as headache, loss of consciousness, sleepiness, and impaired speech or thinking
D. Interventions
   1. Note the time and duration of the seizure.
   2. Assess behavior at the onset of the seizure: if the client experienced an aura, if a change in facial expression occurred, or if a sound or cry occurred from the client.
   3. If the client is standing, place the client on the floor and protect the head and body.
   4. Maintain a patent airway (do not force the jaws open or place anything in the client's mouth).
   5. Administer oxygen.
   6. Prepare to suction fluids from the airway.
   7. Turn the client's head to the side.

BOX 65-15

Types of Seizures

GENERALIZED SEIZURES

Tonic-Clonic

Tonic-clonic seizures may begin with an aura.

The tonic phase involves the stiffening or rigidity of the muscles of the arms and legs and usually lasts 10 to 20 seconds, followed by loss of consciousness.

The clonic phase consists of hyperventilation and jerking of the extremities and usually lasts about 30 seconds.

Full recovery from the seizure may take several hours.

Absence

Brief seizure lasts seconds, and the individual may or may not lose consciousness.

No loss or change in muscle tone occurs.

Seizures may occur several times during a day.

The victim appears to be daydreaming.

This type of seizure is more common in children.

Myoclonic

Myoclonic seizures present as a brief generalized jerking or stiffening of extremities.

The victim may fall to the ground from the seizure.

Atonic or Akinetic (Drop Attacks)

An atonic seizure is a sudden momentary loss of muscle tone.

The victim may fall to the ground as a result of the seizure.

PARTIAL SEIZURES

Simple Partial

The simple partial seizure produces sensory symptoms accompanied by motor symptoms that are localized or confined to a specific area.

The client remains conscious and may report an aura.

Complex Partial

The complex partial seizure is a psychomotor seizure.

The area of the brain most involved is the temporal lobe.

The seizure is characterized by periods of altered behavior that the client is not aware of.

The client loses consciousness for a few seconds.

---

8. Prevent injury during the seizure.
9. Remain with the client.
10. Do not restrain the client.
11. Loosen restrictive clothing.
12. Note the type, character, and progression of the movements during the seizure.
13. Monitor for incontinence.
14. Administer intravenous medications such as diazepam (Valium), phenytoin (Dilantin), and phenobarbital sodium (Luminal) as prescribed to stop the seizure.
15. Document the characteristics of the seizure.
16. Monitor behavior following the seizure, such as the state of consciousness, motor ability, and speech ability.
17. Instruct the client about the importance of life-long medication and the need for follow-up medication blood levels.
18. Instruct the client to avoid alcohol, excessive stress, and fatigue.
19. Encourage the client to contact available community resources, such as the Epilepsy Foundation of America.

XI. CEREBROVASCULAR ACCIDENT (CVA)

A. Description
   1. Cerebrovascular accident is a sudden focal neurological deficit caused by cerebrovascular disease.
   2. Cerebrovascular accident is a syndrome in which the cerebral circulation is interrupted, causing neurological deficits.
   3. Cerebral anoxia lasting longer than 10 minutes causes cerebral infarction with irreversible change.
   4. Surrounding cerebral edema and congestion cause further dysfunction.
   5. Diagnosis is determined by computed tomography scan, electroencephalogram, and cerebral arteriography.
   6. The permanent disability cannot be determined until the cerebral edema subsides.
   7. The order in which function may return is facial, swallowing, lower limb, speech, and arms.
   8. Carotid endarterectomy is a surgical intervention used in stroke management and is targeted at stroke prevention especially in clients with symptomatic carotid stenosis.

B. Causes
   1. Thrombosis
   2. Embolism
   3. Hemorrhage from rupture of a vessel
   4. Transient ischemic attack

C. Risk factors
   1. Atherosclerosis
   2. Hypertension
   3. Anticoagulation therapy
   4. Diabetes mellitus
   5. Stress
   6. Obesity
   7. Oral contraceptives

D. Assessment (Fig. 65-4; Boxes 65-16 and 65-17)
   1. Assessment findings depend on the area of the brain affected.
   2. Lesions in the cerebral hemisphere result in manifestations on the contralateral side, which is the side of the body opposite the cerebrovascular accident.
   3. Airway patency is always a priority.
   4. Pulse (may be slow and bounding)
   5. Respirations (Cheyne-Stokes)
   6. Blood pressure (hypertension)
   7. Headache, nausea, and vomiting

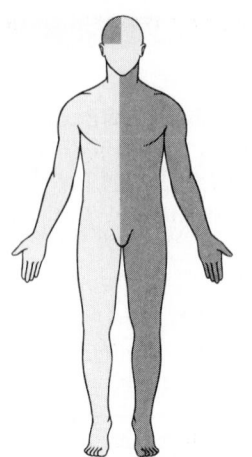
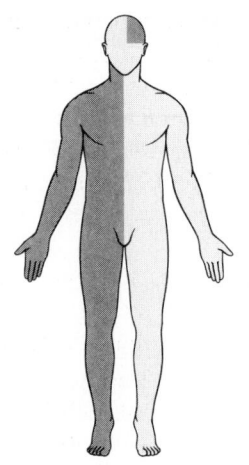

Right-brain damage (stroke on right side of the brain)	Left-brain damage (stroke on left side of the brain)
• Paralyzed left side: hemiplegia	• Paralyzed right side: hemiplegia
• Left-sided neglect	• Impaired speech/language aphasias
• Spatial-perceptual deficits	• Impaired right/left discrimination
• Tends to deny or minimize problems	• Slow performance, cautious
• Rapid performance, short attention span	• Aware of deficits: depression, anxiety
• Impulsive, safety problems	• Impaired comprehension related to language, math
• Impaired judgment	
• Impaired time concepts	

FIG. 65-4   Manifestations of right brain and left brain stroke. (From Lewis, S., Heitkemper, M., & Dirksen, S. [2004]. *Medical-surgical nursing: Assessment and management of clinical problems* [6th ed.]. St. Louis: Mosby.)

BOX 65-16

Neurological Assessment in Cerebrovascular Accident

Changes in level of consciousness
Signs of increasing intracranial pressure
Assessment of cranial nerves V, VII, IX, X, and XII
Cranial nerve V: difficulty with chewing
Cranial nerve VII: facial paralysis or paresis
Cranial nerves IX and X: dysphagia
Cranial nerve IX: absent gag reflex
Cranial nerve XII: impaired tongue movement

BOX 65-17

Assessment Findings in a Cerebrovascular Accident

AGNOSIA
Inability to use an object correctly

APRAXIA
Inability to carry out a purposeful activity

HEMIANOPSIA
Blindness in half of the visual field

HOMONYMOUS HEMIANOPSIA
Blindness in the same visual field of both eyes

NEGLECT SYNDROME (UNILATERAL NEGLECT)
Client unaware of the existence of his or her paralyzed side

PROPRIOCEPTION ALTERATIONS
Altered position sense that places the client at increased risk of injury
Pyramid Point: With visual problems, client must turn the head to scan the complete range of vision.

---

8. Facial drooping
9. Nuchal rigidity
10. Visual changes
11. Ataxia
12. Dysarthria
13. Dysphagia
14. Speech changes
15. Decreased sensation to pressure, heat, and cold
16. Bowel and bladder dysfunctions
17. Paralysis

E. Aphasia
1. Expressive
   a. Damage occurs in Broca's area of the frontal brain.
   b. Client understands what is said but is unable to communicate verbally.
2. Receptive
   a. Injury involves Wernicke's area in the temporoparietal area.
   b. Client is unable to understand the spoken and often the written word.

3. Global or mixed: Language dysfunction occurs in expression and reception.
4. Interventions for aphasia
   a. Provide repetitive directions.
   b. Break tasks down to one step at a time.
   c. Repeat names of objects frequently used.
   d. Use a picture board or communication board.

F. Interventions during the acute phase of CVA
1. Maintain a patent airway and administer oxygen as prescribed.
2. Monitor vital signs.
3. Maintain a blood pressure of 150/100 mm Hg to maintain cerebral perfusion.
4. Suction fluids as prescribed, but never suction nasally and for longer than 10 seconds to prevent increasing ICP.
5. Monitor for increasing ICP because the client is at most risk during the first 72 hours following the CVA.
6. Position the client on the side, with head of bed elevated 15 to 30 degrees as prescribed.

7. Monitor level of consciousness, pupillary response, motor and sensory response, cranial nerve function, and reflexes
8. Maintain a quiet environment, and provide minimal handling of the client to prevent further bleeding.
9. Insert a Foley catheter as prescribed.
10. Administer intravenous fluids as prescribed.
11. Maintain fluid and electrolyte balance.
12. Prepare to administer anticoagulants, antiplatelets, diuretics, antihypertensives, and anticonvulsants as prescribed.
13. Establish a form of communication.

G. Interventions in the postacute phase of a CVA
1. Continue with interventions from the acute phase.
2. Position the client 2 hours on the unaffected side, 20 minutes on the affected side.
3. Position the client in the prone position if prescribed, for 30 minutes 3 times daily.
4. Provide skin, mouth, and eye care.
5. Perform passive range of motion exercises to prevent contractures.
6. Place antiembolism stockings on client.
7. Measure thighs and calves for an increase in size, and assess for positive Homans' sign.
8. Monitor gag reflex and ability to swallow.
9. Provide sips of fluids and slowly advance diet to foods that are easy to chew and swallow.
10. Provide soft and semisoft foods and fluids rather than liquids because the CVA client is better able to tolerate these types of food.
11. When the client is eating, position the client sitting in a chair, or sitting up in bed with the head and neck positioned slightly forward and flexed.
12. Place food in the back of the mouth on the unaffected side to prevent trapping of food in the affected cheek.

H. Interventions in the chronic phase of CVA
1. Neglect syndrome
   a. Client is unaware of the existence of his or her paralyzed side (**unilateral neglect**), which places the client at risk for injury.
   b. Teach the client to touch and use both sides of the body.
2. **Hemianopsia**
   a. Client has blindness in half of the visual field.
   b. **Homonymous hemianopsia** is blindness in the same visual field of both eyes.
   c. Encourage client to turn the head to scan the complete range of vision; otherwise, he or she does not see half of the visual field.
3. Approach the client from the unaffected side.
4. Place the client's personal objects within the visual field.
5. Provide eye care for visual deficits.

6. Place a patch over the affected eye if the client has diplopia.
7. Increase mobility as tolerated.
8. Encourage fluid intake and a high-fiber diet.
9. Administer stool softeners as prescribed.
10. Encourage the client to express feelings.
11. Encourage independence in activities of daily living.
12. Assess the need for assistive devices such as a cane, walker, splints, or braces.
13. Teach transfer technique from bed to chair and chair to bed.
14. Provide gait training.
15. Initiate physical and occupational therapy.
16. Refer client to a speech and language pathologist.

XII. MULTIPLE SCLEROSIS

A. Description
1. Multiple sclerosis is a chronic, progressive, non-contagious, degenerative disease of the CNS characterized by demyelinization of the neurons.
2. Multiple sclerosis usually occurs between the ages of 20 and 40 and consists of periods of remissions and exacerbations.
3. The causes are unknown, but the disease is thought to be a result of an autoimmune response or viral infection.
4. Precipitating factors include pregnancy, fatigue, stress, infection, and trauma.
5. Electroencephalogram findings are abnormal.
6. A lumbar puncture indicates increased gamma-globulin, but the serum globulin level is normal.

B. Assessment
1. Fatigue and weakness
2. Ataxia and vertigo
3. Tremors and spasticity of the lower extremities
4. Parasthesias
5. Blurred vision and diplopia
6. Nystagmus
7. Dysphasia
8. Decreased perception to pain, touch, and temperature
9. Bladder and bowel disturbances, including urgency, frequency, retention, and incontinence
10. Abnormal reflexes, including hyperreflexia, absent reflexes, and a positive **Babinski's reflex**
11. Emotional changes such as apathy, euphoria, irritability, and depression
12. Memory changes and confusion

C. Interventions
1. Provide bed rest during exacerbation.
2. Protect the client from injury by providing safety measures.
3. Place an eye patch on the eye for diplopia.
4. Monitor for potential complications such as urinary tract infections, calculuses, decubitus ulcers, respiratory tract infections, and contractures.

5. Promote regular elimination by bladder and bowel training.
6. Encourage independence.
7. Assist the client to establish a regular exercise and rest program.
8. Instruct the client to balance moderate activity with rest periods.
9. Assess the need for and provide assistive devices.
10. Initiate physical and speech therapy.
11. Instruct the client to avoid fatigue, stress, infection, overheating, and chilling.
12. Instruct the client to increase fluid intake and eat a balanced diet, including low-fat, high-fiber foods and foods high in potassium.
13. Instruct the client in safety measures related to sensory loss, such as regulating the temperature of bath water and avoiding heating pads.
14. Instruct the client in safety measures related to motor loss, such as avoiding the use of scatter rugs and using assistive devices.
15. Instruct the client in the self-administration of prescribed medications (Box 65-18).
16. Provide information about the National Multiple Sclerosis Society.

▲ XIII. MYASTHENIA GRAVIS
A. Description

BOX 65-18

Medications Used with Multiple Sclerosis

BACLOFEN (LIORESAL), DANTROLENE (DANTRIUM), OR DIAZEPAM (VALIUM)
Used to lessen muscle spasticity

BETHANECHOL (URECHOLINE)
Used to prevent urinary retention

CARBAMAZEPINE (TEGRETOL)
Used to treat paresthesia

CORTICOSTEROIDS
Corticotropin (Acthar)
Methylprednisolone Sodium Succinate (Solu-Medrol)
Used to reduce edema and the inflammatory response
Used to decrease the length of time the client's symptoms are exacerbated and to improve the degree of recovery

IMMUNOSUPPRESSIVE MEDICATIONS
Used to treat chronic progressive multiple sclerosis to stabilize the disease process

OXYBUTYNIN CHLORIDE (DITROPAN)
Used to increase bladder capacity

PROPRANOLOL (INDERAL) AND CLONAZEPAM (KLONOPIN)
Used to treat cerebellar ataxia

---

1. Myasthenia gravis is a neuromuscular disease characterized by considerable weakness and abnormal fatigue of the voluntary muscles.
2. A defect in the transmission of nerve impulses at the myoneural junction occurs.
3. Causes include insufficient secretion of acetylcholine, excessive secretion of cholinesterase, and unresponsiveness of the muscle fibers to acetylcholine.

B. Assessment
1. Weakness and fatigue
2. Difficulty chewing
3. Dysphagia
4. Ptosis
5. Diplopia
6. Weak, hoarse voice
7. Difficulty breathing
8. Diminished breath sounds
9. Respiratory paralysis and failure

C. Interventions
1. Monitor respiratory status and ability to cough and deep breathe adequately.
2. Monitor for respiratory failure.
3. Maintain suctioning and emergency equipment at the bedside.
4. Monitor vital signs.
5. Monitor speech and swallowing abilities to prevent aspiration.
6. Encourage the client to sit up when eating.
7. Assess muscle status.
8. Instruct the client to conserve strength.
9. Plan short activities that coincide with times of maximal muscle strength.
10. Monitor for myasthenic and cholinergic crises.
11. Administer anticholinesterase medications as prescribed.
12. Instruct the client to avoid stress, infection, fatigue, and over-the counter medications.
13. Instruct the client to wear a Medic-Alert bracelet.
14. Inform the client about services from the Myasthenia Gravis Foundation.

D. Anticholinesterase medications
1. Action: Increase levels of acetycholine at the myoneural junction
2. Medications
   a. Neostigmine bromide (Prostigmin)
   b. Pyridostigmine bromide (Mestinon, Regonol)
   c. Edrophonium chloride (Tensilon)
3. Side effects
   a. Sweating
   b. Salivation
   c. Nausea
   d. Diarrhea and abdominal cramps
   e. Bradycardia
   f. Hypotension
4. Interventions
   a. Administer medications on time.

b. Administer medication 30 minutes before meals with milk and crackers to reduce gastrointestinal upset.

c. Monitor and record muscle strength.

d. Note that excessive doses lead to cholinergic crisis.

e. Have the antidote (atropine sulfate) available.

E. Myasthenic crisis

1. Description

a. Myasthenic crisis is an acute exacerbation of the disease.

b. The crisis is caused by a rapid, unrecognized progression of the disease, an inadequate amount of medication, infection, fatigue, or stress.

2. Assessment

a. Increased pulse, respirations, and blood pressure

b. Anorexia and cyanosis

c. Bowel and bladder incontinence

d. Decreased urine output

e. Absent cough and swallow reflex

3. Interventions

a. Assess for signs of myasthenic crisis.

b. Increase anticholinesterase medication.

F. Cholinergic crisis

1. Description

a. Cholinergic crisis results in depolarization of the motor end plates.

b. The crisis is caused by overmedication with anticholinesterase.

2. Assessment

a. Abdominal cramps

b. Nausea, vomiting, and diarrhea

c. Blurred vision

d. Pallor

e. Facial muscle twitching

f. Hypotension

g. Pupillary miosis

3. Interventions

a. Hold anticholinesterase medication.

b. Prepare to administer the antidote, atropine sulfate, if prescribed.

▲ G. **Tensilon test**

1. Description: The Tensilon test is performed to diagnose myasthenia gravis and to differentiate between myasthenic crisis and cholinergic crisis.

2. To diagnose myasthenia gravis

a. Edrophonium (Tensilon) injection is administered to the client.

b. Positive for myasthenia gravis: Client shows improvement in muscle strength after the administration of Tensilon.

c. Negative for myasthenia gravis: Client shows no improvement in muscle strength, and strength may even deteriorate after injection of Tensilon.

3. To differentiate crisis

a. Myasthenic crisis: Tensilon is administered, and if strength improves, the client needs more medication.

b. Cholinergic crisis: Tensilon is administered, and if weakness is more severe, the client is overmedicated; administer atropine sulfate, the antidote, as prescribed.

XIV. PARKINSON'S DISEASE ▲

A. Description

1. Parkinson's disease is a degenerative disease caused by the depletion of dopamine, which interferes with the inhibition of excitatory impulses.

2. Parkinson's disease results in a dysfunction of the extrapyramidal system.

3. Parkinson's disease is a slow, progressive disease that results in a crippling disability.

4. The debilitation can result in falls, self-care deficits, failure of body systems, and depression.

5. Mental deterioration occurs late in the disease.

B. Assessment

1. Bradykinesia, abnormal slowness of movement, and sluggishness of physical and mental responses

2. Akinesia

3. Monotonous speech

4. Handwriting that becomes progressively smaller

5. Tremors in hands and fingers at rest (pill rolling)

6. Tremors increasing when fatigued and decreasing with purposeful activity or sleep

7. Rigidity with jerky interrupted movements

8. Restlessness and pacing

9. Blank facial expression—mask-like facies

10. Drooling

11. Difficulty swallowing and speaking

12. Loss of coordination and balance

13. Shuffling steps, stooped position, and propulsive gait

C. Interventions

1. Assess neurological status.

2. Assess ability to swallow and chew.

3. Provide high-calorie, high-protein, high-fiber soft diet with small, frequent feedings.

4. Increase fluid intake to 2000 mL/day.

5. Monitor for constipation.

6. Promote independence along with safety measures.

7. Avoid rushing the client with activities.

8. Assist with ambulation and provide assistive devices.

9. Instruct client to rock back and forth to initiate movement.

10. Instruct the client to wear low-heeled shoes.

11. Encourage the client to lift feet when walking and to avoid prolonged sitting.

12. Provide a firm mattress, and position the client prone, without a pillow, to facilitate proper posture.

13. Instruct in proper posture by teaching the client to hold the hands behind the back to keep the spine and neck erect.
14. Promote physical therapy and rehabilitation.
15. Administer anticholinergic medications as prescribed to treat tremors and rigidity and to inhibit the action of acetylcholine.
16. Administer antiparkinsonian medications to increase the level of dopamine in the CNS.
17. Instruct the client to avoid foods high in vitamin B$_6$ because they block the effects of antiparkinsonian medications.
18. Instruct the client to avoid monoamine oxidase inhibitors because they will precipitate hypertensive crisis.
19. Refer to Chapter 66 regarding medication to treat Parkinson's disease.

XV. TRIGEMINAL NEURALGIA

A. Description
   1. Trigeminal neuralgia is a sensory disorder of the fifth cranial nerve.
   2. Trigeminal neuralgia results in severe, recurrent, sharp, facial pain along the trigeminal nerve.
B. Assessment
   1. Client has pain on the lips, gums, or nose, or across the cheeks.
   2. Situations that stimulate symptoms include cold, washing the face, chewing, or food or fluids of extreme temperatures.
C. Interventions
   1. Instruct the client to avoid hot or cold foods and fluids.
   2. Provide small feedings of liquid and soft foods.
   3. Instruct the client to chew food on the unaffected side.
   4. Administer medications as prescribed (Box 65-19).
D. Surgical interventions
   1. An alcohol injection along the affected portion of the nerve to produce anesthesia of the nerve may provide relief of pain for up to 16 months.
   2. Retrogasserian rhizotomy or total severance of the sensory root of the trigeminal nerve may give relief.
   3. The Jannetta procedure surgically relocates the artery that is compressing the trigeminal nerve.
   4. Electrocoagulation or percutaneous radiofrequency rhizotomy creates a heat lesion.

BOX 65-19

Medications to Treat Trigeminal Neuralgia

Amitriptyline (Elavil)
Baclofen (Lioresal)
Carbamazepine (Tegretol)
Diazepam (Valium)
Phenytoin (Dilantin)

XVI. BELL'S PALSY (FACIAL PARALYSIS)

A. Description
   1. Bell's palsy is caused by a lower motor neuron lesion of the seventh cranial nerve that may result from infection, trauma, hemorrhage, meningitis, or a tumor.
   2. Bell's palsy results in paralysis of one side of the face.
   3. Recovery usually occurs in a few weeks without residual effects.
B. Assessment
   1. Flaccid facial muscles
   2. Inability to raise the eyebrows, frown, smile, close the eyelids, or puff out the cheeks
   3. Upward movement of the eye when attempting to close the eyelid
   4. Loss of taste
C. Interventions
   1. Encourage facial exercises to prevent the loss of muscle tone (a face sling may be prescribed to prevent stretching of weak muscles).
   2. Protect the eyes from dryness and prevent injury.
   3. Promote frequent oral care.
   4. Instruct the client to chew on the unaffected side.

XVII. GUILLAIN-BARRÉ SYNDROME

A. Description
   1. Guillain-Barré syndrome is an acute infectious neuronitis of the cranial and peripheral nerves.
   2. The immune system overreacts to the infection and destroys the myelin sheath.
   3. The syndrome usually is preceded by a mild upper respiratory infection or gastroenteritis.
   4. The recovery is a slow process and can take years.
   5. The major concern is difficulty breathing.
B. Assessment
   1. Paresthesias
   2. Weakness of lower extremities
   3. Gradual progressive weakness of upper extremities and facial muscles
   4. Possible progression to respiratory failure
   5. Cardiac dysrhythmias
   6. Cerebrospinal fluid that reveals an elevated protein level
   7. Abnormal electroencephalogram
C. Interventions
   1. Care is directed toward the treatment of symptoms.
   2. Monitor respiratory status.
   3. Provide respiratory treatments.
   4. Prepare to initiate respiratory support.
   5. Monitor cardiac status.
   6. Assess for complications of immobility.
   7. Provide the client and family with support.

XVIII. AMYOTROPHIC LATERAL SCLEROSIS

A. Description
   1. Amyotrophic lateral sclerosis also is known as Lou Gehrig's disease.

2. Amyotrophic lateral sclerosis is a progressive degenerative disease involving the motor system.

3. The sensory and autonomic systems are not involved, and mental status changes do not result from the disease.

4. The cause of the disease may be related to an excess of glutamate, a chemical responsible for relaying messages between the motor neurons.

5. As the disease progresses, muscle weakness and atrophy develop until a flaccid quadriplegia develops.

6. Eventually the respiratory muscles become affected, leading to respiratory compromise, pneumonia, and death.

7. No cure is known, and the treatment is symptomatic.

B. Assessment
1. Fatigue
2. Fatigue while talking
3. Muscle weakness and atrophy
4. Tongue atrophy
5. Dysphagia
6. Weakness of the hands and arms
7. Fasciculations of the face
8. Nasal quality of speech
9. Dysarthria

C. Interventions
1. Care is directed toward the treatment of symptoms.
2. Monitor respiratory status.
3. Provide respiratory treatments.
4. Prepare to initiate respiratory support.
5. Assess for complications of immobility.
6. Provide the client and family with support.

XIX. ENCEPHALITIS

A. Description
1. Encephalitis is an inflammation of the brain parenchyma and often the meninges.
2. Encephalitis affects the cerebrum, the brainstem, and the cerebellum.
3. Encephalitis most often is caused by a viral agent, although bacteria, fungi, or parasites also may be involved.
4. Viral encephalitis is almost always preceded by a viral infection.

B. Transmission
1. Arboviruses can be transmitted to human beings through the bite of an infected mosquito or tick.
2. Echovirus, coxsackievirus, poliovirus, herpes zoster, and viruses that cause mumps and chickenpox are common enteroviruses associated with encephalitis.
3. Herpes simplex type 1 virus can cause viral encephalitis.
4. The organism that causes amebic meningoencephalitis can enter the nasal mucosa of persons swimming in warm freshwater, ponds, and lakes.

C. Assessment
1. Presence of cold sores, lesions, or ulcerations of the oral cavity
2. History of insect bites and swimming in freshwater
3. Exposure to infectious diseases
4. Travel to areas where the disease in prevalent
5. Fever
6. Nausea and vomiting
7. Stiff neck
8. Changes in level of consciousness and mental status
9. Signs of **increased ICP**
10. Motor dysfunction and focal neurological deficits

D. Interventions
1. Monitor vital and neurological signs.
2. Assess level of consciousness using the **Glasgow Coma Scale.**
3. Assess for mental status changes and personality and behavior changes.
4. Assess for signs of **increased ICP.**
5. Assess for the presence of nuchal rigidity and a positive **Kernig's sign** or **Brudzinski's sign**, indicating meningeal irritation.
6. Assist the client to turn, cough, and deep breathe frequently.
7. Elevate the head of the bed 30 to 45 degrees.
8. Assess for muscle and neurological deficits.
9. Administer acyclovir (Zovirax) as prescribed.
10. Initiate rehabilitation as needed for motor dysfunction or neurological deficits.

XX. WEST NILE VIRUS

A. Description
1. West Nile virus is a potentially serious illness that affects the CNS.
2. The virus is contracted primarily by the bite of an infected mosquito (mosquitoes become carriers when they feed on infected birds).
3. Symptoms typically develop between 3 and 14 days after being bitten by the infected mosquito.
4. Neurological effects can be permanent.

B. Assessment
1. Many individuals will not experience any symptoms.
2. Mild symptoms include fever, headache and body aches, nausea, vomiting, swollen glands, or a rash on the chest, stomach, or back.
3. Severe symptoms include a high fever, headache, neck stiffness, stupor, disorientation, tremors, muscle weakness, vision loss, numbness, paralysis, seizures, or coma.

C. Interventions are supportive; there is no specific treatment for the virus.

D. Prevention
1. Use insect repellents containing DEET (N, N-diethylmeta-toluamide) when outdoors and wear long sleeves and pants and light-colored clothing.
2. Stay indoors at dusk and dawn when mosquitoes are most active.
3. Ensure that mosquito breeding sites are eliminated, such as standing water and water in bird baths, and keep wading pools empty and on their sides when not in use.

▲ XXI. MENINGITIS
A. Description
1. Meningitis is inflammation of the arachnoid and pia mater of the brain and spinal cord.
2. Meningitis is caused by bacterial and viral organisms, although fungal and protozoal meningitis also occurs.
3. Predisposing factors include skull fractures, brain or spinal surgery, sinus or upper respiratory infections, the use of nasal sprays, and individuals with a compromised immune system.
4. Cerebrospinal fluid is analyzed to determine the diagnosis and the type of meningitis.
B. Transmission
1. Transmission is by direct contact, including droplet spread.
2. Transmission occurs in areas of high population density, crowded living areas, and prisons.
C. Assessment
1. Mild lethargy
2. Memory changes
3. Short attention span
4. Personality and behavior changes
5. Severe headache
6. Generalized muscle aches and pains
7. Nausea and vomiting
8. Fever and chills
9. Tachycardia
10. Deterioration in the level of consciousness
11. Photophobia
12. Signs of meningeal irritation such as nuchal rigidity and positive **Kernig's sign** and **Brudzinski's sign**
13. Red, macular rash with meningococcal meningitis
14. Abdominal and chest pain with viral meningitis
D. Interventions
1. Monitor vital signs and neurological signs.
2. Assess for signs of increasing ICP.
3. Initiate seizure precautions.
4. Monitor for seizure activity.
5. Monitor for signs of meningeal irritation.
6. Perform cranial nerve assessment.
7. Assess peripheral vascular status.
8. Maintain isolation precautions as necessary with bacterial meningitis.
9. Maintain urine and stool precautions with viral meningitis.
10. Maintain respiratory isolation for the client with pneumococcal meningitis
11. Elevate the head of the bed 30 degrees, and avoid neck flexion and extreme hip flexion.
12. Prevent stimulation and restrict visitors.
13. Administer analgesics as prescribed.
14. Administer antibiotics as prescribed.

PRACTICE QUESTIONS

1. The client has an impairment of cranial nerve II. Specific to this impairment the nurse would plan to do which of the following to ensure client safety?
   1. Provide a clear path for ambulation without obstacles.
   2. Test the temperature of the shower water.
   3. Speak loudly to the client.
   4. Check the temperature of the food on the dietary tray.
2. The client has a neurological deficit involving the limbic system. Specific to this type of deficit the nurse would document which of the following information related to the client's behavior?
   1. Demonstrates inability to add and subtract; does not know who is president.
   2. Cannot recall what was eaten for breakfast today.
   3. Is disoriented to person, place, and time.
   4. Affect is flat, with periods of emotional lability.
3. The nurse is planning to test the function of the trigeminal nerve (cranial nerve V). The nurse would gather which of the following items to perform the test?
   1. Flashlight, pupil size chart or millimeter ruler
   2. Tuning fork and audiometer
   3. Safety pin, hot and cold water in test tubes, cotton wisp
   4. Snellen's chart, ophthalmoscope
4. The nurse is testing the coordinated functioning of cranial nerves III, IV, and VI. To do this correctly, the nurse would test the
   1. Corneal reflex.
   2. Six cardinal fields of gaze.
   3. Pupil response to light.
   4. Pupil response to light and accommodation.
5. The nurse is assessing the motor function of an unconscious client. The nurse would plan to use which of the following to test the client's peripheral response to pain?
   1. Sternal rub
   2. Pressure on the orbital rim
   3. Squeezing of the sternocleidomastoid muscle
   4. Nail bed pressure
6. The client admitted with a neurological problem indicates to the nurse that magnetic resonance imaging may be done. The nurse interprets that the client may be ineligible for this diagnostic procedure based on the client's history of

1. Hypertension.
2. Chronic obstructive pulmonary disorder.
3. Heart failure.
4. Prosthetic valve replacement.

7. The client is having a lumbar puncture performed. The nurse would plan to place the client in which position for the procedure?
   1. Side-lying, with legs pulled up and head bent down onto chest
   2. Side-lying, with a pillow under the hip
   3. Prone, in slight Trendelenburg's position
   4. Prone, with a pillow under the abdomen

8. The client has just undergone computerized tomography scanning with a contrast medium. The nurse would evaluate that the client understands postprocedure care if the client verbalized to
   1. Eat lightly for the remainder of the day.
   2. Rest quietly for the remainder of the day.
   3. Hold medications for at least 4 hours.
   4. Increase fluid intake for the day.

9. The nurse is assisting with caloric testing of the oculovestibular reflex of an unconscious client. Cold water is injected into the left auditory canal. The client exhibits eye conjugate movements toward the left followed by rapid nystagmus toward the right. The nurse understands that this indicates the client has
   1. A cerebral lesion.
   2. A temporal lesion.
   3. An intact brainstem.
   4. Brain death.

10. The nurse is admitting the client to the short stay unit following a myelogram. A water-based contrast agent was used. The nurse would plan which of the following activity restrictions for the client?
    1. Bedrest for 6 to 8 hours, with the head of bed elevated 15 to 30 degrees
    2. Bedrest for 2 to 4 hours, with the head of bed elevated 15 to 30 degrees
    3. Bedrest for 6 to 8 hours, with the head of bed flat
    4. Bedrest for 2 to 4 hours, with the head of bed flat

11. The nurse is caring for the client with increased intracranial pressure. The nurse would note which of the following trends in vital signs if the intracranial pressure is rising?
    1. Increasing temperature, increasing pulse, increasing respirations, decreasing blood pressure
    2. Increasing temperature, decreasing pulse, decreasing respirations, increasing blood pressure
    3. Decreasing temperature, decreasing pulse, increasing respirations, decreasing blood pressure
    4. Decreasing temperature, increasing pulse, decreasing respirations, increasing blood pressure

12. The nurse is positioning the client with increased intracranial pressure. Which of the following positions would the nurse avoid?
    1. Head turned to the side

2. Head midline
3. Neck in neutral position
4. Head of bed elevated 30 to 45 degrees

13. The client recovering from a head injury is arousable and participating in care. The nurse determines that the client understands measures to prevent elevations in intracranial pressure if the nurse observed the client doing which of the following activities?
    1. Exhaling during repositioning
    2. Isometric exercises
    3. Blowing nose
    4. Coughing vigorously

14. The client has clear fluid leaking from the nose following a basilar skull fracture. The nurse assesses that this is cerebrospinal fluid if the fluid
    1. Clumps together on the dressing and has a pH of 7.
    2. Separates into concentric rings and tests positive for glucose.
    3. Is grossly bloody in appearance and has a pH of 6.
    4. Is clear and tests negative for glucose.

15. The client with a head injury has begun urinating copious amounts of dilute urine through the Foley catheter. The client's urine output for the previous shift was 3000 mL. The nurse implements a new physician order to administer
    1. Desmopressin (DDAVP, Stimate).
    2. Dexamethasone (Decadron).
    3. Ethacrynic acid (Edecrin).
    4. Mannitol (Osmitrol).

16. The nurse is caring for the client in the emergency department following a head injury. The client momentarily lost consciousness at the time of the injury and then regained it. The client now has lost consciousness again. The nurse takes quick action, knowing this is compatible with
    1. Skull fracture.
    2. Concussion.
    3. Subdural hematoma.
    4. Epidural hematoma.

17. The nurse is evaluating the status of the client who had a craniotomy 3 days ago. The nurse would suspect the client is developing meningitis as a complication of surgery if the client exhibits
    1. A positive Brudzinski's sign.
    2. A negative Kernig's sign.
    3. Absence of nuchal rigidity.
    4. A Glasgow Coma Scale score of 15.

18. The client with a cervical spine injury has Crutchfield (cervical) tongs applied in the emergency department. The nurse would avoid which of the following when planning care for this client?
    1. Use of a Roto-rest bed
    2. Assessment of the integrity of the weights and pulleys
    3. Comparing the amount of ordered traction with the amount in use
    4. Removing the weights to reposition the client

19. The nurse has completed discharge instructions for the client with application of a Halo device. The nurse determines that the client needs further clarification of the instructions if the client stated to
   1. Use caution because the device alters balance.
   2. Wash the skin daily under the lamb's wool liner of the vest.
   3. Use a straw for drinking.
   4. Drive only during the daytime.

20. The nurse is caring for the client who suffered a spinal cord injury 48 hours ago. The nurse monitors for gastrointestinal complications by assessing for
   1. A flattened abdomen.
   2. Hematest positive nasogastric tube drainage.
   3. Hyperactive bowel sounds.
   4. A history of diarrhea.

21. A nursing student develops a plan of care for a client with paraplegia who has a Risk for Injury related to spasticity of the leg muscles. The nurse reads the plan and would speak to the student about which incorrect intervention?
   1. Removing potentially harmful objects near the spastic limbs
   2. Performing range of motion to the affected limbs
   3. Use of padded restraints to immobilize the limb
   4. Use of as-needed orders for muscle relaxants such as baclofen (Lioresal)

22. The nurse is caring for the client who has suffered a spinal cord injury. The nurse further assesses the client for other signs of autonomic dysreflexia if the client experiences
   1. Severe, throbbing headache.
   2. Pallor of the face and neck.
   3. Sudden tachycardia.
   4. Severe and sudden hypotension.

23. The family of a client with a spinal cord injury rushes to the nursing station saying that the client needs immediate help. On entering the room, the nurse notes that the client is diaphoretic with a flushed face and neck and complains of a severe headache. The pulse rate is 40 beats per minute and the blood pressure is 230/100 mm Hg. The nurse acts quickly, knowing that the client is experiencing
   1. Spinal shock.
   2. Malignant hypertension.
   3. Pulmonary embolism.
   4. Autonomic dysreflexia

24. The client with a spinal cord injury is prone to experiencing autonomic dysreflexia. The nurse would avoid which of the following measures to minimize the risk of recurrence?
   1. Strict adherence to a bowel retraining program
   2. Limiting bladder catheterization to once every 12 hours
   3. Keeping the linen wrinkle-free under the client
   4. Preventing unnecessary pressure on the lower limbs

25. The nurse is planning care for the client in spinal shock. Which of the following actions would be least helpful in minimizing the effects of vasodilation below the level of the injury?
   1. Monitoring vital signs before and during position changes
   2. Using vasopressor medications as prescribed
   3. Moving the client quickly as one unit
   4. Applying Teds or compression stockings

26. The nurse is caring for a client admitted with spinal cord injury. The nurse minimizes the risk of compounding the injury most effectively by
   1. Keeping the client on a stretcher.
   2. Logrolling the client on a firm mattress.
   3. Logrolling the client on a soft mattress.
   4. Placing the client on a Stryker frame.

27. The nurse is evaluating the neurological signs of the male client in spinal shock following spinal cord injury. Which of the following observations by the nurse indicates that spinal shock persists?
   1. Positive reflexes
   2. Hyperreflexia
   3. Inability to elicit a Babinski's reflex
   4. Reflex emptying of the bladder

28. The nurse is assessing the client who is experiencing seizure activity. The nurse understands that it is unnecessary to determine information about which of the following items as part of routine assessment of seizures?
   1. Duration of the seizure
   2. What the client ate in the 2 hours preceding seizure activity
   3. Seizure progression and type of movements
   4. Changes in pupil size or eye deviation

29. The nurse is planning to institute seizure precautions for a client who is being admitted from the emergency department. Which of the following measures would the nurse avoid in planning for the client's safety?
   1. Placing an airway, oxygen, and suction equipment at the bedside
   2. Padding the side rails of the bed
   3. Putting a padded tongue blade at the head of the bed
   4. Having intravenous equipment ready for insertion of an intravenous catheter

30. The nurse is caring for the client who begins to experience seizure activity while in bed. Which of the following actions by the nurse would be contraindicated?
   1. Loosening restrictive clothing
   2. Removing the pillow and raising padded siderails
   3. Restraining the client's limbs
   4. Positioning the client to the side if possible, with head flexed forward

31. The nurse has given medication instructions to the client receiving phenytoin (Dilantin). The nurse

determines that the client has an adequate understanding if the client states

1. The medication dose may be self-adjusted depending on side effects.
2. Alcohol is not contraindicated while taking this medication.
3. Good oral hygiene is needed, including brushing and flossing.
4. The morning dose of the medication should be taken before a serum drug level is drawn.

32. The nurse is planning care for the client with hemiparesis of the right arm and leg. The nurse incorporates in the care plan to place objects
    1. Within the client's reach on the right side.
    2. Within the client's reach on the left side.
    3. Just out of the client's reach on the right side.
    4. Just out of the client's reach on the left side.

33. The client with a cerebrovascular accident has residual dysphagia. When a diet order is initiated, the nurse avoids doing which of the following?
    1. Giving the client thin liquids
    2. Thickening liquids to the consistency of oatmeal
    3. Placing food on the unaffected side of the mouth
    4. Allowing plenty of time for chewing and swallowing

34. The nurse has instructed the family of a client with cerebrovascular accident who has homonymous hemianopsia about measures to help the client overcome the deficit. The nurse determines that the family understands the measures to use if they stated to
    1. Place objects in the client's impaired field of vision.
    2. Approach the client from the impaired field of vision.
    3. Remind the client to turn the head to scan the lost visual field.
    4. Discourage the client from wearing eyeglasses.

35. The nurse is assessing the adaptation of the client to changes in functional status after a cerebrovascular accident. The nurse assesses that the client is adapting most successfully if the client
    1. Experiences bouts of depression and irritability.
    2. Consistently uses adaptive equipment in dressing self.
    3. Has difficulty with using modified feeding utensils.
    4. Gets angry with family if they interrupt a task.

36. A nursing student is caring for a client with a cerebrovascular accident who is experiencing unilateral neglect. The nurse would intervene if the student planned to use which of the following strategies to help the client adapt to this deficit?
    1. Move the commode and chair to the affected side.
    2. Place the bedside articles on the affected side.
    3. Approach the client from the unaffected side.
    4. Tell the client to scan the environment.

37. The nurse is trying to communicate with a client with cerebrovascular accident and aphasia. Which of the following actions by the nurse would be least helpful to the client?
    1. Speaking to the client at a slower rate
    2. Completing the sentences that the client cannot finish
    3. Looking directly at the client during attempts at speech
    4. Allowing plenty of time for the client to respond

38. The client with diplopia has been taught to use an eye patch to promote better vision and prevent injury. The nurse determines that the client has correct understanding of the use of the patch if the client states to
    1. Use the patch only when vision is especially troublesome.
    2. Wear the patch for 1 hour at a time.
    3. Wear the patch continuously, alternating eyes each day.
    4. Wear the patch continuously, alternating eyes each week.

39. A client receives a dose of edrophonium (Tensilon) intravenously. The client shows improvement in muscle strength for a period of time following the injection. The nurse interprets that this finding is compatible with
    1. Multiple sclerosis.
    2. Amyotrophic lateral sclerosis.
    3. Myasthenia gravis.
    4. Muscular dystrophy.

40. The client with myasthenia gravis is having difficulty speaking. The speech is dysarthritic and has a nasal tone. The nurse would avoid using which of the following communication strategies when working with this client?
    1. Repeating what the client said to verify the message
    2. Encouraging the client to speak quickly
    3. Using a communication board when necessary
    4. Asking yes and no questions when able

41. The client with myasthenia gravis has a Risk for Ineffective Airway Clearance and a Risk for Ineffective Breathing Pattern. The nurse would keep which of the following available at the client's bedside?
    1. Incentive spirometer and cough pillow
    2. Oxygen and metered-dose inhaler
    3. Pulse oximeter and a cardiac monitor
    4. Ambu bag and suction equipment

42. The client has experienced an episode of myasthenic crisis. The nurse would assess whether the client has precipitating factors such as
    1. Too little exercise.
    2. Increased intake of fatty foods.
    3. Omitted doses of medication.
    4. Excess medication.

43. The nurse is teaching the client with myasthenia gravis about prevention of myasthenic and cholinergic crises. The nurse tells the client that this is most effectively done by
    1. Doing all chores early in the day while less fatigued.
    2. Taking medications on time to maintain therapeutic blood levels.
    3. Doing muscle strengthening exercises.
    4. Eating large, well-balanced meals.

44. The home health nurse is visiting the client with myasthenia gravis and is discussing methods to minimize the risk of aspiration during meals because of decreased muscle strength. Which of the following suggestions would the nurse avoid giving to the client?
    1. Sit straight up in the chair while eating.
    2. Cut food into very small pieces, chewing thoroughly.
    3. Swallow when the chin is tipped slightly downward to the chest.
    4. Lift the head while swallowing liquids.

45. The nurse has instructed the client with myasthenia gravis about ways to manage the client's own health at home. The nurse determines that the client needs more information if the client made which of the following statements?
    1. "I should take my medications an hour before mealtime."
    2. "I've made arrangements to get a portable resuscitation bag and home suction equipment."
    3. "Going to the beach will be a nice, relaxing form of activity."
    4. "Here's the Medic-Alert bracelet I obtained."

46. The client with Parkinson's disease has a nursing diagnosis of Risk for Falls related to an abnormal gait documented in the nursing care plan. The nurse assesses the client expecting to observe which type of gait
    1. Broad based and waddling.
    2. Accelerating with walking on toes.
    3. Unsteady and staggering.
    4. Shuffling and propulsive.

47. The client with Parkinson's disease is embarrassed about the symptoms of the disorder, and is bored and lonely. The nurse would plan which of the following approaches as most therapeutic in assisting the client to cope with the disease?
    1. Plan only a few activities for the client during the day.
    2. Assist the client with activities of daily living as much as possible.
    3. Encourage and praise perseverance in exercising and performing activities of daily living.
    4. Cluster activities at the end of the day when the client is most bored.

48. The nurse has given instructions to the client with Parkinson's disease about maintaining mobility. The nurse determines that the client understood the directions if the client stated to
    1. Exercise in the evening to combat fatigue.
    2. Rock back and forth to start movement with bradykinesia.
    3. Sit in soft, deep chairs.
    4. Buy clothes with many buttons to maintain finger dexterity.

49. The nurse has given suggestions to the client with trigeminal neuralgia about strategies to minimize episodes of pain. The nurse determines that the client needs reinforcement of information if the client made which of the following statements?
    1. "I will wash my face with cotton pads."
    2. "I'll have to start chewing on the unaffected side."
    3. "I should rinse my mouth sometimes if toothbrushing is painful."
    4. "I'll try to eat my food either very warm or very cold."

50. The client with Bell's palsy asks the nurse what caused this problem to occur. The nurse's response is based on an understanding that the cause is
    1. Unknown, but possibly includes ischemia, viral infection, or an autoimmune problem.
    2. Unknown, but possibly includes long-term tissue malnutrition and cellular hypoxia.
    3. Primarily genetic in origin and is triggered by exposure to neurotoxins.
    4. Primarily genetic in origin and is triggered by exposure to meningitis.

51. The client with an onset of Bell's palsy is upset and crying about the change in the facial appearance. The nurse plans to support the client emotionally by telling the client that
    1. This is similar to a cerebrovascular accident, but all symptoms will reverse without treatment.
    2. This is not a cerebrovascular accident, and many clients recover in 3 to 5 weeks.
    3. This is caused by a small tumor, which can be removed easily.
    4. This is a temporary problem, with treatment similar to that for migraine headaches.

52. The nurse is reinforcing information given to the client with Bell's palsy about medications that may be used to decrease edema of nerve tissue. The nurse gives the client specific information about which of the following medications?
    1. Acetylsalicylic acid (Aspirin)
    2. Ibuprofen (Motrin)
    3. Dexamethasone (Decadron)
    4. Prednisone (Deltasone)

53. The nurse has given the client with Bell's palsy instructions on preserving muscle tone in the face and preventing denervation. The nurse determines

that the client needs additional information if the client stated to

1. Expose the face to cold and drafts.
2. Massage the face with a gentle upward motion.
3. Wrinkle the forehead, blow out the cheeks, and whistle.
4. Use a device for electrical stimulation of the face.

54. The client is admitted to the hospital with a diagnosis of Guillian-Barré syndrome. The nurse inquires during the nursing admission interview if the client has a history of
1. Back injury or trauma to the spinal cord.
2. Seizures or trauma to the brain.
3. Respiratory or gastrointestinal infection during the previous month.
4. Meningitis during the last 5 years.

55. The client with Guillian-Barré syndrome has ascending paralysis and is intubated and receiving mechanical ventilation. Which of the following strategies would the nurse incorporate in the plan of care to help the client cope with this illness?
1. Giving client full control over care decisions and restricting visitors
2. Providing information, giving positive feedback, and encouraging relaxation
3. Providing intravenously administered sedatives, reducing distractions, and limiting visitors
4. Providing positive feedback and encouraging active range of motion

56. The nurse is admitting a client with Guillian-Barré syndrome to the nursing unit. The client has an ascending paralysis to the level of the waist. Knowing the complications of the disorder, the nurse brings which of the following items into the client's room?
1. Nebulizer and pulse oximeter
2. Flashlight and incentive spirometer
3. Electrocardiogram monitoring electrodes and intubation tray
4. Blood pressure cuff and flashlight

57. The nurse is evaluating the respiratory outcomes for the client with Guillian-Barré syndrome. The nurse would evaluate that which of the following is the least optimal outcome for the client?
1. Adventitious breath sounds
2. Spontaneous breathing
3. Oxygen saturation 98%
4. Vital capacity within normal range

58. The client is admitted with an exacerbation of multiple sclerosis. The nurse is assessing the client for possible precipitating risk factors. Which of the following factors, if stated by the client, would the nurse assess as being unrelated to the exacerbation?
1. A stressful week at work
2. Ingestion of more fruits and vegetables
3. A recent bout of the flu
4. Inability to sleep well

59. The client with multiple sclerosis is experiencing muscle weakness, spasticity, and an ataxic gait. Based on this information, the nurse would formulate which of the following nursing diagnoses for the client?
1. Impaired Physical Mobility
2. Activity Intolerance
3. Impaired Tissue Integrity
4. Self Care Deficit

60. The nurse is planning care for the client with a neurogenic bladder caused by multiple sclerosis. Which of the following plans for fluid administration of at least 2000 mL/day would be most helpful to this client?
1. 400 to 500 mL with each meal, additional fluids in the morning but not after midday
2. 400 to 500 mL with each meal, 500 to 600 mL in the evening before bedtime
3. 400 to 500 mL with each meal, 200 to 250 mL at midmorning, midafternoon, and late afternoon
4. 400 to 500 mL with each meal, with all extra fluid concentrated in the afternoon and evening

CRITICAL THINKING: PRIORITIZING (ORDERED RESPONSE)

The client with a spinal cord injury suddenly experiences an episode of autonomic dysreflexia. After checking the client's vital signs, list in order of priority, the nurse's actions. (Number 1 is the first priority and number 5 is the last priority).

____ Check for bladder distention.

____ Raise the head of the bed.

____ Contact the physician.

____ Loosen tight clothing on the client.

____ Administer an antihypertensive medication.

ANSWERS

1. 1

Rationale: Cranial nerve II is the optic nerve, which governs vision. The nurse can provide safety for the visually impaired client by clearing the path of obstacles when ambulating. Testing the shower water temperature would be useful if there were an impairment of peripheral nerves. Speaking loudly may help overcome a deficit of cranial nerve VIII (vestibulocochlear). Cranial nerve VII (facial) and IX (glossopharyngeal) control taste from the anterior two thirds and posterior third of the tongue, respectively.

Test-Taking Strategy: Use the process of elimination. Recalling that cranial nerve II is the optic nerve will direct you easily to option 1. Review the function of this nerve if you had difficulty with this question.
Level of Cognitive Ability: Application
Client Needs: Safe, Effective Care Environment
Integrated Process: Nursing Process—planning
Content Area: Adult health—neurological
Reference: Phipps, W., Monahan, F., Sands, J., Marek, J., & Neighbors, M. (2003). *Medical-surgical nursing: Health and illness perspectives* (7th ed., pp. 1305-1306). St. Louis: Mosby.

2. 4

Rationale: The limbic system is responsible for feelings (affect) and emotions. Calculation ability and knowledge of current events relates to function of the frontal lobe. The cerebral hemispheres, with specific regional functions, control orientation. Recall of recent events is controlled by the hippocampus.

Test-Taking Strategy: Use the process of elimination. Recall that the limbic system is responsible for feelings and emotions to direct you to option 4. Review the function of the limbic system if you had difficulty with this question.
Level of Cognitive Ability: Application
Client Needs: Psychosocial Integrity
Integrated Process: Communication and Documentation
Content Area: Adult health—neurological
Reference: Black, J., Hawks, J., & Keene, A. (2001). *Medical-surgical nursing: Clinical management for positive outcomes* (6th ed., p. 1858). Philadelphia: W. B. Saunders.

3. 3

Rationale: The trigeminal nerve has a motor and sensory division. The motor division innervates the muscles for chewing (mastication). The sensory division innervates the entire face, scalp, cornea, and nasal and oral cavities. The sensations of pain, temperature, and touch can be assessed using each of the respective items noted in option 3. The corneal reflex (motor division) also can be tested using the cotton wisp. The supplies noted in options 1, 2, and 4 are used for testing cranial nerves III, VIII, and II, respectively.

Test-Taking Strategy: Use the process of elimination. Recalling the function of cranial nerve V will direct you to option 3. Review the function of this nerve if you had difficulty with this question.
Level of Cognitive Ability: Application
Client Needs: Health Promotion and Maintenance
Integrated Process: Nursing Process—assessment

Content Area: Adult health—neurological
Reference: Black, J., Hawks, J., & Keene, A. (2001). *Medical-surgical nursing: Clinical management for positive outcomes* (6th ed., p. 1885). Philadelphia: W. B. Saunders.

4. 2

Rationale: Cranial nerves III (oculomotor), IV (trochlear), and VI (abducens) have only motor components and control, in a coordinated manner, the six cardinal fields of gaze. This is tested by moving an object in six directions (involving horizontal and diagonal movements). Corneal reflex is the function of the trigeminal nerve (cranial nerve V). Pupillary response and accommodation is the function of cranial nerve III (oculomotor) alone.

Test-Taking Strategy: If you look at this question carefully, you will see that each of the incorrect options has to do with pupillary reactions of some type. The correct option is the one that is different from the others. Being able to move the eyes through the six cardinal fields of gaze is a coordinated effort of three cranial nerves. Review cranial nerve testing if you had difficulty with this question.
Level of Cognitive Ability: Application
Client Needs: Health Promotion and Maintenance
Integrated Process: Nursing Process—assessment
Content Area: Adult health—neurological
Reference: Black, J., Hawks, J., & Keene, A. (2001). *Medical-surgical nursing: Clinical management for positive outcomes* (6th ed., pp. 1984-1885). Philadelphia: W. B. Saunders.

5. 4

Rationale: Motor testing in the unconscious client can be done only by testing response to painful stimuli. Nailbed pressure tests a basic peripheral response. Cerebral responses to pain are tested using sternal rub, placing upward pressure on the orbital rim, or squeezing the clavicle or sternocleidomastoid muscle.

Test-Taking Strategy: Note the keywords "peripheral response." The nailbeds are the most distal of all the options and are therefore the most peripheral. Each of the other options may elicit a generalized response, but not a localized one. Review the process of peripheral testing if you had difficulty with this question.
Level of Cognitive Ability: Application
Client Needs: Health Promotion and Maintenance
Integrated Process: Nursing Process—assessment
Content Area: Adult health—neurological
Reference: Black, J., Hawks, J., & Keene, A. (2001). *Medical-surgical nursing: Clinical management for positive outcomes* (6th ed., p. 1887). Philadelphia: W. B. Saunders.

6. 4

Rationale: The client having a magnetic resonance imaging scan has all metallic objects removed because of the magnetic field generated by the device. A careful history is done to determine if any metal objects are inside the client, such as orthopedic hardware, pacemakers, artificial heart valves, aneurysm clips, or intrauterine devices. These may heat up, become dislodged, or malfunction during this procedure. The client may be ineligible if significant risk exists.

Test-Taking Strategy: Use the process of elimination noting the key word "ineligible." You will note that each of the incorrect options is a medical disorder. The correct option is the name of a surgical procedure in which an artificial valve (sometimes metal) is implanted. An important concept regarding magnetic resonance imaging is the avoidance of any metal objects in the vicinity of the machine. Review the contraindications related to this procedure if you had difficulty with this question.
Level of Cognitive Ability: Analysis
Client Needs: Physiological Integrity
Integrated Process: Nursing Process—assessment
Content Area: Adult health—neurological
Reference: Black, J., Hawks, J., & Keene, A. (2001). *Medical-surgical nursing: Clinical management for positive outcomes* (6th ed., pp. 196-197). Philadelphia: W. B. Saunders.

7. 1
Rationale: The client undergoing lumbar puncture is positioned lying on the side, with the legs pulled up to the abdomen, and with the head bent down onto the chest. This position helps to open the spaces between the vertebrae.
Test-Taking Strategy: Use the process of elimination. Recall that a lumbar puncture is the introduction of a needle into the subarachnoid space. The correct option is the only position that flexes the vertebrae for easier needle insertion. Review positioning procedures for a lumbar puncture if you had difficulty with this question.
Level of Cognitive Ability: Application
Client Needs: Physiological Integrity
Integrated Process: Nursing Process—implementation
Content Area: Adult health—neurological
Reference: Black, J., Hawks, J., & Keene, A. (2001). *Medical-surgical nursing: Clinical management for positive outcomes* (6th ed., p. 1897). Philadelphia: W. B. Saunders.

8. 4
Rationale: After computed tomography scanning, the client may resume all usual activities. The client should be encouraged to consume extra fluids to replace those lost with diuresis from the contrast dye.
Test-Taking Strategy: Use the process of elimination. Noting the key words "scanning with a contrast medium" will direct you to option 4. Review the procedure related to computed tomography scanning if you had difficulty with this question.
Level of Cognitive Ability: Analysis
Client Needs: Physiological Integrity
Integrated Process: Teaching/Learning
Content Area: Adult health—neurological
Reference: Ignatavicius, D., & Workman, M. (2002). *Medical-surgical nursing: Critical thinking for collaborative care* (4th ed., p. 892). Philadelphia: W. B. Saunders.

9. 3
Rationale: Caloric testing provides information about differentiating between cerebellar and brainstem lesions. After determining patency of the ear canal, cold or warm water is injected into the auditory canal. A normal response that indicates intact function of cranial nerves III, VI, and VIII is conjugate eye movements toward the side being irrigated, followed by rapid nystagmus to the opposite side. Absent or dysconjugate eye movements indicate brainstem damage.
Test-Taking Strategy: To answer this question correctly, you must understand the purpose and nature of the test. Remember that this test is used as an adjunct to determine brain death. This would limit the choices to options 3 or 4. Knowledge of the test results and their meaning is needed to differentiate between the remaining options. Review this test if you had difficulty with this question.
Level of Cognitive Ability: Analysis
Client Needs: Physiological Integrity
Integrated Process: Nursing Process—analysis
Content Area: Adult health—neurological
Reference: Black, J., Hawks, J., & Keene, A. (2001). *Medical-surgical nursing: Clinical management for positive outcomes* (6th ed., p. 1903). Philadelphia: W. B. Saunders.

10. 1
Rationale: Following a myelogram, the client is placed on bedrest for 6 to 8 hours after the procedure. When a water-based contrast medium is used, the client is positioned with the head of bed elevated 15 to 30 degrees. With use of an oil-based medium, the head of the bed is positioned flat (even though the contrast is aspirated out after the procedure).
Test-Taking Strategy: Use the process of elimination. With a myelogram procedure, remember that the longer the bedrest, the less likelihood of complications. This will assist in eliminating options 2 and 4. If you can remember "oil rises, so keep the head low," you will be able to choose correctly from the remaining options. Review post procedure care following a myelogram, if you had difficulty with this question.
Level of Cognitive Ability: Application
Client Needs: Physiological Integrity
Integrated Process: Nursing Process—planning
Content Area: Adult health—neurological
Reference: Black, J., Hawks, J., & Keene, A. (2001). *Medical-surgical nursing: Clinical management for positive outcomes* (6th ed., p. 1899). Philadelphia: W. B. Saunders.

11. 2
Rationale: A change in vital signs may be a late sign of increased intracranial pressure. Trends include increasing temperature and blood pressure and decreasing pulse and respirations. Respiratory irregularities also may arise.
Test-Taking Strategy: This question looks complex but can be answered logically. If you remember that the temperature rises, then you are able to eliminate options 3 and 4. If you know that the client becomes bradycardic, or know that the blood pressure rises, you are able to select the correct option. Review the signs of increased intracranial pressure if you had difficulty with this question.
Level of Cognitive Ability: Analysis
Client Needs: Physiological Integrity
Integrated Process: Nursing Process—assessment
Content Area: Adult health—neurological
Reference: Black, J., Hawks, J., & Keene, A. (2001). *Medical-surgical nursing: Clinical management for positive outcomes* (6th ed., p. 2027). Philadelphia: W. B. Saunders.

12. 1

Rationale: The head of the client with increased intracranial pressure should be positioned so the head is in a neutral, midline position. The nurse should avoid flexing or extending the neck or turning the head side to side. The head of the bed should be raised to 30 to 45 degrees. Use of proper positions promotes venous drainage from the cranium to keep intracranial pressure down.

Test-Taking Strategy: Use the process of elimination noting the key word "avoid." Select the position that interferes with arterial circulation to the brain or with venous drainage from the brain. The only position that meets one of those criteria is option 1. Review client positioning with intracranial pressure if you had difficulty with this question.

Level of Cognitive Ability: Application
Client Needs: Physiological Integrity
Integrated Process: Nursing Process—implementation
Content Area: Adult health—neurological
Reference: Ignatavicius, D., & Workman, M. (2002). *Medical-surgical nursing: Critical thinking for collaborative care* (4th ed., p. 1003). Philadelphia: W. B. Saunders.

13. 1

Rationale: Activities that increase intrathoracic and intraabdominal pressures cause an indirect elevation of the intracranial pressure. Some of these activities include isometric exercises, Valsalva's maneuver, coughing, sneezing, and blowing the nose. Exhaling during activities such as repositioning or pulling up in bed, opens the glottis, which prevents intrathoracic pressure from rising.

Test-Taking Strategy: Use the process of elimination. Evaluate each of the options in terms of the tension it puts on the body. Doing so will help you eliminate each of the incorrect options systematically. Review the measures that will reduce or prevent increased intracranial pressure if you had difficulty with this question.

Level of Cognitive Ability: Analysis
Client Needs: Physiological Integrity
Integrated Process: Nursing Process—evaluation
Content Area: Adult health—neurological
Reference: Ignatavicius, D., & Workman, M. (2002). *Medical-surgical nursing: Critical thinking for collaborative care* (4th ed., p. 1003). Philadelphia: W. B. Saunders.

14. 2

Rationale: Leakage of cerebrospinal fluid (CSF) from the ears or nose may accompany basilar skull fracture. Cerebrospinal fluid can be distinguished from other body fluids because the drainage will separate into bloody and yellow concentric rings on dressing material, called halo's sign. The fluid also tests positive for glucose.

Test-Taking Strategy: Use the process of elimination and knowledge regarding the characteristics of CSF. Recall that CSF contains glucose, whereas other secretions, such as mucus, do not. Knowing that CSF separates into rings also will help you answer this question. Review testing for CSF fluid if you had difficulty with this question.

Level of Cognitive Ability: Analysis
Client Needs: Physiological Integrity
Integrated Process: Nursing Process—assessment

Content Area: Adult health—neurological
Reference: Ignatavicius, D., & Workman, M. (2002). *Medical-surgical nursing: Critical thinking for collaborative care* (4th ed., p. 929). Philadelphia: W. B. Saunders.

15. 1

Rationale: A complication of head injury is diabetes insipidus, which can occur with insult to the hypothalamus, the antidiuretic hormone storage vesicles, or the posterior pituitary gland. Urine output that exceeds 9 L per day generally requires treatment with desmopressin. Dexamethasone, a glucocorticoid, is administered to treat cerebral edema. This medication already may be ordered for the head-injured client. Ethacrynic acid and mannitol are diuretics, which would be contraindicated.

Test-Taking Strategy: Use the process of elimination recalling that a complication of head injury is diabetes insipidus. Knowing that diabetes insipidus results in excretion of large amounts of dilute urine, you can eliminate options 3 and 4 immediately. From the remaining options, select option 1 because of its action. Review the action and purpose of desmopressin if you had difficulty with this question.

Level of Cognitive Ability: Analysis
Client Needs: Physiological Integrity
Integrated Process: Nursing Process—implementation
Content Area: Pharmacology
Reference: Ignatavicius, D., & Workman, M. (2002). *Medical-surgical nursing: Critical thinking for collaborative care* (4th ed., p. 1005). Philadelphia: W. B. Saunders.

16. 4

Rationale: The changes in neurological signs from an epidural hematoma begin with loss of consciousness as arterial blood collects in the epidural space and exerts pressure. The client regains consciousness as the cerebrospinal fluid is reabsorbed rapidly to compensate for the rising intracranial pressure. As the compensatory mechanisms fail, even small amounts of additional blood cause the intracranial pressure to rise rapidly, and the client's neurological status deteriorates quickly.

Test-Taking Strategy: Use the process of elimination. Begin to answer this question by ruling out skull fracture and concussion as responsible for fluctuating neurological signs. Recall that a subdural hematoma is a collection of venous blood, which may accumulate more slowly and cause a steadier deterioration of neurological signs. This will help you discriminate between epidural and subdural hematomas. Review the clinical manifestations associated with the various types of head injury if you had difficulty with this question.

Level of Cognitive Ability: Analysis
Client Needs: Physiological Integrity
Integrated Process: Nursing Process—assessment
Content Area: Adult health—neurological
Reference: Ignatavicius, D., & Workman, M. (2002). *Medical-surgical nursing: Critical thinking for collaborative care* (4th ed., p. 991). Philadelphia: W. B. Saunders.

17. 1

Rationale: Signs of meningeal irritation compatible with meningitis include nuchal rigidity, positive Brudzinski's sign, and positive Kernig's sign. Nuchal rigidity is characterized by a stiff neck and soreness, which is especially noticeable when the neck is flexed. Kernig's sign is positive when the client feels pain and spasm of the hamstring muscles when the knee and thigh are extended from a flexed, right-angle position. Brudzinski's sign is positive when the client flexes the hips and knees in response to the nurse gently flexing the head and neck onto the chest. A Glasgow Coma Scale score of 15 is a perfect score and indicates the client is awake and alert with no neurological deficits.

Test-Taking Strategy: Use the process of elimination, focusing on the client's diagnosis, meningitis. You can eliminate options 2, 3, and 4 because they are normal findings. Review the signs of meningitis if you had difficulty with this question.

Level of Cognitive Ability: Analysis
Client Needs: Physiological Integrity
Integrated Process: Nursing Process—assessment
Content Area: Adult health—neurological
Reference: Phipps, W., Monahan, F., Sands, J., Marek, J., & Neighbors, M. (2003). *Medical-surgical nursing: Health and illness perspectives* (7th ed., pp. 1359-1360). St. Louis: Mosby.

18. 4

Rationale: Crutchfield (cervical) tongs are applied after drilling holes in the client's skull under local anesthesia. Weights are attached to the tongs, which exert pulling pressure on the longitudinal axis of the cervical spine. Serial x-ray films of the cervical spine are taken, with weights being added gradually until the x-ray film reveals that the vertebral column is realigned. After that, weights may be reduced gradually to a point that maintains alignment. The client with Crutchfield tongs is placed on a Stryker frame or Roto-rest bed. The nurse ensures that weights hang freely, and the amount of weight matches the current order. The nurse also inspects the integrity and position of the ropes and pulleys. The nurse does not remove the weights to administer care.

Test-Taking Strategy: Use the process of elimination noting the key word "avoid." Recalling the basics related to the care of a client in traction will direct you to option 4. Review nursing care related to the client with cervical tongs, if you had difficulty with this question.

Level of Cognitive Ability: Application
Client Needs: Physiological Integrity
Integrated Process: Nursing Process—planning
Content Area: Adult health—neurological
References: Ignatavicius, D., & Workman, M. (2002). *Medical-surgical nursing: Critical thinking for collaborative care* (4th ed., p. 937). Philadelphia: W. B. Saunders.
Lewis, S., Heitkemper, M., & Dirksen, S. (2004). *Medical-surgical nursing: Assessment and management of clinical problems* (6th ed., p. 1620). St. Louis: Mosby.
Phipps, W., Monahan, F., Sands, J., Marek, J., & Neighbors, M. (2003). *Medical-surgical nursing: Health and illness perspectives* (7th ed., pp. 1473, 1478). St. Louis: Mosby.

19. 4

Rationale: The halo device alters balance and can cause fatigue because of its weight. The client should cleanse the skin daily under the vest to protect the skin from ulceration and should use powder or lotions sparingly or not at all. The wool liner should be changed if odor becomes a problem. The client should have food cut into small pieces to facilitate chewing and use straws for drinking. Pin care is done as instructed. The client may not drive because the device impairs the range of vision.

Test-Taking Strategy: Use the process of elimination and note the key words "needs further clarification." Visualize this device to answer correctly. The inability to turn the head without turning the torso would contraindicate driving. Review client education points related to a halo device if you had difficulty with this question.

Level of Cognitive Ability: Analysis
Client Needs: Physiological Integrity
Integrated Process: Teaching/Learning
Content Area: Adult health—neurological
Reference: Lewis, S., Heitkemper, M., & Dirksen, S. (2004). *Medical-surgical nursing: Assessment and management of clinical problems* (6th ed., p. 1629). St. Louis: Mosby.

20. 2

Rationale: After spinal cord injury, the client can develop paralytic ileus, which is characterized by the absence of bowel sounds and abdominal distention. Development of a stress ulcer can be detected by hematest positive nasogastric tube aspirate or stool. A history of diarrhea is irrelevant.

Test-Taking Strategy: Use the process of elimination, focusing on the client's diagnosis and the signs of a gastrointestinal complication. Review this information if you had difficulty with this question.

Level of Cognitive Ability: Application
Client Needs: Physiological Integrity
Integrated Process: Nursing Process—assessment
Content Area: Adult health—neurological
References: Ignatavicius, D., & Workman, M. (2002). *Medical-surgical nursing: Critical thinking for collaborative care* (4th ed., p. 1257). Philadelphia: W. B. Saunders.
Phipps, W., Monahan, F., Sands, J., Marek, J., & Neighbors, M. (2003). *Medical-surgical nursing: Health and illness perspectives* (7th ed., pp. 440, 1409). St. Louis: Mosby.

21. 3

Rationale: Range of motion exercises are beneficial in stretching muscles, which may diminish spasticity. Removing potentially harmful objects is a good safety measure. Use of muscle relaxants also is indicated if the spasms cause discomfort to the client or pose a risk to the client's safety. Use of limb restraints will not alleviate spasticity and could harm the client.

Test-Taking Strategy: Use the process of elimination. Noting the key word "incorrect" should direct you easily to option 3. Review care to the paraplegic client if you had difficulty with this question.

Level of Cognitive Ability: Application
Client Needs: Safe, Effective Care Environment
Integrated Process: Nursing Process—implementation
Content Area: Leadership/Management
Reference: Ignatavicius, D., & Workman, M. (2002). *Medical-surgical nursing: Critical thinking for collaborative care* (4th ed., pp. 934, 936-938). Philadelphia: W. B. Saunders.

22. 1

Rationale: The client with spinal cord injury is at risk for autonomic dysreflexia with an injury above the level of T7.

Autonomic dysreflexia is characterized by severe, throbbing headache; flushing of the face and neck; bradycardia; and sudden, severe hypertension. Other signs include nasal stuffiness, blurred vision, nausea, and sweating. Autonomic dysreflexia is a life-threatening syndrome triggered by a noxious stimulus below the level of the injury.

Test-Taking Strategy: Use the process of elimination. Recalling that a massive sympathetic nervous system response occurs causing the severe hypertension, the throbbing headache, and flushing of the face and neck will direct you to the correct option. Review the signs of autonomic dysreflexia if you had difficulty with this question.
Level of Cognitive Ability: Application
Client Needs: Physiological Integrity
Integrated Process: Nursing Process—assessment
Content Area: Adult health—neurological
Reference: Ignatavicius, D., & Workman, M. (2002). *Medical-surgical nursing: Critical thinking for collaborative care* (4th ed., p. 931). Philadelphia: W. B. Saunders.

23. **4**
Rationale: The client with a spinal cord injury is at risk for autonomic dysreflexia with an injury above the level of T7. Autonomic dysreflexia is characterized by severe, throbbing headache, flushing of the face and neck, bradycardia, and sudden severe hypertension. Other signs include nasal stuffiness, blurred vision, nausea, and sweating. Autonomic dysreflexia is a life-threatening syndrome triggered by a noxious stimulus below the level of the injury.

Test-Taking Strategy: Use the process of elimination. Begin by eliminating options 1 and 3. The client in spinal shock would be hypotensive (not hypertensive), and the client's clinical picture does not correlate with pulmonary embolism. (Knowing also that autonomic dysreflexia does not occur until spinal shock resolves may be useful.) Recalling that malignant hypertension occurs with anesthesia will assist you in eliminating option 2. Review the signs of autonomic dysreflexia if you had difficulty with this question.
Level of Cognitive Ability: Analysis
Client Needs: Physiological Integrity
Integrated Process: Nursing Process—analysis
Content Area: Adult health—neurological
Reference: Phipps, W., Monahan, F., Sands, J., Marek, J., & Neighbors, M. (2003). *Medical-surgical nursing: Health and illness perspectives* (7th ed., pp. 1425-1426). St. Louis: Mosby.

24. **2**
Rationale: The most frequent cause of autonomic dysreflexia is a distended bladder. Straight catheterization should be done every 4 to 6 hours, and Foley catheters should be checked frequently to prevent kinks in the tubing. Constipation and fecal impaction are other causes, so maintaining bowel regularity is important. Other causes include stimulation of the skin from tactile, thermal, or painful stimuli. The nurse administers care to minimize risk in these areas.
Test-Taking Strategy: Use the process of elimination. Remember that autonomic dysreflexia is caused by noxious stimuli to the bowel, bladder, or skin. With this in mind, you can eliminate easily each of the incorrect options. Review the measures

to minimize the risk of autonomic dysreflexia if you had difficulty with this question.
Level of Cognitive Ability: Application
Client Needs: Physiological Integrity
Integrated Process: Nursing Process—implementation
Content Area: Adult health—neurological
References: Ignatavicius, D., & Workman, M. (2002). *Medical-surgical nursing: Critical thinking for collaborative care* (4th ed., p. 935). Philadelphia: W. B. Saunders.
Lewis, S., Heitkemper, M., & Dirksen, S. (2004). *Medical-surgical nursing: Assessment and management of clinical problems* (6th ed., p. 1625). St. Louis: Mosby.

25. **3**
Rationale: Reflex vasodilation below the level of the spinal cord injury places the client at risk for orthostatic hypotension, which may be profound. Measures to minimize this include measuring vital signs before and during position changes, use of a tilt-table with early mobilization, and changing the client's position slowly. Venous pooling can be reduced by using Teds (compression stockings) or pneumatic boots. Vasopressor medications are administered as per protocol.
Test-Taking Strategy: Use the process of elimination. Note the key words "least helpful." Note the word "quickly" in option 3. Knowing that quick position changes and movement would aggravate hypotension will direct you to this opinion. Review care to the client with spinal shock if you had difficulty with this question.
Level of Cognitive Ability: Application
Client Needs: Physiological Integrity
Integrated Process: Nursing Process—planning
Content Area: Adult health—neurological
Reference: Ignatavicius, D., & Workman, M. (2002). *Medical-surgical nursing: Critical thinking for collaborative care* (4th ed., p. 939). Philadelphia: W. B. Saunders.

26. **4**
Rationale: Spinal immobilization is necessary after spinal cord injury to prevent further damage and insult to the spinal cord. Whenever possible, the client is placed on a Stryker frame, which allows the nurse to turn the client to prevent complications of immobility, while maintaining alignment of the spine. If a Stryker frame is not available, a firm mattress with a bedboard under it should be used.
Test-Taking Strategy: Use the process of elimination, focusing on the issue, preventing further injury. This will direct you easily to option 4. If you are unfamiliar with a Stryker frame, review this content.
Level of Cognitive Ability: Application
Client Needs: Safe, Effective Care Environment
Integrated Process: Nursing Process—implementation
Content Area: Adult health—neurological
Reference: Ignatavicius, D., & Workman, M. (2002). *Medical-surgical nursing: Critical thinking for collaborative care* (4th ed., p. 936). Philadelphia: W. B. Saunders.

27. **3**
Rationale: Resolution of spinal shock is occurring when there is return of reflexes (especially flexors to noxious cutaneous

stimuli), a state of hyperreflexia rather than flaccidity, reflex emptying of the bladder, and a positive Babinski's reflex.

Test-Taking Strategy: Recall that spinal shock is characterized by the loss of movement of skeletal muscles, bowel or bladder wall, and depressed reflex action. Return of any of these indicates that spinal shock is beginning to resolve. Note that options 1, 2, and 4 are similar, indicating the presence of reflexes. Review signs of spinal shock if you had difficulty with this question.

Level of Cognitive Ability: Analysis
Client Needs: Physiological Integrity
Integrated Process: Nursing Process—evaluation
Content Area: Adult health—neurological
References: Ignatavicius, D., & Workman, M. (2002). *Medical-surgical nursing: Critical thinking for collaborative care* (4th ed., pp. 889, 931). Philadelphia: W. B. Saunders.
Phipps, W., Monahan, F., Sands, J., Marek, J., & Neighbors, M. (2003). *Medical-surgical nursing: Health and illness perspectives* (7th ed., p. 1311). St. Louis: Mosby.

28. **2**
Rationale: Typically, seizure assessment includes the time the seizure began, part(s) of the body affected, the type of movements and progression of the seizure, changes in pupil size, eye deviation or nystagmus, client condition during the seizure, and postictal status.

Test-Taking Strategy: Use the process of elimination, noting the key word "unnecessary." The option about the client's intake before the seizure suggests concern about vomiting and subsequent aspiration. The nurse is concerned about aspiration, not from vomiting, but from inhalation of the client's own saliva. Because all of the other options are standard assessments, this is the answer to the question. Review nursing assessment during a seizure, if you had difficulty answering this question.

Level of Cognitive Ability: Application
Client Needs: Physiological Integrity
Integrated Process: Nursing Process—assessment
Content Area: Adult health—neurological
Reference: Ignatavicius, D., & Workman, M. (2002). *Medical-surgical nursing: Critical thinking for collaborative care* (4th ed., p. 903). Philadelphia: W. B. Saunders.

29. **3**
Rationale: Seizure precautions may vary from agency to agency, but they generally have some commonalities. Usually an airway, oxygen, and suctioning equipment are kept available at the bedside. The side rails of the bed are padded, and the bed is kept in the lowest position. The client has an intravenous access in place to have a readily accessible route if anticonvulsant medications must be administered. The use of padded tongue blades is highly controversial, and they should not be kept at the bedside. Forcing a tongue blade into the mouth during a seizure more likely will harm the client who bites down during seizure activity. Risks include blocking the airway from improper placement, chipping the client's teeth, and subsequent risk of aspirating tooth fragments. If the client has an aura before the seizure, it may give the nurse enough time to place an oral airway before seizure activity begins.

Test-Taking Strategy: Use the process of elimination noting the key word "avoid." Evaluate this question from the perspective of causing possible harm. No harm can come to the client from any of the options except for the tongue blade. Review seizure precautions, if you had difficulty with this question.

Level of Cognitive Ability: Application
Client Needs: Safe, Effective Care Environment
Integrated Process: Nursing Process—planning
Content Area: Adult health—neurological
Reference: Ignatavicius, D., & Workman, M. (2002). *Medical-surgical nursing: Critical thinking for collaborative care* (4th ed., p. 901). Philadelphia: W. B. Saunders.

30. **3**
Rationale: Nursing actions during a seizure include providing for privacy, loosening restrictive clothing, removing the pillow and raising side rails in bed, and placing the client on one side with the head flexed forward, if possible, to allow the tongue to fall forward and facilitate drainage. The limbs are never restrained because the strong muscle contractions could cause the client harm. If the client is not in bed when seizure activity begins, the nurse lowers the client to the floor if possible, protects the head from injury, and moves furniture that may injure the client. Other aspects of care are as described for the client who is in bed.

Test-Taking Strategy: Use the process of elimination and note the key word "contraindicated." Evaluate this question from the perspective of causing possible harm. No harm can come to the client from any of the options except for restraining the limbs. Remember, avoid restraints. Review care to a client during a seizure, if you had difficulty with this question.

Level of Cognitive Ability: Application
Client Needs: Physiological Integrity
Integrated Process: Nursing Process—implementation
Content Area: Adult health—neurological
Reference: Ignatavicius, D., & Workman, M. (2002). *Medical-surgical nursing: Critical thinking for collaborative care* (4th ed., p. 903). Philadelphia: W. B. Saunders.

31. **3**
Rationale: Typical anticonvulsant medication instructions include taking the dose daily to keep the blood level of the drug constant and having a serum drug level drawn before taking the morning dose. The client is taught not to stop the medication abruptly, to avoid alcohol, to check with the physician before taking over-the-counter medications, to avoid activities where alertness and coordination are required until medication effects are known, to provide good oral hygiene, and to obtain regular dental care. The client should also wear a Medic-Alert bracelet.

Test-Taking Strategy: Use the process of elimination. Using knowledge of general principles related to the medication administration will assist you in eliminating options 1 and 2. From the remaining options, recall that medications generally are not taken just before drawing of therapeutic serum levels because the results would be artificially high. This leaves oral hygiene as the correct option because of the risk of gingival hyperplasia. Review client education related to phenytoin (Dilantin) if you had difficulty with this question.

Level of Cognitive Ability: Analysis
Client Needs: Physiological Integrity
Integrated Process: Teaching/Learning
Content Area: Adult health—neurological
References: Ignatavicius, D., & Workman, M. (2002). *Medical-surgical nursing: Critical thinking for collaborative care* (4th ed., p. 902). Philadelphia: W. B. Saunders.
McKenry, L., & Salerno, E. (2001). *Mosby's pharmacology in nursing* (21st ed., p. 361). St. Louis: Mosby.

32. **2**

Rationale: Hemiparesis is a weakness of the face, arm, and leg on one side. The client with one-sided hemiparesis benefits from having objects placed on the unaffected side and within reach. Other helpful activities with hemiparesis include range of motion exercises to the affected side and muscle strengthening exercises to the unaffected side.

Test-Taking Strategy: Use the process of elimination. Begin to answer by eliminating options 3 and 4 as potentially hazardous to the client. Also, distinguish between hemiparesis and unilateral neglect to answer this question. The client with hemiparesis has weakness on one side, and therefore objects should be placed on the stronger side. With unilateral neglect, objects are placed on the affected side to train the client to attend to that part of the environment. Knowing this, select option 2. Review care to the client with hemiparesis if you had difficulty with this question.

Level of Cognitive Ability: Application
Client Needs: Safe, Effective Care Environment
Integrated Process: Nursing Process—planning
Content Area: Adult health—neurological
Reference: Ignatavicius, D., & Workman, M. (2002). *Medical-surgical nursing: Critical thinking for collaborative care* (4th ed., p. 980). Philadelphia: W. B. Saunders.

33. **1**

Rationale: Before the client with dysphagia is started on a diet, the gag and swallow reflexes must have returned. The client is assisted with meals as needed and is given ample time to chew and swallow. Food is placed on the unaffected side of the mouth. Liquids are thickened to avoid aspiration.

Test-Taking Strategy: Use the process of elimination, noting the key word "avoids." Option 4 is generally a good action for all clients. Option 3 is correct because the client has better sensation and motion on the unaffected side of the mouth. Remember that thickened liquids are easier for the client with impaired facial motion and swallowing ability to manage. Knowing this enables you to choose option 1 as the action to avoid. Review care to the client with residual dysphagia if you had difficulty with this question.

Level of Cognitive Ability: Application
Client Needs: Physiological Integrity
Integrated Process: Nursing Process—implementation
Content Area: Adult health—neurological
Reference: Ignatavicius, D., & Workman, M. (2002). *Medical-surgical nursing: Critical thinking for collaborative care* (4th ed., p. 1189). Philadelphia: W. B. Saunders.

34. **3**

Rationale: Homonymous hemianopsia is loss of one half of the visual field. The client with homonymous hemianopsia should have objects placed in the intact field of vision, and the nurse also should approach the client from the intact side. The nurse instructs the client to scan the environment to overcome the visual deficit and does client teaching from within the intact field of vision. The nurse encourages the use of personal eyeglasses, if they are available.

Test-Taking Strategy: Use the process of elimination. Recalling the definition of homonymous hemianopsia will direct you easily to option 3. Review the concept of homonymous hemianopsia if you are unfamiliar with it.

Level of Cognitive Ability: Analysis
Client Needs: Safe, Effective Care Environment
Integrated Process: Teaching/Learning
Content Area: Adult health—neurological
Reference: Ignatavicius, D., & Workman, M. (2002). *Medical-surgical nursing: Critical thinking for collaborative care* (4th ed., pp. 980-981, 1018). Philadelphia: W. B. Saunders.

35. **2**

Rationale: Clients are evaluated as coping successfully with lifestyle changes after a cerebrovascular accident if they make appropriate lifestyle alterations, use the assistance of others, and have appropriate social interactions. Options 1, 3, and 4 are not adaptive behaviors.

Test-Taking Strategy: Use the process of elimination, focusing on the key words "adapting most successfully." Options 1 and 4 are behaviors that may be expected in the client with a cerebrovascular accident, but they are not adaptive responses. Rather they are a result of the insult to the brain. Options 2 and 3 indicate that the client is trying to adapt, but option 2 has the best outcome. Review care to the client with a cerebrovascular accident if you had difficulty with this question.

Level of Cognitive Ability: Analysis
Client Needs: Psychosocial Integrity
Integrated Process: Nursing Process—evaluation
Content Area: Adult health—neurological
Reference: Ignatavicius, D., & Workman, M. (2002). *Medical-surgical nursing: Critical thinking for collaborative care* (4th ed., pp. 988-989). Philadelphia: W. B. Saunders.

36. **3**

Rationale: Unilateral neglect is an unawareness of the paralyzed side of the body, which increases the client's risk for injury. The nurse's role is to refocus the client's attention to the affected side. The nurse moves personal care items and belongings to the affected side, as well as the bedside chair and commode. The nurse teaches the client to scan the environment to become aware of that half of the body and approaches the client from the affected side to increase awareness further.

Test-Taking Strategy: Use the process of elimination, noting the key word "intervene." Recall that with unilateral neglect, the client loses awareness of the affected side. If you know that the client needs to be trained to attend to that side, you can eliminate each of the incorrect options. Review care to the client with unilateral neglect if you had difficulty with this question.

Level of Cognitive Ability: Application
Client Needs: Physiological Integrity
Integrated Process: Nursing Process—implementation
Content Area: Leadership/Management

References: Ignatavicius, D., & Workman, M. (2002). *Medical-surgical nursing: Critical thinking for collaborative care* (4th ed., pp. 960, 986). Philadelphia: W. B. Saunders.
Phipps, W., Monahan, F., Sands, J., Marek, J., & Neighbors, M. (2003). *Medical-surgical nursing: Health and illness perspectives* (7th ed., p. 1369). St. Louis: Mosby.

37. **2**

Rationale: Clients with aphasia after cerebrovascular accident often fatigue easily and have a short attention span. General guidelines when trying to communicate with the aphasic client include speaking more slowly and allowing adequate response time, listening to and watching attempts to communicate, and trying to put the client at ease with a caring and understanding manner. The nurse would avoid shouting (because the client is not deaf), appearing rushed for a response, and letting family members provide all the responses for the client.
Test-Taking Strategy: Use the process of elimination, noting the key words "least helpful." This question tests a fundamental concept in communicating with the aphasic client. If this question was difficult, review these communication strategies.
Level of Cognitive Ability: Application
Client Needs: Psychosocial Integrity
Integrated Process: Communication and Documentation
Content Area: Adult health—neurological
Reference: Ignatavicius, D., & Workman, M. (2002). *Medical-surgical nursing: Critical thinking for collaborative care* (4th ed., p. 987). Philadelphia: W. B. Saunders.

38. **3**

Rationale: Placing an eye patch over one eye in the client with diplopia removes the second image and restores more normal vision. The patch is alternated each day to maintain the strength of the extraocular muscles of the eyes.
Test-Taking Strategy: Use the process of elimination. Knowing that an eye patch will help diplopia only while it is worn will assist you in eliminating options 1 and 2. Recalling that the extraocular muscles weaken with eye patch use will direct you to option 3. Review instructions for the client with diplopia if you had difficulty with this question.
Level of Cognitive Ability: Analysis
Client Needs: Physiological Integrity
Integrated Process: Teaching/Learning
Content Area: Adult health—neurological
References: Ignatavicius, D., & Workman, M. (2002). *Medical-surgical nursing: Critical thinking for collaborative care* (4th ed., p. 963). Philadelphia: W. B. Saunders.
Lewis, S., Heitkemper, M., & Dirksen, S. (2004). *Medical-surgical nursing: Assessment and management of clinical problems* (6th ed., p. 1542). St. Louis: Mosby.

39. **3**

Rationale: Myasthenia gravis often can be diagnosed based on clinical signs and symptoms. The diagnosis can be confirmed by injecting the client with a dose of edrophonium (Tensilon). This medication inhibits the breakdown of an enzyme in the neuromuscular junction, so more acetylcholine binds onto receptors. If the muscle is strengthened for 3 to 5 minutes after this injection, it confirms a diagnosis of myasthenia gravis. Another medication, neostigmine (Prostigmin) also may be used because the effect lasts for 1 to 2 hours, giving a better analysis. For either medication, atropine sulfate should be available as the antidote.
Test-Taking Strategy: Use the process of elimination. Knowledge of the purpose and expected findings of the Tensilon test is required to answer this question. Review the Tensilon test if you are unfamiliar with it.
Level of Cognitive Ability: Analysis
Client Needs: Physiological Integrity
Integrated Process: Nursing Process—analysis
Content Area: Pharmacology
Reference: Ignatavicius, D., & Workman, M. (2002). *Medical-surgical nursing: Critical thinking for collaborative care* (4th ed., pp. 960-962). Philadelphia: W. B. Saunders.

40. **2**

Rationale: The client has speech that is nasal and dysarthritic because of cranial nerve involvement of the muscles governing speech. The nurse listens attentively and verbally verifies what the client has said, asks questions requiring a yes or no response, and develops alternative communication methods (letter board, picture board, pen and paper, flash cards). Encouraging the client to speak quickly is unsuccessful and counterproductive.
Test-Taking Strategy: Use the process of elimination, noting the key word "avoid." Options 3 and 4 are classic examples of alternative communication methods that are useful and are eliminated first. Because option 1 is also helpful, this leaves option 2 as the correct option. Speaking quickly is difficult for a client with a speech impairment. Review communication strategies for the client with speaking difficulty if this question was difficult.
Level of Cognitive Ability: Application
Client Needs: Psychosocial Integrity
Integrated Process: Communication and Documentation
Content Area: Adult health—neurological
Reference: Ignatavicius, D., & Workman, M. (2002). *Medical-surgical nursing: Critical thinking for collaborative care* (4th ed., p. 963). Philadelphia: W. B. Saunders.

41. **4**

Rationale: The client with myasthenia gravis may experience episodes of respiratory distress if excessively fatigued or if the client develops myasthenic crisis or cholinergic crisis. For this reason, an Ambu bag, intubation tray, and suction equipment should be available at the bedside.
Test-Taking Strategy: Use the process of elimination. Note that each option has two items. For the option to be correct, both parts of the option must be correct. Knowing that the client with myasthenia gravis is at risk for aspiration and respiratory failure helps you select option 4 over each of the others. Additionally, option 4 addresses the maintenance of a patent airway. Review care of the client with myasthenia gravis if you had difficulty with this question.
Level of Cognitive Ability: Application
Client Needs: Physiological Integrity
Integrated Process: Nursing Process—implementation
Content Area: Adult health—neurological
Reference: Ignatavicius, D., & Workman, M. (2002). *Medical-surgical nursing: Critical thinking for collaborative care* (4th ed., p. 962). Philadelphia: W. B. Saunders.

42. **3**

Rationale: Myasthenic crisis often is caused by undermedication and responds to the administration of cholinergic medications such as neostigmine (Prostigmin) and pyridostigmine (Mestinon). Cholinergic crisis (the opposite problem) is caused by excess medication and responds to withholding of medications. Too little exercise and fatty food intake are incorrect. Overexertion and overeating possibly could trigger myasthenic crisis.

Test-Taking Strategy: Use the process of elimination. Recalling that undermedication is a common cause of myasthenic crisis will direct you easily to option 3. Review the causes of myasthenic crisis if you had difficulty with this question.
Level of Cognitive Ability: Application
Client Needs: Physiological Integrity
Integrated Process: Nursing Process—assessment
Content Area: Adult health—neurological
Reference: Ignatavicius, D., & Workman, M. (2002). *Medical-surgical nursing: Critical thinking for collaborative care* (4th ed., pp. 961-962). Philadelphia: W. B. Saunders.

43. **2**

Rationale: Clients with myasthenia gravis are taught to space out activities over the day to conserve energy and restore muscle strength. Taking medications correctly to maintain blood levels that are not too low or too high is important. Muscle strengthening exercises are not helpful and can fatigue the client. Overeating is a cause of exacerbation of symptoms, as is exposure to heat, crowds, erratic sleep habits, and emotional stress.

Test-Taking Strategy: Use the process of elimination. Recalling that the common causes of myasthenic and cholinergic crises are undermedication and overmedication, respectively, will assist you in eliminating each of the incorrect options. No other option would prevent both of those complications. Review measures to prevent myasthenic and cholinergic crises if you are unfamiliar with them.
Level of Cognitive Ability: Application
Client Needs: Physiological Integrity
Integrated Process: Teaching/Learning
Content Area: Adult health—neurological
Reference: Ignatavicius, D., & Workman, M. (2002). *Medical-surgical nursing: Critical thinking for collaborative care* (4th ed., p. 961). Philadelphia: W. B. Saunders.

44. **4**

Rationale: The client avoids swallowing any type of food or drink with the head lifted upward, which could actually cause aspiration by opening the glottis. The client should be advised to sit upright while eating, not to talk with food in the mouth (glottis is open), cut food into very small pieces, chew thoroughly, and tip the chin downward to swallow.

Test-Taking Strategy: Use the process of elimination noting the key word "avoid." If you look at the construct of this question, you will note that options 3 and 4 oppose each other. This makes it likely that one of the two is correct. In examining each of them, option 4 is the better choice. Lifting the head opens the airway, which will increase the risk of aspiration during drinking or eating. Review care to the client with myasthenia gravis if you had difficulty with this question.

Level of Cognitive Ability: Application
Client Needs: Physiological Integrity
Integrated Process: Teaching/Learning
Content Area: Adult health—neurological
Reference: Ignatavicius, D., & Workman, M. (2002). *Medical-surgical nursing: Critical thinking for collaborative care* (4th ed., p. 963). Philadelphia: W. B. Saunders.

45. **3**

Rationale: Most ongoing treatment for myasthenia gravis in done in outpatient settings, and the client needs to be aware of the lifestyle changes needed to maintain independence. Taking medications an hour before mealtime gives greater muscle strength for chewing and is indicated. The client should have portable suction equipment and a portable resuscitation bag available in case of respiratory distress. The client should carry medical identification about the presence of the condition. The client should avoid situations that could worsen the symptoms, including stress, infection, heat, surgery, or alcohol.

Test-Taking Strategy: Use the process of elimination, noting the key words "needs more information." Options 2 and 4 are reasonable courses of action, and so they are eliminated first. To discriminate between the remaining options, recall that premedication an hour before meals gives strength to the muscles (for chewing and swallowing) and that heat and infection (crowds at the beach) trigger myasthenic crisis. Review client education points with myasthenia gravis if you had difficulty with this question.
Level of Cognitive Ability: Analysis
Client Needs: Health Promotion and Maintenance
Integrated Process: Teaching/Learning
Content Area: Adult health—neurological
Reference: Ignatavicius, D., & Workman, M. (2002). *Medical-surgical nursing: Critical thinking for collaborative care* (4th ed., p. 965). Philadelphia: W. B. Saunders.

46. **4**

Rationale: The parkinsonian gait is characterized by short, accelerating, shuffling steps. The client leans forward with the head, hips, and knees flexed, and has difficulty starting and stopping. A dystrophic gait is broad based and waddling. A festinating gait is accelerating with walking on toes. An ataxic gait is staggering and unsteady.

Test-Taking Strategy: Use the process of elimination. Recall that the client has difficulty in initiating movement and bradykinesia. The gait is difficult to start, but it accelerates once it has begun. This will assist in eliminating options 1 and 3. From the remaining options, recall that the client with Parkinson's disease shuffles but does not walk on the toes. Review the characteristics associated with Parkinson's disease if you had difficulty with this question.
Level of Cognitive Ability: Analysis
Client Needs: Physiological Integrity
Integrated Process: Nursing Process—assessment
Content Area: Adult health—neurological
Reference: Phipps, W., Monahan, F., Sands, J., Marek, J., & Neighbors, M. (2003). *Medical-surgical nursing: Health and illness perspectives* (7th ed., p. 1390). St. Louis: Mosby.

47. 3

Rationale: The client with Parkinson's disease tends to become withdrawn and depressed and should become an active participant in personal care to prevent this. Activities should be planned throughout the day to inhibit daytime sleeping and boredom. The nurse gives the client encouragement and praises the client for perseverance. Exercise helps prevent progression of the disease, and self-care improves self-esteem.

Test-Taking Strategy: Use the process of elimination, focusing on the issue. Options 1 and 4 are the least helpful of all available options and are eliminated first. Option 2 is well intentioned but is not therapeutic in helping the client to cope with the disease. Option 3 is the best choice. Review care to the client with Parkinson's disease if you had difficulty with this question.

Level of Cognitive Ability: Application
Client Needs: Psychosocial Integrity
Integrated Process: Nursing Process—planning
Content Area: Adult health—neurological
Reference: Phipps, W., Monahan, F., Sands, J., Marek, J., & Neighbors, M. (2003). *Medical-surgical nursing: Health and illness perspectives* (7th ed., pp. 1395-1397). St. Louis: Mosby.

48. 2

Rationale: The client with Parkinson's disease should exercise in the morning when energy levels are highest. The client should avoid sitting in soft, deep chairs because they are difficult to get up from. The client can rock back and forth to initiate movement. The client should buy clothes with Velcro fasteners and slide-locking buckles to support the ability to dress self.

Test-Taking Strategy: Use the process of elimination. Option 1 is not useful to clients with fatigue from any disorder, so eliminate this option first. Knowing that the client with Parkinson's has difficulty with movement and dexterity helps to eliminate options 3 and 4 next. Review client teaching points with Parkinson's disease if you had difficulty with this question.

Level of Cognitive Ability: Analysis
Client Needs: Physiological Integrity
Integrated Process: Teaching/Learning
Content Area: Adult health—neurological
Reference: Phipps, W., Monahan, F., Sands, J., Marek, J., & Neighbors, M. (2003). *Medical-surgical nursing: Health and illness perspectives* (7th ed., p. 1396). St. Louis: Mosby.

49. 4

Rationale: Facial pain can be minimized by using cotton pads to wash the face and using room-temperature water. The client should chew on the unaffected side of the mouth, eat a soft diet, and take in foods and beverages at room temperature. If toothbrushing triggers pain, sometimes an oral rinse after meals is helpful instead.

Test-Taking Strategy: Use the process of elimination, and note the key words "needs reinforcement of information." Recall that the pain of trigeminal neuralgia is triggered by mechanical or thermal stimuli. Very hot or cold foods are likely to trigger the pain, not relieve it. Review client education points if you had difficulty with this question.

Level of Cognitive Ability: Analysis
Client Needs: Physiological Integrity

Integrated Process: Teaching/Learning
Content Area: Adult health—neurological
Reference: Ignatavicius, D., & Workman, M. (2002). *Medical-surgical nursing: Critical thinking for collaborative care* (4th ed., p. 971). Philadelphia: W. B. Saunders.

50. 1

Rationale: Bell's palsy is a one-sided facial paralysis from compression of the facial nerve. The exact cause is unknown. Possible causes include vascular ischemia, infection, exposure to viruses such as herpes zoster or herpes simplex, autoimmune disease, or a combination of these items.

Test-Taking Strategy: Use the process of elimination. If you know that the cause of Bell's palsy is uncertain, you are able to eliminate options 3 and 4. Recalling that infection, viruses, and the immune system may have an effect in causing this disorder will direct you to option 1. Review the cause of Bell's palsy if you had difficulty with this question.

Level of Cognitive Ability: Comprehension
Client Needs: Physiological Integrity
Integrated Process: Nursing Process—implementation
Content Area: Adult health—neurological
Reference: Lewis, S., Heitkemper, M., & Dirksen, S. (2004). *Medical-surgical nursing: Assessment and management of clinical problems* (6th ed., p. 1605). St. Louis: Mosby.

51. 2

Rationale: Clients with Bell's palsy should be reassured that they have not experienced a cerebrovascular accident and that symptoms often disappear spontaneously in 3 to 5 weeks. The client is given supportive treatment for symptoms. Bell's palsy usually is not caused by a tumor, and the treatment is not similar to that for migraine headaches.

Test-Taking Strategy: Use the process of elimination. Bell's palsy is not similar to cerebrovascular accident, which eliminates option 1 first. Bell's palsy is not caused by an easily removed tumor, nor is it treated like a migraine headache, which eliminates each of the other incorrect options. Review the characteristics of Bell's palsy if you had difficulty with this question.

Level of Cognitive Ability: Application
Client Needs: Psychosocial Integrity
Integrated Process: Caring
Content Area: Adult health—neurological
References: Ignatavicius, D., & Workman, M. (2002). *Medical-surgical nursing: Critical thinking for collaborative care* (4th ed., p. 971). Philadelphia: W. B. Saunders.
Lewis, S., Heitkemper, M., & Dirksen, S. (2004). *Medical-surgical nursing: Assessment and management of clinical problems* (6th ed., p. 1605). St. Louis: Mosby.

52. 4

Rationale: Bell's palsy may be treated with prednisone. The medication reduces inflammation and edema, allowing return of normal circulation to the nerve. The medication may reduce the severity of the palsy, reduce the pain, and preserve substantial, if not all, nerve function. Options 1, 2, and 3 are incorrect.

Test-Taking Strategy: Eliminate options 1 and 2 because they are similar. From the remaining options, it is necessary to know how Bell's palsy may be treated to direct you to

option 4. Review Bell's palsy and the action and purposes of these medications if you had difficulty with this question.
Level of Cognitive Ability: Application
Client Needs: Physiological Integrity
Integrated Process: Teaching/Learning
Content Area: Pharmacology
Reference: Ignatavicius, D., & Workman, M. (2002). *Medical-surgical nursing: Critical thinking for collaborative care* (4th ed., p. 971). Philadelphia: W. B. Saunders.

53. **1**
Rationale: Prevention of muscle atrophy with Bell's palsy is accomplished with the use of facial massage, facial exercises, and electrical stimulation of the nerves. Exposure to cold or drafts is avoided. Local application of heat to the face may improve blood flow and provide comfort.
Test-Taking Strategy: Use the process of elimination, noting the key words "needs additional information." Evaluate each of the options regarding their effect on preserving muscle tone in the face. Option 1 is unrelated to muscle tone and also is contraindicated in clients with this condition. Review teaching points for the client with Bell's palsy if you had difficulty with this question.
Level of Cognitive Ability: Analysis
Client Needs: Physiological Integrity
Integrated Process: Teaching/Learning
Content Area: Adult health—neurological
References: Lewis, S., Heitkemper, M., & Dirksen, S. (2004). *Medical-surgical nursing: Assessment and management of clinical problems* (6th ed., p. 1606). St. Louis: Mosby.
Phipps, W., Monahan, F., Sands, J., Marek, J., & Neighbors, M. (2003). *Medical-surgical nursing: Health and illness perspectives* (7th ed., p. 1433). St. Louis: Mosby.

54. **3**
Rationale: Guillian-Barré syndrome is a clinical syndrome of unknown origin that involves cranial and peripheral nerves. Many clients report a history of respiratory or gastrointestinal infection in the 1 to 4 weeks before the onset of neurological deficits. Occasionally, the syndrome has been triggered by vaccination or surgery.
Test-Taking Strategy: Use the process of elimination and knowledge regarding the causes related to this disorder. If you are unfamiliar with Guillian-Barré syndrome, review this disorder.
Level of Cognitive Ability: Analysis
Client Needs: Physiological Integrity
Integrated Process: Nursing Process—assessment
Content Area: Adult health—neurological
Reference: Ignatavicius, D., & Workman, M. (2002). *Medical-surgical nursing: Critical thinking for collaborative care* (4th ed., p. 954). Philadelphia: W. B. Saunders.

55. **2**
Rationale: The client with Guillian-Barré syndrome experiences fear and anxiety from the ascending paralysis and sudden onset of the disorder. The nurse can alleviate these fears by providing accurate information about the client's condition, giving expert care, giving positive feedback to the client, and

encouraging relaxation and distraction. The family can become involved with selected care activities and provide diversion for the client as well.
Test-Taking Strategy: Use the process of elimination. Option 1 should be eliminated first because it is not practical to think that the client would be given full control over all care decisions. The client who is paralyzed cannot participate in active range of motion, which eliminates option 4. From the remaining options, option 2 is more beneficial in assisting the client to cope than option 3. Review care to the client with Guillian-Barré syndrome if you had difficulty with this question.
Level of Cognitive Ability: Application
Client Needs: Psychosocial Integrity
Integrated Process: Caring
Content Area: Adult health—neurological
Reference: Ignatavicius, D., & Workman, M. (2002). *Medical-surgical nursing: Critical thinking for collaborative care* (4th ed., p. 958). Philadelphia: W. B. Saunders.

56. **3**
Rationale: The client with Guillian-Barré syndrome is at risk for respiratory failure because of ascending paralysis. An intubation tray should be available for use. Another complication of this syndrome is cardiac dysrhythmias, which necessitates the use of electrocardiogram monitoring. Because the client is immobilized, the nurse should assess for deep vein thrombosis and pulmonary embolism routinely.
Test-Taking Strategy: Use the process of elimination. With an ascending paralysis, the client is at risk for involvement of respiratory muscles and subsequent respiratory failure. Option 3 is the only option that includes an intubation tray, which would be needed if the client's status deteriorated to needing intubation and mechanical ventilation. This option most directly addresses airway. Review care to the client with Guillian-Barré syndrome if you had difficulty with this question.
Level of Cognitive Ability: Application
Client Needs: Physiological Integrity
Integrated Process: Nursing Process—implementation
Content Area: Adult health—neurological
References: Ignatavicius, D., & Workman, M. (2002). *Medical-surgical nursing: Critical thinking for collaborative care* (4th ed., p. 956). Philadelphia: W. B. Saunders.
Lewis, S., Heitkemper, M., & Dirksen, S. (2004). *Medical-surgical nursing: Assessment and management of clinical problems* (6th ed., p. 1607). St. Louis: Mosby.
Phipps, W., Monahan, F., Sands, J., Marek, J., & Neighbors, M. (2003). *Medical-surgical nursing: Health and illness perspectives* (7th ed., p. 1402). St. Louis: Mosby.

57. **1**
Rationale: Satisfactory respiratory outcomes include clear breath sounds on auscultation, spontaneous breathing, normal vital capacity, and normal arterial blood gases and pulse oximetry.
Test-Taking Strategy: Use the process of elimination, noting the key words "least optimal." Only one option does not represent full respiratory function. This should help you eliminate each of the incorrect options. Review care to the client with Guillian-Barré syndrome if you had difficulty with this question.
Level of Cognitive Ability: Analysis

Client Needs: Physiological Integrity
Integrated Process: Nursing Process—evaluation
Content Area: Adult health—neurological
Reference: Ignatavicius, D., & Workman, M. (2002). *Medical-surgical nursing: Critical thinking for collaborative care* (4th ed., p. 956). Philadelphia: W. B. Saunders.

58. 2
Rationale: The onset or exacerbation of multiple sclerosis is preceded by a number of different factors, including emotional stress, fatigue, infection, physical injury, and pregnancy. No methods of primary prevention are known. Intake of fruit and vegetables is an unrelated item.
Test-Taking Strategy: Use the process of elimination, and note the key word "unrelated." If you examine each of the options, all but the option 2 involves physiological or psychological stress. Review the precipitating risk factors associated with multiple sclerosis if you had difficulty with this question.
Level of Cognitive Ability: Analysis
Client Needs: Physiological Integrity
Integrated Process: Nursing Process—assessment
Content Area: Adult health—neurological
Reference: Ignatavicius, D., & Workman, M. (2002). *Medical-surgical nursing: Critical thinking for collaborative care* (4th ed., p. 947). Philadelphia: W. B. Saunders.

59. 1
Rationale: Impaired Physical Mobility has been defined by the North American Nursing Diagnosis Association as "a state in which the individual experiences a limitation of ability for independent physical movement." The client's muscle weakness, muscle spasticity, and ataxic gait meet the defining characteristics for this nursing diagnosis. In addition, neuromuscular impairment is listed as a related factor or defining characteristic.
Test-Taking Strategy: Use the process of elimination. Focusing on the data provided in the question will direct you easily to option 1. Review care to the client with multiple sclerosis if you had difficulty with this question.
Level of Cognitive Ability: Analysis
Client Needs: Physiological Integrity
Integrated Process: Nursing Process—analysis
Content Area: Adult health—neurological
References: Lewis, S., Heitkemper, M., & Dirksen, S. (2004). *Medical-surgical nursing: Assessment and management of clinical problems* (6th ed., p. 1568). St. Louis: Mosby.
Phipps, W., Monahan, F., Sands, J., Marek, J., & Neighbors, M. (2003). *Medical-surgical nursing: Health and illness perspectives* (7th ed., p. 1387). St. Louis: Mosby.

60. 3
Rationale: Spacing fluid intake over the day helps the client with a neurogenic bladder to establish regular times for successful voiding. Omitting intake after the evening meal minimizes

incontinence or the need to empty the bladder during the night.
Test-Taking Strategy: Use the process of elimination. Options 2 and 4 should be eliminated first because they could cause or aggravate nocturia. From the remaining options, option 3 provides fluids at times that coincide with toileting schedules for bladder training. Review care to the client with multiple sclerosis if you had difficulty with this question.
Level of Cognitive Ability: Application
Client Needs: Physiological Integrity
Integrated Process: Nursing Process—implementation
Content Area: Adult health—neurological
Reference: Ignatavicius, D., & Workman, M. (2002). *Medical-surgical nursing: Critical thinking for collaborative care* (4th ed., p. 1568). Philadelphia: W. B. Saunders.

CRITICAL THINKING: PRIORITIZING (ORDERED RESPONSE)

Answer: 31425
Rationale: Autonomic dysreflexia is characterized by severe hypertension, bradycardia, severe headache, nasal stuffiness, and flushing. The cause is a noxious stimulus, most often a distended bladder or constipation. Autonomic dysreflexia is a neurological emergency and must be treated promptly to prevent a hypertensive stroke. Immediate nursing actions are to sit the client up in bed in a high-Fowler's position and remove the noxious stimulus. The nurse would loosen any tight clothing and then check for bladder distention. If the client has a Foley catheter, the nurse would check for kinks in the tubing. The nurse also would check for a fecal impaction and disimpact the client if necessary. The physician is contacted especially if these actions do not relieve the signs and symptoms. Antihypertensive medication may be prescribed by the physician to minimize cerebral hypertension.
Test-Taking Strategy: Recalling that this syndrome causes severe hypertension will assist you in determining that elevating the head of the bed is the first action. Next, recalling that the syndrome is caused by a noxious stimulus will assist you in determining that loosening tight clothing and checking for bladder distention would be the next actions. Because loosening any tight clothing would take less time than checking for bladder distention, this action would be taken next. Antihypertensives require a physician's order; therefore calling the physician would be the next action. Review immediate nursing interventions for the client experiencing autonomic dysreflexia if you had difficulty with this question.
Level of Cognitive Ability: Application
Client Needs: Physiological Integrity
Integrated Process: Nursing Process—implementation
Content Area: Adult health—neurological
References: Ignatavicius, D., & Workman, M. (2002). *Medical-surgical nursing: Critical thinking for collaborative care* (4th ed., p. 935). Philadelphia: W. B. Saunders.
Lewis, S., Heitkemper, M., & Dirksen, S. (2004). *Medical-surgical nursing: Assessment and management of clinical problems* (6th ed., p. 162). St. Louis: Mosby.

REFERENCES

Black, J., Hawks, J., & Keene, A. (2001). *Medical-surgical nursing: Clinical management for positive outcomes* (6th ed.). Philadelphia: W. B. Saunders.

Chernecky, C. & Berger, B. (2004). *Laboratory tests and diagnostic procedures* (4th ed.). Philadelphia: W. B. Saunders.

Harkreader, H. & Hogan, M. A. (2004). *Fundamentals of nursing: Caring and clinical judgment* (2nd ed.). Philadelphia: W. B. Saunders.

Ignatavicius, D., & Workman, M. (2002). *Medical-surgical nursing: Critical thinking for collaborative care* (4th ed.). Philadelphia: W. B. Saunders.

Jarvis, C. (2000). *Physical examination and health assessment* (3rd ed.). Philadelphia: W. B. Saunders.

Lewis, S., Heitkemper, M., & Dirksen, S. (2004). *Medical-surgical nursing: Assessment and management of clinical problems* (6th ed.). St. Louis: Mosby.

McKenry, L., & Salerno, E. (2001). *Mosby's pharmacology in nursing* (21st ed.). St. Louis: Mosby.

Perry, A. & Potter, P. (2002). *Clinical nursing skills and techniques* (5th ed.). St. Louis: Mosby.

Phipps, W., Monahan, F., Sands, J., Marek, J., & Neighbors, M. (2003). *Medical-surgical nursing: Health and illness perspectives* (7th ed.). St. Louis: Mosby.

Potter, P. & Perry, A. (2001). *Fundamentals of nursing* (5th ed.). St. Louis: Mosby.

Varcarolis, E. (2002). *Foundations of psychiatric mental health nursing* (4th ed.). Philadelphia: W. B. Saunders.

Neurological Medications

I. ANTIMYASTHENIC MEDICATIONS

A. Description

1. Antimyasthenic medications relieve muscle weakness associated with myasthenia gravis by blocking acetycholine breakdown at the neuromuscular junction.
2. Antimyasthenic medications are used to treat or diagnose myasthenia gravis or to distinguish cholinergic crisis from myasthenic crisis.
3. Neostigmine bromide (Prostigmin), pyridostigmine bromide (Mestinon), ambenonium (Mytelase) are used to control myasthenic symptoms.
4. Edrophonium chloride (Tensilon) is used to diagnose myasthenia gravis and to distinguish cholinergic crisis from myasthenic crisis.

B. Medications (Box 66-1)

C. Side effects: cholinergic crisis (Box 66-2)

D. Interventions

1. Assess neuromuscular status, including reflexes, muscle strength, and gait.
2. Monitor the client for signs and symptoms of medication overdose (cholinergic crisis) and underdose (myasthenic crisis).
3. Instruct the client to take medications on time to prevent weakness because weakness can impair the client's ability to breath and swallow.
4. Instruct the client to take the medication before meals for best absorption.

5. Instruct the client to wear a Medic-Alert bracelet.
6. Note that antimyasthenic therapy is lifelong therapy.
7. Evaluate for medication effectiveness, which is based on the improvement of neuromuscular symptoms or strength without cholinergic signs and symptoms.
8. When administering edrophonium (Tensilon), have emergency resuscitation equipment on hand and atropine sulfate available for cholinergic crisis.

E. Tensilon test

1. Edrophonium (Tensilon) is injected intravenously.
2. The **Tensilon test** can cause ventricular fibrillation and cardiac arrest.
3. Atropine sulfate is the antidote for overdose.
4. Diagnosis of myasthenia gravis: Most myasthenic clients will show a significant improvement in muscle tone within 30 to 60 seconds after injection, and the muscle improvement lasts 4 to 5 minutes.
5. The **Tensilon test** is used to diagnose cholinergic crisis (overdose with anticholinesterase) or myasthenic crisis (undermedication).
   a. In cholinergic crisis, muscle tone does not improve after the administration of Tensilon, and muscle twitching may be noted around the eyes and face.

BOX 66-1

Antimyasthenic Medications

Ambenonium chloride (Mytelase)
Edrophonium chloride (Tensilon, Enlon)
Neostigmine bromide (Prostigmin)
Pyridostigmine bromide (Mestinon)

BOX 66-2

Signs of Cholinergic Crisis

Abdominal cramps
Gastrointestinal disturbances
Hypertension
Increased bronchial secretions
Increased salivation and tearing
Miosis
Nausea, vomiting, diarrhea
Sweating

b. A Tensilon injection makes the client in cholinergic crisis temporarily worse (negative **Tensilon test**).

c. A Tensilon injection temporarily improves the condition when the client is in myasthenic crisis (positive **Tensilon test**).

II. ANTIPARKINSONIAN MEDICATIONS

A. Description

1. Antiparkinsonian medications restore the balance of the neurotransmitters acetylcholine and dopamine in the central nervous system (CNS), decreasing the signs and symptoms of Parkinson's disease.

2. These medications include the dopaminergics, which stimulate the dopamine receptors, and the anticholinergics, which block the cholinergic receptors.

3. Antiparkinsonian medications are used for drug-induced parkinsonism, in which neuroleptic agents block dopamine receptors in the CNS, leading to functional loss of dopamine activity.

4. Antiparkinsonian medications are used for Parkinson's disease, in which dopamine-containing neurons in the basal ganglia are destroyed or deficient, which causes loss of fine motor control.

B. Dopaminergic medications

1. Description

a. Dopaminergic medications stimulate the dopamine receptors.

b. Dopaminergic medications increase the amount of dopamine available in the CNS or enhance neurotransmission of dopamine.

c. Dopaminergic medications are contraindicated in clients with cardiac, renal, or psychiatric disorders.

d. Levodopa taken with a monoamine oxidase inhibitor antidepressant can cause a hypertensive crisis.

2. Medications (Box 66-3)

3. Side effects

a. Dyskinesia

b. Involuntary body movements

c. Tachycardia

d. Nausea and vomiting

e. Urinary retention

f. Constipation

g. Dizziness

h. Orthostatic hypotension

i. Confusion

j. Mood changes

k. Hallucinations

4. Interventions

a. Assess vital signs

b. Assess for risk of injury.

c. Instruct the client to take the medication with food if nausea and vomiting occur.

d. Assess for signs and symptoms of parkinsonism such as rigidity, tremors, akinesia, and

---

BOX 66-3

Medications to Treat Parkinson's Disease

MEDICATIONS AFFECTING THE AMOUNT OF DOPAMINE
Amantadine (Symmetrel)
Bromocriptine (Parlodel)
Carbidopa-levodopa (Sinemet)
Levodopa (Larodopa, Dopar)
Pergolide mesylate (Permax)
Pramipexole (Mirapex)
Ropinirole (Requip)
Selegiline hydrochloride (Carbex, Eldepryl)
Tolcapone (Tasmar)

ANTICHOLINERGICS
Benztropine mesylate (Cogentin)
Biperiden hydrochloride (Akineton)
Ethopropazine hydrochloride (Parsidol)
Procyclidine hydrochloride (Kemadrin)
Trihexyphenidyl hydrochloride (Artane)

CATHECHOL O-METHYLTRANSFERASE (COMT) INHIBITORS
Diphenhydramine hydrochloride (Benadryl)
Entacapone (Comtan)
Tolcapone (Tasmar)

---

bradykinesia; a stooped forward posture; shuffling gait; and masked facies.

e. Monitor for signs of dyskinesia.

f. Instruct the client taking carbidopa-levodopa (Sinemet) to eat low-protein foods because high-protein diets interfere with medication transport to the CNS.

g. Instruct the client to change positions slowly to minimize orthostatic hypotension.

h. Instruct the client not to discontinue the medication abruptly.

i. Instruct the client to report side effects and symptoms of dyskinesia.

j. Instruct the client to avoid alcohol.

k. Monitor the client for improvement in signs and symptoms of parkinsonism without the development of severe side effects from the medications.

l. Inform the client that urine or perspiration may be discolored and that this is harmless, but it may stain the clothing.

m. Advise the client with diabetes mellitus that glucose testing should not be done through urine testing because the results will not be reliable.

n. When administering levodopa, instruct the client to avoid excessive vitamin B_6 intake to prevent medication reactions.

C. Anticholinergic medications

1. Description

a. Anticholinergic medications block the cholinergic receptors in the CNS, thereby suppressing acetylcholine activity.

b. Anticholinergic medications reduce the rigidity and some of the tremors but have a minimal effect on the bradykinesia.

c. Anticholinergic medications are contraindicated in clients with glaucoma.

d. The client with chronic obstructive lung disease can develop dry, thick mucous secretions.

2. Medications (Box 66-3)

3. Side effects

a. Blurred vision

b. Dry mouth and dry secretions

c. Increased pulse rate

d. Constipation

e. Urinary retention

f. Restlessness and confusion

g. Photophobia

4. Interventions

a. Monitor vital signs.

b. Assess for risk of injury.

c. Assess for signs and symptoms of parkinsonism such as rigidity, tremors, akinesia, and bradykinesia; a stooped forward posture; shuffling gait; and masked facies.

d. Monitor the client for improvement in signs and symptoms.

e. Assess the client's bowel and urinary function and monitor for urinary retention and constipation.

f. Monitor for involuntary movements.

g. Encourage the client to avoid alcohol, smoking, caffeine, and aspirin to decrease gastric acidity.

h. Instruct the client to consult with the physician before taking any nonprescription medications.

i. Instruct the client to minimize dry mouth by increasing fluid intake and by using ice chips, hard candy, or gum.

j. Instruct the client to prevent constipation by increasing fluids and fiber in the diet.

k. Instruct the client to use sunglasses in direct sunlight because of possible photophobia.

l. Instruct the client to have routine eye examinations to assess for intraocular pressure.

III. ANTICONVULSANT MEDICATIONS (TABLE 66-1)

A. Description

1. Anticonvulsant medications are used to depress abnormal neuronal discharges and prevent the spread of seizures.

2. Anticonvulsant medications should be used with caution in clients taking anticoagulants, aspirin, sulfonamides, cimetidine (Tagamet), and antipsychotic drugs.

3. Absorption is decreased with the use of antacids, calcium preparations, and antineoplastic medications.

B. Interventions for clients on anticonvulsants

1. Initiate seizure precautions.

2. Monitor urinary output.

3. Monitor liver and renal function tests.

4. Monitor for signs of medication toxicity, which would include CNS depression, ataxia, nausea, vomiting, drowsiness, dizziness, restlessness, and visual disturbances

5. If a seizure occurs, assess seizure activity, including location and duration.

6. Protect the client from hazards in the environment during a seizure.

C. Client education (Box 66-4)

D. Hydantoins (Box 66-5)

1. Hydantoins are used to treat seizures.

2. Phenytoin (Dilantin) also is used to treat dysrhythmias.

3. Phenytoin decreases the effectiveness of some birth control pills.

4. Side effects

TABLE 66-1

Anticonvulsant Medications

Medication	Therapeutic Serum Range
Amobarbital (Amytal)	1-5 mcg/mL
Carbamazepine (Tegretol)	3-14 mcg/mL
Clonazepam (Klonopin)	20-80 ng/mL
Ethosuximide (Zarontin)	40-100 mcg/mL
Ethotoin (Peganone)	10-50 mcg/mL
Lorazepam (Ativan)	50-240 ng/mL
Mephenytoin (Mesantoin)	25-40 mcg/mL
Mephobarbital (Mebaral)	15-40 mcg/mL
Phenobarbital (Luminal)	15-40 mcg/mL
Phenytoin (Dilantin)	10-20 mcg/mL
Primidone (Mysoline)	5-10 mcg/mL
Valproic acid (Depakene)	40-100 mcg/mL

BOX 66-4

Client Education: Anticonvulsants

Take anticonvulsant with food to decrease gastrointestinal irritation, but avoid milk and antacids, which impairs absorption.

If taking liquid medication, shake well before ingesting.

Do not discontinue medication.

Avoid alcohol.

Avoid over-the-counter medications.

Wear a Medic-Alert bracelet.

Use caution when driving or performing activities that require alertness.

Maintain good oral hygiene and use a soft toothbrush.

Instruct client in the importance of preventative dental checkups.

Instruct client in the importance of follow-up with periodic blood studies related to determining toxicity.

Monitor serum glucose levels (diabetes mellitus).

Urine may be a harmless pink-red or red-brown color.

Report symptoms of sore throat, bruising, and nosebleeds, which may indicate a blood dyscrasia.

Inform the physician if adverse reactions occur, such as gingivitis, nystagmus, slurred speech, rash, or dizziness.

a. Gingival hyperplasia (reddened gums that bleed easily)
b. Slurred speech
c. Confusion
d. Depression
e. Nausea and vomiting
f. Constipation
g. Headaches
h. Blood dyscrasias: decreased platelet count and decreased white blood cell count
i. Elevated blood glucose
j. Alopecia
k. Hirsutism
5. Interventions
a. Oral tube feedings may interfere with the absorption of orally administered phenytoin and diminish the effectiveness of the medication; therefore feedings should be scheduled as far as possible from the phenytoin administration.
b. Monitor therapeutic serum levels to assess for toxicity.
c. Monitor for signs of toxicity.
d. When administering phenytoin intravenously, dilute in normal saline because dextrose causes the medication to precipitate.
e. When administering phenytoin intravenously, to treat status epilepticus, infuse no faster than 50 mg per minute; otherwise, hypotension and cardiac dysrhythmias can occur.
f. Instruct the client about the importance of good oral hygiene and regular dental examinations.
g. Instruct the client to consult with the physician before taking other medications to ensure compatibility with anticonvulsants.
E. Barbiturates (Box 66-6)
1. Barbiturates are used for tonic-clonic seizures and acute episodes of seizures caused by status epilepticus.
2. Barbiturates also may be used as adjuncts to anesthesia.
3. Side effects
a. Drowsiness

b. Dizziness
c. Hypotension
d. Respiratory depression
e. Tolerance to the medication
F. Benzodiazepines (Box 66-7)
1. Benzodiazepines are used to treat absence seizures.
2. Diazepam (Valium) is used to treat status epilepticus, anxiety, and skeletal muscle spasms.
3. Clorazepate (Tranxene) is used as adjunctive therapy for partial seizures.
4. Side effects
a. Ataxia
b. Respiratory and cardiac depression
c. Medication tolerance and drug dependency
G. Succinimides (Box 66-8)
1. Succinimides are used to treat absence seizures.
2. Side effects
a. Anorexia, nausea, vomiting
b. Blood dyscrasias
H. Oxazolidinediones (Box 66-9)
1. Oxazolidinediones are used for absence seizures.
2. Side effects
a. Sedation
b. Photophobia
I. Valproates (Box 66-10)
1. Valproates are used to treat tonic-clonic, partial, myoclonic, and psychomotor seizures.

BOX 66-7

Benzodiazepines

Clonazepam (Klonopin)
Clorazepate (Tranxene)
Diazepam (Valium)
Lorazepam (Ativan)

BOX 66-8

Succinimides

Ethosuximide (Zarontin)
Methsuximide (Celontin)
Phensuximide (Milontin)

BOX 66-9

Oxazolidinediones

Paramethadione (Paradione)
Trimethadione (Tridione)

BOX 66-5

Hydantoins

Ethotoin (Peganone)
Fosphenytoin (Cerebyx)
Mephenytoin (Mesantoin)
Phenytoin (Dilantin)

BOX 66-6

Barbiturates

Amobarbital (Amytal)
Mephobarbital (Mebaral)
Phenobarbital
Primidone (Mysoline)

BOX 66-10

Valproates

Valproic acid (Depakene)
Divalproex sodium (Depakote)

2. Side effects
   a. Nausea
   b. Vomiting
   c. Abdominal cramps
   d. Diarrhea
   e. Constipation
   f. Hepatotoxicity
J. Iminostilbenes
   1. Iminostilbenes are used to treat seizure disorders that have not responded to other anticonvulsants (Box 66-11).
   2. Iminostilbenes are used to treat trigeminal neuralgia.
   3. Side effects
      a. Drowsiness
      b. Dizziness
      c. Nausea
      d. Vomiting
      e. Constipation or diarrhea
      f. Visual abnormalities
      g. Dry mouth
      h. Headache

IV. CENTRAL NERVOUS SYSTEM STIMULANTS
A. Description
   1. Amphetamines and caffeine stimulate the cerebral cortex of the brain (Box 66-12).
   2. Analeptics and caffeine act on the brainstem and medulla to stimulate respiration.
   3. Anorexiants act on the cerebral cortex and hypothalamus to suppress appetite (Box 66-13).
   4. Central nervous system stimulants are used to treat narcolepsy and attention deficit hyperactivity disorders.
   5. Central nervous system stimulants are used as adjunctive therapy for exogenous obesity.
   6. Other central nervous system stimulants (Box 66-14).
B. Side effects
   1. Irritability
   2. Restlessness
   3. Tremors
   4. Insomnia
   5. Heart palpitations
   6. Tachycardia
   7. Hypertension
   8. Dry mouth
   9. Anorexia
   10. Weight loss
   11. Diarrhea or constipation
   12. Impotence
   13. Dependence and tolerance
C. Interventions
   1. Monitor vital signs.
   2. Assess mental status.
   3. Assess height, weight, and growth of the child.
   4. Monitor complete blood count and white blood cell and platelet counts before and during therapy.
   5. Monitor for side effects.
   6. Monitor sleep patterns.
   7. Monitor for withdrawal symptoms such as nausea, vomiting, weakness, and headache.
   8. Instruct the client to take the medication before meals.
   9. Instruct the client to avoid foods and beverages containing caffeine to prevent additional stimulation.
   10. Instruct the client to read labels on over-the-counter products because many contain caffeine.
   11. Instruct the client to avoid alcohol.
   12. Instruct the client not to discontinue the medication abruptly.

BOX 66-11

Other Anticonvulsants

Carbamazepine (Tegretol)
Felbamate (Felbatol)
Gabapentin (Neurontin)
Lamotrigine (Lamictal)
Oxcarbazepine (Trileptal)
Tiagabine (Gabitril)
Topiramate (Topamax)
Zonisamide (Zonegran)

BOX 66-12

Amphetamines

Amphetamine sulfate
Dextroamphetamine sulfate (Dexedrine)
Methamphetamine hydrochloride (Desoxyn)
Methylphenidate hydrochloride (Ritalin)
Pemoline (Cylert)

BOX 66-13

Anorexiants

Benzphetamine hydrochloride (Didrex)
Diethylpropion hydrochloride (Tenuate, Tepanil)
Mazindol (Sanorex, Mazanor)
Phendimetrazine (Anorex, Bontril, Melfiat, Obalan)
Phentermine hydrochloride (Fastin, Adipex, Zantril)
Phenylpropanolamine (Acutrim, Dexatrim, Phenyldrine)
Sibutramine (Meridia)

BOX 66-14

Other Central Nervous System Stimulants

Aminophylline
Caffeine
Doxapram (Dopram)
Theophylline

13. Instruct the client to take the last daily dose of the CNS stimulant at least 6 hours before bedtime to prevent insomnia.
14. Monitor for drug dependence and abuse with amphetamines.
15. If a child is taking a CNS stimulant, instruct the parents to notify the school nurse.
16. Monitor for calming effects of CNS stimulants within 3 to 4 weeks on children with attention deficit hyperactivity disorder.
17. Monitor growth in the child on long-term therapy with methylphenidate hydrochloride (Ritalin).

V. NON-NARCOTIC ANALGESICS (BOX 66-15)
A. Nonsteroidal antiinflammatory drugs (NSAIDs)
   1. Description
      a. Nonsteroidal antiinflammatory drugs are aspirin and aspirin-like medications that inhibit the synthesis of prostaglandins.
      b. The medications act as an analgesic to relieve pain, as an antipyretic to reduce body temperature, and as an anticoagulant to inhibit platelet aggregation.
      c. Nonsteroidal antiinflammatory drugs are used to relieve inflammation and pain and to treat rheumatoid arthritis, bursitis, tendinitis, osteoarthritis, and acute gout.
      d. Nonsteroidal antiinflammatory drugs are contraindicated in clients with hypersensitivity or liver or renal disease.
      e. Children with flu symptoms should not take aspirin because of the risk of Reye's syndrome.
      f. Clients taking anticoagulants should not take aspirin.
      g. Aspirin and an NSAID should not be taken together because aspirin decreases the blood level and the effectiveness of the NSAID.
      h. Nonsteroidal antiinflammatory drugs can increase the effects of warfarin (Coumadin), sulfonamides, cephalosporins, and phenytoin (Dilantin).
      i. Hypoglycemia can result if ibuprofen (Motrin) is taken with insulin or an oral hypoglycemic medication.
      j. A high risk of toxicity exists if ibuprofen is taken concurrently with calcium blockers.
      k. Cyclooxygenase-2 inhibitors block the inflammatory pathway selectively at the level of cyclooxygenase-2 and reduce inflammation; these medications do not cause the adverse effects that some NSAIDs cause.
   2. Side effects (Box 66-16)
   3. Interventions
      a. Assess client for allergies.
      b. Obtain a medication history on the client.
      c. Assess for history of gastric upset or bleeding or liver or renal disease.

BOX 66-15

Non-Narcotic Analgesics

ACETAMINOPHEN
Acetaminophen (Tylenol)

ASPIRIN
Aspirin (acetylsalicylic acid) (A.S.A., Aspergum, Bayer, Ecotrin)
Aspirin (acetylsalicylic acid), buffered (Alka-Seltzer, Bufferin)

NONSTEROIDAL ANTIINFLAMMATORY DRUGS
Fenoprofen (Nalfon)
Flurbipofen (Ansaid)
Ibuprofen (Motrin, Advil, Nuprin, Medipren)
Ketoprofen (Orudis)
Naproxen (Anaprox, Naprosyn)
Oxaprozin (Daypro)

CYCLOOXYGENASE-2 INHIBITORS
Celecoxib (Celebrex)

OTHER NONSTEROIDAL ANTIINFLAMMATORY DRUGS
Diclofenac (Voltaren)
Diflunisal (Dolobid)
Etodolac (Lodine)
Indomethacin (Indocin)
Ketorolac tromethamine (Toradol)
Moloxicam (Mobic)
Nabumetone (Relafen)
Piroxicam (Feldene)
Sulindac (Clinoril)
Tolmetin (Tolectin)
Valdecoxib (Bextra)

BOX 66-16

Side Effects of Aspirin and Nonsteroidal Antiinflammatory Drugs

ASPIRIN
Dizziness
Drowsiness
Flushing
Gastrointestinal symptoms
Headaches
Tinnitus
Visual changes

NONSTEROIDAL ANTIINFLAMMATORY DRUGS
Blood dyscrasias
Dizziness
Gastric irritation
Hypotension
Pruritus
Sodium and water retention
Tinnitus

d. Assess the client for gastrointestinal upset during medication administration.

e. Monitor for edema.

f. Monitor serum salicylate (aspirin) level when the client is taking high doses.

g. Monitor for signs of bleeding such as tarry stools, bleeding gums, petechiae, ecchymosis, and purpura.

h. Instruct the client to take the medication with water, milk, or food.

i. Enteric-coated form or buffered form of aspirin can be taken to decrease gastric distress.

j. Instruct the client that enteric-coated tablets cannot be crushed or broken.

k. Advise the client to inform other health care professionals if they are taking high doses of aspirin.

l. Note that aspirin should be discontinued 3 to 7 days before surgery to reduce the risk of bleeding.

m. Instruct the client to avoid alcoholic beverages.

B. Acetaminophen (Tylenol)

1. Description

a. Acetaminophen inhibits prostaglandin synthesis.

b. Acetaminophen is used to decrease pain and fever.

c. Acetaminophen is contraindicated in hepatic or renal disease, alcoholism, and hypersensitivity.

2. Side effects

a. Anorexia, nausea, vomiting

b. Rash

c. Hypoglycemia

d. Oliguria

e. Hepatotoxicity

3. Interventions

a. Monitor vital signs.

b. Assess client for history of liver dysfunction.

c. Monitor for hepatic damage, which includes nausea, vomiting, diarrhea, and abdominal pain.

d. Monitor liver enzyme tests.

e. Instruct the client that self-medication should not be used longer than 10 days for an adult and 5 days for a child.

f. Note that the antidote for acetaminophen is acetylcysteine (Mucomyst).

g. Evaluate for the effectiveness of the medication.

VI. NARCOTIC ANALGESICS

A. Description

1. Narcotic analgesics suppress pain impulses but can suppress respiration and coughing by acting on the respiratory and cough center in the medulla of the brainstem.

2. Narcotic analgesics can produce euphoria and sedation.

3. Narcotic analgesics can cause physical dependence.

4. Narcotic analgesics are used for relief of mild, moderate, or severe pain.

B. Medications (Box 66-17)

1. Codeine sulfate

a. Codeine sulfate also is an effective cough suppressant at low doses.

b. Codeine sulfate can cause constipation.

2. Hydromorphone hydrochloride (Dilaudid)

a. Hydromorphone can decrease respiration.

b. Hydromorphone can cause constipation.

3. Meperidine hydrochloride (Demerol)

a. Meperidine can cause hypotension, dizziness, urinary retention.

b. Meperidine is used for acute pain and as a preoperative medication.

c. Meperidine can increase intracranial pressure in head injuries.

d. Meperidine is contraindicated in clients with head injuries and **increased intracranial pressure**, respiratory disorders, hypotension, shock, and severe hepatic and renal disease and in clients taking monoamine oxidase inhibitors.

e. Meperidine should not be taken with alcohol or sedative hypnotics because it may increase the CNS depression.

4. Morphine sulfate

a. Morphine can cause respiratory depression, orthostatic hypotension, and constipation.

b. Morphine may cause nausea and vomiting because of increased vestibular sensitivity.

c. Morphine is used for acute pain caused by myocardial infarction or cancer, for dyspnea

---

BOX 66-17

Narcotic (Opioid) Analgesics

Buprenorphine hydrochloride (Buprenex)
Butorphanol tartrate (Stadol, Stadol NS)
Codeine sulfate, codeine phosphate
Dezocine (Dalgan)
Fentanyl (Duragesic, Sublimaze)
Hydrocodone (Hycodan)
Hydromorphone hydrochloride (Dilaudid, Hydrostat IR, PMS-Hydromorphone)
Levorphanol tartrate (Levo-Dromoran)
Meperidine hydrochloride (Demerol)
Methadone hydrochloride (Dolophine)
Morphine sulfate
Nalbuphine hydrochloride (Nubain)
Oxycodone (Roxicodone)
Oxycodone hydrochloride with acetaminophen (Percocet)
Oxycodone with aspirin (Percodan)
Oxymorphone hydrochloride (Numorphan)
Pentazocine (Talwin)
Propoxyphene napsylate (Darvon-N)

caused by pulmonary edema, and as a preoperative medication.

   d. Morphine is contraindicated in severe respiratory disorders, head injuries, **increased intracranial pressure,** severe renal disease, or seizure activity.

   e. Morphine is used with caution in clients with shock or blood loss.

5. Oxycodone with aspirin (Percodan)

   a. Percodan should not be taken by a client allergic to aspirin.

   b. Percodan can cause gastric irritation and should be taken with food or plenty of liquids.

6. Propoxyphene hydrochloride (Darvon) and propoxyphene napsylate (Darvon-N)

   a. Darvon compound contains aspirin and should not be taken by a client allergic to aspirin.

   b. Darvocet-N contains acetaminophen.

7. Nalbuphine hydrochloride (Nubain) is preferable for treating the pain of an myocardial infarction because it reduces the oxygen needs of the heart without reducing blood pressure.

8. Methadone hydrochloride (Dolophine)

   a. Dilute doses of oral concentrate with at least 90 mL of water.

   b. Dilute dispersible tablets in at least 120 mL of water, orange juice, or acidic fruit beverage.

   c. Methadone is used as a replacement medication for opiate dependence or to facilitate withdrawal.

9. Hydrocodone (Hycodan) frequently is used for cough suppression.

C. Interventions for narcotic analgesics

1. Monitor vital signs.

2. Assess the client thoroughly before administering pain medication.

3. Initiate nursing measures such as massage, distraction, deep breathing and relaxation exercises, the application of heat or cold as prescribed, and providing care and comfort before administering the narcotic analgesic.

4. Administer medications 30 to 60 minutes before painful activities.

5. Monitor respiratory rate, and if the rate is less than 12 breaths per minute in an adult, withhold the medication unless ventilatory support is being provided.

6. Monitor pulse, and if bradycardia develops, hold the dose and notify the physician.

7. Monitor blood pressure for hypotension.

8. Auscultate breath sounds because narcotic analgesics suppress the cough reflex.

9. Encourage activities such as turning, deep breathing, and incentive spirometry to prevent atelectasis and pneumonia.

10. Monitor level of consciousness.

11. Initiate safety precautions such as side rails, a night light, and supervised ambulation.

12. Monitor intake and output.

13. Assess for urinary retention.

14. Instruct the client to take oral doses with milk or a snack to reduce gastric irritation.

15. Instruct the client to avoid alcohol.

16. Instruct the client to avoid activities that require alertness.

17. Note effectiveness of medication.

18. Have the narcotic antagonist, oxygen, and resuscitation equipment available.

D. Morphine sulfate

1. Side effects

   a. Respiratory depression

   b. Orthostatic hypotension

   c. Urinary retention

   d. Nausea

   e. Vomiting

   f. Constipation

   g. Cough suppression

   h. Reduction in pupillary size

   i. Miosis

2. Interventions

   a. Have naxolone (Narcan) available for overdose.

   b. Assess vital signs.

   c. Note rate and depth of respirations.

   d. Withhold the medication if the respiratory rate is less than 12 breaths per minute; respirations of less than 10 breaths per minute can indicate respiratory distress.

   e. Monitor urinary output, which should be at least 30 mL per hour.

   f. Monitor bowel sounds for decreased peristalsis because constipation can occur.

   g. Monitor for pupil changes because pinpoint pupils can indicate morphine overdose.

   h. Avoid alcohol or CNS depressants because they can cause respiratory depression.

   i. Instruct the client to report dizziness or difficulty breathing.

   j. To administer morphine intravenously, dilute in at least 5 mL of sterile water for injection and administer at a rate of 15 mg or less over 4 to 5 minutes.

E. Meperidine hydrochloride (Demerol)

1. Side effects

   a. Respiratory depression

   b. Hypotension

   c. Tachycardia

   d. Drowsiness

   e. Constipation

   f. Urinary retention

   g. Nausea

   h. Vomiting

   i. Tremors

2. Interventions

   a. Monitor vital signs.

b. Monitor for respiratory depression and hypotension.

c. Have naloxone (Narcan) available for overdose.

d. Monitor for urinary retention.

e. Monitor bowel sounds and for constipation.

f. To administer meperidine intravenously, dilute in at least 5 mL of sterile water or normal saline for injection and administer the dose over 4 to 5 minutes.

VII. NARCOTIC ANTAGONISTS (BOX 66-18)

A. Narcotic antagonists are used to treat respiratory depression from narcotic overdose.

B. Interventions

1. Monitor blood pressure, pulse, and respiratory rate every 5 minutes initially, tapering to every 15 minutes, and then every 30 minutes until client is stable.

2. Place the client on a cardiac monitor and monitor cardiac rhythm.

3. Auscultate breath sounds.

4. Have resuscitation equipment available.

5. Do not leave the client unattended.

6. Monitor the client closely for several hours because when the effects of the antagonist wears off, the client may again display signs of narcotic overdose.

VIII. OSMOTIC DIURETICS (BOX 66-19)

A. Description

1. Osmotic diuretics increase osmotic pressure of the glomerular filtrate, inhibiting reabsorption of water and electrolytes.

2. Osmotic diuretics are used for oliguria and to prevent renal failure.

3. Osmotic diuretics are used to decrease intracranial pressure.

4. Osmotic diuretics are used to decrease intraocular pressure in narrow-angle glaucoma.

5. Mannitol is used with chemotherapy to induce diuresis.

B. Side effects

1. Fluid and electrolyte imbalances

BOX 66-18

Narcotic Antagonists

Nalmefene (Revex)
Naloxone hydrochloride (Narcan)
Naltrexone (ReVia)

BOX 66-19

Osmotic Diuretics

Mannitol (Osmitrol)
Urea (Ureaphil)

---

2. Pulmonary edema from the rapid shifts of fluid

3. Nausea and vomiting

4. Tachycardia from the rapid fluid loss

5. Hyponatremia and dehydration

C. Interventions

1. Monitor vital signs.

2. Monitor weight.

3. Monitor urine output.

4. Monitor electrolytes levels.

5. Monitor lungs and heart sounds for signs of pulmonary edema.

6. Monitor for signs of dehydration.

7. Monitor neurological status.

8. Assess for signs of decreasing intracranial pressure if appropriate.

9. Change the client's position slowly to prevent orthostatic hypotension.

10. Monitor for crystallization in the vial of mannitol before administering the medication; if crystallization is noted, do not administer the medication from that vial.

PRACTICE QUESTIONS

1. The nurse is caring for a client in the emergency room diagnosed with Bell's palsy. The client has been taking acetaminophen (Tylenol), and a Tylenol overdose is suspected. The nurse anticipates that the antidote to be prescribed is

   1. Auranofin (Ridaura).

   2. Fludarabine (Fludara).

   3. Acetylcysteine (Mucomyst).

   4. Pentostatin (Nipent).

2. The client with trigeminal neuralgia tells the nurse that acetaminophen (Tylenol) is taken daily for the relief of generalized discomfort. Which laboratory value would indicate toxicity associated with the medication?

   1. Platelet count of 400,000 cells/μL

   2. Direct bilirubin level of 2 mg/dL

   3. Prothrombin time of 12 seconds

   4. Sodium of 140 mEq/L

3. The client is suspected of having myasthenia gravis. Edrophonium (Tensilon) 2 mg is administered intravenously to determine the diagnosis. Which of the following indicates that the client has myasthenia gravis?

   1. An increase in muscle strength within 30 to 60 seconds following administration of the medication

   2. A decrease in muscle strength within 30 to 60 seconds following administration of the medication

   3. Joint pain following administration of the medication

   4. Feelings of faintness, dizziness, hypotension, and signs of flushing in the client

4. The client with myasthenia gravis becomes increasingly weaker. The physician prepares to identify whether

the client is reacting to an overdose of the medication (cholinergic crisis) or an increasing severity of the disease (myasthenic crisis). An injection of edrophonium (Tensilon) is administered. Which of the following would indicate that the client is in cholinergic crisis?

1. An improvement of the weakness
2. A temporary worsening of the condition
3. No change in the condition
4. Complaints of muscle spasms

5. The client with myasthenia gravis verbalizes complaints of feeling much weaker than normal. The physician plans to implement a diagnostic test to determine whether the client is experiencing a myasthenic crisis. The physician administers edrophonium (Tensilon). Which of the following would indicate that the client is experiencing a myasthenic crisis?

1. Increasing weakness
2. No change in the condition
3. A temporary improvement in the condition
4. An increase in muscle spasms

6. Carbidopa-levodopa (Sinemet) is prescribed for the client with Parkinson's disease. The nurse monitors the client for adverse reactions to the medication. Which of the following would indicate that the client is experiencing an adverse reaction?

1. Pruritus
2. Hypertension
3. Tachycardia
4. Impaired voluntary movements

7. Phenytoin (Dilantin), 100 mg PO 3 times daily, has been prescribed for the client for seizure control. The home health nurse visits the client and provides teaching regarding the medication. Which of the following statements, if made by the client, would indicate effective teaching?

1. "It's okay to break the capsules to make it easier for me to swallow them."
2. "I will use a soft toothbrush to brush my teeth."
3. "If I forget to take my medication, I can wait until the next dose and eliminate that dose."
4. "If my throat becomes sore, it's a normal effect of the medication, and it's nothing to be concerned about."

8. The client is taking phenytoin (Dilantin) for seizure control. A serum drug level is drawn, and the nurse reviews the results. Which of the following would indicate a therapeutic serum drug range?

1. 5 to 10 mcg/mL
2. 10 to 20 mcg/mL
3. 20 to 30 mcg/mL
4. 30 to 40 mcg/mL

9. The nurse is preparing an intravenous infusion of phenytoin (Dilantin) as prescribed by the physician for the client with seizures. Which of the following solutions will the nurse plan to use to dilute this medication?

1. Lactated Ringer's solution
2. 5% dextrose
3. 5% dextrose and ½ normal saline
4. Normal saline solution

10. The home health nurse visits a client who is taking phenytoin (Dilantin) for control of seizures. During the assessment, the nurse notes that the client is taking birth control pills. Which of the following information should the nurse include in the teaching plan?

1. The increased risk of thrombophlebitis while taking phenytoin and birth control pills together
2. The potential decreased effectiveness of the birth control pills while taking phenytoin
3. That the client may stop the medication if it is causing severe gastrointestinal effects
4. That pregnancy should be avoided while taking phenytoin

11. A client with trigeminal neuralgia is being treated with carbamazepine (Tegretol), 400 mg PO daily. Which of the following indicates that the client is experiencing an adverse reaction to the medication?

1. White blood cell count, 3000 cells/μL
2. Blood urea nitrogen, 15 mg/dL
3. Sodium, 140 mEq/L
4. Uric acid, 5 mg/dL

12. The nurse is caring for a client receiving morphine sulfate 10 mg subcutaneously every 4 hours for pain. Because this medication has been prescribed for this client, which nursing action would be included in the plan of care?

1. Monitor the client's temperature.
2. Encourage fluids.
3. Maintain the client in a supine position.
4. Encourage the client to cough and deep breathe.

13. Meperidine hydrochloride (Demerol) is prescribed for the client with pain. Which of the following would the nurse monitor for as a side effect of this medication?

1. Hypertension
2. Bradycardia
3. Diarrhea
4. Urinary retention

14. The nurse is caring for a client with severe back pain. Codeine sulfate has been prescribed for the client. Which of the following does the nurse specifically include in the plan of care while the client is taking this medication?

1. Monitor for hypertension.
2. Monitor fluid balance.
3. Monitor bowel activity.
4. Monitor peripheral pulses.

15. Dantrolene (Dantrium) is prescribed for a client with spinal cord injury for discomfort caused by spasticity. Which of the following laboratory values would the nurse monitor while the client is taking this medication?

1. Sedimentation rate
2. White blood cell count
3. Liver function studies
4. Creatinine

16. The client with epilepsy is taking the prescribed dose of phenytoin (Dilantin) to control seizures. Results of a phenytoin blood level study reveal a level of 35 mcg/mL. Which of the following symptoms would be expected as a result of this laboratory result?
    1. No symptoms because this is a normal therapeutic level
    2. Slurred speech
    3. Tachycardia
    4. Nystagmus

17. Mannitol (Osmitrol) is prescribed for the client with increased intracranial pressure following a head injury. The nurse prepares to administer this medication knowing that the therapeutic action is to
    1. Induce diuresis by raising the osmotic pressure of glomerular filtrate, thereby inhibiting tubular reabsorption of water and solutes.
    2. Induce diuresis by promoting the reabsorption of sodium and water in the loop of Henle.
    3. Prevent the filtration of sodium and water through the kidneys.
    4. Prevent the filtration of sodium and potassium through the kidneys.

18. Dexamethasone (Decadron) IV is prescribed for the client with cerebral edema. The nurse prepares the medication for administration and plans to
    1. Mix the medication in 100 mL of lactated Ringer's solution.
    2. Mix the medication in 1000 mL of 5% dextrose.

3. Prepare an undiluted direct injection of the medication.
4. Dilute the medication in lactated Ringer's solution and administer as a direct injection.

19. The client arrives at the emergency department complaining of back spasms. The client states, "I have been taking two to three aspirin every 4 hours for the last week, and it hasn't helped my back." Aspirin intoxication is suspected, and the nurse assesses the client for which of the following?
    1. Diarrhea
    2. Constipation
    3. Tinnitus
    4. Photosensitivity

20. A client with multiple sclerosis is receiving diazepam (Valium), a centrally acting skeletal muscle relaxant. Which of the following, if noted during assessment of the client, would indicate that the client is experiencing a side effect related to this medication?
    1. Headache
    2. Increased salivation
    3. Urinary retention
    4. Drowsiness

CRITICAL THINKING: FILL IN THE BLANK

The client with myasthenia gravis is receiving pyridostigmine (Mestinon), and the nurse is monitoring the client for signs and symptoms of cholinergic crisis that can occur because of overdose of the medication. The nurse plans to have the antidote for cholinergic crisis available and obtains which medication from the pharmacy?

Answer: _____

ANSWERS

1. **3**

Rationale: The antidote for acetaminophen is acetylcysteine (Mucomyst). The normal therapeutic serum level of acetaminophen is 10 to 20 mcg/mL. A toxic level is greater than 50 mcg/mL, and levels of greater than 200 mcg/mL could indicate hepatotoxicity. Auranofin (Ridaura) is a gold preparation used to treat rheumatoid arthritis. Fludarabine (Fludara) and pentostatin (Nipent) are antineoplastic agents.

Test-Taking Strategy: Use the process of elimination. Eliminate options 2 and 4 first because they are similar (antineoplastic agents). Recalling that auranofin is used to treat rheumatoid arthritis will direct you to option 3. Review the antidote for acetaminophen if you had difficulty with this question.

Level of Cognitive Ability: Analysis
Client Needs: Physiological Integrity
Integrated Process: Nursing Process—analysis
Content Area: Pharmacology
References: Kee, J., & Hayes, E. (2003). *Pharmacology: A nursing process approach* (4th ed., p. 264). Philadelphia: W. B. Saunders.

Lehne, R. (2001). *Pharmacology for nursing care* (4th ed., p. 777). Philadelphia: W. B. Saunders.

2. **2**

Rationale: In adults, overdose of acetaminophen causes liver damage. Option 2 is an indicator of liver function and is the only option that indicates an abnormal laboratory value. The normal direct bilirubin is 0 to 0.3 mg/dL. The normal platelet count is 150,000 to 400,000 cells/μL. The normal prothrombin time is 10 to 13 seconds. The normal sodium is 135 to 145 mEq/L.

Test-Taking Strategy: Use the process of elimination. Knowledge that acetaminophen causes liver damage and knowledge of normal laboratory results will assist you in answering this question. Option 2 is the only abnormal value. Also, of all of the options the bilirubin is the most directly related laboratory value to liver function. Review the effects of toxicity from acetaminophen and normal laboratory values if you had difficulty with this question.

Level of Cognitive Ability: Analysis
Client Needs: Physiological Integrity

Integrated Process: Nursing Process—analysis
Content Area: Pharmacology
References: Hodgson, B., & Kizior, R. (2004). *Saunders nursing drug handbook 2004* (p. 8). Philadelphia: W. B. Saunders.
Kee, J., & Hayes, E. (2003). *Pharmacology: A nursing process approach* (4th ed., pp. 264, 261). Philadelphia: W. B. Saunders.

3. 1
Rationale: Edrophonium is a short-acting acetylcholinesterase inhibitor used as a diagnostic agent. When a client with suspected myasthenia gravis is given 2 mg of the medication intravenously, an increase in muscle strength should be seen in 30 to 60 seconds. If no response occurs, another 4 to 10 mg of edrophonium is given over the next 2 minutes, and muscle strength is tested again. If no increase in muscle strength occurs with this higher dose, the muscle weakness is not caused by myasthenia gravis. Clients receiving injections of this medication commonly demonstrate a drop in blood pressure, feel faint and dizzy, and are flushed.
Test-Taking Strategy: Use the process of elimination. Recalling that the client with myasthenia gravis is treated with medication to improve muscle strength will assist in directing you to option 1. Review this medication as a diagnostic tool for suspected myasthenia gravis if you had difficulty with this question.
Level of Cognitive Ability: Analysis
Client Needs: Physiological Integrity
Integrated Process: Nursing Process—analysis
Content Area: Pharmacology
References: Gutierrez, K., & Queener, S. (2003). *Pharmacology for nursing practice* (p. 147). St. Louis: Mosby.
Lehne, R. (2001). *Pharmacology for nursing care* (4th ed., p. 128). Philadelphia: W. B. Saunders.

4. 2
Rationale: An edrophonium injection makes the client in cholinergic crisis temporarily worse. This in known as a negative Tensilon test.
Test-Taking Strategy: Use the process of elimination. Recalling that a cholinergic crisis indicates an overdose to medication, it seems reasonable that a worsening of the condition will occur when medication is administered. Review cholinergic crisis if you had difficulty with this question.
Level of Cognitive Ability: Analysis
Client Needs: Physiological Integrity
Integrated Process: Nursing Process—analysis
Content Area: Pharmacology
References: Gutierrez, K., & Queener, S. (2003). *Pharmacology for nursing practice* (p. 147). St. Louis: Mosby.
Lehne, R. (2001). *Pharmacology for nursing care* (4th ed., p. 129). Philadelphia: W. B. Saunders.

5. 3
Rationale: Edrophonium is administered to determine whether the client is reacting to an overdose of a medication (cholinergic crisis) or an increasing severity of the disease (myasthenic crisis). When the edrophonium injection is given and the condition improves temporarily, the client is in myasthenic crisis. This is known as a positive Tensilon test.
Test-Taking Strategy: Use the process of elimination. Recall that myasthenic crisis is treated with medication. It seems

reasonable then that the client's condition will improve when medication is administered. Review this diagnostic test and the differences between cholinergic and myasthenic crisis if you had difficulty with this question.
Level of Cognitive Ability: Analysis
Client Needs: Physiological Integrity
Integrated Process: Nursing Process—analysis
Content Area: Pharmacology
References: Gutierrez, K., & Queener, S. (2003). *Pharmacology for nursing practice* (p. 307). St. Louis: Mosby.
Lehne, R. (2001). *Pharmacology for nursing care* (4th ed., p. 129). Philadelphia: W. B. Saunders.

6. 4
Rationale: Dyskinesia and impaired voluntary movement may occur with high levodopa dosages. Nausea, anorexia, dizziness, orthostatic hypotension, bradycardia, and akinesia (the temporary muscle weakness that lasts 1 minute to 1 hour, also know as "on-off phenomena") is a frequent side effect of the medication.
Test-Taking Strategy: Use the process of elimination. Options 2 and 3 are similar and are cardiac related options, so these options can be eliminated first. Note that the question asks for an adverse reaction; therefore select option 4 over option 1 because it is related neurologically. Review the adverse effects of levodopa if you had difficulty with this question.
Level of Cognitive Ability: Analysis
Client Needs: Physiological Integrity
Integrated Process: Nursing Process—analysis
Content Area: Pharmacology
Reference: Hodgson, B., & Kizior, R. (2004). *Saunders nursing drug handbook 2004* (pp. 150-151). Philadelphia: W. B. Saunders.

7. 2
Rationale: Phenytoin is an anticonvulsant. Gingival hyperplasia, bleeding, swelling, and tenderness of the gums can occur with the use of this medication. The client needs to be taught good oral hygiene, gum massage, and the need for regular dentist visits. The client should not skip medication doses because this could precipitate a seizure. Capsules should not be chewed or broken, and they must be swallowed. The client needs to be instructed to report a sore throat, fever, glandular swelling, or any skin reaction because this indicates hematological toxicity.
Test-Taking Strategy: Use the process of elimination. Note the key words "indicate effective teaching." Eliminate option 3 because the client needs to be encouraged to take medications on time. Also, eliminate option 4 because the client needs to report these symptoms to the physician. Remember, capsules should not be broken. Review the client teaching points related to phenytoin if you had difficulty with this question.
Level of Cognitive Ability: Analysis
Client Needs: Physiological Integrity
Integrated Process: Teaching/Learning
Content Area: Pharmacology
Reference: Kee, J., & Hayes, E. (2003). *Pharmacology: A nursing process approach* (4th ed., p. 285). Philadelphia: W. B. Saunders.

8. 2
Rationale: The therapeutic serum drug level range for phenytoin is 10 to 20 mcg/mL.
Test-Taking Strategy: Use the process of elimination. A helpful Pyramid Point is to remember that the theophylline therapeutic range and the acetaminophen therapeutic range are the same as the phenytoin therapeutic range. Remembering this may assist you when answering questions related to these three medications. Review this medication if you had difficulty with this question.
Level of Cognitive Ability: Analysis
Client Needs: Physiological Integrity
Integrated Process: Nursing Process—analysis
Content Area: Pharmacology
References: Hodgson, B., & Kizior, R. (2004). *Saunders nursing drug handbook 2004* (p. 806). Philadelphia: W. B. Saunders. Kee, J., & Hayes, E. (2003). *Pharmacology: A nursing process approach* (4th ed., p. 283). Philadelphia: W. B. Saunders.

9. 4
Rationale: Intravenous infusion of phenytoin should be administered by injection into a large vein. The medication may be diluted in normal saline solution; however, dextrose solution should be avoided because of medication precipitation. The medication is administered as intermittent doses. Continuous intravenous infusions should not be used. Infusion rates of more than 50 mg/min may cause hypotension or cardiac dysrhythmias, especially in older and debilitated clients.
Test-Taking Strategy: Use the process of elimination. In most, but not all, situations, medications can be diluted in normal saline, so this would be the best option to select if you were unfamiliar with the intravenous administration of this medication. Review this procedure if you had difficulty with this question.
Level of Cognitive Ability: Application
Client Needs: Physiological Integrity
Integrated Process: Nursing Process—planning
Content Area: Pharmacology
Reference: Hodgson, B., & Kizior, R. (2004). *Saunders nursing drug handbook 2004* (p. 806). Philadelphia: W. B. Saunders.

10. 2
Rationale: Phenytoin enhances the rate of estrogen metabolism, which can decrease the effectiveness of some birth control pills. Options 1, 3, and 4 are inappropriate instructions.
Test-Taking Strategy: Use the process of elimination. Option 1 would cause anxiety in the client. A client should not be instructed to stop anticonvulsant medication, as indicated in option 3. Pregnancy does not need to be "avoided." Review medication interactions related to phenytoin if you had difficulty with this question.
Level of Cognitive Ability: Application
Client Needs: Health Promotion and Maintenance
Integrated Process: Teaching/Learning
Content Area: Pharmacology
Reference: Lehne, R. (2001). *Pharmacology for nursing care* (4th ed., p. 696). Philadelphia: W. B. Saunders.

11. 1
Rationale: Adverse effects of carbamazepine appear as blood dyscrasias, including aplastic anemia, agranulocytosis,

thrombocytopenia, leukopenia, cardiovascular disturbances, thrombophlebitis, dysrhythmias, and dermatological effects.
Test-Taking Strategy: Use the process of elimination. If you are familiar with normal laboratory values, you will note that the only option that indicates an abnormal value is option 1. Review the signs of adverse reactions related to this medication if you had difficulty with this question.
Level of Cognitive Ability: Analysis
Client Needs: Physiological Integrity
Integrated Process: Nursing Process—analysis
Content Area: Pharmacology
Reference: Lehne, R. (2001). *Pharmacology for nursing care* (4th ed., p. 203). Philadelphia: W. B. Saunders.

12. 4
Rationale: Morphine sulfate suppresses the cough reflex. Clients need to be encouraged to cough and deep breath to prevent pneumonia. Options 1, 2, and 3 are not associated specifically with the use of this medication.
Test-Taking Strategy: Use the process of elimination. The question is asking specifically about a nursing action related to this medication. Recalling that morphine sulfate suppresses the cough reflex and the respiratory reflex will direct you to the correct option. Additionally, use the ABCs—airway, breathing, and circulation—when selecting the correct option. Review the nursing considerations when administering this medication if you had difficulty with this question.
Level of Cognitive Ability: Application
Client Needs: Physiological Integrity
Integrated Process: Nursing Process—planning
Content Area: Pharmacology
Reference: Hodgson, B., & Kizior, R. (2004). *Saunders nursing drug handbook 2004* (p. 692). Philadelphia: W. B. Saunders.

13. 4
Rationale: Side effects of this medication include respiratory depression, orthostatic hypotension, tachycardia, drowsiness and mental clouding, constipation, and urinary retention.
Test-Taking Strategy: Use the process of elimination. You must know the side effects associated with specific narcotic analgesics to answer the question. Review the side effects of this medication if you had difficulty with this question.
Level of Cognitive Ability: Analysis
Client Needs: Physiological Integrity
Integrated Process: Nursing Process—assessment
Content Area: Pharmacology
Reference: Hodgson, B., & Kizior, R. (2004). *Saunders nursing drug handbook 2004* (p. 636). Philadelphia: W. B. Saunders.

14. 3
Rationale: While the client is taking codeine sulfate, the nurse would monitor vital signs and assess for hypotension. The nurse also should increase fluid intake, palpate the bladder for urinary retention, auscultate bowel sounds, and monitor the pattern of daily bowel activity and stool consistency. The nurse should monitor respiratory status and initiate deep breathing and coughing exercises. Additionally, the nurse monitors the effectiveness of the pain medication.
Test-Taking Strategy: Use the process of elimination. Note the key word "specifically" and recall that codeine sulfate can

cause constipation. If you had difficulty with this question, review nursing measures related to the administration of codeine sulfate.
Level of Cognitive Ability: Application
Client Needs: Physiological Integrity
Integrated Process: Nursing Process—planning
Content Area: Pharmacology
References: Kee, J., & Hayes, E. (2003). *Pharmacology: A nursing process approach* (4th ed., pp. 239, 269). Philadelphia: W. B. Saunders.
Lehne, R. (2001). *Pharmacology for nursing care* (4th ed., p. 271). Philadelphia: W. B. Saunders.

15. 3
Rationale: Dantrolene can cause liver damage, and the nurse should monitor the liver function studies. Baseline liver function studies are done before therapy starts, and regular liver function studies are performed throughout therapy. Dantrolene is discontinued if no relief of spasticity is achieved in 6 weeks.
Test-Taking Strategy: Use the process of elimination. Knowledge that this medication is hepatotoxic will direct you to the correct option. If you had difficulty with this question, review the adverse effects of this medication.
Level of Cognitive Ability: Analysis
Client Needs: Physiological Integrity
Integrated Process: Nursing Process—assessment
Content Area: Pharmacology
Reference: Lehne, R. (2001). *Pharmacology for nursing care* (4th ed., p. 217). Philadelphia: W. B. Saunders.

16. 2
Rationale: The therapeutic phenytoin level is 10 to 20 mcg/mL. At greater than 20 mcg/mL, involuntary movements of the eyeballs (nystagmus) appears. At greater than 30 mcg/mL, ataxia and slurred speech occur.
Test-Taking Strategy: Use the process of elimination and knowledge regarding the therapeutic phenytoin level. From this point, you must know the symptoms that would be noted in the client when the phenytoin level is 35 mcg/mL. Review therapeutic levels and associated symptoms if you had difficulty with this question.
Level of Cognitive Ability: Analysis
Client Needs: Physiological Integrity
Integrated Process: Nursing Process—assessment
Content Area: Pharmacology
Reference: Hodgson, B., & Kizior, R. (2004). *Saunders nursing drug handbook 2004* (p. 807). Philadelphia: W. B. Saunders.

17. 1
Rationale: Mannitol is an osmotic diuretic that induces diuresis by raising the osmotic pressure of glomerular filtrate, thereby inhibiting tubular reabsorption of water and solutes. Mannitol is used to reduce intracranial pressure in the client with head trauma.
Test-Taking Strategy: Use the process of elimination. Read the question carefully, noting that it identifies a client with increased intracranial pressure. The only option that suggests an action that will produce diuresis and thus reduce intracranial pressure is option 1. If you had difficulty with this question, review the action of mannitol.

Level of Cognitive Ability: Analysis
Client Needs: Physiological Integrity
Integrated Process: Nursing Process—analysis
Content Area: Pharmacology
Reference: Hodgson, B., & Kizior, R. (2004). *Saunders nursing drug handbook 2004* (p. 625). Philadelphia: W. B. Saunders.

18. 3
Rationale: Dexamethasone may be given by direct intravenous injection or intravenous infusion. Dexamethasone may be mixed with 0.9% sodium chloride or 5% dextrose. If administered as an infusion, a minimum amount of diluting solution is needed.
Test-Taking Strategy: Use the process of elimination. Eliminate option 2 because 1000 mL of solution is a large amount to use to dilute this medication, particularly in a client with cerebral edema. Eliminate options 1 and 4 because they are similar, addressing the use of lactated Ringer's solution. If you had difficulty with this question, review the administration of dexamethasone.
Level of Cognitive Ability: Application
Client Needs: Physiological Integrity
Integrated Process: Nursing Process—planning
Content Area: Pharmacology
References: Hodgson, B., & Kizior, R. (2004). *Saunders nursing drug handbook 2004* (p. 291). Philadelphia: W. B. Saunders.
Kee, J., & Hayes, E. (2003). *Pharmacology: A nursing process approach* (4th ed., p. 728). Philadelphia: W. B. Saunders.

19. 3
Rationale: Mild intoxication with acetylsalicylic acid (aspirin) is called salicylism and is experienced commonly when the daily dosage is more than 4 g. Tinnitus (ringing in the ears) is the most frequent effect noted with intoxication. Hyperventilation may occur because salicylate stimulates the respiratory center. Fever may result because salicylate interferes with the metabolic pathways coupling oxygen consumption and heat production. Options 1, 2, and 4 are not associated specifically with toxicity.
Test-Taking Strategy: Use the process of elimination. Note that the question refers to aspirin intoxication. Option 1 and 2 relate to gastrointestinal symptoms, are similar, and are eliminated first. From the remaining options, you must know that tinnitus occurs. If you had difficulty with this question, review aspirin intoxication.
Level of Cognitive Ability: Analysis
Client Needs: Physiological Integrity
Integrated Process: Nursing Process—assessment
Content Area: Pharmacology
Reference: Hodgson, B., & Kizior, R. (2004). *Saunders nursing drug handbook 2004* (p. 76). Philadelphia: W. B. Saunders.

20. 4
Rationale: Incoordination and drowsiness are common side effects resulting from this medication. Options 1, 2, and 3 are unrelated to the use of this medication.
Test-Taking Strategy: Use the process of elimination. Note that the question addresses a centrally acting skeletal muscle relaxant. This will assist in directing you to option 4. If you had difficulty with this question, review the side effects associated with diazepam (Valium).

Level of Cognitive Ability: Analysis
Client Needs: Physiological Integrity
Integrated Process: Nursing Process—assessment
Content Area: Pharmacology
Reference: Hodgson, B., & Kizior, R. (2004). *Saunders nursing drug handbook 2004* (p. 300). Philadelphia: W. B. Saunders.

CRITICAL THINKING: FILL IN THE BLANK

Answer: Atropine sulfate
Rationale: The antidote for cholinergic crisis is atropine sulfate.

Test-Taking Strategy: Recall that atropine sulfate is an anticholinergic agent. Because the client is at risk for cholinergic crisis, it would seem reasonable that the antidote would have to contain anticholinergic properties. If you are unfamiliar with cholinergic crisis and its antidote, review this information.
Level of Cognitive Ability: Application
Client Needs: Physiological Integrity
Integrated Process: Nursing Process—planning
Content Area: Pharmacology
Reference: Hodgson, B., & Kizior, R. (2004). *Saunders nursing drug handbook 2004* (p. 300). Philadelphia: W. B. Saunders.

REFERENCES

Gutierrez, K., & Queener, S. (2003). *Pharmacology for nursing practice.* St. Louis: Mosby.

Hodgson, B., & Kizior, R. (2004). *Saunders nursing drug handbook 2004.* Philadelphia: W. B. Saunders.

Kee, J., & Hayes, E. (2003). *Pharmacology: A nursing process approach* (4th ed.). Philadelphia: W. B. Saunders.

Lehne, R. (2001). *Pharmacology for nursing care* (4th ed.). Philadelphia: W. B. Saunders.

McKenry, L., & Salerno, E. (2003). *Mosby's pharmacology in nursing* (21st ed.). St. Louis: Mosby.

UNIT XVII

The Adult Client with a Musculoskeletal Disorder

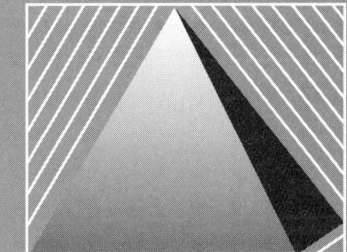

PYRAMID TERMS

casts Plaster or fiberglass mold that provides immobilization of bones and joints after a fracture or injury.

compartment syndrome Increased pressure within one or more compartments causing massive compromise of circulation to an area and causing irreversible neuromuscular damage within 4 to 6 hours of onset if not treated.

external fixation Stabilization of a fracture by the use of an external frame, with multiple pins applied through the bone.

fat embolism An arterial blockage that can occur 24 to 48 hours or within the first 72 hours following a fracture.

internal fixation Stabilization of a fracture that involves the application of screws, plates, pins, or nails to hold the fragments in alignment.

reduction The procedure that restores the bone to proper alignment.

traction Force applied in two directions to reduce and immobilize a fracture.

▶ PYRAMID TO SUCCESS

The Pyramid to Success focuses on the emergency care for a client who sustains a fracture or other musculoskeletal injury, monitoring for complications related to fractures, and interventions if complications occur. Nursing care related to casts and traction is emphasized. Skill related to instructing the client in the use of an assistive device such as a cane, a walker, or crutches is a Pyramid Point. Pyramid Points also include postoperative care following hip surgery or amputation and care of the client with rheumatoid arthritis or osteoporosis. Focus on the points related to the psychosocial effects as a result of the musculoskeletal disorder, such as unexpected body image changes, and the appropriate and available support services needed for the client. The Integrated Processes addressed in this unit include Nursing Process, Caring, Communication and Documentation, and Teaching/Learning.

CLIENT NEEDS
Safe, Effective Care Environment

Asepsis related to wounds
Client rights
Confidentiality regarding disorder and plan of care
Dietary consultation
Establishing priorities
Handling of hazardous and infectious materials
Informed consent for diagnostic treatments and surgical procedures
Physical therapy and occupational therapy referrals
Prevention of injury from accidents
Standard precautions

Health Promotion and Maintenance

Aging process and disease prevention
Expected body image changes
Health promotion related to diet and activity
Home care instructions regarding care related to musculoskeletal disorder
Physical assessment related to the musculoskeletal system
Reinforcement regarding the importance of prescribed therapy

Psychosocial Integrity

Ability to cope with feelings of isolation and loss of independence
Available support systems and use of community resources
Cultural, religious, and spiritual influences
Grief and loss related to mobility limitations and restrictions
Mobilization of coping mechanisms
Sensory and perceptual alterations

Situational role changes as a result of musculoskeletal disorder

Unexpected body image changes as a result of injury or disease

Physiological Integrity

Care related to casts and traction

Complications of a fracture

Complications related to procedures or injuries

Emergency care for a fracture or other injury

Measures to promote comfort

Pharmacological therapy

Postoperative interventions

Promotion of normal elimination patterns

Promotion of self-care measures

Use of assistive devices for mobility such as canes, walkers, and crutches

REFERENCES

Chernecky, C., & Berger, B. (2004). *Laboratory tests & diagnostic procedures* (4th ed.). Philadelphia: W. B. Saunders.

Harkreader, H., & Hogan, M. A. (2004). *Fundamentals of nursing: Caring and clinical judgment* (2nd ed.). Philadelphia: W. B. Saunders.

Ignatavicius, D., & Workman, M. (2002). *Medical-surgical nursing: Critical thinking for collaborative care* (4th ed.). Philadelphia: W. B. Saunders.

Lewis, S., Heitkemper, M., & Dirksen, S. (2004). *Medical-surgical nursing: Assessment and management of clinical problems* (6th ed.). St. Louis: Mosby.

National Council of State Boards of Nursing (Eds.). (2003). *Test Plan for the National Council Licensure Examination for Registered Nurses* (effective date: April 2004). Chicago: Author.

Perry, A., & Potter, P. (2002). *Clinical nursing skills and techniques* (5th ed.). St. Louis: Mosby.

Phipps, W., Monahan, F., Sands, J., Marek, J., & Neighbors, M. (2003). *Medical-surgical nursing: Health and illness perspectives* (7th ed.). St. Louis: Mosby.

Potter, P., & Perry, A. (2001). *Fundamentals of nursing* (5th ed.). St. Louis: Mosby.

Varcarolis, E. M. (2002). *Foundations of psychiatric mental health nursing* (4th ed.). Philadelphia: W. B. Saunders.

Musculoskeletal System

I. ANATOMY AND PHYSIOLOGY

A. Skeleton
1. Axial portion
   a. Cranium
   b. Vertebras
   c. Ribs
2. Appendicular portion
   a. Limbs
   b. Shoulders
   c. Hips

B. Types of bones (Box 67-1)
1. Spongy bone
   a. Spongy bone is located in the ends of long bones and the center of flat and irregular bones.
   b. Spongy bone can withstand forces applied in many directions.
2. Dense (compact) bone
   a. Dense bone covers spongy bone.
   b. Dense bone forms a cylinder around a central marrow cavity.
   c. Dense bone can withstand force predominantly in one direction.
3. Characteristics of the bones
   a. Bones support and protect structures of the body.
   b. Bones provide attachments for muscles, tendons, and ligaments.
   c. Bones contain tissue in the central cavities, which aids in the formation of blood cells.

d. Bones assist in regulating calcium and phosphate concentrations.
4. Bone growth
   a. The length of bone growth results from the ossification of the epiphyseal cartilage at the ends of bones, and bone growth stops between the ages of 18 and 25 years.
   b. The width of bone growth results from the activity of osteoblasts and occurs throughout life but does slow down with aging.
   c. As aging occurs, bone resorption accelerates, decreasing bone mass and predisposing the client to injury.

C. Types of joints (Table 67-1)
1. Characteristics of the joints
   a. Joints allow the movement between bones.
   b. Joints are formed where two bones join.
   c. Joint surfaces are covered with cartilage.
   d. Joints are enclosed in a capsule.
   e. Joints contain a cavity filled with synovial fluid.
   f. Ligaments hold the bone and joint in the correct position.
   g. Articulation is the meeting point of two or more bones.

BOX 67-1

Types of Bones

Long
Short
Flat
Irregular

TABLE 67-1

Types of Joints

Type	Description
Amphiarthrosis	Cartilaginous joints
	Slightly movable joints
Condyloid	Freely movable joints
	Allow frictionless, painless movement
Diarthrosis	Synovial joints
	Ball-and-socket joints
Synarthrosis	Fibrous or fixed joints
	No movement associated with these joints

2. Synovial fluid
   a. Synovial fluid is found in the joint capsule.
   b. Synovial fluid is formed by the synovial membrane, which lines the joint capsule.
   c. Synovial fluid lubricates the cartilage.
   d. Synovial fluid provides a cushion against shocks.
D. Muscles
   1. Characteristics of muscles
      a. Muscles are made up of bundles of muscle fibers.
      b. Muscles provide the force to move bones.
      c. Muscles assist in maintaining posture.
      d. Muscles assist with heat production.
   2. The process of contraction and relaxation
      a. Muscle contraction and relaxation require large amounts of adenosine triphosphate.
      b. Contraction also requires calcium, which functions as a catalyst.
      c. Acetylcholine released by the motor end plate of the motor neuron initiates an action potential.
      d. Acetylcholine then is destroyed by acetylcholinesterase.
      e. Calcium is required to contract muscle fibers and acts as a catalyst for the enzyme needed for the sliding together action of actin and myosin.
      f. Following contraction, adenosine triphosphate transports calcium out to allow actin and myosin to separate and allow the muscle to relax.
   3. Skeletal muscles
      a. Skeletal muscles are attached to two bones and cross at least one joint.
      b. The point of origin is the point of attachment on the bone closest to the trunk.
      c. The point of insertion is the point of attachment on the bone farthest from the trunk.
      d. Skeletal muscles act in groups.
      e. Prime movers contract to produce movement.
      f. Antagonists relax.
      g. Synergists contract to stabilize body movement.
      h. Nerves activate and control the muscles.

II. RISK FACTORS ASSOCIATED WITH MUSCULOSKELETAL DISORDERS (Box 67-2)

III. DIAGNOSTIC TESTS

A. Radiographs
   1. Description: Radiography is a commonly used procedure to diagnose disorders of the musculoskeletal system.
   2. Interventions
      a. Handle injured area carefully.
      b. Administer analgesics as prescribed before the procedure, particularly if the client is in pain.
      c. Remove any radiopaque objects, such as jewelry.
      d. Shield client's testes, ovaries, or pregnant abdomen.
      e. The client must lie still during a radiograph.

BOX 67-2

Risk Factors Associated with Musculoskeletal Disorders

Autoimmune disorders
Calcium deficiency
Degenerative conditions
Falls
Hyperuricemia
Infection
Medications
Metabolic disorders
Neoplastic disorders
Obesity
Postmenopausal states
Trauma and injury

---

   f. Inform the client that exposure to radiation is minimal and not dangerous.
   g. Health care provider is to wear a lead apron if staying in the room with the client.
B. Arthrocentesis
   1. Description
      a. Arthrocentesis involves aspirating synovial fluid, blood, or pus via a needle inserted into a joint cavity.
      b. Medication may be instilled into the joint if necessary to alleviate inflammation.
   2. Interventions
      a. Obtain an informed consent.
      b. Apply a compress bandage postprocedure as prescribed.
      c. Instruct the client to rest the joint for 8 to 24 hours postprocedure.
      d. Instruct the client to notify the physician if a fever or swelling of the joint occurs.
C. Arthrogram
   1. Description
      a. Arthrogram is a radiographic examination of the soft tissues of the joint structures and is used to diagnose trauma to the joint capsule or ligaments.
      b. A local anesthetic is used for the procedure.
      c. A contrast medium or air is injected into the joint cavity, and the joint is moved through range of motion as a series of x-ray films are taken.
   2. Interventions
      a. Instruct the client to fast from food and fluids for 8 hours before the procedure as prescribed.
      b. Assess the client for allergies to iodine or seafood before the procedure.
      c. Obtain an informed consent.
      d. Inform the client of the need to remain as still as possible, except when asked to reposition.
      e. Minimize the use of the joint for 12 hours after the procedure.
      f. Instruct the client that the joint may be edematous and tender for 1 to 2 days after the

procedure and may be treated with ice packs and analgesics as prescribed.

g. Instruct the client that if edema and tenderness last longer than 2 days to notify the physician.

h. If knee arthrography was performed, an Ace wrap over the knee may be prescribed for 3 to 4 days.

i. If air was used for injection, crepitus may be felt in the joint for up to 2 days.

D. Arthroscopy

1. Description

a. Arthroscopy provides an endoscopic examination of various joints.

b. Articular cartilage abnormalities can be assessed, loose bodies can be removed, and the cartilage can be trimmed.

c. A biopsy may be performed during the procedure.

2. Interventions

a. Instruct the client to fast for 8 to 12 hours before the procedure.

b. Obtain an informed consent.

c. Administer pain medication as prescribed postprocedure.

d. An elastic wrap should be worn for 2 to 4 days as prescribed postprocedure.

e. Instruct the client that walking without weight bearing usually is permitted after sensation returns but to limit activity for 1 to 4 days as prescribed following the procedure.

f. Instruct the client to elevate the extremity as often as possible for 2 days following the procedure and to place ice on the site to minimize swelling.

g. Reinforce instructions regarding the use of crutches, which may be used for 5 to 7 days postprocedure for walking.

h. Advise the client to notify the physician if fever or increased knee pain occurs or if edema continues for more than 3 days postprocedure.

E. Bone mineral density measurements

1. Dual energy x-ray absorptiometry

a. Dual energy x-ray absorptiometry measures bone mass of the spine, other bones, and the total body.

b. Radiation exposure is minimal.

c. Dual energy x-ray absorptiometry is used to diagnosis metabolic bone disease and to monitor changes in bone density with treatment.

d. Inform client that procedure is painless.

2. Quantitative ultrasound

a. Quantitative ultrasound evaluates strength, density, and elasticity of various bones using ultrasound rather than radiation.

b. Inform client that the procedure is painless.

F. Bone scan

1. Description

a. Radioisotope is injected intravenously and will collect in areas that indicate abnormal bone metabolism and some fractures, if they exist.

b. The isotope is excreted in the urine and feces within 48 hours and is not harmful to others.

2. Interventions

a. Hold fluids for 4 hours before the procedure.

b. Obtain an informed consent.

c. Remove all jewelry and metal objects.

d. Following the injection of the radioisotope, the client must drink 32 oz of water (if not contraindicated) to promote renal filtering of the excess isotope.

e. From 1 to 3 hours after the injection, have the client void, and then the scanning procedure is performed.

f. Inform the client of the need to lie supine during the procedure and that the procedure is not painful.

g. No special precautions are required after the procedure because a minimal amount of radioactivity exists in the radioisotope.

h. Monitor the injection site for redness and swelling.

i. Encourage oral fluid intake following the procedure.

G. Bone or muscle biopsy

1. Description: Biopsy may be done during surgery or through aspiration or punch or needle biopsy.

2. Interventions

a. Obtain an informed consent.

b. Monitor for bleeding, swelling, hematoma, or severe pain.

c. Elevate the site for 24 hours following the procedure to reduce edema.

d. Apply ice packs as prescribed following the procedure to prevent the development of a hematoma.

e. Monitor for signs of infection following the procedure.

f. Inform the client that mild to moderate discomfort is normal following the procedure.

H. Electromyography

1. Description

a. Electromyography measures electrical potential associated with skeletal muscle contractions.

b. Needles are inserted into the muscle, and recordings of muscular electrical activity are traced on recording paper through an oscilloscope.

2. Interventions

a. Obtain an informed consent.

b. Instruct the client that the needle insertion is uncomfortable.

c. Instruct the client not to take any stimulants or sedatives for 24 hours before the procedure.

d. Inform the client that slight bruising may occur at the needle insertion sites.

I. Myelogram
1. Description: A myelogram requires injection of dye or air into the subarachnoid space followed by radiography to detect abnormalities of the spinal cord and vertebras.
2. Preprocedure interventions
a. Obtain an informed consent.
b. Provide hydration for at least 12 hours before the test.
c. Assess client for allergies to iodine or seafood (shellfish).
d. Premedicate for sedation as prescribed.
3. Postprocedures interventions
a. Obtain vital signs and perform neurological assessment frequently as prescribed.
b. If a water-base dye is used, elevate the head 15 to 30 degrees for 8 hours as prescribed.
c. If an oil-base dye is used, keep the client flat 6 to 8 hours as prescribed.
d. If air is used, keep the head lower than the trunk.
e. Encourage fluids and monitor intake and output.

IV. **INJURIES**
A. Strains
1. Strains are an excessive stretching of a muscle or tendon.
2. Management involves cold and heat applications, exercise with activity limitations, antiinflammatory medications, and muscle relaxants.
3. Surgical repair may be required for a severe strain (ruptured muscle or tendon).
B. Sprains
1. Sprains are an excessive stretching of a ligament, usually caused by a twisting motion.
2. Sprains are characterized by pain and swelling.
3. Management involves rest, ice, and a compression bandage to reduce swelling and provide joint support.
4. Casting may be required for moderate sprains to allow the tear to heal.
5. Surgery may be necessary for severe ligament damage.
C. Rotator cuff injuries
1. Musculotendinous or rotator cuff of the shoulder sustains a tear, usually as a result of trauma.
2. Injury is characterized by shoulder pain and the inability to maintain abduction of the arm at the shoulder (drop arm test).
3. Management involves nonsteroidal antiinflammatory drugs (NSAIDs), physical therapy, sling support, and ice/heat applications.
4. Surgery may be required if medical management is unsuccessful or for those who have a complete tear.

V. **FRACTURES**
A. Description: A fracture is a break in the continuity of the bone caused by trauma, twisting as a result of

muscle spasm or indirect loss of leverage, or bone decalcification and disease that result in osteopenia.
B. Types of fractures (Box 67-3)
C. Assessment of a fracture of an extremity
1. Pain or tenderness over the involved area
2. Loss of function
3. Obvious deformity
4. Crepitation
5. Erythema, edema, ecchymosis
6. Muscle spasm and impaired sensation
D. Initial care of a fracture of an extremity
1. Immobilize affected extremity.
2. If a compound (open) fracture exists, splint the extremity and cover the wound with a sterile dressing.
E. Interventions for a fracture (Box 67-4)
F. **Reduction** restores the bone to proper alignment.
1. Closed **reduction**
a. Closed **reduction** is performed by manual manipulation.
b. Closed **reduction** may be performed under local or general anesthesia.
c. A **cast** may be applied following **reduction**.

BOX 67-3

Types of Fractures

Closed or simple: Skin over the fractured area remains intact.
Comminuted: The bone is splintered or crushed, with three or more fragments.
Complete: The bone is separated completely by a break into two parts.
Compression: A fractured bone is compressed by other bone.
Depressed: Bone fragments are driven inward.
Greenstick: One side of the bone is broken and the other is bent; these fractures occur most commonly in children.
Impacted: A part of the fractured bone is driven into another bone.
Incomplete: The bone is partially broken.
Oblique: The break extends in an oblique direction.
Open or compound: The bone is exposed to air through a break in the skin, and soft tissue injury and infection are common.
Pathological: The fracture results from weakening of the bone structure by pathological processes such as neoplasia or osteomalacia. Also called spontaneous fracture.
Spiral: The break partially encircles bone.
Transverse: The bone is fractured straight across.

BOX 67-4

Interventions for a Fracture

Reduction
Fixation
Traction
Casts

2. Open **reduction**
   a. Open **reduction** involves a surgical intervention.
   b. Fracture may be treated with **internal fixation** devices.
   c. The client may be placed in **traction** or a **cast** following the procedure.
G. Fixation
   1. **Internal fixation** (Fig. 67-1)
      a. **Internal fixation** follows open **reduction**.
      b. **Internal fixation** involves the application of screws, plates, pins, or nails to hold the fragments in alignment.
      c. **Internal fixation** may involve the removal of damaged bone and replacement with a prosthesis.

d. **Internal fixation** provides immediate bone strength.
   e. Risk of infection is associated with the procedure.
   2. **External fixation** (Fig. 67-2)
      a. An external frame is used with multiple pins applied through the bone.
      b. **External fixation** provides more freedom of movement than with **traction**.
H. **Traction** (Fig. 67-3)
   1. Description
      a. **Traction** is the exertion of a pulling force applied in two directions to reduce and immobilize a fracture.
      b. **Traction** provides proper bone alignment and reduces muscle spasms.

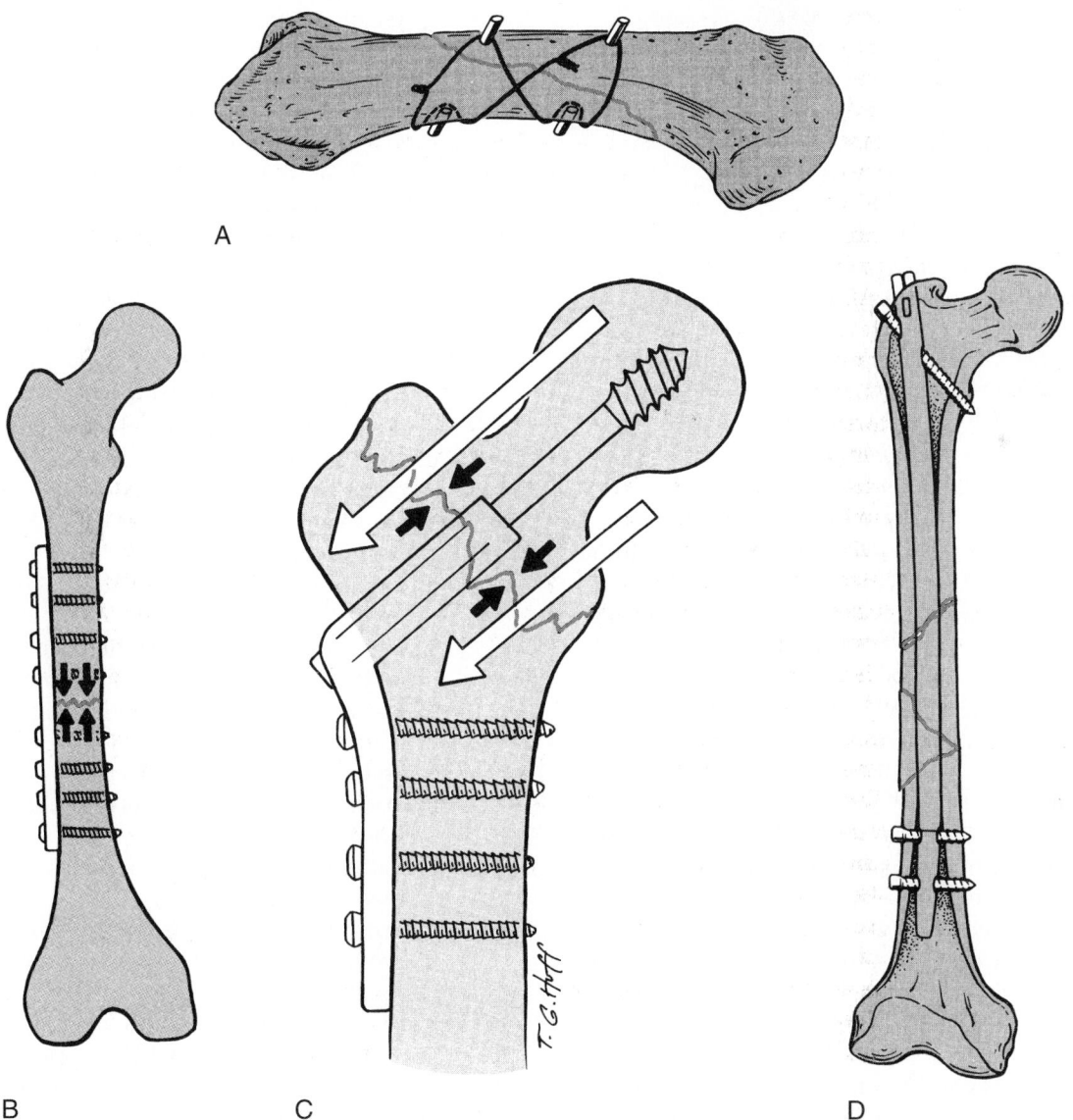

FIG. 67-1 Examples of internal fixation. **A,** Tension band wiring technique using Kirschner wires for fracture of a phalanx. **B,** Compression plate to the lateral aspect of the femur. **C,** Sliding hip screw. **D,** Static locked intramedullary and fixed to proximal and distal fragments of the femur. (From Browner, B. D., et al. [1992]. *Skeletal trauma.* Philadelphia: W. B. Saunders.)

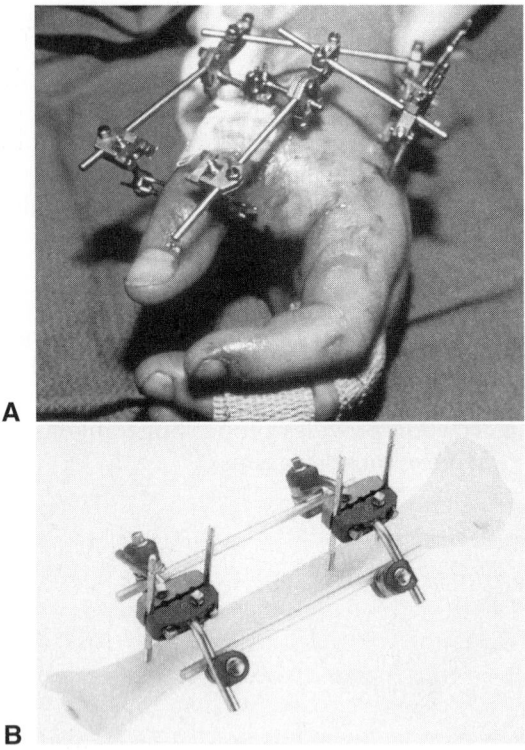

FIG. 67-2 External fixators. **A,** Mini-Hoffman system in use on hand. **B,** Hoffman II on the tibia (standard system). (From Lewis, S., Heitkemper, M., & Dirksen, S. [2004]. *Medical-surgical nursing: Assessment and management of clinical problems* [6th ed., p. 1644]. St. Louis: Mosby.

2. Interventions
   a. Maintain proper body alignment.
   b. Ensure that the weights hang freely and do not touch the floor.
   c. Do not remove or lift the weights without a physician's order
   d. Ensure that pulleys are not obstructed and that ropes in the pulleys move freely
   e. Place knots in the ropes to prevent slipping.
   f. Check the ropes for fraying.
I. Skeletal **traction** (Fig. 67-4)
   1. Description: **Traction** is applied mechanically to the bone with pins, wires, or tongs.
   2. Interventions
      a. Monitor color, motion, and sensation of the affected extremity.
      b. Monitor the insertion sites for redness, swelling, or drainage.
      c. Provide insertion site care as prescribed.
   3. Cervical tongs and a halo fixation device (Refer to Chapter 65 regarding care of the client with these types of devices.)
J. Skin **traction** (Box 67-5)
   1. Description: **Traction** is applied by the use of elastic bandages or adhesive.
   2. Cervical skin **traction** (Fig. 67-3)

a. Cervical skin **traction** relieves muscle spasms and compression in the upper extremities and neck.
   b. Cervical skin **traction** uses a head halter and a chin pad to attach the **traction**.
   c. Use powder to protect the ears from friction rub.
   d. Position the client with the head of the bed elevated 30 to 40 degrees, and attach the weights to a pulley system over the head of the bed.
3. Buck's (extension) skin **traction** (Fig. 67-3)
   a. Buck's skin **traction** is used to alleviate muscle spasms and immobilizes a lower limb by maintaining a straight pull on the limb with the use of weights.
   b. A boot appliance is applied to attach to the **traction**.
   c. Weight is attached to a pulley; allow the weights to hang freely over the edge of bed.
   d. Not more than 8 to 10 lb of weight should be applied.
   e. Elevate the foot of the bed to provide the **traction**.
4. Russell's skin **traction** (Refer to Chapter 43 regarding information related to these types of **traction**.)
5. Pelvic skin **traction** (Fig. 67-3)
   a. Pelvic skin **traction** is used to relieve low back, hip, or leg pain and to reduce muscle spasm.
   b. Apply the **traction** snugly over the pelvis and iliac crest and attach to the weights.
   c. Use measures as prescribed to prevent the client from slipping down in bed.
K. Balanced suspension **traction** (Fig. 67-3)
   1. Description
      a. Balanced suspension **traction** is used with skin or skeletal **traction**.
      b. Balanced suspension **traction** is used to approximate fractures of the femur, tibia, or fibula.
      c. Balanced suspension **traction** is produced by a counterforce other than client.
   2. Interventions
      a. Position the client in low Fowler's on either the side or the back.
      b. Maintain a 20-degree angle from the thigh to the bed.
      c. Protect the skin from breakdown.
      d. Provide pin care if pins are used with the skeletal **traction**.
      e. Clean the pin sites with sterile normal saline and hydrogen peroxide or povidone-iodine (Betadine) as prescribed or per agency procedure.
L. Dunlop's **traction**
   1. Description: Horizontal **traction** is used to align fractures of the humerus; vertical **traction** maintains the forearm in proper alignment.
   2. Interventions: Nursing care is similar to that for Buck's skin **traction**.

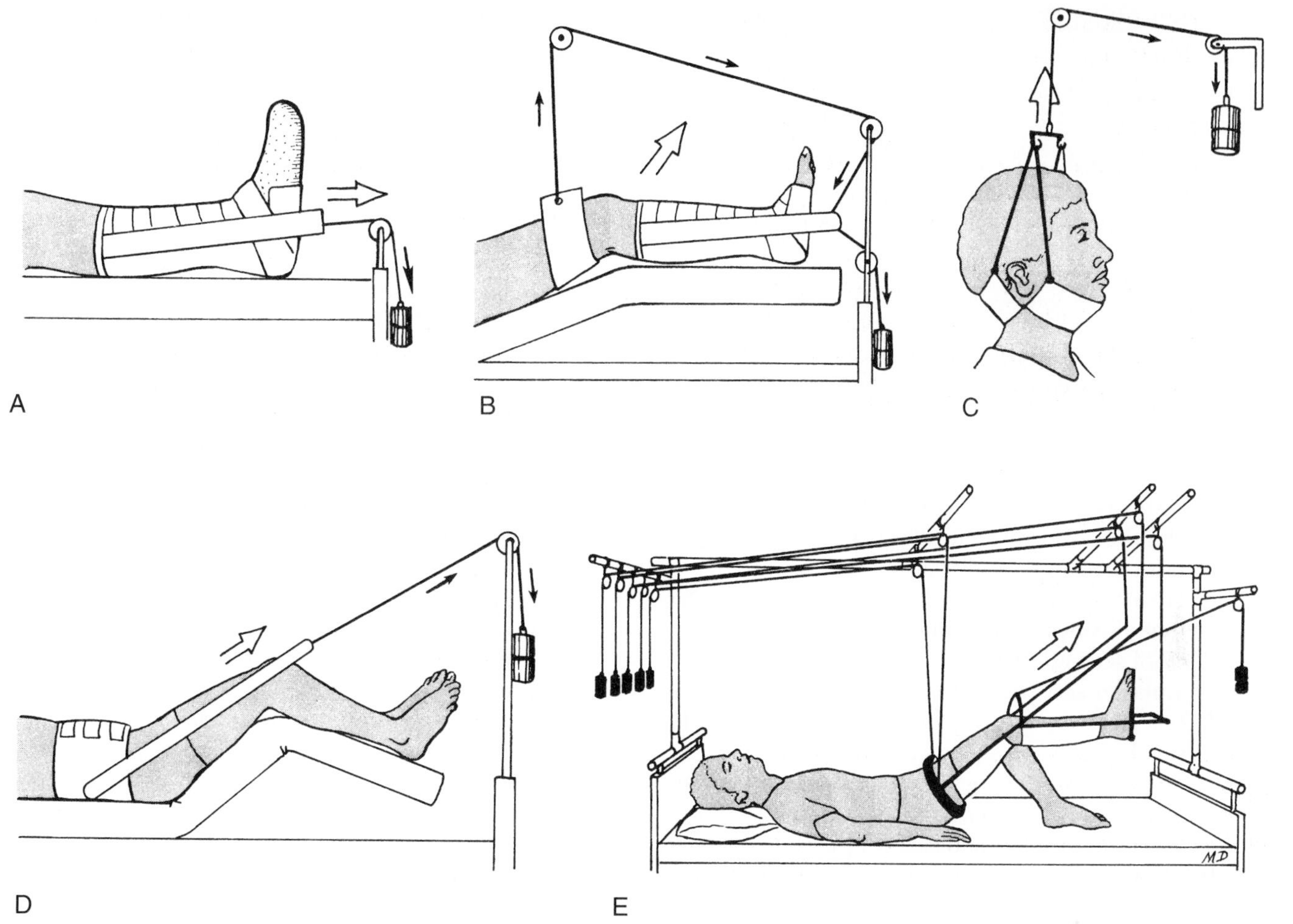

A

B

C

D

E

FIG. 67-3 Examples of common types of traction. **A,** Buck's traction. **B,** Russell's traction. **C,** Head halter traction. **D,** Pelvic traction. **E,** Balanced suspension traction. (From deWit, S. [1998]. *Essentials of medical-surgical nursing* [4th ed.]. Philadelphia: W. B. Saunders.)

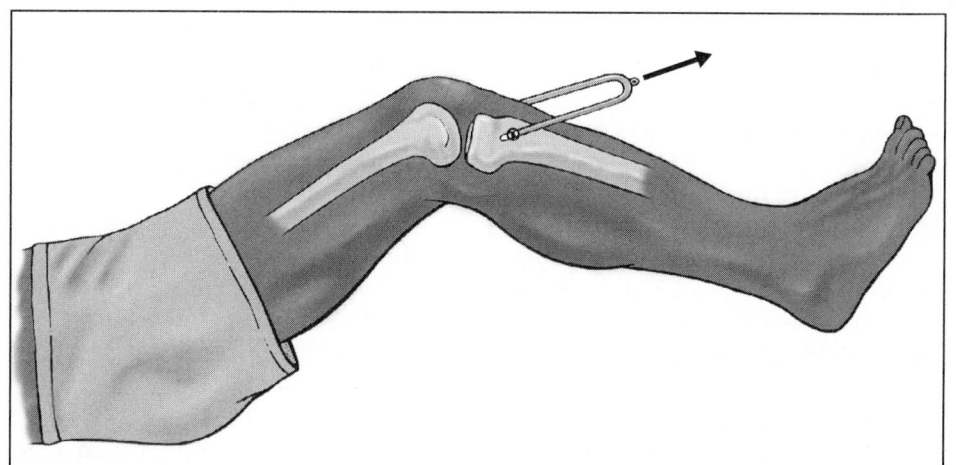

FIG. 67-4 Skeletal traction (Steinmann pin). (From Monahan, F. D., & Neighbors, M. [1998]. *Medical-surgical nursing: Foundations for clinical practice* [2nd ed.]. Philadelphia: W. B. Saunders.)

BOX 67-5

Types of Skin Traction

Buck's traction
Cervical traction
Pelvic traction
Russell's traction

BOX 67-6

Complications of Fractures

Avascular necrosis
Compartment syndrome
Fat emboli
Infection and osteomyelitis
Pulmonary emboli

▲ M. **Casts**
   1. Description: Casts are made of plaster or fiberglass to provide immobilization of bone and joints after a fracture or injury.
   2. Interventions
      a. Keep the **cast** and extremity elevated.
      b. Allow a wet **cast** 24 to 48 hours to dry (synthetic casts dry in 20 minutes).
      c. Handle a wet **cast** with the palms of the hands until dry.
      d. Turn the extremity unless contraindicated so that all sides of the wet **cast** will dry.
      e. Cool setting on a hair dryer can be used to dry a plaster **cast** (heat cannot be used on a plaster **cast** because the **cast** heats up and burns the skin).
      f. The **cast** will change from a dull to a shiny substance when dry.
      g. Examine the skin and **cast** for pressure areas.
      h. Monitor the extremity for circulatory impairment such as pain, swelling, discoloration, tingling, numbness, coolness, or diminished pulse.
      i. Notify the physician immediately if circulatory compromise occurs.
      j. Prepare for bivalving or cutting the **cast** if circulatory impairment occurs.
      k. Petal the **cast;** maintain smooth edges around the **cast** to prevent crumbling of the **cast** material.
      l. Monitor the client's temperature.
      m. Monitor for the presence of a foul odor, which may indicate infection.
      n. Monitor drainage and circle the area of drainage on the **cast.**
      o. Monitor for warmth on the **cast.**
      p. Monitor for wet spots, which may indicate a need for drying or the presence of drainage under the **cast.**
      q. If an open draining area exists on the affected extremity, the physician will make a cut-out portion of the **cast** or a window.
   ▲ r. Instruct the client not to stick objects inside the **cast.**
      s. Teach the client to keep the **cast** clean and dry.
      t. Instruct the client in isometric exercises to prevent muscle atrophy.

▲ VI. **COMPLICATIONS OF FRACTURES (BOX 67-6)**
   A. **Fat embolism**
      1. Description

      a. A **fat embolism** originates in the bone marrow and occurs after a fracture.
      b. Clients with long bone fractures are at the greatest risk for the development of **fat embolism.**
      c. **Fat embolism** can occur within the first 72 hours following the injury.
   2. Assessment
      a. Restlessness
      b. Mental status changes
      c. Tachycardia, tachypnea, and hypotension
      d. Dyspnea
      e. Petechial rash over the upper chest and neck
   3. Interventions
      a. Notify the physician immediately.
      b. Treat symptoms as prescribed to prevent respiratory failure and death.
   B. **Compartment syndrome** ▲
      1. Description
         a. **Compartment syndrome** is increased pressure within one or more compartments, causing massive compromise of circulation to an area.
         b. **Compartment syndrome** leads to decreased perfusion and tissue anoxia.
         c. Within 4 to 6 hours after the onset of **compartment syndrome,** neuromuscular damage is irreversible if not treated.
      2. Assessment
         a. Unrelieved or increased pain
         b. Swelling
         c. Pain with passive motion
         d. Inability to move joints
         e. Loss of sensation (paresthesia)
         f. Pulselessness
      3. Interventions: Notify the physician immediately.
   C. Infection and osteomyelitis
      1. Description: Infection and osteomyelitis can be caused by the interruption of the integrity of the skin; the infection invades bone tissue.
      2. Assessment
         a. Fever
         b. Pain
         c. Erythema in the area surrounding the fracture
         d. Tachycardia
         e. Elevated white blood cell count
      3. Interventions
         a. Notify the physician.
         b. Prepare to initiate aggressive intravenous antibiotic therapy.

D. Avascular necrosis
   1. Description: Avascular necrosis is an interruption in the blood supply to the bony tissue, which results in the death of the bone.
   2. Assessment
      a. Pain
      b. Decreased sensation
   3. Interventions
      a. Notify the physician if pain or decreased sensation occurs.
      b. Prepare the client for removal of necrotic tissue because it serves as a focus for infection.
E. Pulmonary embolism
   1. Description: Pulmonary embolism is caused by immobility precipitated by a fracture.
   2. Assessment
      a. Restlessness and apprehension
      b. Dyspnea and chest pain
      c. Diaphoresis
      d. Arterial blood gas changes
   3. Interventions
      a. Notify the physician if signs of emboli are present.
      b. Prepare to administer anticoagulant therapy.

VII. CRUTCH WALKING

A. Description
   1. An accurate measurement of the client for crutches is important because an incorrect measurement could damage the brachial plexus.
   2. The distance between the axillas and the arm pieces on the crutches should be two to three fingerwidths in the axilla space.
   3. The elbows should be slightly flexed, 20 to 30 degrees, when the client is walking
   4. When ambulating with the client, stand on the affected side.
   5. Instruct the client never to rest the axilla on the axillary bars.
   6. Instruct the client to look up and outward when ambulating and to place the crutches 6 to 10 inches diagonally in front of the foot.
   7. Instruct the client to stop ambulation if numbness or tingling in the hands or arms occurs.
B. Crutch gaits (Fig. 67-5)
C. Assisting the client with crutches to sit and stand
   1. Place the unaffected leg against the front of the chair.
   2. Move the crutches to the affected side, and grasp the arm of the chair with the hand on the unaffected side.

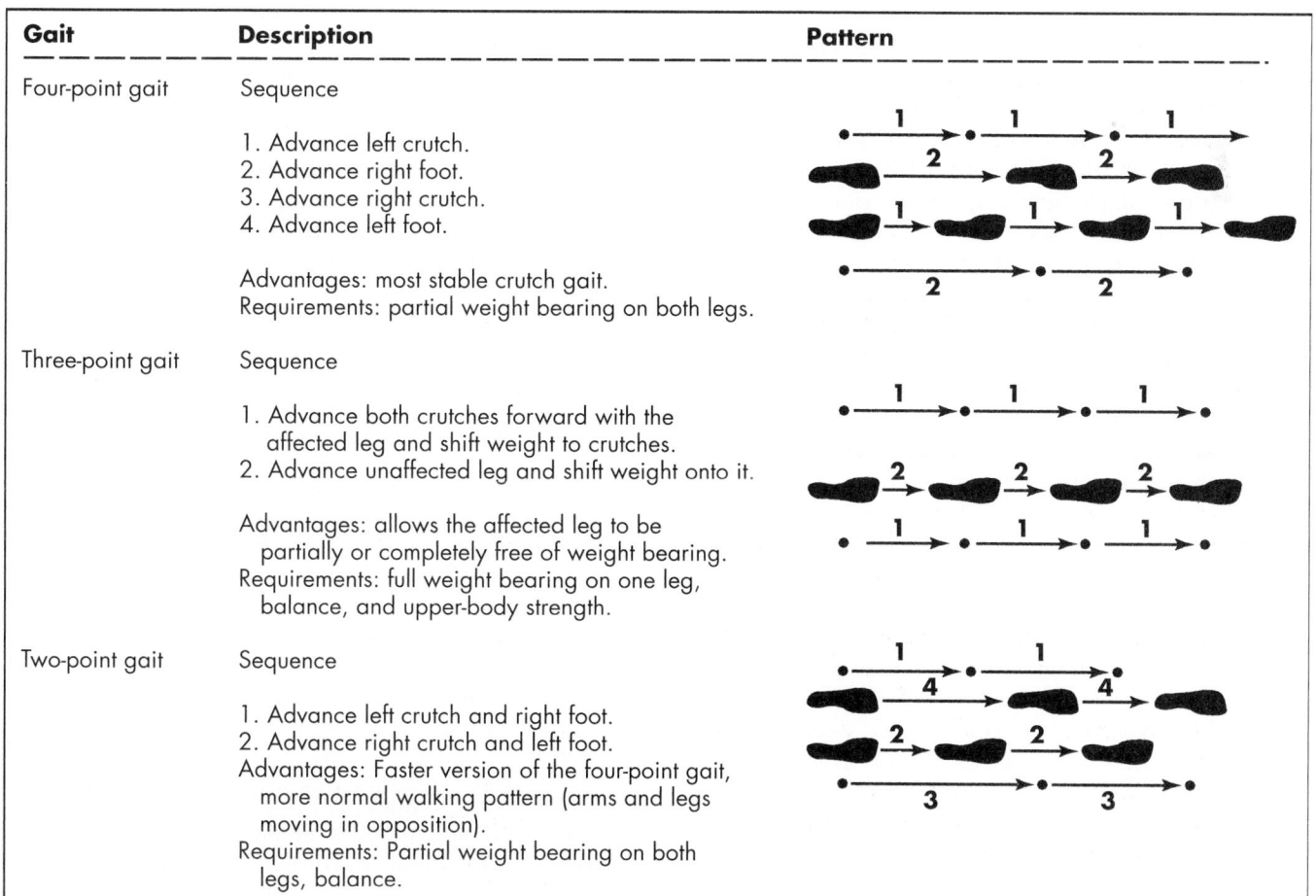

Gait	Description	Pattern
Four-point gait	Sequence 1. Advance left crutch. 2. Advance right foot. 3. Advance right crutch. 4. Advance left foot. Advantages: most stable crutch gait. Requirements: partial weight bearing on both legs.	
Three-point gait	Sequence 1. Advance both crutches forward with the affected leg and shift weight to crutches. 2. Advance unaffected leg and shift weight onto it. Advantages: allows the affected leg to be partially or completely free of weight bearing. Requirements: full weight bearing on one leg, balance, and upper-body strength.	
Two-point gait	Sequence 1. Advance left crutch and right foot. 2. Advance right crutch and left foot. Advantages: Faster version of the four-point gait, more normal walking pattern (arms and legs moving in opposition). Requirements: Partial weight bearing on both legs, balance.	

FIG. 67-5   Crutch gaits. (From deWit, S. [1998]. *Essentials of medical-surgical nursing* [4th ed.]. Philadelphia: W. B. Saunders.)

3. Flex the knee of the unaffected leg to lower self into the chair while placing the affected leg straight out in front.
4. Reverse the steps to move from a sitting to a standing position.

D. Going up and down stairs
1. Up the stairs
   a. The client moves the unaffected leg up first.
   b. The client moves the affected leg and the crutches up.
2. Down the stairs
   a. The client moves the crutches and the affected leg down.
   b. The client moves the unaffected leg down.

VIII. CANES AND WALKERS

A. Description: Canes and walkers are made of a light-weight material with a rubber tip at the bottom.
B. Interventions
1. Stand at the affected side of the client when ambulating.
2. The handle should be at the level of the client's greater trochanter.
3. The client's elbow should be flexed at a 15- to 30-degree angle.
4. Instruct the client to hold the cane 4 to 6 inches to the side of the foot.
5. Instruct the client to hold the cane in the hand on the unaffected side so that the cane and weaker leg can work together with each step.
6. Instruct the client to move the cane at the same time as the affected leg.
7. Instruct the client to inspect the rubber tips regularly for worn places.
C. Hemicanes or quadripod canes
1. Hemicanes or quadripod canes are used for clients who have the use of only one upper extremity.
2. Hemicanes provide more security than a quadripod cane; however, both types provide more security than a single-tipped cane.
3. Position the cane at the client's unaffected side, with the straight, nonangled side adjacent to the body.
4. Position the cane 6 inches from client's side, with the hand grips level with the greater trochanter.
D. Walker
1. Stand adjacent to the client on the affected side.
2. Instruct the client to put all four points of the walker flat on the floor before putting weight on the hand pieces.
3. Instruct the client to move the walker forward and to walk into it.

IX. FRACTURED HIP

A. Types
1. Intracapsular
   a. Bone is broken inside the joint.

b. Skin **traction** is applied preoperatively to immobilize and prevent pain.
c. Treatment includes a total hip replacement or **internal fixation** with replacement of the femoral head with a prosthesis (Fig. 67-6).
d. Avoid hip flexion to prevent displacement.
2. Extracapsular
   a. Fracture can occur at the greater trochanter or can be an intertrochanteric fracture.
   b. Trochanteric fracture is outside the joint.
   c. Preoperative treatment includes balanced suspension **traction** or possibly Buck's extension **traction**.
   d. Avoid hip flexion to prevent displacement.
   e. Surgical treatment includes **internal fixation** with nail plate, screws, or wires
B. Postoperative interventions
1. Maintain leg and hip in proper alignment.
2. Prevent flexion or external or internal rotation.
3. Turn the client from back to unaffected side.
4. Do not position client to the affected side unless prescribed by the physician.
5. Maintain leg abduction to prevent internal or external rotation.
6. Use a trochanter roll to prevent external rotation.
7. Ensure that the hip flexion angle does not exceed 60 to 80 degrees.
8. Elevate the head of the bed 30 to 45 degrees for meals only.
9. Assist the client to ambulate as prescribed by the physician.
10. Avoid weight bearing on the affected leg as prescribed; instruct the client in the use of a walker to avoid weight bearing.
11. Keep the operative leg extended, supported, and elevated when getting client out of bed.

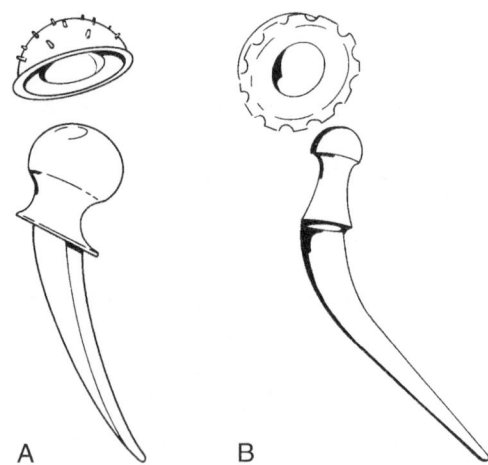

FIG. 67-6   Hip prostheses. **A,** The McKee-Farrar procedure involves replacement of the femoral head and acetabulum with a metal prosthesis. **B,** The Charnley prosthesis involves total prosthetic replacement of the hip joint. (From deWit, S. [1998]. *Essentials of medical-surgical nursing* [4th ed.]. Philadelphia: W. B. Saunders.)

12. Avoid hip flexion greater than 90 degrees and avoid low chairs when out of bed.
13. Monitor the wound for infection or hemorrhage.
14. Monitor circulation and sensation of the affected side.
15. Maintain the Hemovac or Jackson-Pratt drain if in place; maintain compression to facilitate drainage and monitor and record output of drainage.
16. Drainage should decrease in amount continuously, and by 48 hours postoperatively, drainage should be about 30 mL in an 8-hour period.
17. Maintain the use of antiembolism stockings, and encourage the client to flex and extend the feet and ankles.
18. Instruct the client to avoid crossing the legs and activities that require bending over.
19. Physical therapy will begin postoperatively as prescribed by the physician.

X. TOTAL KNEE REPLACEMENT

A. Description: Total knee replacement is implantation of a device to substitute for the femoral condyles and the tibial joint surfaces.
B. Postoperative interventions
  1. Monitor the incision for drainage and infection.
  2. Maintain the Hemovac or Jackson-Pratt drain if in place.
  3. Begin continuous passive motion 24 to 48 hours postoperatively as prescribed to exercise the knee and provide moderate flexion and extension.
  4. Administer analgesics before continuous passive motion to decrease pain.
  5. The leg should not be dangled to prevent dislocation.
  6. Prepare the client for out-of-bed activities as prescribed.
  7. Avoid weight bearing and instruct the client in crutch walking.

XI. HERNIATION: INTERVERTEBRAL DISK

A. Description: Nucleus of the disk protrudes into the annulus, causing nerve compression.
B. Cervical disk
  1. Cervical disk herniation occurs at C5 to C6 and C6 to C7 interspaces.
  2. Herniation causes pain and stiffness in the neck, top of the shoulders, scapula, upper extremities, and head.
  3. Herniation produces paresthesia and numbness of the upper extremities.
  4. Interventions
    a. Provide bed rest to relieve pressure and reduce inflammation and edema.
    b. Provide immobilization as prescribed via cervical collar, **traction,** or brace.
    c. Apply hot, moist compresses as prescribed to increase the blood flow and relax spasms.
    d. Instruct the client to avoid flexing, extending, or rotating the neck.
    e. Instruct the client that while sleeping to avoid the prone position and keep the head, spine, and hip in alignment.
    f. Instruct the client to avoid long periods of sitting.
    g. Instruct the client in the use of analgesics, sedatives, antiinflammatory agents, and corticosteroids as prescribed.
    h. Prepare the client for a corticosteroid injection into the epidural space if prescribed.
    i. Assist the client with the application of a cervical collar or cervical **traction** as prescribed.
  5. Cervical collar
    a. A cervical collar is used for cervical disk herniation.
    b. A cervical collar holds the head in a neutral or slightly flexed position.
    c. The client may have to wear a cervical collar 24 hours a day.
    d. Inspect the skin under the collar for irritation.
    e. When the pain subsides, the client is taught cervical isometric exercises to strengthen the muscles.
C. Lumbar disk
  1. Lumbar disk herniation most often occurs at L4 to L5 or L5 to S1 interspaces.
  2. Postural deformity occurs.
  3. Herniation produces muscle weakness, sensory loss, and alteration of the tendon reflexes.
  4. The client experiences low back pain and muscle spasms with radiation of the pain into one hip and down the leg (sciatica).
  5. Pain is aggravated by bending, lifting, straining, sneezing, and coughing and is relieved by bed rest.
  6. Interventions
    a. Provide bed rest as prescribed.
    b. Apply moist heat and massage as prescribed.
    c. Instruct the client to sleep on the side, with the knees and hips in a position of flexion and with a pillow between the legs.
    d. Apply pelvic **traction** as prescribed to relieve muscle spasms.
    e. Begin ambulation gradually as the inflammation and edema subside.
    f. Instruct the client in the use of muscle relaxants, antiinflammatory medications, and corticosteroids as prescribed.
    g. Instruct the client in the use of a corset or brace as prescribed.
    h. Instruct the client regarding correct posture while sitting, standing, walking, and working.
    i. Instruct the client to lift objects by bending the knees and keeping the back straight, avoiding lifting anything above the elbows.
    j. Instruct the client regarding a weight-control program as prescribed.

k. Instruct the client in an exercise program as prescribed to strengthen abdominal and back muscles.

D. Disk surgery (Box 67-7)
1. Preoperative interventions
a. Reassure the client that surgery will not weaken the back.
b. Instruct the client regarding coughing and deep-breathing exercises.
c. Instruct the client about logrolling and range of motion exercises.
2. Postoperative interventions: cervical disk
a. Monitor for respiratory difficulty.
b. Encourage coughing and deep breathing.
c. Monitor for hoarseness and inability to cough effectively because this may indicate laryngeal nerve damage.
d. Use throat sprays or lozenges for sore throat, and do not use those that may numb the throat so as to avoid choking.
e. Monitor the wound for drainage.
f. Provide a soft diet if the client complains of dysphagia.
g. Monitor for sudden return of radicular pain, which may indicate that the cervical spine has become unstable.
3. Postoperative interventions: lumbar disk
a. Monitor for wound hemorrhage.
b. Monitor sensation and motor ability of the lower extremities as well as color, temperature, and sensation of toes.
c. Monitor for urinary retention, paralytic ileus, and constipation.
d. Initiate measures to prevent constipation, such as a high-fiber diet, increased fluid intake, and stool softeners, as prescribed.
e. When turning and repositioning the client, place the bed in a flat position and a pillow between the legs; turn the client as a unit (logroll) without twisting the client's back.
f. When positioning the client, a pillow is placed under the head with the knees slightly flexed.
g. Avoid extreme knee flexion when the client is lying on the side.
h. To assist the client out of bed, raise the head of the bed while the client lies on the side; the client's head and shoulders are supported by the first nurse, the client pushes self to a sitting position, and the second nurse eases the legs over the side of the bed.
i. Instruct the client to avoid sitting because it places a strain on the surgical site.
j. Administer narcotics and sedatives as prescribed to relieve pain and anxiety.
k. Encourage early ambulation.
l. Assist the client with the use of a back brace or corset if prescribed.

XII. AMPUTATION OF A LOWER EXTREMITY (FIG. 67-7)
A. Description: Amputation is the surgical removal of a lower limb or part of the limb.
B. Postoperative interventions
1. Monitor vital signs.
2. Monitor for infection and hemorrhage.
3. Mark bleeding and drainage on the dressing if it occurs.
4. Keep a tourniquet at the bedside.
5. Monitor for pulmonary emboli.
6. Observe for and prevent contractures.
7. Monitor for signs of necrosis and neuroma.
8. Evaluate for phantom limb sensation and pain; explain sensation and pain to the client, and medicate the client as prescribed.
9. Check the physician's orders regarding positioning.

BOX 67-7

Types of Disk Surgery

Chemolysis: injections to dissolve affected disk
Diskectomy: removal of herniated disk tissue and related matter
Diskectomy with fusion: fusion of vertebras with bone graft
Laminectomy: removal of the lamina
Laminotomy: division of the lamina of a vertebra

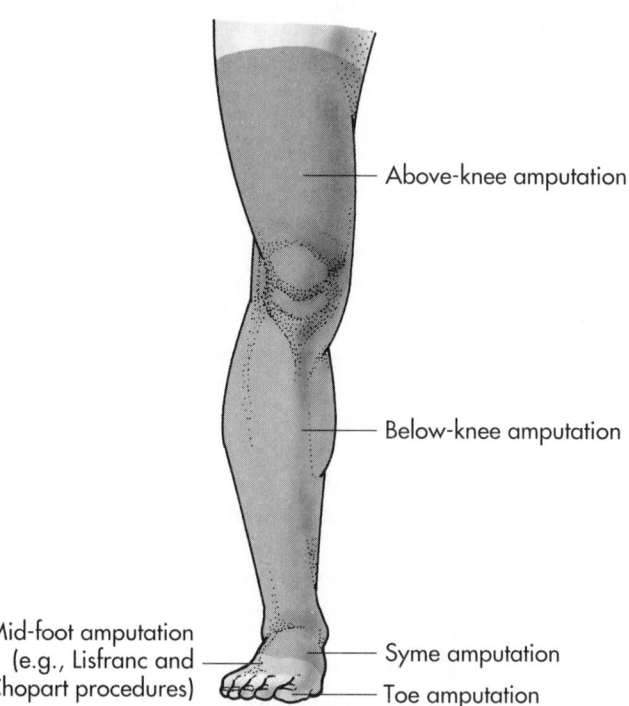

Mid-foot amputation (e.g., Lisfranc and Chopart procedures)
Above-knee amputation
Below-knee amputation
Syme amputation
Toe amputation

FIG. 67-7 Common levels of lower-extremity amputation. (From Ignatavicius, D., Workman, M., & Mishler, M. [1999]. *Medical-surgical nursing across the health care continuum* [3rd ed.]. Philadelphia: W. B. Saunders.)

10. If prescribed, during the first 24 hours, elevate the foot of the bed to reduce edema; then keep the bed flat to prevent hip flexion contractures.

11. Do not elevate the stump itself because elevation can cause flexion contracture of the hip joint.

12. After 24 and 48 hours postoperatively, position the client prone if prescribed, to stretch the muscles and prevent flexion contractures of hip.

13. In the prone position, place a pillow under the abdomen and stump and keep the legs close together to prevent abduction.

14. Maintain application of an Ace wrap or elastic stump shrinker as prescribed to provide stump shrinkage.

15. Remove and rewrap the Ace bandage or elastic stump shrinker 3 or 4 times daily as prescribed.

16. Wash the stump with mild soap and water and apply lanolin to the skin if prescribed.

17. Massage the skin toward the suture line to increase circulation.

18. Prepare for a **cast** application if prescribed to prepare the stump for a prosthesis.

19. Encourage the client to look at the stump.

20. Encourage verbalization regarding loss of the body part, and assist the client to identify coping mechanisms to deal with the loss.

C. Interventions for below-the-knee amputation
   1. Prevent edema.
   2. Do not allow the stump to hang over the edge of the bed.
   3. Do not allow the client to sit for long periods of time so as to prevent contractures.

D. Interventions for above-the-knee amputation
   1. Prevent internal or external rotation of the limb.
   2. Place a sandbag or rolled towel along the outside of the thigh to prevent rotation.

E. Rehabilitation
   1. Instruct the client in crutch walking.
   2. Prepare the stump for a prosthesis.
   3. Prepare the client for fitting of the stump for a prosthesis.
   4. Instruct the client in exercises to maintain range of motion.
   5. Provide psychosocial support to the client.

XIII. RHEUMATOID ARTHRITIS

A. Description
   1. Rheumatoid arthritis is a chronic systemic inflammatory disease (immune complex disorder); the cause may be related to a combination of environmental and genetic factors.
   2. Rheumatoid arthritis leads to destruction of connective tissue and synovial membrane within the joints.
   3. Rheumatoid arthritis weakens and leads to dislocation of the joint and permanent deformity.
   4. Formation of pannus occurs at the junction of synovial tissue and articular cartilage, projecting into the joint cavity and causing necrosis.
   5. Exacerbations are increased by physical or emotional stress.
   6. Risk factors include exposure to infectious agents; fatigue and stress can exacerbate the condition.
   7. Vasculitis can cause malfunction and eventual failure of an organ or system.

B. Assessment
   1. Inflammation, tenderness, and stiffness of the joints
   2. Moderate to severe pain and morning stiffness lasting longer than 30 minutes
   3. Joint deformities, muscle atrophy, and decreased range of motion
   4. Spongy, soft feeling in the joints
   5. Low-grade temperature, fatigue, and weakness
   6. Anorexia, weight loss, and anemia
   7. Elevated sedimentation rate and positive rheumatoid factor
   8. X-ray film showing joint deterioration
   9. Synovial tissue biopsy showing inflammation

C. Rheumatoid factor
   1. A blood test used to diagnose rheumatoid arthritis
   2. Values
      a. Nonreactive: 0 to 39 international units/mL
      b. Weakly reactive: 40 to 79 international units/mL
      c. Reactive: greater than 80 international units/mL

D. Pain
   1. Salicylates (acetylsalicyic acid [aspirin])
      a. Monitor for side effects, including tinnitus, gastrointestinal upset, and prolonged bleeding time.
      b. Administer with meals or a snack.
      c. Monitor for abnormal bleeding or bruising.
   2. Nonsteroidal antiinflammatory drugs (NSAIDs)
      a. These drugs may be prescribed in combination with salicylates if pain and inflammation have not decreased within 6 to 12 weeks following salicylate therapy.
      b. Monitor for side effects such as gastrointestinal upset, central nervous system manifestations, skin rash, hypertension, fluid retention, and changes in renal function.
   3. Corticosteroids: Administer as prescribed during exacerbations or when commonly used agents are ineffective.
   4. Antineoplastic medications: Administer as prescribed in clients with life-threatening rheumatoid arthritis.
   5. Gold salts: Administer as prescribed in combination with salicylates and NSAIDS to induce remission and decrease pain and inflammation.

E. Physical mobility
   1. Preserve joint function.
   2. Provide range of motion exercises to maintain joint motion and muscle strengthening.
   3. Balance rest and activity.

4. Splints may be used during acute inflammation to prevent deformity.
5. Prevent flexion contractures.
6. Apply heat or cold therapy as prescribed to joints.
7. Apply paraffin baths and massage as prescribed
8. Encourage consistency with exercise program.
9. Instruct the client to stop exercise if pain increases.
10. Exercise only to the point of pain.
11. Avoid weight bearing on inflamed joints.

F. Self-care (Box 67-8)
1. Assess the need for assistive devices such as higher toilet seats, chairs, and wheelchairs to facilitate mobility.
2. Collaborate with an occupational therapist to obtain assistive or adaptive devices.
3. Instruct the client in alternative strategies for providing activities of daily living.

G. Fatigue
1. Identify factors that may contribute to fatigue.
2. Monitor for signs of anemia.
3. Administer iron, folic acid, and vitamin supplements as prescribed.
4. Monitor for drug-related blood loss by testing the stool for occult blood.
5. Instruct the client in measures to conserve energy, such as pacing activities and obtaining assistance when possible.

H. Body image disturbance
1. Assess the client's reaction to the body change.
2. Encourage the client to verbalize feelings.
3. Assist the client with self-care activities and grooming.
4. Encourage the client to wear street clothes.

I. Surgical interventions
1. Synovectomy: Surgical removal of the synovia to help maintain joint function

---

BOX 67-8

Client Education for Rheumatoid Arthritis and Degenerative Joint Disease

Assist the client to identify and correct safety hazards in the home.
Instruct the client in the correct use of assistive or adaptive devices.
Instruct the client in energy conservation measures.
Review the prescribed exercise program.
Instruct the client to sit in a chair with a high, straight back.
Instruct the client to use only a small pillow when lying down.
Instruct the client in measures to protect the joints.
Instruct the client regarding the prescribed medications.
Stress the importance of follow-up visits with the health care provider.

---

2. Arthrodesis: Bony fusion of a joint to regain some mobility
3. Joint replacement (arthroplasty): Surgical replacement of diseased joints with artificial joints, which is performed to restore motion to a joint and function to the muscles, ligaments, and other soft tissue structures that control a joint

XIV. OSTEOARTHRITIS (DEGENERATIVE JOINT DISEASE)

A. Description
1. Osteoarthritis is progressive degeneration of the joints as a result of wear and tear.
2. Osteoarthritis causes the formation of bony buildup and the loss of articular cartilage in peripheral and axial joints.
3. Osteoarthritis affects the weight-bearing joints and joints that receive the greatest stress, such as the knees, toes, and lower spine.
4. The cause is unknown but may be trauma, fractures, infections, or obesity.

B. Assessment
1. Joint pain that diminishes after rest and intensifies after activity, noted early in the disease process
2. As the disease progresses, pain occurs with slight motion or even at rest
3. Symptoms are aggravated by temperature change and humidity
4. Crepitus
5. Joint enlargement
6. Presence of Heberden's nodes or Bouchard's nodes
7. Limited range of motion
8. Difficulty getting up after prolonged sitting
9. Skeletal muscle atrophy
10. Inability to perform activities of daily living
11. Compression of the spine as manifested by radiating pain, stiffness, and muscle spasms in one or both extremities

C. Pain
1. Administer NSAIDs, salicylates, and muscle relaxants as prescribed.
2. Prepare the client for corticosteroid injections into joints as prescribed.
3. Place affected joint in a functional position.
4. Immobilize the affected joint with a splint or brace.
5. Avoid large pillows under the head or knees.
6. Provide a bed or foot cradle.
7. Position the client prone twice a day.
8. Instruct the client in the importance of moist heat, hot packs or compresses, and paraffin dips as prescribed.
9. Apply cold applications as prescribed when the joint is acutely inflamed.
10. Encourage adequate rest, recommending 10 hours of sleep at night and a 1- to 2-hour nap in the afternoon.

D. Nutrition
   1. Encourage a well-balanced diet.
   2. Encourage weight loss if necessary.
E. Physical mobility
   1. Reinforce the exercise program and the importance of participating in the program.
   2. Instruct the client that exercises should be active rather than passive and to exercise only to the point of pain.
   3. Instruct the client to stop exercise if pain is increased with exercising.
   4. Instruct the client to decrease the number of repetitions in an exercise when the inflammation is severe.
F. Surgical management
   1. Osteotomy: The bone is cut to correct joint deformity and promote realignment.
   2. Total joint replacement
      a. Total joint replacement is performed when all measures of pain relief have failed.
      b. Hips and knees are replaced most commonly.
      c. Total joint replacement is contraindicated in the presence of infection, advanced osteoporosis, or severe inflammation.

▶ XV. OSTEOPOROSIS
A. Description
   1. Osteoporosis is an age-related metabolic disease.
   2. Bone demineralization results in the loss of bone mass, leading to fragile and porous bones and subsequent fractures.
   3. Greater bone resorption than bone formation occurs.
   4. Osteoporosis occurs most commonly in the wrist, hip, and vertebral column.
   5. Osteoporosis can occur postmenopausally or as a result of a metabolic disorder or calcium deficiency.
   6. Client may be asymptomatic until the bones become so weak that a sudden injury causes a fracture.
   7. Risk factors (Box 67-9)
B. Assessment
   1. Possibly asymptomatic

BOX 67-9

Risk Factors for Osteoporosis

Cigarette smoking
Early menopause
Excessive use of alcohol
Family history
Female gender
Increasing age
Insufficient intake of calcium
Sedentary lifestyle
Thin, small frame
White (European descent) or Asian race

---

   2. Back pain after lifting, bending, or stooping
   3. Back pain that increases with palpation
   4. Pelvic or hip pain, especially with weight bearing
   5. Problems with balance
   6. Decline in height from vertebral compression
   7. Kyphosis of the dorsal spine
   8. Constipation, abdominal distention, and respiratory impairment as a result of movement restriction and spinal deformity
   9. Pathological fractures
   10. Appearance of thin, porous bone on x-ray film
C. Interventions
   1. Assess risk for injury.
   2. Provide a safe and hazard-free environment, and assist the client to identify hazards in the home environment.
   3. Use side rails to prevent falls.
   4. Move the client gently when turning and repositioning.
   5. Encourage ambulation; assist with ambulation if the client is unsteady.
   6. Instruct in the use of assistive devices such as a cane or walker.
   7. Provide range of motion exercises.
   8. Instruct the client in the use of good body mechanics.
   9. Instruct the client in exercises to strengthen abdominal and back muscles to improve posture and provide support for the spine.
   10. Instruct the client to avoid activities that can cause vertebral compression.
   11. Apply a back brace as prescribed during an acute phase to immobilize the spine and provide spinal column support.
   12. Encourage the use of a firm mattress.
   13. Provide a diet high in protein, calcium, vitamins C and D, and iron.
   14. Encourage adequate fluid intake to prevent renal calculuses.
   15. Instruct the client to avoid alcohol and coffee.
   16. Administer estrogen or androgens to decrease the rate of bone resorption as prescribed.
   17. Administer calcium, vitamin D, and phosphorus as prescribed for bone metabolism.
   18. Administer calcitonin as prescribed to inhibit bone loss.
   19. Administer analgesics, muscle relaxants, and anti-inflammatory medications as prescribed.

XVI. GOUT
A. Description
   1. Gout is a systemic disease in which urate crystals deposit in joints and other body tissues.
   2. Gout leads to abnormal amounts of uric acid in the body.
   3. Primary gout results from a disorder of purine metabolism.

4. Secondary gout involves excessive uric acid in the blood that is caused by another disease.

B. Phases

1. Asymptomatic
   a. Client has no symptoms.
   b. Serum uric acid is elevated.
2. Acute: Client has excruciating pain and inflammation of one or more small joints, especially the great toe.
3. Intermittent: Client is asymptomatic period between acute attacks.
4. Chronic
   a. Chronic gout results from repeated episodes of acute gout.
   b. Chronic gout results in deposits of urate crystals under the skin and within the major organs, especially the renal system.

C. Assessment

1. Excruciating pain in the involved joints
2. Swelling and inflammation of the joints
3. Tophi (hard, fairly large, and irregularly shaped deposits in the skin) that may break open and discharge a yellow gritty substance
4. Low-grade fever
5. Malaise and headache
6. Pruritis
7. Presence of renal stones
8. Elevated uric acid levels

D. Interventions

1. Provide a low-purine diet as prescribed.
2. Instruct the client to avoid foods such as organ meats, wines, and aged cheese.
3. Encourage a high fluid intake of 2000 mL to prevent stone formation.
4. Encourage weight-reduction diet if required.
5. Instruct the client to avoid alcohol and starvation diets because they may precipitate a gout attack.
6. Increase urinary pH (above 6) by eating alkaline ash foods such as citrus fruits and juices, milk, and other dairy products.
7. Provide bed rest during the acute attacks.
8. Monitor joint range of motion ability and appearance of joints.
9. Position the joint in mild flexion during acute attack.
10. Elevate the affected extremity.
11. Protect the affected joint from excessive movement or direct contact with sheets or blankets.
12. Provide heat or cold for local treatments to affected joint as prescribed.
13. Administer NSAIDs and antigout medications as prescribed.

PRACTICE QUESTIONS

1. A client is treated in a physician's office after a fall that sprained an ankle. X-ray examination has ruled out a fracture. Before sending the client home, the nurse plans to teach the client to avoid which of the following in the next 24 hours?
   1. Application of a heating pad
   2. Application of an Ace wrap
   3. Resting the foot
   4. Elevating the ankle on a pillow while sitting or lying down

2. A nurse has given dietary instructions to a client to minimize the risk of osteoporosis. The nurse would evaluate that the client understands the recommended dietary changes if the client stated he or she should increase intake of which food?
   1. Rice
   2. Yogurt
   3. Sardines
   4. Chicken

3. A nurse is conducting health screening for osteoporosis. The nurse would interpret that which of the following clients is at greatest risk of developing this disorder?
   1. A 36-year-old man who has asthma
   2. A 25-year-old woman who jogs
   3. A sedentary 65-year-old woman who smokes cigarettes
   4. A 70-year-old man who consumes excess alcohol

4. A home health nurse is planning to teach a client with osteoporosis about home modifications to reduce the risk of falls. Which of the following recommendations would be unnecessary to include in the teaching plan?
   1. Use of staircase railings
   2. Use of night lights
   3. Removing wall-to-wall carpeting
   4. Placing handrails in the bathroom

5. A nurse is reviewing the postprocedure plan of care formulated by a nursing student for a client scheduled for a bone biopsy. The nurse determines that the student needs to read about postprocedure care if which inaccurate intervention is documented?
   1. Monitoring site for swelling, bleeding, or hematoma
   2. Administering narcotic analgesics intramuscularly
   3. Elevating the limb for 24 hours
   4. Monitoring vitals signs every 4 hours

6. A nurse has given instructions to a client returning home after arthroscopy of a knee. The nurse would evaluate that the client understands the instructions if the client states to
   1. Stay off the leg entirely for the rest of the day.
   2. Resume regular exercise the following day.
   3. Refrain from eating food for the remainder of the day.
   4. Report fever or site inflammation to the physician.

7. A nurse is caring for a client who is going to have an arthrogram with a contrast medium. Which assessment by the nurse would be of highest priority?
   1. Allergy to iodine or shellfish

2. Ability of the client to remain still during the procedure

3. Whether the client has any remaining questions about the procedure

4. Whether the client wishes to void before the procedure

8. A client with possible rib fracture has never had a chest radiograph. The nurse would plan to tell the client which of the following items about the procedure?

1. The x-rays stimulate a small amount of pain.

2. Removal of jewelry and any other metal objects is necessary.

3. The client will be asked to breathe in and out as the radiograph is taken.

4. The x-ray technologist will stand next to the client during the procedure.

9. A client has had a bone scan done. The nurse would evaluate that the client understands the elements of follow-up care if the client states that he or she should

1. Report any feelings of nausea or flushing.

2. Ambulate at least 3 times before the end of the day.

3. Eat only small meals for the remainder of the day.

4. Drink plenty of water for 1 to 2 days following the procedure.

10. A client seeks treatment in the emergency room for a lower leg injury. Deformity of the lower aspect of the leg is visible, and the injured leg appears shorter than the other. The area is painful, swollen, and beginning to become ecchymotic. The nurse interprets that this client has experienced a

1. Contusion.

2. Fracture.

3. Sprain.

4. Strain.

11. A nurse is one of several persons who witness a vehicle hit a pedestrian at fairly low speed on a small street. The person is dazed and tries to get up. The leg appears fractured. The nurse would plan to

1. Stay with the person and encourage the person to remain still.

2. Assist the person to get up and walk to the sidewalk.

3. Leave the person for a few moments to call an ambulance.

4. Try to reduce the fracture manually.

12. A nurse is planning to teach a client with a left arm cast about measures to keep the left shoulder from becoming stiff and frozen. Which suggestion would the nurse include in the teaching plan?

1. Lift the left arm up over the head.

2. Lift the right arm up over the head.

3. Make a fist with the hand of the casted arm.

4. Use a sling on the left arm.

13. A client has a fiberglass (nonplaster) cast applied to the lower leg. The client asks the nurse when the client will be able to walk on the cast. The nurse replies that the client will be able to bear weight on the cast

1. Within 20 to 30 minutes of application.

2. In about 8 hours.

3. In 24 hours.

4. In 48 hours.

14. A nurse has given a client with a leg cast instructions on cast care at home. The nurse would evaluate that the client needs further instruction if the client makes which of the following statements?

1. "I should avoid walking on wet, slippery floors."

2. "It's okay to wipe dirt off the top of the cast with a damp cloth."

3. "I'm not supposed to scratch the skin underneath the cast."

4. "If the cast gets wet, I can dry it with a hair dryer turned to the warmest setting."

15. A client with a hip fracture asks the nurse why Buck's extension traction is being applied before surgery. The nurse's response is based on the understanding that Buck's extension traction primarily

1. Provides rigid immobilization of the fracture site.

2. Provides comfort by reducing muscle spasms and provides fracture immobilization.

3. Lengthens the fractured leg to prevent severing of blood vessels.

4. Allows bony healing to begin before surgery.

16. A client in skeletal leg traction with an overbed frame is not allowed to turn from side to side. Which action by the nurse would be most useful in trying to provide good skin care to the client?

1. Ask the client to lift up by digging into the mattress with the unaffected leg.

2. Push down on the mattress of the bed while administering care.

3. Have another nurse turn the client anyway.

4. Ask the client to pull up on a trapeze to lift the hips off the bed.

17. A nurse is evaluating the pin sites of a client in skeletal traction. The nurse would be least concerned with which of the following findings?

1. Purulent drainage

2. Serous drainage

3. Pain at a pin site

4. Inflammation

18. A client immobilized in skeletal leg traction complains of being bored and restless. Based on these complaints, the nurse formulates which of the following nursing diagnoses for this client?

1. Deficient Diversional Activity

2. Powerlessness

3. Self-Care Deficit

4. Impaired Physical Mobility

19. A client has Buck's extension traction applied to the right leg. The nurse would plan which of the following interventions to prevent complications of the device?
    1. Massage the skin of the right leg with lotion every 8 hours.
    2. Give pin care once a shift.
    3. Inspect the skin on the right leg at least once every 8 hours.
    4. Release the weights on the right leg for range of motion exercises daily.

20. A nurse is caring for a client who had skeletal traction applied to the left leg. The client is complaining of severe left leg pain. Which of the following actions should the nurse take first?
    1. Medicate the client with an analgesic.
    2. Provide pin care.
    3. Call the physician.
    4. Check the client's alignment in bed.

21. A nurse is assessing the casted extremity of a client. The nurse would assess for which of the following signs and symptoms indicative of infection?
    1. Coolness and pallor of the extremity
    2. Presence of a "hot spot" on the cast
    3. Diminished distal pulse
    4. Dependent edema

22. A client has sustained a closed fracture and has just had a cast applied to the affected arm. The client is complaining of intense pain. The nurse has elevated the limb, applied an ice bag, and administered an analgesic with little relief. The nurse interprets that this pain may be due to
    1. Impaired tissue perfusion.
    2. The newness of the fracture.
    3. The anxiety of the client.
    4. Infection under the cast.

23. A nurse is admitting a client with multiple trauma to the nursing unit. The client has a leg fracture and had a plaster cast applied. In positioning the casted leg, the nurse should
    1. Keep the leg in a level position.
    2. Keep the leg level for 3 hours and elevate it for 1 hour.
    3. Elevate the leg on pillows continuously for 24 to 48 hours.
    4. Elevate the leg for 3 hours and put it flat for 1 hour.

24. A client is complaining of skin irritation from the edges of a cast applied the previous day. The nurse should take which of the following actions?
    1. Massage the skin at the rim of the cast.
    2. Apply lotion to the skin at the rim of the cast.
    3. Use a rough file to smooth the cast edges.
    4. Petal the cast edges with adhesive tape.

25. A client is being discharged to home after application of a plaster leg cast. The nurse would evaluate that the client understands proper care of the cast if the client states that he or she should
    1. Avoid getting the cast wet.
    2. Use the fingertips to lift and move the leg.
    3. Cover the casted leg with warm blankets.
    4. Use a padded coat hanger end to scratch under the cast.

26. A client being measured for crutches asks the nurse why the crutches cannot rest up underneath the arm for extra support. The nurse's response is based on the understanding that this could result in
    1. Impaired range of motion while the client ambulates.
    2. Skin breakdown in the area of the axilla.
    3. Injury to the brachial plexus nerves.
    4. A fall and further injury.

27. A nurse is planning to teach a client how to stand on crutches. The nurse plans to incorporate into written instructions that the client should be told to place the crutches
    1. 8 inches to the front and side of the client's toes.
    2. 3 inches to the front and side of the client's toes.
    3. 20 inches to the front and side of the client's toes.
    4. 15 inches to the front and side of the client's toes.

28. A nurse has given a client instructions about crutch safety. The nurse determines that the client needs reinforcement of information if the client states
    1. The need to have spare crutches and tips available.
    2. That crutch tips will not slip even when wet.
    3. Not to use someone else's crutches.
    4. That crutch tips should be inspected periodically for wear.

29. A client with right-sided weakness needs to learn how to use a cane. The nurse plans to teach the client to position the cane by holding it with the
    1. Left hand and placing the cane in front of the left foot.
    2. Right hand and placing the cane in front of the right foot.
    3. Left hand and 6 inches lateral to the left foot.
    4. Right hand and 6 inches lateral to the right foot.

30. A nurse is evaluating a client's use of a cane for left-sided weakness. The nurse would intervene and correct the client if the nurse observed that the client
    1. Holds the cane on the right side.
    2. Keeps the cane 6 inches out to the side of the right foot.
    3. Moves the cane when the right leg is moved.
    4. Leans on the cane when the right leg swings through.

31. A client with a fractured femur experiences sudden dyspnea. A set of arterial blood gas tests reveal the following: pH, 7.35; $Paco_2$, 43; Pao_2, 58; HCO_3^-, 23. A nurse interprets that the client probably has experienced fat embolus because of the result of the
    1. $Paco_2$

2. PaO_2

3. HCO_3^-

4. pH

32. A client with a fat embolus is experiencing respiratory distress. The nurse plans to assist with which of the following therapies?
    1. Administration of bronchodilators, intubation, mechanical ventilation
    2. Administration of plasma expanders, low-flow oxygen, and suctioning
    3. Administration of corticosteroids, intubation, mechanical ventilation with positive-end expiratory pressure
    4. Administration of antihypertensives, high-flow oxygen, continuous positive airway pressure mask

33. A nurse is caring for a client being treated for fat embolus after multiple fractures. Which of the following data would the nurse evaluate as the most favorable indication of resolution of the fat embolus?
    1. Arterial oxygen level of 78 mm Hg
    2. Minimal dyspnea
    3. Clear chest radiograph
    4. Oxygen saturation of 85%

34. A nurse is caring for a client who develops compartment syndrome from a severely fractured arm. The client asks the nurse how this can happen. The nurse's response is based on the understanding that
    1. An injured artery causes impaired arterial perfusion through the compartment.
    2. The fascia expands with injury, causing pressure on underlying nerves and muscles.
    3. A bone fragment has injured the nerve supply in the area.
    4. Bleeding and swelling cause increased pressure in an area that cannot expand.

35. A nurse has conducted teaching with a client in an arm cast about signs and symptoms of compartment syndrome. The nurse determines that the client understands the information if the client stated that he or she should report which of the following early symptoms of compartment syndrome?
    1. Pain that is relieved only by oxycodone and aspirin (Percodan)
    2. Pain that increases when the arm is dependent
    3. Cold, bluish-colored fingers
    4. Numbness and tingling in the fingers

36. A nurse is repositioning a client who has returned to the nursing unit after internal fixation of a fractured right hip. The nurse should use a
    1. Pillow to keep the right leg abducted during turning.
    2. Pillow to keep the right leg adducted during turning.
    3. Trochanter roll to prevent external rotation while turning.
    4. Trochanter roll to prevent abduction while turning.

37. A nurse has an order to get a client out of bed to a chair on the first postoperative day after total knee replacement. The nurse would plan to do which of the following to protect the knee joint?
    1. Apply a knee immobilizer before getting the client up and elevate the client's surgical leg while sitting.
    2. Apply an Ace wrap around the dressing and put ice on the knee while sitting.
    3. Lift the client to the bedside chair, leaving the continuous passive motion machine in place.
    4. Obtain a walker to minimize weight bearing by the client on the affected leg.

38. A nurse has completed giving discharge instructions to a client after total knee replacement with a metal prosthesis. The nurse determines that the instructions are not understood fully if the client says he or she should
    1. Report fever, redness, or increased pain.
    2. Ignore changes in the shape of the knee.
    3. Report bleeding gums or tarry stools.
    4. Tell future caregivers about the metal implant.

39. A client with diabetes mellitus has had a right below-the-knee amputation. The nurse would assess specifically for which of the following signs and symptoms because of the history of diabetes?
    1. Edema of the stump
    2. Hemorrhage
    3. Separation of wound edges
    4. Slight redness of incision

40. A client is admitted to the nursing unit after a left below-the-knee amputation following a crush injury to the foot and lower leg. The client tells the nurse "I think I'm going crazy. I can feel my left foot itching." The nurse interprets the client's statement to be
    1. A normal response that indicates the presence of phantom limb sensation.
    2. A normal response that indicates the presence of phantom limb pain.
    3. An abnormal response that indicates that the client needs more psychological support.
    4. An abnormal response that indicates that the client is in denial about the limb loss.

41. A nurse is planning to teach the client with below-the-knee amputation about care to prevent skin breakdown. Which of the following points would the nurse include while developing the teaching plan?
    1. A stump sock must be worn at all times and changed twice a week.
    2. The residual limb is washed gently and dried every other day.
    3. The socket of the prosthesis is washed with a harsh bactericidal agent daily.
    4. The socket of the prosthesis must be dried carefully before using it.

42. A nurse is caring for a client who had an above-the-knee amputation 2 days ago. The residual limb was wrapped with an elastic compression bandage, which has come off. The nurse immediately
    1. Calls the physician.
    2. Rewraps the stump with an elastic compression bandage.
    3. Applies ice to the site.
    4. Applies a dry sterile dressing and elevates it on one pillow.

43. A client is complaining of low back pain that radiates down the left posterior thigh. The nurse further assesses the client to see if the pain is worsened or aggravated by
    1. Bed rest.
    2. Application of heat.
    3. Bending or lifting.
    4. Ibuprofen (Motrin).

44. A client has just undergone spinal fusion after experiencing herniated lumbar disk. The nurse would avoid which of the following to maintain client safety after this procedure?
    1. Logrolling technique for repositioning
    2. Pillows under the length of the legs
    3. Head of bed flat
    4. Overhead trapeze

45. A nurse has taught a client with a herniated lumbar disk about proper body mechanics and other items pertinent to low back care. The nurse determines that the client needs further instruction if the client says he or she should
    1. Get out of bed by sitting straight up and swinging the legs over the side of the bed.
    2. Increase fiber and fluid intake in the diet.
    3. Strengthen the back muscles by swimming or walking.
    4. Bend at the knees to pick up objects.

46. A nurse is caring for a client who has had spinal fusion with insertion of hardware. The nurse would be concerned especially with which of the following assessment findings?
    1. Complaints of discomfort during repositioning
    2. Temperature of 101.6° F orally
    3. Old, bloody drainage outlined on the surgical dressing
    4. Discomfort during coughing and deep breathing exercises

47. A client has several fractures of the lower leg and has been placed in an external fixation device. The client is upset about the appearance of the leg, which is edematous. The nurse formulates which of the following nursing diagnoses for the client?
    1. Disturbed Body Image
    2. Activity Intolerance
    3. Risk for Impaired Physical Mobility
    4. Social Isolation

48. A client has been placed in Buck's extension traction. The nurse can provide for countertraction to reduce shear and friction by
    1. Slightly elevating the head of the bed.
    2. Slightly elevating the foot of the bed.
    3. Providing an overhead trapeze.
    4. Using a footboard.

49. A nurse is caring for a client with a diagnosis of gout. Which of the following laboratory values would the nurse expect to note in the client?
    1. Uric acid level of 8 mg/dL
    2. Calcium level of 9 mg/dL
    3. Phosphorus level of 3 mg/dL
    4. Potassium level of 4 mEq/L

50. A nurse is caring for a client with osteoarthritis. The nurse performs an assessment, knowing that which of the following is a clinical manifestation associated with the disorder?
    1. Morning stiffness
    2. A decreased sedimentation rate
    3. Joint pain that diminishes after rest
    4. Elevated antinuclear antibody levels

CRITICAL THINKING: MULTIPLE RESPONSE

A nurse is preparing a list of cast care instructions for a client who just had a plaster cast applied to his right forearm. Select all instructions that the nurse includes on the list.

____ Keep the cast and extremity elevated.

____ Allow the wet cast 24 to 48 hours to dry.

____ Use a hair dryer set on a warm to hot setting to dry the cast.

____ Tingling and numbness in the extremity is expected.

____ Use a soft padded object that will fit under the cast to scratch the skin under the cast.

____ The cast needs to be kept clean and dry.

ANSWERS

1. 1

Rationale: Soft tissue injuries such as sprains are treated by RICE (*rest*, *ice*, *compression*, and *elevation*) for the first 24 hours after the injury. Ice is applied intermittently for 20 to 30 minutes at a time. Heat is not used in the first 24 hours because it could increase venous congestion, which would increase edema and pain.

Test-Taking Strategy: Use the process of elimination. Note the key word "avoid." Sprains should be rested and elevated, so eliminate options 3 and 4. Use of an Ace wrap is also helpful in reducing the pain and swelling, so eliminate option 2. Review treatment measures for a sprain if you had difficulty with this question.

Level of Cognitive Ability: Application
Client Needs: Physiological Integrity
Integrated Process: Nursing Process—planning
Content Area: Adult health—musculoskeletal
Reference: Ignatavicius, D., & Workman, M. (2002). *Medical-surgical nursing: Critical thinking for collaborative care* (4th ed., p. 1154). Philadelphia: W. B. Saunders.

2. 2

Rationale: A client at risk for osteoporosis needs to increase intake of calcium. The major dietary source of calcium is dairy food, including milk, yogurt, and a variety of cheeses. Calcium also may be added to certain products, such as orange juice, which then is advertised as being "fortified" with calcium. Calcium supplements are available and recommended for those with typically low calcium intake. Options 1, 3, and 4 are not food sources high in calcium.

Test-Taking Strategy: Use the process of elimination. Recall that the client at risk for osteoporosis needs to increase intake of calcium. Knowing that dairy products are high in calcium will direct you to option 2. Review osteoporosis and food sources of calcium if you had difficulty with this question.

Level of Cognitive Ability: Analysis
Client Needs: Physiological Integrity
Integrated Process: Teaching/Learning
Content Area: Adult health—musculoskeletal
Reference: Ignatavicius, D., & Workman, M. (2002). *Medical-surgical nursing: Critical thinking for collaborative care* (4th ed., pp. 1099, 1101). Philadelphia: W. B. Saunders.

3. 3

Rationale: Risk factors for osteoporosis include being female, postmenopausal, of advanced age, low-calcium diet, excessive alcohol intake, being sedentary, and smoking cigarettes. Long-term use of corticosteroids, anticonvulsants, and furosemide (Lasix) also increases risk.

Test-Taking Strategy: Use the process of elimination. Eliminate option 2 first. The 25-year-old woman who jogs (exercise using the long bones) has negligible risk. The 36-year-old man with asthma is eliminated next because his only risk factor might be long-term corticosteroid use. Of the two remaining options, the 65-year-old woman has more risk (age, gender, postmenopausal, sedentary, smoking) than the 70-year-old man (age, alcohol consumption). Review the risk factors associated with osteoporosis if you had difficulty with this question.

Level of Cognitive Ability: Analysis

Client Needs: Health Promotion and Maintenance
Integrated Process: Nursing Process—assessment
Content Area: Adult health—musculoskeletal
Reference: Ignatavicius, D., & Workman, M. (2002). *Medical-surgical nursing: Critical thinking for collaborative care* (4th ed., p. 1095). Philadelphia: W. B. Saunders.

4. 3

Rationale: Home modifications to reduce the risk for falls include use of railings on all staircases, ample lighting, removal of scatter rugs, and placement of hand rails in the bathroom. Removal of wall-to-wall carpeting is not necessary.

Test-Taking Strategy: Note the key word "unnecessary." Begin to answer this question by eliminating options 1 and 4. Both of these items provide physical support to the client and are needed. Use of night lights will enhance vision for the client getting up at night to use the bathroom and also is warranted. Wall-to-wall carpeting does not pose a risk to the client and does not need to be removed. Review home care measures to ensure safety if you had difficulty with this question.

Level of Cognitive Ability: Application
Client Needs: Safe, Effective Care Environment
Integrated Process: Teaching/Learning
Content Area: Adult health—musculoskeletal
Reference: Ignatavicius, D., & Workman, M. (2002). *Medical-surgical nursing: Critical thinking for collaborative care* (4th ed., p. 1102). Philadelphia: W. B. Saunders.

5. 2

Rationale: Nursing care after bone biopsy includes monitoring the site for swelling, bleeding, and hematoma formation. The biopsy site is elevated for 24 hours to reduce edema. The vital signs are monitored every 4 hours for 24 hours. The client usually requires mild analgesics; more severe pain usually indicates that complications are arising.

Test-Taking Strategy: Use the process of elimination. Note the key word "inaccurate." Recalling that this procedure is done under local anesthesia will direct you to option 2. Review nursing care following a bone biopsy if you had difficulty with this question.

Level of Cognitive Ability: Analysis
Client Needs: Physiological Integrity
Integrated Process: Teaching/Learning
Content Area: Adult health—musculoskeletal
Reference: Ignatavicius, D., & Workman, M. (2002). *Medical-surgical nursing: Critical thinking for collaborative care* (4th ed., p. 1090). Philadelphia: W. B. Saunders.

6. 4

Rationale: After arthroscopy, the client usually can walk carefully on the leg once sensation has returned. The client is instructed to avoid strenuous exercise for at least a few days. The client may resume the usual diet. Signs and symptoms of infection should be reported to the physician.

Test-Taking Strategy: Use the process of elimination. Recalling the general client teaching points related to surgical procedures will direct you to option 4. Review client teaching points following arthroscopy if you had difficulty with this question.

Level of Cognitive Ability: Analysis
Client Needs: Physiological Integrity

Integrated Process: Teaching/Learning
Content Area: Adult health—musculoskeletal
Reference: Ignatavicius, D., & Workman, M. (2002). *Medical-surgical nursing: Critical thinking for collaborative care* (4th ed., p. 1091). Philadelphia: W. B. Saunders.

7. **1**

Rationale: Because of the risk of allergy to contrast dye, the nurse places highest priority on assessing whether the client has an allergy to iodine or shellfish. The nurse also reinforces information about the test, tells the client about the need to remain still during the procedure, and encourages the client to void before the procedure for comfort.
Test-Taking Strategy: Use the process of elimination. Note the key words "highest priority." This tells you that more than one or all of the options are correct (in fact, they all are). Use Maslow's hierarchy of needs theory. Although options 2, 3, and 4 compete for priority, option 1 (allergy to iodine or shellfish) takes first preference. The consequence of possible anaphylactic shock (physiological risk) makes this the correct option. Review client preparation for an arthrogram if you had difficulty with this question.
Level of Cognitive Ability: Analysis
Client Needs: Physiological Integrity
Integrated Process: Nursing Process—assessment
Content Area: Delegating/Prioritizing
Reference: Lewis, S., Heitkemper, M., & Dirksen, S. (2004). *Medical-surgical nursing: Assessment and management of clinical problems* (6th ed., p. 1645). St. Louis: Mosby.

8. **2**

Rationale: A radiograph is a photographic image of a part of the body on a special film, which is used to diagnose a wide variety of conditions. Radiography itself is painless; any discomfort would arise from repositioning a painful part for filming. The nurse may want to premedicate a client who is at risk for pain. Any radiopaque objects such as jewelry or other metal must be removed. The client is asked to breathe in deeply and then hold the breath while the chest radiograph is taken. To minimize risk of radiation exposure, the x-ray technologist stands in a separate area protected by a lead wall. The client also wears a lead shield over the gonads.
Test-Taking Strategy: Use the process of elimination. Recalling that radiopaque objects need to be removed will direct you to option 2. Review client preparation for a chest radiograph if you had difficulty with this question.
Level of Cognitive Ability: Application
Client Needs: Physiological Integrity
Integrated Process: Nursing Process—implementation
Content Area: Adult health—musculoskeletal
References: Chernecky, C., & Berger, B. (2001). *Laboratory tests and diagnostic procedures* (3rd ed., p. 337). Philadelphia: W. B. Saunders.
Lewis, S., Heitkemper, M., & Dirksen, S. (2004). *Medical-surgical nursing: Assessment and management of clinical problems* (6th ed., p. 1645). St. Louis: Mosby.

9. **4**

Rationale: No special restrictions are necessary after a bone scan. The client is encouraged to drink large amounts of water

for 24 to 48 hours to flush the radioisotope from the system. The minimal amount of radioactivity of the isotope presents no hazards to the client or staff.
Test-Taking Strategy: Use the process of elimination. Options 2 or 3 serve no purpose, so eliminate these options first. Nausea and flushing could accompany dye injection during a procedure, but this procedure uses radioisotopes. Additionally, the question relates to care after the procedure. Remember that fluids hasten elimination of the isotope from the client's system. Review care following a bone scan if you had difficulty with this question.
Level of Cognitive Ability: Analysis
Client Needs: Physiological Integrity
Integrated Process: Teaching/Learning
Content Area: Adult health—musculoskeletal
References: Chernecky, C., & Berger, B. (2001). *Laboratory tests and diagnostic procedures* (3rd ed., p. 261). Philadelphia: W. B. Saunders.
Lewis, S., Heitkemper, M., & Dirksen, S. (2004). *Medical-surgical nursing: Assessment and management of clinical problems* (6th ed., p. 1645). St. Louis: Mosby.

10. **2**

Rationale: Typical signs and symptoms of fracture include pain, loss of function in the area, deformity, shortening of the extremity, crepitus, swelling, and ecchymosis. Not all fractures lead to the development of every sign. A contusion results from a blow to soft tissue and causes pain, swelling, and ecchymosis. A sprain is an injury to a ligament caused by a wrenching or twisting motion. Symptoms include pain, swelling, and inability to use the joint or bear weight normally. A strain results from a pulling force on the muscle. Symptoms include soreness and pain with muscle use.
Test-Taking Strategy: Use the process of elimination. Within the list of signs and symptoms in the question, note the one stating that one leg is shorter than another. Only a fractured bone (which shortens with displacement) could cause this sign. This makes it easy to eliminate each of the incorrect options. Review signs of a fracture if you had difficulty with this question.
Level of Cognitive Ability: Analysis
Client Needs: Physiological Integrity
Integrated Process: Nursing Process—assessment
Content Area: Adult health—musculoskeletal
Reference: Ignatavicius, D., & Workman, M. (2002). *Medical-surgical nursing: Critical thinking for collaborative care* (4th ed., p. 1130). Philadelphia: W. B. Saunders.

11. **1**

Rationale: With a suspected fracture, the client is not moved unless it is dangerous to remain in that spot. The nurse should remain with the client and have someone else call for emergency help. A fracture is not reduced at the scene. Before the client is moved, the site of fracture is immobilized to prevent further injury.
Test-Taking Strategy: Use the process of elimination. Eliminate options 2 and 4 first because either of these options could result in further injury to the client. Of remaining options the more prudent action would be for the nurse to remain with

the client and have someone else call for emergency assistance. Review care to the client with a fracture if you had difficulty with this question.
Level of Cognitive Ability: Application
Client Needs: Physiological Integrity
Integrated Process: Nursing Process—implementation
Content Area: Adult health—musculoskeletal
Reference: Ignatavicius, D., & Workman, M. (2002). *Medical-surgical nursing: Critical thinking for collaborative care* (4th ed., p. 1132). Philadelphia: W. B. Saunders.
Phipps, W., Monahan, F., Sands, J., Marek, J., & Neighbors, M. (2003). *Medical-surgical nursing: Health and illness perspectives* (7th ed., p. 1469). St. Louis: Mosby.

12. 1
Rationale: Immobility and the weight of a casted arm may cause the shoulder above an arm fracture to become stiff. The shoulder of a casted arm should be lifted over the head periodically as a preventive measure. The use of slings further immobilizes the shoulder and may be contraindicated. Making fists with the left hand provides good isometric exercise to maintain muscle strength. Range of motion of the affected fingers is also a useful general measure. Lifting the right arm is of no particular value.
Test-Taking Strategy: Use the process of elimination. Imagine each of the movements and think about the muscle groups that are moved with each. Options 2 and 4 provide for no movement of the left arm and are eliminated first. Making a fist with the hand on the casted arm provides good isometric exercise to the muscles surrounding the fracture but again does nothing for the shoulder. The only viable option is raising the arm over the head, which provides some range of motion for the shoulder joint. Review teaching points for a client with a casted arm if you had difficulty with this question.
Level of Cognitive Ability: Application
Client Needs: Physiological Integrity
Integrated Process: Teaching/Learning
Content Area: Adult health—musculoskeletal
Reference: Perry A., & Potter, P. (2002). *Clinical nursing skills and techniques* (5th ed., p. 875). St. Louis: Mosby.

13. 1
Rationale: A fiberglass cast is made of water-activated polyurethane materials that are dry to the touch within minutes and reach full rigid strength in about 20 minutes. Because of this, the client can bear weight on the cast within 20 to 30 minutes.
Test-Taking Strategy: Use the process of elimination. Note the key word "nonplaster." Options 3 and 4 should be eliminated first because these time frames are similar to the drying times for plaster casts. Recalling that the nonplaster type of cast is lighter and dries quickly may help you to choose the 20 to 30 minute time frame as correct. Review client teaching points related to a nonplaster cast if you had difficulty with this question.
Level of Cognitive Ability: Application
Client Needs: Physiological Integrity
Integrated Process: Teaching/Learning
Content Area: Adult health—musculoskeletal

Reference: Ignatavicius, D., & Workman, M. (2002). *Medical-surgical nursing: Critical thinking for collaborative care* (4th ed., p. 1134). Philadelphia: W. B. Saunders.

14. 4
Rationale: Client instructions should include avoiding walking on wet, slippery floors to prevent falls. Surface soil on a cast can be removed with a damp cloth. If the cast gets wet, it can be dried with a hair dryer set to a cool setting to prevent skin breakdown. If the skin under the cast itches, cool air from a hair dryer may be used to relieve it. The client should never scratch under a cast because of the risk of skin breakdown and ulcer formation.
Test-Taking Strategy: Use the process of elimination. Note the key words "needs further instruction." Remember never to use a hair dryer on a cast or on the skin under any cast with the dryer set at the warmest setting; only cool settings are used to prevent burns. Review client teaching points about a cast if you had difficulty with this question.
Level of Cognitive Ability: Analysis
Client Needs: Physiological Integrity
Integrated Process: Teaching/Learning
Content Area: Adult health—musculoskeletal
Reference: Ignatavicius, D., & Workman, M. (2002). *Medical-surgical nursing: Critical thinking for collaborative care* (4th ed., p. 1135). Philadelphia: W. B. Saunders.

15. 2
Rationale: Buck's extension traction is a type of skin traction often applied after hip fracture before the fracture is reduced in surgery. Traction reduces muscle spasms and helps to immobilize the fracture. Traction does not lengthen the leg for the purpose of preventing blood vessel severance. Traction also does not allow for bony healing to begin.
Test-Taking Strategy: Use the process of elimination. Focus on the client's diagnosis, hip fracture. Read each option carefully. Noting the words "provides fracture immobilization" will direct you to option 2. Review the purpose of Buck's traction if you had difficulty with this question.
Level of Cognitive Ability: Application
Client Needs: Physiological Integrity
Integrated Process: Nursing Process—implementation
Content Area: Adult health—musculoskeletal
Reference: Ignatavicius, D., & Workman, M. (2002). *Medical-surgical nursing: Critical thinking for collaborative care* (4th ed., p. 1136). Philadelphia: W. B. Saunders.

16. 4
Rationale: If the client in skeletal traction may not turn from side to side, the nurse should have the client pull up on a trapeze and try to lift the hips off the bed for skin care, bedpan use, and linen changes. If the client is unable to pull up on a trapeze, the nurse can push down on the mattress with one hand while administering care with the other.
Test-Taking Strategy: Use the process of elimination. Option 3 is contraindicated because it ignores a medical order. Option 1 is not feasible as stated. The client cannot lift up from the bed using only one foot. Options 2 and 4 are acceptable alternatives. Because the question asks which would be "most useful," the answer is option 4. Providing care to the client

who can lift the hips off the bed by use of a trapeze is easier and more efficient than providing care to one who cannot. Review care to the client in skeletal leg traction if you had difficulty with this question.
Level of Cognitive Ability: Application
Client Needs: Physiological Integrity
Integrated Process: Nursing Process—implementation
Content Area: Adult health—musculoskeletal
References: Ignatavicius, D., & Workman, M. (2002). *Medical-surgical nursing: Critical thinking for collaborative care* (4th ed., p. 1137). Philadelphia: W. B. Saunders.
Phipps, W., Monahan, F., Sands, J., Marek, J., & Neighbors, M. (2003). *Medical-surgical nursing: Health and illness perspectives* (7th ed., p. 1472). St. Louis: Mosby.

17. **2**
Rationale: A small amount of serous oozing is expected at pin insertion sites. Signs of infection such as inflammation, purulent drainage, and pain at the pin site are not expected findings and should be reported to the physician.
Test-Taking Strategy: Use the process of elimination. Note the key words "least concerned." Options 1 and 4 seem to indicate an infectious problem and are eliminated first. From the remaining options, note that the complaint of pain is at "a pin site." Also, because serous drainage is an expected finding, select option 2. Review expected findings in the client with skeletal traction if you had difficulty with this question.
Level of Cognitive Ability: Analysis
Client Needs: Physiological Integrity
Integrated Process: Nursing Process—evaluation
Content Area: Adult health—musculoskeletal
Reference: Ignatavicius, D., & Workman, M. (2002). *Medical-surgical nursing: Critical thinking for collaborative care* (4th ed., p. 1137). Philadelphia: W. B. Saunders.

18. **1**
Rationale: A major defining characteristic of Deficient Diversional Activity is expression of boredom by the client. The question does not identify difficulties with coordination, range of motion, or muscle strength, which would indicate Impaired Physical Mobility. The question also does not relate client feelings of inability to perform activities of daily living (Self-Care Deficit) or lack of control (Powerlessness).
Test-Taking Strategy: Use the process of elimination. When asked about a nursing diagnosis, focus on the information in the question to direct you to the correct option. Review the defining characteristics of Deficient Diversional Activity if you had difficulty with this question.
Level of Cognitive Ability: Analysis
Client Needs: Psychosocial Integrity
Integrated Process: Nursing Process—analysis
Content Area: Adult health—musculoskeletal
Reference: Perry, A., & Potter, P. (2002). *Clinical nursing skills and techniques* (5th ed., p. 827). St. Louis: Mosby.

19. **3**
Rationale: Buck's extension traction is a type of skin traction. The nurse inspects the skin of the limb in traction at least once every 8 hours for irritation or inflammation. Massaging the skin with lotion is not indicated. The nurse never releases the weights of traction unless specifically ordered by the physician. There are no pins to care for with skin traction.
Test-Taking Strategy: Use the process of elimination and the steps of the nursing process to answer this question. Option 3 is the only option that relates to assessment. Review care to the client in Buck's traction if you had difficulty with this question.
Level of Cognitive Ability: Application
Client Needs: Physiological Integrity
Integrated Process: Nursing Process—planning
Content Area: Adult health—musculoskeletal
Reference: Ignatavicius, D, & Workman, M. (2002). *Medical-surgical nursing: Critical thinking for collaborative care* (4th ed., p. 1137). Philadelphia: W. B. Saunders.

20. **4**
Rationale: A client who complains of severe pain may need realignment or may have traction weights ordered that are too heavy. The nurse realigns the client, and if that is ineffective, then calls the physician. Severe leg pain, once traction has been established, indicates a problem. Medicating the client should be done after one has tried to determine and treat the cause of the pain. Providing pin care is unrelated to the problem as described.
Test-Taking Strategy: Use the process of elimination. Note the key word "first." Use the steps of the nursing process to direct you to option 4. This is the only option that addresses assessment. Review care of the client in traction if you had difficulty with this question.
Level of Cognitive Ability: Application
Client Needs: Physiological Integrity
Integrated Process: Nursing Process—implementation
Content Area: Delegating/Prioritizing
Reference: Ignatavicius, D., & Workman, M. (2002). *Medical-surgical nursing: Critical thinking for collaborative care* (4th ed., p. 1137). Philadelphia: W. B. Saunders.

21. **2**
Rationale: Signs and symptoms of infection under a casted area include odor or purulent drainage from the cast or the presence of "hot spots," which are areas of the cast that are warmer than others. The physician should be notified if any of these occur. Signs of impaired circulation in the distal limb include coolness and pallor of the skin, diminished arterial pulse, and edema.
Test-Taking Strategy: Use the process of elimination. Answer this question thinking about what you would expect to note with infection: redness, swelling, heat, and purulent drainage. With this in mind, you can eliminate options 1 and 3 easily. From the remaining options, remember "dependent edema" is not necessarily indicative of infection. Swelling would be continuous. The "hot spot" on the cast could signify infection underneath that area and is the correct answer to the question. Review signs of infection in an extremity with a cast if you had difficulty with this question.
Level of Cognitive Ability: Analysis
Client Needs: Physiological Integrity

Integrated Process: Nursing Process—assessment
Content Area: Adult health—musculoskeletal
Reference: Ignatavicius, D., & Workman, M. (2002). *Medical-surgical nursing: Critical thinking for collaborative care* (4th ed., p. 1136). Philadelphia: W. B. Saunders.

22. **1**
Rationale: Most pain associated with fractures can be minimized with rest, elevation, application of cold, and administration of analgesics. Pain that is not relieved by these measures should be reported to the physician because the pain may result from impaired tissue perfusion, tissue breakdown, or necrosis. Because this is a new closed fracture and cast, infection would not have had time to set in.
Test-Taking Strategy: Use the process of elimination. Focus on the issue, intense pain. Use of the ABCs—airway, breathing, and circulation—will direct you to option 1. Review care to the client with a fracture and new cast if you had difficulty with this question.
Level of Cognitive Ability: Analysis
Client Needs: Physiological Integrity
Integrated Process: Nursing Process—analysis
Content Area: Adult health—musculoskeletal
References: Lewis, S., Heitkemper, M., & Dirksen, S. (2004). *Medical-surgical nursing: Assessment and management of clinical problems* (6th ed., p. 1669). St. Louis: Mosby.
Perry, A., & Potter, P. (2002). *Clinical nursing skills and techniques* (5th ed., p. 871). St. Louis: Mosby.

23. **3**
Rationale: A casted extremity is elevated continuously for the first 24 to 48 hours to minimize swelling and to promote venous drainage. Options 1, 2, and 4 are incorrect.
Test-Taking Strategy: Use the process of elimination. Recalling that edema is a concern and knowledge of the effects of gravity on edema will direct you to option 3. Review care to the client with a new cast if you had difficulty with this question.
Level of Cognitive Ability: Application
Client Needs: Physiological Integrity
Integrated Process: Nursing Process—implementation
Content Area: Adult health—musculoskeletal
Reference: Phipps, W., Monahan, F., Sands, J., Marek, J., & Neighbors, M. (2003). *Medical-surgical nursing: Health and illness perspectives* (7th ed., p. 1471). St. Louis: Mosby.

24. **4**
Rationale: The nurse petals the edges of the cast with tape to minimize skin irritation. If a client has a cast applied and returns home, the client can be taught to do the same.
Test-Taking Strategy: Use the process of elimination. Options 1 and 2 are similar, and neither helps to get rid of the cause of the irritation, so eliminate them first. Imagine the use of a "rough file"; it would create plaster chips and dust that could go underneath the cast. By the process of elimination, the nurse would petal the cast to cushion the skin from the irritating cast material. Review care to the client with a cast if you had difficulty with this question.
Level of Cognitive Ability: Application
Client Needs: Physiological Integrity
Integrated Process: Nursing Process—implementation

Content Area: Adult health—musculoskeletal
Reference: Ignatavicius, D., & Workman, M. (2002). *Medical-surgical nursing: Critical thinking for collaborative care* (4th ed., p. 1134). Philadelphia: W. B. Saunders.

25. **1**
Rationale: A plaster cast must remain dry to keep its strength. The cast should be handled with the palms of the hands, not the fingertips, until fully dry. Air should circulate freely around the cast to help it dry; the cast also gives off heat as it dries. The client should never scratch under the cast; the client may use a hair dryer on the cool setting to eliminate an itch.
Test-Taking Strategy: Use the process of elimination. Knowing that a wet cast can be dented with the fingertips, causing pressure underneath, helps you to eliminate option 2 first. Knowing that the cast needs to dry helps you to eliminate option 3 next. Option 4 is dangerous to skin integrity and is also eliminated. Remember that plaster casts, once they have dried after application, should not become wet. Review care to the client with a cast if you had difficulty with this question.
Level of Cognitive Ability: Analysis
Client Needs: Physiological Integrity
Integrated Process: Teaching/Learning
Content Area: Adult health—musculoskeletal
Reference: Perry, A., & Potter, P. (2002). *Clinical nursing skills and techniques* (5th ed., p. 872). St. Louis: Mosby.

26. **3**
Rationale: Crutches are measured so that the tops are 2 to 3 fingerbreadths from the axillas. This ensures that the client's axillas are not resting on the crutch or bearing the weight of the crutch, which could result in injury to the nerves of the brachial plexus.
Test-Taking Strategy: Use the process of elimination. Recalling the risk associated with brachial nerve plexus injury will direct you to option 3. Review the complications associated with the use of crutches if you had difficulty with this question.
Level of Cognitive Ability: Comprehension
Client Needs: Physiological Integrity
Integrated Process: Teaching/Learning
Content Area: Adult health—musculoskeletal
Reference: Ignatavicius, D., & Workman, M. (2002). *Medical-surgical nursing: Critical thinking for collaborative care* (4th ed., p. 1140). Philadelphia: W. B. Saunders.

27. **1**
Rationale: The classic tripod position is taught to the client before one gives instructions on gait. The crutches are placed anywhere from 6 to 10 inches in front and to the side of the client, depending on the client's body size. This provides a wide enough base of support to the client and improves balance.
Test-Taking Strategy: Use the process of elimination. Three inches (option 2) and 20 inches (option 3) seem excessively short and long, respectively, and are eliminated first. Visualize the descriptions in the options. Eight inches seems more in keeping with the normal length of a stride than 15 inches for someone with crutches. Review the points related to client instructions for the use of crutches if you had difficulty with this question.

Level of Cognitive Ability: Application
Client Needs: Physiological Integrity
Integrated Process: Nursing Process—planning
Content Area: Adult health—musculoskeletal
References: Ignatavicius, D., & Workman, M. (2002). *Medical-surgical nursing: Critical thinking for collaborative care* (4th ed., p. 1140). Philadelphia: W. B. Saunders.
Potter, P., & Perry, A. (2001). *Fundamentals of nursing* (5th ed., p. 1010). St. Louis: Mosby.

28. 2
Rationale: Crutch tips should remain dry. Water could cause slipping by decreasing the surface friction of the rubber tip on the floor. If crutch tips get wet, the client should dry them with a cloth or paper towel. The client should use only crutches measured for the client. The tips should be inspected for wear, and spare crutches and tips should be available if needed.
Test-Taking Strategy: Use the process of elimination. Note the key words "needs reinforcement of information." Remember that crutch tips can slip when they get wet, posing a possible threat to the unsuspecting client. Review client teaching points related to safety and the use of crutches if you had difficulty with this question.
Level of Cognitive Ability: Analysis
Client Needs: Physiological Integrity
Integrated Process: Teaching/Learning
Content Area: Adult health—musculoskeletal
Reference: Potter, P., & Perry, A. (2001). *Fundamentals of nursing* (5th ed., p. 1009). St. Louis: Mosby.

29. 3
Rationale: The client is taught to hold the cane on the side opposite from the weakness. The reason is that with normal walking, the opposite arm and leg move together (called reciprocal motion). The cane is placed 4 to 6 inches lateral to the fifth toe.
Test-Taking Strategy: Use the process of elimination. Knowing that the cane is held at the client's side, not in front, helps you to eliminate options 1 and 2 first. Knowing that the preferred method is to have the cane positioned on the stronger side helps you to choose option 3 over option 4. Review client teaching points related to the use of a cane if you had difficulty with this question.
Level of Cognitive Ability: Application
Client Needs: Physiological Integrity
Integrated Process: Teaching/Learning
Content Area: Adult health—musculoskeletal
References: Ignatavicius, D., & Workman, M. (2002). *Medical-surgical nursing: Critical thinking for collaborative care* (4th ed., p. 1140). Philadelphia: W. B. Saunders.
Potter, P., & Perry, A. (2001). *Fundamentals of nursing* (5th ed., p. 1008). St. Louis: Mosby.

30. 3
Rationale: The cane is held on the stronger side to minimize stress on the affected extremity and provide a wide base of support. The cane is held 4 to 6 inches lateral to the fifth toe. The cane is moved forward with the affected leg. The client leans on the cane for added support while the stronger side swings through.

Test-Taking Strategy: Use the process of elimination. Note the key word "intervene." Knowing that the cane is held on the stronger side helps you eliminate options 1 and 2 first. Recalling that the client moves the cane with the weaker leg and leans on it for support when the stronger leg swings through will direct you to option 3. Review client instructions about the use of a cane if you had difficulty with this question.
Level of Cognitive Ability: Application
Client Needs: Safe, Effective Care Environment
Integrated Process: Nursing Process—implementation
Content Area: Adult health—musculoskeletal
References: Perry, A., & Potter, P. (2002). *Clinical nursing skills and techniques* (5th ed., p. 858). St. Louis: Mosby.
Potter, P., & Perry, A. (2001). *Fundamentals of nursing* (5th ed., p. 1008). St. Louis: Mosby.

31. 2
Rationale: A key feature of fat embolism is a significant degree of hypoxemia, with a PaO_2 often less than 60 mm Hg. Options 1, 3, and 4 are normal blood gas results.
Test-Taking Strategy: Use the process of elimination. Recall that fat embolus causes significant hypoxemia. Also note that the values of the $PaCO_2$, HCO_3^-, and pH are normal. Review the clinical manifestations of fat embolism if you had difficulty with this question.
Level of Cognitive Ability: Analysis
Client Needs: Physiological Integrity
Integrated Process: Nursing Process—analysis
Content Area: Adult health—musculoskeletal
Reference: Phipps, W., Monahan, F., Sands, J., Marek, J., & Neighbors, M. (2003). *Medical-surgical nursing: Health and illness perspectives* (7th ed., p. 1486). St. Louis: Mosby.

32. 3
Rationale: Respiratory failure is the most common cause of death after fat embolus. The client may be intubated and mechanically ventilated with positive end-expiratory pressure to treat the significant hypoxemia and pulmonary edema. Corticosteroids are given to treat inflammatory lung reactions and control cerebral edema.
Test-Taking Strategy: Use the process of elimination. Fat embolus does not cause bronchoconstriction or bronchospasm, which may help to eliminate option 1. The question makes no mention of hypovolemia, so the plasma expanders in option 2 have no use. From the remaining options you need to know that corticosteroids are used for the inflammatory lung reaction and that hypertension may not be part of the clinical picture. Review the complications associated with fat embolism and the manifestations of respiratory failure if you had difficulty with this question.
Level of Cognitive Ability: Application
Client Needs: Physiological Integrity
Integrated Process: Nursing Process—planning
Content Area: Adult health—musculoskeletal
Reference: Phipps, W., Monahan, F., Sands, J., Marek, J., & Neighbors, M. (2003). *Medical-surgical nursing: Health and illness perspectives* (7th ed., p. 1486). St. Louis: Mosby.

33. 3
Rationale: A clear chest radiograph is a good indicator that fat embolus is resolving. When fat embolism occurs, the chest

radiograph has a "snowstorm" appearance. Eupnea, not minimal dyspnea, is a normal sign. Arterial oxygen levels should be 80 to 100 mm Hg. Oxygen saturation should be greater than 95%.
Test-Taking Strategy: Use the process of elimination. Note the key words "most favorable indication." Knowing that the arterial oxygen and oxygen saturation levels are below normal helps you to eliminate options 1 and 4. Dyspnea, even at a minimal level, is not normal, so eliminate option 2. Review the expected outcomes in a client being treated for fat embolism if you had difficulty with this question.
Level of Cognitive Ability: Analysis
Client Needs: Physiological Integrity
Integrated Process: Nursing Process—evaluation
Content Area: Adult health—musculoskeletal
Reference: Phipps, W., Monahan, F., Sands, J., Marek, J., & Neighbors, M. (2003). *Medical-surgical nursing: Health and illness perspectives* (7th ed., p. 1486). St. Louis: Mosby.

34. 4
Rationale: Compartment syndrome is caused by bleeding and swelling within a compartment, which is lined by fascia and does not expand. The bleeding and swelling put pressure on the nerves, muscles, and blood vessels in the compartment, triggering the symptoms. Options 1, 2, and 3 are inaccurate descriptions of compartment syndrome.
Test-Taking Strategy: Use the process of elimination. Note the name of the syndrome and the relationship of the name to the description in option 4. Review the pathophysiology related to compartment syndrome if you had difficulty with this question.
Level of Cognitive Ability: Comprehension
Client Needs: Physiological Integrity
Integrated Process: Nursing Process—implementation
Content Area: Adult health—musculoskeletal
Reference: Phipps, W., Monahan, F., Sands, J., Marek, J., & Neighbors, M. (2003). *Medical-surgical nursing: Health and illness perspectives* (7th ed., p. 1487). St. Louis: Mosby.

35. 4
Rationale: The earliest symptom of compartment syndrome is paresthesia (numbness and tingling in the fingers). Other symptoms include pain unrelieved by narcotics, pain that increases with limb elevation, and pallor and coolness to the distal limb. Cyanosis is a late sign.
Test-Taking Strategy: Use the process of elimination. Note the key word "early." Knowing that compartment syndrome is characterized by insufficient circulation and ischemia caused by pressure will direct you to option 4. Review the early signs of compartment syndrome if you had difficulty with this question.
Level of Cognitive Ability: Analysis
Client Needs: Physiological Integrity
Integrated Process: Teaching/Learning
Content Area: Adult health—musculoskeletal
Reference: Ignatavicius, D., & Workman, M. (2002). *Medical-surgical nursing: Critical thinking for collaborative care* (4th ed., p. 1127). Philadelphia: W. B. Saunders.

36. 1
Rationale: Following internal fixation of a hip fracture, the client is turned to the affected side or the unaffected side as prescribed by the surgeon. Before moving the client, the nurse places a pillow between the client's legs to keep the affected leg in abduction. The nurse then repositions the client while maintaining proper alignment and abduction. A trochanter roll is useful in preventing external rotation, but it is used once the client has been repositioned. A trochanter roll is not used while the client is being turned.
Test-Taking Strategy: Use the process of elimination. Visualizing each description in the options and recalling that the affected leg needs to remain abducted will direct you to option 1. Review care to the client after internal fixation if you had difficulty with this question.
Level of Cognitive Ability: Application
Client Needs: Physiological Integrity
Integrated Process: Nursing Process—implementation
Content Area: Adult health—musculoskeletal
Reference: Ignatavicius, D., & Workman, M. (2002). *Medical-surgical nursing: Critical thinking for collaborative care* (4th ed., p. 1145). Philadelphia: W. B. Saunders.

37. 1
Rationale: The nurse assists the client to get out of bed after putting a knee immobilizer on the affected joint for stability. The surgeon orders the weight-bearing limits on the affected leg. To minimize edema, the leg is elevated while the client is sitting in the chair. The continuous passive motion machine is used while the client is in bed.
Test-Taking Strategy: Use the process of elimination. A compression dressing should already be in place on the wound, so you can eliminate option 2. Because the continous passive motion machine is used while the client is in bed, eliminate option 3. From the remaining options, recalling that ambulation is not started until the second postoperative day will direct you to option 1. Also, a knee immobilizer is most appropriate to protect a knee joint. Review care to the client following total knee replacement if you had difficulty with this question.
Level of Cognitive Ability: Application
Client Needs: Physiological Integrity
Integrated Process: Nursing Process—planning
Content Area: Adult health—musculoskeletal
Reference: Ignatavicius, D., & Workman, M. (2002). *Medical-surgical nursing: Critical thinking for collaborative care* (4th ed., p. 1153). Philadelphia: W. B. Saunders.

38. 2
Rationale: After total knee replacement, the client should report signs and symptoms of infection and any changes in the shape of the knee. Any of these could indicate developing complications. With a metal implant, the client must be on anticoagulant therapy and should report adverse effects of this therapy, including bleeding from a variety of sources. With a metal implant, the client must notify caregivers, because certain diagnostic tests (magnetic resonance imaging) will need to be avoided, and the client will need antibiotic prophylaxis for invasive procedures.
Test-Taking Strategy: Note the key words "not understood." The client has a metal prosthesis, which indicates that the client is receiving anticoagulant therapy. This would make options 3 and 4 correct. Reporting signs and symptoms of

infection is important, so eliminate option 1. Recalling that changes in the shape of the knee could indicate developing complications with the prosthesis will direct you to option 2. Review client teaching points after this surgical procedure if you had difficulty with this question.

Level of Cognitive Ability: Analysis
Client Needs: Physiological Integrity
Integrated Process: Teaching/Learning
Content Area: Adult health—musculoskeletal
Reference: Lewis, S., Heitkemper, M., & Dirksen, S. (2004). *Medical-surgical nursing: Assessment and management of clinical problems* (6th ed., p. 1688). St. Louis: Mosby.

39. 3
Rationale: Clients with diabetes mellitus are more prone to wound infection and delayed wound healing because of the disease. Postoperative stump edema and hemorrhage are complications in the immediate postoperative period that apply to any client with an amputation. Slight redness of the incision is considered normal, as long as it is dry and intact.
Test-Taking Strategy: Use the process of elimination. Recalling that diabetes mellitus increases the client's chances of developing infection and delayed wound healing will direct you to option 3. Review the complications associated with an amputation in the client with diabetes mellitus if you had difficulty with this question.

Level of Cognitive Ability: Application
Client Needs: Physiological Integrity
Integrated Process: Nursing Process—assessment
Content Area: Adult health—musculoskeletal
Reference: Ignatavicius, D., & Workman, M. (2002). *Medical-surgical nursing: Critical thinking for collaborative care* (4th ed., p. 1149). Philadelphia: W. B. Saunders.

40. 1
Rationale: Phantom limb sensations are felt in the area of the amputated limb. These sensations can include itching, warmth, and cold. The sensations are due to intact peripheral nerves in the area amputated. Whenever possible, the client should be prepared for these sensations. The client may also feel painful sensations in the amputated limb, called phantom limb pain. The origin of the pain is less well understood, but the client should be prepared for this too whenever possible.
Test-Taking Strategy: Use the process of elimination. Knowing that sensation and pain may be felt in the residual limb helps you to eliminate options 3 and 4 first because the sensations are not abnormal responses. Select option 1 because the client has described an itching sensation, but has not complained of pain in the residual limb. Review expected findings following amputation if you had difficulty with this question.

Level of Cognitive Ability: Analysis
Client Needs: Psychosocial Integrity
Integrated Process: Nursing Process—assessment
Content Area: Adult health—musculoskeletal
References: Ignatavicius, D., & Workman, M. (2002). *Medical-surgical nursing: Critical thinking for collaborative care* (4th ed., p. 1147). Philadelphia: W. B. Saunders.
Phipps, W., Monahan, F., Sands, J., Marek, J., & Neighbors, M. (2003). *Medical-surgical nursing: Health and illness perspectives* (7th ed., p. 782). St. Louis: Mosby.

41. 4
Rationale: A stump sock must be worn at all times to absorb perspiration and is changed daily. The residual limb is washed, dried, and inspected for breakdown twice each day. The socket of the prosthesis is cleansed with a mild detergent and rinsed and dried carefully each day. A harsh bactericidal agent would not be used.
Test-Taking Strategy: Use the process of elimination. Eliminate options 1 and 2 because of the lengthy time frames. Eliminate option 3 because of the word "harsh." Review client teaching related to skin care following an amputation if you had difficulty with this question.

Level of Cognitive Ability: Application
Client Needs: Health Promotion and Maintenance
Integrated Process: Teaching/Learning
Content Area: Adult health—musculoskeletal
References: Ignatavicius, D., & Workman, M. (2002). *Medical-surgical nursing: Critical thinking for collaborative care* (4th ed., p. 1151). Philadelphia: W. B. Saunders.
Phipps, W., Monahan, F., Sands, J., Marek, J., & Neighbors, M. (2003). *Medical-surgical nursing: Health and illness perspectives* (7th ed., pp. 781, 783). St. Louis: Mosby.

42. 2
Rationale: If the client with an amputation has a cast or elastic compression bandage that slips off, the nurse must wrap the stump immediately with another elastic compression bandage. Otherwise, excessive edema will form rapidly that could cause a significant delay in rehabilitation. If the client had a cast that slipped off, the nurse would have to call the physician so that a new one could be applied. Elevation on one pillow is not going to impede the development of edema greatly once compression is released. Ice would be of limited value in controlling edema from this cause. If the physician were called, the order likely would be to reapply the compression dressing anyway.
Test-Taking Strategy: Use the process of elimination. Recalling that excessive edema can form rapidly will direct you to option 2. Review care to the client after amputation if you had difficulty with this question.

Level of Cognitive Ability: Application
Client Needs: Physiological Integrity
Integrated Process: Nursing Process—implementation
Content Area: Adult health—musculoskeletal
Reference: Ignatavicius, D., & Workman, M. (2002). *Medical-surgical nursing: Critical thinking for collaborative care* (4th ed., p. 1150). Philadelphia: W. B. Saunders.

43. 3
Rationale: Low back pain that radiates into one leg (sciatica) is consistent with herniated lumbar disk. The nurse assesses the client to see whether the pain is aggravated by events that increase intraspinal pressure, such as bending, lifting, sneezing, and coughing, or by lifting the leg straight up while supine (straight leg raising test).
Test-Taking Strategy: Use the process of elimination. Recall that bed rest, heat (or sometimes ice), and nonsteroidal anti-inflammatory agents usually relieve back pain, whereas bending, lifting, and straining aggravate it. Review the causes of back pain and the factors that alleviate or aggravate pain if you had difficulty with this question.

Level of Cognitive Ability: Application
Client Needs: Physiological Integrity
Integrated Process: Nursing Process—assessment
Content Area: Adult health—musculoskeletal
Reference: Ignatavicius, D., & Workman, M. (2002). *Medical-surgical nursing: Critical thinking for collaborative care* (4th ed., p. 926). Philadelphia: W. B. Saunders.

44. 4
Rationale: After a client has spinal fusion, the head of bed is generally kept flat. The client is logrolled from side to side as ordered. Pillows may be placed under the entire length of the legs by surgeon preference to relieve tension on the lower back. The use of an overhead trapeze is contraindicated because its use could promote twisting of the spine after surgery.
Test-Taking Strategy: Use the process of elimination. Note the key word "avoid." After spinal surgery the nurse uses positioning techniques and aids that will keep the spine in good alignment. Thus options 1 and 3 are indicated. From the remaining options, recall that using pillows under the length of the legs promotes slight flexion of the spine while avoiding pressure on the popliteal space (which predisposes to thrombophlebitis). Using an overbed trapeze could allow the client to twist the spine, which is directly contraindicated. Review care to the client after spinal fusion if you had difficulty with this question.
Level of Cognitive Ability: Application
Client Needs: Safe, Effective Care Environment
Integrated Process: Nursing Process—implementation
Content Area: Adult health—musculoskeletal
References: Ignatavicius, D., & Workman, M. (2002). *Medical surgical nursing: Critical thinking for collaborative care* (4th ed., p. 929). Philadelphia: W. B. Saunders.
Lewis, S., Heitkemper, M., & Dirksen, S. (2004). *Medical-surgical nursing: Assessment and management of clinical problems* (6th ed., p. 1704). St. Louis: Mosby.

45. 1
Rationale: Clients are taught to get out of bed by sliding near the edge of the mattress. The client then rolls onto one side and pushes up from the bed using one or both arms. The client keeps the back straight, and swings the legs over the side. Increasing fluid intake and dietary fiber helps prevent straining at stool, thereby preventing increases in intraspinal pressure. Walking and swimming are excellent exercises for strengthening lower back muscles. Proper body mechanics includes bending at the knees, not the waist, to lift objects.
Test-Taking Strategy: Use the process of elimination. Note the key words "needs further instruction." Recall that the client with low back pain should avoid events that increase intraspinal pressure. This will direct you to option 1. Review client teaching about body mechanics if you had difficulty with this question.
Level of Cognitive Ability: Analysis
Client Needs: Physiological Integrity
Integrated Process: Teaching/Learning
Content Area: Adult health—musculoskeletal
References: Ignatavicius, D., & Workman, M. (2002). *Medical-surgical nursing: Critical thinking for collaborative care* (4th ed., p. 930). Philadelphia: W. B. Saunders.

Phipps, W., Monahan, F., Sands, J., Marek, J., & Neighbors, M. (2003). *Medical-surgical nursing: Health and illness perspectives* (7th ed., p. 1579). St. Louis: Mosby.

46. 2
Rationale: The nursing assessment conducted after spinal surgery is similar to that done after other surgical procedures. For this specific type of surgery the nurse assesses the neurovascular status of the lower extremities, watches for signs and symptoms of infection, and inspects the surgical site for evidence of cerebrospinal fluid leakage (drainage is clear and tests positive for glucose). A mild temperature is expected after insertion of hardware, but a temperature of 101.6° F should be reported.
Test-Taking Strategy: Use the process of elimination. Note the key words "concerned especially." Thus you are looking for the option that has the greatest deviation from normal. Options 1 and 4 are expected after surgery, and although the nurse tries to minimize discomfort, the client is likely to have some discomfort even with proper analgesic use. The words "old" and "outlined" in option 3 indicate that this is not a new occurrence. This leaves the temperature of 101.6° F, which is excessive and should be reported. Review the signs of complications following this surgical procedure if you had difficulty with this question.
Level of Cognitive Ability: Analysis
Client Needs: Physiological Integrity
Integrated Process: Nursing Process—assessment
Content Area: Adult health—musculoskeletal
References: Ignatavicius, D., & Workman, M. (2002). *Medical-surgical nursing: Critical thinking for collaborative care* (4th ed., p. 930). Philadelphia: W. B. Saunders.
Phipps, W., Monahan, F., Sands, J., Marek, J., & Neighbors, M. (2003). *Medical-surgical nursing: Health and illness perspectives* (7th ed., p. 1579). St. Louis: Mosby.

47. 1
Rationale: The client experiences a Disturbed Body Image related to a change in the structure and function of the affected leg. No data in the question support a diagnosis of (actual) Activity Intolerance or Social Isolation. The client does have an actual (not at risk for) Impaired Physical Mobility because of the fixation device.
Test-Taking Strategy: Use the process of elimination. Note the key words "upset about the appearance." This should direct you to option 1. Review the defining characteristics for Disturbed Body Image if you had difficulty with this question.
Level of Cognitive Ability: Analysis
Client Needs: Psychosocial Integrity
Integrated Process: Nursing Process—analysis
Content Area: Adult health—musculoskeletal
Reference: Ignatavicius, D., & Workman, M. (2002). *Medical-surgical nursing: Critical thinking for collaborative care* (4th ed., p. 1131). Philadelphia: W. B. Saunders.

48. 2
Rationale: The part of the bed under an area in traction usually is elevated to aid in countertraction. For the client in Buck's extension traction (which is applied to a leg), the foot of the bed is elevated.

Test-Taking Strategy: Use the process of elimination. Recalling the principles of traction and countertraction will assist you in eliminating option 3. Knowing that Buck's extension traction is applied to the leg helps to eliminate option 1. From the remaining options, option 4 places undue pressure on the client's unaffected foot. Furthermore, a footboard is not used for the purpose of providing countertraction. Review the principles of traction and countertraction if you had difficulty with this question.
Level of Cognitive Ability: Application
Client Needs: Physiological Integrity
Integrated Process: Nursing Process—implementation
Content Area: Adult health—musculoskeletal
References: Ignatavicius, D., & Workman, M. (2002). *Medical-surgical nursing: Critical thinking for collaborative care* (4th ed., p. 1136). Philadelphia: W. B. Saunders.
Phipps, W., Monahan, F., Sands, J., Marek, J., & Neighbors, M. (2003). *Medical-surgical nursing: Health and illness perspectives* (7th ed., p. 1472). St. Louis: Mosby.

49. 1
Rationale: In addition to the presence of clinical manifestations, gout is diagnosed by the presence of persistent hyperuricemia of greater than 7 mg/dL. Options 2, 3, and 4 indicate normal laboratory values. Additionally, the presence of uric acid in an aspirated sample of synovial fluid confirms the diagnosis.
Test-Taking Strategy: Use the process of elimination and knowledge of normal laboratory values. Recalling that increased uric acid levels occur in gout and noting that option 1 is the only abnormal value will assist you in answering the question. Review the manifestations of gout and the normal uric acid level if you had difficulty with this question.
Level of Cognitive Ability: Analysis
Client Needs: Physiological Integrity
Integrated Process: Nursing Process—assessment
Content Area: Adult health—musculoskeletal
References: Chernecky, C., & Berger, B. (2001). *Laboratory tests and diagnostic procedures* (3rd ed., p. 1042). Philadelphia: W. B. Saunders.
Ignatavicius, D., & Workman, M. (2002). *Medical-surgical nursing: Critical thinking for collaborative care* (4th ed., p. 358). Philadelphia: W. B. Saunders.

50. 3
Rationale: The stiffness and joint pain that occur in osteoarthritis diminishes after rest and intensifies with activity. No specific laboratory findings are useful in diagnosing osteoarthritis. The client may have a normal or slightly elevated sedimentation rate. Morning stiffness lasting longer than 30 minutes occurs in rheumatoid arthritis. Elevated white blood cell counts, platelet counts, and antinuclear antibodies occur in rheumatoid arthritis.
Test-Taking Strategy: Use the process of elimination and knowledge about the differences between osteoarthritis and rheumatoid arthritis to answer this question. Review the characteristics of osteoarthritis if you had difficulty with the question.
Level of Cognitive Ability: Analysis
Client Needs: Physiological Integrity
Integrated Process: Nursing Process—assessment
Content Area: Adult health—musculoskeletal
References: Ignatavicius, D., & Workman, M. (2002). *Medical-surgical nursing: Critical thinking for collaborative care* (4th ed., p. 329). Philadelphia: W. B. Saunders.
Phipps, W., Monahan, F., Sands, J., Marek, J., & Neighbors, M. (2003). *Medical-surgical nursing: Health and illness perspectives* (7th ed., p. 1523). St. Louis: Mosby.

CRITICAL THINKING: MULTIPLE RESPONSE
Answer:
Keep the cast and extremity elevated.
Allow the wet cast 24 to 48 hours to dry.
The cast needs to be kept clean and dry.
Rationale: A plaster cast takes 24 to 48 hours to dry (synthetic casts dry in 20 minutes). The cast and extremity are elevated to prevent swelling and circulatory compromise. A wet cast is handled with the palms of the hand until it is dry, and the extremity is turned (unless contraindicated) so that all sides of the wet cast will dry. A cool setting on the hair dryer can be used to dry a plaster cast (heat cannot be used on a plaster cast because the cast heats up and burns the skin). The cast needs to be kept clean and dry, and the client is instructed not to stick anything under the cast because of the risk of breaking skin integrity. The client is instructed to monitor the extremity for circulatory impairment such as pain, swelling, discoloration, tingling, numbness, coolness, or diminished pulse. The physician is notified immediately if circulatory impairment occurs.
Test-Taking Strategy: Focus on the issue, a plaster cast. Recalling that edema occurs following a fracture and recalling the complications associated with a cast will assist you in answering the question. Review cast care instructions if you had difficulty with this question.
Level of Cognitive Ability: Application
Client Needs: Physiological Integrity
Integrated Process: Teaching/Learning
Content Area: Adult health—musculoskeletal
Reference: Ignatavicius, D., & Workman, M. (2002). *Medical-surgical nursing: Critical thinking for collaborative care* (4th ed., p. 1135). Philadelphia: W. B. Saunders.

REFERENCES

Black, J., Hawks, J., & Keene, A. (2001). *Medical-surgical nursing: Clinical management for positive outcomes* (6th ed.). Philadelphia: W. B. Saunders.

Chernecky, C., & Berger, B. (2001). *Laboratory tests and diagnostic procedures* (3rd ed.). Philadelphia: W. B. Saunders.

Harkreader, H., & Hogan, M. A. (2004). *Fundamentals of nursing: Caring and clinical judgment* (2nd ed.). Philadelphia: W. B. Saunders.

Ignatavicius, D., & Workman, M. (2002). *Medical-surgical nursing: Critical thinking for collaborative care* (4th ed.). Philadelphia: W. B. Saunders.

Jarvis, C. (2000). *Physical examination & health assessment* (3rd ed.). Philadelphia: W. B. Saunders.

Lewis, S., Heitkemper, M., & Dirksen, S. (2004). *Medical-surgical nursing: Assessment and management of clinical problems* (6th ed.). St. Louis: Mosby.

Perry, A., & Potter, P. (2002). *Clinical nursing skills and techniques* (5th ed.). St. Louis: Mosby.

Phipps, W., Monahan, F., Sands, J., Marek, J., & Neighbors, M. (2003). *Medical-surgical nursing: Health and illness perspectives* (7th ed.). St. Louis: Mosby.

Potter, P., & Perry, A. (2001). *Fundamentals of nursing* (5th ed.). St. Louis: Mosby.

Musculoskeletal Medications

I. SKELETAL MUSCLE RELAXANTS (BOX 68-1)

A. Description
1. Skeletal muscle relaxants act directly on the neuromuscular junction or indirectly on the central nervous system (CNS).
2. Centrally acting muscle relaxants depress neuron activity in the spinal cord or brain.
3. Peripherally acting muscle relaxants act directly on the skeletal muscles.
4. Skeletal muscle relaxants are used to prevent or relieve muscle spasms, to treat spasticity associated with spinal cord disease or lesions, for painful musculoskeletal conditions, and for chronic debilitating disorders such as multiple sclerosis, cerebrovascular accident, or cerebral palsy.
5. Skeletal muscle relaxants are contraindicated in clients with severe liver, renal, or heart disease.
6. Skeletal muscle relaxants should not be taken with CNS depressants such as barbiturates, narcotics, and alcohol; sedatives; hypnotics; or tricyclic antidepressants.

B. Side effects
1. Dizziness and hypotension
2. Drowsiness
3. Dry mouth
4. Gastrointestinal upset
5. Photosensitivity
6. Liver toxicity

C. Interventions
1. Obtain a medical history.
2. Monitor vital signs.
3. Monitor for CNS side effects.
4. Assess for risk of injury.
5. Assess involved joints and muscles for pain and mobility.
6. Monitor liver function tests because hepatotoxicity can occur.
7. Monitor renal function studies.
8. Instruct the client to take the medication with food to decrease gastrointestinal upset.
9. Instruct the client to report side effects.
10. Instruct the client to avoid alcohol and CNS depressants.
11. Instruct the client to avoid activities requiring alertness.

D. Nursing considerations
1. Baclofen (Lioresal)
   a. Baclofen causes CNS effects such as drowsiness, dizziness, weakness, and fatigue and nausea, constipation, and urinary retention.
   b. Administer with caution in the client with a seizure disorder.
   c. Baclofen can be administered by the physician through intrathecal infusion using an implantable pump.
2. Dantrolene (Dantrium)
   a. Dantrolene acts directly on skeletal muscles to relieve spasticity.

BOX 68-1

Skeletal Muscle Relaxants

Baclofen (Lioresal)
Carisoprodol (Soma)
Chlorphenesin carbamate (Maolate)
Chlorzoxazone (Paraflex, Parafon Forte, Relaxazone)
Cyclobenzaprine (Flexeril)
Dantrolene (Dantrium)
Diazepam (Valium)
Metaxalone (Skelaxin)
Methocarbamol (Robaxin)
Orphenadrine (Disipal)
Orphenadrine extended release (Norflex)
Tizanidine (Zanaflex)

b. Liver damage is the most serious adverse effect.

c. Liver function tests should be monitored before the initiation of treatment and during treatment.

d. Dantrolene can cause gastrointestinal bleeding, urinary frequency, impotence, photosensitivity, and rash.

e. Instruct the client to wear protective clothing when in the sun.

f. Instruct the client to notify the physician if rash, bloody or tarry stool, or yellow discoloration of the skin or eyes occurs.

g. Instruct the client with an implantable pump to maintain medication refill appointments to prevent the pump from emptying and experiencing sudden withdrawal symptoms (which could be life threatening).

3. Cyclobenzaprine (Flexeril)

a. Cyclobenzaprine is contraindicated in clients who have received monoamine oxidase inhibitors within 14 days of initiation of cyclobenzaprine therapy and in clients with cardiac disorders.

b. Cyclobenzaprine should be used with caution in clients with a history of urinary retention, angle-closure glaucoma, or increased intraocular pressure.

c. Cyclobenzaprine should be used only for short-term (2 to 3 weeks) therapy.

4. Methocarbamol (Robaxin)

a. Parenteral form is contraindicated in clients with renal impairment.

b. Parenteral form can cause hypotension, bradycardia, anaphylaxis, and seizures.

c. Methocarbamol may cause urine to turn brown, black, or green.

d. Inform the client to notify the physician if blurred vision, nasal congestion, urticaria, or rash occurs.

5. Chlorzoxazone (Paraflex, Parafon Forte, Relaxazone)

a. Monitor client for hypersensitivity reactions such as urticaria, redness or itching, and possibly angioedema.

b. Chlorzoxazone may cause malaise and urine discoloration.

6. Carisoprodol (Soma)

a. Advise the client to take the medication with food to prevent gastrointestinal upset.

b. Instruct the client to report any rash or hypersensitivity to the physician.

II. ANTIGOUT MEDICATIONS (BOX 68-2)

A. Description

1. Antigout medications decrease inflammation.

2. Antigout medications reduce uric acid production and increase uric acid excretion to prevent or relieve gout or to manage hyperuricemia.

BOX 68-2

Antigout Medications

Allopurinol (Zyloprim)
Colchicine
Probenecid (Benemid)

---

3. Antigout medications should be used cautiously in clients with gastrointestinal, renal, cardiac, or hepatic disease.

4. Allopurinol (Zyloprim) can increase the effect of warfarin (Coumadin) and oral hypoglycemic agents.

B. Side effects

1. Headaches

2. Nausea, vomiting, and diarrhea

3. Blood dyscrasias such as bone marrow depression

4. Flushed skin and skin rash

5. Uric acid kidney stones

6. Sore gums

7. Metallic taste

C. Interventions

1. Assess serum uric acid levels.

2. Monitor intake and output.

3. Maintain a fluid intake of at least 2000 to 3000 mL a day to avoid kidney stones.

4. Monitor complete blood cell count and renal and liver function studies.

5. Instruct the client to avoid alcohol and caffeine because these products can increase uric acid levels.

6. Instruct the client not to take large doses of vitamin C while taking allopurinol (Zyloprim) because kidney stones may occur.

7. Encourage the client to comply with therapy to prevent elevated uric acid levels, which can trigger a gout attack.

8. Instruct the client to avoid foods high in purine, such as wine, alcohol, organ meats, sardines, salmon, scallops, and gravy.

9. Instruct the client to take the medication with food.

10. Instruct the client to report side effects to the physician.

11. Advise the client to have a yearly eye examination because visual changes can occur from prolonged use of allopurinol.

12. Caution the client not to take aspirin with these medications because this could trigger a gout attack.

13. Concurrent use of aspirin causes elevated uric acid levels; the client should be instructed to take acetaminophen (Tylenol).

III. ANTIARTHRITIC MEDICATIONS (BOX 68-3)

A. Acetylsalicylic acid (aspirin) and nonsteroidal anti-inflammatory medications (Refer to Chapter 66.)

B. Gold therapy
  1. Description
    a. Gold therapy is referred to as chrysotherapy or heavy-metal therapy.
    b. Gold therapy depresses migration of leukocytes and suppresses prostaglandin activity.
    c. Gold therapy reduces inflammation by decreasing enzyme release and altering the immune response.
    d. Gold therapy is used primarily for palliative relief of symptoms in rheumatoid arthritis.
    e. Box 68-4 lists contraindications.
  2. Side effects
    a. Dizziness
    b. Urticaria and rash
    c. Erythema and dermatitis
    d. Alopecia
    e. Stomatitis
    f. Diarrhea
    g. Hepatitis
    h. Metallic taste in the mouth
    i. Blood dyscrasias such as bone marrow suppression
    j. Photosensitivity reactions
    k. Gold toxicity
  3. Interventions
    a. Obtain the client's medical history.
    b. Monitor for blood dyscrasias before and during therapy.
    c. Monitor for proteinuria and hematuria before and during therapy.

    d. When administering the gold injection, monitor the client for 30 minutes after injection for possible allergic reaction.
    e. Instruct the client to maintain good oral hygiene.
    f. Instruct the client to use sunscreen and protective clothing to prevent photosensitivity reactions.
    g. Teach the client about the signs and symptoms of gold toxicity, which include pruritis, skin rash, metallic taste, stomatitis, and diarrhea.
    h. If toxicity occurs, dimercaprol (BAL in oil) may be prescribed to enhance gold excretion.

IV. MEDICATIONS TO PREVENT AND TREAT OSTEOPOROSIS
A. Calcium and vitamin D supplementation
B. Estrogen replacement therapy after menopause may be prescribed to prevent osteoporosis.
C. Calcitonin (Calcimar)
  1. Calcitonin is secreted by the thyroid gland and inhibits osteoclastic bone resorption.
  2. When calcitonin is taken, calcium supplementation is necessary to prevent secondary hyperparathyroidism.
D. Biphosphonates (Box 68-5)
  1. Biphosphonates inhibit osteoclast-mediated bone resorption, thereby increasing total bone mass.
  2. Common side effects are anorexia, weight loss, and gastritis.
  3. Alendronate (Fosamax)
    a. Precautions need to be taken with administration to prevent gastrointestinal side effects (especially esophageal irritation) and increase absorption.
    b. Alendronate should be taken with a full glass of water after rising in the morning.
    c. Client should not eat or drink anything for 30 minutes following administration and should not lie down after taking the medication.
E. Selective estrogen receptor modulators
  1. Selective estrogen receptor modulators mimic the effect of estrogen in bone by reducing bone resorption.
  2. Raloxifene (Evista): Most common side effects are leg cramps and hot flashes.

BOX 68-3

Antiarthritic Medications

Auranofin (Ridaura)
Aurothioglucose (Solganal)
Azathioprine (Imuran)
Etanercept (Enbrel)
Gold sodium thiomalate (Myochrysine)
Hydroxychloroquine sulfate (Plaquenil)
Leflunomide (Arava)
Penicillamine (Cuprimine)

BOX 68-4

Contraindications to Gold Therapy

Colitis
Congestive heart failure
Eczema
Hemorrhagic conditions
Recent radiation therapy
Renal or hepatic dysfunction
Systemic lupus erythematosus
Uncontrolled diabetes mellitus
Urticaria

BOX 68-5

Biphosphonates Used to Treat Osteoporosis

Alendronate (Fosamax)
Clodronate (Bonefos)
Etidronate (Didronel)
Pamidronate (Aredia)
Risedronate (Actonel)
Tiludronate (Skelid)

F. Teriparatide (Forteo)
   1. Teriparatide stimulates new bone formation.
   2. Teriparatide is a portion of the human parathyroid hormone and works by increasing the action of osteoblasts.
   3. Teriparatide is used to treat osteoporosis in men and postmenopausal women who are at high risk for having a fracture.

PRACTICE QUESTIONS

1. Allopurinol (Zyloprim) has been prescribed for a client. The nurse prepares to administer this medication, knowing that which of the following information is accurate about this medication?
   1. Allopurinol is used for the lysis of thrombi obstructing coronary arteries.
   2. Allopurinol prevents calcium ion entry across cell membranes of the cardiac smooth muscle
   3. Allopurinol decreases sympathetic outflow from the central nervous system.
   4. Allopurinol decreases uric acid production and reduces uric acid concentrations in the serum and urine.

2. A community health nurse visits a client at home. The client is taking allopurinol (Zyloprim) 400 mg PO daily. The nurse instructs the client
   1. That the effect of the medication will occur immediately.
   2. To drink 3000 mL of fluid per day.
   3. To take the medication on an empty stomach.
   4. That if swelling of the lips occurs, this is a normal expected response.

3. Colchicine is prescribed for a client with a diagnosis of gout. The nurse reviews the client's record knowing that this medication would be contraindicated in which of the following disorders?
   1. Renal failure
   2. Hypothyroidism
   3. Diabetes mellitus
   4. Myxedema

4. A home health nurse is caring for a client who is taking probenecid (Benemid). The client has been instructed to restrict the diet to low-purine foods. Which of the following foods would the nurse instruct the client to avoid?
   1. Potatoes
   2. Ice cream
   3. Spinach
   4. Scallops

5. A physician prescribes auranofin (Ridaura) for a client with rheumatoid arthritis. Which of the following would indicate to the nurse that the client is experiencing toxicity related to the medication?
   1. Constipation
   2. A metallic taste in the mouth

3. Ringing in the ears
4. Joint pain

6. Alendronate (Fosamax) is prescribed for a client with osteoporosis. The nurse instructs the client to
   1. Take the medication at bedtime.
   2. Take the medication with a full glass of water after rising in the morning.
   3. Take the medication in the morning with breakfast.
   4. To lie down for 30 minutes after taking the medication.

7. A film-coated form of diflunisal (Dolobid), a nonsteroidal antiinflammatory medication, has been prescribed for a client to treat chronic rheumatoid arthritis. The client calls the clinic nurse because of difficulty swallowing the tablets. Which of the following instructions would the nurse provide to the client?
   1. Crush the tablets and mix with food.
   2. Open the tablet and mix the contents with food.
   3. Swallow the tablets with large amounts of water or milk.
   4. Notify the physician for a medication change.

8. Baclofen (Lioresal) is prescribed for a client with multiple sclerosis. The nurse monitors the client, knowing that the primary therapeutic effect of this medication is which of the following?
   1. Increased muscle tone
   2. Decreased muscle spasms
   3. Decreased local pain and tenderness
   4. Increased range of motion

9. A nurse is monitoring a client receiving baclofen (Lioresal) for side effects related to the medication. Which of the following would indicate that the client is experiencing a side effect?
   1. Drowsiness
   2. Diarrhea
   3. Polyuria
   4. Muscular excitability

10. A nurse is providing discharge instructions to a client receiving baclofen (Lioresal). Which of the following would be included in the teaching plan?
    1. Restrict fluid intake.
    2. Avoid the use of alcohol.
    3. Stop the medication if diarrhea occurs.
    4. Notify the physician if fatigue occurs.

11. An adult client with muscle spasms is taking an oral maintenance dose of baclofen (Lioresal). Which of the following represents a safe maintenance dose for this medication?
    1. 15 mg qid
    2. 25 mg qid
    3. 30 mg qid
    4. 40 mg qid

12. A client with acute muscle spasms has been taking baclofen (Lioresal). The client calls the clinic nurse because of continuous feelings of weakness and fatigue and asks the nurse about discontinuing the

medication. Which of the following responses to the client would be most appropriate?
1. "It is best that you taper the dose if you intend to stop the medication."
2. "Weakness and fatigue commonly occur and will diminish with continued medication use."
3. "It is all right to stop the medication if you think that you can tolerate the muscle spasms."
4. "You should never stop the medication."

13. Dantrolene sodium (Dantrium) is prescribed for the client experiencing flexor spasms. The nurse monitors the client, knowing that which of the following is the therapeutic action of this medication?
1. Dantrolene acts within the spinal cord to suppress hyperactive reflexes.
2. Dantrolene acts on the central nervous system to suppress spasms.
3. Dantrolene acts directly on the skeletal muscle to relieve spasticity.
4. Dantrolene depresses spinal reflexes.

14. A nurse is analyzing the laboratory studies on a client receiving dantrolene sodium (Dantrium). Which of the following laboratory tests would identify an adverse effect associated with the administration of this medication?
1. Blood urea nitrogen
2. Creatinine
3. Liver function tests
4. Platelet count

15. A physician is planning to administer a skeletal muscle relaxant to a client with a spinal cord injury. The medication is going to be administered intrathecally (within the spinal column). Which of the following medications would the nurse expect to be prescribed and administered by this route?
1. Cyclobenzaprine hydrochloride (Flexeril)
2. Chlorzoxazone (Paraflex)
3. Dantrolene sodium (Dantrium)
4. Baclofen (Lioresal)

16. A nurse is reviewing the record of a client who has been prescribed baclofen (Lioresal). Which of the following disorders, if noted in the client's history, would alert the nurse to contact the physician?
1. Coronary artery disease
2. Diabetes mellitus
3. Seizure disorders
4. Hyperthyroidism

17. Cyclobenzaprine hydrochloride (Flexeril) is prescribed for a client for muscle spasms. The nurse is reviewing the client's record. Which of the

following disorders, if noted in the record, would indicate a need to contact the physician about the administration of this medication?
1. Glaucoma
2. Hypothyroidism
3. Emphysema
4. Diabetes mellitus

18. A client is to receive a prescription for methocarbamol (Robaxin). The nurse provides instructions to the client about the medication. Which of the following client statements would indicate a need for further education?
1. "My urine may turn brown or green."
2. "If my vision becomes blurred, I don't need to be concerned about it."
3. "I might get some nasal congestion from this medication."
4. "This medication is prescribed to help relieve my muscle spasms."

19. A nurse is administering an intravenous dose of methocarbamol (Robaxin) to a client with multiple sclerosis. For which of the following adverse effects would the nurse monitor?
1. Hypertension
2. Tachycardia
3. Rapid pulse
4. Bradycardia

20. A nurse is reviewing a physician's orders for an adult client who has been admitted to the hospital following a back injury. Carisoprodol (Soma) is prescribed for the client to relieve the muscle spasms. The physician has prescribed 350 mg to be administered 4 times a day. The nurse determines that this dosage is
1. The normal adult dosage.
2. A lower than normal dosage.
3. A higher than normal dosage.
4. A dosage requiring further clarification.

CRITICAL THINKING: FILL IN THE BLANK

A nurse is caring for a hospitalized client who is taking allopurinol (Zyloprim) for a history of gout. The nurse reviews the physician's orders and notes that the physician has prescribed the following medications: pentazocine (Talwin), warfarin sodium (Coumadin), and ergonovine maleate (Ergotrate). Which of these prescribed medications would the nurse question?

Answer: _____

ANSWERS

1. 4

Rationale: Allopurinol (Zyloprim) is an antigout medication. Allopurinol decreases uric acid production by inhibiting xanthine oxidase, an enzyme, and reduces uric acid concentrations in serum and urine.

Test-Taking Strategy: Use the process of elimination. Note that options 1 and 2 are similar in that they address a cardiac situation. Knowledge that this medication is in the antigout classification will assist in directing you to the correct option. If you had difficulty with this question, review the action of allopurinol (Zyloprim).

Level of Cognitive Ability: Comprehension
Client Needs: Physiological Integrity
Integrated Process: Nursing Process—planning
Content Area: Pharmacology
Reference: Hodgson, B., & Kizior, R. (2004). *Saunders nursing drug handbook 2004* (p. 23). Philadelphia: W. B. Saunders.

2. 2

Rationale: Clients taking allopurinol are encouraged to drink 3000 mL of fluid a day. A full therapeutic effect may take 1 or more weeks. Allopurinol is to be given with, or immediately after, meals or milk. A client who develops a rash, irritation of the eyes, or swelling of the lips or mouth should contact the physician because this may indicate hypersensitivity.

Test-Taking Strategy: Use the process of elimination. Option 4 can be eliminated easily because it indicates hypersensitivity, which is not a normal expected response. From the remaining options, recalling that this medication is used to treat gout will direct you to option 2. If you had difficulty with this question, review the client instructions related to allopurinol.

Level of Cognitive Ability: Application
Client Needs: Physiological Integrity
Integrated Process: Teaching/Learning
Content Area: Pharmacology
Reference: Hodgson, B., & Kizior, R. (2004). *Saunders nursing drug handbook 2004* (p. 24). Philadelphia: W. B. Saunders.

3. 1

Rationale: Colchicine is contraindicated in clients with severe gastrointestinal, renal, hepatic, or cardiac disorders and in clients with blood dyscrasias. Clients with impaired renal function may exhibit myopathy and neuropathy manifested as generalized weakness. This medication should be used with caution in clients with impaired hepatic function, the older client, and the debilitated.

Test-Taking Strategy: Use the process of elimination. Note that options 2, 3, and 4 are endocrine-related disorders. Option 1, the correct option, is different from the others. Review the contraindications associated with this medication if you had difficulty with this question.

Level of Cognitive Ability: Analysis
Client Needs: Physiological Integrity
Integrated Process: Nursing Process—analysis
Content Area: Pharmacology
Reference: Kee, J., & Hayes, E. (2003). *Pharmacology: A nursing process approach* (4th ed., p. 387). Philadelphia: W. B. Saunders.

4. 4

Rationale: Uric acid is produced when purine is catabolized. Probenecid is a medication used for clients with gout to inhibit the reabsorption of uric acid by the kidney and promote excretion of uric acid in the urine. Clients are instructed to modify their diets and limit excessive purine intake. High-purine foods to avoid or limit include organ meats, roe, sardines, scallops, anchovies, broth, mincemeat, herring, shrimp, mackerel, gravy, yeast, wine, and alcohol.

Test-Taking Strategy: Use the process of elimination. Options 1 and 3 are high-nutrient foods, so eliminate these options first. From this point, use your knowledge about the purpose of the medication, the treatment for gout, and food sources high in purine to select the correct option. If you had difficulty with this question, review foods that are high in purine.

Level of Cognitive Ability: Application
Client Needs: Physiological Integrity
Integrated Process: Teaching/Learning
Content Area: Pharmacology
References: Hodgson, B., & Kizior, R. (2004). *Saunders nursing drug handbook 2004* (p. 834). Philadelphia: W. B. Saunders. Kee, J., & Hayes, E. (2003). *Pharmacology: A nursing process approach* (4th ed., p. 389). Philadelphia: W. B. Saunders.

5. 2

Rationale: Auranofin is the one gold preparation that is given orally rather than by injection. Gastrointestinal reactions including diarrhea, abdominal pain, nausea, and loss of appetite are common early in therapy but usually subside in the first 3 months. Early symptoms of toxic reactions include a rash, purple blotches, pruritus, mouth lesions, and a metallic taste in the mouth.

Test-Taking Strategy: Recalling that auranofin is a gold preparation will assist you in answering the question. Noting that the question is asking for a toxic effect will direct you to option 2. Remember that gold is a metal. If you had difficulty with this question, review toxicity related to gold compounds.

Level of Cognitive Ability: Analysis
Client Needs: Physiological Integrity
Integrated Process: Nursing Process—assessment
Content Area: Pharmacology
Reference: Kee, J., & Hayes, E. (2003). *Pharmacology: A nursing process approach* (4th ed., p. 384). Philadelphia: W. B. Saunders.

6. 2

Rationale: Precautions need to be taken with administration of alendronate to prevent gastrointestinal side effects (especially esophageal irritation) and increase absorption of the medication. The medication needs to be taken with a full glass of water after rising in the morning. The client should not eat or drink anything for 30 minutes following administration and should not lie down after taking the medication.

Test-Taking Strategy: Knowledge regarding the administration of alendronate is needed to answer this question. Review this medication if you had difficulty with this question.

Level of Cognitive Ability: Application
Client Needs: Physiological Integrity
Integrated Process: Teaching/Learning
Content Area: Pharmacology

Reference: Lewis, S., Heitkemper, M., & Dirksen, S. (2004). *Medical-surgical nursing: Assessment and management of clinical problems* (6th ed., p. 1711). St. Louis: Mosby.

7. **3**

Rationale: Dolobid may be given with water, milk, or meals. The tablets should not be crushed or broken open.

Test-Taking Strategy: Use the process of elimination. Eliminate option 4 first as the least likely option. Note the words "film-coated" to eliminate options 1 and 2. Additionally, these options are similar in that they suggest breaking the tablets. If you had difficulty with this question, review the procedure for administration.

Level of Cognitive Ability: Application
Client Needs: Physiological Integrity
Integrated Process: Teaching/Learning
Content Area: Pharmacology
References: Hodgson, B., & Kizior, R. (2004). *Saunders nursing drug handbook 2004* (pp. 308-309). Philadelphia: W. B. Saunders.
Kee, J., & Hayes, E. (2003). *Pharmacology: A nursing process approach* (4th ed., p. 379). Philadelphia: W. B. Saunders.

8. **2**

Rationale: Baclofen is a skeletal muscle relaxant and acts at the spinal cord level to decrease the frequency and amplitude of muscle spasms in clients with spinal cord injuries or debilitating diseases such as multiple sclerosis.

Test-Taking Strategy: Use the process of elimination. Knowledge that this medication is a skeletal muscle relaxant will direct you easily to option 2. Review this medication if you had difficulty with this question.

Level of Cognitive Ability: Analysis
Client Needs: Physiological Integrity
Integrated Process: Nursing Process—evaluation
Content Area: Pharmacology
Reference: Hodgson, B., & Kizior, R. (2004). *Saunders nursing drug handbook 2004* (p. 92). Philadelphia: W. B. Saunders.

9. **1**

Rationale: Baclofen is a skeletal muscle relaxant and frequently causes drowsiness, dizziness, weakness, and fatigue. Baclofen also can cause nausea, constipation, and urinary retention. Clients should be warned about the possible reactions.

Test-Taking Strategy: Use the process of elimination. Knowledge that baclofen is a skeletal muscle relaxant used to treat muscle spasticity will direct you easily to option 1. If you had difficulty with this question, review the side effects of this medication.

Level of Cognitive Ability: Analysis
Client Needs: Physiological Integrity
Integrated Process: Nursing Process—assessment
Content Area: Pharmacology
Reference: Hodgson, B., & Kizior, R. (2004). *Saunders nursing drug handbook 2004* (p. 93). Philadelphia: W. B. Saunders.

10. **2**

Rationale: Baclofen is a skeletal muscle relaxant. The client should be cautioned against the use of alcohol and other CNS depressants because baclofen potentiates the depressant activity of these agents. Constipation rather than diarrhea is an adverse effect. Restriction of fluids is not necessary, but the client should be warned that urinary retention can occur. Fatigue is related to a CNS effect that is most intense during the early phase of therapy and diminishes with continued medication use. The client does not need to notify the physician about fatigue.

Test-Taking Strategy: Use the process of elimination. Knowledge that baclofen is a skeletal muscle relaxant will direct you easily to option 2. If you were unsure of the correct option, use general principles related to medication administration. Alcohol should be avoided with the use of medications. Review client teaching points related to this medication if you had difficulty with this question.

Level of Cognitive Ability: Application
Client Needs: Physiological Integrity
Integrated Process: Teaching/Learning
Content Area: Pharmacology
References: Hodgson, B., & Kizior, R. (2004). *Saunders nursing drug handbook 2004* (p. 93). Philadelphia: W. B. Saunders.
Kee, J., & Hayes, E. (2003). *Pharmacology: A nursing process approach* (4th ed., p. 369). Philadelphia: W. B. Saunders.

11. **1**

Rationale: Baclofen is dispensed in tablets of 10 and 20 mg for oral use. Dosages are low initially and then are increased gradually. Maintenance doses range from 15 to 20 mg administered 3 to 4 times a day.

Test-Taking Strategy: Knowledge about the normal adult maintenance dosage is required to answer this question. This may be a difficult question, and if you are unfamiliar with this maintenance dosage, review this content.

Level of Cognitive Ability: Analysis
Client Needs: Physiological Integrity
Integrated Process: Nursing Process—analysis
Content Area: Pharmacology
References: Hodgson, B., & Kizior, R. (2004). *Saunders nursing drug handbook 2004* (p. 93). Philadelphia: W. B. Saunders.
Kee, J., & Hayes, E. (2003). *Pharmacology: A nursing process approach* (4th ed., p. 367). Philadelphia: W. B. Saunders.

12. **2**

Rationale: The client should be instructed that symptoms such as drowsiness, weakness, and fatigue are more intense in the early phase of therapy and diminish with continued medication use. The client should be instructed never to withdraw abruptly or stop the medication because abrupt withdrawal can cause visual hallucinations, paranoid ideation, and seizures. For the nurse to inform the client that these symptoms will subside and to encourage the client to continue the use of the medication is the best option.

Test-Taking Strategy: Use the process of elimination. Note the key words "most appropriate." Eliminate option 4 first because it is an extreme nursing response. Next, eliminate options 1 and 3 because these responses do not represent the scope of nursing practice. Review the effects of this medication if you had difficulty with this question.

Level of Cognitive Ability: Application
Client Needs: Physiological Integrity

Integrated Process: Nursing Process—implementation
Content Area: Pharmacology
Reference: Kee, J., & Hayes, E. (2003). *Pharmacology: A nursing process approach* (4th ed., p. 369). Philadelphia: W. B. Saunders.

13. 3
Rationale: Dantrolene (Dantrium) acts directly on skeletal muscle to relieve muscle spasticity. The primary action is the suppression of calcium release from the sarcoplasmic reticulum. This in turn decreases the ability of the skeletal muscle to contract.
Test-Taking Strategy: Use the process of elimination. Options 1, 2, and 4 are similar in that they address the central nervous system and the depression of reflexes. Therefore eliminate these options. Review the action of this medication if you had difficulty with this question.
Level of Cognitive Ability: Analysis
Client Needs: Physiological Integrity
Integrated Process: Nursing Process—assessment
Content Area: Pharmacology
References: Hodgson, B., & Kizior, R. (2004). *Saunders nursing drug handbook 2004* (p. 273). Philadelphia: W. B. Saunders.
Kee, J., & Hayes, E. (2003). *Pharmacology: A nursing process approach* (4th ed., p. 368). Philadelphia: W. B. Saunders.

14. 3
Rationale: Dose-related liver damage is the most serious adverse effect of dantrolene. To reduce the risk of liver damage, tests of liver function should be performed before treatment and throughout the treatment interval. Dantrolene is administered in the lowest effective dosage for the shortest time necessary.
Test-Taking Strategy: Use the process of elimination. Eliminate options 1 and 2 because these tests assess kidney function. From the remaining options, you must recall that this medication affects liver function. Review this medication if you had difficulty with this question.
Level of Cognitive Ability: Analysis
Client Needs: Physiological Integrity
Integrated Process: Nursing Process—analysis
Content Area: Pharmacology
Reference: Hodgson, B., & Kizior, R. (2004). *Saunders nursing drug handbook 2004* (p. 274). Philadelphia: W. B. Saunders.

15. 4
Rationale: Baclofen is the only skeletal muscle relaxant that can be administered intrathecally within the spinal column.
Test-Taking Strategy: Knowledge about intrathecal administration of muscle relaxants is required to answer this question. If you are unfamiliar with this form of therapy, review this content.
Level of Cognitive Ability: Analysis
Client Needs: Physiological Integrity
Integrated Process: Nursing Process—analysis
Content Area: Pharmacology
Reference: Gutierrez, K., & Queener, S. (2003). *Pharmacology for nursing practice* (p. 320). St. Louis: Mosby.

16. 3
Rationale: Clients with seizure disorders may have a lowered seizure threshold when baclofen is administered. Concurrent

therapy may require an increase in the anticonvulsive medication.
Test-Taking Strategy: Use the process of elimination and knowledge about the contraindications and the cautions associated with the administration of baclofen. If you are unfamiliar with these contraindications and cautions, review this content.
Level of Cognitive Ability: Analysis
Client Needs: Physiological Integrity
Integrated Process: Nursing Process—analysis
Content Area: Pharmacology
References: Gutierrez, K., & Queener, S. (2003). *Pharmacology for nursing practice* (p. 321). St. Louis: Mosby.
Hodgson, B., & Kizior, R. (2004). *Saunders nursing drug handbook 2004* (p. 93). Philadelphia: W. B. Saunders.

17. 1
Rationale: Because cyclobenzaprine (Flexeril) has anticholinergic effects, it should be used with caution in clients with a history of urinary retention, glaucoma, and increased intraocular pressure. Cyclobenzaprine should be used only for a short term (2 to 3 weeks).
Test-Taking Strategy: Use the process of elimination. Knowledge that this medication has anticholinergic effects will direct you to option 1. If you are unfamiliar with this medication and the contraindications associated with its administration, review this content.
Level of Cognitive Ability: Analysis
Client Needs: Physiological Integrity
Integrated Process: Nursing Process—analysis
Content Area: Pharmacology
Reference: Hodgson, B., & Kizior, R. (2004). *Saunders nursing drug handbook 2004* (p. 255). Philadelphia: W. B. Saunders.

18. 2
Rationale: The client needs to be told that the urine may turn brown, black, or green. Other adverse effects include blurred vision, nasal congestion, urticaria, and rash. The client needs to be instructed that if these adverse effects occur to notify the physician.
Test-Taking Strategy: Use the process of elimination. Note the key words "need for further education." This will assist in directing you to option 2. If you had difficulty with this question, review this medication.
Level of Cognitive Ability: Analysis
Client Needs: Physiological Integrity
Integrated Process: Teaching/Learning
Content Area: Pharmacology
References: Gutierrez, K., & Queener, S. (2003). *Pharmacology for nursing practice* (p. 321). St. Louis: Mosby.
Lehne, R. (2001). *Pharmacology for nursing care* (4th ed., p. 216). Philadelphia: W. B. Saunders.

19. 4
Rationale: Intravenous administration of methocarbamol can cause hypotension and bradycardia. The nurse needs to monitor for these side effects.
Test-Taking Strategy: Use the process of elimination. Eliminate options 2 and 3 first because they are similar. Knowledge about the specific side effects related to the intravenous use of

this medication will direct you to option 4. Review this medication if you had difficulty with this question.
Level of Cognitive Ability: Analysis
Client Needs: Physiological Integrity
Integrated Process: Nursing Process—analysis
Content Area: Pharmacology
Reference: Gutierrez, K., & Queener, S. (2003). *Pharmacology for nursing practice* (p. 323). St. Louis: Mosby.

20. 1
Rationale: The normal adult dosage for carisoprodol (Soma) is 350 mg PO 3 to 4 times daily.
Test-Taking Strategy: Use the process of elimination. This question may be difficult if you are not familiar with the normal medication dosage. Review this medication if you had difficulty with this question.
Level of Cognitive Ability: Analysis
Client Needs: Physiological Integrity
Integrated Process: Nursing Process—analysis
Content Area: Pharmacology
Reference: Kee, J., & Hayes, E. (2003). Pharmacology: *A nursing process approach* (4th ed., p. 367). Philadelphia: W. B. Saunders.

CRITICAL THINKING: FILL IN THE BLANK
Warfarin sodium (Coumadin)
Rationale: Allopurinol is an antigout medication that may increase the effects of orally administered anticoagulants. Warfarin sodium is an anticoagulant, and if this medication were prescribed for the client, the nurse would verify the order. Ergonovine maleate is an antimigraine medication. Pentazocine is an opioid analgesic.
Test-Taking Strategy: Recalling the interactive effect between allopurinol and warfarin sodium will assist you in answering the question. If you had difficulty with this question, review the medication interactions associated with this medication.
Level of Cognitive Ability: Analysis
Client Needs: Physiological Integrity
Integrated Process: Nursing Process—implementation
Content Area: Pharmacology
Reference: Kee, J., & Hayes, E. (2003). *Pharmacology: A nursing process approach* (4th ed., p. 387). Philadelphia: W. B. Saunders.

REFERENCES

Gutierrez, K., & Queener, S. (2003). *Pharmacology for nursing practice.* St. Louis: Mosby.

Hodgson, B., & Kizior, R. (2004). *Saunders nursing drug handbook 2004.* Philadelphia: W. B. Saunders.

Kee, J., & Hayes, E. (2003). *Pharmacology: A nursing process approach* (4th ed.). Philadelphia: W. B. Saunders.

Lehne, R. (2001). *Pharmacology for nursing care* (4th ed.). Philadelphia: W. B. Saunders.

Lewis, S., Heitkemper, M., & Dirksen, S. (2004). *Medical-surgical nursing: Assessment and management of clinical problems* (6th ed.). St. Louis: Mosby.

The Adult Client with an Immune Disorder

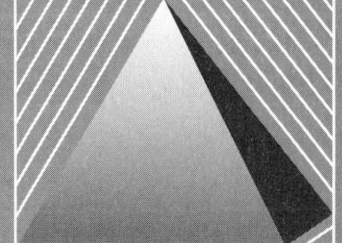

PYRAMID TERMS

acquired immunity Immunity received passively from the mother's antibodies, animal serum, or from the production of antibodies in response to a disease. Immunization produces active acquired immunity.

allergy An abnormal, individual response to certain substances that normally do not trigger such an exaggerated reaction

cellular response A delayed response against slowly developing bacterial infections; also called delayed hypersensitivity.

humoral response An immediate response that provides protection against acute, rapidly developing bacterial and viral infections.

immune deficiency The absence or inadequate production of immune bodies.

natural immunity Immunity present at birth; also called innate immunity.

▶ PYRAMID TO SUCCESS

Pyramid Points focus on the effects of and complications associated with an immune deficiency. Specific focus relates to the nursing care related to the disorder, the impact of the treatment or disorder, and client adaptation. Acquired immunodeficiency syndrome is a pyramid focus, along with protecting the client from infection and preventing the transmission of infection to other individuals. Psychosocial issues relate to social isolation and the body image disturbances that can occur as a result of the immune disorder. The Integrated Processes addressed in this unit include Nursing Process, Caring, Communication and Documentation, and Teaching/Learning.

▶ CLIENT NEEDS
Safe, Effective Care Environment

Advance directives
Advocacy related to client's decisions
Asepsis
Client rights
Confidentiality regarding diagnosis
Consultation with members of the health care team
Establishing priorities
Handling of hazardous and infectious materials
Informed consent for treatments and procedures
Preventing infection
Standard and other precautions

Health Promotion and Maintenance

Client lifestyle choices
Expected body image changes
Health promotion programs
Health screening measures
Immunizations
Prevention of disease related to infection

Psychosocial Integrity

Ability to cope, adapt, and problem solve during illness or stressful events
Assistance in mobilizing appropriate support and resource systems
Assisting the client and family to cope
Grief and loss related to death and the dying process
Promotion of a positive environment to maintain optimal quality of life
Religious, spiritual, and cultural preferences

Physiological Integrity

Diagnostic tests and laboratory values
Managing pain
Medical emergencies
Monitoring for the expected and unexpected responses to treatments
Promotion of nutrition
Protecting the client from infection
Provision of basic care and comfort

REFERENCES

Chernecky, C., & Berger, B. (2004). *Laboratory tests & diagnostic procedures* (4th ed.). Philadelphia: W. B. Saunders.

Harkreader, H., & Hogan, M. A. (2004). *Fundamentals of nursing: Caring and clinical judgment* (2nd ed.). Philadelphia: W. B. Saunders.

Ignatavicius, D., & Workman, M. (2002). *Medical-surgical nursing: Critical thinking for collaborative care* (4th ed.). Philadelphia: W. B. Saunders.

Lewis, S., Heitkemper, M., & Dirksen, S. (2004). *Medical-surgical nursing: Assessment and management of clinical problems* (6th ed.). St. Louis: Mosby.

National Council of State Boards of Nursing (Eds.). (2003). *Test Plan for the National Council Licensure Examination for Registered Nurses* (effective date: April 2004). Chicago: Author.

Perry, A., & Potter, P. (2002). *Clinical nursing skills and techniques* (5th ed.). St. Louis: Mosby.

Phipps, W., Monahan, F., Sands, J., Marek, J., & Neighbors, M. (2003). *Medical-surgical nursing: Health and illness perspectives* (7th ed.). St. Louis: Mosby.

Potter, P., & Perry, A. (2001). *Fundamentals of nursing* (5th ed.). St. Louis: Mosby.

Varcarolis, E. M. (2002). *Foundations of psychiatric mental health nursing* (4th ed.). Philadelphia: W. B. Saunders.

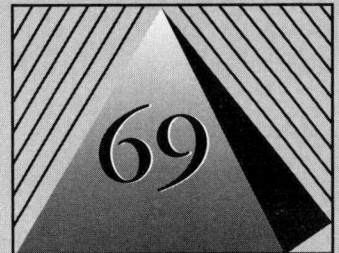

Immune Disorders

I. FUNCTIONS OF THE IMMUNE SYSTEM
A. The immune system provides protection against invasion from outside the body, such as microorganisms.
B. The immune system protects the body from internal threats.
C. The immune system maintains the internal environment by removing dead or damaged cells.

II. IMMUNE RESPONSE
A. T lymphocytes and B lymphocytes
   1. Lymphocytes migrate to lymphoid tissue where they wait to form sensitized lymphocytes for cellular immunity or antibodies for humoral immunity.
   2. Some B lymphocytes lie dormant until a specific antigen enters the body, at which time they greatly increase in number and are available for defense.
   3. T lymphocytes are responsible for rejection of transplanted tissue.
   4. T and B lymphocytes are necessary for a normal immune response.
B. **Humoral response**
   1. **Humoral response** is immediate.
   2. **Humoral response** provides protection against acute, rapidly developing bacterial and viral infections.
C. **Cellular response**
   1. **Cellular response** is delayed and also is called delayed hypersensitivity.
   2. **Cellular response** is active against slowly developing bacterial infections.
   3. **Cellular response** also is involved in autoimmune response, some allergic reactions, and rejection of foreign cells.

III. IMMUNITY
A. **Natural immunity**
   1. **Natural immunity** also is called innate immunity.
   2. **Natural immunity** is present at birth.
B. **Acquired immunity**
   1. **Acquired immunity** is received passively from the mother's antibodies, animal serum, or from the production of antibodies in response to a disease.
   2. Immunization produces active **acquired immunity**.

IV. IMMUNIZATIONS (REFER TO CHAPTER 47 REGARDING IMMUNIZATIONS.)

V. LABORATORY STUDIES
A. Antinuclear antibody
   1. Antinuclear antibody is a blood test used in the differential diagnosis of rheumatic diseases and to detect antinucleoprotein factors and patterns associated with certain autoimmune diseases.
   2. The test is positive at a titer of 1:20 or 1:40, depending on the laboratory.
   3. A positive result does not necessarily confirm a disease.
B. Anti-dsDNA antibody test
   1. The anti-dsDNA (double-stranded DNA) antibody test is a blood test done specifically to identify or differentiate DNA antibodies found in systemic lupus erythematosus (SLE) or other rheumatic diseases.
   2. The test supports a diagnosis, monitors disease activity and response to therapy, and establishes a prognosis for SLE.
   3. Values
      a. Negative: less than 70 units by enzyme-linked immunosorbent assay
      b. Borderline: 70 to 200 units
      c. Positive: greater than 200 units
C. Refer to Chapter 11 for testing related to acquired immunodeficiency syndrome (AIDS).

VI. IMMUNE DEFICIENCY

A. Description
  1. **Immune deficiency** is the absence or inadequate production of immune bodies.
  2. **Immune deficiency** can be congenital (primary) or acquired (secondary).
  3. Treatment depends on the inadequacy of immune bodies and its primary cause.
B. Assessment
  1. Factors that decrease immune function
  2. Frequent infections
  3. Nutritional status
  4. Medication history such as use of corticosteroids
  5. History of alcohol or drug abuse
C. Interventions
  1. Protect client from infection.
  2. Promote balanced, adequate nutrition.
  3. Use strict aseptic technique for all procedures.
  4. Provide psychosocial care regarding lifestyle changes and role changes.
  5. Instruct the client in measures to prevent infection.

▲ VII. HYPERSENSITIVITY AND ALLERGY

A. Description
  1. An **allergy** is an abnormal, individual response to certain substances that normally do not trigger such an exaggerated reaction.
  2. In some types of allergies, a reaction occurs on a second and subsequent contact with the allergen.
  3. Skin testing may be done to determine the allergen.
B. Assessment
  1. History of exposure to allergens
  2. Itching, tearing, and burning of eyes
  3. Itching and burning of the skin
  4. Rashes
  5. Nose twitching, nasal stuffiness
C. Interventions
  1. Identification of the specific allergen.
  2. Management of the symptoms with antihistamines, antiinflammatory agents, or corticosteroids
  3. Ointments, creams, wet compresses, and soothing baths for local reactions
  4. Desensitization programs

▲ VIII. ANAPHYLAXIS

A. Description
  1. Anaphylaxis is a serious and dramatic allergic reaction with the release of histamine from the damaged cells.
  2. Anaphylaxis can cause shock and death if not treated immediately.
B. Assessment
  1. Identification of the allergy
  2. Difficulty breathing
  3. Difficulty swallowing
  4. Complaints of a swollen tongue
  5. Facial edema and swelling of the lips
  6. Skin redness
  7. Presence of a rash
C. Interventions
  1. Establish a patent airway.
  2. Prepare for the administration of epinephrine (Adrenalin), diphenhydramine hydrochloride (Benadryl), or corticosteroids.
  3. Provide measures to control shock.
  4. Provide emotional support.
  5. Instruct the client to wear a Medic-Alert bracelet.
  6. Instruct the client in the use of prescribed medication such as epinephrine (Epi Pen) for immediate treatment of a reaction.

IX. LATEX ALLERGY

A. Description
  1. Latex **allergy** is a hypersensitivity to latex.
  2. The source of the allergic reaction is thought to be due to the proteins in the natural rubber latex or the various chemicals used in the manufacturing process of the latex from a liquid substance into the finished product.
  3. Symptoms of the **allergy** can range from mild contact dermatitis to moderately severe symptoms of rhinitis, conjunctivitis, urticaria, and bronchospasm to severe life-threatening anaphylaxis.
B. Common routes of exposure (Box 69-1)
  1. Cutaneous: natural latex gloves
  2. Percutaneous and parenteral: intravenous lines and catheters; hemodialysis equipment
  3. Mucosal: use of latex condoms, catheters, airways, and nipples

---

BOX 69-1

Products That May Contain Natural Rubber Latex

Ace bandages (brown)
Adhesive or elastic bandages
Ambu bag
Balloons
Blood pressure cuff (tubing and bladder)
Catheter leg bag straps
Catheters
Condoms
Diaphragms
Elastic pressure stockings
Electrocardiogram pads
Feminine hygiene pads
Gloves
Intravenous catheters, tubing, and rubber injection ports
Levin tubes
Pads for crutches
Prepackaged enema kits
Rubber stoppers on medication vials
Stethoscopes
Syringes

Note: Most health care agencies use as many non-latex products as possible.

4. Aerosol: aerosolization of powder from latex gloves can occur when gloves are dispensed from the box or when gloves are removed from the hands

C. At-risk individuals
 1. Health care workers
 2. Individuals who work in manufacturing latex products
 3. Females
 4. Individuals with spina bifida
 5. Individuals who wear gloves frequently such as food handlers, hairdressers, and auto mechanics.
 6. Individuals allergic to kiwis, bananas, pineapples, tropical fruits, avocados, potatoes, and chestnuts.

D. Assessment
 1. Anaphylactic hypersensitivity
   a. Rapid onset
   b. Urticaria, wheezing, dyspnea, laryngeal edema, bronchospasm, tachycardia, angioedema, hypotension, and cardiac arrest
 2. Delayed-type hypersensitivity: symptoms of contact dermatitis such as pruritus, edema, erythema, vesicles, papules, and crusting and thickening of the skin

E. Interventions (Box 69-2)
 1. Ask the client about a known **allergy** to latex when performing the initial assessment.
 2. Identify risk factors to a latex **allergy** in the client.
 3. Individuals with an **allergy**
   a. Avoid latex products.
   b. Obtain an emergency medical kit that contains antihistamines and epinephrine.
   c. Wear a Medic-Alert bracelet.
   d. Inform health care providers and local and paramedic ambulance companies about the **allergy.**
   e. Advise the individual to place a warning label in the car window to alert police and paramedics of the **allergy,** in case of a car accident.
   f. Provide information about local support groups and resources of alternative products.

X. AUTOIMMUNE DISEASE

A. Description
 1. Body is unable to recognize its own cells as a part of itself.
  2. Autoimmune disease can affect collagenous tissue.

B. Systemic lupus erythematosus (SLE)
 1. Description

BOX 69-2

Interventions for the Client with a Latex Allergy

Use nonlatex gloves and latex-safe supplies.
Keep a latex safe supply cart near the client's room.
Apply a cloth barrier to the client's arm under a blood pressure cuff.
Use latex-free syringes, medication containers (glass ampules), and latex-safe intravenous equipment.

---

a. Systemic lupus erythematosus is a chronic progressive systemic inflammatory disease that can cause major organs and systems to fail.
b. Connective tissue and fibrin deposits collect in blood vessels on collagen fibers and on organs.
c. The deposits lead to necrosis and inflammation in blood vessels, lymph nodes, gastrointestinal tract, and pleura.
d. No cure for the disease is known.

2. Causes
 a. The cause of SLE is unknown, and SLE is thought to be due to a defect in the immunological mechanisms or from genetic origin.
 b. Precipitating factors include medications, stress, genetic factors, sunlight or ultraviolet light, and pregnancy.

3. Assessment
 a. Precipitating factors as sunlight, stress, medications, and pregnancy
 b. Dry scaly raised rash on the face or upper body
 c. Fever
 d. Weakness, malaise, and fatigue
 e. Anorexia
 f. Weight loss
 g. Photosensitivity
 h. Joint pain
 i. Erythema of the palms
 j. Butterfly erythema of the face
 k. Anemia
 l. Positive antinuclear antibodies test and lupus erythematosus preparation
 m. Elevated sedimentation rate

4. Interventions
 a. Monitor skin integrity and provide frequent oral care.
 b. Instruct the client to clean skin with a mild soap, avoiding harsh and perfume substances.
 c. Assist with the use of ointments and creams for rash as prescribed.
 d. Identify factors contributing to fatigue.
 e. Administer iron, folic acid, or vitamin supplements as prescribed if anemia occurs.
 f. Provide a high-vitamin and high-iron diet.
 g. Provide a high-protein diet if there is no evidence of kidney disease.
 h. Instruct in measures to conserve energy, such as pacing activities and balancing rest with exercise.
 i. Administer topical or systemic corticosteroids, salicylates, and nonsteroidal antiinflammatory drugs as prescribed for pain and inflammation.
 j. Administer hydroxychloroquine sulfate (Plaquenil) as prescribed to decrease the inflammatory response.
 k. Instruct the client to avoid exposure to sunlight and ultraviolet light.

l. Monitor for proteinuria and red cell casts in the urine.

m. Monitor for bruising, bleeding, and injury.

n. Assist with plasmapheresis as prescribed to remove autoantibodies and immune complexes from the blood before organ damage occurs.

o. Monitor for signs of organ involvement such as pleuritis, nephritis, pericarditis, coronary artery disease, hypertension, neuritis, anemia, and peritonitis.

p. Note that lupus nephritis occurs early in the disease process.

q. Provide supportive therapy as major organs become affected.

r. Provide emotional support and encourage the client to verbalize feelings.

s. Provide information regarding support groups and encourage use of community resources.

C. Scleroderma (progressive systemic sclerosis)

1. Description

a. Scleroderma is a chronic connective tissue disease similar to SLE that is characterized by inflammation, fibrosis, and sclerosis.

b. Scleroderma affects the connective tissue throughout the body.

c. Scleroderma causes fibrotic changes involving the skin, synovial membranes, esophagus, heart, lungs, kidneys, and gastrointestinal tract.

d. Treatment is directed toward forcing the disease into remission and slowing its progress.

2. Assessment

a. Pain

b. Stiffness and muscle weakness

c. Pitting edema of the hands and fingers that progresses to the rest of the body

d. Taut and shiny skin that is free from wrinkles

e. Skin tissue is tight, hard, and thick and loses its elasticity

f. Masklike hard skin that adheres to underlying structures

g. Dysphagia

h. Decreased range of motion

i. Joint contractures

j. Inability to perform activities of daily living

3. Interventions

a. Encourage activity as tolerated.

b. Maintain a constant room temperature.

c. Provide small frequent meals, eliminating foods that stimulate gastric secretions such as spicy foods, caffeine, and alcohol.

d. Advise the client to sit up for 1 to 2 hours after meals if esophageal involvement exists.

e. Provide supportive therapy as the major organs become affected.

f. Administer corticosteroids as prescribed for inflammation.

g. Provide emotional support and encourage the use of resources as necessary.

D. Polyarteritis nodosa

1. Description

a. Polyarteritis nodosa is a collagen disease that causes inflammation of the arteries and thickening and impairment of the circulation.

b. Treatment is similar to treatment for SLE.

c. Polyarteritis nodosa affects middle-aged men and involves every body system.

d. The cause is unknown, and the prognosis is poor.

e. Renal disorders and cardiac involvement are the most frequent causes of death.

2. Assessment

a. Malaise and weakness

b. Low-grade fever

c. Severe abdominal pain

d. Bloody diarrhea

e. Weight loss

f. Elevated sedimentation rate

3. Interventions

a. Provide supportive care as required.

b. Provide a well-balanced diet.

c. Administer corticosteroids and analgesics to control pain and inflammation.

d. Provide emotional support and encourage the client to verbalize feelings.

e. Initiate support services for the client.

E. Pemphigus vulgaris

1. Description

a. Pemphigus vulgaris is a rare disease that occurs predominately between middle and old age.

b. The cause is unknown, and the disorder is potentially fatal.

c. Initial lesions occur on the oral mucosa and then progress to a generalized distribution.

d. Treatment is aimed at suppressing the immune response that causes blister formation.

2. Assessment

a. Lesions that appear as fragile flaccid bullae

b. Partial thickness wounds that bleed, weep, and form crusts when bullae are disrupted

c. Debilitation, malaise, and pain

d. Chewing and swallowing difficulties

e. Nikolsky's sign: separation of the epidermis caused by rubbing the skin

f. Leukocytosis, eosinophilia, foul-smelling discharge from skin

3. Interventions

a. Provide supportive care.

b. Provide oral hygiene and increase fluid intake.

c. Soothe oral lesions.

d. Assist with oatmeal or potassium permanganate baths as prescribed for relief of symptoms.

e. Administer topical or systemic antibiotics as prescribed for secondary infections.

f. Administer corticosteroids and cytotoxic agents as prescribed to bring about remission.

XI. GOODPASTURE'S SYNDROME

A. Description
1. Goodpasture's syndrome is an autoimmune disorder; autoantibodies are made against the glomerular basement membrane and neutrophils.
2. Goodpasture's syndrome is most common in males and young adults, and the exact cause is unknown.
3. The lungs and the kidneys are affected primarily, and the disorder usually is not diagnosed until significant pulmonary or renal involvement occurs.

B. Assessment
1. Clinical manifestations indicating pulmonary and renal involvement
2. Shortness of breath
3. Hemoptysis
4. Decreased urine output
5. Edema and weight gain
6. Hypertension and tachycardia

C. Interventions
1. Focus on suppressing the autoimmune response with medications such as corticosteroids and plasmapheresis (filtration of the plasma to remove some proteins) to remove the autoantibodies.
2. Provide supportive therapy for pulmonary and renal involvement.

▲ XII. ACQUIRED IMMUNODEFICIENCY SYNDROME

A. Description
1. Acquired immunodeficiency syndrome (AIDS) is an infectious disease characterized by severe deficits in cellular function.
2. The syndrome is manifested clinically by opportunistic infection and unusual neoplasms.
3. The cause is human immunodeficiency virus
4. The disease has a long incubation period, sometimes up to 10 years or more.
5. Manifestations may not appear until late in the infection.

B. AIDS-related complex
1. AIDS-related complex is similar to AIDS.
2. AIDS-related complex is two or more symptoms or two or more laboratory findings characteristic of immunodeficiency.
3. Client is not as ill as the client with AIDS.
4. AIDS-related complex may lead to AIDS.

C. High-risk groups
1. Male homosexuals or bisexuals
2. Intravenous drug abusers
3. Persons receiving blood transfusions (hemophiliacs, surgical clients)
4. Those individuals with frequent exposure to blood and body fluids
5. Heterosexual contact with high-risk individuals
6. Babies born to infected mothers

D. Assessment
1. Malaise, weight loss
2. Lymphadenopathy of at least 3 months
3. Leukopenia
4. Diarrhea
5. Fatigue
6. Night sweats
7. Presence of opportunistic Infections
8. *Pneumocystis carinii* pneumonia (major source of mortality)
9. Kaposi's sarcoma: purplish/red lesions of internal organs and skin
10. Fungal infections
11. Candidiasis
12. Cytomegalovirus

E. Interventions
1. Provide respiratory support.
2. Administer respiratory treatments as prescribed.
3. Administer oxygen as prescribed.
4. Maintain fluid and electrolyte balance.
5. Monitor for signs of infection.
6. Prevent the spread of infection.
7. Initiate standard and other precautions as necessary.
8. Provide comfort as necessary.
9. Provide meticulous skin care.
10. Provide adequate nutritional support as prescribed.
11. Refer to Chapters 25 and 46 for additional information on AIDS.

PRACTICE QUESTIONS

1. A client is suspected of having systemic lupus erythematous. The nurse monitors the client, knowing that which of the following is a characteristic sign of systemic lupus erythematous?
   1. Rash on the face across the bridge of the nose and on the cheeks
   2. Fatigue
   3. Fever
   4. Elevated red blood cell count

2. The nurse provides home care instructions to a client with systemic lupus erythematous and tells the client about the methods to manage fatigue. Which statement by the client indicates a need for further instructions?
   1. "I should avoid long periods of rest."
   2. "I should sit whenever possible."
   3. "I should take a hot bath in the evening."
   4. "I should do a moderate amount of low-impact exercises when I am not fatigued."

3. The client has requested and undergone testing for human immunodeficiency virus. The client now asks what will be done next because the results of two enzyme-linked immunosorbent assays have been positive. The nurse's response is based on the understanding that
   1. The client probably will have a bone marrow biopsy done.

2. A Western blot will be done to confirm these findings.

3. A CD4 cell count will be done to measure T-helper lymphocyte

4. The client will be diagnosed definitively as positive for human immunodeficiency virus at this point.

4. The nurse is caring for the client with acquired immunodeficiency syndrome. The nurse detects early infection with *Pneumocystis carinii* by monitoring the client for which clinical manifestation?
   1. Dyspnea on exertion
   2. Dyspnea at rest
   3. Fever
   4. Cough

5. The client with acquired immunodeficiency syndrome has a concurrent diagnosis of histoplasmosis. The nurse notes, during the assessment, that the client has enlarged lymph nodes. The nurse interprets that
   1. The client has disseminated histoplasmosis infection.
   2. This is a side effect of the medications given to treat acquired immunodeficiency syndrome.
   3. This indicates that the histoplasmosis is resolving.
   4. The client probably has another infection that is developing.

6. The nurse is caring for the client with acquired immunodeficiency syndrome who is experiencing night fever and night sweats. Which nursing intervention would be the least helpful in managing this symptom?
   1. Keep a change of bed linens nearby in case they are needed.
   2. Administer an antipyretic after the client spikes the fever.
   3. Make sure the pillow has a plastic cover.
   4. Keep liquids at the bedside.

7. The client exposed to human immunodeficiency virus (HIV) about 3 months ago has seroconverted to an HIV-positive status. The nurse anticipates that the client will experience which of the following at this time?
   1. Oral lesions
   2. Purplish skin lesions
   3. Chronic cough
   4. No signs and symptoms

8. The client with acquired immunodeficiency syndrome has raised, dark purplish–colored lesions on the trunk of the body. The nurse anticipates that which of the following procedures will be done to confirm whether these lesions are due to Kaposi's sarcoma?
   1. Enzyme-linked immunosorbent assay
   2. Western blot

3. Skin biopsy
4. Lung biopsy

9. The nurse participating in a health fair is setting up a booth on prevention of human immunodeficiency virus transmission. A poster is planned that will list sexual behaviors in one of two columns, rated "safe" and "not safe." Which of the following behaviors would the nurse place in the "not safe" column?
   1. Use of latex condoms
   2. Use of natural skin condoms
   3. Abstinence
   4. Mutual monogamy

10. The client with acquired immunodeficiency syndrome is experiencing nausea and vomiting. The nurse would make which of the following dietary alterations for this client to enhance nutritional intake?
    1. Avoid dairy products and red meat.
    2. Plan large, nutritious meals.
    3. Add spices to food for added flavor.
    4. Serve foods while they are warm.

11. The client with acquired immunodeficiency syndrome has a respiratory infection from *Pneumocystis carinii* and a nursing diagnosis of Impaired Gas Exchange written in the plan of care. Which of the following indicates that the expected outcome of care has not yet been achieved?
    1. Client is free of complaints of shortness of breath.
    2. Client expectorates secretions easily.
    3. Client has clear breath sounds.
    4. Client limits fluid intake.

12. A client with pemphigus vulgaris is being seen in the clinic regularly. The nurse plans care based on which of the following descriptions of this condition?
    1. The presence of skin vesicles found along the nerve caused by a virus
    2. An autoimmune disease that causes blistering in the epidermis
    3. The presence of red, raised papules and large plaques covered by silvery scales
    4. The presence of tiny red vesicles

13. The nurse is providing dietary instructions to the client with systemic lupus erythematosus. Which of the following dietary items would the nurse instruct the client to avoid?
    1. Cantaloupe
    2. Broccoli
    3. Turkey
    4. Steak

14. The client is brought to the emergency room and is experiencing an anaphylaxis reaction from eating shellfish. The nurse implements which immediate action?
    1. Administering epinephrine (Adrenalin)
    2. Administering a corticosteroid

3. Maintaining a patent airway

4. Instructing the client on the importance of obtaining a Medic-Alert bracelet

15. The nurse is assisting in planning care for a client with a diagnosis of immune deficiency. The nurse would incorporate which of the following as a priority in the plan of care?

   1. Providing emotional support to decrease fear
   2. Protecting the client from infection
   3. Encouraging discussion about lifestyle changes
   4. Identifying factors that decreased the immune function

16. A client calls the nurse in the emergency room and tells the nurse that he was just stung by a bumble bee while gardening. The client is afraid of a severe reaction because the client's neighbor experienced such a reaction just 1 week ago. The most appropriate nursing action is to

   1. Ask the client if he ever sustained a bee sting in the past.
   2. Tell the client to call an ambulance for transport to the emergency room.
   3. Advise the client to soak the site in hydrogen peroxide.
   4. Tell the client not to worry about the sting unless difficulty with breathing occurs.

17. The nurse is assisting in administering immunizations at a health care clinic. The nurse understands that an immunization will provide

   1. Natural immunity from disease.
   2. Acquired immunity from disease.
   3. Innate immunity from disease.
   4. Protection from all diseases.

18. The nurse is assigned to care for a client with systemic lupus erythematosus. The nurse plans care knowing that this disorder is

   1. A local rash that occurs as a result of allergy.
   2. An inflammatory disease of collagen contained in connective tissue.
   3. A disease caused by overexposure to sunlight.
   4. A disease caused by the continuous release of histamine in the body.

19. The nurse is assigned to care for a client admitted to the hospital with a diagnosis of systemic lupus erythematosus. The nurse reviews the physician's orders, expecting to note that which of the following medications is prescribed?

   1. Antibiotic
   2. Narcotic analgesic
   3. Antidiarrheal
   4. Corticosteroid

20. The nurse administers an injection to a client with a diagnosis of acquired immunodeficiency syndrome. After administering the medication, the nurse disposes of the used needle by

1. Placing it in a puncture-resistant container.
2. Laying the needle and syringe on the bedside table and carefully recapping the needle.
3. Asking the client to recap the needle.
4. Recapping the needle before placing it in a puncture-resistant container.

21. The community health nurse is conducting a research study and is identifying clients in the community at risk for latex allergy. Which client population is at most risk for developing this type of allergy?

   1. The homeless
   2. Individuals living in a group home
   3. Children in day care centers
   4. Hairdressers

22. The clinic nurse is providing home care instructions to a client who has been diagnosed with a latex allergy. The nurse most appropriately instructs the client to avoid

   1. Outdoor activities as much as possible.
   2. Going to parties.
   3. The use of condoms.
   4. Sunlight.

23. The home care nurse is performing an assessment on a client who has been diagnosed with an allergy to latex. In determining the client's risk factors associated with the allergy, the nurse questions the client about an allergy to which food item?

   1. Milk
   2. Bananas
   3. Yogurt
   4. Eggs

24. The home care nurse is assigned to visit a client who returned to home from the emergency room following treatment for a sprained ankle. The nurse notes that the client was sent home with crutches that have rubber axillary pads and needs instructions regarding crutch walking. On admission assessment, the nurse discovers that the client has an allergy to latex. Before providing instructions regarding crutch walking, the nurse most appropriately

   1. Contacts the physician.
   2. Covers the crutch pads with cloth.
   3. Tells the client that the crutches must be removed from the house immediately.
   4. Calls the local medical supply store and asks for a cane to be delivered.

25. The home care nurse is ordering dressing supplies for a client who has an allergy to latex. The nurse asks the medical supply personnel to deliver which of the following?

   1. Adhesive bandages
   2. Elastic bandages
   3. Cotton pads and silk tape
   4. Brown Ace bandages

CRITICAL THINKING: FILL IN THE BLANK

The home care nurse is assigned to visit a client who has a diagnosis of hypertension. The client was just discharged from the hospital to home. On assessment of the client, the nurse discovers that the client has an allergy to latex. The nurse realizes that the blood pressure equipment contains latex. What action will the nurse take regarding obtaining the client's blood pressure?

Answer: _____

ANSWERS

1. **1**
Rationale: Skin lesions or rash on the face across the bridge of the nose and on the cheeks is a characteristic sign of systemic lupus erythematosus (SLE). Fever and fatigue may occur potentially before and during exacerbation. Anemia is most likely to occur in SLE.
Test-Taking Strategy: Use the process of elimination. Note the key words "characteristic sign." Recalling the characteristic butterfly rash associated with SLE will direct you to option 1. If you are unfamiliar with this disorder, review this content.
Level of Cognitive Ability: Analysis
Client Needs: Physiological Integrity
Integrated Process: Nursing Process—assessment
Content Area: Adult health—immune
Reference: Phipps, W., Monahan, F., Sands, J., Marek, J., & Neighbors, M. (2003). *Medical-surgical nursing: Health and illness perspectives* (7th ed., p. 1547). St. Louis: Mosby.

2. **3**
Rationale: To help reduce fatigue in the client with systemic lupus erythematosus, the nurse should instruct the client to sit whenever possible, to avoid hot baths, to schedule moderate low-impact exercises when not fatigued, and to maintain a balanced diet. The client is instructed to avoid long periods of rest because it promotes joint stiffness.
Test-Taking Strategy: Note the key words "need for further instructions" and focus on the issue "fatigue." By the process of elimination, you should be directed easily to option 3 as the action that would exacerbate fatigue. If you had difficulty with this question, review measures to prevent fatigue in a client with systemic lupus erythematosus.
Level of Cognitive Ability: Analysis
Client Needs: Health Promotion and Maintenance
Integrated Process: Teaching/Learning
Content Area: Adult health—immune
Reference: Lewis, S., Heitkemper, M., & Dirksen, S. (2004). *Medical-surgical nursing: Assessment and management of clinical problems* (6th ed., p. 1743). St. Louis: Mosby.

3. **2**
Rationale: If the results of two enzyme-linked immunosorbent assays are positive, the Western blot is done to confirm the findings. If the result of the Western blot is positive, then the client is considered to be positive for human immunodeficiency virus and to be infected with the human immunodeficiency virus. Options 1, 3, and 4 are incorrect.
Test-Taking Strategy: Knowledge of the procedural steps in diagnosing human immunodeficiency virus is needed to answer this question. If you are unfamiliar with these diagnostic tests, review this content.
Level of Cognitive Ability: Analysis

Client Needs: Physiological Integrity
Integrated Process: Nursing Process—assessment
Content Area: Adult health—immune
Reference: Phipps, W., Monahan, F., Sands, J., Marek, J., & Neighbors, M. (2003). *Medical-surgical nursing: Health and illness perspectives* (7th ed., p. 1621). St. Louis: Mosby.

4. **4**
Rationale: The client with *Pneumocystis carinii* infection usually has a cough as the first symptom, which begins as nonproductive and then progresses to productive. Later signs include fever, dyspnea on exertion, and finally dyspnea at rest.
Test-Taking Strategy: Use the process of elimination, noting the key word "early." Although all of these symptoms may appear at some point in the client with *P. carinii* infection, knowing that the cough appears first helps to you eliminate each of the other options. Review the early signs of *P. carinii* infection if you had difficulty with this question.
Level of Cognitive Ability: Analysis
Client Needs: Physiological Integrity
Integrated Process: Nursing Process—assessment
Content Area: Adult health—immune
Reference: Ignatavicius, D., & Workman, M. (2002). *Medical-surgical nursing: Critical thinking for collaborative care* (4th ed. p. 371). Philadelphia: W. B. Saunders.

5. **1**
Rationale: Histoplasmosis usually starts as a respiratory infection in the client with acquired immunodeficiency syndrome and then becomes a disseminated infection, with enlargement of lymph nodes, spleen, and liver. Options 2, 3, and 4 are incorrect.
Test-Taking Strategy: Knowing that lymph nodes may enlarge with generalized infection helps you eliminate options 2 and 3. Because the question contains no information that indicates that option 4 is true, option 1 is the correct option by the process of elimination. Review disseminated infections in the client with acquired immunodeficiency syndrome if you had difficulty with this question.
Level of Cognitive Ability: Analysis
Client Needs: Physiological Integrity
Integrated Process: Nursing Process—analysis
Content Area: Adult health—immune
Reference: Ignatavicius, D., & Workman, M. (2002). *Medical-surgical nursing: Critical thinking for collaborative care* (4th ed., p. 373). Philadelphia: W. B. Saunders.

6. **2**
Rationale: For clients with acquired immunodeficiency syndrome who experience night fever and night sweats, the nurse may offer the client an antipyretic of choice before the client goes to sleep. Keeping a change of bed linens and night

clothes nearby for use is also helpful. The pillow should have a plastic cover, and a towel may be placed over the pillowcase if diaphoresis is profuse. The client should have liquids at the bedside to drink.

Test-Taking Strategy: Use the process of elimination, noting the key words "least helpful." Options 1 and 3 are helpful from an environmental viewpoint, so eliminate them first as answers to this question. Knowing that liquids will help prevent dehydration will assist you in eliminating this option next. Because night fever and sweats occur serially, giving the antipyretic before sleep as a prophylactic measure is most helpful. Review care to the client with acquired immunodeficiency syndrome if you had difficulty with this question.

Level of Cognitive Ability: Application
Client Needs: Physiological Integrity
Integrated Process: Nursing Process—implementation
Content Area: Adult health—immune
References: Ignatavicius, D., & Workman, M. (2002). *Medical-surgical nursing: Critical thinking for collaborative care* (4th ed., p. 373). Philadelphia: W. B. Saunders.
Lewis, S., Heitkemper, M., & Dirksen, S. (2004). *Medical-surgical nursing: Assessment and management of clinical problems* (6th ed., p. 278). St. Louis: Mosby.

7. **4**

Rationale: The client in Stage 1 (seroconversion) acute human immunodeficiency virus (HIV) infection has laboratory documentation of HIV-positive status but is asymptomatic. Following introduction of the infection and seroconversion in Stage 1, the client may remain asymptomatic for 6 months to in excess of 10 years (Stage 2, chronic asymptomatic status). The client's T4 cell count is normal during these two stages. The client will begin to show symptoms in Stage 3, symptomatic stage, when the T4 cell count drops to less than 500 cells/μL. At this time, the client experiences opportunistic infections, including oral lesions (thrush) and skin lesions (Kaposi's sarcoma). The client also may experience signs of respiratory infection in Stage 3.

Test-Taking Strategy: Use the process of elimination. Read the question carefully noting the 3-month period between exposure and seroconversion. This will direct you to option 4. Review the clinical manifestations associated with HIV if you had difficulty with this question.

Level of Cognitive Ability: Analysis
Client Needs: Physiological Integrity
Integrated Process: Nursing Process—assessment
Content Area: Adult health—immune
Reference: Phipps, W., Monahan, F., Sands, J., Marek, J., & Neighbors, M. (2003). *Medical-surgical nursing: Health and illness perspectives* (7th ed., p. 1656). St. Louis: Mosby.

8. **3**

Rationale: The skin biopsy is the procedure of choice to diagnose Kaposi's sarcoma, which frequently complicates the clinical picture of the client with acquired immunodeficiency syndrome. Lung biopsy would confirm *Pneumocystis carinii* infection. The enzyme-linked immunosorbent assay and Western blot are tests to diagnose human immunodeficiency virus status.

Test-Taking Strategy: Use the process of elimination. Eliminate options 1 and 2, which are used to diagnose whether the

client is human immunodeficiency virus positive. Knowledge of the meaning of Kaposi's sarcoma, or attention to the words "lesions" and "trunk" will help you to choose correctly between the remaining options. Review the diagnostic testing to confirm Kaposi's sarcoma if you had difficulty with this question.

Level of Cognitive Ability: Analysis
Client Needs: Physiological Integrity
Integrated Process: Nursing Process—analysis
Content Area: Adult health—immune
Reference: Ignatavicius, D., & Workman, M. (2002). *Medical-surgical nursing: Critical thinking for collaborative care* (4th ed., p. 374). Philadelphia: W. B. Saunders.

9. **2**

Rationale: Abstinence is the safest way to avoid human immunodeficiency virus infection. Another reliable method is participation in a mutually monogamous relationship. The use of latex condoms is considered safe because the latex prevents the transmission of the human immunodeficiency virus as long as the condom is used properly and remains in place. The use of "natural skin" condoms is not considered safe because the pores in the condom are large enough for the virus to pass through.

Test-Taking Strategy: Use the process of elimination, noting the issue of the question, sexual behaviors that are not safe. Recalling that condoms not made of latex will not protect the individual from sexually transmitted diseases will direct you to option 2. Review these preventive measures if you had difficulty with this question.

Level of Cognitive Ability: Application
Client Needs: Health Promotion and Maintenance
Integrated Process: Teaching/Learning
Content Area: Adult health—immune
Reference: Phipps, W., Monahan, F., Sands, J., Marek, J., & Neighbors, M. (2003). *Medical-surgical nursing: Health and illness perspectives* (7th ed., p. 1858). St. Louis: Mosby.

10. **1**

Rationale: The client with acquired immunodeficiency syndrome who has nausea and vomiting should avoid fatty products such as diary products and red meat. Meals should be small and frequent to lessen the chance of vomiting. The client should avoid spices and odorous foods because they aggravate nausea. Foods are best tolerated cold or at room temperature.

Test-Taking Strategy: Use the process of elimination and basic principles for treating nausea and vomiting to answer this question. Doing so will guide you to option 1. Review nutritional support for the client with acquired immunodeficiency syndrome if you had difficulty with this question.

Level of Cognitive Ability: Application
Client Needs: Physiological Integrity
Integrated Process: Nursing Process—implementation
Content Area: Adult health—immune
Reference: Ignatavicius, D., & Workman, M. (2002). *Medical-surgical nursing: Critical thinking for collaborative care* (4th ed., p. 383). Philadelphia: W. B. Saunders.

11. **4**

Rationale: The status of the client with a diagnosis of Impaired Gas Exchange would be evaluated against the standard outcome criteria for this nursing diagnosis. These would include that the client states that breathing is easier, coughs up secretions effectively, and has clear breath sounds. The client should not limit fluid intake because fluids are needed to decrease the viscosity of secretions for expectoration.

Test-Taking Strategy: Use the process of elimination and note the key words "expected outcome" and "has not yet been achieved." This will direct you easily to option 4. Review care to the client with acquired immunodeficiency syndrome if you had difficulty with this question.

Level of Cognitive Ability: Analysis
Client Needs: Physiological Integrity
Integrated Process: Nursing Process—evaluation
Content Area: Adult health—immune
Reference: Phipps, W., Monahan, F., Sands, J., Marek, J., & Neighbors, M. (2003). *Medical-surgical nursing: Health and illness perspectives* (7th ed., p. 1678). St. Louis: Mosby.

12. 2
Rationale: Pemphigus vulgaris is an autoimmune disease that causes blistering in the epidermis. The client has large flaccid blisters (bullae). Because the blisters are in the epidermis, they have a thin covering of skin and break easily, leaving large denuded areas of skin. On initial examination, clients may have crusting areas instead of intact blisters. Option 1 describes herpes zoster, option 3 describes psoriasis, and option 4 describes eczema.

Test-Taking Strategy: Use the process of elimination. Recalling that pemphigus vulgaris is an autoimmune disorder will direct you easily to option 2. If you had difficulty with this question, review the characteristics of this disorder.

Level of Cognitive Ability: Comprehension
Client Needs: Physiological Integrity
Integrated Process: Nursing Process—planning
Content Area: Adult health—immune
Reference: Ignatavicius, D., & Workman, M. (2002). *Medical-surgical nursing: Critical thinking for collaborative care* (4th ed., p. 1551). Philadelphia: W. B. Saunders.

13. 4
Rationale: The client with systemic lupus erythematosus is at risk for cardiovascular disorders such as coronary artery disease and hypertension. The client is advised of lifestyle changes to reduce these risks, which include smoking cessation and prevention of obesity and hyperlipidemia. The client is advised to reduce salt, fat, and cholesterol intake.

Test-Taking Strategy: Use the process of elimination. Note the key word "avoid" in the question. Knowledge regarding the risks associated with systemic lupus erythematosus will assist you in answering this question. Use knowledge regarding basic nutritional components of food items to help direct you to option 4. If you had difficulty with this question, review therapeutic management of systemic lupus erythematosus.

Level of Cognitive Ability: Application
Client Needs: Health Promotion and Maintenance
Integrated Process: Teaching/Learning
Content Area: Adult health—immune
Reference: Lewis, S., Heitkemper, M., & Dirksen, S. (2004). *Medical-surgical nursing: Assessment and management of clinical problems* (6th ed., p. 1739). St. Louis: Mosby.

14. 3
Rationale: The immediate action would be to maintain a patent airway. The client then would receive epinephrine. Corticosteroids also may be prescribed. The client will need to be instructed about obtaining and wearing a Medic-Alert bracelet, but this is not the immediate action.

Test-Taking Strategy: Focus on the key word "immediate." This key word tells you that you need to prioritize your nursing actions. Use the ABCs—airway, breathing, and circulation—to answer the question. Airway is always the priority. Review care to the client experiencing an anaphylaxis reaction if you had difficulty with this question.

Level of Cognitive Ability: Application
Client Needs: Physiological Integrity
Integrated Process: Nursing Process—implementation
Content Area: Delegating/Prioritizing
References: Ignatavicius, D., & Workman, M. (2002). *Medical-surgical nursing: Critical thinking for collaborative care* (4th ed., p. 399). Philadelphia: W. B. Saunders.
Lewis, S., Heitkemper, M., & Dirksen, S. (2004). *Medical-surgical nursing: Assessment and management of clinical problems* (6th ed., p. 251). St. Louis: Mosby.

15. 2
Rationale: The client with immune deficiency has inadequate or the absence of immune bodies and is at risk for infection. The priority nursing intervention would be to protect the client from infection. Options 1, 3, and 4 may be components of care but are not the priority.

Test-Taking Strategy: Use Maslow's hierarchy of needs theory to answer the question. Remember that physiological needs are the priority. This will direct you easily to option 2. Review the care of a client with immune deficiency if you had difficulty with this question.

Level of Cognitive Ability: Application
Client Needs: Physiological Integrity
Integrated Process: Nursing Process—planning
Content Area: Delegating/Prioritizing
Reference: Lewis, S., Heitkemper, M., & Dirksen, S. (2004). *Medical-surgical nursing: Assessment and management of clinical problems* (6th ed., p. 277). St. Louis: Mosby.

16. 1
Rationale: In some types of allergies, a reaction occurs only on second and subsequent contacts with the allergen. The most appropriate action therefore would be to ask the client if he ever received a bee sting in the past. Option 2 is unnecessary. Option 3 is not appropriate advise. The client should not be told "not to worry."

Test-Taking Strategy: Use the steps of the nursing process to answer the question. Option 1 is the only option that addresses assessment. Review information related to allergic reactions if you had difficulty with this question.

Level of Cognitive Ability: Application
Client Needs: Physiological Integrity
Integrated Process: Nursing Process—implementation
Content Area: Adult health—immune
Reference: Lewis, S., Heitkemper, M., & Dirksen, S. (2004). *Medical-surgical nursing: Assessment and management of clinical problems* (6th ed., p. 246). St. Louis: Mosby.

17. 2

Rationale: Acquired immunity can occur by receiving an immunization that causes antibodies to a specific pathogen to form. Natural (innate) immunity is present at birth. No immunization protects the client from all diseases.

Test-Taking Strategy: Use the process of elimination and knowledge regarding immunity to disease to answer the question. Eliminate option 4 first because of the absolute word "all." Next eliminate options 1 and 3 because they are similar. Review natural and acquired immunity, if you had difficulty with this question.

Level of Cognitive Ability: Comprehension
Client Needs: Physiological Integrity
Integrated Process: Nursing Process—implementation
Content Area: Adult health—immune
Reference: Phipps, W., Monahan, F., Sands, J., Marek, J., & Neighbors, M. (2003). *Medical-surgical nursing: Health and illness perspectives* (7th ed., p. 190). St. Louis: Mosby.

18. 2

Rationale: Systemic lupus erythematosus is an inflammatory disease of collagen contained in connective tissue. Options 1, 3, and 4 are not associated with this disease.

Test-Taking Strategy: Use the process of elimination. Eliminate option 1 because systemic lupus erythematosus is a systemic disorder, not a local one. Next eliminate option 4 because of its similarity to option 1. From the remaining options, select option 2 because of its systemic characteristic. If you are unfamiliar with disorder, review its characteristics.

Level of Cognitive Ability: Comprehension
Client Needs: Physiological Integrity
Integrated Process: Nursing Process—planning
Content Area: Adult health—immune
Reference: Ignatavicius, D., & Workman, M. (2002). *Medical-surgical nursing: Critical thinking for collaborative care* (4th ed., p. 352). Philadelphia: W. B. Saunders.

19. 4

Rationale: Treatment of systemic lupus erythematosus is based on the systems involved and symptoms. Treatment normally consists of antiinflammatory drugs, corticosteroids, and immunosuppressants. Options 1, 2, and 3 are not a standard component of medication therapy.

Test-Taking Strategy: Use the process of elimination. Recalling that systemic lupus erythematosus is an inflammatory disorder will direct you to option 4. If you are unfamiliar with the treatments normally prescribed in this disease, review this content.

Level of Cognitive Ability: Analysis
Client Needs: Physiological Integrity
Integrated Process: Nursing Process—analysis
Content Area: Adult health—immune
References: Ignatavicius, D., & Workman, M. (2002). *Medical-surgical nursing: Critical thinking for collaborative care* (4th ed., p. 335). Philadelphia: W. B. Saunders.
Lewis, S., Heitkemper, M., & Dirksen, S. (2004). *Medical-surgical nursing: Assessment and management of clinical problems* (6th ed., p. 1550). St. Louis: Mosby.

20. 1

Rationale: The correct procedure for needle disposal is to dispose of uncapped needles and sharps in a hard-wall, puncture-resistant container immediately after use. Needles are not recapped.

Test-Taking Strategy: Use the process of elimination and principles related to the safe disposal of needles and syringes to answer the question. Note that options 2, 3, and 4 are similar in that they all address recapping the needle. Review these principles, if you had difficulty with this question.

Level of Cognitive Ability: Application
Client Needs: Safe, Effective Care Environment
Integrated Process: Nursing Process—implementation
Content Area: Adult health—immune
Reference: Potter, P., & Perry, A. (2001). *Fundamentals of nursing* (5th ed., p. 948). St. Louis: Mosby.

21. 4

Rationale: Individuals at risk for developing a latex allergy include health care workers; individuals who work with manufacturing latex products; females; individuals with spina bifida; individuals who wear gloves frequently such as food handlers, hairdressers, and auto mechanics; and individuals allergic to kiwis, bananas, pineapples, passion fruits, avocados, and chestnuts.

Test-Taking Strategy: Focus on the issue, a latex allergy. Recalling the cause and the source of the allergic reaction will direct you easily to option 4. Review the cause of this type of allergy and the individuals at risk if you had difficulty with this question.

Level of Cognitive Ability: Analysis
Client Needs: Health Promotion and Maintenance
Integrated Process: Nursing Process—assessment
Content Area: Adult health—immune
References: Ignatavicius, D., & Workman, M. (2002). *Medical-surgical nursing: Critical thinking for collaborative care* (4th ed., pp. 400-401). Philadelphia: W. B. Saunders.
Phipps, W., Monahan, F., Sands, J., Marek, J., & Neighbors, M. (2003). *Medical-surgical nursing: Health and illness perspectives* (7th ed., p. 412). St. Louis: Mosby.

22. 3

Rationale: Mucosal exposure to latex can occur on contact with latex condoms. The nurse most appropriately would provide instructions to the client about the need to avoid the use of condoms unless they are latex free. No reason exists for the client to avoid outdoor activities or sunlight or to avoid parties; however, the client should be informed that certain forms of balloons are made of latex.

Test-Taking Strategy: Use the process of elimination. Note the key word "avoid." Eliminate option 1 and 4 first because they are similar. From the remaining options, focusing on the issue will direct you to option 3. Review home care instructions for the client with a latex allergy if you had difficulty with this question.

Level of Cognitive Ability: Application
Client Needs: Health Promotion and Maintenance
Integrated Process: Teaching/Learning
Content Area: Adult health—immune

Reference: Ignatavicius, D., & Workman, M. (2002). *Medical-surgical nursing: Critical thinking for collaborative care* (4th ed., pp. 400-401). Philadelphia: W. B. Saunders.

23. **2**

Rationale: Individuals who are allergic to bananas, avocados, tropical fruits, kiwis, potatoes, and chestnuts are at risk for developing a latex allergy. This is thought to be due to a possible cross-reaction between the food and the latex allergen. Options 1, 3, and 4 are unrelated to latex allergy.

Test-Taking Strategy: Use the process of elimination and knowledge regarding the food items related to a latex allergy. Eliminate options 1, 3, and 4 because they are similar and relate to dairy products. Review the food items that are associated with a risk for latex allergy if you had difficulty with this question.

Level of Cognitive Ability: Analysis
Client Needs: Physiological Integrity
Integrated Process: Nursing Process—assessment
Content Area: Adult health—immune
Reference: Phipps, W., Monahan, F., Sands, J., Marek, J., & Neighbors, M. (2003). *Medical-surgical nursing: Health and illness perspectives* (7th ed., p. 412). St. Louis: Mosby.

24. **2**

Rationale: The rubber pads used on crutches may contain latex. If the client requires the use of crutches, the nurse can cover the pads with a cloth to prevent cutaneous contact. Option 3 is inappropriate and may alarm the client. The nurse cannot order a cane for a client. Additionally, this type of assistive device may not be appropriate considering this client's injury. No reason exists to contact the physician at this time.

Test-Taking Strategy: Use the process of elimination and knowledge regarding the alternative resources for a client with an allergy to latex. No data in the question support the need to contact the physician. The nurse should not prescribe assistive devices for the client. Option 3 is not a therapeutic action. Review care to the client with a latex allergy if you had difficulty with this question.

Level of Cognitive Ability: Application
Client Needs: Physiological Integrity
Integrated Process: Nursing Process—implementation
Content Area: Adult health—immune

Reference: Harkreader, H., & Hogan, M. A. (2004). *Fundamentals of nursing: Caring and clinical judgment* (2nd ed., p. 1221). Philadelphia: W. B. Saunders.

25. **3**

Rationale: Cotton pads and plastic or silk tape are latex-free products. The items identified in options 1, 2, and 4 are products that contain latex.

Test-Taking Strategy: Use the process of elimination and knowledge regarding the products that contain latex to answer this question. Eliminate options 2 and 4 first because they are similar. Noting the key words "cotton" and "silk" in option 3 will assist in answering correctly from the remaining options. Review the list of products that contain latex if you had difficulty with this question.

Level of Cognitive Ability: Application
Client Needs: Physiological Integrity
Integrated Process: Nursing Process—implementation
Content Area: Adult health—immune
Reference: Phipps, W., Monahan, F., Sands, J., Marek, J., & Neighbors, M. (2003). *Medical-surgical nursing: Health and illness perspectives* (7th ed., p. 412). St. Louis: Mosby.

CRITICAL THINKING: FILL IN THE BLANK

Answer: Obtain the blood pressure by placing the equipment over the client's clothing.

Rationale: A blood pressure cuff and a stethoscope contain latex. If available, a nylon or vinyl cuff that is latex free can be used to obtain the blood pressure. An alternative to this method is to wrap stockinette over the equipment or obtain the blood pressure by placing the equipment over the client's clothing.

Test-Taking Strategy: Recall that a source of exposure to latex is cutaneous. Avoiding skin contact with the blood pressure equipment will prevent a reaction. Covering the skin will prevent cutaneous contact. Review interventions for the client with a latex allergy if you had difficulty with this question.

Level of Cognitive Ability: Application
Client Needs: Physiological Integrity
Integrated Process: Nursing Process—implementation
Content Area: Adult health—immune
Reference: Harkreader, H., & Hogan, M. A. (2004). *Fundamentals of nursing: Caring and clinical judgment* (2nd ed., p. 1221). Philadelphia: W. B. Saunders.

REFERENCES

Harkreader, H., & Hogan, M. A. (2004). *Fundamentals of nursing: Caring and clinical judgment* (2nd ed.). Philadelphia: W. B. Saunders.

Ignatavicius, D., & Workman, M. (2002). *Medical-surgical nursing: Critical thinking for collaborative care* (4th ed.). Philadelphia: W. B. Saunders.

Lewis, S., Heitkemper, M., & Dirksen, S. (2004). *Medical-surgical nursing: Assessment and management of clinical problems* (6th ed.). St. Louis: Mosby.

Phipps, W., Monahan, F., Sands, J., Marek, J., & Neighbors, M. (2003). *Medical-surgical nursing: Health and illness perspectives* (7th ed.). St. Louis: Mosby.

Potter, P., & Perry, A. (2001). *Fundamentals of nursing* (5th ed.). St. Louis: Mosby.

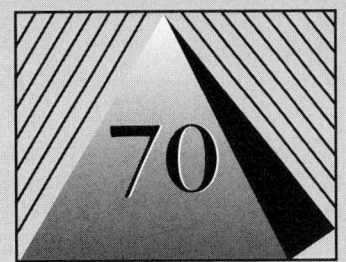

Immunological Medications

I. HUMAN IMMUNODEFICIENCY VIRUS AND ACQUIRED IMMUNODEFICIENCY SYNDROME (BOX 70-1)

A. Medications include nucleoside reverse transcriptase inhibitors, nonnucleoside reverse transcriptase inhibitors, nucleotide reverse transcriptase inhibitors, protease inhibitors, and fusion inhibitors.

B. Other medications include those that are used to treat complications or opportunistic infections that develop.

C. Nucleoside reverse transcriptase inhibitors, nonnucleoside reverse transcriptase inhibitors, and nucleotide reverse transcriptase inhibitors work by inhibiting the activity of reverse transcriptase.

D. Protease inhibitors work by interfering with the activity of the enzyme protease.

BOX 70-1

Medications for Human Immunodeficiency Virus and Acquired Immunodeficiency Syndrome

NUCLEOSIDE REVERSE TRANSCRIPTASE INHIBITORS
Abacavir (Ziagen)
Didanosine (Videx)
Lamivudine (Epivir)
Lamivudine and zidovudine combination (Combivir)
Lamivudine, zidovudine, and abacavir combination (Trizivir)
Stavudine (d4t, Zerit)
Zalcitabine (ddC, HIVID)
Zidovudine (Ritrovir, AZT)

NONNUCLEOSIDE REVERSE TRANSCRIPTASE INHIBITORS
Delaviridine (Rescriptor)
Efavirenz (Sustiva)
Nevirapine (Viramune)

NUCLEOTIDE REVERSE TRANSCRIPTASE INHIBITOR
Tenofovir DF (Viread)

PROTEASE INHIBITORS
Amprenavir (Agenerase)
Indinavir (Crixivan)
Lopinavir and ritonavir combination (Kaletra)
Nelfinavir (Viracept)
Ritonavir (Norvir)
Saquinavir (Fortovase)

FUSION INHIBITOR
Enfuvirtide (Fuzeon)

ANTIINFLAMMATORY MEDICATION
Sulfasalazine (Azulfidine)

ANTIINFECTIVE MEDICATIONS
Metronidazole (Flagyl)
Pentamidine isethionate (Pentam 300)

ANTIFUNGAL MEDICATIONS
Amphotericin B (Fungizone)
Fluconazole (Diflucan)
Ketoconazole (Nizoral)

ANTIVIRAL MEDICATIONS
Acyclovir (Zovirax)
Foscarnet (Foscavir)
Ganciclovir (Cytovene)

ANTIFUNGAL, ANTIINFECTIVE, ANTIPROTOZOAL
Dapsone (Avlosulfon)

ANTIMALARIAL, ANTIPROTOZOAL
Pyrimethamine (Daraprim)

E. Fusion inhibitors work by inhibiting the binding of human immunodeficiency virus to cells.

F. Nucleoside reverse transcriptase inhibitors
   1. Abacavir (Ziagen) can cause nausea; monitor for hypersensitivity reaction, including fever, nausea, vomiting, diarrhea, lethargy, malaise, sore throat, shortness of breath, cough, and rash.
   2. Didanosine (Videx) can cause nausea, diarrhea, peripheral neuropathy, hepatotoxicity, and pancreatitis.
   3. Lamivudine (Epivir) causes nausea and nasal congestion.
   4. Stavudine (d4t, Zerit) can cause peripheral neuropathy and pancreatitis.
   5. Zidovudine (Ritrovir, AZT) can cause nausea, vomiting, anemia, leukopenia, myopathy, fatigue, and headache.
   6. Zalcitabine (ddC, HIVID) can cause oral ulcers, peripheral neuropathy, hepatotoxicity, and pancreatitis.

G. Nonnucleoside reverse transcriptase inhibitors
   1. Nevirapine (Viramune) can cause rash, Stevens-Johnson syndrome, hepatitis, and increased transaminase levels.
   2. Delaviridine (Rescriptor) can cause rash, liver function changes, and pruritis.
   3. Efavirenz (Sustiva) can cause rash, dizziness, confusion, difficulty concentrating, dreams, and encephalopathy.

H. Nucleotide reverse transcriptase inhibitor: Tenofovir DF (Viread) can cause nausea and vomiting.

I. Protease inhibitors
   1. Amprenavir (Agenerase)
      a. Amprenavir can cause nausea, vomiting, headache, altered taste sensations, perioral paresthesia, rashes, and increased liver function studies.
      b. Oral solution contains an alcohol that can interact with metronidazole (Flagyl) and can cause feelings of inebriation.
   2. Indinavir (Crixivan) can cause nausea, diarrhea, hyperbilirubinemia, nephritis, and kidney stones.
   3. Lopinavir and ritonavir combination (Kaletra) can cause nausea, diarrhea, altered taste sensations, circumoral paresthesia, and hepatitis.
   4. Nelfinavir (Viracept) can cause nausea, flatulence, and diarrhea.
   5. Ritonavir (Norvir) can cause nausea, vomiting, diarrhea, altered taste sensations, circumoral paresthesia, hepatitis, and increased triglyceride levels.
   6. Saquinavir (Fortovase) can cause nausea, diarrhea, photosensitivity, and headache.

J. Fusion inhibitor: Enfuvirtide (Fuzeon) can cause skin irritation at injection site, fatigue, nausea, insomnia, and peripheral neuropathy.

K. Antiinflammatory medications
   1. Sulfasalazine (Azulfidine)

a. Sulfasalazine is used to treat toxoplasmosis or nocardiasis.
b. Sulfasalazine is administered orally.
c. Sulfasalazine can cause renal toxicity.
d. Sulfasalazine suppresses bone marrow function.
e. Sulfasalazine increases photosensitivity.
f. Monitor urine output and complete blood count.
g. Monitor the client for sore throat, pallor, purpura, jaundice, and weakness.
h. Encourage fluid intake.
i. Advise the client to avoid exposure to the sun.

L. Antiinfective medications
   1. Pentamidine isethionate (Pentam 300)
      a. Pentamidine is used to treat *Pneumocystis carinii* pneumonia.
      b. Pentamidine is administered intramuscularly or intravenously.
      c. Pentamidine can cause nephrotoxicity.
      d. Monitor blood pressure and heart rate (may cause hypotension).
      e. Monitor for hypoglycemia.
      f. Pentamidine is hepatotoxic and immunosuppressive.
      g. Monitor liver function tests and complete blood count.
   2. Metronidazole (Flagyl)
      a. Metronidazole is used to treat cryptosporidiosis and giardiasis.
      b. Metronidazole is administered orally or intravenously.
      c. Administer metronidazole with food or milk.
      d. Monitor for dry mouth, dizziness, or fungal infection.
      e. Instruct the client to avoid alcohol during treatment.

M. Antifungal medications
   1. Ketoconazole (Nizoral)
      a. Ketoconazole is used to treat candidiasis, coccidioidomycosis, or histoplasmosis.
      b. Ketoconazole is administered orally.
      c. Administer ketoconazole with food or milk.
      d. Instruct the client to avoid antacids for 2 hours after taking the medication because gastric acid is needed to activate the medication.
      e. Ketoconazole is hepatotoxic.
      f. Monitor hepatic function and liver function studies.
      g. Instruct the client to avoid exposure to the sun because the medication increases photosensitivity.
      h. Instruct the client to avoid alcohol during treatment.
   2. Fluconazole (Diflucan)
      a. Fluconazole is used to treat candidiasis.
      b. Fluconazole is administered orally.
      c. Fluconazole is hepatotoxic.

d. Monitor for abdominal pain, fever, and diarrhea.

e. Monitor hepatic function and liver function studies.

3. Amphotericin B (Fungizone)

a. Amphotericin B is used to treat candidiasis and other fungal infections.

b. Amphotericin B is administered intravenously.

c. Amphotericin B is nephrotoxic.

d. Amphotericin B can cause thrombophlebitis.

e. Amphotericin B suppresses bone marrow function.

f. Monitor renal function.

g. Monitor infusion site.

h. Monitor complete blood count.

N. Antiviral medications

1. Ganciclovir (Cytovene)

a. Ganciclovir is used to treat cytomegalovirus retinitis.

b. Ganciclovir is administered orally or intravenously.

c. Ganciclovir suppresses bone marrow function.

d. Monitor neutrophil and platelet count.

e. Administer ganciclovir with food.

2. Acyclovir (Zovirax)

a. Acyclovir is used to treat herpes simplex, herpes zoster, or varicella zoster.

b. Acyclovir may be administered orally or intravenously.

c. Acyclovir is nephrotoxic.

d. Monitor renal function.

e. Encourage fluid intake.

f. Acyclovir is irritating to the blood vessel when administered intravenously.

3. Foscarnet (Foscavir)

a. Foscarnet is used to treat cytomegalovirus retinitis in clients infected with human immunodeficiency virus.

b. Foscarnet is administered intravenously.

c. Foscarnet is nephrotoxic.

d. Monitor renal function.

II. SYSTEMIC LUPUS ERYTHEMATOSUS (BOX 70-2)

A. Description: Medications are used to control symptoms and to prevent or control serious complications that occur as a result of organ damage by the inflammatory process.

B. Azathioprine (Imuran)

1. Azathioprine has a glucocorticoid-sparing effect.

BOX 70-2

Systemic Lupus Erythematosus

Azathioprine (Imuran)
Corticosteroids, such as prednisone (Deltasone)
Cyclophosphamide (Cytoxan)
Hydroxychloroquine sulfate (Plaquenil)
Nonsteroidal antiinflammatory drugs

---

2. Azathioprine potentiates the immunosuppressive action of glucocorticoids and thereby allows a lower dosage of glucocorticoid to have a greater immunosuppressive action.

3. Monitor complete blood count and liver function tests.

C. Cyclophosphamide (Cytoxan)

1. Cyclophosphamide provides immunosuppressive treatment of diffuse proliferative nephritis and other organ inflammation unresponsive to glucocorticoids.

2. Cyclophosphamide is reserved for use in severe cases because of the adverse side effects.

D. Hydroxychloroquine sulfate (Plaquenil)

1. Hydroxychloroquine is an antimalarial drug used to prevent the recurrence of an exacerbation.

2. An eye examination should be performed initially and 6 months after treatment.

3. Administer hydroxychloroquine with meals or a glass of milk.

E. Prednisone (Deltasone)

1. Prednisone is used at high doses to treat exacerbations and at low doses to control symptoms when other medications do not work.

2. Refer to Chapter 54 for information on glucocorticoids.

F. Nonsteroidal antiinflammatory drugs

1. Nonsteroidal antiinflammatory drugs are used to control fever and arthralgia.

2. Refer to Chapter 66 for information on nonsteroidal antiinflammatory drugs.

III. IMMUNIZATIONS (REFER TO CHAPTER 47.)

PRACTICE QUESTIONS

1. Dapsone (Avlosulfon) is prescribed for a client with acquired immunodeficiency syndrome to treat toxoplasmosis. The nurse reinforces medication instructions and tells the client to

1. Discontinue the medication if nausea and vomiting develops.

2. Plan to take the medication every 6 hours around the clock.

3. Contact the physician if fever or a sore throat occurs.

4. Report to the clinic weekly for the injections.

2. Pyrimethamine (Daraprim) has been added to the medication regimen for the client with acquired immunodeficiency syndrome. On review of the client's record, the nurse notes this new prescription and plans care knowing that this has been prescribed to treat

1. Toxoplasmosis.

2. Cardiac irregularities.

3. Kaposi's sarcoma.

4. Nausea and vomiting.

3. Saquinavir (Fortovase) is prescribed for the client who is human immunodeficiency virus seropositive.

The nurse reinforces medication instructions and tells the client to

1. Take the medication on an empty stomach.
2. Eat low-calorie foods.
3. Eat foods that are low in fat.
4. Avoid sun exposure.

4. The clinic nurse is providing medication instructions to a client who will be receiving hydroxychloroquine sulfate (Plaquenil) to treat systemic lupus erythematosus. The nurse instructs the client about the importance of returning to the clinic in 6 months for which of the following?

1. Dental examination
2. Eye examination
3. Chest radiograph
4. Sigmoidoscopy

5. The client who is human immunodeficiency virus seropositive has been taking Stavudine (d4t, Zerit). The nurse monitors which of the following most closely while the client is taking this medication?

1. Appetite
2. Gait
3. Gastrointestinal function
4. Level of consciousness

6. The client who is human immunodeficiency virus seropositive has been taking zalcitabine (ddC, HIVID) as a component of treatment. The nurse plans to monitor which of the following most closely while the client is taking this medication?

1. Liver function studies
2. Platelet count
3. Red blood cell count
4. Glucose level

7. The nurse is assigned to care for a client with cytomegalovirus retinitis and acquired immunodeficiency syndrome who is receiving foscarnet (Foscavir). The nurse checks the latest results of which of the following laboratory studies while the client is taking this medication?

1. Serum albumin
2. Serum creatinine
3. CD4 cell count
4. Lymphocyte count

8. The client with acquired immunodeficiency syndrome and *Pneumocystis carinii* infection has been receiving pentamidine (Pentam 300). The client develops a temperature of 101° F. The nurse does further monitoring of the client, knowing that this sign would most likely indicate

1. The dose of the medication is too low.
2. The client is experiencing toxic effects of the medication.
3. The client has developed inadequacy of thermoregulation.
4. The result of another infection caused by leukopenic effects of the medication.

9. The client with acquired immunodeficiency syndrome has begun therapy with zidovudine (Retrovir, AZT). The nurse carefully monitors which of the following laboratory results during treatment with this medication?

1. Complete blood count
2. Blood urea nitrogen
3. Blood culture
4. Blood glucose level

10. The nurse is reviewing the results of serum laboratory studies drawn on a client with acquired immunodeficiency syndrome who is receiving didanosine (Videx). The nurse interprets that the client may have the medication discontinued by the physician if which of the following significantly elevated results is noted?

1. Serum creatinine
2. Serum amylase
3. Blood glucose
4. Serum protein

CRITICAL THINKING: FILL IN THE BLANK

The client who is human immunodeficiency virus seropositive has been taking ritonavir (Norvir). The client returns to the clinic for follow-up laboratory blood tests. The nurse reviews the client's record and expects to note a physician's order for which specific laboratory blood test?

Answer: _____

ANSWERS

1. **3**

Rationale: Dapsone may be prescribed to treat toxoplasmosis. The medication is taken orally daily. The medication suppresses bone marrow activity, and the complete blood cell count is monitored closely. If the client develops fever, sore throat, purpura, or jaundice, the physician is notified. Medications are available to treat nausea and vomiting, and the client should not discontinue the medication if these symptoms occur but should contact the physician.

Test-Taking Strategy: Use the process of elimination. Eliminate option 1 first because the nurse would not tell the client to discontinue the medication. Next, eliminate options 2 and 4, knowing that the medication is administered orally daily. Review this medication if you had difficulty with this question.

Level of Cognitive Ability: Application
Client Needs: Physiological Integrity
Integrated Process: Teaching/Learning
Content Area: Adult health—immune

Reference: Lehne, R. (2001). *Pharmacology for nursing care* (4th ed., p. 990). Philadelphia: W. B. Saunders.

2. 1

Rationale: Pyrimethamine (Daraprim) is an antimalarial and an antiprotozoal medication used to treat toxoplasmosis or *Pneumocyctis carinii* pneumonia. Pyrimethamine is not used to treat nausea, vomiting, cardiac irregularities, or Kaposi's sarcoma.

Test-Taking Strategy: Use the process of elimination. If you knew that this medication was an antimalarial and an antiprotozoal medication, then you easily would be directed to option 1. Review this medication if you had difficulty with this medication.

Level of Cognitive Ability: Analysis
Client Needs: Physiological Integrity
Integrated Process: Nursing Process—planning
Content Area: Adult health—immune
Reference: Lehne, R. (2001). *Pharmacology for nursing care* (4th ed., p. 1095). Philadelphia: W. B. Saunders.

3. 4

Rationale: Saquinavir is an antiretroviral (protease inhibitor) used with other antiretroviral medications to manage human immunodeficiency virus infection. Saquinavir is administered with meals and is best absorbed if the client consumes high-calorie, high-fat meals. Saquinavir can cause photosensitivity, and the nurse should instruct the client to avoid sun exposure.

Test-Taking Strategy: Use the process of elimination. Options 2 and 3 can be eliminated first, knowing that these dietary measures likely would not be prescribed for this client. From the remaining options, you must know that this medication can cause photosensitivity. Review this medication if you had difficulty with this question.

Level of Cognitive Ability: Application
Client Needs: Physiological Integrity
Integrated Process: Teaching/Learning
Content Area: Adult health—immune
Reference: Hodgson, B., & Kizior, R. (2004). *Saunders nursing drug handbook 2004* (p. 905). Philadelphia: W. B. Saunders.

4. 2

Rationale: Ocular toxicity is an adverse reaction to the use of hydroxychloroquine sulfate. An eye examination should be performed when medication therapy is started and after 6 months of therapy. Options 1, 3, and 4 are unrelated to the use of this medication.

Test-Taking Strategy: To answer this question, you must recall that this medication causes retinopathy. If you are unfamiliar with this medication, review its toxic effects.

Level of Cognitive Ability: Application
Client Needs: Physiological Integrity
Integrated Process: Teaching/Learning
Content Area: Adult health—immune
Reference: Lehne, R. (2001). *Pharmacology for nursing care* (4th ed., p. 796). Philadelphia: W. B. Saunders.

5. 2

Rationale: Stavudine is an antiretroviral used to manage human immunodeficiency virus infection in clients who do not respond to or who cannot tolerate conventional therapy. The medication can cause peripheral neuropathy, and the nurse should monitor the client's gait closely and ask the client about paresthesia.

Test-Taking Strategy: Knowledge that this medication causes peripheral neuropathy is needed to answer this question. If you are not familiar with this medication and the important assessment measures, review this content.

Level of Cognitive Ability: Application
Client Needs: Physiological Integrity
Integrated Process: Nursing Process—assessment
Content Area: Adult health—immune
Reference: Lehne, R. (2001). *Pharmacology for nursing care* (4th ed., p. 1035). Philadelphia: W. B. Saunders.

6. 1

Rationale: Zalcitabine is an antiretroviral (nucleoside reverse transcriptase inhibitor) used to manage human immunodeficiency virus infection with other antiretrovirals. Zalcitabine also has been used as a single agent in clients who are intolerant of other regimens. Zalcitabine can cause serious liver damage, and liver function studies should be monitored closely. Options 2, 3, and 4 are not associated specifically with the use of this medication.

Test-Taking Strategy: Recalling that this medication is hepatotoxic will direct you to option 1. If you are unfamiliar with this medication, review this content.

Level of Cognitive Ability: Application
Client Needs: Physiological Integrity
Integrated Process: Nursing Process—assessment
Content Area: Adult health—immune
Reference: Hodgson, B., & Kizior, R. (2004). *Saunders nursing drug handbook 2004* (p. 1067). Philadelphia: W. B. Saunders.

7. 2

Rationale: Foscarnet (Foscavir) is toxic to the kidneys. Serum creatinine is monitored before therapy, 2 to 3 times per week during induction therapy, and at least weekly during maintenance therapy. Foscarnet also may cause decreased levels of calcium, magnesium, phosphorus, and potassium. Thus these levels also are measured with the same frequency.

Test-Taking Strategy: Use the process of elimination. Recalling that this medication is nephrotoxic will direct you easily to option 2. Review this medication if you are unfamiliar with it.

Level of Cognitive Ability: Application
Client Needs: Physiological Integrity
Integrated Process: Nursing Process—assessment
Content Area: Adult health—immune
Reference: Hodgson, B., & Kizior, R. (2004). *Saunders nursing drug handbook 2004* (pp. 444-445). Philadelphia: W. B. Saunders.

8. 4

Rationale: Frequent side effects of this medication include leukopenia, thrombocytopenia, and anemia. The client should be monitored routinely for signs and symptoms of infection. Options 1, 2, and 3 are inaccurate interpretations.

Test-Taking Strategy: Use the process of elimination focusing on the key words "develops a temperature." Note the relationship between these key words and option 4. Review the side effects of this medication if you had difficulty with this question.

Level of Cognitive Ability: Application
Client Needs: Physiological Integrity
Integrated Process: Nursing Process—analysis
Content Area: Adult health—immune
Reference: Gutierrez, K., & Queener, S. (2003). *Pharmacology for nursing practice* (p. 519). St. Louis: Mosby.

9. **1**
Rationale: A common side effect of this medication therapy is agranulocytopenia and anemia. The nurse monitors the complete blood count results for these changes. Options 2, 3, and 4 are unrelated to the use of this medication.
Test-Taking Strategy: Recalling that zidovudine (AZT) causes leukopenia will direct you to option 1. Review this medication if you had difficulty with this question.
Level of Cognitive Ability: Application
Client Needs: Physiological Integrity
Integrated Process: Nursing Process—assessment
Content Area: Adult health—immune
Reference: Hodgson, B., & Kizior, R. (2004). *Saunders nursing drug handbook 2004* (p. 1073). Philadelphia: W. B. Saunders.

10. **2**
Rationale: A serum amylase level that is increased 1.5 to 2 times normal may signify pancreatitis in the client with acquired immunodeficiency syndrome and is potentially fatal. The medication may have to be discontinued. The medication is also hepatotoxic and can result in liver failure.

Test-Taking Strategy: Recalling that this medication can cause damage to the pancreas and is hepatotoxic will direct you to the correct option. Review this medication if you had difficulty with this question.
Level of Cognitive Ability: Analysis
Client Needs: Physiological Integrity
Integrated Process: Nursing Process—assessment
Content Area: Adult health—immune
Reference: Hodgson, B., & Kizior, R. (2004). *Saunders nursing drug handbook 2004* (p. 307). Philadelphia: W. B. Saunders.

CRITICAL THINKING: FILL IN THE BLANK
Answer: Triglyceride level
Rationale: Ritonavir (Norvir) is an antiretroviral (protease inhibitor) used with other antiretroviral medications to manage human immunodeficiency virus infection. Ritonavir can increase the triglyceride level and therefore this level should be monitored. Liver function studies also are monitored.
Test-Taking Strategy: You must be familiar with the adverse effects related to this medication to answer this question. Remember that ritonavir increases the triglyceride level. If you are unfamiliar with this medication, review this information.
Level of Cognitive Ability: Analysis
Client Needs: Physiological Integrity
Integrated Process: Nursing Process—analysis
Content Area: Adult health—immune
Reference: Hodgson, B., & Kizior, R. (2004). *Saunders nursing drug handbook 2004* (p. 892). Philadelphia: W. B. Saunders.

REFERENCES

Gutierrez, K., & Queener, S. (2003). *Pharmacology for nursing practice.* St. Louis: Mosby.

Hodgson, B., & Kizior, R. (2004). *Saunders nursing drug handbook 2004.* Philadelphia: W. B. Saunders.

Lehne, R. (2001). *Pharmacology for nursing care* (4th ed.). Philadelphia: W. B. Saunders.

Lewis, S., Heitkemper, M., & Dirksen, S. (2004). *Medical-surgical nursing: Assessment and management of clinical problems* (6th ed.). St. Louis: Mosby.

McKenry, L., & Salerno, E. (2003). *Mosby's pharmacology in nursing* (21st ed.). St. Louis: Mosby.

The Adult Client with a Mental Health Disorder

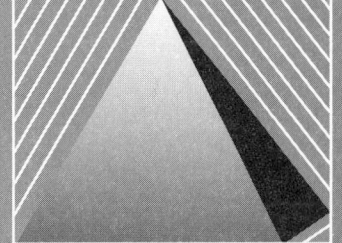

PYRAMID TERMS

abuse   An act of misuse, deceit, or exploitation; the wrong or improper use or action toward another individual that results in injury, damage, maltreatment, or corruption.

addiction   A state of dependence or compulsive use. In relation to drug dependence, addiction incorporates the concepts of loss of control with respect to the use of a drug, taking the drug despite related problems and complications, and a tendency to relapse.

coping mechanisms   Methods of adjusting to environmental stress without altering one's own goals or purposes. Methods can include conscious and unconscious mechanisms.

crisis   A temporary state of disequilibrium in which an individual's usual coping mechanisms or problem-solving methods fail. Crisis can result in personality growth or personality disorganization.

defense mechanisms   A coping mechanism (protective defense) of the ego that attempts to protect the individual from feelings of inadequacy and worthlessness and to prevent awareness of anxiety. When anxiety is too painful, the individual copes by using defense mechanisms to protect the ego and decrease anxiety.

milieu   The physical and social environment in which an individual lives. Milieu therapy focuses on positive physical and social environmental manipulation to produce positive change.

restraints   Physical restraints include any manual method or mechanical device, material, or equipment that inhibits free movement. Chemical restraints include the administration of medications for the specific purpose of inhibiting a specific behavior or movement.

seclusion   Placing a client alone in a specially designed room for protection and close supervision. Seclusion is the last measure in a process to maximize safety to the client and others.

suicide   The ultimate act of self-destruction in which an individual purposefully ends his or her own life.

suicide attempt   Any willfull, self-inflicted, or life-threatening attempt by an individual that has not lead to death.

PYRAMID TO SUCCESS

The Pyramid to Success focuses on the therapeutic nurse-client relationship, client rights, hospital admission procedures, the ethical and legal issues related to the care of the client with a mental health disorder, grief and loss, and end-of-life issues. Pyramid Points focus on the use of restraints, seclusion, and electroconvulsive therapy. Focus on care to the client with an addiction, such as an eating disorder or drug or alcohol disorder. Additional focus areas include anxiety, depression, suicide, abuse and violence, rape crisis interventions, posttraumatic stress disorders, obsessive-compulsive disorders, schizophrenia, and bipolar disorders. Pyramid Points address the use of medications prescribed for the client with a mental health disorder, particularly lithium and the benzodiazepines. The Integrated Processes addressed in this unit include Nursing Process, Caring, Communication and Documentation, and Teaching/Learning.

CLIENT NEEDS
Safe, Effective Care Environment

Client advocacy
Client rights
Confidentiality
Establishing priorities
Informed consent related to treatments, such as restraints, seclusion, and electroconvulsive therapy
Legal responsibilities related to reporting incidences of violence and abuse
Psychiatric consultations and referrals
Provision of safety to client and others
Use of restraints and seclusion

Health Promotion and Maintenance

Health promotion programs related to addictions
Individual lifestyle choices
Psychosocial assessment techniques

Psychosocial Integrity

Abuse/neglect
Behavioral interventions
Chemical dependency

Coping mechanisms
Counseling techniques
Crisis intervention
Domestic violence
End-of-life issues
Grief and loss
Religious, cultural, and spiritual influences on health
Sexual abuse/rape
Stress management
Support systems
Therapeutic nurse-client relationship
Therapeutic milieu

Physiological Integrity

Abusive and self-destructive behavior
Alterations in body systems related to addictions
Elimination
Expected and untoward effects of medications
Laboratory values related to medication therapy
Medication administration
Nutrition
Pathophysiology related to mental health disorders

Personal hygiene measures
Potential complications related to medications and electroconvulsive therapy
Rest and sleep

REFERENCES

Carson, V. (2000). *Mental health nursing: The nurse-patient journey* (2nd ed.). Philadelphia: W. B. Saunders.

Chernecky, C., & Berger, B. (2004). *Laboratory tests & diagnostic procedures* (4th ed.). Philadelphia: W. B. Saunders.

Harkreader, H., & Hogan, M. A. (2004). *Fundamentals of nursing: Caring and clinical judgment* (2nd ed.). Philadelphia: W. B. Saunders.

Keltner, N., Schwecke, L., & Bostrom, C. (2003). *Psychiatric nursing* (4th ed.). St. Louis: Mosby.

Lewis, S., Heitkemper, M., & Dirksen, S. (2004). *Medical-surgical nursing: Assessment and management of clinical problems* (6th ed.). St. Louis: Mosby.

National Council of State Boards of Nursing (Eds.). (2003). *Test Plan for the National Council Licensure Examination for Registered Nurses* (effective date: April 2004). Chicago: Author.

Potter, P., & Perry, A. (2001). *Fundamentals of nursing* (5th ed.). St. Louis: Mosby.

Stuart, G., & Laraia, M. (2001). *Principles and practice of psychiatric nursing* (7th ed.). St. Louis: Mosby.

Varcarolis, E. M. (2002). *Foundations of psychiatric mental health nursing* (4th ed.). Philadelphia: W. B. Saunders.

Foundations of Psychiatric Mental Health Nursing

I. MENTAL HEALTH

A. Mental health is a lifelong process of successful adaptation to a changing internal and external environment.

B. The individual is in contact with reality and the environment and possesses the ability to love, work, and resolve conflicts within a framework of reasonability.

C. The individual has psychobiological resilience.

II. PSYCHIATRIC/MENTAL HEALTH ILLNESS

A. Description
1. Psychiatric illness is loss of the ability to respond to the environment in ways that are in accord with oneself or the expectations of society.
2. Psychiatric illness is characterized by thought or behavior patterns that impair functioning and cause the individual distress.

B. Personality characteristics
1. Person is unaccepting of self and dislikes self.
2. Person has an unrealistic perception of strengths and weaknesses.
3. Thoughts and perceptions may not be reality based.
4. Person is unable to find meaning and purpose in life.
5. Person lacks direction and productivity in life.
6. Person has difficulty in meeting own needs.
7. Person depends on others for thought and actions.

C. Adaptations to stress
1. Person feels out of control with self and with the environment.
2. Person has a negative perception of the environment.
3. Person has ineffective **coping mechanisms.**

D. Interpersonal relationships
1. Person is unable to love and care for others.
2. Person is unable to feel loved by others or accept feelings from others.

III. COPING AND DEFENSE MECHANISMS

A. **Coping mechanisms**
1. Coping involves any effort to decrease the stress response.
2. **Coping mechanisms** can be constructive or destructive, task oriented in relation to direct problem solving, or defense oriented, regulating the response to protect oneself.
3. Destructive **coping mechanisms** often cause a mental health disorder because the person avoids the problem that causes the disorder.
4. Neurotic or psychotic behaviors typically can result when **coping mechanisms** become destructive.

B. **Defense mechanisms** (Box 71-1)
1. A defense mechanism is a coping mechanism (protective defense) of the ego that attempts to protect the individual from feelings of inadequacy and worthlessness and to prevent awareness of anxiety.
2. When anxiety is too painful, the individual copes by using **defense mechanisms** to protect the ego and decrease anxiety.

C. Interventions
1. Assess the client's use of the defense mechanism.
2. Determine whether the use of the defense mechanism characterizes unhealthy adjustment.
3. Facilitate appropriate use of **defense mechanisms.**
4. Avoid criticizing the behavior and the use of **defense mechanisms.**
5. Assist the client to identify the source of the anxiety.
6. Assist the client to explore methods to reduce the anxiety.

BOX 71-1

Types of Defense Mechanisms

COMPENSATION
Putting forth extra effort to achieve in areas where one has a real or imagined deficiency

CONVERSION
The expression of emotional conflicts through physical symptoms

DENIAL
Disowning consciously intolerable thoughts and impulses

DISPLACEMENT
Feelings toward one person are directed to another who is less threatening, thereby satisfying an impulse with a substitute object

DISSOCIATION
The blocking off of an anxiety-provoking event or period of time from the conscious mind

FANTASY
Gratification by imaginary achievements and wishful thinking

FIXATION
Never advancing to the next level of emotional development and organization; the persistence in later life of interests and behavior patterns appropriate to an earlier age

IDENTIFICATION
The unconscious attempt to change oneself to resemble an admired person

INSULATION
Withdrawing into passivity and becoming inaccessible so as to avoid further threatening situations

INTELLECTUALIZATION
Excessive reasoning to avoid feeling; the thinking is disconnected from feelings, and situations are dealt with at a cognitive level

INTROJECTION
A type of identification in which the individual incorporates the traits or values of another into self

ISOLATION
Response in which a person blocks feelings associated with an unpleasant experience

PROJECTION
Transferring one's internal feelings, thoughts, and unacceptable ideas and traits to someone else

RATIONALIZATION
An attempt to make unacceptable feelings and behavior acceptable by justifying the behavior

REACTION FORMATION
Developing conscious attitudes and behaviors and acting out behaviors opposite to what one really feels

REGRESSION
Returning to an earlier developmental stage to express an impulse to deal with reality

REPRESSION
An unconscious process in which the client blocks undesirable and unacceptable thoughts from conscious expression.

SUBLIMATION
Replacement of an unacceptable need, attitude, or emotion with one more socially acceptable

SUBSTITUTION
The replacement of a valued unacceptable object with an object that is more acceptable to the ego

SUPPRESSION
The conscious, deliberate forgetting of unacceptable or painful thoughts, ideas, and feelings

SYMBOLIZATION
The conscious use of an idea or object to represent another actual event or object; many times the meaning is not clear because the symbol may be representative of something unconscious

UNDOING
Engaging in behavior that is considered to be opposite of a previous unacceptable behavior, thought, or feeling.

▲ **IV. THE NURSE-CLIENT RELATIONSHIP**
  A. Principles
    1. Maintain genuineness, respect, an empathic understanding, and concreteness with the client.
    2. Care for the client in a holistic manner.
    3. Assess religious and spiritual practices of the client because these practices may give the client hope, comfort, and support with healing.
    4. Assess cultural beliefs and values including emotion-producing situations, how emotions are expressed, and what the appropriate social response to expressed emotions may be.
    5. Maintain appropriate limits.
    6. Maintain honest and open communication.
    7. Encourage expression of the client's feelings.
    8. Assist the client to develop resources.
  B. Phases of a therapeutic nurse-client relationship
    1. Preinteraction phase
      a. The preinteraction phase begins before the nurse's first contact with the client.

b. The nurse's task is self-exploration about his or her values and feelings for caring for the client.

2. Orientation or introductory phase
   a. Establish boundaries, acceptance, and trust with the client.
   b. Identify the expectations of the relationship (establishing a contract).
   c. Determine why the client sought help and whether it was voluntary.
   d. Assess the anxiety in the client.
   e. Define goals with the client.
   f. Prepare the client for termination and separation of the relationship.

3. Working phase
   a. Promote an attitude of acceptance.
   b. Assist the client to express feelings.
   c. Identify problems (theme identification).
   d. Promote insight and the use of constructive **coping mechanisms.**
   e. Increase the client's independence.

4. Termination or separation phase
   a. Prepare the client for termination and separation on initial contact.
   b. Evaluate progress and achievement of goals.
   c. Identify and deal with termination and separation issues.
   d. Encourage the client to discuss feelings about termination.
   e. Do not promise the client that the relationship will be continued.
   f. Refer and transfer the client to other support systems.

V. THERAPEUTIC COMMUNICATION PROCESS

A. Principles
   1. Communication includes verbal and nonverbal expression.
   2. Successful communication includes appropriateness, efficiency, flexibility, and feedback.
   3. Anxiety in the nurse or client impedes communication.
   4. Communication needs to be goal directed within a professional framework.

B. Therapeutic and nontherapeutic communication techniques (Box 71-2)

VI. *DIAGNOSTIC AND STATISTICAL MANUAL OF MENTAL HEALTH DISORDERS*

A. The *Diagnostic and Statistical Manual of Mental Health Disorders* classifies medical diagnoses according to the American Psychiatric Association.

B. The manual is a system used in clinical, research, and educational settings, in which diagnostic criteria are inclusive for each diagnosis but allow for individualized differences within a pattern of behavior.

BOX 71-2

Therapeutic and Nontherapeutic Communication Techniques

THERAPEUTIC TECHNIQUES
Clarifying and validating
Encouraging formulation of a plan of action
Focusing and refocusing
Giving information and presenting reality
Listening
Maintaining neutral responses
Maintaining silence
Providing acknowledgment and feedback
Providing nonverbal encouragement
Reflecting
Restating
Sharing perceptions
Summarizing
Using broad openings and open-ended questions

NONTHERAPEUTIC TECHNIQUES
Asking the client "Why?"
Being defensive or challenging the client
Changing the subject
Giving advice or approval or disapproval
Making stereotypical comments
Making value judgments
Placing the client's feelings on hold
Providing false reassurance

C. The manual includes a list of culture-bound syndromes that may or may not be associated with a particular diagnostic category.

D. Knowledge of the criteria for a particular psychiatric diagnosis will assist the nurse in making a clinical decision about a nursing diagnosis.

VII. TYPES OF MENTAL HEALTH ADMISSIONS AND DISCHARGES

A. Voluntary admission
   1. Any citizen of lawful age may apply in writing (usually on a standard admission form) for admission to the hospital.
   2. The client, or the client's guardian if the client is too ill, voluntarily seeks assistance.
   3. Client agrees to accept treatment.
   4. Civil rights are retained fully by the client (Box 71-3)
   5. Client is free to sign out of the hospital.

B. Involuntary admission
   1. Involuntary admission may be necessary when a person is mentally ill, is a danger to self or others, or is in need of psychiatric treatment or physical care.
   2. Involuntary admission is a status in which a person who has the legal capacity to consent to mental health treatment refuses to do so and is detained involuntarily for treatment by the state.

BOX 71-3

Client Rights

Right to accessible health care
Right to coordination and continuity of health care
Right to courteous and individualized health care
Right to information about the qualifications, names, and titles of personnel delivering care
Right to refuse observation by those not directly involved in care
Right to privacy and confidentiality
Right to informed consent
Right to treatment
Right to refuse treatment
Right to treatment in the least restrictive setting
Right not to be subjected to unnecessary restraints
Right to habeas corpus; may request a hearing at any time to be released from the hospital
Right to information about diagnosis, prognosis, and treatment
Right to information on the charges of service
Right to communicate with people outside the hospital through written correspondence, telephone, and personal visits
Right to keep clothing and personal effects
Right to be employed
Right to religious freedom
Right to execute wills
Right to retain licenses, privileges, or permits established by the law, such as a driver's or professional license

3. The client who is admitted involuntarily does not lose his or her right of informed consent.
4. The length of time for hospitalization is specified by the state and varies from state to state.
5. The client is considered legally competent until he or she has been declared incompetent through a legal proceeding.
6. If the nurse believes that a client lacks competency, action should be initiated to have a legal guardian appointed from the court.
7. Categories
   a. Evaluation and emergency care
   b. Certification for observation and treatment
   c. Extended or indeterminate commitment
C. Release from the hospital
   1. Description
      a. Release depends on the client's admission status.
      b. The client who sought voluntary admission has the right to demand and receive release.
      c. Some states provide for conditional release of voluntary clients, which enables the treating physician or administrator to order continued treatment on an outpatient basis if the clinical needs of the client would warrant further care.
   2. Conditional release
      a. Conditional release usually requires outpatient treatment for a specified period of time to determine the client's compliance with medication protocol, ability to meet basic needs, and ability to reintegrate into the community.
      b. A voluntary client who is released conditionally cannot be reinstitutionalized without the client's consent, unless the institution complies with the procedures for involuntary admission.
      c. An involuntary client who is released conditionally may be reinstitutionalized while the commitment is still in effect without recommencement of formal admission procedures.
   3. Discharge
      a. Discharge (unconditional release) is the termination of the client-institution relationship.
      b. This release may be ordered by the psychiatrist, court, or administration.
      c. The administration officer of an institution has the discretion to discharge clients.
      d. In most states, clients can institute a court proceeding to seek a judicial discharge (writ of habeas corpus).
      e. Discharge planning and follow-up care are important for the continued well-being of the client with a mental health disorder.
      f. After-care case managers are needed to facilitate the client's adaptation back into the community and to provide early referral if the treatment plan is not followed.

PRACTICE QUESTIONS

1. Unresolved feelings related to loss most likely may be recognized during which phase of the therapeutic nurse-client relationship?
   1. Orientation
   2. Working
   3. Termination
   4. Trusting

2. A client with a diagnosis of major depression who attempted suicide says to the nurse, "I should have died. I've always been a failure. Nothing ever goes right for me." The most therapeutic response to the client is
   1. "I don't see you as a failure."
   2. "Feeling like this is all part of being ill."
   3. "You've been feeling like a failure for a while?"
   4. "You have everything to live for."

3. The community health nurse visits a client at home. The client states, "I haven't slept at all the last couple of nights." Which response by the nurse illustrates the most therapeutic communication technique for this client?
   1. "Go on ..."
   2. "Sleeping?"
   3. "The last couple of nights?"
   4. "You're having difficulty sleeping?"

4. The nurse is performing an admission assessment on a client and is attempting to obtain subjective data

regarding the client's sexual/reproductive status. The client states, "I don't want to discuss this; it's private and personal." Which statement, if made by the nurse, indicates that the nurse is therapeutic?

1. "I hate being asked these sorts of questions too."

2. "I am a professional nurse, and as such I'll have you know that all information is kept confidential."

3. "I know that some of these questions are difficult for you, but as a professional nurse, I must legally respect your confidentiality."

4. "This is difficult for you to speak about, but I am trying to perform a complete assessment and I need this information."

5. The nurse is caring for a Native American client who says, "I don't want you to touch me. I'll take care of myself!" Which nursing response is most therapeutic?

1. "Okay. If that's what you want. I'll just leave this cup for you to collect your urine in. After breakfast, I will take more blood from you."

2. "If you didn't want our care, why did you come here?"

3. "Why are you being so difficult? I only want to help you."

4. "It sounds as though you want to take care of yourself. Let's work together so you can do things for yourself."

6. A client admitted to the mental health unit is experiencing Disturbed Thought Processes. The client believes that the food is being poisoned. Which communication technique does the nurse plan to use to encourage the client to eat?

1. Using open-ended questions and silence

2. Offering opinions about the necessity of adequate nutrition

3. Identifying the reasons that the client may not want to eat

4. Focusing on self-disclosure regarding food preferences

7. The nurse is working with a client who has sought counseling after trying to rescue a neighbor involved in a house fire. In spite of the client's efforts, the neighbor died. Which action does the nurse engage in with the client during the working phase of the nurse-client relationship?

1. Exploring the client's potential for self-harm

2. Exploring the client's ability to function

3. Inquiring about the client's perception or appraisal of the neighbor's death

4. Inquiring about and examining the client's feelings that may block adaptive coping

8. A client who has just been sexually assaulted is quiet and calm. The nurse analyzes this behavior as indicating which defense mechanism?

1. Denial

2. Projection

3. Rationalization

4. Intellectualization

9. The nurse completes the initial assessment of a client admitted to the mental health unit. The nurse analyzes the data obtained on assessment and determines that which of the following presents a priority concern?

1. The presence of bruises on the client's body

2. The client's report of not eating or sleeping

3. The client's report of suicidal thoughts

4. The significant other's disapproving of the treatment

10. Laboratory work is prescribed on a client who has been experiencing delusions. When the nurse approaches the client to obtain a specimen of the client's blood, the client begins to shout "You're all vampires. Let me out of here!" The most appropriate nursing response is which of the following?

1. "I am not going to hurt you; I am going to help you!"

2. "What makes you think that I am a vampire?"

3. "I'll leave and come back later for your blood."

4. "It must be frightful to think others want to hurt you."

11. An inebriated client is brought to the emergency department by the local police. The client is told that the physician will be in to see the client in about 30 minutes. The client becomes loud and offensive and wants to be seen by the physician immediately. The most appropriate nursing intervention is which of the following?

1. Attempt to talk with the client to deescalate behavior.

2. Watch the behavior escalate before intervening.

3. Inform the client that the client will be asked to leave if the behavior continues.

4. Offer to take the client to an examination room until the client can be treated.

12. A client is admitted to a mental health unit for treatment of psychotic behavior. The client is at the locked exit door and is shouting, "Let me out. There's nothing wrong with me. I don't belong here." The nurse analyzes this behavior as

1. Projection.

2. Denial.

3. Regression.

4. Rationalization.

13. A home health nurse is talking to the spouse of a client taking an antidepressant. The spouse says, "Now that my husband is responding to the antidepressant, the suicidal risk is over and you can stop making these home visits." After analyzing this statement, which of the following is the most appropriate nursing response?

1. "I agree with you. Clients who want to kill themselves are only suicidal for a limited time. No one can feel self-destructive forever."

2. "I need to continue with my visits. Your comment reflects a lack of knowledge that this disease runs in families."

3. "I agree with you. The suicidal threats were really attention seeking. Continuing to visit would reinforce your husband's use of manipulation."

4. "I need to continue with my visits. Most suicides occur within 3 months after improvement begins because the client now has the energy to carry out the suicidal intentions."

14. The supervisor reprimands the nurse in charge of the nursing unit because the charge nurse has not adhered to the unit budget. Later that afternoon, the charge nurse accuses the nursing staff of wasting supplies. This behavior is an example of
   1. Denial.
   2. Repression.
   3. Suppression.
   4. Displacement.

15. The client says to the nurse, "I 'm going to die, and I wish my family would stop hoping for a cure! I get so angry when they carry on like this! After all, I'm the one who's dying." The most therapeutic response by the nurse is
   1. "You're feeling angry that your family continues to hope for you to be cured?"
   2. "I think we should talk more about your anger with your family."
   3. "Well, it sounds like you're being pretty pessimistic. After all, years ago people died of pneumonia."
   4. "Have you shared your feelings with your family?"

16. The nurse employed in a mental health unit is assigned to care for a client admitted to the unit 2 days ago. On review of the client's record, the nurse notes that the admission was a voluntary admission. Based on this type of admission, the nurse anticipates which of the following?
   1. The client will resist treatment measures.
   2. The client's family will resist treatment measures.
   3. The client will be angry and will refuse care.
   4. The client will participate in the planning of the care and treatment plan.

17. A nurse enters a client's room, and the client is demanding release from the hospital. The nurse reviews the client's record and notes that the client was admitted 2 days ago for treatment of an anxiety disorder and that the admission was a voluntary admission. Which of the following actions will the nurse take?
   1. Tell the client that discharge is not possible at this time.
   2. Call the client's family.
   3. Contact the physician.
   4. Persuade the client to stay a few more days.

18. A client is admitted to the mental health unit. On admission assessment the nurse notes that the client is admitted by involuntary status. Based on this type of admission, the nurse would most likely expect that the client
   1. Presents a harm to self.
   2. Requested the admission.
   3. Consented to the admission.
   4. Provided written application to the facility for admission.

19. The nurse is caring for a client who is scheduled for electroconvulsive therapy. The nurse notes that an informed consent has not been obtained for the procedure. On review of the record, the nurse notes that the admission was an involuntary hospitalization. Based on this information, the nurse determines
   1. That an informed consent does not need to be obtained.
   2. That an informed consent should be obtained from the family.
   3. That an informed consent needs to be obtained from the client.
   4. That the physician will obtain the informed consent.

20. Following a group therapy session, a client approaches a nurse and verbalizes a need for seclusion because of uncontrollable feelings. The most appropriate nursing action would be to
   1. Inform the client that seclusion has not been prescribed.
   2. Obtain an informed consent.
   3. Call the client's family.
   4. Place the client in seclusion immediately.

21. The nurse is providing care to a client admitted to the hospital with a diagnosis of acute anxiety disorder. The nurse is conversing with the client. The client says to the nurse, "I have a secret that I want to tell you. You won't tell anyone about it, will you?" The most appropriate nursing response is which of the following?
   1. "No, I won't tell anyone."
   2. "I cannot promise to keep a secret."
   3. "If you tell me the secret, I will tell it to your doctor."
   4. "If you tell me the secret, I will need to document it in your record."

22. The nurse employed in a mental health clinic is greeted by a neighbor in a local grocery store. The neighbor says to the nurse, "How is Carol doing? She is my best friend and is seen at your clinic every week." The most appropriate nursing response is which of the following?
   1. "I'm not suppose to discuss this, but because you are my neighbor, I can tell you that she is doing great!"
   2. "I'm not suppose to discuss this, but because you are my neighbor, I can tell you that she really has some problems!"

3. "If you want to know about Carol, you need to ask her yourself."
4. "I cannot discuss any client situation with you."

23. The client was admitted involuntarily to the mental health unit because of episodes of extremely violent behavior. The client is demanding to be discharged from the hospital. The nurse does not allow the client to leave. Which of the following represent the legal ramifications associated with the nurse's behavior?
    1. The nurse will be charged with imprisonment.
    2. The nurse will be charged with assault.
    3. The nurse will be charged with slander.
    4. No charge will be made against the nurse because the nurse's actions are reasonable.
24. The nurse is preparing the client for the termination phase of the nurse-client relationship. The nurse prepares to implement which nursing task that is most appropriate for this phase?
    1. Identifying expected outcomes
    2. Planning short-term goals
    3. Making appropriate referrals
    4. Developing realistic solutions
25. During the termination phase of the nurse-client relationship, the clinic nurse observes that the client continuously demonstrates bursts of anger. The most appropriate interpretation of the behavior is that the client

1. Requires further treatment and is not ready to be discharged.
2. Is displaying typical behaviors that can occur during termination.
3. Needs to be admitted to the hospital.
4. Needs to be referred to the psychiatrist as soon as possible.

CRITICAL THINKING: MULTIPLE RESPONSE

The nurse in the mental health unit reviews the therapeutic and nontherapeutic communication techniques with a nursing student. Select all therapeutic communication techniques.

____ Making value judgments

____ Listening

____ Giving advice or approval or disapproval

____ Maintaining neutral responses

____ Providing false reassurance

____ Restating

____ Asking the client, "Why?"

____ Providing acknowledgment and feedback

ANSWERS

1. **3**

Rationale: In the termination phase the relationship comes to a close. Ending treatment sometimes may be traumatic for clients who have come to value the relationship and the help. Because loss is an issue, any unresolved feelings related to loss may resurface during this phase. Options 1, 2, and 4 are incorrect.
Test-Taking Strategy: Note the key words "unresolved," "loss," and "recognized" in the question. Considering the phases of the therapeutic nurse-client relationship will direct you to option 3. Review these phases and the nursing implications if you had difficulty with this question.
Level of Cognitive Ability: Analysis
Client Needs: Psychosocial Integrity
Integrated Process: Caring
Content Area: Mental health
Reference: Fortinash, K., & Holoday-Worret, P. (2000). *Psychiatric mental health nursing* (2nd ed., p. 19). St. Louis: Mosby.

2. **3**

Rationale: Responding to the feelings expressed by a client is an effective therapeutic communication technique. The correct option is an example of the use of restating. Options 1, 2, and 4 block communication because they minimize the client's experience and do not facilitate exploration of the client's expressed feelings.
Test-Taking Strategy: Use the process of elimination and therapeutic communication techniques to direct you to

the option that directly addresses the client feelings and concerns. Also, option 3 is the only option that is stated in the form of a question and is open ended and thus will encourage the verbalization of feelings. Review therapeutic communication techniques if you had difficulty with this question.
Level of Cognitive Ability: Application
Client Needs: Psychosocial Integrity
Integrated Process: Communication and Documentation
Content Area: Mental health
References: Fortinash, K., & Holoday-Worret, P. (2000). *Psychiatric mental health nursing* (2nd ed., p. 159). St. Louis: Mosby.
Stuart, G., & Laraia, M. (2001). *Principles & practice of psychiatric nursing* (7th ed., p. 31). St. Louis: Mosby.

3. **4**

Rationale: Option 4 uses the therapeutic communication technique of restatement. Although restatement is a technique that has a prompting component to it, it repeats the client's major theme, which assists the nurse to obtain a more specific perception of the problem from the client. Options 1, 2, and 3 are not therapeutic responses.
Test-Taking Strategy: Use the process of elimination. Option 1 is a general lead and allows the client to direct the discussion. Option 2 uses reflection that simply repeats the client's last words to prompt further discussion. Option 3 focuses on the number of nights rather than the specific problem of sleep. Option 4 will provide the perception of the problem from the

client's perspective. Review therapeutic communication techniques if you had difficulty with this question.
Level of Cognitive Ability: Application
Client Needs: Psychosocial Integrity
Integrated Process: Communication and Documentation
Content Area: Mental health
References: Fortinash, K., & Holoday-Worret, P. (2000). *Psychiatric mental health nursing* (2nd ed., p. 159). St. Louis: Mosby.
Stuart, G., & Laraia, M. (2001). *Principles & practice of psychiatric nursing* (7th ed., p. 30). St. Louis: Mosby.

4. 3
Rationale: Option 3 is the only option that identifies a therapeutic response. In option 1 the nurse's feelings are the focus. This response clearly ignores the fact that the issue is about the client and the client's discomfort, not about the nurse. In option 2 the nurse becomes pompous and a tad angry and supercilious, which is not therapeutic. In option 4, the nurse begins correctly with an empathic stance but then becomes demanding.
Test-Taking Strategy: Use of the process of elimination and therapeutic communication techniques will direct you to option 3. Review therapeutic communication techniques if you had difficulty with this question.
Level of Cognitive Ability: Analysis
Client Needs: Psychosocial Integrity
Integrated Process: Communication and Documentation
Content Area: Mental health
Reference: Varcarolis, E. (2002). *Foundations of psychiatric mental health nursing* (4th ed., p. 258). Philadelphia: W. B. Saunders.

5. 4
Rationale: Native Americans may view touch differently from other Americans. The most therapeutic response is the one that reflects the client's feelings and empowers the client by offering self-control over one's own care. In option 1 the nurse uses avoidance and information giving. Option 2 is an aggressive and nontherapeutic communication technique. Option 3 labels the client's behavior and is likely to provoke anger from the client.
Test-Taking Strategy: Use the process of elimination and knowledge regarding the use of therapeutic communication techniques. Focus on the client's cultural heritage and the client's feelings to direct you to option 4. Review therapeutic communication techniques and cultural considerations if you had difficulty with this question.
Level of Cognitive Ability: Application
Client Needs: Psychosocial Integrity
Integrated Process: Communication and Documentation
Content Area: Mental health
Reference: Fortinash, K., & Holoday-Worret, P. (2000). *Psychiatric mental health nursing* (2nd ed., p. 112). St. Louis: Mosby.

6. 1
Rationale: Open-ended questions and silence are strategies used to encourage clients to discuss their problem. Options 2 and 3 are not helpful to the client because they do not encourage

the client to express feelings. The nurse should not offer opinions and should encourage the client to identify the reasons for the behavior. Option 4 is not a client centered intervention.
Test-Taking Strategy: Use the process of elimination. Eliminate options 2 and 3 first because they do not support client expression of feelings. Eliminate option 4 next because it is not a client-centered response. Focusing on the client's feelings will direct you easily to option 1. Review therapeutic communication techniques if you had difficulty with this question.
Level of Cognitive Ability: Application
Client Needs: Psychosocial Integrity
Integrated Process: Communication and Documentation
Content Area: Mental health
Reference: Stuart, G., & Laraia, M. (2001). *Principles & practice of psychiatric nursing* (7th ed., p. 472). St. Louis: Mosby.

7. 4
Rationale: The client must first deal with feelings and negative responses before the client is able to work through the meaning of the crisis. Option 4 pertains directly to the client's feelings. Options 1, 2, and 3 do not directly address the client's feelings.
Test-Taking Strategy: Focus on the issue of the question, the working phase of the nurse client relationship. Use the process of elimination focusing on this issue and on the option that focuses on the feelings of the client. Review the phases of the nurse-client relationship if you had difficulty with this question.
Level of Cognitive Ability: Application
Client Needs: Psychosocial Integrity
Integrated Process: Caring
Content Area: Mental health
Reference: Stuart, G., & Laraia, M. (2001). *Principles & practice of psychiatric nursing* (7th ed., pp. 592, 667). St. Louis: Mosby.

8. 1
Rationale: Denial is refusal to admit to a painful reality and may be a response by a victim of sexual abuse. Projection is transferring one's internal feelings, thoughts, and unacceptable ideas and traits to someone else. Rationalization is justifying the unacceptable attributes about oneself. Intellectualization is the excessive use of abstract thinking or generalizations to decrease painful thinking.
Test-Taking Strategy: Use the process of elimination. Note the key words "calm" and "quiet." These behaviors indicate denial in a sexually abused victim. If you had difficulty with this question, review content related to the sexually abused victim and defense mechanisms.
Level of Cognitive Ability: Analysis
Client Needs: Psychosocial Integrity
Integrated Process: Nursing Process—analysis
Content Area: Mental health
Reference: Stuart, G., & Laraia, M. (2001). *Principles & practice of psychiatric nursing* (7th ed., pp. 236, 483). St. Louis: Mosby.

9. 3
Rationale: The client's thoughts are important when verbalized. A client's report of suicidal thoughts is of highest priority. Options 1, 2, and 4 will affect the treatment of the client but are not of greatest importance at this time.
Test-Taking Strategy: The client is the focus of the question; therefore eliminate option 4. Use the process of elimination

and principles related to prioritizing to select the correct option. The life-threatening concern is identified in option 3. Review the techniques of assessment and analysis of assessment data from a client with a mental health disorder if you had difficulty with this question.
Level of Cognitive Ability: Analysis
Client Needs: Psychosocial Integrity
Integrated Process: Nursing Process—analysis
Content Area: Delegating/Prioritizing
Reference: Fortinash, K., & Holoday-Worret, P. (2000). *Psychiatric mental health nursing* (2nd ed., p. 664). St. Louis: Mosby.

10. 4
Rationale: Option 4 helps the client to focus on the emotion underlying the delusion but does not argue with it. Option 3 avoids the client. Option 2 places the client in a position that requires a response. Option 1 is an attempt to convince the client to believe another thought. This response may cause the client to hold the delusion more strongly.
Test-Taking Strategy: Use the process of elimination and therapeutic communication techniques to answer the question. Option 4 is the only option that recognizes the client's need and focuses on the client's feelings. Review therapeutic communication techniques if you had difficulty with this question.
Level of Cognitive Ability: Application
Client Needs: Psychosocial Integrity
Integrated Process: Caring
Content Area: Mental health
Reference: Stuart, G., & Laraia, M. (2001). *Principles & practice of psychiatric nursing* (7th ed., pp. 33, 423). St. Louis: Mosby.

11. 4
Rationale: Safety of the client, other clients, and staff is of prime concern. Option 1 is not appropriate, given the fact that the client is inebriated and may not be able to be reasoned with. Option 2 is inaccurate because waiting to intervene could cause the client to become even more agitated and a threat to others. Option 3 would aggravate an already agitated individual further. Option 4 is in effect an isolation technique that allows for separation from others and provides a less stimulating environment where the client can maintain dignity.
Test-Taking Strategy: Focus on the issue, an inebriated client. Use this information and the process of elimination in selecting the correct option. Option 4 most directly addresses the situation and the behavior and feelings of the client. Review therapeutic communication techniques if you had difficulty with this question.
Level of Cognitive Ability: Application
Client Needs: Psychosocial Integrity
Integrated Process: Nursing Process—implementation
Content Area: Mental health
References: Fortinash, K., & Holoday-Worret, P. (2000). *Psychiatric mental health nursing* (2nd ed., p. 11). St. Louis: Mosby.
Varcarolis, E. (2002). *Foundations of psychiatric mental health nursing* (4th ed., p. 681). Philadelphia: W. B. Saunders.

12. 2
Rationale: Denial is refusal to admit to a painful reality, which is treated as if it does not exist. In projection a person unconsciously rejects emotionally unacceptable features and attributes them to other persons, objects, or situations. In regression the client returns to an earlier, more comforting, although less mature way of behaving. Rationalization is justifying illogical or unreasonable ideas, actions, or feelings by developing acceptable explanations that satisfy the teller and the listener.
Test-Taking Strategy: Use the process of elimination. The key words in the question that should direct you to the correct option are "There's nothing wrong with me." Select the option that recognizes the client's attempt to avoid looking at the reality of the situation. If you had difficulty with this question, review defense mechanisms.
Level of Cognitive Ability: Analysis
Client Needs: Psychosocial Integrity
Integrated Process: Nursing Process—analysis
Content Area: Mental health
Reference: Fortinash, K., & Holoday-Worret, P. (2000). *Psychiatric mental health nursing* (2nd ed., p. 10). St. Louis: Mosby.

13. 4
Rationale: Most suicides occur within 3 months after the beginning of the improvement, when the client has the energy to carry out the suicidal intentions. Options 1, 2, and 3 are incorrect.
Test-Taking Strategy: Use the process of elimination and knowledge regarding the facts about suicide to answer the question. Recalling that a critical time for a suicidal client is when the client has energy will direct you to option 4. Review the concepts related to suicide and therapeutic communication techniques if you had difficulty with this question.
Level of Cognitive Ability: Application
Client Needs: Physiological Integrity
Integrated Process: Communication and Documentation
Content Area: Mental health
Reference: Fortinash, K., & Holoday-Worret, P. (2000). *Psychiatric mental health nursing* (2nd ed., p. 662). St. Louis: Mosby.

14. 4
Rationale: Ego defense mechanisms are operations outside of a person's awareness that the ego calls into play to protect against anxiety. Displacement is the discharging of pent-up feelings on persons less threatening than those who initially aroused the emotion. Denial is the blocking out of painful or anxiety-inducing events or feelings. Repression is unconsciously keeping unacceptable feelings out of awareness. Suppression is consciously keeping unacceptable feelings and thoughts out of awareness.
Test-Taking Strategy: Use the process of elimination. Read the behavior identified in the question to assist you in determining the type of ego defense mechanism or behavior used. If you had difficulty with this question, review defense mechanisms.
Level of Cognitive Ability: Analysis
Client Needs: Psychosocial Integrity
Integrated Process: Nursing Process—analysis

Content Area: Mental health
Reference: Fortinash, K., & Holoday-Worret, P. (2000). *Psychiatric mental health nursing* (2nd ed., p. 10). St. Louis: Mosby.

15. 1
Rationale: Restating is the therapeutic communication technique in which the nurse repeats what the client says to show understanding and to review what was said. Option 1 uses the therapeutic technique of restating. In option 2 the nurse attempts to use focusing, but the attempt to discuss central issues is premature. In option 3 the nurse makes a judgment and is nontherapeutic in the one-to-one relationship. In option 4 the nurse is attempting to assess the client's ability to discuss feelings openly with family members.
Test-Taking Strategy: Use therapeutic communication techniques to answer the question. Option 1 is the only option that identifies the use of a therapeutic technique and focuses on the client's feelings. Review these techniques if you had difficulty with this question.
Level of Cognitive Ability: Application
Client Needs: Psychosocial Integrity
Integrated Process: Communication and Documentation
Content Area: Mental health
Reference: Varcarolis, E. (2002). *Foundations of psychiatric mental health nursing* (4th ed., pp. 255, 830). Philadelphia: W. B. Saunders.

16. 4
Rationale: Generally, the client seeks voluntary admission. A voluntary admission permits a client to make a written application for admission. If the client seeks voluntary admission, the most likely expectation is that the client will participate in the treatment program. Options 1, 2, and 3 are not characteristics of this type of admission.
Test-Taking Strategy: Use the process of admission. Note the key words "voluntary admission." This should direct you to option 4. Additionally, note that options 1, 2, and 3 are similar. Review the various types of hospital admission processes if you had difficulty with this question.
Level of Cognitive Ability: Analysis
Client Needs: Psychosocial Integrity
Integrated Process: Nursing Process—analysis
Content Area: Mental health
References: Fortinash, K., & Holoday-Worret, P. (2000). *Psychiatric mental health nursing* (2nd ed., p. 84). St. Louis: Mosby.
Stuart, G., & Laraia, M. (2001). *Principles & practice of psychiatric nursing* (7th ed., p. 162). St. Louis: Mosby.

17. 3
Rationale: Generally, the client seeks voluntary admission. Voluntary clients have the right to demand and obtain release. If the client is a minor, the release may be contingent on the consent of the parents or guardian. The nurse needs to be familiar with the state and facility policies and procedures. Many states require that the client submit a written release notice to the facility staff, who reevaluate the client's condition for possible conversion to involuntary status, according to criteria established by laws. The best nursing action is to contact the physician.

Test-Taking Strategy: Use the process of elimination. Noting the type of hospital admission will assist in eliminating option 1. To "persuade" a client to stay in the hospital is inappropriate. Option 2 should be eliminated simply based on the issue of client rights and the issue of confidentiality. Review the various types of hospital admission and discharge processes if you had difficulty with this question.
Level of Cognitive Ability: Application
Client Needs: Psychosocial Integrity
Integrated Process: Nursing Process—implementation
Content Area: Mental health
Reference: Varcarolis, E. (2002). *Foundations of psychiatric mental health nursing* (4th ed., p. 171). Philadelphia: W. B. Saunders.

18. 1
Rationale: Involuntary admission is made without the client's consent. Involuntary admission is necessary when a person is a danger to self or others or is in need of psychiatric treatment. Options 2, 3, and 4 describe the process of voluntary admission.
Test-Taking Strategy: Use the process of elimination. Note the key words "involuntary status." This should direct you easily to option 1. Also, note that options 2, 3, and 4 are similar. Review the process of involuntary admission if you had difficulty with this question.
Level of Cognitive Ability: Analysis
Client Needs: Psychosocial Integrity
Integrated Process: Nursing Process—analysis
Content Area: Mental health
Reference: Stuart, G., & Laraia, M. (2001). *Principles & practice of psychiatric nursing* (7th ed., p. 163). St. Louis: Mosby.

19. 3
Rationale: Clients who are admitted involuntarily do not lose their right to informed consent. Clients must be considered legally competent until they have been declared incompetent through a legal proceeding. The informed consent needs to be obtained from the client.
Test-Taking Strategy: Knowledge regarding the hospital admission processes and client's rights is necessary to answer this question. If you had difficulty with this question, focus on the issue of client rights to direct you to option 3. Review client rights if you had difficulty with this question.
Level of Cognitive Ability: Analysis
Client Needs: Safe, Effective Care Environment
Integrated Process: Nursing Process—analysis
Content Area: Mental health
Reference: Stuart, G., & Laraia, M. (2001). *Principles & practice of psychiatric nursing* (7th ed., pp. 173, 162). St. Louis: Mosby.

20. 2
Rationale: A client may request to be secluded or restrained. Federal laws require the consent of the client, unless an emergency situation exists in which an immediate risk to the client or others can be documented. The use of seclusion and restraint is permitted only on the written order of a physician, which must be reviewed and renewed every 24 hours and which also must specify the type of restraint to be used.

Test-Taking Strategy: Use the process of elimination and knowledge regarding the issue of clients rights to direct you to option 2. The nurse has no reason to call the family at this time; therefore eliminate option 3. Knowing that a physician's written order is necessary will assist you in eliminating option 4. Option 1 is not the best option because this information, if given to a client experiencing uncontrollable feelings, may cause escalation of the feelings. Review the nursing implications regarding seclusion and restraint if you had difficulty with this question.
Level of Cognitive Ability: Application
Client Needs: Psychosocial Integrity
Integrated Process: Nursing Process—implementation
Content Area: Mental health
Reference: Fortinash, K., & Holoday-Worret, P. (2000). *Psychiatric mental health nursing* (2nd ed., p. 89). St. Louis: Mosby.

21. **2**
Rationale: The nurse should never promise to keep a secret. Secrets are appropriate in a social relationship but not in a therapeutic one. The nurse needs to be honest with the client and tell the client that a promise cannot be made to keep the secret. Options 1, 3, and 4 are inappropriate responses.
Test-Taking Strategy: Use the process of elimination. Option 1 can be eliminated easily because it is inappropriate. Options 3 and 4 are not only inappropriate but also are to an extent threatening and may even block further communication. Review therapeutic communication techniques and nurse client relationships if you had difficulty with this question.
Level of Cognitive Ability: Application
Client Needs: Psychosocial Integrity
Integrated Process: Communication and Documentation
Content Area: Mental health
Reference: Fortinash, K., & Holoday-Worret, P. (2000). *Psychiatric mental health nursing* (2nd ed., p. 170). St. Louis: Mosby.

22. **4**
Rationale: A nurse is required to maintain confidentiality regarding the client and the client's care. Confidentiality is basic to the therapeutic relationship and is a client's right. The most appropriate response to the neighbor is option 4. Option 3 is correct in a sense; however, it is a rather blunt statement. Options 1 and 2 identify statements that do not maintain client confidentiality. Option 4 is most direct and correct.
Test-Taking Strategy: Focus on the issue of the question, maintaining confidentiality. This should assist you easily in eliminating options 1 and 2. From the remaining options, select option 4 over option 3 because it is most direct and correct. Option 3 is a rather blunt and rude statement. Review confidentiality issues if you had difficulty with this question.
Level of Cognitive Ability: Application
Client Needs: Safe, Effective Care Environment
Integrated Process: Nursing Process—implementation
Content Area: Mental health
Reference: Fortinash, K., & Holoday-Worret, P. (2000). *Psychiatric mental health nursing* (2nd ed., p. 170). St. Louis: Mosby.

23. **4**
Rationale: False imprisonment is an act with the intent to confine a person to a specific area. A nurse can be charged with false imprisonment if the nurse prohibits a client from leaving the hospital if the client was admitted voluntarily and if no agency or legal policies exist for detaining the client. However, if the client was admitted involuntarily or had agreed to an evaluation before discharge, the nurse's actions are reasonable.
Test-Taking Strategy: Noting the key words "admitted involuntarily" will assist you in eliminating option 1 and direct you to option 4. Options 2 and 3 are unrelated to the issue of the question and can be eliminated easily. Review the issues related to false imprisonment and hospital admissions if you had difficulty with this question.
Level of Cognitive Ability: Analysis
Client Needs: Safe, Effective Care Environment
Integrated Process: Nursing Process—analysis
Content Area: Mental health
Reference: Stuart, G., & Laraia, M. (2001). *Principles & practice of psychiatric nursing* (7th ed., p. 163). St. Louis: Mosby.

24. **3**
Rationale: Tasks of the termination phase include evaluating client performance, evaluating achievement of expected outcomes, evaluating future needs, making appropriate referrals, and dealing with the common behaviors associated with termination. Options 1, 2, and 4 identify the tasks of the working phase of the relationship.
Test-Taking Strategy: Use the process of elimination. Noting the key words "termination phase" should direct you easily to option 3. If you are unfamiliar with the appropriate tasks of the phases of the nurse-client relationship, review this content.
Level of Cognitive Ability: Application
Client Needs: Psychosocial Integrity
Integrated Process: Nursing Process—planning
Content Area: Mental health
Reference: Fortinash, K., & Holoday-Worret, P. (2000). *Psychiatric mental health nursing* (2nd ed., p. 519). St. Louis: Mosby.

25. **2**
Rationale: In the termination phase of a relationship it is normal for a client to demonstrate a number of regressive behaviors that can be disturbing to the nurse. Typical behaviors include return of symptoms, anger, withdrawal, and minimizing the relationship. The anger that the client is experiencing is a normal behavior during the termination phase and does not necessarily indicate the need for hospitalization or treatment.
Test-Taking Strategy: Note the key words "termination phase." This alone may assist in directing you to option 2. Additionally, note the similarity between options 1, 3, and 4. These options address the need for further supervised treatment. If you are unfamiliar with the client behaviors associated with the termination phase, review this content.
Level of Cognitive Ability: Analysis
Client Needs: Psychosocial Integrity
Integrated Process: Nursing Process—analysis

Content Area: Mental health
Reference: Fortinash, K., & Holoday-Worret, P. (2000). *Psychiatric mental health nursing* (2nd ed., p. 518). St. Louis: Mosby.

CRITICAL THINKING: MULTIPLE RESPONSE

Answer:
Listening
Maintaining neutral responses
Restating
Providing acknowledgment and feedback
Rationale: Some of the therapeutic communication techniques include listening, maintaining silence, maintaining neutral responses, using of broad openings and open-ended questions, focusing and refocusing, restating, clarifying and validating, sharing perceptions, reflecting, providing acknowledgment and feedback, giving information and presenting reality, encouraging formulation of a plan of action, providing nonverbal encouragement, and summarizing.
Test-Taking Strategy: Focus on the issue, therapeutic communication techniques. This will assist you in selecting the correct answers. Review therapeutic and nontherapeutic techniques if you had difficulty with this question.
Level of Cognitive Ability: Comprehension
Client Needs: Psychosocial Integrity
Integrated Process: Teaching/Learning
Content Area: Mental health
Reference: Harkreader, H., & Hogan, M. A. (2004). *Fundamentals of nursing: Caring and clinical judgment* (2nd ed., pp. 251-252). Philadelphia: W. B. Saunders.

REFERENCES

Fortinash, K., & Holoday-Worret, P. (2000). *Psychiatric mental health nursing* (2nd ed.). St. Louis: Mosby.

Harkreader, H., & Hogan, M. A. (2004). *Fundamentals of nursing: Caring and clinical judgment* (2nd ed.). Philadelphia: W. B. Saunders.

Keltner, N., Schwecke, L., & Bostrom, C. (2003). *Psychiatric nursing* (4th ed.). St. Louis: Mosby.

Stuart, G., & Laraia, M. (2001). *Principles & practice of psychiatric nursing* (7th ed.). St. Louis: Mosby.

Varcarolis, E. (2002). *Foundations of psychiatric mental health nursing* (4th ed.). Philadelphia: W. B. Saunders.

Models of Care

I. MILIEU THERAPY

A. Description
1. **Milieu** is the physical and social environment in which an individual lives.
2. **Milieu** therapy provides a safe environment that is adapted to the individual client's needs and also provides greater comfort and freedom of expression than the client has experienced in the past.
3. **Milieu** therapy is staffed by persons trained to provide support and understanding and individual attention.
4. All members contribute to the planning and functioning of the setting.
5. The power hierarchy is diminished because all members are viewed as significant and valuable members of the community.

B. Focus
1. The focus of **milieu** therapy is positive environmental manipulation, physical and social, to effect a positive change.
2. The focus is client's rights through involvement in setting goals, freedom of movement, and informal relationships with staff.
3. The focus is group and social interaction.
4. The focus is use of community meetings, activity groups, social skills groups, and physical exercise programs.

II. PSYCHOTHERAPY

A. Description
1. Psychotherapy is use of a group of techniques to modify feelings, attitudes, and behaviors in clients.
2. Therapist uses verbal and nonverbal means of communication to build a relationship with the client.

B. Focus
1. The basic concept involves understanding.
2. The focus is on issues of importance to the client, purpose of the interaction, identification of the roles of the therapist and client, and the use of primarily verbal means of communication.
3. Nonverbal techniques include silence, body language, facial expressions, and respect for personal space.

C. Levels of psychotherapy (Box 72-1)
1. Supportive therapy
   a. Supportive therapy allows the client to express feelings, explore alternatives, and make decisions in a safe, caring environment.
   b. Supportive therapy may be needed briefly or over a period of years.
   c. No plan exists to introduce new methods of coping; instead the therapist reinforces the client's existing **coping mechanisms.**
2. Reeducative therapy
   a. Reeducative therapy involves learning new ways of perceiving and behaving.
   b. The client explores alternatives in a planned, systematic way and requires a longer period than supportive therapy.
   c. The client enters into a contract that specifies desired changes of behavior.
   d. Reeducative therapy includes short-term psychotherapy, reality therapy, cognitive restructuring, and behavior modification.

BOX 72-1

Levels of Psychotherapy

Supportive therapy
Reeducative therapy
Reconstructive therapy

3. Reconstructive therapy
   a. Reconstructive therapy involves deep psychotherapy or psychoanalysis.
   b. Reconstructive therapy may require 2 to 5 years of therapy or more and focuses on all aspects of the client's life.
   c. Emotional and cognitive restructuring of self takes place.
   d. Positive outcomes include a greater understanding of self and others, more emotional freedom, and the development of potential abilities.

III. BEHAVIOR AND BEHAVIOR MODIFICATION
A. Behavior therapy
   1. Behavior therapy is an approach to bring about behavioral change.
   2. Behavior therapy includes a group of diversified approaches for dealing with maladaptive behavior.
   3. The belief is that most behaviors are learned.
   4. Maladaptive behavior is a way of dealing with stress, and the therapy is an approach to bring about a change in the behavior.
B. Self-control therapy
   1. Self-control therapy is a combination of cognitive and behavioral approaches.
   2. A basic theme is that talking to oneself can direct and control actions more effectively.
   3. Self-control therapy is useful to deal with stress.
C. Desensitization
   1. Desensitization is the reduction of intense reactions to a stimulus by repeated exposure to the stimulus in a weaker and milder form.
   2. Gradually over a period of time, exposure is increased until the fear of the object or situation has ceased.
D. Aversion therapy
   1. Negative reinforcement is a technique to change behavior.
   2. A stimulus attractive to the client is paired with an unpleasant event in hopes of endowing the stimulus with negative properties.
E. In modeling, the therapist acts as a role model for specified identified behaviors and the client learns through imitation.
F. Operant conditioning entails rewarding a client for desired behaviors and is the basis for behavior modification.

IV. COGNITIVE THERAPY
A. Cognitive therapy is an active, directive, time-limited, structured approach used to treat a variety of psychiatric disorders.
B. Therapeutic techniques are designed to identify reality testing and correct distorted conceptualization and the dysfunctional belief underlying these cognitions.

C. The client learns to master problems in situations that the client previously considered insuperable by evaluating and correcting thinking.
D. The cognitive therapist helps the client to think and act more realistically and adaptively about psychological problems so as to reduce symptoms.
E. Various cognitive and behavioral strategies are used in cognitive therapy.

V. GROUP DEVELOPMENT AND GROUP THERAPY
A. Stages of group development (Box 72-2)
   1. Initial stage
      a. Group development involves superficial rather that open and trusting communication.
      b. Members become acquainted with each other and search for similarity between themselves and other group members.
      c. Members may be unclear about the purpose or goals of the group.
      d. A certain amount of structuring of group norms, roles, and responsibilities take place.
   2. Working stage
      a. During this stage, the real work of the group is accomplished.
      b. Members are familiar with each other, the group leader, and the group roles, and they feel free to approach their problems and to attempt to solve their problems.
      c. Conflict and cooperation surface during the group's work.
   3. Termination stage
      a. The group evaluates the experience and explores members' feelings about it and the impending separation.
      b. The termination stage provides an opportunity for members who have difficulty with termination to learn to deal more realistically and comfortably with this normal part of human experience.
B. Psychoanalytical group psychotherapy
   1. Therapist holds a main position.
   2. Each client in the group has a relationship with the therapist.
   3. Communication is focused on three levels: unconscious, semiconscious, and conscious information.
C. Transactional analysis
   1. The three ego states of the individual—the parent, the child, and the adult—are examined in transactional analysis groups.

BOX 72-2

Stages of Group Development

Initial stage
Working stage
Termination stage

2. The goal is that individuals in the group will communicate from the proper ego states for the situation and the responses of others, thereby lessening conflict and promoting mature relationships.

D. Rational emotive therapy: The therapist designs activities to eliminate the irrational ideas of the members of the group.

E. Rogerian therapy
   1. The therapist's goal is the help the members express their feelings toward one another during group sessions.
   2. The therapist's role is one of encouraging the expression of feelings, clarifying these feelings with clients, and accepting clients and their feelings nonjudgmentally.

F. Gestalt therapy
   1. Emphasis is on the "here and now."
   2. Gestalt therapy emphasizes self-expression, self-exploration, and self-awareness in the present.
   3. The client and therapist focus on everyday problems and try to solve them.
   4. The individual becomes aware of the total self and the surrounding environment.
   5. Awareness of the problem renders the client capable of change.
   6. The therapist's role is to help the members express their feelings and grow from their experiences.

G. Interpersonal group therapy promotes the individual's comfort with others in the group, which then transfers to other relationships.

H. Self-help or support groups (See box 72-3 for examples.)
   1. Support groups are based on the premise that persons who have experienced a similar problem are able to help others who have the same problem.
   2. Support groups prevent the individual member from feeling lonely and isolated.

BOX 72-3

Self-help or Support Groups

Adult Children of Alcoholics
Al-Alon
Alcoholics Anonymous
Co-dependents Anonymous
Gamblers Anonymous
Narcotics Anonymous
Overeaters Anonymous
Bereavement
Health conditions, such as cancer
Parents without partners
Recovery groups, such as for those who have
   experienced trauma
Smoking cessation
Unexpected body image changes, such as mastectomy or
   colostomy

---

3. Support groups help members decrease levels of stress and increase levels of self-acceptance.
4. Members are better able to deal with the problems that they brought to the group and develop new or more effective patterns of behavior.

I. Family therapy
   1. Family therapy is a specific intervention mode based on the premise that the members, with the presenting symptoms, signal the presence of pain in the entire family.
   2. The therapist works to assist the family members to identify and express their thoughts and feelings; define family roles and rules; try new, more productive styles of relating; and restore strength to the family.

PRACTICE QUESTIONS

1. An 18-year-old woman is admitted to an inpatient unit with the diagnosis of anorexia nervosa. A cognitive behavioral approach is used as part of her treatment plan. The nurse understands that the purpose of this approach is to
   1. Help the client identify and examine dysfunctional thoughts and beliefs.
   2. Emphasize social interaction with clients who withdraw.
   3. Provide a supportive environment.
   4. Examine intrapsychic conflicts and past issues.

2. The nurse is preparing to provide reminiscence therapy for a group of clients. Which of the following clients would the nurse select for this group?
   1. A client who exhibits profound depression with moderate cognitive impairment
   2. A catatonic, immobile client with moderate cognitive impairment
   3. An undifferentiated schizophrenic client with moderate cognitive impairment
   4. A client with mild depression who demonstrates normal cognition

3. A client with major depression is considering cognitive therapy. The client says to the nurse "How does this treatment work?" The nurse responds and tells the client that
   1. " This type of treatment helps you examine how your thoughts and feelings contribute to your difficulties."
   2. "This type of treatment helps you examine how your past life has contributed to your problems."
   3. "This type of treatment helps you confront your fears by gradually exposing you to them."
   4. "This type of treatment will help you relax and develop new coping skills."

4. The client asks the nurse about milieu therapy. The nurse responds knowing that the primary locus of milieu therapy can best be described as which of the following?

1. A form of behavior modification therapy
2. A cognitive approach to changing behavior
3. A living, learning, or working environment
4. A behavioral approach to changing behavior

5. The nurse is caring for a client with a phobia who is being treated for the condition. The client is introduced to short periods of exposure to the phobic object while in a relaxed state. The nurse understands that this form of behavior modification can best be described as
   1. Systematic desensitization.
   2. Self-control therapy.
   3. Milieu therapy.
   4. Aversion therapy.

6. A client with an eating disorder is planning to attend group meetings with Overeaters Anonymous, and the nurse describes this group to the client. The nurse determines that the client needs additional information if the client states which of the following about this self-help group?
   1. "People who have a similar problem are able to help others."
   2. "It is designed to serve people who have a common problem."
   3. "The members provide support to each other."
   4. "The leader is a nurse or psychiatrist."

7. The client is preparing to attend a Gambler's Anonymous meeting for the first time. The prototype used by this group is the 12-step program developed by Alcoholics Anonymous. The nurse tells the client that the first step in the 12-step program is which of the following?
   1. Stating that the gambling will be stopped
   2. Discontinuing relationships with friends who are gamblers
   3. Substituting gambling for other activities
   4. Admitting to having a problem

8. The nurse is conducting a group therapy session, and a client with a manic disorder is monopolizing the group. The most appropriate nursing action is which of the following?
   1. Suggest that the client stop talking and try listening to others.
   2. Ask the client to leave.
   3. Tell the client to stop monopolizing the group.
   4. Refer the client to another group.

9. The nurse is planning to formulate a psychotherapy group. Several clients are interested in attending the session. The nurse plans the group, knowing that the maximum number of group members to include in this group is
   1. 10.
   2. 12.
   3. 14.
   4. 16.

10. A nurse employed in a mental health unit of a hospital is the leader of a group psychotherapy session. The nurse's role in the termination stage of group development is to
    1. Encourage members to become acquainted with one another.
    2. Acknowledge the contributions of each group member.
    3. Encourage accomplishment of the group's work.
    4. Encourage problem-solving.

CRITICAL THINKING: FILL IN THE BLANK

The nurse is providing information to a client about the use of disulfiram (Antabuse) for the treatment of alcohol abuse. The nurse understands that this form of treatment works on the principle of which therapy?

Answer: _____

ANSWERS

1. 1

Rationale: Cognitive behavioral therapy is used to help clients identify and examine dysfunctional thoughts and to identify and examine values and beliefs that maintain these thoughts. Option 2, 3, and 4 are incorrect.

Test-Taking Strategy: Use the process of elimination. Note the key words "cognitive behavioral." Focusing on these key words should direct you to option 1. If you are unfamiliar with this type of therapy and its purpose, review this content.

Level of Cognitive Ability: Comprehension
Client Needs: Psychosocial Integrity
Integrated Process: Nursing Process—planning
Content Area: Mental health
Reference: Fortinash, K., & Holoday-Worret, P. (2000). *Psychiatric mental health nursing* (2nd ed., p. 463). St. Louis: Mosby.

2. 4

Rationale: Reminiscence therapy is best for clients who meet the following criteria: normal to mild cognitive impairment; mild to moderate depression; and withdrawn, socially isolated, understimulated behavior.

Test-Taking Strategy: Use the process of elimination, focusing on the type of therapy addressed in the question. Options 1, 2, and 3 describe clients whose cognitive impairment would not be improved with this form of therapy. If you had difficulty with this question, review the characteristics of reminiscence therapy.

Level of Cognitive Ability: Application
Client Needs: Psychosocial Integrity
Integrated Process: Nursing Process—implementation
Content Area: Mental health
Reference: Stuart, G., & Laraia, M. (2001). *Principles & practice of psychiatric nursing* (7th ed., p. 339). St. Louis: Mosby.

3. 1

Rationale: Cognitive therapy frequently is used with clients who have depression. This type of therapy is based on exploring the client's subjective experience. Cognitive therapy includes examining the client's thoughts and feelings about situations and how these thoughts and feelings contribute to and perpetuate the client's difficulties and mood.

Test-Taking Strategy: Focusing on the word "cognitive" will assist you in selecting the correct option. Look for a similar word used in the question and repeated in one of the options. Option 1 uses the word "thought" in describing the treatment. Review this form of therapy if you had difficulty with this question.

Level of Cognitive Ability: Application
Client Needs: Psychosocial Integrity
Integrated Process: Nursing Process—implementation
Content Area: Mental health
References: Fortinash, K., & Holoday-Worret, P. (2000). *Psychiatric mental health nursing* (2nd ed., p. 287). St. Louis: Mosby.
Varcarolis, E. (2002). *Foundations of psychiatric mental health nursing* (4th ed., p. 459). Philadelphia: W. B. Saunders.

4. 3

Rationale: Milieu therapy, or "therapeutic community," has as its focus a living, learning, or working environment. Such therapy may be based on any number of therapeutic modalities from structured behavioral therapy to spontaneous, humanistically oriented approaches. Although milieu may include behavioral approaches, option 3 describes its primary focus.

Test-Taking Strategy: Use the process of elimination. Note that options 1, 2, and 4 are similar and that option 3 identifies a global description. Review milieu therapy if you had difficulty with this question.

Level of Cognitive Ability: Comprehension
Client Needs: Psychosocial Integrity
Integrated Process: Nursing Process—implementation
Content Area: Mental health
Reference: Varcarolis, E. (2002). *Foundations of psychiatric mental health nursing* (4th ed., p. 43). Philadelphia: W. B. Saunders.

5. 1

Rationale: Systematic desensitization is a form of therapy used when the client is introduced to short periods of exposure to the phobic object while in a relaxed state. Gradually exposure is increased until the anxiety about or fear of the object or situation has ceased. Options 2, 3, and 4 are incorrect.

Test-Taking Strategy: Use the process of elimination. Focus on the key words "introduced to short periods of exposure." This should assist in directing you to the correct option. If you had difficulty with this question, review systematic desensitization.

Level of Cognitive Ability: Comprehension
Client Needs: Psychosocial Integrity
Integrated Process: Nursing Process—implementation
Content Area: Mental health
Reference: Fortinash, K., & Holoday-Worret, P. (2000). *Psychiatric mental health nursing* (2nd ed., pp. 52-53). St. Louis: Mosby.

6. 4

Rationale: The sponsor of a self-help group is an experienced member of the group. A nurse or psychiatrist may be asked by the group to serve as a resource but would not be the leader of the group. Options 1, 2, and 3 are characteristics of a self-help group.

Test-Taking Strategy: Use the process of elimination and focus on the issue, self-help group. Note the key words "needs additional information" in the stem of the question. Note that options 1, 2, and 3 are similar. This should direct you easily to option 4, the correct option. Review the characteristics of a self-help group if you had difficulty with this question.

Level of Cognitive Ability: Analysis
Client Needs: Psychosocial Integrity
Integrated Process: Teaching/Learning
Content Area: Mental health
Reference: Varcarolis, E. (2002). *Foundations of psychiatric mental health nursing* (4th ed., p. 942). Philadelphia: W. B. Saunders.

7. 4

Rationale: The first step in the 12-step program is to admit that a problem exists. Options 1 and 2 are unrealistic as a first step in the process to recovery. Although option 3 may be a strategy, it is not the first step.

Test-Taking Strategy: Use the process of elimination. Note the key words "first step" in the question. This will assist in directing you to option 4. If you are unfamiliar with the 12-step program, review this content.

Level of Cognitive Ability: Application
Client Needs: Psychosocial Integrity
Integrated Process: Nursing Process—implementation
Content Area: Mental health
Reference: Varcarolis, E. (2002). *Foundations of psychiatric mental health nursing* (4th ed., p. 942). Philadelphia: W. B. Saunders.

8. 1

Rationale: If a client is monopolizing the group, the nurse must be direct and decisive. The best action is to suggest that the client stop talking and try listening to others. Although option 3 may be a direct response, option 1 is a more specific and direct statement. Options 2 and 4 are inappropriate.

Test-Taking Strategy: Use the process of elimination. Eliminate options 2 and 4 first because they are similar. Use therapeutic communication techniques to assist in directing you to option 1. If you had difficulty with this question, review therapeutic communication techniques for the client with a manic disorder.

Level of Cognitive Ability: Application
Client Needs: Psychosocial Integrity
Integrated Process: Nursing Process—implementation
Content Area: Mental health
References: Stuart, G., & Laraia, M. (2001). *Principles & practice of psychiatric nursing* (7th ed., p. 34). St. Louis: Mosby.
Varcarolis, E. (2002). *Foundations of psychiatric mental health nursing* (4th ed., p. 943). Philadelphia: W. B. Saunders.

9. 1

Rationale: The ideal number of clients in a psychotherapy group ranges from 7 to 10. Having more than 10 members is not recommended because the group will subdivide, which is counterproductive. Too large a group also can create more opportunities for acting out as opposed to working through issues.

Test-Taking Strategy: Knowledge regarding the general guidelines related to establishing a psychotherapy group is required to answer this question. If you are unfamiliar with these guidelines, review this content.
Level of Cognitive Ability: Comprehension
Client Needs: Psychosocial Integrity
Integrated Process: Nursing Process—planning
Content Area: Mental health
Reference: Varcarolis, E. (2002). *Foundations of psychiatric mental health nursing* (4th ed., p. 946). Philadelphia: W. B. Saunders.

10. 2
Rationale: In the termination stage the group leader's task is to acknowledge the contributions of each member and the experience of the group as a whole. In this stage the group members prepare for separation and assist each other to prepare for the future. Option 1 identifies the orientation stage. Options 3 and 4 identify the tasks of the working stage.
Test-Taking Strategy: Use the process of elimination. Eliminate options 3 and 4 first because they are similar. From the remaining options, note the relationship between the words "termination stage" in the question and option 2. Review the stages of group development if you had difficulty with this question.

Level of Cognitive Ability: Application
Client Needs: Psychosocial Integrity
Integrated Process: Nursing Process—implementation
Content Area: Mental health
Reference: Varcarolis, E. (2002). *Foundations of psychiatric mental health nursing* (4th ed., p. 934). Philadelphia: W. B. Saunders.

CRITICAL THINKING: FILL IN THE BLANK
Answer: Aversion therapy
Rationale: Aversion therapy, also known as aversion conditioning or negative reinforcement, is a technique used to change behavior. In this therapy a stimulus attractive to the client is paired with an unpleasant event in hopes of endowing the stimulus with negative properties.
Test-Taking Strategy: Focus on the issue, the use of disulfiram (Antabuse) to treat alcohol abuse. Recalling the purpose and use of disulfiram will assist you in identifying the purpose of aversion therapy. If you had difficulty with this question, review this form of therapy.
Level of Cognitive Ability: Comprehension
Client Needs: Psychosocial Integrity
Integrated Process: Teaching/Learning
Content Area: Mental health
References: Stuart, G., & Laraia, M. (2001). *Principles & practice of psychiatric nursing* (7th ed., p. 669). St. Louis: Mosby. Varcarolis, E. (2002). *Foundations of psychiatric mental health nursing* (4th ed., pp. 42-43). Philadelphia: W. B. Saunders.

REFERENCES

Fortinash, K., & Holoday-Worret, P. (2000). *Psychiatric mental health nursing* (2nd ed.). St. Louis: Mosby.

Stuart, G., & Laraia, M. (2001). *Principles & practice of psychiatric nursing* (7th ed.). St. Louis: Mosby.

Varcarolis, E. (2002). *Foundations of psychiatric mental health nursing* (4th ed.). Philadelphia: W. B. Saunders.

Mental Health Disorders

I. ANXIETY

A. Description
1. Anxiety is a subjective, individual experience.
2. Anxiety is a normal response to stress.
3. Anxiety is a feeling of apprehension, uneasiness, uncertainty, or dread.
4. Anxiety occurs as a result of threats that may be misperceived or misinterpreted.
5. Anxiety occurs as a result of a threat to identity or self-esteem.
6. Anxiety may result when values are threatened.
7. Anxiety may precede new experiences.

B. Types of anxiety
1. Normal: a healthy type of anxiety
2. Acute: precipitated by imminent loss or change that threatens the sense of security
3. Chronic: anxiety that the individual has lived with for a long time

C. Levels of anxiety
1. Mild
   a. Mild anxiety is associated with the tension of everyday life.
   b. The individual is alert.
   c. The perceptual field is increased.
   d. Mild anxiety can be motivating, produce growth and creativity, and increase learning.
2. Moderate
   a. The focus is on immediate concerns.
   b. Moderate anxiety narrows the perceptual field.
   c. Selective inattentiveness occurs.
   d. Learning and problem-solving still take place.
3. Severe
   a. Severe anxiety is a feeling that something bad is about to happen.
   b. A significant reduction in perceptual field occurs.

c. Focus is on specific details or scattered details.
d. All behavior is directed at relieving the anxiety.
e. Learning and problem-solving are not possible.
f. The individual needs direction to focus.
4. Panic
   a. Panic is associated with dread and terror and a sense of impending doom.
   b. The personality is disorganized.
   c. The individual is unable to communicate or function effectively.
   d. Increased motor activity occurs.
   e. Loss of rational thoughts with distorted perception occurs.
   f. Inability to concentrate occurs.
   g. If prolonged, panic can lead to exhaustion and death.

D. Interventions: general nursing measures
1. Recognize the anxiety.
2. Establish trust.
3. Protect the client.
4. Do not attack **coping mechanisms.**
5. Do not force the client into situations that provoke anxiety.
6. Decrease stimulation in the environment.
7. Modify the environment by setting limits or limiting the interaction with others.
8. Provide creative outlets.
9. Provide activities that limit the amount of time for destructive behavior.
10. Promote relaxation techniques.
11. Administer antianxiety medications as prescribed.

E. Interventions: mild to moderate levels
1. Help the client identify the anxiety.
2. Encourage the client to talk about feelings and concerns.
3. Help the client identify thoughts and feelings that occurred before the onset of anxiety.

4. Encourage problem solving.
5. Encourage gross motor exercise.
F. Interventions: severe to panic levels
   1. Reduce the anxiety quickly.
   2. Use a calm manner.
   3. Always remain with the client.
   4. Minimize environmental stimuli.
   5. Provide clear, simple statements.
   6. Use a low-pitched voice.
   7. Attend to the physical needs of the client.
   8. Provide gross motor activity.
   9. Administer antianxiety medications as prescribed.

II. GENERALIZED ANXIETY DISORDER

A. Description
   1. Generalized anxiety disorder is an unrealistic anxiety in which the cause usually can be identified.
   2. Physical symptoms occur.
B. Assessment
   1. Restlessness and inability to relax
   2. Episodes of trembling and shakiness
   3. Chronic muscular tension
   4. Dizziness
   5. Inability to concentrate
   6. Chronic fatigue and sleep problems
   7. Inability to recognize the connection between the anxiety and physical symptoms
   8. Focused on the physical discomfort
C. Panic disorder
   1. Description
      a. The cause usually cannot be identified.
      b. Panic disorder produces a sudden onset with feelings of intense apprehension and dread.
      c. Severe, recurrent, intermittent anxiety attacks lasting 5 to 30 minutes occur.
   2. Assessment
      a. Choking sensation
      b. Labored breathing
      c. Pounding heart
      d. Chest pain
      e. Dizziness
      f. Nausea
      g. Blurred vision
      h. Numbness or tingling of the extremities
      i. A sense of unreality and helplessness
      j. A fear of being trapped
      k. A fear of dying
   3. Interventions
      a. Attend to physical symptoms.
      b. Assist the client to identify the thoughts that aroused the anxiety and identify the basis for these thoughts.
      c. Assist the client to change the unrealistic thoughts to more realistic thoughts.
      d. Use cognitive restructuring.
      e. Administer antianxiety medications as prescribed.

III. POSTTRAUMATIC STRESS DISORDER

A. Description: After experiencing a psychologically traumatic event, outside the range of usual experience, the individual reexperiences the event via recurrent and intrusive dreams or flashbacks.
B. Stressors
   1. A natural disaster
   2. A terrorist attack
   3. Combat experiences
   4. Victim of rape
   5. Accidents
   6. Victim of crime or violence
   7. Victim of sexual, physical, and emotional **abuse**
   8. Reexperiencing the event as flashbacks
C. Assessment
   1. Emotional numbness
   2. Detachment
   3. Depression
   4. Anxiety
   5. Sleep disturbances and nightmares
   6. Flashbacks of the event
   7. Hypervigilance
   8. Guilt about surviving the event
   9. Poor concentration and avoidance of activities that trigger the memory of the event
D. Interventions
   1. Promote desensitization through gradual exposure to the event or situations similar to the event.
   2. Instruct the client in relaxation techniques.
   3. Provide individual therapy that addresses loss of control issues or anger.
   4. Encourage use of support groups.
   5. Encourage use of hypnotherapy.

IV. PHOBIAS

A. Description
   1. A phobia is an irrational fear of an object or situation that persists although the person may recognize it as unreasonable.
   2. A phobia is associated with panic level anxiety if the object, situation, or activity cannot be avoided.
   3. **Defense mechanisms** commonly used include repression and displacement.
B. Types (Box 73-1)
C. Interventions
   1. Stay with the client when the anxiety is high to promote safety and security.
   2. Identify the basis of the anxiety.
   3. Allow the client to verbalize feelings about the anxiety-producing object or situation; frequently talking about the feared object is the first step in the desensitization process.
   4. Promote desensitization by gradually introducing the individual to the feared object or situation in small doses.

BOX 73-1

Types of Phobias

Acrophobia	Fear of heights
Agoraphobia	Fear of open spaces
Astraphobia	Fear of electrical storms
Claustrophobia	Fear of closed spaces
Hematophobia	Fear of blood
Hydrophobia	Fear of water
Monophobia	Fear of being alone
Mysophobia	Fear of dirt or germs
Nyctophobia	Fear of darkness
Pyrophobia	Fear of fires
Social phobia	Fear of situations in which one might be embarrassed or criticized and the fear of making a fool of oneself
Xenophobia	Fear of strangers
Zoophobia	Fear of animals

---

5. Teach relaxation techniques such as breathing exercises, muscle relaxation exercises, and visualization of pleasant situations.
6. Do not force the client to have contact with the phobic object or situation.

V. OBSESSIVE-COMPULSIVE DISORDER

A. Obsessions: preoccupation with persistent intrusive thoughts and ideas
B. Compulsions
   1. A compulsion is a repeated performance of rituals or purposeless behaviors designed to prevent some event, divert unacceptable thoughts, and decrease anxiety.
   2. Obsessions and compulsions often occur together and can disrupt normal activities.
   3. Anxiety occurs when one resists obsessions or compulsions and from being powerless to resist the thoughts or rituals.
   4. Obsessive thoughts can involve issues of violence, aggression, sexual behavior, orderliness, or religion and uncontrollably can interrupt conscious thoughts and the ability to function.
C. Compulsive behavior patterns
   1. Compulsive behavoir patterns decrease the anxiety.
   2. The patterns are associated with the obsessive thoughts.
   3. The patterns neutralize the thought.
   4. During stressful times, the ritualistic behavior increases.
   5. **Defense mechanisms** include repression, displacement, and undoing.
D. Interventions
   1. Identify the situations that precipitate the behavior.
   2. Do not interrupt the compulsive behaviors.
   3. Allow time for the client to perform the compulsive rituals.
   4. Provide for client safety related to the behaviors.

BOX 73-2

Types of Somatoform Disorders

Conversion disorder
Hypochondriasis
Somatization disorder

---

5. Implement a schedule for the client that distracts from the behaviors.
6. Set limits on the rituals that may interfere with the client's physical well-being to protect the client from physical harm.
7. Encourage the client to verbalize concerns.
8. Establish a written contract that will assist the client to decrease the frequency of compulsive behaviors gradually.

VI. SOMATOFORM DISORDERS

A. Description (Box 73-2)
   1. Somatoform disorders are characterized by persistent worry or complaints regarding physical illness without supporting physical findings.
   2. The client focuses on the physical signs and symptoms and is unable to control the signs and symptoms.
   3. The physical signs and symptoms increase with psychosocial stressors.
   4. The anxiety is redirected into a somatic concern.
B. Somatization disorder
   1. Description
      a. The client has multiple physical complaints involving multiple body systems.
      b. The emotional stress can result from anxiety, fear, depression, worry, or repressed anger.
      c. The client may unconsciously use somatization for secondary gains such as increased attention and decreased responsibilities.
   2. Assessment
      a. Physical complaints of pain, denial of emotional problems, signs of anxiety, fear, and low self-esteem
      b. Psychosexual symptoms
      c. Secondary gain
C. Hypochondriasis
   1. Description
      a. Hypochondriasis is the preoccupation with fears of having a serious disease.
      b. No evidence of physical illness exists.
      c. Hypochondriasis causes a significantly impaired social and occupational functioning.
   2. Assessment
      a. Preoccupation with physical functioning
      b. Frequent somatic complaints
      c. Complaints of fatigue and insomnia
      d. Anxiety
      e. Difficulty expressing feelings

f. Extensive use of home remedies or nonprescription medications

g. Repeatedly visiting the doctor

h. Secondary gain

▲ D. Conversion disorder

1. Description

a. Conversion disorder is a physical symptom or a deficit suggesting loss or altered body function related to psychological conflict or a neurological disorder.

b. Conversion disorder is an expression of a psychological conflict or need.

c. The most common conversion symptoms are blindness, deafness, paralysis, and the inability to talk.

d. Conversion disorder has no organic cause.

e. Symptoms are not produced intentionally by the client.

f. Symptoms are related directly to conflict and decrease anxiety.

2. Assessment

a. "La belle indifference": unconcerned with symptoms

b. Physical limitation or disability

c. Feelings of guilt, anxiety, or frustration

d. Low self-esteem and feelings of inadequacy

e. Unexpressed anger or conflict

f. Secondary gain

E. Interventions

1. Obtain a nursing history and assess for physical problems.

▲ 2. Do not reinforce the sick role.

3. Discourage verbalization about physical symptoms by not responding with positive reinforcement.

4. Explore with the client the needs being met by the physical symptoms.

5. Assist the client to identify alternative ways of meeting needs.

6. Assist the client to relate feelings and conflicts to the physical symptoms.

▲ 7. Allow a specific time period to discuss physical complaints because the client will feel less threatened if this behavior is limited rather than stopped completely

▲ 8. Convey understanding that the physical symptoms are real to the client.

9. Assure the client that physical illness has been ruled out.

10. Explore the source of anxiety and stimulate verbalization of anxiety.

11. Encourage the use of relaxation techniques as the anxiety increases.

12. Implement pain-reduction measures as required.

13. Report and assess any new physical complaint.

▲ 14. Encourage diversional activities to decrease the client's focus on self.

15. Provide positive feedback for accomplishments to increase self-esteem.

16. Assist the client in recognizing their own feelings and emotions.

17. Establish a written contract with the client that will redirect the client's thoughts and feelings.

18. Administer antianxiety medications as prescribed.

VII. DISSOCIATIVE DISORDER

A. Description

1. Dissociative disorder is a disruption in integrative functions of memory, consciousness, or identity.

2. Dissociative disorder is associated with exposure to an extremely traumatic event.

B. Dissociative identity disorder (multiple personality)

1. Description

a. Two or more fully developed distinct and unique personalities exist within the person.

b. Personalities may take full control of the client, one at a time.

c. The personalities may or may not be aware of each other.

2. Assessment

a. The client may have an inability to recall important information (unrelated to ordinary forgetfulness).

b. Transition from one personality to the other is related to stress and is sudden.

c. Dissociation is used as a method of distancing and defending self from anxiety and traumatizing experiences.

C. Dissociative amnesia

1. Description

a. Dissociative amnesia is the inability to recall important personal information because it is anxiety provoking.

b. Memory impairment may be partial or almost complete.

2. Assessment

a. Localized: The client blocks out all memories about a specified period.

b. Selective: The client recalls some but not all memories about a specified period.

c. Generalized: Client has loss of all memory about past life.

D. Dissociative fugue

1. Description

a. The client assumes a new identity in a new environment.

b. The disorder may occur suddenly.

2. Assessment

a. Client may drift from place to place.

b. Client develops few social relationships.

c. When the fugue lifts, the client returns home and is unable to recall the fugue state.

E. Depersonalization disorder
   1. Description: an altered self-perception in which one's own reality is temporarily lost or changed
   2. Assessment
      a. Feelings of detachment
      b. Intact reality testing
F. Interventions
   1. Develop a trusting relationship with the client.
   2. Encourage verbal expression of painful experiences, anxieties, and concerns.
   3. Explore methods of coping.
   4. Identify sources of conflict.
   5. Focus on the client's strengths and skills.
   6. Orient the client.
   7. Provide nondemanding simple routines.
   8. Allow the client to progress at his or her own pace.
   9. Use stress-reduction techniques.
   10. Plan for individual, group, and/or family psychotherapy to integrate dissociated aspects of personality or memory and to expand self-awareness.

VIII. BIPOLAR DISORDER

A. Description (Box 73-3)
   1. Bipolar disorder is characterized by episodes of mania and depression with periods of normal mood and activity in between.
   2. The medication of choice is lithium carbonate, which can be toxic and therefore requires the regular monitoring of serum lithium levels.
B. Interventions for mania (Box 73-4)

BOX 73-3

Assessment of Bipolar Disorder

MANIA
Becomes angry quickly
Delusional self-confidence
Distracted by environmental stimuli
Extroverted personality
Flight of ideas
Grandiose and persecutory delusions
High and unstable affect
Inability to eat or sleep because of involvement in more important things
Inability to sleep yet still active
Inappropriate affect
Inappropriate dress
Initiation of activity
Pressured speech
Restlessness
Sexually promiscuous

Significant decrease in appetite
Unlimited energy
Urgent motor activity

DEPRESSION
Decrease in activities of daily living
Decreased emotion and physical activity
Easily fatigued
Inability to make decisions
Internalizing hostility
Introverted personality
Lack of energy
Lack of initiative
Lack of self-confidence
Lack of sexual interest
Withdrawn from groups

BOX 73-4

Dealing with Inappropriate Behaviors

AGGRESSIVE BEHAVIOR
Assist the client in identifying feelings of frustration and aggression.
Encourage the client to talk out instead of acting out feelings of frustration.
Assist the client in identifying precipitating events or situations that lead to aggressive behavior.
Describe the consequences of the behavior on self and others.
Assist in identifying previous coping mechanisms.
Assist the client in problem-solving techniques to cope with frustration or aggression.

DEESCALATION TECHNIQUES
Maintain safety for the client, other clients, and self.
Maintain a large personal space and use a nonaggressive posture.
Use a calm approach and communicate with a calm, clear tone of voice (be assertive not aggressive).

Determine what the client considers to be his or her need.
Avoid verbal struggles.
Provide the client with clear options that deal with the client's behavior.
Assist the client with problem-solving and decision making regarding the options.

MANIPULATIVE BEHAVIOR
Set clear, consistent, realistic, and enforceable limits and communicate expected behaviors.
Be clear about the consequences associated with exceeding set limits and follow through with the consequences in a nonpunitive manner if necessary.
Discuss the client's behavior in a nonjudgmental and nonthreatening manner.
Avoid power struggles with the client (avoid arguing with the client).
Assist the client in developing means of setting limits on own behavior.

1. Remove hazardous objects from the environment.
2. Assess the client closely for fatigue.
3. Use comfort measures to promote sleep.
4. Provide frequent rest periods.
5. Monitor the client's sleep patterns.
6. Provide a private room if possible.
7. Administer a hypnotic or sedative medication as prescribed.
8. Encourage the client to ventilate feelings.
9. Use calm, slow interactions.
10. Help the client focus on one topic during the conversation.
11. Ignore or distract the client from grandiose thinking.
12. Present reality to the client.
13. Do not argue with the client.
14. Limit group activities and assess the client's tolerance level.
15. Provide high-calorie finger foods and fluids.
16. Supervise the client's choice of clothing.
17. Reduce environmental stimuli.
18. Set limits on inappropriate behaviors.
19. Provide physical activities and outlets for tension.
20. Avoid competitive games.
21. Provide gross motor activities such as walking and writing.
22. Provide structured activities or one to one activities with the nurse.
23. Provide simple and direct explanations for routine procedures.
24. Supervise the administration of medication.

IX. SCHIZOPHRENIA

A. Description
1. Schizophrenia is a group of mental disorders characterized by psychotic features, inability to trust others, disordered thought processes, and disrupted interpersonal relationships.
2. Disturbances in affect, mood, behavior, and thought processes occur.

B. Assessment
1. Physical characteristics
   a. Disheveled appearance
   b. Body image distortions
   c. Preoccupied with somatic complaints
   d. Neglects eating, sleeping, and elimination
2. Motor activity (Box 73-5)
   a. Catatonic posturing: holding bizarre postures for long periods of time
   b. Catatonic excitement: moving excitedly with no environmental stimuli present
   c. Possible total immobilization
   d. Inability to respond to commands or responding only to commands
   e. Waxy flexibility
   f. Repetitive or stereotyped movements

BOX 73-5

Abnormal Motor Behaviors

DESCRIPTION
Abnormal motor behavior or activity displayed by the mentally ill client and occurring as a result of a psychiatric disorder

TYPES OF ABNORMAL MOTOR BEHAVIORS
Akathisia
Displaying motor restlessness and muscular quivering; the client is unable to sit or lie quietly
Echolalia
Repeating the speech of another person
Echopraxia
Repeating the movements of another person
Parkinson-like Symptoms
Making masklike faces, drooling, and having shuffling gait, tremors, and muscular rigidity
Waxy Flexibility
Having one's arms or legs placed in a certain position and holding that same position for hours
Dyskinesia
Impairment of the power of voluntary movements

---

   g. Motor activity that may be increased as evidenced by agitation, pacing, inability to sleep, loss of appetite and weight, and impulsiveness
   h. Possible inability to initiate activity, known as anergia
3. Emotional characteristics
   a. Mistrust
   b. View of the world as threatening and unsafe
   c. Feelings not easily interpreted
   d. Ambivalence manifested as compulsive rituals, negativism, and overcompliance
   e. Display of feelings of helplessness, anxiety, anger, guilt, and depression and decreased self-esteem
4. Compulsive rituals: attempt to solve conflicting feelings by constant, repetitive activity, which may be stereotyped or seem meaningless
5. Overcompliance: attempt to deny responsibility for any action by doing only what another exactly instructs
6. Affective disturbances
   a. Flat affect or inappropriate affect
   b. Altered thought processes
7. Thought processes (Box 73-6)
   a. Impaired reality testing
   b. Fragmentation of thoughts
   c. Blocking
   d. Loose associations
   e. Autistic thinking
   f. Perception of environment in a totally self-centered way
   g. Neologisms
   h. Magical thinking

BOX 73-6
Abnormal Thought Processes

DESCRIPTION
Abnormal thought processes displayed by the mentally ill client and occurring as a result of a psychiatric disorder

BLOCKING
A sudden cessation of a thought in the middle of a sentence; the client is unable to continue the train of thought; often sudden new thoughts come up unrelated to the topic

CIRCUMSTANTIALITY
Before getting to the point or answering a question, the individual gets caught up in countless details and explanations

CONFABULATION
Filling a memory gap with detailed fantasy believed by the teller; the purpose of confabulation is to maintain self-esteem; seen in organic conditions such as Korsakoff's psychosis

FLIGHT OF IDEAS
A constant flow of speech in which the individual jumps from one topic to another in rapid succession; a connection between topics exists, although it is sometimes difficult to identify; seen in manic states

LOOSENESS OF ASSOCIATION
Haphazard, illogical, and confused thinking and interrupted connections in thought; seen mostly in schizophrenic disorders

NEOLOGISMS
Words that an individual makes up that only have meaning for the individual; often part of a delusional system

WORD SALAD
A mixture of words and phrases that have no meaning

BOX 73-7
Delusions

DESCRIPTION
A false belief held to be true even when there is evidence to the contrary

TYPES
Grandeur
The false belief that one is a powerful and important person
Jealousy
The false belief that one's partner or mate is going out with other persons
Persecution
The thought that one is being singled out for harm by others

INTERVENTIONS
Ask the client to describe the delusion.
Be open and honest in interactions to reduce suspiciousness.
Focus the conversation on reality-based topics rather than on the delusion.
Encourage the client to express feelings and focus on the feelings that the delusions generate.
If the client obsesses on the delusion, set firm limits on the amount of time for talking about the delusion.
Do not dispute with the client or try to convince the client that the delusions are false.
Validate if part of the delusion is real.

---

i. Inability to conceptualize meaning in words or thoughts
j. Inability to organize facts logically
k. Delusions
8. Types of delusions (Box 73-7)
   a. Loss of reference in which the client believes that certain events, situations, or interactions are related directly to self
   b. Delusions of persecution in which the client believes that he or she is being harassed, threatened, or persecuted by some powerful force
   c. Delusions of grandeur in which the client attaches special significance to self in relation to others or the universe and has an exaggerated sense of self that has no basis in reality
   d. Somatic delusions in which the client believes that his or her body is changing or responding in an unusual way, which has no basis in reality
9. Perceptual distortions
   a. Illusions that may be brief experiences with a misinterpretation or misperception of reality
   b. Hallucinations such as perceiving objects, sensations, or images with no basis in reality (Box 73-8)
10. Language and communication disturbances (Box 73-9)
    a. Related to disorders in thought process
    b. Inability to organize language
    c. Difficulty communicating clearly
    d. Inappropriate responses to a situation
    e. A single word or phrase that may represent the whole meaning of the conversation such that the client may feel that he or she has communicated adequately
    f. Development of a private language
C. Types of schizophrenia (Box 73-10)
   1. Paranoid schizophrenia
      a. Suspiciousness
      b. Hostility
      c. Delusions
      d. Auditory hallucinations
      e. Anxiety and anger

BOX 73-8
Hallucinations

DESCRIPTION
A sense perception for which no external stimuli exist; can have an organic or functional cause

TYPES
Auditory
Hearing voices when none are present
Gustatory
Experiencing taste in the absence of stimuli
Olfactory
Smelling smells that do not exist
Tactile
Feeling touch sensations in the absence of stimuli
Visual
Seeing things that are not there

INTERVENTIONS
Ask the client directly about the hallucination.
Avoid reacting to the hallucination as if it were real.
Decrease stimuli or move the client to another area.
Do not negate the client's experience.
Focus on reality based topics.
Attempt to engage the client's attention through a concrete activity.
Respond verbally to anything real that the client talks about.
Avoid touching the client.
Monitor for signs of increasing anxiety or agitation, which may indicate that the hallucinations are increasing.

BOX 73-9
Language and Communication Disturbances

Clang association	Repetition of words or phrases that are similar in sound but in no other way
Echolalia	Repetition of words or phrases heard from another person
Mutism	Absence of verbal speech
Neologism	A new word devised that has special meaning only to the client
Pressured speech	Speaking as if the words are being forced out quickly
Verbigeration	Purposeless repetition of words or phrases
Word salad	Form of speech in which words or phrases are connected meaninglessly

BOX 73-10
Types of Schizophrenia

Catatonic
Disorganized
Paranoid
Residual
Undifferentiated

    f. Aloofness
    g. Persecutory themes
    h. Violence
  2. Disorganized schizophrenia
    a. Extreme social withdrawal
    b. Disorganized speech or behavior
    c. Flat or inappropriate affect
    d. Silliness unrelated to speech
    e. Stereotyped behaviors
    f. Grimacing mannerisms
    g. Inability to perform activities of daily living
  3. Catatonic schizophrenia
    a. Significant psychomotor disturbances
    b. Immobility
    c. Stupor
    d. Waxy flexibility
    e. Excessive purposeless motor activity
    f. Echolalia
    g. Automatic obedience
    h. Stereotyped or repetitive behavior
  4. Undifferentiated schizophrenia
    a. Undifferentiated schizophrenia does not meet the criteria for paranoid, disorganized, or catatonic schizophrenia.
    b. Delusions and hallucinations

    c. Disorganized speech
    d. Disorganized or catatonic behavior
    e. Flat affect
    f. Social withdrawal
  5. Residual schizophrenia
    a. Diagnosed as schizophrenic in the past
    b. Time limited between attacks but may last for many years
    c. The client exhibits considerable social isolation and withdrawal and impaired role functioning
D. Interventions: Refer to Box 73-11.
E. Interventions: active hallucinations
  1. Monitor for hallucination cues.
  2. Intervene with one-on-one contact.
  3. Decrease stimuli or move the client to another area.
  4. Avoid conveying to the client that others also are experiencing the hallucination.
  5. Respond verbally to anything real that the client talks about.
  6. Avoid touching the client.
  7. Encourage the client to express feelings.
  8. During a hallucination, attempt to engage the client's attention through a concrete activity.
  9. Accept and do not joke about or judge the client's behavior.
  10. Provide easy activities and a structured environment with routine activities of daily living.

BOX 73-11

Interventions for Schizophrenia

Assess the client's physical needs.

Set limits on the client's behaviors when it interferes with others and becomes disruptive.

Maintain a safe environment.

Initiate one-on-one interaction and progress to small groups as tolerated.

Spend time with the client even if client is unable to respond.

Monitor for altered thought processes.

Maintain ego boundaries and avoid touching the client.

Limit the time of interaction with the client.

Avoid an overly warm approach; a neutral approach is less threatening.

Do not make promises to the client that cannot be kept.

Establish daily routines.

Assist the client to improve grooming and accept responsibility for personal care.

Sit with the client in silence if necessary.

Provide short, brief and frequent contact with the client.

Tell the client when you are leaving.

Tell the client when you do not understand.

Do not "go along" with the client's delusions or hallucinations.

Provide simple concrete activities such as puzzles or word games.

Reorient the client as necessary.

Help the client establish what is real and unreal.

Stay with the client if the client is frightened.

Speak to the client in a simple direct and concise manner.

Reassure the client that the environment is safe.

Remove the client from group situations if the client's behavior is too bizarre, disturbing, or dangerous to others.

Set realistic goals.

Initially do not offer choices to the client, and gradually assist the client in making own decisions.

Use canned or packaged food, especially with the paranoid schizophrenic client.

Provide a radio or tape player at night for insomnia.

Explain to the client everything that is being done.

Set limits on the client's behavior if the client is unable to do so.

Decrease excessive stimuli in the environment.

Monitor for suicide risk.

Assist the client to use alternative means to express feelings through music or art therapy or writing.

---

11. Monitor for signs of increasing fear, anxiety, or agitation.
12. Provide **seclusion** as necessary.
13. Administer medications as prescribed.

F. Interventions: delusions
  1. Interact based on reality.
  2. Encourage the client to express feelings.
  3. Do not dispute with the client or try to convince the client that delusions are false.
  4. Initially initiate activities on a one-on-one basis.
  5. Alter hospital routines as necessary, such as using canned or packaged food or food from home.
  6. Recognize accomplishments and provide positive feedback for successes.

X. PARANOID DISORDERS

A. Description
  1. The client demonstrates suspiciousness and mistrust of others.
  2. The client often is viewed by others as hostile, stubborn, and defensive.
  3. Paranoid disorder is a concrete, pervasive delusional system characterized by persecutory and grandiose beliefs.

B. Behaviors
  1. Suspicious and mistrustful
  2. Emotionally distant
  3. Distortion of reality
  4. Poor insight
  5. Hypervigilance

6. Low self-esteem
7. Highly sensitive, difficulty in admitting own error, and taking pride in being correct
8. Hypercritical and intolerant of others
9. Hostile, aggressive, and quarrelsome
10. Evasive
11. Concrete thinking

C. Delusions
  1. Delusions serve a purpose in establishing identity and self-esteem.
  2. Client may have grandiose and persecutory delusions.
  3. Process of delusion includes denial, projection, and rationalization.
  4. As trust in others increases, the need for delusions decreases.

D. Types of paranoid disorders (Box 73-12)
  1. Paranoid personality
     a. Suspicious
     b. Nonpsychotic
     c. No hallucinations or delusions
     d. No symptoms of schizophrenia

BOX 73-12

Types of Paranoid Disorders

Paranoid personality
Paranoid state
Paranoia
Paranoid schizophrenia

2. Paranoid state
   a. Onset abrupt in response to stress and subsides when stress decreases
   b. No hallucinations but experiences paranoid delusions
   c. May be sensitive and suspicious before the development of delusions
   d. Psychotic state
   e. No symptoms of schizophrenia
3. Paranoia
   a. Client appears normal except for delusional system
   b. Single, highly organized delusional system
   c. Not bizarre
   d. No hallucinations
   e. Reserved and sensitive before onset
   f. Psychotic state
   g. No symptoms of schizophrenia
4. Paranoid schizophrenia
   a. Before the onset client becomes cold, withdrawn, distrustful, resentful, argumentative, sarcastic, and defiant.
   b. Bizarre, numerous, and changeable delusions occur.
   c. Delusions become less logical as the client becomes more disorganized.
   d. Persecutory hallucinations occur.
   e. Psychotic state ensues.
   f. All symptoms of schizophrenia are present.
E. Interventions (Box 73-13)

XI. PERSONALITY DISORDERS
A. Description
   1. Personality disorders include various inflexible maladaptive behavior patterns or traits that may impair functioning and relationships.
   2. The individual usually remains in touch with reality and typically has a lack of insight into his or her behavior.
   3. Stress exacerbates manifestations of the personality disorder.
   4. In severe cases the personality disorder may deteriorate to a psychotic state.
B. Characteristics
   1. Poor impulse control
      a. Acting out to manage internal pain
      b. Forms of acting out include physical and verbal attacks, manipulation, substance **abuse**, promiscuous sexual behaviors, and **suicide attempts**
   2. Mood characteristics
      a. Experience abandonment and depression
      b. Moods that include rage, guilt, fear, and emptiness
   3. Impaired judgment
      a. Difficulty with problem solving

BOX 73-13

Interventions for Paranoid Disorders

Assess for suicide risk.
Diminish suspicious behavior.
Avoid direct eye contact.
Establish a trusting relationship.
Promote increased self-esteem.
Remain calm, nonthreatening, and nonjudgmental.
Provide continuity of care.
Respond honestly to the client.
Follow through on commitments made to the client.
Acknowledge the client's feelings but tell the client that you do not share the client's interpretation of an event.
Provide a daily schedule of activities.
Assist the client to identify diversionary activities.
Gradually introduce the client to groups.
Refocus conversation to reality-based topics.
Use role playing to help the client identify thoughts and feelings.
Provide positive reinforcement for successes.
Do not argue with delusions.
Use concrete, specific words.
Do not be secretive with the client.
Do not whisper in the client's presence.
Assure the client that he or she will be safe.
Involve the client in noncompetitive tasks.
Provide the client opportunity to complete small tasks.
Monitor eating, drinking, sleeping, and elimination patterns.
Limit physical contact.
Monitor for agitation and decrease stimuli as needed.

---

   b. Inability to perceive the consequences of behavior
   4. Impaired reality testing: distortion of reality and often projection of own feelings onto others
   5. Impaired object relations: rigid and inflexible, with difficulty in intimate relationships
   6. Impaired self-perception: distorted self-perception and experience of self-hate or self-idealization
   7. Impaired thought processes
      a. Concrete or diffuse thinking
      b. Difficulty concentrating
      c. Impaired memory
   8. Impaired stimulus barrier
      a. Inability to regulate incoming sensory stimuli
      b. Increased excitability
      c. Excessive response to noise and light
      d. Poor attention span
      e. Agitated
      f. Insomnia
C. Schizoid personality disorder
   1. Description: characterized by an inability to form warm, close social relationships
   2. Assessment
      a. Social detachment and lack of close relationships
      b. Interest in solitary activities

c. Aloof and indifferent

d. Restricted expression of emotions

e. Lack of interest in others

D. Schizotypal personality disorder

1. Description: exhibition of abnormal or highly unusual thoughts, perceptions, speech, and behavior patterns

2. Assessment

a. Suspicious

b. Paranoia

c. Magical thinking

d. Odd thinking and speech

e. Relationship deficits

E. Paranoid personality disorder

1. Description: characterized by suspiciousness and mistrust of others

2. Assessment

a. Suspicious and distrusting

b. Argumentative

c. Hostile aloofness

d. Rigid, critical, and controlling of others

e. Grandiosity

F. Histrionic personality disorder

1. Description

a. Characterized by overly dramatic and intensely expressive behavior

b. Client is lively and dramatic and enjoys being the center of attention

c. Interpersonal relations may be poor

2. Assessment

a. Attention seeking

b. Need to be the center of attention

c. Sexually seductive or provocative

d. Self-dramatizing and theatrical

e. Overly concerned with appearance

f. Romantic fantasies and control of partners

g. Easily bored

h. Display of dependency

G. Narcissistic personality disorder

1. Description

a. Characterized by an increased sense of self-importance

b. Client is preoccupied with fantasies and unlimited success and has a constant need for attention and admiration

2. Assessment

a. Grandiosity

b. Need for admiration and inflation of accomplishments

c. Overestimation of abilities and underestimation of contributions of others

d. Lack of empathy and sensitivity to needs of others

H. Avoidant personality disorder

1. Description: characterized by social withdrawal and extreme sensitivity to potential rejection

2. Assessment

a. Feelings of inadequacy

b. Hypersensitive to reactions of others and poor reaction to criticism

c. Social inhibition

d. Lack of support system

I. Dependent personality disorder

1. Description

a. The individual lacks self-confidence and the ability to function independently.

b. Person passively allows others to make decisions and assume responsibility for major areas in the person's life.

2. Assessment

a. Person has difficulty making decisions.

b. Person lacks autonomy.

c. Person cannot tolerate being alone and always must have a close relationship.

d. Person needs others to assume responsibility and make decisions.

J. Obsessive-compulsive personality disorder

1. Description: the client has difficulty expressing warm and tender emotions and reflects perfectionism, stubbornness, the need to control others, and a devotion to work

2. Assessment

a. Orderliness and perfectionism

b. Overly conscientious

c. Inflexible and preoccupied with details and rules

d. Devoted to work and lacks leisure activities and friendships

e. Miserly and stubborn

f. Hoards worthless objects

K. Antisocial personality disorder

1. Description

a. A pattern of irresponsible and antisocial behavior

b. Characterized by selfishness, inability to maintain lasting relationships, poor sexual adjustment, failure to accept social norms, irritability, and aggressiveness

2. Assessment

a. Perception of the world as hostile

b. Superficial charm and hostility

c. No shame or guilt

d. Self-centered

e. Unreliable

f. Easily bored

g. Poor work history

h. Inability to tolerate frustration

i. View others as objects to be manipulated

j. Poor judgment

k. Impulsive

L. Borderline personality disorder

1. Description

a. Characterized by instability in interpersonal relationships, mood, and self-image

b. Behavior may be impulsive and unpredictable

2. Assessment
   a. Unclear identity
   b. Unstable and intense
   c. Extreme shifts in mood
   d. Easily angered
   e. Easily bored
   f. Argumentative
   g. Depression
   h. Self-destructive behavior
   i. Manipulation
   j. Inability to tolerate anxiety
   k. Chronic feelings of emptiness and fear of being alone
   l. Splitting

M. Passive-aggressive personality disorder
   1. Description
      a. Characterized by passively expressing covert aggression rather than dealing with it directly
      b. Behavior can interfere with social and work activities
   2. Assessment
      a. Procrastination
      b. Stubbornness
      c. Intentional inefficiency
      d. Forgetfulness
      e. Dependency

N. Interventions
   1. Maintain safety against self-destructive behaviors.
   2. Allow the client to make choices and be as independent as possible.
   3. Encourage the client to discuss feelings rather than act them out.
   4. Provide consistency in response to the client's acting-out behaviors.
   5. Discuss expectations and responsibilities with the client.
   6. Discuss the consequences that will follow certain behaviors.
   7. Inform the client that harm to self, others, and property is unacceptable.
   8. Identify splitting behavior.
   9. Assist the client to deal directly with anger.
   10. Develop a written contract with the client.
   11. Encourage the client to keep a journal recording daily feelings.
   12. Encourage the client to participate in group activities, and praise nonmanipulative behavior.
   13. Set and maintain limits to decrease manipulative behavior.
   14. Remove the client from group situations in which attention-seeking behaviors occur.
   15. Provide realistic praise for positive behaviors in social situations.

XII. COGNITIVE IMPAIRMENT DISORDERS
A. Autism: Refer to Chapter 35.

B. Attention deficit hyperactivity disorder: Refer to Chapter 35.
C. Tourette's disorder: Refer to Chapter 35.
D. Dementia and Alzheimer's disease
   1. Dementia
      a. Dementia is an organic syndrome with progressive deterioration in intellectual functioning.
      b. Long- and short-term memory loss occurs with impairment in judgment, abstract thinking, problem-solving ability, and behavior.
      c. Dementia results in a self-care deficit.
      d. The most common type of dementia is Alzheimer's disease.
   2. Alzheimer's disease (Box 73-14)
      a. Alzheimer's disease is an irreversible form of senile dementia from nerve cell deterioration.
      b. Individuals with Alzheimer's disease experience cognitive deterioration and progressive loss of ability to carry out activities of daily living.
      c. The client experiences a steady decline in physical and mental functioning and usually requires nursing home placement in the final stages of the illness.
   3. Interventions
      a. Identify and reinforce retained skills.
      b. Provide continuity of care.
      c. Orient client to the environment.
      d. Furnish environment with familiar possessions.
      e. Acknowledge the client's feelings.
      f. Assist the client and family members to manage memory deficits and behavior changes.
      g. Encourage the family members to express feelings about caregiving.
      h. Provide the caregiver support and identify the resources and support groups available.
      i. Monitor activities of daily living.
      j. Remind client how to perform self-care activities.
      k. Maintain independence.
      l. Provide consistent routines.
      m. Provide exercise such as walking with an escort.
      n. Avoid activities that tax the memory.
      o. Allow plenty of time to complete a task.
      p. Use constant encouragement in a step-by-step approach.

BOX 73-14

Alzheimer's Disease

Agnosia	Failure to recognize or identify objects despite intact sensory function
Amnesia	Loss of memory caused by brain degeneration
Aphasia	Language disturbance in understanding and expressing the spoken word
Apraxia	Inability to perform motor activities despite intact motor function

q. Provide activities that distract and occupy time, such as listening to music, coloring, and watching television.

r. Provide mental stimulation with simple games or activities.

4. Wandering
   a. Provide a safe environment.
   b. Prevent unsafe wandering.
   c. Provide close supervision.
   d. Close and secure doors.
   e. Use identification bracelets and electronic surveillance.

5. Communication
   a. Adapt to the communication level of the client.
   b. Use a firm volume and a low-pitched voice to communicate.
   c. Stand directly in front of the client and maintain eye contact.
   d. Call the client by name and identify self; wait for a response.
   e. Use a calm and reassuring voice.
   f. Use pantomime gestures if the client is unable to understand spoken words.
   g. Use slow, clear, verbal communication techniques.
   h.. Use short words and simple sentences.
   i. Ask only one question at a time and give one direction at a time.
   j. Repeat questions if necessary but do not rephrase.

6. Impaired judgment
   a. Remove throw rugs, toxic substances, and dangerous electrical appliances from the environment.
   b. Reduce hot water heater temperature.

7. Altered thought processes
   a. Call the client by name.
   b. Orient the client frequently.
   c. Use familiar objects in the room.
   d. Place a calendar and clock in a visible place.
   e. Maintain familiar routines.
   f. Allow the client to reminisce.
   g. Make tasks simple.
   h. Allow time for the client to complete a task.
   i. Provide positive reinforcement for positive behaviors.

8. Altered sleep patterns
   a. Allow client to wander in a safe place until client becomes tired.
   b. Prevent shadows in the room.
   c. Avoid the use of hypnotics because they cause confusion and aggravate the sundown effect.

9. Agitation
   a. Assess the precipitant of the agitation.
   b. Reassure the client.
   c. Remove items that can be hazardous during the time of agitation.

d. Approach the client slowly and calmly from the front and then speak, gesture, and move slowly.

e. Remove the client to a less stressful environment.

f. Use touch gently.

g. Do not argue with the client or restrain the client.

h. Distract the client with questions about the problem and gradually turn the attention to something else.

XIII. PSYCHOSEXUAL ALTERATIONS

A. Sexuality
   1. One's sense of being a sexual individual
   2. Includes how one looks, behaves, and relates to others

B. Sexual expression (Box 73-15)

C. Alterations in sexual behavior
   1. Transsexualism: feeling that one's sex is inappropriate and desiring to acquire sexual characteristics of the opposite sex
   2. Exhibitionism: sexual urges and fantasies and exposure of genitals to strangers
   3. Fetishism: using nonliving objects for sexual gratification
   4. Pedophelia: desiring sexual activity with a child under age 13
   5. Sexual masochism: sexual gratification that involves receiving pain
   6. Sexual sadism: sexual gratification that involves inflicting pain
   7. Voyeurism: sexual gratification through observing others disrobing or engaging in sexual activity
   8. Zoophilia: intense sexual arousal or desire for sexual contact with animals
   9. Frotteurism: intense sexual arousal or desire when rubbing against a nonconsenting person

D. Interventions
   1. Assess sexual history and precipitating event for sexual disorder.
   2. Encourage the client to explore personal beliefs.
   3. Provide a nonjudgmental attitude.
   4. Provide supportive psychotherapy.

BOX 73-15

Sexual Expression

Bisexuality	Sexual attraction to and activity with both sexes
Heterosexuality	Male-female sexual relationships
Homosexuality	Sexual attraction to a member of the same sex
Transvestism	Obsession with wearing clothing of the opposite sex

PRACTICE QUESTIONS

1. The nurse is planning activities for a client who has bipolar disorder with aggressive social behavior. Which of the following activities would be most appropriate for this client?
   1. Ping pong
   2. Writing
   3. Chess
   4. Basketball

2. A client is admitted to the hospital with a diagnosis of major depression, severe, single episode. The nurse assesses the client and identifies a nursing diagnosis of imbalanced nutrition related to poor nutritional intake. The most appropriate nursing intervention related to this diagnosis is
   1. Explain to the client the importance of a good nutritional intake.
   2. Weigh the client 3 times per week before breakfast.
   3. Report the nutritional concern to the psychiatrist and obtain a nutritional consultation as soon as possible.
   4. Consult with the nutritionist, offer the client several small meals per day, and schedule brief nursing interactions with the client during these times.

3. In planning activities for the depressed client, especially during the early stages of hospitalization, which of the following plans is best?
   1. Provide an activity that is quiet and solitary to avoid increased fatigue, such as working on a puzzle or reading a book.
   2. Plan nothing until the client asks to participate in milieu.
   3. Offer the client a menu of daily activities and insist the client participate in all of them.
   4. Provide a structured daily program of activities and encourage the client to participate.

4. The depressed client verbalizes feelings of low self-esteem and self-worth typified by statements such as "I'm such a failure … I can't do anything right!" The best nursing response would be
   1. To tell the client that this is not true; that we all have a purpose in life.
   2. To remain with the client and sit in silence; this will encourage the client to verbalize feelings.
   3. To reassure the client that you know how the client is feeling and that things will get better.
   4. To identify recent behaviors or accomplishments that demonstrate skill ability.

5. A client with a diagnosis of major depression, recurrent with psychotic features is admitted to the mental health unit. To create a safe environment for the client, the nurse most importantly devises a plan of care that deals specifically with the client's
   1. Disturbed Thought Processes.
   2. Imbalanced Nutrition.
   3. Self-Care Deficit.
   4. Deficient Knowledge.

6. A depressed client is ready for discharge. The nurse feels comfortable that the client has a good understanding of the disease process when the client states
   1. "I'll never let this happen to me again. I won't let my boss or my job or my family get to me!"
   2. "It's important for me to eat well, exercise, and to take my medication. If I begin to lose my appetite or not sleep well, I've got to get in to see my doctor."
   3. "I've learned I am a good person and that I am worthy of giving and receiving love. I don't need anyone, I have myself to rely on!"
   4. "I don't know what happened to me. I've always been able to make decisions for myself and for my business. I don't ever want to feel so weak or vulnerable again!"

7. The nurse assesses a client with the admitting diagnosis of bipolar affective disorder, mania. The symptom presented by the client that requires the nurse's immediate intervention is the client's
   1. Outlandish behaviors and inappropriate dress.
   2. Grandiose delusions of being a royal descendent of King Arthur.
   3. Nonstop physical activity and poor nutritional intake.
   4. Constant, incessant talking that includes sexual innuendoes and teasing the staff.

8. The nurse reviews the activity schedule for the day and plans which activity for the manic client?
   1. Brown-bag luncheon and a book review
   2. Tetherball
   3. Paint-by-number activity
   4. Deep breathing and progressive relaxation group

9. A client who is delusional says to the nurse, "The federal guards were sent to kill me." The nurse's best response is
   1. "The guards are not out to kill you."
   2. "I don't believe this is true."
   3. "I don't know anything about the guards. Do you feel afraid that people are trying to hurt you?"
   4. "What makes you think the guards were sent to hurt you?"

10. A woman comes into the emergency room in a severe state of anxiety following a car accident. The most appropriate nursing intervention is to
    1. Remain with the client.
    2. Put the client in a quiet room.
    3. Teach the client deep breathing.
    4. Encourage the client to talk about their feelings and concerns.

11. A male client with delirium becomes disoriented and confused in his room at night. The best initial nursing intervention is to
    1. Use a night light and turn off the television.

2. Keep the television and a soft light on during the night.

3. Move the client next to the nurse's station.

4. Play soft music during the night, and maintain a well-lit room.

12. A hospitalized client is being considered for electroconvulsive therapy. The client appears calm, but the family is anxious. The client's mother begins to cry and states, "My son's brain will be destroyed. How can the doctor do this to him?" The nurse's best response is

1. "It sounds as though you need to speak to the psychiatrist."

2. "Your son has decided to have this treatment. You should be supportive to him."

3. "Perhaps you'd like to see the electroconvulsive therapy room and speak to the staff."

4. "It sounds as though you have some concerns about the electroconvulsive therapy procedure. Why don't we sit down together and discuss any concerns you may have."

13. The nurse is performing an assessment on a client with dementia. Which data gathered during the assessment would indicate a manifestation associated with dementia?

1. Presence of personal hygienic care

2. Improvement in sleeping

3. Absence of sundown syndrome

4. Confabulation

14. The community health nurse visits a client who recently retired. The client states, "Lately I'm getting forgetful about things. Do you think I'm getting Alzheimer's disease?" Which response by the nurse would be most therapeutic?

1. "Tell me more about your forgetfulness. It isn't unusual for forgetfulness to occur if memory is not exercised. Are you staying socially active?"

2. "Oh, I'm certain it's not Alzheimer's disease because there's no family history of it."

3. "Now, I'm not going to discuss this with you because I think you're just normal."

4. "I am so forgetful too. I have to make out lists now to go shopping."

15. The nurse is discharging a client with a history of command hallucinations to harm self or others. The nurse provides instructions to the client about interventions for hallucinations and anxiety and determines that the client understands the instructions if the client states

1. "My medications won't make me anxious."

2. "I can call my therapist when I'm hallucinating so that I can talk about my feelings and plans and not hurt anyone."

3. "I'll go to support group and talk so that I don't hurt anyone."

4. " I won't get anxious or hear things if I get enough sleep and eat well."

16. The nurse develops a nursing diagnosis of self-care deficit for an older client with dementia. Which of the following is the most appropriate goal for this client?

1. The client will be admitted to a long-term care facility to have activities of daily living needs met.

2. The client will function at the highest level of independence possible.

3. The client will complete all activities of daily living independently within a 1 hour time frame.

4. The nursing staff will attend to all the client's activities of daily living needs during the hospital stay.

17. The nurse observes that a client is pacing, agitated, and presenting aggressive gestures. The client's speech pattern is rapid, and affect is belligerent. Based on these observations, the nurse's immediate priority of care is to

1. Provide safety for the client and other clients on the unit.

2. Offer the client a less stimulated area to calm down and gain control.

3. Provide the clients on the unit with a sense of comfort and safety.

4. Assist the staff in caring for the client in a controlled environment.

18. The nurse is caring for a male client diagnosed with catatonic stupor. The client is lying on the bed with the body pulled into a fetal position. The most appropriate nursing intervention is which of the following?

1. Leave the client alone and intermittently check on him.

2. Take the client into the dayroom with other clients so they can help watch him.

3. Sit beside the client in silence with occasional open-ended questions.

4. Ask direct questions to encourage talking.

19. The client is admitted to the mental health unit with a diagnosis of schizophrenia. A nursing diagnosis formulated for the client is disturbed thought process, related to paranoia. In formulating nursing interventions with the members of the health care team, the nurse provides instructions to

1. Avoid laughing or whispering in front of the client.

2. Increase socialization of the client with peers.

3. Have the client sign a release of information to appropriate parties so that adequate data can be obtained for assessment purposes.

4. Begin to educate the client about social supports in the community.

20. A client is admitted to the mental health unit with a diagnosis of depression. The nurse develops a plan of care for the client and includes which most appropriate activity in the plan?

1. Reading and writing most of the day
2. Nothing until the client asks to participate in milieu
3. Several activities that the client can choose from
4. A structured program of activities for the client to participate in

21. When planning the discharge of a client with chronic anxiety, the nurse directs the goals at promoting a safe environment at home. The most appropriate maintenance goal should focus on which of the following?
    1. Continued contact with a crisis counselor
    2. Identifying anxiety-producing situations
    3. Ignoring feelings of anxiety
    4. Eliminating all anxiety from daily situations

22. The client is unwilling to go out of the house for fear of "doing something crazy in public." Because of this fear the client remains homebound except when accompanied outside by the spouse. Based on this data, the nurse determines that the client is experiencing
    1. Social phobia.
    2. Agoraphobia.
    3. Claustrophobia.
    4. Hypochondriasis.

23. A nurse is conducting a group therapy session. During the session, a client with mania consistently talks and dominates the group session and her behavior is disrupting group interactions. The nurse would initially
    1. Ask the client to leave the group session.
    2. Tell the client that she will not be able to attend any future group sessions.
    3. Tell the client that she needs to allow other client's in the group time to talk.
    4. Ask another nurse to escort the client out of the group session.

24. A client is admitted to a medical nursing unit with a diagnosis of acute blindness. Many tests are performed, and there seems to be no organic reason why this client cannot see. The nurse later learns that the client became blind after witnessing a hit-and-run car accident, when a family of three was killed. The nurse suspects that the client may be experiencing a
    1. Psychosis.
    2. Conversion disorder.
    3. Dissociative disorder.
    4. Repression.

25. The manic client announces to everyone in the day-room that a stripper is coming to perform this evening. When the nurse firmly states that this will not happen, the manic client becomes verbally abusive and threatens physical violence to the nurse. Based on the analysis of this situation, the nurse determines that the most appropriate action would be to
    1. With assistance, escort the manic client to her room and administer haloperidol (Haldol) as prescribed if needed.
    2. Tell the client that smoking privileges are revoked for 24 hours.
    3. Orient the client to time, person, and place.
    4. Tell the client that the behavior is not appropriate.

CRITICAL THINKING: MULTIPLE RESPONSE

Select all nursing interventions for a hospitalized client with mania who is exhibiting manipulative behavior.

____ Communicate expected behaviors to the client.

____ Enforce rules and inform the client that he or she will not be allowed to attend therapy groups.

____ Ensure that the client knows that he or she is not in charge of the nursing unit.

____ Be clear with the client regarding the consequences of exceeding limits set regarding behavior.

____ Assist the client in testing out alternative behaviors for obtaining needs.

ANSWERS

1. 2
Rationale: Solitary activities that require a short attention span with mild physical exertion are the most appropriate activities for a client who is exhibiting aggressive behavior. Writing (journaling), walks with staff, and finger painting are activities that minimize stimuli and provide a constructive release for tension. Competitive games should be avoided because they can stimulate aggression and increase psychomotor activity.
Test-Taking Strategy: Use the process of elimination. Options 1, 3, and 4 are similar in that they are activities that the client cannot do alone. Option 2 identifies a solitary activity. Review

care to the client with aggressive behavior if you had difficulty with this question.
Level of Cognitive Ability: Application
Client Needs: Physiological Integrity
Integrated Process: Nursing Process—planning
Content Area: Mental health
Reference: Varcarolis, E. (2002). *Foundations of psychiatric mental health nursing* (4th ed., p. 517). Philadelphia: W. B. Saunders.

2. 4
Rationale: Change in appetite is one of the major symptoms of depression. Other symptoms include a depressed mood,

increased fatigue, feelings of worthlessness, diminished ability to think or indecisiveness, and psychomotor agitation or retardation. Option 1 is incorrect because the client is experiencing poor concentration; hence even if the client does understand the rationale, the client still may not be able to complete tasks. Weighing the client does not address how to increase nutritional intake. Reporting to the psychiatrist and the nutritionist is to some degree correct but lacks the method as to how one might increase food intake.
Test-Taking Strategy: Use the process of elimination focusing on the issue, poor nutritional status. Option 4 is the only option that addresses the imbalanced nutrition concretely and designs a method in which the client feasibly will increase the nutritional intake. Review care to the client with depression if you had difficulty with this question.
Level of Cognitive Ability: Application
Client Needs: Physiological Integrity
Integrated Process: Nursing Process—implementation
Content Area: Mental health
References: Fortinash, K., & Holoday-Worret, P. (2000). *Psychiatric mental health nursing* (2nd ed., p. 287). St. Louis: Mosby.
Varcarolis, E. (2002). *Foundations of psychiatric mental health nursing* (4th ed., p. 468). Philadelphia: W. B. Saunders.

3. 4
Rationale: A depressed person experiences a depressed mood and often is withdrawn. The person also experiences difficulty concentrating, loss of interest or pleasure, low energy, fatigue, and feelings of worthlessness and poor self-esteem. The plan of care needs to provide successful experiences in a stimulating yet structured environment. Options 1 and 2 provide little or no structure. Option 3 is a forceful and absolute approach.
Test-Taking Strategy: Use the process of elimination. Recall that the depressed client requires a structured/stimulating program. Eliminate options 1 and 2 because these provide little or no structure and stimulation. Option 3 is eliminated because of the word "all." Review care to the client with depression if you had difficulty with this question.
Level of Cognitive Ability: Application
Client Needs: Psychosocial Integrity
Integrated Process: Nursing Process—planning
Content Area: Mental health
Reference: Varcarolis, E. (2002). *Foundations of psychiatric mental health nursing* (4th ed., p. 487). Philadelphia: W. B. Saunders.

4. 4
Rationale: Feelings of low self-esteem and worthlessness are common symptoms of the depressed client. An effective plan of care to enhance the client's personal self-esteem is to provide experiences for the client that are challenging but will not be met with failure. Reminders of the client's past accomplishments or personal successes are ways to interrupt the client's negative self-talk and distorted cognitive view of self. Silence may be interpreted as agreement. Options 1 and 3 give advice and devalue the client's feelings.
Test-Taking Strategy: Use the process of elimination and therapeutic communication techniques. Focus on the client's diagnosis. You can eliminate options 1 and 3 easily. From the

remaining options, focusing on the client's diagnosis will direct you to option 4. Review care to the client with depression if you had difficulty with this question.
Level of Cognitive Level: Application
Client Needs: Psychosocial Integrity
Integrated Process: Nursing Process—implementation
Content Area: Mental health
Reference: Varcarolis, E. (2002). *Foundations of psychiatric mental health nursing* (4th ed., pp. 462, 467). Philadelphia: W. B. Saunders.

5. 1
Rationale: Major depression, recurrent, with psychotic features alerts the nurse that in addition to the criteria that designates the diagnosis of major depression, one also must deal with the client's psychosis. Psychosis is defined as a state in which a person's mental capacity to recognize reality and to communicate and relate to others is impaired, thus interfering with the person's capacity to deal with the demands of life. Altered thought processes generally indicate a state of increased anxiety in which hallucinations and delusions prevail. Although all of the nursing diagnoses may be appropriate because the client is experiencing psychosis, option 1 is the correct option.
Test-Taking Strategy: Use the process of elimination. All of the nursing diagnoses listed may be appropriate for a client diagnosed with major depression. The key to the correct option lies with the words "psychotic features" in which the client often suffers with altered thought processes, such as hallucinations and delusions. Review appropriate nursing diagnoses for major depression and psychotic features if you had difficulty with this question.
Level of Cognitive Ability: Analysis
Client Needs: Safe, Effective Care Environment
Integrated Process: Nursing Process—planning
Content Area: Mental health
Reference: Stuart, G., & Laraia, M. (2001). *Principles & practice of psychiatric nursing* (7th ed., p. 362). St. Louis: Mosby.

6. 2
Rationale: The exact cause of depression is not known but is believed to be related to a biochemical disruption of neurotransmitters in the brain. Diet, exercise, and medication are recognized treatment for the disease process. Options 1, 3, and 4 offer no insight into the disease process. In addition, options 1 and 4 reflect possible blaming or personal failure; option 3, an unwillingness to reach out to others.
Test-Taking Strategy: Use the process of elimination, looking for the global option. Option 2 is the only option that incorporates a holistic treatment approach, good nutrition, exercise, and medication, as well as the client's knowledge of the signs of possible relapse. Review concepts related to depression if you had difficulty with this question.
Level of Cognitive Ability: Analysis
Client Needs: Health Promotion and Maintenance
Integrated Process: Nursing Process—evaluation
Content Area: Mental health
Reference: Fortinash, K., & Holoday-Worret, P. (2000). *Psychiatric mental health nursing* (2nd ed., p. 276). St. Louis: Mosby.

7. 3

Rationale: Mania is a mood characterized by excitement, euphoria, hyperactivity, excessive energy, decreased need for sleep, and impaired ability to concentrate or complete a single train of thought. Mania is a period when the mood is predominantly elevated, expansive, or irritable. All options reflect a client's possible symptomatology. Option 3, however, clearly presents a problem that compromises one's physiological integrity and needs to be addressed immediately.

Test-Taking Strategy: Note the key word "immediate" and use Maslow's hierarchy of needs theory to assist you in answering the question. Option 3 is the only option that reflects a physiological need. Review care to the client with mania if you had difficulty with this question.

Level of Cognitive Ability: Analysis
Client Needs: Physiological Integrity
Integrated Process: Nursing Process—assessment
Content Area: Delegating/Prioritizing
Reference: Stuart, G., & Laraia, M. (2001). *Principles & practice of psychiatric nursing* (7th ed., p. 351). St. Louis: Mosby.

8. 2

Rationale: A person who is experiencing mania is overactive and full of energy, lacks concentration, and has poor impulse control. The client needs an activity that will allow use of excess energy yet not endanger others during the process. Options 1, 3, and 4 are relatively sedate activities that require concentration, a quality that is lacking in the manic state. Such activities may lead to increased frustration and anxiety for the client. Tetherball is an exercise that uses the large muscle groups of the body and is a great way to expend the increased energy this client is experiencing.

Test-Taking Strategy: Use the process of elimination. Eliminate options 1, 3, and 4 because they are similar and relatively sedate activities. Review the appropriate interventions for a manic client if you had difficulty with this question.

Level of Cognitive Ability: Application
Client Needs: Psychosocial Integrity
Integrated Process: Nursing Process—planning
Content Area: Mental health
Reference: Stuart, G., & Laraia, M. (2001). *Principles & practice of psychiatric nursing* (7th ed., p. 376). St. Louis: Mosby.

9. 3

Rationale: For the nurse to empathize with the client's experience is most therapeutic. Disagreeing with delusions may make the client more defensive, and the client may cling to the delusions even more. Encouraging discussion regarding the delusion is inappropriate.

Test-Taking Strategy: Use therapeutic communication techniques. Eliminate options 1 and 2 because they are similar and are statements that disagree with the client. Option 4 is encouraging discussion regarding the delusion. Review communication techniques with the client experiencing delusions if you had difficulty with this question.

Level of Cognitive Ability: Application
Client Needs: Psychosocial Integrity
Integrated Process: Communication and Documentation
Content Area: Mental health

Reference: Varcarolis, E. (2002). *Foundations of psychiatric mental health nursing* (4th ed., p. 254). Philadelphia: W. B. Saunders.

10. 1

Rationale: If a client with severe anxiety is left alone, the client may feel abandoned and become overwhelmed. Placing the client in a quiet room is also important, but the nurse must stay with the client. Teaching the client deep breathing or relaxation is not possible until the anxiety decreases. Encouraging the client to discuss concerns and feelings would not take place until the anxiety has decreased.

Test-Taking Strategy: Use the process of elimination. Note the key words "severe state" and "most appropriate." Eliminate options 3 and 4 first knowing that these actions are not possible when the client is in a severe state of anxiety. From the remaining options, the most appropriate action is to remain with the client. Review care to the client with severe anxiety if you had difficulty with this question.

Level of Cognitive Ability: Application
Client Needs: Psychosocial Integrity
Integrated Process: Nursing Process—implementation
Content Area: Mental health
Reference: Fortinash, K., & Holoday-Worret, P. (2000). *Psychiatric mental health nursing* (2nd ed., p. 250). St. Louis: Mosby.

11. 1

Rationale: Provision of a consistent daily routine and a low stimulating environment is important when the client is disorientated. Noise, including radio and television, may add to the confusion and disorientation. Moving the client next to the nurses' station is not the initial action.

Test-Taking Strategy: Use the process of elimination. Note the key word "initial" in the stem of the question. Eliminate options 2 and 4 first because they are similar. Focusing on the key word will direct you easily to option 1. Review measures related to the client who is disoriented and confused if you had difficulty with this question.

Level of Cognitive Ability: Application
Client Needs: Psychosocial Integrity
Integrated Process: Nursing Process—implementation
Content Area: Mental health
References: Fortinash, K., & Holoday-Worret, P. (2000). *Psychiatric mental health nursing* (2nd ed., p. 411). St. Louis: Mosby.
Varcarolis, E. (2002). *Foundations of psychiatric mental health nursing* (4th ed., p. 598). Philadelphia: W. B. Saunders.

12. 4

Rationale: In option 4 the nurse encourages the client and the family to verbalize fears and concertns. Options 1, 2, and 3 avoid dealing with concerns and are blocks to communication.

Test-Taking Strategy: Use the process of elimination and therapeutic communication techniques. Option 4 is the only therapeutic option. Options 1, 2, and 3 are blocks to communication. Review these therapeutic techniques if you had difficulty with this question.

Level of Cognitive Ability: Application
Client Needs: Psychosocial Integrity

Integrated Process: Communication and Documentation
Content Area: Mental health
Reference: Stuart, G., & Laraia, M. (2001). *Principles & practice of psychiatric nursing* (7th ed., p. 611). St. Louis: Mosby.

13. 4
Rationale: The clinical picture of dementia varies from the development of mild cognitive defects to severe, life-threatening alterations in neurological functioning. For the client to use confabulation or the fabrication of events or experiences to fill in memory gaps is not unusual. Often, lack of inhibitions on the part of the client may constitute the first indication of anything being "wrong" to the client's significant others (the client may undress in front of persons or demonstrate slovenly table manners where once the client was well mannered). As the dementia progresses, the client will have episodes of wandering or sundowning.
Test-Taking Strategy: Use the process of elimination. Knowledge regarding the manifestations associated with dementia is required to answer this question. Focusing on the issue, a manifestation will direct you to option 4. If you had difficulty with this question, review the manifestations associated with dementia.
Level of Cognitive Ability: Analysis
Client Needs: Psychosocial Integrity
Integrated Process: Nursing Process—assessment
Content Area: Mental health
Reference: Stuart, G., & Laraia, M. (2001). *Principles & practice of psychiatric nursing* (7th ed., p. 466). St. Louis: Mosby.

14. 1
Rationale: The most effective communication technique is the one in which the nurse is giving information. Regarding memory functioning, the normal older adult who ages will find that the time required for memory scanning is longer for recent and remote memory recall. Dementia of the Alzheimer's type involves a disorder that is characterized by a syndrome of symptomatology the onset of which is slow and insidious with a generally progressive and deteriorating course. In option 2 the nurse gives false reassurance, which devalues the client's feelings and discourages the client from expressing feelings. In option 3 the nurse is rejecting the client by refusing to consider the client's ideas or demonstrating ridicule or contempt for the client's ideas or behavior. In option 4 the nurse makes a social, not a professional, comment and belittles the client's concerns, which will discourage the expression of feelings.
Test-Taking Strategy: Use the process of elimination and knowledge of therapeutic communication techniques. Option 1 is the only option that identifies the use of a therapeutic communication technique. Review these techniques if you had difficulty with this question.
Level of Cognitive Ability: Application
Client Needs: Psychosocial Integrity
Integrated Process: Communication and Documentation
Content Area: Mental health
References: Fortinash, K., & Holoday-Worret, P. (2000). *Psychiatric mental health nursing* (2nd ed., p. 395). St. Louis: Mosby.

Stuart, G., & Laraia, M. (2001). *Principles & practice of psychiatric nursing* (7th ed., p. 34). St. Louis: Mosby.

15. 2
Rationale: The risk for impulsive and aggressive behavior may increase if a client is receiving command hallucinations to harm self or others. The nurse should ask the client whether the client has intentions to hurt himself or herself or others. Talking about auditory hallucinations can interfere with subvocal muscular activity associated with a hallucination. Options 1, 3, and 4 will aid in wellness but are not specific interventions for hallucinations, if they occur.
Test-Taking Strategy: Use the process of elimination. Options 1, 3 and 4 are interventions that a client can do to aid wellness. Option 2 is a specific agreement to seek help and evidences self-responsible commitment and control over one's own behavior. Review teaching points for a client with a history of hallucinations if you had difficulty with this question.
Level of Cognitive Ability: Analysis
Client Needs: Psychosocial Integrity
Integrated Process: Teaching/Learning
Content Area: Mental health
Reference: Varcarolis, E. (2002). *Foundations of psychiatric mental health nursing* (4th ed., p. 544). Philadelphia: W. B. Saunders.

16. 2
Rationale: All clients, regardless of age, need to be encouraged to perform at the highest level of independence possible. Independence contributes to the client's sense of control and sense of well-being. Option 1 is incorrect because one does not know what the "self-care deficit" entails. To assume that the client requires long-term care on such little data would be erroneous. Options 3 and 4 are absolute statements.
Test-Taking Strategy: Use the process of elimination. Eliminate options 3 and 4 first because of the absolute word "all." From the remaining options, select option 2 because it is the global option. Review care to the client with dementia if you had difficulty with this question.
Level of Cognitive Ability: Application
Client Needs: Health Promotion and Maintenance
Integrated Process: Nursing Process—planning
Content Area: Mental health
Reference: Fortinash, K., & Holoday-Worret, P. (2000). *Psychiatric mental health nursing* (2nd ed., p. 400). St. Louis: Mosby.

17. 1
Rationale: Safety to the client and other clients is the priority. Option 1 is the only option that addresses the client and other clients' safety needs. Option 2 addresses the client's needs. Option 3 addresses other clients' needs. Option 4 is not client-centered.
Test-Taking Strategy: Note the key words "immediate priority" and use Maslow's hierarchy of needs theory to prioritize. Note the words "agitated, aggressive, and belligerent." Safety is the key issue. Option 1 is the global option and addresses the safety of all. Review nursing interventions to provide safety to clients if you had difficulty with this question.

Level of Cognitive Ability: Application
Client Needs: Safe, Effective Care Environment
Integrated Process: Nursing Process—implementation
Content Area: Delegating/Prioritizing
Reference: Stuart, G., & Laraia, M. (2001). *Principles & practice of psychiatric nursing* (7th ed., p. 748). St. Louis: Mosby.

18. **3**
Rationale: Clients who are withdrawn may be immobile and mute and may require consistent, repeated approaches. Communication with withdrawn clients requires much patience from the nurse. Interventions include the establishment of interpersonal contact. The nurse facilitates communication with the client by sitting in silence, asking open-ended questions, and pausing to provide opportunities for the client to respond.
Test-Taking Strategy: Eliminate option 1 because the client would not be left alone. Option 2 relies on other clients to care for this client, and this is an inappropriate expectation. Asking direct questions to this client is not therapeutic. Option 3 provides for client supervision and communication as appropriate. Review care to the client with catatonic stupor if this question was difficult.
Level of Cognitive Ability: Application
Client Needs: Psychosocial Integrity
Integrated Process: Nursing Process—implementation
Content Area: Mental health
Reference: Varcarolis, E. (2002). *Foundations of psychiatric mental health nursing* (4th ed., p. 560). Philadelphia: W. B. Saunders.

19. **1**
Rationale: Disturbed thought process related to paranoia is the client's problem, and the plan of care must address this problem. The client is experiencing paranoia and is distrustful and suspicious of others. The members of the health care team need to establish a rapport and trust with the client. Hence laughing or whispering in front of the client would be counterproductive. Options 2, 3, and 4 ask the client to trust on a multitude of levels. These options are actions that are too intrusive for a client who is paranoid.
Test-Taking Strategy: Use the process of elimination and knowledge regarding this disorder to answer the question. Noting that the client has paranoia will direct you to option 1. Review this disorder if you had difficulty with this question.
Level of Cognitive Ability: Application
Client Needs: Psychosocial Integrity
Integrated Process: Nursing Process—implementation
Content Area: Mental health
Reference: Stuart, G., & Laraia, M. (2001). *Principles & practice of psychiatric nursing* (7th ed., p. 433). St. Louis: Mosby.

20. **4**
Rationale: A client with depression often suffers a depressed mood and is withdrawn. The person also experiences difficulty concentrating, loss of interest or pleasure, low energy, fatigue, and feelings of worthlessness and poor self-esteem. The plan of care needs to provide successful experiences in a stimulating yet structured environment. Options 1, 2, and 3 are too "restrictive" and offer little or no structure and stimulation.

Test-Taking Strategy: Use the process of elimination. Recall that the depressed client requires a structured and stimulating program in a safe environment. Option 4 is the only option that will provide a safe and effective environment. Review care to the client with depression if you had difficulty with this question.
Level of Cognitive Ability: Application
Client Needs: Psychosocial Integrity
Integrated Process: Nursing Process—planning
Content Area: Mental health
References: Fortinash, K., & Holoday-Worret, P. (2000). *Psychiatric mental health nursing.* (2nd ed., p. 279). St. Louis: Mosby.
Stuart, G., & Laraia, M. (2001). *Principles & practice of psychiatric nursing* (7th ed., p. 276). St. Louis: Mosby.

21. **2**
Rationale: Recognizing situations that produce anxiety allows the client to prepare to cope with anxiety or avoid a specific stimulus. Counselors will not be available for all anxiety producing situations, and this option does not encourage the development of internal strengths. Ignoring feelings will not resolve anxiety. Elimination of all anxiety from life is impossible.
Test-Taking Strategy: Use the process of elimination. Eliminate option 4 first because of the word "all." Eliminate option 3 next because feelings should not be ignored. From the remaining options, select option 2 because this option is more client centered and provides the preparation for the client to deal with anxiety should it occur. Review home care planning for the client with chronic anxiety if you had difficulty with this question.
Level of Cognitive Ability: Application
Client Needs: Safe, Effective Care Environment
Integrated Process: Nursing Process—planning
Content Area: Mental health
References: Fortinash, K., & Holoday-Worret, P. (2000). *Psychiatric mental health nursing* (2nd ed., p. 250). St. Louis: Mosby.
Stuart, G., & Laraia, M. (2001). *Principles & practice of psychiatric nursing* (7th ed., p. 295). St. Louis: Mosby.

22. **2**
Rationale: Agoraphobia is a fear of open spaces and the fear of being trapped in a situation from which there may not be an escape. Agoraphobia includes the possibility of experiencing a sense of helplessness or embarrassment if an attack occurs. Avoidance of such situations usually results in reduction of social and professional interactions. Social phobia focuses more on a specific situations such as the fear of speaking, performing, or eating in public. Claustrophobia is a fear of closed places. Clients with hypochondriacal symptoms focus their anxiety on physical complaints and are preoccupied with their health.
Test-Taking Strategy: Use the process of elimination. Focusing on the key words "remains homebound" will direct you to option 2. If you had difficulty with this question, review phobia types and associated client behaviors.
Level of Cognitive Ability: Analysis
Client Needs: Psychosocial Integrity

Integrated Process: Nursing Process—assessment
Content Area: Mental health
Reference: Varcarolis, E. (2002). *Foundations of psychiatric mental health nursing* (4th ed., p. 311). Philadelphia: W. B. Saunders.

23. **3**

Rationale: Manic clients may be talkative and can dominate group meetings or therapy sessions by their excessive talking. If this occurs, the nurse initially would set limits on the client's behavior. Initially asking the client to leave the session or asking another person to escort the client out of the session is inappropriate. This may agitate the client and further escalate the client's behavior. Option 2 is also an inappropriate initial action because it violates a client's right to receive treatment and is a threatening action.

Test-Taking Strategy: Use the process of elimination and note the key word "initially." Eliminate options 1 and 4 first because they are similar. Next, eliminate option 2 because it violates the client's right to receive treatment and is a threatening action. Remember that setting firm limits with the client initially is best. Review care to a client with mania if you had difficulty with this question.
Level of Cognitive Ability: Application
Client Needs: Psychosocial Integrity
Integrated Process: Nursing Process—implementation
Content Area: Mental health
References: Stuart, G., & Laraia, M. (2001). *Principles & practice of psychiatric nursing* (7th ed., p. 366). St. Louis: Mosby. Varcarolis, E. (2002. *Foundations of psychiatric mental health nursing* (4th ed., p. 504). Philadelphia: W. B. Saunders.

24. **2**

Rationale: A conversion disorder is the alteration or loss of a physical function that cannot be explained by any known pathophysiological mechanism. A conversion disorder is thought to be an expression of a psychological need or conflict. In this situation the client witnessed an accident that was so psychologically painful that the client became blind. A dissociative disorder is a disturbance or alteration in the normally integrative functions of identity, memory, or consciousness. Psychosis is a state in which a person's mental capacity to recognize reality, communicate, and relate to others is impaired, thus interfering with the person's capacity to deal with life demands. Repression is a coping mechanism in which unacceptable feelings are kept out of awareness.

Test-Taking Strategy: Use the process of elimination. The key to the correct option lies in the fact that the client presents no organic reason to account for the blindness; hence a conversion disorder. If you had difficulty with this question, review defense mechanisms and the concepts associated with a conversion disorder.
Level of Cognitive Ability: Analysis
Client Needs: Psychosocial Integrity
Integrated Process: Nursing Process—analysis
Content Area: Mental health

Reference: Fortinash, K., & Holoday-Worret, P. (2000). *Psychiatric mental health nursing* (2nd ed., p. 245). St. Louis: Mosby.

25. **1**

Rationale: The client is at risk for injury to self and others and therefore should be escorted out of the dayroom. Antipsychotic medications are useful to manage the manic client. Hyperactive and agitated behavior usually responds to haloperidol (Haldol). Option 2 may increase the agitation that already exists in this client. Orientation will not halt the behavior. Telling the client that the behavior is not appropriate already has been attempted by the nurse.

Test-Taking Strategy: Use the process of elimination and Maslow's hierarchy of needs theory to answer the question. Look for the option that promotes safety of the client, other clients, and staff. If you had difficulty with this question, review the appropriate interventions in dealing with a manic client.
Level of Cognitive Ability: Analysis
Client Needs: Psychosocial Integrity
Integrated Process: Nursing Process—implementation
Content Area: Mental health
Reference: Fortinash, K., & Holoday-Worret, P. (2000). *Psychiatric mental health nursing* (2nd ed., p. 350). St. Louis: Mosby.

CRITICAL THINKING: MULTIPLE RESPONSE

Answer:
Communicate expected behaviors to the client.
Be clear with the client regarding the consequences of exceeding limits set regarding behavior.
Assist the client in testing out alternative behaviors for obtaining needs.

Rationale: Interventions for dealing with the client exhibiting manipulative behavior include setting clear, consistent, and enforceable limits on manipulative behaviors; being clear with the client regarding the consequences of exceeding limits set; following through with the consequences in a nonpunitive manner; and assisting the client in identifying personal strengths and in testing out alternative behaviors for obtaining needs. Enforcing rules and informing the client that he or she will not be allowed to attend therapy groups is a violation of a client's rights. Ensuring that the client knows that he or she is not in charge of the nursing unit is inappropriate; power struggles need to be avoided.

Test-Taking Strategy: Focus on the issue, manipulative behavior. Recalling clients' rights and that power struggles need to be avoided will assist in selecting the correct interventions. Review care to the client with manipulative behavior if you had difficulty with this question.
Level of Cognitive Ability: Application
Client Needs: Psychosocial Integrity
Integrated Process: Nursing Process—implementation
Content Area: Mental health
Reference: Varcarolis, E. (2002). *Foundations of psychiatric mental health nursing* (4th ed., p. 394). Philadelphia: W. B. Saunders.

REFERENCES

Carson, V. (2000). *Mental health nursing: The nurse-patient journey* (2nd ed.). Philadelphia: W. B. Saunders.

Fortinash, K., & Holoday-Worret, P. (2000). *Psychiatric mental health nursing* (2nd ed.). St. Louis: Mosby.

Keltner, N., Schwecke, L., & Bostrom, C. (2003). *Psychiatric nursing* (4th ed.). St. Louis: Mosby.

Stuart, G., & Laraia, M. (2001). *Principles & practice of psychiatric nursing* (7th ed.). St. Louis: Mosby.

Varcarolis, E. (2002). *Foundations of psychiatric mental health nursing* (4th ed.). Philadelphia: W. B. Saunders.

Addictions

I. EATING DISORDERS

A. Description: Eating disorders are characterized by uncertain self-identification and grossly disturbed eating habits.

B. Compulsive overeating
   1. Compulsive overeating is bingelike overeating without purging.
   2. Food consumption is out of the individual's control and occurs in a stereotyped fashion.
   3. Client may be repulsed by eating, and the eating relieves tension but does not produce pleasure.
   4. Client is aware that eating patterns are abnormal and feels depressed after eating.
   5. Client eats secretly during a binge and consumes high-calorie and easily digestible food.
   6. Client repeatedly tries to diet but without success.
   7. Client lacks interest in exercise programs and feels helpless and hopeless about weight.
   8. When experiencing guilt, anger, depression, boredom, loneliness, inadequacy, or ambivalence, client responds by eating.

C. Anorexia nervosa
   1. Description
      a. The onset often is associated with a stressful life event.
      b. The client intensely fears obesity.
      c. Body image is distorted, and the client has a disturbed self-concept.
      d. Client is preoccupied with foods that prevent weight gain and a phobia against foods that produce weight gain.
      e. The eating disorder can be life-threatening.
      f. Death can occur from starvation, **suicide**, or electrolyte imbalance.
   2. Assessment
      a. Refusal to eat and appetite loss
      b. Appetite denial

   c. Feelings of lack of control
   d. Self-induced vomiting and self-administered enemas
   e. Compulsive exercising
   f. Overachiever and perfectionist
   g. Decreased temperature, pulse, and blood pressure
   h. Weight loss
   i. Gastrointestinal disturbances
   j. Constipation
   k. Electrolyte imbalances
   l. Scaly, dry skin
   m. Sleep disturbances
   n. Hormone deficiencies
   o. Amenorrhea for at least 3 consecutive menstrual periods
   p. Teeth and gum deterioration
   q. Cyanosis and numbness of extremities
   r. Esophageal varices from vomiting
   s. Bone degeneration

D. Bulimia nervosa
   1. Description
      a. The client indulges in eating binges followed by purging behaviors.
      b. Most clients remain within a normal weight range but feel that their lives are dominated by the eating-related conflict.
   2. Assessment
      a. Preoccupied with body shape and weight
      b. Consumption of high-calorie food in secret; guilt about secretive eating
      c. Binge, purge syndrome
      d. Attempts to lose weight through diets, vomiting, enemas, cathartics, and amphetamines or diuretics
      e. Need to control yet experiences feelings of powerlessness or loss of control
      f. Low self-esteem
      g. Poor interpersonal relationships

h. Mood swings
i. Self-mutilating behavior; suicidal thoughts and attempts at **suicide**
j. Electrolyte imbalances
k. Loss of tooth enamel and dental decay
l. Stomach ulcers and rectal bleeding
m. Esophageal varices from vomiting
n. Cardiac disease and hypertension

E. Interventions: clients with an eating disorder
1. Assess the client's nutritional status.
2. Establish a contract with the client concerning the diet plan for the day.
3. Assist the client in identifying precipitators to the eating disorder.
4. Encourage the client to state feelings about the eating behavior.
5. Be accepting and nonjudgmental, expressing neither approval nor disapproval of the behavior.
6. Encourage behavior modification techniques.
7. Provide praise and positive reinforcement for accomplishments.
8. Supervise client during mealtimes and for a specified period after meals.
9. Set a time limit for each meal.
10. Provide a pleasant, relaxed environment for eating.
11. Monitor for signs of physical complications related to the eating disorder.
12. Record intake and output.
13. Weigh the client daily at the same time, using the same scale, after the client voids.
14. When weighing the client, ensure that the client is wearing the same clothing as when the previous weight was taken.
15. Monitor and restore fluid and electrolyte balance.
16. Monitor elimination patterns.
17. Assess and limit the client's activity level.
18. Encourage the client to participate in diversional activities.
19. Assess the client's suicidal potential.
20. Administer antidepressant medication as prescribed.
21. Encourage psychotherapy as prescribed.
22. Refer the client to support groups.

II. SUBSTANCE ABUSE DISORDERS

A. Description: Substance **abuse** disorders cause behavioral changes associated with regular substance **abuse** that affects the central nervous system.
B. Substance dependence (Box 74-1)
1. Substance dependence is a pattern of repeated use of a substance, which usually results in tolerance, withdrawal, and compulsive drug-taking behavior.
2. Client takes substances in larger amounts and over longer periods of time than was intended.
3. Client has the desire to cut down but has unsuccessful efforts to decrease or discontinue use.

BOX 74-1

CAGE Screening Test

C: Have you ever felt the need to *cut* down on your drinking/drug use?
A: Have you ever been *annoyed* at criticism of your drinking/drug use?
G: Have you ever felt *guilty* about something you have done when you have been drinking or taking drugs?
E: Have you ever had an *eye opener,* drinking or taking drugs first thing in the morning to get going or to avoid withdrawal symptoms?

---

4. Daily activities revolve around the use of a substance.
C. Substance tolerance is the need for increased amounts of the substance to achieve the desired effect.
D. Substance **abuse**
1. Client recurrently uses substances.
2. Client experiences recurrent, significant harmful consequences related to the use of substances.
3. Client has legal problems related to substance **abuse.**
E. Substance withdrawal
1. Physiological and substance-specific cognitive symptoms occur.
2. Substance withdrawal occurs when blood levels decrease in an individual with prolonged heavy use of a substance.
F. Precipitating factors of substance **abuse**
1. Rebellion and peer group pressure in adolescence
2. Pleasure-seeking experience as the substance decreases physical and emotional pain
3. Group influence and peer pressure
4. Depression
5. Loss and grieving
G. Dysfunctional behaviors of substance **abuse**
1. Insensitive to self and others
2. Manipulative
3. Impulsiveness
4. Anger, including physical and verbal **abuse**
5. Avoidance of relationships, with physical and emotional distancing
6. Sense of self-importance and requiring special treatment
7. Denial; blaming everything but the substance
8. Codependence; modifying self-behaviors and response to others
9. Low self-esteem
10. Depression

III. ALCOHOL ABUSE

A. Description
1. Alcohol is a central nervous system depressant affecting all body tissues.
2. Physical dependence is a biological need for alcohol to avoid physical withdrawal symptoms.

3. Psychological dependence is a craving for the subjective effect of alcohol.
B. Risk factors
   1. Biological predisposition
   2. Depressed and highly anxious characteristics
   3. Low self-esteem
   4. Poor self-control
   5. History of rebelliousness, poor school performance, delinquency
   6. Poor parental relationships
C. Assessment
   1. Slurred speech
   2. Uncoordinated movements
   3. Unsteady gait
   4. Restlessness
   5. Belligerence
   6. Confusion
   7. Sneaking drinks, drinking in the morning, and experiencing blackouts
   8. Binge drinking
   9. Arguments about drinking
   10. Missing work
   11. Increased tolerance to alcohol
   12. Intoxication, with blood alcohol levels of 0.1% (100 mg alcohol per deciliter of blood) or higher
D. Psychological symptoms
   1. Depression
   2. Hostility
   3. Suspiciousness
   4. Rationalization
   5. Irritability
   6. Isolation
   7. Decrease in inhibitions
   8. Decrease in self-esteem
   9. Denial that a problem exists
E. Complications associated with chronic alcohol use
   1. Vitamin deficiencies
      a. Vitamin B deficiency causing peripheral neuropathies
      b. Thiamine deficiency causing Korsakoff's syndrome
   2. Alcoholic-induced persistent amnesiac disorder causing severe memory problems
   3. Wernicke's encephalopathy, causing confusion, ataxia, and abnormal eye movements
   4. Hepatitis; cirrhosis of the liver
   5. Esophagitis and gastritis
   6. Pancreatitis
   7. Anemias
   8. Immune system dysfunctions
   9. Brain damage
   10. Peripheral neuropathy
   11. Cardiac disorders

IV. ALCOHOL WITHDRAWAL
A. Description

1. Early signs develop within a few hours after cessation of alcohol intake.
2. These signs peak after 24 to 48 hours and then rapidly disappear, unless the withdrawal progresses to alcohol withdrawal delirium.
B. Withdrawal (Box 74-2)
C. Withdrawal delirium (Box 74-3)
   1. Withdrawal delirium is a medical emergency.
   2. Death has occurred from myocardial infarction, fat emboli, peripheral vascular collapse, electrolyte imbalance, aspiration pneumonia, or **suicide.**
   3. The state of delirium usually peaks 48 to 72 hours after cessation or reduction of intake (although can occur later) and lasts 2 to 3 days.
D. Interventions
   1. Provide care in a nonjudgmental manner.
   2. Check the client frequently.
   3. Monitor vital signs and neurological signs (hourly for the client with delirium).
   4. Provide a quiet, nonstimulating environment; encourage a family member (one at a time) to stay with the client to minimize anxiety.
   5. Orient the client frequently.
   6. Explain all treatments and procedures in a quiet and simple manner.

BOX 74-2
Early Signs of Alcohol Withdrawal

Anorexia (nausea and vomiting may occur)
Anxiety
Easily startled
Hyperalertness
Hypertension
Insomnia
Irritability
Jerky movements
Possibly experiences hallucinations, illusions, or vivid nightmares
Possibly reports a feeling of "shaking inside"
Seizures (usually appear 7 to 48 hours after cessation of alcohol)
Tachycardia
Tremors

BOX 74-3
Manifestations of Alcohol Withdrawal Delirium

Agitation
Anorexia
Anxiety
Delirium
Diaphoresis
Disorientation with fluctuating levels of consciousness
Fever (temperature of 100° to 103° F)
Hallucinations and delusions
Insomnia
Tachycardia and hypertension

7. Initiate seizure precautions.
8. Administer sedating or anticonvulsant medication as prescribed.
9. Provide small, frequent, high-carbohydrate foods (administer antiemetic before meals as needed).
10. Monitor intake and output.
11. Administer vitamins (multivitamin, vitamin B complex including thiamine, and vitamin C)
12. Assist client with activities of daily living and assist with ambulation if stable.
13. Allow client to express fears.

E. Disulfiram (Antabuse) therapy
1. Description
   a. Disulfiram is an alcohol deterrent used for alcoholic dependence.
   b. The medication sensitizes the client to alcohol, so a disulfiram-alcohol reaction occurs if alcohol is ingested.
   c. The client must abstain from alcohol for at least 12 hours before the initial dose is administered.
   d. Adverse effects usually begin within minutes to a half hour after consuming alcohol and may last 30 to 120 minutes.
   e. The client must avoid drinking alcohol for 14 days after disulfiram therapy has been discontinued; otherwise, the client is at risk for disulfiram-alcohol reaction.
2. Adverse reactions
   a. Facial flushing
   b. Sweating
   c. Throbbing headache
   d. Neck pain
   e. Nausea and vomiting
   f. Hypotension
   g. Tachycardia
   h. Respiratory distress
3. Client education
   a. Educate as to the effects of the medication.
   b. Ensure that the client agrees to abstain from alcohol and any alcohol-containing substances.

c. Instruct the client that the effects of the medication may occur for several days after discontinuance.
d. Instruct the client to avoid the use of substances that contain alcohol, such as cough medicines, rubbing compounds, vinegar, mouthwashes, and aftershave lotions.

F. Dealing with the client who abuses alcohol (Box 74-4 and 74-5)

V. DRUG DEPENDENCY

A. Central nervous system depressants
1. Central nervous system depressants can include alcohol, benzodiazepines, and barbiturates and act as a depressant, sedative, and hypnotic.
2. Intoxication (Box 74-6)
3. Overdose can produce cardiovascular or respiratory depression, coma, shock, convulsions, and death.
4. Overdose: If client is awake, induce vomiting and administer activated charcoal; if client is comatose, clear airway, intubate, provide gastric lavage with activated charcoal, use seizure precautions, prepare for possible dialysis, and administer flumazenil (Romazicon) intravenously.
5. Withdrawal effects include nausea, vomiting, tachycardia, diaphoresis, irritability, tremors, insomnia, seizures; withdrawal must be treated with a carefully titrated similar drug (abrupt withdrawal can lead to death).

B. Central nervous system stimulants
1. Central nervous system stimulants can include amphetamines, cocaine, and crack.

BOX 74-5

Therapies for Substance Abuse Clients and Their Families

Behavior therapy, aversion conditioning with disulfiram (Antabuse)
Hospitalization
Psychotherapy (individual, group, family)
Support groups such as Alcoholics Anonymous; Narcotics Anonymous; Pills Anonymous; Al-Anon, Al-a-Teen, or Narc-Anon (for family members and friends of alcoholics or addicts); and Adult Children of Alcoholics
Transitional living programs (halfway houses)

BOX 74-4

Dealing with the Client Who Abuses Alcohol

Direct the client's focus to the substance abuse problem.
Identify with the client those situations that precipitate angry feelings.
Set limits on manipulative behavior and verbal and physical abuse.
Hold the client firmly to reasonable limits, consistently reinforcing rules, with reasonable consequences for breaking rules.
Hold the client accountable for all behaviors.
Assist the client to explore strengths and weaknesses.
Encourage time-out if the client is losing control.
Encourage the client to participate in group therapy and support groups.

BOX 74-6

Intoxication: Central Nervous System Depressants

Drowsiness
Hypotension
Impairment of memory, attention, judgment, and social or occupational functioning
Incoordination and unsteady gait
Irritability
Slurred speech

2. Intoxication (Box 74-7)
3. Overdose can produce respiratory distress, ataxia, hyperpyrexia, seizures, coma, cerebrovascular accident, myocardial infarction, and death.
4. Overdose is treated with antipsychotics and management of associated effects.
5. Withdrawal effects include fatigue, depression, agitation, apathy, anxiety, insomnia, disorientation, lethargy, and craving; withdrawal is treated with antidepressants, dopamine agonist, or bromocriptine (Parlodel).

C. Opioids
1. Opioids can include opium, heroin, meperidine (Demerol), morphine sulfate, codeine sulfate, methadone (Dolophine), hydromorphone (Dilaudid), or fentanyl (Sublimaze).
2. Intoxication (Box 74-8)
3. Overdose can produce respiratory depression, coma, shock, seizures, and death.
4. Overdose is treated with a narcotic antagonist such as naloxone (Narcan).
5. Withdrawal effects include yawning, insomnia, irritability, rhinorrhea, diaphoresis, cramps, nausea and vomiting, muscle aches, chills, fever, lacrimation, and diarrhea; withdrawal is treated by methadone tapering or medication detoxification.

D. Hallucinogens
1. Hallucinogens can include lysergic acid diethylamide (LSD), mescaline (peyote), or psilocybin (mushrooms), or phencyclidine (PCP).
2. Intoxication (Box 74-9)

3. Overdose effects of LSD, peypote, and psilocybin include psychosis, brain damage, and death; effects of PCP include psychosis, hypertensive crisis, hyperthermia, seizures, and respiratory arrest.
4. Treatment (LSD, peypote, psilocybin) involves low environmental stimuli (speak slowly, clearly, and in a low voice) and medications to treat anxiety.
5. Treatment (PCP) involves possible gastric lavage (if alert), acidifying urine to assist in excreting drug, and interventions to treat behavioral disturbances, hyperthermia, hypertension, and respiratory distress.

E. Inhalants
1. Inhalants can include gases or liquids such as butane, paint thinner, paint and wax removers, airplane glue, nail polish remover, and nitrous oxide.
2. Intoxication (Box 74-10)
3. Overdose can cause damage to the nervous system and death.
4. Treatment: Interventions include treating affected body systems.

F. Marijuana (*Cannabis sativa*)
1. Marijuana generally is smoked but can be ingested.
2. Marijuana causes euphoria, detachment, relaxation, talkativeness, slowed perception of time, anxiety, or paranoia.

BOX 74-7

Intoxication: Central Nervous System Stimulants

Dilated pupils
Euphoria
Hypertension
Impairment of judgment and social or occupational
  functioning
Insomnia
Nausea and vomiting
Paranoia, delusions, hallucinations
Potential for violence
Tachycardia

BOX 74-8

Intoxication: Opioids

Constricted pupils
Decreased respirations
Drowsiness
Euphoria
Hypotension
Impairment of memory, attention, and judgment
Psychomotor retardation
Slurred speech

BOX 74-9

Intoxication: Hallucinogens

Agitation and belligerence
Anxiety and depression
Bizarre behavior, regressive behavior, or violent
  behavior
Blank stare
Diaphoresis
Dilated pupils
Elevated vital signs including blood pressure
Hallucinations
Impairment of judgment and social and occupational
  functioning
Incoordination
Muscular rigidity and chronic jerking
Paranoia
Seizures
Tachycardia
Tremors

BOX 74-10

Intoxication: Inhalants

Enhancement of sexual pleasure
Euphoria
Excitation followed by drowsiness, light-headedness,
  disinhibition, and agitation
Giggling and laughter

3. Long-term dependence can result in lethargy, difficulty concentrating, and memory loss.

G. Other recreational drugs
   1. Other recreational drugs can include ecstasy, GHB (gamma-hydroxybutyrate), and ketamine.
   2. Effects include euphoria, increased energy, increased self-confidence, and increased sociability.
   3. Adverse effects include hyperthermia, rhabdomyolysis, renal failure, hepatotoxicity, depression, panic attacks, psychosis, cardiovascular collapse, and death.

H. Interventions: withdrawal
   1. Initiate seizure precautions.
   2. Hydrate the client.
   3. Monitor vital signs every hour.
   4. Monitor intake and output.
   5. Orient client frequently.
   6. Maintain minimal stimuli.
   7. Approach client in an accepting and nonjudgmental manner.
   8. Direct client's focus to the substance **abuse** problem.
   9. Identify with client situations that precipitate angry feelings.
   10. Limit the client's blame-placing or rationalizing to explain the substance **abuse** problem.
   11. Assist client to use assertive techniques rather than manipulation to meet needs.
   12. Set limits on manipulative behavior and verbal and physical **abuse**.
   13. Hold client firmly to reasonable limits, consistently reinforcing rules, with reasonable consequences for breaking rules.
   14. Hold client accountable for all behaviors.
   15. Assist client to explore strengths and weaknesses.
   16. Encourage time-out if client is losing control.
   17. Encourage client to participate in unit activities.
   18. Encourage client to participate in group therapy and support groups.
   19. Box 74-11 delineates nursing care for clients.

BOX 74-11

Withdrawal: Nursing Care

Obtain information regarding the drug type and amount consumed.
Assess vital signs.
Remove unnecessary objects from the environment.
Provide one-to-one supervision if necessary.
Provide a quiet, calm environment with minimal stimuli.
Maintain client orientation.
Ensure client's safety by implementing seizure precautions.
Use restraints, if necessary and prescribed, to prevent client from harming self and others.
Provide for physical needs.
Provide food and fluids as tolerated.
Administer medications as prescribed to decrease withdrawal symptoms.
Collect blood and urine samples for drug screening.

PRACTICE QUESTIONS

1. The nurse is caring for a female client who was admitted to the mental health unit recently for anorexia nervosa. The nurse enters the client's room and notes that the client is engaged in rigorous push-ups. Which nursing action is most appropriate?
   1. Allow the client to complete her exercise program.
   2. Tell the client that she is not allowed to exercise rigorously.
   3. Interrupt the client and offer to take her for a walk.
   4. Interrupt the client and weigh her immediately.

2. The nurse is caring for a client with anorexia nervosa. The nurse is monitoring the behavior of the client and understands that the client with anorexia nervosa manages anxiety by
   1. Always reinforcing self-approval.
   2. Having the need always to make the right decision.
   3. Engaging in immoral acts.
   4. Observing rigid rules and regulations.

3. The nurse is reviewing a nursing plan of care formulated by a nursing student for a hospitalized client with bulimia nervosa. The nurse would question which intervention listed in the plan?
   1. Monitoring intake and output
   2. Monitoring electrolyte levels
   3. Observing for excessive exercise
   4. Checking for the presence of laxatives and diuretics in the client's room

4. The nurse is monitoring a client who abuses alcohol for signs of alcohol withdrawal. Which of the following would alert the nurse to the potential for delirium tremors?
   1. Hypertension, changes in level of consciousness, hallucinations
   2. Hypotension, ataxia, hunger
   3. Stupor, agitation, muscular rigidity
   4. Hypotension, coarse hand tremors, agitation

5. The spouse of a client admitted to the mental health unit for alcohol withdrawal says to the nurse, "I should get out of this bad situation." The most helpful response by the nurse would be
   1. "I agree with you. You should get out of this situation."
   2. "What do you find difficult about this situation."
   3. "Why don't you tell your husband about this."
   4. "This is not the best time to make that decision."

6. The home health nurse visits a client at home and determines that the client is dependent on drugs. Which of the following assessment questions would assist the nurse to provide appropriate nursing care?
   1. "Why did you get started on these drugs?"

2. "How long did you think you could take these drugs without someone finding out?"

3. "How much do you use and what effect does it have on you?"

4. The nurse does not ask any questions in fear that the client is in denial and will throw the nurse out of the home.

7. The client with a diagnosis of anorexia nervosa, who is in a state of starvation, is in a two-bed room. A newly admitted client will be assigned to this client's room. Which of the following clients would be an appropriate choice as this client's roommate?

   1. A client with pneumonia
   2. A client receiving diagnostic tests
   3. A client who could benefit from the client's assistance at mealtime
   4. A client who thrives on managing others

8. A female client with anorexia nervosa is a member of a predischarge group/support group. The client verbalizes that she would like to buy some new clothes, but her finances are limited. Group members brought some used clothes to the client to replace the client's old clothes. The client believed that the new clothes were much too tight and reduced her calorie intake to 800 calories daily. The nurse analyzes this behavior as

   1. Normal behavior.
   2. Indicative of the client's ambivalence about hospital discharge.
   3. Evidence of the client's altered/distorted body image.
   4. Regression as the client is moving toward the community.

9. The nurse determines that the wife of an alcoholic client is benefiting from attending an Al-Anon group when the nurse hears the wife say

   1. "My attendance at the meetings has helped me to see that I provoke my husband's violence."
   2. "I no longer feel that I deserve the beatings my husband inflicts on me."
   3. "I can tolerate my husband's destructive behaviors now that I know they are common with alcoholics."
   4. "I enjoy attending the meetings because they get me out of the house and away from my husband."

10. The client has been hospitalized and is participating in substance abuse therapy group sessions. On discharge the client has consented to participate in Alcoholics Anonymous (AA) community groups. The nurse is monitoring the client's response to the substance abuse sessions. Which statement by the client best indicates that the client has developed effective coping response styles and has processed information effectively for self use?

    1. "I know I'm ready to be discharged. I feel like I can say 'no' and leave a group of friends if they are drinking … 'No Problem.'"
    2. "This group has really helped a lot. I know it will be different when I go home. But I'm sure that my family and friends will all help me like the people in this group have … They'll all help me … I know they will … They won't let me go back to old ways."
    3. "I'm looking forward to leaving here. I know that I will miss all of you. So, I'm happy and I'm sad, I'm excited and I'm scared. I know that I have to work hard to be strong and that everyone isn't going to be as helpful as you people."
    4. "I'll keep all my appointments; go to all my AA groups; I'll do everything I'm supposed to … Nothing will go wrong that way."

11. A hospitalized client with a history of alcohol abuse tells that nurse, "I am leaving now. I have to go. I don't want anymore treatment. I have things that I have to do right away." The client has not been discharged. In fact, the client is scheduled for an important diagnostic test to be performed in 1 hour. After the nurse discusses the client's concerns with the client, the client dresses and begins to walk out of the hospital room. The most appropriate nursing action is to

    1. Restrain the client until the physician can be reached.
    2. Call security to block all exit areas.
    3. Tell the client that the client cannot return to this hospital again if the client leaves now.
    4. Call the nursing supervisor.

12. The nurse is preparing to perform an admission assessment on a client with a diagnosis of bulimia nervosa, and a nursing student will be observing the nurse. The nurse asks the student about the expected assessment findings and determines that the student needs to research the disorder further if the student states that which of the following is a characteristic finding?

    1. Loss of tooth enamel
    2. Dental decay
    3. Electrolyte imbalances
    4. Body weight well below ideal range

CRITICAL THINKING: FILL IN THE BLANK

A client who has been drinking alcohol regularly admits to having "a problem." The client is asking for assistance with the problem. The nurse would support the client to attend which self-help community groups?

Answer: _____

ANSWERS

1. 3

Rationale: Clients with anorexia nervosa frequently are preoccupied with rigorous exercise and push themselves beyond normal limits to work off caloric intake. The nurse must provide for appropriate exercise and place limits on rigorous activities. Options 1, 2, and 4 are inappropriate nursing actions.

Test-Taking Strategy: Use the process of elimination. Focus on the key words "most appropriate." Also focus on the need for the nurse to set firm limits with clients who have this disorder. If you had difficulty with this question, review interventions for the client with anorexia nervosa.

Level of Cognitive Ability: Application
Client Needs: Physiological Integrity
Integrated Process: Nursing Process—implementation
Content Area: Mental health
Reference: Stuart, G., & Laraia, M. (2001). *Principles & practice of psychiatric nursing* (7th ed., p. 540). St. Louis: Mosby.

2. 4

Rationale: Clients with anorexia nervosa have the desire to please others. Their need to be correct or perfect interferes with rational decision-making processes. These clients are moralistic. Rules and rituals help the clients manage their anxiety.

Test-Taking Strategy: Use the process of elimination and focus on the issue, managing anxiety. Eliminate options 1 and 2 because of the absolute word "always." Option 3 is not characteristic of the client with anorexia. Review the characteristics associated with this disorder if you had difficulty with this question.

Level of Cognitive Ability: Analysis
Client Needs: Psychosocial Integrity
Integrated Process: Nursing Process—assessment
Content Area: Mental health
Reference: Fortinash, K., & Holoday-Worret, P. (2000). *Psychiatric mental health nursing* (2nd ed., p. 458). St. Louis: Mosby.

3. 3

Rationale: Excessive exercise is a characteristic of anorexia nervosa, not a characteristic of clients with bulimia. Frequent vomiting, in addition to laxative and diuretic abuse, may lead to dehydration and electrolyte imbalance. Assessing for dehydration and electrolyte imbalance are important nursing actions. Option 3 is the only option that is not a characteristic of bulimia.

Test-Taking Strategy: Use the process of elimination. Note the key words "the nurse would question" in the stem of the question. Options 1, 2, and 4 are similar and directly or indirectly infer concern about fluid and electrolyte balance. Option 3 is different from the other options. Review the characteristics associated with bulimia nervosa if you had difficulty with this question.

Level of Cognitive Ability: Analysis
Client Needs: Physiological Integrity
Integrated Process: Teaching/Learning
Content Area: Mental health
Reference: Fortinash, K., & Holoday-Worret, P. (2000). *Psychiatric mental health nursing* (2nd ed., pp. 454, 456). St. Louis: Mosby.

4. 1

Rationale: Some of the symptoms associated with delirium tremors typically are anxiety, insomnia, anorexia, hypertension, disorientation, hallucinations, changes in level of consciousness, agitation, fever, and delusions.

Test-Taking Strategy: Use the process of elimination. Review each option carefully to ensure that all of the symptoms in the option are correct. Eliminate options 2 and 4 first, knowing that hypertension rather than hypotension occurs. From the remaining options, recalling that the client who is stuporous is not likely to exhibit delirium tremors will direct you to option 1. Review these symptoms if you had difficulty with this question.

Level of Cognitive Ability: Analysis
Client Needs: Physiological Integrity
Integrated Process: Nursing Process—assessment
Content Area: Mental health
Reference: Varcarolis, E. (2002). *Foundations of psychiatric mental health nursing* (4th ed., p. 750). Philadelphia: W. B. Saunders.

5. 2

Rationale: The most helpful response is one that encourages the client to problem solve. Giving advice implies that the nurse knows what is best and also can foster dependency. The nurse should not agree with the client, nor should the nurse request that the client provide explanations.

Test-Taking Strategy: Use therapeutic communication techniques. Eliminate option 3 because of the word "Why," which should be avoided in communication. Eliminate option 1 because the nurse is agreeing with the client. Eliminate option 4 because this option places the client's feelings on hold. Option 2 is the only option that addresses the client's feelings. Review therapeutic communication techniques if you had difficulty with this question.

Level of Cognitive Ability: Application
Client Needs: Psychosocial Integrity
Integrated Process: Communication and Documentation
Content Area: Mental health
Reference: Varcarolis, E. (2002). *Foundations of psychiatric mental health nursing* (4th ed., p. 258). Philadelphia: W. B. Saunders.

6. 3

Rationale: Whenever the nurse employs an assessment for a client who is dependent on drugs, it is best for the nurse to attempt to elicit information by being nonjudgmental and direct. Option 1 is incorrect because it is judgmental and off focus and reflects the nurse's bias. Option 2 is incorrect because it is judgmental, insensitive, and aggressive, which is nontherapeutic. Option 4 is incorrect because it indicates passivity on the nurse's part and uses rationalization to avoid the therapeutic nursing intervention.

Test-Taking Strategy: Use the process of elimination and therapeutic communication techniques to answer the question. Also focus on the issue "provide appropriate nursing care." Review assessment of a client who is a substance abuser if you had difficulty with this question.

Level of Cognitive Ability: Analysis
Client Needs: Psychosocial Integrity
Integrated Process: Nursing Process—assessment
Content Area: Mental health

Reference: Varcarolis, E. (2002). *Foundations of psychiatric mental health nursing* (4th ed., p. 258). Philadelphia: W. B. Saunders.

7. 2

Rationale: The client receiving diagnostic tests is an acceptable roommate. The client with anorexia nervosa is most likely experiencing hematological complications, such as leukopenia. Having a roommate with pneumonia would place the client with anorexia nervosa at risk for infection. The client with anorexia nervosa should not be put in a situation in which the client is able to focus on the nutritional needs of others or being managed by others because this may contribute to sublimation and suppression of personal hunger.

Test-Taking Strategy: Use the process of elimination and note the key words "in a state of starvation." Recalling the characteristics associated with anorexia nervosa will direct you to option 2. Review care of the client with anorexia nervosa if you have difficulty with this question.

Level of Cognitive Ability: Analysis
Client Needs: Safe, Effective Care Environment
Integrated Process: Nursing Process—planning
Content Area: Mental health
Reference: Fortinash, K., & Holoday-Worret, P. (2000). *Psychiatric mental health nursing* (2nd ed., p. 508). St. Louis: Mosby.

8. 3

Rationale: Altered/distorted body image is a concern with clients with anorexia nervosa. Although the client may struggle with ambivalence and show regressed behavior, the client's coping pattern relates to the basic issue of distorted body image. The nurse should address this need in the support group.

Test-Taking Strategy: Use the process of elimination, focusing on the information provided in the question, which is related directly to an altered body image. This should direct you to the correct option. Review the needs of the client with anorexia nervosa if you had difficulty with this question.

Level of Cognitive Ability: Analysis
Client Needs: Psychosocial Integrity
Integrated Process: Nursing Process—analysis
Content Area: Mental health
Reference: Fortinash, K., & Holoday-Worret, P. (2000). *Psychiatric mental health nursing* (2nd ed., pp. 459-460). St. Louis: Mosby.

9. 2

Rationale: Al-Anon support groups are a protected, supportive opportunity for spouses and significant others to learn what to expect and to obtain excellent pointers about successful behavioral changes. Option 2 is the most healthy response because it exemplifies an understanding that the alcoholic partner is responsible for his behavior and cannot be allowed to blame family members for loss of control. In option 1 the nonalcoholic partner should not feel responsible when the spouse loses control. Option 3 indicates that the wife remains codependent. Option 4 indicates that the group is viewed as an escape, not a place to work on issues.

Test-Taking Strategy: Use the process of elimination. Identify the client of the question and identify the option that most directly addresses the issue of the question, benefiting from attending an Al-Anon group. This will direct you to option 2. Review the purpose of this group if you had difficulty with this question.

Level of Cognitive Ability: Analysis
Client Needs: Psychosocial Integrity
Integrated Process: Nursing Process—analysis
Content Area: Mental health
Reference: Fortinash, K., & Holoday-Worret, P. (2000). *Psychiatric mental health nursing* (2nd ed., p. 381). St. Louis: Mosby.

10. 3

Rationale: In the defense mechanism of denial the person denies reality. Option 1 identifies denial. In option 2 the client is relying heavily on others, and the client's focus of control is external. In option 4 the client is concrete and procedure oriented; again the client denies that "nothing will go wrong that way" if the client follows all the directions. In option 3 the client is expressing real concern and ambivalence about discharge from the hospital. The client also demonstrates reality in the statement.

Test-Taking Strategy: Use the process of elimination. Focus on the issue and select the option that identifies the most realistic client verbalization. Review the expected client outcomes from group therapy if you had difficulty with this question.

Level of Cognitive Ability: Analysis
Client Needs: Psychosocial Integrity
Integrated Process: Nursing Process—analysis
Content Area: Mental health
Reference: Fortinash, K., & Holoday-Worret, P. (2000). *Psychiatric mental health nursing* (2nd ed., p. 380). St. Louis: Mosby.

11. 4

Rationale: A nurse can be charged with false imprisonment if a client is made to believe wrongfully that the client cannot leave the hospital. Most health care facilities have documents that the client is asked to sign that relate to the client's responsibilities when the client leaves against medical advice. The client should be asked to sign this document before leaving. The nurse should request that the client wait to speak to the physician before leaving, but if the client refuses to do so, the nurse cannot hold the client against the client's will. Restraining the client and calling security to block exits constitutes false imprisonment. Any client has a right to health care and cannot be told otherwise.

Test-Taking Strategy: Use the process of elimination. Keeping the concept of false imprisonment in mind, eliminate options 1 and 2 because they are similar. Eliminate option 3, knowing that any client has a right to health. From the options presented, the best action is option 4. Review the points related to false imprisonment if you had difficulty with this question.

Level of Cognitive Ability: Application
Client Needs: Safe, Effective Care Environment
Integrated Process: Nursing Process—implementation
Content Area: Mental health
Reference: Stuart, G., & Laraia, M. (2001). *Principles & practice of psychiatric nursing* (7th ed., p. 165). St. Louis: Mosby.

12. 4

Rationale: Clients with bulimia nervosa initially may not appear to be physically or emotionally ill. They are often at or slightly below ideal body weight. On further inspection the client demonstrates dental decay and loss of tooth enamel if the client has been inducing vomiting. Electrolyte imbalances are present.

Test-Taking Strategy: Use the process of elimination. Eliminate options 1 and 2 because they are similar. From the remaining options, recall that in anorexia nervosa the body weight is normally below 85% of ideal body weight. Option 4 is a characteristic sign of anorexia nervosa not bulimia nervosa. Review the characteristics of these disorders if you had difficulty with this question.

Level of Cognitive Ability: Analysis
Client Needs: Psychosocial Integrity
Integrated Process: Teaching/Learning
Content Area: Mental health
Reference: Fortinash, K., & Holoday-Worret, P. (2000). *Psychiatric mental health nursing* (2nd ed., p. 458). St. Louis: Mosby.

CRITICAL THINKING: FILL IN THE BLANK

Answer: Alcoholics Anonymous
Rationale: Alcoholics Anonymous is a major self-help organization for the treatment of alcoholism.
Test-Taking Strategy: Focus on the issue and the client's problem identified in the question. Familiarize yourself with the purpose of specific support groups if you had difficulty with this question.
Level of Cognitive Ability: Application
Client Needs: Psychosocial Integrity
Integrated Process: Nursing process—implementation
Content Area: Mental health
Reference: Fortinash, K., & Holoday-Worret, P. (2000). *Psychiatric mental health nursing* (2nd ed., p. 380). St. Louis: Mosby.

REFERENCES

Carson, V. (2000). *Mental health nursing: The nurse-patient journey* (2nd ed.). Philadelphia: W. B. Saunders.

Fortinash, K., & Holoday-Worret, P. (2000). *Psychiatric mental health nursing* (2nd ed.). St. Louis: Mosby.

Keltner, N., Schwecke, L., & Bostrom, C. (2003). *Psychiatric nursing* (4th ed.). St. Louis: Mosby.

Stuart, G., & Laraia, M. (2001). *Principles & practice of psychiatric nursing* (7th ed.). St. Louis: Mosby.

Varcarolis, E. (2002). *Foundations of psychiatric mental health nursing* (4th ed.). Philadelphia: W. B. Saunders.

Crisis Theory and Intervention

I. CRISIS INTERVENTION

A. Description
1. **Crisis** is a temporary state of severe emotional disorganization caused by failure of **coping mechanisms** and lack of support.
2. Decision making and problem solving are inadequate.
3. Treatment is immediate, supportive, and directly responsive to the immediate **crisis** to assist the client and the family through the stressful situation.

B. Phases of a **crisis**
1. Phase 1: External precipitating event
2. Phase 2
   a. Perception of threat
   b. Increase in anxiety
   c. Client may cope or resolve **crisis**.
3. Phase 3
   a. Failure of coping
   b. Increasing disorganization
   c. Emergence of physical symptoms
   d. Relationship problems
4. Phase 4
   a. Mobilization of internal and external resources
   b. Resolutions related to precrisis functioning that include functioning at a higher level, at the same level, or at a lower level

C. Types of crises (Box 75-1)

D. **Crisis** intervention
1. Treatment is immediate, supportive, and directly responsive to the immediate **crisis.**
2. Interventions are goal directed,
3. Feelings of the client are acknowledged.
4. Intervention provides opportunities for expression and validation of feelings.
5. Connections are made between the meaning of the event and the **crisis.**

6. Client explores alternative **coping mechanisms** and tries out new behaviors.

II. GRIEF

A. Grief is the emotional responses to a loss, a process that an individual must experience to finally accept the reality of loss.
B. Grief usually involves moving through a series of stages or tasks to help resolve the grief (Box 75-2).

BOX 75-1

Types of Crises

Maturational	Relates to developmental stages and associated role changes
Situational	Arises from an external source and is associated with a life event that upsets an individual or a group's psychological equilibrium
Adventitious	Relates to a crisis of disaster or an event that is not a part of everyday life and is unplanned and accidental

---

BOX 75-2

The Grief Response

STAGE 1: SHOCK AND DISBELIEF
Survivor may have feelings of numbness, difficulties with decision making, emotional outbursts, denial, and isolation.

STAGE 2: EXPERIENCING THE LOSS
Survivor may feel angry at the loved one who died or may feel guilt about the death.
Bargaining and or depression also may occur in this stage.

STAGE 3: REINTEGRATION
Survivor begins to reorganize his or her life and accepts the reality of the loss.

C. Feelings associated with grief can include anger, frustration, loneliness, sadness, guilt, regret, or peace.

D. Healing can occur when the pain of the loss has lessened and the survivor has adapted to life without the deceased; the survivor will continue to experience memories of the deceased.

E. Types of grief
   1. Normal grief: Physical, emotional, cognitive, or behavioral reactions can occur; the process of resolution can take months to years.
   2. Anticipatory grief occurs before the loss and is associated with an acute, chronic, or terminal illness.
   3. Disenfranchised grief occurs when a loss is experienced and cannot be acknowledged openly (societal norms do not define the loss as a loss within its traditional definition).
   4. Dysfunctional grief occurs with prolonged emotional instability and a lack of progression to successful coping with the loss.
   5. Children's grief is based on their developmental level (Box 75-3).

▶ **III. LOSS**
A. Loss is the absence of something desired or previously thought to be available.
B. Actual loss can be identified by others and can arise in response to or in anticipation of a situation.

BOX 75-3

Children's Grief

BIRTH TO 1 YEAR
Infant has no concept of death.
Infant reacts to the loss of mother or caregiver.

1 TO 2 YEARS
Child may see death as reversible.
Grief response occurs only to the death of the significant person in the child's life.
Child may scream, withdraw, or become disinterested in environment.

2 TO 5 YEARS
Child may see death as reversible.
Child has a sense of loss and is concerned about who will provide care.
Regression or aggressive behavior may occur.

5 TO 9 YEARS
Child begins to see death as permanent.
Child may feel responsible for the occurrence.
Child has difficulty concentrating.

PREADOLESCENT THROUGH ADOLESCENCE
Adolescent sees death as permanent.
Adolescent experiences a strong emotional reaction.
Adolescent may regress

BOX 75-4

Communication Process

Determine how much the client and family want to know.
Determine whether there is a spokesperson for the family.
Be aware of cultural and religious beliefs and how they may affect the communication process; consider personal space issues, eye contact, and touch.
Obtain an interpreter if necessary.
Allow opportunity for informed choices.
Assist with the decision-making process if asked; use problem solving to assist in decision making, and avoid interjecting personal views or opinions.
Encourage expression of feelings, concerns, and fears.
Be honest and truthful, and let the client and family know that you will not abandon them.
Ask the client and family about their expectations and needs.
Be a sensitive listener; sit in silence if necessary and appropriate.
Extend touch and hold the client's or family member's hand if appropriate.
Encourage reminiscing.
If you do not know what to do in a particular situation, seek assistance.
If you do not know what to say to a client or family who is talking about death, listen attentively and use therapeutic communication techniques such as open-ended questions or reflection.
Acknowledge your own feelings; let the client and family know that the topic of conversation is a difficult one and that you do not know what to say.
Realize that it is acceptable to cry with the client and family during the grief process.

C. Perceived loss is experienced by one person and cannot be verified by others.

D. Anticipatory loss is experienced before the loss occurs.

E. Mourning
   1. Mourning is the outward and social expression of loss.
   2. Mourning may be dictated by cultural and religious beliefs.

F. Bereavement
   1. Bereavement includes the inner feelings and the outward reactions of the survivor.
   2. Bereavement includes grief and mourning.

IV. NURSE'S ROLE: GRIEF AND LOSS ▲
A. The nurse's role includes the client, family members, and significant other.
B. The nurse communicates with the client, family members, and significant other (Box 75-4).
C. Allow ongoing opportunities for fully informed choices.
D. Facilitate the grief process; assess grief and assist the survivor to feel the loss and complete the tasks of the grief process.

E. Consider the survivor's culture, religion, family structure, individual life experiences, coping skills, and support systems.

F. Grief affects survivors physically, psychologically, socially, and spiritually; therefore a multidisciplinary team approach including a bereavement specialist facilitates the grief process.

▲ V. END-OF-LIFE

A. Description: End of life refers to issues related to death and dying.

B. Cultural and religious issues (Box 75-5; also refer to Chapter 6 for additional information regarding cultural and religious issues)

1. Hispanic and Latino groups
   a. Primary language is Spanish.
   b. Predominant religion is Roman Catholic.
   c. Prayer and folk remedies are common, as is the use of religious objects.
   d. Members may avoid eye contact as a sign of respect.
   e. Members tend not to complain of pain.
   f. The family generally makes decisions and may withhold the diagnosis or prognosis from the client.
   g. Extended family members often are involved in end-of-life care (pregnant women may be prohibited from caring for the dying or attending funerals).
   h. Several family members may be at the dying client's bedside.
   i. Vocal expression of grief and mourning is acceptable and expected.
   j. Members may refuse procedures that alter the body, such as organ donation or autopsy.
   k. Members may prefer to die at home.

2. African Americans
   a. Members discuss issues with the spouse or older family member (elders are held in high respect).
   b. Family is highly valued and is central to the care of the terminally ill.
   c. Pain is reported openly.
   d. Open displays of emotion are common and accepted.
   e. Organ and blood donation usually is not allowed.
   f. Members may prefer to die at home.

3. Chinese American
   a. Eye contact often is avoided because it represents disrespect to persons in authority.
   b. Personal distance should be maintained.
   c. Affection between family members rarely is exhibited in public.
   d. Members may not report pain.
   e. Family members may make decisions about care and often do not tell the client the diagnosis or prognosis.
   f. Dying at home may be considered bad luck.

BOX 75-5

Religion and End-of-Life Care

CHRISTIANITY

Catholic and Orthodox Religions
Priest anoints the sick.
Other sacraments before death include reconciliation and holy communion.

Protestant
No last rites are given (anointing of the sick is accepted by some groups).
Prayers are given to offer comfort and support.

Church of Jesus Christ of Latter-Day Saints (Mormons)
Cleric may administer a sacrament if the client requests.

Jehovah Witness
Members do not believe in sacraments.
Members will be excommunicated if they receive a blood transfusion.

ISLAM
Second-degree male relatives such as cousins or uncles should be the contact person and determine whether the client and/or family should be given information about the client.
Client may choose to face Mecca (west or southwest in the United States).
The head should be elevated above the body.
Discussions about death usually are not welcomed.
Stopping medical treatment is against Allah's (Arabic word for God) will.
Grief may be expressed through slapping or hitting the body.
If possible, only a same-sex Muslim should handle the body after death; if not possible, non-Muslims should wear gloves so as not to touch the body.

JUDAISM
Prolongation of life is important (a client on life support must remain so until death).
A dying person should not be left alone (a rabbi's presence is desired).
Autopsy and cremation are forbidden.

HINDUISM
Rituals include tying a thread around the neck or wrist of the dying person, sprinkling the person with special water, or placing a leaf of basil on the person's tongue.
After death, the sacred threads are not removed and the body is not washed.

BUDDHISM
A shrine to Buddha may be placed in the client's room.
Time for meditation at the shrine is important and should be respected.
Clients may refuse medications that may alter their awareness (such as opioids).
After death, a monk may recite prayers for 1 hour (need not be done in the presence of the body).

4. Native American
   a. Eye contact is avoided.
   b. Personal distance needs to be maintained.
   c. Family meetings may be held to make decisions about end-of-life and the type of treatments that should be pursued.
   d. Members may not report pain.
   e. Some tribes avoid contact with the dying (may prefer to die in the hospital).
C. Legal and ethical issues
   1. Outcomes related to care during illness and the dying experience should be based on the client's wishes.
   2. Issues for consideration may include organ and tissue donations, advance directives or other legal documents, withholding or withdrawing treatment, and cardiopulmonary resuscitation.
D. Palliative care
   1. Palliative care focuses on caring interventions and symptom management rather than cure for diseases that no longer respond to treatment.
   2. A pain-controlled and symptom-controlled environment is established (the dying client should be as pain free and as comfortable as possible).
   3. Hospice care provides support and care for clients in the last phases of incurable diseases so that they might live as fully and as comfortable as possible; client and family needs are the focus of any intervention.
E. Near-death physiological manifestations
   1. As death approaches, metabolism is reduced and the body gradually slows down until all function ends.
   2. Sensory organs: Client experiences blurred vision, decreased sense of taste and smell, decreased pain and touch perception, and loss of blink reflex, and client appears to stare (hearing is believed to be the last sense lost).
   3. Respirations
      a. Respirations may be rapid, slow, shallow, and irregular.
      b. Respirations may be noisy and wet sounding (death rattle).
      c. Cheyne-Stokes respiration is alternating periods of apnea and deep, rapid breathing.
   4. Circulation
      a. Heart rate slows, and blood pressure falls progressively.
      b. Skin is cool to touch, and extremities become pale, mottled, and cyanotic.
      c. Skin is waxlike very near death.
   5. Urinary output gradually decreases; incontinence may occur.
   6. Gastrointestinal motility and peristalsis diminish, leading to constipation, gas accumulation, and distension; a bowel movement may occur before death or at the time of death.

7. Musculoskeletal system: Client gradually loses ability to move, has difficulty speaking and swallowing, and loses the gag reflex.
F. Death
   1. Death occurs when all vital organs and body systems cease to function.
   2. Generally respirations cease first, and then the heart beat stops a few minutes thereafter.
G. Brain death occurs when the cerebral cortex stops functioning or is irreversibly damaged.
H. Nursing care
   1. Assessment of the client
      a. Assessment should be limited to obtaining essential data.
      b. Frequency of assessment depends on the client's stability (at least every 8 hours); as changes occur, assessment needs to be done more frequently.
      c. Avoid repeated, unnecessary assessments on the dying client.
   2. Physical care (Box 75-6)
   3. Psychosocial care
      a. Monitor for anxiety and depression.
      b. Monitor for fear (Box 75-7).
      c. Encourage the client and family to express feelings.
      d. Provide support and advocacy for the client and family.
      e. Provide privacy for the client and family.
      f. Provide a private room for the client.
      g. Maintain respect and dignity for the client.
   4. Postmortem care (Box 75-8)
      a. Maintain respect and dignity for the client.
      b. Determine whether the client is an organ donor; if so, follow appropriate procedures related to the donation.
      c. Consider cultural rituals, state laws, and agency procedures when performing postmortem care.
      d. Prepare the body for immediate viewing by the family.
      e. Provide privacy and time for the family to be with the deceased person.

VI. DEPRESSION

A. Description
   1. Depression affects feelings, thoughts, and behaviors.
   2. Depression can occur after a loss, including loss of self-esteem, the end of a significant relationship, the death of a loved one, or a traumatic event.
   3. The loss is followed by grief and mourning and if this process does not resolve, depression results.
   4. Depression may be mild, moderate, or severe.
   5. Treatment includes counseling, antidepressant medication, and electroconvulsive therapy.
B. Mild depression
   1. Triggered by an external event, and the experience follows the normal grief reaction
   2. Lasts less than 2 weeks

3. Feeling sad
4. Feeling let down or disappointed
5. Mild alterations in sleep patterns
6. Feeling less alert
7. Irritability
8. Disinterested in spending time with others
9. Increased use of alcohol or drugs

C. Moderate depression
1. Persists over time
2. The person experiences a sense of change and often seeks help.
3. Despondent and gloomy
4. Dejected
5. Low self-esteem

6. Helplessness and powerlessness
7. May experience intense anxiety and anger
8. Diurnal variation: The person may feel better at a certain time of the day, such as in the morning.
9. Slow thought processes and difficulty in concentrating
10. Rumination: persistent thinking about and discussion of a particular subject
11. Negative thinking and suicidal thoughts
12. Sleep disturbances
13. Social withdrawal
14. Anorexia, weight loss, and fatigue
15. Somatic complaints
16. Menstrual changes
17. Increased use of alcohol or drugs

D. Severe depression
1. Intense and pervasive
2. Despair and hopelessness
3. Guilt and worthlessness
4. Flat affect
5. May show agitation and pace about
6. Poor posture and unkempt appearance
7. Decreased speech

BOX 75-6

Physical Care to the Dying Client

PAIN
Administer pain medication.
Do not delay or deny pain medication.

DYSPNEA
Elevate the head of the bed or position on the side.
Administer supplemental oxygen.
Suction fluids from airway as needed.

SKIN
Assess color and temperature.
Assess for breakdown.
Implement measures to prevent breakdown.

DEHYDRATION
Maintain regular oral care.
Encourage taking of ice chips and sips of fluid.
Do not force the client to eat or drink.
Use moist cloths to provide moisture to the mouth.
Apply lubricant to the lips and oral mucous membranes.

ANOREXIA, NAUSEA, AND VOMITING
Provide antiemetics before meals.
Have family members provide the client's favorite foods.
Provide frequent small portions of favorite foods.

ELIMINATION
Monitor urinary and bowel elimination.
Place absorbent pads under the client and check frequently.

WEAKNESS AND FATIGUE
Provide rest periods.
Assess tolerance for activities.
Provide assistance and support as needed for maintaining bed or chair positions.

RESTLESSNESS
Maintain a calm soothing environment.
Do not restrain.
Limit the number of visitors at the client's bedside.
Allow a family member to stay with the client.

BOX 75-7

Fear Associated with Dying

FEAR OF PAIN
Fear of pain may occur based on anxieties related to dying.
Do not delay or deny pain relief measures to a terminally ill client.

FEAR OF LONELINESS AND ABANDONMENT
Allow family members to stay with the client.
Holding hands and touching (if culturally acceptable) and listening to the client are important.

FEAR OF MEANINGLESS
Client may feel hopeless and powerless.
Encourage life reviews and focus on the client's positive aspects of their life.

Adapted from Lewis, S., Heitkemper, M., & Dirksen, S. (2004). *Medical-surgical nursing: Assessment and management of clinical problems* (6th ed., p. 168). St. Louis: Mosby.

BOX 75-8

General Postmortem Procedures

Close the client's eyes.
Replace dentures.
Wash the body.
Place pads under the perineum.
Remove tubes and dressings.
Straighten the body and place a pillow under the head in preparation for family viewing.

8. Self-destructive thoughts; however, client may lack energy to act on thought
9. Social withdrawal
10. Poor concentration and overwhelmed by simple tasks
11. Severe psychomotor retardation
12. Anorexia and considerable weight loss
13. Constipation and urinary retention
14. Lack of sexual interest
15. Terminal insomnia
16. Diurnal variation: The person feels worse in the morning and better as the day goes on.
17. Delusions and hallucinations

E. Interventions
1. Altered Thought Processes
   a. Encourage client to discuss losses or changes in life situation.
   b. Encourage client to express sadness or anger and allow adequate time for verbal responses.
   c. Assist client in developing short-term goals.
   d. Encourage the use of problem solving and positive thinking.
   e. Limit decision making.
   f. Spend short periods of time throughout the day with the client.
   g. Be on time when a schedule is planned with the client.
   h. Sit in silence with clients who are not verbalizing.
   i. Use simple, concrete words when communicating.
   j. Avoid a cheerful attitude.
2. Risk for Self-Harm
   a. Assess for **suicide** clues and intervene to provide safety precautions as necessary.
   b. Ask client directly, "Have you thought of hurting yourself?"
   c. Assess lethality of plans.
   d. Do not leave client alone for extended periods.
   e. If the client has a suicidal plan, place on a one-to-one supervision.
   f. Form a suicidal contract with the client.
3. Activity Intolerance
   a. Encourage daily exercise.
   b. Assist with activities of daily living if the client is unable to perform them.
   c. Begin with one-to-one activities.
   d. Provide activities for easy mastery to increase self-esteem and assist to alleviate guilt feelings.
   e. Provide activities that do not require a great deal of concentration (simple card games, drawing).
   f. Engage in gross motor activities (walking).
   g. Eventually bring the client into small group activities and then large groups.
4. Altered Nutrition
   a. Ensure adequate nutrition.
   b. Offer small, high-calorie, high-protein snacks and fluids throughout the day.
   c. Stay with the client during meals.
   d. Weigh client weekly.
   e. Assess bowel patterns for constipation.
5. Sleep Pattern Disturbance
   a. Ensure adequate sleep.
   b. Provide rest periods after activities.
   c. Encourage the client to dress and stay out of bed during the day.
   d. Provide relaxation measures at bedtime.
   e. Decrease environmental stimuli at bedtime.
   f. Spend time with the client before bedtime.

VII. ELECTROCONVULSIVE THERAPY

A. Description
1. Electroconvulsive therapy is an effective treatment for depression that consists of inducing a grand mal (tonic-clonic) seizure by passing an electrical current through electrodes that are attached to the temples.
2. The administration of a muscle relaxant minimizes seizure activity, preventing damage to long bones and cervical vertebrae.
3. The usual course is 6 to 12 treatments given 2 to 3 times per week.
4. Maintenance electroconvulsive therapy once a month may help to decrease the relapse rate for the client with recurrent depression.
5. Electroconvulsive therapy is not a permanent cure.
6. Electroconvulsive therapy is not necessarily effective in the client with dysrhythmic depression or the client with depression and personality disorders, those with drug dependence, or those with depression brought on by situational or social difficulties.
7. At-risk clients include those with recent myocardial infarction, cerebrovascular accident, or cerebral vascular malformation or clients with an intracranial mass lesion.

B. Uses of electroconvulsive therapy
1. Clients with major depressive and bipolar depressive disorders especially when psychotic symptoms are present such as delusions of guilt, somatic delusions, and delusions of infidelity
2. Clients who have depression with significant psychomotor retardation and stupor
3. Manic clients whose conditions are resistant to lithium and antipsychotic medications and in clients who are rapid cyclers (a client with a bipolar disorder who has many episodes of mood swings close together)
4. Clients with schizophrenia (especially catatonia), those with schizoaffective syndromes, and psychotic clients

Electroconvulsive Therapy: Indications for Use

Antidepressant medications have no effect.
A need exists for a rapid, definitive response such as when a client is suicidal or homicidal.
The client is in extreme agitation or stupor.
The risks of other treatments outweigh the risk of electroconvulsive therapy.
The client has a history of poor medication response, a history of good electroconvulsive therapy response, or both.
The client prefers electroconvulsive therapy as a treatment.

C. Indications for use of electroconvulsive therapy (Box 75-9)

D. Preprocedure
 1. Explain the procedure to the client.
 2. Encourage the client to discuss feelings, including myths regarding electroconvulsive therapy.
 3. Teach the client and family what to expect.
 4. Informed consent must be obtained when voluntary clients are being treated.
 5. For involuntary clients, when informed consent cannot be obtained, permission may be obtained from the next of kin, although in some states the permission for electroconvulsive therapy must be obtained from the court.
 6. Maintain NPO status of client after midnight or at least 4 hours before treatment.
 7. Take baseline vital signs.
 8. Ask the client to void.
 9. Have client remove hairpins, contact lenses, and dentures.
 10. Administer preoperative medication if prescribed; glycopyrrolate (Robinul) or atropine sulfate may be prescribed to prevent the potential for aspiration and to minimize bradydysrhythmias in response to electrical stimulants.

E. During the procedure
 1. Place a blood pressure cuff on one of the client's arms.
 2. Insert an intravenous line and attach electroencephalogram and electrocardiogram electrodes.
 3. Place a pulse oximeter onto the client's finger.
 4. Monitor blood pressure throughout the treatment.
 5. Medications administered may include a short-acting anesthetic such as methohexital sodium (Brevital), thiopental sodium (Pentothal) and a muscle relaxant such as succinylcholine (Anectine)
 6. Administer 100% oxygen by mask via positive pressure throughout the procedure.
 7. Place an airway or bite block to prevent biting of the tongue.
 8. Administer electrical stimulus; the seizure should last 30 to 60 seconds.

F. Postprocedure
 1. The client will be transported to a recovery room with the blood pressure cuff and pulse oximeter in place, where oxygen, suction, and other emergency equipment is available.
 2. Once the client is awake, talk to the client and take vital signs.
 3. The client may be confused; provide frequent orientation (brief, distinct, and simple) and reassurance.
 4. Client returns to the nursing unit when a 90% oxygen saturation level is maintained, vital signs are stable, and mental status is satisfactory.
 5. Assess the gag reflex before giving the client fluids, food, or medication.

G. Potential side effects
 1. Major side effects are confusion, disorientation, and short-term memory loss.
 2. The client may be confused and disorientated on awakening.
 3. Memory deficits may occur, but memory usually recovers completely, although some clients have memory loss lasting up to 6 months.

VIII. SUICIDAL BEHAVIOR

A. Description
 1. Suicidal clients characteristically have feelings of worthlessness, guilt, and hopelessness that are so overwhelming that they feel unable to go on with life and unfit to live.
 2. The nurse caring for a depressed client always considers the possibility of **suicide**.

B. High-risk groups
 1. Those with a history of previous **suicide attempts**
 2. Family history of **suicide attempts**
 3. Adolescents
 4. Older clients
 5. Disabled or terminally ill adults
 6. Clients with personality disorders
 7. Clients with organic brain syndrome or dementia
 8. Depressed or psychotic clients
 9. Substance abusers

C. Clues (Box 75-10)

D. Assessment (Box 75-11)

E. Interventions
 1. Initiate **suicide** precautions.
 2. Remove harmful objects.
 3. Do not leave the client alone.
 4. Provide a one-to-one supervision at all times.
 5. Provide a nonjudgmental, caring attitude.
 6. Develop a contract that is written, dated, and signed and that indicates alternative behavior at times of suicidal thoughts.
 7. Encourage the client to talk about feelings and to identify positive aspects about self.
 8. Encourage active participation in own care.

BOX 75-10

Suicidal Clues

Giving away personal, special, and prized possessions
Canceling social engagements
Making out or changing a will
Taking out or changing insurance policies
Positive or negative changes in behavior
Poor appetite
Sleeping difficulties
Feelings of hopelessness
Difficulty in concentrating
Loss of interest in activities
Client statements that indicate an intent to attempt suicide
Sudden calmness or improvement in a depressed client
Client questions about poisons, guns, or other lethal objects

BOX 75-11

Suicidal Client: Assessment

THE PLAN

Does the client have a plan?
What is the plan, how lethal is the plan, and how likely is death to occur?
Does the client have the means to carry out the plan?

CLIENT HISTORY OF ATTEMPTS

What suicide attempts occurred in the past and what were the outcomes?
Was the client accidentally rescued?
Have the past attempts and methods been the same, or have methods increased in lethality?

PSYCHOSOCIAL

Is the client alone or alienated from others?
Is hostility or depression present?
Do hallucinations exist?
Is substance abuse present?
Has client had any recent losses or physical illness?
Has client had any environmental or lifestyle changes?

9. Keep client active by assigning simple tasks.
10. Check that visitors do not leave harmful objects in the client's room.
11. Identify support systems.
12. Do not allow the client to leave the unit unless accompanied by a staff member.
13. Continue to assess the client's **suicide** potential.

IX. ABUSIVE BEHAVIORS

A. Anger
  1. Anger is a feeling of annoyance that may be displaced onto an object or person.
  2. Anger is used to avoid anxiety and gives a feeling of power in situations in which the person feels out of control.

B. Aggression can be harmful and destructive when not controlled.
C. Violence is the physical force that is threatening to the safety of self and others.
D. Assessment
  1. History of violence or self-harm
  2. Poor impulse control and low tolerance of frustration
  3. Defiant and argumentative
  4. Raising of voice
  5. Making verbal threats
  6. Pacing and agitation
  7. Muscle rigidity
  8. Flushed face
  9. Glaring at others
E. Interventions
  1. Maintain safety for the client, other client's, and self.
  2. Use a calm approach and communicate with a calm, clear tone of voice (be assertive not aggressive and avoid verbal struggles)
  3. Maintain a large personal space and use a nonaggressive posture.
  4. Listen actively and acknowledge the client's anger.
  5. Determine what the client considers to be his or her need.
  6. Provide the client with clear options that deal with the client's behavior, set limits on behavior, and make the client aware of the consequences of anger and violence.
  7. Discuss the use of **restraints** or seclusion if the client is unable to control angry behavior that may lead to violence.
  8. Assist the client with problem solving and decision making regarding the options.
F. **Restraints** and seclusion
  1. Description
    a. Physical **restraints:** any manual method or mechanical device, material, or equipment that inhibits free movement
    b. **Seclusion:** the last step in a process to maximize safety for a client and others, in which a client is placed alone in a specially designed room for protection and close supervision
    c. Chemical **restraints:** medications given for a specific purpose of inhibiting a specific behavior or movement and that have an impact on the client's ability to relate to the environment
  2. Use of **restraints** and **seclusion**
    a. **Restraints** and **seclusion** should never be used as punishment or for the convenience of the health care staff.
    b. The least restrictive means of restraint for the shortest duration should be used.
    c. **Restraints** and **seclusion** are used when behavior is physically harmful to the client or others.

d. **Restraints** and **seclusion** are used when the disruptive behavior presents a danger to the facility.

e. **Restraints** and **seclusion** are used when alternative or less restrictive measures are insufficient in protecting the client or others from harm.

f. **Restraints** and **seclusion** are used when the client anticipates that a controlled environment would be helpful and requests seclusion.

g. **Restraints** require a written order of a physician, which must be reviewed and renewed every 24 hours and which also must specify the type of restraint to be used.

h. In an emergency, the charge nurse may place a client in **restraints** or **seclusion** and obtain a written or verbal order as soon as possible thereafter.

i. Laws require the consent of the client unless an emergency situation exists and can be documented.

j. The client must be removed from **restraints** or **seclusion** when safer and quieter behavior is observed.

k. While in **restraints** or **seclusion,** the client must be protected from all sources of harm.

l. The nurse must document the behavior leading to **restraints** or **seclusion** and the time the client is placed in and released from **restraints** or **seclusion.**

m. The client in **restraints** or **seclusion** needs constant one-to-one supervision; physical, safety, and comfort needs must be assessed every 15 to 30 minutes, and these observations are also documented.

X. FAMILY VIOLENCE

A. Description

1. The violence begins with threats or verbal or physical minor assaults (tension-building), and the victim attempts to comply with the requests of the abuser.
2. The abuser loses control and becomes destructive and harmful (acute battering) while the victim attempts to protect himself or herself.
3. Following the battering, the abuser then becomes loving and attempts to make peace (calmness and a diffusion of tension).
4. The abuser believes that violence is normal and that the victim is responsible for the **abuse.**
5. Outsiders are usually not aware of what is happening in the family.
6. Family members are isolated socially and lack autonomy and trust among each other; caring and intimacy in the family are absent.
7. Family members expect other members of the family to meet their needs, but none are able to do so.
8. The abuser threatens to abandon the family.

BOX 75-12

Types of Violence

PHYSICAL VIOLENCE
Infliction of physical pain or bodily harm

SEXUAL VIOLENCE
Any form of sexual contact without consent

EMOTIONAL VIOLENCE
Infliction of mental anguish

PHYSICAL NEGLECT
Failure to provide health care to prevent or treat physical or emotional illnesses

DEVELOPMENTAL NEGLECT
Failure to provide physical and cognitive stimulation needed to prevent developmental deficits

EDUCATIONAL NEGLECT
Depriving a child of education

ECONOMIC EXPLOITATION
Illegal or improper exploitation of money, funds, or other resources for one's personal gain

---

B. Types of violence (Box 75-12)

C. The vulnerable person

1. The vulnerable person is the one in the family unit against whom violence is perpetrated.
2. Those most vulnerable are children and older adults.
3. Every battered person is a crime victim.

D. Characteristics of abusers

1. Impaired self-esteem
2. Strong dependency needs
3. Narcissistic and suspicious
4. History of **abuse** during childhood
5. Perceive victims as their property and believe that they are entitled to **abuse** them

E. Characteristics of victims

1. Victims feel trapped, dependent, helpless, and powerless.
2. Victims are depressed.
3. Victims have low self-esteem and blame themselves for the violence.

F. Interventions

1. Report suspected or actual cases of child **abuse** or **abuse** to the older adult to appropriate authorities (follow state and agency guidelines).
2. Assess for evidence of physical injuries.
3. Ensure privacy and confidentiality during the assessment and provide a nonjudgmental and empathetic approach to foster trust; reassure the victim that he or she has not done anything wrong.

4. Assist the victim to develop self-protective abilities and other problem-solving abilities.
5. Develop a safety plan (a fast escape if the violence returns) and ensure that the victim is aware of safe houses and shelters in the community.
6. Assess suicidal potential of the victim.
7. Assess the potential for homicide.
8. Assess for the use of drugs and alcohol.
9. Determine family coping patterns and support systems.
10. Provide support and assistance in coping with contacting the legal system.
11. Assist in resolving family dysfunction with prescribed therapies.
12. Encourage individual therapy for victims that promotes coping with the trauma and prevents further psychological conflict.
13. Provide individual therapy for abusers that focuses on preventing violent behavior and repairing relationships.
14. Encourage psychotherapy, counseling, group therapy, and support groups to assist family members to develop coping strategies.
15. Assist the family to identify an access to community and personal resources.
16. Maintain accurate and thorough medical health records.

▲ **XI. CHILD ABUSE (REFER TO CHAPTER 35.)**
A. Description: Child **abuse** involves physical, emotional, or sexual **abuse** and also can involve neglect.
B. Assessment
1. Physical **abuse**
   a. Unexplained bruises, burns, or fractures
   b. Bald spots on scalp
   c. Apprehensiveness in child
   d. Extreme aggressiveness or withdrawal
   e. Fear of parents
   f. Lack of crying when approached by a stranger
2. Physical neglect
   a. Inadequate weight gain
   b. Poor hygiene
   c. Consistent hunger (begs or steals food)
   d. Inconsistent school attendance
   e. Constant fatigue
   f. Reports of lack of child supervision
   g. Delinquency
3. Emotional **abuse**
   a. Speech disorders
   b. Habit disorders, such as sucking, biting, rocking
   c. Learning disorders
   d. Self-harm behaviors
4. Sexual **abuse**
   a. Difficulty walking or sitting
   b. Torn, stained, or bloody underclothing
   c. Pain, swelling, or itching of the genitals

d. Bruises, bleeding, or lacerations in the genital or anal area
   e. Poor peer relations
   f. Delinquency
   g. Changes in sleep patterns
   h. Self-harm behaviors
5. Shaken baby syndrome
   a. **Abuse** can cause intracranial hemorrhage leading to cerebral edema and death.
   b. Baby often has respiratory problems.
   c. Nurse would note full bulging fontanelles and a head circumference greater than expected.
C. Interventions
1. Assess injuries; support the child during a thorough physical assessment.
2. Report cases of suspected **abuse** to appropriate authorities (follow state and agency guidelines).
3. Remove the child from the abusive environment and plan to place the child in an environment that is safe (contact child protective services), thereby preventing further injury.
4. Move slowly and avoid any loud noises when near the child.
5. Communicate with the child at the child's eye level.
6. Reassure the child that he or she is not "bad" and is not responsible for the abuser's behavior.
7. Document accurately and completely all information related to the suspected **abuse**.
8. Assist the parents' in identifying stressors and alternative ways to express feelings.
9. Provide education to the parents, and refer parents to **crisis** hotlines and community support systems such as Parents Anonymous (a group for parents who have abused or fear that they may **abuse** their child physically) or Parents United International, Inc. (a group devoted to helping sexually abused families).

XII. ABUSE TO THE OLDER ADULT
A. Description
1. **Abuse** to an older adult involves physical, emotional, or sexual **abuse** and also can involve neglect or economic exploitation.
2. Individuals at most risk include those who are dependent because of their immobility or altered mental status.
3. Factors that contribute to **abuse** and neglect include long-standing family violence, caregiver stress, and the individual's increasing dependence on others.
4. Victims may attempt to dismiss injuries as accidental, and abusers may prevent victims from receiving proper medical care to avoid discovery.
5. Victims often are isolated socially by their abusers.
B. Assessment
1. Physical **abuse**
   a. Sprains, dislocations, or fractures
   b. Abrasions, bruises, or lacerations

c. Pressure sores

d. Puncture wounds

e. Burns

2. Sexual **abuse**

a. Torn or stained underclothing

b. Discomfort or bleeding in the genital area

c. Difficulty in walking or sitting

d. Unexplained genital infections or disease

3. Emotional **abuse**

a. Confusion

b. Fearful and agitated

c. Changes in appetite and weight

d. Withdrawn and loss of interest in self and social activities

4. Neglect

a. Disheveled appearance

b. Dressed inadequately or inappropriately

c. Dehydration and malnutrition

d. Lacking physical needs, such as glasses, hearing aids, and dentures

5. Skin breaks

6. Signs of medication overdose

7. Economic exploitation

a. Inability to pay bills and fearful when discussing finances

b. Confused, inaccurate, or no knowledge of finances

C. Interventions

1. Assess for physical injuries and treat physical injuries.

2. Report cases of suspected **abuse** to appropriate authorities (follow state and agency guidelines).

3. Remove the older adult from the abusive environment and contact elderly protective services.

4. Explore alternative living arrangements that are least restrictive and disruptive to the victim.

5. Obtain assistance for financial matters.

6. Provide referrals to emergency community resources.

7. Assess the need for respite care and arrange counseling and treatment for the abuser.

▲ XIII. RAPE AND SEXUAL ASSAULT

A. Description

1. Rape is engaging another person in a sexual act and/or sexual intercourse through the use of force and without the consent of the sexual partner.

2. The victim is not required by law to report the rape or assault.

3. The victim often is blamed by others and often receives no support from significant others.

4. Acquaintance rapes involve someone known to the victim.

5. Statutory rape is the act of sexual intercourse with a person under the age of legal consent even if the minor consents.

6. Marital rape

a. Husbands of abused women believe it is their right to have sex whenever they want.

b. Victims describe forced vaginal intercourse or anal intercourse, being physically abused during sex, having objects inserted into their vagina and anus, or being forced to have sex with their animals or while their children are present.

B. Assessment

1. Female client

a. Obtain the date of the last menstrual period.

b. Determine form of birth control used and last act of intercourse before rape.

c. Determine duration of intercourse, orifices violated, and penile penetration.

d. Determine use of condom by perpetrator.

2. Shame, embarrassment, and humiliation

3. Anger and revenge

4. Fear of telling others for fear of not being believed

C. Rape trauma syndrome

1. Sleep disturbances, nightmares

2. Loss of appetite

3. Fears, anxiety, phobias, suspicion

4. Decrease in activities and motivation

5. Disruptions in relationships with partner, family, friends

6. Self-blame, guilt, shame

7. Lowered self-esteem, feelings of worthlessness

8. Somatic complaints

D. Interventions

1. Perform the assessment in a quiet, private area.

2. Stay with the victim.

3. Assess the victim's stress level before performing treatments and procedures.

4. Victim should not shower, bathe, douche (female), or change clothing until an examination is performed.

5. Obtain written consent for the examination, photographs, laboratory tests, release of information, and laboratory samples.

6. Assist with the female pelvic examination and obtaining specimens to detect semen (the pelvic examination may trigger a flashback of the attack); a shower and fresh clothing should be made available to the client after the examination.

7. Preserve any evidence.

8. Treat physical injuries and provide client safety.

9. Document all events in the care of the victim.

10. Reinforce to the victim that surviving the assault is most important; if the victim survived the rape, then he or she did exactly what was necessary to stay alive.

11. Refer to **crisis** intervention and support groups.

PRACTICE QUESTIONS

1. The nurse is reviewing the assessment data of a client admitted to the mental health unit. The nurse notes

that the admission nurse has documented that the client is experiencing anxiety as a result of a situational crisis. The nurse determines that this type of crisis could be caused by
1. A fire that destroyed the client's home.
2. A recent rape episode experienced by the client.
3. The death of a loved one.
4. Witnessing a murder.

2. The nurse is conducting an initial assessment on a client in crisis. When assessing the client's perception of the precipitating event that led to the crisis, the most appropriate question to ask is
1. "What leads you to seek help now?"
2. "Who is available to help you?"
3. "What do you usually do to feel better?"
4. "With whom do you live?"

3. The nurse is developing a plan of care for the client in a crisis state. When developing the plan, the nurse considers which of the following?
1. Presenting symptoms in a crisis situation are similar for all individuals experiencing a crisis.
2. A crisis state indicates that the individual is suffering from an emotional illness.
3. A crisis state indicates that the individual is suffering from an mental illness.
4. A client's response to a crisis is individualized and what constitutes a crisis for one person may not constitute a crisis for another person.

4. The nurse observes that a client with a potential for violence is agitated, pacing up and down the hallway, and is making aggressive and belligerent gestures at other clients. Which statement would be most appropriate to make to this client?
1. "What is causing you to become agitated?"
2. "You need to stop that behavior now!"
3. "You will need to be restrained if you do not change your behavior."
4. "You will need to be placed in seclusion!"

5. During a conversation with a depressed client on an inpatient unit, the client says to the nurse, "My family would be better off without me." The nurse's best response is
1. "Everyone feels this way when they are depressed."
2. "Have you talked to your family about this."
3. "You sound very upset. Are you thinking of hurting yourself."
4. "You will feel better once your medication begins to work."

6. The nurse has been observing a client closely who has been displaying aggressive behaviors. The nurse observes that the behavior displayed by the client is escalating. Which nursing intervention is least helpful to this client at this time?
1. Acknowledge the client's behavior.
2. Maintain a safe distance with the client.
3. Assist the client to an area that is quiet.
4. Initiate confinement measures.

7. Which behavior observed by the nurse indicates a suspicion that a depressed female adolescent client may be suicidal?
1. The client becomes angry while speaking on the telephone and slams the receiver down on the hook.
2. The client runs out of the therapy group, swearing at the group leader, and runs to her room.
3. The client gets angry with her roommate when the roommate borrows the client's clothes without asking.
4. The client gives away a prized compact disc and a cherished autograph picture of the performer.

8. A client is admitted to the mental health unit following a serious suicidal attempt by hanging. The nurse's most important aspect of care is to maintain client safety. This is accomplished best by
1. Assigning a staff member to the client who will remain with the client at all times.
2. Admitting the client to a seclusion room where all potentially dangerous articles are removed.
3. Removing the client's clothing and placing the client in a hospital gown.
4. Requesting that a peer remain with the client at all times.

9. The police arrive at the emergency room with a client who has seriously lacerated both wrists. The initial nursing action is to
1. Examine and treat the wound sites.
2. Secure and record a detailed history.
3. Encourage and assist the client to ventilate feelings.
4. Administer an antianxiety agent.

10. The nursing care plan indicates a nursing diagnosis of risk for self-directed violence, suicidal ideations with a plan. An expected outcome of this plan of care would be that the client
1. Develops adequate coping and problem solving skills.
2. Displays less anxiety and agitation.
3. Establishes a relationship with staff and peers.
4. Denies suicidal ideation and identifies options to deal with stressors.

11. The nurse receives a telephone call from a male client who states that he wants to kill himself and has a bottle of sleeping pills in front of him. The best nursing action is to
1. Insist that the client give you his name and address so that you can get the police there immediately.
2. Keep the client talking and allow the client to ventilate feelings.
3. Use therapeutic communication techniques, especially the reflection of feelings.
4. Keep the client talking and signal to another staff member to trace the call so that appropriate help can be sent.

12. A client is admitted to the hospital with a nursing diagnosis of dysfunctional grieving related to the

loss of a spouse. The client progresses well and is approaching discharge. Which of the following is an appropriate outcome for this nursing diagnosis?

1. The client verbalizes stages of grief and plans to attend a community grief group.
2. The client verbalizes connections between significant losses and low self-esteem.
3. The client verbalizes decreased desire for self-harm and discusses two alternatives to suicide.
4. The client reports three additional coping strategies.

13. The client in a severe major depressive episode is unable to address activities of daily living (ADLs). The most appropriate nursing intervention is to

1. Feed, bathe, and dress the client as needed until the client can perform these activities independently.
2. Structure the client's day so that adequate time can be devoted to the client's assuming responsibility for the ADLs.
3. Offer the client choices and consequences for the failure to comply with the expectation of maintaining ADLs.
4. Have the client's peers confront the client about how the noncompliance in addressing ADLs affects the milieu.

14. The nurse is preparing a hospitalized client with a diagnosis of depression for discharge. In evaluating the coping strategies learned during hospitalization, the nurse would recognize which of the following statements, if made by the client, as an indication that further teaching needs to occur?

1. "I have learned ways to deal with the stresses in my life."
2. "I know that I won't become depressed again."
3. "I know that I can't be all things to all people."
4. "I need to take my medications just as prescribed."

15. The nurse is monitoring a client who is in seclusion. The nurse determines that the client is safe to come out of seclusion when the client states

1. "I am no longer a threat to myself or others."
2. "I need to go to the bathroom."
3. "I want to be alone for a while in my own room."
4. "I can't breathe in here. The walls are closing in on me."

16. The nurse is preparing a discharge plan for the client who attempted suicide. The plan of care should focus on which of the following?

1. Follow-up appointments
2. Contracts and immediate available crisis resources
3. Encouraging the family always to be with the client
4. Providing the hospital telephone number

17. An older male client who is a victim of elder abuse and the family have been attending weekly counseling sessions. Which of the following statements, if made by the abusive family member, would

indicate that the abuser has learned positive coping skills?

1. "I will be more careful to make sure that my father's needs are met."
2. "I am so sorry and embarrassed that the abusive event occurred. It won't happen again."
3. "I feel better able to care for my father now that I know where to obtain assistance."
4. "Now that my father is moving into my home, I will need to change my ways."

18. The moderately depressed client who was hospitalized 2 days ago suddenly begins smiling and reporting that the crisis is over. The client says to the nurse, "I'm finally cured." The nurse interprets this behavior as a cue to modify the treatment plan by

1. Allowing the client off unit privileges as needed.
2. Suggesting a reduction of medication.
3. Allowing increased "in room" activities.
4. Increasing the level of suicide precautions.

19. The nurse is planning care for a client being admitted to the nursing unit who attempted suicide. Which of the following priority nursing interventions will the nurse include in the plan of care?

1. Check whereabouts of the client every 15 minutes.
2. Suicide precautions with 30 minute checks
3. One-to-one suicide precautions
4. Ask the client to report suicidal thoughts immediately.

20. The emergency room nurse is caring for a client who has been identified as a victim of physical abuse. In planning care for the client, which of the following is the priority nursing action?

1. Adhering to the mandatory abuse reporting laws
2. Obtaining treatment for the abusing family member
3. Notifying the case worker of the family situation
4. Removing the client from any immediate danger

21. The emergency room nurse is caring for an adult client who is a victim of family violence. Which priority instruction would be included in the discharge instructions?

1. Explaining the importance of leaving the violent situation
2. Information regarding shelters
3. Instructions regarding self-defense classes
4. Instructions regarding calling the police

22. A female victim of a sexual assault is being seen in the crisis center. The client states that she still feels "as though the rape just happened yesterday" even though it has been a few months since the incident. The most appropriate nursing response is which of the following?

1. "What do you think that you can do to alleviate some of your fears about being raped again"?
2. "Tell me more about the incident that causes you to feel like the rape just occurred."

3. "It will take some time to get over these feelings about your rape."
4. "You need to try to be realistic. The rape did not just occur."

23. The nurse in the emergency department is caring for a young female victim of sexual assault. The client's physical assessment is complete and physical evidence has been collected. The nurse notes that the client is withdrawn, confused, and at times physically immobile. These behaviors are interpreted by the nurse as
    1. Evidence that the client is a high suicide risk.
    2. Indicative of the need for hospital admission.
    3. Signs of depression.
    4. Normal reactions to a devastating event.
24. The nurse has been working with a victim of rape in a clinic setting for the past 4 weeks. Which of the following is unrealistic as a short-term initial goal?
    1. The client will resolve feelings of fear and anxiety related to the rape trauma.
    2. Physical wounds will heal.
    3. The client will verbalize feelings about the event.
    4. The client will participate in the treatment plan.
25. A client comes to the clinic after losing all personal belongings in a hurricane. The nurse develops a nursing diagnosis of Ineffective Coping. Which of the following is the least realistic goal for this client?

1. The client will identify a realistic perception of stressors.
2. The client will develop adaptive coping patterns.
3. The client will express and share feelings regarding the present crisis.
4. The client will stop blaming himself or herself for the lack of insurance.

CRITICAL THINKING: MULTIPLE RESPONSE

A nurse is preparing to care for a dying client, and several family members are at the client's bedside. Select the therapeutic techniques that the nurse will use when communicating with the family.

___ Be honest and truthful and let the client and family know that you will not abandon them.

___ Explain everything that is happening to all family members.

___ Encourage expression of feelings, concerns, and fears.

___ Extend touch and hold the client's or family member's hand if appropriate.

___ Make the decisions for the family.

___ Discourage reminiscing.

ANSWERS

1. 3
Rationale: A situational crisis arises from external rather than internal sources. External situations that could precipitate crisis include loss of or change of a job, the death of a loved one, abortion, a change in financial status, divorce, the addition of new family members, pregnancy, and severe illness. Options 1, 2, and 4 identify adventitious crisis. An adventitious crisis is not a part of every day life, is unplanned, or accidental.
Test-Taking Strategy: Use the process of elimination. Eliminate options 1, 2, and 4 because they are similar types of occurrences. If you had difficulty with this question, review the types of crisis.
Level of Cognitive Ability: Analysis
Client Needs: Psychosocial Integrity
Integrated Process: Nursing Process—analysis
Content Area: Mental health
Reference: Fortinash, K., & Holoday-Worret, P. (2000). *Psychiatric mental health nursing* (2nd ed., p. 596). St. Louis: Mosby.

2. 1
Rationale: A nurse's initial task when assessing a client in crisis is to assess the individual or family and the problem. The more clearly the problem can be defined, the better the chance a solution can be found. Option 1 will assist in determining data related to the precipitating event that led to the crisis.

Options 2 and 4 assess situational supports. Option 3 assesses personal coping skills.
Test-Taking Strategy: Use the process of elimination. Note the key words "precipitating event." Focus on these key words when selecting the correct option. Eliminate options 2 and 4 because this data will determine support systems. Eliminate option 3 because this question would be asked when determining coping skills. Review assessment techniques for the client in crisis if you had difficulty with this question.
Level of Cognitive Ability: Application
Client Needs: Psychosocial Integrity
Integrated Process: Nursing Process—assessment
Content Area: Mental health
Reference: Fortinash, K., & Holoday-Worret, P. (2000). *Psychiatric mental health nursing* (2nd ed., p. 127). St. Louis: Mosby.

3. 4
Rationale: Although each crisis response can be described in similar terms as far as presenting symptoms are concerned, what constitutes a crisis for one person may not constitute a crisis for another person because each is a unique individual. Being in the crisis state does not mean that the client is suffering from an emotional or mental illness.
Test-Taking Strategy: Use the process of elimination. Eliminate option 1 because of the word "all." Next eliminate options 2 and 3 because a crisis does not indicate "illness." Review the characteristics of a crisis state if you had difficulty with this question.

Level of Cognitive Ability: Analysis
Client Needs: Psychosocial Integrity
Integrated Process: Nursing Process—planning
Content Area: Mental health
Reference: Fortinash, K., & Holoday-Worret, P. (2000). *Psychiatric mental health nursing* (2nd ed., pp. 592, 598). St. Louis: Mosby.

4. 1

Rationale: The best statement is to ask the client what is causing the agitation. This will assist the client to become aware of the behavior and may assist the nurse in planning appropriate interventions for the client. Option 2 is demanding behavior that could cause increased agitation in the client. Options 3 and 4 are threats to the client and are inappropriate.
Test-Taking Strategy: Use the process of elimination. Eliminate option 2 because of the demand that it places on the client. Eliminate options 3 and 4 because they indicate threats to the client. Review appropriate nursing actions for the agitated client if you had difficulty with this question.
Level of Cognitive Ability: Application
Client Needs: Psychosocial Integrity
Integrated Process: Communication and Documentation
Content Area: Mental health
References: Fortinash, K., & Holoday-Worret, P. (2000). *Psychiatric mental health nursing* (2nd ed., p. 268). St. Louis: Mosby.
Varcarolis, E. (2002). *Foundations of psychiatric mental health nursing* (4th ed., p. 677). Philadelphia: W. B. Saunders.

5. 3

Rationale: Clients who are depressed may be at risk for suicide. For the nurse to assess suicidal ideation and plan is critical. Ask the client directly if a plan for self-harm exists. Options 1, 2, and 4 do not deal directly with the client's feelings.
Test-Taking Strategy: Using therapeutic communication techniques will assist in directing you to the correct option. Option 3 is the only option that deals directly with the client's feelings. Additionally, clients at risk for suicide need to be assessed directly regarding the potential for self-harm. Review care to the client at risk for suicide if you had difficulty with this question.
Level of Cognitive Ability: Application
Client Needs: Psychosocial Integrity
Integrated Process: Communication and Documentation
Content Area: Mental health
Reference: Stuart, G., & Laraia, M. (2001). *Principles & practice of psychiatric nursing* (7th ed., pp. 35, 353). St. Louis: Mosby.

6. 4

Rationale: During the escalation period, the client's behavior is moving toward loss of control. Nursing actions include taking control, maintaining a safe distance, acknowledging behavior, moving the client to a quiet area, and medicating the client if appropriate. To initiate confinement measures during this period is not appropriate. Initiation of confinement measures is most appropriate during the crisis period.
Test-Taking Strategy: Note the key words "behavior," "escalating," and "least helpful." Recalling that the least restrictive

measures should be used will direct you to option 4. Review care to the client with aggressive behavior if you had difficulty with this question.
Level of Cognitive Ability: Application
Client Needs: Psychosocial Integrity
Integrated Process: Nursing Process—implementation
Content Area: Mental health
Reference: Fortinash, K., & Holoday-Worret, P. (2000). *Psychiatric mental health nursing* (2nd ed., p. 172). St. Louis: Mosby.

7. 4

Rationale: A depressed, suicidal client often gives away that which is of value as a way of saying good-bye and wanting to be remembered. Options 1, 2, and 3 deal with anger and acting-out behaviors that are often typical of any adolescent.
Test-Taking Strategy: Use the process of elimination. Eliminate options 1, 2, and 3 because they are similar. Option 4 is different and an action that could indicate that the client may be "saying good-bye." Review behaviors that indicate a suicide intent if you had difficulty with this question.
Level of Cognitive Ability: Analysis
Client Needs: Psychosocial Integrity
Integrated Process: Nursing Process—assessment
Content Area: Mental health
References: Fortinash, K., & Holoday-Worret, P. (2000). *Psychiatric mental health nursing* (2nd ed., p. 432). St. Louis: Mosby.
Stuart, G., & Laraia, M. (2001). *Principles & practice of psychiatric nursing* (7th ed., pp. 787-788). St. Louis: Mosby.

8. 1

Rationale: Hanging is a serious suicide attempt. The plan of care must reflect action that will ensure the client safety. Constant observation status (one-to-one) with a staff member who is never less than an arm's length away is the best selection. Seclusion should not be the initial intervention, and the least restrictive measure should be used. Placing the client in a hospital gown and requesting that a peer remain with the client will not ensure a safe environment.
Test-Taking Strategy: Use the process of elimination. Eliminate option 2 because seclusion should not be the initial intervention. Eliminate option 4 next because the responsibility to safeguard a client is not the peer's responsibility. Eliminate option 3 because removing one's clothing will not maximize all possible safety strategies. Review nursing interventions for the client at risk for suicide if you had difficulty with this question.
Level of Cognitive Ability: Analysis
Client Needs: Safe, Effective Care Environment
Integrated Process: Nursing Process—implementation
Content Area: Mental health
References: Stuart, G., & Laraia, M. (2001). *Principles & practice of psychiatric nursing* (7th ed., p. 391). St. Louis: Mosby.
Varcarolis, E. (2002). *Foundations of psychiatric mental health nursing* (4th ed., p. 651). Philadelphia: W. B. Saunders.

9. 1

Rationale: The initial nursing action is to assess and treat the self-inflicted injuries. Injuries from lacerated wrists can lead to

a life-threatening situation. Other interventions may follow after the client has been treated medically.
Test-Taking Strategy: Use Maslow's hierarchy of needs theory to prioritize. Physiological needs come first. Option 1 addresses the physiological need. Review care to the client who attempted suicide if you had difficulty with this question.
Level of Cognitive Ability: Application
Client Needs: Physiological Integrity
Integrated Process: Nursing Process—implementation
Content Area: Delegating/Prioritizing
Reference: Fortinash, K., & Holoday-Worret, P. (2000). *Psychiatric mental health nursing* (2nd ed., pp. 664-665). St. Louis: Mosby.

10. **4**
Rationale: A suicidal client may have numerous diagnoses that encompass inadequate coping skills, anxiety, and strained interpersonal relationships. The question, however, directly and clearly designates that the problems that need to be dealt with are the "Risk for self-directed violence" and the client's "suicidal ideations with a plan." The expected outcome is that the client no longer has suicidal ideations and has identified options to deal with stress. Options 1, 2, and 3 are not related directly to the nursing diagnosis as stated in the question.
Test-Taking Strategy: When presented with a question that identifies a nursing diagnosis, use the information in the question to assist in directing you to the correct option. Option 4 is the only option that offers a resolution to the problem of "suicidal ideations with a plan" in that the client denies the "suicidal ideation and identifies ideations options." Review the appropriate plan of care for a suicidal client if you had difficulty with this question.
Level of Cognitive Ability: Analysis
Client Needs: Psychosocial Integrity
Integrated Process: Nursing Process—evaluation
Content Area: Mental health
Reference: Stuart, G., & Laraia, M. (2001). *Principles & practice of psychiatric nursing* (7th ed., p. 647). St. Louis: Mosby.

11. **4**
Rationale: In a crisis the nurse must take an authoritative, active role to promote the client's safety. A bottle of sleeping pills in front of a client who verbalizes he wants to kill himself is a "crisis." The client's safety is of prime concern. Keeping the client on the telephone and getting help to the client is the best intervention. Insisting that the client provide his name may anger the client and he might hang up. Option 2 lacks the authoritative action stance of securing the client's safety. Using therapeutic communication techniques is important, but overuse of "reflection" may sound uncaring or superficial and is lacking direction/solutions to the immediate problem of the client's safety.
Test-Taking Strategy: Use the process of elimination focusing on the issue, the client's safety. Option 4 is the global option that most directly addresses safety of the client. Review care to the suicidal client if you had difficulty with this question.
Level of Cognitive Ability: Application
Client Needs: Safe, Effective Care Environment
Integrated Process: Nursing Process—implementation

Content Area: Mental health
Reference: Varcarolis, E. (2002). *Foundations of psychiatric mental health nursing* (4th ed., p. 255). Philadelphia: W. B. Saunders.

12. **1**
Rationale: The question is focused on the nursing diagnosis of dysfunctional grieving. The only option that deals with grief is option 1. Options 2, 3, and 4 are unrelated to this nursing diagnosis.
Test-Taking Strategy: When presented with a question that identifies a nursing diagnosis, use the information in the question to assist in directing you to the correct option. Option 1 is the only option that is focused on the nursing diagnosis of dysfunctional grieving. Additionally, note the word "grieving" in the question and the word "grief" in the correct option. Review expected outcomes for the client experiencing dysfunctional grieving if you had difficulty with this question.
Level of Cognitive Ability: Analysis
Client Needs: Psychosocial Integrity
Integrated Process: Nursing Process—evaluation
Content Area: Mental health
Reference: Fortinash, K., & Holoday-Worret, P. (2000). *Psychiatric mental health nursing* (2nd ed., p. 692). St. Louis: Mosby.
Varcarolis, E. (2002). *Foundations of psychiatric mental health nursing* (4th ed., p. 844). Philadelphia: W. B. Saunders.

13. **1**
Rationale: The symptoms of major depression includes depressed mood, loss of interest or pleasure, changes in appetite and sleep patterns, psychomotor agitation or retardation, fatigue, feelings of worthlessness/guilt, diminished ability to think or concentrate, and recurrent thoughts of death. Often the client does not have the energy or interest to complete activities of daily living. Options 2 and 3 may lead to increased feelings of worthlessness if the client fails to meet expectations. Option 4 will increase the client's feelings of poor self-esteem and unworthiness.
Test-Taking Strategy: Use the process of elimination. Note the key words "severe major depressive episode." Remember that severely depressed clients are unable to perform even the simplest of activities of daily living. Review care to the client with severe depression if you had difficulty with this question.
Level of Cognitive Ability: Application
Client Needs: Physiological Integrity
Integrated Process: Nursing Process—implementation
Content Area: Mental health
Reference: Varcarolis, E. (2002). *Foundations of psychiatric mental health nursing* (4th ed., p. 463). Philadelphia: W. B. Saunders.

14. **2**
Rationale: Depression may be a recurring illness for some persons. The client needs to understand the symptoms and recognize when treatment needs to begin again. Options 1, 3, and 4 indicate that the client has learned some coping skills, such as setting limits and taking medications. Option 2 is an unrealistic statement, indicating that further teaching is needed.
Test Taking Strategy: Use the process of elimination, noting the key words "further teaching needs to occur." Review expected

outcomes for the client with depression if you had difficulty with this question.

Level of Cognitive Ability: Analysis
Client Needs: Psychosocial Integrity
Integrated Process: Teaching/Learning
Content Area: Mental health
Reference: Fortinash, K., & Holoday-Worret, P. (2000). *Psychiatric mental health nursing* (2nd ed., p. 276). St. Louis: Mosby.

15. **1**
Rationale: The client in seclusion must be assessed at regular intervals (usually every 15 to 30 minutes) for physical needs, safety, and comfort. Option 2 indicates a physical need that could be met with a urinal or bedpan, if necessary; it does not indicate that the client has calmed down enough to leave the seclusion room. Option 3 could be an attempt to manipulate the nurse. No indication is given that the client will exercise self-control when alone in the room. Option 4 indicates the need for supportive communication or possibly medication as needed; it does not necessitate discontinuing seclusion.
Test-Taking Strategy: The issue of the question specifically relates to safety. Use the process of elimination and focus on the issue to direct you to option 1. Review seclusion procedures if you had difficulty with this question.
Level of Cognitive Ability: Analysis
Client Needs: Safe, Effective Care Environment
Integrated Process: Nursing Process—evaluation
Content Area: Mental health
References: Fortinash, K., & Holoday-Worret, P. (2000). *Psychiatric mental health nursing* (2nd ed., p. 89). St. Louis: Mosby. Varcarolis, E. (2002). *Foundations of psychiatric mental health nursing* (4th ed., p. 509). Philadelphia: W. B. Saunders.

16. **2**
Rationale: Crisis times may occur between appointments. Contracts facilitate the client feeling a responsibility for keeping a promise. This gives the client control. Option 3 is unrealistic. Providing telephone numbers will not assure available and immediate crisis intervention.
Test-Taking Strategy: Use the process of elimination. The issue of the question relates to the availability of immediate resources for the client if needed. Eliminate option 3 first because this is unrealistic. Options 1 and 4 will not necessarily provide immediate resources. Also note the word "immediate" in the correct option. Review care to the client who attempted suicide if you had difficulty with this question.
Level of Cognitive Ability: Application
Client Needs: Psychosocial Integrity
Integrated Process: Nursing Process—planning
Content Area: Mental health
References: Fortinash, K., & Holoday-Worret, P. (2000). *Psychiatric mental health nursing* (2nd ed., pp. 672, 665). St. Louis: Mosby.
Stuart, G., & Laraia, M. (2001). *Principles & practice of psychiatric nursing* (7th ed., p. 396). St. Louis: Mosby.

17. **3**
Rationale: Elder abuse is sometimes the result of family members who are being expected to care for their aging parents.

This care can cause the family to become overextended, frustrated, or financially depleted. Knowing where to turn in the community for assistance in caring for aging family members can bring the much needed relief. These alternatives are a positive alternative coping strategy, which many families use.
Test-Taking Strategy: Use the process of elimination. Note the key words "positive coping skills." Option 3 identifies a means of coping with the issues. The other options identify statements of good faith or promises, which may or may not be kept in the future. Only option 3 outlines a definitive plan for how to handle the pressure associated with the father's care. Review coping mechanisms if you had difficulty with this question.
Level of Cognitive Ability: Analysis
Client Needs: Psychosocial Integrity
Integrated Process: Nursing Process—evaluation
Content Area: Mental health
Reference: Varcarolis, E. (2002). *Foundations of psychiatric mental health nursing* (4th ed., p. 714). Philadelphia: W. B. Saunders.

18. **4**
Rationale: A client who is moderately depressed and has only been in the hospital 2 days is unlikely to have such a dramatic cure. When a depression suddenly lifts, it is likely that the client may have made the decision to harm himself or herself. Suicide precautions are necessary to keep the client safe.
Test-Taking Strategy: Use the process of elimination. Options 1 and 2 support the client's notion that a cure has occurred. Option 3 allows the client to increase isolation and that would present a threat to the client's safety. Safety is of the utmost importance; therefore option 4 is the correct option. Review care to the client with depression if you had difficulty with this question.
Level of Cognitive Ability: Analysis
Client Needs: Safe, Effective Care Environment
Integrated Process: Nursing Process—planning
Content Area: Mental health
Reference: Fortinash, K., & Holoday-Worret, P. (2000). *Psychiatric mental health nursing* (2nd ed., p. 666). St. Louis: Mosby.

19. **3**
Rationale: One-to-one suicide precautions are required for the client who has attempted suicide. Options 1 and 2 may be appropriate, but not at the present time considering the situation. Option 4 also may be an appropriate nursing intervention, but the priority is identified in option 3. The best intervention is constant supervision so that the nurse may intervene as needed if the client attempts to cause harm to self.
Test-Taking Strategy: Use the process of elimination noting the key words "attempted suicide." Option 3 is the only option that provides a safe environment. Review interventions for the suicidal client if you had difficulty with this question.
Level of Cognitive Ability: Application
Client Needs: Safe, Effective Care Environment
Integrated Process: Nursing Process—implementation
Content Area: Mental health
Reference: Varcarolis, E. (2002). *Foundations of psychiatric mental health nursing* (4th ed., p. 651). Philadelphia: W. B. Saunders.

20. 4

Rationale: Whenever the abused client remains in the abusive environment, priority must be placed on ascertaining whether the person is in any immediate danger. If so, emergency action must be taken to remove the person from the abusing situation. Options 1, 2, and 3 may be appropriate interventions but are not the priority.

Test Taking Strategy: Use Maslow's hierarchy of needs theory, remembering that if a physiological need is not present, then safety is the priority. This guide should direct you to option 4, the only option that directly addresses client safety. Review care to the client who is a victim of physical abuse if you had difficulty with this question.

Level of Cognitive Ability: Application
Client Needs: Safe, Effective Care Environment
Integrated Process: Nursing Process—planning
Content Area: Delegating/Prioritizing
Reference: Fortinash, K., & Holoday-Worret, P. (2000). *Psychiatric mental health nursing* (2nd ed., p. 629). St. Louis: Mosby.

21. 2

Rationale: Tertiary prevention of family violence includes assisting the victim once the abuse has already occurred. The nurse should provide the client with information regarding where to obtain help. This includes a specific plan for removing self from the abuser, information as to escaping, hotlines, and the location of shelters. An abused person is usually reluctant to call the police. Teaching the victim to fight back is not the appropriate action for the victim when dealing with a violent person.

Test-Taking Strategy: Note the key word "priority." Focus on the issue of the question, which relates to providing the client with a safe environment. Use Maslow's hierarchy of needs theory to assist in directing you to option 2. If you had difficulty with this question, review the nursing measures for caring for a victim of family violence.

Level of Cognitive Ability: Application
Client Needs: Safe, Effective Care Environment
Integrated Process: Nursing Process—implementation
Content Area: Delegating/Prioritizing
Reference: Fortinash, K., & Holoday-Worret, P. (2000). *Psychiatric mental health nursing* (2nd ed., p. 629). St. Louis: Mosby.

22. 2

Rationale: Option 2 allows the client to express her ideas and feelings more fully, and portrays a nonhurried, nonjudgmental, supportive attitude. Clients need to be reassured that their feelings are normal and that they may express their concerns freely in a safe, caring environment. Option 1 places the problem solving totally on the client. Option 3 places the client's feelings on hold. Option 4 immediately blocks communication.

Test-Taking Strategy: Use the process of elimination. Option 2 is the only option that addresses the client's feelings. Always address the client's feelings first. Review therapeutic communication techniques if you had difficulty with this question.

Level of Cognitive Ability: Application
Client Needs: Psychosocial Integrity
Integrated Process: Caring

Content Area: Mental health
Reference: Varcarolis, E. (2002). *Foundations of psychiatric mental health nursing* (4th ed., pp. 258, 723). Philadelphia: W. B. Saunders.

23. 4

Rationale: During the acute phase of the rape crisis, the client can display a wide range of emotional and somatic responses. The symptoms noted indicate a normal reaction to an intensely difficult crisis event.

Test-Taking Strategy: Use the process of elimination and knowledge regarding client responses to devastating events to answer the question. Focus on the symptoms noted in the question to direct you to option 4. If you had difficulty with this question, review normal and abnormal client responses to dealing with devastating crisis events.

Level of Cognitive Ability: Analysis
Client Needs: Psychosocial Integrity
Integrated Process: Nursing Process—analysis
Content Area: Mental health
Reference: Varcarolis, E. (2002). *Foundations of psychiatric mental health nursing* (4th ed., p. 727). Philadelphia: W. B. Saunders.

24. 1

Rationale: Short-term goals include the beginning stages of dealing with the rape trauma. Clients will be expected initially to keep appointments, participate in care, begin to explore feelings, and begin to heal any physical wounds that were inflicted at the time of the rape.

Test-Taking Strategy: Use the process of elimination. Note the key words "unrealistic" and "short-term initial goal." Use the process of elimination, considering each option and the reality of the option statement being achieved short term. Note the word "resolve" in option 1. This word should provide you with the clue that this option is a long-term goal. Review expected outcomes in the plan of care for the client who has been raped if you had difficulty with this question.

Level of Cognitive Ability: Analysis
Client Needs: Psychosocial Integrity
Integrated Process: Nursing Process—planning
Content Area: Mental health
Reference: Varcarolis, E. (2002). *Foundations of psychiatric mental health nursing* (4th ed., p. 729). Philadelphia: W. B. Saunders.

25. 4

Rationale: Options 1, 2, and 3 identify a positive movement toward increased self-esteem and problem solving. Option 4 places undue pressure on the client by implying that the client was negligent and contributed to the loss.

Test-Taking Strategy: Use the process of elimination. Note the key words "least realistic." The words "realistic" and "adaptive," and the words "express and share feelings" in options 1, 2, and 3 respectively, identify positive goals. This should assist in directing you to option 4. Additionally, nothing in the question indicates that the client lacked insurance, as option 4 reflects. Review expected outcomes for the client who experienced a crisis if you had difficulty with this question.

Level of Cognitive Ability: Analysis
Client Needs: Psychosocial Integrity
Integrated Process: Nursing Process—planning

Content Area: Mental health
Reference: Stuart, G., & Laraia, M. (2001). *Principles & practice of psychiatric nursing* (7th ed., p. 68). St. Louis: Mosby.

CRITICAL THINKING: MULTIPLE RESPONSE

Answer:
Be honest and truthful and let the client and family know that you will not abandon them.
Encourage expression of feelings, concerns, and fears.
Extend touch and hold the client's or family member's hand if appropriate.
Rationale: The nurse must determine whether there is a spokesperson for the family and how much the client and family want to know. The nurse needs to allow the family and client the opportunity for informed choices and assist with the decision-making process if asked. The nurse should encourage expression of feelings, concerns, and fears, as well as reminiscing. The nurse needs to be honest and truthful and let the client and family know that they will not be abandoned. Extend touch and hold the client's or family member's hand if appropriate.
Test-Taking Strategy: Recalling therapeutic communication techniques and client and family rights will assist you in answering this question. Review these techniques and care to the dying client if you had difficulty with this question.
Level of Cognitive Ability: Application
Client Needs: Psychosocial Integrity
Integrated Process: Caring
Content Area: Mental health
Reference: Potter, P., & Perry, A. (2001). *Fundamentals of nursing* (5th ed., pp. 462, 629-630). St. Louis: Mosby.

REFERENCES

Fortinash, K., & Holoday-Worret, P. (2000). *Psychiatric mental health nursing* (2nd ed.). St. Louis: Mosby.

Keltner, N., Schwecke, L., & Bostrom, C. (2003). *Psychiatric nursing* (4th ed.). St. Louis: Mosby.

Potter, P., & Perry, A. (2001). *Fundamentals of nursing* (5th ed.). St. Louis: Mosby.

Stuart, G., & Laraia, M. (2001). *Principles & practice of psychiatric nursing* (7th ed.). St. Louis: Mosby.

Varcarolis, E. (2002). *Foundations of psychiatric mental health nursing* (4th ed.). Philadelphia: W. B. Saunders.

Psychiatric Medications

I. SELECTIVE SEROTONIN REUPTAKE INHIBITORS (BOX 76-1)

A. Description
1. Selective serotonin reuptake inhibitors inhibit serotonin uptake.
2. Selective serotonin reuptake inhibitors produce an antidepressant response.

B. Side effects
1. Nausea, vomiting, cramping, and diarrhea
2. Dry mouth
3. Central nervous system (CNS) stimulation
4. Photosensitivity
5. Insomnia/somnolence
6. Nervousness
7. Headache, dizziness
8. Seizure activity
9. Weight loss or gain

C. Interventions
1. Monitor vital signs.
2. Monitor weight.
3. Initiate safety precautions, particularly if dizziness occurs.

BOX 76-1

Reuptake Inhibitors

SELECTIVE SEROTONIN REUPTAKE INHIBITORS
Citalopram (Celexa)
Escitalopram (Lexapro)
Fluoxetine (Prozac)
Fluvoxamine (Luvox)
Paroxetine hydrochloride (Paxil)
Sertraline hydrochloride (Zoloft)

ATYPICAL REUPTAKE INHIBITORS
Buproprion hydrochloride (Wellbutrin)
Venlafaxine hydrochloride (Effexor)

4. Administer with a snack or with meals to reduce the risk of dizziness and light-headedness.
5. Monitor the suicidal client, especially during improved mood and increased energy levels.
6. Instruct the client taking fluoxetine (Prozac) to take the medication early in the day to avoid interference with sleep.
7. For the client on long-term therapy, monitor liver and renal function tests.
8. Monitor white blood cell and neutrophil counts and discontinue the medication, as prescribed, if levels fall below normal.
9. If priapism (painful, prolonged penile erection) occurs, discontinue the medication immediately and notify the physician.
10. Inform the client about the possibility of decreased libido.
11. Instruct the client to change positions slowly to avoid a hypotensive effect.
12. Instruct the client to avoid alcohol.
13. Instruct the client to report any visual changes to the physician.

II. TRICYCLIC ANTIDEPRESSANTS (BOX 76-2)

A. Description
1. Tricyclic antidepressants block the reuptake of norepinephrine and serotonin at the presynaptic neuron.
2. Tricyclic antidepressants are used to treat depression.
3. Tricyclic antidepressants may reduce seizure threshold.
4. Tricyclic antidepressants may reduce effectiveness of antihypertensive agents.
5. Concurrent use with alcohol or antihistamines can cause CNS depression.
6. Concurrent use with monoamine oxidase inhibitors can cause hypertensive crisis.

BOX 76-2

Tricyclic Antidepressants

Amitriptyline hydrochloride (Elavil)
Amoxapine (Asendin)
Clomipramine (Anafranil)
Desipramine hydrochloride (Norpramin)
Doxepin hydrochloride (Sinequan)
Imipramine hydrochloride (Tofranil)
Maprotiline (Ludiomil)
Mirtazapine (Remeron)
Nortriptyline hydrochloride (Aventyl)
Protriptyline hydrochloride (Vivactil)
Trazodone (Desyrel)
Trimipramine maleate (Surmontil)

B. Side effects
   1. Anticholinergic effects
   2. Dry mouth
   3. Decreased gastrointestinal motility and constipation
   4. Difficulty voiding
   5. Dilated pupils and blurred vision
   6. Photosensitivity
   7. Cardiovascular disturbances
   8. Tachycardia, dysrhythmias
   9. Orthostatic hypotension
   10. Sedation
   11. Weight gain
   12. Anxiety, restlessness, and irritability
   13. Decreased or increased libido with ejaculatory and erection disturbances
C. Interventions
   1. Instruct the client that the medication may take several weeks to produce the desired effect (client response may not occur until 2 to 4 weeks after the first dose).
   2. Monitor the suicidal client, especially during improved mood and increased energy levels.
   3. Instruct the client to change positions slowly to avoid a hypotensive effect.
   4. Monitor pattern of daily bowel activity.
   5. Assess for urinary retention.
   6. For the client on long-term therapy, monitor liver and renal function tests.
   7. Administer with food or milk if gastrointestinal distress occurs.
   8. Administer the entire daily oral dose at one time, preferably at bedtime.
   9. Instruct the client to avoid alcohol and nonprescription medications to prevent adverse medication interactions.
   10. Instruct the client to avoid driving and other activities requiring alertness.
   11. When the medication is discontinued, it should be tapered gradually.

BOX 76-3

Monoamine Oxidase Inhibitors

Isocarboxazid (Marplan)
Phenelzine sulfate (Nardil)
Tranylcypromine sulfate (Parnate)

III. MONOAMINE OXIDASE INHIBITORS (BOX 76-3)

A. Description
   1. Monoamine oxidase inhibitors inhibit the enzyme monoamine oxidase, which is present in the brain, blood platelets, liver, spleen, and kidneys.
   2. Inhibition of monoamine oxidase metabolizes amines, norepinephrine, and serotonin, and the concentration of these amines increases.
   3. Monoamine oxidase inhibitors are used for depression in the client who has not responded to other antidepressant therapies, including electroconvulsive therapy.
   4. Concurrent use with amphetamines, antidepressants, dopamine, epinephrine, guanethidine, levodopa, methyldopa, nasal decongestants, norepinephrine, reserpine, tyramine-containing foods, and vasoconstrictors may cause hypertensive crisis.
   5. Concurrent use with narcotic analgesics may cause hypertension, hypotension, coma, or seizures.
B. Side effects
   1. Orthostatic hypotension
   2. Restlessness
   3. Insomnia
   4. Dizziness
   5. Weakness, lethargy
   6. Gastrointestinal upset
   7. Dry mouth
   8. Weight gain
   9. Peripheral edema
   10. Anticholinergic effects
   11. CNS stimulation, including anxiety, agitation, and mania
   12. Delay in ejaculation
C. Hypertensive crisis
   1. Hypertension
   2. Occipital headache radiating frontally
   3. Neck stiffness and soreness
   4. Nausea and vomiting
   5. Sweating
   6. Fever and chills
   7. Clammy skin
   8. Dilated pupils
   9. Palpitations, tachycardia, or bradycardia
   10. Constricting chest pain
   11. Antidote for hypertensive crisis: 5 to 10 mg phentolamine (Regitine) intravenous injection
D. Interventions
   1. Monitor blood pressure frequently for hypertension.
   2. Monitor for signs of hypertensive crisis.

3. If palpitations or frequent headaches occur, discontinue the medication and notify the physician.
4. Administer with food if gastrointestinal distress occurs.
5. Instruct the client that the medication effect may be noted during the first week of therapy, but maximum benefit may take up to 3 weeks.
6. Instruct the client to report headache, neck stiffness, or neck soreness immediately.
7. Instruct the client to change positions slowly to prevent orthostatic hypotension.
8. Instruct the client to avoid caffeine or over-the-counter preparations such as weight-reducing pills or medications for hay fever and colds.
9. Monitor for client compliance with medication administration.
10. Instruct the client to carry a Medic-Alert card indicating that a monoamine oxidase inhibitor medication is prescribed.
11. Avoid administering the medication in the evening because insomnia may result.
12. Monoamine oxidase inhibitors should be tapered and discontinued 7 to 14 days before surgery.
13. When the medication is discontinued, it should be discontinued gradually.
14. Instruct the client to avoid foods that require bacteria/molds for their preparation/preservation or those that contain tyramine (Box 76-4).

▲ IV. MOOD STABILIZERS (BOX 76-5)
A. Description
   1. Mood stabilizers affect cellular transport mechanism, alter the presynaptic and postsynaptic events affecting serotonin, and thus enhance serotonin function.

BOX 76-4

Foods to Avoid that Contain Tyramine

Avocados
Bananas
Beef or chicken liver
Brewer's yeast
Broad beans
Caffeine such as coffee, tea, or chocolate
Cheese, especially aged, except cottage cheese
Figs
Meat extracts and tenderizers
Overripe fruit
Papaya
Pickled herring
Raisins
Red wine, beer, sherry
Sausage, bologna, pepperoni, salami
Sour cream
Soy sauce
Yogurt

---

2. Concurrent use with diuretics, fluoxetine (Prozac), methyldopa, or nonsteroidal antiinflammatory medications increases lithium reabsorption by the kidney or inhibits lithium excretion, either of which increases the risk of lithium toxicity.
3. Acetazolamide (Diamox), aminophylline, phenothiazines, or sodium bicarbonate may increase renal excretion of lithium, reducing its effectiveness.
4. The therapeutic dose is only slightly less than the amount producing toxicity.
5. The therapeutic drug serum level of lithium is 0.6 to 1.2 mEq/L.
6. The causes of an increase in the lithium level include decreased sodium intake; fluid and electrolyte loss associated with severe sweating, dehydration, diarrhea, or diuretic therapy; and illness or overdose
7. Serum lithium levels should be checked every 1 to 2 months or whenever any behavioral change suggests an altered serum level.
8. Blood samples to check serum lithium levels should be drawn in the morning, 12 hours after the last dose was taken.

B. Side effects
   1. Polyuria
   2. Polydipsia
   3. Anorexia, nausea
   4. Dry mouth
   5. Mild thirst
   6. Weight gain
   7. Abdominal bloating
   8. Soft stools or diarrhea
   9. Fine hand tremors
   10. Inability to concentrate
   11. Muscle weakness
   12. Lethargy
   13. Fatigue
   14. Headache
   15. Hair loss

C. Interventions
   1. Monitor the suicidal client, especially during improved mood and increased energy levels.

BOX 76-5

Mood Stabilizers

LITHIUM PREPARATIONS
Lithium carbonate (Eskalith, Lithane, Lithobid)
Lithium citrate (Cibalith-Si)

OTHER MOOD STABILIZERS
Carbamazepine (Tegretol)
Divalproex sodium (Depakote)
Gabapentin (Neurontin)
Lamotrigine (Lamictal)
Oxcarbazepine (Trileptal)
Topiramate (Topamax)

2. Administer the medication with food to minimize gastrointestinal irritation.
3. Instruct the client to maintain a fluid intake of 6 to 8 glasses of water a day.
4. Instruct the client to avoid excessive amounts of coffee, tea, or cola, which have a diuretic effect.
5. Instruct the client to maintain an adequate salt intake.
6. Do not administer diuretics while the client is taking lithium.
7. Instruct the client to avoid alcohol.
8. Instruct the client to avoid over-the-counter medications.
9. Instruct the client that the client may take a missed dose within 2 hours of the scheduled time; otherwise, the client should skip the missed dose and take the next dose at the scheduled time.
10. Instruct the client not to adjust the dosage without consulting the physician because lithium should be tapered off and not discontinued abruptly.
11. Instruct the client of the signs and symptoms of lithium toxicity.
12. Instruct the client to notify the physician if polyuria, prolonged vomiting, diarrhea, or fever occur.
13. Instruct the client that the therapeutic response to the medication will be noted in 1 to 3 weeks.
14. Monitor electrocardiogram, renal function tests, and thyroid tests.

D. Lithium toxicity
1. Description
   a. Lithium toxicity cccurs when ingested lithium cannot be detoxified and excreted by the kidneys.
   b. Symptoms of toxicity begin to appear when the serum lithium level is at 1.5 mEq/L to 2 mEq/L.
2. Mild toxicity
   a. Serum lithium level at 1.5 mEq/L
   b. Apathy
   c. Lethargy
   d. Diminished concentration
   e. Mild ataxia
   f. Coarse hand tremors
   g. Slight muscle weakness
3. Moderate toxicity
   a. Serum lithium level of 1.5 mEq/L to 2.5 mEq/L
   b. Nausea, vomiting
   c. Severe diarrhea
   d. Mild to moderate ataxia and incoordination
   e. Slurred speech
   f. Tinnitus
   g. Blurred vision
   h. Muscle twitching
   i. Irregular tremor
4. Severe toxicity

   a. Serum lithium level above 2.5 mEq/L
   b. Nystagmus
   c. Muscle fasciculations
   d. Deep tendon hyperreflexia
   e. Visual or tactile hallucinations
   f. Oliguria or anuria
   g. Impaired level of consciousness
   h. Tonic-clonic seizures or coma leading to death
5. Interventions for lithium toxicity
   a. Hold lithium and notify the physician.
   b. Monitor vital signs and level of consciousness.
   c. Monitor cardiac status.
   d. Prepare to obtain lithium level; electrolytes, blood urea nitrogen, and creatinine level; and complete blood cell count.
   e. Monitor for suicidal tendencies and institute suicide precautions.

V. ANTIANXIETY OR ANXIOLYTIC MEDICATIONS
A. Description
1. Antianxiety medications depress the CNS, thereby increasing the effects of gamma-aminobutyric acid, which produces relaxation and may depress the limbic system.
2. Benzodiazepines have anxiety-reducing (anxiolytic), sedative-hypnotic, muscle-relaxing and anticonvulsant actions (Box 76-6).
B. Side effects
1. Daytime sedation
2. Ataxia
3. Dizziness
4. Headaches
5. Blurred or double vision
6. Hypotension
7. Tremor
8. Amnesia
9. Slurred speech
10. Urinary incontinence

BOX 76-6

Benzodiazepines

Alprazolam (Xanax)
Chlordiazepoxide (Librium)
Clonazepam (Klonopin)
Clorazepate (Tranxene)
Diazepam (Valium)
Estazolam (ProSom)
Flurazepam (Dalmane)
Halazepam (Paxipam)
Lorazepam (Ativan)
Oxazepam (Serax)
Prazepam (Centrax)
Quazepam (Doral)
Temazepam (Restoril)
Triazolam (Halcion)

11. Constipation

12. Paradoxical CNS excitement

C. Acute toxicity

1. Somnolence

2. Confusion

3. Diminished reflexes and coma

4. Flumazenil (Romazicon), a benzodiazepine antagonist administered intravenously, will reverse benzodiazepine intoxication in 5 minutes.

5. The client being treated for an overdose of a benzodiazepine may experience agitation, restlessness, discomfort, and anxiety.

D. Interventions

1. Monitor for motor responses such as agitation, trembling, and tension.

2. Monitor for autonomic responses such as cold clammy hands and sweating.

3. Monitor for paradoxical CNS excitement during early therapy, particularly in older and debilitated individuals.

4. Monitor for visual disturbances because the medications can worsen glaucoma.

5. Monitor liver and renal function tests and complete blood cell counts.

6. Reduce the medication dose as prescribed for the older adult clients and for the client with impaired liver function.

7. Initiate safety precautions because the older adult client is at risk for falling when taking the medication for sleep or anxiety.

8. Assist with ambulation if drowsiness or light-headedness occurs.

9. Instruct the client that drowsiness usually disappears during continued therapy.

10. Instruct the client to avoid tasks that require alertness until the response to the medication is established.

11. Instruct the client to avoid alcohol.

12. Instruct the client not to take other medications without consulting the physician.

13. Instruct the client not to stop the medication abruptly (can result in seizure activity).

E. Withdrawal

1. To lessen withdrawal symptoms, the dosage of a benzodiazepine should be tapered gradually over 2 to 6 weeks.

2. Abrupt or too rapid withdrawal results in the following:

a. Restlessness

b. Irritability

c. Insomnia

d. Hand tremors

e. Abdominal or muscle cramps

f. Sweating

g. Vomiting

h. Seizures

VI. MEDICATIONS FOR INSOMNIA AND ANXIETY (BOX 76-7)

A. Description

1. These medications depress the reticular activating system by promoting the inhibitory synaptic action of the neurotransmitter gamma-aminobutyric acid.

2. These medications are used for short-term treatment of insomnia or for sedation to relieve anxiety, tension, and apprehension.

B. Side effects

1. Confusion

2. Irritability

3. Allergic reactions

4. Agranulocytosis

5. Thrombocytopenia purpura

6. Megaloblastic anemia

C. Overdose

1. Tachycardia

2. Hypotension

3. Cold and clammy skin

4. Dilated pupils

5. Weak and rapid pulse

6. Signs of shock

7. Depressed respirations

8. Absent reflexes

9. Coma and death may result from respiratory and cardiovascular collapse

D. Withdrawal

1. Severe withdrawal symptoms begin within 24 hours after the medication is discontinued in an individual with severe drug dependence.

2. Gradual withdrawal is used to detoxify a dependent person.

3. Anxiety

4. Insomnia

5. Nightmares

6. Daytime agitation

7. Tremors

BOX 76-7

Barbiturates and Sedative-Hypnotic Anxiolytics

BARBITURATES

Amobarbital (Amytal)

Aprobarbital (Alurate)

Butabarbital (Butisol)

Pentobarbital (Nembutal)

Phenobarbital (Luminal)

Secobarbital (Seconal)

SEDATIVE-HYPNOTIC ANXIOLYTICS

Buspirone (BuSpar)

Chloral hydrate (Noctec)

Hydroxyzine hydrochloride (Atarax)

Zaleplon (Sonata)

Zolpidem tartrate (Ambien)

8. Delirium
9. Seizures
E. Interventions
   1. Administer lower doses as prescribed for the older client.
   2. Medications should be used with caution in the client who has suicidal tendencies or has a history of drug **addiction.**
   3. Maintain safety by supervising ambulation and using side rails at night.
   4. Instruct the client to take medication as directed.
   5. Instruct the client to avoid driving or operating hazardous equipment if drowsiness, dizziness, or unsteadiness occurs.
   6. Instruct the client to avoid alcohol.
   7. For insomnia, instruct the client to take the medication 30 minutes before bedtime.
   8. Instruct the client that a hangover effect may occur in the morning.
   9. Instruct the client not to discontinue the medication abruptly.
   10. Instruct the client taking chloral hydrate to take the medication with food and a full glass of water, fruit juice, or ginger ale to improve the taste and to prevent gastric irritation.

VII. ANTIPSYCHOTIC MEDICATIONS (BOX 76-8)
A. Description
   1. Antipsychotic medications improve the thought processes and the behavior of the client with psychotic symptoms, especially the client with schizophrenia.

BOX 76-8

Antipsychotic Medications

TYPICAL ANTIPSYCHOTICS
Chlorpromazine hydrochloride (Thorazine)
Fluphenazine hydrochloride (Prolixin)
Perphenazine (Trilafon)
Thioridazine hydrochloride (Mellaril)
Thiothixene hydrochloride (Navane)
Trifluoperazine (Stelazine)
Triflupromazine hydrochloride (Vesprin)

ATYPICAL ANTIPSYCHOTICS
Aripiprazole (Abilify)
Clozapine (Clozaril)
Haloperidol (Haldol)
Loxapine (Loxitane)
Molindone hydrochloride (Moban)
Olanzapine (Zyprexa)
Quetiapine (Seroquel)
Risperidone (Risperdal)
Ziprasidone (Geodon)

---

2. Antipsychotic medications block dopamine receptors in the brain, thereby reducing the psychotic symptoms.
3. Antipsychotic medications block the chemoreceptor trigger zone and vomiting center in the brain, producing an antiemetic effect.
4. Phenothiazines lower the seizure threshold.
5. Antipsychotic medications should not be given with other antipsychotic or antidepressant medications.

B. Side effects
   1. Anticholinergic effects
   2. Dry mouth
   3. Increased heart rate
   4. Urinary retention
   5. Constipation
   6. Hypotension
   7. Drowsiness
   8. Blood dyscrasias agranulocytosis
   9. Pruritis
   10. Photosensitivity
C. Extrapyramidal syndrome
   1. Parkinsonism
      a. Tremors
      b. Masklike facies
      c. Rigidity
      d. Shuffling gait
   2. Dystonia
      a. Facial grimacing
      b. Abnormal or involuntary eye movements
   3. Akathisia
      a. Restlessness
      b. Constant moving about
   4. Tardive dyskinesia
      a. Protrusion of the tongue
      b. Chewing motion
      c. Involuntary movement of the body and extremities
D. Interventions
   1. Monitor vital signs.
   2. Monitor for extrapyramidal syndrome.
   3. Monitor for symptoms of neuroleptic malignant syndrome.
   4. Monitor urine output.
   5. Monitor serum glucose.
   6. Note that the client taking an antipsychotic medication may require long-term medication for parkinsonian symptoms.
   7. Administer the medication with food or milk to decrease gastric irritation.
   8. For oral use, the liquid form might be preferred because some clients hide tablets to avoid taking them.
   9. Note that the absorption rate is faster with the liquid form.
   10. Avoid skin contact with the liquid concentrate to prevent contact dermatitis.

11. Protect the liquid concentrate from light.
12. Dilute the liquid concentrate with fruit juice.
13. Inform the client that a full therapeutic effect of the medication may not be evident for 3 to 6 weeks following initiation of therapy; however, an observable therapeutic response may be apparent after 7 to 10 days.
14. Inform the client that phenothiazines may cause a harmless change in urine color to pinkish to red-brown.
15. Instruct the client to use sunscreen, hats, and protective clothing when outdoors.
16. Instruct the client to avoid alcohol or other CNS depressants.
17. Instruct the client to change positions slowly to avoid orthostatic hypotension.
18. Instruct the client to report signs of agranulocytosis, including sore throat, fever, and malaise.
19. Instruct the client to report signs of liver dysfunction, including jaundice, malaise, fever, right upper abdominal pain.
20. When discontinuing antipsychotics, the medication dosage should be reduced gradually to avoid sudden reoccurrence of psychotic symptoms.

▶ VIII. NEUROLEPTIC MALIGNANT SYNDROME

A. Description
   1. Neuroleptic malignant syndrome is a potentially fatal syndrome that may occur at any time during therapy with neuroleptic medications (antipsychotic or antischizophrenic medications).
   2. Although rare, neuroleptic malignant syndrome more commonly occurs at the initiation of therapy, after the client is changed from one medication to another, after a dosage increase, or when a combination of medications is used.
B. Assessment
   1. Dyspnea or tachypnea
   2. Tachycardia or irregular pulse rate
   3. Fever
   4. High or low blood pressure
   5. Increased sweating
   6. Loss of bladder control
   7. Skeletal muscle rigidity
   8. Pale skin
   9. Excessive weakness or fatigue
   10. Altered level of consciousness
   11. Seizures
   12. Severe extrapyramidal side effects
   13. Difficulty swallowing
   14. Excessive salivation
   15. Oculogyric crisis
   16. Dyskinesia
   17. Elevated white blood cell count
   18. Elevated liver function tests
   19. Elevated creatinine phosphokinase level

C. Interventions
   1. Notify the physician.
   2. Monitor vital signs.
   3. Initiate safety and seizure precautions.
   4. Discontinue the neuroleptic medication.
   5. Monitor level of consciousness.
   6. Administer antipyretics as prescribed.
   7. Use a cooling blanket to lower the body temperature.
   8. Monitor electrolytes and administer fluids intravenously as prescribed.

IX. MEDICATIONS TO TREAT ATTENTION DEFICIT HYPERACTIVITY DISORDER (BOX 76-9)

A. Children with attention deficit hyperactivity disorder may require medication to reduce hyperactive behavior and lengthen attention span.
B. Medications that are most effective in controlling this disorder are CNS stimulants.
C. Central nervous system stimulants, which increase agitation and activity in adults, have a calming effect on children with attention deficit hyperactivity disorder and increase alertness and sensitivity to stimuli.
D. Interventions
   1. Monitor for CNS side effects.
   2. Instruct the client/parents that over-the-counter medications need to be avoided.
   3. Instruct the client/parents that the last dose of the day should be taken at least 6 hours before bedtime (14 hours for extended-released forms) to prevent insomnia.
   4. Monitor height and weight (particularly in children).
   5. Reinforce that several weeks of therapy may be necessary before the therapeutic effect is noted.
   6. Instruct the client/parents that a drug-free period may be prescribed to allow growth of the child if the medication has caused growth retardation.

X. MEDICATIONS TO TREAT ALZHEIMER'S DISEASE

A. Acetylcholinesterase inhibitors may be used to treat Alzheimer's disease to improve cognitive functions in the early stages.

BOX 76-9

Medications to Treat Attention Deficit Hyperactivity Disorder

Amphetamine
Atomoxetine (Strattera)
Dextroamphetamine (Dexedrine)
Dextroamphetamine and amphetamine (Adderall XR)
Methamphetamine (Desoxyn)
Methylphenidate hydrochloride (Concerta)
Methylphenidate (Ritalin)
Pemoline (Cylert)

B. Donepezil (Aricept)
1. Donepezil is a reversible inhibitor of acetyl-cholinesterase.
2. Donepezil is used to treat mild to moderate dementia of Alzheimer's disease.
3. Common side effects include nausea and diarrhea.
4. Donepezil can slow the heart rate through its vagotonic effect.
C. Tacrine (Cognex)
1. Tacrine is a centrally acting acetylcholinesterase inhibitor.
2. Tacrine is used to treat mild to moderate dementia of Alzheimer's disease.
3. Side effects include ataxia, loss of appetite, nausea, vomiting, and diarrhea.
4. An adverse effect is hepatotoxicity; liver function studies need to be monitored.

PRACTICE QUESTIONS

1. A client receiving lithium carbonate (Lithobid) complains of loose, watery stools, and difficulty walking. The nurse would expect the serum lithium level to be which of the following?
   1. 0.7 mEq/L
   2. 1 mEq/L
   3. 1.3 mEq/L
   4. 1.8 mEq/L
2. The nurse is teaching a client who is being started on imipramine hydrochloride (Tofranil) about the medication. The nurse informs the client that the maximum desired effects may
   1. Start during the first week of administration.
   2. Start during the second week of administration.
   3. Not occur for 2 to 3 weeks of administration.
   4. Not occur until after 2 months of administration.
3. A client receiving thioridazine hydrochloride (Mellaril) complains of feeling "faint" when trying to get out of bed in the morning. The nurse recognizes this complaint as a symptom of
   1. Psychosomatic disorder.
   2. Cardiac dysrhythmias.
   3. Respiratory insufficiency.
   4. Postural hypotension.
4. The client receiving tricyclic antidepressants arrives at the mental health clinic. Which observation would indicate that the client is following the medication plan correctly?
   1. Client reports sleeping 12 hours per night and 3 to 4 hours during the day.
   2. Client arrives at the clinic neat and appropriate in appearance.
   3. Client reports not going to work for this past week.
   4. Client complains of not being able to "do anything" anymore.
5. The nurse is performing a follow-up teaching session with a client discharged 1 month ago. The client is taking fluoxetine (Prozac). What information would be important for the nurse to obtain during this client visit regarding the side effects related to the medication?
   1. Problems with excessive sweating
   2. Gastrointestinal dysfunctions
   3. Cardiovascular symptoms
   4. Problems with mouth dryness
6. The client who has been taking buspirone hydrochloride (BuSpar) for 1 month returns to the clinic for a follow-up assessment. The nurse determines that the medication is effective if the absence of which manifestation(s) has occurred?
   1. Alcohol withdrawal symptoms
   2. Paranoid thought process
   3. Rapid heartbeat or anxiety
   4. Thought broadcasting or delusions
7. A client taking lithium carbonate (Eskalith) reports vomiting, abdominal pain, diarrhea, blurred vision, tinnitus, and tremors. The lithium level is 2.5 mEq/L. The nurse interprets this level as
   1. Normal.
   2. Slightly above normal.
   3. Excessively below normal.
   4. Toxic.
8. A hospitalized client is prescribed chloral hydrate (Noctec). The nurse includes which action in the plan of care?
   1. Monitor apical heart rate every 2 hours.
   2. Monitor blood pressure every 4 hours.
   3. Instruct the client to call for ambulation assistance.
   4. Clear a path to the bathroom at bedtime.
9. The home health nurse visits the client. The client gives the nurse a bottle of clomipramine hydrochloride (Anafranil). The nurse notes that the medication has not been taken by the client in 2 months. What behaviors observed in the client would validate noncompliance with this medication?
   1. Frequent hand washing with hot, soapy water
   2. Complaints of hunger and fatigue
   3. A pulse rate fewer than 60 beats per minute
   4. Complaints of insomnia
10. The mental health clinic nurse is discussing the activities of the past week with a client receiving amitriptyline hydrochloride (Elavil). The nurse evaluates that the medication is most effective for this client if the client reports which of the following?
    1. Ability to get to work on time each day
    2. Having difficulty concentrating on an activity
    3. Sleeping 14 to 16 hours a day
    4. Decrease in appetite
11. The client with schizophrenia has been started on medication therapy with haloperidol (Haldol). The nurse determines that the client is experiencing the intended effects of the medication if which of the following client behaviors is observed?
    1. Decreased appetite and food intake

2. Taking sips of water for dry mouth
3. Presence of a fixed stare
4. Absence of delusional statements

12. The hospitalized client has begun taking bupropion (Wellbutrin) as an antidepressant agent. The nurse monitors this client for which adverse effect that indicates that the client is taking an excessive amount of medication?
    1. Dizziness when getting upright
    2. Seizure activity
    3. Increased weight
    4. Constipation

13. The client has been started on medication therapy with alprazolam (Xanax). When the nurse teaches the client that the medication should not be discontinued abruptly, the client asks why. The nurse incorporates which of the following in formulating a reply?
    1. Rebound central nervous system excitation could occur, causing feelings of restlessness and irritability.
    2. Abruptly stopping the medication will make the medication much less effective if it must be restarted.
    3. The client is likely to become resistant to medication effects.
    4. The client is likely to suffer irreversible damage to the kidneys.

14. The client's medication sheet contains an order for sertraline hydrochloride (Zoloft). To ensure safe administration of the medication, the nurse would administer the dose
    1. Evenly spaced around the clock.
    2. At the same time each evening.
    3. On an empty stomach.
    4. As needed when the client complains of depression.

15. The client with schizophrenia has been started on medication therapy with clozapine (Clozaril). The nurse assesses the results of which laboratory study to monitor for adverse effects from this medication?
    1. White blood cell count
    2. Platelet count
    3. Blood glucose
    4. Liver function studies

16. A client is scheduled for discharge and will be taking phenobarbital sodium (Luminal) for an extended period of time. The nurse would place highest priority on teaching the client which of the following points that directly relates to client safety?

1. Avoid drinking alcohol while taking this medication.
2. Take the medication only with meals.
3. Take medication at the same time each day.
4. Use a dose container to help prevent missed doses.

17. The 26-year-old female client with schizophrenia has been prescribed chlorpromazine (Thorazine). The client calls the mental health clinic and tells the nurse that her urine has become dark. The client has no other urinary symptoms. The nurse tells the client
    1. To increase intake of acid-ash foods and liquids.
    2. To seek treatment for urinary tract infection.
    3. That this is an expected side effect of the medication.
    4. That this indicates medication toxicity.

18. A client is receiving fluphenazine hydrochloride (Prolixin) daily. The nurse would teach the client to do which of the following to minimize common side effects of this medication?
    1. Have the blood pressure checked once a week.
    2. Monitor the temperature daily.
    3. Eat snacks at midmorning and at bedtime.
    4. Use hard sour candy or sugarless gum.

19. The nurse is describing the medication side effects to a client who is taking oxazepam (Serax). The nurse incorporates in discussions with the client the need to
    1. Take antidiarrheal agents if diarrhea occurs.
    2. Rest if the heart begins to beat rapidly.
    3. Consume a low-fiber diet.
    4. Increase fluids and bulk in the diet.

20. The nurse is administering thioridazine hydrochloride (Mellaril) in oral concentrate form. The nurse prepares this medication by mixing it in which of the following just before giving it to the client?
    1. Tea
    2. Fruit juice
    3. Pudding
    4. Applesauce

CRITICAL THINKING: FILL IN THE BLANK

A hospitalized client is started on phenelzine sulfate (Nardil) for the treatment of depression. At lunchtime a tray is delivered to the client that contains yogurt, tossed salad, crackers, and oatmeal cookies. Which of these food items will the nurse remove from the client's tray?

Answer: _____

ANSWERS

1. 4

Rationale: The therapeutic serum level of lithium is 0.6 to 1.2 mEq/L. A serum lithium level of 1.8 mEq/L indicates moderate toxicity. Serum lithium concentrations of 1.5 to 2.5 mEq/L may produce vomiting, diarrhea, ataxia, incoordination, muscle twitching, and slurred speech.

Test-Taking Strategy: Focusing on the client's symptoms will assist in answering this question. Review the normal lithium level and signs of toxicity if you had difficulty with this question.

Level of Cognitive Ability: Analysis
Client Needs: Physiological Integrity
Integrated Process: Nursing Process—analysis
Content Area: Pharmacology
Reference: Hodgson, B., & Kizior, R. (2004). *Saunders nursing drug handbook 2004* (p. 607). Philadelphia: W. B. Saunders.

2. 3

Rationale: The maximum therapeutic effects of imipramine hydrochloride may not occur for 2 to 3 weeks after the antidepressant therapy has been initiated.

Test-Taking Strategy: Focus on the key word "maximum." Recalling that it takes 2 to 3 weeks for a maximum therapeutic effect to occur with most antidepressants will direct you to option 3. Review this medication if you had difficulty with this question.

Level of Cognitive Ability: Application
Client Needs: Physiological Integrity
Integrated Process: Teaching/Learning
Content Area: Pharmacology
Reference: Hodgson, B., & Kizior, R. (2004). *Saunders nursing drug handbook 2004* (p. 528). Philadelphia: W. B. Saunders.

3. 4

Rationale: Thioridazine hydrochloride (Mellaril), an antipsychotic, can cause postural hypotension. The client needs to be taught to get out of bed slowly and to rise from a sitting position slowly because of this untoward effect related to the medication. Options 1, 2, and 3 are not related to this medication.

Test-Taking Strategy: Use the process of elimination. Note the key words "feeling 'faint.'" This should direct you to option 4. Review the side effects of this medication if you had difficulty with this question.

Level of Cognitive Ability: Analysis
Client Needs: Physiological Integrity
Integrated Process: Nursing Process—assessment
Content Area: Pharmacology
Reference: Hodgson, B., & Kizior, R. (2004). *Saunders nursing drug handbook 2004* (p. 974). Philadelphia: W. B. Saunders.

4. 2

Rationale: Depressed individuals will sleep for long periods, are not able to go to work, and feel as if they cannot "do anything." Once they have had some therapeutic effect from their medication, they will report resolution of many of these complaints and demonstrate an improvement in their appearance.

Test-Taking Strategy: Use the process of elimination. The client's behaviors or reports identified in options 1, 3, and 4 are symptoms of depression. The improvement in appearance indicates a therapeutic response to the medication, thus compliance with the medication regimen. Review the expected effect of a tricyclic antidepressant if you had difficulty with this question.

Level of Cognitive Ability: Analysis
Client Needs: Physiological Integrity
Integrated Process: Nursing Process—evaluation
Content Area: Pharmacology
Reference: Lehne, R. (2001). *Pharmacology for nursing care* (4th ed., p. 327). Philadelphia: W. B. Saunders.

5. 2

Rationale: The most common side effects related to this medication include central nervous system and gastrointestinal system dysfunction. Fluoxetine affects the gastrointestinal system by causing nausea and vomiting, cramping, and diarrhea. Excessive sweating, dry mouth, and cardiovascular symptoms are not side effects associated with this medication.

Test-Taking Strategy: Use the process of elimination. Recalling that this medication causes gastrointestinal problems will direct you to option 2. Review the side effects related to this medication if you had difficulty with this question.

Level of Cognitive Ability: Analysis
Client Needs: Physiological Integrity
Integrated Process: Nursing Process—assessment
Content Area: Pharmacology
Reference: Hodgson, B., & Kizior, R. (2004). *Saunders nursing drug handbook 2004* (p. 427). Philadelphia: W. B. Saunders.

6. 3

Rationale: Buspirone hydrochloride is not recommended for the treatment of drug or alcohol withdrawal, thought disorders, or schizophrenia. Buspirone hydrochloride most often is indicated for the treatment of anxiety.

Test-Taking Strategy: Use the process of elimination. Recalling that buspirone hydrochloride is an antianxiety medication will direct you to the correct option. Review the action and use of this medication if you had difficulty with this question.

Level of Cognitive Ability: Analysis
Client Needs: Physiological Integrity
Integrated Process: Nursing Process—evaluation
Content Area: Pharmacology
Reference: Hodgson, B., & Kizior, R. (2004). *Saunders nursing drug handbook 2004* (p. 427). Philadelphia: W. B. Saunders.

7. 4

Rationale: Maintenance serum levels of lithium are 0.6 to 1.2 mEq/L. Symptoms of toxicity begin to appear at levels of 1.5 mEq/L to 2 mEq/L. Lithium toxicity requires immediate medical attention with lavage and possible peritoneal dialysis or hemodialysis.

Test-Taking Strategy: Use the process of elimination. Recalling that the high end of the maintenance level is 1.2 mEq/L will direct you to option 4. Review the maintenance level and signs of toxicity if you had difficulty with this question.

Level of Cognitive Ability: Analysis
Client Needs: Physiological Integrity
Integrated Process: Nursing Process—analysis
Content Area: Pharmacology
Reference: Hodgson, B., & Kizior, R. (2004). *Saunders nursing drug handbook 2004* (p. 607). Philadelphia: W. B. Saunders.

8. 3

Rationale: Chloral hydrate is a sedative. This medication does not affect cardiac function. Blood pressure changes are not significant with the use of this medication. The client should call for assistance to the bathroom at night. Additionally, the client may experience residual daytime sedation; therefore the nurse also should instruct the client to call for ambulation assistance during the daytime hours.

Test-Taking Strategy: Use the process of elimination. Recalling that this medication is a sedative will direct you easily to option 3. Review nursing considerations related to this medication if you had difficulty with this question.

Level of Cognitive Ability: Application
Client Needs: Safe, Effective Care Environment
Integrated Process: Nursing Process—planning
Content Area: Pharmacology
Reference: Hodgson, B., & Kizior, R. (2004). *Saunders nursing drug handbook 2004* (p. 196). Philadelphia: W. B. Saunders.

9. 1

Rationale: Clomipramine hydrochloride is a tricyclic antidepressant used to treat obsessive compulsive disorder. Weight gain and tachycardia are side effects of this medication. Sedation sometimes occur and insomnia is a seldom side effect.

Test-Taking Strategy: Recalling that this medication is a tricyclic antidepressant used to treat obsessive compulsive disorder will direct you to option 1. Review the purpose and use of this medication if you had difficulty with this question.

Level of Cognitive Ability: Analysis
Client Needs: Physiological Integrity
Integrated Process: Nursing Process—evaluation
Content Area: Pharmacology
Reference: Hodgson, B., & Kizior, R. (2004). *Saunders nursing drug handbook 2004* (p. 228). Philadelphia: W. B. Saunders.

10. 1

Rationale: Amitriptyline is a tricyclic antidepressant. Depressed individuals sleep for extended periods, have a change in appetite, are unable to go to work, and have difficulty concentrating. They also may experience increased fatigue, feelings of guilt or worthlessness, loss of interest in activities, and possible suicidal tendencies. Once they have had some therapeutic effect from their medication, they will report resolution of many of these complaints and demonstrate an improvement in their appearance.

Test-Taking Strategy: Use the process of elimination. Note the key words "most effective." The symptoms stated in options 2, 3, and 4 are symptoms of depression. The ability to report to work indicates a therapeutic response to the medication. Review the action and expected effects of amitriptyline if you had difficulty with this question.

Level of Cognitive Ability: Analysis
Client Needs: Physiological Integrity
Integrated Process: Nursing Process—evaluation
Content Area: Pharmacology
Reference: Hodgson, B., & Kizior, R. (2004). *Saunders nursing drug handbook 2004* (p. 50). Philadelphia: W. B. Saunders.

11. 4

Rationale: Haloperidol (Haldol) is an antipsychotic used to manage psychotic disorder. Hallucinations, delusions, and altered thought processes are characteristics of a psychotic disorder and should decrease with effective treatment. Fixed stare (option 3) and dry mouth (option 2) are side effects of therapy. Option 1 is unrelated to this medication.

Test-Taking Strategy: Use the process of elimination. Recalling that this medication is an antipsychotic will direct you to option 4. Review the purpose of this medication if you had difficulty with this question.

Level of Cognitive Ability: Analysis
Client Needs: Physiological Integrity
Integrated Process: Nursing Process—evaluation
Content Area: Pharmacology
Reference: Hodgson, B., & Kizior, R. (2004). *Saunders nursing drug handbook 2004* (p. 489). Philadelphia: W. B. Saunders.

12. 2

Rationale: The nurse monitors for signs of toxicity. Seizure activity is common in bupropion dosages greater than 450 mg daily. This medication does not cause significant orthostatic blood pressure changes. Weight gain is an occasional side effect, whereas constipation is a common side effect of this medication.

Test-Taking Strategy: Use the process of elimination. Note the key words "adverse effect" and "excessive amount." These key words will direct you to option 2. Review this medication if you had difficulty with this question.

Level of Cognitive Ability: Analysis
Client Needs: Physiological Integrity
Integrated Process: Nursing Process—assessment
Content Area: Pharmacology
Reference: Hodgson, B., & Kizior, R. (2004). *Saunders nursing drug handbook 2004* (p. 129). Philadelphia: W. B. Saunders.

13. 1

Rationale: The abrupt withdrawal of alprazolam could result in seizure activity from rebound central nervous system excitation. All clients receiving this medication should be warned of this danger. The other options are incorrect.

Test-Taking Strategy: Use the process of elimination. Remember that options that are similar are not likely to be correct. With this in mind, eliminate options 2 and 3 first. From the remaining options, recalling the adverse effects will direct you to option 1. If this question was difficult, review the adverse effects associated with this medication.

Level of Cognitive Ability: Application
Client Needs: Physiological Integrity
Integrated Process: Teaching/Learning
Content Area: Pharmacology
Reference: Hodgson, B., & Kizior, R. (2004). *Saunders nursing drug handbook 2004* (p. 29). Philadelphia: W. B. Saunders.

14. 2

Rationale: Sertraline (Zoloft) is classified as an antidepressant. Sertraline generally is administered once every 24 hours. It may be administered in the morning or evening, but evening administration may be preferable because drowsiness is a side effect. The medication may be administered without food or with food if gastrointestinal distress occurs. Sertraline is not ordered for use as needed.

Test-Taking Strategy: Use the process of elimination. Recalling that this medication is administered daily will direct you to

option 2. Review this medication if you had difficulty with this question.
Level of Cognitive Ability: Application
Client Needs: Physiological Integrity
Integrated Process: Nursing Process—implementation
Content Area: Pharmacology
Reference: Kee, J., & Hayes, E. (2003). *Pharmacology: A nursing process approach* (4th ed., p. 312). Philadelphia: W. B. Saunders.

15. 1
Rationale: The client taking clozapine may experience agranulocytosis, which is monitored by reviewing the results of the white blood cell count. Treatment is interrupted if the white blood cell count drops below 3000 cells/mm³. Agranulocytosis could be fatal if undetected and untreated. The other options are not related specifically to the use of this medication.
Test-Taking Strategy: Use the process of elimination. Recalling that this medication causes agranulocytosis will direct you to option 1. Review the adverse effects of this medication if you had difficulty with this question
Level of Cognitive Ability: Analysis
Client Needs: Physiological Integrity
Integrated Process: Nursing Process—assessment
Content Area: Pharmacology
References: Hodgson, B., & Kizior, R. (2004). *Saunders nursing drug handbook 2004* (, p. 237). Philadelphia: W. B. Saunders. Kee, J., & Hayes, E. (2003). *Pharmacology: A nursing process approach* (4th ed., p. 295). Philadelphia: W. B. Saunders.

16. 1
Rationale: Phenobarbital sodium is an anticonvulsant and a hypnotic agent. The client should avoid taking any other central nervous system depressants (such as alcohol) while taking this medication. The medication may be given without regard to meals. Taking the medication at the same time each day enhances compliance and maintains more stable blood levels of the medication. Using a dose container or "pill box" may be helpful for some clients.
Test Taking Strategy: Use the process of elimination. Focus on the issue, client safety. Note the key words "highest priority." This tells you that more than one or all of the options may be partially or totally correct and that you must prioritize your answer. Remember, alcohol should not be consumed when one is taking a hypnotic. Review client teaching points related to this medication if you had difficulty with this question.
Level of Cognitive Ability: Application
Client Needs: Safe, Effective Care Environment
Integrated Process: Teaching/Learning
Content Area: Pharmacology
Reference: Hodgson, B., & Kizior, R. (2004). *Saunders nursing drug handbook 2004* (p. 801). Philadelphia: W. B. Saunders.

17. 3
Rationale: Chlorpromazine is an antipsychotic medication. A side effect of this medication is that the color of urine may darken. The client should be aware that this effect is harmless. The other options are incorrect.
Test-Taking Strategy: Use the process of elimination. Eliminate options 1 and 2 first because the question states

that the client exhibits no other symptoms of urinary tract infection. From the remaining options, you must know the side effects of this medication. Review the side effects of this medication if you had difficulty with this question.
Level of Cognitive Ability: Application
Client Needs: Physiological Integrity
Integrated Process: Nursing Process—implementation
Content Area: Pharmacology
Reference: Hodgson, B., & Kizior, R. (2004). *Saunders nursing drug handbook 2004* (p. 204). Philadelphia: W. B. Saunders.

18. 4
Rationale: Dry mouth is a common side effect. Frequent mouth rinsing with water, sucking on hard candy, and chewing sugarless gum will alleviate this common side effect. Hypotension and hypertension are rare side effects of fluphenazine. Mild leukopenia may occur, but the temperature does not need to be taken daily. Weight gain is a common side effect, and frequent snacks will worsen the problem.
Test Taking Strategy: Use the process of elimination, noting the key words "common side effects." Eliminate options 1 and 2 because they are assessments rather than interventions. As such, they cannot "minimize" a side effect. From the remaining options, you must recall that a dry mouth is a side effect. Review the common side effects related to this medication if you had difficulty with this question.
Level of Cognitive Ability: Application
Client Needs: Physiological Integrity
Integrated Process: Teaching/Learning
Content Area: Pharmacology
Reference: Kee, J., & Hayes, E. (2003). *Pharmacology: A nursing process approach* (4th ed., p. 298). Philadelphia: W. B. Saunders.

19. 4
Rationale: Oxazepam causes constipation, and the client is instructed to increase fluid intake and bulk (high fiber) in the diet. If the heart begins to beat fast, the physician is notified because this could indicate overdose. Additionally, diarrhea could indicate an incomplete intestinal obstruction, and if this occurs, the physician is notified.
Test-Taking Strategy: Use the process of elimination. Recalling that constipation is a side effect of this medication will direct you to option 4. Review the side effects and adverse effects of oxazepam if you had difficulty with this question.
Level of Cognitive Ability: Application
Client Needs: Physiological Integrity
Integrated Process: Teaching/Learning
Content Area: Pharmacology
Reference: Gutierrez, K., & Queener, S. (2003). *Pharmacology for nursing practice* (p. 251). St. Louis: Mosby.

20. 2
Rationale: The oral concentrate form of thioridazine (Mellaril) should be diluted in water or fruit juice just before administration to the client. The other options are incorrect.
Test-Taking Strategy: Knowledge regarding the nursing considerations related to the administration of thioridazine is required to answer this question. If you are unfamiliar with this medication, review the concepts related to the administration of this medication.

Level of Cognitive Ability: Application
Client Needs: Physiological Integrity
Integrated Process: Nursing Process—implementation
Content Area: Pharmacology
Reference: Kee, J., & Hayes, E. (2003). *Pharmacology: A nursing process approach* (4th ed., p. 297). Philadelphia: W. B. Saunders.

CRITICAL THINKING: FILL IN THE BLANK

Answer: Yogurt
Rationale: Phenelzine sulfate is a monoamine oxidase inhibitor. The client should avoid taking in foods that are high in tyramine. Use of these foods could trigger a potentially fatal hypertensive crisis. Foods to avoid include yogurt, aged cheeses, smoked or processed meats, red wines, and fruits such as avocados, raisins, or figs.

Test-Taking Strategy: Recall that phenelzine sulfate is a monoamine oxidase inhibitor and that foods high in tyramine needed to be avoided. Next, from the food items listed in the question, identify the food that contains tyramine. Review the food items to avoid with monoamine oxidase inhibitors if you had difficulty with this question.
Level of Cognitive Ability: Application
Client Needs: Physiological Integrity
Integrated Process: Nursing Process—implementation
Content Area: Pharmacology
Reference: Hodgson, B., & Kizior, R. (2004). *Saunders nursing drug handbook 2004* (p. 799). Philadelphia: W. B. Saunders.

REFERENCES

Gutierrez, K., & Queener, S. (2003). *Pharmacology for nursing practice.* St. Louis: Mosby.

Hodgson, B., & Kizior, R. (2004). *Saunders nursing drug handbook 2004.* Philadelphia: W. B. Saunders.

Kee, J., & Hayes, E. (2003). *Pharmacology: A nursing process approach* (4th ed.). Philadelphia: W. B. Saunders.

Lehne, R. (2001). *Pharmacology for nursing care* (4th ed.). Philadelphia: W. B. Saunders.

McKenry, L., & Salerno, E. (2003). *Mosby's pharmacology in nursing* (21st ed.). St. Louis: Mosby.

Comprehensive Test

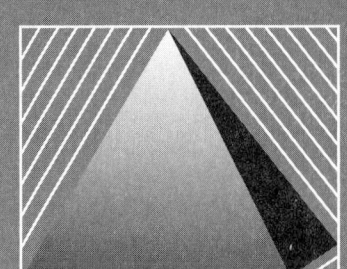

1. The nurse is assessing the child with a suspected diagnosis of appendicitis. In assessing the intensity and progression of the pain, the nurse palpates the child at McBurney's point. In performing this assessment, the nurse knows that McBurney's point is located midway between the
   1. Right anterior inferior iliac crest and the umbilicus.
   2. Left anterior superior iliac crest and the umbilicus.
   3. Right anterior superior iliac crest and the umbilicus.
   4. Left anterior superior iliac crest and the umbilicus.

2. The nurse is caring for a client with a burn injury to the lower legs. Nitrofurazone (Furacin) is prescribed to be applied to the sites of injury. The nurse documents which of the following in the plan of care as the appropriate method to apply this medication?
   1. Apply saline-soaked dressings over the medication.
   2. Apply 1-inch film directly to the burn sites.
   3. Apply $\frac{1}{16}$-inch film directly to the burn sites.
   4. Apply $\frac{1}{2}$-inch film directly to the burn sites after cleansing the wounds.

3. A client suspected of having an abdominal tumor is scheduled for a computerized tomography scan with dye injection. The nurse tells the client that
   1. The test may be painful.
   2. The dye injected may cause a warm, flushing sensation.
   3. Fluids will be restricted following the test.
   4. The test takes about 2 hours.

4. The nurse is caring for a client whose magnesium level is 3.5 mg/dL. Which assessment sign/symptom would the nurse most likely expect to note in the client based on this magnesium level?
   1. Tetany
   2. Twitches
   3. Positive Trousseau's sign
   4. Loss of deep tendon reflexes

5. The nurse is caring for a client with a diagnosis of hyperthyroidism. Laboratory studies are performed, and the serum calcium level is 12 mg/dL. Which medication would the nurse anticipate to be prescribed for the client?
   1. Calcium gluconate
   2. Calcium chloride
   3. Calcitonin (Calcimar)
   4. Large doses of vitamin D

6. The nurse prepares to administer sodium polystyrene sulfonate (Kayexalate) to the client. Before administering the medication, the nurse reviews the action of the medication and understands that it releases
   1. Bicarbonate in exchange primarily for sodium ions.
   2. Sodium ions in exchange primarily for bicarbonate ions.
   3. Sodium ions in exchange primarily for potassium ions.
   4. Potassium ions in exchange primarily for sodium ions.

7. Which of the following clients is least likely at risk for the development of third spacing?
   1. The client with cirrhosis
   2. The client with diabetes mellitus
   3. The client with liver failure
   4. The client with renal failure

8. The nurse is preparing to care for a client following a gastroscopy procedure. The nurse includes which most appropriate component in the nursing care plan?
   1. Place the client in a supine position to provide comfort.
   2. Monitor the client's vital signs every hour for 4 hours.
   3. Provide saline gargles immediately on return to the unit to aid in comfort.
   4. Check the gag reflex by using a tongue depressor to stroke the back of client's throat.

9. Intravenous Ringer's lactate solution is prescribed for the postoperative client. The nursing instructor asks the nursing student who is caring for the client about the tonicity of the prescribed intravenous solution. The nursing student responds correctly by stating that this solution is
   1. Isotonic.
   2. Normotonic.
   3. Hypotonic.
   4. Hypertonic.

10. The nurse reviews the arterial blood gas results of a client with Guillain-Barré syndrome. The pH is 7.35 and the P_{CO_2} is 50 mm Hg. The nurse interprets that this client is experiencing which acid-base imbalance?
    1. Respiratory acidosis
    2. Respiratory alkalosis
    3. Metabolic acidosis
    4. Metabolic alkalosis

11. The client is admitted 24 hours following an aspirin overdose. The nurse assesses this client for which signs and symptoms indicating the acid-base disturbance that can occur in the client?
    1. Bradycardia and hyperactivity
    2. Restlessness, confusion, and a positive Trousseau's sign
    3. Headache, nausea, vomiting, and diarrhea
    4. Bradypnea, dizziness, and paresthesias

12. The adult client with hepatic encephalopathy has a serum ammonia level of 95 mcg/dL and receives treatment with lactulose (Chronulac). The nurse would evaluate that the client had the best and most realistic response, if the serum ammonia level changed to which of the following after medication administration?
    1. 80 mcg/dL
    2. 60 mcg/dL
    3. 10 mcg/dL
    4. 5 mcg/dL

13. The client who suffered a crush injury to the leg has a highly positive urine myoglobin level. The nurse assesses this particular client carefully for signs of
1. Cerebrovascular accident.
2. Acute tubular necrosis.
3. Respiratory failure.
4. Myocardial infarction.

14. The adult male client admitted to the hospital with shock has received fluid volume replacement. The nurse evaluates that the client has had adequate fluid resuscitation if the client's repeat hematocrit level has decreased to which of the following values in the normal range?
1. 56%
2. 48%
3. 39%
4. 34%

15. The nurse is formulating a plan of care for a client receiving enteral feedings. Which nursing diagnosis is of highest priority for this client?
1. Imbalanced Nutrition, Less Than Body Requirements
2. Risk for Aspiration
3. Risk for Deficient Fluid Volume
4. Diarrhea

16. A client who has a gastrostomy tube for feeding refuses to participate in the plan of care, will not make eye contact, and does not speak to the family or visitors. The nurse assesses that this client is using which type of coping mechanism?
1. Self-control
2. Problem-solving
3. Accepting responsibility
4. Distancing

17. The nurse conducting a weight loss program prepares to monitor a client's weight loss. What method would assess the effectiveness of weight loss most accurately?
1. Daily weights
2. Serum protein levels
3. Calorie counts
4. Daily intake and output

18. The clinic nurse is monitoring a client with anorexia nervosa. Which statement if made by a client would indicate to the nurse that treatment has been effective?
1. "I no longer have a weight problem."
2. "I don't want to starve myself anymore."
3. "I'll eat until I don't feel hungry."
4. "My friends and I went out to lunch today."

19. The nurse is teaching the postgastrectomy client about measures to prevent dumping syndrome. Which statement by the client indicates a need for further teaching?
1. "I need to lie down after eating."
2. "I need to drink liquids with meals."
3. "I need to eat small meals six times daily."

4. "I need to avoid concentrated sweets."

20. A client has been diagnosed with pernicious anemia. In planning care for the client, the nurse anticipates that the client will be treated with
1. Thiamine.
2. Iron.
3. Vitamin B_{12}.
4. Folic acid.

21. An older postoperative client has been tolerating a full liquid diet, and the nurse plans to advance the diet to solid food as prescribed. Which assessment is most important for the nurse to make before advancing the diet to solids?
1. Food preferences
2. Cultural preferences
3. Presence of bowel sounds
4. Ability to chew

22. The client with diabetes mellitus has been instructed in the dietary exchange system. The client asks the nurse if bacon is allowed in the diet. Which nursing response is most appropriate?
1. "Bacon is much too high in fat."
2. "Bacon is not allowed."
3. "One strip of bacon may be eaten if you eliminate one teaspoon of butter."
4. "Bacon may be eaten if you eliminate one meat item from your diet."

23. The client with heart disease is provided instructions regarding a low-fat diet. The nurse determines that the client understands the diet if the client states that a food item to avoid is
1. Apples.
2. Oranges.
3. Avocado.
4. Cherries.

24. A client with liver cancer who is receiving chemotherapy tells the nurse that some foods on the meal tray taste bitter. The nurse would try to limit which food that is most likely to cause this taste for the client?
1. Beef
2. Potatoes
3. Custard
4. Cantaloupe

25. A nursing student is caring for a client who has been admitted to the hospital with malnutrition. The student is reviewing the results of the various laboratory tests performed on the client with the nursing instructor. Which statement if made by the nursing student indicates an understanding of the interpretation of the results?
1. "An elevated creatinine level indicates respiratory problems."
2. "A normal hemoglobin level indicates that iron and protein intake is sufficient."
3. "An elevated albumin level indicates a definite dehydration."

4. "A normal red blood cell level indicates adequate vitamin B$_6$ intake."

26. The nurse notes that the infant with a diagnosis of hydrocephalus has a head that is heavier than the average infant. The nurse determines that special safety precautions are needed when moving the infant. Which statement would the nurse include in the discharge teaching with the parents to reflect this safety need?
    1. "When picking up your infant, support the infant's neck and head with the open palm of your hand."
    2. "Feed your infant in a side-lying position."
    3. "Place a helmet on your infant when in bed."
    4. "Hyperextend your infant's head with a rolled blanket under the neck area."

27. The nurse is performing an admission assessment on a child with a seizure disorder. The nurse is interviewing the child's parents to determine their adjustment to caring for their child who has a chronic illness. Which statement if made by the parents would indicate a need for further teaching?
    1. "Our child is involved in a swim program with neighbors and friends."
    2. "Our child sleeps in our bedroom at night."
    3. "Our babysitter just completed cardiopulmonary resuscitation training."
    4. "We worry about injuries when our child has a seizure."

28. The nurse is reviewing the results of a serum level drawn from a child who is receiving carbamazepine (Tegretol) for the control of seizures. The results indicate a level of 10 mcg/mL. The nurse analyzes the results and anticipates that the physician will prescribe
    1. An increase of the dose of the medication.
    2. A decrease of the dose of the medication.
    3. Discontinuation of the medication.
    4. Continuation of the presently prescribed dosage.

29. The nursing student is asked to describe the corpus of the uterus. Which of the following responses, if made by the student, indicates an understanding of the anatomy of the uterus?
    1. "The corpus is the lower portion of the uterus."
    2. "The corpus is the upper part of the uterus."
    3. "The corpus is the area where the cervix meets the external os."
    4. "The corpus is the area where the vagina meets the uterus."

30. The nurse instructs a client with diabetes mellitus about blood glucose monitoring and monitoring for signs of hypoglycemia. The nurse informs the client that hypoglycemia is a blood glucose level of less than
    1. 120 mg/dL.
    2. 110 mg/dL.
    3. 90 mg/dL.
    4. 60 mg/dL.

31. The client newly diagnosed with diabetes mellitus is instructed by the physician to obtain glucagon for emergency home use. The client asks the home care nurse about the purpose of the medication. The nurse instructs the client that the purpose of the medication is to treat
    1. Hypoglycemia from insulin overdose.
    2. Hyperglycemia from insufficient insulin.
    3. Lipoatrophy from insulin injections.
    4. Lipohypertrophy from inadequate insulin absorption.

32. The nurse is providing care to a Cuban American client who is terminally ill. Numerous family members are present most of the time, and many of the family members are emotional. The most appropriate action is to
    1. Restrict the number of family members visiting at one time.
    2. Inform the family that emotional outbursts are to be avoided.
    3. Request permission to move the client to a private room and allow the family members to visit.
    4. Contact the physician to speak to the family regarding their behaviors.

33. The nurse is instructing a postpartum client with endometritis about preventing the spread of infection to the newborn infant. The nurse would tell the client that
    1. Hands should be washed thoroughly before holding the infant.
    2. The newborn infant will not be allowed in the mother's room at all.
    3. There is no danger of the newborn contracting the disease.
    4. Visitors are not allowed to hold the baby.

34. A client presents to the emergency department with upper gastrointestinal bleeding and is in moderate distress. In planning care, which nursing action would be the first priority for this client?
    1. Thorough investigation of precipitating events
    2. Insertion of a nasogastric tube and hematest of emesis
    3. Complete abdominal examination
    4. Assessment of vital signs

35. The nurse is caring for a client with possible cholelithiasis who is being prepared for an intravenous cholangiogram, and the nurse teaches the client about the procedure. Which client statement indicates that the client understands the purpose of this test?
    1. "They are going to 'look at' my gallbladder and ducts."
    2. "This procedure will drain my gallbladder."
    3. "My gallbladder will be irrigated."
    4. "They will put medication in my gallbladder."

36. The nurse provides instructions to a malnourished client regarding iron supplementation during

pregnancy. Which statement if made by the client would indicate an understanding of the instructions?

1. "The iron is best absorbed if taken with orange juice."
2. "Meat does not provide iron and should be avoided."
3. "Iron supplements will give me diarrhea."
4. "My body has all the iron it needs, and I don't need to take supplements."

37. The nurse has given discharge instructions to the client who has underwent vein ligation and stripping early in the day. The nurse evaluates that the client understands activity and positioning limitations if the client states that it is most appropriate to

1. Lie down with the legs elevated and avoid sitting.
2. Cross the legs at the ankle only, but not at the knee.
3. Sit in the chair 3 times a day for 3 hours at a time.
4. Walk upright for as much as possible each day.

38. Octreotide acetate (Sandostatin) is prescribed for the client with acromegaly. The nurse monitors the client, knowing that which side effect is associated with the administration of this medication?

1. Constipation
2. Polyuria
3. Abdominal pain
4. Hypotension

39. Levothyroxine (Synthroid) is prescribed for a client diagnosed with hypothyroidism. The nurse reviews the client's record and notes that the client presently is taking warfarin (Coumadin). The nurse contacts the physician, anticipating that the physician will prescribe which of the following?

1. An increased dosage of warfarin.
2. A decreased dosage of warfarin.
3. An increased dosage of levothyroxine.
4. A decreased dosage of levothyroxine.

40. The nurse is teaching the client with emphysema about positions that help breathing during dyspneic episodes. The nurse instructs the client to avoid which of the following positions, which will aggravate breathing?

1. Sitting up with the elbows resting on knees
2. Standing and leaning against a wall
3. Lying on the back in low Fowler's position
4. Sitting up and leaning on a table

41. The client is about to undergo a lumbar puncture. The nurse describes to the client that which of the following positions will be used during the procedure?

1. Side-lying with the legs pulled up and the head bent down onto the chest
2. Side-lying with a pillow under the hip
3. Prone with a pillow under the abdomen
4. Prone in slight Trendelenburg's position

42. The nurse recognizes that which of the following interventions is unlikely to facilitate effective communication between the dying client and his or her family?

1. The nurse encourages the client and family to identify and discuss feelings openly.
2. The nurse makes decisions for the client and family to relieve them of unnecessary demands.
3. The nurse assists the client and family in carrying out spiritually meaningful practices.
4. The nurse maintains a calm attitude and one of acceptance when the family or client expresses anger.

43. The client with acute pancreatitis is experiencing severe pain from the disorder. The nurse determines that the client understood suggestions for positioning to reduce pain if the client avoided

1. Leaning forward.
2. Drawing the legs up to the chest.
3. Sitting up.
4. Lying flat.

44. The client has had surgery to repair a fractured left hip. The nurse obtains which of the following most important items from the unit storage area to use when repositioning the client from side to side in bed?

1. Abductor splint
2. Adductor splint
3. Bed pillow
4. Overhead trapeze

45. The nurse is preparing to care for a client who has undergone a myelogram using a oil-based contrast agent. The nurse plans to position the client on bedrest for

1. 6 to 8 hours with the head of bed flat.
2. 6 to 8 hours with the head of bed elevated 15 to 30 degrees.
3. 2 to 4 hours with the head of bed flat.
4. 2 to 4 hours with the head of bed elevated 15 to 30 degrees.

46. The nurse has given activity guidelines to the client with chronic lower back pain. The nurse determines that the client understood the instructions if the client states to avoid which of the following positions?

1. Lying on the side with knees and hips bent
2. Lying prone
3. Standing with one foot on a step or stool
4. Sitting using a lumbar roll or pillow

47. The nurse has just admitted to the nursing unit a client with a basilar skull fracture who is at risk for increased intracranial pressure. Pending specific physician orders, the nurse would avoid placing the client in which of the following positions?

1. Neck in neutral position
2. Head of bed elevated 30 to 45 degrees
3. Flat with head turned to the side
4. Head midline

48. The nurse reviews the arterial blood gas results of an assigned client and notes that the laboratory report indicates a pH of 7.30, P_{CO_2} of 58 mm Hg, P_{O_2} of 80 mm Hg, and a HCO_3 of 27 mEq/L. The nurse interprets that the client has which acid-base disturbance?
   1. Metabolic acidosis
   2. Metabolic alkalosis
   3. Respiratory acidosis
   4. Respiratory alkalosis

49. Cortisone acetate (Cortone) is prescribed for a client with adrenal insufficiency. The nurse provides instructions to the client regarding the medication. Which statement if made by the client indicates a need for further instruction?
   1. "I will eat a good breakfast every day."
   2. "I will avoid people with colds."
   3. "I will limit my sodium intake."
   4. "I will stop the medication when I feel better."

50. The hospitalized client with diabetes mellitus received NPH insulin in the morning. The nurse monitors the client for hypoglycemia, knowing that the peak action occurs
   1. 2 to 4 hours after administration.
   2. 6 to 14 hours after administration.
   3. 14 to 18 hours after administration.
   4. 18 to 24 hours after administration.

51. The nurse has admitted a client to the clinical nursing unit following modified right radical mastectomy for the treatment of breast cancer. The nurse plans to place the right arm in which of the following positions?
   1. Elevated above shoulder level
   2. Elevated on a pillow
   3. Level with the right atrium
   4. Dependent to the right atrium

52. On the second postpartum day, a woman complains of burning on urination, urgency, and frequency of urination. A urinalysis is collected, and the results indicate the presence of a urinary tract infection. The nurse instructs the new mother regarding measures to take for the treatment of the infection. Which of the following statements if made by the mother would indicate a need for further instructions?
   1. "The prescribed medication must be taken until it is completed."
   2. "My fluid intake should be increased to at least three thousand milliliters daily."
   3. "I need to urinate frequently throughout the day."
   4. "I should consume foods and fluids that will increase urine alkalinity."

53. The registered nurse is beginning a new job in a clinic and is attending an orientation session. Following the orientation session, another new employee asks the registered nurse to describe case management, a component of the discussions in the orientation session, because the employee did not understand the concept clearly. The registered nurse responds that
   1. "Case management requires an experienced nurse because it represents a primary health prevention focus and is managed by a single nurse."
   2. "Case management saves money for the institution because client's with similar problems are treated in the same manner."
   3. "Case management is an important concept, but it doesn't promote appropriate use of personnel."
   4. "Case management will maximize hospital revenues and at the same time provide optimal outcome of client care."

54. The nurse provides dietary instructions to a client with diabetes mellitus regarding the prescribed diabetic diet. Which statement if made by the client indicates a need for further teaching?
   1. "I need to drink diet soft drinks."
   2. "I'll eat a balanced meal plan."
   3. "I need to purchase special dietetic foods."
   4. "I'll snack on fruit instead of cake."

55. The client received 20 units of NPH insulin subcutaneously at 8 AM. The nurse should assess the client for a hypoglycemic reaction at
   1. 10 AM
   2. 11 AM
   3. 5 PM
   4. 11 PM

56. The community health nurse is working with disaster relief in a local community following a hurricane that ruined many homes in the community. The nurse is working to find housing for the survivors and is organizing counseling services. These actions of the nurse represent which type of level of prevention?
   1. The primary level of prevention
   2. The secondary level of prevention
   3. The tertiary level of prevention
   4. The fourth level of prevention

57. A pregnant woman in her second trimester calls the prenatal clinic nurse to report a recent exposure to a child with rubella. Which of the following responses by the nurse would be most appropriate and supportive to the woman?
   1. "There is no need to be concerned if you don't have a fever or rash within the next two days."
   2. "Be sure to tell the doctor on your next prenatal visit, but there is little risk in the second trimester."
   3. "You should avoid all school-aged children during pregnancy."
   4. "You were wise to call. I will check your rubella titer screening results, and we can identify immediately whether future interventions are needed."

58. The breast-feeding mother of an infant with lactose intolerance asks the nurse about dietary measures. The nurse tells the mother to avoid
   1. Hard cheeses

2. Green, leafy vegetables

3. Dried beans

4. Egg yolk

59. A client with diabetes mellitus is told that amputation of the leg is necessary to sustain life. The client is upset and states to the nurse, "This is all the doctor's fault! I have done everything that the doctor has asked me to do!" The nurse interprets the client's statement as

1. An expected coping mechanism.

2. A need to notify the hospital lawyer.

3. An expression of guilt on the part of the client.

4. An ineffective coping mechanism.

60. A client brought to the emergency room is dead on arrival. The family of the client tells the physician that the client had a terminal cancer. The emergency room physician examines the client and asks the nurse to contact the medical examiner regarding an autopsy. The family of the client tells the nurse that they do not want an autopsy performed. Which of the following responses to the family is most appropriate?

1. "It is required by federal law. Why don't we talk about it, and why don't you tell me why you don't want the autopsy done?"

2. "The decision is made by the medical examiner."

3. "I will contact the medical examiner regarding your request."

4. "An autopsy is mandatory for any client who is dead on arrival."

61. A pregnant woman who is positive for human immunodeficiency virus (HIV) delivers a newborn infant, and the nurse provides instructions to help the mother regarding the newborn infant care. Which statement by the client indicates the need for further instructions?

1. "I will be sure to wash my hands before and following bathroom use."

2. "Support groups are available to assist me with understanding my diagnosis of HIV."

3. "I need to breast-feed, especially for the first six weeks postpartum."

4. "My newborn infant should be on antiviral medications for the first six weeks after delivery."

62. A pregnant woman has a positive history of genital herpes but has not had lesions during this pregnancy. The nurse should plan to provide which of the following information to the client?

1. "You will be isolated from your newborn infant following delivery."

2. "You will be evaluated at the time of delivery for herpetic genital tract lesions, and if lesions are present, a cesarean delivery will be needed."

3. "There is little risk to your newborn infant during this pregnancy, birth, and following delivery."

4. "Vaginal deliveries can reduce neonatal infection risks even if you have an active lesion at birth."

63. A 7-year-old child is diagnosed with viral conjunctivitis. Antibiotic eye drops are prescribed for the child. The mother asks the nurse when the child can return to school. The most appropriate response is

1. "The child can return to school immediately."

2. "The child should be kept home until the antibiotic eye drops have been administered for twenty-four hours."

3. "The child should be kept home until the antibiotic eye drops have been administered for seventy-two hours."

4. "The child cannot return to school until seen by the physician in one week."

64. An adolescent is diagnosed with conjunctivitis, and the nurse provides information to the adolescent about the use of contact lenses. Which statement by the client indicates the need for further information?

1. "My contact lens can be worn if they are cleaned as directed."

2. "I should not wear my contact lens."

3. "New contact lenses should be obtained."

4. "My old contact lenses should be discarded."

65. A pregnant client is seen in the health care clinic and asks the nurse what causes the breasts to change in size and appearance during pregnancy. The nurse plans to base the response on which of the following?

1. The breast changes are due to the secretion of estrogen and progesterone.

2. The breasts become stretched because of the weight gain.

3. The increased metabolic rate causes the breasts to become larger.

4. Cortisol secreted by the adrenal glands play a factor in increasing the size and appearance of the breasts.

66. The nurse is caring for a client receiving bolus feedings via a Levin-type nasogastric tube. As the nurse is finishing the feeding, the client asks for the bed to be positioned flat to sleep. The nurse understands that the most appropriate position for this client at this time is which of the following?

1. Head of bed flat with the client in the supine position for at least 30 minutes

2. Head of bed elevated 30 to 45 degrees with the client in the right lateral position for 60 minutes

3. Head of bed elevated 45 to 60 degrees with the client in the supine position for 90 minutes

4. Head of bed in semi-Fowler position with the client in the left lateral position for 60 minutes

67. Before administering an intermittent tube feeding through a nasogastric tube, the nurse assesses for gastric residual. The nurse understands that this procedure is important to

1. Confirm proper nasogastric tube placement.

2. Observe gastric contents.

3. Assess fluid and electrolyte status.

4. Evaluate absorption of the last feeding.

68. A 4-year-old child is diagnosed with otitis media. The mother asks the nurse about the causes of this illness. The nurse responds, knowing that which of the following is an unassociated risk factor related to otitis media?
    1. Household smoking
    2. Bottle-feeding
    3. Exposure to illness in other children
    4. A history of urinary tract infections

69. The pediatric nurse assists the physician in performing a lumbar puncture on a 3-year-old child with leukemia suspected of having central nervous system metastasis. The nurse places the child in which position for this procedure?
    1. Prone with the knees flexed to the abdomen and the head bent with the chin resting on the chest
    2. Modified Sims' position
    3. Lateral recumbent with the knees flexed to the abdomen and the head bent with the chin resting on the chest
    4. Lithotomy position

70. A client with diabetes mellitus is self-administering NPH insulin from a vial that is kept at room temperature. The client asks the nurse about the length of time an unrefrigerated vial of insulin will maintain its potency. The most appropriate response to the client is which of the following?
    1. 2 weeks
    2. 1 month
    3. 2 months
    4. 6 months

71. The nurse is caring for a client scheduled for a transphenoidal hypophysectomy. The preoperative teaching instructions would include which most important statement?
    1. "Your hair will need to be shaved."
    2. "Deep breathing and coughing will be needed after surgery."
    3. "Toothbrushing will not be permitted for at least two weeks following surgery."
    4. "You will receive spinal anesthesia."

72. The nurse caring for a client with Addison's disease would expect to note which of the following on assessment of the client?
    1. Obesity
    2. Edema
    3. Hypotension
    4. Hirsutism

73. The nurse is conducting a prepared child birth class and is instructing pregnant women about the method of effleurage. The nurse instructs the women to perform the procedure by
    1. Contracting and then consciously relaxing different muscle groups.
    2. Contracting an area of the body such as an arm or leg and then concentrating on letting tension go from the rest of the body.

    3. Massaging the abdomen during contractions using both hands in a circular motion.
    4. Instructing the significant other to stroke or massage a tightened muscle by the use of touch.

74. During a routine prenatal visit, the client complains of gums that bleed easily with brushing. The nurse performs an assessment and then teaches the client about proper nutrition to minimize this problem. Which statement if made by the client indicates an understanding of the proper nutrition to minimize this problem?
    1. "I will eat three servings of cracked wheat bread each day."
    2. "I will eat fresh fruits and vegetables for snacks and for dessert each day."
    3. "I will drink eight ounces of water with each meal."
    4. "I will eat two saltine crackers before I get up each morning."

75. A 6-year-old child has just been diagnosed with localized Hodgkin's disease, and chemotherapy is planned to begin immediately. The mother of the child asks the nurse why radiation therapy was not prescribed as a part of the treatment. The most appropriate and supportive response to the mother is
    1. "I'm not sure. I'll discuss it with the physician."
    2. "The child is too young to have radiation therapy."
    3. "It's very costly, and chemotherapy works just as well."
    4. "The physician would prefer that you discuss treatment options with the oncologist."

76. A diagnostic work-up is being performed on a 1-year-old child suspected of having a diagnosis of neuroblastoma. The nurse reviews the results of the diagnostic tests and understands that which finding is related most specifically to this type of tumor?
    1. Elevated vanillylmandelic acid urinary levels
    2. The presence of blast cells in the bone marrow
    3. Projectile vomiting occurring most often in the morning
    4. Positive Babinski's sign

77. The nurse is developing a postoperative plan of care for a 40-year-old male Filipino client scheduled for an appendectomy. The nurse most appropriately includes in the plan of care to
    1. Inform the client the he will need to ask for pain medication when needed.
    2. Offer pain medication when nonverbal signs of discomfort are identified.
    3. Offer pain medication regularly as prescribed.
    4. Allow the client to maintain control and request pain medication on his own.

78. The nurse provides instructions regarding home care to the parents of a 3-year-old child hospitalized with hemophilia. Which statement if made by a parent indicates a need for further instructions?
    1. "We will supervise the child closely."
    2. "We will pad corners of the furniture."

3. "We will remove household items that can fall over easily."

4. "We will avoid having the child receive immunizations and cancel the scheduled dental appointments."

79. The nurse is planning to instruct the Mexican American client about nutrition and dietary restrictions. When developing the plan, the nurse is aware that this ethnic group
   1. Enjoys food that lacks color, flavor, and texture.
   2. Primarily eats raw fish.
   3. Enjoys eating red meat.
   4. Views food as a primary form of socialization.

80. The registered nurse is planning the client assignments for the day. Which of the following is the most appropriate assignment for the nursing assistant?
   1. A client with bladder cancer who will be receiving chemotherapy
   2. A client on bedrest who requires range of motion exercises every 4 hours
   3. A new diabetic mellitus client scheduled for discharge
   4. A client scheduled to receive a blood transfusion

81. Propythiouracil (PTU) is prescribed for the client with hyperthyroidism. The nurse provides instructions to the client regarding the medication and informs the client to notify the physician if which of the following signs occur?
   1. Drowsiness
   2. Sore throat
   3. Increased urination
   4. Dry mouth

82. A client who has been taking iodine solution (Lugol's solution, potassium iodide solution) is admitted to the emergency room and an iodine overdose is suspected. Gastric lavage is initiated to remove the iodine from the stomach. In addition to treatment with gastric lavage, the nurse anticipates that which of the following will be administered?
   1. Calcium gluconate
   2. Vitamin K
   3. Acetylcysteine (Mucomyst)
   4. Sodium thiosulfate

83. The nurse is interviewing a 16-year-old client during her initial prenatal clinic visit. The client is beginning week 18 of her first pregnancy. Which statement if made by the client indicates an immediate need for further investigation?
   1. "I don't like my face anymore. I always look like I have been crying."
   2. "I don't like my breasts anymore. These silver lines are ugly."
   3. "I don't like my stomach anymore. That brown line is disgusting."
   4. "I don't like my figure anymore. My clothes are all too tight."

84. The client seen in the health care clinic has tested positive for gonorrhea. The nurse anticipates that which medication will be prescribed for the client based on this finding?
   1. Ceftriaxone (Rocephin)
   2. Penicillin G benzathine (Bicillin)
   3. Acyclovir (Zovirax)
   4. Azithromycin (Zithromax)

85. The client is brought into the emergency room in ventricular fibrillation. The advanced cardiac life support nurse prepares to defibrillate by placing conductive gel pads on which part of the chest?
   1. To the upper and lower half of the sternum
   2. To the right of the sternum just below the clavicle and to the left of the precordium
   3. To the right shoulder and in the back of the left shoulder
   4. Parallel between the umbilicus and the right nipple

86. A rubella vaccine is prescribed to be administered to a 2-day postpartum client. The nurse preparing to administer the vaccine develops a list of the potential risks associated with this vaccine. The nurse reviews the list with the client and cautions the client to avoid
   1. Sunlight for 3 days.
   2. Scratching the injection site.
   3. Pregnancy for 2 to 3 months after the vaccination.
   4. Sexual intercourse for 2 to 3 months after the vaccination.

87. The client has undergone mastectomy. The nurse interprets that the client is making the best adjustment to the loss of the breast if which of the following behaviors is observed?
   1. Participating in the care of the surgical drain
   2. Reading postoperative care booklet
   3. Refusing to look at the wound
   4. Asking for pain medication when needed

88. The client is preparing for discharge from the hospital after radical vulvectomy. The nurse plans to teach this client that which of the following activities is acceptable after discharge because it will not precipitate complications?
   1. Sexual activity
   2. Walking
   3. Sitting for lengthy periods
   4. Driving a car

89. The child with croup is being discharged from the hospital. The nurse provides instructions to the mother and advises the mother to bring the child to the emergency room if the child
   1. Appears tired.
   2. Takes fluids poorly.
   3. Is irritable.
   4. Develops stridor.

90. The emergency room nurse is caring for a child suspected of epiglottitis and has ensured that the child

has a patent airway. The next priority in the care of this child would be to
1. Prepare the child for a chest radiograph.
2. Assist the physician with intubation.
3. Prepare the child for tracheotomy.
4. Prepare to administer epinephrine.

91. The nurse reviews the plan of care for a client at 37 weeks of gestation who has sickle cell anemia. The nurse determines that which nursing diagnosis listed on the nursing care plan will receive the highest priority?
1. Activity Intolerance
2. Disturbed Body Image
3. At risk for pain
4. Deficient Fluid Volume

92. The mother arrives at the clinic with her 3-year-old child. The mother tells the nurse that the child has had a fever and a cough for the past 2 days and that this morning the child began to wheeze. Viral pneumonia is diagnosed. Based on the diagnosis, the nurse anticipates that which of the following will be a component of the treatment plan?
1. Orally administered antibiotics
2. Hospitalization and intravenously administered antibiotics
3. Supportive treatment
4. Intravenous fluid administration

93. A mother of a child with cystic fibrosis asks the clinic nurse about the disease. The nurse tells the mother that cystic fibrosis is
1. A disease that causes the formation of multiple cysts in the lungs.
2. A chronic multisystem disorder affecting the exocrine glands.
3. Transmitted as an autosomal dominant trait.
4. A disease that causes dilation of the passageways of many organs.

94. Minoxidil solution (Rogaine) is prescribed for the client to treat hair loss. The nurse tells the client that the usual dosage for this medication is
1. 1 mL applied 6 times daily.
2. 1 mL applied at bedtime.
3. 1 mL applied 2 times a day.
4. 1 mL applied 4 times a day.

95. Collagenase (Santyl) is prescribed for a client with a severe burn to the hand. The home care nurse provides instructions to the client regarding the use of the medication. Which client statement indicates an accurate understanding of the use of this medication?
1. "I will apply the ointment once a day and leave it open to the air."
2. "I will apply the ointment once a day and cover it with a sterile dressing."
3. "I will apply the ointment twice a day and leave it open to the air."
4. "I will apply the ointment at bedtime and in the morning and cover it with a sterile dressing."

96. The mother of an infant diagnosed with Hirschsprung's disease asks the nurse about the disorder. The nurse tells the mother that this disease is a
1. Congenital aganglionosis or megacolon.
2. Complete small intestinal obstruction.
3. Condition that causes the pyloric valve to remain open.
4. Severe inflammation of the gastrointestinal tract.

97. The nurse is preparing to care for a newborn infant who will be returning from surgery with a colostomy that was created for imperforate anus. When the newborn infant returns from surgery, the nurse assesses the stoma and notes that it is red and edematous. Which of the following is the most appropriate nursing intervention?
1. Call the physician.
2. Document the findings.
3. Apply ice immediately.
4. Elevate the buttocks.

98. The nurse is developing a plan of care for a preterm newborn infant and is addressing measures to provide skin care. The nurse develops measures knowing that the preterm newborn infant's skin appears
1. Reddened, thin, and gelatinous with decreased amounts of subcutaneous fat and open posture.
2. Thin and gelatinous with increased subcutaneous fat.
3. Thin and gelatinous with increased amounts of brown fat.
4. With fine downy hair on a thin epidermal and dermal layer with increased amount of brown fat.

99. The nurse in the labor room is performing an initial assessment on a newborn infant. On assessment of the newborn infant's head, the nurse notes that the ears are low set. Which of the following nursing actions would be most appropriate?
1. Cover the ears with gauze pads.
2. Document the findings.
3. Arrange for hearing testing.
4. Notify the physician.

100. The clinic nurse is assessing the status of jaundice in a child with hepatitis. Which anatomical area will provide the best data regarding the presence of jaundice?
1. The nailbeds
2. The skin in the abdominal area
3. The skin in the sacral area
4. The membranes in the ear canal

101. A prenatal client with a history of heart disease has been instructed on care at home. Which statement if made by the client would indicate that the client understands her needs?
1. "There is no restriction on people who visit me."
2. "I should avoid stressful situations."

3. "My weight gain is not important."

4. "I should rest on my right side."

102. A prenatal client has acquired the sexually transmitted infection human papillomavirus. When planning care, which of the following interventions would the nurse anticipate would be prescribed because of its safety during pregnancy?

1. Cryotherapy

2. Use of cytotoxic agents

3. Treatment with imiquimod

4. Treatment with podophyllin

103. The home care nurse is assigned to visit a Mexican American client to perform an admission assessment. On initial meeting of the client, the nurse would

1. Greet the client with a handshake.

2. Avoid touching the client.

3. Avoid any affirmative nods during the conversations with the client.

4. Smile and use humor throughout the entire admission assessment.

104. Russell's traction is prescribed for a child with a lower leg fracture. The mother of the child asks the nurse about the purpose of the traction. The nurse explains to the mother that this type of traction primarily provides

1. Reduction or realignment of a fracture site.

2. Keeps the child from moving around in bed.

3. Provides a form of restraint for the child.

4. Will relieve the child's pain.

105. The home care nurse's assignment is to visit a new mother at home 24 to 48 hours after discharge. Which of the following would the nurse expect to note in a healthy mother who is breast-feeding her newborn infant?

1. A mother breast-feeding with the infant in a tummy to tummy position without signs of cracked nipples; the baby demonstrates bursts of sucking followed by a pause and swallow.

2. A mother breast-feeding the infant with the infant's head turned toward her breast, with the body flat in her arms; mother with sore nipples and infant with a suck blister.

3. A mother complaining of breast engorgement with the infant demonstrating difficulty in latching onto the breast.

4. A mother with cracked nipples feeding the infant with a supplemental bottle.

106. The nurse is assigned to care for a client who is in traction. The nurse prepares a plan of care for the client and includes which nursing action in the plan?

1. Monitor the weights to be sure that they are resting on a firm surface.

2. Check the weights to be sure that they are off of the floor.

3. Make sure that the knots are at the pulleys.

4. Make sure the head of the bed is kept at a 45- to 90-degree angle.

107. A nurse is setting up the physical environment for an interview with a client and plans to obtain subjective data regarding the client's health. Select all interventions that are appropriate.

___ Set the room temperature at a comfortable level.

___ Provide seating for the client so that the client faces a strong light.

___ Ensure that the distance between the client and nurse is at least 6 feet.

___ Place a chair for the client across from the nurse's desk.

___ Remove distracting objects from the interviewing area.

___ Ensure comfortable seating at eye level for the client and nurse.

108. The private duty nurse has been caring for a terminally ill client whose death is imminent. The nurse has developed a close relationship with the family of the client. Which of the following nursing interventions will the nurse avoid in dealing with the family during this difficult time?

1. Making the decisions for the family

2. Encouraging family discussion of concerns

3. Encouraging family requested clergy visits

4. Accepting the family's expressions of anger

109. The nurse is reviewing the record of a pregnant client and notes that the physician has documented the presence of Chadwick's sign. The nurse understands that the hormone responsible for the development of this sign is which of the following?

1. Human chorionic gonadotropin

2. Estrogen

3. Progesterone

4. Prolactin

110. The nurse is caring for an older client who has been placed in Buck's extension traction following a hip fracture. On assessment of the client the nurse notes that the client is disoriented. The most appropriate nursing intervention is to

1. Ask the family to stay with the client.

2. Apply restraints to the client.

3. Ask the laboratory to perform electrolyte studies.

4. Reorient the client frequently and place a clock and a calendar in the client's room.

111. The nurse is preparing a plan of care for the client in skin traction. The nurse includes in the plan that a priority intervention is to assess the client frequently for

1. The presence of bowel sounds.

2. Signs of infection around the pin sites.

3. Signs of skin breakdown.

4. Urinary incontinence.

112. A contraction stress test is scheduled for the pregnant client, and the client asks the nurse about the test. The nurse tells the client that
    1. Small amounts of oxytocin (Pitocin) are administered during internal fetal monitor to stimulate uterine contractions.
    2. An external fetal monitor is attached, and the woman ambulates on a treadmill until contractions begin.
    3. The uterus is stimulated to contract by the use of small amounts of oxytocin (Pitocin) or by nipple stimulation.
    4. Uterine contractions are stimulated by Leopold's maneuvers.

113. The mother arrives at a well-baby clinic with her 1-month-old infant. She expresses concern because one of the infant's eyes appears to be crossed. The most appropriate and supportive response by the nurse is which of the following?
    1. "The infant will probably need surgery."
    2. "This condition is probably permanent."
    3. "It bears watching because the other eye may do the same thing."
    4. "This is normal in the young infant but should not be present after about age four months."

114. The physician prescribes "patching" for a child with strabismus of the right eye, and the nurse instructs the mother regarding this procedure. Which of the following will the nurse include in the instructions?
    1. Place the patch on the right eye.
    2. Place the patch on both eyes.
    3. Place the patch on the left eye.
    4. Alternate the patch from the right to the left eye hourly.

115. A nonstress test is performed on a client who is pregnant, and the results of the test indicate nonreactive findings. The physician prescribed a contraction stress test. The test is performed, and the nurse notes that the physician has documented the results as negative. The nurse interprets this finding as indicating
    1. A high risk for fetal demise.
    2. A normal test result.
    3. The need for a cesarean delivery.
    4. An abnormal test result.

116. The nurse has developed a plan of care for a client who is in traction and documents a nursing diagnosis of Self-Care Deficit. The nurse evaluates the plan of care and determines that which of the following observations indicates a successful outcome?
    1. The client allows the nurse to complete the care daily.
    2. The client allows the family to assist in the care.
    3. The client refuses care.
    4. The client assists in self-care as much as possible.

117. The home care nurse is visiting a client who is in a body cast. The nurse is performing an assessment and is assessing the psychosocial adjustment of the client to the cast. The nurse most appropriately would assess
    1. The type of transportation available for follow-up care.
    2. The ability to perform activities of daily living.
    3. The need for sensory stimulation.
    4. The amount of home care support available.

118. The maternity nurse is providing an in-service educational session to nursing students regarding the process of conception. The nurse instructs the nursing students that fertilization of a mature ovum occurs in which of the following areas?
    1. Uterus
    2. Ovary
    3. Distal third of the fallopian tube
    4. Wall of the myometrium

119. The nurse is preparing to teach a client how to use crutches safely. Before initiating the teaching, the nurse performs an assessment on the client. The priority nursing assessment should include which of the following?
    1. The client's fear related to the use of the crutches
    2. The client's understanding of the need for increased mobility
    3. The client's vital signs, muscle strength, and previous activity level of the client
    4. The client's feelings about the restricted mobility

120. The nurse is assessing for Kernig's sign in a child with a suspected diagnosis of meningitis. The nurse performs this test by
    1. Bending the head towards the knees and hips and assessing for pain.
    2. Tapping the facial nerve and assessing for spasm.
    3. Compressing the upper arm and assessing for tetany.
    4. Raising the leg with the knee flexed and then extending the leg at the knee and assessing for pain.

121. The physician has written an order to start progressive ambulation as tolerated on a hospitalized client who experiences periods of confusion because of bedrest and prolonged confinement to the hospital room. Which nursing intervention would be most appropriate when planning to implement the physician's order and in addressing the needs of the client?
    1. Help the client to ambulate in the room for short distances frequently.
    2. Help the client to ambulate to the bathroom in the client's room 3 times a day
    3. Progressively increase ambulation in the hall 3 times a day.
    4. Assist with range of motion exercises 3 times a day to increase strength.

122. A client is seen in the health care clinic, and a vitamin K deficiency is suspected. On assessment of the client the nurse would expect to note which of the following if this vitamin deficiency were present?
    1. Client complaints of night blindness
    2. Signs of clotting problems
    3. Scaly skin
    4. Client complaints of skeletal pain

123. The nurse is caring for a postterm, small-for-gestational-age newborn infant immediately after admission to the nursery. The priority nursing action would be to monitor
    1. Urinary output.
    2. Total bilirubin levels.
    3. Blood glucose levels.
    4. Hemoglobin and hematocrit levels.

124. The nurse is performing an initial assessment on a large-for-gestational-age newborn infant. Which physical assessment technique would the nurse perform to assess for the evidence of birth trauma?
    1. Palpate the clavicles for a fracture.
    2. Auscultate the heart for a cardiac defect.
    3. Blanch the skin for evidence of jaundice.
    4. Perform the Ortolani maneuver for hip dislocation.

125. Somatropin (Humatrope), a growth hormone, is prescribed for a client. The nurse reviews the assessment data in the client's health record, knowing that the medication is contraindicated in which of the following conditions?
    1. A child with growth hormone deficiency
    2. A child with pituitary dwarfism
    3. A 20-year-old with growth failure
    4. A child with growth failure

126. The nurse is caring for a client who is receiving growth hormone replacement therapy. The nurse monitors the client for which side effect of this therapy?
    1. Hyperglycemia
    2. Hyperthyroidism
    3. Hypoglycemia
    4. Hypocalciuria

127. The nurse is assessing a client with a diagnosis of goiter. Which of the following would the nurse expect to note during the assessment of the client?
    1. Client complaints of slow wound healing
    2. Client complaints of chronic fatigue
    3. An enlarged thyroid gland
    4. The presence of heart damage

128. A fasting blood glucose screening is performed on a pregnant client. The results indicate that the blood glucose is 140 mg/dL. Which of the following would the nurse anticipate to be prescribed for the mother?
    1. Administration of an oral hypoglycemic agent
    2. Administration of NPH insulin daily

    3. A 3-hour glucose tolerance test
    4. A sliding scale regular insulin dose

129. The pregnant client seen in the health care clinic has tested positive for human immunodeficiency virus. Based on this information, the nurse determines that
    1. The client has the herpes simplex virus.
    2. Human immunodeficiency virus antibodies are detected on the enzyme-linked immunosorbent assay.
    3. The neonate definitely will develop this disease after birth.
    4. This client has contacted an airborne disease.

130. During a wellness fair, an adult client admits to a nurse of not eating a well-balanced diet. According to the Food Guide Pyramid, which of the following instructions would the nurse provide to the client?
    1. "Your diet should consist of six to eleven servings of bread, cereal, pasta, or rice a day."
    2. "Your diet should consist of two to four servings of vegetables a day."
    3. "Your diet should consist of four to five servings of milk, yogurt or cheese a day."
    4. "Your diet should consist of four to six servings of meat, poultry, fish, dry beans, or nuts a day."

131. An 85-year-old client is hospitalized for a right fractured hip. During the postoperative period, the client's appetite is poor and the client refuses to get out of bed. Which nursing statement would be most appropriate to make to the client?
    1. "It is important for you to get out of bed so that calcium will go back into the bone."
    2. "We need to increase your calcium intake because you are spending too much time in bed."
    3. "We need to give you iodine so that it will help in hemoglobin synthesis."
    4. "You need to remember to turn yourself in bed every two hours to keep from getting so stiff."

132. Lindane (Kwell) is prescribed for the treatment of scabies. The nurse reviews the client's record, knowing the medication therapy is contraindicated if the client is
    1. A 42-year-old woman.
    2. An older client.
    3. A 6-year-old child.
    4. A 52-year-old man with hypertension.

133. DuoDerm is prescribed for a client with a leg ulcer. The home health nurse is preparing a plan of care for the client and most appropriately documents to
    1. Change the DuoDerm daily.
    2. Apply the DuoDerm over a dry sterile dressing.
    3. Change the DuoDerm weekly.
    4. Apply the DuoDerm over a normal saline-soaked dressing.

134. A nurse develops a plan of care for a client being admitted to the hospital with a diagnosis of cerebral aneurysm who will be placed on aneurysm precautions. The nurse includes which intervention in the plan?
    1. Provide the client with a low-fiber diet.
    2. Keep the room lights on to ensure client orientation to the environment.
    3. Place the client in a semiprivate room to provide stimulation.
    4. Restrict visitors to close family or significant others and keep visits short.

135. Glyburide (DiaBeta) 2.5 mg orally daily is prescribed for a client. The nurse tells the client
    1. To take the medication in the morning before breakfast.
    2. To expect his skin color to change from pink to yellow and to expect pale-colored stools.
    3. That the medication is used to prevent foot infections.
    4. That if an altered taste sensation occurs, to contact the physician immediately.

136. A nurse employed on a medical unit in a hospital receives a telephone call from the admission office and is told that a client with a diagnosis of mycoplasmal pneumonia will be admitted to the nursing unit. The nurse prepares for the admission and obtains the necessary supplies to place the client on which type of transmission-based precautions?
    Answer: _____

137. A nurse manager is providing an educational session to nursing staff members about the phases of viral hepatitis. The nurse manager tells the staff that which clinical manifestation(s) are primarily characteristic of the preicteric phase?
    1. Right upper quadrant pain
    2. Fatigue, anorexia, and nausea
    3. Jaundice, dark-colored urine, and clay-colored stools
    4. Pruritis

138. The registered nurse is planning assignments for the clients on a nursing unit. The registered nurse needs to assign four clients and has a registered nurse, a licensed practical (vocational) nurse, and two nursing assistants on a nursing team. Which of the following clients would the nurse most appropriately assign the licensed practical (vocational) nurse?
    1. The client who requires a 24-hour urine collection
    2. An older client requiring assistance with a bed bath and frequent ambulation
    3. A client on a mechanical ventilator requiring frequent assessment and suctioning
    4. A client with an abdominal wound requiring wound irrigations and dressing changes every 3 hours

139. A nursing instructor asks the nursing student to describe the definition of a critical path. Which of the following statements, if made by the student, indicates a need for further understanding regarding critical paths?
    1. "They are developed through the collaborative efforts of all members of the health care team."
    2. "They provide an effective way to monitor care and for reducing or controlling the length of hospital stay for the client."
    3. "They are developed based on appropriate standards of care."
    4. "They are nursing care plans and use the steps of the nursing process."

140. The nurse is caring for an 18-month-old child who has been vomiting. The most appropriate position for the child during naps and sleep time is
    1. Side-lying position.
    2. Prone with the face turned to the side.
    3. Supine.
    4. Prone with the head elevated.

141. The parents of a child with a cleft lip are concerned and ask the nurse when the lip will be repaired. The nurse supportively tells the parents that
    1. Cleft lip repair usually is performed between 6 months and 2 years of age.
    2. Cleft lip repair usually is performed by 6 months of age.
    3. Cleft lip repair usually is performed during the first weeks of life.
    4. Cleft lip cannot be repaired.

142. The nurse is assessing the client for signs of postpartum depression. Which of the following, if noted in the new mother, would indicate the need for further assessment related to this form of depression?
    1. The mother is caring for the infant in a loving manner.
    2. The mother constantly complains of tiredness and fatigue.
    3. The mother demonstrates an interest in the surroundings.
    4. The mother looks forward to visits from the father of the newborn.

143. A postpartum client is attempting to breast-feed for the first time. The nurse notes that the client has inverted nipples. What nursing action can the nurse take to assist the client in breast-feeding the newborn infant?
    1. Provide breast shells and assist the mother with using a breast pump before each feeding to make the nipples easier for the newborn infant to grasp.
    2. Have the mother grasp the nipples between the thumb and forefinger and tug firmly to get the nipple to protrude.

3. Massage the breast, applying gentle pressure on the areola.

4. Take a cool shower, allowing the water to run over the breasts because this will encourage the nipples to protrude.

144. The nurse instructs the client in breast self-examination. The nurse tells the client to lie down and to examine the left breast. The nurse instructs the client that while examining the left breast to place a pillow
1. Under the right shoulder.
2. Under the left shoulder.
3. Under the small of the back.
4. Under the right scapula.

145. The nurse is teaching breast self-examination to a client who had a hysterectomy. The most appropriate instruction regarding when the breast self-examination should be performed is
1. 7 to 10 days after menses.
2. Just before menses begins.
3. At ovulation time.
4. At a specific day of the month and on that same day every month thereafter.

146. The nursing instructor asks the nursing student to describe Montgomery's tubercles of the breast. The student indicates an understanding of this anatomical structure if the student states that the Montgomery's tubercles are
1. Sebaceous glands that are located in the areola.
2. Lobes of glandular tissue that secrete milk.
3. Small sacs that contain acinar cells to secrete milk.
4. Ducts containing milk from all areas of the breast.

147. The 32-year-old female client has a history of fibrocystic disorder of the breasts. The nurse interviewing the client asks whether the breast lumps are more noticeable
1. In the spring months.
2. In the autumn.
3. After menses.
4. Before menses.

148. A 1-year-old child is diagnosed with intussusception, and the mother of the child asks the nurse to describe the disorder. The nurse tells the mother that this disorder is
1. An acute bowel obstruction.
2. A condition when a proximal segment of the bowel prolapses into a distal segment of the bowel.
3. A condition when a distal segment of the bowel prolapses into a proximal segment of the bowel.
4. A condition that causes an acute inflammatory process in the bowel.

149. A 3-year-old child is seen in the health care clinic, and a diagnosis of encopresis is made. The nurse reviews the assessment findings expecting to note documentation of which sign of this disorder?
1. Nausea and vomiting
2. Diarrhea
3. Evidence of soiled clothing
4. Malaise and anorexia

150. The nurse is teaching the client who had laryngectomy for laryngeal cancer how to use an artificial larynx. The nurse tells the client to
1. Insert the device into the tracheostomy.
2. Hold the device alongside the neck.
3. Hold the device over the upper portion of the sternum.
4. Swallow air into the esophagus to make speech.

151. A client is scheduled for a Papanicolaou's smear at the next scheduled clinic visit. The nurse provides instructions to the client regarding preparation for this test. The nurse tells the client that
1. The test can be performed during menstruation.
2. Fluids are restricted on the day of the test.
3. The test is painless.
4. Vaginal douching is required 2 hours before the test.

152. A nurse witnesses an accident on a highway and stops to provide assistance to the victim. The nurse notes that the client sustained a head injury and a compound fracture to the left leg. The nurse provides the appropriate care before transport of the victim to the hospital by ambulance. The client develops a severe bone infection at the site of the fracture that requires amputation of the leg and files suit against the nurse who provided care at the scene of the accident. Which of the following is accurate regarding the nurse's immunity from this suit?
1. The Good Samaritan law will protect the nurse.
2. The Good Samaritan law will not protect the nurse.
3. The Good Samaritan law will provide immunity from suit even if the nurse accepted compensation for the care provided.
4. The Good Samaritan law protects laypersons and not professional health care providers.

153. A client is seen in the clinic for complaints of thirst, frequent urination, and headaches. Following diagnostic studies, diabetes insipidus in diagnosed. Lypressin (Diapid) is prescribed. The nurse instructs the client that the medication is prescribed to
1. Relieve the headaches.
2. Increase water reabsorption.
3. Decrease the production of the antidiuretic hormone.
4. Stimulate the production of aldosterone.

154. Somatrem (Protropin) is prescribed for the client with pituitary dwarfism. The nurse explains to the

client that the expected outcome of the medication is

1. Growth that begins in 4 to 5 years.
2. An increase in height that will begin in late adulthood.
3. An immediate increase in growth.
4. Growth spurts that occur every 2 years.

155. The nurse manager attends a conference, and the topic of discussion is leadership styles. The nurse is seeking a leadership style that will best empower staff toward excellence. Which leadership style would the nurse select to achieve this goal?
    1. Autocratic
    2. Situational
    3. Democratic
    4. Laissez-faire

156. A community health nurse is working with disaster relief following a tornado. The nurse's goal with the overall community is to prevent as much injury and death as possible from the uncontrollable event. Finding safe housing for survivors, providing support to families, organizing counseling, and securing physical care when needed are examples of which type of prevention?
    1. The primary level of prevention
    2. The secondary level of prevention
    3. The tertiary level of prevention
    4. Aggregate care prevention

157. The nursing instructor asks the nursing student about the physiology related to the cessation of ovulation that occurs during pregnancy. Which of the following responses, if made by the student, indicates an understanding of this physiological process?
    1. "Ovulation ceases during pregnancy because the circulating levels of estrogen and progesterone are high."
    2. "Ovulation ceases during pregnancy because the circulating levels of estrogen and progesterone are low."
    3. "The low levels of estrogen and progesterone increase the release of the follicle-stimulating hormone and the luteinizing hormone."
    4. "The high levels of estrogen and progesterone promote the release of the follicle-stimulating hormone and luteinizing hormone."

158. The nurse is developing a plan of care for an adolescent who is hospitalized and is placed in skeletal traction. The nurse incorporates interventions in the plan of care that address the psychosocial development of the adolescent. What is the chief developmental task of the adolescent according to Erik Erikson?
    Answer: _____

159. Etidronate (Didronel), an antihypercalcemic medication, is prescribed for the client. The nurse instructs the client to take the medication

1. 2 hours before meals.
2. With meals.
3. With milk.
4. With an antacid.

160. The client was hospitalized for a cervical radiation implant. The implant is removed, and the nurse provides home care instructions to the client. Which statement made by the client indicates a need for further instructions?
    1. "Cream may be used to relieve dryness or itching."
    2. "Foul-smelling vaginal discharge is a sign of an infection."
    3. "Sexual intercourse may be resumed after seven to ten days."
    4. "Some vaginal bleeding is expected for one to three months."

161. The nurse teaches skin care to the client receiving external radiation therapy. Which of the following statements, if made by the client, would indicate the need for further instruction?
    1. "I will handle the area gently"
    2. "I will avoid the use of deodorants"
    3. "I will limit sun exposure to one hour daily"
    4. "I will wear loose fitting clothing"

162. The nurse manager is planning to implement a change in the nursing unit from team nursing to primary nursing. The nurse anticipates resistance to the change during the change process. The primary technique that the nurse would use in implementing this change is which of the following?
    1. Introduce the change gradually.
    2. Confront the individuals involved in the change process.
    3. Use coercion to implement the change.
    4. Manipulate the participants in the change process.

163. Insulin lispro (Humalog), a rapid-acting form of insulin, is prescribed for the client. The client is instructed to administer the insulin before meals. The nurse instructs the client to administer the insulin
    1. Immediately before eating.
    2. 30 minutes before eating.
    3. 45 minutes before eating.
    4. 60 minutes before eating.

164. The emergency room nurse is caring for a client admitted with diabetic ketoacidosis. The physician prescribes intravenous insulin. The nurse plans to prepare which type of insulin for the client?
    1. NPH
    2. Regular
    3. Lente
    4. Ultralente

165. A physician's order reads "levothyroxine (Synthroid), 150 mcg PO daily." The medication

label reads "Synthroid, 0.1 mg per tablet." A nurse administers how many tablet(s) to the client?

Answer: _____

166. Metformin (Glucophage) is prescribed for the client with type 2 diabetes mellitus. The nurse tells the client that the most common side effect of the medication is
    1. Hypoglycemia.
    2. Gastrointestinal disturbances.
    3. Weight gain.
    4. Flushing and palpitations.

167. The nurse encourages the pregnant client who is human immunodeficiency virus positive to report any signs of vaginal discharge or perineal tenderness to the health care provider immediately. The client asks the nurse about the importance of this action and the nurse responds by telling the client that this is necessary to
    1. Relieve anxiety for the pregnant client.
    2. Eliminate the need for further unnecessary screenings.
    3. Assist in identifying potential infections that may need to be treated.
    4. Minimize the financial cost of caring for an human immunodeficiency virus–positive client.

168. The pregnant client who is anemic tells the nurse that she is concerned about her baby's condition following delivery. Which nursing response would best support the client?
    1. "You will not have any problems if you follow all the advice the doctor has given you."
    2. "Your baby will need to spend a few days in the neonatal intensive care unit following delivery."
    3. "Don't worry about your baby; complications are rare."
    4. "The effects of anemia on your baby are difficult to predict, but let's review your plan of care to assure you are providing the best nutrition and growth potential."

169. The diabetic nurse specialist conducts a teaching session to a group of nursing students regarding sulfonylureas, oral hypoglycemic medications used for type 2 diabetes mellitus. The nurse specialist tells the students that the primary action of these medications is to
    1. Decrease glucose production by the liver.
    2. Inhibit carbohydrate digestion.
    3. Promote insulin secretion by the pancreas.
    4. Decrease insulin resistance.

170. The client with diabetes mellitus calls the clinic and tells the nurse that he has been nauseated during the night. The client asks the nurse if the morning insulin dose should be administered. Which of the following is the most appropriate nursing response?
    1. Omit the insulin.
    2. Administer half of the prescribed dose.

    3. Administer the full dose as prescribed.
    4. Wait until noon before making a decision.

171. The client with Cushing's syndrome verbalizes concern to the nurse regarding the appearance of the buffalo hump that has developed. Which statement by the nurse is most appropriate?
    1. "This is permanent, but looks are deceiving and not that important."
    2. "Don't be concerned; this problem can be covered with clothing."
    3. "Try not to worry about it; there are other things to be concerned about."
    4. "Usually these physical changes slowly improve following treatment."

172. The nurse is caring for a client following thyroidectomy. The nurse notes that calcium gluconate is prescribed for the client. The nurse determines that this medication has been prescribed to
    1. Treat thyroid storm.
    2. Prevent cardiac irritability.
    3. Stimulate release of parathyroid hormone.
    4. Treat hypocalcemic tetany.

173. Select all interventions that apply to the care of a child who is having a seizure.
    ___ Insert an oral airway.
    ___ Place the child in a supine position.
    ___ Loosen clothing around the child's neck.
    ___ Restrain the child.
    ___ Time the seizure.
    ___ Stay with the child.
    ___ Move furniture or other items away from the child.

174. The client with type 1 diabetes mellitus is to begin an exercise program, and the nurse is providing instructions to the client regarding the program. Which of the following does the nurse include in the teaching plan?
    1. Exercise is best performed during peak times of insulin.
    2. Administer insulin after exercising.
    3. Take a blood glucose test before exercising.
    4. Try to exercise before mealtime.

175. The nursery room nurse is assessing a newborn infant who was born to a mother who abuses alcohol. Which of the following assessment findings would the nurse expect to note?
    1. Lethargy
    2. Higher than normal birth weight
    3. Irritability
    4. A greater than normal appetite when feeding

176. The postpartum nurse teaches a mother how to provide a bath to the newborn infant and observes the mother performing the procedure. Which of the following indicates a need to provide additional instructions?
    1. The mother plans to bathe the newborn infant after a feeding.

2. The mother fills a clean basin or sink with 2 to 3 inches of water and the checks the temperature using the wrist.

3. The mother states to never leave the newborn infant in the tub of water alone.

4. The mother states to gather all supplies before starting the bath.

177. A 13-year-old child is diagnosed with an Ewing's sarcoma of the femur. Following a course of radiation and chemotherapy, it has been decided that leg amputation is necessary. Following the amputation, the child becomes frightened because of aching and cramping felt in the missing limb. Which nursing statement would be most appropriate to assist in alleviating the child's fear?

1. "This aching and cramping is normal and temporary and will subside."

2. "This normally occurs after the surgery, and we will teach you ways to deal with it."

3. "The pain medication that I give you will take these feelings away."

4. "This pain is not real pain, and relaxation exercises will help it go away."

178. Oral iron supplements are prescribed for the 6-year-old child with iron deficiency anemia. The nurse instructs the mother to administer the iron with which of the following food items?

1. Water

2. Milk

3. Apple juice

4. Tomato juice

179. A client with diabetes mellitus is being discharged following treatment for hyperglycemic hyperosmolar nonketotic syndrome precipitated by acute illness. The client tells the nurse, "I will call the doctor next time I can't eat for more than a day or so." Which of the following statements reflects the most appropriate analysis of this client's level of knowledge?

1. The client needs immediate education before discharge.

2. The client's statement is accurate, but knowledge should be evaluated further.

3. The client's statement is inaccurate, and the client should be scheduled for outpatient diabetic counseling.

4. The client requires follow-up teaching regarding the administration of insulin.

180. The client with type 1 diabetes mellitus is having trouble remembering the types, duration, and onset of the action of insulin. The client tells the nurse that the family members have not been supportive. The nurse's best response to the client is

1. "You can't always depend on your family to help."

2. "Let me go over the types of insulin with you again."

3. "It's not really necessary for you to remember this."

4. "What is it that you don't understand?"

181. A nursing student is asked to describe the size of the uterus in a nonpregnant client. The student responds correctly by stating that the uterus in a nonpregnant client

1. Weighs about 2 oz.

2. Weighs about 2.2 lb.

3. Has a capacity of about 50 mL.

4. Is round and weighs about 1000 g.

182. Fludrocortisone (Florinef) is prescribed for the client with Addison's disease. The nurse prepares to administer the medication knowing that the primary action of this medication is to

1. Enhance the reabsorption of sodium and chloride ions in the distal tubules of the kidney.

2. Promote the retention of potassium in the distal tubules of the kidney.

3. Promote the retention of hydrogen ions in the distal tubules of the kidney.

4. Promote the excretion of water in the distal tubules of the kidney.

183. The nurse is performing an assessment on a pregnant client at 16 weeks of gestation. On assessment, the nurse would expect that the fundus of the uterus would be located at which of the following areas?

1. Midway between the symphysis pubis and the umbilicus

2. At the umbilicus

3. Just above the symphysis pubis

4. At the level of the xiphoid process

184. The nursing instructor asks the nursing student to identify the priorities of care for an assigned client. The student correctly identifies the client needs that are the priority by telling the nursing instructor that

1. Actual or life-threatening concerns are the priority.

2. Time constraints related to the client's needs are the priority.

3. Obtaining needed supplies to care for the client is the priority.

4. Completing care in a reasonable time frame is the priority.

185. The nurse is employed in a prenatal clinic and is performing prenatal assessments on clients who are in their first trimester of pregnancy. The nurse is concerned with identifying clients who may be at risk for the development of postpartum complications. Which of the following clients would be least likely at risk for the development of thromboembolitic disorders in the postpartum period?

1. A 39-year-old woman who reports that she smokes.

2. A 37-year-old woman in her fourth pregnancy who is overweight.

3. A 26-year-old woman with a family history of thrombophlebitis.

4. A woman who is 22 years old with a first pregnancy and who states that oral contraceptives taken in the past have caused thrombophlebitis.

186. A client arrives at the clinic complaining of fatigue, a lack of energy, constipation, and depression. Following diagnostic studies, hypothyroidism is diagnosed and levothyroxine (Synthroid) is prescribed. The nurse instructs the client that the expected outcome of the medication is to
   1. Increase energy levels.
   2. Achieve normal thyroid hormone levels.
   3. Increase blood glucose levels.
   4. Alleviate depression.

187. A client diagnosed with hypothyroidism is taking levothyroxine (Synthroid). The client returns to the clinic 1 week after beginning the medication and tells the nurse that the medication has not helped. The most appropriate nursing response to the client is based on which of the following?
   1. A higher dosage is required.
   2. The medication may need to be changed.
   3. Full therapeutic effect may take 1 to 3 weeks.
   4. Full therapeutic effect may take up to 4 months.

188. The nurse has provided instructions for the postpartum mother at risk for thrombosis regarding measures to prevent the occurrence. Which of the following statements if made by the mother indicates a need for further education?
   1. "I should perform regularly scheduled exercise such as walking."
   2. "I should avoid prolonged standing or sitting in one position."
   3. "I should avoid using pillows under my knees to prevent pressure in the back of my knee area."
   4. "I should apply my antiembolism stockings after my shower in the morning."

189. The nurse is preparing to administer an intravenous insulin injection. The vial of regular insulin has been refrigerated. On inspection of the vial, the nurse finds the medication frozen. The nurse should
   1. Wait for the insulin to thaw at room temperature.
   2. Check the temperature settings of the refrigerator.
   3. Discard the insulin and obtain another vial.
   4. Rotate the vial between the hands until the medications becomes liquid.

190. In the prenatal clinic the nurse is interviewing a new client and obtaining health history information. The nurse plans to do which of the following to elicit accurate responses to the area of questions that refer to sexually transmitted diseases?
   1. Establish a therapeutic relationship.

2. Use specific close-ended questions.

3. Omit this area of questions because it is highly personal.

4. Apologize for the embarrassment that these questions will cause the client.

191. The clinic nurse is teaching a pregnant client about the warning signs in pregnancy. Which of the following, if identified as a warning sign by the client, would indicate a need for further education?
   1. Visual disturbances
   2. Rapid weight gain
   3. Generalized or facial edema
   4. The presence of irregular, painless contractions

192. The nurse is preparing to discharge a client who has had a parathyroidectomy. The discharge instructions include medication administration of oral calcium supplements that the client will need daily. Which statement by the nurse would be appropriate regarding the oral calcium supplement therapy?
   1. Store the tablets in the refrigerator to maintain potency.
   2. Check the pulse daily, and if it is fewer than 60 beats per minute, do not take the tablets.
   3. Take the tablets following a meal.
   4. Avoid sunlight because the medication can cause skin color change.

193. The nurse is providing instructions to a client with hypophosphatemia. The nurse instructs the client to avoid
   1. Fish.
   2. Chicken.
   3. Organ meats.
   4. Cheese.

194. A nurse is assessing the learning readiness of a client newly diagnosed with diabetes mellitus. Which client behavior indicates to the nurse that the client is not ready to learn?
   1. The client complains of fatigue whenever the nurse plans a teaching session.
   2. The client asks if the spouse can attend the teaching session.
   3. The client asks for written materials about diabetes mellitus before class.
   4. The client asks appropriate questions about what will be taught.

195. A young male client with type 1 diabetes mellitus tells the nurse that he might lose his job because he has been having frequent hypoglycemic reactions. His boss thinks that he is drunk during these episodes and that he has been drinking on the job. Which action by the nurse would best assist this client to meet his needs?
   1. Contact the local employment office to help him find another job.
   2. Ask the client if he indeed has been drinking at work.

3. Examine factors with the client that may be causing frequent hypoglycemic episodes.

4. Ask the client what he does to treat his hypoglycemia.

196. The nurse in the newborn nursery is assessing a neonate who was born of a mother addicted to cocaine. Which of the following would the nurse expect to note in the neonate?
    1. Tremors
    2. Bradycardia
    3. Flaccid muscles
    4. Extreme lethargy

197. Thyroid replacement therapy is prescribed for the client diagnosed with hypothyroidism. The client asks the nurse when the medication will no longer be needed. The most appropriate nursing response is which of the following?
    1. "You will need to ask your physician."
    2. "Most clients require medication therapy for about 1 year."
    3. "It depends on the results of the laboratory values."
    4. "The medication will need to be continued for life."

198. A community health nurse is preparing a poster for an educational session for a group of women and will be discussing the risk factors associated with breast cancer. Select the risk factors for breast cancer that the nurse will list on the poster.
    ___ Family history of breast cancer
    ___ Age greater than 40 years
    ___ Early menarche
    ___ Early menopause
    ___ Previous cancer of the breast, uterus, or ovaries
    ___ Multiparity
    ___ First child born before the age of 30 years
    ___ High-dose radiation exposure to chest

199. The nurse is performing a physical assessment on a client during her first prenatal visit to the clinic. The nurse takes the client's temperature and notes that the temperature is 99.2° F. Based on this finding, which nursing action is most appropriate?
    1. Document the temperature.
    2. Retake the temperature by the rectal route.
    3. Notify the physician.
    4. Inform the client that the temperature is elevated and antibiotics may be required.

200. The physician orders a 24-hour urine collection for vanillylmandelic acid. The community health nurse visits the client at home and instructs the client in the procedure for the collection of the urine. Which statement if made by the client would indicate a need for further instruction?
    1. "I will start the collection in two days. Starting now, I cannot eat or drink any tea, chocolate, vanilla, or fruit until the test is completed."

2. "When I start the collection, I will urinate and discard that specimen."

3. "I will pour the urine in the collection bottle each time I urinate and refrigerate the urine."

4. "I can take medication if I need to during the collection."

201. The client with pheochromocytoma is scheduled for surgery and says to the nurse, "I'm not sure that surgery is the best thing to do?" The most appropriate response by the nurse is which of the following?
    1. "You have concerns about the surgical treatment for your condition?"
    2. "There is no reason to worry. Your doctor is a wonderful surgeon."
    3. "You are very ill. Your physician has made the correct decision."
    4. "I think you are making the right decision to have the surgery."

202. The nurse has inserted a nasogastric tube to the level of the oropharynx and has repositioned the client's head in a flexed-forward position. The client has been asked to begin swallowing. The nurse starts slowly to advance the nasogastric tube with each swallow. The client begins to cough, gag, and choke. Which nursing action would least likely result in proper tube insertion and promote client relaxation?
    1. Continuing to advance the tube to the desired distance
    2. Pulling the tube back slightly
    3. Checking the back of the pharynx using a tongue blade and flashlight
    4. Instructing the client to breathe slowly and take sips of water

203. The maternity nurse is describing the ovarian cycle to a group of nursing students. The instructor asks a nursing student to identify the phases of the cycle. Which of the following, if identified as a phase of the cycle by the nursing student, indicates a need to further research this area?
    1. Follicular phase
    2. Ovulatory phase
    3. Luteal phase
    4. Proliferative phase

204. A client is seen in the health care clinic and is diagnosed with mild anemia. The anemia is believed to result from the menstrual period. The woman asks the nurse how much blood is lost during a menstrual period. The nurse plans to base the response on which of the following amounts of blood lost during this time?
    1. 40 mL
    2. 60 mL
    3. 80 mL
    4. 100 mL

205. The nurse is caring for a client with acute pancreatitis and is monitoring the client for paralytic

ileus. Which assessment data would alert the nurse to this occurrence?

1. Firm, nontender mass palpable at the lower right costal margin
2. Severe, constant pain with rapid onset
3. Inability to pass flatus
4. Loss of anal sphincter control

206. The nurse inspects the color of the drainage from a nasogastric tube on a postoperative client about 24 hours following a laparotomy. Which of the following findings would indicate the need to notify the physician?

1. Light yellowish brown drainage
2. Dark red drainage
3. Dark brown drainage
4. Green-tinged drainage

207. The nurse is preparing to discontinue a client's nasogastric tube. The client is positioned properly, and the tube has been flushed with 15 mL of air to clear secretions. Before removing the tube, the nurse makes which statement to the client?

1. "Take a deep breath when I tell you and breathe normally while I remove the tube."
2. "Take a deep breath when I tell you and bear down while I remove the tube."
3. "Take a deep breath when I tell you and slowly exhale while I remove the tube."
4. "Take a deep breath when I tell you and hold it while I remove the tube."

208. The nurse is caring for a client with a nasogastric tube connected to continuous suction. During the assessment, the nurse observes that the client is mouth breathing, has dry mucous membranes, and has a foul breath odor. In planning care, which of the following would be most appropriate to maintain the integrity of this client's oral mucosa?

1. Offer small sips of water frequently.
2. Encourage sucking on sour, hard candy.
3. Brush teeth frequently; use mouthwash and water.
4. Use lemon-glycerin swabs to provide oral hygiene.

209. A client with a small-bowel obstruction asks the nurse to explain the purpose of the nasogastric tube and continuous gastric suction. After the teaching is completed, the nurse determines that the client understands if the client states that the purpose of the continuous gastric suction is to

1. Provide nourishment.
2. Relieve the bronchi of mucus.
3. Withdraw gastric contents for laboratory analysis.
4. Remove gas and fluids from the stomach and intestine.

210. The client with a history of lung disease is at risk for developing respiratory acidosis. The nurse assesses this client for which signs and symptoms characteristic of this disorder?

1. Bradycardia and hyperactivity
2. Decreased respiratory rate and depth
3. Headache, restlessness, and confusion
4. Bradypnea, dizziness, and paresthesias

211. The nurse is caring for a client with a resolved intestinal obstruction who has a nasogastric tube in place. The client has tolerated the tube being clamped every 2 hours for 1 hour. The physician has now ordered the nasogastric tube to be removed. Before removing the tube, the nurse assesses for

1. Proper nasogastric tube placement.
2. Normal serum electrolyte levels.
3. The presence of bowel sounds in all four quadrants.
4. Normal pH of the gastric aspirate.

212. The nurse has administered about half of the enema solution when the client complains of pain and cramping. Which nursing action is the most appropriate?

1. Raise the enema bag so that the solution can be completed quickly.
2. Clamp the tubing for 30 seconds and restart the flow at a slower rate.
3. Reassure the client and continue the flow.
4. Discontinue the enema and notify the physician.

213. The nurse is preparing to administer an enema. The nurse positions the client in the

1. Left lateral position with the right leg acutely flexed.
2. Right Sims' position.
3. Dorsal recumbent position.
4. Right lateral position with the left leg acutely flexed.

214. The nurse aspirates 40 mL of undigested formula from the client's nasogastric tube. Before administering an intermittent tube feeding, the nurse understands that the 40 mL of gastric aspirate should be

1. Discarded properly and recorded as output on the client's intake and output record.
2. Poured into the nasogastric tube through a syringe with the plunger removed.
3. Mixed with the formula and poured into the nasogastric tube through a syringe with the plunger removed.
4. Diluted with water and injected into the nasogastric tube by putting pressure on the plunger.

215. The client experiencing a great deal of stress and anxiety is being taught to use self-control therapy. Which statement by the client indicates a need for further teaching about the therapy?

1. "An advantage of this technique is that I can use it anywhere."
2. "This form of therapy can be applied to new situations."

3. "Talking to oneself is a basic component to this form of therapy."

4. "This therapy provides a negative reinforcement when the stimulus is produced."

216. A nurse is preparing a list of home care instructions regarding stoma and laryngectomy care to a client who had a laryngectomy. Select all instructions that would be included in the list.
   ____ Avoid wearing high-collar clothing.
   ____ Avoid swimming and use care when showering.
   ____ Keep the humidity in the home low.
   ____ Avoid exposure to persons with infections.
   ____ Restrict fluid intake.
   ____ Obtain a Medic-Alert bracelet.
   ____ Prevent debris from entering the stoma.

217. A nurse obtains the vital signs on an older client and notes that the client's heart rate is 60 beats per minute and the respiratory rate is 24 breaths per minute. The nurse most appropriately would
   1. Recheck the heart rate and respiratory rate in 30 minutes.
   2. Contact the physician to report the heart rate and respiratory rate.
   3. Document the findings.
   4. Check the client for signs of infection.

218. An infant returns to the nursing unit following surgery for a diagnosis of esophageal atresia with tracheoesophageal fistula. The infant is receiving fluids intravenously, and a gastrostomy tube is in place. Following assessment, the nurse positions the infant and
   1. Connects the gastrostomy to the feeding pump.
   2. Attaches the gastrostomy tube to low suction.
   3. Tapes the gastrostomy tube to the bed linens.
   4. Elevates the gastrostomy tube.

219. A depressed client is found unconscious on the floor in the day room. The nurse finds several empty bottles of a prescribed tricyclic antidepressant lying near the client. The immediate action of the nurse is to
   1. Call the resuscitation team because this incident presents a medical emergency.
   2. Induce vomiting and notify the physician for further orders.
   3. Ask the secretary to call the physician.
   4. Try to figure out the number of pills taken.

220. The client is scheduled for an upper gastrointestinal endoscopy. Which assessment is essential to include in the plan of care following the procedure?
   1. Monitoring for rectal bleeding
   2. Assessing pulses
   3. Monitoring urine output
   4. Assessing for the presence of the gag reflex

221. The nurse is preparing to insert a nasogastric tube into a client. What nursing measure will best facilitate easy insertion of the tube?

1. Placing the nasogastric tube in warm water
2. Removing the tube if any resistance to insertion is met
3. Asking the client to swallow as the tube is being advanced
4. Hyperextending the head to insert the tube

222. A physician orders 2000 mL of 5% dextrose and ½ normal saline to infuse over 24 hours. The drop factor is 15 drops per 1 mL. A nurse sets the flow rate at how many drops per minute?
   Answer: _____

223. The client is returned to the nursing unit following thoracic surgery with chest tubes in place. During the first few hours postoperatively, the nurse assesses for drainage and expects to note that it is
   1. Serous.
   2. Serosanguinous.
   3. Bloody.
   4. Bloody with frequent small clots.

224. The client has had radical neck dissection and begins to hemorrhage at the incision site. Which action by the nurse would be contraindicated?
   1. Lowering the head of the bed to a flat position.
   2. Applying manual pressure over the site.
   3. Monitoring the client's airway.
   4. Calling the physician immediately.

225. The nurse has an order to begin administering foscarnet (Foscavir) to the client with cytomegalovirus retinitis and acquired immunodeficiency syndrome. The nurse assesses the latest results of which laboratory study before administering the dose?
   1. Serum albumin
   2. Serum creatinine
   3. CD4 cell count
   4. Lymphocyte count

226. The client with tuberculosis asks the nurse about precautions to take after discharge to prevent infection of others. The nurse develops a response to the client's question based on the understanding that
   1. The client should maintain enteric precautions only.
   2. The disease is transmitted by droplet nuclei.
   3. Clothing and sheets should be bleached after each use.
   4. Deep pile carpet should be removed from the home.

227. The nurse is caring for the client after pulmonary angiography with catheter insertion via the left groin. The nurse assesses for allergic reaction to the contrast medium by noting the presence of
   1. Hematoma in the left groin.
   2. Discomfort in the left groin.
   3. Stridor.
   4. Hypothermia.

228. A sexually active 20-year-old client has developed viral hepatitis. Which of the following statements

if made by the client would indicate a need for further teaching?

1. "A condom should be used for sexual intercourse."
2. "I can never drink alcohol again."
3. "I won't go back to work right away."
4. "My close friends should get the vaccine."

229. A nurse would include which interventions in the plan of care for a client with hypothyroidism (myxedema)?

____ Instruct the client about thyroid replacement therapy.

____ Encourage the client to consume fluids and high-fiber foods in the diet.

____ Provide a cool environment for the client.

____ Instruct the client to consume a high-fat diet.

____ Instruct the client to contact the physician if episodes of chest pain occur.

____ Inform the client that iodine preparations will be prescribed to treat the disorder.

230. The nurse is administering a dose of isoproterenol hydrochloride (Isuprel) to a client. The nurse monitors for which of the following side effects of this medication?

1. Increased pulse and blood pressure
2. Drowsiness
3. Hyperglycemia
4. Hypokalemia

231. The nurse is preparing to care for a client who will be weaned from a cuffed tracheostomy tube. The nurse is planning to use a tracheostomy plug and plans to insert it into the opening in the outer cannula. Which of the following nursing interventions is required before plugging the tube?

1. Place the inner cannula into the tube.
2. Deflate the cuff on the tube.
3. Ensure that the client is able to swallow.
4. Ensure that the client is able to speak.

232. Cinoxacin (Cinobac), a urinary antiseptic, is prescribed for the client. The nurse checks the client's record knowing that this medication is used with caution in which of the following disorders?

1. Hepatic disease
2. Renal disease
3. Diabetes insipidus
4. Congestive heart failure

233. Bethanechol chloride (Urecholine) is prescribed for the client. The nurse instructs the client to take the medication

1. With meals.
2. 2 hours after meals.
3. With a snack in the afternoon.
4. At bedtime with crackers and cheese.

234. The client is diagnosed with glaucoma. Which of the following assessment data gathered by the nurse identifies a risk factor associated with this eye disorder?

1. A history of migraine headaches
2. Frequent urinary tract infections
3. Cardiovascular disease
4. Frequent upper respiratory infections

235. The client with retinal detachment is admitted to the nursing unit in preparation for a scleral buckling procedure. Which of the following would the nurse anticipate to be prescribed?

1. Bathroom privileges only
2. Elevating the head of the bed to 45 degrees
3. Placing an eye patch over the client's affected eye
4. Wearing dark glasses to read or watch television

236. The nurse is caring for a client who is on strict bedrest. The nurse develops a plan of care and develops goals related to the prevention of deep vein thrombosis and pulmonary emboli. Which of the following nursing actions would be most helpful to prevent these disorders from developing?

1. Applying a heating pad to the lower extremities
2. Encouraging active range of motion exercises
3. Placing a pillow under the knees
4. Restricting fluids

237. The nurse is caring for a suicidal client. The most appropriate nursing intervention in dealing with this client is to

1. Demonstrate confidence in the client's ability to deal with stressors.
2. Provide hope and reassurance that the problems will resolve themselves.
3. Display an attitude of detachment, confrontation, and efficiency.
4. Provide authority, action, and participation.

238. The client with tuberculosis, whose status is being monitored in an ambulatory care clinic, asks the nurse when it is permissible to return to work. The nurse replies that the client may resume employment when

1. Three sputum cultures are negative.
2. Five sputum cultures are negative.
3. A sputum culture and a chest x-ray film are negative.
4. A sputum culture and a Mantoux test are negative.

239. The nurse is admitting a client to the nursing unit who is suspected of having tuberculosis. The nurse plans to admit the client to a room that has

1. Ultraviolet light and three air exchanges per hour.
2. 10 air exchanges per hour and venting to the outside.
3. Venting to the outside and ultraviolet light.
4. Venting to the outside, six air exchanges per hour, and ultraviolet light.

240. Methenamine mandelate (Mandelamine) is prescribed for the client with a gram-positive urinary tract infection. Which of the following conditions, if noted in the client's record, would alert the

nurse to question the order for this prescribed medication?
1. Cirrhosis of the liver
2. Diabetes mellitus
3. Peripheral vascular disease
4. Hypothyroidism

241. Laboratory analysis of a urine for culture and sensitivity reveals a gram-negative bacterial infection. The client is treated with nalidixic acid (NegGram). Which of the following existing disorders in the client would alert the nurse to question the prescription for this medication?
1. Diabetes mellitus
2. Seizure disorder
3. Coronary artery disease
4. Peptic ulcer disease

242. A client comes to the emergency room following an assault and is extremely agitated, is trembling, and is hyperventilating. The most appropriate initial nursing action would be to
1. Encourage the client to discuss the assault.
2. Place the client in a quiet room alone to decrease stimulation.
3. Remain with the client until the anxiety decreases.
4. Begin to teach relaxation techniques.

243. A nasogastric tube has been inserted into a client, and the physician prescribes that the tube be attached to intermittent suction. The nurse attaches the suction, noting that the pressure should not exceed
1. 10 mm Hg.
2. 20 mm Hg.
3. 25 mm Hg.
4. 30 mm Hg.

244. The client is diagnosed with a gastrointestinal bleed, and the bleeding has been controlled. Antacids are prescribed to be administered every hour. The nurse administers the antacids and plans to maintain an approximate gastric pH of
1. 3.
2. 6.
3. 9.
4. 15.

245. The nurse provides instructions regarding the administration of cyclosporine (Sandimmune) to a client. Which of the following statements, if made by the client, would indicate the need for further instruction?
1. "I need to mix the concentrate well and drink it immediately."
2. "After taking the medication, I need to rinse the container with diluent and drink it to ensure that I have taken the complete dose."
3. "I will purchase a dropper from the pharmacist to calibrate the amount of medication that I need."

4. "I will mix the concentrate with orange juice to improve the taste."

246. The nurse is caring for a client admitted to the hospital with a suspected diagnosis of acute appendicitis. Which of the following laboratory results would the nurse expect to note if the client indeed has appendicitis?
1. Leukopenia with a shift to the right
2. Leukocytosis with a shift to the right
3. Leukocytosis with a shift to the left
4. Leukopenia with a shift to the left

247. The client with acute pancreatitis is experiencing severe pain from the disorder. The nurse would teach the client to avoid which of the following positions that could aggravate the pain?
1. Sitting up
2. Lying flat
3. Leaning forward
4. Flexing the left leg

248. A client is admitted to the hospital with acute viral hepatitis. Which of the following signs or symptoms would the nurse expect to note based on this diagnosis?
1. Spider angiomas
2. Fatigue
3. Pale urine
4. Weight gain

249. A woman comes into the emergency room following an assault. She exhibits hyperventilation, pacing, rapid speech, and headache. The nurse assesses the level of anxiety to be
1. Panic.
2. Severe.
3. Moderate.
4. Psychotic.

250. The nurse is caring for the client who has been taking hydrocodone (Hycodan) for the last 3 months. The nurse assesses the client for which of the following side effects of this medication?
1. Psychological and physical dependence
2. Tachycardia and hypertension
3. Diarrhea and abdominal cramping
4. Increased respiratory rate and bronchospasm

251. Cromolyn sodium (Intal) is prescribed for the client with allergic asthma. The nurse understands that this medication acts to
1. Inhibit the release of mediators from mast cells after exposure to an antigen.
2. Promote the migration of eosinophils into the inflammatory site.
3. Increase the number of eosinophils.
4. Dilate the bronchi.

252. The clinic nurse is preparing to evaluate the peripheral vision of a client by the confrontational method. Which of the following describes the accurate procedure to perform this test?

1. The examiner and the client cover the same eyes and stare at each other's uncovered eye, and a small object is brought into the visual field.
2. The examiner and the client cover the eyes directly opposite to one another and stare at each other's uncovered eye, and a small object is brought into the visual field.
3. The client is asked to discriminate numbers from a chart composed of colored dots.
4. The room is darkened and the client is asked to identify colored blocks and shapes when they appear in the visual field.

253. The nurse prepares to administer acetylcysteine (Mucomyst) to the client with an overdose of acetaminophen (Tylenol). Which of the following is appropriate when administering this antidote?
    1. Mixing the medication in a flavored ice drink and allowing the client to drink the medication.
    2. Administering the medication intravenously, mixed in 50 mL of normal saline and piggybacked through the main intravenous line
    3. Administering the medication intramuscularly in the gluteal muscle
    4. Administering the medication subcutaneously in the deltoid muscle

254. The client is receiving baclofen (Lioresal) for muscle spasms caused by a spinal cord injury. The nurse monitors the client for which side effect related to this medication?
    1. Photosensitivity
    2. Slurred speech
    3. Hypertension
    4. Muscle pain

255. A client in the labor room delivers a 7-lb girl. The obstetrician hands the newborn infant to the delivery room nurse. Prioritize and number the nursing actions in caring for the newborn infant in the order in which they would be performed. (Number 1 would indicate the first action.)
    ___ Performs an Apgar score
    ___ Checks the newborn infant's temperature
    ___ Hands the newborn infant to the father
    ___ Dries the infant

256. A transcutaneous electrical nerve stimulation is prescribed for a client with pain, and the nurse instructs the client about the purpose of the transcutaneous electrical nerve stimulation unit. Which statement by the client indicates the need for further instructions?
    1. "Electrodes are attached to the skin."
    2. "The unit relieves pain."
    3. "The unit will reduce the needs for analgesics."
    4. "Hospitalization is required because the unit is not portable."

257. The nurse is developing a plan of care for the client experiencing anxiety following the loss of a job. The client is verbalizing concerns regarding the ability to meet role expectations and financial obligations. The most appropriate nursing diagnosis for this client is
    1. Dysfunctional Family Process.
    2. Disturbed Thought Process.
    3. Risk for anxiety.
    4. Ineffective Coping.

258. The nurse is monitoring the chest tube drainage system in a client with a chest tube. The nurse notes intermittent bubbling in the water seal compartment. Which of the following is the most appropriate action?
    1. Change the chest tube drainage system.
    2. Document the findings.
    3. Check for an airleak.
    4. Notify the physician.

259. The nurse is preparing to perform an otoscopic examination on an adult client. The nurse does which of the following to perform this examination?
    1. Pulls the pinna up and back before inserting the speculum
    2. Pulls the earlobe down and back before inserting the speculum
    3. Uses the smallest speculum available to decrease the discomfort of the examination
    4. Tilts the clients head forward and down before inserting the speculum

260. Cinoxacin (Cinobac) is prescribed for the client with a urinary tract infection. The clinic nurse is instructing the client regarding the administration of the medication. The nurse tells the client to take the medication
    1. 1 hour before meals.
    2. With meals.
    3. At bedtime.
    4. In the morning before breakfast.

261. The client who has just suffered a large flail chest is experiencing severe pain and dyspnea. The client's central venous pressure is rising, and the arterial blood pressure is falling. The nurse interprets that the client is experiencing
    1. Mediastinal flutter.
    2. Mediastinal shift.
    3. Hypovolemic shock.
    4. Fat embolism.

262. The nurse is caring for the client who is suspected of having lung cancer. The nurse assesses the client for which most frequent early symptom of lung cancer?
    1. Hemoptysis
    2. Cough
    3. Hoarseness
    4. Pleuritic pain

263. A client arrives in the emergency room in a crisis state. The client demonstrates signs of profound anxiety and is unable to focus on anything but the

object of the crisis and the impact on self. The initial nursing assessment would focus on
1. The object of the crisis.
2. The presence of support systems.
3. The physical condition of the client.
4. The client's coping mechanisms.

264. After performing an initial abdominal assessment on a client with a diagnosis of cholelithiasis, the nurse documents that the bowel sounds are normal. Which of the following descriptions best describes "normal bowel sounds?"
1. Waves of loud gurgles auscultated in all four quadrants.
2. High-pitched, loud rushes auscultated especially in one or two quadrants.
3. Relatively high-pitched clicks or gurgles auscultated in all four quadrants.
4. Low-pitched swishing auscultated in one or two quadrants.

265. A nurse is calculating a client's fluid intake for an 8-hour period. The client drank 8 oz of tea and 4 oz of orange juice for breakfast, 4 oz of water at 10 AM and at 1 PM when taking his medications, and 6 oz of iced tea at lunch. At 8 AM and again at 2 PM, the client received his antibiotics intravenously in 50 mL of normal saline. What is the client's total intake in milliliters?
Answer: _____

ANSWERS

1. 3
Rationale: McBurney's point is midway between the right anterior superior iliac crest and the umbilicus. McBurney's point is usually the location of greatest pain in the child with appendicitis.
Test-Taking Strategy: Use the process of elimination. Knowledge that the appendix is located in the right side of the abdomen will assist you in eliminating options 2 and 4. From this point, attempt to visualize this assessment procedure. This will assist in directing you to option 3. Review the location of McBurney's point if you had difficulty with this question.
Level of Cognitive Ability: Comprehension
Client Needs: Health Promotion and Maintenance
Integrated Process: Nursing Process—assessment
Content Area: Child health
Reference: James, S., Ashwill, J., & Droske, S. (2002). *Nursing care of children: Principles & practice* (2nd ed., p. 560). Philadelphia: W. B. Saunders.

2. 3
Rationale: Nitrofurazone (Furacin) is applied topically to the burn and has a broad spectrum of antibiotic activity. Nitrofurazone is used in burns in which bacterial resistance to other agents is a real or potential problem. A film of $1/16$ inch is applied directly to the burn. Saline-soaked dressings are not used.
Test-Taking Strategy: Use the process of elimination. Option 1 can be eliminated because infection is a major concern with the burn client and a wet dressing can harbor bacteria more easily. Recalling that a thin film is required will direct you easily to option 3. Review the use of this medication for burn therapy if you had difficulty with this question.
Level of Cognitive Ability: Application
Client Needs: Physiological Integrity
Integrated Process: Communication and Documentation
Content Area: Pharmacology
Reference: McKenry, L., & Salerno, E. (2003). *Mosby's pharmacology in nursing* (21st ed., p. 1135). St. Louis: Mosby.

3. 2
Rationale: The computed tomography scan causes no pain and can take 15 to 60 minutes to perform. The dye may cause a warm flushing sensation when injected. Fluids are encouraged following the procedure. If an iodine dye is used, the client should be asked about allergies to seafood or iodine.
Test-Taking Strategy: Use the process of elimination. Note the key words "dye injection" in the question. This should provide you with the clue that the issue relates to the dye. If you are unfamiliar with this diagnostic test, review the important teaching points related to it.
Level of Cognitive Ability: Application
Client Needs: Physiological Integrity
Integrated Process: Nursing Process—implementation
Content Area: Adult health—oncology
Reference: Chernecky, C., & Berger, B. (2001). *Laboratory tests and diagnostic procedures* (3rd ed., p. 378). Philadelphia: W. B. Saunders.

4. 4
Rationale: The normal magnesium level is 1.6 to 2.6 mg/dL. A client with a magnesium level of 3.5 mg/dL is experiencing hypermagnesemia. Assessment signs/symptoms include neurological depression, drowsiness and lethargy, loss of deep tendon reflexes, respiratory insufficiency, bradycardia, and hypotension. Tetany, twitches, and a positive Trousseau's sign are seen in a client with hypomagnesemia.
Test-Taking Strategy: First you must determine that the client is experiencing hypermagnesemia. Next, use the process of elimination, noting that options 1, 2, and 3 are similar in that they reflect neurological excitability. If you had difficulty with this question, review the assessment signs/symptoms found in magnesium imbalances.
Level of Cognitive Ability: Analysis
Client Needs: Physiological Integrity
Integrated Process: Nursing Process—assessment
Content Area: Fundamental skills
Reference: Chernecky, C., & Berger, B. (2001). *Laboratory tests and diagnostic procedures* (3rd ed., p. 708). Philadelphia: W. B. Saunders.

5. 3
Rationale: The normal serum calcium level is 8.6 to 10 mg/dL. This client is experiencing hypercalcemia. Calcium gluconate and calcium chloride are medications used to treat tetany that occurs from acute hypocalcemia. In hypercalcemia, large

doses of vitamin D need to be avoided. Calcitonin (Calcimar), a thyroid hormone, decreases the plasma calcium level by increasing the incorporation of calcium into the bones, thus keeping calcium out of the serum.
Test-Taking Strategy: First, you need to determine that the client is experiencing hypercalcemia. With this knowledge, you can eliminate options 1 and 2 easily because you would not administer medication that would add calcium to the body. Remembering that excessive vitamin D is a causative factor of hypercalcemia will assist you in eliminating option 4. If you had difficulty with this question, review the treatment for hypercalcemia.
Level of Cognitive Ability: Analysis
Client Needs: Physiological Integrity
Integrated Process: Nursing Process—planning
Content Area: Pharmacology
Reference: McKenry, L., & Salerno, E. (2003). *Mosby's pharmacology in nursing* (21st ed., p. 837). St. Louis: Mosby.

6. **3**
Rationale: Sodium polystyrene sulfonate is a cation exchange resin used to treat hyperkalemia. The resin passes through the intestine or is retained in the colon. The resin releases sodium ions in exchange for primarily potassium ions. The therapeutic effect occurs 2 to 12 hours after oral administration and longer after rectal administration.
Test-Taking Strategy: Use the process of elimination. Looking closely at the name of the medication (Kayexalate) may provide you with assistance regarding the action of the medication. If you had difficulty with this question, review the action of this important medication.
Level of Cognitive Ability: Comprehension
Client Needs: Physiological Integrity
Integrated Process: Nursing Process—planning
Content Area: Pharmacology
Reference: McKenry, L., & Salerno, E. (2003). *Mosby's pharmacology in nursing* (21st ed., p. 756.). St. Louis: Mosby

7. **2**
Rationale: Fluid that shifts into the interstitial spaces and remains there is referred to as third space fluid. Common sites for third spacing include the abdomen, pleural cavity, peritoneal cavity, and the pericardial sac. Third space fluid is physiologically useless because it does not circulate to provide nutrients for the cells. Risk factors include clients with liver or kidney disease, major trauma, burns, sepsis, wound healing or major surgery, malignancy, gastrointestinal malabsorption, malnutrition, and alcoholic or older clients.
Test-Taking Strategy: Use the process of elimination and note the key words "least likely." Eliminate options 1 and 4 first because fluid balance disturbances likely will occur with these conditions. From the remaining options, liver failure is the option that is most acute and therefore is most similar to options 1 and 4. Review the risk factors associated with third spacing if you had difficulty with this question.
Level of Cognitive Ability: Analysis
Client Needs: Physiological Integrity
Integrated Process: Nursing Process—assessment
Content Area: Fundamental skills

Reference: Phipps, W., Monahan, F., Sands, J., Marek, J., & Neighbors, M. (2003). *Medical-surgical nursing: Health and illness perspectives* (7th ed., p. 245). St. Louis: Mosby.

8. **4**
Rationale: Before the gastroscopy procedure, medication is given to prevent a gag reflex. On return from the procedure the nurse must test the client's gag reflex to assure that it is present to prevent aspiration of contents. The client must be placed in a side-lying or semi-Fowler position to avoid aspiration. Vital signs should be taken every 30 minutes for 2 hours to detect abnormalities. Saline gargles must be administered only when the gag reflex has been confirmed.
Test-Taking Strategy: Use the process of elimination. Use of the ABCs—airway, breathing, and circulation—will assist you in answering the question. Option 4 is the only option that addresses airway. If you had difficulty with this question, review the care to the client following a gastroscopy procedure.
Level of Cognitive Ability: Application
Client Needs: Physiological Integrity
Integrated Process: Nursing Process—planning
Content Area: Adult health—gastrointestinal
Reference: Chernecky, C., & Berger, B. (2001). *Laboratory tests and diagnostic procedures* (3rd ed., p. 552). Philadelphia: W. B. Saunders.

9. **1**
Rationale: Ringer's lactate solution is an isotonic solution. Other isotonic solutions include 5% dextrose in water (5% D/W), 0.9% normal saline (NS), and 5% dextrose in 0.225% saline (5% D/¼ NS); whereas 0.45% saline (½ NS) is hypotonic, and 10% dextrose in water (10% D/W), 5% dextrose in 0.9% saline (5% D/NS), and 5% dextrose in 0.45% saline (5% D/½ NS) are hypertonic solutions.
Test-Taking Strategy: Use the process of elimination and knowledge regarding the tonicity of the various intravenous solutions. If you had difficulty with this question, review this content.
Level of Cognitive Ability: Comprehension
Client Needs: Physiological Integrity
Integrated Process: Teaching/Learning
Content Area: Fundamental skills
Reference: Ignatavicius, D., & Workman, M. (2002). *Medical-surgical nursing: Critical thinking for collaborative care* (4th ed., p. 166). Philadelphia: W. B. Saunders.

10. **1**
Rationale: The normal pH is 7.35 to 7.45. The normal P_{CO_2} is 35 to 45 mm Hg. In respiratory acidosis the pH is low and the P_{CO_2} is elevated. This is an expected finding in a client with a neuromuscular disorder such as Guillian-Barré syndrome because the client may retain carbon dioxide because of ventilatory failure as paralysis ensues.
Test-Taking Strategy: Remember that in a respiratory imbalance you will find an opposite response between the pH and the P_{CO_2}. Also remember that the pH is down in an acidotic condition. Recalling this information will allow you to eliminate each of the incorrect options. Review interpretation of blood gas results if you had difficulty with this question.
Level of Cognitive Ability: Analysis

Client Needs: Physiological Integrity
Integrated Process: Nursing Process—analysis
Content Area: Fundamental skills
Reference: Chernecky, C., & Berger, B. (2001). *Laboratory tests and diagnostic procedures* (3rd ed., p. 227). Philadelphia: W. B. Saunders.

11. **3**
Rationale: The client who ingests a large amount of aspirin (acetylsalicylic acid) is at risk for developing metabolic acidosis 24 hours after the poisoning. If metabolic acidosis occurs, the client may exhibit hyperpnea with Kussmaul's respirations, headache, nausea, vomiting, diarrhea, fruity smelling breath because of improper fat metabolism, central nervous system depression, twitching, convulsions, and hyperkalemia. In the early hours following aspirin overdose, the client may exhibit respiratory alkalosis as a compensatory mechanism. By 24 hours after overdose, however, the compensatory mechanism fails, and the client reverts to metabolic acidosis.
Test-Taking Strategy: Knowledge about the clinical manifestations of metabolic acidosis will direct you to option 3. Use the process of elimination, recalling the significant gastrointestinal symptoms that can occur in this disorder. Review the clinical manifestations of metabolic acidosis if this question was difficult.
Level of Cognitive Ability: Analysis
Client Needs: Physiological Integrity
Integrated Process: Nursing Process—assessment
Content Area: Fundamental skills
Reference: Hodgson, B., & Kizior, R. (2004). *Saunders nursing drug handbook 2004* (p. 85). Philadelphia: W. B. Saunders.

12. **2**
Rationale: The normal serum ammonia level is 35 to 65 mcg/dL. In the client with hepatic encephalopathy the serum level is not likely to drop below normal, nor is it likely to drop into the low-normal range. The most optimal yet realistic change would be to 60 mcg/dL, which falls into the high-normal range. A level of 80 mcg/dL represents insufficient effect of the medication.
Test-Taking Strategy: Use the process of elimination and knowledge of the normal serum ammonia level. Option 2 is the only option that identifies a normal ammonia level. Review this test and the desirable effects of this medication if you had difficulty with this question.
Level of Cognitive Ability: Analysis
Client Needs: Physiological Integrity
Integrated Process: Nursing Process—evaluation
Content Area: Adult health—gastrointestinal
Reference: Chernecky, C., & Berger, B. (2001). *Laboratory tests and diagnostic procedures* (3rd ed., p. 150). Philadelphia: W. B. Saunders.

13. **2**
Rationale: The normal urine myoglobin level is negative. After extensive muscle destruction or damage, myoglobin is released into the bloodstream where it is cleared from the body by the kidneys. When a large amount of myoglobin is being cleared from the body, a risk exists of the renal tubules being clogged with myoglobin, causing acute tubular necrosis. This is one form of acute renal failure.

Test-Taking Strategy: Use the process of elimination. Note the relationship of the word "urine" in the question and "acute tubular necrosis" in the correct option. Review the significance of myoglobin in the urine if you had difficulty with this question.
Level of Cognitive Ability: Analysis
Client Needs: Physiological Integrity
Integrated Process: Nursing Process—assessment
Content Area: Adult health—renal
Reference: Chernecky, C, & Berger, B. (2001). *Laboratory tests and diagnostic procedures* (3rd ed., p. 757). Philadelphia: W. B. Saunders.

14. **2**
Rationale: The normal hematocrit level for an adult male is 42% to 52%. The client who is in shock has an elevated level because of hemoconcentration. The client's level may be expected to drift back down to within the normal range once fluid volume has been restored adequately. Thus option 2 is the only correct option. Option 1 is too high, whereas options 3 and 4 are low.
Test-Taking Strategy: Use the process of elimination. Recalling that the normal hematocrit level is 42% to 52% will direct you to option 2. Because this is a common laboratory study, it would be useful to have this one committed to memory.
Level of Cognitive Ability: Analysis
Client Needs: Physiological Integrity
Integrated Process: Nursing Process—evaluation
Content Area: Fundamental skills
Reference: Chernecky, C., & Berger, B. (2001). *Laboratory tests and diagnostic procedures* (3rd ed., p. 372). Philadelphia: W. B. Saunders.

15. **2**
Rationale: Any condition in which gastrointestinal motility is slowed or esophageal reflux is possible places a client at risk for aspiration. Options 1 and 4 may be appropriate nursing diagnoses but are not of highest priority. Option 3 is not as likely to occur in this client.
Test-Taking Strategy: Note the key words "highest priority." Use the ABCs: airway, breathing, and circulation. Option 2 addresses airway management. Options 1, 3, and 4 are possible problems, but not as high a priority as airway maintenance.
Level of Cognitive Ability: Analysis
Client Needs: Physiological Integrity
Integrated Process: Nursing Process—planning
Content Area: Delegating/Prioritizing
Reference: Lewis, S., Heitkemper, M., & Dirksen, S. (2004). *Medical-surgical nursing: Assessment and management of clinical problems* (6th ed., p. 985). St. Louis: Mosby.

16. **4**
Rationale: Self-control is demonstrated by stoicism and hiding feelings. Problem solving involves making plans and verbalizing what will be done. Accepting responsibility places the responsibility for a situation on one's self. Distancing is an unwillingness or inability to discuss events.
Test-Taking Strategy: Note the key words "refuses," "will not," and "does not." These words indicate ineffective coping. Option 4, distancing, is the one option that correlates with

these key words. If you had difficulty with this question, review coping mechanisms.
Level of Cognitive Ability: Analysis
Client Needs: Psychosocial Integrity
Integrated Process: Nursing Process—assessment
Content Area: Adult health—gastrointestinal
Reference: Black, J., Hawks, J., & Keene, A. (2001). *Medical-surgical nursing: Clinical management for positive outcomes* (6th ed., pp. 26, 408). Philadelphia: W. B. Saunders.

17. 1
Rationale: The most accurate measurement of weight loss is daily weighing of the client at the same time, in the same clothes, and using the same scale. Options 2, 3, and 4 assist in measuring nutrition and hydration status rather than actual loss of pounds.
Test-Taking Strategy: Note the key words "most accurately." Also note the issue of the question and the similar words in the question and the correct option. If you had difficulty with this question, review the methods of monitoring weight loss.
Level of Cognitive Ability: Comprehension
Client Needs: Physiological Integrity
Integrated Process: Nursing Process—assessment
Content Area: Fundamental skills
Reference: Potter, P., & Perry, A. (2001). *Fundamentals of nursing* (5th ed., p. 739). St. Louis: Mosby.

18. 4
Rationale: In anorexia nervosa the client tries to establish identity and control by self-imposed starvation. Options 1, 2, and 3 are verbalizations of the client's intentions. Option 4 is a measurable action that can be verified.
Test-Taking Strategy: Note the key words "that treatment has been effective." With this in mind, use the process of elimination and select the option that is measurable. Option 4 is the only measurable action.
Level of Cognitive Ability: Analysis
Client Needs: Psychosocial Integrity
Integrated Process: Nursing Process—evaluation
Content Area: Fundamental skills
Reference: Fortinash, K., & Holoday-Worret, P. (2000). *Psychiatric mental health nursing* (2nd ed., pp. 452, 455, 458). St. Louis: Mosby.

19. 2
Rationale: The client with dumping syndrome should be placed on a low carbohydrate and moderate protein and fat diet. The client should lie down after eating and should avoid drinking liquids with meals. Frequent small meals are encouraged, and the client should avoid concentrated sweets.
Test-Taking Strategy: Note the key words "need for further teaching" in the stem of the question. Think about this disorder and use the process of elimination, selecting option 2 as the item that will contribute to the problems associated with dumping syndrome. If you had difficulty with this question, review the diet associated with this syndrome.
Level of Cognitive Ability: Analysis
Client Needs: Physiological Integrity
Integrated Process: Teaching/Learning
Content Area: Adult health—gastrointestinal

Reference: Williams, S., & Schlenker, E. (2003). *Essentials of nutrition & diet therapy* (8th ed., p. 558). St. Louis: Mosby.

20. 3
Rationale: Vitamin B_{12} deficiency is caused by Pernicious anemia. Treatment consists of monthly injections of vitamin B_{12}. Thiamine is prescribed most often for the client with alcoholism. Iron is administered for iron deficiency anemia, and folic acid is administered for folic-acid deficiency.
Test-Taking Strategy: Knowledge regarding the relationship between pernicious anemia and vitamin B_{12} is required to answer this question. Review the treatment for this disorder if you had difficulty with this question.
Level of Cognitive Ability: Analysis
Client Needs: Physiological Integrity
Integrated Process: Nursing Process—planning
Content Area: Adult health—gastrointestinal
Reference: McKenry, L., & Salerno, E. (2003). *Mosby's pharmacology in nursing* (21st ed., p. 1162). St. Louis: Mosby.

21. 4
Rationale: Modification of a client's diet of solid food to a soft or mechanical chopped diet may be necessary if the client has difficulty chewing. Food and cultural preferences should be ascertained on admission. Bowel sounds should have been assessed previously and be present before introducing any diet.
Test-Taking Strategy: Note the key words "tolerating a full liquid diet." Eliminate options 1 and 2 first because they are similar. Eliminate option 3 next because the client has been tolerating a full liquid diet; therefore bowel sounds must have been present. The issue relates to consistency of food. Option 4 is the only option that addresses a factor affecting food consistency. If necessary, review these dietary factors
Level of Cognitive Ability: Analysis
Client Needs: Physiological Integrity
Integrated Process: Nursing Process—assessment
Content Area: Fundamental skills
Reference: Jarvis, C. (2000). *Physical examination & health assessment* (3rd ed., p. 382). Philadelphia: W. B. Saunders.

22. 3
Rationale: Bacon is a component of the fat group in the exchange system. One teaspoon of butter is equal to 1 tsp margarine, 1 tsp of any oil, 1 tbs of salad dressing, 1 strip of bacon, 5 large olives, or 10 whole peanuts.
Test-Taking Strategy: Note the key words "most appropriate" in the stem of the question. Eliminate options 1 and 2 because they are similar. Select option 3 over option 4, knowing that bacon is an item of the fat group. Review foods in the exchange system if you had difficulty with this question.
Level of Cognitive Ability: Application
Client Needs: Physiological Integrity
Integrated Process: Teaching/Learning
Content Area: Adult health—endocrine
Reference: Potter, P., & Perry, A. (2001). *Fundamentals of nursing* (5th ed., p. 1376). St. Louis: Mosby.

23. 3
Rationale: Fruits and vegetables, except avocado, olives, and coconut, contain minimal amounts of fat.

Test-Taking Strategy: Use the process of elimination. Options 1 and 2 can be eliminated easily based on general knowledge regarding nutrition. From the remaining two options, remember that avocado is high in fat content. Review the food items high in fat content if you had difficulty with this question.
Level of Cognitive Ability: Analysis
Client Needs: Health Promotion and Maintenance
Integrated Process: Nursing Process—evaluation
Content Area: Adult health—cardiovascular
Reference: Grodner, M., Anderson, S., & DeYoung, S. (2000). *Foundations and clinical applications of nutrition: A nursing approach* (p. 850). St. Louis: Mosby.

24. **1**
Rationale: Chemotherapy may cause distortion of taste. Frequently beef and pork are reported to taste bitter or metallic. The nurse can promote client nutrition by assisting the client to choose alternative sources of protein in the diet. Options 2, 3, and 4 are not likely to cause distortion of taste.
Test-Taking Strategy: The issue of the question is optimal management of a change in taste sensation. To answer this question accurately, you must be familiar with the most troublesome foods. If you had difficulty with this question, review interventions related to nutrition in the client receiving chemotherapy.
Level of Cognitive Ability: Application
Client Needs: Physiological Integrity
Integrated Process: Nursing Process—implementation
Content Area: Adult health—oncology
Reference: Williams, S., & Schlenker, E. (2003). *Essentials of nutrition & diet therapy* (8th ed., pp. 599-600). St. Louis: Mosby.

25. **2**
Rationale: Normal hemoglobin levels indicate that iron and protein intake is sufficient. Elevated creatinine levels indicate kidney problems, which is not considered a nutritional disorder. Elevated albumin levels may indicate dehydration falsely. A normal red blood cell level indicates adequate vitamin B_{12} intake.
Test-Taking Strategy: Knowledge regarding the interpretation of the common laboratory test findings is required to answer this question. Review these common laboratory tests if you had difficulty with this question.
Level of Cognitive Ability: Analysis
Client Needs: Physiological Integrity
Integrated Process: Nursing Process—analysis
Content Area: Fundamental skills
Reference: Potter, P., & Perry, A. (2001). *Fundamentals of nursing* (5th ed., p. 1350). St. Louis: Mosby.

26. **1**
Rationale: Hydrocephalus is a condition characterized by an enlargement of the cranium because of an abnormal accumulation of cerebrospinal fluid within the cerebral ventricular system. This characteristic causes the increase in the weight of the infant's head. The infant may experience significant head enlargement. Care must be exercised to see that the head is well supported when the infant is fed or moved to prevent extra strain on the infant's neck, and measures must be taken to prevent the development of pressure areas. Supporting the infant's head and neck, when picking up the infant, will prevent hyperextension of the neck area and keep the infant from falling backward. The infant should be fed with the head elevated for proper motility of food processing. A helmet could suffocate an unattended infant during rest and sleep times, and hyperextension of the infant's head can put pressure on the neck vertebras, causing injury.
Test-Taking Strategy: Use the process of elimination and focus on the issue of the question, moving the infant with an enlarged head size. Visualize each of the options to assist in directing you to option 1, the safe measure. If you had difficulty with this question, review care to the infant with hydrocephalus.
Level of Cognitive Ability: Application
Client Needs: Safe, Effective Care Environment
Integrated Process: Teaching/Learning
Content Area: Child health
Reference: Murray, S., McKinney, E., & Gorrie, T. (2002). *Foundations of maternal-newborn nursing* (3rd ed., p. 867). Philadelphia: W. B. Saunders.

27. **2**
Rationale: Parents are concerned especially about seizures that might go undetected at night time. The nurse needs to decrease parental overprotection and should suggest the use of a baby monitor for nighttime. Options 1 and 3 identify parental understanding of the disorder. Option 4 is a common concern. The parents need to be reminded that as the child grows, they cannot always observe their child but that their knowledge of seizure activity and care are appropriate to minimize complications.
Test-Taking Strategy: Note the key words "need for further teaching." Use the process of elimination, recalling that parental overprotection needs to be discouraged. Option 2 identifies a need to provide the parents with an alternate manner to monitor for night seizures. Review parental home care instructions for the child with a seizure disorder if necessary.
Level of Cognitive Ability: Analysis
Client Needs: Health Promotion and Maintenance
Integrated Process: Nursing Process—evaluation
Content Area: Child health
Reference: James, S., Ashwill, J., & Droske, S. (2002). *Nursing care of children: Principles & practice* (2nd ed., p. 973). Philadelphia: W. B. Saunders.

28. **4**
Rationale: When carbamazepine is administered, blood level samples need to be drawn periodically to check for the child's absorption of the medication. The amount of the medication prescribed is based on the blood level achieved. The therapeutic serum range of carbamazepine is 5 to 12 mcg/mL. The nurse would anticipate that the physician would continue the presently prescribed dosage.
Test-Taking Strategy: You must know the therapeutic serum drug level of carbamazepine to answer the question. Recalling that the therapeutic level is 5 to 12 mcg/mL will direct you to option 4 because a result of 10 mcg/mL is within the therapeutic range. If you had difficulty with this question, learn the therapeutic serum drug level of carbamazepine.
Level of Cognitive Ability: Analysis
Client Needs: Physiological Integrity

Integrated Process: Nursing Process—analysis
Content Area: Pharmacology
Reference: Hodgson, B., & Kizior, R. (2004). *Saunders nursing drug handbook 2004* (pp. 148-150). Philadelphia: W. B. Saunders.

29. 2
Rationale: The uterus has three divisions: the corpus, isthmus, and the cervix. The upper division is the corpus or the body of the uterus. The uppermost part of the uterine corpus, above the area where the fallopian tubes enter the uterus, is the fundus of the uterus. Options 1, 3, and 4 are incorrect.
Test-Taking Strategy: Eliminate options 3 and 4 because they are similar. From the remaining options, knowledge regarding the divisions of the uterus is required to answer this question. If you had difficulty with this question, review the anatomical structure of the uterus.
Level of Cognitive Ability: Comprehension
Client Needs: Physiological Integrity
Integrated Process: Teaching/Learning
Content Area: Maternity/Antepartum
Reference: Murray, S., McKinney, E., & Gorrie, T. (2002). *Foundations of maternal-newborn nursing* (3rd ed., p. 63). Philadelphia: W. B. Saunders.

30. 4
Rationale: Hypoglycemia is a blood glucose level of less than 50 to 60 mg/dL.
Test-Taking Strategy: Recalling the normal blood glucose level will assist in eliminating options 1, 2, and 3. If you are unfamiliar with the normal blood glucose level or the concept of hypoglycemia, review this content.
Level of Cognitive Ability: Application
Client Needs: Health Promotion and Maintenance
Integrated Process: Teaching/Learning
Content Area: Adult health—endocrine
References: Chernecky, C., & Berger, B. (2001). *Laboratory tests and diagnostic procedures* (3rd ed., p. 560). Philadelphia: W. B. Saunders.
Ignatavicius, D., & Workman, M. (2002). *Medical-surgical nursing: Critical thinking for collaborative care* (4th ed., p. 1478). Philadelphia: W. B. Saunders.

31. 1
Rationale: Glucagon is used to treat hypoglycemia resulting from insulin overdose. The family of the client is instructed in how to administer the medication. In an unconscious client, arousal usually occurs within 5 to 20 minutes of glucagon injection. Once consciousness has been regained, carbohydrates should be given orally. Lipoatrophy and lipohypertrophy result from insulin injections.
Test-Taking Strategy: Use the process of elimination. Noting the word "glucagon" will assist you in determining that the medication contains some form of glucose. This relationship should direct you easily to option 1. Review the purpose of this medication if you are unfamiliar with it.
Level of Cognitive Ability: Application
Client Needs: Physiological Integrity
Integrated Process: Teaching/Learning
Content Area: Pharmacology
Reference: McKenry, L., & Salerno, E. (2003). *Mosby's pharmacology in nursing* (21st ed., pp. 877-878). St. Louis: Mosby.

32. 3
Rationale: In the Cuban American culture, loud crying and other physical manifestations of grief are considered socially acceptable. Of the options provided, option 3 is the only option that identifies a culturally sensitive approach on the part of the nurse. Options 1, 2, and 4 are inappropriate nursing interventions.
Test-Taking Strategy: Focus on the client(s) of the question, which are the family members. Use the process of elimination and therapeutic nursing interventions, recalling the characteristics of the culture and the importance of cultural sensitivity. This will direct you easily to option 3. If you had difficulty with this question, review the characteristics of this culture.
Level of Cognitive Ability: Application
Client Needs: Psychosocial Integrity
Integrated Process: Caring
Content Area: Fundamental skills
Reference: Potter, P., & Perry, A. (2001). *Fundamentals of nursing* (5th ed., pp. 405, 456). St. Louis: Mosby.

33. 1
Rationale: Transmission of infectious diseases can occur through contaminated items such as hands and bed linens in clients with endometritis. An important method of preventing infection is to break the chain of infection. Hand washing is one of the most effective methods of preventing the transmission of infectious diseases. The newborn infant is allowed in the mother's room and visitors are allowed to hold the newborn infant as long as hand washing and other protective measures are instituted.
Test-Taking Strategy: Use the process of elimination. Eliminate options 2, 3, and 4 because of the absolute terms "at all," "no," and "not." Review content related to the transmission of infection if you had difficulty with this question.
Level of Cognitive Ability: Application
Client Needs: Safe, Effective Care Environment
Integrated Process: Teaching/Learning
Content Area: Maternity/Postpartum
References: Lowdermilk, D., & Perry, S. (2003). *Maternity nursing* (6th ed., p. 704). St. Louis: Mosby.
Murray, S., McKinney, E., & Gorrie, T. (2002). *Foundations of maternal-newborn nursing* (3rd ed., p. 965). Philadelphia: W. B. Saunders.

34. 4
Rationale: The priority nursing action is to assess the vital signs. This data would indicate the amount of blood loss that has occurred and also provides a baseline by which to monitor the progress of treatment. The client may not be able to provide subjective data until the immediate physical needs are met. Although an abdominal examination and an assessment of the precipitating events may be necessary, these actions are not the priority.
Test-Taking Strategy: Note the key words "first priority." Use the process of elimination and the ABCs—airway, breathing, and circulation. This will direct you to option 4. Review care to the client with gastrointestinal bleeding if you had difficulty with this question.
Level of Cognitive Ability: Application

Client Needs: Physiological Integrity
Integrated Process: Nursing Process—implementation
Content Area: Delegating/Prioritizing
Reference: Lewis, S., Heitkemper, M., & Dirksen, S. (2004). *Medical-surgical nursing: Assessment and management of clinical problems* (6th ed., p. 1024). St. Louis: Mosby.

35. **1**
Rationale: An intravenous cholangiogram is for diagnostic purposes. The cholangiogram outlines the gallbladder and the ducts, so gallstones that have moved into the ductal system can be detected. Radiographs are used to visualize the biliary duct system after intravenous injection of radiopaque dye. This test is diagnostic and does not involve irrigation, instillation of medications, or draining of the gallbladder.
Test-Taking Strategy: Use the process of elimination. Eliminate option 2, 3, and 4 because they are similar. If you are unfamiliar with this procedure, review its purpose.
Level of Cognitive Ability: Analysis
Client Needs: Physiological Integrity
Integrated Process: Teaching/Learning
Content Area: Adult health—gastrointestinal
Reference: Chernecky, C., & Berger, B. (2001). *Laboratory tests and diagnostic procedures* (3rd ed., p. 652). Philadelphia: W. B. Saunders.

36. **1**
Rationale: Iron is needed to allow for transfer of adequate iron to the fetus and to permit expansion of the maternal red blood cell mass. During pregnancy, the relative excess of plasma causes a decrease in the hemoglobin concentration and hematocrit, known as physiologic anemia of pregnancy. This is a normal adaptation during pregnancy. Meats are an excellent source of iron. Iron supplements usually cause constipation. Iron is best absorbed if taken with a vitamin C substance.
Test-Taking Strategy: Use the process of elimination, focusing on the key words "understanding of the instructions." Knowledge of basic principles related to nutrition during pregnancy will assist you in eliminating options 2 and 4. From the remaining options, remember that iron causes constipation. Review client teaching points related to iron supplementation if you had difficulty with this question.
Level of Cognitive Ability: Analysis
Client Needs: Physiological Integrity
Integrated Process: Teaching/Learning
Content Area: Maternity/Antepartum
Reference: Lowdermilk, D., & Perry, S. (2003). *Maternity nursing* (6th ed., p. 249). St. Louis: Mosby.

37. **1**
Rationale: The client who has had vein ligation and stripping should avoid standing or sitting for prolonged periods. The client should remain lying down unless performing a specific activity for the first few days following the procedure. Prolonged standing and sitting increases the risk of edema in the legs by decreasing blood return to the heart. The client should avoid crossing the legs at any level for the same reason.
Test-Taking Strategy: Use the process of elimination and principles associated with gravity and blood flow to answer this question. Eliminate option 2 first because of the absolute term

"only." Knowing that prolonged standing or sitting is harmful helps you eliminate options 3 and 4. Review client instructions following a vein ligation and stripping if you had difficulty with this question.
Level of Cognitive Ability: Analysis
Client Needs: Health Promotion and Maintenance
Integrated Process: Nursing Process—evaluation
Content Area: Adult health—cardiovascular
Reference: Lewis, S., Heitkemper, M., & Dirksen, S. (2004). *Medical-surgical nursing: Assessment and management of clinical problems* (6th ed., p. 936). St. Louis: Mosby.

38. **3**
Rationale: Octreotide acetate (Sandostatin) is used to reduce growth hormone levels in clients with acromegaly. The most common side effects of octreotide include diarrhea, nausea, gallstone formation, and abdominal discomfort. Hypertension, although rare, may occur. Polyuria is not associated with this medication.
Test-Taking Strategy: Knowledge regarding the side effects associated with octreotide is required to answer the question. Review these side effects if you had difficulty with this question.
Level of Cognitive Ability: Analysis
Client Needs: Physiological Integrity
Integrated Process: Nursing Process—assessment
Content Area: Pharmacology
Reference: Hodgson, B., & Kizior, R. (2004). *Saunders nursing drug handbook 2004* (p. 745). Philadelphia: W. B. Saunders.

39. **2**
Rationale: Levothyroxine (Synthroid) accelerates the degradation of vitamin K–dependent clotting factors. As a result, the effects of warfarin (Coumadin) are enhanced. Therefore if thyroid hormone replacement therapy is instituted in a client who has been taking warfarin, the dosage of warfarin should be reduced.
Test-Taking Strategy: Use the process of elimination, recalling that levothyroxine enhances the effects of warfarin. Review these medication interactions if you had difficulty with this question.
Level of Cognitive Ability: Analysis
Client Needs: Physiological Integrity
Integrated Process: Nursing Process—analysis
Content Area: Pharmacology
Reference: Lehne, R. (2001). *Pharmacology for nursing care* (4th ed., p. 640). Philadelphia: W. B. Saunders.

40. **3**
Rationale: The client should use the positions outlined in options 1, 2, and 4. These allow for maximal chest expansion. The client should not lie on the back because it reduces movement of a large area of the client's chest wall. Sitting is better than standing whenever possible. If no chair is available, then leaning against a wall while standing allows accessory muscles to be used for breathing and not posture control.
Test-Taking Strategy: Use the process of elimination, noting the key words "dyspneic episodes" and "avoid." Also note that options 1, 2, and 4 are similar in that they address upright positions. If you had difficulty with this question, review client teaching points related to emphysema.

Level of Cognitive Ability: Application
Client Needs: Physiological Integrity
Integrated Process: Teaching/Learning
Content Area: Adult health—respiratory
Reference: Ignatavicius, D., & Workman, M. (2002). *Medical-surgical nursing: Critical thinking for collaborative care* (4th ed., pp. 547-548). Philadelphia: W. B. Saunders.

41. 1
Rationale: The client undergoing lumbar puncture is positioned lying on the side with the legs pulled up to the abdomen and with the head bent down onto the chest. This position helps to open the spaces between the vertebras and allows for easier needle insertion by the physician. Each of the other options identifies incorrect positions for this procedure.
Test-Taking Strategy: Use the process of elimination. Recalling that a lumbar puncture is the introduction of a needle into the subarachnoid space will direct you to option 1. You can reason that the position of the client must facilitate the puncture and that the correct option is the only position that flexes the vertebras and widens the spaces between them. Review care to the client undergoing a lumbar puncture if you had difficulty with this question.
Level of Cognitive Ability: Application
Client Needs: Physiological Integrity
Integrated Process: Nursing Process—implementation
Content Area: Adult health—neurological
Reference: Chernecky, C., & Berger, B. (2001). *Laboratory tests and diagnostic procedures* (3rd ed., p. 694). Philadelphia: W. B. Saunders.

42. 2
Rationale: Maintaining effective and open communication among family members affected by death and grief is of the greatest importance. Option 1 describes encouraging discussion of feelings and is likely to enhance communications. Option 3 is also an effective intervention, because spiritual practices give meaning to life and have an impact on how persons react to crisis. Option 4 is also an effective technique because the client and family need to know that someone will be there who is supportive and nonjudgmental. Option 2 describes the nurse removing autonomy and decision making from the client and family, who already are experiencing feelings of loss of control in that they cannot change the process of dying. This is an ineffective intervention, which can impair communication further.
Test-Taking Strategy: Use the process of elimination, noting the key words "unlikely to facilitate." Understanding that persons in crisis usually feel helpless and unable to control their circumstances can assist you in identifying option 2 as a response that further removes control. Review these therapeutic interventions if you had difficulty with this question.
Level of Cognitive Ability: Comprehension
Client Needs: Psychosocial Integrity
Integrated Process: Caring
Content Area: Fundamental skills
Reference: Fortinash, K., & Holoday-Worret, P. (2000). *Psychiatric mental health nursing* (2nd ed., pp. 680-681). St. Louis: Mosby.

43. 4
Rationale: The pain of pancreatitis is aggravated by lying supine or by walking because the pancreas is located retroperitoneally, and the edema and inflammation intensify the irritation of the posterior peritoneal wall with these positions or movements. The fetal position (with the legs drawn up to the chest) may decrease the abdominal pain of pancreatitis. Positions such as sitting up, leaning forward, and flexing the legs (especially the left leg) also will alleviate some of the pain associated with pancreatitis.
Test-Taking Strategy: Use the process of elimination and note the key word "avoided." Use your critical thinking skills to visualize the anatomy of the pancreas and the potential effects from stretching associated with the various positions identified in the options. Also remember that options that are similar are not likely to be correct. This will help you to eliminate options 1, 2, and 3. Review care to the client with pancreatitis if you had difficulty with this question.
Level of Cognitive Ability: Analysis
Client Needs: Physiological Integrity
Integrated Process: Nursing Process—evaluation
Content Area: Adult health—gastrointestinal
Reference: Ignatavicius, D., & Workman, M. (2002). *Medical-surgical nursing: Critical thinking for collaborative care* (4th ed., p. 1344). Philadelphia: W. B. Saunders.

44. 1
Rationale: Following surgery to repair a fractured hip, an abductor splint is used to maintain the affected extremity in good alignment when the client is turned side to side. An overhead trapeze and bed pillow also may be used in the postoperative period, but they are not the priority items to be used in repositioning.
Test-Taking Strategy: Use the process of elimination, noting the key words "most important." Also focus on the issue, repositioning the client from side to side in the postoperative period. Use principles of client safety and knowledge of this surgical procedure to direct you to option 1. Review care to the client with a fractured hip if you had difficulty with this question.
Level of Cognitive Ability: Application
Client Needs: Physiological Integrity
Integrated Process: Nursing Process—implementation
Content Area: Adult health—musculoskeletal
Reference: Lewis, S., Heitkemper, M., & Dirksen, S. (2004). *Medical-surgical nursing: Assessment and management of clinical problems* (6th ed., p. 1677). St. Louis: Mosby.

45. 1
Rationale: If an oil-based dye is used during a myelogram, the dye is removed at the end of the procedure. The client is positioned flat in bed for 6 to 8 hours after the dye is removed. When a water-based contrast medium is used, the client is positioned with the head of bed elevated for at least 8 hours to keep the dye from irritating the cerebral meninges.
Test-Taking Strategy: Use the process of elimination. Note the key words "oil-based contrast agent." Use knowledge regarding care to the client following this procedure to direct you to option 1. Review this procedure if you had difficulty with this question.
Level of Cognitive Ability: Application

Client Needs: Physiological Integrity
Integrated Process: Nursing Process—planning
Content Area: Adult health—neurological
Reference: Chernecky, C., & Berger, B. (2001). *Laboratory tests and diagnostic procedures* (3rd ed., p. 757). Philadelphia: W. B. Saunders.

46. **2**

Rationale: The client should avoid positions or activities that place strain on the lower back. The client should not sleep on the abdomen (prone) or on the side if the hips and knees are straight. The client should not lean forward without bending the knees, stand in one position for lengthy amounts of time, or lift anything above elbow level. For the client to stand with a foot elevated on a stool or sit using a form of lumbar support may be helpful.
Test-Taking Strategy: Use the process of elimination, noting the key word "avoid." Use knowledge of body mechanics and low back injury to answer the question. If you had difficulty with this question, review client teaching points related to lower back pain.
Level of Cognitive Ability: Analysis
Client Needs: Health Promotion and Maintenance
Integrated Process: Teaching/Learning
Content Area: Adult health—musculoskeletal
Reference: Lewis, S., Heitkemper, M., & Dirksen, S. (2004). *Medical-surgical nursing: Assessment and management of clinical problems* (6th ed., pp. 1700-1701). St. Louis: Mosby.

47. **3**

Rationale: The head of the client at risk for or with increased intracranial pressure should be positioned so the head is in a neutral, midline position. The nurse should avoid flexing or extending the neck or turning the head side to side. The head of bed should be raised to 30 to 45 degrees. Use of proper positions promotes venous drainage from the cranium to keep intracranial pressure down.
Test-Taking Strategy: Use the process of elimination, noting the key words "at risk for increased intracranial pressure" and "avoid." Visualize each of the positions identified in the options and identify the position that is detrimental to the client with increased intracranial pressure. This would be the position that interferes with arterial circulation to the brain or with venous drainage from the brain. The only position that meets one of those criteria is option 3. Review care to the client at risk for or with increased intracranial pressure if you had difficulty with this question.
Level of Cognitive Ability: Application
Client Needs: Physiological Integrity
Integrated Process: Nursing Process—implementation
Content Area: Adult health—neurological
Reference: Ignatavicius, D., & Workman, M. (2002). *Medical-surgical nursing: Critical thinking for collaborative care* (4th ed., p. 1004). Philadelphia: W. B. Saunders.

48. **3**

Rationale: The normal pH is 7.35 to 7.45. The normal P_{CO_2} is 35 to 45 mm Hg. In respiratory acidosis the pH is low and the P_{CO_2} is elevated. Options 1, 2, and 4 are incorrect interpretations of the values identified in the question.

Test-Taking Strategy: Remember that in a respiratory imbalance you will find an opposite response between the pH and the P_{CO_2}. Also remember that the pH is down in an acidotic condition. Recalling this information will allow you to eliminate each of the incorrect options. Review interpretation of blood gas results if you had difficulty with this question.
Level of Cognitive Ability: Analysis
Client Needs: Physiological Integrity
Integrated Process: Nursing Process—analysis
Content Area: Fundamental skills
Reference: Chernecky, C., & Berger, B. (2001). *Laboratory tests and diagnostic procedures* (3rd ed., p. 227). Philadelphia: W. B. Saunders.

49. **4**

Rationale: To prevent acute adrenal insufficiency, glucocorticoids should not be discontinued abruptly. These medications can cause sodium and water retention and the loss of potassium, and clients should be instructed to limit sodium intake and consume potassium-rich foods. Additionally, adequate dietary intake is important. These medications can increase the risk of infection, and the client should avoid contact with persons who are ill.
Test-Taking Strategy: Use the process of elimination. Note the key words "indicate a need for further instruction." You should be able to eliminate options 1, 2, and 3 easily, remembering that the client should not stop these medications, or in fact any medication, without physician approval. Review the administration of glucocorticoids if you had difficulty with this question.
Level of Cognitive Ability: Analysis
Client Needs: Physiological Integrity
Integrated Process: Teaching/Learning
Content Area: Pharmacology
Reference: Hodgson, B., & Kizior, R. (2003). *Saunders nursing drug handbook 2003* (p. 282). Philadelphia: W. B. Saunders.

50. **2**

Rationale: NPH insulin is an intermediate-acting insulin. The onset of action for NPH insulin is 1 to 2 hours, and it peaks in 6 to 14 hours, and its duration of action is 24 hours.
Test-Taking Strategy: Read the question carefully, noting that the question is asking about NPH insulin. Knowledge regarding the onset of action, peak, and duration of action is required to answer the question. Review these points regarding NPH and regular insulin if you had difficulty with this question.
Level of Cognitive Ability: Application
Client Needs: Physiological Integrity
Integrated Process: Nursing Process—implementation
Content Area: Pharmacology
Reference: Lehne, R. (2001). *Pharmacology for nursing care* (4th ed., p. 617). Philadelphia: W. B. Saunders.

51. **2**

Rationale: The client's operative arm should be positioned so that it is elevated on a pillow and not exceeding shoulder elevation. This promotes optimal drainage from the limb without impairing the circulation to the arm. If the arm is positioned flat (option 3) or dependent (option 4), this could increase the edema in the arm, which is contraindicated because of lymphatic disruption caused by surgery.

Test-Taking Strategy: Use the process of elimination. Read each option carefully and attempt to visualize the positions identified in the options. Using the principles of circulation and gravity will direct you easily to option 2. Option 2 is the option that avoids the two extremes of height in positioning the limb affected by surgery. Review care to the client following mastectomy if you had difficulty with this question.

Level of Cognitive Ability: Application
Client Needs: Physiological Integrity
Integrated Process: Nursing Process—planning
Content Area: Adult health—oncology
Reference: Ignatavicius, D., & Workman, M. (2002). *Medical-surgical nursing: Critical thinking for collaborative care* (4th ed., p. 1744). Philadelphia: W. B. Saunders.

52. 4
Rationale: The woman with a urinary tract infection must be encouraged to take the medication for the entire time it is prescribed. The woman also should be instructed to drink at least 3000 mL of fluid each day to flush the infection from the bladder and to urinate frequently throughout the day. Foods and fluids that acidify the urine need to be encouraged.

Test-Taking Strategy: Use the process of elimination. Note the key words "indicate a need for further instructions." Recall that foods and fluids that acidify the urine should be consumed rather that foods and fluids that cause urine alkalinity. If you had difficulty with this question, review nursing considerations for the client with a urinary tract infection.

Level of Cognitive Ability: Analysis
Client Needs: Physiological Integrity
Integrated Process: Teaching/Learning
Content Area: Maternity/Postpartum
Reference: McKenry, L., & Salerno, E. (2003). *Mosby's pharmacology in nursing* (21st ed., pp. 791-792). St. Louis: Mosby.

53. 4
Rationale: Case management represents an interdisciplinary health care delivery system to promote appropriate use of hospital personnel and material resources to maximize hospital revenues while providing for optimal outcome of client care. Options 1, 2, and 3 are inaccurate statements regarding case management.

Test-Taking Strategy: Use the process of elimination and knowledge regarding the characteristics of case management. Review the characteristics of case management if you had difficulty with this question.

Level of Cognitive Ability: Application
Client Needs: Safe, Effective Care Environment
Integrated Process: Teaching/Learning
Content Area: Leadership/Management
Reference: Potter, P., & Perry, A. (2001). *Fundamentals of nursing* (5th ed., p. 44). St. Louis: Mosby.

54. 3
Rationale: The nurse must emphasize to the client and family that they are not eating a diabetic diet but rather a balanced meal plan. Adherence to nutrition principles is an important component of diabetic management, and an individualized meal plan should be developed for the client. The client does not need to purchase special dietetic foods.

Test-Taking Strategy: Use the process of elimination. Note the key words "indicates a need for further teaching." Careful reading of this question and the options will direct you easily to the correct option. Review dietary instructions for the client with diabetes mellitus if you had difficulty with this question.

Level of Cognitive Ability: Analysis
Client Needs: Health Promotion and Maintenance
Integrated Process: Teaching/Learning
Content Area: Adult health—endocrine
Reference: Williams, S., & Schlenker, E. (2003). *Essentials of nutrition & diet therapy* (8th ed., p. 509). St. Louis: Mosby.

55. 3
Rationale: NPH is an intermediate-acting insulin. The onset of action of NPH insulin is 1 to 2 hours, it peaks in 6 to 14 hours, and its duration of action is 24 hours. Hypoglycemic reactions most likely occur during peak time.

Test-Taking Strategy: Use the process of elimination and knowledge regarding the onset, peak, and duration of action for NPH Insulin. Recalling that peak action is between 4 to 12 hours will direct you easily to option 3. Review the characteristics of NPH insulin if you had difficulty with this question.

Level of Cognitive Ability: Analysis
Client Needs: Physiological Integrity
Integrated Process: Nursing Process—assessment
Content Area: Adult health—endocrine
Reference: Lehne, R. (2001). *Pharmacology for nursing care* (4th ed., p. 617). Philadelphia: W. B. Saunders.

56. 3
Rationale: Tertiary prevention involves the reduction of the amount and degree of disability, injury, and damage following a crisis. Primary prevention means keeping the crisis from ever occurring, and secondary prevention focuses on reducing the intensity and duration of the crisis during the crisis itself. No fourth prevention level exists.

Test-Taking Strategy: Identify the scenario in the question and the role of the nurse in the question. Focus on these nursing roles and use knowledge regarding the various levels of prevention to answer the question. If you had difficulty with this question, review the levels of prevention.

Level of Cognitive Ability: Comprehension
Client Needs: Safe, Effective Care Environment
Integrated Process: Nursing Process—implementation
Content Area: Leadership/Management
Reference: Fortinash, K., & Holoday-Worret, P. (2000). *Psychiatric mental health nursing* (2nd ed., p. 22). St. Louis: Mosby.

57. 4
Rationale: Rubella virus is spread by aerosol droplet transmission through the upper respiratory tract and has an incubation period of 14 to 21 days. The risk of maternal and subsequent fetal infection during the second trimester includes hearing loss and congenital anomalies. Rubella titer determination is a standard antenatal test for childbearing women during their initial screening and entry into the health care delivery system. Option 4 helps to clarify maternal concerns with accurate

information based on the acquisition of rubella infection and potential fetal side effects.

Test-Taking Strategy: Use the process of elimination and knowledge regarding the transmission of rubella virus to the fetus. Use of therapeutic communication techniques also will direct you to option 4. Option 4 addresses the client's concerns. Review concepts related to exposure to rubella during pregnancy if you had difficulty with this question.

Level of Cognitive Ability: Application
Client Need: Psychosocial Integrity
Integrated Process: Nursing Process—implementation
Content Area: Maternity/Antepartum
Reference: Murray, S., McKinney, E., & Gorrie, T. (2002). *Foundations of maternal-newborn nursing* (3rd ed., p. 724). Philadelphia: W. B. Saunders.

58. 1

Rationale: Breast-feeding mothers need to be encouraged to limit dairy products. Cheese is a dairy product. Alternative calcium sources that can be consumed by the mother include egg yolk; green, leafy vegetables; dried beans; cauliflower; and molasses.

Test-Taking Strategy: Use the process of elimination. Note the key word "avoid" in the stem of the question. Knowledge that lactose is the sugar found in dairy products will direct you easily to option 1. Review the dietary management for the infant with lactose intolerance if you had difficulty with this question.

Level of Cognitive Ability: Application
Client Needs: Health Promotion and Maintenance
Integrated Process: Nursing Process—implementation
Content Area: Maternity/Postpartum
Reference: Murray, S., McKinney, E., & Gorrie, T. (2002). *Foundations of maternal-newborn nursing* (3rd ed., pp. 205, 578). Philadelphia: W. B. Saunders.

59. 1

Rationale: The nurse needs to be aware of the effective and ineffective coping mechanisms that can occur in a client when loss is anticipated. The expression of anger is known to be a normal response to impending loss, and the anger may be directed toward the self, God or other spiritual being, or toward the caregivers. Notifying the hospital lawyer is inappropriate. Guilt may or may not be a component of the client's feelings, and the data in the question do not provide indication that guilt is present.

Test-Taking Strategy: Focus on the data provided in the question. Note that options 1 and 4 address coping mechanisms. This provides you with the clue that one of these options may be the correct response. Additionally, knowledge of the stages of grief associated with loss will direct you easily to option 1. Review these stages and expected client responses if you had difficulty with this question.

Level of Cognitive Ability: Analysis
Client Needs: Psychosocial Integrity
Integrated Process: Nursing Process—analysis
Content Area: Mental Health
Reference: Fortinash, K., & Holoday-Worret, P. (2000). *Psychiatric mental health nursing* (2nd ed., p. 718). St. Louis: Mosby.

60. 3

Rationale: An autopsy is required by state law in certain circumstances, including the sudden death of a client and a death that occurs under suspicious circumstances. A client may have provided oral or written instructions regarding an autopsy following death. If an autopsy is not required by law, these oral or written requests will be granted. If no oral or written instructions were provided, state law determines who has the authority to consent for an autopsy. Most often the decision rests with the surviving relative or next of kin.

Test-Taking Strategy: Note the key words "most appropriate." Use knowledge regarding the laws and issues surrounding autopsy and therapeutic communication techniques to answer the question. Eliminate options 1 and 4 because these statements are not completely accurate. From the remaining options, option 3 is the most therapeutic and appropriate response to the family. Review the issues and laws surrounding autopsy if you had difficulty with this question.

Level of Cognitive Ability: Application
Client Needs: Safe, Effective Care Environment
Integrated Process: Caring
Content Area: Fundamental skills
Reference: Potter, P., & Perry, A. (2001). *Fundamentals of nursing* (5th ed., pp. 436-637). St. Louis: Mosby.

61. 3

Rationale: The mode of perinatal transmission of human immunodeficiency virus (HIV) to the fetus or neonate of an HIV-positive woman can occur during the antenatal, intrapartal, or postpartum periods. Transmission of HIV can occur during breast-feeding. Therefore HIV-positive clients should be encouraged to bottle-feed their neonates. Frequent hand washing is encouraged. Support groups and community agencies can be identified to assist the parents with the newborn infant's home care, the impact of the diagnosis of HIV infection, and available financial resources. Newborn infants of HIV-positive clients are recommended to receive antiviral medications for the first 6 weeks of life.

Test-Taking Strategy: Use the process of elimination. Note the key word "need for further instructions" in the stem of the question. Recalling that breast-feeding is discouraged in the HIV-positive woman will direct you easily to the correct option. Review home care measures for the HIV-positive client if you had difficulty with this question.

Level of Cognitive Ability: Analysis
Client Need: Safe, Effective Care Environment
Integrated Process: Teaching/Learning
Content Area: Maternity/Postpartum
Reference: Murray, S., McKinney, E., & Gorrie, T. (2002). *Foundations of maternal-newborn nursing* (3rd ed., p. 728). Philadelphia: W. B. Saunders.

62. 2

Rationale: With active herpetic genital lesions, cesarean delivery can reduce neonatal infection risks. In the absence of active genital lesions, vaginal delivery is indicated unless there are other indications for cesarean delivery. Maternal isolation is not necessary, but potentially exposed newborn infants should have cultures taken on the day of delivery.

Test-Taking Strategy: Use the process of elimination. Knowledge regarding the transmission of genital herpes to the newborn infant is required to answer this question. If you had difficulty with this question, review this content area.
Level of Cognitive Ability: Application
Client Need: Safe, Effective Care Environment
Integrated Process: Nursing Process—implementation
Content Area: Maternity/Antepartum
Reference: Murray, S., McKinney, E., & Gorrie, T. (2002). *Foundations of maternal-newborn nursing* (3rd ed., p. 725). Philadelphia: W. B. Saunders.

63. 2
Rationale: Viral conjunctivitis is extremely contagious. The child should be kept home from school or day care until the child has received antibiotic eye drops for 24 hours.
Test-Taking Strategy: Use the process of elimination. Recalling that viral conjunctivitis is highly contagious will assist you in eliminating option 1. Eliminate option 4 next because this time frame is lengthy. From the remaining options, knowledge regarding the action of antibiotics will assist in directing you to option 2. Review infection control measures related to viral conjunctivitis if you had difficulty with this question.
Level of Cognitive Ability: Application
Client Needs: Safe, Effective Care Environment
Integrated Process: Teaching/Learning
Content Area: Child health
Reference: James, S., Ashwill, J., & Droske, S. (2002). *Nursing care of children: Principles & practice* (2nd ed., p. 1048). Philadelphia: W. B. Saunders.

64. 1
Rationale: If the child wears contact lenses, the child should be instructed to discontinue wearing them until the infection had cleared completely. Securing new contact lenses will eliminate the chance of reinfection from contaminated contact lenses and also will lessen the risk of a corneal ulceration.
Test-Taking Strategy: Use the process of elimination. Note the key words "need for further information" in the stem of the question. Options 2, 3, and 4 are similar in that they relate to avoiding the use of contact lenses during infection. If you had difficulty with this question, review treatment measures for conjunctivitis.
Level of Cognitive Ability: Application
Client Needs: Safe, Effective Care Environment
Integrated Process: Teaching/Learning
Content Area: Child health
Reference: James, S., Ashwill, J., & Droske, S. (2002). *Nursing care of children: Principles & practice* (2nd ed., p. 1048). Philadelphia: W. B. Saunders.

65. 1
Rationale: During pregnancy, the breasts change in size and appearance. The increase in size is due to the effects of estrogen and progesterone. Estrogen stimulates the growth of mammary ductal tissue, and progesterone promotes the growth of lobes, lobules, and alveoli. A delicate network of veins is often visible just beneath the surface of the skin. Options 2, 3, and 4 are incorrect.

Test-Taking Strategy: Use the process of elimination. Knowledge regarding the physiological changes that occur during pregnancy is required to answer this question. If you are unfamiliar with the effects of hormones and the changes that occur, review this content.
Level of Cognitive Ability: Comprehension
Client Needs: Physiological Integrity
Integrated Process: Nursing Process—planning
Content Area: Maternity/Antepartum
Reference: Lowdermilk, D., & Perry, S. (2003). *Maternity nursing* (6th ed., p. 174). St. Louis: Mosby.

66. 2
Rationale: Aspiration is a possible complication associated with nasogastric tube feeding. The head of the bed is elevated 30 to 45 degrees for at least 30 minutes following bolus tube feeding to prevent vomiting and aspiration. The right lateral position uses gravity to facilitate gastric retention to prevent vomiting. The flat supine position is to be avoided for the first 30 minutes after a tube feeding.
Test-Taking Strategy: Use the process of elimination. Note that each answer has three components: the level of elevation of the head, the client's position, and the duration. You can eliminate option 1 immediately because this position could result in aspiration. Option 2 and 4 are the same elevation, but the right lateral position is the correct position, and 60 minutes is the correct duration. Eliminate option 3 because of the supine position and the longer duration. Review care to the client receiving a bolus tube feeding if you had difficulty with this question.
Level of Cognitive Ability: Application
Client Needs: Physiological Integrity
Integrated Process: Nursing Process—implementation
Content Area: Adult health—gastrointestinal
Reference: Ignatavicius, D., & Workman, M. (2002). *Medical-surgical nursing: Critical thinking for collaborative care* (4th ed., p. 1210). Philadelphia: W. B. Saunders.

67. 4
Rationale: All the stomach contents are aspirated and measured before administering a tube feeding. This procedure measures the gastric residual. The gastric residual is assessed to confirm whether undigested formula from a previous feeding remains and thereby evaluates absorption of the last feeding. Assessment of gastric residual is important because administration of a tube feeding to a full stomach could result in overdistention, thus predisposing the client to regurgitation and possible aspiration. Options 1, 2, and 3 do not relate to the purpose of assessing residual.
Test-Taking Strategy: Use the process of elimination. Focusing on the issue, the purpose of assessing residual, will direct you to option 4. Review the purpose of this procedure if you had difficulty with this question
Level of Cognitive Ability: Comprehension
Client Needs: Physiological Integrity
Integrated Process: Nursing Process—assessment
Content Area: Adult health—gastrointestinal
Reference: Lewis, S., Heitkemper, M., & Dirksen, S. (2004). *Medical-surgical nursing: Assessment and management of clinical problems* (6th ed., p. 984). St. Louis: Mosby.

68. 4

Rationale: Factors that increase the risk of otitis media include exposure to illness in other children in day care centers, household smoking, bottle-feeding, and congenital conditions such as Down syndrome and cleft palate. The use of a pacifier beyond age 6 months also has been identified as a risk factor. Allergies also are thought to precipitate otitis media.

Test-Taking Strategy: Use the process of elimination. Note the key word "unassociated" in the stem of the question. Careful reading of each of the options will direct you quickly to option 4. If you had difficulty with this question, review the risk factors associated with otitis media.

Level of Cognitive Ability: Analysis

Client Needs: Health Promotion and Maintenance

Integrated Process: Nursing Process—assessment

Content Area: Child health

Reference: James, S., Ashwill, J., & Droske, S. (2002). *Nursing care of children: Principles & practice* (2nd ed., p. 630). Philadelphia: W. B. Saunders.

69. 3

Rationale: A lateral recumbent position with the knees flexed to the abdomen and the head bent with the chin resting on the chest is assumed for a lumbar puncture. This position separates the spinal processes and facilitates needle insertion into the subarachnoid space. Options 1, 2, and 4 are incorrect positions.

Test-Taking Strategy: Use the process of elimination. Note the key word "lumbar" in the question. Visualize each of the descriptions of positions described in the options and focus on the key word to direct you to option 3. Review this procedure if you are unfamiliar with it.

Level of Cognitive Ability: Application

Client Needs: Physiological Integrity

Integrated Process: Nursing Process—implementation

Content Area: Child health

Reference: Chernecky, C., & Berger, B. (2001). *Laboratory tests and diagnostic procedures* (3rd ed., p. 694). Philadelphia: W. B. Saunders.

70. 2

Rationale: An insulin vial in current use can be kept at room temperature for up to 1 month without significant loss of activity. Direct sunlight and heat must be avoided.

Test-Taking Strategy: Use the process of elimination. Note the key word "unrefrigerated" in the stem of the question. This word will assist in directing you to the correct option. If you are unfamiliar with the concepts related to insulin stability, review this information.

Level of Cognitive Ability: Application

Client Needs: Physiological Integrity

Integrated Process: Teaching/Learning

Content Area: Pharmacology

Reference: Lehne, R. (2001). *Pharmacology for nursing care* (4th ed., p. 617). Philadelphia: W. B. Saunders.

71. 3

Rationale: Based on the location of the surgical procedure, spinal anesthesia would not be used. Additionally, the hair would not be shaved. Although coughing (vigorous coughing is avoided) and deep breathing is important, specific to this procedure is avoiding toothbrushing to prevent disruption of the surgical site.

Test-Taking Strategy: Consider the anatomical location and the surgical procedure itself to eliminate options 1 and 4. Next, note the key words "most important." Because of the anatomical location of the surgery, option 3 is most important. Review this surgical procedure if you had difficulty with this question.

Level of Cognitive Ability: Application

Client Needs: Physiological Integrity

Integrated Process: Teaching/Learning

Content Area: Adult health—endocrine

Reference: Lewis, S., Heitkemper, M., & Dirksen, S. (2004). *Medical-surgical nursing: Assessment and management of clinical problems* (6th ed., p. 1305). St. Louis: Mosby.

72. 3

Rationale: Common manifestations of Addison's disease include postural hypotension from fluid loss, syncope, muscle weakness, anorexia, nausea and vomiting, abdominal cramps, weight loss, depression, and irritability. Options 1, 2, and 4 are not specific to this disorder.

Test-Taking Strategy: Use the process of elimination and knowledge regarding the clinical manifestations associated with Addison's disease to answer this question. If you had difficulty with this question, review the clinical manifestations of this disorder.

Level of Cognitive Ability: Analysis

Client Needs: Physiological Integrity

Integrated Process: Nursing Process—assessment

Content Area: Adult health—endocrine

Reference: Ignatavicius, D., & Workman, M. (2002). *Medical-surgical nursing: Critical thinking for collaborative care* (4th ed., p. 403). Philadelphia: W. B. Saunders.

73. 3

Rationale: Effleurage is massage of the abdomen during contractions. Women learn to do effleurage using both hands in a circular motion. Progressive relaxation involves contracting and then consciously releasing different muscle groups. Neuromuscular disassociation helps the woman relax her body even when one group of muscles is strongly contracted. In this procedure the woman contracts an area such as an arm or leg then concentrates on letting tension go from the rest of the body. Touch relaxation helps the woman to learn to loosen taut muscles when she is touched by her partner.

Test-Taking Strategy: Use the process of elimination, focusing on the issue, effleurage. You must know the procedure for this technique to answer the question correctly. If you had difficulty with this question or are unfamiliar with this cutaneous stimulation technique, review this technique.

Level of Cognitive Ability: Application

Client Needs: Physiological Integrity

Integrated Process: Teaching/Learning

Content Area: Maternity/Antepartum

Reference: Lowdermilk, D., & Perry, S. (2003). *Maternity nursing* (6th ed., p. 280). St. Louis: Mosby.

74. **2**

Rationale: Fresh fruits and vegetables will provide vitamins and minerals needed for healthy gums. Cracked wheat bread may abrade the tender gums; drinking water with meals has no direct effect on gums; saltine crackers before arising helps decrease nausea.

Test-Taking Strategy: Use the process of elimination and focus on the issue of the question. Eliminate options 1 and 4 first because these measures could produce irritation to any fragile gums. From the remaining options, eliminate option 3, remembering that drinking water with meals has no direct effect on gums. Review measures that promote dental health during pregnancy if you had difficulty with this question.

Level of Cognitive Ability: Analysis
Client Needs: Physiological Integrity
Integrated Process: Teaching/Learning
Content Area: Maternity/Antepartum
Reference: Lowdermilk, D., & Perry, S. (2003). *Maternity nursing* (6th ed., p. 248). St. Louis: Mosby.

75. **2**

Rationale: Radiation therapy usually is delayed until a child is 8 years of age whenever possible to prevent retardation of bone growth and soft tissue development. Options 1, 3, and 4 are inappropriate responses to the mother.

Test-Taking Strategy: Note the age of the child in the question. Additionally, use therapeutic communication techniques and knowledge regarding the effects of radiation to answer this question. Options 1 and 4 are nontherapeutic and place the mother's inquiry on hold. From the remaining options, use the child's age as a guide in directing you to option 2. Review the effects of radiation therapy if you had difficulty with this question.

Level of Cognitive Ability: Application
Client Needs: Physiological Integrity
Integrated Process: Nursing Process—implementation
Content Area: Child health
Reference: James, S., Ashwill, J., & Droske, S. (2002). *Nursing care of children: Principles & practice* (2nd ed., p. 795). Philadelphia: W. B. Saunders.

76. **1**

Rationale: Neuroblastoma is a solid tumor found only in children. Neuroblastoma arises from neural crest cells that normally develop into the sympathetic nervous system and the adrenal medulla. Typically, the tumor compresses adjacent normal tissue and organs. Neuroblastoma cells may excrete catecholamines and their metabolites. Urine samples will indicate elevated vanillylmandelic acid levels. The presence of blast cells in the bone marrow occurs in leukemia. Projectile vomiting occurring most often in the morning and a positive Babinski's sign are clinical manifestations of a brain tumor.

Test-Taking Strategy: Use the process of elimination. If you are unfamiliar with this type of tumor, recall that blast cells are noted in leukemia and eliminate option 2. Next, eliminate options 3 and 4, noting that these manifestations are found in the child with a brain tumor. Review the manifestations associated with neuroblastoma if you had difficulty with this question.

Level of Cognitive Ability: Analysis
Client Needs: Physiological Integrity
Integrated Process: Nursing Process—assessment
Content Area: Child health
Reference: Chernecky, C., & Berger, B. (2001). *Laboratory tests and diagnostic procedures* (3rd ed., p. 1054). Philadelphia: W. B. Saunders.

77. **3**

Rationale: Filipinos view pain as part of living an honorable life. The client may appear stoic and be tolerant of a high degree of pain. Health care providers need to offer and in fact encourage pain relief interventions for the Filipino client who does not complain of pain despite physiological indicators. Option 3 is the most appropriate intervention to include in the plan of care.

Test-Taking Strategy: Note the key words "most appropriately." Use the process of elimination and knowledge of cultural responses to pain in the Filipino client to answer this question. If you had difficulty with this question, review these cultural differences.

Level of Cognitive Ability: Application
Client Needs: Physiological Integrity
Integrated Process: Nursing Process—planning
Content Area: Fundamental skills
Reference: Potter, P., & Perry, A. (2001). *Fundamentals of nursing* (5th ed., p. 1290). St. Louis: Mosby.

78. **4**

Rationale: The nurse needs to stress the importance of immunizations, dental hygiene, and routine well-child care. Options 1, 2, and 3 are appropriate. The nurse also should instruct the parents in the measures to implement in the event of blunt trauma, especially trauma involving the joints, and to apply prolonged pressure to superficial wounds until the bleeding has stopped.

Test-Taking Strategy: Use the process of elimination. Note the key words "indicates a need for further instructions." Knowledge that bleeding is a concern in this disorder will assist you in eliminating options 1, 2, and 3, which include measures of protection and safety for the child. If you had difficulty with this question, review home care instructions for the child with hemophilia.

Level of Cognitive Ability: Analysis
Client Needs: Health Promotion and Maintenance
Integrated Process: Teaching/Learning
Content Area: Child health
Reference: Wong, D., Perry, S., & Hockenberry, M. (2002). *Maternal child nursing care* (2nd ed., p. 1368). St. Louis: Mosby.

79. **4**

Rationale: Mexican foods are rich in color, flavor, texture, and spiciness. In the Mexican American culture, any occasion is seen as a time to celebrate with food and enjoy the companionship of family and friends. Because food is a primary form of socialization in the Mexican culture, Mexican Americans may have difficulty adhering to a prescribed diet. Asian Americans eat raw fish, rice, and soy sauce. European Americans prefer carbohydrates and red meat.

Test-Taking Strategy: Use the process of elimination and knowledge regarding the food practices and preferences and the meaning of food in the Mexican American culture. If you had difficulty with this question, review the food preferences associated with this culture.
Level of Cognitive Ability: Comprehension
Client Needs: Physiological Integrity
Integrated Process: Nursing Process—planning
Content Area: Fundamental skills
Reference: Williams, S. (2001). *Basic nutrition & diet therapy* (11th ed., p. 220). St Louis: Mosby.

80. 2
Rationale: The nurse must determine the most appropriate assignment based on the skills of the staff member and the needs of the client. In this case, the most appropriate assignment for a nursing assistant would be to care for a client on bed rest who requires range of motion exercises. The nursing assistant is trained in this procedure. The client receiving chemotherapy and the client receiving a blood transfusion require the assessment skills that a licensed nurse has. The client with diabetes mellitus who is being discharged will require predischarge review of diabetic management instructions and potentially coordination of necessary home care services.
Test-Taking Strategy: Note the key words "most appropriate" in the stem of the question. Use the process of elimination and recall the principles of delegation and supervision of the work of others in answering the question. Work that is delegated to others must be done consistent with the individual's level of expertise and licensure or lack of licensure. Review the principles of delegation if you had difficulty with this question.
Level of Cognitive Ability: Application
Client Needs: Safe, Effective Care Environment
Integrated Process: Nursing Process—planning
Content Area: Delegating/Prioritizing
Reference: Potter, P., & Perry, A. (2001). *Fundamentals of nursing* (5th ed., p. 359). St. Louis: Mosby.

81. 2
Rationale: An adverse effect of propylthiouracil (PTU) is agranulocytosis. The client needs to be informed of the early signs of this adverse effect, which includes fever or sore throat. Drowsiness is an occasional side effect of the medication. Increased urination and dry mouth are unrelated to this medication.
Test-Taking Strategy: Use the process of elimination. Recalling that agranulocytosis is an adverse effect of propylthiouracil (PTU) will direct you to option 2. Review the adverse effects of this medication if you had difficulty with this question.
Level of Cognitive Ability: Application
Client Needs: Physiological Integrity
Integrated Process: Teaching/Learning
Content Area: Pharmacology
Reference: Lehne, R. (2001). *Pharmacology for nursing care* (4th ed., p. 643). Philadelphia: W. B. Saunders.

82. 4
Rationale: Iodine solution can cause iodine toxicity. Iodine is corrosive, and overdose will injure the gastrointestinal tract.

Symptoms include abdominal pain, vomiting, and diarrhea. Swelling of the glottis may result in asphyxiation. Treatment consists of gastric lavage to remove iodine from the stomach and administration of sodium thiosulfate to reduce iodine to iodide. Calcium gluconate is used for acute hypocalcemia. Acetylcysteine (Mucomyst) is the antidote for acetaminophen (Tylenol) overdose. Vitamin K is the antidote for warfarin (Coumadin).
Test-Taking Strategy: Use the process of elimination. Knowledge of the specific antidotes for medication overdose is required to answer this question. You should be able to eliminate options 1, 2, and 3 easily because these medications should be familiar to you. If you are unfamiliar with iodine overdose, review this content.
Level of Cognitive Ability: Analysis
Client Needs: Physiological Integrity
Integrated Process: Nursing Process—analysis
Content Area: Pharmacology
Reference: Lehne, R. (2001). *Pharmacology for nursing care* (4th ed., p. 644). Philadelphia: W. B. Saunders.

83. 1
Rationale: In option 1, there is an implication of periorbital and facial edema that could indicate pregnancy-induced hypertension. Because the question identifies an adolescent who has not sought early prenatal care, she is at higher risk for the development of pregnancy-induced hypertension. Options 2, 3, and 4 also deal with body image, and although these comments should not be ignored, the need for follow-up is not urgent.
Test-Taking Strategy: Use the process of elimination. Note the week of the first prenatal visit (week 18). Also note the key words "immediate need." Although all of the options identify a potential alteration in body image, option 1 is the only option that identifies data that could indicate a complication of the pregnancy. Review assessment signs related to pregnancy-induced hypertension if you had difficulty with this question.
Level of Cognitive Ability: Analysis
Client Needs: Physiological Integrity
Integrated Process: Nursing Process—analysis
Content Area: Maternity/Antepartum
Reference: Murray, S., McKinney, E., & Gorrie, T. (2002). *Foundations of maternal-newborn nursing* (3rd ed., p. 143). Philadelphia: W. B. Saunders.

84. 1
Rationale: Treatment for gonorrhea consists of antibiotic therapy with ceftriaxone 125 mg intramuscularly once plus doxycycline 100 mg PO bid for 7 days; therefore option 1 is correct. Option 2 is the treatment for syphilis, option 3 is the treatment for genital herpes simplex virus, and option 4 is the treatment for chlamydia.
Test-Taking Strategy: The issue of the question is the specific medication required to treat the disease. Review content regarding gonorrhea and the medication used to treat this sexually transmitted disease if you had difficulty with this question!
Level of Cognitive Ability: Analysis
Client Needs: Physiological Integrity

Integrated Process: Nursing Process—analysis
Content Area: Pharmacology
Reference: Lowdermilk, D., & Perry, S. (2003). *Maternity nursing* (6th ed., p. 639). St. Louis: Mosby.

85. **2**
Rationale: The advanced cardiac life support nurse would place one gel pad to the right of the sternum just below the clavicle and the other gel pad to the left of the precordium. The nurse then would place the electrode paddles over the pads. Options 1, 3, and 4 identify incorrect positions.
Test-Taking Strategy: Use the process of elimination, considering the anatomical location of the heart. This will assist easily to eliminate options 1, 3, and 4. If you had difficulty with this question, review the correct placement of pads for defibrillation.
Level of Cognitive Ability: Application
Client Needs: Physiological Integrity
Integrated Process: Nursing Process—implementation
Content Area: Adult health—cardiovascular
Reference: Lewis, S., Heitkemper, M., & Dirksen, S. (2004). *Medical-surgical nursing: Assessment and management of clinical problems* (6th ed., p. 875). St. Louis: Mosby.

86. **3**
Rationale: Rubella vaccine is a live attenuated virus that evokes an antibody response that provides immunity for 15 years. Because rubella is a live vaccine, it will act as the virus and is potentially teratogenic in the organogenesis phase of fetal development. The client needs to be informed about the potential effects that this vaccine may have and the need to avoid becoming pregnant for a period of 2 to 3 months after receiving the vaccine. Abstinence from sexual intercourse is not necessary, unless another form of effective contraception is not being used. The vaccine may cause local or systemic reactions, but all are mild and short-lived. Sunlight has no effect on the person who is vaccinated.
Test-Taking Strategy: Use the process of elimination. Recalling that rubella is a live vaccine will direct you easily to option 3. Review the risks associated with the administration of this vaccine if you had difficulty with this question.
Level of Cognitive Ability: Application
Client Needs: Safe, Effective Care Environment
Integrated Process: Nursing Process—implementation
Content Area: Maternity/Postpartum
Reference: Lowdermilk, D., & Perry, S. (2003). *Maternity nursing* (6th ed., p. 399). St. Louis: Mosby.

87. **1**
Rationale: The client demonstrates the best adaptation by participating in personal care, which would include care of surgical drains that would be in place for a short time after discharge. Asking for pain medication is also an action-oriented option, but it does not relate to acceptance of the loss of the breast. Reading the postoperative care booklet is useful but is not the best of the options presented here. Refusing to look at the wound indicates no adaptation to the loss.
Test-Taking Strategy: Use the process of elimination. Note the key word "best." This tells you that more than one or all of the options may be partially or totally correct. Note that option 1

is the most action-oriented activity. Review psychosocial adaptation to the loss of a breast if you had difficulty with this question.
Level of Cognitive Ability: Analysis
Client Needs: Psychosocial Integrity
Integrated Process: Nursing Process—evaluation
Content Area: Adult health—oncology
Reference: Lewis, S., Heitkemper, M., & Dirksen, S. (2004). *Medical-surgical nursing: Assessment and management of clinical problems* (6th ed., p. 1375). St. Louis: Mosby.

88. **2**
Rationale: The client should resume activity slowly, but walking is a beneficial activity. The client should know to rest when fatigue occurs. Activities to be avoided include driving, heavy housework, wearing tight clothing, crossing the legs, and prolonged standing or sitting. Sexual activity is prohibited for 4 to 6 weeks after surgery.
Test-Taking Strategy: Use the process of elimination. Note the key words "not precipitate complications." With this in mind, evaluate each of the options in terms of the stress or harm it could cause to the perineal area. Review home care measures following vulvectomy if you had difficulty with this question.
Level of Cognitive Ability: Application
Client Needs: Physiological Integrity
Integrated Process: Teaching/Learning
Content Area: Adult health—oncology
Reference: Black, J., Hawks, J., & Keene, A. (2001). *Medical-surgical nursing: Clinical management for positive outcomes* (6th ed., p. 1077). Philadelphia: W. B. Saunders.

89. **4**
Rationale: The mother should be instructed to bring the child to the emergency room if the child develops stridor at rest, cyanosis, severe agitation or fatigue, and moderate to severe retractions or is unable to take fluids orally.
Test-Taking Strategy: Use the ABCs—airway, breathing and circulation—to answer the question. If you had difficulty with this question, review home care instructions for the child with croup.
Level of Cognitive Ability: Application
Client Needs: Physiological Integrity
Integrated Process: Teaching/Learning
Content Area: Child health
Reference: James, S., Ashwill, J., & Droske, S. (2002). *Nursing care of children: Principles & practice* (2nd ed., p. 643). Philadelphia: W. B. Saunders.

90. **1**
Rationale: When epiglottitis is suspected, the priorities are to maintain a patent airway and to obtain a chest x-ray film to confirm the diagnosis. If epiglottitis is present, the child is taken promptly to the operating room for tracheal intubation or immediate surgical airway. Epinephrine is not used to treat epiglottitis.
Test-Taking Strategy: Use the process of elimination. Note the key word "suspected" in the question. This should assist in directing you to option 1. Confirmation of the diagnosis is necessary to determine the appropriate management. If you

had difficulty with this question, review the treatment of this life threatening condition.
Level of Cognitive Ability: Analysis
Client Needs: Physiological Integrity
Integrated Process: Nursing Process—implementation
Content Area: Child health
References: James, S., Ashwill, J., & Droske, S. (2002). *Nursing care of children: Principles & practice* (2nd ed., p. 644). Philadelphia: W. B. Saunders.
Wong, D., Perry, S., & Hockenberry, M. (2002). *Maternal child nursing care* (2nd ed., p. 1201). St. Louis: Mosby.

91. 4
Rationale: For the client with sickle cell anemia, dehydration will precipitate sickling of the red blood cells. Sickling can lead to life-threatening consequences for the pregnant woman and for the fetus, such as an interruption of blood flow to the placenta. Options 1, 2, and 3 also may be appropriate nursing diagnoses for the client with sickle cell anemia but are not the priority.
Test-Taking Strategy: Use Maslow's hierarchy of needs theory, remembering that physiological needs come first. Using this principle, eliminate options 1 and 2. From the remaining options, select option 4 because it identifies an actual rather than an "at risk for" nursing diagnosis. Review sickle cell anemia if you had difficulty with this question.
Level of Cognitive Ability: Analysis
Client Needs: Physiological Integrity
Integrated Process: Nursing Process—analysis
Content Area: Delegating/Prioritizing
Reference: Murray, S., McKinney, E., & Gorrie, T. (2002). *Foundations of maternal-newborn nursing* (3rd ed., p. 719). Philadelphia: W. B. Saunders.

92. 3
Rationale: With viral pneumonia, treatment is supportive. More severely ill children may be hospitalized and given oxygen, chest physiotherapy, and intravenous fluids. Antibiotics are not given. Bacterial pneumonia, however, is treated with antibiotic therapy.
Test-Taking Strategy: Use the process of elimination. Note the key word "viral" in the question. Recalling that antibiotics are not effective in treating viruses will assist you in eliminating options 1 and 2. No data in the question support the need for intravenous fluid administration. Option 3 is also the most global response. Review the care of a child with viral pneumonia if you had difficulty with this question.
Level of Cognitive Ability: Analysis
Client Needs: Physiological Integrity
Integrated Process: Nursing Process—analysis
Content Area: Child health
Reference: James, S., Ashwill, J., & Droske, S. (2002). *Nursing care of children: Principles & practice* (2nd ed., p. 651). Philadelphia: W. B. Saunders.

93. 2
Rationale: Cystic fibrosis is a chronic multisystem disorder affecting the exocrine glands. The mucus produced by these glands (particularly those of the bronchioles, small intestine, and the pancreatic and bile ducts) is abnormally thick, causing obstruction of the small passageways of these organs. Cystic fibrosis is transmitted as an autosomal recessive trait.
Test-Taking Strategy: Use the process of elimination. Recalling that this is a multisystem disorder will direct you to option 2. Additionally, option 2 is the most global option. Review this disorder if you are unfamiliar with it.
Level of Cognitive Ability: Analysis
Client Needs: Physiological Integrity
Integrated Process: Teaching/Learning
Content Area: Child health
Reference: James, S., Ashwill, J., & Droske, S. (2002). *Nursing care of children: Principles & practice* (2nd ed., p. 674). Philadelphia: W. B. Saunders.

94. 3
Rationale: A 2% minoxidil solution is used for topical treatment of baldness. The usual dosage is 1 mL applied 2 times a day.
Test-Taking Strategy: Use the process of elimination. Eliminate options 1 and 4 because of the excessiveness of application. From the remaining options, you must know the usual dosage for this medication. Review this medication if you had difficulty with this question.
Level of Cognitive Ability: Application
Client Needs: Physiological Integrity
Integrated Process: Teaching/Learning
Content Area: Pharmacology
Reference: Lehne, R. (2001). *Pharmacology for nursing care* (4th ed., p. 1159). Philadelphia: W. B. Saunders.

95. 2
Rationale: Collagenase (Santyl) is used to promote débridement of dermal lesions and severe burns. Collagenase is applied once daily and covered with a sterile dressing.
Test-Taking Strategy: Use the process of elimination. Note the key words "indicates an accurate understanding" in the stem of the question. Eliminate options 3 and 4 first because they are similar. From the remaining options, recalling that the client with a burn is at risk for infection will direct you to option 2, the option that indicates covering the wound. Review this medication if you are unfamiliar with it.
Level of Cognitive Ability: Analysis
Client Needs: Physiological Integrity
Integrated Process: Teaching/Learning
Content Area: Pharmacology
Reference: Lehne, R. (2001). *Pharmacology for nursing care* (4th ed., p. 1145). Philadelphia: W. B. Saunders.

96. 1
Rationale: Hirschsprung's disease, also known as congenital aganglionosis or megacolon, is the result of an absence of ganglion cells in the rectum and to varying degrees upward in the colon. Options 2, 3, and 4 are incorrect.
Test-Taking Strategy: Use the process of elimination and knowledge regarding the pathophysiology associated with Hirschsprung's disease to answer this question. If you are unfamiliar with this disorder, review the pathophysiology associated with it.
Level of Cognitive Ability: Application
Client Needs: Physiological Integrity

Integrated Process: Teaching/Learning
Content Area: Child health
Reference: James, S., Ashwill, J., & Droske, S. (2002). *Nursing care of children: Principles & practice* (2nd ed., p. 572). Philadelphia: W. B. Saunders.

97. 2
Rationale: A fresh colostomy stoma will be red and edematous, but this will decrease with time. The colostomy site then will be pink without evidence of abnormal drainage, swelling, or skin breakdown. The nurse would document these findings because this is a normal expectation. Options 1, 3, and 4 are inappropriate interventions.
Test-Taking Strategy: Use the process of elimination. Note the key words "returns from surgery." You would expect redness and edema at this time. Review postoperative colostomy assessment if you had difficulty with this question.
Level of Cognitive Ability: Application
Client Needs: Physiological Integrity
Integrated Process: Nursing Process—implementation
Content Area: Child health
Reference: James, S., Ashwill, J., & Droske, S. (2002). *Nursing care of children: Principles & practice* (2nd ed., pp. 381, 546). Philadelphia: W. B. Saunders.

98. 1
Rationale: The skin of a newborn infant plays a significant role in thermoregulation and as a barrier against infection. The skin of a preterm newborn infant is immature in contrast to a term newborn infant. The skin of a preterm newborn is thin and gelatinous, with decreased amounts of subcutaneous fat, brown fat, and glycogen stores. In addition, preterm newborn infants lose heat because of the high body surface area in relation to their weight and because their posture is more relaxed with less flexion. For these reasons, preterm newborn infants are less able to generate heat, which places the preterm newborn at risk for increased heat loss and increased fluid requirements.
Test-Taking Strategy: Use the process of elimination. Focus on the issue, preterm newborn infant. Options 2, 3, and 4 are similar and address an "increased" amount of fat. Review the characteristics of a preterm newborn infant if you had difficulty with this question.
Level of Cognitive Ability: Comprehension
Client Needs: Physiological Integrity
Integrated Process: Nursing Process—planning
Content Area: Maternity/Postpartum
Reference: Murray, S., McKinney, E., & Gorrie, T. (2002). *Foundations of maternal-newborn nursing* (3rd ed., p. 506). Philadelphia: W. B. Saunders.

99. 4
Rationale: Low or oddly placed ears are associated with a variety of congenital defects and should be reported immediately. Although the findings would be documented, the most appropriate action would be to notify the physician. Options 1, 2, and 3 are inaccurate and inappropriate nursing actions.
Test-Taking Strategy: Use the process of elimination. Knowledge regarding the normal assessment findings in a newborn infant is required to answer this question. Knowledge that low set ears is an abnormal finding will direct you easily to option 4. Review normal assessment findings in a newborn if you had difficulty with this question.
Level of Cognitive Ability: Application
Client Needs: Physiological Integrity
Integrated Process: Nursing Process—implementation
Content Area: Maternity/Postpartum
Reference: Lowdermilk, D., & Perry, S. (2003). *Maternity nursing* (6th ed., p. 471). St. Louis: Mosby.

100. 1
Rationale: Jaundice, if present, is best assessed in the sclera, nailbeds, and mucous membranes. Generalized jaundice will appear in the skin throughout the body. Option 4 is not an appropriate area to assess for the presence of jaundice.
Test-Taking Strategy: Use the process of elimination. Note the key word "best" in the stem of the question. You can eliminate options 2 and 3 first because they are similar and jaundice present in the skin is generalized. From the remaining options, recalling that discoloration can be assessed best in the nailbeds will direct you to option 1. Review assessment findings related to jaundice if you had difficulty with this question.
Level of Cognitive Ability: Analysis
Client Needs: Health Promotion and Maintenance
Integrated Process: Nursing Process—assessment
Content Area: Child health
Reference: James, S., Ashwill, J., & Droske, S. (2002). *Nursing care of children: Principles & practice* (2nd ed., p. 237). Philadelphia: W. B. Saunders.

101. 2
Rationale: Stress causes increased heart workload, and the client should be instructed to avoid stress. To avoid infections, individuals with active infections should not be allowed to visit the client. Otherwise restrictions are not required. Too much weight gain can place further demands on the heart. Resting should be on the left side to promote blood return.
Test-Taking Strategy: Use the process of elimination. Note the key words "heart disease" and "the client understands her needs" in the question. Using principles related to the therapeutic management of cardiac disease in general will assist in directing you to option 2. If you had difficulty with this question, review the measures for the pregnant client with cardiac disease.
Level of Cognitive Ability: Analysis
Client Needs: Health Promotion and Maintenance
Integrated Process: Teaching/Learning
Content Area: Maternity/Antepartum
Reference: Lowdermilk, D., & Perry, S. (2003). *Maternity nursing* (6th ed., p. 587). St. Louis: Mosby.

102. 1
Rationale: Cryotherapy is a procedure that is safe to perform on the pregnant client. Cytotoxic agents are contraindicated during pregnancy because of their toxic effects. Imiquimod and podophyllin are agents used to treat human papillomavirus; however, their use in pregnancy is contraindicated.
Test-Taking Strategy: Use the process of elimination. Eliminate options 2, 3, and 4 because they are similar in that they are identify pharmacological measures. Review the treatment

modalities for human papilloma virus in the pregnant client if you had difficulty with this question.

Level of Cognitive Ability: Analysis
Client Needs: Physiological Integrity
Integrated Process: Nursing Process—planning
Content Area: Maternity/Antepartum
Reference: Lowdermilk, D., & Perry, A. (2003). *Maternity nursing* (6th ed., p. 94). St. Louis: Mosby.

103. 1
Rationale: To demonstrate respect, compassion, and understanding, health care providers should greet Mexican American clients with a handshake. On establishing rapport, providers may demonstrate further approval and respect through touch, smiling, and affirmative nods of the head. Given the diversity of dialects and the nuances of language, culturally congruent use of humor is difficult to accomplish and therefore should be avoided.
Test-Taking Strategy: Use the process of elimination and knowledge regarding the cultural communication patterns of the Mexican American. Review the characteristics of this cultural group if you had difficulty with this question.
Level of Cognitive Ability: Application
Client Needs: Psychosocial Integrity
Integrated Process: Nursing Process—implementation
Content Area: Fundamental skills
Reference: Jarvis, C. (2000). *Physical examination and health assessment* (3rd ed., p. 72). Philadelphia: W. B. Saunders.

104. 1
Rationale: Russell's traction uses skin traction to realign a fracture in the lower extremity and immobilize the hip and knee in a flexed position. Keeping the hip flexion at the prescribed angle is important to prevent fracture malalignment. The traction also may relieve pain by reducing muscle spasms, but this is not the primary reason for this traction. The child still can move in bed with some restriction as a result of the traction. Traction is never used to restrain a child.
Test-Taking Strategy: Use the process of elimination and eliminate options 2 and 3 first because they are similar. Recalling the purpose of this type of traction and noting the key word "primarily" will assist in directing you to option 1. If you had difficulty with this question, review Russell's traction.
Level of Cognitive Ability: Application
Client Needs: Physiological Integrity
Integrated Process: Nursing Process—implementation
Content Area: Child health
Reference: James, S., Ashwill, J., & Droske, S. (2002). *Nursing care of children: Principles & practice* (2nd ed., p. 857). Philadelphia: W. B. Saunders.

105. 1
Rationale: The infant should be positioned completely facing the mother with head, neck, and spine aligned. Poor positioning increases the number of attempts for latching on. Option 2 is incorrect because it demonstrates improper positioning. Options 3 and 4 are the result of improper positioning. Additionally, options 2, 3, and 4 identify complications (sore nipples, breast engorgement, cracked nipples).

Test-Taking Strategy: Use the process of elimination. Options 2, 3, and 4 are similar and identify complications (sore nipples, breast engorgement, cracked nipples). Option 1 is the only option that identifies a normal expectation. Review normal expectations of a mother who is breast-feeding if you had difficulty with this question.
Level of Cognitive Ability: Analysis
Client Needs: Health Promotion and Maintenance
Integrated Process: Nursing Process—assessment
Content Area: Maternity/Postpartum
Reference: Lowdermilk, D., & Perry, A. (2003). *Maternity nursing* (6th ed., p. 624). St. Louis: Mosby.

106. 2
Rationale: To achieve proper traction, weights need to be free-hanging with knots kept away from the pulleys. Weights are not to be kept resting on a firm surface. The head of the bed is usually kept low to provide countertraction.
Test-Taking Strategy: Use the process of elimination. Attempt to visualize the traction, recalling that there must be weight to exert the pull from the traction setup. This concept will assist in eliminating options 1 and 3. Recalling that countertraction is needed will assist in eliminating option 4. Review care to the client in traction if you had difficulty with this question.
Level of Cognitive Ability: Application
Client Needs: Physiological Integrity
Integrated Process: Nursing Process—planning
Content Area: Adult health—musculoskeletal
Reference: Black, J., Hawks, J., & Keene, A. (2001). *Medical-surgical nursing: Clinical management for positive outcomes* (6th ed., p. 610). Philadelphia: W. B. Saunders.

107. Answer:
Set the room temperature at a comfortable level.
Remove distracting objects from the interviewing area.
Ensure comfortable seating at eye level for the client and nurse.
Rationale: When preparing the physical environment for an interview, the nurse would set the room temperature at a comfortable level. The nurse would provide sufficient lighting for the client and nurse to see each other. The nurse would avoid having the client face a strong light because the client would have to squint into the full light. Distracting objects and equipment should be removed from the interview area. The nurse should arrange seating so that the nurse and client are seated comfortably at eye level and the nurse avoids facing the client across a desk or table because this creates a barrier. The nurse should set the distance between himself or herself and the client at 4 to 5 feet. If the nurse places the client any closer, the nurse will be invading the client's private space and may create anxiety in the client. If the nurse places the client farther away, the nurse may be seen as distant and aloof by the client.
Test-Taking Strategy: Read each intervention carefully. Use the guidelines for preparing the physical environment for conducting an interview to select the appropriate interventions. Review these guidelines if you had difficulty with this question.
Level of Cognitive Ability: Application
Client Needs: Health Promotion and Maintenance
Integrated Process: Nursing Process—planning
Content Area: Fundamental skills

Reference: Jarvis, C. (2000). *Physical examination and health assessment* (3rd ed., pp. 59-60). Philadelphia: W. B. Saunders.

108. 1
Rationale: Maintaining effective and open communication among family members affected by death and grief is of utmost importance. The nurse needs to maintain and enhance communication and preserve the family's sense of self-direction and control. Option 1 removes autonomy and decision making from the family at a time when they already are experiencing feelings of loss of control. This is an ineffective intervention that can impair communication. Option 2 is likely to enhance communications. Option 3 is an effective intervention because spiritual practices give meaning to life and have an impact on how persons react to crisis. Option 4 is also an effective technique, and family needs to know that someone will be there who is supportive and nonjudgmental.
Test-Taking Strategy: Note the key word "avoid" in the stem of the question. Use the process of elimination, focusing on therapeutic communication techniques to direct you to option 1. Review therapeutic techniques for individuals in crisis if you had difficulty with this question.
Level of Cognitive Ability: Application
Client Needs: Psychosocial Integrity
Integrated Process: Caring
Content Area: Fundamental skills
Reference: Potter, P., & Perry, A. (2001). *Fundamentals of nursing* (5th ed., pp. 630-631). St. Louis: Mosby.

109. 2
Rationale: The cervix undergoes significant changes following conception. The most obvious changes occur in color and consistency. In response to the increasing levels of estrogen, the cervix becomes congested with blood, resulting in the characteristic bluish color that extends to include the vagina and labia. This discoloration, referred to as Chadwick's sign, is one of the earliest signs of pregnancy.
Test-Taking Strategy: Use the process of elimination. Knowledge regarding physiological changes and the hormones responsible for these changes is required to answer this question. If you are unfamiliar with these physiological changes, review this context.
Level of Cognitive Ability: Comprehension
Client Needs: Physiological Integrity
Integrated Process: Nursing Process—assessment
Content Area: Maternity/Antepartum
Reference: Murray, S., McKinney, E., & Gorrie, T. (2002). *Foundations of maternal-newborn nursing* (3rd ed., p. 121). Philadelphia: W. B. Saunders.

110. 4
Rationale: An inactive older person may become disoriented because of lack of sensory stimulation. The most appropriate nursing intervention would be to reorient the client frequently and to place objects such as a clock and a calendar in the client's room to maintain orientation. The family can assist with orientation of the client, but it is not appropriate to ask the family to stay with the client. Prescribing laboratory studies is not the within the scope of nursing practice. Restraints may cause further disorientation and should not be applied unless specifically prescribed, and agency policies and procedures should be followed before the application of restraints.
Test-Taking Strategy: Use the process of elimination. Note the key words "most appropriate." Eliminate option 3 first because it is not within the scope of nursing practice to prescribe laboratory studies. Next, eliminate option 2 because restraints may add to the disorientation that the client is experiencing. Placing the responsibility of the client on the family is not appropriate; therefore eliminate option 1. Note the relationship between the words "disoriented" in the question and "reorient" in the correct option. Review the measures related to caring for a client who is disoriented if you had difficulty with this question.
Level of Cognitive Ability: Application
Client Needs: Psychosocial Integrity
Integrated Process: Nursing Process—implementation
Content Area: Adult health—musculoskeletal
Reference: Ebersole, P., & Hess, P. (2001). *Geriatric nursing & healthy aging* (p. 142). St. Louis: Mosby.

111. 3
Rationale: Skin traction is achieved by Ace wraps, boots, or slings that apply a direct force on the client's skin. Traction is maintained with 5 to 8 lb of weight, and this type of traction can cause skin breakdown. Skin traction has no pin sites. Urinary incontinence is not related to the use of skin traction. Although constipation can occur as a result of immobility and that assessment of bowel sounds may be a component of the assessment, this intervention is not the priority assessment.
Test-Taking Strategy: Use the process of elimination. Note the key word "priority" in the stem of the question. Eliminate option 2 first because skin traction has no pin sites. Visualizing the traction setup and knowledge of the complications associated with this type of traction will direct you easily to option 3. Review the complications associated with skin traction and the priority nursing interventions if you had difficulty with this question.
Level of Cognitive Ability: Application
Client Needs: Physiological Integrity
Integrated Process: Nursing Process—planning
Content Area: Adult health—musculoskeletal
Reference: Lewis, S., Heitkemper, M., & Dirksen, S. (2004). *Medical-surgical nursing: Assessment and management of clinical problems* (6th ed., p 1659). St. Louis: Mosby.

112. 3
Rationale: A contraction stress test assesses placental oxygenation and function, determines fetal ability to tolerate labor, determines fetal well-being, and is performed if the nonstress test is abnormal. The fetus is exposed to the stressor of contractions to assess the adequacy of placental perfusion under simulated labor conditions. An external fetal monitor is applied to the mother and a 20- to 30-minute baseline strip is recorded. The uterus is stimulated to contract by the administration of a dilute dose of oxytocin (Pitocin) or by having the mother use nipple stimulation until three palpable contractions with a duration of 40 seconds or more in a 10-minute period have been achieved. Frequent maternal blood pressure readings are done, and the client is monitored closely while increasing doses of oxytocin are given. Options 1, 2, and 4 are inaccurate.

Test-Taking Strategy: Use the process of elimination. Eliminate option 1 because of the words "internal fetal monitor." Eliminate option 2 because a treadmill is not used to stimulate contractions. From the remaining options, recalling that the uterus is stimulated to contract by use of small amounts of oxytocin (Pitocin) or by nipple stimulation will direct you to option 3. If you had difficulty answering this question, review the contraction stress test.
Level of Cognitive Ability: Application
Client Needs: Physiological Integrity
Integrated Process: Nursing Process—implementation
Content Area: Maternity/Antepartum
Reference: Chernecky, C., & Berger, B. (2001). *Laboratory tests and diagnostic procedures* (3rd ed., pp. 505-506). Philadelphia: W. B. Saunders.

113. 4

Rationale: Strabismus, also called lazy eye, is a condition in which the eyes are not aligned because of lack of coordination of the extraocular muscles. Strabismus is normal in the young infant but should not be present after about age 4 months. Options 1, 2, and 3 are not appropriate responses to the mother of a 1-month-old infant.
Test-Taking Strategy: Use the process of elimination and note the key words "1-month-old infant" and "most appropriate." Also use therapeutic communication techniques. Options 1, 2, and 3 may cause fear and concern in the mother. If you had difficulty with this question, review this disorder.
Level of Cognitive Ability: Application
Client Needs: Psychosocial Integrity
Integrated Process: Caring
Content Area: Child health
Reference: James, S., Ashwill, J., & Droske, S. (2002). *Nursing care of children: Principles & practice* (2nd ed., pp. 1044-1046). Philadelphia: W. B. Saunders.

114. 3

Rationale: Patching may be used to treat strabismus to strengthen the weak eye. In this treatment the "good" eye is patched. This encourages the child to use the weaker eye. Patching is most successful when done during the preschool years. The schedule for patching is individualized and is prescribed by the ophthalmologist.
Test-Taking Strategy: Use the process of elimination. Remembering that this condition is a "lazy eye" will direct you to the correct option. Patching the unaffected eye to strengthen the muscles in the affected eye makes sense. Review the procedure for patching if you had difficulty with this question.
Level of Cognitive Ability: Application
Client Needs: Physiological Integrity
Integrated Process: Teaching/Learning
Content Area: Child health
Reference: James, S., Ashwill, J., & Droske, S. (2002). *Nursing care of children: Principles & practice* (2nd ed., p. 1046). Philadelphia: W. B. Saunders.

115. 2

Rationale: Contraction stress test results may be interpreted as negative (normal), positive (abnormal), or equivocal. A negative test result indicates that no late decelerations occurred in

the fetal heart rate, although the fetus was stressed by three contractions of at least 40 seconds' duration in a 10-minute period. Repetitive late decelerations render the test results positive.
Test-Taking Strategy: Use the process of elimination, noting that options 1, 3, and 4 are similar in that they indicate an abnormal test result finding. If you had difficulty with this question and are unfamiliar with the interpretation of the results of a contraction stress test, review this content.
Level of Cognitive Ability: Analysis
Client Needs: Physiological Integrity
Integrated Process: Nursing Process—analysis
Content Area: Maternity/Antepartum
References: Chernecky, C., & Berger, B. (2001). *Laboratory tests and diagnostic procedures* (3rd ed., pp. 505-506). Philadelphia: W. B. Saunders.
Lowdermilk, D., & Perry, A. (2003). *Maternity nursing* (6th ed., p. 562). St. Louis: Mosby.

116. 4

Rationale: A successful outcome for the nursing diagnosis of Self-Care Deficit is for the client to do as much of the self-care as possible. The nurse should promote independence in the client and allow the client to perform as much self-care as is optimal considering the client's condition. The nurse would determine that the outcome is unsuccessful if the client refused care or allows others to do the care.
Test-Taking Strategy: Use the process of elimination. Focusing on the key words "successful outcome" will assist in eliminating the incorrect options. Additionally, note that options 1 and 2 are similar and should be eliminated. Review successful outcomes related to the nursing diagnosis of Self-Care Deficit if you had difficulty with this question.
Level of Cognitive Ability: Analysis
Client Needs: Physiological Integrity
Integrated Process: Nursing Process—evaluation
Content Area: Adult health—musculoskeletal
Reference: Ignatavicius, D., & Workman, M. (2002). *Medical-surgical nursing: Critical thinking for collaborative care* (4th ed., p. 128). Philadelphia: W. B. Saunders.

117. 3

Rationale: A psychosocial assessment of the client who is immobilized most appropriately would include the need for sensory stimulation. This assessment also should include factors such as body image, past and present coping skills, and the coping methods used during the period of immobilization. Although transportation, home care support, and the ability to perform activities of daily living are components of an assessment, they are not as specifically related to psychosocial adjustment as is the need for sensory stimulation.
Test-Taking Strategy: Use the process of elimination and focus on the key words "psychosocial" and "most appropriately." Option 2 can be eliminated first because it relates to physiological integrity rather than psychosocial integrity. Next eliminate options 1 and 4 because they are related most closely to physical supports rather than psychosocial needs of the client. Review the components of a psychosocial assessment if you had difficulty with this question.
Level of Cognitive Ability: Analysis

Client Needs: Psychosocial Integrity
Integrated Process: Nursing Process—assessment
Content Area: Adult health—musculoskeletal
Reference: Potter, P., & Perry, A. (2001). *Fundamentals of nursing* (5th ed., p. 1497). St. Louis: Mosby.

118. **3**
Rationale: The mature ovum is transported through the fallopian tube by the muscular action of the tube and the movement of the cilia within the tube. Fertilization normally occurs in the distal third of the fallopian tube near the ovaries. The ovum, fertilized or not, enters the uterus about 3 days after its release from the ovary. Options 1, 2, and 4 are incorrect.
Test-Taking Strategy: Use the process of elimination. Knowledge regarding the process of fertilization is required to answer this question. Remember that fertilization occurs in the fallopian tube. Review the process of fertilization if you are unfamiliar with it.
Level of Cognitive Ability: Comprehension
Client Needs: Physiological Integrity
Integrated Process: Teaching/Learning
Content Area: Fundamental skills
Reference: Lowdermilk, D., & Perry, A. (2003). *Maternity nursing* (6th ed., p. 150). St. Louis: Mosby.

119. **3**
Rationale: Vitals signs provide a baseline to determine how well the client will tolerate activity. Assessing muscle strength will help determine whether the client has enough strength for crutch walking and if muscle-strengthening exercises are necessary. Previous activity level will provide information related to the tolerance of activity. Options 1, 2, and 4 are also a component of the assessment, but physiological needs take precedence over psychosocial needs.
Test-Taking Strategy: Note the key word "priority" in the stem of the question. Use Maslow's hierarchy of needs theory to prioritize. Remember that physiological needs take precedence over psychosocial needs. This should direct you easily to option 3. Review assessment of the client's readiness to use crutches if you had difficulty with this question.
Level of Cognitive Ability: Analysis
Client Needs: Physiological Integrity
Integrated Process: Nursing Process—assessment
Content Area: Delegating/Prioritizing
Reference: Potter, P., & Perry, A. (2001). *Fundamentals of nursing* (5th ed., pp. 1006-1008). St. Louis: Mosby.

120. **4**
Rationale: To test for Kernig's sign, the leg is raised with the knee flexed. Then the leg is extended at the knee. If any resistance is noted or pain is felt, the result is a positive Kernig's sign. This is a common finding in meningitis. Brudzinski's sign occurs when flexion of the head causes flexion of the hips and knees. Chvostek's sign, seen in tetany, is a spasm of the facial muscles elicited by tapping the facial nerve in the region of the parotid gland. Trousseau's sign is a sign for tetany in which carpal spasm can be elicited by compressing the upper arm and causing ischemia to the nerves distally.
Test-Taking Strategy: Knowledge regarding the appropriate procedure to elicit Kernig's sign is required to answer the question.

Use the process of elimination and assessment techniques to direct you to option 4. If you had difficulty with this question, review these signs, their significance, and the procedures to elicit these signs.
Level of Cognitive Ability: Application
Client Needs: Health Promotion and Maintenance
Integrated Process: Nursing Process—assessment
Content Area: Child health
Reference: James, S., Ashwill, J., & Droske, S. (2002). *Nursing care of children: Principles & practice* (2nd ed., p. 977). Philadelphia: W. B. Saunders.

121. **3**
Rationale: The cause of the confusion in this situation is due to bedrest and decreased sensory stimulation from prolonged confinement. Therefore helping the client to ambulate in the hall is best. This will increase sensory stimulation and may decrease confusion. Options 1 and 2 will not address the client's need for sensory stimulation. Option 4 is an action that should have been performed in preparation for ambulation while the client was on bedrest.
Test-Taking Strategy: Use the process of elimination. Focus on the issue "confusion because of bedrest and prolonged confinement." Eliminate option 4 first because this action should have been performed in preparation for ambulation while the client was on bedrest. Next eliminate options 1 and 2 because they are similar in that they address helping the client to ambulate in the hospital room. Review interventions related to promoting sensory stimulation if you had difficulty with this question.
Level of Cognitive Ability: Application
Client Needs: Psychosocial Integrity
Integrated Process: Nursing Process—planning
Content Area: Fundamental skills
Reference: Potter, P., & Perry, A. (2001). *Fundamentals of nursing* (5th ed., p. 1653). St. Louis: Mosby.

122. **2**
Rationale: Vitamin K is associated with the production of prothrombin, which helps the blood properly clot. Vitamin A deficiency is associated with night blindness. Vitamin B_2 (riboflavin) deficiency is associated with scaly skin. Vitamin D deficiency can cause skeletal pain.
Test-Taking Strategy: Knowledge regarding the clinical manifestations associated with a vitamin K deficiency is required to answer this question. Recalling that vitamin K is the antidote for warfarin (Coumadin), an anticoagulant medication, will assist in directing you to option 2. Review the clinical manifestations associated with vitamin K deficiency if you had difficulty with this question.
Level of Cognitive Ability: Analysis
Client Needs: Physiological Integrity
Integrated Process: Nursing Process—assessment
Content Area: Fundamental skills
Reference: Lehne, R. (2001). *Pharmacology for nursing care* (4th ed., p. 885). Philadelphia: W. B. Saunders.

123. **3**
Rationale: The most common metabolic complication in the small-for-gestational-age (SGA) newborn infant is

hypoglycemia, which can produce central nervous system abnormalities and mental retardation if not corrected immediately. Urinary output, although important, is not the highest priority action because the postterm SGA infant typically is dehydrated because of placental dysfunction. Hemoglobin and hematocrit levels are monitored because the postterm SGA infant exhibits polycythemia, although this also does not require immediate attention. The polycythemia contributes to increased bilirubin levels, usually beginning on the second day after delivery.

Test-Taking Strategy: Use the process of elimination and knowledge regarding the SGA newborn infant. Recalling that the most common metabolic complication in the SGA newborn infant is hypoglycemia will direct you to option 3. Review the SGA newborn content if you had difficulty with this question.
Level of Cognitive Ability: Application
Client Needs: Physiological Integrity
Integrated Process: Nursing Process—implementation
Content Area: Delegating/Prioritizing
Reference: Lowdermilk, D., & Perry, A. (2003). *Maternity nursing* (6th ed., p. 487). St. Louis: Mosby.

124. **1**
Rationale: Because of the newborn infant's large size, an increased risk for shoulder dystocia exists. Shoulder dystocia may result in fractured clavicles and brachial plexus palsy. Other complications related to birth trauma include facial paralysis, phrenic nerve palsy, depressed skull fractures, hematomas, and bleeding. Option 2 would not be related to birth trauma even though an increase in cardiac defects occurs in the large-for-gestational-age newborn infant, such as transposition of the great vessels. Jaundice would not be present initially. Hip dislocation is a congenital disorder and is not caused by birth trauma.
Test-Taking Strategy: Use the process of elimination focusing on the key words "birth trauma." Think of trauma is an injury. Option 1 is the only option that identifies an injury. Review the risks associated with delivery of a large-for-gestational-age newborn infant if you had difficulty with this question.
Level of Cognitive Ability: Analysis
Client Needs: Health Promotion and Maintenance
Integrated Process: Nursing Process—assessment
Content Area: Maternity/Postpartum
Reference: Lowdermilk, D., & Perry, A. (2003). *Maternity nursing* (6th ed., p. 684). St. Louis: Mosby.

125. **3**
Rationale: Somatropin (Humatrope) should not be administered during or after epiphyseal closure. Efficacy of therapy declines as the client grows older and is usually lost entirely by age 20 to 24 years.
Test-Taking Strategy: Use the process of elimination and note the key word "contraindicated." Note the similarity between options 1, 2, and 4. These options relate to growth failure. Note the difference in option 3, for it identifies a particular age of a client. Review the contraindications associated with the administration of somatropin if you had difficulty with this question.

Level of Cognitive Ability: Analysis
Client Needs: Physiological Integrity
Integrated Process: Nursing Process—assessment
Content Area: Pharmacology
Reference: Lehne, R. (2001). *Pharmacology for nursing care* (4th ed., p. 652). Philadelphia: W. B. Saunders.

126. **1**
Rationale: Hyperglycemia can occur from the administration of growth hormone, particularly in a client with diabetes mellitus. Growth hormone therapy is associated with a decline in thyroid function. Hypercalciuria can occur particularly during the first 2 to 3 months of therapy. Glucose and thyroid hormone levels should be monitored.
Test-Taking Strategy: Knowledge regarding the side effects associated with growth hormone replacement therapy is required to answer the question. Review these side effects if you are unfamiliar with them.
Level of Cognitive Ability: Analysis
Client Needs: Physiological Integrity
Integrated Process: Nursing Process—assessment
Content Area: Pharmacology
Reference: Lehne, R. (2001). *Pharmacology for nursing care* (4th ed., p. 652). Philadelphia: W. B. Saunders.

127. **3**
Rationale: An enlarged thyroid gland occurs in the client with goiter because an excessive amount of thyroxine occurs in the thyroid gland, causing it to enlarge. Slow wound healing can occur with zinc deficiency. Chronic fatigue occurs with iron deficiency. Heart damage can occur with selenium deficiency. Additionally, heart damage would not likely be noted during the nursing assessment. Further diagnostic tests, in addition to the assessment, would be necessary to determine heart damage.
Test-Taking Strategy: Use the process of elimination. Thinking about the anatomical location of a goiter will direct you easily option 3. Review the manifestations associated with this disorder if you had difficulty with this question.
Level of Cognitive Ability: Analysis
Client Needs: Physiological Integrity
Integrated Process: Nursing Process—assessment
Content Area: Adult health—endocrine
Reference: Black, J., Hawks, J., & Keene, A. (2001). *Medical-surgical nursing: Clinical management for positive outcomes* (6th ed., p. 1090). Philadelphia: W. B. Saunders.

128. **3**
Rationale: A maternal glucose level is performed to screen for gestational diabetes. If the results of the glucose level are above the normal level, a glucose tolerance test is performed. Options 1, 2, and 4 would not be prescribed based solely on the maternal glucose levels. Further follow-up would be implemented.
Test-Taking Strategy: Use the process of elimination. Eliminate options 1, 2, and 4 because they are similar in that they identify the administration of medication to treat the elevated blood glucose. Option 3 is the only option that identifies further evaluation of the client. Review measures to evaluate

and treat elevated blood glucose levels in a pregnant client, if you had difficulty with this question.
Level of Cognitive Ability: Analysis
Client Needs: Physiological Integrity
Integrated Process: Nursing Process—analysis
Content Area: Maternity/Antepartum
Reference: Lowdermilk, D., & Perry, A. (2003). *Maternity nursing* (6th ed., p. 147). St. Louis: Mosby.

129. **2**
Rationale: Diagnosis of human immunodeficiency virus (HIV) infection depends on serological studies to detect HIV antibodies. The most commonly used test is the enzyme-linked immunosorbent assay. Options 1 and 4 are incorrect because HIV infection primarily occurs through the exchange of body fluids. Option 3 is incorrect. A neonate born to an HIV-positive mother is at risk for developing the virus.
Test-Taking Strategy: Use the process of elimination. Eliminate option 3 first because of the absolute word "definitely." Next eliminate options 1 and 4 because HIV infection primarily occurs through the exchange of body fluids. Review the significance of an HIV test in a pregnant client if you had difficulty with this question.
Level of Cognitive Ability: Analysis
Client Needs: Physiological Integrity
Integrated Process: Nursing Process—analysis
Content Area: Maternity/Antepartum
Reference: Lowdermilk, D., & Perry, A. (2003). *Maternity nursing* (6th ed., p. 168). St. Louis: Mosby.

130. **1**
Rationale: The Food Guide Pyramid is a guide for healthy clients to get the proper amounts of nutrition. A nutritious diet for a healthy client should consist of 55% to 58% of foods containing carbohydrates. Six to 11 servings of the bread, cereal, pasta, or rice is the correct amount. The correct number of servings of vegetables is 3 to 5. The correct number of servings of milk, yogurt, or cheese is 2 to 3. The correct servings of meat, poultry, fish, dry beans, or nuts is 2 to 3. Additionally, 2 to 4 servings from the fruit group is recommended.
Test-Taking Strategy: Knowledge regarding the components of the Food Guide Pyramid is required to answer this question. If you had difficulty with this question and are unfamiliar with the components of the Food Guide Pyramid, review this dietary food guide.
Level of Cognitive Ability: Application
Client Needs: Physiological Integrity
Integrated Process: Teaching/Learning
Content Area: Fundamental skills
Reference: Jarvis, C. (2000). *Physical examination and health assessment* (3rd ed., p. 138). Philadelphia: W. B. Saunders.

131. **1**
Rationale: Early ambulation in the postoperative period is important because if a client does not increase activity, the bones will suffer from loss of calcium. Increasing calcium intake would cause elevated amounts of calcium in the blood that could lead to kidney stones. Iron, not iodine, is recommended for hemoglobin synthesis because oxygen is necessary for wound healing. Clients who are not turned in bed will develop

pressure ulcers. A client who is immobile and is 85-years-old needs to be turned every 2 hours by the nursing staff. The client should not be expected to turn without help.
Test-Taking Strategy: Use the process of elimination. Option 4 should be eliminated first because in this statement the nurse is not accepting responsibility for the client's care. Next eliminate option 3 because iodine is not useful in hemoglobin synthesis. From the remaining options, select option 1 over option 2 because of the importance of the client to get out of bed. Review the complications associated with immobility if you had difficulty with this question.
Level of Cognitive Ability: Application
Client Needs: Physiological Integrity
Integrated Process: Nursing Process—implementation
Content Area: Fundamental skills
Reference: Leuckenotte, A. (2000). *Gerontologic nursing* (2nd ed., p. 728). St. Louis: Mosby.

132. **3**
Rationale: Lindane can penetrate the intact skin and can cause seizures if absorbed in sufficient quantities. Clients at highest risk for seizures are premature infants, children, and clients with preexisting seizure disorders. Lindane should not be used on pediatric clients unless safer medications have failed to control infection.
Test-Taking Strategy: Use the process of elimination. Remembering that the medication can cause seizures will direct you to option 3. Review the contraindications associated with the use of this medication if you had difficulty with this question.
Level of Cognitive Ability: Analysis
Client Needs: Physiological Integrity
Integrated Process: Nursing Process—analysis
Content Area: Pharmacology
Reference: Lehne, R. (2001). *Pharmacology for nursing care* (4th ed., p. 1099). Philadelphia: W. B. Saunders.

133. **3**
Rationale: DuoDerm contains hydroactive particles embedded in a polymer base that are softened by wound moisture and act as a protective gel over healing tissue. DuoDerm is applied directly to the wound and can be left in place up to 7 days.
Test-Taking Strategy: Use the process of elimination. Recall the purpose of this type of dressing to assist in directing you to option 3. Review the nursing interventions associated with the use of a protective dressing if you had difficulty with this question.
Level of Cognitive Ability: Application
Client Needs: Physiological Integrity
Integrated Process: Nursing Process—implementation
Content Area: Pharmacology
Reference: McKenry, L., & Salerno, E. (2003). *Mosby's pharmacology in nursing* (21st ed., p. 447). St. Louis: Mosby.

134. **4**
Rationale: The client with a cerebral aneurysm is placed on aneurysm precautions to maintain a stable perfusion pressure and prevent bleeding. Additionally, any activity that will increase intracranial pressure is avoided. The client is placed in a quiet private room. Bed rest with the head of the bed elevated about 30 degrees is usually prescribed. Some physicians may allow bathroom privileges; if the client is allowed these

privileges, then the nurse must stress the importance of not bending over. Visitors are restricted to close family or significant others and visits are kept short. The client's room is kept slightly darkened and bright lights are avoided. Straining while moving bowels is avoided, and stool softeners are usually prescribed. A low-fiber diet is avoided because it could lead to constipation.
Test-Taking Strategy: Use the process of elimination and focus on the client's diagnosis. Recalling that stimulation is avoided, as is any activity that will increase intracranial pressure, will direct you to option 4. Review the components of aneurysm precautions if you had difficulty with this question.
Level of Cognitive Ability: Application
Client Needs: Physiological Integrity
Integrated Process: Nursing Process—planning
Content Area: Adult Health—neurological
Reference: Phipps, W., Monahan, F., Sands, J., Marek, J. & Neighbors, M. (2003). *Medical-surgical nursing: health and illness perspectives* (7th ed., p. 1385). St. Louis: Mosby.

135. **1**
Rationale: Glyburide is a second generation sulfonylurea used to treat diabetes mellitus. The client is instructed to take a single daily dose 15 to 30 minutes before breakfast. Cholestatic jaundice is an adverse reaction. If the client develops signs of jaundice (skin color changes or pale-colored stools), the physician needs to be notified. The medication is not used to prevent foot infections. Altered taste sensation is a frequent side effect and does not warrant physician notification.
Test-Taking Strategy: Focus on the name of the medication. This will assist in determining its medication classification and that the medication is used to treat diabetes mellitus. This will assist in eliminating option 3. Recalling that signs of jaundice need to be reported to the physician will assist in eliminating option 2. From the remaining options, recalling that medications to treat diabetes mellitus are administered in the morning will direct you to option 1. Review this medication if you had difficulty with this question.
Level of Cognitive Ability: Application
Client Needs: Physiological Integrity
Integrated Process: Teaching/Learning
Content Area: Pharmacology
Reference: Hodgson, B., & Kizior, R. (2004). *Saunders nursing drug handbook 2004* (p. 480). Philadelphia: W. B. Saunders.

136. *Answer:* Droplet precautions
Rationale: Droplet precautions are required for a client with mycoplasmal pneumonia because this type of pneumonia is transmitted by droplet nuclei larger than 5 μm. Barrier protection includes placing the client in a private room or with a cohort client. The nurse wears a mask when in the client's room.
Test-Taking Strategy: Focus on the diagnosis of the client, and recall that pneumonia is transmitted by droplets larger than 5 μm. If you are unfamiliar with transmission-based precautions, review these isolation procedures.
Level of Cognitive Ability: Application
Client Needs: Safe, Effective Care Environment
Integrated Process: Nursing Process—planning
Content Area: Fundamental skills
Reference: Potter, P., & Perry, A. (2001). *Fundamentals of nursing* (5th ed., pp. 858-859). St. Louis: Mosby.

137. **2**
Rationale: In the preicteric phase, the client has nonspecific complaints of fatigue, anorexia, nausea, cough, and joint pain. Options 1,3, and 4 are clinical manifestations that occur in the icteric phase. In the posticteric phase, jaundice decreases, the color of urine and stool return to normal, and the client's appetite improves.
Test-Taking Strategy: Note the key word "preicteric." This will assist in eliminating options 1, 3, and 4. Also note that option 2 identifies vague and nonspecific complaints. Review the clinical manifestations associated with the phases of viral hepatitis if you had difficulty with this question.
Level of Cognitive Ability: Application
Client Needs: Safe, Effective Care Environment
Integrated Process: Teaching/Learning
Content Area: Leadership/Management
Reference: Phipps, W., Monahan, F. Sands, J., Marek, J. & Neighbors, M. (2003). *Medical-surgical nursing: health and illness perspectives* (7th ed., p. 1161). St. Louis: Mosby.

138. **4**
Rationale: When delegating nursing assignments, the nurse needs to consider the skills and educational level of the nursing staff. Collecting a 24-hour urine and frequent ambulation can be provided most appropriately by the nursing assistant, considering the clients identified in each of the options. The client on the mechanical ventilator requiring frequent assessment and suctioning should be cared for most appropriately by the registered nurse. The licensed practical (vocational nurse) is skilled in wound irrigations and dressing changes, and the client needing such care would be assigned to this staff member.
Test-Taking Strategy: Use the principles related to delegation and assignments, and consider the education and skills of each health care provider. Note the key word "assessment" in option 3. This should alert you that this client should be assigned to the registered nurse. You can eliminate options 1 and 2 easily because a nursing assistant can perform these tasks easily. This should assist in directing you to option 4. If you had difficulty with this question, review the principles related to delegation and assignment making.
Level of Cognitive Ability: Application
Client Needs: Safe, Effective Care Environment
Integrated Process: Nursing Process—planning
Content Area: Delegating/Prioritizing
Reference: Potter, P., & Perry, A. (2001). *Fundamentals of nursing* (5th ed., p. 336). St. Louis: Mosby.

139. **4**
Rationale: Critical paths are not specifically nursing care plans; however, they can take the place of a nursing care plan and actually map out the desired clinical progress of a client during admission. Options 1, 2, and 3 appropriately describe the use of a critical path.
Test-Taking Strategy: Use the process of elimination and knowledge regarding the definition and purpose of critical paths to direct you to option 4. Note the key words in the question "a need for further understanding." If you had difficulty with this question, review critical paths.
Level of Cognitive Ability: Comprehension
Client Needs: Safe, Effective Care Environment

Integrated Process: Teaching/Learning
Content Area: Leadership/Management
Reference: Potter, P., & Perry, A. (2001). *Fundamentals of nursing* (5th ed., p. 342). St. Louis: Mosby.

140. **1**
Rationale: The vomiting child should be placed in an upright or side-lying position to prevent aspiration. Options 2, 3, and 4 will place the child at risk for aspiration if vomiting occurs.
Test-Taking Strategy: Use the process of elimination. Eliminate options 2 and 4 first because they are similar. Additionally, these positions would place the child at risk for aspiration if vomiting occurred. Visualize the remaining two positions. Option 3 is also inappropriate and would cause aspiration. Review appropriate positioning techniques if you had difficulty with this question.
Level of Cognitive Ability: Application
Client Needs: Physiological Integrity
Integrated Process: Nursing Process—implementation
Content Area: Child health
Reference: James, S., Ashwill, J., & Droske, S. (2002). *Nursing care of children: Principles & practice* (2nd ed., p. 526). Philadelphia: W. B. Saunders.

141. **3**
Rationale: Cleft lip repair usually is performed during the first few weeks of life. Early repair may improve bonding and makes feeding much easier. Revisions may be required at a later age. Options 1, 2, and 4 are incorrect.
Test-Taking Strategy: Use the process of elimination. Option 4 can be eliminated easily first. Eliminate options 1 and 2 next, because they are similar. Review the management of cleft lip repair if you had difficulty with this question.
Level of Cognitive Ability: Application
Client Needs: Psychosocial Integrity
Integrated Process: Caring
Content Area: Child health
Reference: James, S., Ashwill, J., & Droske, S. (2002). *Nursing care of children: Principles & practice* (2nd ed., p. 535). Philadelphia: W. B. Saunders.

142. **2**
Rationale: Postpartum depression is not the normal depression that many new mothers experience from time to time. The woman experiencing depression shows less interest in her surroundings and a loss of her usual emotional response toward the family. The woman is also unable to show pleasure or love and may have intense feelings of unworthiness, guilt, and shame. The woman often expresses a sense of loss of self. Generalized fatigue, complaints of ill health, and difficulty in concentrating are also present. The mother would have little interest in food and may experience sleep disturbances.
Test-Taking Strategy: Focus on the issue of the question to assist in answering. Note the key words "need for further assessment." Use the process of elimination noting that options 1, 3, and 4 identify positive maternal behaviors. If you had difficulty with this question, review the clinical manifestations of postpartum depression.
Level of Cognitive Ability: Analysis
Client Needs: Psychosocial Integrity

Integrated Process: Nursing Process—analysis
Content Area: Maternity/Postpartum
Reference: Murray, S., McKinney, E., & Gorrie, T. (2002). *Foundations of maternal-newborn nursing* (3rd ed., p. 796). Philadelphia: W. B. Saunders.

143. **1**
Rationale: Wearing breast shells and using a breast pump before each feeding will make it easier for the newborn infant to grasp the nipple. True inverted nipples will retract if the areola is pressed between the thumb and forefinger, making option 2 incorrect. Option 3 is an appropriate instruction for the mother experiencing engorgement. Option 4 will only make the mother cold, and it has no effect on inverted nipples.
Test-Taking Strategy: Use the process of elimination. Focus on the key words "inverted nipples" to assist in directing you to option 1. Review the concepts related to breast-feeding if you had difficulty with this question.
Level of Cognitive Ability: Application
Client Needs: Health Promotion and Maintenance
Integrated Process: Nursing Process—implementation
Content Area: Maternity/Postpartum
Reference: Murray, S., McKinney, E., & Gorrie, T. (2002). *Foundations of maternal-newborn nursing* (3rd ed., pp. 582-584). Philadelphia: W. B. Saunders.

144. **2**
Rationale: The nurse would instruct the client to lie down and place a towel or pillow under the shoulder on the side of the breast to be examined. If the left breast is to be examined, the pillow would be placed under the left shoulder.
Test-Taking Strategy: Use the process of elimination. Attempt to visualize this procedure to select the correct option. Remember to examine the left breast, the pillow is placed under the left; to examine the right breast, the pillow is placed under the right. If you are unfamiliar with the procedure for performing breast self-examination, review this important self-examination.
Level of Cognitive Ability: Application
Client Needs: Health Promotion and Maintenance
Integrated Process: Teaching/Learning
Content Area: Adult health—oncology
Reference: Potter, P., & Perry, A. (2001). *Fundamentals of nursing* (5th ed., p. 795). St. Louis: Mosby.

145. **4**
Rationale: If the client has had a hysterectomy or is no longer menstruating, the breast self-exmination should be performed on the same day every month. Options 1 and 2 are inappropriate because the client who had a hysterectomy would not be menstruating. Not performing the breast self-exmination at ovulation time is best because of the hormonal changes that occur.
Test-Taking Strategy: Use the process of elimination. Note the key word "hysterectomy" in the question to eliminate options 1 and 2. Eliminate option 3 because of the hormonal changes that occur at this time. If you are unfamiliar with the procedure for performing breast self-examination, review this important self-examination.
Level of Cognitive Ability: Application
Client Needs: Health Promotion and Maintenance
Integrated Process: Teaching/Learning

Content Area: Adult health—oncology
Reference: Potter, P., & Perry, A. (2001). *Fundamentals of nursing* (5th ed., p. 795). St. Louis: Mosby.

146. 1
Rationale: Montgomery's tubercles are sebaceous glands located in the areola. They are inactive and not obvious except during pregnancy and lactation, when they enlarge and secrete a substance that keeps the nipple soft. Within each breast are lobes of glandular tissue that secrete milk. Alveoli are small sacs that contain acinar cells to secrete milk. The alveoli drain into lactiferous ducts, which connect to drain milk from all areas of the breast.
Test-Taking Strategy: Use the process of elimination and knowledge regarding the anatomy and physiology of the breast to answer this question. If you are unfamiliar with the anatomy of the female breast, review these structures.
Level of Cognitive Ability: Comprehension
Client Needs: Physiological Integrity
Integrated Process: Teaching/Learning
Content Area: Fundamental skills
Reference: Ignatavicius, D., & Workman, M. (2002). *Medical-surgical nursing: Critical thinking for collaborative care* (4th ed., p. 1709). Philadelphia: W. B. Saunders.

147. 4
Rationale: The nurse assesses the client with fibrocystic breast disorder for worsening of symptoms (breast lumps, painful breasts, and possible nipple discharge) before the onset of menses. This is associated with cyclical hormone changes.
Test-Taking Strategy: Use the process of elimination. Note the key words "more noticeable," which imply a predictable variation in symptoms. Use knowledge of the effects of various hormones in the body to select the correct option. Review the characteristics of fibrocystic breast disease if you had difficulty with this question.
Level of Cognitive Ability: Application
Client Needs: Physiological Integrity
Integrated Process: Nursing Process—assessment
Content Area: Adult health—oncology
Reference: Ignatavicius, D., & Workman, M. (2002). *Medical-surgical nursing: Critical thinking for collaborative care* (4th ed., p. 1735). Philadelphia: W. B. Saunders.

148. 2
Rationale: Intussusception occurs when a proximal segment of the bowel prolapses into a distal segment of the bowel. Intussusception is a common cause of acute bowel obstruction in infants and young children. Intussusception is not an inflammatory process.
Test-Taking Strategy: Use the process of elimination. Recalling that this condition is a telescoping of the bowel will assist you in eliminating options 1 and 4. Use the principles of gravity to assist in directing you to the correct option. Review this disorder if you had difficulty with this question.
Level of Cognitive Ability: Application
Client Needs: Physiological Integrity
Integrated Process: Teaching/Learning
Content Area: Child health

Reference: James, S., Ashwill, J., & Droske, S. (2002). *Nursing care of children: Principles & practice* (2nd ed., p. 570). Philadelphia: W. B. Saunders.

149. 3
Rationale: Encopresis is defined as fecal incontinence and is a major concern if the child is constipated. Signs include evidence of soiled clothing, scratching or rubbing the anal area because of irritation, fecal odor without apparent awareness by the child, and social withdrawal.
Test-Taking Strategy: Use the process of elimination and knowledge regarding the definition of encopresis to direct you to option 3. Review the assessment findings in this disorder if you had difficulty with this question.
Level of Cognitive Ability: Analysis
Client Needs: Physiological Integrity
Integrated Process: Nursing Process—assessment
Content Area: Child health
Reference: James, S., Ashwill, J., & Droske, S. (2002). *Nursing care of children: Principles & practice* (2nd ed., p. 552). Philadelphia: W. B. Saunders.

150. 2
Rationale: The artificial larynx is an electronic device that assists the client after laryngectomy to produce speech. The two types are one that is held at the side of the neck and one that is inserted into the mouth. The vibration produces a mechanical-sounding speech that is monotone but is intelligible.
Test-Taking Strategy: Use the process of elimination. Focus on the key words "artificial larynx." To answer this question accurately, you must be generally familiar with these devices. Review the available devices that assist with speech if you had difficulty with this question.
Level of Cognitive Ability: Application
Client Needs: Physiological Integrity
Integrated Process: Teaching/Learning
Content Area: Adult health—oncology
Reference: Lewis, S., Heitkemper, M., & Dirksen, S. (2004). *Medical-surgical nursing: Assessment and management of clinical problems* (6th ed., p. 589). St. Louis: Mosby.

151. 3
Rationale: A Papanicolaou's smear is usually painless. The test cannot be performed during menstruation. The client needs to be instructed to avoid douching for at least 24 hours before the test. No reason exists to restrict fluids on the day of the test.
Test-Taking Strategy: Use the process of elimination. Eliminate option 2 first as an unlikely preparation measure. Eliminate options 1 and 4 next because menstruation and douching will affect the results of the test. Review client preparation for a Papanicolaou's test if you had difficulty with this question.
Level of Cognitive Ability: Application
Client Needs: Physiological Integrity
Integrated Process: Nursing Process—implementation
Content Area: Adult health—oncology
Reference: Chernecky, C., & Berger, B. (2001). *Laboratory tests and diagnostic procedures* (3rd ed., pp. 786-787). Philadelphia: W. B. Saunders.

152. 1

Rationale: A Good Samaritan law is passed by a state legislator to encourage nurses and other health care providers to provide care to a person when an accident, emergency, or injury occurs, without fear of being sued for the care provided. Its protection lies in the inability of the injured person to sue the nurse or other health care provider the care provided at the scene of the accident or during the emergency, even if further injury occurred because of the health care provider's care. Called immunity from suit, this protection usually applies only if all of the conditions of the law are met, such as the heath care provider receives no compensation for the care provided, and the care given is not willfully and wantonly negligent.

Test-Taking Strategy: Use the process of elimination. Eliminate options 2 and 4 because they are similar. No data in the question are given regarding the issue of compensation; therefore the best option is option 1. Review the Good Samaritan law if you had difficulty with this question.

Level of Cognitive Ability: Comprehension
Client Needs: Safe, Effective Care Environment
Integrated Process: Nursing Process—implementation
Content Area: Fundamental skills
Reference: Potter, P., & Perry, A. (2001). *Fundamentals of nursing* (5th ed., p. 429). St. Louis: Mosby.

153. 2

Rationale: Lypressin is an antidiuretic hormone used to treat diabetes insipidus. Lypressin promotes renal conservation of water by acting on the collecting ducts of the kidney to increase the permeability to water, which results in increased water reabsorption. Options 1, 3, and 4 are not actions of the medication.

Test-Taking Strategy: Note the diagnosis identified in the question. Recalling the pathophysiology associated with the disorder will assist in the process of elimination and in directing you to the correct option. Review the action of lypressin if you had difficulty with this question.

Level of Cognitive Ability: Application
Client Needs: Physiological Integrity
Integrated Process: Teaching/Learning
Content Area: Pharmacology
Reference: Lehne, R. (2001). *Pharmacology for nursing care* (4th ed., p. 654). Philadelphia: W. B. Saunders.

154. 3

Rationale: Somatrem (Protropin) is a growth hormone used to treat dwarfism. When treatment is started, height may be increased by as much as 6 inches. To monitor treatment, height and weight should be measured monthly. Options 1, 2, and 4 are incorrect.

Test-Taking Strategy: Use the process of elimination. Options 1, 2, and 4 are similar in that each identifies lengthy and specific time frames related to the expected outcome of the medication. Review the expected outcome of somatrem if you had difficulty with this question.

Level of Cognitive Ability: Application
Client Needs: Physiological Integrity
Integrated Process: Teaching/Learning
Content Area: Pharmacology

Reference: Lehne, R. (2001). *Pharmacology for nursing care* (4th ed., pp. 651-652). Philadelphia: W. B. Saunders.

155. 3

Rationale: Democratic styles best empower staff toward excellence because this style of leadership allows nurses an opportunity to grow professionally. The autocratic style is task orientated and directive. Situational leadership style uses a style depending on the situation and events. Laissez-faire allows staff to work without assistance, direction, or supervision.

Test-Taking Strategy: Note the key words "empower staff toward excellence." Use the process of elimination and knowledge of the characteristics of the various leadership styles to direct you to option 3. If you had difficulty with this question, review the various leadership styles.

Level of Cognitive Ability: Comprehension
Client Needs: Safe, Effective Care Environment
Integrated Process: Nursing Process—planning
Content Area: Leadership/Management
Reference: Potter, P., & Perry, A. (2001). *Fundamentals of nursing* (5th ed., p. 69). St. Louis: Mosby.

156. 3

Rationale: Tertiary prevention involves the reduction of the amount and degree of disability, injury, and damage following a crisis. Primary prevention means keeping the crisis from ever occurring, and secondary prevention focuses on reducing the intensity and duration of a crisis during the crisis itself. No aggregate care prevention level exists.

Test-Taking Strategy: Identify the nurse's role in the question. Also, noting the key words "following a towards" will direct you to option 3. If you had difficulty with this question, take time to review the levels of prevention.

Level of Cognitive Ability: Comprehension
Client Needs: Safe, Effective Care Environment
Integrated Process: Nursing Process—planning
Content Area: Leadership/Management
Reference: Varcarolis, E. (2002). *Foundations of psychiatric mental health nursing* (4th ed., p. 627). Philadelphia: W. B. Saunders.

157. 1

Rationale: Ovulation ceased during pregnancy because the circulating levels of estrogen and progesterone are high, inhibiting the release of follicle-stimulating hormones and luteinizing hormones that are necessary for ovulation. Options 2, 3, and 4 are incorrect.

Test-Taking Strategy: Use the process of elimination. Knowledge regarding the hormonal changes that occur during the menstrual cycle and during pregnancy is required to answer this question. If you are unfamiliar with these physiological changes, review this content.

Level of Cognitive Ability: Comprehension
Client Needs: Physiological Integrity
Integrated Process: Teaching/Learning
Content Area: Fundamental skills
Reference: Murray, S., McKinney, E., & Gorrie, T. (2002). *Foundations of maternal-newborn nursing* (3rd ed., p. 122). Philadelphia: W. B. Saunders.

158. *Answer:* Identity vs. Role Confusion
Rationale: Adolescence is a period of major physical changes. The adolescent is aware of these changes and is concerned with the way he or she appears to others. Adolescents are trying to learn who they are. Role confusion occurs when the adolescent is unable to see himself or herself as separate or unique from others and does not establish a direction or career goal in life.
Test-Taking Strategy: You must know the psychosocial stages of development according to Erik Erikson to answer this question. Review this theory if you are unfamiliar with it.
Level of Cognitive Ability: Comprehension
Client Needs: Psychosocial Integrity
Integrated Process: Nursing Process—planning
Content Area: Child health
Reference: James, S., Ashwill, J., & Droske, S. (2002). *Nursing care of children: Principles & practice* (2nd ed., p. 71). Philadelphia: W. B. Saunders.

159. **1**
Rationale: Etidronate (Didronel) should be taken on an empty stomach 2 hours before meals. Etidronate should not be taken within 2 hours of taking vitamins, mineral supplements, antacids, or medications high in calcium, magnesium, iron, or albumin.
Test-Taking Strategy: Use the process of elimination. Eliminate options 2, 3, and 4 because they are similar. Note that each of these options suggests administering the medication with another substance. Option 1 is the only option that reflects administering the medication on an empty stomach. Review concepts related to the administration of this medication if you had difficulty with this question.
Level of Cognitive Ability: Application
Client Needs: Physiological Integrity
Integrated Process: Teaching/Learning
Content Area: Pharmacology
Reference: Hodgson, B., & Kizior, R. (2004). *Saunders nursing drug handbook 2004* (p. 390). Philadelphia: W. B. Saunders.

160. **2**
Rationale: Foul-smelling vaginal discharge is expected and will occur for some time following removal of a cervical radiation implant. Options 1, 3, and 4 are accurate discharge instructions.
Test-Taking Strategy: Use the process of elimination. Note the key words "need for further instructions." Knowledge regarding the client teaching points related to radiation implants is required to answer the question. Review these points if you had difficulty with this question.
Level of Cognitive Ability: Application
Client Needs: Health Promotion and Maintenance
Integrated Process: Teaching/Learning
Content Area: Adult health—oncology
Reference: Ignatavicius, D., & Workman, M. (2002). *Medical-surgical nursing: Critical thinking for collaborative care* (4th ed., p. 1774). Philadelphia: W. B. Saunders.

161. **3**
Rationale: The client needs to be instructed to avoid exposure to the sun. Options 1, 2, and 4 are accurate measures in the care of a client receiving external radiation therapy.

Test-Taking Strategy: Use the process of elimination. Note the key words "need for further instruction." Eliminate option 1 because of the word "gently" and option 4 because of the word "loose." From the remaining options, recalling that sun exposure is to be avoided will assist you in answering the question. Review skin care measures for the client receiving external radiation if you had difficulty with this question.
Level of Cognitive Ability: Analysis
Client Needs: Health Promotion and Maintenance
Integrated Process: Teaching/Learning
Content Area: Adult health—oncology
Reference: Ignatavicius, D., & Workman, M. (2002). *Medical-surgical nursing: Critical thinking for collaborative care* (4th ed., p. 429). Philadelphia: W. B. Saunders.

162. **1**
Rationale: The primary technique one can use to handle resistance to change during the change process is to introduce the change gradually. Confrontation is an important strategy used to meet resistance when it occurs. Coercion is another strategy that can be used to decrease resistance to change but is not always a successful technique for managing resistance. Manipulation usually involves a covert action such as leaving out pieces of vital information that the participants might negatively receive. Manipulation is not the best method of implementing a change.
Test-Taking Strategy: Use the process of elimination and knowledge regarding techniques used to handle resistance during the change process to direct you to option 1. Note the key words "primary technique" in the question. If you had difficulty with this question, review the techniques that can be used to deal with resistance during the change process.
Level of Cognitive Ability: Application
Client Needs: Safe, Effective Care Environment
Integrated Process: Nursing Process—planning
Content Area: Leadership/Management
Reference: Potter, P., & Perry, A. (2001). *Fundamentals of nursing* (5th ed., pp. 72-73). St. Louis: Mosby.

163. **1**
Rationale: The effect of insulin lispro begins within 15 minutes of subcutaneous injection, peaks in $1/2$ to $1^1/_2$ hours, and has a duration of action of 4 to 5 hours. Insulin lispro acts more rapidly that regular insulin and has a shorter duration of action. Because of its rapid onset, insulin lispro can be administered immediately before eating. In contrast, regular insulin generally is administered 30 to 60 minutes before meals.
Test-Taking Strategy: Use the process of elimination. Note the key words "rapid-acting." This will assist you in eliminating options 3 and 4. From the remaining options, remember that the question is asking about lispro, not regular, insulin. This should direct you to option 1. Review the characteristics of insulin lispro if you had difficulty with this question.
Level of Cognitive Ability: Application
Client Needs: Physiological Integrity
Integrated Process: Teaching/Learning
Content Area: Pharmacology
Reference: Hodgson, B., & Kizior, R. (2004). *Saunders nursing drug handbook 2004* (p. 537). Philadelphia: W. B. Saunders.

164. **2**

Rationale: Because regular insulin forms a true solution, it is safe for intravenous use. Regular insulin is the only type of insulin that can be administered intravenously.

Test-Taking Strategy: Remember that regular insulin is the only type of insulin that can be administered intravenously. If you had difficulty with this question, review the different types of insulin and their methods of administration.

Level of Cognitive Ability: Application

Client Needs: Physiological Integrity

Integrated Process: Nursing Process—planning

Content Area: Pharmacology

Reference: Hodgson, B., & Kizior, R. (2004). *Saunders nursing drug handbook 2004* (p. 591). Philadelphia: W. B. Saunders,.

165. *Answer:* 1.5 tablets

Rationale: You must convert 150 mcg to milligrams. In the metric system, to convert smaller to larger, divide by 1000 or move the decimal three places to the left. Therefore 150 mcg equals 0.15 mg. Next, use the formula to calculate the correct dose.

Formula:

$$\frac{Desired}{Available} \times Tablet = Tablets\ per\ dose$$

$$\frac{0.15\ mg}{0.1\ mg} \times 1\ Tablet = 1.5\ Tablets$$

Test-Taking Strategy: In this medication calculation problem, you first must convert micrograms to milligrams. Next, follow the formula for the calculation of the correct dose. Label each figure, including the answer. Recheck your work, and make sure that the answer makes sense. If you had difficulty with this question, review medication calculation problems.

Level of Cognitive Ability: Application

Client Needs: Physiological Integrity

Integrated Process: Nursing Process—implementation

Content Area: Fundamental skills

Reference: Potter, P., & Perry, A. (2001). *Fundamentals of nursing* (5th ed., p. 898). St. Louis: Mosby.

166. **2**

Rationale: The most common side effect of metformin (Glucophage) is gastrointestinal disturbances including decreased appetite, nausea, and diarrhea. These generally subside over time. This medication does not cause weight gain; in fact, clients lose an average of 7 to 8 lb because the medication causes nausea and decreased appetite. Although hypoglycemia can occur, it is not the most common side effect.

Test-Taking Strategy: Use the process of elimination, noting the key words "most common side effect." Review these side effects if you had difficulty with this question.

Level of Cognitive Ability: Application

Client Needs: Physiological Integrity

Integrated Process: Teaching/Learning

Content Area: Pharmacology

Reference: Hodgson, B., & Kizior, R. (2003). *Saunders nursing drug handbook 2003* (p. 716). Philadelphia: W. B. Saunders.

167. **3**

Rationale: The human immunodeficiency virus–positive client may be at high risk for superimposed infections during pregnancy. Among these include *Candida* infections, genital herpes, and anogenital condyloma. Early reporting of symptoms may alert the members of the health care team that further assessment and testing is needed to diagnose and manage additional maternal and fetal physiological risks. Options 1, 2, and 4 represent possible outcomes of early recognition of infection but are not the priority of care when promoting maternal-fetal well-being.

Test-Taking Strategy: Focus on the issue of the question and use Maslow's hierarchy of needs theory. Option 3 is the only option that addresses physiological integrity. Review teaching points related to the pregnant client with human immunodeficiency virus if you had difficulty with this question.

Level of Cognitive Ability: Application

Client Needs: Health Promotion and Maintenance

Integrated Process: Nursing Process—implementation

Content Area: Maternity/Antepartum

Reference: Murray, S., McKinney, E., & Gorrie, T. (2002). *Foundations of maternal-newborn nursing* (3rd ed., pp. 722, 724, 728). Philadelphia: W. B. Saunders.

168. **4**

Rationale: The effects of maternal iron deficiency anemia on the developing fetus and neonate are unclear. In general, the fetus is believed to receive adequate maternal stores of iron, even if a deficiency is present. Neonates of severely anemic mothers have been reported to experience reduced red blood cell volume, hemoglobin, and iron stores. Options 1 and 3 provide a false reassurance to the client. Option 2 will cause further concern in the client. Option 4 provides the most realistic support for the client and allows the nurse an opportunity to review the client's plan of care to clarify information and reassure the mother.

Test-Taking Strategy: Use the process of elimination and therapeutic communication techniques to answer the question. Eliminate options 1 and 3 because these options provide a false reassurance to the client. Eliminate option 2 next because this response will cause further concern in the client. If you had difficulty with this question, review therapeutic communication technique and the effects of maternal anemia on the fetus.

Level of Cognitive Ability: Application

Client Needs: Psychosocial Integrity

Integrated Process: Caring

Content Area: Maternity/Antepartum

Reference: Lowdernick, D. & Perry, S. *Maternity of women's health care* (8th ed. p. 918) St. Louis: Mosby.

169. **3**

Rationale: Sulfonylureas promote insulin secretion by the pancreas and also may increase tissue response to insulin. Biguanides decrease glucose production by the liver. Alpha-glucosidase inhibitors inhibit carbohydrate digestion. Thiazolidinediones decrease insulin resistance.

Test-Taking Strategy: Knowledge regarding the specific action of the sulfonylureas is required to answer this question. Review this classification of medications if you had difficulty with this question.

Level of Cognitive Ability: Analysis

Client Needs: Physiological Integrity

Integrated Process: Nursing Process—analysis
Content Area: Pharmacology
Reference: Lehne, R. (2001). *Pharmacology for nursing care* (4th ed., p. 624). Philadelphia: W. B. Saunders.

170. 3
Rationale: When the client with diabetes mellitus becomes ill, control is more difficult. Insulin is not omitted, and the client is encouraged to consume liquid carbohydrates if unable to eat regular meals. The client is instructed to notify the physician if vomiting or diarrhea occurs or if the illness progresses past 2 days.
Test-Taking Strategy: Use the process of elimination. You can eliminate options 1, 2, and 4 easily because it is not within the legal parameters of nursing responsibilities to adjust or alter medication dosages. If you had difficulty with this question, review the client teaching points related to the administration of insulin on "sick days."
Level of Cognitive Ability: Application
Client Needs: Health Promotion and Maintenance
Integrated Process: Nursing Process—implementation
Content Area: Pharmacology
Reference: McKenry, L., & Salerno, E. (2003). *Mosby's pharmacology in nursing* (21st ed., p. 871). St. Louis: Mosby.

171. 4
Rationale: The client with Cushing's syndrome should be reassured that most physical changes resolve with treatment. Options 1, 2, and 3 are not therapeutic responses.
Test-Taking Strategy: Use the process of elimination. If you are unfamiliar with this disorder, you can eliminate options 1, 2, and 3 easily because these statements are not therapeutic responses to a client. Review the effects of treatment in a client with Cushing's syndrome if you had difficulty with this question.
Level of Cognitive Ability: Application
Client Needs: Psychosocial Integrity
Integrated Process: Caring
Content Area: Adult health—endocrine
Reference: Lewis, S., Heitkemper, M., & Dirksen, S. (2004). *Medical-surgical nursing: Assessment and management of clinical problems* (6th ed., pp. 1328-1329). St. Louis: Mosby.

172. 4
Rationale: Hypocalcemia can develop after thyroidectomy if the parathyroid glands are removed accidentally during surgery. Manifestations develop 1 to 7 days after surgery. If the client develops numbness and tingling around the mouth, fingertips, or toes; muscle spasms; or twitching, the physician is notified immediately. Calcium gluconate should be kept at the bedside.
Test-Taking Strategy: Use the process of elimination. Noting the name of the medication (calcium gluconate) should direct you easily to option 4. Calcium would be given if hypocalcemia tetany occurs. Review care to the client following thyroidectomy if you had difficulty with this question.
Level of Cognitive Ability: Analysis
Client Needs: Physiological Integrity
Integrated Process: Nursing Process—analysis
Content Area: Adult health—endocrine

Reference: Lehne, R. (2001). *Pharmacology for nursing care* (4th ed., p. 806). Philadelphia: W. B. Saunders.

173. *Answer:*
Loosen clothing around the child's neck.
Time the seizure.
Stay with the child.
Move furniture or other items away from the child.
Rationale: During a seizure, the nurse places the child on his or her side in a lateral position. Positioning on the side will prevent aspiration because saliva will drain out the corner of the child's mouth. The child is not restrained because this could cause injury to the child. The nurse would loosen clothing around the child's neck and ensure a patent airway. Nothing is placed into the child's mouth during a seizure because this action may cause injury to the child's mouth, gums, or teeth. The nurse would stay with the child to reduce the risk of injury and allow for observation and timing of the seizure.
Test-Taking Strategy: Visualize this clinical situation. Recalling that airway patency and safety is the priority will assist in determining the appropriate interventions. Review care to the child experiencing a seizure if you had difficulty with this question.
Level of Cognitive Ability: Application
Client Needs: Physiological Integrity
Integrated Process: Nursing Process—implementation
Content Area: Child health
Reference: James, S., Ashwill, J., & Droske, S. (2002). *Nursing care of children: Principles & practice* (2nd ed., p. 973). Philadelphia: W. B. Saunders.

174. 3
Rationale: A blood glucose test performed before exercising provides the client with information regarding the need to consume a snack before exercising. Exercising during the peak times of insulin or before mealtime places the client at risk for hypoglycemia. Insulin should be administered as prescribed.
Test-Taking Strategy: Focus on the issue, the occurrence of a hypoglycemia reaction. Use the process of elimination, keeping this issue in mind, and the action of insulin to eliminate options 1, 2, and 4. Review client instructions for implementing an exercise program if you had difficulty with this question.
Level of Cognitive Ability: Application
Client Needs: Health Promotion and Maintenance
Integrated Process: Teaching/Learning
Content Area: Adult health—endocrine
Reference: Potter, P., & Perry, A. (2001). *Fundamentals of nursing* (5th ed., p. 1014). St. Louis: Mosby.

175. 3
Rationale: Characteristic behaviors of the newborn infant with fetal alcohol syndrome (FAS) are similar to the behaviors common to the drug-exposed newborn infant. These behaviors include irritability, tremors, poor feeding, and hypersensitivity to stimuli. Newborn infants with FAS are smaller at birth and may fail to thrive. Head circumference and weight are most affected.
Test-Taking Strategy: Use the process of elimination. Recalling that the behaviors of the newborn infant with FAS similar to behaviors common to the drug-exposed newborn infant will assist in directing you to option 3. If you had difficulty

with this question, review characteristics in the newborn infant with FAS.

Level of Cognitive Ability: Analysis
Client Needs: Physiological Integrity
Integrated Process: Nursing Process—assessment
Content Area: Maternity/Postpartum
Reference: Murray, S., McKinney, E., & Gorrie, T. (2002). *Foundations of maternal-newborn nursing* (3rd ed., p. 640). Philadelphia: W. B. Saunders.

176. 1
Rationale: Bathing a newborn infant after a feeding is not advisable because handling may cause regurgitation. Because bathing is thought to be relaxing to the infant, before feeding may be the best time. Options 2, 3, and 4 are appropriate interventions in teaching the mother how to bathe a newborn.
Test-Taking Strategy: Use the process of elimination. Note the key words "need to provide additional instructions." Recalling that handling the baby may cause regurgitation will assist in directing you to option 1. Review teaching points regarding bathing of a newborn if you had difficulty with this question.
Level of Cognitive Ability: Analysis
Client Needs: Health Promotion and Maintenance
Integrated Process: Teaching/Learning
Content Area: Maternity/Postpartum
Reference: Murray, S., McKinney, E., & Gorrie, T. (2002). *Foundations of maternal-newborn nursing* (3rd ed., pp. 558, 568). Philadelphia: W. B. Saunders.

177. 1
Rationale: Following amputation, phantom limb pain is a temporary condition that some children may experience. This sensation of burning, aching, or cramping in the missing limb is most distressing to the child. The child needs to be reassured that the condition is normal and only temporary. Options 2, 3 and 4 are not appropriate responses to the child.
Test-Taking Strategy: Use therapeutic communication techniques. Note that the issue of the question relates to alleviating the child's fear. Option 1 is the only option that will alleviate fear. Options 2, 3, and 4 infer that this pain may be permanent.
Level of Cognitive Ability: Application
Client Needs: Psychosocial Integrity
Integrated Process: Caring
Content Area: Child health
Reference: Wong, D., Perry, S., & Hockenberry, M. (2002). *Maternal child nursing care* (2nd ed., p. 1560). St. Louis: Mosby.

178. 4
Rationale: Vitamin C (ascorbic acid) increases the absorption of iron by the body. The mother should be instructed to administer the medication with a citrus fruit or juice high in vitamin C. From the options presented, option 4 is the option that identifies the item highest in vitamin C.
Test-Taking Strategy: Use the process of elimination. Recalling that vitamin C increases the absorption of iron will assist you in eliminating options 1 and 2. From the remaining options, select option 4 because this food item contains the highest

amount of vitamin C. Review foods high in vitamin C if you had difficulty with this question.
Level of Cognitive Ability: Application
Client Needs: Physiological Integrity
Integrated Process: Teaching/Learning
Content Area: Child health
Reference: James, S., Ashwill, J., & Droske, S. (2002). *Nursing care of children: Principles & practice* (2nd ed., p. 746). Philadelphia: W. B. Saunders.

179. 1
Rationale: If the client becomes ill and cannot retain fluids or food for a period of 4 hours, the physician should be notified. The client's statement in this question indicates a need for immediate education to prevent hyperglycemic hyperosmolar nonketotic syndrome, a life-threatening emergency.
Test-Taking Strategy: Use the process of elimination and focus on the issue. Eliminate option 2 first because the client's statement is inaccurate. Eliminate option 3 next because the client requires immediate education. Eliminate option 4 because hyperglycemic hyperosmolar nonketotic syndrome most commonly occurs with type 2 diabetes mellitus and insulin is not the issue of the question. Review diabetic management during times of illness if you had difficulty with this question.
Level of Cognitive Ability: Analysis
Client Needs: Health Promotion and Maintenance
Integrated Process: Nursing Process—analysis
Content Area: Adult health—endocrine
Reference: Ignatavicius, D., & Workman, M. (2002). *Medical-surgical nursing: Critical thinking for collaborative care* (4th ed., p. 1483). Philadelphia: W. B. Saunders.

180. 2
Rationale: Reinforcement of knowledge and behaviors is vital to the success of the client's self-care. Options 1, 3, and 4 do not address the need for client instructions and are not therapeutic responses.
Test-Taking Strategy: Use the process of elimination and therapeutic communication techniques. Option 1 devalues a client's family, option 3 places the client's issue on "hold," and option 4 requests an explanation from the client. Option 2 validates and clarifies previous information. Review therapeutic communication techniques if you had difficulty with this question.
Level of Cognitive Ability: Application
Client Needs: Psychosocial Integrity
Integrated Process: Communication and Documentation
Content Area: Adult health—endocrine
Reference: Lewis, S., Heitkemper, M., & Dirksen, S. (2004). *Medical-surgical nursing: Assessment and management of clinical problems* (6th ed., p. 1290). St. Louis: Mosby.

181. 1
Rationale: Before conception, the uterus is a small, pear-shaped cavity contained entirely in the pelvic cavity. Before pregnancy, the uterus weighs about 60 g (2 oz) and has a capacity of about 10 mL (one third of an ounce). At the end on pregnancy, the uterus weighs about 1000 g (2.2 lb) and has a sufficient capacity for the fetus, placenta, and amniotic fluid, a total of approximately 500 to 1500 mL.

Test-Taking Strategy: Use the process of elimination and knowledge regarding the structure of the uterus to answer this question. Note the key word "nonpregnant" and attempt to visualize each of the items identified in the options. Review the anatomical structure of the uterus, if you had difficulty with this question.
Level of Cognitive Ability: Comprehension
Client Needs: Physiological Integrity
Integrated Process: Teaching/Learning
Content Area: Fundamental skills
Reference: Murray, S., McKinney, E., & Gorrie, T. (2002). *Foundations of maternal-newborn nursing* (3rd ed., p. 63). Philadelphia: W. B. Saunders.

182. 1
Rationale: Fludrocortisone (Florinef) has mineralocorticoid activity and also has a modest glucocorticoid effect. Fludrocortisone acts primarily on the distal tubules of the kidneys, enhancing the reabsorption of sodium and chloride ions and the excretion of potassium and hydrogen ions. Fludrocortisone promotes water retention.
Test-Taking Strategy: Use the process of elimination and knowledge regarding the action of fludrocortisone. If you are unfamiliar with this medication, try to recall the pathophysiology associated with Addison's disease to assist you in answering the question. Review this medication action if you are unfamiliar with it.
Level of Cognitive Ability: Comprehension
Client Needs: Physiological Integrity
Integrated Process: Nursing Process—planning
Content Area: Pharmacology
Reference: Hodgson, B., & Kizior, R. (2003). *Saunders nursing drug handbook 2003* (p. 466). Philadelphia: W. B. Saunders.

183. 1
Rationale: At 12 weeks of gestation the uterus extends out of the maternal pelvis and can be palpated above the symphysis pubis. At 16 weeks the fundus reaches midway between the symphysis pubis and the umbilicus. At 20 weeks the fundus is located at the umbilicus. By 36 weeks, the fundus reaches its highest level at the xiphoid process.
Test-Taking Strategy: Use the process of elimination and knowledge regarding the patterns of uterine growth to answer this question. Focus on the weeks of gestations identified in the question to assist in directing you to the correct option. If you are unfamiliar with the patterns of uterine growth during pregnancy, review this content.
Level of Cognitive Ability: Comprehension
Client Needs: Health Promotion and Maintenance
Integrated Process: Nursing Process—assessment
Content Area: Maternity/Antepartum
Reference: Murray, S., McKinney, E., & Gorrie, T. (2002). *Foundations of maternal-newborn nursing* (3rd ed., p. 425). Philadelphia: W. B. Saunders.

184. 1
Rationale: Setting priorities means deciding which client needs or problems require immediate action and which ones could be delayed until a later time because they are not urgent. Client problems that involve actual or life-threatening

concerns are always considered first. Although time constraints, obtaining needed supplies, and completing care in a reasonable time frame are components of time management, these items are not the priority in planning care for the client based on the options provided.
Test-Taking Strategy: Use the process of elimination and principles related to prioritizing to answer the question. Noting the key word "life-threatening" in option 1 will assist in directing you to this option. Review the principles related to prioritizing if you had difficulty with this question.
Level of Cognitive Ability: Application
Client Needs: Safe, Effective Care Environment
Integrated Process: Nursing Process—planning
Content Area: Delegating/Prioritizing
Reference: Potter, P., & Perry, A. (2001). *Fundamentals of nursing* (5th ed., p. 323). St. Louis: Mosby.

185. 3
Rationale: Certain factors create a risk for the development of thromboembolitic disorders. These factors include smoking, varicose veins, obesity, a history of thrombophlebitis, women older than 35 years or who have had more than three pregnancies, and women who had a cesarean birth. From the options presented, a 26-year-old woman with a family history of thrombophlebitis is least likely to develop thromboembolitic disorders in the postpartum period.
Test-Taking Strategy: Use the process of elimination. Note the key words "least likely" in the stem of the question. Knowing that a woman older than 35 years of age is at risk will assist you in eliminating options 1 and 2. From the remaining options, select option 3 because the woman described in option 4 actually has a history of thrombophlebitis. If you had difficulty with this question, review the predisposing factors and risks associated with thromboembolitic disorders.
Level of Cognitive Ability: Analysis
Client Needs: Health Promotion and Maintenance
Integrated Process: Nursing Process—assessment
Content Area: Maternity/Antepartum
Reference: Murray, S., McKinney, E., & Gorrie, T. (2002). *Foundations of maternal-newborn nursing* (3rd ed., p. 784). Philadelphia: W. B. Saunders.

186. 2
Rationale: Laboratory determinations of serum thyroid-stimulating hormone are an important means of evaluation. Successful therapy will cause elevated thyroid-stimulating hormone levels to fall. These levels will begin their decline within hours of the onset of therapy and will continue to drop as plasma levels of thyroid hormone build up. If an adequate dosage is administered, thyroid-stimulating hormone levels will remain suppressed for the duration of the therapy.
Test-Taking Strategy: Use the process of elimination. Note the key words "expected outcome." Relate the diagnosis hypothyroidism with "thyroid" hormone levels in the correct option. If you had difficulty with this question, review the therapeutic effect of levothyroxine (Synthroid).
Level of Cognitive Ability: Application
Client Needs: Physiological Integrity
Integrated Process: Teaching/Learning
Content Area: Pharmacology

Reference: Lehne, R. (2001). *Pharmacology for nursing care* (4th ed., pp. 640-641). Philadelphia: W. B. Saunders.

187. 3
Rationale: Levothyroxine (Synthroid) is used to treat hypothyroidism. Although therapy with levothyroxine may begin with small doses that are increased gradually, the most appropriate response is to inform the client that full therapeutic effect may take 1 to 3 weeks.
Test-Taking Strategy: Use the process of elimination. Eliminate options 1 and 2 first because they are similar. Next, eliminate option 4 because the time frame is lengthy. If you had difficulty with this question, review the therapeutic effects of this medication.
Level of Cognitive Ability: Application
Client Needs: Physiological Integrity
Integrated Process: Teaching/Learning
Content Area: Pharmacology
Reference: Lehne, R. (2001). *Pharmacology for nursing care* (4th ed., p. 640). Philadelphia: W. B. Saunders.

188. 4
Rationale: The nurse should instruct the client to apply antiembolism stockings before the client rises in the morning to prevent the venous congestion that will begin as soon as the mother gets up. Circulation can be improved with a regular schedule of activity, preferably walking, and the nurse should instruct the mother to avoid prolonged standing or sitting in one position. The nurse also should encourage the mother to maintain a fluid intake of at least 2500 mL a day to prevent dehydration and consequent sluggish circulation.
Test-Taking Strategy: Use the process of elimination. Note the key words "need for further education." Knowledge regarding the application of antiembolism stockings will assist in directing you to option 4. If you had difficulty with this question, review measures to prevent thrombosis in the postpartum woman.
Level of Cognitive Ability: Analysis
Client Needs: Health Promotion and Maintenance
Integrated Process: Teaching/Learning
Content Area: Maternity/Postpartum
Reference: Murray, S., McKinney, E., & Gorrie, T. (2002). *Foundations of maternal-newborn nursing* (3rd ed., p. 785). Philadelphia: W. B. Saunders.

189. 3
Rationale: Insulin should not be frozen. If the nurse notes that the vial of insulin is frozen, the nurse should discard the insulin and obtain a new vial. Options 1, 2, and 4 are incorrect actions.
Test-Taking Strategy: Use the process of elimination. Eliminate options 1 and 4 because they are similar. From the remaining options, option 3 is related most directly to the issue of the question. Review insulin storage principles if you had difficulty with this question.
Level of Cognitive Ability: Application
Client Needs: Physiological Integrity
Integrated Process: Nursing Process—implementation
Content Area: Adult health—endocrine
Reference: Lehne, R. (2001). *Pharmacology for nursing care* (4th ed., p. 620). Philadelphia: W. B. Saunders.

190. 1
Rationale: The initial assessment interview establishes the therapeutic relationship between the nurse and the pregnant woman. The interview is planned, purposeful communication that focuses on specific content. Options 2, 3, and 4 are incorrect and would not lend themselves to eliciting accurate information from the client.
Test-Taking Strategy: Use the process of elimination, focusing on the issue of the question. Remember that establishing a therapeutic relationship is most meaningful. Review therapeutic communication techniques and care to the client with a sexually transmitted disease if you had difficulty with this question.
Level of Cognitive Ability: Application
Client Needs: Psychosocial Integrity
Integrated Process: Caring
Content Area: Maternity/Antepartum
Reference: Lowdermilk, D, & Perry, A. (2003). *Maternity nursing* (6th ed., p. 89). St. Louis: Mosby.

191. 4
Rationale: Visual disturbances, rapid weight gain, and generalized or facial edema are warning signs in pregnancy. Braxton Hicks contractions are the normal, irregular, painless contractions of the uterus that may occur throughout the pregnancy. Additional warning signs in pregnancy include vaginal bleeding, premature rupture of the membranes, preterm uterine contractions that are normal and regular, change in or absence of fetal activity, severe headache, epigastric pain, persistent vomiting, abdominal pain, and signs of infection.
Test-Taking Strategy: Use the process of elimination, noting the key words "need for further education." Recalling that Braxton Hicks contractions are irregular, painless contractions will assist in directing you to option 4. If you had difficulty with this question, review the warning signs in pregnancy.
Level of Cognitive Ability: Analysis
Client Needs: Health Promotion and Maintenance
Integrated Process: Teaching/Learning
Content Area: Maternity/Antepartum
Reference: Lowdermilk, D., & Perry, A. (2003). *Maternity nursing* (6th ed., pp. 218, 222). St. Louis: Mosby.

192. 3
Rationale: Oral calcium supplements need to be administered with food to enhance absorption and to decrease gastrointestinal irritation. Options 1, 2, and 4 are unrelated to oral calcium therapy.
Test-Taking Strategy: Use the process of elimination, focusing on the medication being addressed in the question. Recalling that oral calcium supplements need to be administered with food will direct you to option 3. Review the administration of oral calcium supplements if you had difficulty with this question.
Level of Cognitive Ability: Application
Client Needs: Physiological Integrity
Integrated Process: Teaching/Learning
Content Area: Adult health—endocrine
Reference: Hodgson, B., & Kizior, R. (2003). *Saunders nursing drug handbook 2003* (p. 158). Philadelphia: W. B. Saunders.

193. **4**

Rationale: Diet therapy for hypophosphatemia consists primarily of an increased intake of phosphorus-rich foods while decreasing the intake of calcium-rich foods. Options 1, 2, and 3 identify food items allowed, whereas option 4 should be avoided because it is a calcium-rich food.

Test-Taking Strategy: Note the key word "avoid." Recalling that the client with hypophosphatemia needs to decrease the intake of calcium-rich foods will direct you to option 4. If you had difficulty with the question, review the dietary measures for the client with hypophosphatemia.

Level of Cognitive Ability: Application
Client Needs: Physiological Integrity
Integrated Process: Teaching/Learning
Content Area: Fundamental skills
Reference: Ignatavicius, D., & Workman, M. (2002). *Medical-surgical nursing: Critical thinking for collaborative care* (4th ed., p. 191). Philadelphia: W. B. Saunders.

194. **1**

Rationale: Physical symptoms can interfere with an individual's ability to learn and also can indicate to the teacher that the learner lacks motivation to learn, if the symptoms repeatedly recur when teaching is initiated. Options 2, 3, and 4 identify active client participation in learning.

Test-Taking Strategy: Use the process of elimination and note the key words "not ready to learn." Options 2, 3, and 4 identify the client as actively seeking information. Option 1 suggest avoidance on the part of the client. Review teaching/learning concepts if you had difficulty with this question.

Level of Cognitive Ability: Analysis
Client Needs: Psychosocial Integrity
Integrated Process: Teaching/Learning
Content Area: Adult health—endocrine
Reference: Ignatavicius, D., & Workman, M. (2002). *Medical-surgical nursing: Critical thinking for collaborative care* (4th ed., p. 1485). Philadelphia: W. B. Saunders.

195. **3**

Rationale: Hypoglycemic reactions present adrenergic symptoms of tremor, shakiness, and nervousness that are similar to the signs of alcohol intoxication. The best strategy to assist the client to meet his needs is to decrease the episodes of hypoglycemia by first identifying and then eliminating those factors that precipitate this event. Options 1 and 2 are inappropriate. Option 4 is not related directly to the issue of the question.

Test-Taking Strategy: Use the process of elimination and therapeutic communication techniques. Option 1 presumes that the problem is unavoidable and thus the client is at fault. Option 2 presumes that the client may be drinking, and option 4 avoids the issue of the question. Review therapeutic communication techniques if you had difficulty with this question.

Level of Cognitive Ability: Analysis
Client Needs: Psychosocial Integrity
Integrated Process: Nursing Process—implementation
Content Area: Adult health—endocrine
Reference: Lewis, S., Heitkemper, M., & Dirksen, S. (2004). *Medical-surgical nursing: Assessment and management of clinical problems* (6th ed., p. 1295). St. Louis: Mosby.

196. **1**

Rationale: Clinical symptoms at birth in neonates exposed to cocaine in utero include tremors, tachycardia, irritability, muscular rigidity, hypertension, and exaggerated startle reflex. These infants are difficult to console and exhibit an inability to respond to voices or environmental stimuli. They are often poor feeders and have episodes of diarrhea.

Test-Taking Strategy: Use the process of elimination. Think about the effects of the drug to assist in directing you to the correct option. Also note the similarity between options 2, 3, and 4. If you had difficulty with this question, review the effects of cocaine on the fetus and neonate.

Level of Cognitive Ability: Analysis
Client Needs: Physiological Integrity
Integrated Process: Nursing Process—assessment
Content Area: Maternity/Postpartum
Reference: Lowdermilk, D., & Perry, A. (2003). *Maternity nursing* (6th ed., pp. 770-772). St. Louis: Mosby.

197. **4**

Rationale: For most clients with hypothyroidism, replacement therapy must be continued for life. Treatment provides symptomatic relief but does not produce a cure. The client should be told that although therapy will cause symptoms to improve, these improvements do not constitute a reason to interrupt or discontinue the medication. Options 2 and 3 are incorrect. Option 1 places the client's question on hold.

Test-Taking Strategy: Use the process of elimination. Eliminate option 1 first because it places the client's question on hold. Next eliminate options 2 and 3 because they are similar. Review this disorder and the medication therapy associated with it if you had difficulty with this question.

Level of Cognitive Ability: Application
Client Needs: Physiological Integrity
Integrated Process: Teaching/Learning
Content Area: Pharmacology
Reference: Lehne, R. (2001). *Pharmacology for nursing care* (4th ed., p. 639). Philadelphia: W. B. Saunders.

198. *Answer:*

Family history of breast cancer
Age greater than 40 years
Early menarche
Previous cancer of the breast, uterus, or ovaries
High-dose radiation exposure to chest

Rationale: Risk factors for breast cancer include family history of breast cancer; age greater than 40 years; early menarche or late menopause or both; previous cancer of the breast, uterus, or ovaries; nulliparity or first child born after age 30 years; and high-dose radiation exposure to chest.

Test-Taking Strategy: Focus on the issue, the risk factors associated with breast cancer. Thinking about the physiology associated with the reproductive system and the most common causes of cancer will assist you in answering the question. Review these risk factors if you had difficulty with this question.

Level of Cognitive Ability: Analysis
Client Needs: Physiological Integrity
Integrated Process: Nursing Process—assessment
Content Area: Adult health—oncology

Reference: Ignatavicius, D., & Workman, M. (2002). *Medical-surgical nursing: Critical thinking for collaborative care* (4th ed., p. 1737). Philadelphia: W. B. Saunders.

199. **1**
Rationale: The normal temperature during pregnancy is 36.2° to 37.6° C (98° to 99.6° F). A temperature higher than this may suggest infection that might require medical management. Options 2, 3, and 4 are unnecessary.
Test-Taking Strategy: Use the process of elimination. Recalling that the normal body temperature in the prenatal period is 98° to 99.6° F will direct you to option 1. Review the normal vital signs during pregnancy if you had difficulty with this question.
Level of Cognitive Ability: Application
Client Needs: Physiological Integrity
Integrated Process: Nursing Process—implementation
Content Area: Maternity/Antepartum
Reference: Murray, S., McKinney, E., & Gorrie, T. (2002). *Foundations of maternal-newborn nursing* (3rd ed., p. 143). Philadelphia: W. B. Saunders.

200. **4**
Rationale: Because a 24-hour urine collection is a timed quantitative determination, it is essential that the client start the test with an empty bladder. Therefore the client is instructed to void, discard the first urine, note the time, and start the test. The 24-hour urine specimen collection bottle must be kept on ice or refrigerated. In a vanillylmandelic acid collection, the client is instructed to avoid tea, chocolate, vanilla, and all fruits for 2 days before urine collection begins. Clients also are reminded not to take medications for 2 to 3 days before or during the test unless prescribed.
Test-Taking Strategy: Use the process of elimination. Note the key words "a need for further instructions." Use knowledge regarding the basic procedure for collecting a 24-hour urine sample to answer the question. Review this procedure if you had difficulty with this question.
Level of Cognitive Ability: Analysis
Client Needs: Physiological Integrity
Integrated Process: Teaching/Learning
Content Area: Adult health—endocrine
Reference: Chernecky, C., & Berger, B. (2001). *Laboratory tests and diagnostic procedures* (3rd ed., p. 1057). Philadelphia: W. B. Saunders.

201. **1**
Rationale: Paraphrasing is restating the client's messages in the nurse's own words. Option 1 addresses the therapeutic communication technique of paraphrasing. In option 2 the nurse is offering a false reassurance, and this type of response will block communication. Option 3 also represents a communication block in that it reflects a lack of the client's right to an opinion. In option 4 the nurse is expressing approval, which can be harmful to a nurse-client relationship.
Test-Taking Strategy: Use the process of elimination and therapeutic communication techniques. Select the option that will enhance communication. Always address the client's concerns and feelings. Review therapeutic communication techniques if you had difficulty with this question.

Level of Cognitive Ability: Application
Client Needs: Psychosocial Integrity
Integrated Process: Caring
Content Area: Adult health—endocrine
Reference: Varcarolis, E. (2002). *Foundations of psychiatric mental health nursing* (4th ed., p. 258). Philadelphia: W. B. Saunders.

202. **1**
Rationale: As the nasogastric tube is passed through the oropharynx, the gag reflex is stimulated, which may cause coughing, gagging, or choking. Instead of passing through to the esophagus, the nasogastric tube may coil around itself in the oropharynx, or it may enter the larynx and obstruct the airway. Because the tube may enter the larynx and obstruct the airway, pulling the tube back slightly will remove it from the larynx; advancing the tube might position it in the trachea. Swallowing closes the epiglottis over the trachea and helps move the tube into the esophagus. Slow breathing helps the client relax to reduce the gag response. The nurse should check the back of the client's throat to note if the tube has coiled. The tube may be advanced after the client relaxes.
Test-Taking Strategy: Use the process of elimination. Note the key words "least likely." Options 2, 3, and 4 aim at assessing and promoting relaxation whereas option 1 could result in an unsafe malposition of the nasogastric tube into the trachea. Review the procedure for inserting a nasogastric tube if you had difficulty with this question.
Level of Cognitive Ability: Application
Client Needs: Physiological Integrity
Integrated Process: Nursing Process—implementation
Content Area: Adult health—gastrointestinal
Reference: Potter, P., & Perry, A. (2001). *Fundamentals of nursing* (5th ed., pp. 1274, 1467). St. Louis: Mosby.

203. **4**
Rationale: The ovarian cycle consists of three phases: the follicular phase, ovulatory phase, and luteal phase. The proliferative phase is a phase of the endometrial cycle.
Test-Taking Strategy: Use the process of elimination. Note the key words "indicates a need to further research." Also focus on the issue of the question, the ovarian cycle. Review the phases of the ovarian cycle if you had difficulty with this question.
Level of Cognitive Ability: Comprehension
Client Needs: Physiological Integrity
Integrated Process: Teaching/Learning
Content Area: Fundamental skills
Reference: Murray, S., McKinney, E., & Gorrie, T. (2002). *Foundations of maternal-newborn nursing* (3rd ed., p. 68). Philadelphia: W. B. Saunders.

204. **1**
Rationale: During a menstrual period, a woman loses about 40 mL of blood. Because of the recurrent loss of blood, many women become mildly anemic during their reproductive years, especially if their diets are low in iron.
Test-Taking Strategy: Use the process of elimination. Knowledge regarding the menstrual phase of the menstrual cycle and the amount of blood lost during a menstrual period is required to answer this question. If you are unfamiliar with the menstrual phase, review this content area.

Level of Cognitive Ability: Comprehension
Client Needs: Physiological Integrity
Integrated Process: Nursing Process—planning
Content Area: Fundamental skills
Reference: Murray, S., McKinney, E., & Gorrie, T. (2002). *Foundations of maternal-newborn nursing* (3rd ed., p. 69). Philadelphia: W. B. Saunders.

205. **3**
Rationale: An inflammatory reaction such as acute pancreatitis can cause paralytic ileus, the most common form of non-mechanical obstruction. Inability to pass flatus is a clinical manifestation of paralytic ileus. Option 1 is the description of the physical finding of liver enlargement. The liver is usually enlarged in cases of cirrhosis or hepatitis. Although this client may have an enlarged liver, an enlarged liver is not a sign of paralytic ileus or intestinal obstruction. Pain is associated with paralytic ileus, but the pain usually presents as a more constant generalized discomfort. Pain that is severe, constant, and rapid in onset more likely is caused by strangulation of the bowel. Loss of sphincter control is not a sign of paralytic ileus.
Test-Taking Strategy: Use the process of elimination. Noting the word "paralytic" will assist in directing you to option 3. Review the clinical manifestations of paralytic ileus if you had difficulty with this question.
Level of Cognitive Ability: Analysis
Client Needs: Physiological Integrity
Integrated Process: Nursing Process—assessment
Content Area: Adult health—gastrointestinal
Reference: Phipps, W., Monahan, F., Sands, J., Marek, J., & Neighbors, M. (2003). *Medical-surgical nursing: Health and illness perspectives* (7th ed., p. 440). St. Louis: Mosby.

206. **2**
Rationale: For the first 12 hours following a laparotomy, the nasogastric tube drainage may be dark brown to dark red. Later the drainage should change to a light yellowish brown. The presence of bile may cause a greenish tinge. The physician should be notified if dark red drainage is noted.
Test-Taking Strategy: Focus on the issue "need to notify the physician." Use the process of elimination and recall that bleeding is a concern in the postoperative client. This concept will direct you easily to option 2. Review the signs of postoperative complications following a laparotomy if you had difficulty with this question.
Level of Cognitive Ability: Analysis
Client Needs: Physiological Integrity
Integrated Process: Nursing Process—analysis
Content Area: Adult health—gastrointestinal
Reference: Ignatavicius, D., & Workman, M. (2002). *Medical-surgical nursing: Critical thinking for collaborative care* (4th ed., pp. 297, 1227). Philadelphia: W. B. Saunders.

207. **3**
Rationale: The client should take a deep breath because the client's airway will be obstructed temporarily during tube removal. The nurse then tells the client to exhale slowly and withdraws the tube during exhalation. Bearing down could inhibit the removal of the tube. Breathing normally could

result in aspiration of gastric secretions during inhalation. Holding the breath does not facilitate tube removal.
Test-Taking Strategy: Use the process of elimination. Attempt to visualize the process of tube removal to direct you to option 3. Remember that exhaling slowly will facilitate the process of removal. Review the procedure for removal of a nasogastric tube if you had difficulty with this question.
Level of Cognitive Ability: Application
Client Needs: Physiological Integrity
Integrated Process: Nursing Process—implementation
Content Area: Adult health—gastrointestinal
Reference: Potter, P., & Perry, A. (2001). *Fundamentals of nursing* (5th ed., p. 1479). St. Louis: Mosby.

208. **3**
Rationale: After a nasogastric tube is in place, mouth care is important. With one naris occluded, the client tends to mouth breathe, drying the mucous membranes. Small sips of water are contraindicated when the client is receiving gastric suction. Hard candy would increase the salivation but would not be useful in cleaning the oral cavity. Lemon-glycerin swabs have a drying and irritating effect on the mucous membranes.
Test-Taking Strategy: Focus on the issue, maintaining the integrity of the oral mucosa. Options 1, 2, and 4 are unrelated to this issue and can be eliminated easily. Review the basic measures related to maintaining the integrity of oral mucosa if you had difficulty with this question.
Level of Cognitive Ability: Application
Client Needs: Health Promotion and Maintenance
Integrated Process: Nursing Process—planning
Content Area: Fundamental skills
Reference: Potter, P., & Perry, A. (2001). *Fundamentals of nursing* (5th ed., p. 1097). St. Louis: Mosby.

209. **4**
Rationale: Treatment of intestinal obstruction is directed toward decompression of the intestine by removal of gas and fluid. Nasogastric tubes may be used to decompress the bowel. Continuous gastric suction does not provide nourishment. Option 2 is the purpose for tracheal suctioning. Although gastric contents may be sent for laboratory analysis, it is not the main purpose for continuous gastric suction.
Test-Taking Strategy: Use the process of elimination. Option 2 can be eliminated first because it is unrelated to a gastrointestinal disorder. Eliminate option 1 next, recalling that a client with a bowel obstruction is NPO. From the remaining options, focusing on the client's diagnosis will direct you to option 4. Review the treatment for a client with a bowel obstruction if you had difficulty with this question.
Level of Cognitive Ability: Analysis
Client Needs: Physiological Integrity
Integrated Process: Teaching/Learning
Content Area: Adult health—gastrointestinal
Reference: Potter, P., & Perry, A. (2001). *Fundamentals of nursing* (5th ed., p. 1353). St. Louis: Mosby.

210. **3**
Rationale: When the client is experiencing respiratory acidosis, in an attempt to compensate the respiratory rate and depth increase. The client also experiences headache, restlessness,

mental status changes such as drowsiness and confusion, visual disturbances, diaphoresis, cyanosis as the hypoxia becomes more acute, hyperkalemia, a rapid and irregular pulse, and dysrhythmias.

Test-Taking Strategy: Use the process of elimination and knowledge of the signs and symptoms of respiratory acidosis to answer the question. Remember that restlessness and confusion occurs in respiratory acidosis. If this question was difficult, review the clinical manifestations associated with respiratory acidosis.

Level of Cognitive Ability: Analysis
Client Needs: Physiological Integrity
Integrated Process: Nursing Process—assessment
Content Area: Fundamental skills
Reference: Potter, P., & Perry, A. (2001). *Fundamentals of nursing* (5th ed., p. 1204). St. Louis: Mosby.

211. **3**
Rationale: Distention, vomiting, and abdominal pain are a few of the symptoms associated with intestinal obstruction. Nasogastric tubes may be used to remove gas and fluid from the stomach, thus relieving distention and vomiting. Bowel sounds return to normal as the obstruction is resolved and normal bowel function is restored. Discontinuing the nasogastric tube before normal bowel function returns may result in a return of the symptoms, necessitating reinsertion of the nasogastric tube. Serum electrolyte levels, tube placement, and pH of gastric aspirate are important assessments for the client with a nasogastric tube in place but would not assist in determining the readiness for removing the nasogastric tube.

Test-Taking Strategy: Use the process of elimination. Eliminate options 1 and 4 first because they are similar. Assessing the pH of gastric aspirate is one method of assessing tube placement. From the remaining options, focus on the issue and the client's diagnosis to direct you to option 3. Review abdominal assessment in the client with an intestinal obstruction if you had difficulty with this question.

Level of Cognitive Ability: Analysis
Client Needs: Physiological Integrity
Integrated Process: Nursing Process—assessment
Content Area: Adult health—gastrointestinal
Reference: Potter, P., & Perry, A. (2001). *Fundamentals of nursing* (5th ed., p. 1479). St. Louis: Mosby.

212. **2**
Rationale: The enema fluid should be administered slowly. If the client complains of fullness or pain, the flow is stopped for 30 seconds and restarted at a slower rate. Slow enema administration and stopping the flow temporarily, if necessary, will decrease the likelihood of intestinal spasm and premature ejection of the solution. The higher the solution container is held above the rectum, the faster the flow and the greater the force in the rectum. The nurse does not need to discontinue the enema and notify the physician at this time. Although client reassurance is important, continuing the flow is inappropriate.

Test-Taking Strategy: Use the process of elimination. Eliminate options 1 and 3 first because they are similar. From the remaining options, focusing on the issue will direct you to option 2. Review the procedure for administering an enema if you had difficulty with this question.

Level of Cognitive Ability: Application
Client Needs: Physiological Integrity
Integrated Process: Nursing Process—implementation
Content Area: Fundamental skills
Reference: Potter, P., & Perry, A. (2001). *Fundamentals of nursing* (5th ed., p. 1464). St. Louis: Mosby.

213. **1**
Rationale: The sigmoid and descending colon are located on the left side. Therefore the left lateral position uses gravity to facilitate the flow of solution into the sigmoid and descending colon. Acute flexion of the right leg allows for adequate exposure of the anus. Options 2, 3, and 4 are incorrect positions.

Test-Taking Strategy: Knowledge of the anatomy of the rectum will assist you in eliminating options 2 and 4. Attempt to visualize the remaining positions to eliminate option 3. Review the procedure for administering an enema if you had difficulty with this question.

Level of Cognitive Ability: Application
Client Needs: Physiological Integrity
Integrated Process: Nursing Process—implementation
Content Area: Fundamental skills
Reference: Potter, P., & Perry, A. (2001). *Fundamentals of nursing* (5th ed., p. 1463). St. Louis: Mosby.

214. **2**
Rationale: After checking residual feeding contents, the gastric contents are reinstilled into the stomach by removing the syringe bulb or plunger and pouring the gastric contents into the syringe and through the nasogastric tube. Gastric contents should be reinstilled to maintain the client's electrolyte balance. The gastric contents should be poured into the nasogastric tube through a syringe without a plunger and not injected by putting pressure on the plunger. Gastric contents do not need to be mixed with water nor should the contents be discarded.

Test-Taking Strategy: Use the process of elimination. Eliminate option 4 because of the words "putting pressure." Recalling that gastric contents need to be reinstilled to maintain electrolyte balance will assist you in eliminating options 1 and 3. Review care to the client with a nasogastric tube and nasogastric tube feedings if you had difficulty with this question.

Level of Cognitive Ability: Application
Client Needs: Physiological Integrity
Integrated Process: Nursing Process—implementation
Content Area: Adult health—gastrointestinal
Reference: Potter, P., & Perry, A. (2001). *Fundamentals of nursing* (5th ed., p. 1478). St. Louis: Mosby.

215. **4**
Rationale: Option 4 describes aversion therapy. Options 1, 2, and 3 are characteristics of self-control therapy.

Test-Taking Strategy: Use the process of elimination. Note the key words "need for further teaching" in the stem of the question. Think about the issue "self-control." This issue should direct you easily to option 4. If you are unfamiliar with self-control therapy, review this content.

Level of Cognitive Ability: Analysis
Client Needs: Psychosocial Integrity
Integrated Process: Teaching/Learning
Content Area: Mental health

Reference: Varcarolis, E. (2002). *Foundations of psychiatric mental health nursing* (4th ed., pp. 271–278). Philadelphia: W. B. Saunders.

216. *Answer:*
Avoid swimming and use care when showering.
Avoid exposure to persons with infections.
Obtain a Medic-Alert bracelet.
Prevent debris from entering the stoma.
Rationale: The nurse would teach the client how to care for the stoma depending on the type of laryngectomy performed. Most interventions focus on protection of the stoma and the prevention of infection. Interventions include to avoid swimming and use care when showering, avoid exposure to persons with infections, prevent debris from entering the stoma, and obtaining a Medic-Alert bracelet. Additional interventions include wearing a stoma guard or high-collar clothing to cover the stoma, increasing the humidity in the home, and increasing fluid intake to 3000 mL/day to keep the secretions thin.
Test-Taking Strategy: Recalling that most interventions focus on protection of the stoma and the prevention of infection will assist you in identifying the client instructions for home care. Review these instructions if you had difficulty with this question.
Level of Cognitive Ability: Application
Client Needs: Physiological Integrity
Integrated Process: Teaching/Learning
Content Area: Adult health—oncology
Reference: Ignatavicius, D., & Workman, M. (2002). *Medical-surgical nursing: Critical thinking for collaborative care* (4th ed., p. 525). Philadelphia: W. B. Saunders.

217. **3**
Rationale: Respiratory rates are generally higher in older adults, with a normal rate of 16 to 25 breaths per minute. The heart rate also decreases with age. Therefore because the data in the question indicate normal findings, the nurse would document the heart rate and respiratory rate. Options 1, 2, and 4 are unnecessary based on the data in the question.
Test-Taking Strategy: Focus on the data in the question. Recalling the normal respiratory rate in an older client and recalling that the heart rate decreases as a client ages will direct you to option 3. Review age-related changes in the cardiac and respiratory system if you had difficulty with this question.
Level of Cognitive Ability: Application
Client Needs: Health Promotion and Maintenance
Integrated Process: Nursing Process—implementation
Content Area: Fundamental skills
Reference: Lueckenotte, A. (2000). *Gerontologic nursing* (2nd ed., pp. 448, 486). St. Louis: Mosby.

218. **4**
Rationale: In the immediate postoperative period the gastrostomy tube is elevated, allowing gastric contents to pass to the small intestine and air to escape. This promotes comfort and decreases the risk of leakage at the anastomosis. Options 1, 2, and 3 are incorrect.
Test-Taking Strategy: Option 3 can be eliminated easily because this action could cause accidental removal of the tube. Option 2 can be eliminated next with the concept that suction on a surgical site could disrupt the repair. Recalling that feedings are

not initiated in the immediate postoperative period will assist in directing you to the correct option. Review postoperative nursing care if you had difficulty with this question.
Level of Cognitive Ability: Application
Client Needs: Physiological Integrity
Integrated Process: Nursing Process—implementation
Content Area: Child health
Reference: Murray, S., McKinney, E., & Gorrie, T. (2002). *Foundations of maternal-newborn nursing* (3rd ed., pp. 540-541). Philadelphia: W. B. Saunders.

219. **1**
Rationale: Tricyclic antidepressants can be fatal when taken as an overdose, regardless of the amount ingested. Serious, life-threatening symptoms can develop after an overdose. Immediate emergency medical attention and cardiac monitoring is necessary with an overdose of tricyclic antidepressants.
Test-Taking Strategy: Use the process of elimination. Note the key word "immediate" in the stem of the question. Options 2, 3, and 4 would delay measures in providing immediate treatment. Additionally, vomiting is not induced in a client who is unconscious. Review care to the client with an overdose if you had difficulty with this question.
Level of Cognitive Ability: Application
Client Needs: Physiological Integrity
Integrated Process: Nursing Process—implementation
Content Area: Mental health
Reference: Varcarolis, E. (2002). *Foundations of psychiatric mental health nursing* (4th ed., pp. 473-474). Philadelphia: W. B. Saunders.

220. **4**
Rationale: Following the procedure, the client remains NPO until the gag reflex returns, which is usually in 1 to 2 hours. Options 1, 2, and 3 are not specific assessments related to this procedure.
Test-Taking Strategy: Use the process of elimination. Note the key words "upper gastrointestinal endoscopy." The only option that relates to the anatomical location of this procedure is option 4. Review postprocedure care following endoscopy if you had difficulty with this question.
Level of Cognitive Ability: Application
Client Needs: Physiological Integrity
Integrated Process: Nursing Process—planning
Content Area: Adult health—gastrointestinal
Reference: Potter, P., & Perry, A. (2001). *Fundamentals of nursing* (5th ed., p. 1454). St. Louis: Mosby.

221. **3**
Rationale: To best facilitate insertion, when the tube reaches the pharynx, the client is encouraged to lower the head slightly, swallow, and if allowed, to take sips of water. The nasogastric tube would be iced so that it is stiff to ease insertion. If the tube meets resistance, the tube is withdrawn slightly and repassed. Option 3 is the only option that would facilitate insertion.
Test-Taking Strategy: Use the process of elimination. Focus on the issue, facilitating easy insertion of the nasogastric tube. Next, visualize the procedure to direct you to option 3. Review this procedure if you had difficulty with this question.
Level of Cognitive Ability: Application

Client Needs: Physiological Integrity
Integrated Process: Nursing Process—implementation
Content Area: Adult health—gastrointestinal
Reference: Potter, P., & Perry, A. (2001). *Fundamentals of nursing* (5th ed., p. 1476). St. Louis: Mosby.

222. *Answer:* 21 drops per minute
Rationale: Use the intravenous flow rate formula.
Formula:

$$\frac{\text{Total volume} \times \text{Drop factor}}{\text{Time in minutes}} = \text{Drops per minute}$$

$$\frac{2000 \text{ mL} \times 15 \text{ gtt}}{1440 \text{ minutes}} = \frac{30,000}{1440} = 20.8, \text{ or } 21 \text{ gtt per minute}$$

Test-Taking Strategy: Use the formula for calculating intravenous flow rates when answering the question. Be careful with the multiplication and division. Using the formula carefully will direct you to the correct option. Review intravenous infusion rates if you had difficulty with this question.
Level of Cognitive Ability: Application
Client Needs: Physiological Integrity
Integrated Process: Nursing Process—implementation
Content Area: Fundamental skills
Reference: Potter, P., & Perry, A. (2001). *Fundamentals of nursing* (5th ed., p. 1229). St. Louis: Mosby.

223. **3**
Rationale: In the first few hours after surgery, the drainage from the chest tube is bloody. After several hours, the drainage becomes serosanguineous. The client should not experience frequent clotting. Proper chest tube function should allow for drainage of blood before it has the chance to clot in the chest or the tubing.
Test-Taking Strategy: Recall that following thoracic surgery, there may be considerable capillary oozing for some hours in the postoperative period. This would lead you to choose the bloody drainage over serous or serosanguineous. Knowing that patent chest tubes do not allow blood to collect in the pleural space eliminates the option of blood with clots. Review the assessment measures required in the care of a client with a chest tube if you had difficulty with this question.
Level of Cognitive Ability: Analysis
Client Needs: Physiological Integrity
Integrated Process: Nursing Process—assessment
Content Area: Adult health—respiratory
Reference: Potter, P., & Perry, A. (2001). *Fundamentals of nursing* (5th ed., p. 1174). St. Louis: Mosby.

224. **1**
Rationale: If the client begins to hemorrhage from the surgical site following radical neck dissection, the nurse elevates the head of the bed to maintain airway patency and prevent aspiration. The nurse applies pressure over the bleeding site and calls the physician immediately.
Test-Taking Strategy: Use the process of elimination, noting the key word "contraindicated." Options 2 and 3 are indicated if the client is hemorrhaging. Calling the physician also is indicated immediately, whereas lowering the head of bed does not help with airway maintenance. Review the nursing actions for the client who begins to hemorrhage if you had difficulty with this question.

Level of Cognitive Ability: Application
Client Needs: Physiological Integrity
Integrated Process: Nursing Process—implementation
Content Area: Adult health—respiratory
Reference: Lewis, S., Heitkemper, M., & Dirksen, S. (2004). *Medical-surgical nursing: Assessment and management of clinical problems* (6th ed., p. 583). St. Louis: Mosby.

225. **2**
Rationale: Foscarnet (Foscavir) is toxic to the kidneys. Serum creatinine is monitored before therapy, 2 to 3 times per week during induction therapy, and at least weekly during maintenance therapy. Foscarnet also may cause decreased levels of calcium, magnesium, phosphorus, and potassium. Thus these levels also are measured with the same frequency.
Test-Taking Strategy: Use the process of elimination. Recalling that foscarnet is nephrotoxic will direct you to option 2. Review the adverse effects of this medication if you had difficulty with this question.
Level of Cognitive Ability: Analysis
Client Needs: Physiological Integrity
Integrated Process: Nursing Process—assessment
Content Area: Adult health—immune
Reference: Hodgson, B., & Kizior, R. (2003). *Saunders nursing drug handbook 2003* (p. 493). Philadelphia: W. B. Saunders.

226. **2**
Rationale: Tuberculosis is spread by droplet nuclei, or the airborne route. The disease is not carried on objects such as clothing, eating utensils, linens, or furniture. Bleaching of clothing and linens is unnecessary, although the client and family members should use good hand-washing technique. Removing carpeting from the home is not necessary.
Test-Taking Strategy: Knowing that tuberculosis is not carried on inanimate objects helps you to eliminate options 3 and 4 first. To discriminate between options 1 and 2, recall that the disease is transmitted by the airborne route. If you had difficulty with this question, review the transmission mode of tuberculosis.
Level of Cognitive Ability: Application
Client Needs: Safe, Effective Care Environment
Integrated Process: Teaching/Learning
Content Area: Adult health—respiratory
Reference: Ignatavicius, D., & Workman, M. (2002). *Medical-surgical nursing: Critical thinking for collaborative care* (4th ed., pp. 586-587). Philadelphia: W. B. Saunders.

227. **3**
Rationale: Signs of allergic reaction to the contrast dye include early signs such as localized itching and edema, which then are followed by more severe symptoms such as respiratory distress, stridor, and decreased blood pressure.
Test-Taking Strategy: Focus on the issue, an allergic reaction. Hypothermia is an unrelated event and is eliminated first. Discomfort is expected, and is eliminated next. Hematoma formation is a complication of the procedure but does not indicate allergic reaction and therefore is eliminated. The remaining option is stridor, which is a sign of a severe allergic reaction and possible anaphylaxis. Review the signs of an allergic reaction to the contrast medium if you had difficulty with this question.

Level of Cognitive Ability: Analysis
Client Needs: Physiological Integrity
Integrated Process: Nursing Process—assessment
Content Area: Adult health—respiratory
Reference: Chernecky, C., & Berger, B. (2001). *Laboratory tests and diagnostic procedures* (3rd ed., p. 873). Philadelphia: W. B. Saunders.

228. 2

Rationale: To prevent transmission of hepatitis, a condom is advised during sexual intercourse, as well as vaccination of the partner. Alcohol should be avoided for 1 year because it is detoxified in the liver and may interfere with recovery. Rest is especially important until laboratory studies show that the liver function has returned to normal. The client's activity is increased gradually.
Test-Taking Strategy: Use the process of elimination focusing on the key words "need for further teaching." Noting the absolute word "never" in option 2 will direct you to this option. Review client instructions regarding hepatitis if you had difficulty with this question.
Level of Cognitive Ability: Analysis
Client Needs: Physiological Integrity
Integrated Process: Teaching/Learning
Content Area: Adult health—gastrointestinal
Reference: Lewis, S., Heitkemper, M., & Dirksen, S. (2004). *Medical-surgical nursing: Assessment and management of clinical problems* (6th ed., p. 1114). St. Louis: Mosby.

229. Answer:

Instruct the client about thyroid replacement therapy.
Encourage the client to consume fluids and high-fiber foods in the diet.
Instruct the client to contact the physician if episodes of chest pain occur.
Rationale: The clinical manifestations of hypothyroidism are the result of decreased metabolism from low levels of thyroid hormone. Interventions are aimed at replacement of the hormones and providing measures to support the signs and symptoms related to a decreased metabolism. The nurse encourages the client to consume a well-balanced diet that is low in fat for weight reduction and high in fluids and high-fiber foods to prevent constipation. The client often has cold intolerance and requires a warm environment. The client would notify the physician if chest pain occurs because it could be an indication of overreplacement of thyroid hormone. Iodine preparations are used to treat hyperthyroidism. These medications decrease blood flow through the thyroid gland and reduce the production and release of thyroid hormone.
Test-Taking Strategy: Focus on the client's diagnosis, hypothyroidism. Recalling that in this disorder the client has a decreased metabolic rate will assist in determining the appropriate interventions. Review interventions for the client with hypothyroidism and hyperthyroidism if you had difficulty with this question.
Level of Cognitive Ability: Application
Client Needs: Physiological Integrity
Integrated Process: Nursing Process—implementation
Content Area: Adult health—endocrine

References: Ignatavicius, D., & Workman, M. (2002). *Medical-surgical nursing: Critical thinking for collaborative care* (4th ed., pp. 1427, 1434). Philadelphia: W. B. Saunders.
Phipps, W., Monahan, F., Sands, J., Marek, J., & Neighbors, M. (2003). *Medical-surgical nursing: Health and illness perspectives* (7th ed., p. 901). St. Louis: Mosby.

230. 1

Rationale: Isoproterenol is an adrenergic bronchodilator. Side effects can include tachycardia, hypertension, chest pain, dysrhythmias, nervousness, restlessness, and headache, among others. The nurse monitors for these effects during therapy.
Test-Taking Strategy: Use the process of elimination. Recall that this medication is an adrenergic agent. Thus isoproterenol causes bronchodilation but also increases pulse and blood pressure because of its cardiovascular effects. With this in mind, you can eliminate each of the incorrect options. Remembering that tachycardia is a side effect should assist you in selecting the option that identifies an increased pulse, option 1. Review the side effects of this medication if you had difficulty with this question.
Level of Cognitive Ability: Analysis
Client Needs: Physiological Integrity
Integrated Process: Nursing Process—assessment
Content Area: Pharmacology
Reference: Hodgson, B., & Kizior, R. (2003). *Saunders nursing drug handbook 2003* (p. 618). Philadelphia: W. B. Saunders.

231. 2

Rationale: Plugging a tracheostomy tube usually is done by inserting the tracheostomy plug (decanullation stopper) into the opening of the outer cannula. This closes off the tracheostomy and air flow, and respiration occurs normally through the nose and mouth. When plugging a cuffed tracheostomy tube, the cuff must be deflated. If the cuff remains inflated, ventilation cannot occur and respiratory arrest could result. The inner cannula is removed before plugging the tracheostomy tube.
Test-Taking Strategy: Note the key word "required" in the question. This should assist in directing you to the option that addresses a priority physiological need. Use the process of elimination to direct you to option 2 because an inflated cuff would cause airway obstruction. Review this procedure if you had difficulty with this question.
Level of Cognitive Ability: Application
Client Needs: Physiological Integrity
Integrated Process: Nursing Process—implementation
Content Area: Adult health—respiratory
Reference: Lewis, S., Heitkemper, M., & Dirksen, S. (2004). *Medical-surgical nursing: Assessment and management of clinical problems* (6th ed., p. 576). St. Louis: Mosby.

232. 2

Rationale: Cinoxacin should be administered with caution in clients with renal impairment. The dosage should be reduced, and failure to do so could result in accumulation of cinoxacin to toxic levels.
Test-Taking Strategy: Use the process of elimination. Knowledge that this medication is used with caution in clients with renal impairment will direct you to option 2. If you are

unfamiliar with this medication, review its cautions and contraindications.

Level of Cognitive Ability: Analysis
Client Needs: Physiological Integrity
Integrated Process: Nursing Process—analysis
Content Area: Pharmacology
Reference: McKenry, L., & Salerno, E. (2003). *Mosby's pharmacology in nursing* (21st ed., p. 1006). St. Louis: Mosby.

233. **2**
Rationale: Administration of urecholine with food can cause nausea and vomiting in the client. To avoid this problem, doses should be administered orally 1 hour before meals or 2 hours after meals.
Test-Taking Strategy: Use the process of elimination. Note that options 1, 3, and 4 are similar in that they suggest administering the medication with a food item. Review client teaching points related to this medication if you had difficulty with this question.
Level of Cognitive Ability: Application
Client Needs: Physiological Integrity
Integrated Process: Teaching/Learning
Content Area: Pharmacology
Reference: Lehne, R. (2001). *Pharmacology for nursing care* (4th ed., p. 117). Philadelphia: W. B. Saunders.

234. **3**
Rationale: Hypertension, cardiovascular disease, diabetes mellitus, and obesity are associated with the development of glaucoma. Options 1, 2, and 4 do not identify risk factors associated with this eye disorder.
Test-Taking Strategy: Use the process of elimination. Focusing on the issue, a risk factor associated with glaucoma, will direct you to option 3. If you had difficulty with this question, review the risk factors associated with this disorder.
Level of Cognitive Ability: Analysis
Client Needs: Health Promotion and Maintenance
Integrated Process: Nursing Process—assessment
Content Area: Adult health—eye
Reference: Ignatavicius, D., & Workman, M. (2002). *Medical-surgical nursing: Critical thinking for collaborative care* (4th ed., p. 1035). Philadelphia: W. B. Saunders.

235. **3**
Rationale: The nurse places an eye patch over the client's affected eye to reduce eye movement. Some clients may need bilateral patching. Depending on the location and size of the retinal break, activity restrictions may be needed immediately. These restrictions are necessary to prevent further tearing or detachment and to promote drainage of any subretinal fluid. The nurse positions the client as prescribed by the physician.
Test-Taking Strategy: Use the process of elimination. Remember that the eye needs to be protected and rested. This should direct you option 3. If you had difficulty with this question, review care to the client with retinal detachment.
Level of Cognitive Ability: Analysis
Client Needs: Physiological Integrity
Integrated Process: Nursing Process—analysis
Content Area: Adult health—eye

Reference: Ignatavicius, D., & Workman, M. (2002). *Medical-surgical nursing: Critical thinking for collaborative care* (4th ed., p. 1041). Philadelphia: W. B. Saunders.

236. **2**
Rationale: Persons at greatest risk for pulmonary emboli are immobilized clients. Basic preventive measures include early ambulation, leg elevation, active leg exercises, elastic stockings, and intermittent pneumatic calf compression. Keeping the client well hydrated is essential because dehydration predisposes to clotting. A pillow under the knees may cause venous stasis. Heat should not be applied without a physician's prescription.
Test-Taking Strategy: Use the process of elimination and basic principles related to the care of the immobile client to answer this question. If you are unfamiliar with these basic measures, review this content.
Level of Cognitive Ability: Application
Client Needs: Physiological Integrity
Integrated Process: Nursing Process—planning
Content Area: Adult health—respiratory
Reference: Potter, P., & Perry, A. (2001). *Fundamentals of nursing* (5th ed., p. 1516). St. Louis: Mosby.

237. **4**
Rationale: A crisis is an acute, time-limited state of disequilibrium resulting from situational, developmental, or societal sources of stress. A person in this state such as a suicidal client is temporarily unable to cope with or adapt to the stressor by using previous coping mechanisms. One who intervenes in this situation (the nurse) "takes over" for the client who is not in control and devises a plan (action) to secure and maintain the client's safety. Once this has occurred, the nurse works collaboratively with the client (participates) in developing new coping and problem-solving strategies.
Test-Taking Strategy: Use the process of elimination. The client who experiences a "suicidal crisis" is in a state of acute disequilibrium. Remember that in a "crisis," an authority figure must emerge to take action. Review care to the client in crisis if you had difficulty with this question.
Level of Cognitive Ability: Application
Client Needs: Psychosocial Integrity
Integrated Process: Nursing Process—implementation
Content Area: Mental health
Reference: Fortinash, K., & Holoday-Worret, P. (2000). *Psychiatric mental health nursing* (2nd ed., p. 672). St. Louis: Mosby.

238. **1**
Rationale: The client must have sputum cultures performed every 2 to 4 weeks after initiation of antituberculosis drug therapy. The client may return to work when the results of three sputum cultures are negative because the client is considered noninfectious at that point.
Test-Taking Strategy: Use the process of elimination. Knowing that a positive Mantoux test never reverts to negative helps you eliminate option 4. From the remaining options, you must know that three negative sputum cultures are required. If this question was difficult, review these concepts related to tuberculosis.

Level of Cognitive Ability: Application
Client Needs: Safe, Effective Care Environment
Integrated Process: Nursing Process—implementation
Content Area: Adult health—respiratory
Reference: Ignatavicius, D., & Workman, M. (2002). *Medical-surgical nursing: Critical thinking for collaborative care* (4th ed., p. 587). Philadelphia: W. B. Saunders.

239. **4**
Rationale: The client is admitted to a private room that has at least six air exchanges per hour and that has negative pressure in relation to surrounding areas. The room should be vented to the outside and should have ultraviolet lights installed.
Test-Taking Strategy: Use the process of elimination. Knowing that the air must vent to the outside helps to eliminate option 1. Knowing that ultraviolet light is useful in killing these organisms helps you to eliminate option 2. From the remaining options, recall that there must be an air flow system that allows for at least six air exchanges per hour. If you had difficulty with this question, review the care to the hospitalized client with tuberculosis.
Level of Cognitive Ability: Application
Client Needs: Safe, Effective Care Environment
Integrated Process: Nursing Process—planning
Content Area: Adult health—respiratory
Reference: Potter, P., & Perry, A. (2001). *Fundamentals of nursing* (5th ed., pp. 859-860). St. Louis: Mosby.

240. **1**
Rationale: Methenamine mandelate (Mandelamine) is contraindicated in clients with renal or hepatic disease or clients with severe dehydration. The nurse would question the physician's prescription for this medication in the client with cirrhosis of the liver.
Test-Taking Strategy: Use the process of elimination. Knowledge that this medication is contraindicated in hepatic disease will direct you easily to option 1. If you are unfamiliar with this medication and its contraindications, review this content.
Level of Cognitive Ability: Analysis
Client Needs: Physiological Integrity
Integrated Process: Nursing Process—analysis
Content Area: Pharmacology
Reference: Lehne, R. (2001). *Pharmacology for nursing care* (4th ed., p. 976). Philadelphia: W. B. Saunders.

241. **2**
Rationale: Nalidixic acid (NegGram) is used for acute and chronic urinary tract infections, especially gram-negative bacterial infections. The medication is contraindicated in clients with a history of seizures. Nalidixic acid is used with caution in clients with liver or renal disorders.
Test-Taking Strategy: Use the process of elimination and knowledge regarding the contraindications associated with this medication to answer the question. Review this medication if you had difficulty with this question.
Level of Cognitive Ability: Analysis
Client Needs: Physiological Integrity
Integrated Process: Nursing Process—analysis
Content Area: Pharmacology
Reference: Lehne, R. (2001). *Pharmacology for nursing care* (4th ed., p. 976). Philadelphia: W. B. Saunders.

242. **3**
Rationale: This client is in a severe state of anxiety. When a client is in a severe or panic state of anxiety, it is critical for the nurse to remain with the client. Processing the anxiety at this point will increase the client's level of anxiety further. The client in a severe state of anxiety would not be able to learn relaxation techniques.
Test-Taking Strategy: Use the process of elimination and note the key words "most appropriate initial." The best action in this situation is to remain with the client. If you are unfamiliar with the symptoms of the different levels of anxiety and the interventions that are indicated, review this information.
Level of Cognitive Ability: Application
Client Needs: Psychosocial Integrity
Integrated Process: Nursing Process—implementation
Content Area: Mental health
Reference: Fortinash, K., & Holoday-Worret, P. (2000). *Psychiatric mental health nursing* (2nd ed., pp. 595, 599). St. Louis: Mosby.

243. **3**
Rationale: When a nasogastric tube is attached to suction, it may be continuous or intermittent, with a pressure not exceeding 25 mm Hg. The specific pressure and the intervals are prescribed by the physician. Options 1, 2, and 4 are incorrect.
Test-Taking Strategy: Knowledge regarding the restrictions related to the amount of pressure with suction on a gastrointestinal tube is required to answer this question. If you are unfamiliar with the care of a client with a nasogastric tube attached to suction, review this content.
Level of Cognitive Ability: Analysis
Client Needs: Physiological Integrity
Integrated Process: Nursing Process—implementation
Content Area: Adult health—gastrointestinal
Reference: Lewis, S., Heitkemper, M., & Dirksen, S. (2004). *Medical-surgical nursing: Assessment and management of clinical problems* (6th ed., p. 1778). St. Louis: Mosby.

244. **2**
Rationale: During the first few days after hemorrhage, gastric pH should be increased to between 5.5 and 7 and maintained at this level to control secretory activity. Ranitidine (Zantac) or cimetidine (Tagamet) may be prescribed in addition to antacids to accomplish this. The use of antacids complements the effectiveness of histamine H_2-receptor antagonists for maintaining the pH level of gastric secretions.
Test-Taking Strategy: Use the process of elimination and knowledge regarding the treatment goals following gastrointestinal bleeding to answer this question. Remembering that gastric secretions are acidic will assist you in eliminating option 1. Options 3 and 4 identify an alkaline pH. Therefore option 2 is the best choice. Review care to the client with gastrointestinal bleeding if you had difficulty with this question.
Level of Cognitive Ability: Application
Client Needs: Physiological Integrity
Integrated Process: Nursing Process—planning
Content Area: Adult health—gastrointestinal
Reference: Ignatavicius, D., & Workman, M. (2002). *Medical-surgical nursing: Critical thinking for collaborative care* (4th ed., p. 1419). Philadelphia: W. B. Saunders.

Lewis, S., Heitkemper, M., & Dirksen, S. (2004). *Medical-surgical nursing: Assessment and management of clinical problems* (6th ed., p. 1419). St. Louis: Mosby.

245. 3
Rationale: The client needs to be instructed to dispense the oral liquid into a glass container using a specially calibrated pipette. The client should not use any other type of dropper to calibrate the amount of prescribed medication. The medication is mixed with milk, chocolate milk, or orange juice.
Test-Taking Strategy: Use the process of elimination. Note the key words "indicate the need for further instruction." Knowledge regarding the administration of the oral concentrate will direct you to option 3. Review the client instructions regarding administering this medication if you had difficulty with this question.
Level of Cognitive Ability: Analysis
Client Needs: Physiological Integrity
Integrated Process: Teaching/Learning
Content Area: Pharmacology
Reference: Lehne, R. (2001). *Pharmacology for nursing care* (4th ed., p. 749). Philadelphia: W. B. Saunders.

246. 3
Rationale: Laboratory findings do not establish the diagnosis of appendicitis, but often a moderate elevation of the white blood cell count (leukocytosis) to 10,000 to 18,000 cells/mm³ occurs with a "shift to the left" (an increased number of immature white blood cells.).
Test-Taking Strategy: Use the process of elimination. Knowledge that an inflammatory process causes a rise in the white blood cell count will assist you in eliminating options 1 and 4. From the remaining options, you must understand the significance of a "shift to the left." If you are unfamiliar with the meaning of "shift to the left," review this content.
Level of Cognitive Ability: Analysis
Client Needs: Physiological Integrity
Integrated Process: Nursing Process—assessment
Content Area: Adult health—gastrointestinal
Reference: Chernecky, C., & Berger, B. (2001). *Laboratory tests and diagnostic procedures* (3rd ed., pp. 439, 442). Philadelphia: W. B. Saunders.

247. 2
Rationale: Positions such as sitting up, leaning forward, and flexing the legs (especially the left leg) may alleviate some of the pain associated with pancreatitis. The pain is aggravated by lying supine or walking because the pancreas is located retroperitoneally, and the edema and inflammation intensify the irritation of the posterior peritoneal wall with these positions.
Test-Taking Strategy: Note the key word "avoid." Use the process of elimination and your critical thinking skills to visualize the pancreas and the potential effects from stretching associated with the various positions listed. Remember also that options that are similar are not likely to be correct. This will help you to eliminate at least options 1 and 3. Review pain reduction measures for the client with pancreatitis if you had difficulty with this question.
Level of Cognitive Ability: Application
Client Needs: Physiological Integrity

Integrated Process: Teaching/Learning
Content Area: Adult health—gastrointestinal
Reference: Lewis, S., Heitkemper, M., & Dirksen, S. (2004). *Medical-surgical nursing: Assessment and management of clinical problems* (6th ed., p. 1138). St. Louis: Mosby.

248. 2
Rationale: Common signs of acute viral hepatitis include weight loss, dark urine, and fatigue. The client is anorexic, possibly from a toxin produced by the diseased liver, and finds food distasteful. The urine darkens because of excess bilirubin being excreted by the kidneys. Fatigue occurs during all phases of hepatitis. Spider angiomas—small, dilated blood vessels—are common in cirrhosis of the liver.
Test-Taking Strategy: Use the process of elimination. Recalling the function of the liver will direct you to the correct option. If you had difficulty with this question, review content associated with hepatitis.
Level of Cognitive Ability: Application
Client Needs: Physiological Integrity
Integrated Process: Nursing Process—assessment
Content Area: Adult health—gastrointestinal
Reference: Lewis, S., Heitkemper, M., & Dirksen, S. (2004). *Medical-surgical nursing: Assessment and management of clinical problems* (6th ed., p. 1108). St. Louis: Mosby.

249. 2
Rationale: The client who has severe anxiety may be hyperventilating complaining of a headache, has loud or rapid speech, and purposeless activity. The client symptoms in the question do not relate to options 1, 3, and 4.
Test-Taking Strategy: Use the process of elimination. Note the client's symptoms in the question to answer the question correctly. Review the signs and symptoms associated with each level of anxiety if you had difficulty with this question.
Level of Cognitive Ability: Analysis
Client Needs: Psychosocial Integrity
Integrated Process: Nursing Process—assessment
Content Area: Mental health
Reference: Fortinash, K., & Holoday-Worret, P. (2000). *Psychiatric mental health nursing* (2nd ed., p. 250). St. Louis: Mosby.

250. 1
Rationale: Hydrocodone is an opioid analgesic that also has antitussive properties. Side effects of this medication include physical and psychological dependence, bradycardia and hypotension, respiratory depression, nausea, vomiting, constipation, sedation, and confusion.
Test-Taking Strategy: Use the process of elimination. Recalling that this medication is an opioid analgesic will direct you to option 1. If this question was difficult, review information on the implications of opioid use and the side effects of this medication.
Level of Cognitive Ability: Application
Client Needs: Psychosocial Integrity
Integrated Process: Nursing Process—assessment
Content Area: Pharmacology
Reference: Hodgson, B., & Kizior, R. (2003). *Saunders nursing drug handbook 2003* (p. 554). Philadelphia: W. B. Saunders.

251. 1
Rationale: Cromolyn sodium (Intal) is an antiasthmatic, antiallergic, and a mast cell stabilizer that inhibits the release of mediators from mast cells after exposure to an antigen. Cromolyn also can interrupt the migration of eosinophils into the inflammatory site and decrease the number of eosinophils. These actions decrease airway hyperresponsiveness in some clients with asthma. Cromolyn has no bronchodilating action.
Test-Taking Strategy: Use the process of elimination. Eliminate options 2 and 3 first because they are similar. From the remaining options, knowing that cromolyn sodium (Intal) has no bronchodilating action is helpful. Also note the relationship between the words "antigen" in the correct option and "allergic" in the question. Review the action of this medication if you had difficulty with this question.
Level of Cognitive Ability: Analysis
Client Needs: Physiological Integrity
Integrated Process: Nursing Process—analysis
Content Area: Pharmacology
Reference: McKenry, L., & Salerno, E. (2003). *Mosby's pharmacology in nursing* (21st ed., p. 724). St. Louis: Mosby.

252. 2
Rationale: The confrontational method assumes that the examiner has normal peripheral vision. The client sits facing the examiner about 2 feet away. The eyes of the client and the examiner should be at the same level. The examiner and the client cover the eyes directly opposite to one another and stare at each other's uncovered eye. A small object is brought from the peripheral visual field and tests the superior, temporal, inferior, and nasal field. The client states when he or she sees the object.
Test-Taking Strategy: Use the process of elimination. Eliminate option 3 because this option describes the test for color vision. Option 4 does not describe a confrontational test and addresses testing color. Visualize the process of testing as you read through options 1 and 2. This may assist you in selecting the correct option. If you had difficulty with this question, review this assessment test.
Level of Cognitive Ability: Application
Client Needs: Health Promotion and Maintenance
Integrated Process: Nursing Process—assessment
Content Area: Adult health—eye
Reference: Jarvis, C. (2000). *Physical examination and health assessment* (3rd ed., p. 308). Philadelphia: W. B. Saunders.

253. 1
Rationale: Because acetylcysteine has a pervasive flavor of rotten eggs, it must be disguised in a flavored ice drink and preferably is drunk through a straw to minimize contact with the mouth. Acetylcysteine is the antidote for acetaminophen. Acetylcysteine is a solution that also is used as a mucolytic agent, administered via nebulization. Acetylcysteine is not administered intravenously, intramuscularly, or subcutaneously.
Test-Taking Strategy: Use the process of elimination. Knowing that the medication is a solution that also is used for nebulization treatments will assist you in selecting the option that indicates an oral route. Note that options 2, 3, and 4 are similar and indicate parenteral administration and that option 1, the correct option, indicates oral administration. Review this medication if you had difficulty with this question.
Level of Cognitive Ability: Application
Client Needs: Physiological Integrity
Integrated Process: Nursing Process—implementation
Content Area: Pharmacology
Reference: Lehne, R. (2001). *Pharmacology for nursing care* (4th ed., p. 778). Philadelphia: W. B. Saunders.

254. 2
Rationale: Side effects of baclofen include drowsiness, dizziness, weakness, and nausea. Occasional side effects include headache, paresthesia of the hands and feet, constipation or diarrhea, anorexia, hypotension, confusion, and nasal congestion. Paradoxical central nervous system excitement and restlessness can occur along with slurred speech, tremor, dry mouth, nocturia, and impotence.
Test-Taking Strategy: Use the process of elimination. Option 2 is the option that is associated most closely with a neurological disorder. If you had difficulty with this question, review the side effects related to baclofen.
Level of Cognitive Ability: Analysis
Client Needs: Physiological Integrity
Integrated Process: Nursing Process—assessment
Content Area: Pharmacology
Reference: Lehne, R. (2001). *Pharmacology for nursing care* (4th ed., p. 217). Philadelphia: W. B. Saunders.

255. 1342
Rationale: The first assessment of the newborn is done immediately after birth by using the Apgar score. The Apgar score permits rapid assessment of the need for resuscitation. The nurse verifies that respirations have been established, dries the infant, and assesses the temperature. The infant may be wrapped in a warm blanket and placed in the arms of the mother or given to the father or partner to hold. The nurse also would place identification bracelets on the newborn infant and mother. In some settings the father or partner also wears an identification bracelet.
Test-Taking Strategy: Use the ABCs—airway, breathing, and circulation—to assist you in determining that checking the Apgar score is the first priority. Next, visualize the nursing actions from the items presented. Drying the infant and checking the temperature address physiological needs and are attended to before other needs. Review immediate care to the newborn infant if you had difficulty with this question.
Level of Cognitive Ability: Application
Client Needs: Health Promotion and Maintenance
Integrated Concept: Nursing Process—implementation
Content Area: Maternity/Intrapartum
Reference: Lowdermilk, D., & Perry, S. (2004). *Maternity women's health care* (8th ed., p. 708). St. Louis: Mosby.

256. 4
Rationale: The transcutaneous electrical nerve stimulation unit is a portable unit, and the client controls the system for relieving pain and reducing the need for analgesics. The system is attached to the skin of the body by electrodes. Hospitalization is not required.

Test-Taking Strategy: Use the process of elimination. Note the words "need for further instructions" in the stem of the question. You should be directed to option 4 because it would not be a cost-effective pain management technique if the client required hospitalization. Review the principles related to the transcutaneous electrical nerve stimulation unit if you had difficulty with this question.
Level of Cognitive Ability: Analysis
Client Needs: Physiological Integrity
Integrated Process: Teaching/Learning
Content Area: Pharmacology
Reference: Potter, P., & Perry, A. (2001). *Fundamentals of nursing* (5th ed., p. 1308). St. Louis: Mosby.

257. **4**
Rationale: Ineffective coping may be evidenced by inability to meet basic needs, inability to meet role expectations, alteration in social participation, use of inappropriate defense mechanisms, or impairment of usual patterns of communication. Disturbed thought processes are evidenced by altered attention span, distractibility or disorientation to time, place, person, and events. Dysfunctional family process may exist when the family has difficulty adapting or responding to the changes or traumatic experience of the member in crisis.
Test-Taking Strategy: Use the data presented in the question to direct you to the correct option. Option 3 can be eliminated easily because the client presently is experiencing anxiety. Eliminate option 1 because no data in the question address the family. Similarly, no data suggest disturbed thought processes, so eliminate this option also, leaving option 4 as the correct option. Review nursing diagnoses for the client experiencing anxiety if you had difficulty with this question.
Level of Cognitive Ability: Analysis
Client Needs: Psychosocial Integrity
Integrated Process: Nursing Process—analysis
Content Area: Mental health
Reference: Stuart, G., & Laraia, M. (2001). *Principles & practice of psychiatric nursing* (7th ed., pp. 230, 281). St. Louis: Mosby.

258. **2**
Rationale: Bubbling in the water seal compartment is caused by air passing out of the pleural space into the fluid in the chamber. Intermittent bubbling is normal and indicates that the system is accomplishing one of its purposes; that is, removing air from the pleural space. Continuous bubbling during inspiration and expiration indicates that an air leak exists. If this occurs, the leak must be corrected.
Test-Taking Strategy: Focus on the key words "intermittent bubbling" and "water seal compartment." Recalling that intermittent bubbling is normal will direct you to option 2. If you are unfamiliar with chest tube drainage systems, review this content.
Level of Cognitive Ability: Application
Client Needs: Physiological Integrity
Integrated Process: Nursing Process—implementation
Content Area: Adult health—respiratory
Reference: Lewis, S., Heitkemper, M., & Dirksen, S. (2004). *Medical-surgical nursing: Assessment and management of clinical problems* (6th ed., p. 623). St. Louis: Mosby.

259. **1**
Rationale: The nurse tilts the client's head slightly away and holds the otoscope upside down as if it were a large pen. The pinna is pulled up and back and the nurse visualizes the external canal while slowly inserting the speculum. Options 2, 3, and 4 are incorrect.
Test-Taking Strategy: Use the process of elimination. Note that the question addresses to adult client. Use basic knowledge regarding the administration of ear medications to select the correct option. In the adult the pinna is pulled up and back. Review the procedure for performing an otoscopic examination if you had difficulty with this question.
Level of Cognitive Ability: Application
Client Needs: Health Promotion and Maintenance
Integrated Process: Nursing Process—assessment
Content Area: Adult health—ear
Reference: Jarvis, C. (2000). *Physical examination and health assessment* (3rd ed., pp. 355-356). Philadelphia: W. B. Saunders.

260. **2**
Rationale: Cinoxacin (Cinobac) is a urinary antiseptic and is administered with meals to decrease gastrointestinal side effects. The normal dosage is 1 g per day administered in 2 to 4 divided doses for a period of 7 to 14 days.
Test-Taking Strategy: Use the process of elimination. Eliminate options 1 and 4 first because they are similar. From the remaining options, recalling that this medication is administered more than once daily will direct you to option 2. Review this medication if you had difficulty with this question.
Level of Cognitive Ability: Application
Client Needs: Physiological Integrity
Integrated Process: Teaching/Learning
Content Area: Pharmacology
Reference: Clark, J., Queener, S., & Karb, V. (2000). *Pharmacologic basis of nursing practice* (6th ed., p. 521). St. Louis: Mosby.

261. **1**
Rationale: The client with severe flail chest will have significant paradoxical chest movement. This causes the mediastinal structures to swing back and forth with respiration. This movement can affect hemodynamics. Specifically, the client's central venous pressure rises, the filling of the right side of the heart is impaired, and the arterial blood pressure falls. This is referred to as mediastinal flutter.
Test-Taking Strategy: Use the process of elimination. Because the question makes no mention of hemorrhage or bleeding, eliminate hypovolemic shock first. Knowing that these signs and symptoms are not compatible with fat embolism helps you eliminate that option next. From the remaining options, knowing that mediastinal shift is a result of tension pneumothorax helps you to choose mediastinal flutter as the correct option. Review the complications of a flail chest if you had difficulty with this question.
Level of Cognitive Ability: Analysis
Client Needs: Physiological Integrity
Integrated Process: Nursing Process—analysis
Content Area: Adult health—respiratory
Reference: Phipps, W., Monahan, F., Sands, J., Marek, J., & Neighbors, M. (2003). *Medical-surgical nursing: Health and illness perspectives* (7th ed., p. 606). St. Louis: Mosby.

262. 2
Rationale: Cough is the most frequent early symptom of lung cancer, which begins as nonproductive and hacking and progresses to productive. In the smoker who already has a cough, a change in the character and frequency of cough usually occurs. Wheezing and blood-streaked sputum (hemoptysis) are later signs. Pain is a late sign and is usually pleuritic. Hoarseness indicates that the affected tissue is in the upper airway.
Test-Taking Strategy: Use the process of elimination. Begin to answer this question by eliminating pain and hemoptysis because these reasonably would be later signs. To discriminate between cough and hoarseness, think about location. Hoarseness would indicate that the affected tissue is in the upper airway, whereas cough would indicate lower airway. Because the question is asking about lung cancer, which is lower airway, the answer must be cough. Review the frequent early symptoms of lung cancer if you had difficulty with this question.
Level of Cognitive Ability: Application
Client Needs: Physiological Integrity
Integrated Process: Nursing Process—assessment
Content Area: Adult health—respiratory
Reference: Lewis, S., Heitkemper, M., & Dirksen, S. (2004). *Medical-surgical nursing: Assessment and management of clinical problems* (6th ed., p. 561). St. Louis: Mosby.

263. 3
Rationale: The initial nursing assessment of a client in a crisis state is to evaluate the physical condition of the client, the potential for self-harm, and the potential for harm to others. Once this has been determined and appropriate interventions have been initiated, the nurse then would proceed with the mental health interview.
Test-Taking Strategy: Use Maslow's hierarchy of needs theory to answer the question. Physiological needs take priority over other needs. Option 3 is the only option that addresses a physiological need. Review care to the client in crisis if you had difficulty with this question.
Level of Cognitive Ability: Analysis
Client Needs: Physiological Integrity
Integrated Process: Nursing Process—assessment
Content Area: Delegating/Prioritizing
Reference: Fortinash, K., & Holoday-Worret, P. (2000). *Psychiatric mental health nursing* (2nd ed., p. 598). St. Louis: Mosby.

264. 3
Rationale: Although frequency and intensity of bowel sounds varies depending on the phase of digestion, normal bowel sounds are high-pitched clicks or gurgles. Loud gurgles (borborygmi) indicate hyperperistalsis. Bowel sounds will be more high pitched and loud (hyperresonance) when the intestines are under tension, such as in intestinal obstruction. A swishing or buzzing sound represents turbulent blood flow associated with a bruit. Bruits are not normal sounds.
Test-Taking Strategy: Use the process of elimination. Normally, bowel sounds are audible in all four quadrants; therefore eliminate options 2 and 4. From the remaining options, use knowledge regarding normal findings to direct you to option 3. Review abdominal assessment if you had difficulty with this question.
Level of Cognitive Ability: Comprehension
Client Needs: Health Promotion and Maintenance
Integrated Process: Nursing Process—assessment
Content Area: Adult health—gastrointestinal
Reference: Lewis, S., Heitkemper, M., & Dirksen, S. (2004). *Medical-surgical nursing: Assessment and management of clinical problems* (6th ed., p. 957). St. Louis: Mosby.

265. Answer: 880 mL
Rationale: The client consumed a total of 26 oz of fluid (12 oz at breakfast, 8 oz with medications, and 6 oz at lunch). This equals 780 mL (1 oz = 30 mL). The client also received a total of 100 mL of intravenous fluid (50 mL at 8 AM and 50 mL at 2 PM). Therefore the total intake is 880 mL.
Test-Taking Strategy: Focus on the issue, the client's intake in milliliters. Read the question carefully, noting the client's oral intake in ounces, and then convert the total ounces to milliliters. Remember that 1 oz equals 30 mL. Once you have done this, remember to add the 100 mL of intravenous fluid to the oral total. Review procedures for calculating intake and output if you had difficulty with this question.
Level of Cognitive Ability: Comprehension
Client Needs: Physiological Integrity
Integrated Process: Nursing Process—assessment
Content Area: Fundamental skills
Reference: Harkreader, H., & Hogan, M. A. (2004). *Fundamentals of nursing: Caring and clinical judgment* (2nd ed., pp. 580-582). Philadelphia: W. B. Saunders.

REFERENCES

Black, J., Hawks, J., & Keene, A. (2001). *Medical-surgical nursing: Clinical management for positive outcomes* (6th ed.). Philadelphia: W. B. Saunders.

Chernecky, C., & Berger, B. (2001). *Laboratory tests and diagnostic procedures* (3rd ed.). Philadelphia: W. B. Saunders.

Clark, J., Queener, S., & Karb, V. (2000). *Pharmacologic basis of nursing practice* (6th ed.). St. Louis: Mosby.

Ebersole, P., & Hess, P. (2001). *Geriatric nursing & healthy aging.* St. Louis: Mosby.

Fortinash, K., & Holoday-Worret, P. (2000). *Psychiatric mental health nursing* (2nd ed.). St. Louis: Mosby.

Grodner, M., Anderson, S., & DeYoung, S. (2000). *Foundations and clinical applications of nutrition: A nursing approach.* St. Louis: Mosby.

Harkreader, H., & Hogan, M. A. (2004). *Fundamentals of nursing: Caring and clinical judgment* (2nd ed.). Philadelphia: W. B. Saunders.

Hodgson, B., & Kizior, R. (2003). *Saunders nursing drug handbook 2003.* Philadelphia: W. B. Saunders.

Hodgson, B., & Kizior, R. (2004). *Saunders nursing drug handbook 2004.* Philadelphia: W. B. Saunders.

Ignatavicius, D., & Workman, M. (2002). *Medical-surgical nursing: Critical thinking for collaborative care* (4th ed.). Philadelphia: W. B. Saunders.

James, S., Ashwill, J., & Droske, S. (2002). *Nursing care of children: Principles & practice* (2nd ed.). Philadelphia: W. B. Saunders.

Jarvis, C. (2000). *Physical examination & health assessment* (3rd ed.). Philadelphia: W. B. Saunders.

Lehne, R. (2001). *Pharmacology for nursing care* (4th ed.). Philadelphia: W. B. Saunders.

Leuckenotte, A. (2000). *Gerontologic nursing* (2nd ed.). St. Louis: Mosby.

Lewis, S., Heitkemper, M., & Dirksen, S. (2004). *Medical-surgical nursing: Assessment and management of clinical problems* (6th ed.). St. Louis: Mosby.

Lowdermilk, D., & Perry, S. (2004). *Maternity & women's health care* (8th ed.). St. Louis: Mosby.

Lowdermilk, D., & Perry, S. (2003). *Maternity nursing* (6th ed.). St. Louis: Mosby.

McKenry, L., & Salerno, E. (2003). *Mosby's pharmacology in nursing* (21st ed.). St. Louis: Mosby.

Murray, S., McKinney, E., & Gorrie, T. (2002). *Foundations of maternal-newborn nursing* (3rd ed.). Philadelphia: W. B. Saunders.

Phipps, W., Monahan, F., Sands, J., Marek, J., & Neighbors, M. (2003). *Medical-surgical nursing: Health and illness perspectives* (7th ed.). St. Louis: Mosby.

Potter, P., & Perry, A. (2001). *Fundamentals of nursing* (5th ed.). St. Louis: Mosby.

Stuart, G., & Laraia, M. (2001). *Principles and practice of psychiatric nursing* (7th ed.). St. Louis: Mosby.

Varcarolis, E. (2002). *Foundations of psychiatric mental health nursing* (4th ed.). Philadelphia: W. B. Saunders.

Williams, S. (2001). *Basic nutrition & diet therapy* (11th ed.). St Louis: Mosby.

Williams, S., & Schlenker, E. (2003). *Essentials of nutrition & diet therapy* (8th ed.). St. Louis: Mosby.

Wong, D., Perry, S., & Hockenberry, M. (2002). *Maternal child nursing care* (2nd ed.). St. Louis: Mosby.

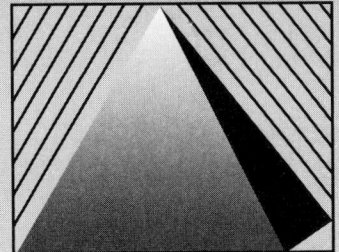

General Bibliography

Agency for Healthcare Research and Quality. www.ahcpr.gov/

American Academy of Family Physicians. http://www.aafp.org

American Academy of Pediatrics. http://www.aap.org

American Cancer Society. http://www.cancer.org

American Heart Association. (1997-1999). Pediatric basic life support. In *Basic life support for health care providers*. Dallas, TX: Author.

American Heart Association. (2001). *Basic life support for health care providers*. Dallas, TX: Author.

American Heart Association & International Liaison Committee on Resuscitation. (2000). *Guidelines 2000 for cardiopulmonary resuscitation and emergency cardiovascular care*. Dallas, TX: Author.

American Lung Association. www.lungusa.org.

American SIDS Institute. www.sids.org

Asthma and Allergy Foundation of America. www.aafa.org.

Black, J., Hawks, J., & Keene, A. (2001). *Medical-surgical nursing: Clinical management for positive outcomes* (6th ed.). Philadelphia: W. B. Saunders.

Brent, N. (2001). *Nurses and the law* (2nd ed.). Philadelphia: W. B. Saunders.

Carson, V. (2000). *Mental health nursing: The nurse-patient journey* (2nd ed.). Philadelphia: W. B. Saunders.

Celiac Sprue Association/United States of America. www.csaceliacs.org

Centers for Disease Control and Prevention. (2004). *Recommended childhood and adolescent immunization schedule* (2004). Retrieved January 16, 2004, from http://www.cdc.gov/nip

Centers for Disease Control and Prevention. (2004). *Smallpox pre-vaccination information packet*. Atlanta: Author. Retrieved August 12, 2003, from http://www.bt.cdc.gov/agent/smallpox/vaccination/infopacket.asp

Centers for Disease Control and Prevention. http://www2.cdc.gov/mmwr/

Chernecky, C., & Berger, B. (2001). *Laboratory tests and diagnostic procedures* (3rd ed.). Philadelphia: W. B. Saunders.

Chernecky, C., & Berger, B. (2004). *Laboratory tests and diagnostic procedures* (4th ed.). Philadelphia: W. B. Saunders.

Clark, J., Queener, S., & Karb, V. (2000). *Pharmacologic basis of nursing practice* (6th ed.). St. Louis: Mosby.

Clemen-Stone, S., McGuire, S., & Eigsti, D. (2002). *Comprehensive community family* (6th ed.). St. Louis: Mosby.

Commission on Graduates of Foreign Nursing Schools. http://www.cgfns.org

Cooley's Anemia Foundation. http://www.thalassemia.org

Cystic Fibrosis Foundation. http://www.CFF.org

Ebersole, P., & Hess, P. (2001). *Geriatric nursing & healthy aging*. St. Louis: Mosby.

Educational Testing Service, Princeton, New Jersey. http://toefl@ets.org.

Elkin, M., Perry, A., & Potter, P. (2004). *Nursing interventions & clinical skills* (3rd ed.). St. Louis: Mosby.

Fortinash, K., & Holoday-Worret, P. (2000). *Psychiatric mental health nursing* (2nd ed.). St. Louis: Mosby.

Fulginiti, V., & Department of Health and Human Services (2003). *Pocket guide for the smallpox vaccine adverse effects*. Atlanta: Centers for Disease Control and Prevention. Retrieved January 17, 2003, from www.smallpox/basics/index.asp

Giger, J., & Davidhizar, R. (2004). *Transcultural nursing: Assessment & intervention* (4th ed.). St. Louis: Mosby.

Gutierrez, K., & Queener, S. (2003). *Pharmacology for nursing practice*. St. Louis: Mosby.

Harkreader, H., & Hogan, M. A. (2004). *Fundamentals of nursing: Caring and clinical judgment* (2nd ed.). Philadelphia: W. B. Saunders.

Herlihy, B., & Maebius, N. (2003). *The human body in health and illness* (2nd ed.). Philadelphia: W. B. Saunders.

Hill, S., & Bauer, B. (2000). *Mental health nursing*. Philadelphia: W. B. Saunders.

Hodgson, B., & Kizior, R. (2003). *Saunders nursing drug handbook 2003*. Philadelphia: W. B. Saunders.

Hodgson, B., & Kizior, R. (2004). *Saunders nursing drug handbook 2004*. Philadelphia: W. B. Saunders.

Ignatavicius, D., & Workman, M. (2002). *Medical surgical nursing: Critical thinking for collaborative care* (4th ed.). Philadelphia: W. B. Saunders.

Immunization Action Coalition. http://www.immunize.org

International English Language Testing System. ielts@ceii.org; http://www.ielts.org

James, S., Ashwill, J., & Droske, S. (2002). *Nursing care of children: Principles & practice* (2nd ed.). Philadelphia: W. B. Saunders.

Jarvis, C. (2000). *Physical examination & health assessment* (3rd ed.). Philadelphia: W. B. Saunders.

Joint Commission on Accreditation of Healthcare Organizations. (2004). *2004 national patient safety goals*. Oakbrook Terrace, IL: Author. Retrieved March 1, 2004, from http://www.jcaho.org/accredited+organizations/patient+safety/04+npsg/04_faqs.htm

Kee, J., & Hayes, E. (2003). *Pharmacology: A nursing process approach* (4th ed.). Philadelphia: W. B. Saunders.

Kee, J., & Marshall, S. (2000). *Clinical calculations: With applications to general and specialty areas* (4th ed.). Philadelphia: W. B. Saunders.

Kee, J., & Marshall, S. (2004). *Clinical calculations: With applications to general and specialty areas* (5th ed.). Philadelphia: W. B. Saunders.

Keltner, N., Schwecke, L., & Bostrom, C. (2003). *Psychiatric nursing* (4th ed.). St. Louis: Mosby.

Lehne, R. (2001). *Pharmacology for nursing care* (4th ed.). Philadelphia: W. B. Saunders.

Lewis, S., Heitkemper, M., & Dirksen, S. (2004). *Medical-surgical nursing: Assessment and management of clinical problems* (6th ed.). St. Louis: Mosby.

Linton, A., & Maebius, N. (2003). *Introduction to medical-surgical nursing* (3rd ed.). Philadelphia: W. B. Saunders.

Lowdermilk, D., & Perry, S. (2003). *Maternity nursing* (6th ed.). St. Louis: Mosby.

Lowdermilk, D., & Perry, S. (2004). *Maternity & women's health care* (8th ed.). St. Louis: Mosby.

Lowdermilk, D., Perry, S., & Bobak, I. (2000). *Maternity & women's health care* (7th ed.). St. Louis: Mosby.

Lueckenotte, A. (2000). *Gerontologic nursing* (2nd ed.). St. Louis: Mosby.

Malarkey, L., & McMorrow, M. (2000). *Nurse's manual of laboratory tests and diagnostic procedures* (2nd ed.). Philadelphia: W. B. Saunders.

Matteson, P. (2001). *Women's health during the childbearing years: A community-based approach.* St. Louis: Mosby.

McKenry, L., & Salerno, E. (2003). *Mosby's pharmacology in nursing* (21st ed.). St. Louis: Mosby.

McKinney, E., Ashwill, J., Murray, S., James, S., Gorrie, T., & Droske, S. (2000). *Maternal-child nursing.* Philadelphia: W. B. Saunders.

Mosby's medical, nursing, & allied health dictionary (6th ed.). (2002). St. Louis: Mosby.

Murray, S., McKinney, E., & Gorrie, T., (2002). *Foundations of maternal-newborn nursing* (3rd ed.). Philadelphia: W. B. Saunders.

National Brain Tumor Foundation. http://www.braintumor.org

National Council of State Boards of Nursing (Eds.). (2000). *Draft: Test Plan for the National Council Licensure Examination for Registered Nurses.* Chicago: Author.

National Council of State Boards of Nursing (Eds.). (2003). *Test Plan for the National Council Licensure Examination for Registered Nurses* (effective date: April 2004). Chicago: Author.

National Council of State Boards of Nursing. http://www.ncsbn.org

O'Neill, P. (2002). *Caring for the older adult.* Philadelphia: W. B. Saunders.

Peckenpaugh, N. (2003). *Nutrition essentials and diet therapy* (9th ed.). Philadelphia: W. B. Saunders.

Perry, A., & Potter, P. (2002). *Clinical nursing skills & techniques* (5th ed.). St. Louis: Mosby.

Phipps, W., Monahan, F., Sands, J., Marek, J., & Neighbors, M. (2003). *Medical-surgical nursing: Health and illness perspectives* (7th ed.). St. Louis: Mosby.

Potter, P., & Perry, A. (2001). *Fundamentals of nursing* (5th ed.). St. Louis: Mosby.

Riley, J. (2000). *Communication in nursing* (4th ed.). St. Louis: Mosby.

Riordan, J., Bibb, D., Miller, M., & Rawlins, T. (2001). Predicting breastfeeding duration using the LATCH breastfeeding assessment tool. *Journal of Human Lactation, 17*(1), 20-23.

Skidmore-Roth, L. (2001). *Mosby's handbook of herbs & natural supplements.* St. Louis: Mosby.

Stanhope, M., & Lancaster, J. (2002). *Foundations of community health nursing: Community-oriented practice.* St. Louis: Mosby.

Stuart, G., & Laraia, M. (2001). *Principles and practice of psychiatric nursing* (7th ed.). St. Louis: Mosby.

Thompson, J., Mcfarland, G., Hirsch, J., & Tucker, S. (2002). *Mosby's clinical nursing* (5th ed.). St. Louis: Mosby.

U.S. Department of Health and Human Services. (2003). *Smallpox vaccine: What you need to know.* Atlanta: Centers for Disease Control and Prevention, National Immunization Program.

Varcarolis, E. M. (2002). *Foundations of psychiatric mental health nursing* (4th ed.). Philadelphia: W. B. Saunders.

Williams, S. (2001). *Basic nutrition & diet therapy* (11th ed.). St Louis: Mosby.

Williams, S., & Schlenker, E. (2003). *Essentials of nutrition & diet therapy* (8th ed.). St. Louis: Mosby.

Wong, D., & Hockenberry, M. (2003). *Nursing care of infants and children* (7th ed.). St. Louis: Mosby.

Wong, D., Hockenberry-Eaton, M. (2000). *Wong's essentials of pediatric nursing* (6th ed.). St. Louis: Mosby.

Wong, D., Perry, S., & Hockenberry, M. (2002). *Maternal child nursing care* (2nd ed.). St. Louis: Mosby.

Yoder-Wise, P. (2003). *Leading and managing in nursing* (3rd ed.). St. Louis: Mosby.

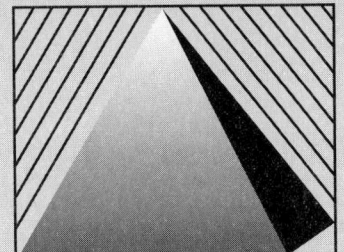

Index

Page numbers followed by b indicate boxes; f, figures;
t, tables.

1217